MELLONI'S ILLUSTRATED MEDICAL DICTIONARY

FOURTH EDITION

IDA G. DOX, PhD

Medical Communication Specialist (retired)
Georgetown University School of Medicine
Washington, DC

B. JOHN MELLONI, PhD

Expert in Biomedical Communication (retired)
National Library of Medicine
National Institutes of Health
Bethesda, Maryland

Professorial Lecturer in Human Anatomy (retired)
Georgetown University School of Medicine
Washington, DC

Co-Director of the Archives of Medical Visual Resources
The Francis A. Countway Library of Medicine
Harvard University Medical School
Boston, Massachusetts

GILBERT M. EISNER, MD, FACP

Clinical Professor of Medicine
Georgetown University School of Medicine
Washington, DC

Clinical Professor of Medicine
George Washington University School of Medicine
Washington, DC

Senior Attending Physician
Washington Hospital Center
Washington, DC

JUNE L. MELLONI, PhD

Educational Consultant and Evaluator of Instructional Programs in the Medical Sciences
Potomac Falls, Virginia

MELLONI'S ILLUSTRATED MEDICAL DICTIONARY

FOURTH EDITION

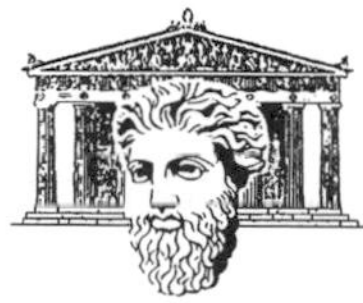

The Parthenon Publishing Group
International Publishers in Medicine, Science & Technology

A CRC PRESS COMPANY
BOCA RATON LONDON NEW YORK WASHINGTON, D.C.

The Fourth Edition of *Melloni's Illustrated Medical Dictionary* is published by:

The Parthenon Publishing Group
23–25 Blades Court
Deodar Road
London
SW15 2NU, UK

The first and second editions of this book were published by Williams and Wilkins, and the third by The Parthenon Publishing Group.

FOURTH EDITION

ISBN: 1-85070-094-X

British Library Cataloguing-in-Publication Data available on request

Library of Congress Cataloging-in-Publication Data
Melloni's illustrated medical dictionary / Ida G. Dox...[et al.]. - 4th ed.
p.; cm.
Rev. ed. of: Melloni's illustrated medical dictionary / Ida G. Dox, B. John Melloni, Gilbert M. Eisner, 3rd ed. c1993
ISBN 1-85070-094-X (alk. paper)
1. Medicine - Dictionaries. I. Title: Illustrated Medical Dictionary. II. Dox, Ida. III. Melloni, Biagio John.
[DNLM: 1. Medicine—Dictionary—English. W 13 M5271 2001]
R121.D76 2001
610'.3—dc21

2001045162

Contents

Preface vii
Prefixes, suffixes, and combining forms ix
How to use this dictionary xiii
Vocabulary 1–740
Plates
- Apparatus 28
- Arch 30
- Arteries of the body 35
- Bones of the body 80
- Breast 93
- Limb buds 95
- Bursa 99
- Cast, Cartilage 109
- Cerebrum, Cerebellum 119
- Blood circulation 128
- Cochlea 133
- Spinal cord 143
- Disks 173
- Duct 178, 180
- Inner ear 186
- Pathogenesis of embolism 192
- Development of the human embryo 193
- Fertilization 215
- Fissure, Fistula, Filum 221
- Foramen 227
- Foramina at base of cranium and structures transmitted through them 228–229
- Forceps 231
- Fossa 233
- Fractures 235, 236
- Girdle (pelvic and shoulder), Glands 246
- Mammary gland 248
- Thyroid gland 249
- Graft 255
- Heart 262
- Implant, Impetigo 293
- Joints 312–314
- Labyrinth 324
- Tissue layers 329
- Ligaments 336–345
- Mandible 364
- Maneuvers 365
- Musculoskeletal System 393
- Central and Peripheral Nervous System 427
- Nodes 453
- Nucleus 458
- Common sites of coronary occlusion 463

Sensory organs 471
Nerve pathways 489
Surgical scissors 574
Signs 586–587
Sinuses 589
Skeletal System 591
Speculums 599
Sphincter muscles 601
Spine 603
Splints 605
Sutures 622
Cardiovascular System 628
Musculoskeletal System 629
Tendons and tenoplasty 641–642
Tests 644–647
Tongue 665
Teeth 667
Tract 670
Tubes 682
DNA typing 688
Valves 701
Major veins of the human body 705

Tables

Amino acids 4–5
Table of Arteries 36–57
Table of Bones 81–89
Range of human hearing 157
Classification of Diabetes Mellitus 165
Equivalent Measures and Weights 203
Eruption of deciduous and permanent teeth 204
Exotoxins produced by some bacteria 208
Classification of hyperlipoproteinemia 281
Incubation periods of various diseases 295
Classification of overweight and obesity 295
Results of Laboratory tests in common jaundice disorders 311
Some differential features of infectious mononucleosis 389
Table of Muscles 394–415
Table of Nerves 428–447
Electromagnetic spectrum 548
Apgar score 577
Synovianalysis 625
International System of Units and Measures 631
Periodic table of elements 634
Normal values of blood plasma 700
Table of Veins 706–720
Vitamins 728

Abbreviations 741
Illustration credits 763
The authors 764

Preface

An understandable dictionary that provides accurate, clear and comprehensive definitions of words is an indispensable tool of learning. In the health sciences, development of applicable new technologies constantly presents opportunities for advances, with a consequent increase in related vocabulary. The fourth edition of the award-winning *Melloni's Illustrated Medical Dictionary* undertakes to provide a clear understanding of current vocabulary originating from such advances.

Melloni's Illustrated Medical Dictionary has remained in print since 1979, when the first edition was published. The present edition retains the philosophy and structure of the original book. This thoroughly updated fourth edition was expanded with over 4000 new entries of up-to-date information (especially in genetics, immunology, oncology, gynecology and radiology), bringing the total number to over 30 000 entries. We also increased the number of line drawings by 500 (including many full-page plates), for a total of over 3000 illustrations with color highlights. We are convinced that these single-concept, "road map" illustrations not only enhance comprehension of the defined term but solidify retention of that information. To increase the usefulness of the dictionary, we added hundreds of abbreviations to the previous list in recognition of their common usage in preference to the full terms they represent. Finally, in our commitment to improve the functional aspect of the book, we heeded the recommendation of many readers and expanded the pronunciation guide, placing each pronunciation next to the corresponding term. Overall, we prepared this dictionary with a constant regard for the accuracy, clarity and conciseness of current medical terminology so that dedicated individuals learning to provide the very best health care to those in need of their services can benefit from a vocabulary of great extent and richness.

We appreciate the excellent suggestions from readers who took the time to write. We especially thank Edward Stim, MD, for his helpful comments. We also thank the staff of Cellmark Diagnostics for providing information about the process of producing DNA typing. Additional suggestions for the increased usefulness of the book are appreciated and encouraged. Please address them to Ida G. Dox, PhD, 9308 Renshaw Drive, Bethesda, MD 20817, USA.

IGD
BJM
GME
JLM

Prefixes, suffixes, and combining forms

A

a-, an- without, lacking
ab- away from
abdomin-, abdomino- abdomen
acanth-, acantho- thorns, spines
acr-, acro- extremity, tip, end, summit
actin-, actino- ray
ad- to, motion toward, proximity
-ad direction toward
aden- gland
adip-, adipo- fat
aer-, aero- air or gas
all- other, different
ambi- both
amido- presence of the amide radical
amino- presence of the radical NH_2
andro- male sex
antero- before
anthropo- human
anti- against, counteraction
-ase enzyme
-ate neutralized or esterified acid
azo- presence of the nitrogen group –N:N–

B

bi-, bin- two, twice
bio- life
bis- twice, doubled
-blast immature
blasto- early stage
bronch-, bronchi-, broncho- bronchus, trachea

C

cac-, caci-, caco- bad, ill
cardi-, cardio- heart
cario- caries
cent-, centi- one hundredth (10^{-2})
cephal-, cephalo- head
cerebr-, cerebri-, cerebro- brain
cheil-, cheilo- lips
chlor- green
chol-, chole-, cholo- bile
choledoch-, choledocho- common bile duct
chondro- cartilage
chorio- membrane
chrom-, chromat-, chromato-, chromo- color
chrys-, chryso- gold
chyl-, chylo- chyle
cine- movement
circum- on all sides
cis- location on the same or the near side
-clysis injection
colp-, colpo- vagina
con- together
contra- against
crani-, cranio- skull
cryo- cold
crypt-, crypto- hidden
cyan-, cyano- blue
cycl-, cyclo- circle, cycle
cyst-, cysto- bladder

D

dacry-, dacryo- tears
dactyl-, dactylo- finger, toe
deca-, deka- ten
deci- one-tenth
dehydr-, dehydro- compound from which hydrogen has been removed
demi- half
dendr-, dendri-, dendro-, tree-shaped
deoxy-, desoxy- compound derived by removal of one oxygen atom from another compound
derm-, derma-, dermat-, dermato- skin
desm-, desmo- ligament, fibrous band
deutero-, deuti-, deuto- second, secondary
dextro- on or toward the right
di- two
dia- through, throughout
diazo- a compound containing the –N=N– or –N(N+ group
didym-, didymo- testis
-didymus, -dymus conjoined twin
dihydro- addition of two hydrogen atoms
dipl-, diplo- double
dis- separation, removal
disc- disk
disco- placenta
dolicho- long
dors-, dorsi-, dorso- back
-dymus conjoined twins
dynamo- power, energy
dys- faulty, bad, improper

E

echin-, echino- spring
-ectasia, lectasis expansion
ect-, ecto- outer, external
-ectomy removal
eleo- oil
elytro- vagina
-emia blood
en- in, into, within
encephal-, encephalo- brain
end-, endo- inside, within
-ene presence of a carbon-carbon double bond
enter-, entero- intestines
entomo- insect
epi- upon
epiplo- omentum
erythr-, erythro- red
etio- cause
eu- good, well, normal
ex- out of, away from
exo- external, outward extra- outside
extra- outside

F

-facient produces, brings about
femto- one quadrillionth (10^{-15})
ferri- containing iron in its highest valence (3)
ferro- divalent ion Fe^{++} in a compound
fibr-, fibro- fiber
fiss- split
-fuge avoid, flee

G

galac-, galacta-, galacto- milk
galvano- direct electric current
gameto- gamete
gastr-, gastro- stomach
gem- twin substitutions of a single atom
-gen produce, originate
gen-, geno- producing
-genic causing
ger-, gerat-, gero-, geronto- old age
giga- one billion
gigant-, giganto- exceedingly large, excessive growth
gingivo- gums
gloss-, glosso- tongue
glyc-, glyco- sugar
gnath-, gnatho- jaw
-gnosis recognition
gonad-, gonado- testis, ovary
-gram something recorded
-graph record, something printed
gyn-, gyne-, gyneco-, gyno- female sex

H

hect- one hundred
hemangio- blood vessel
hem-, hemi- half
hem-, hema-, hemat-, hemato-, hemo- blood
hepat-, hepato- liver
herado- heredity
heter-, hetero- other, different
hexa- six
hist-, histio-, histo- tissue
hol-, holo- whole
homeo-, homo- same, similar
hyal-, hyalo- glass, resembling glass
hydr-, hydro- water, hydrogen
hydroxy- presence of a hydrogen group (OH)
hygro- wet, moist
hyper- above, beyond, excessive
hypn-, hypno- sleep, hypnosis
hyp-, hypo- below, under, deficient
hypsi-, hypso- height
hyster-, hystero- uterus

I

i- immunoreactive
-ia, -iasis pathologic condition
-iatrics, -iatry medical treatment
-ic 1. chemical element that has the higher valence of two possible states 2. acid

-ics science, practice, treatment
-id 1. skin rash 2. family relationship 3. small specimen
-ide binary compound
ideo- idea
idio- peculiar to, individual
ileo- ileum
ilio- ilium
immuno- immunity
in- 1. without 2. inside 3. intensive action
infra- below, beneath
inter- between, among
intra- within
intro- in, into
irido- iris
ischio- ischium
-ism 1. abnormal condition 2. characteristic quality 3. process
is-, iso- identical, equal
-ite resembling, of the nature of
-itis inflammation

J

jeluno- jejunum
juxta- near

K

kal-, kali- potassium
kary-, karyo- nucleus of a living cell
kerato- cornea, thorny tissue
ket-, keto- presence of a ketone group (=CO)
kilo- one thousand
kin-, kine-, kineto- motion
koilo- concave
krymo-, kryo- cold

L

labio- lips
lact-, lacto- milk
laparo- abdomen
laryng-, laryngo- larynx
leio- smooth
-lepsis, -lepsy seizure
lept-, lepto- slender, thin
leuc-, leuco- white, colorless
leuk-, leuko- white, colorless
levo- on or toward the left
-lexis, -lexy speech
lien-, lieno- spleen
linguo- tongue
lip-, lipo- lipid, fat
lith-, litho- stone
-logy study
lymph-, lympho- lymph
lysis dissolution, rupture, separation

M

macr-, macro- large
-mania mental aberration
mast-, masto- breast
mega- 1. one million 2. large
megal-, megalo-, -megaly large
mel- 1. limb 2. cheek 3. honey
melan-, melano- black
mening-, meningo- membrane
meno- menstruation
mento- chin
-mer smallest unit of a repeating chemical structure
mercapto- presence of a thiol group
mero- part, segment
mes-, meso- middle, intermediate
met-, meta- 1. behind 2. occurring later in a series 3. transformation 4. the 1,3 position in the benzene ring 5. a less hydrous acid
metr- uterus
micro- 1. small 2. one millionth
micromicro- one trillionth (10^{-12})
milli- one thousandth (10^{-3})
millimicro- one billionth (10^{-9})
mono- single
morpho- form, figure, structure
multi- many
myco-, myo- fungus
myelo- 1. bone marrow 2. spinal cord
my-, myo- muscle
myring-, myringo- tympanic membrane
myx-, myxo- mucus

N

nano- 1. small 2. one billionth (10^{-9})
narco- stupor
naso- nose
necr-, necro- dead
nemato- threadlike
neo- new
nephr-, nephro- kidney
neur-, neuro- nerve, nervous system
nitro- presence of the univalent group NO_2 in a compound
nitroso- presence of the radical –NO in a compound
noci- 1. injury 2. a harmful agent or influence
nor- 1. nitrogen without a radical 2. a change from a branched-chain compound to a straight-chain compound
noso- disease
nucle-, nucleo- 1. nucleus 2. nucleic acid

O

octa- eight
odont-, odonto- tooth
odyn-, odynia- pain
-oid resemblance, same shape
-ol alcohol, phenol
oleo- oil
olig-, oligo- few, little
-ology see -logy
-oma tumor or neoplasm
omo- shoulder
omphal-, omphalo- umbilicus
onco-, oncho- tumor
-onium postively charged ion
onych-, onycho-, onyx- fingernail, toenail
oo- egg, ovary
oophor-, oophoro- ovary
oothec-, ootheco- ovary
ophthalm-, ophthalmo- eye
-opia vision
orchi-, orchid-, orchio- testis
ortho- 1. straight, normal 2. correction 3. an acid in the highest form of hydration 4. adjacent carbon positions in a benzene ring
-ose 1. carbohydrate 2. a substance resulting from digestion of a protein
-osis 1. abnormal, diseased 2. increase 3. process
osmo- 1. osmosis 2. odor
ost-, oste-, osteo- bone
ostomy see -stomy
ot-, oto- ear
-otomy see -tomy
-ous occurring in its lowest valency
ovari-, ovario- ovary
ovi-, ovo- egg
oxa- an oxygen bridge
oxo- oxygen
oxy- 1. pointed 2. acute 3. shield 4. presence of oxygen in a molecule

P

pachy- thick
-pagus conjoined twins
palato- palate
pale-, paleo- ancient, prehistoric
pan- all
pancreat-, pancreatico-, pancreato-, pancreo- pancreas
para- 1. alongside, accessory, deviation from normal 2. compound derived from two symmetrically arranged substitutions in the benzene ring
parieto- wall of a body cavity
patho-, -pathy disease
ped-, pedi-, pedo- 1. child 2. foot
-penia deficiency
per- 1. throughout 2. highest possible amount of a specified chemical element or radical
peroxy- presence of an additional oxygen atom
-phage, phago- something that eats or destroys
pharyng-, pharyngo- pharynx
phleb-, phlebo- vein
-phobia irrational or abnormal fear
phon-, phono- sound, voice
-phoresis transmission
-phoria constant tendency of an eye to turn from the normal position during binocular vision
-phos light
phot-, photo- light
-phrenia, phreno- 1. diaphragm 2. mind
physi-, physio- natural, physical
physo- 1. tendency to swell 2. air, gas
phyt-, phyto- plants
pico- one trillionth (10^{-12})
pili-, pilo- hair
plani-, plano- flatness
-plasia formation
-plasty shaping, repair of
platy- flatness
pleio- many
pleo- more
pleur-, pleuro- 1. side 2. pleura 3. rib
-ploid multiple in form
pluri- several
pneo- breath, respiration
pneum-, pneuma-, pneumat-, pneumato- 1. pressure of air or gas 2. breath, breathing
pneumo-, pneumon-, pneumono- lungs

pod-, podo- foot
-poesis, -poiesis production, make
poikilo- varied, irregular
polio- gray matter of nervous system
poly- 1. many 2. excessive
post- 1. behind 2. subsequent to
pre- before in time or space
pro- before
proct-, procto- anus, rectum
prostat-, prostato- prostate
prot-, proto- first in a series
pseud-, pseudo- false, deceptive resemblance
psych-, psycho- mind, mental process
psychro- cold
-ptosis downward displacement
ptyal-, ptyalo- saliva
pyel-, pyalo- renal pelvis
pyo- pus
pyro- tire

Q

quadr-, quadri- four
quinque- five

R

rachi-, rachio- spine
radio- radiation emission
re- again, against, behind
recto- rectum
reno- kidney
retro- behind
rhabd-, rhabdo- 1. rod-shaped 2. striated
-rhage-, -rhagia profuse flow
rheo- flow, current
rhin-, rhino- nose
rhod-, rhodo- reddish-rose color
-rrhaphy a joining by sutures
-rrhea, -rrhoea discharge
-rrhexis rupture

S

sacr-, sacro- sacrum
salping-, salpingo- tube
sarco- flesh
scat-, scato- feces
schist-, schisto- split, cleft
schiz-, schizo- division, cleavage
scirrh-, scirrho- hard
scler-, sclero
-scope observe, inspect
-scopy observation, inspection
scoto- darkness
semi- partly
ser-, sero- serum
sial-, sialo- saliva, salivary gland
sidero- iron
somat-, somatico-, somato- body
spermat-, spermato- semen
spermio-, spermo- semen, spermatozoa
spheno- wedge-shaped
sphygm-, sphygmo- pulse
spiro- 1. coil-shaped 2. breathing
splanch-, splanchno- viscera
splen-, spleno- spleen
spodo- waste material
spondyl-, spondylo- vertebra, vertebral column
spor-, sporo- spore
staphyl-, staphylo- bunch of grapes
stearo- fat
steat-, steato- fat
steno- narrowness, constriction
stereo- three-dimensionality
sterno- sternum
steth-, stetho- chest
stomat-, stomato-, stomo- mouth, opening
-stomy surgical opening
strepto- twisted, curved, flexible
stylo- point
sub- under, less than
sulf-, sulfo- presence of a sulfur atom (the spelling sulph- is no longer used)
super- 1. above, superior 2. excess
supra- above
sympath-, sympatheto-, sympathico-, sympatho- sympathetic nervous system
syn- together, joined
syring-, syringo- tube

T

tachy- rapid, accelerated
tel-, tele- distance
tel-, telo- 1. final form 2. an end
teno-, tenon- tendon
tera- one trillion
terato- deformed fetus
tetr-, tetra- four
therm-, thermo- heat
thi-, thio- replacement of oxygen by sulfur
-thiol presence of a thiol group (–SH)
thorac-, thoraco- chest
throm-, thrombo- blood clot, thrombus
-thymia the mind, emotions
thymo- 1. thymus 2. the mind, soul, emotions
thyr-, thyro- thyroid gland
-tome cutting instrument
tomo- a section
-tomy cutting, incising
tox-, toxic-, toxico- poison
trachel-, trachelo- the neck
tracheo- the trachea
trans 1. Across, through, beyond 2. located on opposite sides of a molecule 3. transfer of a chemical group from one compound to another
tri- three
trich-, trichi-, tricho- hair
tris- in chemistry, three of the constituents that follow
troph-, tropho- nutrition
-trophy nutrition
-tropia abnormal deviation in the line of vision
-tropic 1. turning toward 2. having an affinity for
tuber- swelling
typhlo- cecum

U

ultra- surpassing of a specific range
uni- single
ure-, urea-, ureo- urea, urine
uretero- ureter
ureth-, urethro- urethra
uri-, uric-, urico- uric acid
urin-, urine- urine
uro- urine

V

vago- vagus nerve
varic-, varico- varix, varicosity
vas- vessel, fluid-conveying duct
vasculo-, vaso- blood vessels
vene- poison
veni-, veno- veins
ventr-, ventro- abdomen
ventriculo- ventricle
vesic-, vesica- 1. bladder 2. blister
vivi- alive, living

X

xanth-, xantho- yellow
xeno- different
xer-, xero- dryness

Y

-yl in chemistry, a radical, especially a univalent hydrocarbon radical
-ylene a bivalent hydrocarbon radical

Z

zo-, zoo- animals
zyg-, zygo- a yoke, especially a joining together in the manner of a yoke
-zygous a zygotic constitution
-zym-, zymo- enzyme
-zyme enzyme

How to use this dictionary

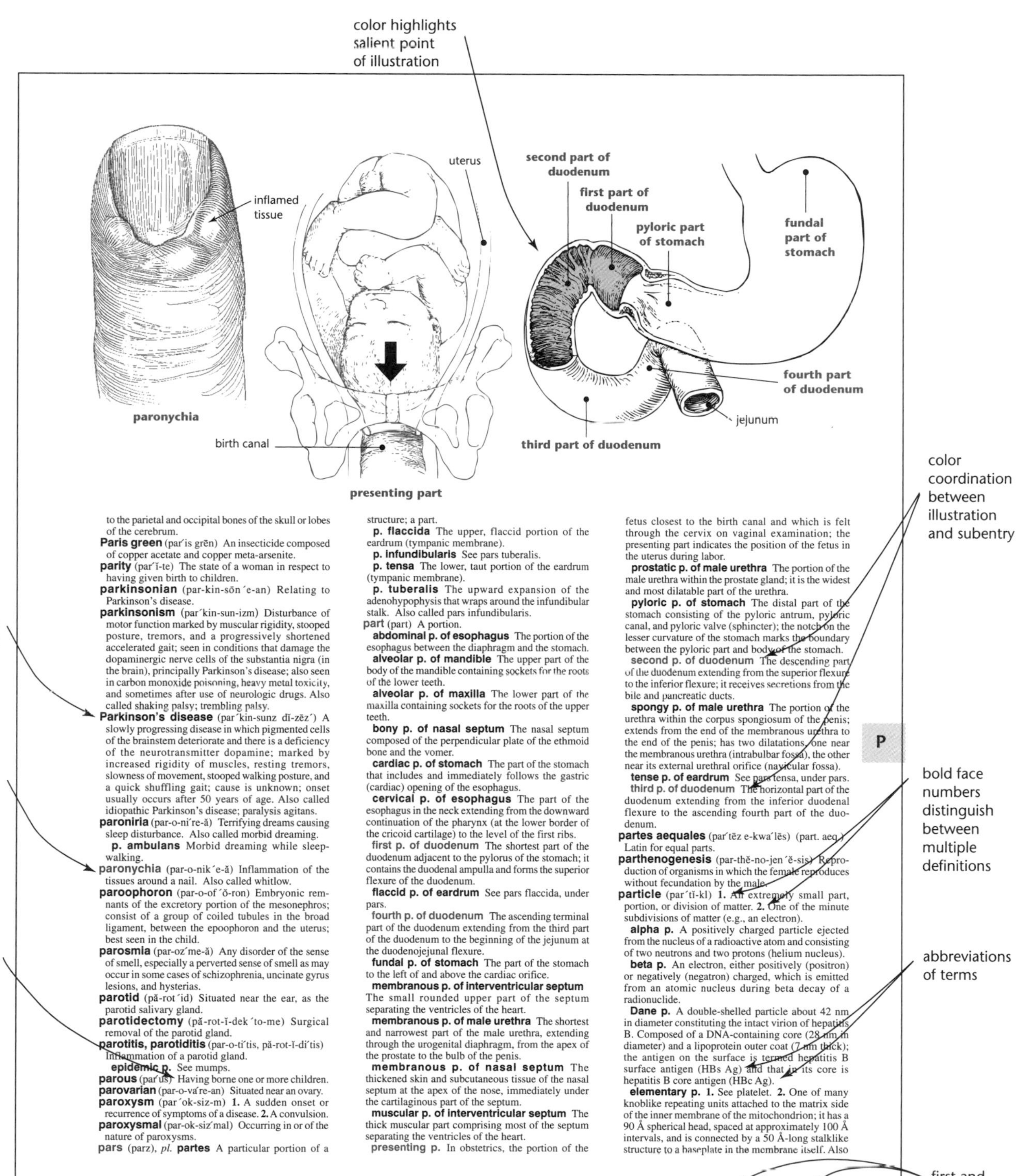

to the parietal and occipital bones of the skull or lobes of the cerebrum.

Paris green (par′is grēn) An insecticide composed of copper acetate and copper meta-arsenite.

parity (par′ĭ-te) The state of a woman in respect to having given birth to children.

parkinsonian (par-kin-sŏn′e-an) Relating to Parkinson's disease.

parkinsonism (par′kin-sun-izm) Disturbance of motor function marked by muscular rigidity, stooped posture, tremors, and a progressively shortened accelerated gait; seen in conditions that damage the dopaminergic nerve cells of the substantia nigra (in the brain), principally Parkinson's disease; also seen in carbon monoxide poisoning, heavy metal toxicity, and sometimes after use of neurologic drugs. Also called shaking palsy; trembling palsy.

Parkinson's disease (par′kin-sunz dĭ-zēz′) A slowly progressing disease in which pigmented cells of the brainstem deteriorate and there is a deficiency of the neurotransmitter dopamine; marked by increased rigidity of muscles, resting tremors, slowness of movement, stooped walking posture, and a quick shuffling gait; cause is unknown; onset usually occurs after 50 years of age. Also called idiopathic Parkinson's disease; paralysis agitans.

paroniria (par-o-ni′re-ă) Terrifying dreams causing sleep disturbance. Also called morbid dreaming.

p. ambulans Morbid dreaming while sleep-walking.

paronychia (par-o-nik′e-ă) Inflammation of the tissues around a nail. Also called whitlow.

paroophoron (par-o-of′ŏ-ron) Embryonic remnants of the excretory portion of the mesonephros; consist of a group of coiled tubules in the broad ligament, between the epoophoron and the uterus; best seen in the child.

parosmia (par-oz′me-ă) Any disorder of the sense of smell, especially a perverted sense of smell as may occur in some cases of schizophrenia, uncinate gyrus lesions, and hysterias.

parotid (pă-rot′id) Situated near the ear, as the parotid salivary gland.

parotidectomy (pă-rot-ĭ-dek′to-me) Surgical removal of the parotid gland.

parotitis, parotiditis (par-o-ti′tis, pă-rot-ĭ-di′tis) Inflammation of a parotid gland.

epidemic p. See mumps.

parous (par′us) Having borne one or more children.

parovarian (par-o-va′re-an) Situated near an ovary.

paroxysm (par′ok-siz-m) **1.** A sudden onset or recurrence of symptoms of a disease. **2.** A convulsion.

paroxysmal (par-ok-siz′mal) Occurring in or of the nature of paroxysms.

pars (parz), *pl.* **partes** A particular portion of a structure; a part.

p. flaccida The upper, flaccid portion of the eardrum (tympanic membrane).

p. infundibularis See pars tuberalis.

p. tensa The lower, taut portion of the eardrum (tympanic membrane).

p. tuberalis The upward expansion of the adenohypophysis that wraps around the infundibular stalk. Also called pars infundibularis.

part (part) A portion.

abdominal p. of esophagus The portion of the esophagus between the diaphragm and the stomach.

alveolar p. of mandible The upper part of the body of the mandible containing sockets for the roots of the lower teeth.

alveolar p. of maxilla The lower part of the maxilla containing sockets for the roots of the upper teeth.

bony p. of nasal septum The nasal septum composed of the perpendicular plate of the ethmoid bone and the vomer.

cardiac p. of stomach The part of the stomach that includes and immediately follows the gastric (cardiac) opening of the esophagus.

cervical p. of esophagus The part of the esophagus in the neck extending from the downward continuation of the pharynx (at the lower border of the cricoid cartilage) to the level of the first ribs.

first p. of duodenum The shortest part of the duodenum adjacent to the pylorus of the stomach; it contains the duodenal ampulla and forms the superior flexure of the duodenum.

flaccid p. of eardrum See pars flaccida, under pars.

fourth p. of duodenum The ascending terminal part of the duodenum extending from the third part of the duodenum to the beginning of the jejunum at the duodenojejunal flexure.

fundal p. of stomach The part of the stomach to the left of and above the cardiac orifice.

membranous p. of interventricular septum The small rounded upper part of the septum separating the ventricles of the heart.

membranous p. of male urethra The shortest and narrowest part of the male urethra, extending through the urogenital diaphragm, from the apex of the prostate to the bulb of the penis.

membranous p. of nasal septum The thickened skin and subcutaneous tissue of the nasal septum at the apex of the nose, immediately under the cartilaginous part of the septum.

muscular p. of interventricular septum The thick muscular part comprising most of the septum separating the ventricles of the heart.

presenting p. In obstetrics, the portion of the fetus closest to the birth canal and which is felt through the cervix on vaginal examination; the presenting part indicates the position of the fetus in the uterus during labor.

prostatic p. of male urethra The portion of the male urethra within the prostate gland; it is the widest and most dilatable part of the urethra.

pyloric p. of stomach The distal part of the stomach consisting of the pyloric antrum, pyloric canal, and pyloric valve (sphincter); the notch on the lesser curvature of the stomach marks the boundary between the pyloric part and body of the stomach.

second p. of duodenum The descending part of the duodenum extending from the superior flexure to the inferior flexure; it receives secretions from the bile and pancreatic ducts.

spongy p. of male urethra The portion of the urethra within the corpus spongiosum of the penis; extends from the end of the membranous urethra to the end of the penis; has two dilatations, one near the membranous urethra (intrabulbar fossa), the other near its external urethral orifice (navicular fossa).

tense p. of eardrum See pars tensa, under pars.

third p. of duodenum The horizontal part of the duodenum extending from the inferior duodenal flexure to the ascending fourth part of the duodenum.

partes aequales (par′tēz e-kwa′lēs) (part. aeq.) Latin for equal parts.

parthenogenesis (par-thĕ-no-jen′ĕ-sis) Reproduction of organisms in which the female reproduces without fecundation by the male.

particle (par′tĭ-kl) **1.** An extremely small part, portion, or division of matter. **2.** One of the minute subdivisions of matter (e.g., an electron).

alpha p. A positively charged particle ejected from the nucleus of a radioactive atom and consisting of two neutrons and two protons (helium nucleus).

beta p. An electron, either positively (positron) or negatively (negatron) charged, which is emitted from an atomic nucleus during beta decay of a radionuclide.

Dane p. A double-shelled particle about 42 nm in diameter constituting the intact virion of hepatitis B. Composed of a DNA-containing core (28 nm in diameter) and a lipoprotein outer coat (7 nm thick); the antigen on the surface is termed hepatitis B surface antigen (HBs Ag) and that in its core is hepatitis B core antigen (HBc Ag).

elementary p. **1.** See platelet. **2.** One of many knoblike repeating units attached to the matrix side of the inner membrane of the mitochondrion; it has a 90 Å spherical head, spaced at approximately 100 Å intervals, and is connected by a 50 Å-long stalklike structure to a baseplate in the membrane itself. Also

487

Paris green ■ particle

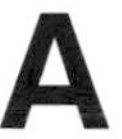

A

α Alpha. For terms beginning with α, see under specific term.

abaissement (ă-bās-mawn´) French for a lowering or depression.

abandonment (ă-ban´don-ment) Termination of the physician-patient relationship unilaterally by the physician under circumstances that require continuing medical care, without giving the patient reasonable time to secure the services of another physician or when alternative sources for medical care are unavailable.

abarognosis (a-bar-og-no´sis) Loss of ability to perceive weight.

abarthrosis (ab-ar-thro´sis) See diarthrosis.

abarticular (ab-ar-tik´u-lar) Not affecting, or far from, a joint.

abarticulation (ab-ar-tik-u-la´shun) **1.** Dislocation. **2.** Diarthrosis.

abasia (ă-ba´zhă) Inability to walk due to impaired motor coordination.

abasic, abatic (ă-ba´sik, ă-bat´ik) Relating to abasia.

abaxial, abaxile (ab-ak´sē-ăl, ab-ak´sīl) Not located on the axis of the body or any structure.

abdomen (ab´dŏ-men, ab-do´men) The part of the body between the thorax and pelvis; contains the viscera. Also called belly.

acute a. An incapacitating condition characterized by intense abdominal pain, which may or may not be associated with fever, nausea, vomiting, and shock.

burst a. See evisceration (2).

abdominal (ab-dom´ĭ-nal) Pertaining to the abdomen.

abdominalgia (ab-dom-ĭ-nal´jă) Pain in the abdomen.

periodic a. Disorder of unknown cause, marked by abdominal pain, recurring fever, inflamed peritoneum, and sometimes purpura. Also called Mediterranean fever; benign paroxysmal peritonitis.

abdominocentesis (ab-dom-ĭ-no-sen-te´sis) See peritoneocentesis.

abdominoplasty (ab-dom´ĭ-no-plas-tē) Removal of loose skin and subcutaneous tissue from the abdominal wall.

abdominoposterior (ab-dom-ĭ-no-pos-te´re-or) Denoting a position of the fetus in the uterus in which its abdomen is turned toward the mother's back.

abdominoscopy (ab-dom-ĭ-nos´ko-pe) Examination of the abdomen, especially visual examination of the abdominal organs.

abdominovaginal (ab-dom-ĭ-no-vag´ ĭ-nal) Relating to the abdomen and vagina.

abdominovesical (ab-dom-ĭ-no-ves´ĭ-kl) Relating to the abdomen and urinary bladder.

abducens (ab-du´senz) Denoting the sixth cranial nerve.

abducent (ab-du´sent) Denoting structures that serve to abduct a part.

abduct (ab-dukt´) To draw away from the median line of the body or from an adjacent part or limb.

abduction (ab-duk´shun) Movement of a part away from the middle line; act of turning outward.

abductor (ab-duk´tor) A structure, such as a muscle, that draws a part away from an axis of the body; opposite of adductor.

abembryonic (ab-em-bre-on´ik) Located away from the embryo.

aberrant (ab-er´ant) Deviating from the normal or expected course, as a duct taking an unusual direction.

aberration (ab-er-a´shun) **1.** A deviation from the normal. **2.** Unequal refraction of light rays passing through a lens, resulting in the formation of an imperfect image.

chromatic a. Aberration resulting from unequal refraction of wavelengths; typical example is a display of colors around an object viewed through a simple lens. Also called newtonian aberration; color aberration.

chromosome a. A departure from the normal number of chromosomes or chromosome structure; e.g., in Down syndrome there are 47 chromosomes, in Turner syndrome there are 45.

color a. See chromatic aberration.

newtonian a. See chromatic aberration.

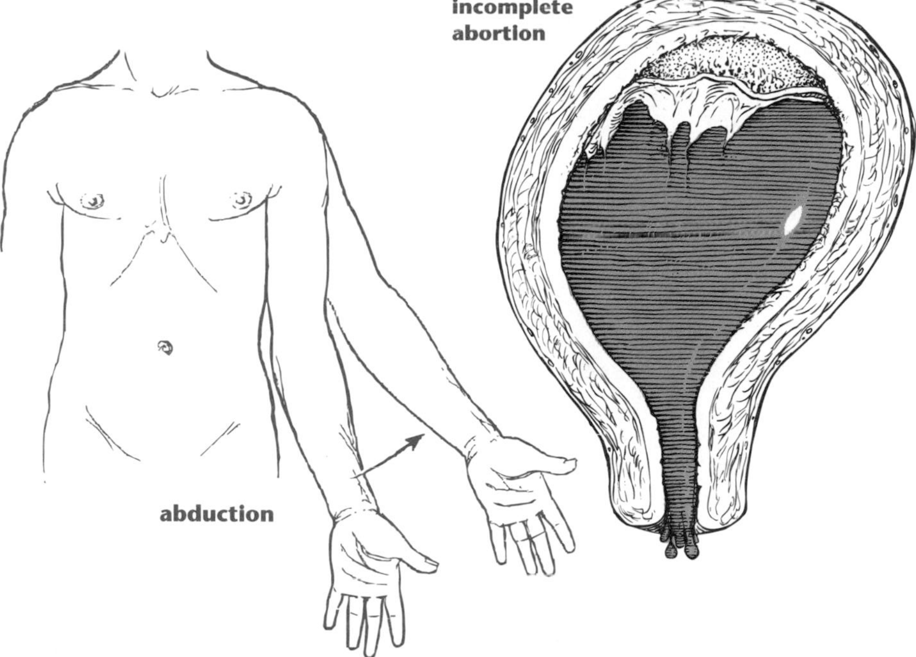

abetalipoproteinemia (a-ba-tă-lip-o-pro-te-ne´me-ă) An autosomal recessive inherited disorder marked by pigmentary degeneration of the retina, presence of large numbers of acanthocytes in the blood, and absence of low-density lipoproteins (LDLs) in the plasma; may be associated with excessive fat in the feces and progressive neurologic disease.

abient (ab´e-ent) Having the tendency to avoid, or move away from, a stimulus.

ability (ă-bil´ĭ -te) The physical or mental competence to function.

impaired urinary concentrating a. Inability to concentrate solutes in the urine; characteristic of diseases affecting the inner portion of the kidney (e.g., pyelonephritis, polycystic kidney disease, sickle cell disease).

abiogenesis (ab-e-o-jen´ĕ-sis) The origin of living matter from nonliving matter; a theory of spontaneous generation.

abiology (a-bi-ol´o-je) The study of nonliving or inorganic things.

abiosis (ab-e-o´sis) Lifelessness; absence of life.

abiotrophy (ab-e-ot´ro-fe) General term denoting degenerative changes of tissues due to genetic causes.

abirritant (ab-ir´rĭ-tant) **1.** Relieving irritation. **2.** A substance having this property.

ablate (ab-lāt´) To remove.

ablatio placentae (ab-la´she-o plă-sen´tē) See abruptio placentae.

ablation (ab-la´shun) **1.** Detachment. **2.** Removal or eradication by surgery or freezing.

ablepharia, ablepharon (ă-blef-ă´re-ă, ă-blef´ă-ron) Congenital absence of the eyelids, partial or total.

ablepharous (ă-blef´ă-rus) Without eyelids.

abluent (ab´loo-ent) A substance that has cleansing properties.

ablution (ab-loo´shun) The act of cleansing.

ablutomania (ab-loo-to-ma´ne-ă) Abnormal concern with cleanliness.

abneural (ab-noor´al) Away from the central nervous system or from the dorsal aspect.

abnormal (ab-nor´mal) Not normal; departing from the usual position, structure, or condition.

abnormality (ab-nor-mal´ĭ-te) The condition or state of being abnormal.

ABO blood group International classification of human blood types according to their compatibility in transfusion; typed as A, B, AB, or O. Also called ABO factors.

aboral (ab-o´ral) Distant from or opposite to the mouth.

abort (ă-bort´) **1.** To expel or to remove the products of conception before the fetus reaches the age of viability. **2.** To arrest the usual course of a disease. **3.** To cause cessation of development.

aborticide (ă-bor´tĭ-sīd) See abortifacient.

abortient (ă-bor´shent) **1.** Aborting. **2.** An abortifacient; a drug that produces abortion.

abortifacient (ă-bor-tĭ-fa´shent) Anything that produces abortion. Also called aborticide.

abortigenic (ă-bor-tĭ-gen´ik) Abortifacient.

abortion (ă-bor´shun) **1.** Expulsion or extraction of all or any part of the products of conception (placenta, membranes, and embryo or fetus) before the end of 20 complete weeks (139 days) of gestation calculated from the first day of the last normal menstrual period, or a fetal weight of less than 500 g. **2.** The arrest of any process.

accidental a. Abortion resulting from injury.

ampullar a. Abortion resulting from implantation of the fertilized egg within the ampulla of the fallopian (uterine) tube.

complete a. Expulsion of fetus (or embryo), placenta, and membranes, ending with cessation of both pain and copious bleeding.

elective a. Induced abortion performed at the request of the pregnant woman, but not due to impaired maternal health or fetal disease and before fetal viability is reached. Also called voluntary abortion.

eugenic a. See therapeutic abortion.

habitual a. A sequence of three or more spontaneous abortions occurring consecutively before 20 weeks of gestation, with the fetus weighing less than 500 g; may be due to fetal or maternal factors (e.g., genetic error, hormonal abnormalities, anatomic anomalies of reproductive tract, infection, systemic disease, immunologic factors). Sometimes causes are unknown. Also called recurrent abortion; recurrent spontaneous abortion.

incomplete a. Abortion in which some of the products of conception (usually a portion of the placenta) remain within the uterus, causing profuse uterine bleeding.

induced a. Intentionally caused abortion; may be therapeutic or nontherapeutic. See also elective abortion; therapeutic abortion.

inevitable a. Bleeding of intrauterine origin before 20 completed weeks of gestation with continuous and progressive dilatation of the cervix.

infected a. Abortion accompanied by fever, generalized pelvic discomfort, purulent discharge, or elevated white blood cell count; caused by infection of the genital organs with pathogenic microorganisms. Distinguished from septic abortion.

justifiable a. See therapeutic abortion.

missed a. Death of an embryo or fetus before completion of the 20th week of gestation with

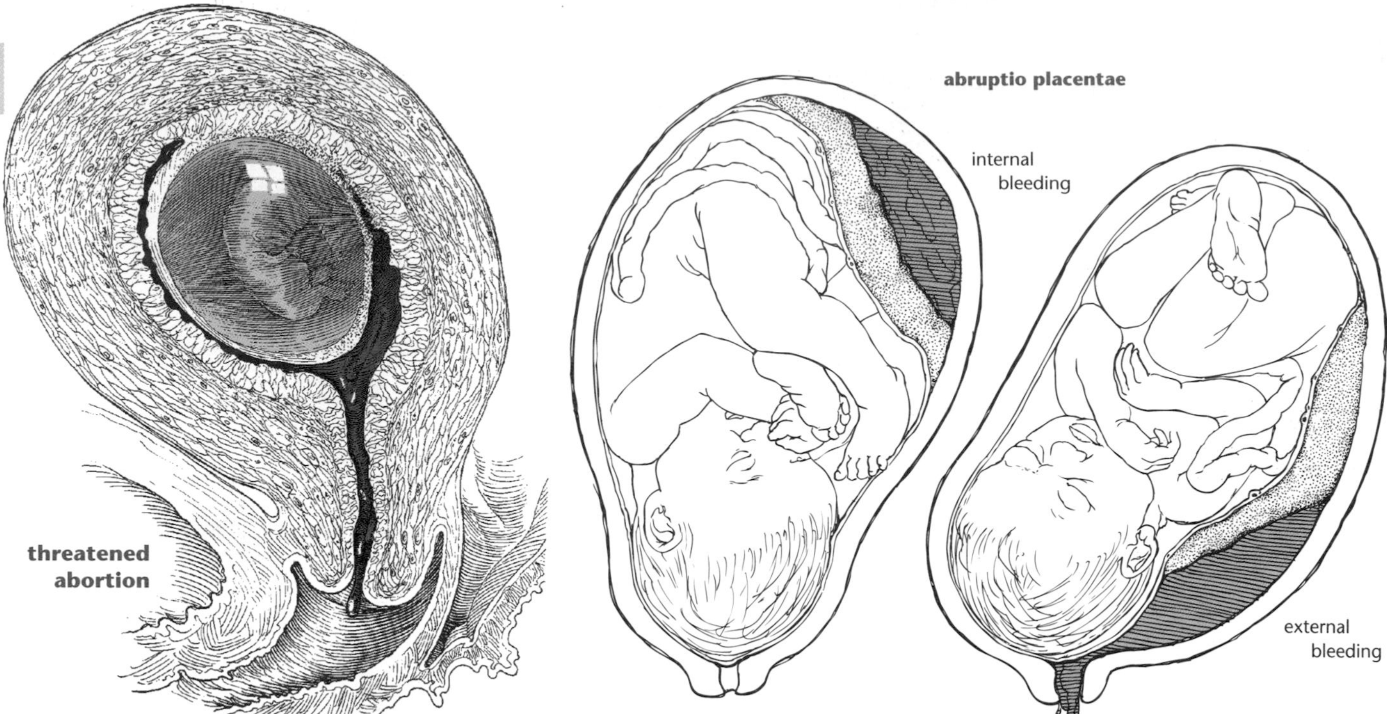

retention of all the products of conception for several weeks; manifested by absence of fetal heartbeat, regression of breast changes, decrease of uterine size, and weight loss.

natural a. See spontaneous abortion.

nontherapeutic a. Abortion induced without a medical reason.

partial-birth a. (PBA) Common term for termination of a late pregnancy with a breech presentation. Labor is induced by conventional methods; the cervix is widely dilated and delivery is expedited by evacuating the cranial contents with a suction catheter, then compressing the cranium. See also dilatation and evacuation (D&E).

recidive a. The occurrence of two consecutive spontaneous abortions before 20 weeks of gestation, with the fetus weighing less than 500 g.

recurrent a. See habitual abortion.

recurrent spontaneous a. See habitual abortion.

septic a. Infected abortion accompanied by life-threatening dissemination of microorganisms and toxic substances throughout the maternal blood circulation; marked by a malodorous discharge, pelvic and abdominal pain, suprapubic tenderness, and peritonitis. Distinguished from infected abortion.

spontaneous a. Abortion resulting from natural causes, without deliberate mechanical or medicinal interference, and occurring before the fetus can survive outside the uterus. Also called fetal loss; miscarriage; natural abortion.

therapeutic a. Abortion performed before the time of fetal viability for medical or psychiatric reasons. Also called eugenic abortion; justifiable abortion.

threatened a. Slight or heavier bloody vaginal discharge, occurring during the first 20 weeks of pregnancy, with or without cramplike pain and low backache, without expulsion of the products of conception, and without dilatation of the cervix.

tubal a. Spontaneous termination of an ectopic pregnancy implanted within a fallopian (uterine) tube; may be expelled into the peritoneal cavity through the end of the tube or, less frequently, may pass into the peritoneal cavity through a rupture of the tubal wall at the implantation site.

voluntary a. See elective abortion.

abortive (ă-bor′tiv) **1.** Causing abortion. **2.** Cutting short, arresting; said of a disease. **3.** Failing to reach completion; partially developed.

aboulia (ă-boo′le-ă) See abulia.

abrachia (ă-bra′ke-ă) Absence of arms.

abrade (ă-brād′) To rub or wear away the external layer by friction, as to scrape away the epidermis from a part; to excoriate.

abrasion (ă-bra′zhun) **1.** A superficial injury, in which the skin or mucous membrane is scraped away. **2.** The process of wearing down of a tooth by friction; usually applied to excessive wear such as that caused by the use of an abrasive dentifrice.

mechanical a. See dermabrasion.

abrasive (ă-bra′siv) **1.** Producing abrasion. **2.** A material used in dentistry for grinding or polishing.

abreaction (ab-re-ak′shun) A form of psychotherapy, called catharsis by Freud, in which emotional release is attained by recalling a forgotten (repressed), painful experience.

abruptio placentae (ab-rup′she-o plă-sen′tē) Premature separation of the normally implanted placenta from its uterine attachment after the 20th week of gestation. Also called placental abruption; ablatio placentae; accidental hemorrhage.

abruption (ab-rup′shun) A tearing away; detachment.

placental a. See abruptio placentae.

abscess (ab′ses) Localized accumulation of pus.

acute a. One of short duration, producing a throbbing pain and fever. Also called hot abscess.

alveolar a. Abscess in a tooth socket usually caused by bacteria spreading from dental caries; causes severe throbbing pain and swelling. Also called dentoalveolar abscess; periodontal abscess.

amebic a. One occurring as a complication of amebic dysentery, usually in the liver, and containing a brown pasty fluid.

appendicular a. An abscess in the area of the vermiform appendix.

breast a. See mammary abscess.

canalicular a. Abscess connected to a milk (lactiferous) duct within a breast, causing a purulent discharge from the nipple.

chronic a. A long-standing collection of pus without inflammation. Also called cold abscess.

cold a. See chronic abscess.

dentoalveolar a. See alveolar abscess.

extradural a. Abscess situated between the skull and the outer covering of the brain (dura mater).

gingival a. A localized, painful, inflammatory lesion of the gingiva, usually arising from a periodontal pocket.

gummatous a. Abscess formed subsequent to the softening and breaking down of a gumma, the characteristic tumor of tertiary syphilis. Also called syphilitic abscess.

hot a. See acute abscess.

iliac a. See psoas abscess.

mammary a. Single or multiple abscesses of the breast substance, affecting usually one breast; most commonly caused by *Staphylococcus aureus*, or occasionally by streptococci. Organisms gain entry through cracks on the nipple, most frequently during lactation, or in skin conditions such as eczema. Destroyed breast tissue may be replaced by fibrous tissue with resulting nipple retraction, which may be mistaken for a tumor. Also called breast abscess.

metastatic a. Secondary abscess caused by organisms carried in the bloodstream from a primary abscess.

orbital a. An abscess within the ocular orbit, frequently an extension of purulent sinusitis.

palmar a. A collection of pus in the palm of the hand, resulting from a puncture injury.

pelvic a. An abscess located in the pelvic cavity, usually in the rectouterine pouch, often occurring as a complication of abdominal or pelvic inflammatory disease.

periapical a. An abscess occurring in the alveolus near the apex of a tooth root, usually due to death of the tooth pulp.

periodontal a. See alveolar abscess.

peritonsillar a. Acute suppurative inflammation of the tonsils and surrounding tissues.

periurethral a. One involving the tissues around the urethra, causing strained, painful urination.

psoas a. One occurring in the sheath of the psoas muscle secondary to tuberculosis of the lower spine or to regional enteritis. Also called iliac abscess.

pulp a. One within the pulp cavity of a tooth.

stitch a. An abscess around a suture.

subdiaphragmatic a. An abscess between the diaphragm and the liver or between the diaphragm and the spleen and stomach. Also called subphrenic abscess.

subphrenic a. See subdiaphragmatic abscess.

syphilitic a. See gummatous abscess.

tubo-ovarian a. Abscess involving a fallopian (uterine) tube and its corresponding ovary, usually associated with inflammation of the tube; often seen in patients with a history of pelvic infection; symptoms include a tender pelvic mass, pelvic and abdominal pain, and fever.

abscissa (ab-sis′ă) The horizontal coordinate which, together with a vertical one (ordinate), forms a frame of reference for the plotting of data.

absence (ab′sens) A brief loss of consciousness. See also childhood absence epilepsy, under epilepsy.

absolute (ab′so-lūt) Complete; unrestricted; unadulterated.

absorb (ab-sorb′) **1.** To take in as through pores or interstices. **2.** To incorporate or take up gases, liquid, light rays, or heat. **3.** To neutralize an acid.

absorbable (ab-sorb′ă-bl) Capable of being absorbed.

absorbent (ab-sor′bent) Anything that can incorporate a substance into itself.

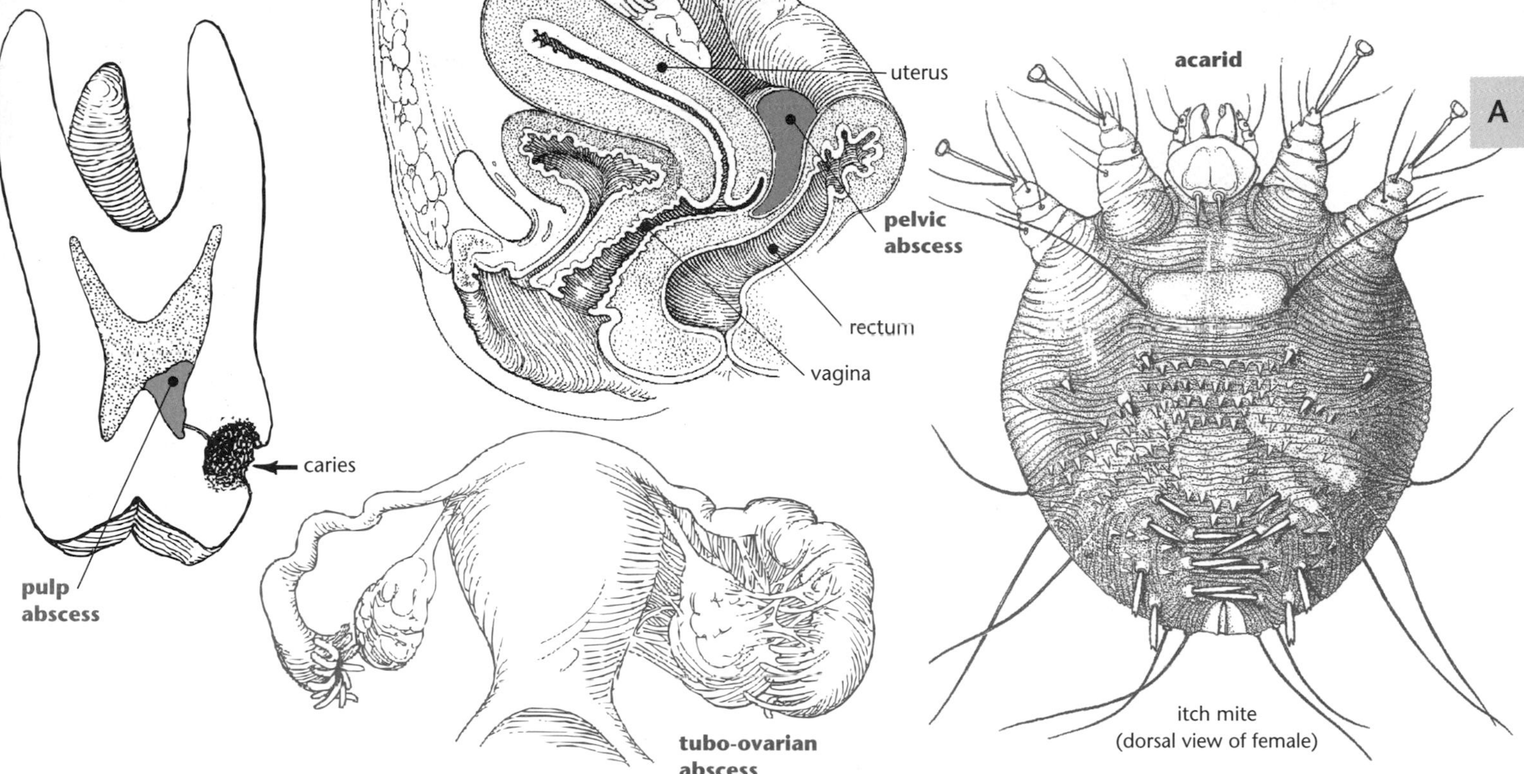

absorptiometer (ab-sorp-she-om´ĕ-ter) **1.** Instrument for measuring the solubility of gas in a liquid. **2.** Device for measuring the layer of absorbed liquid between two glass plates; used as a hematoscope in blood analysis.

absorptiometry (ab-sorp-she-om´ĕ-tre) **1.** Any procedure for measuring absorption of waves or particles. **2.** In radiology, the measurement of the amount of radiation emitted by a radioisotope that is completely dispersed throughout a tissue.

dual-photon a. A method of quantitating bone mineral content by comparing the transmission of two photoelectric energy peaks emitted by gandolinium 153 through bone and soft tissues; used to measure bone density of the spine and hip for diagnosis of osteoporosis and in following therapy response.

absorption (ab-sorp´shun) **1.** The taking up of substances by the skin or other tissues. **2.** The taking up of part or all of the energy of incident radiation by the medium through which radiation passes, resulting in reduction of radiation intensity.

abstergent (ab-ster´jent) Cleansing or purgative.

abstinence (ab´stĭ-nens) A refraining from the indulgence in something, as sexual intercourse or stimulants, by one's own choice. Also called self-denial.

abstract (ab´strakt) **1.** A preparation containing the soluble elements of a drug mixed with lactose. **2.** A summary of a book or literary article.

abulia (ă-bu´le-ă) Pronounced diminution of will power; inability to make decisions. Also written aboulia.

abuse (ă-būs´) **1.** Improper use, particularly excessive use of anything. **2.** Maltreatment.

child a. An act or omission, which is not accidental, committed by a parent, caregiver, or other adult or significantly older child that harms, or threatens to harm, a child's physical or mental health or welfare; the abuse may be emotional, physical, or sexual.

drug a. The excessive and persistent use (usually by self-administration) of any drug without due regard for accepted medical practice. Also called substance abuse.

emotional child a. Acts or omissions usually on the part of parents or other caregivers that cause serious behavioral, cognitive, emotional, or mental disorders in the child; may involve ignoring the child's needs and emotional and developmental growth; and isolating, terrorizing, and corrupting the child by engagement in antisocial behavior. Emotional abuse usually accompanies other forms of abuse and neglect. Also called psychological child abuse.

physical child a. Abuse that results in physical injury, usually perpetrated in the name of discipline.

psychological child a. See emotional child abuse.

sexual child a. Any sexual activity perpetrated by an adult or older child with or upon a child, or the sexual exploitation of a child for the gratification or profit of the other.

substance a. See drug abuse, following definition of drug.

abutment (ă-but´ment) **1.** A supporting structure. **2.** In dentistry, a natural tooth or root used to anchor and support a partial denture appliance.

intermediate a. A natural tooth, without other natural teeth in proximal contact, which is used as an abutment, in addition to the primary or terminal abutments.

acacia (ă-ka´she-ă) The dried gummy exudate from a tropical tree of the genus *Acacia*; used in the preparation of medicinal drugs. Also called gum arabic.

acalculia (ă-kal-ku´le-ă) A form of aphasia characterized by inability to do simple arithmetic.

acantha (ă-kan´thă) A spinous process.

acanthamebiasis (ă-kan-thă-me-bi´ă-sis) Infection with *Acanthamoeba castellani*, a free-living ameba found in moist soil and water; may cause fatal inflammation of the brain and its membranes (meningoencephalitis).

acanthesthesia (ă-kan-thes-the´ză) Condition in which there is a sensation of pressure with a sharp point.

acanthion (ă-kan´the-on) A projection on the anterior nasal spine.

Acanthocephala (ă-kan-tho-sef´ă-lă) A phylum of parasitic worms having a proboscis with hooked spines for attachment to the digestive tract of host.

acanthocephaliasis (ă-kan-tho-sef-ă-li´ă-sis) Infestation with parasites of the phylum Acanthocephala.

Acanthocheilonema (ă-kan-tho-ki-lo-ne´mă) Genus of parasitic worms now classified under the genus *Mansonella*.

acanthocheilonemiasis (ă-kan-tho-ki-lo-ne-mi´ă-sis) See mansonellosis.

acanthocyte (ă-kan´tho-sīt) An abnormal red blood cell having several protoplasmic projections that give it a thorny appearance.

acanthocytosis (ă-kan-tho-si-to´sis) Familial condition marked by the presence in the blood of large numbers of acanthocytes.

acanthoid (ă-kan´thoid) Having the shape of a spine; spinous.

acantholysis (ak-an-thol´ĭ-sis) Disintegration of the epidermis.

acanthoma (ak-an-tho´mă) Carcinoma of the epidermis.

acanthosis (ak-an-tho´sis) Thickening of the prickle-cell layer of the skin.

a. nigricans A benign hyperpigmented skin lesion associated with a variety of disorders of the endocrine system, such as Cushing's syndrome, pituitary tumors, and polycystic ovary syndrome. Often there is an underlying insulin resistance.

acapnia (ă-kap´ne-ă) See hypocapnia.

acari (ak´ă-ri) Plural of acarus.

acariasis (ak-ă-ri´ă-sis) **1.** Any disease caused by mites. **2.** Infestation with mites.

sarcoptic a. See scabies.

acaricide (ă-kar´ĭ-sīd) Any agent that destroys mites.

acarid (ak´ă-rid) A mite or tick; any member of the order Acarina.

Acaridae (ă-kar´ĭ-de) A family of small mites (order Acarina), some of which cause skin eruptions in humans.

Acarina (ak-ă-rī´nă) An order of the class Arachnida, which includes mites and ticks.

acarinosis (ă-kar-ĭ-no´sis) See acariasis.

acarodermatitis (ak-ă-ro-der-mă-ti´tis) A skin rash caused by mites.

acaroid (ak´ă-roid) Resembling a mite.

acarology (ak-ă-rol´o-je) The study of mites and ticks.

acarophobia (ak-ă-ro-fo´be-ă) Abnormal fear of mites (acari), or of small particles.

acarus (ak´ă-rus), *pl.* **ac´ari** A mite or tick.

acaryote (ă-kār´e-ōt) See akaryocyte.

acatalasemia (a-kat-ă-la-se´me-ă) See acatalasia.

acatalasia (a-kat-ă-la´ză) Genetic disorder marked by deficiency of the enzyme catalase; manifestations range from mild (ulcers of tooth sockets) to severe (recession of tooth sockets and gangrene of the gums). Two principal types have been identified: a Japanese type, in which the small amount of residual catalase is physiochemically normal, suggesting a mutation of a regulator (controller) gene; and a Swiss type, in which the catalase is abnormal, suggesting a structural gene mutation. Formerly called acatalasemia.

acatamathesia (a-kat-ă-mă-the´ză) Loss of the power of understanding.

acataphasia (a-kat-ă-fa´ză) Loss of the power to formulate one's thoughts correctly.

acaudal, acaudate (a-kaw´dal, a-kaw´dāt) Without a tail.

accelerant (ak-sel´er-ant) See accelerator.

acceleration (ak-sel-er-a´shun) Increased speed of action, as of pulse or respiration.

accelerator (ak-sel´er-a-tor) Anything (drug,

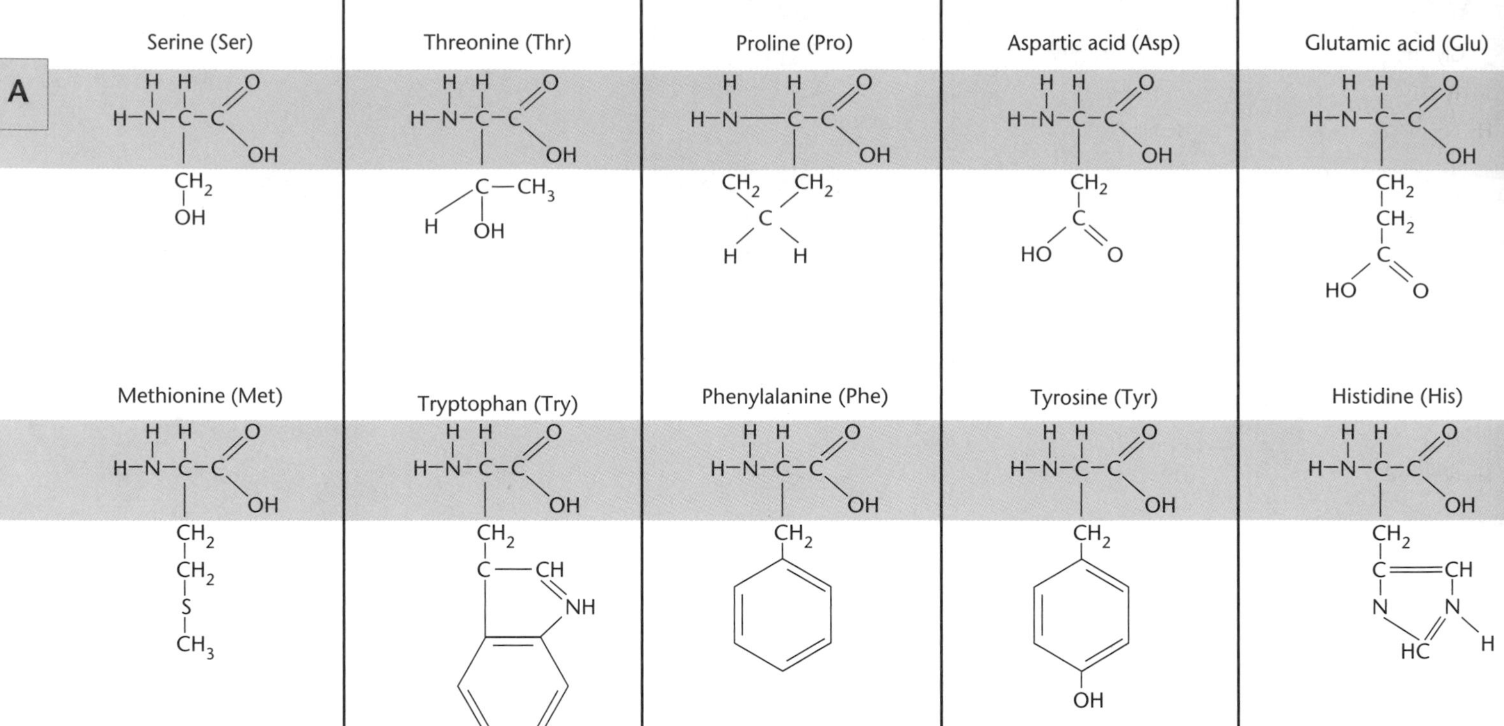

device, nerve, or muscle) that increases speed of action or function. Also called accelerant.

accentuator (ak-sen-chu-a´tor) A substance that increases the action of a tissue stain.

acceptor (ak-sep´tor) A substance that unites with a chemical group or ion of another substance (the donor), thus allowing a chemical reaction to proceed.

accessory (ak-ses´o-re) Supplementary; having a subordinate function to a similar but more important structure.

accessory sign (ak-ses´o-re sīn) Any sign that usually, but not always, accompanies a disease.

accident (ak´sĭ-dent) An unexpected, unintentional, undesirable event, or an unforeseen complication in the course of a disease.

cerebrovascular a., cerebral vascular a. (CVA) See stroke.

acclimatization, acclimation (ă-kli-mă-ti-za´shun, ak-li-ma´shun) Adjustment of an individual or plant to a new environment.

accolé form (ak-ōlā form) See under form.

accommodation (ă-kom-o-da´shun) Alteration in the convexity of the lens of the eye to attain maximal sharpness of a retinal image of an object, distant or near.

accommodative (ă-kom´o-da-tiv) Relating to accommodation.

accouchement (ah-ko͞osh-maw´) French for childbirth or labor.

accrementition (ak-re-men-tish´un) **1.** Reproduction by budding. **2.** Growth by gradual external addition.

accretio cordis (ă-kre´she-o kor´dis) Adhesion of the pericardium to adjacent structures, such as the chest wall, pleura, or diaphragm.

accretion (ă-kre´shun) Slow accumulation of deposits, as on the surface of a tooth.

acellular (a-sel´u-lar) Having no cells.

acenesthesia (ă-sen-es-the´ză) Loss of the normal sense of physical existence.

acentric (ă-sen´trik) **1.** Not centrally located. **2.** Denoting a chromosome fragment lacking a centromere.

acephalia (ă-sĕ-fa´le-ă) See acephaly.

acephalocyst (ă-sef-ă-lo´sist) A cyst filled with liquid that is one of the stages in the development of a sterile tapeworm; it does not give origin to daughter cysts which contain tapeworm heads (scoleces).

acephaly (ă-sef´ă-le) Congenital absence of the head. Also called acephalia.

acervuline (ă-ser´vu-līn) Occurring in cluster forms.

acervulus (ă-ser´vu-lus) See brain sand granules, under granule.

acetabular (as-ĕ-tab´u-lar) Relating to the acetabulum.

Acetabularia (as-ĕ-tab-u-la´re-ă) A genus (phylum Chlorophyta) of single-celled algae which may grow as tall as 10 cm and which possess a distinctive cap; used in the study of molecular biology.

acetabulectomy (as-ĕ-tab-u-lek´to-me) Surgical removal of the acetabulum.

acetabuloplasty (as-ĕ-tab´u-lo-plas-te) Surgical restoration of the acetabulum.

acetabulum (as-ĕ-tab´u-lum) The cup-shaped cavity in the lateral surface of the hipbone in which the head of the femur articulates. Also called hip socket.

acetaldehyde (as-et-al´dĕ-hīd) A colorless liquid, CH_3CHO, with a pungent odor; an intermediate in yeast fermentation of carbohydrate and in alcohol metabolism in man. Also called acetic aldehyde.

acetamide (ă-set´ă-mīd) A colorless crystalline substance, CH_3CONH_2; an amine of acetic acid, used as a solvent.

acetaminophen (ă-set-ă-me´no-fen) *N*-Acetyl-*p*-aminophenol; a white crystalline compound, used to relieve pain and fever. It lacks anti-inflammatory properties and has been known to produce harmful effects to the liver. Also called paracetamol.

acetanilid (as-et-an´ĭ-lid) A white crystalline substance, obtained from the action of acetic acid upon aniline; formerly used to relieve pain and fever.

acetate (as´ĕ-tāt) Any acetic acid salt.

acetazolamide (as-et-ă-zol-ă-mīd) A diuretic that inhibits the action of carbonic anhydrase in the kidney, promoting the loss of bicarbonate and sodium; the effect is to produce a mild acidosis and to alkalinize the urine; used in glaucoma to reduce intraocular pressure; Diamox®.

acetic (ă-se´tik, ă-set´ik) Relating to, or containing, vinegar.

acetic acid (ă-se´tik as´id) A colorless, organic acid with a pungent odor.

glacial a. a. A caustic liquid containing 99.5% acetic acid; used to remove corns and warts.

acetify (ă-set´ĭ-fi) To convert to vinegar or acetic acid.

acetoacetic acid (ă-se-to-ă-se´tik) A colorless syrupy acid, CH_3COH_2COOH; one of the ketone bodies, occurring in excessive quantities in the urine of poorly controlled diabetics.

Acetobacter (ă-se-to-bak´ter) A genus of bacteria (family Pseudomonadaceae) having elongated or rod-shaped forms, sometimes flagellated; important in the production of vinegar.

acetolysis (as-ĕ-tol´ĭ-sis) The splitting of an organic compound by the introduction of the elements of acetic acid.

acetomorphine (as-ĕ-to-mor´fēn) See heroin.

acetone (as´ĕ-tōn) A colorless, volatile, extremely flammable liquid with an ethereal odor, CH_3COCH_3; generally used as an organic solvent.

acetonemia (as-ĕ-to-ne´me-ă) The presence of relatively large amounts of acetone or acetone bodies in the blood, as occurs when there is incomplete oxidation of large amounts of fat, as in ketoacidosis or starvation.

acetonemic (as-ĕ-to-ne´mik) Characterized by acetonemia.

acetonuria (as-ĕ-to-nu´re-ă) The presence of acetone in the urine; it occurs in poorly controlled diabetes mellitus and in starvation from incomplete oxidation of fats.

acetophenetidin (as-ĕ-to-fĕ-net´ĭ-din) See phenacetin.

acetum (ă-se´tum), *pl.* **ace´ta** **1.** Vinegar. **2.** A solution of a drug made with acetic acid.

acetyl (as´ĕ-til) A radical or combining form of acetic acid, CH_3CO.

***N*-acetylaspartate** (ăs-ĕ-til-as-par´tāt) A derivative of aspartate (a salt of aspartic acid); found in the brain. Used as a marker in magnetic imaging in procedures of the nervous system.

acetylation (ă-set-ĭ-la´shun) The introduction of a radical group of acetic acid (acetyl) into an organic compound.

acetylcholine (as-ĕ-til-ko´lēn) (ACh) The acetic acid ester of choline, $CH_3COOCH_2C_2N(CH_3)_3OH$; the chemical transmitter of the nerve impulse across a synapse; also released by the endings of parasympathetic nerves (cholinergic nerves) upon stimulation; produces cardiac slowing, vasodilatation, increased gastrointestinal activity, and other parasympathetic effects; it is hydrolyzed and inactivated by the enzyme cholinesterase; available as acetylcholine bromide and acetylcholine chloride.

acetylcholinesterase (as´ĕ-til-ko-lĭ-nes´tĕ-rās) An enzyme present throughout body tissues that promotes the hydrolysis of acetylcholine; it acts to remove acetylcholine discharged at the neuromuscular junction, thus preventing it from reexciting the muscle.

acetyl coenzyme A, acetyl-CoA (as´ĕ-til ko-en´zīm ā, as´ĕ-til-ko-ā) An important metabolic intermediate of the tricarboxylic acid cycle; formed when an acetyl group is attached to coenzyme A by a thioester bond during oxidation of fatty acid, amino acids, or pyruvate.

acetylcysteine (as-ĕ-til-sis´te-ēn) An agent used in the treatment of some bronchopulmonary disorders to reduce the viscosity of mucus; Mucomyst®.

acetylene (ă-set´ĭ-lēn) A colorless, flammable, explosive gas, C_2H_2, with a disagreeable garlic odor; made by the action of water on calcium carbide; formerly used as an anesthetic.

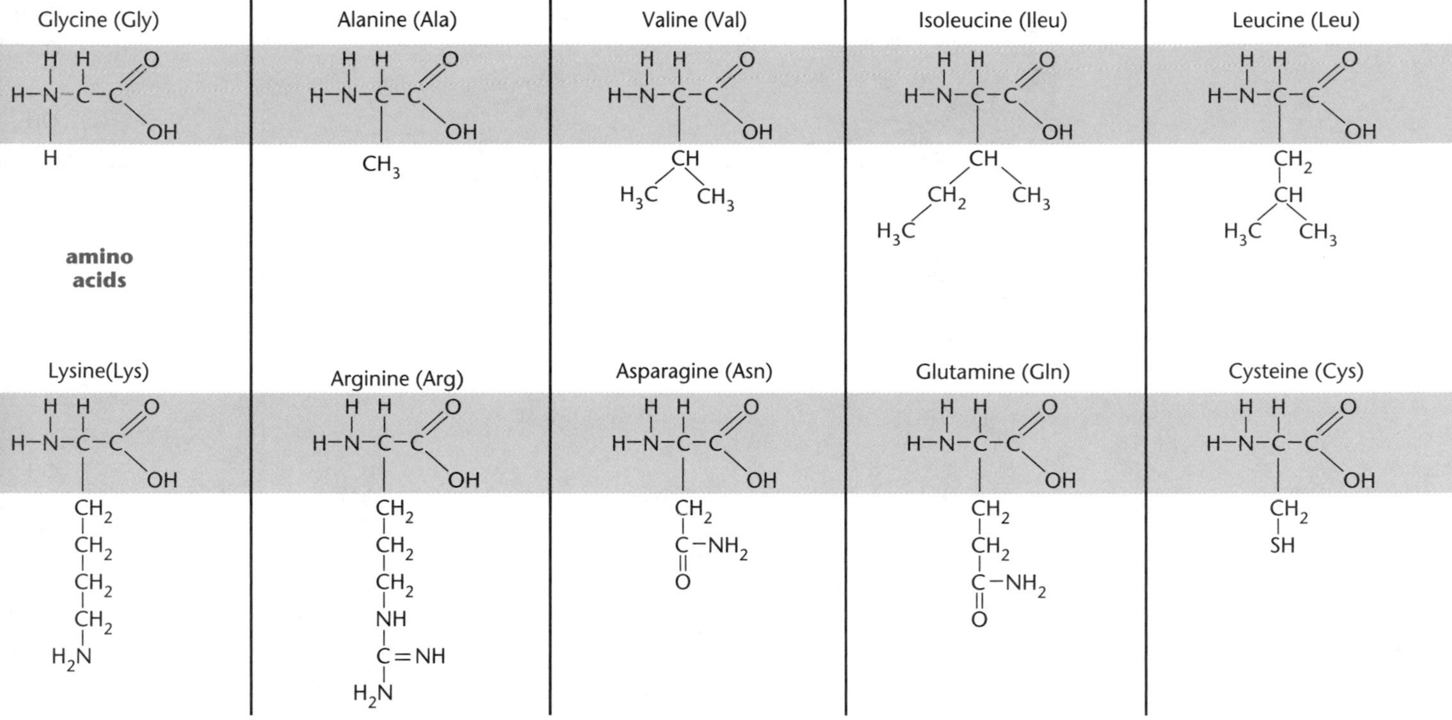

Glycine (Gly) | Alanine (Ala) | Valine (Val) | Isoleucine (Ileu) | Leucine (Leu)

amino acids

Lysine(Lys) | Arginine (Arg) | Asparagine (Asn) | Glutamine (Gln) | Cysteine (Cys)

acetylsalicylic acid (ă-se´til-sal-ă-sil-ik as´id) An antipyretic, analgesic agent of value in the treatment of arthritis and other inflammatory conditions; it inhibits prostaglandin synthesis. Also called aspirin.

acetylstrophanthidin (as-ĕ-til-stro-fan´thĭ-din) A synthetic cardiac glycoside with the most rapid onset of action of all the digitalis preparations.

achalasia (ak-ă-la´ză) Failure to relax; referring especially to sphincter muscles of the esophagus.

ache (āk) A dull pain.

acheiria (ă-ki´re-ă) Congenital lack of one or both hands.

Achilles (ă-kil´ēz) A mythical Greek hero who was invulnerable except in the heel.

A. bursa See bursa of calcaneal tendon, under bursa.

A. tendon See calcaneal tendon, under tendon.

achillodynia (ak-ĭ-lo-din´e-ă) Pain in or about the calcaneal tendon (Achilles tendon). Also called achillobursitis.

achillorrhaphy (ak-ĭ-lor´ă-fe) Repair of a torn calcaneal tendon (Achilles tendon).

achillotenotomy (ă-kil-o-te-not´ŏ-me) See achillotomy.

achillotomy (ăk-ĭ-lot´ŏ-me) Surgical division of the calcaneal tendon (Achilles tendon). Also called achillotenotomy.

plastic a. Elongation of the calcaneal tendon by plastic surgery.

achlorhydria (ă-klor-hi´dre-ă) Absence of hydrochloric acid in the stomach.

achlophobia (ă-klo-fo´biă) A morbid fear of darkness.

acholia (ă-ko´le-ă) Deficiency of bile.

acholic (ă-kol´ik) Lacking bile.

acholuria (ă-ko-lu´re-ă) Absence of bile pigments in the urine.

achondrogenesis (ă-kon-dro-jen´ĕ-sis) **1.** Dwarfism marked by extremely short limbs, rudimentary digits, and large head. **2.** A lethal form marked by lack of ossification in ribs, spine, and pelvis.

achondroplasia, achondroplasty (ă-kon-dro-pla´ză, ă-kon´dro-plas-te) Congenital abnormality in the process of ossification in cartilage, resulting in dwarfism and deformity. Also called osteosclerosis congenita.

achordate, achordal (a-kor´dāt, a-kor´dal) Without a notochord; denoting animal forms classified below the chordates.

achoresis (ak-o-re´sis) Reduction of the capacity of a hollow organ (e.g., bladder) associated with permanent contraction.

achromasia (ak-ro-ma´se-ă) **1.** Absence of normal pigmentation of skin. **2.** Lack of staining reaction in a cell.

achromate (ak´ro-māt) See monochromat.

achromatic (ak-ro-mat´ik) **1.** Colorless. **2.** Refracting light without separating it into its component colors. **3.** Staining poorly.

achromatin (ă-kro´mă-tin) The part of the cell nucleus that is only faintly stained by dyes.

achromatopia (ă-kro-mă-top´e-ă) See achromatopsia.

achromatophilia (ă-kro-mă-to-fil´e-ă) The condition of being resistant to the action of stains.

achromatopsia (ă-kro-mă-top´se-ă) Total color blindness. Also called achromatopia.

achromatosis (ă-kro-mă-to´sis) See achromia.

achromatous (ă-kro´mă-tus) Colorless.

achromia (ă-kro´me-ă) Lack of natural pigmentation, as in the iris or the skin. Also called achromatosis.

achromocyte (ă-kro´mo-sīt) A red blood cell that is devoid of color due to losing most of its hemoglobin. Also called ghost corpuscle; phantom corpuscle; shadow corpuscle.

achromoderma (ă-kro-mŏ-dĕr´mă) See leukoderma.

achromotrichia (ă-kro-mo-trik´ē-ă) Lack or loss of color in the hair.

achylia (ă-ki´le-ă) **1.** Absence of chyle (intestinal digestive secretions). **2.** Absence of stomach secretions.

achylous (ă-ki´lus) **1.** Without gastric juice. **2.** Without chyle.

acicular (ă-sik´u-lar) Needle-shaped; said of some crystals.

acid (as´id) A compound capable of donating a hydrogen ion (proton) to a base and combining with a cation to form a salt; any substance that turns litmus indicators red. For individual acids, see specific names.

amino a. Any organic acid containing one or more amino groups (NH_2) and a carboxyl group (CO_2H) and forming the basic structural units of proteins. Individual amino acid molecules are linked together by chemical bonds between the amino and carboxyl groups to form chains of molecules (polypeptides); polypeptides, in turn, link together to form a protein molecule. Amino acids that cannot be made by the body and must be obtained from the diet are called essential; those that can be made by the body from other amino acids are termed nonessential.

bile a.'s Steroid acids important in digestion and absorption of fats.

binary a. Acid made up of only two elements (e.g., hydrochloric acid).

dibasic a. An acid containing molecules with two displaceable hydrogen ions.

essential fatty a. (EFA) A polyunsaturated fatty acid indispensable for nutrition; its absence causes a specific deficiency disorder and it cannot be fabricated by the body (must be obtained from the diet); e.g., linoleic acid and linolenic acid. Originally called vitamin F.

fatty a.'s A large group of organic acids, especially those present in fat, made up of molecules containing a carboxyl group (COOH) at the end of a long hydrocarbon chain; the number of carbon atoms ranges from 2 to 34. Usually classified as *saturated* (those containing the maximum quantity of hydrogen) and *unsaturated* (whose carbon atoms contain some sites unoccupied by hydrogen); the latter are further classified as *monounsaturated* and *polyunsaturated.*

inorganic a. An acid composed of molecules that do not contain carbon atoms (e.g., hydrochloric acid, boric acid).

monobasic a. An acid containing molecules with one displaceable hydrogen ion.

nonessential fatty a. The main form of circulating lipid.

nonesterified fatty a. (NEFA) The main form of circulating fatty acid used for energy.

omega-3 fatty a., ω-3 fatty a. Monounsaturated fatty acid in which the double bond occurs at the third carbon from the end (omega) of the carbon chain.

organic a. An acid composed of molecules containing carbon atoms (e.g., ascorbic acid, amino acid).

polybasic a. An acid containing molecules with three or more displaceable hydrogen ions.

polyunsaturated fatty a. Any unsaturated fatty acid with two or more double bonds; e.g., linoleic acid (two double bonds) and arachidonic acid (four double bonds).

resin a.'s A class of organic compounds derived from certain plant resins (e.g., abietic acid and pimaric acid). Also called rosin acids.

rosin a.'s See resin acids.

saturated fatty a. A fatty acid in which the carbon chain is connected by single bonds, and is incapable of accepting any more hydrogen, i.e., all the available valence bonds of the carbon chain are filled with hydrogen atoms (e.g., stearic acid and palmitic acid).

unsaturated fatty a. A fatty acid in which the carbon chain has at least one double bond, and is capable of accepting additional hydrogen atoms (e.g., oleic acid).

acidemia (as-ĭ-de´me-a) An increase in the hydrogen ion concentration of the blood; a decrease of the normal pH (7.42) of the blood. COMPARE:

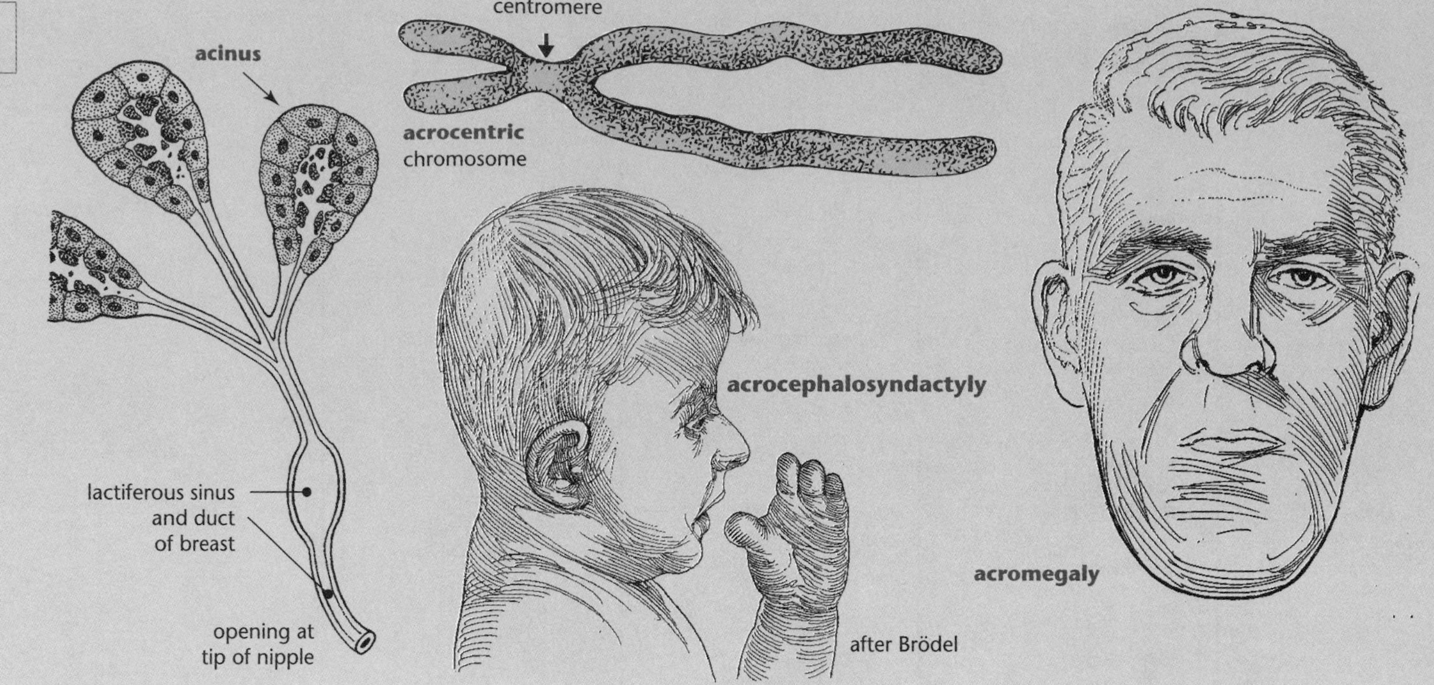

acidosis.
acid-fast (as´id-fast) Denoting bacteria that, once stained with acids such as basic fuchsin, are not decolorized by acid-alcohol.
acidifiable (as-sid´ĭ-fi-ă-bl) Capable of being made acid.
acidify (as-sid´ĭ-fi) **1.** To make acid. **2.** To become acid.
acidity (ă-sid´ĭ-te) **1.** The quality or state of being acid. **2.** The acid content of a fluid.
acidophil (as´id-o-fil) See eosinophilic leukocyte, under leukocyte.
acidophilic (as´i-do-fil'ik) **1.** Tending to stain readily with acid dyes. **2.** Tending to thrive in a highly acid medium.
acidosis (as-ĭ-do´sis) A process tending to produce an increase in hydrogen ion concentration in body fluids; if uncompensated, it produces a lowering of pH. Commonly used synonymously with acidemia.
carbon dioxide a. See respiratory acidosis.
compensated a. Condition in which the pH of blood is kept normal through respiratory or renal mechanisms, even though the blood bicarbonate may be out of the usual range.
hyperchloremic a. See renal tubular acidosis.
lactic a. Accumulation of lactic acid in the body causing decreased bicarbonate concentration.
metabolic a. Acidosis occurring in metabolic disorders in which acid (excluding carbonic acid, H_2CO_3) accumulates in, or bicarbonate is lost from, extracellular fluids.
renal tubular a. (RTA) Acidosis caused by defective elimination of acid or by excessive loss of bicarbonate by the kidneys; characterized by an elevated plasma chloride and a lowered concentration of plasma bicarbonate. Also called hyperchloremic acidosis.
respiratory a. Acidosis caused by failure to eliminate carbon dioxide (CO_2) adequately; the retained CO_2 in the blood yields carbonic acid (H_2CO_3) and its dissociation increases the hydrogen ion concentration; retention of CO_2 may occur because of a ventilatory problem, as in advanced pulmonary disease. Also called carbon dioxide acidosis.
acidotic (as-ĭ-dot´ik) Relating to acidosis.
acidulous (ă-sid´u-lus) Slightly sour or acid.
aciduria (as-ĭ-du´re-ă) Abnormal amounts of acids in the urine.
orotic a. Genetic disorder associated with defective metabolism of pyrimidine, resulting in megaloblastic anemia, retarded physical and mental growth, and excretion of orotic acid in the urine.
aciduric (as-ĭ-du´rik) Capable of living under acid conditions; said of some bacteria.
acidyl (as´ĭ-dil) A term used to denote any acid radical.
acinar (as´ĭ-nar) Relating to an acinus.
acini (as´ĭ-ni) Plural of acinus.
acinitis (as-ĭ-ni´tis) Inflammation of an acinus.
acinous (as´ĭ-nus) Resembling a bunch of grapes or made up of minute sacs (acini).
acinus (as´ĭ-nus), *pl.* **ac´ini** (as´ĭ-ni) **1.** A minute saclike dilatation. **2.** The smallest division of a gland.
aclasis (ă´klă-sis) Continuity of structure provided by pathologic tissue which arises from, and is continuous with, normal tissue.
acleistocardia (ă-klīs-to-kar´de-ă) Condition in which the foramen ovale of the heart fails to close.
acme (ak´me) Stage in the course of a disease marked by greatest intensity; a crisis.
acmesthesia (ak-mes-the´zhă) Sensation of a pinprick in the skin.
acne (ak´ne) An eruption caused by inflammation of the sebaceous glands When used alone, the term usually denotes acne vulgaris.
a. ciliaris Acne on the free edges of the eyelids.
common a. See acne vulgaris.
conglobate a. Severe skin condition marked by numerous abscesses and cysts with interconnecting tracts and pronounced scarring.
a. medicamentosa Acne that is aggravated by certain drugs.
a. rosacea See rosacea.
a. vulgaris Chronic acne, occurring commonly on the face, chest, and back of adolescents and young adults. Also called common acne; acne.
acneform, acneiform (ak´ne-form, ak-ne´ĭ-form) Resembling acne.
acokanthera (ak-o-kan-the´ră) A poisonous substance extracted from the leaves and stems of *Acokanthera ouabaio*; used by some natives of Africa as an arrow poison.
acolous (ak´ō-lus) Without limbs.
acomia (ă-ko´me-ă) See baldness.
aconative (ă-kon´ă-tiv) Without volition.
***cis*-aconitic acid** (sĭs-ak-ō-nit´ik as´id) A production of dehydration of citric acid; an intermediate in the tricarboxylic acid cycle.
acorea (ă-ko-re´ă) Congenital absence of the pupil of the eye.
acoustic (ă-kōōs´tik) Relating to sound or to the sense of hearing.
acousticophobia (ă-kōōs-tĕ-ko-fo´be-ă) Abnormal fear of sounds.
acoustics (ă-kōōs´tiks) The branch of science concerned with the study of sound, its generation, propagation, and perception.
acquired (ă-kwīrd´) Developed after birth, in contrast to congenital or hereditary.
acquired immune deficiency syndrome See AIDS.
acral (ak´ral) Relating to the extremities or peripheral parts.
acrania (ă-kra´ne-ă) Congenital absence of a portion of the skull.
acrid (ak´rid) Pungent or sharp to the taste or smell.
acridine (ak´rĭ-din) A coal tar derivative, $C_{13}H_9N$, occurring in colorless crystals and having a strong, irritating odor. Also called dibenzopyridine.
acritical (ă-krit´ĭ-kal) Without a crisis.
acroagnosis (ak-ro-ag-no´sis) Absence of sensory recognition of a limb.
acroanesthesia (ak-ro-an-es-the´zhă) Lack of sensation in the extremities.
acroataxia (ak-ro-ă-taks´ĭ-ă) Lack of muscular coordination of the fingers and toes.
acrocentric (ak-ro-sen´trik) Denoting a chromosome with a centromere situated close to one end.
acrocephalosyndactyly (ak-ro-sef-ă-lo-sin-dak´tĭ-le) Congenital malformation consisting of a high-domed skull and complete or partial webbing of the digits. An autosomal dominant inheritance. Also called Apert syndrome.
acrocephaly (ak-ro-sef´ă-le) See oxycephaly.
acrochordon (ak-ro-kor´don) A small, soft, pedunculated growth, occurring usually on the neck or eyelids.
acrocyanosis (ak-ro-si-ă-no´sis) A chronic circulatory disorder intensified by cold and emotion, and characterized by cold, cyanotic, sweaty hands and feet; the skin is a mottled blue and red.
acrodermatitis (ak-ro-der-mă-ti´tis) Inflammation of the skin of the hands or feet.
a. chronica atrophicans Dermatitis of the extremities accompanied by atrophy of the skin.
a. vesiculosa tropica Dermatitis of the fingers, occurring in hot climates, in which the skin becomes glossy with numerous small vesicles.
acrodolichomelia (ak-ro-dol-ĕ-ko-me´le-ă) Abnormal largeness of hands and feet.
acrodynia (ak-ro-din´e-ă) A disorder affecting infants and young children, marked by irritability, stomatitis, loss of teeth, insomnia, and redness of the fingers, toes, cheeks, nose, and buttocks. Also called pink disease; erythredema.
acroesthesia (ak-ro-es-the´zhă) **1.** Abnormally increased sensitivity. **2.** Pain in the extremities.
acrogeria (ak-ro-jĕr´e-ă) Premature aging of the skin of the hands and feet.
acrognosis (ak-rog-no´sis) Sensory perception of the limbs and their parts in relation to one another.
acrohyperhidrosis (ak-ro-hī-per-hī-dro´sis) Abnormally increased sweating of the hands and feet.
acrokeratosis verruciformis (ak-ro-ker-ă-to´sis

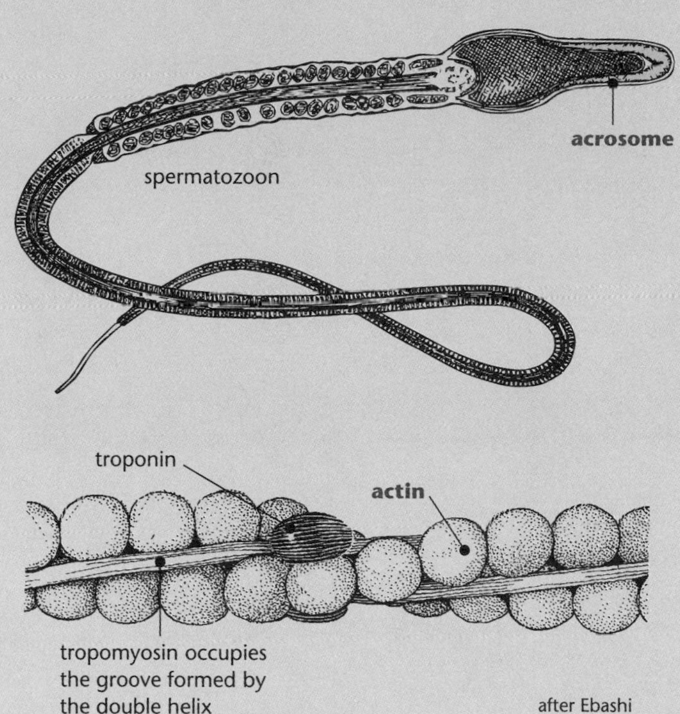

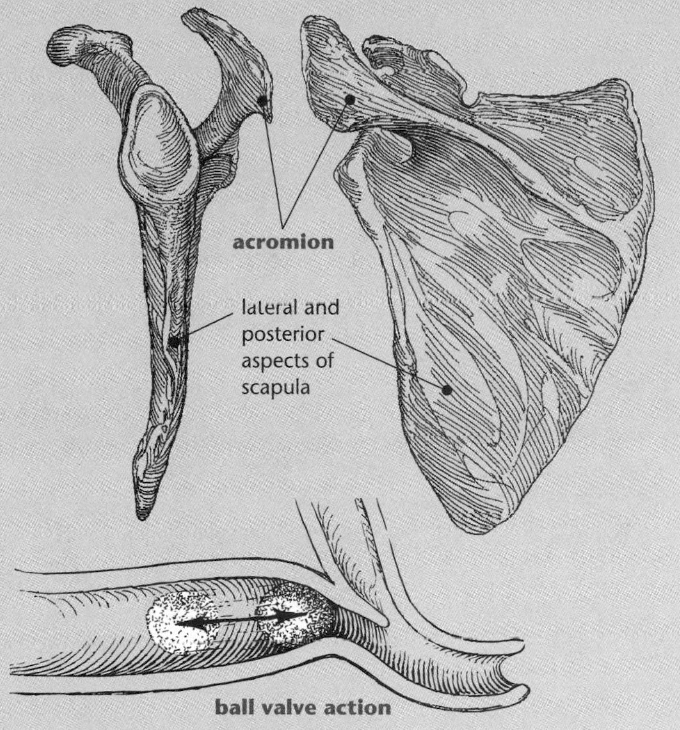

vĕ-rū-si-form´is) A condition marked by warty growths on the hands and feet.

acromegalic (ak-ro-mĕ-gal´ik) Relating to acromegaly.

acromegaly (ak-ro-meg´ă-le) A disease marked by progressive enlargement of the head, face, hands, feet, and internal organs due to a disorder of the pituitary gland, with overproduction of growth hormone after the normal growth period has ended.

acromelalgia (ak-ro-mĕl-al´jă) Disease affecting the extremities, especially the feet; marked by dilatation of blood vessels, headache, vomiting, and redness, pain, and swelling of the toes and fingers.

acrometagenesis (ak-ro-met-ă-jen´e-sis) Congenital deformity of the extremities.

acromial (ă-kro´me-al) Relating to the acromion.

acromicria (ak-ro-mik´re-ă) Abnormal smallness of bones of the head, hands, and feet.

acromioclavicular (ă-kro-me-o-klă-vik´u-lar) Relating to the acromion and clavicle.

acromiocoracoid (ă-kro-me-o-kor´ă-koid) Relating to the acromion and coracoid process.

acromiohumeral (ă-kro-me-o-hu´mer-al) Relating to the acromion and humerus.

acromion (ă-kro´me-on) The flattened process extending laterally from the spine of the scapula and forming the most prominent point of the shoulder.

acromioscapular (ă-kro-me-o-skap´u-lar) Pertaining to the acromion and the body of the scapula (shoulder blade).

acromiothoracic (ă-kro-me-o-tho-ras´ik) Relating to the acromion of the scapula (shoulder blade) and the thorax. Also called thoracicoacromial.

acromphalus (ă-krom´fă-lus) Abnormal protuberance of the navel.

acromycosis (ak-ro-mi-ko´sis) Any disease of the limbs caused by a fungus.

acromyotonia (ak-ro-mi-o-to´ne-ă) Rigidity of the hands or feet, resulting in spasmodic deformity.

acropachy (ak´ro-pak-e) Thickening (clubbing) of the tips of fingers and toes with proliferation of bone tissue and swelling.

acroparesthesia (ak-ro-par-es-the´zhă) A vasomotor-trophic disorder marked by attacks of numbness and prickly or tingling sensations in the extremities, chiefly the tips of the fingers and toes.

acrophobia (ak-ro-fo´be-ă) Morbid fear of high places.

acroposthitis (ak-ro-pos-thi´tis) Inflammation of the prepuce.

acrosclerosis (ak-ro-skle-ro´sis) Thickening of the skin and subcutaneous tissue of the hands and feet due to swelling and thickening of fibrous tissue; scleroderma of the hands and feet.

acrosome (ak´ro-sōm) The dense structure covering the anterior half of the head of a spermatozoon; it contains the enzyme hyaluronidase, which aids the penetration of the egg by the sperm during fertilization.

acroteric (ak-ro-ter´ik) Relating to the outermost parts of the body (e.g., ears, tip of nose, tips of fingers and toes).

acrotic (ă-krot´ik) Pulseless.

acrotrophodynia (ak-ro-trof-o-din´e-ă) Neuritis of the extremities as a result of prolonged exposure to dampness and cold temperatures.

acrylic (ă-kril´ik) Denoting any derivative of acrylic acid, used in the construction of dental and medical prostheses. See also resin.

actin (ak´tin) A muscle protein that, together with myosin, is responsible for muscular contraction.

acting out (ak´ting owt) An expression of an unconscious wish or conflict in action rather than words. Often used imprecisely to denote any kind of disapproved or impulsive behavior.

actinic (ak-tin´ik) Referring to those rays of the electromagnetic spectrum that produce chemical effects.

actinism (ak´tĭ-niz-m) The property of radiation that produces chemical changes or activity.

actinium (ak-tin´e-um) A radioactive element, symbol Ac, atomic number 89, atomic weight 227; found in uranium ores and possessing no stable isotopes.

Actinobacillus (ak-tĭn-o-bă-sil´lus) A genus of small, gram-negative, aerobic bacteria (family Pasteurellaceae); may cause disease in cattle, hogs, and humans.

actinodermatitis (ak-tin-o-der-mă-ti´tis) See photodermatitis.

actinogenesis (ak-tin-o-jen´ĕ-sis) See radiogenesis.

actinolite (ak-tin´o-līt) Any substance that undergoes marked changes in the presence of light.

actinometer (ak-tĭ-nom´ĕ-ter) Any of several instruments for measuring the intensity and chemical effects of actinic rays.

Actinomyces (ak-tĭ-no-mi´sēz) A genus of nonmotile, nonacidfast bacteria (family Actinomycetaceae), occurring in groups of radiating club-shaped rods superficially resembling fungi.

A. israelii A species that is the causal agent of human actinomycosis.

A. odontolyticus Anaerobic species, a natural inhabitant of the human oral cavity; has been isolated from deep dental caries.

Actinomycetaceae (ak-tĭ-no-mi-sĕ-ta´se-e) A family of bacteria (order Actinomycetales) having filamentous shapes with a tendency to branch and resembling both bacteria and fungi; some varieties are pathogenic.

actinomycin (ak-tĭ-no-mi´sin) An antibacterial substance found in some soil bacteria.

actinomycosis (ak-tĭ-no-mi-ko´sis) Contagious disease marked by multiple, painful swellings that progress to form abscesses and suppurating openings in the skin of the jaw and neck; caused by *Actinomyces israelii.* If untreated, infection may extend via the bloodstream, to the lungs and intestinal tract. Also called lumpy jaw.

actinophage (ak-tin´o-fāj) Any virus that destroys bacteria of the genus *Actinomyces.*

actinotherapy (ak-tĭ-no-ther´ă-pe) The treatment of disease, especially of the skin, with ultraviolet light.

action (ak´shun) **1.** The performance of an act, movement, or function. **2.** The transmission of energy.

ball valve a. The periodic or intermittent blockage of a tubular structure by a foreign body.

cumulative a. See cumulative effect, under effect.

sparing a. The lowering of the requirement for an essential food factor in the diet caused by the presence of another food factor which, by itself, is not essential.

specific dynamic a. (SDA) The increase in heat production during digestion; it is greater for protein than for fat or carbohydrate.

synergistic a. The coordinated activity of two or more structures or drugs whereby the combined effect is greater than the sum of the effects produced by their actions alone.

activation (ak-tĭ-va´shun) **1.** Stimulation of development (e.g., in the ovum). **2.** The act of making radioactive.

activator (ak´tĭ-va-tor) **1.** A substance that stimulates the action of another. **2.** An agent that accelerates a reaction.

allosteric a. An activator that enhances enzyme activity when bound to a site other than the active site of the enzyme molecule.

intrinsic sympathomimetic a. (ISA) A drug that has the ability to activate adrenergic receptors, producing effects similar to those of the sympathetic nervous system.

plasminogen a. A peptide-splitting enzyme that converts plasminogen to the clot-dissolving enzyme plasmin by breaking up a single bond in plasminogen.

tissue-plasminogen a. (tPA, TPA) An enzyme made by genetic engineering techniques that is capable of dissolving blood clots, such as those obstructing coronary arteries, by producing plasminogen; used to treat myocardial infarction.

active (ak´tiv) Capable of functioning or changing;

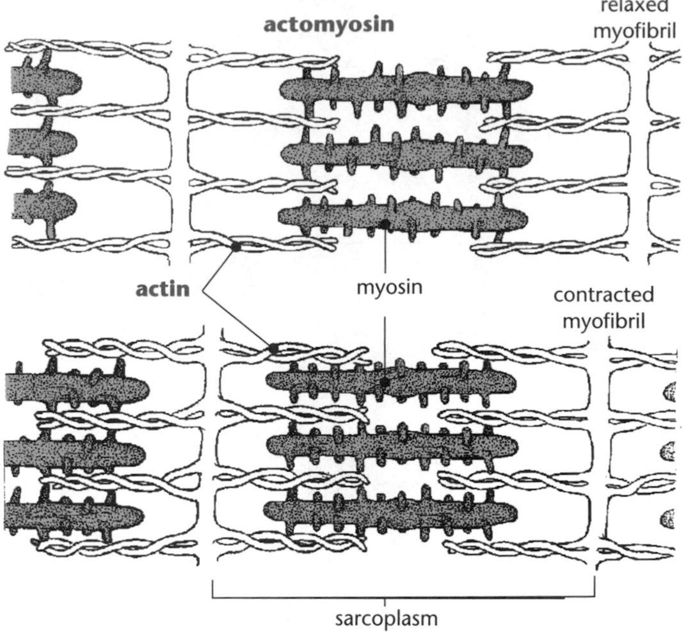

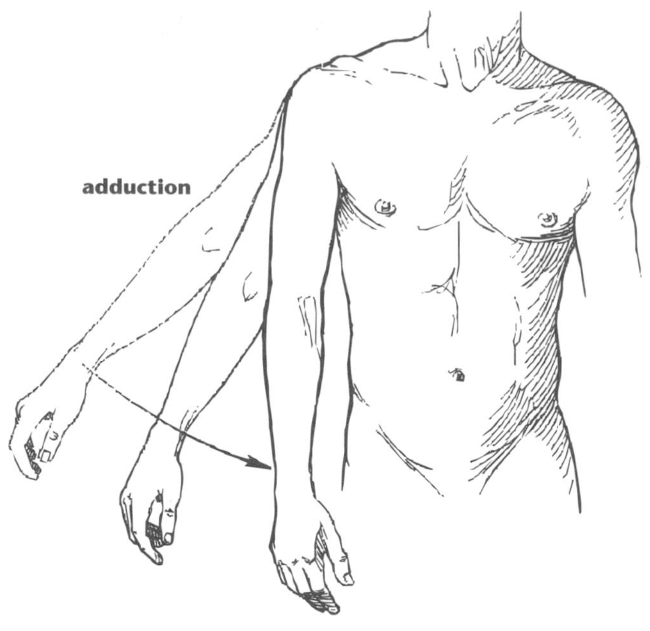

requiring energy, as contrasted to passive.

activity (ak-tiv´ĭ-te) **1.** The condition of being active. **2.** The intensity of a radioactive element. **3.** The release of electrical energy by nerve tissue.

actomyosin (ak-to-mi´o-sin) A unique contractile protein with a linear molecular shape, formed by the union of actin and myosin; responsible for the contraction of muscle fibers.

acuity (ă-ku´ĭ-te) Acuteness, distinctness.

resolution a. See visual acuity.

visual a. (VA) Detailed central vision; dependent on the size and sharpness of the image on the retina, the sensitivity of the nerves, and the interpretative ability of the brain. Also called resolution acuity.

aculeate (ă-ku´le-āt) Thorny; covered with sharp points.

acupressure (ak´u-presh-er) Brief compression of a nerve with the fingers at a special point (pressure point) to relieve pain elsewhere in the body.

acupuncture (ak´u-pungk-cher) A modality developed in China for certain types of anesthesia and treatment of various disorders by insertion of fine stainless steel needles into specific areas of the body; it is thought to work through the body's autonomic nervous system. Also called neuronyxis.

acusector (ak-u-sek´tor) A needle through which a high frequency current is passed; used in electrosurgery as a scalpel.

acusis (ă-kyū́sis) Normal hearing.

acute (ă-kyūt´) Denoting a disease or symptoms of abrupt onset or lasting a relatively short period of time; opposite of chronic.

Acute Physiology and Chronic Health Evaluation System (APACHE) A scoring system designed to assess the severity of illness of patients in intensive care units (ICUs); used for comparison of hospital ICUs to identify different standards of care and to allocate resources.

acyanoblepsia (ă-si-ă-no-blep´se-ă) Inability to see the color blue. Also called blue blindness.

acyanotic (ă-si-ă-not´ik) Not marked by cyanosis.

acyclic (a-si´klik) **1.** In chemistry, denotes an organic compound with an open chain structure. **2.** Not occurring during the series of events that recur regularly.

acyclovir (a-si´klo-vir) Antiviral agent for the treatment of herpes simplex and related viral infections.

acyl (as´il) Any radical derived from an organic acid by removal of the hydroxyl group.

acylation (as-ĕ-la´shun) Introduction of an acyl radical into a compound.

acystia (ă-sis´te-ă) Congenital absence of the urinary bladder.

Acystosporidia (ā-sis-to-spō-rid´e-ă) An order of parasitic sporozoa that includes the genus *Plasmodium*, the malarial parasite.

adactyly (a-dak´tĭ-le) Congenital absence of fingers or toes.

Adam's apple (ad´amz ăp´l) See laryngeal prominence, under prominence.

Adams-Stokes syndrome (ad´amz-stōks sin´drōm) A syndrome characterized by fainting and sometimes convulsions due to prolonged asystole; seen usually when there is a failure of effective contraction in the course of complete heart block or when heart block supervenes on a sinus rhythm; sometimes Cheynes-Stokes respiration may occur. Also called Stokes-Adams syndrome; Morgagni-Adams-Stokes syndrome.

adaptation (ad-ap-ta´shun) **1.** Adjustment of the pupil of the eye to variations in the intensity of light. **2.** Alteration by which an organism becomes fit for a new environment. **3.** Decreased response of a sense organ to repeated stimuli.

dark a. Eye adjustment to reduced illumination (sensitivity to light is increased).

light a. Eye adjustment to increased illumination (sensitivity to light is reduced).

adder (ad´er) See European viper, under viper.

addict (ad´ikt) One who has strong psychologic and physiologic dependence upon some practice which has progressed beyond voluntary control.

addiction (ă-dik´shun) Strong habituation to some practice, beyond voluntary control.

drug a. See drug dependence, under dependence.

addisonian (ad´ĭ-so´ne-an) **1.** Characterized by features of Addison's disease. **2.** Relating to Addison's disease.

Addison's disease (ad´ĭ-sonz dĭ-zēz´) Primary adrenocortical insufficiency; adrenocortical insufficiency caused by destruction of the adrenal cortex, a disease characterized by chronic deficiency of hormones concerned with mineral metabolism and glycostasis; findings include striking skin pigmentation, anemia, hypotension with small heart, severe dental caries, and stiffness of the cartilages of the ear; hyponatremia is present and, later, there may be azotemia and hyperkalemia. Also called primary chronic adrenocortical insufficiency.

additive (ad´ĭ-tiv) **1.** Any substance that is added to another material to fulfil a specific purpose, i.e., to improve it, strengthen it, etc. **2.** The quality of two drugs (e.g., epinephrine and norepinephrine) that act on the same receptors whereby doses of one drug can substitute for those of the other, in proportion to their relative potency.

adducent (ă-du´sent) Bringing toward or together; performing adduction; applied to certain muscles.

adducin (ă-du´sin) A protein that binds to actin (the protein of muscle fibrils) and spectrin (the protein of cell membranes) to form the actin-spectrin network; a part of the cytoskeleton of cells.

adduct (ă-dukt´) To pull or draw toward the median line of the body.

adduction (ă-duk´shun) The act of adducting or the condition of being adducted.

adductor (ă-duk´tor) A structure, such as a muscle, that draws a part toward an axis of the body; opposite of abductor.

adenalgia (ad-e-nal´jă) Pain in a gland. Also called adenodynia.

adenase (ad´ĕ-nās) An enzyme that converts adenine into hypoxanthine; present in the liver, pancreas, and spleen.

adendritic (ă-den-drit´ik) Denoting a nerve call without dendrites, such as certain cells in the spinal ganglia.

adenectomy (ad-ĕ-nek´to-me) Surgical removal of a gland.

adenectopia (ad-ĕ-nek-to´pe-ă) Presence of a gland, or glandular tissue, in other than its normal anatomic position.

adenine (ad´ĕ-nēn) A white, crystalline purine derivative, $C_5H_5N_5$, one of the constituents of ribonucleic acid (RNA) and deoxyribonucleic acid (DNA).

a. arabinoside (Ara-A) A substance that acts intracellularly to inhibit viral replication; used in the treatment of some viral infections such as those caused by cytomegalovirus.

a. nucleotide See adenylic acid.

adenitis (ad-ĕ-ni´tis) Inflammation of a gland.

adenoacanthoma (ad-ĕ-no-ak-an-tho´mă) A malignant tumor (most commonly of the uterus) that is made up of malignant glandular tissue, but most of the cells exhibit benign squamous differentiation.

adenoblast (ad´ĕ-no-blast) Embryonic cell from which glandular tissue develops.

adenocarcinoma (ad-ĕ-no-kar-sĭ-no´mă) Malignant tumor derived from epithelial cells or arranged in a glandlike pattern.

clear cell a. of vagina A rare type of vaginal cancer occurring in young females, between the ages of 10 and 35 years, whose mothers were treated with diethylstilbestrol (DES) during pregnancy in cases of threatened miscarriage (spontaneous abortion).

papillary a. See papillary carcinoma, under carcinoma.

renal a. The most common type of cancer of the kidney, especially among people over 60 years of age; arises in the kidney substance (parenchyma) and may spread via the bloodstream to the lungs, bone, liver, and brain. Also called clear cell carcinoma of kidney; Grawitz' tumor; hypernephroma; renal cell carcinoma.

villoglandular papillary a. A circumscribed

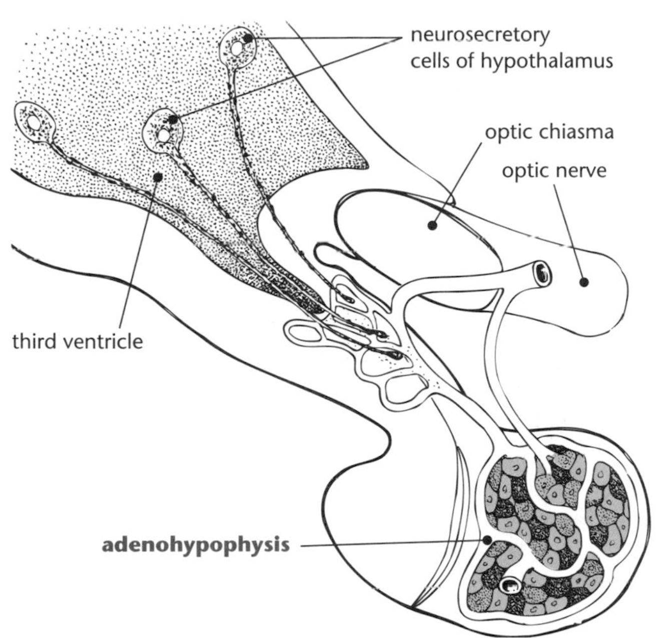

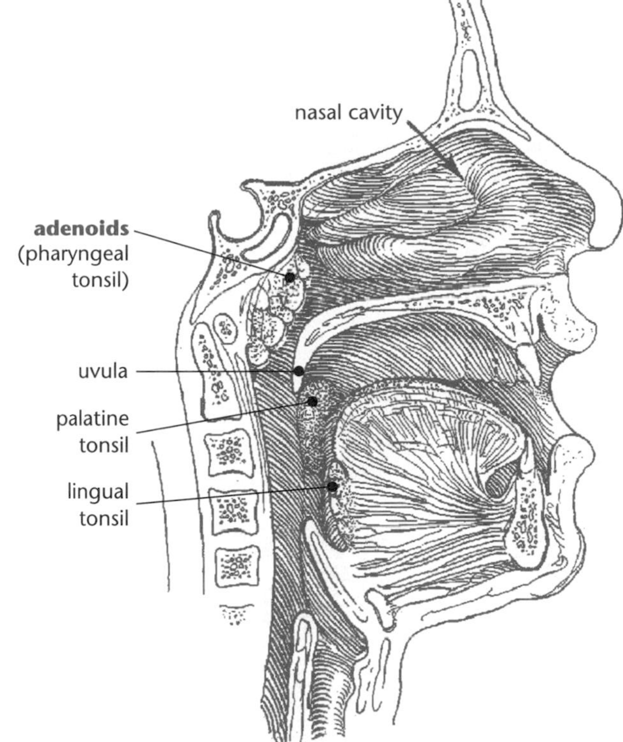

adenocarcinoma of the uterine cervix, usually occurring at a young age (average 33 years); typically, it has a surface papillary component of variable thickness; the invasive portion of the tumor is composed of elongated branching glands separated by a fibrous framework; spread by lymphatic or blood circulation is rare.

adenocystoma (ad-ĕ-no-sis-to´mă) A benign, epithelial, glandlike tumor associated with cysts.

adenocyte (ad´ĕ-no-sīt) The secretory cell of a gland.

adenodiastasis (ad-ĕ-no-dī-as´ta-sis) The presence of glands or glandular tissue in other than their normal sites.

adenofibroma (ad-ĕ-no-fi-bro´mă) A benign tumor made up of connective tissue with some glandular elements.

adenofibrosis (ad-ĕ-no-fi-bro´sis) Formation of a fibrous tissue in a gland.

adenohypophysial (ad-ĕ-no-hi-po-fiz´e-al) Of or relating to the anterior portion of the pituitary gland (hypophysis).

adenohypophysis (ad-ĕ-no-hi-pof´ĭ-sis) The anterior, glandular portion of the pituitary gland (hypophysis); it produces the following hormones: prolactin, follicle stimulating (FSH), luteinizing (LH), adrenocorticotropic (ACTH), thyroid-stimulating (TSH), melanocyte stimulating (MSH), and growth (GH) hormones.

adenoid (ad´ĕ-noid) **1.** Resembling a gland. **2.** Pharyngeal tonsil.

adenoidectomy (ad-ĕ-noid-ek´to-me) Surgical removal of the adenoids.

adenoiditis (ad-ĕ-noid-i´tis) Inflammation of the pharyngeal tonsil.

adenoids (ad´ĕ-noids) Enlargement of the pharyngeal tonsil.

adenolipoma (ad-ĕ-no-lĭ-po´mă) Benign tumor of fat tissue containing some glandular elements.

adenolipomatosis (ad-ĕ-no-lĭ-po-mă-to´sis) Condition marked by the presence of several subcutaneous adenolipomas, especially in the neck, axilla, and groin.

adenolymphocele (ad-ĕ-no-lim´fo-sēl) Cystic enlargement of a lymph node.

adenolymphoma (ad-ĕ-no-lim-fo´mă) A benign (noncancerous) tumor of salivary glands, most commonly seen in the parotid gland (unilaterally); composed of cysts lined with epithelial cells and filled with retained secretions. Also called Warthin's tumor.

adenoma (ad-ĕ-no´mă) Benign tumor of epithelial tissue with a glandlike structure.

bronchial a. Former term for a group of low-grade malignant tumors arising in the bronchi. They include carcinoid and mucoepidermoid tumors.

chromophobic a. See null-cell adenoma.

follicular a. Benign tumor of the thyroid gland with pouch-like dilatations (acini); these may vary from small and rudimentary to large and cystic containing abundant colloid.

growth hormone-producing a. Pituitary adenoma containing cells that secrete excessive growth hormone; may cause gigantism in children and acromegaly in adults.

hepatic a. Tumor of the liver occurring most commonly in association with prolonged use of oral contraceptives and anabolic steroids; when occurring in pregnant women, it has a tendency to rupture, causing sudden pain and hemorrhage into the abdominal cavity. Also called hepatocellular adeno-ma.

hepatocellular a. See hepatic adenoma.

islet cell a. Tumor of the pancreas made up of tissue similar in structure to that of the islets of Langerhans.

null-cell a.'s Pituitary adenomas composed of cells that give negative results on tests for hormone secretion; some may contain functioning cells and may be associated with conditions caused by oversecretion of pituitary hormones. Also called chromophobic adenomas.

pleomorphic a. See mixed tumor of salivary gland, under tumor.

sebaceous a. Tumor of the face made up of sebaceous glands appearing as a collection of reddish and yellowish papules; associated with mental deficiency.

tubular a. Benign, usually pedunculated, polyp of the colon mucosa; risk of its becoming cancerous correlates with size.

villous a. Benign, potentially malignant, tumor of the mucosa of the large intestine.

adenomatoid (ad-ĕ-no´mă-toid) Resembling an adenoma.

adenomatosis (ad-ĕ-no-mă-to´sis) Condition marked by the formation of multiple glandular tumors.

familial endocrine a., type I See multiple endocrine neoplasia, type 1, under neoplasia.

familial endocrine a., type II See multiple endocrine neoplasia, type 2, under neoplasia.

adenomatous (ad-ĕ-nom´ă-tus) Relating to an adenoma or a glandular overgrowth.

adenomyoma (ad-ĕ-no-mi-o´mă) See focal adenomyosis, under adenomyosis.

adenomyosis (ad-ĕ-no-mi-o´sis) The abnormal, but benign, ingrowth of the inner lining of the uterus (endometrium) into the uterine musculature. Also called endometriosis interna.

diffuse a. Adenomyosis involving much or all of the uterus.

focal a. Adenomyosis that concentrates in one area and forms a nodular mass resembling a fibroid. Also called adenomyoma.

adenopathy (ad-ĕ-nop´ă-the) Disease of glands, especially of the lymph nodes.

adenosarcoma (ad-ĕ-no-sar-ko´mă) A malignant tumor containing glandular tissue.

adenose (ad´ĕ-nōs) Relating to a gland.

adenosine (ă-den´o-sēn) An organic compound, $C_{10}H_{13}N_5O_4$, derived from nucleic acids; composed of adenine and a pentose sugar.

a. diphosphate (ADP) A product of the hydrolysis, and the substrate for the biosynthesis, of adenosine triphosphate (ATP).

a. monophosphate (AMP) See adenylic acid.

a. 3´,5´-cyclic monophosphate (cAMP) A mediator of many hormone actions in mammals, acting as an intracellular (sometimes extracellular) "second messenger." Also called cyclic adenylic acid; cyclic AMP; cyclic phosphate.

a. triphosphatase (ATPase) An enzyme, present in muscle tissue, that promotes the splitting off of a phosphate group from adenosine triphosphate.

a. triphosphate (ATP) Organic compound present in all cells; upon hydrolysis, it yields the energy required by a multitude of biologic processes.

adenosis (ad-ĕ-no´sis)–Any disease of glands, especially one affecting the lymph nodes.

adenotome (ad´ĕ-no-tōm)–A surgical instrument for the removal of adenoids.

adenotonsillectomy (ad-ĕ-no-ton-sil-lek´to-me)–Surgical removal of adenoids and tonsils.

Adenoviridae (ad-ĕ-no-vir´ĭ-dē)–A family of viruses (70 to 90 nm in diameter) that contain double-stranded DNA and develop in cell nuclei of mammals and birds; some members have been extensively used in experimental studies of cancer;–includes viruses causing epidemic keratoconjunctivitis, pharyngitis, tonsillitis, and pneumonia.–

adenovirus (ad-ĕ-no-vi´rus)–A virus of the family Adenoviridae.

adenyl (ad´ĕ-nil)–A–radical, $C_5H_4N_4$, that is a constituent of adenine.

adenylate cyclase (ă-den´ĭ-lāt sī´klās) An enzyme located in cell membranes which, in the presence of magnesium, converts adenosine triphosphate (ATP) to 35-cyclic AMP (cAMP); the enzyme is activated by a hormone interacting with a specific receptor (first messenger) on the cell membrane; the cyclic AMP acts as a second messenger within the cell.

adenylic acid (ad-ĕ-nil´ik as´id) One of the hydrolysis products of all nucleic acids, occurring in all tissues and participating in high-energy phosphate transfer. Also called adenosine monophosphate

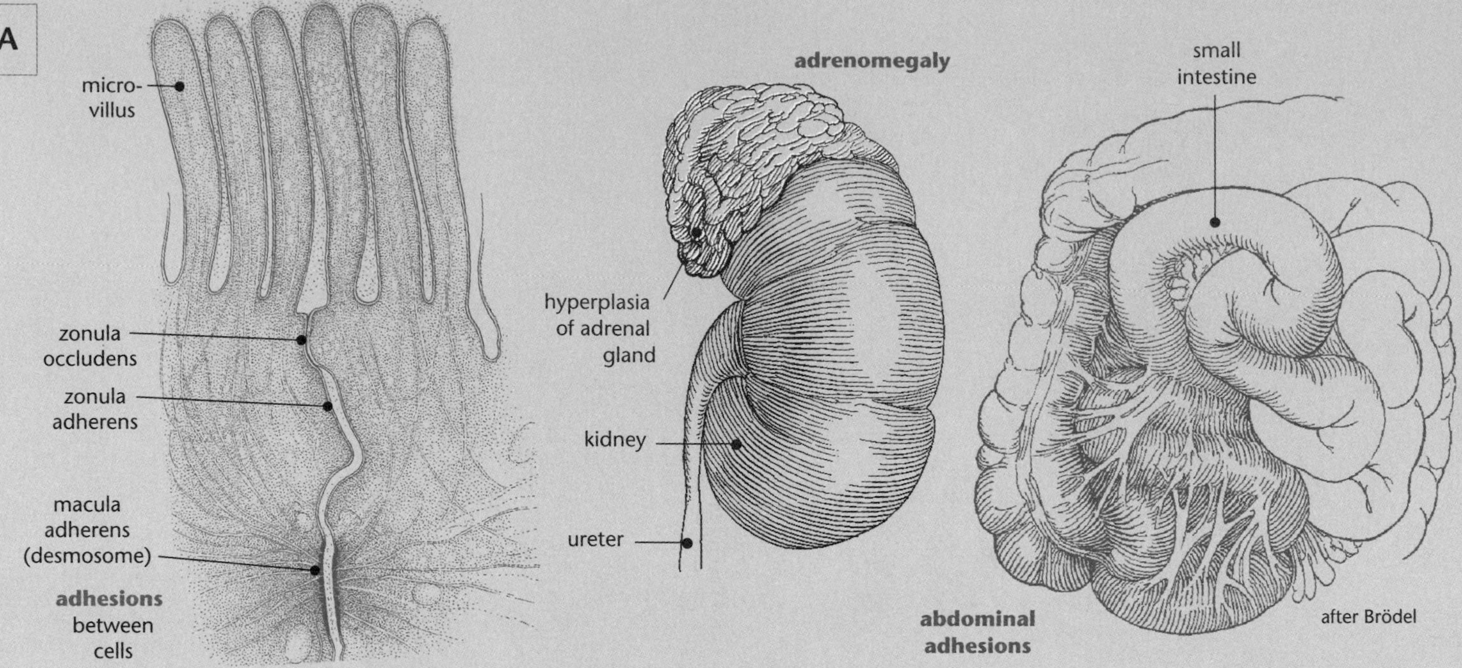

(AMP); adenine nucleotide.

cyclic a. a. See adenosine 3′,5′′-cyclic monophosphate, under adenosine.

adhesins (ad-he′zins) Projections on the surface of bacteria by means of which the microorganism attaches to specific receptors on the host cell.

adhesiolysis (ad-he-ze-o-lĭ′sis) See adhesiotomy.

adhesion (ad-he′zhun) **1.** The union of two surfaces. **2.** A fibrous band that abnormally unites two parts.

posttraumatic uterine a.'s Formation of adhesions within the uterine cavity, usually caused by scraping off of the inner uterine lining (curettage), resulting in reduced or absent menstrual flow and, frequently, infertility. Also called Asherman's syndrome.

primary a.'s See healing by first intention, under healing.

secondary a. See healing by second intention, under healing.

adhesiotomy (ad-he-ze-ot′o-me) Surgical division of adhesions. Also called adhesiolysis.

adiadochokinesia, adiadochokinesis (ă-di-ă-do-ko-ki-ne′zhă, ă-di-ă-do-ko-kin-ē′sis) Inability to perform rapid alternating movements (e.g., pronation and supination).

adiaphoresis (ă-di-ă-fo-rē′sis) Deficiency of perspiration.

adiaphoretic (ă-di-ă-fo-ret′ik) Characterized by or causing adiaphoresis.

adipic acid (ă-dip′ik as′id) Acid formed by the oxidation of fats.

adipocele (ad′ĭ-po-sēl) See lipocele.

adipocere (ad′ĭ-po-sēr) A waxy substance formed on decomposing dead bodies under humid conditions. Commonly called grave wax.

adipokinin (ad-ĭ-po-ki′nin) Pituitary hormone serving to mobilize stored fat.

adipometer (ad-ĭ-pom′ĕ-ter) Instrument for measuring the thickness of a skin fold to estimate amount of subcutaneous fat.

adiponecrosis (ad-ĭ-po-ne-kro′sis) See fat necrosis, under necrosis.

adipose (ad′ĭ-pōs) Related to fat.

adiposis (ad-ĭ-po′sis) Excessive accumulation of fat in the body, either local or general.

adiposity (ad-ĭ-pos′ĭ-te) Obesity; excessive accumulation of fat in the body.

aditus (ad′ĭ-tus) A general anatomic term denoting approach or entrance to an organ.

adjustment (ă-just′ment) **1.** Modification made on a completed denture after its insertion in the mouth. **2.** In chiropractic, manipulation of the spine for restoring normal nerve function. **3.** In psychology, the adaptation of the individual to the social environment.

adjuvant (aj′ĕ-vant, ă-joo′vant) **1.** Assisting. **2.** A substance that enhances the action of another.

Freund's complete a. A mixture of mineral oil, plant waxes, and killed tubercle bacilli; used with antigen to increase antibody production.

Freund's incomplete a. Freund's complete adjuvant minus the tubercle bacilli.

adnerval (ad-ner′val) Near or in the direction of a nerve.

adnexa (ad-nek′să) Appendages; accessory structures.

a. uteri The ovaries and uterine tubes.

adolescence (ad-o-les′ens) General term for the period between childhood and adulthood. It overlaps puberty. See also puberty.

adolescent (ad-o-les′ent) **1.** Relating to adolescence. **2.** A person during the period of adolescence.

adoral (ad-o′ral) Toward or near the mouth.

adrenal (ă-dre′nal) **1.** Near the kidney. **2.** The adrenal gland. See under gland.

adrenalectomy (ă-dre-nal-ek′to-me) Surgical removal of the adrenal glands.

adrenaline (ă-dren′ă-lin) See epinephrine.

adrenarche (ad-ren-ar′ke) Physiologic change in which the function of the adrenal cortex is increased, occurring at approximately the age of nine years.

premature a. Early puberty induced by hyperactivity of the adrenal cortex.

adrenergic (ad-ren-er′jik) **1.** Relating to nerve fibers of the sympathetic nervous system that, upon stimulation, release the chemical transmitter norepinephrine (and possibly small amounts of epinephrine) at their post-ganglionic endings. **2.** Relating to drugs that mimic the action of the sympathetic nervous system. See also alpha-adrenergic receptor and beta-adrenergic receptor, under receptor.

adrenoceptor (ă-dre-no-sep′tor) See adrenergic receptor, under receptor.

adrenocortical (ad-re-no-kor′tĭ-kal) Relating to the adrenal cortex.

adrenocorticomimetic (ad-re-no-kor-tĭ-ko-mi-met′ik) Having a function similar to that of the adrenal cortex.

adrenocorticotropic, adrenocorticotrophic (ad-re-no-kor-tĭ-ko-trop′ik, ad-re-no-kor-tĭ-ko-trof′ik) Stimulating the function or growth of the cortex of the adrenal gland.

adrenocorticotropin (ad-re-no-kor-tĭ-ko-trop′in) See adrenocorticotropic hormone, under hormone.

adrenogenic (ad-ren-o-jen′ik) Produced or originating in the adrenal glands.

adrenoleukodystrophy (ă-dre-no-loo-ko-dis′tro-fe) (ALD) An inherited disorder initially manifested by cerebral symptoms, such as mild muscular weakness and spastic paralysis of the lower limbs, or by decreased hormone secretion from the adrenal cortex; progresses to blindness, aphasia, or dementia due to myelin degeneration in the white matter of the brain. The defective gene is carried on the X chromosome (an X-linkage).

adrenolytic (ă-dre-no-lit′ik) Inhibiting the action of epinephrine (adrenaline) at nerve endings.

adrenomegaly (ă-dre-no-meg′ă-le) Enlargement of the adrenal glands.

adrenomimetic (ă-dre-no-mi-met′ik) Having an action similar to that of epinephrine and norepinephrine.

adrenoprival (ad-re′no-pri-văl) Absence of adrenal function.

adrenosterone (ad-re-no′ster-ōn) A male sex hormone (androgen), $C_{19}H_{24}O_3$, present in the adrenal cortex.

adrenotropin (ă-dre-no-trop′in) See adrenocorticotropic hormone, under hormone.

adsorb (ad-sorb′) To attach one substance to the surface of another.

adsorbate (ad-sor′bāt) A substance adhered to the surface of another by adsorption.

adsorbent (ad-sor′bent) A substance that attracts and holds on its surface another substance.

adsorption (ad-sorp′shun) The process by which gas molecules or small particles in solution are attracted by, and attached to, the surface of another substance.

adulterant (ă-dul′ter-ant) Anything added to a substance which makes it impure or inferior.

adulteration (ă-dul-ter-a′shun) The deliberate addition of an unnecessary or cheap ingredient to a preparation, thus rendering it below the standard specified on the label.

adult polycystic kidney disease (ă-dult pol-e-sis′tik kid′ne dĭ-zēz′) (adult PCKD) Inherited disease due in most cases (greater than 90%) to an abnormality in chromosome 6; characterized by the presence of multiple, gradually enlarging cysts in both kidneys, which compress the normal tissue, leading to renal insufficiency and often causing hematuria (blood in the urine) and hypertension; may be accompanied by minute aneurysms in the brain.

adult respiratory distress syndrome (ă-dult′ re-spi′ră-to-re dĭ-stres′ sin′drōm) (ARDS) Condition occurring shortly after trauma; characterized by edema of the alveoli and surrounding tissues, acute respiratory failure, and shock; precipitated by microembolism and loss of surfactant. Also called posttraumatic pulmonary insufficiency; pump lung; shock lung; wet lung.

advancement (ad-vans′ment) Surgical procedure

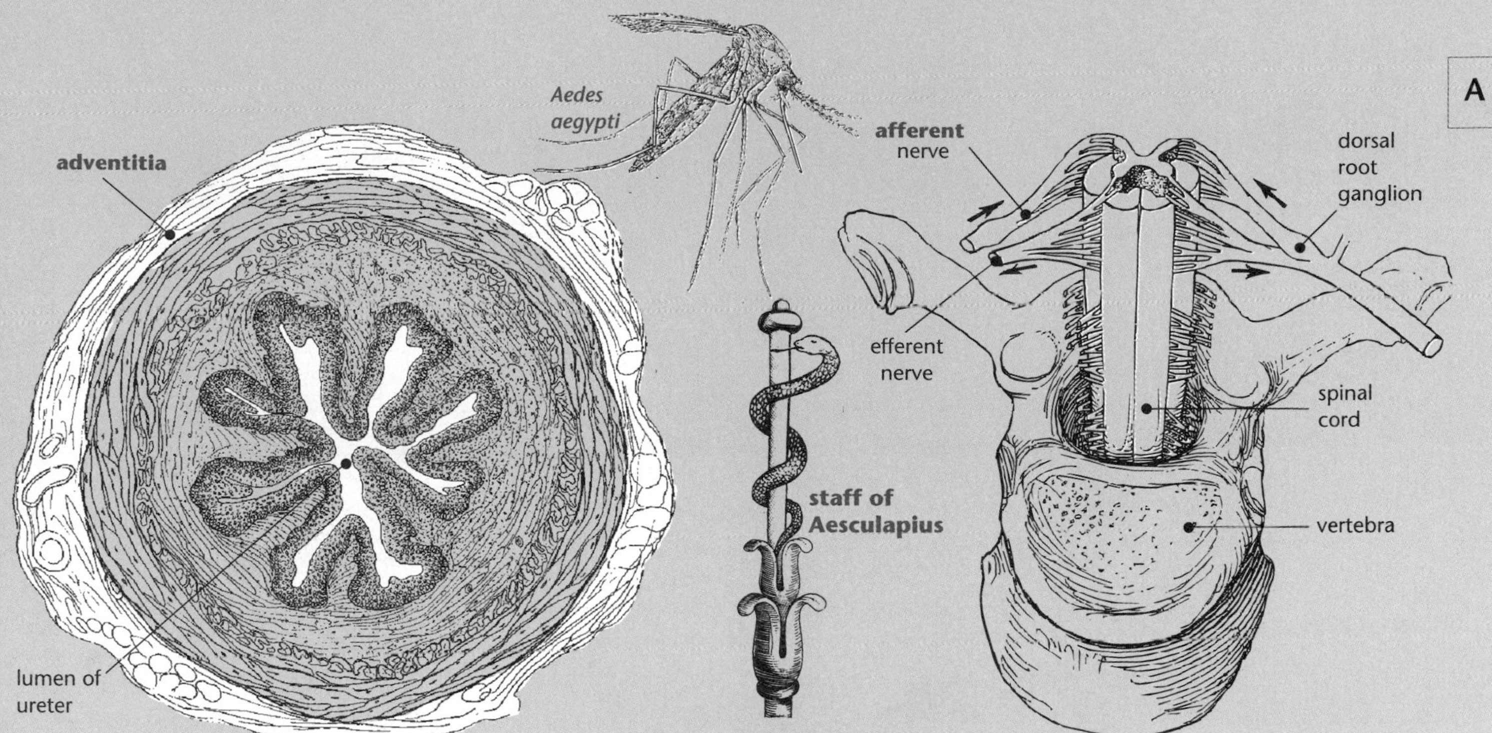

in which the tendon of a muscle is detached and reattached at an advanced point; used to correct strabismus.

adventitia (ad-ven-tish´e-ă) The outer, loose connective tissue covering of a structure such as a blood vessel, thoracic duct, or ureter.

adventitial (ad-ven-tish´al) Relating to adventitia, especially of a blood vessel.

adynamia (ă-di-na´me-ă) Weakness; asthenia.

Aedes (ā-ē´dēz) A genus of small mosquitoes often found in tropical and subtropical areas.

A. aegypti The tiger mosquito with black and yellow markings, carrier of yellow fever and dengue and possibly filariasis and encephalitis.

aerated (ār´āt-ed) Containing air, carbon dioxide, or oxygen.

aeration (ār-a´shun) **1.** The act of airing. **2.** The saturation of a fluid with a gas. **3.** The oxygenation of blood in the lungs.

aerobe (ār´ōb) Any organism capable of living in the presence of air.

facultative a. Microorganism that can live with or without air.

obligate a. Microorganism that needs air to survive.

aerobic (ār-o´bik) Relating to an oxygen-containing environment or to an aerobe.

aerobiosis (ār-o-bi-o´sis) Life in an oxygen-containing environment.

aerodontalgia (ār-o-don-tal´jă) Toothache brought on by reduction of atmospheric pressure.

aerogenic, aerogenous (ār-o-jen´ik, ār-o-jen´us) Gas producing, such as certain bacteria.

aeropathy (ār-op´ă-the) Disease caused by drastic changes in atmospheric pressure (e.g., barotitis media, decompression sickness).

aerophagia, aerophagy (ār-o-fa´jă, ār-of´ă-je) The swallowing of air; usually accompanies emotional disorders.

aerophil, aerophile (ār´o-fil, ār-o-fīl´) Air loving; an organism that requires air for proper growth.

aerophobia (ār-o-fo´be-ă) Abnormal fear of drafts or of fresh air.

aerosinusitis (ār-o-si-nus-i´tis) Inflammatory condition of paranasal sinuses caused by difference between pressures within the sinuses and that of the atmosphere. Also called barosinusitis.

aerosol (ār´o-sol) Relatively stable suspension of liquids or solids in air, oxygen, or inert gases dispersed in the form of a fine mist, usually for therapeutic purposes.

aerotitis media (ār-o-ti´tis me´de-ă) See barotitis media.

Aesculapius (es-ku-la´pe-us) The Roman god of healing.

staff of A. A rod encircled by a single snake; symbol of the medical profession and emblem of the American Medical Association, as well as other medical associations throughout the world.

afebrile (a-feb´ril) Without fever.

affect (af´ekt) **1.** Feeling or emotion. **2.** The outward manifestation of one's feelings.

affective (ă-fek´tiv) Referring to affect.

afferent (af´er-ent) Conveying a fluid or a nerve impulse toward an organ or area.

afferent loop syndrome (af´er-ent lo͞op sin´drōm) Chronic partial obstruction of the duodenum and jejunum following gastrojejunostomy, often resulting in distention and pain after eating.

affinity (ă-fin´ĭ-te) **1.** In chemistry, the attractive force of two substances for each other. **2.** In immunology, the binding strength between a receptor and a ligand.

afibrinogenemia (ă-fi-brin-o-jě-ne´me-ă) Marked deficiency of fibrinogen in the blood.

aflatoxin (af-lă-tok´sin) Toxin produced by the fungus *Aspergillus flavus*; found in improperly stored grains and peanuts; causes liver cancer.

afterbirth (af´ter-berth) The placenta and fetal membranes expelled from the uterus after childbirth. Also called secundines.

afterdischarge (af-ter-dis´charj) The discharge of impulses from a reflex center after stimulation has ceased.

afterimage (af-ter-im´ij) The continued visual sensation or image after cessation of the stimulus.

afterload (af´ter-lōd) In cardiac muscle, the force against which the ventricle ejects once contraction of the muscle fibers begins; for the left ventricle this is equivalent to aortic diastolic pressure.

afterpains (af´ter-pānz) Cramps due to uterine contractions after delivery.

aftersensation (af-ter-sen-sa´shun) Sensation persisting after the stimulus that caused it has been removed.

agalactia (ă-gă-lak´she-ă) Condition in which milk in the breasts is absent after childbirth.

agalactorrhea (ă-gă-lak-to-re´ă) Absence or arrest of milk flow.

agammaglobulinemia (a-gam-ă-glob-u-lĭ-ne´me-ă) Extremely low levels of gamma globulin in the blood, inability to form antibody, and frequent attacks of infectious diseases.

agar (ag´ar) A gelatinous material prepared from seaweed; used as a culture medium for bacteria.

blood a. Bouillon solidified with 1% agar and mixed with blood.

chocolate a. Agar mixed with fresh blood and then heated, which gives it a chocolate brown color; used as a culture medium for *Neisseria*.

Endo a. A medium containing agar, lactose, peptone, dipotassium phosphate, sodium sulfite, basic fuchsin, and distilled water; used for bacteriologic testing of water.

French proof a. See Sabouraud's agar.

MacConkey a. A medium containing bile salts, lactose, peptone, neutral red, and crystal violet; used to identify gram-negative bacilli and mark them as fermenters.

Sabouraud's a. Bouillon solidified with 1% agar, mixed with 1% Chassaing's peptone and 4% maltose or mannite; used for growth of fungi. Also called French proof agar.

Thayer-Martin a. Agar composed of beef infusion, peptone, and starch with 5% chocolate sheep blood and antibiotics; used for transport and primary isolation of *Neisseria gonorrhoeae* and *Neisseria meningitidis*. Also called Thayer-Martin medium.

age (āj) The period of time during which a person has lived.

bone a. Age as determined by x-ray studies of the degree of development in the ossification centers (epiphyses) of long bones, such as those of the extremities. Also called skeletal age.

calendar a. See chronologic age.

childbearing a. The time in a woman's life between puberty and menopause.

chronologic a. Age expressed in calendar units (days, weeks, months, years) from the date of birth. Also called calendar age.

developmental a. (a) Age determined by the degree of anatomic development from the time of implantation. (b) (DA) Age determined by the degree of emotional, mental, anatomic, and physiologic maturity.

gestational a. Age of an embryo or a fetus, timed in weeks beginning with the first day of the mother's last menstruation. Also called menstrual age.

menstrual a. See gestational age.

mental a. The age level of intellectual ability as measured by standardized tests.

physiologic a. Age expressed in terms of function.

skeletal a. See bone age.

agenesis, agenesia (ă jen´ĕ-sis, a-jĕ-ne´zhă) Absence of a body part.

agenosomia (ă-jen-o-so´me-ă) Congenital absence or defective development of the genitals and protrusion of the abdominal organs through an incomplete abdominal wall.

agent (a´jent) Anything capable of producing an effect upon an organism.

adrenergic blocking a. Drug that slows the stimulating effects of sympathetic nerves, epinephrine, norepinephrine, and other adrenergic amines

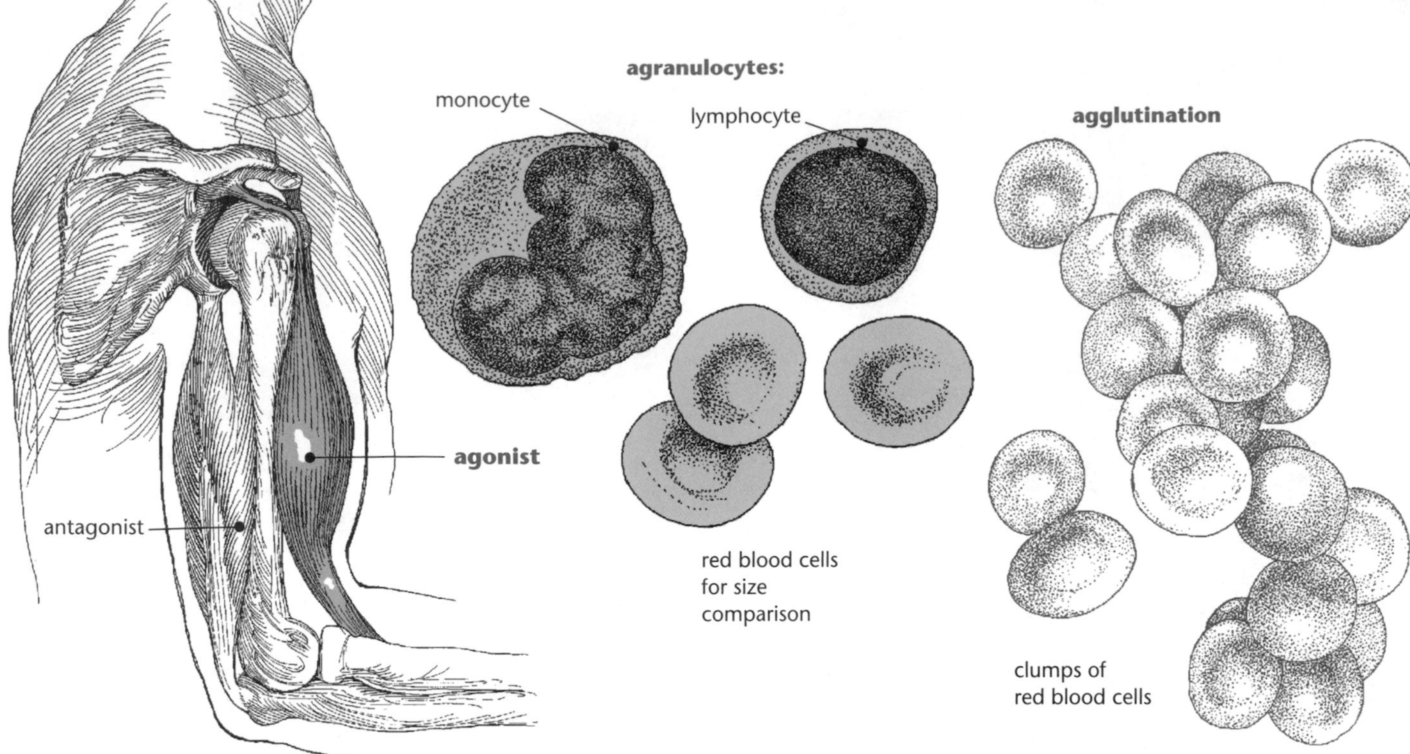

by blocking receptor sites of cells.

alkylating a. Any compound, such as nitrogen mustard, that contains alkyl groups and is toxic to cells (both normal and malignant); used to treat cancer.

alpha-adrenergic blocking a. α-adrenergic blocking agent; one that blocks alpha receptors at effector organs (e.g., phentolamine, phenoxybenzamine, terazosin, doxazosin). Also called alpha-blocker.

beta-adrenergic blocking a. β-adrenergic blocking agent; one that blocks beta receptors at effector organs; e.g., propranolol (nonselective) metoprolol and atenolol (β_1 selective). Also called beta-blocker.

blocking a. A drug that interferes with the function of the autonomic nervous system by blocking transmission at a receptor site on a cell surface, a synapse, or a neuromuscular junction. Also called blocker.

calcium channel-blocking a. Any of a class of drugs that block the entry of calcium into cardiac and smooth muscle cells; also slow nerve impulses through heart muscle. Used to treat hypertension, angina pectoris, and cardiac arrhythmias. Commonly called calcium channel blocker.

contrast a. See contrast medium, under medium.

delta a. See hepatitis D virus, under virus.

Eaton a. See *Mycoplasma pneumoniae*, under *Mycoplasma.*

inotropic a.'s A class of drugs that affect the force of muscle contraction, either positively or negatively.

Norwalk a. See Norwalk virus, under virus.

sclerosing a. Any compound used in the treatment of varicose veins.

Agent Orange (a´jent ŏr´inj) Herbicide containing the carcinogenic chemical dioxin.

ageusia (ă-goo´zhă) Absence of taste perception.

agglutination (ă-gloo-tĭ-na´shun) **1.** The clumping of cells or microorganisms when exposed to a specific immune serum. **2.** The process of joining together in the healing of a wound.

group a. The clumping together of several related varieties of bacteria in the presence of serum specific for one of that group.

agglutinin (ă-gloo´tĭ-nin) An antibody that causes particulate antigens, such as bacteria or other cells, to adhere to one another, forming clumps.

cold a. Agglutinin that causes clumping of human group O red blood cells at temperatures from 0 to 5°C.

incomplete a. Antibody that binds to antigen but does not produce agglutination. Also called incomplete antibody.

agglutinogen (ag-loo-tin´o-gen)An antigenic substance that stimulates the formation of a particular antibody (agglutinin) that causes clumping of cells containing the antigen.

agglutinogenic (ă-gloo-tĭ-no-jen´ik) Causing the production of an agglutinin.

agglutinoid (ă-gloo´tĭ-noid) An agglutinin that has lost its ability to produce clumping but can still combine with its corresponding agglutinogen.

aglomerular (ă-glo-mĕr´u-lăr) Having no glomeruli.

aglycon, aglycone (a-gli´kon, a-gli´kōn) The noncarbohydrate group of a glycoside.

agnogenic (ag-no-jen´ik) Of unknown cause.

agnosia (ag-no´zhă) Loss of ability to comprehend the meaning of sensory stimulation, such as auditory, visual, olfactory, tactile, and gustatory sensations. Failure to recognize objects or to appreciate their form by touch; caused by a lesion in the contralateral parietal lobe of the brain. Also called astereognosis; stereoanesthesia.

auditory a. Inability to recognize different sounds; usually due to a lesion in the auditory cortex of the temporal lobe of the brain.

tactile a. Failure to recognize objects or to appreciate their form by touch; caused by a lesion in the contralateral parietal lobe of the brain. Also called asterognosis; stereoanesthesia.

visual a. Inability to recognize objects by sight; usually due to a lesion in the visual association areas of the brain.

agonal (ag´o-năl) Relating to the moment just before death.

agonist (ag´o-nist) **1.** Denoting a muscle that initiates and maintains a particular movement, against another muscle (antagonist) that opposes such action. **2.** Denoting a chemical that interacts with specific receptors on the cell membrane, thereby initiating a cellular reaction.

agoraphobia (ag-o-ră-fo´be-ă) Intense and abnormal fear of being alone or in public places from which escape might be difficult or help not readily available.

agranulocytes (a-gran´u-lo-sīts) A group of relatively nongranular white blood cells; includes lymphocytes and monocytes. Also called agranular leukocytes.

agranulocytosis (a-gran-u-lo-si-to´sis) A state marked by a great reduction of granular white blood cells in peripheral blood. Term is often used to describe a syndrome marked by reduced polymorphonuclear leukocytes, infected ulcers in the mouth, throat, intestinal tract, and sometimes the skin; the acute form is most frequently drug induced but may be seen in acute leukemia; the chronic form is of unknown cause. Also called agranulocytic angina.

agraphia (ă-graf´e-ă) Loss of the previously possessed ability to write due to a cerebral lesion.

ahaustral (a-haws´tral) Denoting the x-ray appearance of the colon in ulcerative colitis, i.e., smooth, without the characteristic sacculations or pouches (haustra).

AIDS (acquired immune deficiency syndrome) The clinical state caused by infection with a strain of the human immunodeficiency virus (currently, HIV1 or HIV2). The HIV infection, acquired by sexual contact or from contaminated blood products or body parts, progresses as follows: *Acute stage*, viruses enter lymphocytes (helper T cells) and, from this point on, the infected person can transmit the disease to others. About three to five weeks later, symptoms may develop (fever, muscle and joint pain, rash, hives, diarrhea), lasting two to three weeks before disappearing. T cells produce antibodies to kill the virus from the beginning, but they cannot be detected in blood tests until about three months later. *Asymptomatic stage*, the infected person may have no symptoms for several years but the virus population increases and destroys T cells, slowly at first, rapidly later; the immune system becomes compromised. A helper T cell population ($CD4^+$ T cell count) of less than 500 cells/mm^3 is a bad prognostic sign. Defenses begin to fail and symptoms, formerly called AIDS-related complex or ARC, begin to appear (weight loss, fatigue, fever, diarrhea, swollen lymph nodes). *Full-blown AIDS* (advanced HIV disease), final stage of the disease, immune defenses break down completely and secondary (opportunistic) diseases attack the body (*Pneumo-cystis carinii* pneumonia; Kaposi's sarcoma, nervous system diseases; and fungal, bacterial, and parasitic infections). Death usually follows a few years later. Those at greatest risk for contacting AIDS are homosexual and bisexual men and intravenous drug users who share needles. Others include infants born to HIV-infected women and those who receive blood (in transfusion) or body parts (in transplants). See also HIV infection, under infection; HIV disease.

air (ār) The mixture of gases that make up the earth's atmosphere.

alveolar a. See alveolar gas, under gas.

residual a. See residual volume, under volume.

tidal a. See tidal volume, under volume.

air hunger The panicky, shallow, and uncoordinated breathing of patients with chronic obstructive pulmonary disease (COPD); a gasping for air.

akaryocyte (a-kar´e-o-sīt) A cell without a nucleus, such as a red blood cell. Also called acaryote.

akinesia (a-kī-ne´zhă) Loss or impairment of voluntary muscular action.

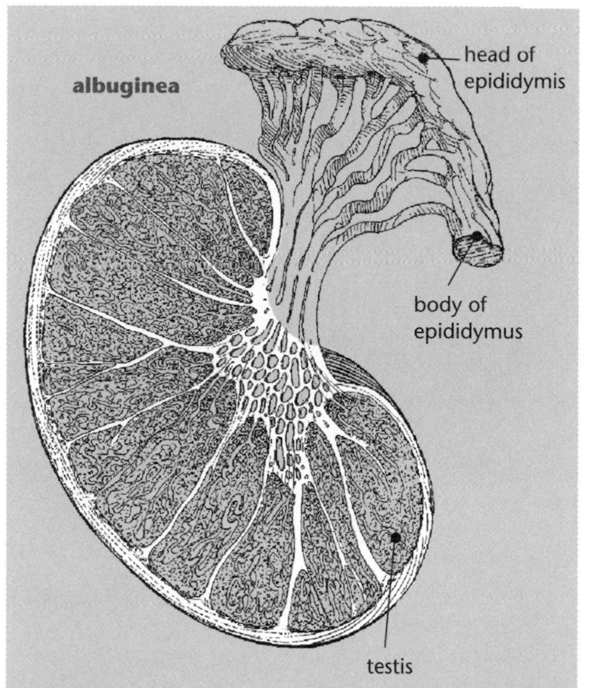

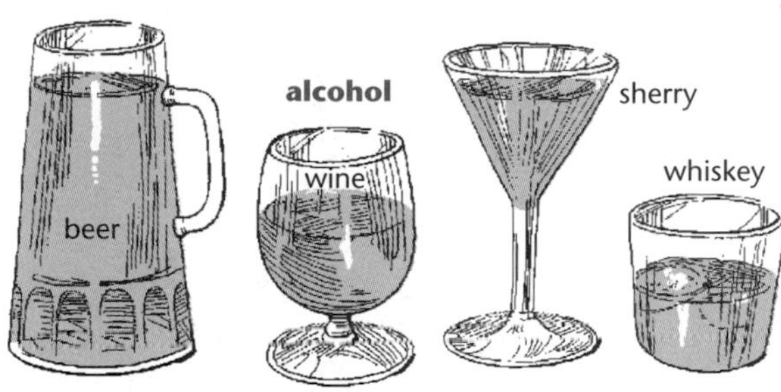

8 oz of beer, 4 oz of wine, 2 oz of sherry, and 1 oz of whiskey contain approximately equal amounts of alcohol

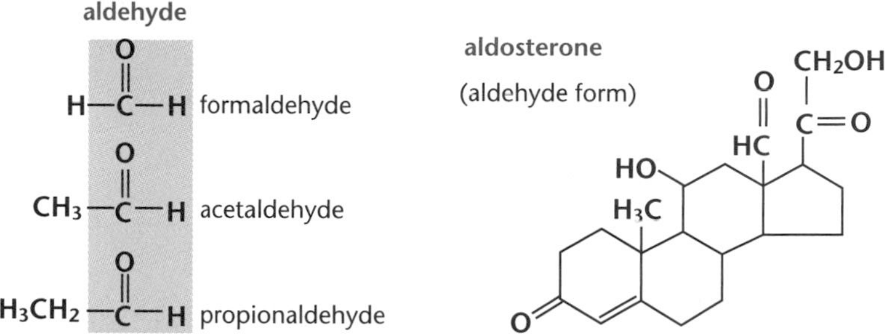

akinesthesia (ă-kin-es-the´zhă) Lack of perception of movement.

ala (ālă), *pl.* **a´lae** **1.** Any winglike structure. **2.** Axilla.

alanine (al´ă-nēn) (Ala) An amino acid of the pyruvic acid family; found widely in proteins.

alanine aminotransferase (al´ă-nēn ă-me-no-trans´fĕr-ās) (ALT) An enzyme that transfers amino groups from an alpha-amino acid to (usually) a 2-keto acid. Also called glutamic pyruvic transaminase (GPT).

alar (ālar) Of or relating to any winged structure or to the armpit.

alastrim (ă-las´trim) A contagious eruptive disease resembling a mild form of smallpox. Also called variola minor.

Albers-Schönberg disease (ahl-berz-shŏrn´bĕrg dĭ-zēz´) See osteopetrosis.

albinism (al´bĭ-niz-m) Absence of pigment in the skin, hair, and irises; may be partial or complete. Also called congenital leukoderma.

albino (al-bi´no) A person marked by albinism.

Albright's syndrome (awl´brīts sin´drōm) A polyostotic fibrous dysplasia of bone marked by dense overgrowth of bone and cystic transformation, most commonly involving several areas of the skeleton; accompanied by pigment spots on the skin and sexual precocity (principally in females).

albuginea (al-bu-jin´e-ă) A thick connective tissue capsule surrounding the testis and ovary.

albumin, albumen (al-bu´min, al-bu´mĕn) A protein in many animal and vegetable tissues, including human plasma, soluble in water and coagulable by heat; a principal constituent of egg white.

Bence Jones a. See Bence Jones protein, under protein.

radioiodinated serum a. (RISA), **iodinated** ^{131}**I serum a.** Human serum albumin iodinated with ^{131}I which emits beta and gamma radiation; used for determining blood and plasma volumes and cardiac output, and for detection of brain tumors.

albuminoid (al-bu´mĭ-noid) **1.** Resembling albumin. **2.** See scleroprotein.

albuminuria (al-bu-mĭ-nu´re-ă) Urinary excretion of albumin in excess of the normal daily amount. See also proteinuria.

alcaptonuria, alkaptonuria (al-kap-to-nu´re-ă) A hereditary condition in which homogentisic acid (alkapton) is not broken down to simpler compounds in the body but is excreted in the urine, which gives it a dark brown color when exposed to air.

alcohol (al´ko-hol) **1.** Any of various compounds that are hydroxyl derivatives of hydrocarbons. **2.** A colorless, flammable liquid, obtained from fermentation of sugars and starches with yeast and produced synthetically from ethylene or acetylene. Unless modified, "alcohol" most commonly refers to ethyl alcohol or ethanol, which is used as a solvent, preservative, topical disinfectant, and in the preparation of drugs, and is the form of alcohol found in intoxicating beverages (beer, wine, and spirits). Also called grain alcohol; ethyl alcohol; ethanol.

absolute a. Alcohol containing not more than 1% of water (by weight).

acid a. 70% ethyl alcohol containing 1% hydrochloric acid.

denatured a. Alcohol that has been rendered unfit to drink by the addition of other chemicals.

methyl a. See methanol.

rubbing a. A mixture of about 70% of absolute alcohol and varying quantities of water, denaturants, and perfumed oils.

wood a. See methyl alcohol.

alcohol dehydrogenase (al´ko-hol de-hi´dro-jen-ās) (ADH) An enzyme present in the liver that promotes the dehydrogenation of ethyl alcohol to acetaldehyde.

alcoholic (al-ko-hol´ik) **1.** Relating to or containing alcohol. **2.** Denoting a person addicted to alcohol.

alcoholism (al´ko-hol-ism) Pathologic condition marked by a pattern of alcohol intake accompanied by physical and psychological dependence. Can be recognized: when it causes impairment of social or occupational functioning, by the need to increase amounts of alcohol intake to achieve desired effects (tolerance), and by severe physical (withdrawal) symptoms when alcohol intake is stopped or reduced. Also called alcohol abuse; alcohol dependence.

paroxysmal a. See periodic drinking bouts, under bout.

aldehyde (al´dĕ-hīd) Any of a group of organic compounds obtained from oxidation of the primary alcohols and containing the group –CHO.

aldehyde dehydrogenase (al´dĕ-hīd de-hi´dro-jen-ās) An enzyme, important in the metabolism of ethyl alcohol, which promotes the oxidation of acetaldehyde to acetic acid.

aldolase (al´do-lās) An enzyme in muscle extract that catalyzes the reversible cleavage of fructose 1,6-diphosphate to yield dihydroxyacetone phosphate and glyceraldehyde.

aldopentose (al-do-pen´tōs) A sugar containing five carbon atoms and the aldehyde group –CHO.

aldosterone (al-dos´ter-ōn) Steroid hormone secreted by the outer layer (cortex) of the adrenal gland; its main function is to regulate sodium and potassium concentration; causes retention of sodium by enhancing sodium reabsorption in the kidney, intestinal tract, and sweat and salivary glands; sodium reabsorption is usually accompanied by increased secretion of potassium ions.

aldosteronism (al-dos´ter-on-iz-m) Condition caused by excessive adrenal production of aldosterone, usually resulting in lowered levels of potassium in the blood, muscular weakness, and hypertension. Also called hyperaldosteronism.

primary a. Aldosteronism caused by a primary disorder of the adrenal gland (e.g., a tumor). Also called Conn's syndrome.

secondary a. Aldosteronism resulting from excessive stimulation of the adrenal gland, frequently associated with fluid-retaining disorders.

Aldrich syndrome (awl´drich sin´drōm) See Wiskott-Aldrich syndrome.

aldrin (al´drin) A highly toxic chlorinated hydrocarbon used as an insecticide.

aleukemia (a-loo-ke´me-ă) Deficiency of white cells in the blood.

aleukemic (a-loo-ke´mik) Relating to aleukemia.

alexia (ă-lek´se-ă) Inability to grasp the meaning of written or printed words. Also called visual aphasia.

alexithymia (ă-lek-sĭ-thi´me-ă) Inability to interpret one's emotions.

algesia (al-je´zhă) Increased sensitivity to pain.

algesimeter (al-je-sim´ĕ-ter) Instrument for measuring the threshold of perception and degree of intensity of a painful stimulus on the skin. Also called odynometer.

algesthesia (al-jes-the´zhă) Perception of pain.

alginate (al´jĭ-nāt) An irreversible hydrocolloid salt of alginic acid that is extracted from marine kelp; used primarily for making dental impressions, particularly for partial dentures.

alginic acid (al-jin´ik as´id) Colloidal polysaccharide obtained from marine kelp; used in the making of alginate, a widely used dental impression material.

algophobia (al-go-fo´be-ă) Morbid fear of pain.

algorithm (al´gŏ-rith-m) Any procedure (either mechanical or through step-by-step instructions) designed to solve a particular type of problem.

alignment (ă-līn´ment) In dentistry, the line along which the teeth, natural or artificial, are arranged.

aliment (al´ĭ-ment) Food.

alimentary (al-ĭ-men´tar-e) Relating to food or nutrition.

alimentation (al-ĭ-men-ta´shun) The process of providing nourishment. Also called feeding.

enteral tube a. See nasogastric feeding, under feeding.

total parenteral a. See total parenteral nutrition, under nutrition.

aliphatic (al-ĭ-fat´ik) Relating to the fatty series of hydrocarbon compounds in which the carbon atoms are arranged in open chains rather than closed rings. Also called fatty; oily.

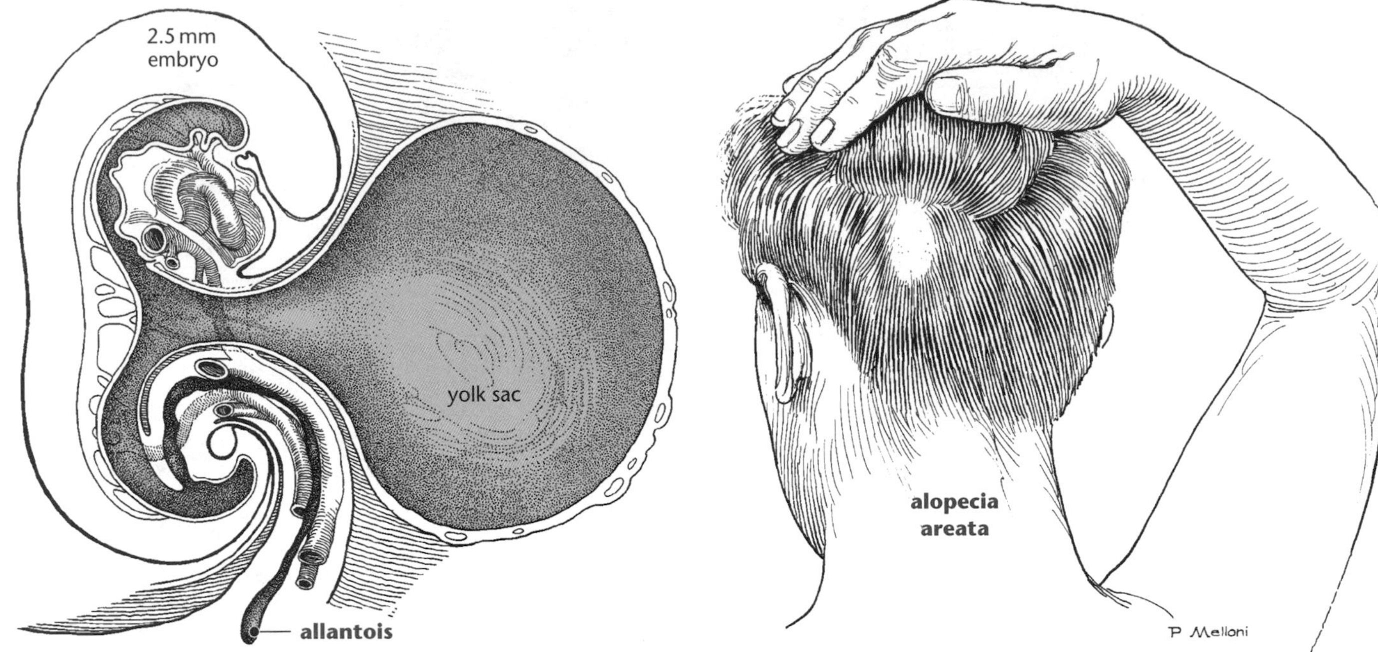

aliquot (al´ĭ-kwot) A portion (e.g., one of the equal parts into which a solution or a solid may be divided).
alkalemia (al-kă-le´me-ă) Decrease in the hydrogen ion concentration of the blood; an increase of pH beyond normal (in man, a pH greater than 7.43). COMPARE: alkalosis.
alkalescent (al-kă-les´ent) Becoming alkaline.
alkali (al´kă-li), *pl.* **al´kalis, al´kalies** Any of a group of basic compounds capable of combining with fatty acids to form soaps.
alkalimetry (al-kă-lim´ĕ-tre) Measurement of the degree of alkalinity present in a substance.
alkaline (al´kă-līn, al´kă-līn) Relating to an alkali (base).
alkalinity (al´kă-lin´ĭ-te) The state of being alkaline.
alkalize, alkalinize (al´kă-līz, al´kă-lin-īz) To make alkaline.
alkaloid (al´kă-loid) A class of compounds present in certain plants that strongly affect human physiology; e.g., morphine (opium poppy), quinine (cinchona bark), reserpine (snake root), caffeine (tea leaves and coffee beans), cocaine (coca leaves), LSD (ergot fungus), nicotine (tobacco leaves).
alkalosis (al-kă-lo´sis) A process tending to produce a decrease in hydrogen ion concentration in the body fluids; if uncompensated, it leads to a rise in pH. Commonly used synonymously with alkalemia.
hypokalemic a. Alkalosis characterized by a low serum potassium concentration; characteristic of the most commonly seen form of metabolic alkalosis.
metabolic a. The state resulting from excessive retention of alkali or excessive loss of acid; common causes include prolonged vomiting or gastric drainage, diuretic therapy, and excessive adrenal corticosteroid secretion or administration; characterized by an elevation of the plasma bicarbonate concentration and a tendency to an alkaline arterial pH; when the arterial pH is actually more alkaline than normal, the condition should, strictly speaking, be called alkalemia.
respiratory a. The state resulting from hyperventilation and reduction of pCO_2 in body fluids.
alkalotic (al-kă-lot´ik) Relating to alkalosis.
alkapton (al-kap´ton) See homogentisic acid.
allantoic acid (al-an-to´ik as´ĭd) Substance formed from the degradation of allantoin.
allantoin (ă-lan´to-in) A nitrogenous crystalline substance, $C_4H_6N_4O_3$; present in allantoic fluid, fetal urine, and some plants.
allantois (ă-lan´to-is) A diverticulum extending from the hindgut of the embryo; appears at about the 16th day of development.
allele (ă-lēl´) One of two or more genes that occupy the same position on homologous chromosomes and determine the heredity of a particular trait. Also called allelic gene. Also spelled allel.
allelic (ă-le´lik) Relating to two or more different genes that occupy the same position in homologous chromosomes.
allelism (ă-le´liz-m) The existence of two or more contrasting genes that occupy the same position in homologous chromosomes.
allergen (al´er-jen) A substance that stimulates an allergic reaction in the body.
allergenic (al-er-jen´ik) Capable of stimulating an allergic reaction.
allergic disease (ă-ler´jik dĭ-zēz´) Disease resulting from allergy or any response stimulated by an allergen; can range from superficial lesions (e.g., urticaria) to deep-seated lesions (e.g., polyarteritis nodosa).
allergic salute (ă-ler´jik să-lo͞ot´) Rubbing of the tip of the nose in a characteristic transverse or upward motion, commonly seen in children afflicted with allergic rhinitis.
allergoid (al´er-goid) A chemically modified allergen that produces antibody of the IgG but not the IgE class, thus reducing allergic symptoms.
allergy (al´er-je) Altered reactivity to a substance, which can result in pathologic reactions upon subsequent exposure to that particular substance. Also called hypersensitivity.
contact a. See contact dermatitis, under dermatitis.
drug a. Unusual sensitivity to a drug or chemical.
alloantibody (al-o-an´tĭ-bod-e) An antibody from one individual that reacts with an antigen present in another individual of the same species. Also called isoantibody.
alloantigen (al-o-an´tĭ-jĕn) Antigen produced by one individual that incites the formation of antibodies in another individual of the same species. Also called homologous antigen; isoantigen.
alloarthroplasty (al-o-ar´thro-plas-te) Surgical construction of an artificial joint.
allochromasia (al-o-kro-ma´zhă) Change in the color of skin or hair.
allocortex (al-o-kor´teks) The primitive part of the cerebral cortex, such as the olfactory cortex, which is not laminated.
allogamy (al-og´ă-me) Fertilization by the union of the ovum from one organism with the spermatozoon from another. Also called cross-fertilization.
allogenic, allogeneic (al-o-jen´ik, al-o-jĕ-ne´ik) Denoting genetically dissimilar individuals of the same species; used in organ or cell transplantation.
allograft (al´o-graft) A graft derived from a genetically dissimilar individual of the same species. Also called allogeneic graft.
allolalia (al-o-la-li´ă) Any speech defect that originates in the brain.
allomerism (ă-lom´er-iz-m) The state of having different chemical composition but the same crystalline form.
allomorphism (al-o-mor´fiz-m) A change in the shape of cells caused by mechanical factors.
alloplasia (al-o-pla´zhă) See heteroplasia.
alloplast (al´o-plast) A presumably inert material used as an implant.
alloploid (al´o-ploid) An organism arising from the combination of two or more sets of chromosomes from different ancestral species. Also called allopolyploid.
all or none (awl or nun) See Bowditch's law, under law.
allosome (al´o-sōm) A chromosome that differs from the ordinary chromosome (autosome); a sex chromosome.
allosterism, allostery (al´o-ster-iz-m, al-o-ster´e) Alteration of an enzymes activity by regulatory molecules that are noncompetitively bound to sites other than the active or catalytic site of the enzyme molecule.
allotransplantation (al-o-trans-plan-ta´shun) The transplantation of tissue from one individual to another of the same species but without the identical genetic makeup.
allotype (al´o-tīp) Any of several antigenic determinants that differ among individuals of the same species.
alloxan (al´ok-san) A reddish, crystalline substance, $C_4H_2N_2O$; a product of oxidation of uric acid; capable of destroying the islets of Langerhans and, hence, inducing experimental diabetes in laboratory animals.
alloy (al´oi) A mixture of two or more metals.
alochia (ă-lo´ke-ă) Absence of vaginal discharges (lochia) after childbirth.
aloe (al´o) The juice from the leaves of *Aloe vera* (family Liliaceae); a common ingredient of skin preparations due to its soothing and healing properties.
aloform (al-o-form) A wing-shaped structure, such as the pterygoid bone of the skull.
alogia (ă-lo´je-ă) See aphasia.
alopecia (al-o-pe´she-ă) Hair loss; may be partial or complete, permanent or temporary.
androgenetic a. Progressive, diffuse loss of scalp hair in men, thought to result from a genetic predisposition. May occur in women associated with elevated androgen levels resulting from ovarian or adrenal gland dysfunction or tumor. Also called alopecia hereditaria.
a. areata Complete loss of hair in patches, chiefly on the scalp.

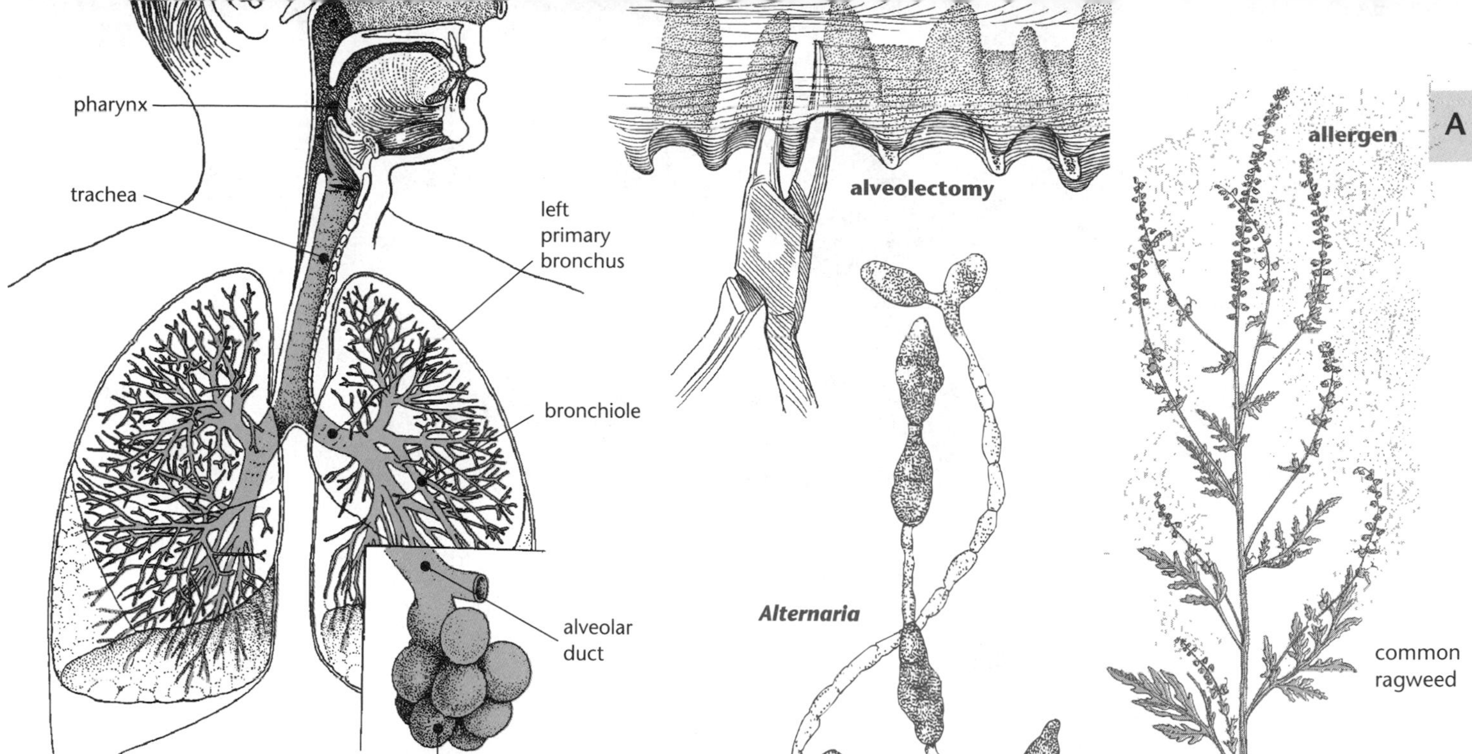

a. capitis totalis Complete hair loss from the scalp.
drug-induced a. Reversible hair loss caused by administration of certain drugs.
a. hereditaria See androgenetic alopecia.
nonscarring a. Alopecia in which only the hair shafts are destroyed; hair follicles remain intact.
scarring a. Alopecia marked by fibrosis, inflammation, and loss of hair follicles.
a. senilis Loss of hair normally occurring in old age. Also called senile alopecia.
a. totalis Total loss of hair from all parts of the body. Also called alopecia universalis.
a. universalis See alopecia totalis.
alpha (al′fă) **1.** The first letter of the Greek alphabet, α; used to denote the first in order of importance. **2.** In chemistry, denotes a location immediately adjacent to the functional group of atoms in a molecule. For terms beginning with alpha, see under specific term.
alpha-blocker (al′fă blok′er) See alpha-adrenergic blocking agent, under agent.
alpha-fetoprotein (al′fă fe-to-pro′tēn) (AFP) Plasma protein produced in the fetal liver and the yolk sac (until this structure degenerates normally at about 12 weeks of gestation). AFP reaches peak levels in fetal blood at about 13 weeks of gestation; then levels decrease, gradually at first and rapidly after 32 weeks. Considerably raised levels of AFP in the amniotic fluid and maternal serum after 14 weeks of gestation may indicate developmental defects (e.g., spina bifida); moderately elevated levels may represent false-positive test results. In other adults, AFP is produced in certain abnormal tissues (e.g., liver cancer, endodermal sinus tumors of the ovary, and testicular cancer). Used also to monitor response to antitumor therapy.
Alphavirus (al′fă-vi-rus) A genus of arthropod-borne viruses (family Togaviridae) including those causing encephalitis. Formerly classified as arbovirus, group A.
Alport syndrome (al′port sin′drōm) Hereditary nephritis associated with nerve deafness. See also hereditary nephritis, under nephritis.
alter (awl′ter) To castrate a male animal.
alternans (awl-ter′nanz) Alternating.
electrical a. Regular alternating variation in the wave amplitude of the electrocardiogram.
Alternaria (awl-ter-na′re-ă) A genus of soil molds having dark-colored conidia; prevalent in air and usually considered to be a common laboratory contaminant; a common allergen in bronchial asthma.
alum (al′um) Any double sulfate of a trivalent metal (aluminum, iron, etc.) and a univalent metal (sodium, potassium, etc.); used as an astringent.
aluminum (ă-loo′mĭ-num) A silvery white, metallic element of extremely light weight; symbol Al, atomic number 13, atomic weight 26.97; its compounds are used therapeutically as antacids and astringents.
a. chloride hexahydrate A white or yellowish-white powder, $Al\ Cl_3{\cdot}6H_2O$; used in 10 to 25% solution as an antiperspirant, a deodorant, or astringent.
a. hydroxide, a. hydrate A white tasteless powder, $Al\ (OH)_3$; used externally as a drying powder because it takes up water, and internally as an antacid. Also called hydrated alumina.
a. hydroxide gel A preparation containing from 3.6 to 4.4% of aluminum oxide (Al_2O_3) in the form of aluminum hydroxide; used to reduce stomach acidity; also prepared in tablet form, which is the dried aluminum hydroxide gel.
alveoalgia (al-ve-o-lal′jă) See dry socket, under socket.
alveolar (al-ve′o-lar) Relating to an alveolus.
alveolectomy (al-ve-o-lek′tŏ-me) Surgical removal of diseased tissue from the alveolar process, following the removal of teeth, in preparation for the fitting of a dental prosthesis.
alveoli (al-ve′o-li) Plural of alveolus.
alveolingual (al-ve-o-ling′gwal) Relating to the surface of the alveolar process adjacent to the tongue.
alveolitis (al-ve-o-li′tis) Inflammation of alveoli.
alveolotomy (al-ve-o-lot′ŏ-me) The surgical opening of a tooth socket for drainage and treatment purposes.
alveolus (al-ve′o-lus), *pl.* **alve′oli** **1.** A small cavity or saclike dilatation. **2.** One of the honeycomb pits in the mucous membrane of the stomach.
dental a. See tooth socket, under socket.
pulmonary a. One of the minute, balloonlike air sacs at the end of a bronchiole in the lungs. Exchange of the gases or respiration takes place through the alveolar walls.
alveus (al′ve-us) **1.** A canal. **2.** The layer of white fibers in the brain that covers the area of the hippocampus adjacent to the lateral ventricle.
Alzheimer's disease (awltz′hi-merz dĭ-zēz′) Disease manifested by impairment of higher intellectual function that progresses to profound dementia over a 5- to 10-year period; it rarely begins before the age of 50, but thereafter increases steadily with advancing age. Early clinical symptoms and signs include memory loss (particularly of recent events), decreased ability to concentrate and solve problems, and mild emotional instability progressing to disorientation, confusion, hallucinations, paranoid delusions, and eventual inability to carry out daily activities and personal care. The brain undergoes gross and microscopic changes. Also called Alzheimer's dementia.
amalgam (ă-mal′gam) An alloy of mercury and other metals, used in dentistry for filling cavities in the teeth.
amalgamate (ă-mal′gă-māt) To make an amalgam by dissolving a metal in mercury.
amalgamation (ă-mal-gă-ma′shun) The process of dissolving a metal in mercury to form an alloy.
amalgamator (ă-mal′gă-māt-or) In dentistry, a device for mixing amalgam mechanically.
Amanita (am-ă-ni′tă) A genus of fungi.
A. phalloides A. Poisonous mushroom which, upon ingestion, causes severe gastrointestinal symptoms, followed by damage to the kidneys, liver, and central nervous system. Also called death cup; death angel.
amantadine hydrochloride (ă-man′tă-dēn hi-dro-klōr′id) An antiviral agent used in preventing illness in individuals exposed to respiratory infection from influenza virus; also used in treating Parkinson's disease; Symmetrel®.
amaurosis (am-aw-ro′sis) Complete loss of vision.
central a. Blindness caused by disease of the central nervous system.
a. fugax Temporary blindness lasting a few minutes.
toxic a. Blindness due to inflammation of the optic nerve caused by the presence in the system of a poisonous agent such as alcohol, tobacco, lead, etc.
amaurotic (am-aw-rot′ik) Relating to blindness.
ambenonium chloride (am-be-no ′ne-um klōr′īd) A chemical compound that inhibits the production of the enzyme cholinesterase; used in the treatment of chronic progressive muscular weakness (myasthenia gravis); Mytelase Chloride®.
ambidextrous (am-bĭ-dek′strus) Being equally skillful with both hands.
ambisexual (am-bĭ-seks′u-al) **1.** Relating to both sexes. **2.** See bisexual.
ambisexuality (am-bĭ-sek′shoo-ăl-ĭ-te) The state of being ambisexual.
ambivalence (am-biv′ă-lens) The existence of contrasting emotional feelings, such as love and hate, about a person or object.
amblyacousia (am-ble-a-koo′sĭ-ă) A slight degree of hearing impairment.
amblyopia (am-ble-o′pe-ă) Diminished vision in one eye without a detectable lesion or disease of the eye. Sometimes used synonymously with suppression amblyopia.
suppression a. Involuntary suppression of vision in one eye, specifically in the retinal area with the greatest visual acuity; occurs when the images formed by the two eyes are so different that they cannot be fused into one image; the difference may be due to unequal refraction (consequently the two

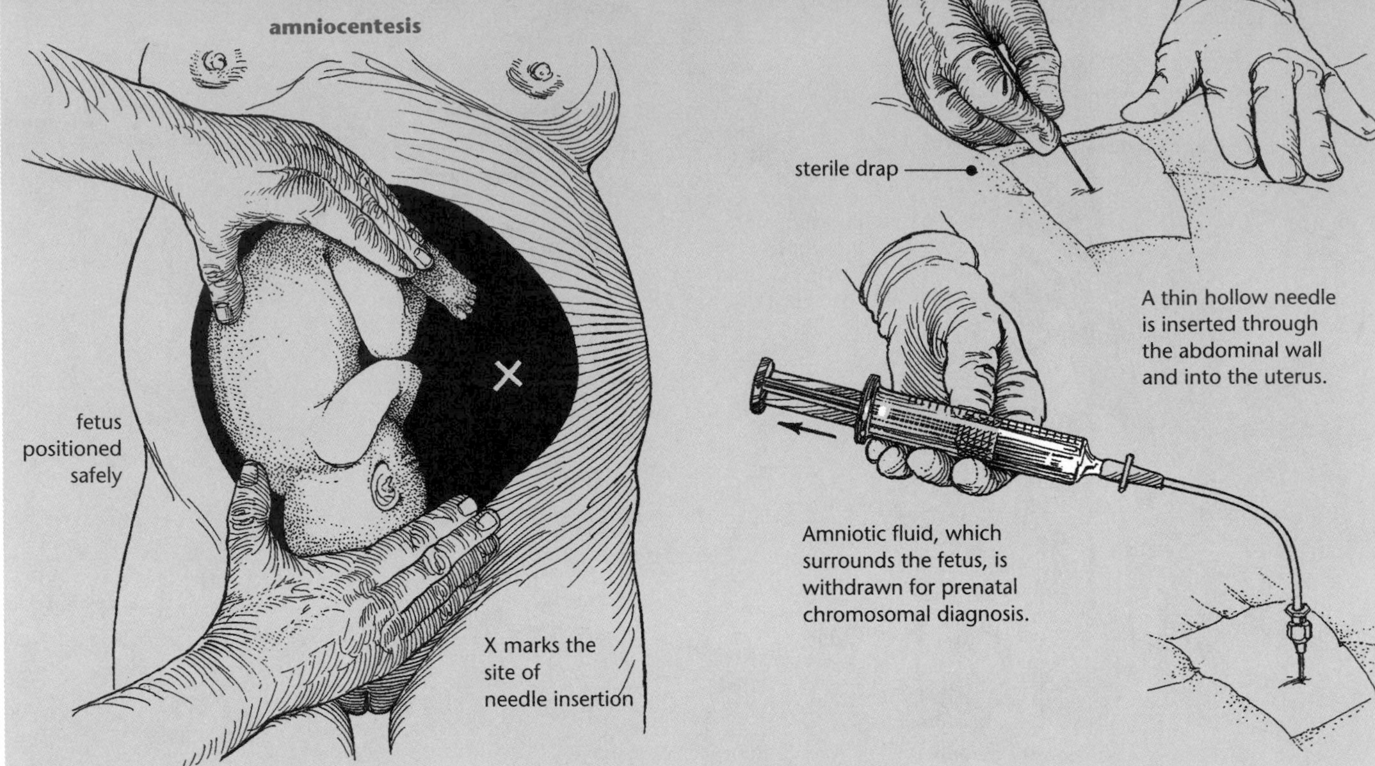
amniocentesis
sterile drap
A thin hollow needle is inserted through the abdominal wall and into the uterus.
fetus positioned safely
Amniotic fluid, which surrounds the fetus, is withdrawn for prenatal chromosomal diagnosis.
X marks the site of needle insertion

images are of a different size), or when each eye points in a different direction.

amblyoscope (am´ble-o-skōp) A device consisting primarily of two angled tubes which can be made to swivel to different degrees of convergence or divergence; used for training an amblyopic eye to share equally with the other eye in binocular vision.

Ambrosia (am-bro´zhă) A genus of coarse annual weeds commonly known as ragweed; it produces large quantities of windborn pollen.

A. elatior Common ragweed that produces highly allergenic pollen capable of causing hay fever and asthma in some individuals; pollination period is from August through October.

ambulatory, ambulant (am´bu-lă-to-re, am´bu-lant) Capable of walking about; said of a patient who is not confined to bed.

ameba (ă-me´bă), *pl.* **ame´bae, ame´bas** Any protozoan of the genus *Amoeba.*

amebiasis (am-e-bi´ă-sis) The condition of being infected with *Amoeba histolytica.*

amebic (ă-me´bik) Pertaining to amebas.

amebicide (ă-me-bĭ-sīd) Anything that destroys amebas.

ameboid (ă-me´boid) Resembling an ameba.

ameboma (am-e-bo´mă) Tumor-like mass sometimes formed in the wall of the colon due to chronic infestation with amebas.

ameiosis (a-mi-o´sis) A type of cell division in which gametes are formed without reduction in chromosome number.

amelanotic (ă-mel-ă-not´ik) Denoting certain types of unpigmented skin growths.

amelia (ă-me´le-ă) Congenital absence of a limb or limbs.

amelification (ă-mel-ĭ-fi-ka´shun) The development of tooth enamel.

amelioration (ă-mēl-yo-ra´shun) Improvement; lessening of the severity of symptoms.

ameloblast (ă-mel´o-blast) Epithelial cell in the developing tooth that produces layers of matrix which become calcified to form rods of tooth enamel; when it completes its function of enamel formation, the ameloblast becomes part of the enamel cuticle (Nasmyth's membrane). Also called enamel cell.

ameloblastoma (ă-mel-o-blas-to´mă) Tumor derived from epithelial tissue characteristic of the enamel organ, occurring mainly in the molar region of the mandible.

ameloblastosarcoma (ă-mel-o-blas-to-sar-ko´mă) Malignant neoplasm derived from odontogenic tissue and containing a large number of ameloblasts.

amelogenesis (am-ĕ-lo-jen´ĕ-sis) Formation and development of tooth enamel. Also called enamelogenesis.

a. imperfecta Hereditary defect of tooth enamel; may be deficient in quantity or defective in structure, resulting in an easily eroded enamel. Also called enamelogenesis imperfecta.

amenorrhea (ă-men-o-re´ă) Absence of menstruation.

athletic a., stress a. Amenorrhea associated with intense exercise; may lead to reduced levels of estrogen and, ultimately, premature osteoporosis.

primary a. Failure of menstruation to begin by the age of 16 years.

secondary a. Cessation of menstruation for at least 3 months in a woman who has menstruated in the past.

amenorrheal, amenorrheic (ă-men-o-re´al, ă-men-o-re´ik) Relating to amenorrhea.

ametropia (am-ĕ-tro´pe-ă) A refractive disorder of the eye in which parallel rays of light do not focus on the retina, but either in front of it (myopia) or behind it (hyperopia).

axial a. Ametropia caused by the lengthening of the eyeball on the optic axis.

amide (am´īd) An organic compound derived from ammonia by the substitution of an acyl radical for hydrogen.

amination (am-ĭ-na´shun) The formation of an amine.

amine (ă-mēn´) Any of a group of organic compounds derived from ammonia by replacement of one or more hydrogen atoms by hydrocarbon radicals.

aminoacetic acid (ă-me-no-ă-se´tik as´id) See glycine.

amino acid (ă-me´no as´id) See under acid.

aminoacidemia (ă-me-no-as-ĭ-de´me-ă) The presence of amino acids in the blood as a result of congenital metabolic disease.

aminoaciduria (am-ĭ-no-as-ĭ-du´re-ă) The presence of excessive amounts of amino acids in the urine, or the presence of amino acids not usually found in the urine.

p-aminobenzoic acid (ă-me-no-ben-zo´ik as´id) (PABA) Para-aminobenzoic acid; a factor of the vitamin B complex; it is an essential growth factor for bacteria.

γ-aminobutyric acid (ă-me-no-bu-ter´ik as´id) (GABA, γ-Abu) Gamma-aminobutyric acid; a substance in the brain, especially in the basal ganglia and neocortex, that plays a role in cortical transmission.

ε-aminocaproic acid (ă-me-no-kă-pro´ik as´id) (EACP) Epsilon-aminocaproic acid; compound that inhibits dissolution of fibrin in the blood; used to prevent bleeding (e.g., in hemophilia and after surgery).

aminoglycoside (am-ĭ-no-gli-ko´sīd) An antibiotic containing amino sugars linked by glycoside; it blocks protein synthesis in bacterial ribosomes.

p-aminohippuric acid (ă-me-no-hĭ-pūr´ik as´id) (PAH) Para-aminohippuric acid; a substance used in clearance studies to determine the total amount of plasma flowing through the kidney.

δ-aminolevulinic acid (ă-me-no-lev-u-lin´ik as´id) (ALA) Delta-aminolevulinic acid; an intermediate in the biosynthesis of porphyrin; excessive levels are found in urine in intermittent acute porphyria.

aminopeptidase (ă-me-no-pep´tĭ-dās) Any of several enzymes promoting the breakdown of peptides; those in intestinal secretions aid in protein digestion.

aminophylline (am-ĭ-nof´ĭ-lin) A xanthine derivative containing 85% anhydrous theophylline and 15% ethylenediamine; used to treat asthma.

p-aminosalicylic acid (ă-me-no-sal-ĭ-sil´ik as´id) (PAS, PASA) Para-aminosalicylic acid; a crystalline compound which retards the growth of bacteria; used as an adjunct in the treatment of tuberculosis.

aminotransferase (ă-me-no-trans´fer-ās) An enzyme transferring an amino group generally from an amino acid to a 2-keto acid. Also called transaminase.

amitosis (am-ĭ-to´sis) Direct division of a cell simply by elongation and division of the nucleus and cytoplasm into two new cells, unlike the ordinary process of cell reproduction (mitosis).

ammonia (ă-mo´ne-ă) A colorless, volatile, pungent, alkaline gas, NH_3, soluble in water, forming ammonia water; formed in the body as a product of protein metabolism; usually converted to urea by the liver or excreted by the kidney to facilitate H^+ (hydrogen ion) excretion.

ammoniacal (am-o-ni´ă-kal) Relating to ammonia.

ammoniated (ă-mo´ne-āt-ed) Combined with or containing ammonia.

ammonium (ă-mo´ne-um) The chemical radical NH_4.

a. chloride A white crystalline compound, NH_4Cl; used as an expectorant and as an acidifying agent. Also called sal ammoniac.

amnesia (am-ne´zhă) Impairment of memory.

anterograde a. Inability to recall events after injury or disease.

retrograde a. Amnesia for events preceding injury or disease.

amnesiac (am-ne´se-ak) An individual suffering from loss of memory.

amnesic (am-ne´sik) Relating to amnesia.

amnestic (am-nes´tik) Causing amnesia.

amniocentesis (am-ne-o-sen-te´sis) Withdrawal of amniotic fluid through the abdominal wall using a

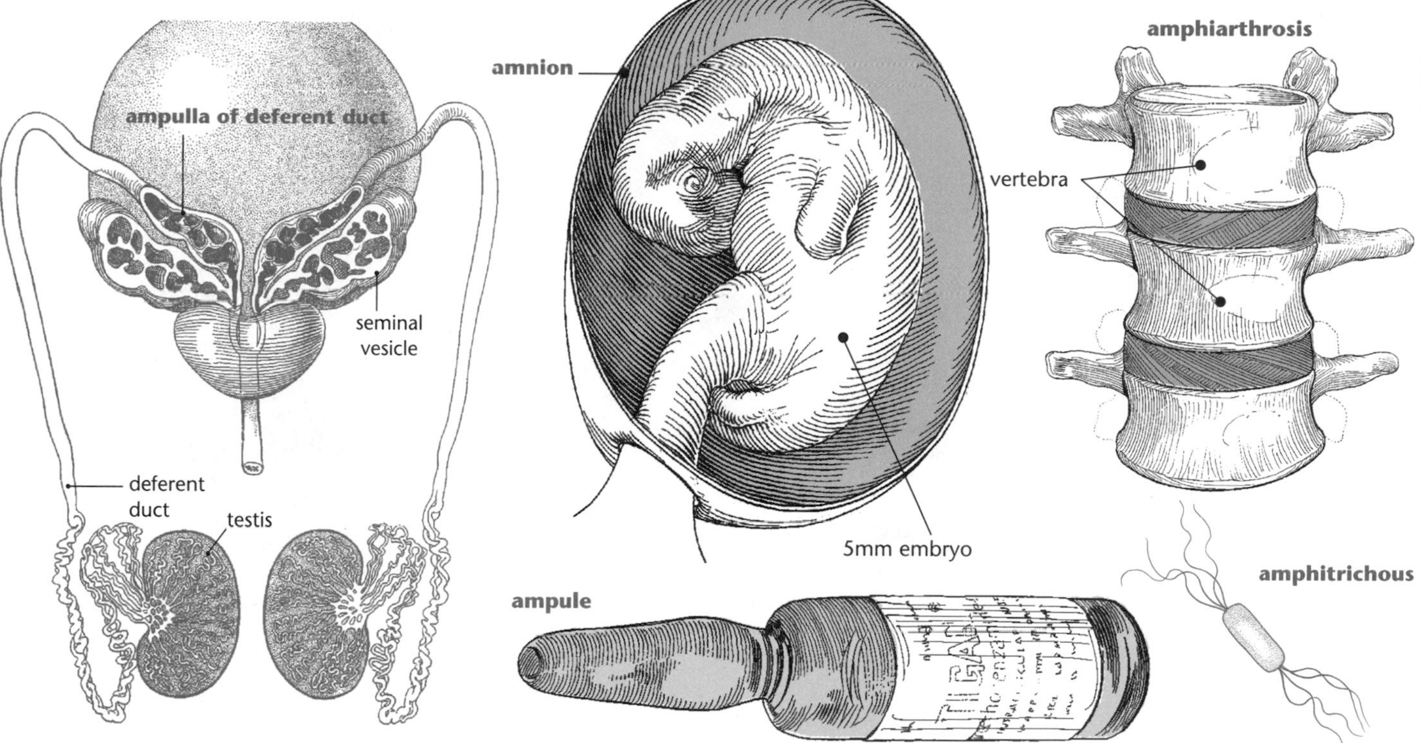

needle and syringe.

amniochorion (am-ne-o-kor´e-on) The amnion and chorion considered together; after the third month of gestation, the two membranes come in close contact and become the avascular sac containing the fetus and amniotic fluid. Commonly called bag of waters.

amnion (am´ne-on) The thin, tough, innermost layer of the membranous sac that surrounds the embryo and fills with amniotic fluid as the pregnancy advances. See also amniochorion.

amnionitis (am-ne-o-ni´tis) Inflammation of the amnion.

amniorrhea (am-ne-o-re´ă) The premature escape of amniotic fluid.

amniorrhexis (am-ne-o-rek´sis) Rupture of the amniotic membrane.

amnioscopy (am-ne-os´kŏ-pe) Direct observation of the amniotic fluid, through the intact amniotic sac, with an endoscope introduced through the cervical canal.

amniotomy (am-ne-ot´o-me) Surgical rupture of the fetal membranes for the purpose of inducing labor.

Amoeba (ă-me´bă) A genus of one-celled protozoans existing in water, soil, or as parasites, having a changeable shape, and moving by means of pseudopodia; some species cause disease in man.

amorphia, amorphism (ă-mor´fe-ă, ă-mor´ ¶z-m) The state or condition of being without a definite form.

amorphous (ă-mor´fus) Lacking a definite shape or structure.

ampere (am´pēr) (A) The unit of electric current strength, equal to the current yielded by 1 volt of electromotive force against 1 ohm of resistance.

amphetamine (am-fet´ă-min) Any of a group of synthetic chemicals that stimulate the central nervous system; pharmacologically classified as sympathomimetic amines. Slang names include: speed; uppers; bennies.

amphiarthrosis (am-fe-ar-thro´sis) A joint or articulation that allows only slight motion (e.g., between the bodies of the vertebrae). Also called amphiarthrodial joint.

amphipathic (am-fĭ-path´ik) Relating to molecules possessing groups with characteristically different properties (e.g., molecules that are hydrophobic at one end and hydrophilic at the other end).

amphitrichous, amphitrichate (am-fit´rĭ-kus, am-fit´rĭ-kāt) Having flagella or a flagellum at both ends, as in certain microorganisms.

amphixenosis (am-fiks en-ō´sis) A transmissible disease caused by a microorganism that can inhabit either human or animal as its maintenance host. COMPARE: anthropozoonosis; zooanthroponosis.

amphophil, amphophile (am´fo-fil, am´fo-fīl) Denoting certain cells that stain readily with either acid or basic dyes.

amphoric (am-for´ik) The quality of a sound sometimes heard in auscultation, described as that produced by blowing over the mouth of a bottle.

amplification (am-plĭ-fĭ-ka´shun) An increase in magnitude, as of a sensory perception.

gene a. The increased reduplication of a gene, especially in aberrant (often malignant) cells.

amplitude (am´plĭ-tood) One of three measurements of the vibration of a sound wave (others are frequency and wavelength); the vertical vibrations that reflect the intensity of sound.

ampule, ampoule, ampul (am´pūl) A small glass container sealed to preserve the sterile condition of its contents, which are used primarily for sub-cutaneous, intramuscular, or intravenous injections.

ampulla (am-pul´ă), *pl.* **ampul´lae** A saclike dilatation of a canal, as seen in the semicircular canals of the inner ear.

a. of deferent duct, a. of vas deferens The dilatation of the duct just before it is joined by the duct of the seminal vesicle.

hepatopancreatic a. The short dilated tube formed by the union of the pancreatic and bile ducts just before they empty into the duodenum. Also called ampulla of Vater.

phrenic a. The normal expansion of the lower end of the esophagus.

a. of uterine tube The wide, tortuous portion of the fallopian (uterine) tube; constitutes nearly one-half of the entire tube.

a. of Vater See hepatopancreatic ampulla.

ampullitis (am-pul-lī´tis) Inflammation of an ampulla, especially of the dilated end of the deferent duct that conveys sperm from the epididymis to the ejaculatory duct.

amputation (am-pu-ta´shun) Removal of a limb or any appendage of the body.

Lisfranc's a. Amputation of the foot between the tarsus and metatarsus. Also called Lisfranc's operation.

root a. Surgical removal of the apical portion of the root of a tooth.

Syme's a. Removal of the foot at the ankle joint; both malleoli are removed. Also called Syme's operation.

amputee (am-pu-te´) A person with one or more amputated limbs.

amygdala (ă-mig´dă-lă), *pl.* **amyg´dalae** **1.** Any almond-shaped anatomic structure, such as a tonsil. **2.** One of two ovoid masses of gray matter, located in the temporal lobe of the brain, at the terminal portion of the inferior horn of the lateral ventricle. Also called amygdaloid nuclear complex.

amygdalase (ă-mig´dă-lās) A glucoside-splitting enzyme.

amygdaloid (ă-mig´dă-loid) Almond-shaped.

amyl (am´ĭl) The univalent organic radical C_5H_{11}.

a. nitrate A flammable and volatile yellow liquid, $C_5H_{11}NO_2$; used as a motor depressant and (formerly) as an inhaler to relieve pain in angina pectoris.

amylase (am´ĭ-lās) An enzyme that promotes the splitting of starches.

α-a. See α-1,4-glucan-4-glucanohydrolase.

β-a. See α-1,4-glucan maltohydrolase.

amylin (am´ĭ-lĭn) The insoluble constituent or cellulose of starch.

amylogenesis (am-ĭ-lo-jen´ĕ-sis) Starch formation.

amyloid (am´ĭ-loid) **1.** Resembling starch. **2.** An abnormal protein-polysaccharide complex deposited extracellularly in various organs or tissues as a product of certain disease processes.

amyloidosis (am-ĭ-loi-do´sis) Accumulation of an abnormal protein, amyloid, in various tissues of the body.

primary a. Amyloidosis that is not caused by another disease, usually involving the tongue, intestinal tract, lungs, skin, and skeletal and heart muscles.

secondary a. Amyloidosis resulting from a chronic disease (e.g., tuberculosis, rheumatoid arthritis, osteomyelitis) and usually affecting the liver, kidneys, and spleen.

amylopectin (am-ĭ-lo-pek´tin) A polysaccharide found in the insoluble component of starch.

amylophagia (am-ĭ-lo-fa´jă) Abnormal craving for starch. Also called starch eating.

amylopsin (am-ĭl-op´sin) The starch-splitting enzyme present in pancreatic juice.

amylose (am´ĭ-lōs) The relatively soluble component of starch.

amyotonia (a-mi-o-to´ne-ă) Lack of muscular tone.

a. congenita Amyotonia occurring in infants, affecting only the musculature innervated by spinal nerves. Also called Oppenheim's syndrome.

amyotrophic (a-mi-o-trof´ik) Relating to muscular degeneration or atrophy.

amyotrophy (a-mi-ot´rŏ-fe) Wasting or degeneration of muscles.

neuralgic a. Condition of unknown cause and spontaneous recovery, marked by pain around a shoulder followed by weakness of the arm muscles innervated by nerves of the brachial plexus. Also called brachial plexus neuropathy; neuralgic amyotrophy; shoulder-hand syndrome.

progressive spinal a. See progressive muscular atrophy, under atrophy.

anabolic (an-ă-bol´ik) Promoting or exhibiting

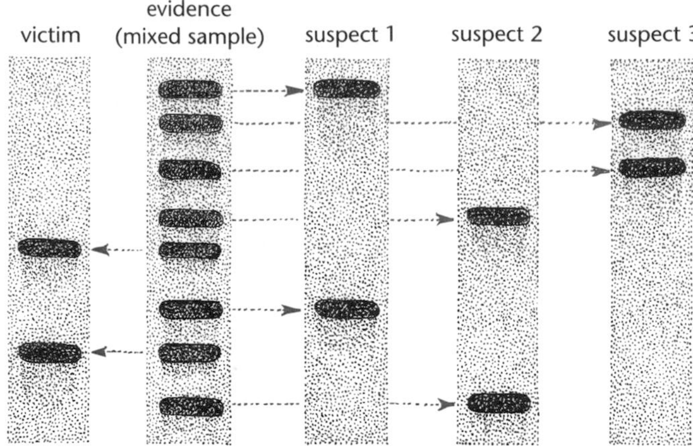

Each single locus probe produces a pattern of at most two bands per person. An eight band pattern indicates the sample was from at least four individuals. Matching of the suspects' band patterns with those of the evidence confirms their involvement.

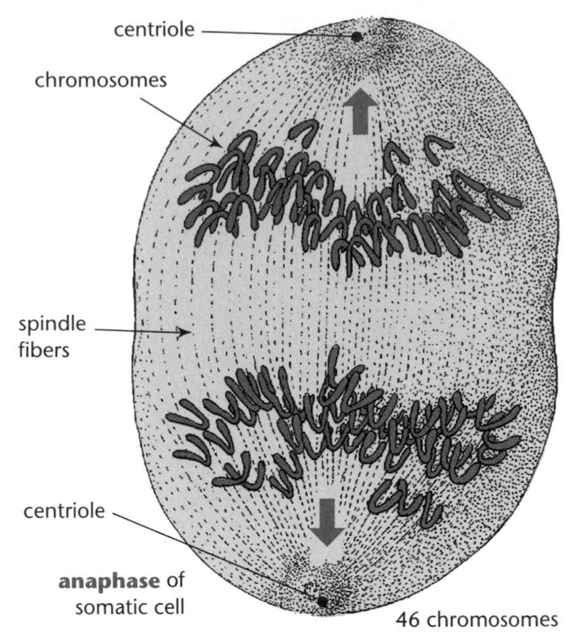

anaphase of somatic cell

anabolism.

anabolism (a-nab´ŏ-liz-m) The process by which living tissues build complex compounds from substances of a simple constitution; an energy-consuming constructive metabolic process; the reverse of catabolism.

anabolistic (a-nab´o-lis-tic) Having constructive metabolic properties, such as the ability to build complex molecules out of simple ones.

anacidity (an-ă-sid´ĭ-te) Lack of acidity; especially, lack of hydrochloric acid in the gastric juice.

anaclitic (an-ă-klit´ik) Having a psychologic dependence on others, as the normal dependence of an infant on its mother or mother substitute.

anacrotic (an-ă-krot´ik) Having an abnormal pulse, evidenced in a pulse tracing in which the ascending line of the curve has a small additional wave or shoulder, as in aortic stenosis. Also called anadicrotic.

anacusis, anakusis (an-ă-koo´sis) Total deafness.

anadicrotic (an-ă-dī-krot´ik) See anacrotic.

anaerobe (an´ĕ-rōb) A microorganism that can live and grow in the complete, or almost complete, absence of free oxygen.

facultative a. A microorganism that thrives in either the presence or absence of free oxygen.

obligate a. A microorganism unable to grow or live in the presence of free oxygen.

anaerobic (an-ĕ-ro´bik) Growing in the absence of oxygen.

anaerogenic (an-ĕ-ro-jen´ik) Producing no gas; applied to bacteria.

anal (a´nal) Relating to the anus.

analeptic (an-ă-lep´tik) A central nervous system stimulant; a restorative medication.

analgesia (an-al-je´zhă) Loss of pain sensation; a condition in which stimuli that normally produce pain are perceived but are not interpreted as pain; may result from disease interrupting pain pathways in the central or peripheral nervous system, or may be induced by drugs (e.g., administration of certain inhalation anesthetics in concentrations lower than those required for surgical anesthesia).

patient-controlled a. (PCA) Reduction of acute pain by self-administration of a predetermined dose of a narcotic drug as established by the physician (e.g., in a postoperative period).

analgesic (an-al-je´zik) **1.** Relieving pain. **2.** A medication that relieves pain without affecting consciousness; the most commonly used analgesic is aspirin (acetylsalicylic acid).

analgia (an-al´jă) Absence of pain.

analog (an´ă-log) **1.** An organ or part similar in function to one in another organism of a different species but different in structure or development. **2.** A chemical compound similar in structure to another but dissimilar in composition.

analogous (a-nal´ŏ-gus) Similar in function or appearance, but not in origin or development.

analphalipoproteinemia (an-al-fa-lip-o-pro-te-ne´me-ă) See Tangier disease.

analysand (ă-nal´ĭ-sand) A patient who is being psychoanalyzed.

analysis (ă-nal´ĭ-sis), *pl.* **anal´yses** **1.** The separation of a substance into its simple constituents. **2.** Psychoanalysis.

decision a. Analysis that involves identifying all available choices for patient care, and the potential outcome of each choice. A model of the decision is plotted to represent the strategies available and to calculate the likelihood that each outcome will occur if a particular strategy is used.

discriminant a. Statistical technique using discrete dependent variables for separating sets of observed values and allocating new values.

Fourier a. A mathematical method of converting a function of time or space into a function of frequency; used in reconstruction of images in computed tomography (CT) and magnetic resonance imaging (MRI).

gastric a. Aspiration and study of the stomach contents; may be performed in the basal state, after a test meal, or after administration of a secretion-promoting agent.

gravimetric a. Determination by weight of the exact proportions of the components of a substance.

Northern blot a. Identification of RNA fragments that have been electrophoretically separated and transferred (blotted) onto nitrocellular or other type of paper or nylon membrane. Specific RNA fragments can then be detected by radioactive probes.

qualitative a. Determination of the nature of the constituents of a substance.

quantitative a. Determination of the quantity, as well as the nature, of the components of a substance.

regression a. A statistical method for finding the relationship between sets of scores on a pair of variables.

semen a. Examination of a semen sample to determine male fertility in an infertile marriage or to substantiate the success of vasectomy.

Southern blot a. A procedure (first developed by E. M. Southern) for separating and identifying DNA sequences; DNA fragments are separated by electrophoresis and transferred (blotted) onto a special filter on which specific fragments can then be detected by radioactive probes.

spectrum a. Determination of the components of a gas by means of a spectroscope.

a. of variance (ANOVA) A statistical method for comparing the means of multiple variables to assess the influence of independent factors on the means, or to determine whether factors associated with any of the variables contribute to the variation.

volumetric a. Quantitative analysis by volume.

Western blot a. A method of identifying proteins or peptides that have been electrophoretically separated and transferred (blotted) onto nitrocellulose or nylon membrane. The blots are then detected by radiolabeled antibody probes. Also called immunoblotting.

analyst (an´ă-list) **1.** One who performs an analysis. **2.** See psychoanalyst.

analyzer (an´ă-li-zer) **1.** A polarizing filter used to determine the direction of polarization of a beam of light. **2.** One of two filters in an instrument used for the study of a polarized beam of light (polariscope).

breath a. A simple device for detecting whether or not a person is intoxicated; the subject blows into a balloon and if the proportion of alcohol in the breath is sufficiently high, a chemical reactant in the device changes color.

wave a. An apparatus by means of which complex wave forms are separated into their component frequencies.

anamnesis (an-am-ne´sis) **1.** The act of recalling to memory. **2.** The history of a patient's illness.

anaphase (an´ă-fāz) The third stage of cell division by mitosis, during which the two chromatids of each chromosome separate and migrate along the spindle fibers toward opposite poles.

anaphoresis (an-ă-fŏ-re´sis) **1.** The motion of electrically charged particles in solution toward a positive pole or anode. **2.** Reduction of sweat secretion.

anaphylactic (an-ă-fĭ-lak´tik) Characterized by a markedly abnormal or extreme sensitivity to a biologically foreign protein.

anaphylactogenic (an-ă-fĭ-lak-to-jen´ik) **1.** Producing an exaggerated or severe reaction to the presence of a protein that is foreign to the body. **2.** Anything that reduces immunity.

anaphylactoid (an-ă-fĭ-lak´toid) Resembling anaphylaxis.

anaphylatoxin (an-ă-fĭ-lă-tok´sin) A small peptide split from the third (C3) or fifth (C5) component of complement; it causes smooth muscle contraction and increased permeability of blood vessels.

anaphylaxis (an-ă-fĭ-lak´sis) An immediate severe hypersensitivity (allergic) reaction to an antigen (allergen) to which the person was previously exposed.

exercise-induced a. A shock-like syndrome associated with vigorous exercise; the first symptoms are usually itching and swelling, especially of the neck.

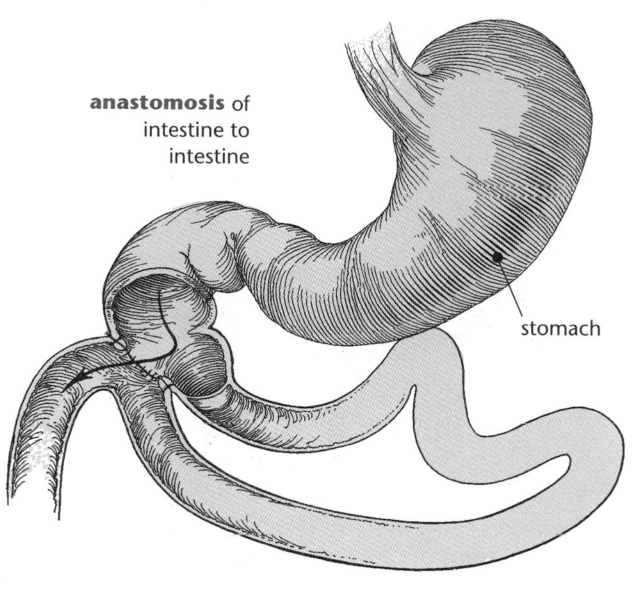

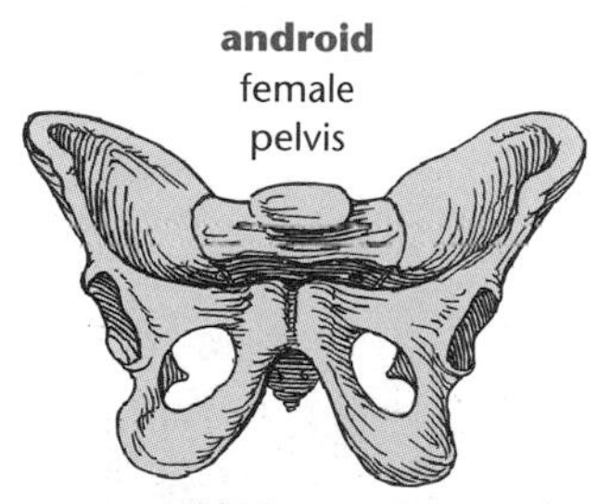

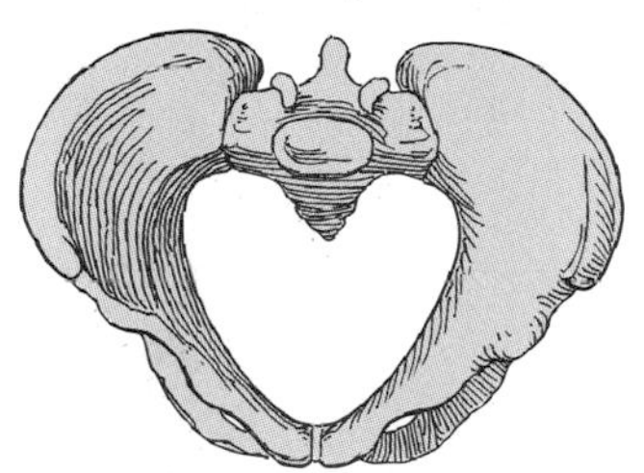
responsible for most cases of severe difficulty in childbirth

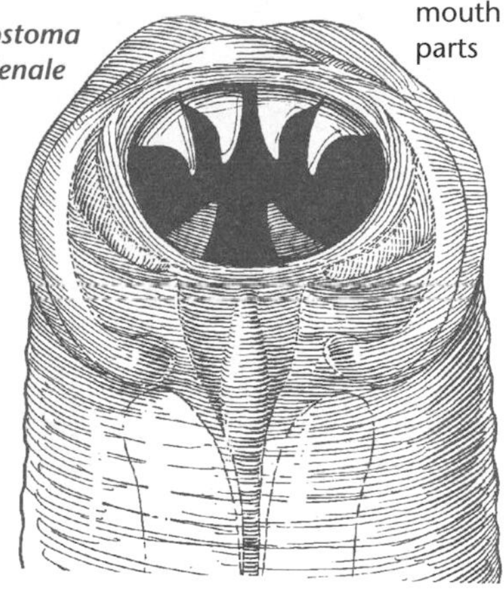

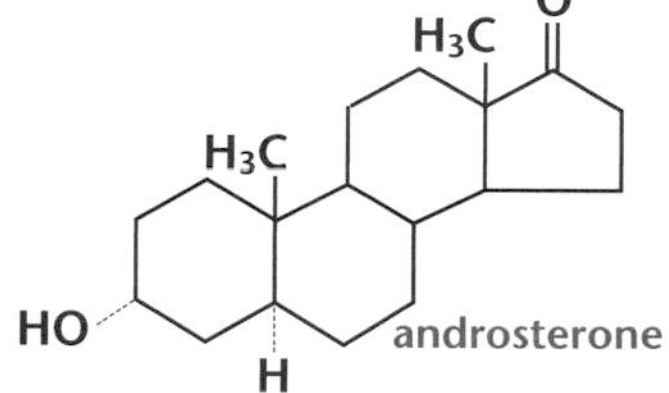

local a. An immediate hypersensitivity reaction occurring in a specific target organ (e.g., skin, nasal mucous membrane).

anaplasia (an-ă-pla´zhă) **1.** The loss of normal differentiation of cells, as in tumor cells. **2.** A reversion of cells to an embryonic state in which reproductive activity is very pronounced.

anaplastic (an-ă-plas´tik) **1.** Relating to anaplasia.

anarthria (an-ar´thre-ă) Loss of ability to articulate properly.

anasarca (an-ă-sar´kă) Generalized massive edema in subcutaneous tissue; may be due to cardiac, renal, or hepatic disease, and to starvation.

anastomose (ă-nas´tŏ-mōs) **1.** To open one into the other; said of blood vessels. **2.** To create by surgery a channel between tubular structures, such as intestines or blood vessels.

anastomosis (ă-nas-tŏ-mo´sis), *pl.* **anastomo´ses** **1.** A connection between tubular structures. **2.** The surgical or pathologic formation of a channel between tubular structures, such as blood vessels or intestines.

intestinal a. See enteroenterostomy.

microvascular a. Anastomosis of minute blood vessels performed under a surgical microscope.

portacaval a. See portal-systemic anastomosis.

portal-systemic a. Anastomoses between the portal and systemic circulations, occurring naturally or created surgically. Also called portacaval anastomosis.

Roux-en-Y a. Operation in which a divided segment of small intestine is used to bypass an obstruction of the upper digestive tract; the distal end of the intestinal segment is connected to a structure above the lesion (e.g., to the stomach or esophagus) and the proximal end is sutured to the small intestine at a suitable distance below the obstruction; the resulting Y-shaped anastomosis provides passage of digestive contents without backward flow.

anastomotic (ă-nas-tŏ-mot´ik) Relating to an anastomosis.

anatomic, anatomical (an-ă-tom´ik, an-ă-tom´ĭ-kal) **1.** Relating to anatomy. **2.** Relating to structure as opposed to function.

anatomist (ă-nat´ŏ-mist) A specialist in anatomy.

anatomy (ă-nat´ŏ-me) The science of the body structure of an organism and its parts.

comparative a. The study of the bodies of different animals in relation to one another.

dental a. The branch of anatomy concerned with the external and internal structure of teeth and the surrounding tissues.

developmental a. See embryology.

gross a. Study of structures as seen without the aid of a microscope.

microscopic a. See histology.

pathologic a. See anatomic pathology, under pathology.

surface a. Study of the outer configuration of the body in relation to underlying and deep structures.

topographic a. The study of the location of the various organs and parts of the body and their relations to one another and to the surface of the body.

anchorage (ang´kor-ij) **1.** The surgical fixation of a prolapsed organ. **2.** In dentistry, a tooth or part of a tooth to which a bridge, crown, filling, etc. is attached; in orthodontics, the teeth used as support for an appliance.

ancillary (an´sil-lār-e) Subordinate; auxiliary.

anconitis (ang-ko-ni´tis) Inflammation of the elbow joint.

ancrod (an´krod) A fibrinogen-splitting substance obtained from the venom of the pit viper, *Agkistrodon rhodostoma*; used as an anticoagulant of blood.

Ancylostoma (an-kĭ-los´tŏ-mă, an-sĭ-los´tŏ-mă) A genus of nematode parasites that attach themselves to the mucosa of the duodenum where they suck the blood of the host, causing anemia; they enter the body of man in the larval stage, usually through the skin of the feet and ankles.

A. duodenale A variety of hookworm characterized by the presence of two pairs of teeth; species predominate in southern Europe, coastal North Africa, northern India, and Japan. Also called Old World hookworm; *Uncinaria duodenalis*.

ancylostomiasis (an-kĭ-los-to-mi´ă-sis) Hookworm disease; infestation with the parasite *Ancylostoma duodenale* or *Necator americanus*, causing anemia by the destruction of red blood cells; in children the infection may result in mental and physical retardation. Also called mountain anemia; uncinariasis.

cutaneous a. The appearance of small itchy vesicles at the site of entrance of the *Ancylostoma* larvae, usually on the feet, prior to the manifestation of intestinal symptoms. Also called ancylostomiasis dermatitis; ground itch.

androblastoma (an-dro-blas-to´mă) See Sertoli-Leydig tumor, under tumor.

androgen (an´dro-jen) A hormone that stimulates the development of male sex characteristics.

androgenic (an-dro-jen´ik) Relating to an androgen or producing male characteristics.

androgynous (an-droj´ĭ-nus) Relating to female pseudohermaphroditism (a true female with masculine characteristics).

android (an´droid) Manlike.

andropathy (an-drop´ă-the) Any disease peculiar to the male sex.

androsterone (an-dros´ter-ōn) An androgen (male sex hormone) derived from testosterone metabolism.

anechoic (an-ĕ-ko´ik) Denoting absence of echoes in an area studied with ultrasonography.

anectasis (an-ek´tă-sis) See primary atelectasis, under atelectasis.

anemia (ă-ne´me-ă) Any condition in which the concentration of hemoglobin in the blood is below the normal for the age and sex of the patient; usually there is also a reduction in the number of red blood cells per mm^3 and in the volume of packed red blood cells per 100 ml of blood. Anemia decreases the oxygen-carrying capacity of the blood.

Addison's a., addisonian a. See pernicious anemia.

aplastic a. Anemia due to failure of bone marrow to produce the normal number of red blood cells for discharge into the bloodstream; usually associated with a reduction of all cellular components of the blood.

congenital hypoplastic a. Anemia occurring in infants, resulting from underdevelopment of bone marrow; may be associated with minor congenital abnormalities. Also called erythrogenesis imperfecta.

congenital spherocytic a. See spherocytosis.

Cooley's a. See beta thalassemia, under thalassemia.

crescent cell a. See sickle cell anemia.

folic acid deficiency a. Anemia occurring in pregnant women secondary to folic acid deficiency; marked by the presence of large embryonic red blood cells in bone marrow; it disappears after delivery but may recur in subsequent pregnancies.

hemolytic a. Anemia resulting from abnormal destruction of red blood cells in the body.

hypochromic a. Anemia marked by a reduction of hemoglobin content of red blood cells, i.e., reduced mean corpuscular hemoglobin concentration (MCHC).

hypochromic microcytic a. Anemia marked by a decrease of hemoglobin content of red blood cells, as in iron deficiency anemia.

hypoplastic a. Anemia resulting from inadequately functioning bone marrow.

iron deficiency a. Anemia developed when insufficient iron is available to the bone marrow where red blood cells are formed; characterized by low concentration of hemoglobin and smaller than normal red blood cells. May be caused by dietary deficiency; increased demand for iron (in growing children, pregnant and lactating women); malabsorption due to other conditions; or chronic blood loss (hookworm disease, peptic ulcers, colon cancer, long-term aspirin ingestion).

macrocytic a. Any anemia in which the average size of circulating blood cells is greater than normal,

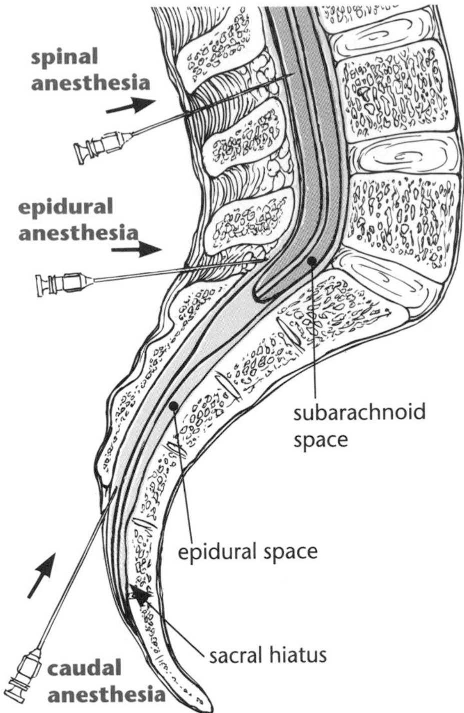

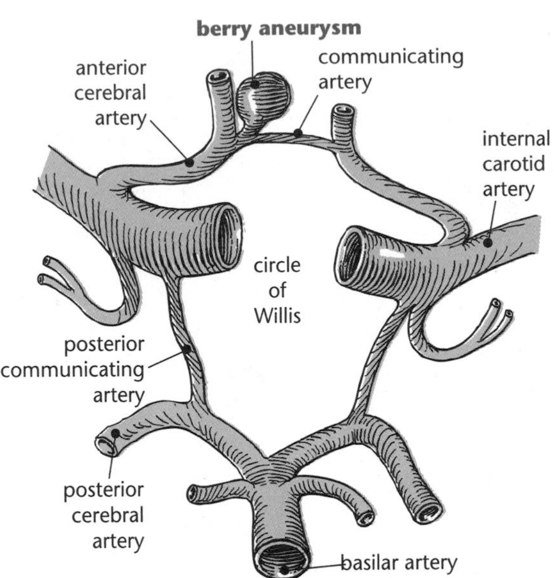

angina pectoris

Typical distribution of pain due to atherosclerotic narrowing of the coronary arteries or transient arterial spasm.

i.e., the mean corpuscular volume (MCV) is increased. See also megaloblastic anemia.

Marchiafava-Micheli a. See paroxysmal nocturnal hemoglobinuria, under hemoglobinuria.

megaloblastic a. Any anemia usually caused by deficiency of vitamin B_{12} or folic acid; characterized by macrocytic erythrocytes and an increased number of megaloblasts in the bone marrow; includes pernicious anemia and folic acid deficiency anemia.

myelophthisic a., myelopathic a. See leukoerythroblastosis.

normochromic a. Anemia in which hemoglobin concentration in red blood cells is within the normal range, i.e., the mean corpuscular hemoglobin concentration (MCHC) is from 32 to 36%.

nutritional a. Anemia resulting from lack of some essential materials in the diet, such as iron or vitamins.

pernicious a. (PA) Anemia due to vitamin B_{12} deficiency; usually caused by absence of stomach acid and intrinsic factor, which are essential for absorption of vitamin B_{12}; may also result from surgical removal of the terminal ileum where absorption takes place; occurs mostly after the age of 50 years and is frequently associated with neurologic damage. Also called addisonian anemia; Addison's anemia.

sickle cell a. Hereditary chronic anemia in which a large number of red blood cells are crescent-shaped and contain an abnormal hemoglobin (hemoglobin S). Also called crescent cell anemia; sickle cell disease.

sideroblastic a., sideroachrestic a. Anemia in which the young erythrocytes in bone marrow contain iron (sideroblasts) and the iron content of reticuloendothelial tissues is increased.

anemic (ă-ne´mik) Pertaining to anemia.

anencephaly (an-en-sef´ă-le) Congenital developmental defect consisting of absence of the vault of the skull, with an exposed, poorly developed, degenerated brain, resulting from the failure of the neural tube to close in the cephalic area; the affected infant usually dies within a few days after birth.

anephric (a-nef´rik) Without kidneys.

anergic (an-er´jik) **1.** Relating to a diminished or absent response to specific antigens. **2.** Marked by abnormal lack of energy.

anergy (an´er-je) **1.** A form of immunologic tolerance in which lymphocytes become functionally unresponsive. **2.** Inability to react; sluggishness.

aneroid (an´er-oid) Not using or containing fluid.

anesthesia (an-es-the´zhă) Partial or total loss of sensation, with or without loss of consciousness, due to injury or disease, or induced by the administration of a drug.

caudal a. Anesthesia produced by the injection of an anesthetic solution into the caudal part of the spinal canal.

continuous spinal a. Continuous intermittent injection of local anesthetic via a catheter into the spinal subarachnoid space.

crossed a. Anesthesia on one side of the body caused by a lesion on the opposite side of the brain.

epidural a. Anesthesia produced by the injection of an anesthetic agent into the extradural space.

field block a. Anesthesia produced by injecting the anesthetic solution in such a way as to create a wall around the operative field.

general a. A state of unconsciousness and complete loss of sensation produced by the administration of an anesthetic, either by inhalation, intravenously, or (rarely) intramuscularly. Also called surgical anesthesia.

local a. Anesthesia of a limited area of the body.

nerve block a. Anesthesia produced by injecting the anesthetic solution around and near peripheral nerves.

paracervical block a. Injection of an anesthetic solution at the 4- and 8-o'clock positions of the cervicovaginal junction to block nerve impulse transmission along the sensory fibers of the hypogastric plexus. Also called paracervical block.

rectal a. General anesthesia produced by introducing the anesthetic solution into the rectum.

regional a. Any of four types of anesthesia: spinal, epidural, caudal, or nerve block.

saddle block a. Anesthesia of the area of the buttocks, perineum, and inner thighs produced by injection of the anesthetic agent low in the dural sac.

spinal a. (a) Anesthesia of the lower part of the body produced by injecting an anesthetic agent in the subarachnoid space around a specified portion of the spinal cord. Also called subarachnoid block anesthesia. (b) Anesthesia due to injury or disease of the spinal cord.

subarachnoid block a. See spinal anesthesia (a).

surgical a. See general anesthesia.

anesthesiologist (an-es-the-ze-ol´o-jist) A physician who specializes in anesthesiology.

anesthesiology (an-es-the-ze-ol´o-je) The branch of science concerned with the study and administration of anesthesia.

anesthetic (an-es-thet´ik) A drug that produces anesthesia.

anesthetist (ă-nes´thĕ-tist) A person (physician, nurse, or technician) who administers anesthesia.

anesthetize (ă-nes thĕ-tīz) To render insensible with an anesthetic.

aneuploid (an´u-ploid) An organism having an abnormal number of chromosomes.

aneuploidy (an-u-ploi´de) The state of having an abnormal number of chromosomes.

aneurysm (an´u-riz-m) An abnormal sac-like bulging of the wall of an artery or of a heart chamber.

berry a. A small berry-like sacculation of a cerebral artery, usually at the circle of Willis at the base of the brain.

cardiac a. Dilatation of the ventricular wall of the heart. Also called mural aneurysm; ventricular aneurysm.

dissecting a. Aneurysm in which blood forces its way between the layers of an arterial wall, causing them to separate; the blood may enter through an intimal tear or by interstitial hemorrhage; occurs especially in the aorta.

false a. A blood clot within the wall of an artery.

fusiform a. A spindle-shaped dilatation of an artery.

mural a. See cardiac aneurysm.

mycotic a. Aneurysm caused by growth of microorganisms within the vessel wall.

traumatic a. Aneurysm formed as a consequence of physical injury of the vessel wall.

ventricular a. See cardiac aneurysm.

aneurysmal (an-u-riz´mal) Relating to an aneurysm.

aneurysmectomy (an-u-riz-mek´to-me) Excision of an aneurysm.

angiectasia, angiectasis (an-je-ek-tā́ze-ă, an-je-ek-tă´sis) Dilatation of a blood vessel or a lymph vessel.

angiitis, angitis (an-jē-ī´tis, an-jī´tis) Inflammation of a blood or lymph vessel.

hypersensitivity a. Inflammation of a blood vessel as a manifestation of an allergic reaction to a specific substance.

angina (an-jī´nă, an´jĭ-nă) A severe strangling pain.

abdominal a. Pain in the abdomen after eating a meal; results from reduced circulation to the intestines. Also called intestinal angina.

agranulocytic a. See agranulocytosis.

crescendo a. See unstable angina.

intestinal a. See abdominal angina.

Ludwig's a. Painful inflammation and pus formation in the area of the submaxillary gland, usually resulting from a tooth infection.

a. pectoris Constricting pain in the chest due to insufficient blood supply to the heart muscle, usually precipitated by effort and relieved rapidly by rest or nitrites; the pain is usually retrosternal and frequently radiates to the precordium, the left shoulder and arm, or the neck.

Prinzmetal's a. See variant angina.

unstable a. Severe chest pain that increases in frequency or duration, starts at rest or during sleep, or

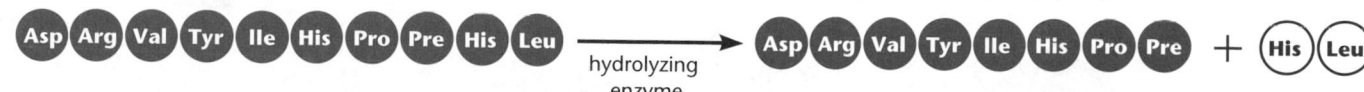

angiotensin I (decapeptide)

Asp Arg Val Tyr Ile His Pro Pre His Leu → hydrolyzing enzyme → Asp Arg Val Tyr Ile His Pro Pre + His Leu

angiotensin II (octapeptide)

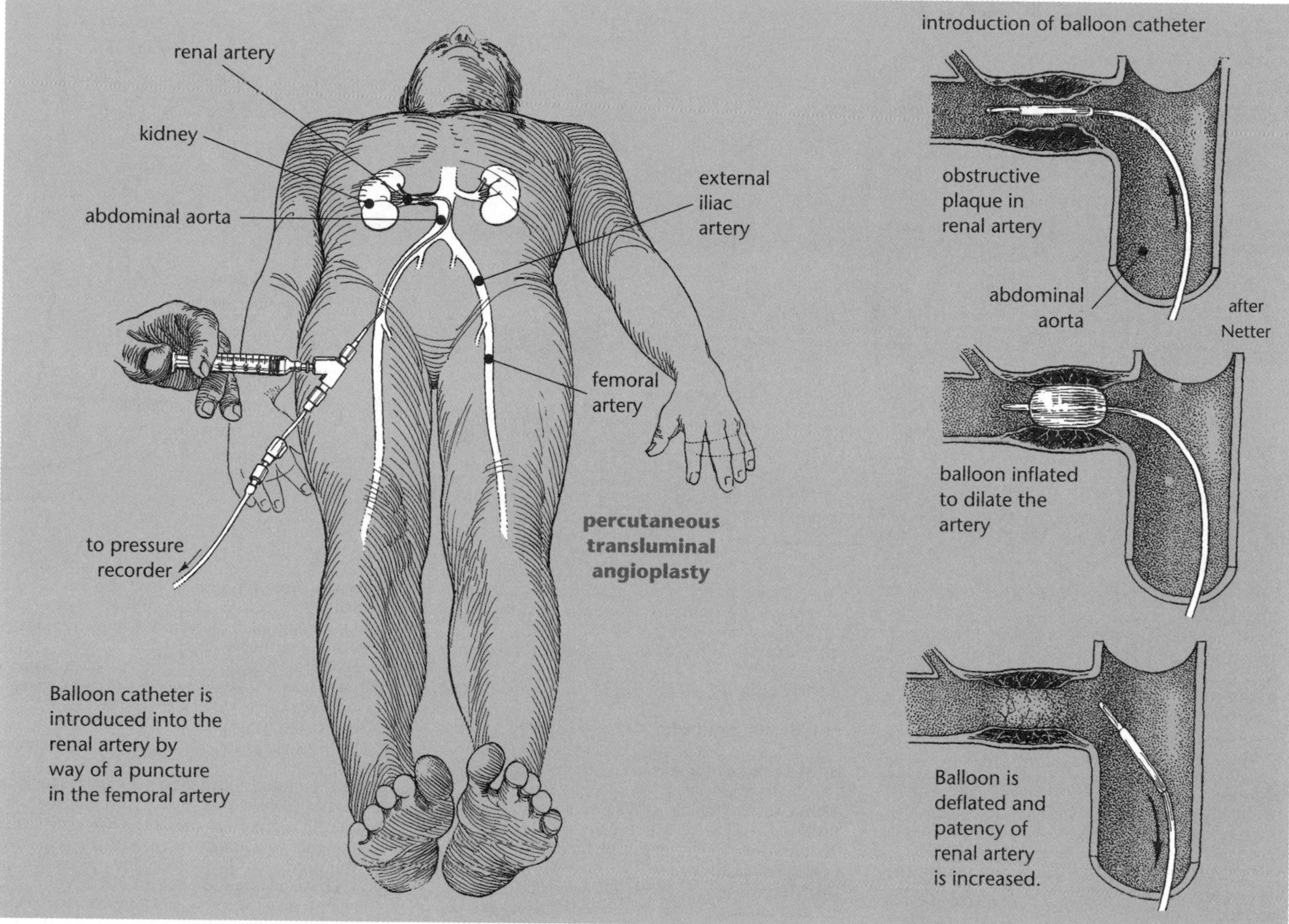

recurs after myocardial infarction or bypass surgery. Also called crescendo angina.

variant a. A type of angina pectoris characterized by pain occurring at rest, believed to be caused by spasms of the coronary arteries. Also called Prinzmetal's angina.

Vincent's a. See fusospirochetal pharyngitis, under pharyngitis.

anginal (an-jĭ'nal, an'jĭ-nal) Relating to angina.

angioblast (an'je-o-blast) **1.** Embryonic tissue from which blood cells and blood vessels are formed. **2.** A vessel-forming cell.

angioblastoma (an-je-o-blas-to'mă) See hemangioblastoma.

angiocardiography (an-je-o-kar-de-og'ră-fe) X-ray examination of the heart and great vessels following the intravenous injection of radiopaque material.

angiocardiopathy (an-je-o-kar-de-op'ă-the) Any disease of the heart and blood vessels.

angioedema (an-je-o-ĕ-de'mă) Allergic reaction manifested by well-demarcated localized swellings of the skin and subcutaneous tissues.

angiogenesis (an-je-o-jen'ĕ-sis) The formation of blood vessels.

angiogram (an'je-o-gram) Radiograph obtained in angiography.

angiography (an-je-og'ră-fe) X-ray visualization of blood vessels after injection of a radiopaque material.

coronary a. Angiography of the arteries supplying the heart muscle.

fluorescein a. Photographic visualization of the passage of fluorescein through blood vessels within the eye after an intravenous fluorescein injection.

magnetic resonance a., MR a. Visualization of blood vessels by means of magnetic resonance (MR) sequences that enhance the signal from circulating blood while suppressing signals from other tissues.

selective a. The injection of radiopaque solution through a catheter into the vessels of the specific area of the body to be studied.

angiohypertonia (an-je-o-hi-per-to'ne-ă) See vasospasm.

angioid (an'je-oid) Resembling blood vessels. See also angioid streaks, under streak.

angiokeratoma (an-je-o-ker-ă-to'mă) A skin disorder consisting of a varying number of multiple violet or purple lesions. Also called telangiectatic wart.

angiokeratosis (an-je-o-ker-ă-to'sis) The occurrence of angiokeratoma.

angiokinesis (an-je-o-kĭ-ne'sis) See vasomotion.

angiology (an-je-ol'ŏ-je) The study of blood and lymph vessels.

angioma (an-je-o'mă) A tumor composed of dilated blood vessels (hemangioma) or lymph vessels (lymphangioma).

cavernous a. See cavernous hemangioma, under hemangioma.

cherry a. See senile hemangioma, under hemangioma.

spider a. See spider telangiectasia, under telangiectasia.

angiomatosis (an-je-o-mă-to'sis) Condition marked by the presence of multiple angiomas.

bacillary a. Opportunistic infection usually occurring in patients with immune deficiency syndrome (AIDS); caused by the rickettsial bacterium *Rochalimaea henselae;* symptoms and signs range from fever and skin nodules to hemorrhagic cysts in the liver.

cerebelloretinal a. See von Hippel-Lindau disease.

angiomatous (an-je-om'ă-tus) Resembling a tumor made up of dilated vessels (angioma).

angiopathy (an-je-op'ă-the) Disease of blood vessels or lymphatics.

angioplasty (an'je-o-plas-te) Surgical reconstruction of a blood vessel.

percutaneous transluminal a. (PTA) Enlargement of the lumen of a narrowed artery (coronary or renal) with a balloon-tip catheter; the catheter is introduced through the skin into the vessel to the narrowed segment where the balloon is inflated, thus dilating the lumen.

angiopoietic (an-je-o-poi-et'ik) Relating to the formation of blood vessels.

angiospasm (an'je-o-spaz-m) See vasospasm.

angiostatin (an-je-o-stă'tin) An internal fragment of plasminogen that is a specific inhibitor of proliferating endothelial cells.

angiostenosis (an-je-o-stĕ-no'sis) Constriction or narrowing of one or more blood vessels.

angiotensin (an-je-o-ten'sin) Peptide formed by the action of the enzyme renin on a globulin in blood plasma; renin splits off from its substrate a decapeptide, angiotensin I (AI), which is changed by a converting enzyme to the octapeptide angiotensin II (AII), a potent vasoconstrictor and stimulator of the synthesis and release of the hormone aldosterone; a heptapeptide, angiotensin III (AIII), has also been found that is a stimulator of aldosterone synthesis and release but has little or no vaso-constrictor activity.

angiotensinogen (an-je-o-ten-sin'o-jen) An alpha$_2$-globulin, also known as renin substrate; it has no pressor activity in the intact form but is acted upon by the enzyme renin, which splits off a decapeptide unit (angiotensin I). Also called renin substrate.

angiotome (an'je-o-tōm) A segment of the vascular system of the embryo.

angiotrophic (an-je-o-trof'ik) Relating to nutrition

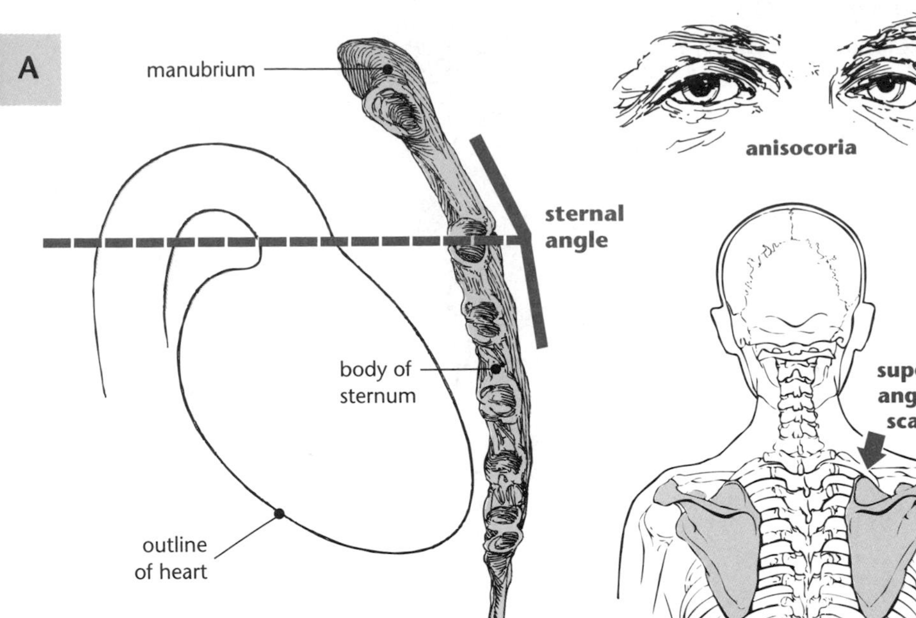

of blood and lymphatic vessels. Also called vasotrophic.

angle (ang´gl) The figure formed by two lines or planes diverging from a common point; the space between two lines or planes diverging from a common point.

acromial a. The palpable point where the lateral border of the acromion joins, and becomes continuous with, the spine of the scapula.

anterior chamber a. The angle formed at the junction of the iris and cornea. Also called iridocorneal angle; filtration angle; angle of the iris.

carrying a. The angle made by the axes of the arm and forearm when the forearm is extended.

cavosurface a. The angle formed by the junction of the wall of a prepared cavity and the surface of a tooth.

cerebellopontine a. The space at the junction of the cerebellum and pons. Also called pontine angle.

a. of convergence The angle between the line of vision and the median line.

costophrenic a. The angle formed between the ribs and the lateral-most portion of the diaphragm; seen in radiographs of the chest.

critical a. The angle of incidence (angle made with the perpendicular by a light ray passing from one medium to another) which results in a refracted ray; if the angle of incidence is greater than 90°, the ray is reflected.

filtration a. See anterior chamber angle.

inferior a. of scapula The angle formed by the junction of the lateral and medial borders of the scapula (shoulder blade).

iridocorneal a. See anterior chamber angle.

a. of iris See anterior chamber angle.

a. of jaw The angle formed by the lower edge of the body of the mandible and the posterior edge of the ramus.

line a. The angle formed by the junction of any two surfaces of a tooth

a. of Louis See sternal angle.

medial a. See superior angle of scapula.

point a. The meeting of three tooth surfaces at a point, forming a corner.

pontine a. See cerebellopontine angle.

sternal a. The angle or ridge on the anterior surface of the sternum (breastbone) at the junction of its body and manubrium. Also called angle of Louis.

superior a. of scapula The angle formed by the junction of the superior and medial borders of the scapula (shoulder blade). Formerly called medial angle.

angstrom, Angström (ang´strem) (Å, A) A unit of length equal to a ten-thousandth of a micron; 10^{-7} mm; used especially to measure the length of light waves or other electromagnetic radiation and cytologic ultrastructures.

anhedonia (an-he-do´ne-ă) Inability to experience pleasure.

anhidrosis (an-hĭ-dro´sis) Marked deficiency of sweat.

anhidrotic, anidrotic (an-hĭ-drot´ik, an-ĭ-drot´ik) Anything that diminishes secretion of sweat.

anhydrase (an-hi´drās) An enzyme that promotes the removal of water from a compound.

anhydrous (an-hi´drus) Without water.

aniline (an´ĭ-lēn, an´ĭ-lin) An oily, colorless or brown compound derived from benzene; used in the preparation of dyes.

anion (an´i-on) A negatively charged ion that is characteristically attracted to the positively charged anode; indicated as a superior minus sign (e.g., Cl^-).

anionic (an-i-on´ik) Relating to a negatively charged ion.

aniridia (an-ĭ-rid´e-ă) Complete or partial absence of the iris.

anisakiasis (an-i-să-ki´ă-sis) Infection of the lining of the stomach and small intestine by larvae of the family Anisakidae, parasites of marine fish. In humans, infection occurs through ingestion of undercooked or raw fish (e.g., sushi) containing third-stage larval nematodes; it can produce severe gastrointestinal inflammation and symptoms like those of ulcer, appendicitis, or tumor.

aniseikonia (an-i-si-ko´ne-ă) A defect of vision in which the image of an object seen by one eye is of a different size than the one seen by the other eye.

anisochromasia (an-i-so-kro-ma´zha) Condition in which only the periphery of the red blood cells is colored while the central portion is almost colorless, as in certain types of anemias caused by iron deficiency.

anisocoria (an-i-so-ko´re-ă) Condition in which the pupils of the two eyes differ in size.

anisocytosis (an-i-so-si-to´sis) Abnormal variation in size of the red blood cells.

anisometropia (an-i-so-mĕ-tro´pe-ă) Difference in the refractive power of the two eyes.

ankle (ang´kl) The joint between the foot and the leg formed by the articulation of the tibia and fibula above with the talus below; the area of this joint.

ankyloblepharon (ang-kĭ-lo-blef´ă-ron) Adhesion of the upper and lower eyelids.

ankyloglossia (ang-kĭ-lo-glos´e-ă) See tongue-tie.

ankylosed (ang´kĭ-lōzd) Denoting an abnormally immobilized joint.

ankylosis (ang-kĭ-lo´sis) Abnormal immobility and fixation of a joint. Also called frozen joint.

artificial a. See arthrodesis.

bony a. See synostosis.

dental a. Fixation of a tooth to its socket as a result of ossification of the surrounding membranes.

false a. See fibrous ankylosis.

fibrous a. Ankylosis caused by the presence of fibrous bands between the bones forming the joint. Also called false ankylosis; pseudoankylosis.

true a. See synostosis.

ankylotic (ang-kĭ-lot´ik) Marked by or relating to ankylosis.

anlage (an´laj), *pl.* **anla´gen** In embryology, the earliest stage of a developing organ or structure, when cells begin to group in a definite pattern; a theoretical stage earlier than primordium.

anneal (ă-nēl´) **1.** The slow cooling procedure that brings about the reassociation of single-stranded segments of DNA from bacterial or viral sources. The single strands result from denaturation or "melting" of DNA in solution when its temperature is raised above the melting temperature. Useful in classification of bacteria and viruses. **2.** To soften a metal by controlled heating and cooling; the process imparts a degree of adaptability to the metal.

annealing (ă-nēl´ĭng) In dentistry, the heating of gold leaf to remove contaminants prior to its insertion into a cavity.

annexin (ă-nek´sin) Any of a family of phospholipid-binding proteins that are Ca^{++} dependent and may act as mediators of calcium activity within cells.

a. II A fibrin-dissolving protein receptor; overproduction leads to hemorrhage.

a. V Annexin with anticoagulant properties; has a role in preventing blood clots in the placenta.

annular (an´u-lar) Circular or ring-shaped.

annulus (an´u-lus) See anulus.

anode (an´ōd) The positive pole of a galvanic battery. Also called positive electrode.

anodontia (an-o-don´she-ă) Congenital absence of one or more teeth.

anodyne (an´o-dīn) An agent that has pain-relieving qualities.

anogenital (ă-no-jen´ĭ-tal) Relating to the anus and genitalia.

anomaly (ă-nom´ă-le) Anything marked by considerable deviation from the normal.

developmental a. Anomaly occurring or originating during intrauterine life.

Ebstein's a. Distortion and downward displacement of the tricuspid valve, resulting in impaired function of the right ventricle.

Pelger-Huët nuclear a. Inherited anomaly of neutrophilic leukocytes characterized by nonlobulation of their nuclei.

anomia (ă-no´me-ă) Inability to name, or to recall

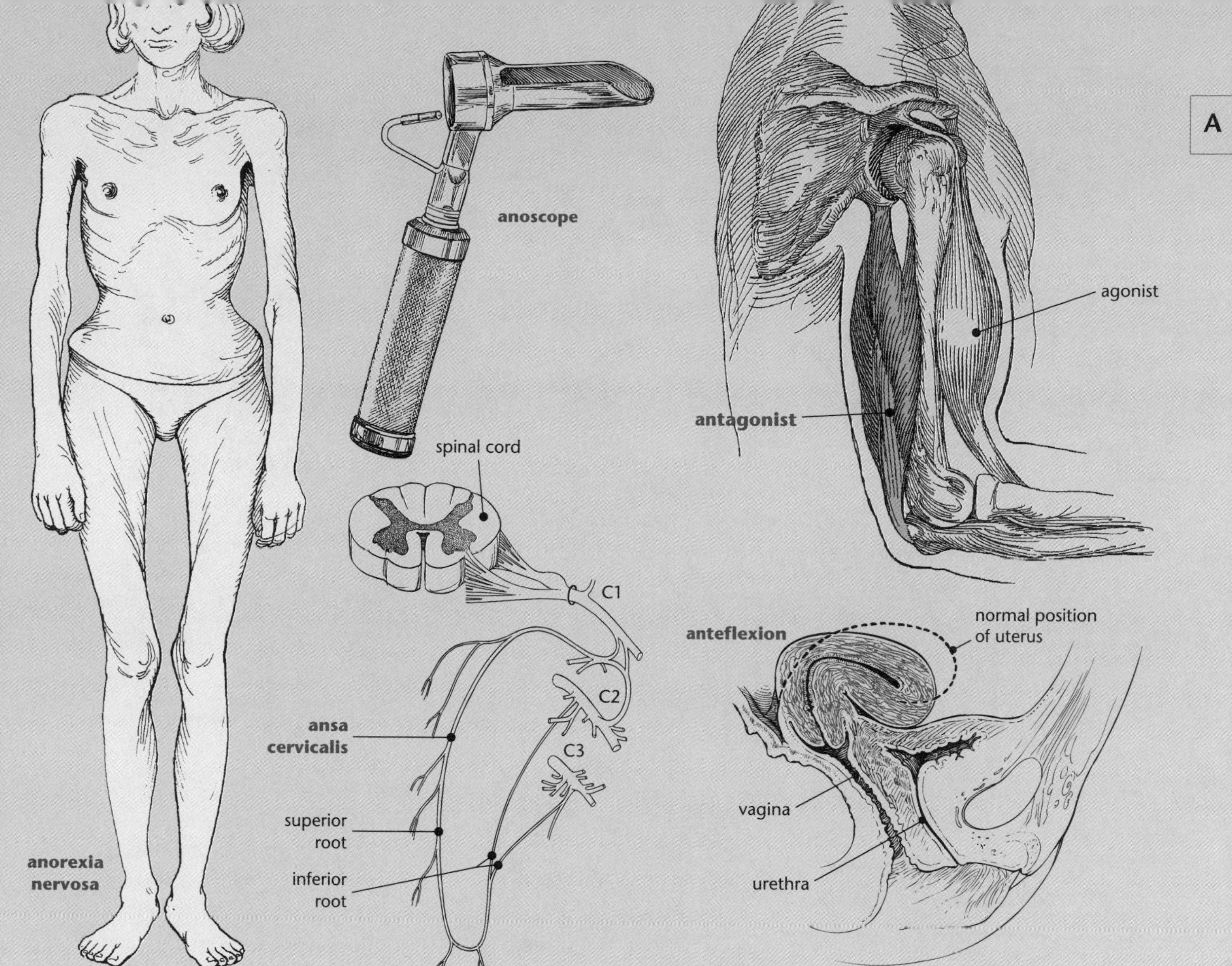

the names of objects. Also called optic aphasia.

Anopheles (ă-nof´ĕ-lēz) A genus of mosquitoes of the family Culicidae, some members of which transmit the malaria parasite to man.

anophthalmia (an-of-thal´me-ă) Congenital absence of a true eyeball.

anopsia (an-op´sĭ-ă) **1.** Failure to use one eye, as in strabismus. **2.** Hypertropia.

anorchism (an-or´kiz-m) Congenital absence of one or both testes.

anorectic, anorexic (an-o-rek´tik, an-o-rek´sĭk) **1.** Having no appetite. **2.** An agent that tends to depress appetite.

anorexia (an-o-rek´se-ă) Loss of appetite.

a. nervosa Condition marked by great loss of appetite leading to emaciation and metabolic derangement, attended by serious neurotic symptoms centered around an inordinate fear of becoming fat; occurs predominantly in young women.

anorexiant (an-o-rek´se-ant) Anything that results in appetite loss (anorexia).

anoscope (a´no-skōp) An instrument for inspecting the anus and lower rectum.

anosigmoidoscopy (a-no-sig-moi-dos´kŏ-pe) Visual examination of the anus, rectum, and sigmoid colon with the aid of a viewing instrument (endoscope).

anosmia (an-oz´me-ă) Absence of the sense of smell.

anosognosia (a-no-sog-no´zhă) Unawareness, real or assumed, of one's own physical illness or disability.

ANOVA Acronym for analysis of variance, see under analysis.

anovular, anovulatory (an-ov´u-lar, an-ov´u-lă-to-re) Denoting a menstrual period not accompanied by ovulation.

anoxemia (an-ok-se´me-ă) Deficiency of oxygen in the arterial blood. Also called hypoxemia.

anoxia (ă-nok´se-ă) Absence, or almost complete absence, of oxygen.

ansa (an´să), *pl.* **an´sae** Any looplike structure.

a. cervicalis A nerve loop in the cervical plexus consisting of fibers from the first three cervical nerves, some of which accompany the hypoglossal nerve for a short distance. Also called ansa hypoglossi.

a. hypoglossi See ansa cervicalis.

ant (ant) An insect of the family Formicidae.

fire a. An aggressive South American ant (genus *Solenopsis*), now commonly seen in the southern United States, whose sting can cause severe allergic reactions, including difficulty in breathing, sweating, nausea, itching, and periods of unconsciousness; it is the only insect in the United States whose sting produces a pustule (a pus-containing eruption).

antacid (ant-as´id) An agent that reduces the acidity of the gastric juice or other secretions (e.g., aluminum hydroxide, magnesium hydroxide, calcium carbonate).

antagonism (an-tag´o-niz-m) Mutual resistance or opposition as between muscles, drugs, bacteria, etc.

antagonist (an-tag´o-nist) **1.** Any structure or substance that opposes or counteracts the action of another structure or substance. **2.** In pharmacology, a chemical that occupies a receptor site on the cell membrane but does not initiate the biologic reaction associated with occupation of the site by an agonist; in effect, an antagonist interferes with the formation of an agonist-receptor complex, the mechanism by which most pharmacologic effects are produced.

competitive a. A drug that interacts reversibly with the same set of receptors as the active drug (agonist) to form a complex, but the complex does not elicit a biologic response and can be displaced from these receptor sites by increasing concentrations of the active drug.

antebrachial (an-te-bra´ke-al) Relating to the forearm.

antecardium (an-te-kar´de-um) See precordium.

antecibum (an-te-si´bum) (a.c.) Latin for before meals.

antecubital (an-te-ku´bĭ-tal) Located in front of the elbow.

anteflexion (an-te-flek´shun) An abnormal forward bending of an organ.

antemortem (an-te-mor´tem) Before death.

antenatal (an-te-na´tal) See prenatal.

antepartum (an-te-par´tum) In obstetrics, before the onset of labor.

anterior (an-te´re-or) **1.** In front. **2.** Toward the belly.

anterior tibial compartment syndrome (an-te´re-or tib´e-al kom-part´ment sin´drōm) Inflammation and necrosis of leg muscles within the anterior fascial compartment resulting from blood vessel insufficiency, secondary to specific vessel disease or injury or to segmental spasm of the anterior tibial artery.

anteroinferior (an-ter-o-in-fēr´e-or) Located in front and below.

anterolateral (an-ter-o-lat´er-al) In front and to one side.

anteromedial (an-ter-o-me´de-al) In front and toward the middle.

anteroposterior (an-ter-o-pos-tēr´e-or) **1.** Relating to both front and back. **2.** Directed from the front to the back.

anterosuperior (an-ter-o-su-pēr´e-or) In front and above.

anteversion (an-te-ver´zhun) The leaning forward

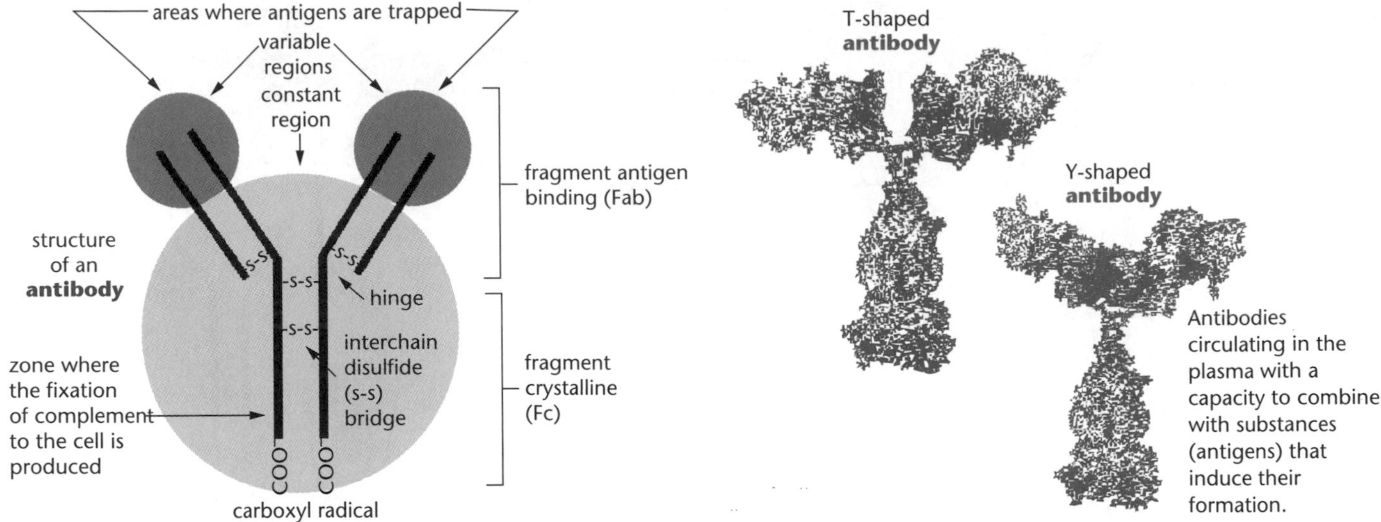

SCHEMATIC REPRESENTATION OF COMPARATIVE STRUCTURES OF 5 CLASSES OF **ANTIBODIES**

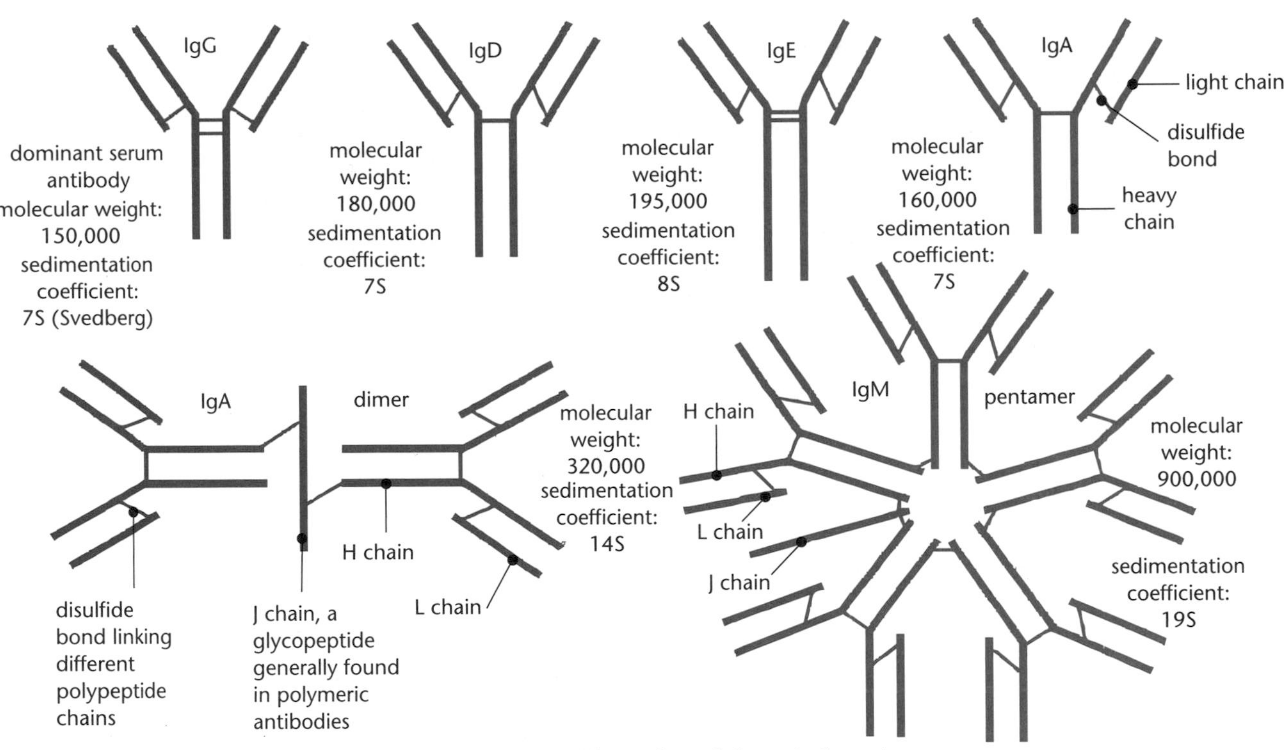

of an organ, such as the uterus, as a whole, without bending.

anteverted (an-te-vert´ed) Tilted forward.

anthelix (ant´he-liks) See antihelix.

anthelmintic, anthelminthic (ant-hel-min´tik, ant-hel-min´thik) Destructive to parasitic worms.

anthracemia (an-thra-sē´me-ă) The presence of *Bacillus anthracis* in the blood.

anthraconecrosis (an-thra-ko-nĕ-kro´sis) Degeneration and transformation of tissue into a dry black mass. Also called black gangrene.

anthracosilicosis (an-thra-ko-sil-ĭ-ko´sis) Fibrous hardening of the lungs due to continuous inhalation of coal dust.

anthracosis (an-thra-ko´sis) Disease caused by accumulation of carbon in the lungs.

anthracotic (an-thra-kot´ik) Marked by anthracosis.

anthrax (an´thraks) Acute contagious disease caused by *Bacillus anthracis*, a bacillus infecting chiefly farm animals. The disease has a strong occupational relationship to industries dealing with animals and their products (farming, leather, and textile industries). It occurs chiefly in countries lacking disease control programs. Also called carbuncular fever.

cutaneous a. Skin anthrax marked by the appearance of a reddish blister that, two or three days later, turns into a large bleeding pustule with a black crust resembling a piece of charcoal. Systemic involvement varies from mild to severe. Also called malignant pustule.

intestinal a. A usually fatal form of anthrax marked by headache, fever, vomiting, bloody diarrhea, prostration and, frequently, hemorrhage from mucous membranes.

pulmonary a. A rare but severe (often fatal) form of anthrax of the lungs marked by chills, fever, rapid breathing, cough, pain in the back and legs, and extreme prostration; caused by inhalation of dust containing spores of the bacillus. Also called woolsorters' disease.

anthrone (an´thrōn) A substance used as a reagent to detect the presence of carbohydrates.

anthropogeny, anthropogenesis (an-thro-poj´ĕ-ne, an-thro-pō-jen´ĕ-sis) The scientific study of man's origin and development, both individual and racial.

anthropology (an-thro-pol´ō-jē) The branch of science concerned with the origin, development, and behavior of humans.

anthropometry (an-thro-pom´ĕ-tre) The study of comparative measurements of the human body for use in anthropologic classification.

anthropozoonosis (an-thro-po-zo-o-no´sis) Human disease caused by microorganisms that are maintained in nature by animals (e.g., trichinosis, rabies).

antiadhesin (an-tĭ-ad-he´zin) An antibody that interacts with components of the bacterial cell surface to prevent adhesion of the bacterium to mucous membranes.

antiandrogen (an-te-an´drŏ-jen) A substance that can diminish the effects of masculinizing (androgenic) hormones.

antiarrhythmic (an-te-ă-rith´mik) Alleviating or preventing irregular heartbeats (arrhythmia).

antibacterial (an-tĭ-bak-te´re-al) Destructive to or preventing the growth of bacteria.

antibiosis (an-tĭ-bi-o´sis) The association of two organisms whereby one is affected detrimentally.

antibiotic (an-tĭ-bi-ot´ik) A substance derived from plants, fungi, or bacteria or produced synthetically, that destroys or inhibits the growth of microorganisms.

broad-spectrum a. An antibiotic which is effective against a variety of microorganisms, particularly against both gram-negative and gram-positive bacteria.

antibody (an´tĭ-bod-e) (Ab) A three-lobed globulin containing two short and two long chains of protein, found in the blood and other body fluids, that can be incited by the presence of antigen (microorganisms, foreign proteins, etc.); it has a destructive influence on the antigen that stimulated its formation, thus

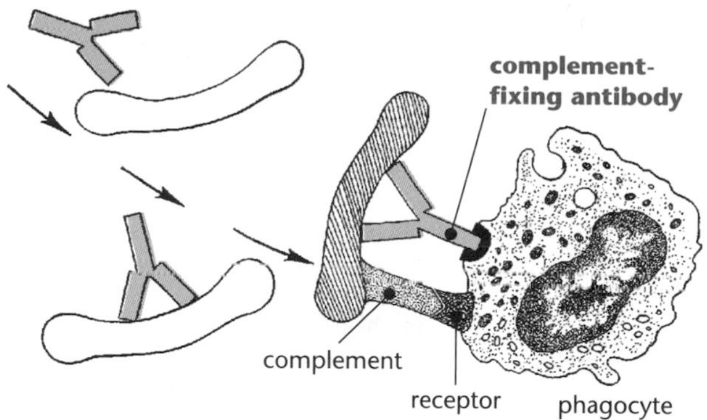

TOXIN	ANTIDOTE
cadmium	calcium disodium edetate (EDTA)
cobalt	calcium disodium edetate (EDTA)
copper	calcium disodium edetate (EDTA)
warfarin	vitamin K
heparin	protamine
lead	calcium disodium edetate (EDTA)
morphine	naloxone
nickel	calcium disodium edetate (EDTA)
nicotene	potassium permanganate
organic phosphate in insecticides	atropine
quinine	potassium permanganate
strychnine	potassium permanganate

A

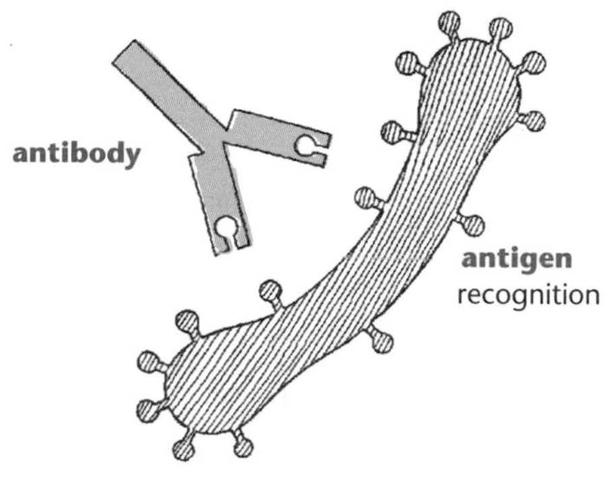

producing immunity; the structure has considerable flexibility and is hinged, so that it can pivot from a taut T-shape to a forked Y-shape.

anticardiolipin a. Antibody that reacts with cardiolipin (a phospholipid present in cell membranes); may be elevated in patients with systemic lupus erythematosus (SLE). Associated with increased incidence of thrombosis, fetal loss, and other abnormalities.

α_1-antichymotripsin A protein that inhibits the action of the digestive enzyme chymotrypsin.

antinuclear a. (ANA) An antibody that acts against components of cell nuclei; found in systemic lupus erythematosus and certain collagen diseases.

antiphospholipid a.'s A group of antibodies (e.g., anticardiolipin antibodies, lupus anticoagulant, VDRL) acting against phosphorylated polysaccharide esters of fatty acids, thought to be markers of a hypercoagulable state of the blood.

antisperm a.'s (ASAs) Antibodies (predominantly IgA type) that immobilize spermatozoa or interfere in any way with spermatozoan activity. They are found in the serum of both males and females and act locally (in the testicles and the vagina); level of their activity fluctuates.

blocking a. Antibody that, by combining with antigen, stops further activity of that antigen.

complement-fixing a., CF a. Antibody that, when combined with antigen, activates complement.

incomplete a. See incomplete agglutinin, under agglutinin.

monoclonal a.'s (MAB, MoAb) Antibodies that are chemically and immunologically homogeneous, artificially produced in the laboratory to react with specific antigens; used as probes in cell biology and biochemistry and, experimentally, to treat certain forms of cancer.

natural a.'s Antibodies occurring naturally in the body without apparent antigenic stimulation from infection or immunization.

neutralizing a. Antibody that, by binding to an infective agent, limits its infectivity.

anticholinergic (an-tĭ-ko-lin-er´jik) Inhibiting the action of a parasympathetic nerve.

anticholinesterase (an-tĭ-ko-lin-es´ter-ās) An agent that inhibits the action of cholinesterase.

α_1-antichymotrypsin (an-tĭ-ki-mo-trip´sin) A protein that inhibits the action of the digestive enzyme chymotrypsin.

anticoagulant (an-tĭ-ko-ag´u-lant) Any substance that prevents coagulation of blood.

anticodon (an-tĭ-ko´don) The three-base sequence of transfer RNA that pairs with a codon in messenger RNA.

anticomplement (an-tĭ-kom´ple-ment) A substance that neutralizes the action of complement (material in normal serum that helps to destroy pathogens).

anticonvulsant (an-tĭ-kon-vul´sant) Any substance that serves to prevent or arrest convulsion.

antidepressant (an-tĭ-de-pres´sant) **1.** Counteracting depression. **2.** An agent that tends to alleviate depression. Also called psychic energizer; thymoleptic.

antidiuretic (an-tĭ-di-u-ret´ik) An agent that causes reduction of urine formation.

antidotal (an-tĭ-do´tal) Relating to an antidote.

antidote (an´tĭ-dōt) An agent that counteracts the effects of an ingested poison, either by inactivating it or by opposing its action following absorption.

antidromic (an-tĭ-drom´ik) Transmitting a nerve impulse in a reverse direction of the normal.

antiemetic (an-te-ĕ-met´ik) **1.** Preventing or arresting nausea. **2.** A drug that prevents or relieves nausea and vomiting by exerting its effects on the vestibular apparatus of the ear, the chemoreceptor trigger zone, the cerebral cortex, or the vomiting center of the brain.

antienzyme (an-te-en´zīm) A substance that neutralizes the action of an enzyme.

antifibrinolysin (an-tĭ-fi-bri-nol´ĭ-sin) A substance that retards the disintegration of fibrin in blood clots.

antigen (an´tĭ-jen) (Ag) Any material capable of triggering in an individual the production of specific antibody or the formation of a specific population of lymphocytes (a type of white blood cell) that react with that material. Antigens may be proteins, toxins, microorganisms, or tissue cells. Whether any material is an antigen in a person depends on whether the material is foreign to the person, the genetic make-up of the person, and the dose of the material. See also CA 15-3; CA 19-9; CA 125.

carcinoembryonic a. (CEA) A glycoprotein component of normal embryonic gastrointestinal tissues; usually found in the adult only in certain carcinomas, especially colonic carcinoma.

CD4 a. A glycoprotein on the membrane of helper T lymphocytes.

CD8 a. A glycoprotein on the membrane of suppressor T lymphocytes.

endogenous a. Any antigen found within an individual.

exogenous a. Any antigen originating from the individual's environment (e.g., pollen).

hepatitis-associated a. (HAA) See hepatitis B surface antigen.

hepatitis B core a. (HBcAg) Antigen of the DNA core of the hepatitis B virus (Dane particle), present in hepatocyte nuclei of patients with hepatitis B.

hepatitis B surface a. (HBsAg) Antigen of the outer lipoprotein coat of the hepatitis B virus (Dane particle), found in the serum and the hepatocyte protoplasm of patients with hepatitis B; persistence of HBsAg in the blood indicates an infectious carrier state.

heterogenetic a. See heterologous antigen.

heterologous a. An antigen that reacts with an antibody whose formation was induced by another antigen. Also called heterogenetic antigen.

histocompatibility a.'s Any of the genetically determined antigens that induce an immune response (rejection) when transplanted from the donor into a genetically different recipient; they are present on nucleated cells of most tissues. Also called transplantation antigens.

HL-A a.'s Original name for human lymphocyte histocompatibility antigens; A stands for locus A (a specific area on a chromosome); currently, HLA is the system designation and locus A is HLA-A. See human lymphocyte antigens.

homologous a. See alloantigen.

human lymphocyte a.'s (HLA) Designation for cell surface proteins that are the gene products of four linked loci (sites) on the sixth human chromosome. These loci are known as A, B, C and D; more than 50 alleles (variations of the gene) are located at loci HLA-A and HLA-B. Human lymphocyte antigens are responsible for rejection of tissue transplants and for certain diseases.

Kveim a. A spleen extract prepared from a sarcoidosis patient, used as a skin test for diagnosis of sarcoidosis.

oncofetal a.'s Antigens present normally in the fetus (e.g., alpha-fetoprotein, carcinoembryonic antigens); associated with tumors in the adult, serving as tumor markers for various cancers.

prostate-specific a. (PSA) A glycoprotein secreted by the cytoplasm of epithelial prostate cells; its normal function is to aid in the liquefaction of semen; normal values in young adults range between 0 and 4 nanograms per milliliter; it occurs in higher levels in the serum of men with benign prostatic hypertrophy. Determinations of serum PSA levels may be of value in the diagnosis and staging of prostatic cancer.

T a. Antigen present in nuclei of cells infected by certain tumor viruses; thought to be an early virus-specific protein.

transplantation a.'s See histocompatibility antigens.

tumor-associated a. (TAA) Antigen found on cells undergoing neoplastic transformation.

tumor-specific a. (TSA) Any antigen that can be detected only on the surface of tumor cells and not on

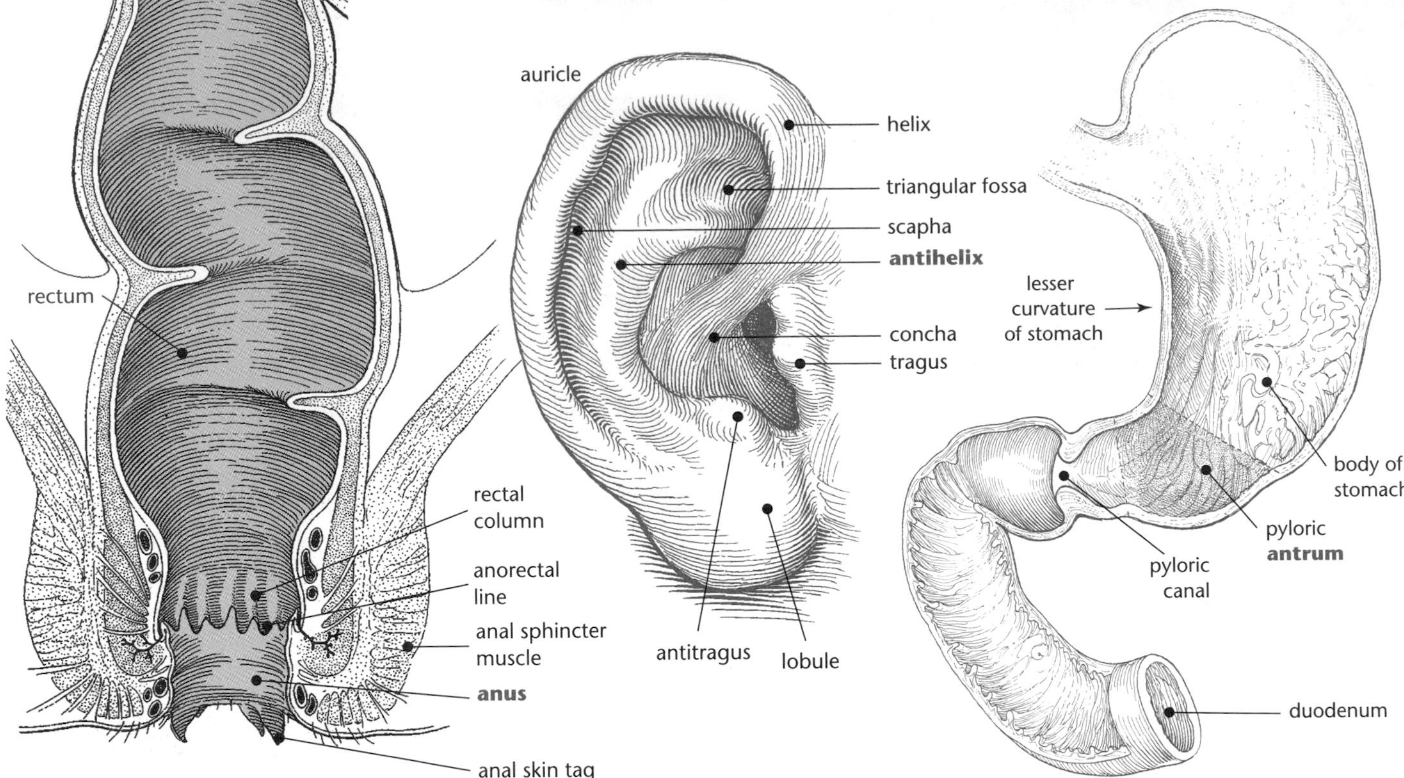

the normal host cells.

antigenic (an-tĭ-jen´ik) Having the properties of an antigen; capable of inciting the formation of antibody. Also called immunogenic.

antigenicity (an-tĭ-je-nis´ĭ-te) The state of being antigenic. Also called immunogenicity.

antihelix (an-te-he´liks) The curved prominence on the external ear parallel to and in front of the helix. Also called anthelix.

antihelminthic (an-tĭ-hel-minth´ik) See anthelmintic.

antihemagglutinin (an-tĭ-he-mă-gloo´tĭ-nin) A substance that checks the action of hemagglutinin.

antihemolysin (an-tĭ-he-mol´ĭ-sin) An agent that inhibits the action of a hemolysin, thus reducing destruction of red blood cells.

antihidrotic (an-tĭ-hi-drot´ik) See antiperspirant.

antihistamine (an-tĭ-his´tă-mēn) Any of several drugs used to counteract the action of histamine in the treatment of allergic symptoms.

antihistaminic (an-tĭ-his-tă-min´ik) Tending to neutralize the action of histamine; said of an agent having such an effect and used to relieve the symptoms of allergy.

antihypertensive (an-tĭ-hi-per-ten´siv) Anything that reduces the blood pressure.

anti-idiotype (an-te-id´e-o-tīp) An antibody that detects, and is directed to, an antigenic determinant (idiotope) in the variable region of an antibody molecule of the same animal species.

anti-inflammatory (an-te-in-flam´ă-to-re) Relieving inflammation.

antimalarial (an-tĭ-mă-lar´e-ăl) Denoting an agent that prevents or cures malaria.

antimetabolite (an-tĭ-mĕ-tab´o-līt) Any substance that interferes with the body's utilization of another substance that is essential for normal physiologic functioning.

antimitotic (an-tĭ-mi-tot´ik) Anything that arrests mitosis.

antimonic (an-tĭ-mon´ik) Relating to antimony.

antimony (an´tĭ-mo-ne) A toxic, irritating, grayish, metallic element; symbol Sb, atomic number 51, atomic weight 121.77.

antimuscarinic (an-tĭ-mus-kă-rin´ik) Counteracting the neurologic effects of muscarine and similar alkaloids.

antimycotic (an-tĭ-mi-kot´ik) See fungicide.

antinatriferic (an-tĭ-nă-trif´er-ik) Inhibiting the transport of sodium.

antinauseant (an-tĭ-naw´ze-ant) **1.** Preventing nausea. **2.** An agent having such properties.

antineoplastic (an-ti-ne-o-plas´tik) Interfering with the growth of a tumor.

antinuclear (an-tĭ-noo´kle-ar) Destructive to a cell nucleus.

antioxidant (an-te-ok´sĭ-dant) A substance that prevents oxidation.

antiperistalsis (an-tĭ-per-ĭ-stal´sis) Reverse peristaltic action of the intestines by which their contents are forced upwards.

antiperspirant (an-ti-per´spi-rant) Arresting the secretion of sweat. Also called antihidrotic; antisudorific.

antiphagocytic (an-tĭ-fag-o-sit´ik) Inhibiting phagocytosis (ingestion and digestion by white blood cells).

antiport (an´tĭ-port) A protein embedded in the cell membrane that serves to transport an intracellular substance across the membrane in exchange for an extracellular substance.

antiprothrombin (an-tĭ-pro-throm´bin) A substance that inhibits the conversion of prothrombin into thrombin, thus preventing coagulation of blood.

antipruritic (an-tĭ-proo-rit´ik) Relieving itching.

antipsychotic (an-tĭ-si-kot´ik) See neuroleptic.

antipyretic (an-tĭ-pi-ret´ik) **1.** Tending to reduce fever. **2.** Any agent that reduces fever.

antirachitic (an-tĭ-ra-kit´ik) Tending to cure rickets.

antirheumatic (an-tĭ-roo-mat´ik) **1.** Delaying the progression of rheumatic disorders. **2.** Any agent possessing such properties.

antiscorbutic (an-tĭ-skor-bu´tik) Curing or preventing scurvy.

antisecretory (an-tĭ-sĕ-kre´to-re) Inhibiting secretions.

antisense (an-tĭ-sens´) See antisense strand, under strand.

antiseptic (an-tĭ-sep´tik) A compound capable of killing or inhibiting the growth of microorganisms when applied to living tissues, without significantly harming the tissue.

antiserum (an-tĭ-se´rum) A human or animal serum containing specific antibodies.

antispasmodic (an-tĭ-spaz-mod´ik) An agent that prevents or relieves involuntary muscular contractions.

antistreptolysin O (an-tĭ-strep-tol´ĭ-sin ō) (ASO) An antibody against a hemolysin produced by beta-hemolytic streptococci; a high or rising titer indicates recent beta hemolytic streptococcus infection.

antisudorific (an-tĭ-soo-dor-if´ik) See antiperspirant.

antithrombin (an-tĭ-throm´bin) A substance that counteracts the action of thrombin, thus preventing coagulation of blood.

antitoxin (an-tĭ-tok´sin) Antibody produced in the blood and other body fluids in response to the poison of a microorganism, usually bacterial exotoxins.

antitragus (an-tĭ-tra´gus) A projection on the external ear opposite the tragus and behind the opening of the external auditory canal.

antitreponemal (an-tĭ-trep-o-ne´mal) Destructive to treponemes (bacteria of the genus *Treponema*).

antitrypsin (an-tĭ-trip´sin) A substance that inhibits the action of the proteolytic enzyme trypsin.

antitussive (an-tĭ-tus´iv) Tending to relieve cough.

antivitamin (an-tĭ-vi´tă-min) Any substance that prevents the biologic functioning of a vitamin.

antivivisection (an-tĭ-viv-ĭ-sek´shŭn) Opposition to experimentation on living animals.

antral (an´tral) Relating to an antrum (body cavity).

antrectomy (an-trek´tŏ-me) Surgical removal of an antrum, especially of the stomach.

antroscope (an´trŏ-skōp) An instrument for inspecting the interior of a maxillary sinus.

antrostomy (an-tros´kŏ-pe) The formation of a permanent opening into any antrum (e.g., the maxillary sinus) for draining purposes.

antrotomy (an-trot´ŏ-me) Incision into an antrum.

antrum (an´trum) A body chamber or cavity.

follicular a. The fluid-filled cavity within the developing ovarian follicle.

pyloric a. The dilated pyloric end of the stomach; it marks the beginning of the pyloric canal.

tympanic a. A cavity in the mastoid part of the temporal bone extending from the middle ear chamber and communicating with the mastoid air cells.

anulus (an´u-lus), *pl.* **an´uli** Latin for a ring-shaped structure. See also ring; circle.

a. fibrosus disci intervertebralis See fibrous ring of intervertebral disk, under ring.

a. inguinalis profundus See deep inguinal ring, under ring.

a. inguinalis superficialis See superficial inguinal ring, under ring.

a. tendinous communis See common tendinous ring, under ring.

anuresis (an-u-re´sis) Total retention of urine in the bladder; failure to urinate.

anuretic (an-u-ret´ik) Relating to anuresis.

anuria (an-u´re-ă) Complete suppression of urine; in clinical use, denoting less than 100 ml urine daily for an adult of average size.

anuric (an-u´rik) Relating to anuria.

anus (a´nus) The lower opening of the digestive tract.

imperforate a. Congenital absence of the anal orifice.

anxiety (ang-zi´ĕ-te) A state of apprehension, uneasiness, dread of impending danger, and fear out of proportion to the real threat, commonly accompanied by physical symptoms. See also generalized anxiety disorder, under disorder.

castration a. See castration complex, under

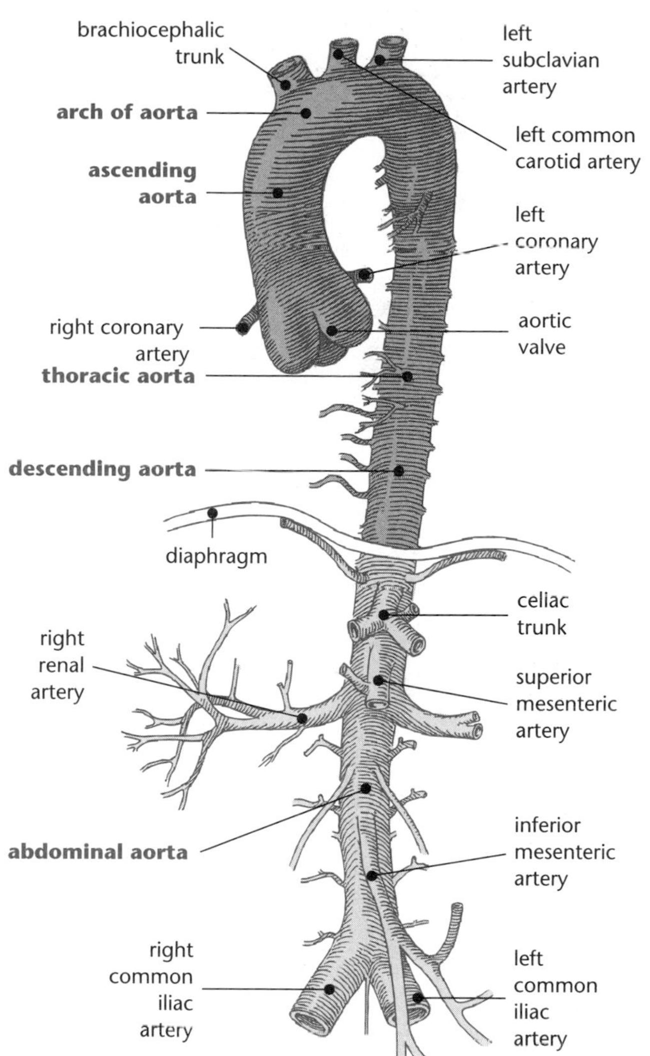

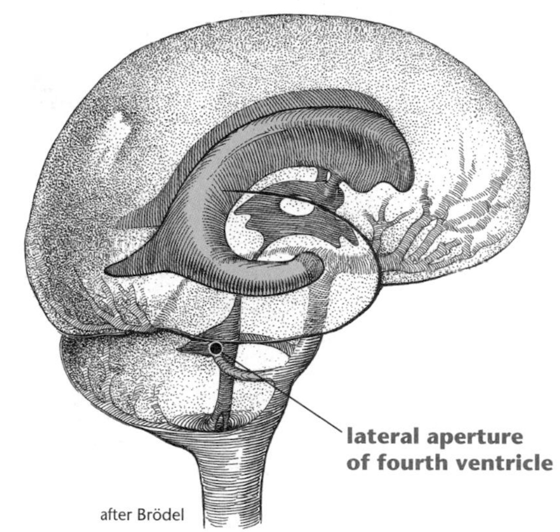

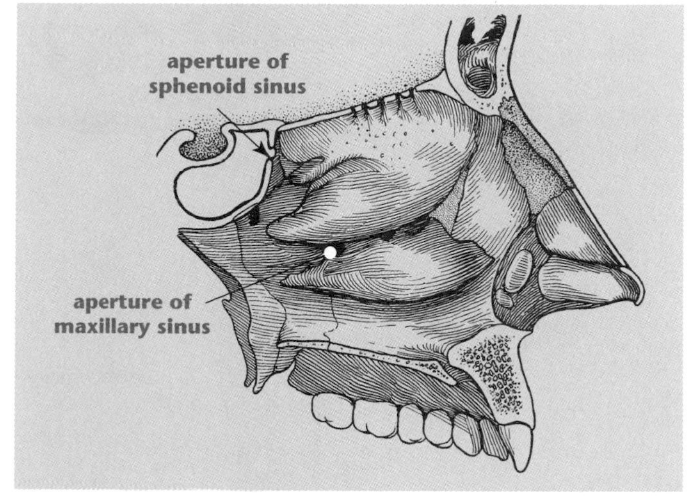

complex.

separation a. Exaggerated apprehension and distress upon separation from a needed person.

anxiety neurosis (ang-zi´ĕ-te nōō-ro´sis) See generalized anxiety disorder, under disorder.

anxiety syndrome (ang-zi´ĕ-te sin´drōm) Rapid heart beat, difficulty in breathing, and profuse sweating accompanied by panic.

aorta (a-or´tă) The largest blood vessel in the body; the main trunk of the systemic arterial circulation, arising from the upper part of the left ventricle from which it receives blood for delivery to all tissues except the lungs.

abdominal a. The terminal part of the descending aorta from the diaphragm to the level of the fourth lumbar vertebra, where it divides into the common iliac arteries.

arch of the a. The curvature by which the aorta changes its course from cephalad to caudad and from which arise the brachiocephalic trunk, left common carotid artery, and left subclavian artery.

ascending a. The first part of the aorta from its origin at the heart to the beginning of the aortic arch.

descending a. The part of the aorta from the end of the aortic arch in the chest to its bifurcation in the abdomen.

overriding a. Developmental anomaly in which the aorta straddles the ventricular septum, thereby receiving ejected blood from both right and left ventricles of the heart.

thoracic a. The portion of the descending aorta from the end of the aortic arch to the diaphragm.

aortic (a-or´tik) Relating to the aorta.

aortic arch syndrome (a-or´tik arch sin´drōm) See Takayasu's arteritis, under arteritis.

aortitis (a-or-ti´tis) Inflammation of one or more of the layers of the wall of the aorta.

rheumatoid a. Aortitis associated with rheumatoid arthritis.

aortogram (a-or´to-gram) X-ray image of the aorta obtained in aortography.

aortography (a-or-tog´ră-fe) Radiographic visualization of the aorta after the injection of a radiopaque medium into the vessel.

retrograde a. Aortography after forcing the radiopaque material through one of the aortic branches, in a direction opposite the bloodstream.

translumbar a. Roentgenography after injection of the radiopaque material into the abdominal aorta.

aortoiliac occlusive disease (a-or-to-il´e-ak ŏ-kloo´siv dĭ-zēz´) Gradual obstruction of the terminal portion of the aorta by atherosclerosis; associated clinical features include intermittent claudication of the lower back, buttocks, thighs, or calves, and atrophy of the limbs; there may also be trophic changes and impotence.

aortopathy (a-or-top´ă-the) Disease of the aorta.

aortotomy (a-or-tot´ŏ-me) Incision into the aorta.

apathy (ap´ă-the) Indifference; lack of emotion.

apatite (ap´ă-tīt) A calcium phosphate present in bone and teeth.

aperiodic (a-pēr-e-od´ik) Occurring irregularly.

aperistalsis (ă-per-ĭ-stal´sis) Absence of the normal contractions of the intestines.

Apert syndrome (ah-pĕr´ sin´drōm) See acrocephalosyndactyly.

apertognathia (ă-per-tog-na´the-ă) See open bite, under bite.

aperture (ap´er-chur) **1.** An opening, hole, or gap. **2.** An opening, usually adjustable, in an optical instrument which limits the amount of light passing through the lens.

inferior a. of minor pelvis See pelvic plane of outlet, under plane.

lateral a. of fourth ventricle One of two lateral openings on the roof of the fourth ventricle of the brain, communicating with the subarachnoid cavity. Also called foramen of Luschka.

a. of maxillary sinus A large, irregular aperture through which the maxillary sinus communicates with the nasal cavity.

median a. of fourth ventricle An opening in the midline of the roof of the fourth ventricle of the brain, communicating with the subarachnoid cavity. Also called foramen of Magendi.

a. of sphenoid sinus An orifice in the anterior wall of the sphenoid sinus through which the sinus opens into the nasal cavity.

superior a. of minor pelvis See pelvic plane of inlet, under plane.

apex (a´peks), *pl.* **a´pices** The tip or pointed end of a conical structure, such as the heart or lung.

orbital a. The posterior part of the orbit.

root a. The tip of the root of a tooth.

Apgar score (ap´gar skōr) See under score.

aphagia (ă-fa´jă) Refusal or inability to eat.

aphakia (ă-fa´ke-ă) Absence of the lens of the eye.

aphalangia (a-fă-lan´jă) Absence of toes and fingers.

aphasia (ă-fa´zhă) A general term for language disorders (reading, writing, speaking, or comprehension of written or spoken words) due to brain dysfunction, not a result of disease of the vocal organs or of intellectual deficiency.

anomic a. Inability to remember words.

auditory a. A form of aphasia in which the individual distinguishes words from other sounds but does not understand them. Also called word deafness.

Broca's a. See expressive aphasia.

expressive a. Any of several aphasias marked by impaired ability to speak or write, although comprehension of spoken and written language and ability to conceptualize are relatively intact; speech output is labored, ungrammatical, telegraphic, and poorly articulated; the patient is aware of, and visibly frustrated by, the deficit. The brain damage involves chiefly the dominant inferior frontal convolution (Broca's area). Also called motor aphasia; Broca's aphasia; nonfluent aphasia.

fluent a. See receptive aphasia.

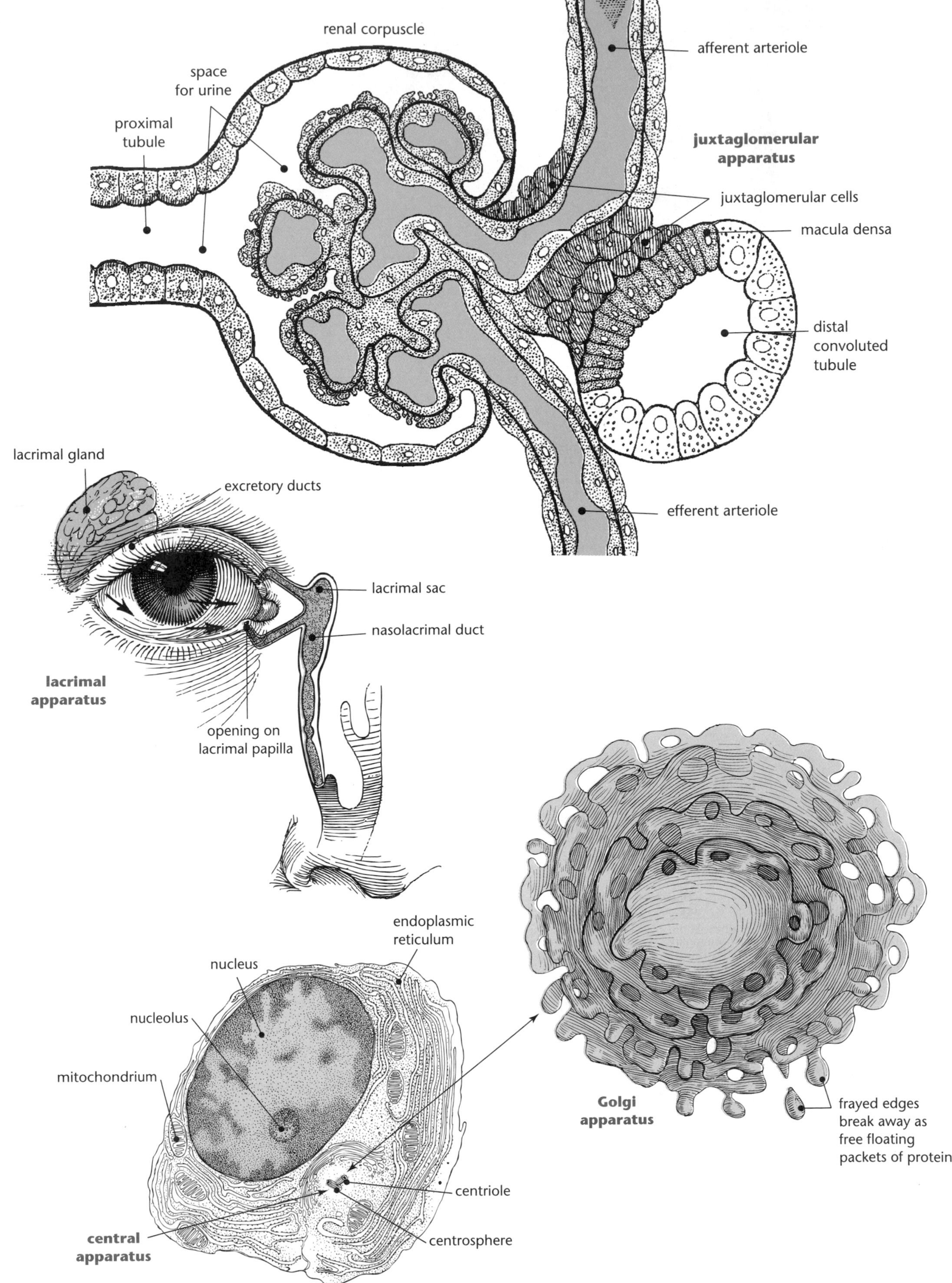
renal corpuscle
space for urine
proximal tubule
afferent arteriole
juxtaglomerular apparatus
juxtaglomerular cells
macula densa
distal convoluted tubule
efferent arteriole
lacrimal gland
excretory ducts
lacrimal sac
nasolacrimal duct
lacrimal apparatus
opening on lacrimal papilla
endoplasmic reticulum
nucleus
nucleolus
mitochondrium
Golgi apparatus
frayed edges break away as free floating packets of protein
centriole
centrosphere
central apparatus

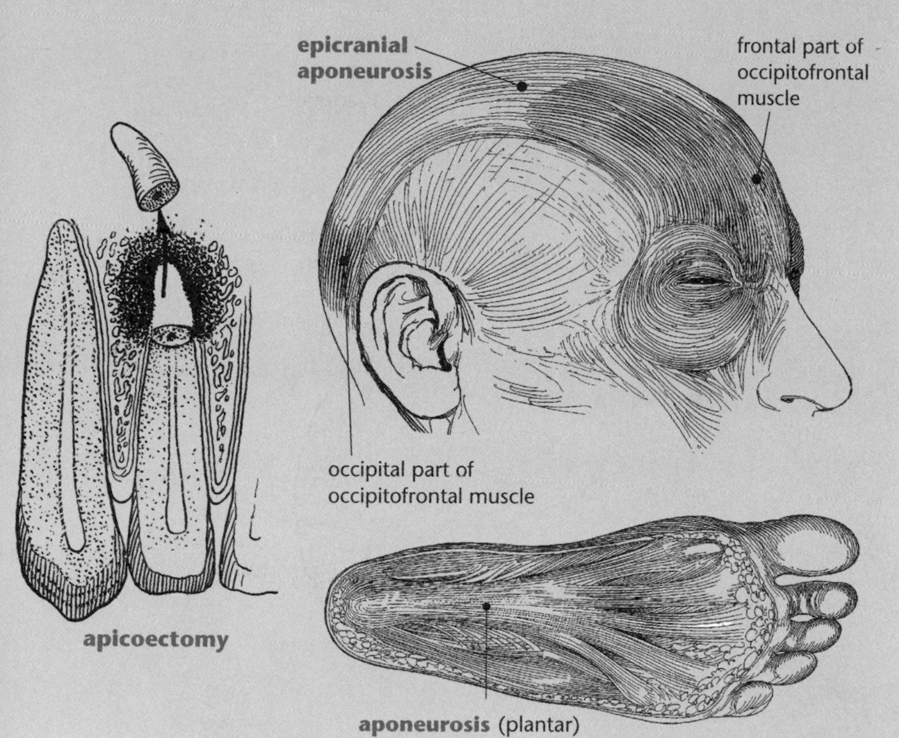

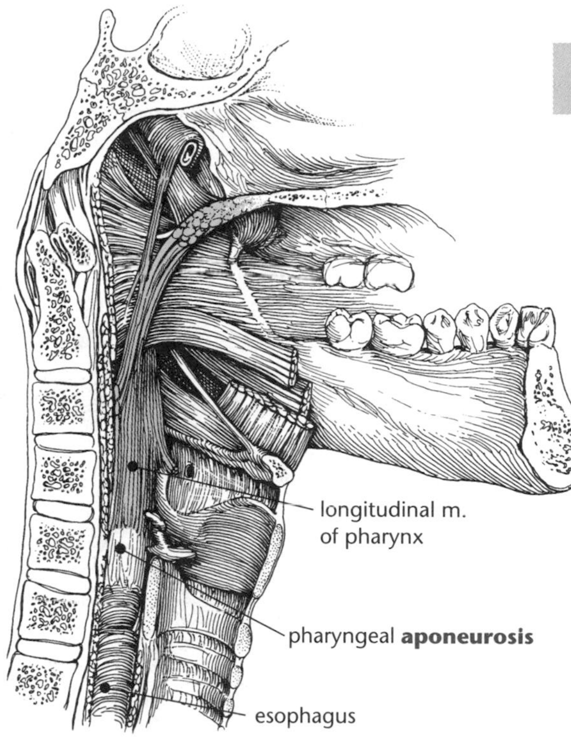

global a. Complete loss of ability to communicate in written or spoken language.
motor a. See expressive aphasia.
nominal a. A form of expressive aphasia marked by inability to name objects or persons. Also called anomia.
nonfluent a. See expressive aphasia.
optic a. Inability to name an object recognized by sight. Also called anomia.
receptive a. Diminished comprehension of written and spoken language. The patient seems unaware of the deficit. Brain damage involves the area in or near the superior temporal gyrus (Wernicke's area). Also called sensory aphasia; Wernicke's apasia; fluent aphasia.
sensory a. See receptive aphasia.
visual a. See alexia.
Wernicke's a. See receptive aphasia.
aphasiac, aphasic (ă-fa´zē-ak, ă-fa´zik) Relating to aphasia.
apheresis (af-ĕ-re´sis) Removal of blood from a donor and reinfusion after selected blood components are removed and retained. Also called pheresis.
aphonia (a-fo´ne-ă) Loss of the voice.
hysterical a. Inability to speak due to psychological factors.
aphonic (a-fon´ik) Relating to aphonia.
aphrodisiac (af-ro-diz´e-ak) Any agent that intensifies sexual desire.
aphtha (af´thă), *pl.* **aph´thae** A small white superficial ulcer of mucous membranes, commonly seen in the mouth.
aphthous (af´thus) Relating to aphthae.
apical (ap´ĭ-kal) Relating to the apex of a structure, such as the tip of the root of a tooth, the top of a lung, or the apex of the heart.
apicoectomy (a-pĭ-ko-ek´to-me) Surgical removal of the tip of a tooth root. Also called apicectomy.
apicostomy (a-pĭ-kos´to-me) Surgical formation of an opening through the alveolar bone to the tip of a tooth root.
apituitarism (ă-pĭ-too´ĭ-tar-iz-m) State in which the pituitary gland (hypophysis) has ceased to function.
aplanasia (ap-lan-ā´zhă) Absence of spherical or monochromatic aberration. Also called aplanatism.
aplanatic (ap-lă-nat´ik) Denoting an optical system or lens free from spherical or monochromatic aberration.
aplasia (ă-pla´zhă) **1.** Complete or partial failure of a tissue or an organ to develop. **2.** In hematology, defective development, or failure to regenerate.
congenital thymic a. See DiGeorge's syndrome.
aplastic (ă-plas´tik) **1.** Pertaining to defective development. **2.** Relating to defective regenerative processes.
apnea (ap-ne´ă) Cessation of respiration.
sleep a. Episodes of apnea during sleep and lasting more than 15 seconds; may be central, associated with cessation of respiratory drive, or obstructive, caused by obstruction of airflow at the nose or mouth.
apocrine (ap´o-krin) Relating to a gland in which some of the apical portion of the gland is discharged along with the secretory product; seen in axillary sweat glands.
apodia (ă-po´de-ă) Congenital absence of feet.
apoenzyme (ap-o-en´zīm) A protein that requires a coenzyme to function as an enzyme; the protein portion of an enzyme.
apoferritin (ap-o-fer´ĭ-tin) A protein of the small intestine; it combines with iron to form ferritin, which is thought to regulate the absorption of iron in the intestinal tract.
apolar (a-po´lar) Without poles or processes, as certain nerve cells.
apolipoprotein (ap-o-lip-o-pro´tēn) (apo) The protein constituent of lipoproteins such as HDL (high density lipoprotein) and LDL (low density lipoprotein), which circulate normally in blood plasma; classified according to function into four groups: A, B, C, E (D is now A-III).
a. A-I Apolipoprotein that activates the liver enzyme LCAT (lecithin-cholesterol acyltransferase); found in HDL and in chylomicrons (minute fat particles in chyle); apo A-I deficiency is associated with low levels of HDL and Tangier disease.
a. B The main protein of LDL, found also in VLDL (very low density lipoprotein) and IDL (intermediate density lipoprotein); elevated levels of apo B occur in individuals with hyperlipoproteinemia.
apomorphine hydrochloride (ap-o-mor´fēn hi-dro-klor´īd) A white crystalline derivative of morphine; used as an emetic, expectorant, and hypnotic.
aponeurorrhaphy (ap-o-nōō-ror´ă-fe) See fasciorrhaphy.
aponeurosis (ap-o-nōō-ro´sis) A pearly white, iridescent, fibrous sheet, composed of closely packed, mostly parallel collagenous bundles; serves as a connection between a muscle and its attachment.
epicranial a. The aponeurosis of the scalp; it covers the upper part of the skull, connecting the frontal and occipital bellies of the occipitofrontal muscle. Also called galea aponeurotica.
apoplexy (ap´o-plek-se) Rupture of a vessel into an organ.
labyrinthine a. A single, abrupt episode of vertigo accompanied by nausea and vomiting; the sense of equilibrium is permanently lost in one ear; tinnitus and hearing loss do not occur. Occlusion of the labyrinthine branch of the internal auditory artery is thought to be the cause.
pituitary a. Sudden onset of headache and vision loss caused by a sudden increase in size of a pituitary tumor due to hemorrhage or infarction.
uteroplacental a. See Couvelaire uterus, under uterus.
apoptosis (ap-op-to´sis) Cell death mediated by enzymatic degradation of DNA; unlike necrosis, it is not associated with inflammation. Also called programmed cell death.
appallic syndrome (ă-pol´ik sin´drōm) See persistent vegetative state, under state.
apparatus (ap-ă-ră´tus) **1.** A group of instruments or devices used together or in succession to perform a specific task. **2.** A group of organs or structures that collectively perform a common function.
Benedict-Roth a. Device for estimating basal metabolic rate by measuring the amount of oxygen used during quiet breathing. Also called Benedict-Roth calorimeter.
central a. The centrosome and centrosphere.
Golgi a. An organelle in a cell consisting of a bowl-shaped, reticular network of saccules, vesicles, and vacuoles; in most cells it is located near the nucleus; it temporarily stores and packages secretory products. Also called Golgi body; Golgi complex.
juxtaglomerular a. (JGA) The juxtaglomerular body (granular epithelioid cells in the terminal part of the afferent arteriole of the kidney) together with the macula densa (the thickened epithelial cells in the wall of the distal convoluted tubule where it contacts the afferent arteriole).
lacrimal a. The tear-forming and tear-conducting system, consisting of the lacrimal gland and ducts and associated structures.
Tiselius a. A device used to separate proteins from solution and to determine the molecular weight and the isoelectric point.
Van Slyke a. Apparatus used to measure the amount of respiratory gases in blood.
Warburg's a. Apparatus used to measure the oxygen consumption of incubated tissue slices.
appendage (ă-pen´dij) Any part in close but subordinate relation to a main structure. Also called appendix.
atrial a. See auricle (2).
epiploic a. See under appendix.
testicular a. A minute, oval, cystlike body on the upper end of the testis, an embryonic vestige. Also called hydatid of Morgagni; Morgagni's appendix.
vesicular a. of uterine tube A fluid-filled cystlike structure attached to the fimbriated end of the uterine tube, an embryonic vestige. Also called hydatid of Morgagni; Morgagni's appendix.
appendectomy (ap-en-dek´tŏ-me) Surgical

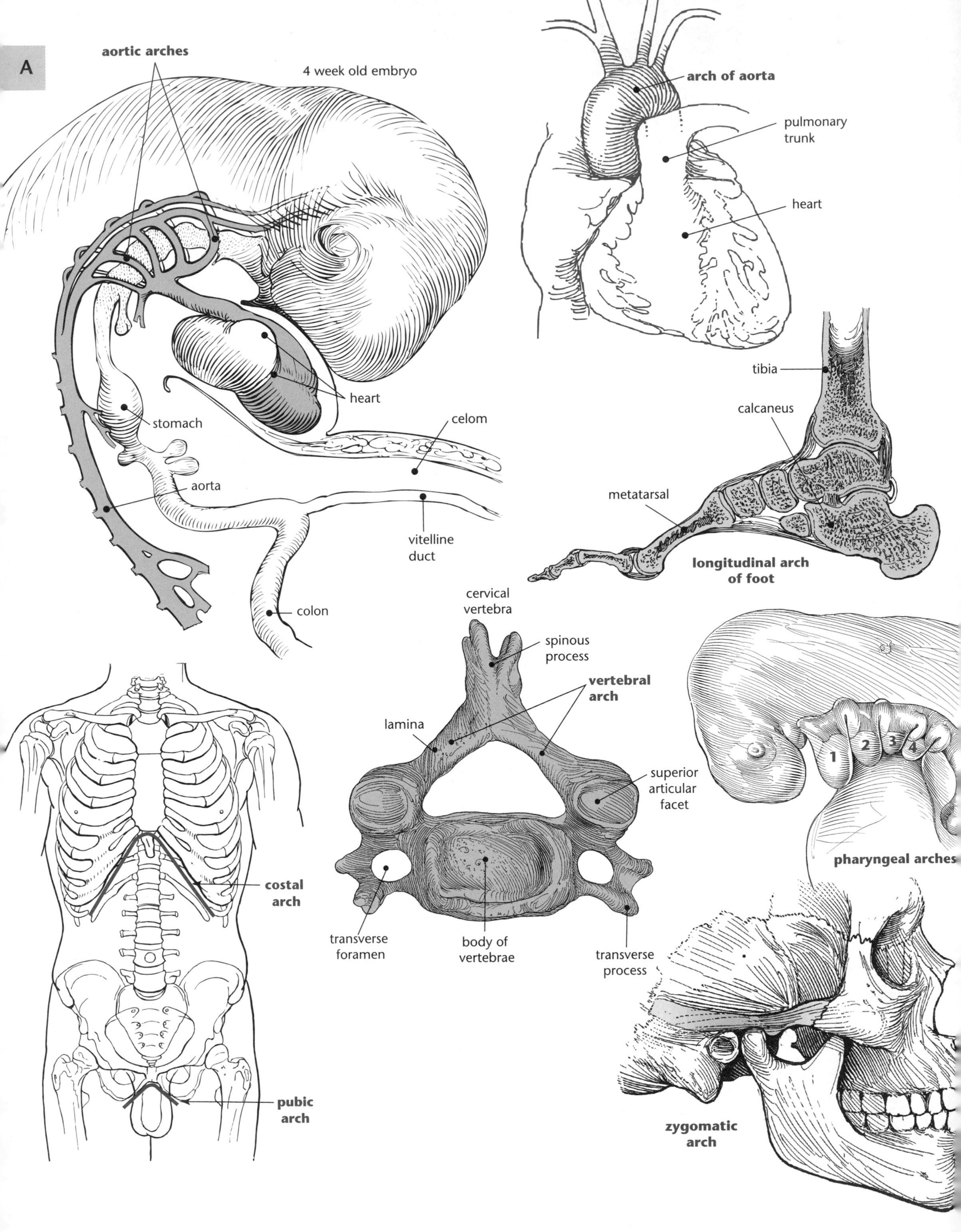
aortic arches
4 week old embryo
heart
stomach
celom
aorta
vitelline duct
colon
arch of aorta
pulmonary trunk
heart
tibia
calcaneus
metatarsal
longitudinal arch of foot
cervical vertebra
spinous process
vertebral arch
lamina
superior articular facet
transverse foramen
body of vertebrae
transverse process
costal arch
pubic arch
1
2
3
4
pharyngeal arches
zygomatic arch

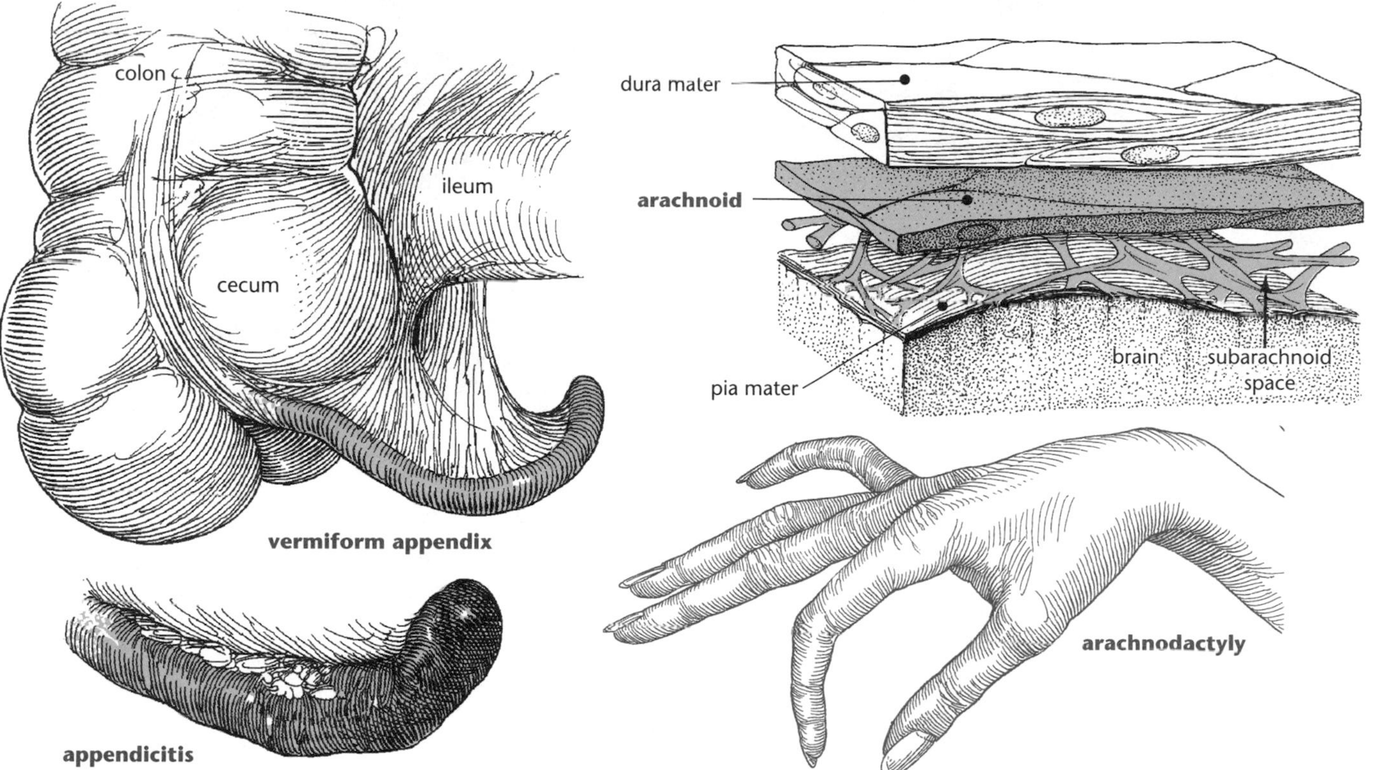

A

removal of an appendix, especially the vermiform appendix.
appendiceal (ap-en-dis´e-al) Of or relating to an appendix.
appendicitis (ă-pen-dĭ-si´tis) Inflammation of the vermiform appendix.
appendicolithiasis (ă-pen-dĭ-ko-lĭ-thi´ă-sis) The presence of stones in the vermiform appendix.
appendicular (ap-en-dik´u-lar) Relating to the appendix.
appendix (ă-pen´diks), *pl.* **appen´dices** An appendage, especially the vermiform appendix.
a. ceci See vermiform appendix.
epiploic a. One of several small peritoneal sacs extending from the serous coat of the large intestine, except the rectum. Also called epiploic appendage.
Morgagni's a. (a) See testicular appendage, under appendage. (b) See vesicular appendage of uterine tube, under appendage.
vermiform a. The slender, worm-shaped tubular structure extending from the blind end of the cecum.
apperception (ap-er-sep´shun) Comprehension based on previous knowledge or memories of past experiences.
appersonation, appersonification (ă-per-so-na´shun, ap-er-son-ĭ-fĭ-ka´shun) Delusion marked by assuming the character of another individual.
appetite (ap´ĕ-tīt) The natural desire for food.
applanation (ap-lă-na´shun) Flattening of a small area of the cornea with a special tonometer to measure the force applied and, thereby, the pressure within the eyeball.
appliance (ă-pli´ans) **1.** Device designed for a particular function (e.g., to stabilize a fractured bone). **2.** A device for moving or for splinting teeth.
applicator (ap-lĭ-ka´tor) A slender rod of wood or plastic with a small cluster of cotton attached to one end; used for making local applications of medicine.
apposition (ap-ŏ-zish´un) The placing in contact of two adjacent and opposing surfaces.
apraxia (ă-prak´se-ă) Inability to execute purposeful movements in absence of paralysis, due to a defect in cortical integration.
verbal a. Speech disorder in which one speech sound is substituted for the desired syllable or word.
apraxic, apractic (ă-prak´sik, ă-prak´tik) Relating to apraxia.
aptyalia (ap-ti-a´le-ă) See asialia.
APUD Acronym for amine precursor uptake and decarboxylation; denoting a system of cells, scattered throughout the body, that secrete a variety of peptide hormones and amines. Also called APUD system; neuroendocrine system.
apyretic (a-pi-ret´ik) Without fever.
apyrexia (a-pi-rek´se-ă) Absence of fever.
apyrexial (a-pi-rek´se-al) Relating to apyrexia.
aqua (ak´wă, ā´kwă), *pl.* **aq´uae** Latin for water.
aquaporin (ak-wă-por´in) (AQP) A water channel present in the kidney and other tissues.
a. 1 (AQP 1) Protein found in red blood cells and some segments of the renal tubules; functions as a molecular water channel. Also called CHIP (channel-forming integral protein).
a. 2 (AQP 2) The water channel in renal collecting ducts; responds to vasopressin (an antidiuretic hormone).
aquatic (ă-kwat´ik) Relating to or living in water.
aqueduct (ak´we-dukt) A canal.
cerebral a. A small canal connecting the third and fourth ventricles of the brain. Also called aqueduct of Sylvius.
a. of Sylvius See cerebral aqueduct.
vestibular a. A thin bony canal leading from the medial wall of the vestibule of the inner ear to the posterior surface of the petrous portion of the temporal bone, where it communicates with the cerebrospinal space; it houses the endolymphatic duct.
aqueous (a´kwe-us) Watery.
aqueous humor (a´kwe-us hu´mor) See under humor.
arabinose (ă-rab´ĭ-nōs) (Ara) A sugar of the pentose class (i.e., its molecule has five carbon atoms); obtained from cherry-tree gum, mesquite gum, or prepared synthetically from D-glucose; used in culture media.
arabinoside (ar-ă-bin´o-sīd) A nucleoside that has arabinose as its sugar component.
arabinosylcytosine (ă-rab-ĭ-no-sil-si´to-sēn) A chemocytotherapeutic agent used as part of a combination regimen in the treatment of ovarian carcinoma and certain leukemias. Also called cytarabine.
arachidonic acid (ă-rak-ĭ-don´ik as´id) A polyunsaturated fatty acid, $C_{20}H_{32}O_2$; a precursor of prostaglandins, essential in nutrition; present abundantly in the amniochorion, decidua, and amniotic fluid.
arachnid (ă-rak´nid) Any member of the class Arachnida.
Arachnida (ă-rak´nĭ-dă) A class of arthropods (subphylum Chelicerata) that characteristically have four pairs of legs; includes spiders, scorpions, mites, and ticks.
arachnidism (ă-rak´nĭ-diz-m) Systemic poisoning following the bite of a spider, especially of the black widow and brown recluse spiders.
arachnodactyly (ă-rak-no-dak´tĭ-le) Hereditary condition marked by excessive length and slenderness of the bones of the fingers and toes; may be accompanied by relaxed joint ligaments and is usually associated with a connective tissue disorder.
arachnoid (ă-rak´noid) **1.** Having the appearance of a cobweb. **2.** The middle of the three membranes covering the brain and spinal cord, between the dura mater and the pia mater; separated from the pia mater by the subarachnoid space.
arachnoidal (ar-ak-noi´dăl) Relating to the middle of the three membranes covering the brain and spinal cord (arachnoid).
arachnoiditis (ă-rak-noi-di´tis) Inflammation of the arachnoid.
adhesive a. Inflammation of the arachnoid and adjacent pia mater, sometimes causing obliteration of the subarachnoid space.
arachnophobia (ă-rak-no-fo´be-ă) An inordinate fear of spiders.
arborescent (ar-bo-res´ent) Treelike; branching.
arborization (ar-bor-ĭ-za´shun) Denoting the branching of nerve fibers and capillaries.
cervical mucus a. See ferning.
arborize (ar´bor-ize) To ramify or branch.
arbovirus (ar´bo-vi-rus) Any arthropod-borne virus of the genera *Alphavirus* and *Flavivirus* (family Togaviridae).
arc (ark) **1.** Anything shaped like an arch or a bow. **2.** The luminous line formed by the electric current crossing a gap between two electrodes.
mercury a. An electric discharge through mercury vapor in a vacuum tube, producing ultraviolet rays.
reflex a. The path followed by a nerve impulse in the production of a reflex act.
arch (arch) Any of several curved structures of the body.
aortic a.'s of the embryo A series of six arterial channels encircling the embryonic pharynx (gut) in the mesenchyme of the pharyngeal arches; they are never present all at the same time.
a. of the aorta The curved portion of the aorta between the ascending and descending parts of the thoracic aorta. Also called aortic arch.
branchial a. See pharyngeal arch.
cortical a.'s of kidney The portion of kidney substance (cortex) located between the bases of the pyramids and the renal capsule.
costal a. An arch formed by the borders of the inferior aperture of the thorax, comprised of the costal cartilages of ribs seven to ten.
dental a. (a) The composite structure of the natural teeth and the alveolar ridge. (b) The curved contour of the remains of the alveolar ridge after the loss of some or all of the natural teeth.
a.'s of foot The two sets of arches (longitudinal and transverse) formed by the bones of the foot.
longitudinal a. The anteroposterior arch of the

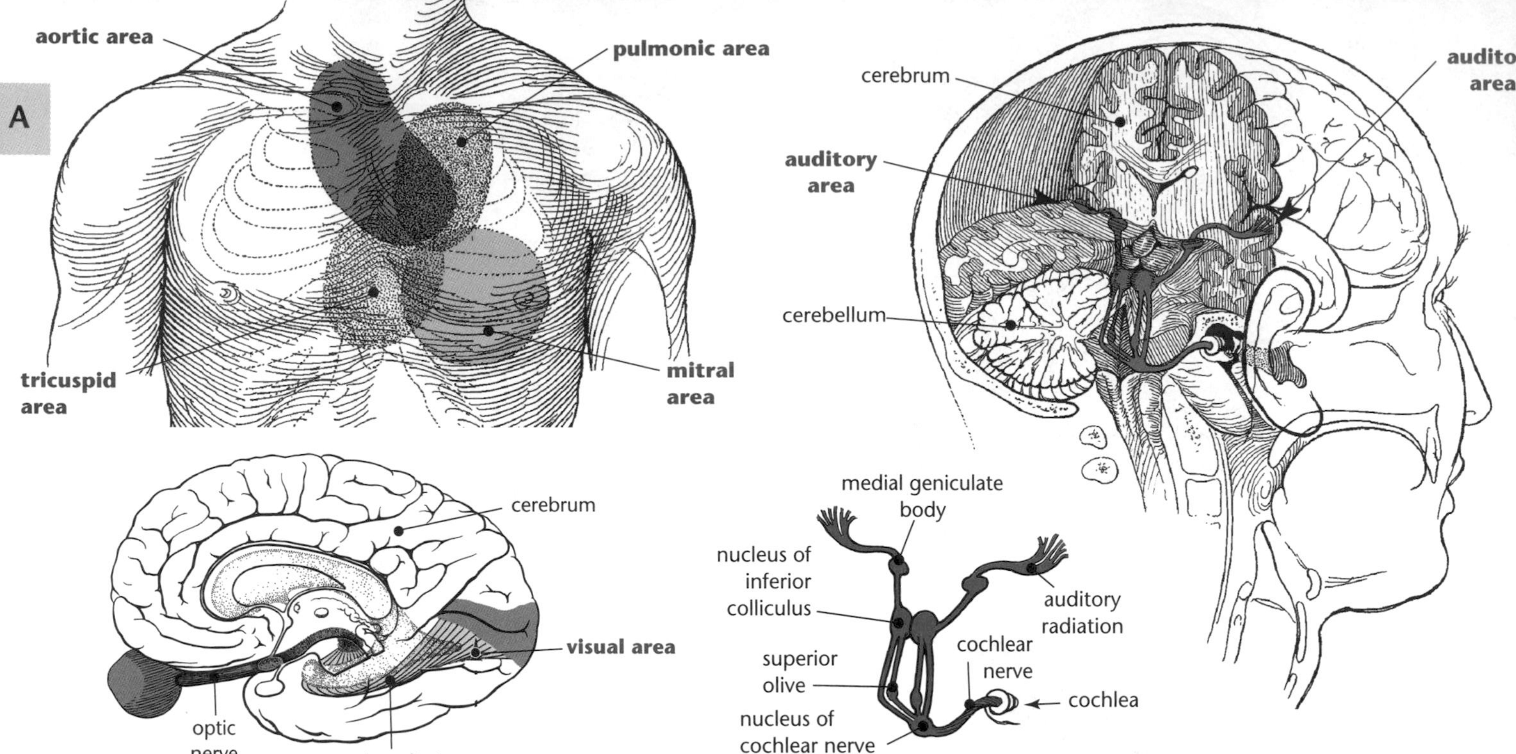

foot, formed by the seven tarsal and five metatarsal bones and the ligaments binding them together.

neural a. See vertebral arch.

palatoglossal a. One of two folds of mucous membrane extending from the posterior edge of the soft palate to the side of the tongue; forms the anterior margin of the tonsillar fossa. Also called anterior pillar of fauces.

palatopharyngeal a. One of two folds of mucous membrane passing downward from the posterior edge of the soft palate to the lateral wall of the pharynx; forms the posterior margin of the tonsillar fossa. Also called posterior pillar of fauces.

pharyngeal a. One of a series of five mesodermal arches (bars) in the neck region of the embryo from which several structures of the head and neck develop. Formerly called branchial arch.

pubic a. Arch on the pelvis formed by the convergence of the inferior rami of the ischium and pubic bones on either side.

superciliary a. An arched prominence above the upper margin of the orbit.

tendinous a. of pelvis A condensation of parietal pelvic fascia arching from the posterior surface of the pubis to the spine of the ischium.

transverse a. The arch of the foot formed by the proximal parts of the metatarsal bones anteriorly and the distal row of the tarsal bones posteriorly.

vertebral a., neural a. The arch on the dorsal side of a vertebra which, with the vertebral body, forms the foramen in which the spinal cord is lodged.

zygomatic a. The arch formed by the zygomatic process of the temporal bone and the temporal process of the zygomatic bone.

archenteron (ar-ken´ter-on) The primitive digestive cavity of the embryo at the gastrula stage. Also called primary gut.

arctation (ark-ta´shun) Stricture; narrowing.

arcuate (ar´ku-āt) Arched.

arcus (ar´kus), *pl.* **ar´cus** Any arch-shaped structure; an arch.

a. juvenilis A gray white ring around the cornea, occurring in the young.

a. senilis An opaque grayish ring around the cornea, occurring in the aged. Also called gerontoxon.

area (ar´e-ă) A distinct part of a surface or space.

aortic a. Area on the chest over the cartilage of the second right rib.

apical a. Area about (a) The tip of the root of a tooth. (b) The apex of a lung. (c) The chest wall corresponding to the apex of the heart (normally the apex beat is in approximately the fifth left intercostal space in the midclavicular line).

auditory a. Region of the cerebral cortex concerned with hearing, occupying the transverse temporal gyri and the superior temporal gyrus.

Broca's speech a. Area comprising the triangular and opercular portions of the inferior frontal gyrus; it governs the motor aspects of speech and is better developed in the left hemisphere of right-handed persons.

Brodmann's a.'s The 47 areas of the cerebral cortex mapped out according to the arrangement of their cellular components.

a. of cardiac dullness Normally a small triangular area on the lower left side of the sternum which, on percussion of the chest, produces a dull sound; it corresponds to the portion of the heart not covered by lung tissue.

basal seat a. The portion of oral structures that is available to support a denture.

controlled a. In radiography, the space in a room containing the radiation source.

a. cribrosa Area of the renal papilla containing 20 or more pores through which the urine oozes into the minor calyces.

frontal a. Portion of the cerebral cortex in front of the central sulcus (fissure of Rolando).

Little's a. A highly vascular area of the anterior portion of the nasal septum; frequent site of nosebleed.

macular a. The part of the retina that contains a yellow pigment, is used for central vision, and appears to be free of vessels when viewed with an ophthalmoscope.

mirror a. The reflecting surface of the lens of the eye and the cornea when illuminated with the slit lamp.

mitral a. The chest area over the apex of the heart (approximately the fifth intercostal space in the midclavicular line) where the sound produced by the left atrioventricular (mitral) valve is usually heard most clearly.

motor a. Portion of the cerebral cortex composed of the anterior wall of the central sulcus (fissure of Rolando) and adjacent portions of the precentral gyrus; its stimulation with electrodes causes contraction of voluntary muscles. Also called precentral cortex area; primary motor area.

parolfactory area of Broca See subcallosal area.

postcentral a., postrolandic a. The sensory area of the cerebral cortex, just posterior to the central sulcus (fissure of Rolando); it receives sensory stimuli from the whole body.

posterior palatal seal a. The soft tissue along the junction of the soft and hard palate on which pressure can be applied by a denture to help its retention.

precentral cortex a. See motor area.

premotor a. Area immediately in front of the motor area, concerned with integrated movements.

primary motor a. See motor area.

pulmonic a. Area of the chest at the second left intercostal space where flow sounds across the pulmonary valves are usually heard best.

skip a.'s Areas of the intestinal lining that are relatively uninvolved in the process of Crohn's disease.

subcallosal a. An area of the cortex in the medial aspect of each cerebral hemisphere, located immediately in front of the lamina terminalis and caudoventral to the subcallosal gyrus. Also called parolfactory area of Broca.

tricuspid a. Area of auscultation for murmurs originating from the right atrioventricular valve (tricuspid); the lower left sternal area.

visual a. Area of the occipital lobe of the cerebral cortex concerned with vision; consists of two parts. *Sensory* or *striate part*, occupies the walls of the calcarine sulcus (occasionally extending around the occipital pole onto the lateral surface of the hemisphere); concerned with recognition of size, form, motion, color, illumination, and transparency. *Psychic* or *parastriate part*, surrounds the sensory portion; associates visual impressions and past experiences for recognition and identification.

areata (ar-e-a´tă) Denoting circumscribed areas or patches.

areflexia (ă-re-flek´se-ă) Absence of reflexes.

Arenaviridae (ă-re-nă-vir´ĭ-de) Family of viruses (50 to 300 nm in diameter) that contain single-stranded RNA, multiply in cytoplasm, and appear sandy on electronmicroscopy; includes viruses causing lymphocytic choriomeningitis and Lassa fever. Also called arenavirus group.

Arenavirus (ă-re´nă-vi-rus) Genus of viruses (family Arenaviridae) that includes the Lassa and the lymphocytic choriomeningitis viruses. Also called lymphocytic choriomeningitis group.

areola (ă-re´o-lă) **1.** One of the minute spaces in a tissue. **2.** A circular pigmented area around a central point, such as the pigmented area around the nipple on the breast.

areolar (ă-re´o-lar) Relating to an areola.

argentaffin, argentaffine (ar-jen´tă-fin, ar-jen´tă-fēn) Denoting cells that have an affinity for silver salts.

argentaffinoma (ar-jen-taf-ĭ-no´mă) See carcinoid tumor, under tumor

argentation (ar-jen-ta´shun) Staining with a silver salt such as silver nitrate.

argentous (ar-jen´tus) Relating to silver, denoting a compound containing silver in its lower valence.

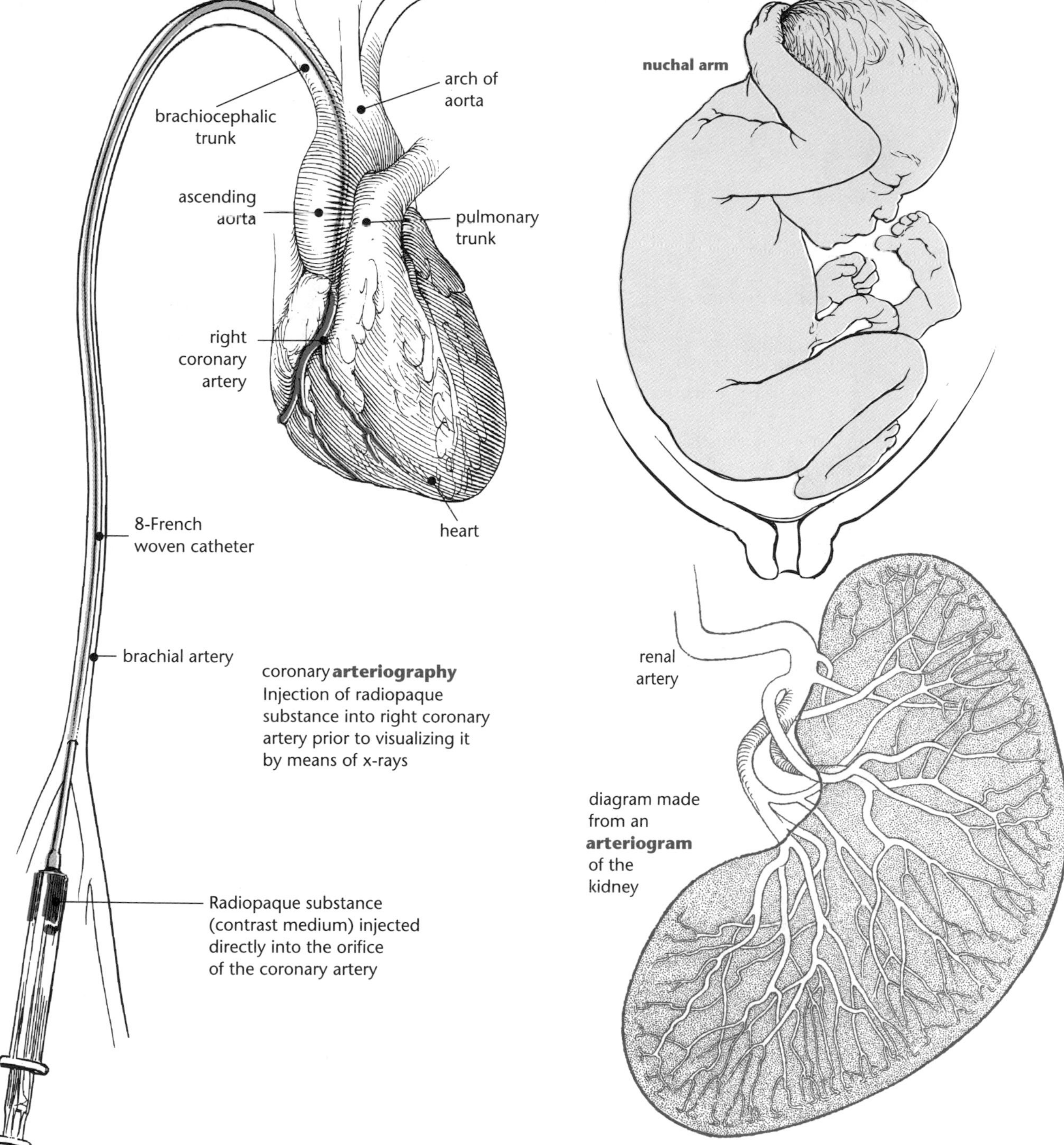

A

argentum (ar-jen´tum) Latin for silver.
arginase (ar´jĭ-nās) A liver enzyme that promotes the splitting of the amino acid arginine into urea and ornithine.
arginine (ar´jĭ-nēn) (Arg) An essential amino acid, $C_6H_{14}N_4O_2$, derived from the hydrolysis of protein.
argon (ar´gon) A colorless, odorless, gaseous element constituting about 1% of the earth's atmosphere; symbol Ar, atomic number 18, atomic weight 39.6.
argyria (ar-jir´e-ă) Chronic silver poisoning causing a permanent grayish discoloration of the skin, conjunctiva, cornea, and internal organs due to the prolonged use of preparations containing silver compounds.
argyrosis (ar-jĭ-ro´sis) See argyria.
ariboflavinosis (a-ri-bo-fla-vĭ-no´sis) See hyporiboflavinosis.
arm (arm) The upper limb of the human body, especially between the shoulder and the elbow.
nuchal a. A fetal arm that is positioned around the back of the neck; sometimes seen in breech deliveries.
armpit (arm´pit) See axilla.
Arnold-Chiari syndrome (ăr-nold-ke-ăr´e sin´drōm) See Arnold-Chiari malformation, under malformation.
arrest (ă-rest´) To prevent or stop function, progress, growth, or motion.
cardiac a. Acute failure of the heart to provide adequate circulation to the brain and other vital organs.
cardioplegic a. The purposeful stopping of all cardiac activity in a patient so that operative procedures may be performed on the heart.
cardiopulmonary a. Failure of circulation and pulmonary ventilation.
deep hypothermic a. Stoppage of all cardiac activities by cooling of the heart.
sinus a. Condition in which the sinoatrial (S-A) node of the heart fails to send impulses to the atria, resulting in a temporary cessation of cardiac contraction.
arrhenoblastoma (ă-re-no-blas-to´mă) An uncommon benign tumor of the ovary that secretes male hormones (androgens), causing masculinization; occurs in young women.
arrhythmia (ă-rith´me-ă) Irregularity, especially of the heart beat.
sinus a. A variation in the rhythm of the heart beat usually related to breathing (slower during expiration, more rapid during inspiration). Also called juvenile arrhythmia because it is commonly found in children.
arrhythmic (ă-rith´mik) Without rhythm.
arrhythmogenic (ă-rith-mo-jen´ik) Causing irregular heartbeats.
arsenic (ar´sĕ-nik) A highly poisonous metallic element; symbol As, atomic number 33, atomic weight 74.9; some of its compounds are used in medicine.
arsenous (ar´sĕ-nus) Relating to arsenic; denoting a compound of arsenic in a low valence.
arsphenamine (ars-fen´ă-mēn) An organic compound of the arseno-type; its discovery by Ehrlich in 1907 represented a major advance in the treatment of syphilis. Also called Salvarsan®; diarsenol.
arteria (ar-te´re-ă), *pl.* **arte´riae** Latin for artery.
arterial (ar-tēr´e-al) Relating to the arteries.
arteriectomy (ar-tĕ-re-ek´tŏ-me) Surgical removal of a segment of an artery.
arteriogram (ar-te´re-o-gram) X-ray image of an artery or arteries obtained in arteriography.
arteriography (ar-te-re-og´ră-fe) **1.** Radiographic visualization of an artery or arteries after injection

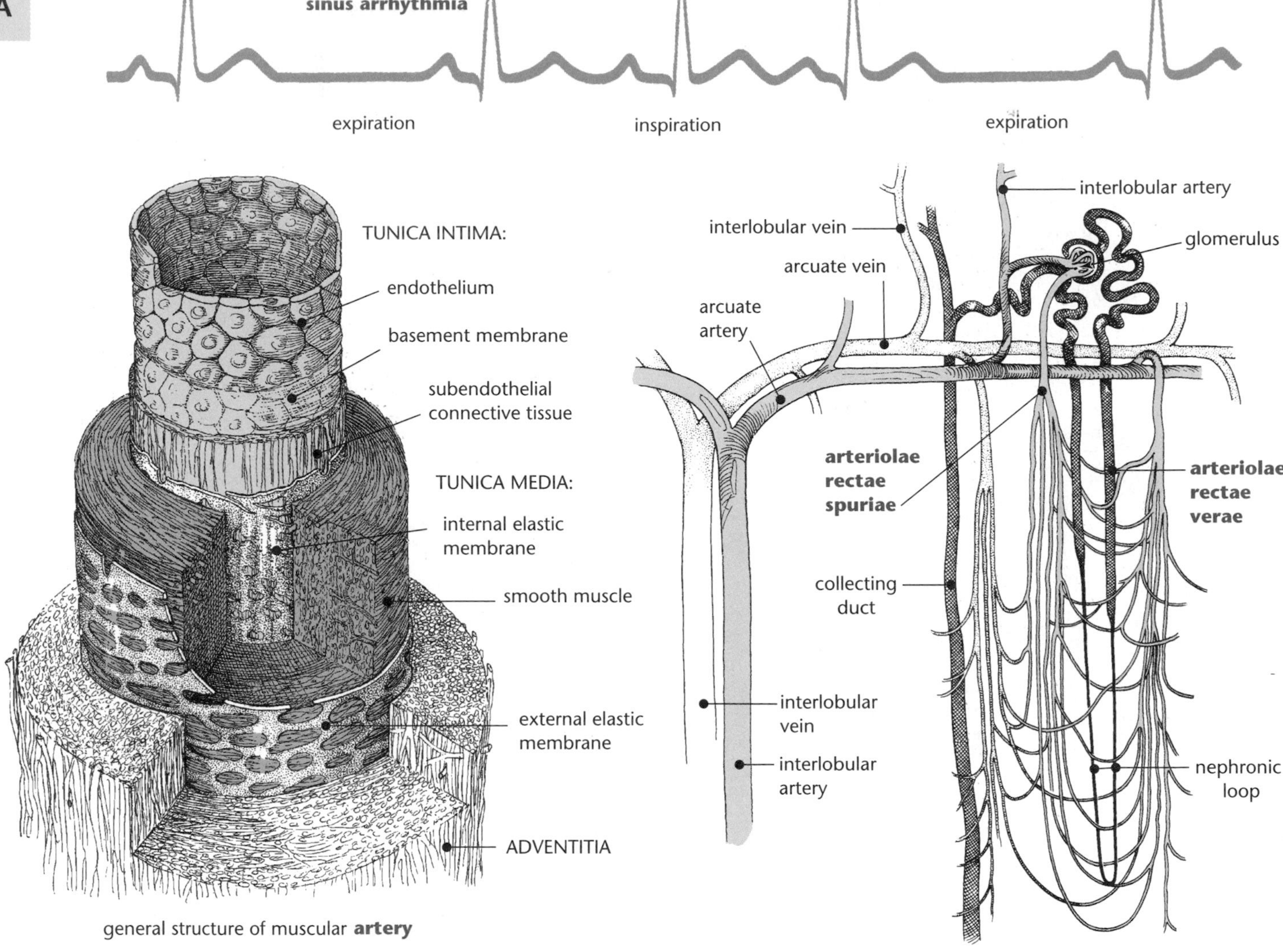

general structure of muscular **artery**

of a radiopaque substance. **2.** A treatise on the arteries. **3.** Sphygmography.

arteriola (ar-tēr-e-o´lă), *pl.* **arterio´lae** Latin for arteriole.

arteriolae rectae spuriae Straight vessels arising from the juxtaglomerular efferent arterioles of the kidney; they run parallel to the nephronic (Henle's) loop. Also called vasa recta spuria.

arteriolae rectae verae The true vasa recta; straight vessels arising directly from the arcuate arteries of the kidney; they run parallel to the nephronic (Henle's) loop.

arteriolar (ar-tēr-e-o´lar) Relating to an arteriole or arterioles.

arteriole (ar-tēr´e-ōl) The smallest subdivision of the arterial tree preceding the capillary; it has muscular walls which, by contracting and relaxing, can alter the flow of blood into body tissues.

afferent glomerular a. A branch of the interlobular artery of the kidney conveying blood to the glomerulus.

efferent glomerular a. Arteriole carrying blood from the glomerular capillary network to the capillary bed of the proximal convoluted tubule.

arteriolitis (ar-tēr-e-o-li´tis) Inflammation of the arterioles.

arteriolonecrosis (ar-tēr-e-o-lo-nĕ-kro´sis) Degeneration or destruction of arterioles, as in malignant hypertension.

arteriolonephrosclerosis (ar-tēr-e-o-lo-nĕ-fro-sklĕ-ro´sis) See arteriolar nephrosclerosis, under nephrosclerosis.

arteriolosclerosis (ar-te-re-o-lo-skle-ro´sis) Hardening of arterioles and small arteries associated with high blood pressure (hypertension); marked by diffuse wall thickening, narrowing of the lumen, and resultant deficiency of blood supply to affected parts. Also called arteriolar sclerosis.

hyaline a. A form occurring typically in elderly people, especially those with mild hypertension and diabetes mellitus.

hyperplastic a. A form characteristically occurring in acute, severe elevations in blood pressure (malignant hypertension).

arteriomotor (ar-tēr-e-o-mo´tor) Causing contraction or dilatation of arteries.

arterionecrosis (ar-tēr-e-o-nĕ-kro´sis) Death of arterial tissues.

arterioplasty (ar-tēr-e-o-plas´te) Replacement of a segment of an artery.

arteriorrhaphy (ar-tēr-e-or´ă-fe) Suture of an artery.

arteriorrhexis (ar-tēr-e-o-rek´sis) Rupture of an artery.

arteriosclerosis (ar-tēr-e-o-sklĕ-ro´sis) Disease of arteries resulting in thickening and loss of elasticity of the arterial walls. Also called arterial sclerosis; hardening of the arteries.

Mönckeberg's a. A form of arteriosclerosis marked by the formation of ringlike calcifications in the middle layer of arterial walls, especially of small arteries. Also called medial calcific sclerosis; medial calcinosis.

a. obliterans Arteriosclerotic narrowing of the lumen of arteries supplying the extremities.

arteriosclerotic (ar-tēr-e-o-sklĕ-rot´ik) Relating to or marked by arteriosclerosis.

arteriospasm (ar-tēr´e-o-spaz-m) Spasm of an artery.

arteriostenosis (ar-tēr-e-o-stĕ-no ´sis) Constriction of an artery or arteries.

arteriotomy (ar-tēr-e-ot´ŏ-me) Incision into the lumen of an artery.

arteriovenous (ar-te-re-o-ve´nus) Relating to both arteries and veins.

arteritis (ar-tĕ-ri´tis) Inflammation of an artery.

a. deformans Chronic inflammation of the inner layer of an artery (intima).

giant cell a. See temporal arteritis.

a. obliterans Inflammation of the inner layer of an artery causing the closure of the artery's lumen.

Takayasu's a. Uncommon disease of medium- and large-sized arteries, characterized by inflammation of the vessels and narrowing of their lumen; it affects all arteries but has a strong predilection for the aortic arch and its branches; most commonly involves the subclavian arteries, followed by the aortic arch, ascending aorta, carotid arteries, and femoral arteries. Symptoms include fever, night sweats, joint pain, appetite and weight loss, and general malaise; pulses are usually absent in the involved arteries. The condition is most prevalent in adolescent girls and young women. Also called aortic arch syndrome; pulseless disease; Takayasu's syndrome.

temporal a. (TA) Inflammation of medium- and large-sized arteries most frequently involving the temporal arteries; associated with polymyalgia rheumatica and, if untreated, may lead to blindness; manifestations include headache, fever, elevated erythrocyte sedimentation rate, and anemia; cause is unknown. Also called giant cell arteritis.

artery (ar´ter-e) A vessel that transports blood away from the heart to different parts of the body; in the normal state after birth, all arteries conduct oxygenated blood except the pulmonary arteries which transport unoxygenated blood from the heart to the lungs.

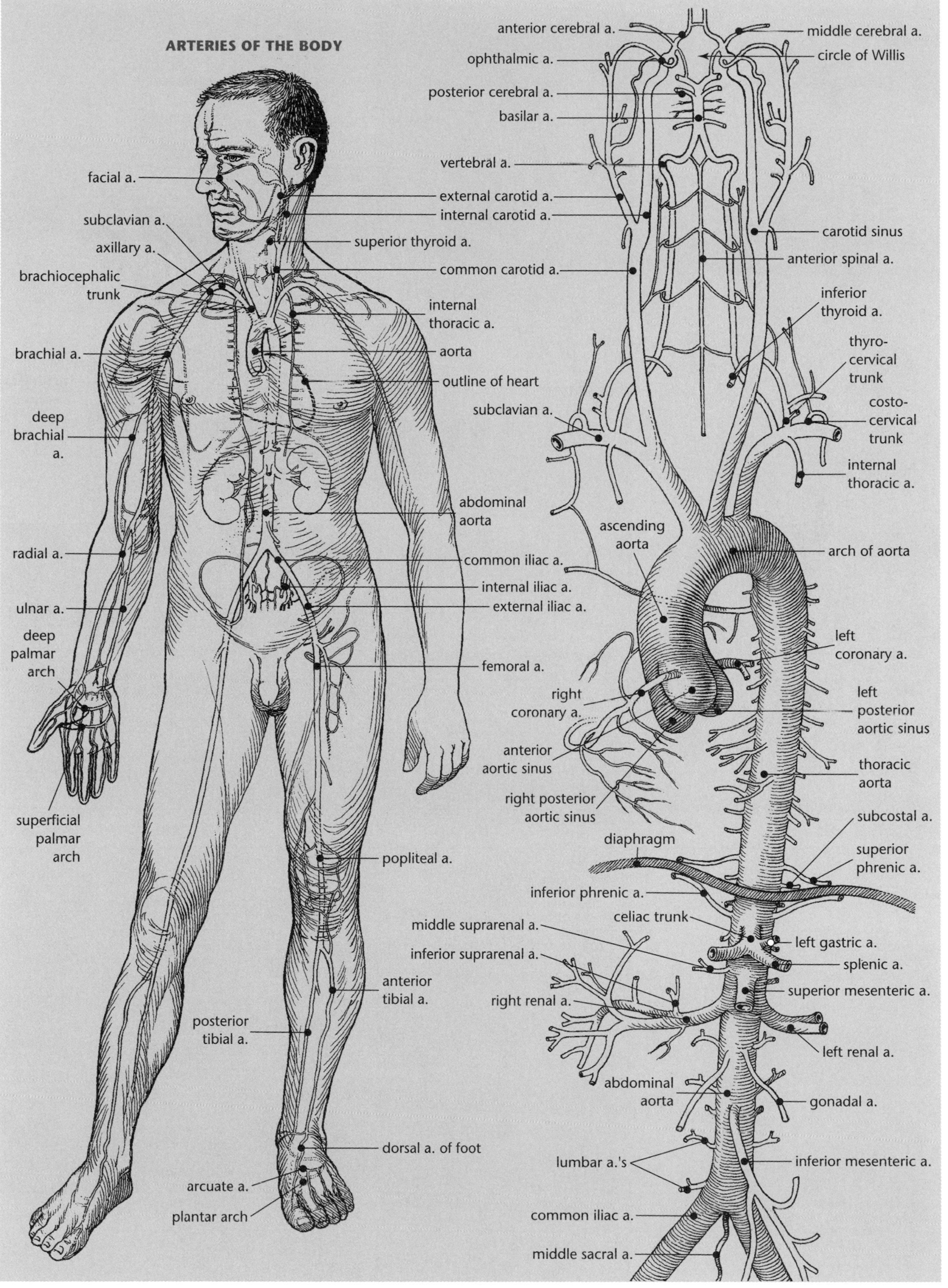
ARTERIES OF THE BODY
facial a.
subclavian a.
axillary a.
brachiocephalic trunk
brachial a.
deep brachial a.
radial a.
ulnar a.
deep palmar arch
superficial palmar arch
external carotid a.
internal carotid a.
superior thyroid a.
common carotid a.
internal thoracic a.
aorta
outline of heart
abdominal aorta
common iliac a.
internal iliac a.
external iliac a.
femoral a.
popliteal a.
anterior tibial a.
posterior tibial a.
dorsal a. of foot
arcuate a.
plantar arch
anterior cerebral a.
ophthalmic a.
posterior cerebral a.
basilar a.
vertebral a.
middle cerebral a.
circle of Willis
carotid sinus
anterior spinal a.
inferior thyroid a.
thyro-cervical trunk
subclavian a.
costo-cervical trunk
internal thoracic a.
ascending aorta
arch of aorta
left coronary a.
right coronary a.
left posterior aortic sinus
anterior aortic sinus
right posterior aortic sinus
thoracic aorta
subcostal a.
diaphragm
superior phrenic a.
inferior phrenic a.
celiac trunk
middle suprarenal a.
left gastric a.
inferior suprarenal a.
splenic a.
superior mesenteric a.
right renal a.
left renal a.
abdominal aorta
gonadal a.
lumbar a.'s
inferior mesenteric a.
common iliac a.
middle sacral a.

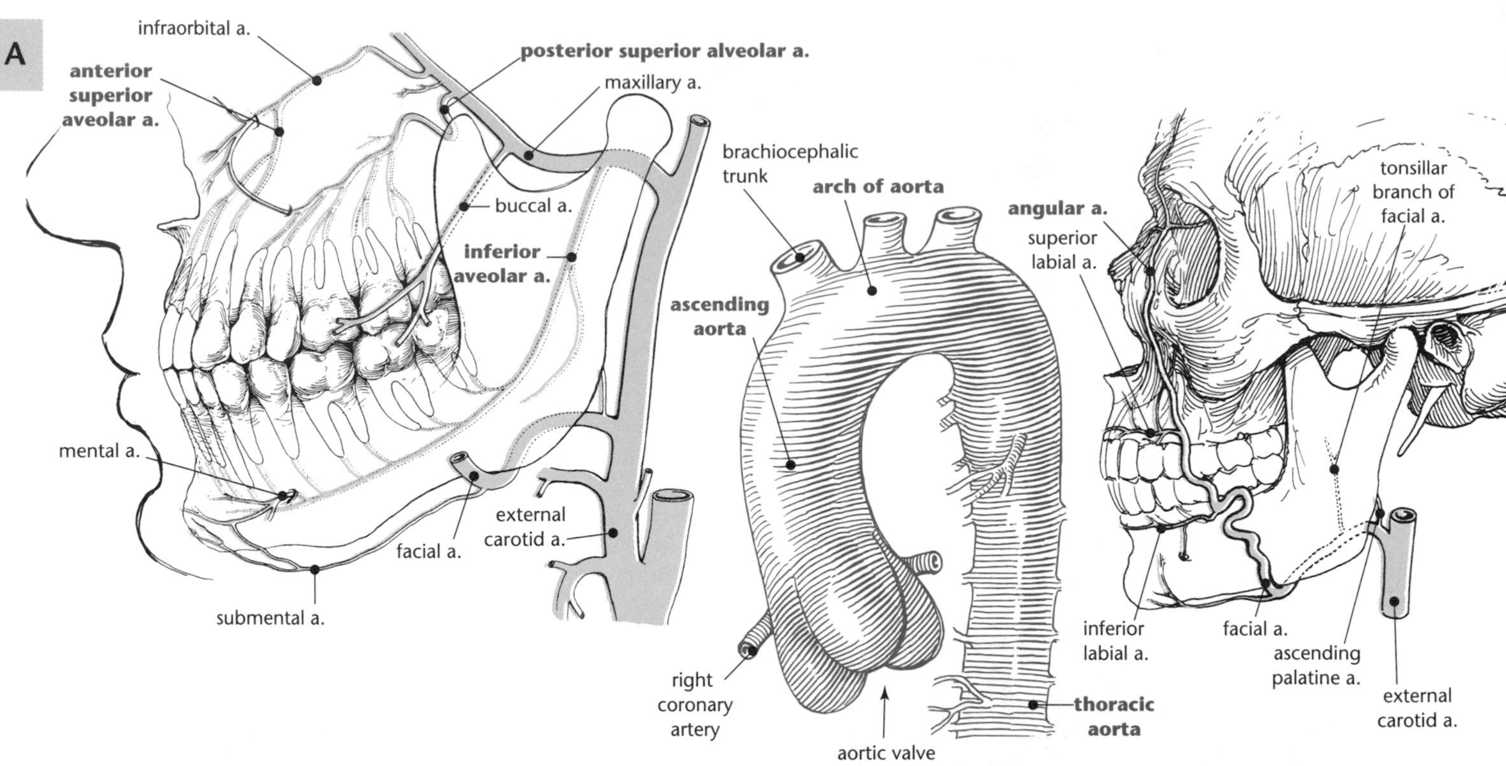

ARTERY	ORIGIN	BRANCHES	DISTRIBUTION
alveolar a., anterior superior anterior dental a. *a. alveolaris superior anterior*	infraorbital a.	dental, peridental	incisor and cuspid teeth of upper jaw, mucous membrane of maxillary sinus
alveolar a., inferior inferior dental a. mandibular a. *a. alveolaris inferior*	maxillary a.	mental, mylohyoid, dental, peridental	mandible and mandibular teeth, gums, lower lip, chin, mylohyoid muscle
alveolar a., posterior superior posterior superior dental a. *a. alveolaris superior posterior*	maxillary a.	dental, antral, alveolar, muscular	molar and bicupsid teeth of upper jaw, mucosa of maxillary sinus, gums
angular a. *a. angularis*	facial a.	muscular, lacrimal	muscle und skin of side of nose, lacrimal sac
aorta *aorta*	left ventricle at aortic valves		see specific branches
ascending aorta *aorta ascendens*	left ventricle at aortic valves	right coronary, left coronary	
arch of aorta *arcus aortae*	continuation of ascending aorta at level of the upper border of the right second sternocostal articulation	brachiocephalic trunk, left common carotid, left subclavian; continues as thoracic aorta at fourth thoracic vertebra	
thoracic aorta *aorta throacica*	continuation of arch of aorta at fourth thoracic vertebra	*visceral portion:* pericardial, bronchial, esophageal, mediastinal; *parietal portion:* posterior intercostal, subcostal, superior phrenic; continues as abdominal aorta at the aortic hiatus of diaphragm	
abdominal aorta *aorta abdominalis*	continuation of thoracic aorta at the aortic hiatus of diaphragm, usually at level of last thoracic vertebra	*visceral portion:* celiac, superior mesenteric, inferior mesenteric, middle suprarenal, renal, testicular, ovarian; *parietal portion:* inferior phrenic, lumbar, middle sacral; continues as common iliac arteries at fourth lumbar vertebra	
appendicular a. *a. appendicularis*	ileocolic a.	none	vermiform appendix
arch, deep palmar		see palmar arch, deep	
arch, plantar		see plantar arch	

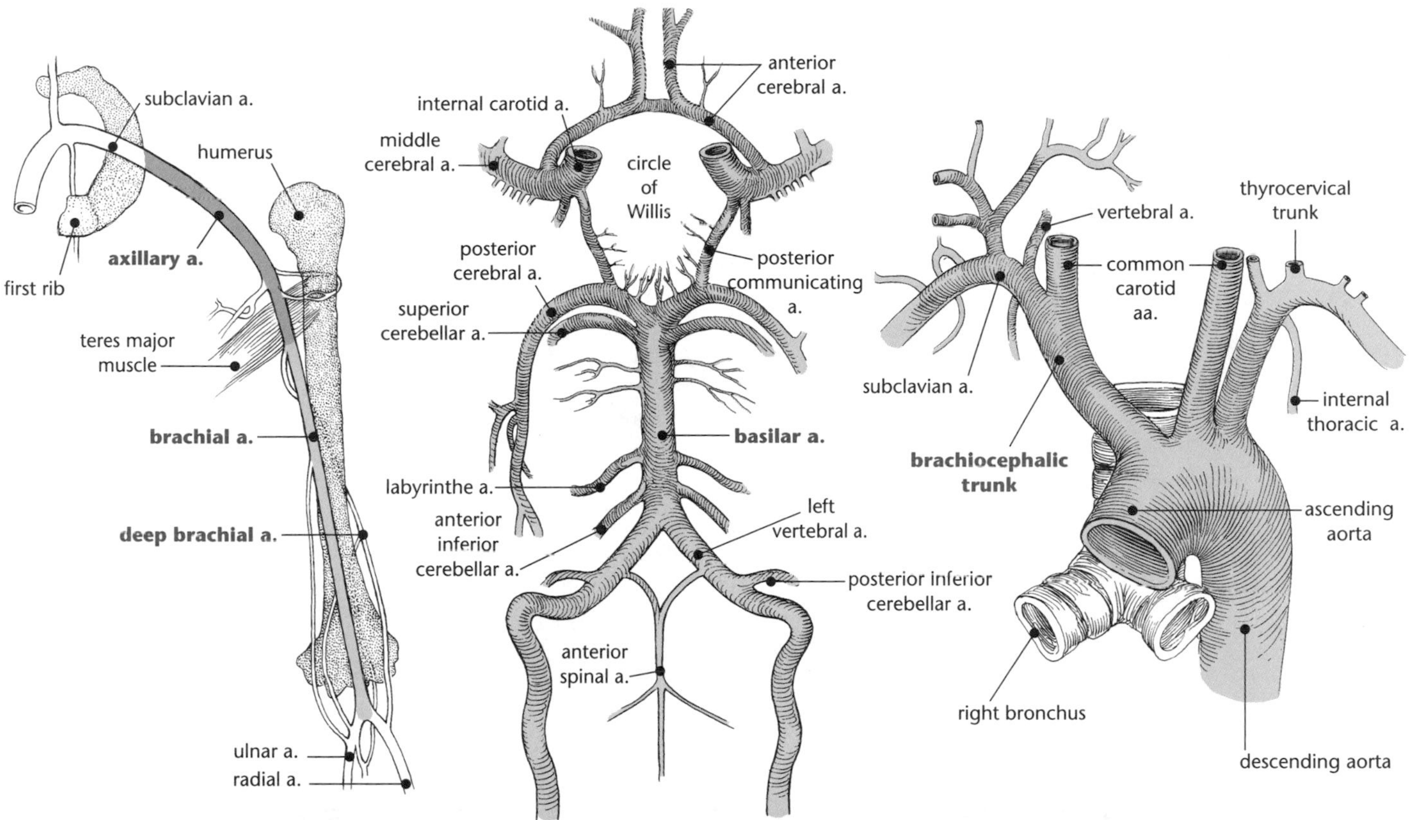

ARTERY	ORIGIN	BRANCHES	DISTRIBUTION
arch, superficial palmar		see palmar arch, superficial	
arcuate a. of foot metatarsal a. *a. arcuata pedis*	dorsal a. of foot	second, third, and fourth metatarsal arteries	foot, sides of toes
arcuate a.'s of kidney *aa. arcuatae renis*	interlobar a.	interlobular arteries	parenchyma of kidney
auditory a., internal		see labyrinthine artery	
auricular a., deep *a. auricularis profunda*	maxillary a.	temporomandibular	cuticular lining of external auditory canal, outer surface of tympanic membrane, temporomandibular joint
auricular a., posterior *a. auricolaris posterior*	external carotid a.	stylomastoid, auricular, occipital, parotid	middle ear, mastoid air cells, auricle, parotid gland, digastric, stapedius and neck muscles
axillary a. *a. axillaris*	continuation of subclavian a. beginning at outer border of first rib	*first part:* highest thoracic; *second part:* thoracoacromial, lateral thoracic; *third part:* subscapular, posterior humeral circumflex, anterior humeral circumflex	pectoral muscles, muscles of shoulder and upper arm, acromion, shoulder joint, sternoclavicular joint, breast
basilar a. *a. basilaris*	from union of right and left vertebral arteries	pontine, labyrinthine, anterior inferior cerebellar, superior cerebellar, posterior cerebral	pons, inner ear, cerebellum, pineal body, ventricles, posterior part of cerebrum
brachial a. *a. brachialis*	continuation of axillary a. at lower border of tendon of teres major muscle	deep brachial, nutrient of humerus, superior ulnar collateral, inferior ulnar collateral, muscular	muscles of shoulder, arm, forearm, and hand; elbow joint
brachial a., deep *superior profunda a.* *a. profunda brachii*	brachial a.	nutrient, deltoid middle col lateral, radial collateral, muscular	humerus, elbow joint, muscles of upper arm including triceps and deltoid
brachiocephalic trunk innominate a. *truncus brachiocephalicus*	beginning of arch of aorta	right common carotid, right subclavian, lowest thyroid thymic, bronchial	right side of head, neck and upper arm, thyroid and thymus glands, and bronchus
bronchial a.'s *aa. bronchiales*	*right side:* first aortic intercostal; *left side:* thoracic aorta	none	bronchial tubes, alveolar tissue of lungs, bronchial lymph nodes, esophagus

A

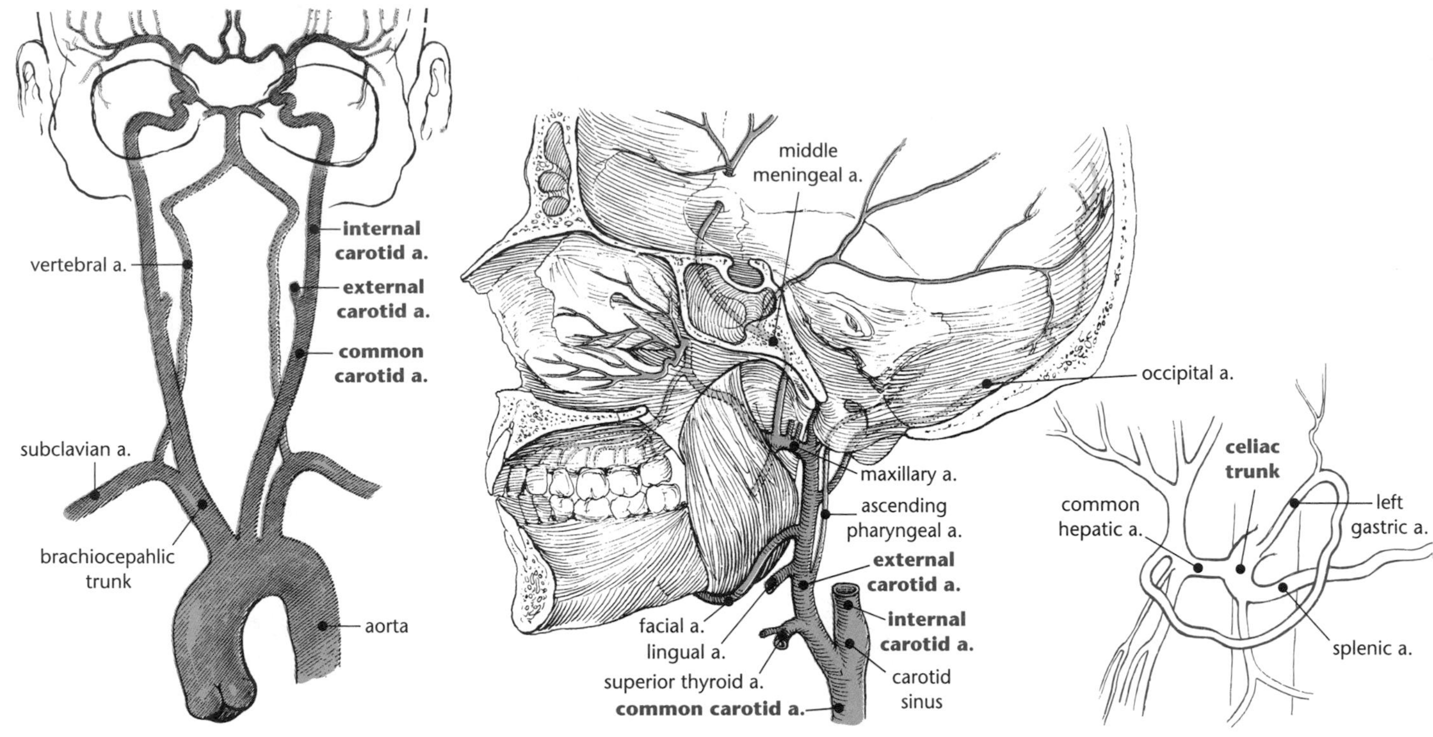

ARTERY	ORIGIN	BRANCHES	DISTRIBUTION
buccal a. buccinator a. *a. buccalis*	maxillary a.	muscular	buccinator muscle, mucosa of maxillary gums, mucosa and skin of cheeks
a. of bulb of penis *a. bulbi penis*	internal pudendal a.	bulbourethral	bulb of penis, posterior part of corpus spongiosum, bulbourethral gland
a. of bulb of vaginal vestibule *a. bulbi vestibuli vaginae*	internal pudendal a.	none	bulb of vestibule, greater vestibular glands
calcaneal a's., medial internal calcaneal a's.. *rami calcanei mediales*	posterior tibial a.	none cles on tibial side of sole	skin and fat in back of calcaneal tendon and heel; mus-
capsular a.'s, middle		see suprarenal arteries, middle	
carotid a., common *a. carotis communis*	*right side:* bifurcation of the brachiocephalic trunk; *left side:* highest part of arch of aorta	external carotid, internal carotid	head
carotid a., external *a. carotis externa*	common carotid a.	*anterior part:* facial, superior thyroid, lingual; *posterior part:* occipital, posterior auricular; *medial part:* ascending pharyngeal; *terminal part:* superficial temporal, maxillary	anterior aspect of face and neck, side of head, skull, dura mater, posterior part of scalp
carotid a., internal *a. carotis interna*	common carotid a.	*cervical part:* carotid sinus; *petrous part:* caroticotympanic, pterygoid canal; *cavernous part:* cavernous sinus, tentorial, inferior hypophyseal, meningeal, trigeminal, and trochlear; *cerebral part:* superior hypophyseal, ophthalmic, anterior choroidal, anterior and middle cerebral, posterior communicating	middle ear, brain, hypophysis, trigeminal ganglion, meninges, orbit, choroid plexus
celiac trunk celiac artery *truncus celiacus*	abdominal aorta, just caudal to aortic hiatus of diaphragm	left gastric, common hepatic, splenic	esophagus, stomach, duodenum, spleen, pancreas, liver, gallbladder, greater omentum, common bile duct

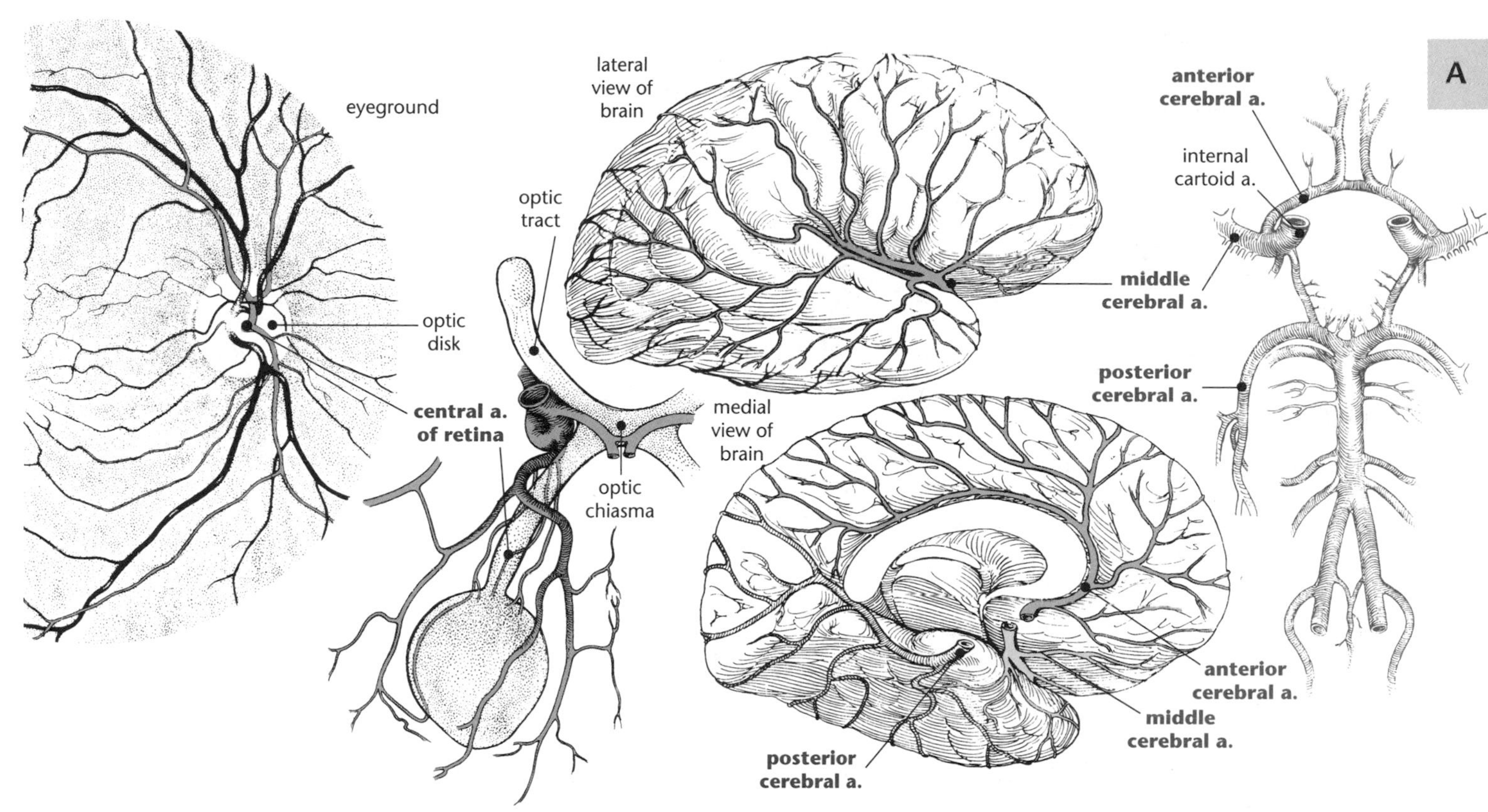

ARTERY	ORIGIN	BRANCHES	DISTRIBUTION
central a. of retina *a. centralis retinae*	ophthalmic a. or lacrimal a.	superior, inferior	retina
cerebellar a., anterior inferior *a. cerebelli inferior anterior*	basilar a.	labyrinthine, posterior spinal	anterior part of inferior surface at cerebellum
cerebellar a., posterior inferior *a. cerebelli inferior posterior*	vertebral a.	medial, lateral	inferior surface of cerebellum, medulla oblongata, choroid plexus at fourth ventricle
cerebellar a., superior *a. cerebelli superior*	basilar a. near its termination	none	superior surface of cerebellum, vermis of cerebellum, pineal body, pia mater, pons, superior medullary velum, choroid plexus at third ventricle
cerebral a., anterior *a. cerebri anterior*	internal carotid a. at the medial extremity of the lateral cerebral sulcus	*precommunicating part:* anterior communicating short, long (recurrent), and anterocentral; *postcommunicating part:* medial, frontobasal, callosomarginal, paracentral, precuneal, parietooccipital	hypothalamus, caudate nucleus, internal capsule, choroid plexus, lateral ventricle, corpus striatum, corpus callosum, frontal lobe, parietal lobe
cerebral a., middle *a. cerebri media*	internal carotid a.	*sphenoidal part:* anterolateral central; *insular part:* insula, lateral frontobasal, anterior, medial, and posterior temporal; *terminal part:* central, precentral, and postcentral sulcus, anterior and posterior parietal, angular gyrus	lentiform nucleus, internal capsule, caudate nucleus, corpus striatum, insula, motor, premotor, sensory, and auditory areas, lateral surface at cerebral hemisphere
cerebral a., posterior *a. cerebri posterior*	terminal bifurcation of basilar a.	*precommunicating part:* posteromedial central; *postcommunicating part:* posterolateral central, thalamus, peduncular, posteromedial, and posterolateral choroidal;	thalmus, third ventricle, globus pallidus, cerebral peduncle, colliculi, pineal body, medial and lateral geniculate bodies, uncus, parahippocampal, medial and lateral

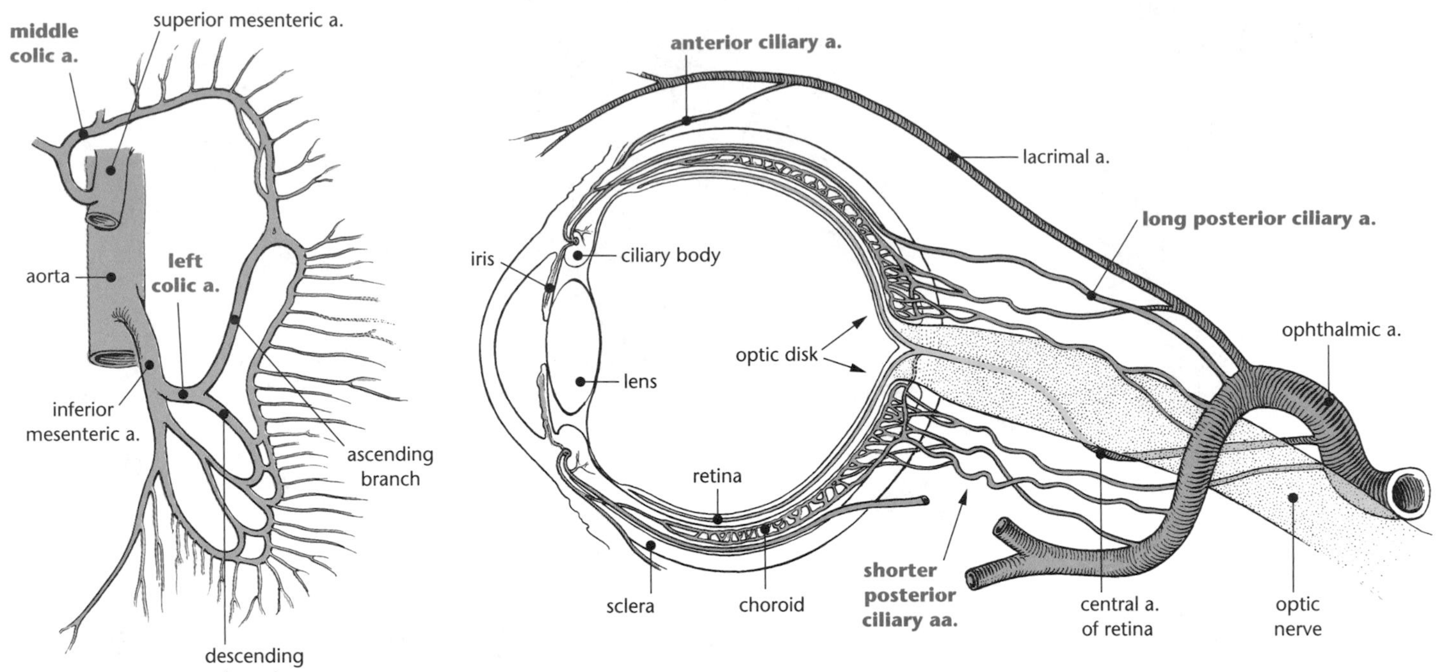

ARTERY	ORIGIN	BRANCHES	DISTRIBUTION
cervical a., ascending *a. cervicalis ascendens*	inferior thyroid a.	spinal	muscles of neck, vertebral canal, vertebrae
cervical a., deep *a. cervicalis profunda*	costocervical trunk	spinal, muscular	spinal card, deep neck muscles
cervical a., superficial *a. cervicalis superficialis*	thyrocervical trunk	ascending, descending	trapezius and neighboring muscles
cervical a., transverse *a. transversa colli* *a. transversa cervicis*	thyrocervical trunk	superficial cervical, dorsal scapular	trapezius, levator m. of scapula, supraspinous m.
choroid a., anterior *a. choroidea anterior*	internal carotid a.	choroid plexus, optic tract, lateral geniculate body, internal capsule, cerebral peduncle, caudate nucleus, hypothalamus and surrounding area	internal capsule, choroid plexus of the inferior horn of lateral ventricle, optic tract, cerebral peduncle, base of brain, lateral geniculate body, caudate nucleus
choroid a., posterior *a. choroidea posterior*	posterior cerebral a.	medial, lateral	choroid plexuses of lateral and third ventricles
ciliary a.'s, anterior *aa. ciliares anteriores*	ophthalmic a.	episcleral, conjunctical, iridic	conjunctiva, iris
ciliary a.'s, long posterior (two in number) *aa. ciliares posteriores longae*	ophthalmic a.	iris, muscular	iris, ciliary body of eye
ciliary a.'s, short posterior (6–12 in number) *aa. ciliares posteriores breves*	ophthalmic a. or one of its branches	none	choroid layer and ciliary processes of eyeball
circumflex a., anterior humeral		see humeral circumflex artery, anterior	
circumflex a., lateral femoral		see femoral circumflex artery, lateral	
circumflex a., medial femoral		see femoral circumflex artery, medial	
circumflex a., posterior humeral		see humeral circumflex artery, posterior	
circumflex a., scapular		see scapular circumflex artery	
circumflex iliac a., deep **circumflex iliac a., superficial**		see iliac circumflex artery, deep see iliac circumflex artery, superficial	
clitoris, deep a. of *a. profunda clitoridis*	internal pudendal a.	none	corpus cavernosum of clitoris
clitoris, dorsal a. of *a. dorsalis clitoridis*	internal pudendal a.	none	glans and prepuce of clitoris
coccygeal a.		see sacral artery, middle	
colic a., left *a. colica sinistra*	inferior mesenteric a.	ascending, descending	descending colon, left part of transverse colon

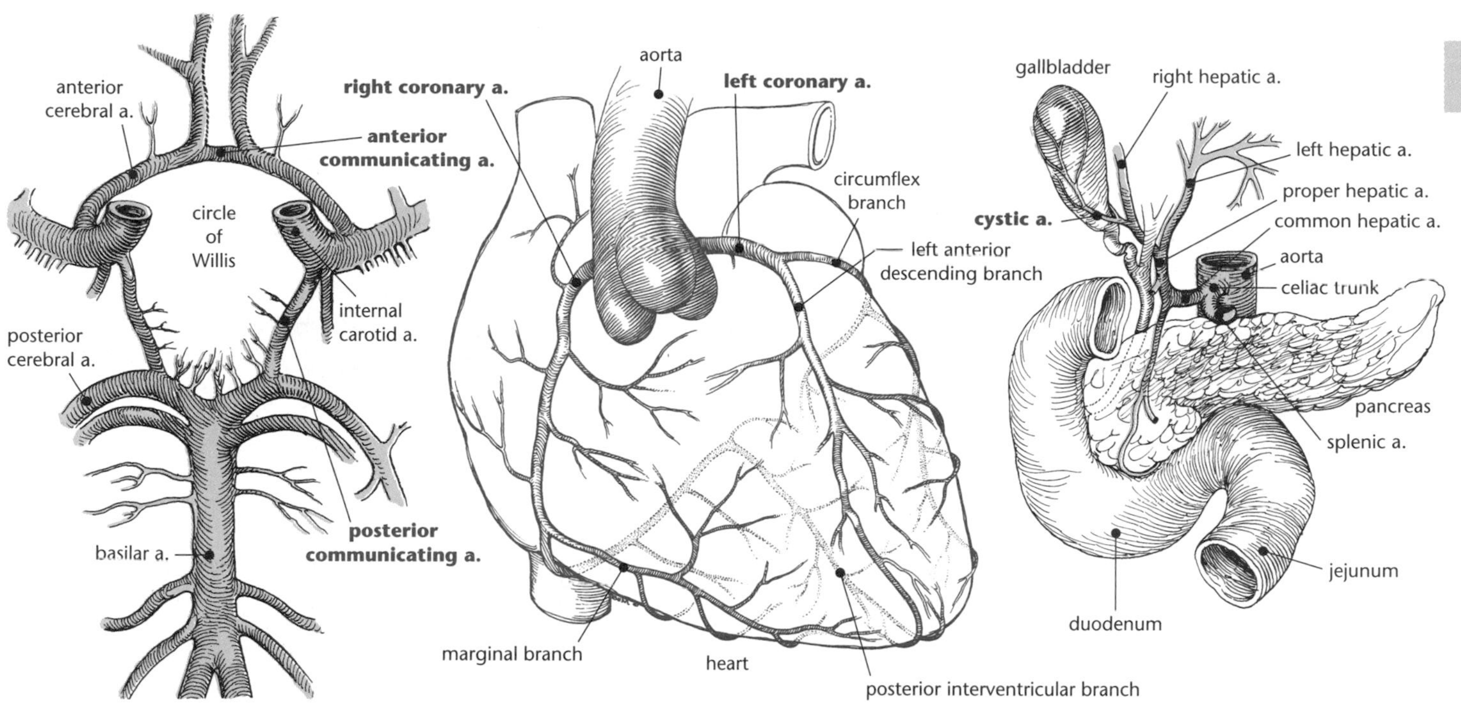

ARTERY	ORIGIN	BRANCHES	DISTRIBUTION
colic a., middle *a. colica media*	superior mesenteric a., just caudal to the pancreas	right, left	transverse colon
colic a., right *a. colica dextra*	superior mesenteric a. or ileocolic a.	descending, ascending	ascending colon
collateral a., inferior ulnar anastomotica magna a. *a. collateralis ulnaris inferior*	brachial a., about 5 cm proximal to elbow	posterior, anterior, anastomotic	triceps, elbow joint, round pronator muscle
collateral a., middle *a. collateralis media*	deep brachial a.	muscular, anastomotic	elbow joint, triceps and anconeus muscles
collateral a., radial *a. collateralis radialis*	continuation of deep brachial a.	muscular, anastomotic	triceps, elbow joint, brachioradial and brachial muscles
collateral a., superior ulnar inferior profunda a. *a. collateralils ulnaris superior*	brachial a., distal to middle of arm	muscular, articular, anastomotic	elbow joint, triceps muscle of arm
communicating a., anterior *a. communicans anterior cerebri*	anterior cerebral a. (connects the two anterior cerebral arteries)	anteromedial	anterior perforated substance of the brain
communicating a., posterior *a. communicans posterior cerebri*	connects the internal carotid a. with posterior cerebral a.	hypophyseal	base of brain between infundibulum and optic tract; internal capsule, anterior third of thalamus; third ventricle
conjunctival a.'s ,anterior *aa. conjunctivales anteriores*	anterior ciliary a.'s	none	conjunctiva
conjunctiva a.'s, posterior *aa. conjunctivales posteriores*	peripheral tarsal arch	none	conjunctiva
coronary a., left *a. coronaria sinistra*	aorta at left aortic sinus	sinoatrial nodal, anterior interventricular (anterior descending), left atrial, circumflex	sinoatrial node, interventricular septum, left atrium, left and right ventricles
coronary a., right *a. coronaria dextra*	aorta at right aortic sinus	marginal, sinoatrial nodal, right atrial, posterior interventricular (posterior descending), atrioventricular nodal	sinoatrial node, atrioventricular node, right atrium, interventricular septum, right and left ventricles
costocervical trunk superior intercostal a. *truncus costocervicalis*	subclavian a.	deep cervical; continues as the highest intercostal a.	deep neck muscles, first and second intercostal spaces, vertebral column
cremasteric a. exernal spermatic a. *a. cremasterica*	inferior epigastric a.	none	cremaster muscle, coverings of spermatic cord
cystic a. *a. cystico*	right hepatic a.	superficial, deep	gallbladder

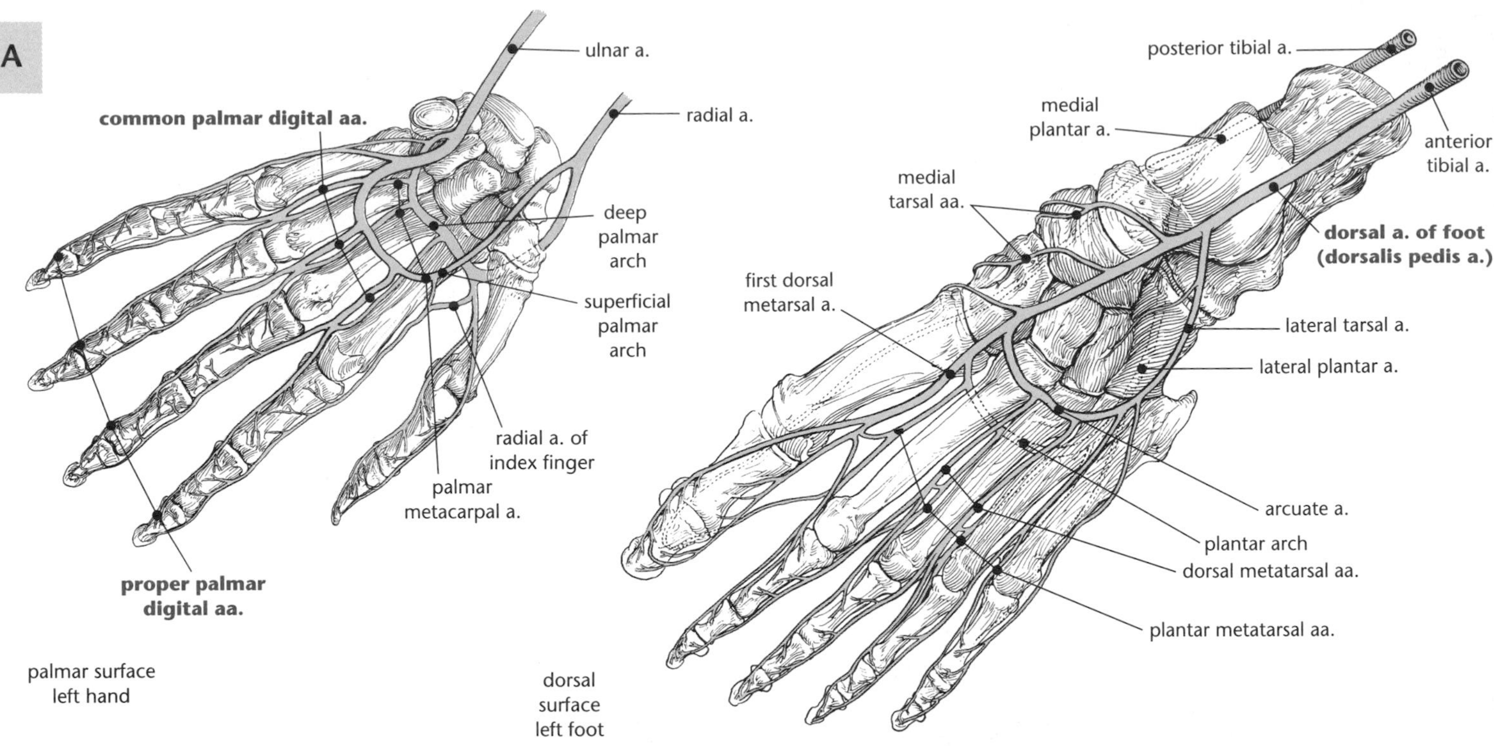

ARTERY	ORIGIN	BRANCHES	DISTRIBUTION
deep a. of clitoris		see clitoris, deep artery of	
deep a. of penis		see penis, deep artery of	
deferential a. a. of ductus deferens *a. ductus deferentis*	umbilical a. (embryonic), superior vesical a.	ureteric	ductus deferens, bladder, seminal vesicles, ureter, testicle
dental a., anterior		see alveolar artery, anterior superior	
dental a., inferior		see alveolar artery, inferior	
dental a., posterior		see alveolar artery, posterior superior	
diaphragmatic a., inferior		see phrenic artery	
digital a.'s, collateral		see digital arteries, paper palmar	
digital a.'s, common palmar (three in number) volar digital a.'s *aa. digitales palmares communes*	superficial palmar arch	proper palmar, digital	fingers
digital a.'s, common plantar *aa. digitales plaantares communes*	plantar metatarsal a.'s	proper plantar, digital	toes
digital a.'s of foot, common		see metatarsal arteries, plantar	
digital a.'s, proper palmar collateral digital a.'s *aa. digitales palmares propriae*	common palmar digital a.'s	dorsal	the sides of each finger, matrix of fingernails
digital a.'s, proper plantar *aa. digitales plantares propriae*	common plantar digital a.'s	none	toes
dorsal a. of clitoris		see clitoris, dorsal artery of	
dorsal a. of foot dorsalis pedis a. dorsal pedal a. *a. dorsalis pedis* (anastomoses with lateral plantar a. to form plantar arterial arch)	continuation of anterior tibial a. at ankle joint	lateral tarsal, medial tarsal, arcuate, dorsal metatarsal, deep plantar, dorsal digital (continues to first intermetatarsal space where it divides into first dorsal metatarsal and deep plantar arteries)	foot
dorsal a. of penis		see penis, dorsal artery of	
dorsalis pedis a.		see dorsal artery of foot	
a. of ductus deferens		see deferential artery	
duodenal a.		see pancreaticoduodenal artery, inferior	
epigastric a., deep		see epigastric artery, inferior	

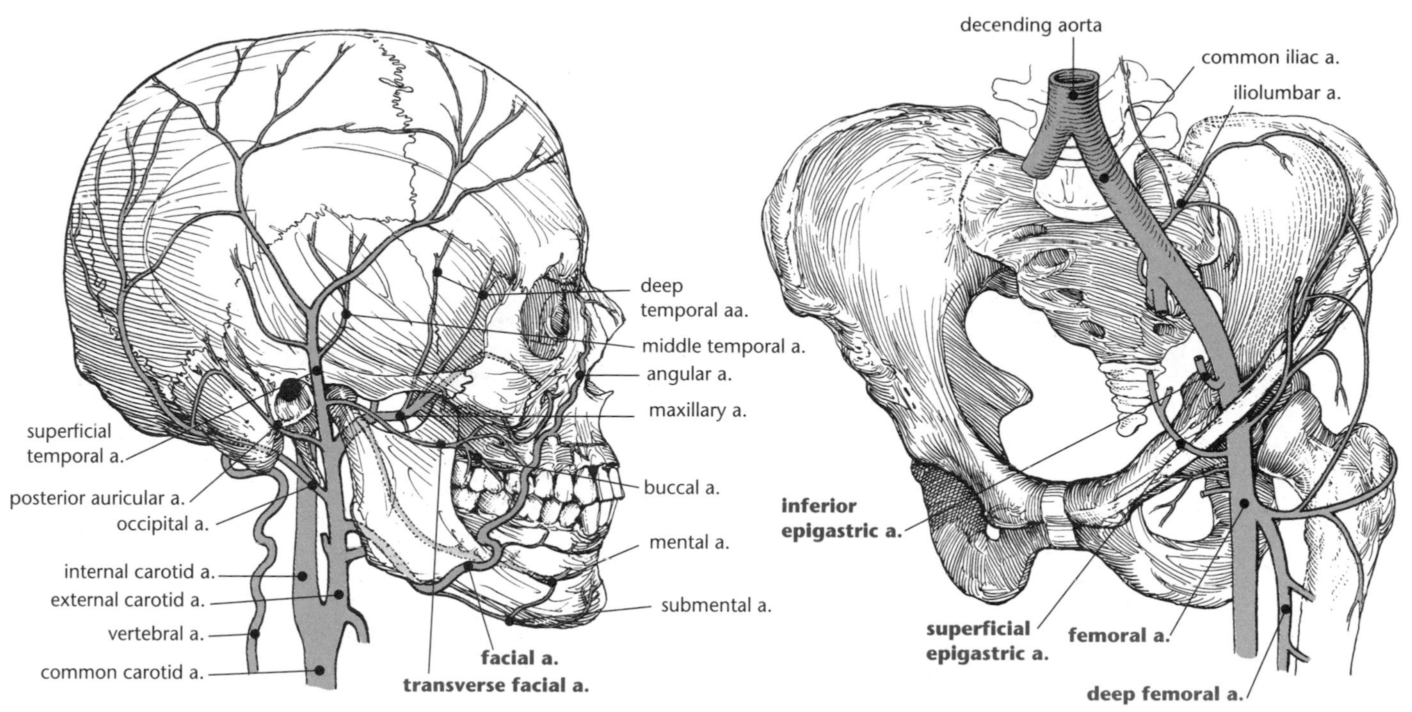

ARTERY	ORIGIN	BRANCHES	DISTRIBUTION
epigastric a., inferior deep epigastric a. *a. epigastrica inferior*	external iliac, immediately above inguinal ligament	cremasteric, pubic, muscular, round ligament of uterus	cremaster and abdominal muscles peritoneum, skin
epigastric a., superficial *a. epigastrica superficialis*	femoral a. about 1 cm below inguinal ligament	none	lower part of abdominal wall, superficial lingual lymph nodes, skin
epigastric a., superior *a. epigastrica superior*	internal thoracic a.	cutaneous, muscular, peritoneal, phrenic, hepatic	skin, muscles and fascia of upper part of abdominal wall; diaphragm, peritoneum, faliciform ligament of liver
episcleral a. *a. episcleralis*	anterior ciliary a.	none	iris, ciliary body, sclera, conjunctiva
esophageal a.'s (four to five in number) *aa. esophagei*	thoracic aorta; inferior thyroid and left gastric a.'s	none	esophagus
ethmoidal a., anterior *a. ethmoidalis anterior*	ophthalmic a.	meningeal, nasal	anterior and middle ethmoid air cells, frontal sinus, dura mater, nasal cavity
ethmoidal a., posterior *a. ethmoidalis posterior*	ophthalmic a.	meningeal, nasal	posterior ethmoid air cells, dura mater, nasal cavity
facial a. external maxillary a. *a. facialis*	external carotid a.	*cervical portion:* ascending palatine, tonsillar, glandular, submental; *facial portion:* inferior labial, superior labial, lateral nasal, angular, muscular	face, tonsil, palate, labial glands and muscles of lips submandibular gland, ala and dorsum of nose, muscles of expression
facial a., deep		see maxillary artery	
facial a., transverse *a. transversa faciei*	superficial temporal a. while still in parotid glaisd	glandular, muscular, cutaneous	parotid gland and duct, masseter muscle, skin of face
femoral a. *a. femoralis*	continuation of external iliac a. immediately distal to inguinal ligament	superficial epigastric, superficial circumflex iliac, external pudendal, descending genicular, deep femoral, muscular	integument of abdominal wall, groin, and perineum; muscles of thigh, external genitals, inguinal lymph nodes
femoral a., deep profunda femoris a. *a. profunda femoris*	femoral a.	medial femoral circumflex, lateral femoral circumflex, perforating muscular	muscles of thigh, hip joint, head and shaft of femur, gluteal muscles

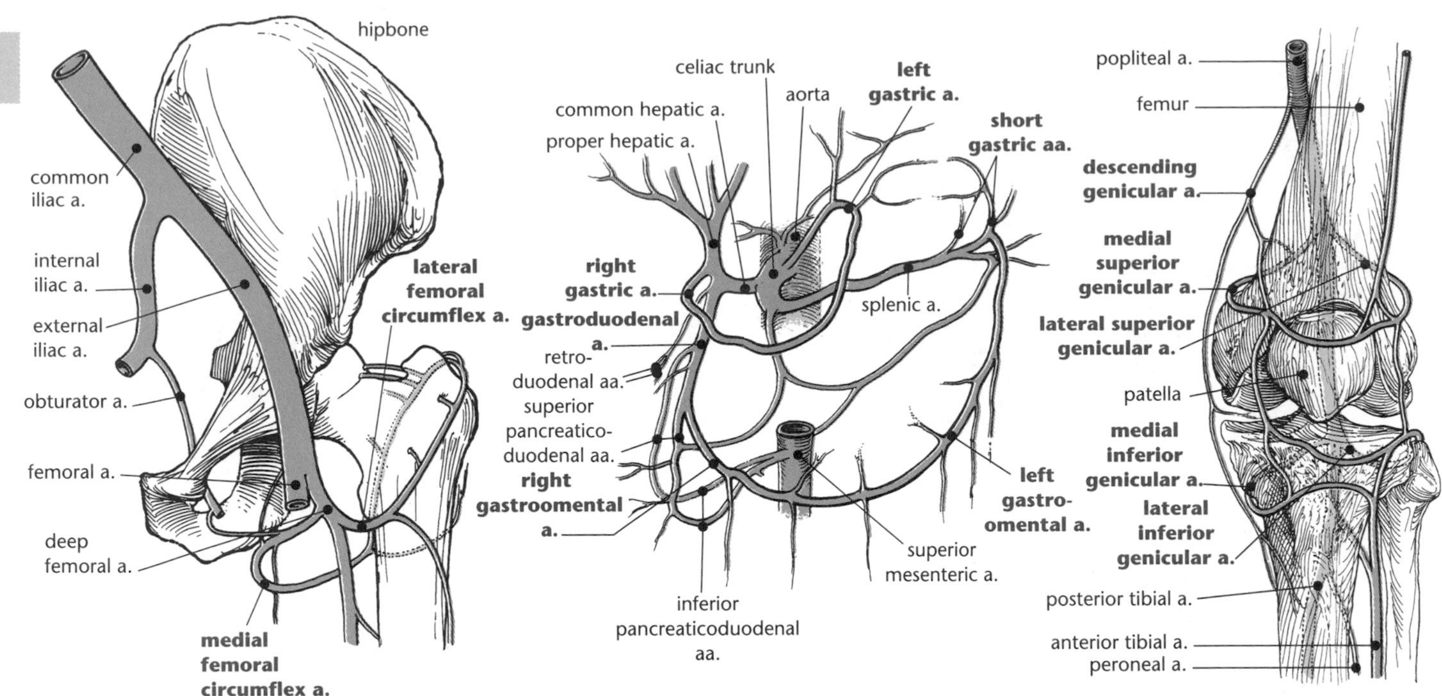

ARTERY	ORIGIN	BRANCHES	DISTRIBUTION
femoral circumflex a., lateral lateral circumflex a. of thigh *a. circumflexa femoris lateralis*	deep femoral a.	ascending, descending, transverse	hip joint, thigh muscles
femoral circumflex a., medial osedial circumflex a. of thigh *a. circumflexa femoris medialis*	deep femoral a.	deep, ascending, transverse, acetabular	hip joint, thigh muscles
fibular a.		see peroneal artery	
frontal a.		see supratrochlear artery	
gastric a., left *a. gastrica sinistra*	celiac trunk	esophageal, pyloric, cardiac (stomach)	lesser curvature of stomach, abdominal part of esophagus; left lobe of liver (at times)
gastric a., right *a. gastrica dextra*	common hepatic a. or proper hepatic a.	none	pyloric end of stomach along lesser curvature
gastric a.'s, short *aa. gastricae breves*	splenic a.	none	fundus of stomach
gastroduodenal a. *a. gastroduodenalis*	common hepatic a.	right gastroepiploic, superior pancreaticoduodenal, retro-duodenal, pancreatic	stomach, duodenum, pan-creas, greater omentum
gastroomental a., left gastroepiploic a., left *a. gastroomentalis sinistra*	splenic a.	gastric, omental (epiploic)	stomach, greater omentum
gastroomental a., right gastroepiploic a., right *a. gastroomentalis dextra*	gastroduodenal a.	gastric, omental (epiploic)	stomach, greater omentum
genicular a., descending descending a. of the knee highest genic-ular a. *a. genus descenden's*	femoral a.	saphenous, articular, muscu-lar	knee joint and adjacent muscles
genicular a., highest		see genicular artery, descending	
genicular a., lateral inferior a. genus lateralis inferior	popliteal a.	none	knee joint, gastrocnemius muscle
genicular a., lateral superior *a. genus lateralis superior*	popliteal a.	none	lower part of femur, knee joint, patella, contiguous muscles
genicular a., medial inferior *a. genus medialis inferior*	popliteal a.	none	proximal end of tibia, knee joint
genicular a. medial superior *a. genus medialis superior*	popliteal a.	none	femur, knee joint, patella contiguous muscles

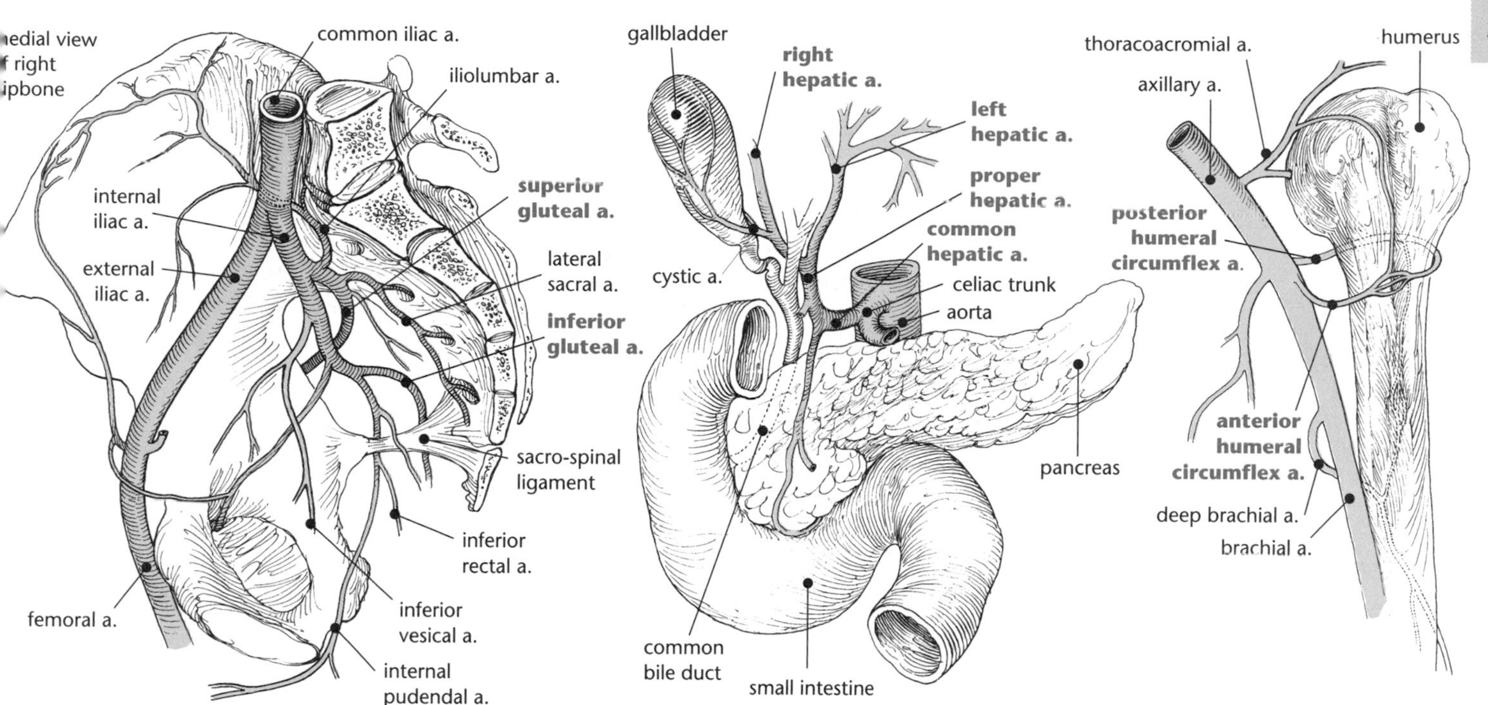

ARTERY	ORIGIN	BRANCHES	DISTRIBUTION
genicular a., middle azygos articular a. *a. genus media*	popliteal a.	none	cruciate ligaments and synovial membrane of knee joint
gluteal a., inferior *a. glutea inferior*	internal iliac a.	sciatic, coccygeal, muscular, articular, cutaneous	muscles at the buttock and back of thigh
gluteal a., superior *a. glutea superior*	internal iliac a.	superficial, deep, nutrient, articular	muscles of hip and buttock; ilium, skin on dorsal surface of sacrum, hip joint
hemorrhoidal a., inferior		see rectal artery, inferior	
hemorrhoidal a., middle		see rectal artery, middle	
hemorrhoidal a., superior		see rectal artery, superior	
hepatic a., common *a. hepatica communis*	celiac trunk	gastroduodenal, proper hepatic, right gastric	stomach, greater omentum, pancreas, duodenum, liver, gallbladder
hepatic a., left *a. hepatica sinista*	proper hepatic a.	caudate lobe, medial segmental, lateral segmental	liver
hepatic a., proper *a. hepatica propria*	common hepatic a.	left hepatic, right hepatic, right gastric	liver, gallbladder, pyloric part at stomach
hepatic a., right *a. hepatica dextra*	proper hepatic a.	cystic, caudate lobe, anterior (left) segmental, posterior (right) segmental	liver and gallbladder
humeral circumflex a., anterior *a. circumflexa humeri anterior*	axillary a.	ascending, descending	head of humerus, shoulder joint, long head of biceps, muscle of arm, deltoid, coracobrachial, tendon of greater pectoral muscle
humeral circumflex a., posterior *a. circumflexa humeri posterior*	axillary a. at distal border of subscapular muscle	muscular, articular, nutrient, descending, acromial	shoulder joints, neck of humerus, deltoid, teres major, teres minor, and triceps muscles
hyaloid a. *a. hyaloidea* (usually disappears in the last month of intrauterine life)	central a. of retina	none	vitreous body, lens of eye
hypogastric a.		see iliac artery, internal	
ileal a.'s *aa. ilei*	superior mesenteric a.	none	ileum

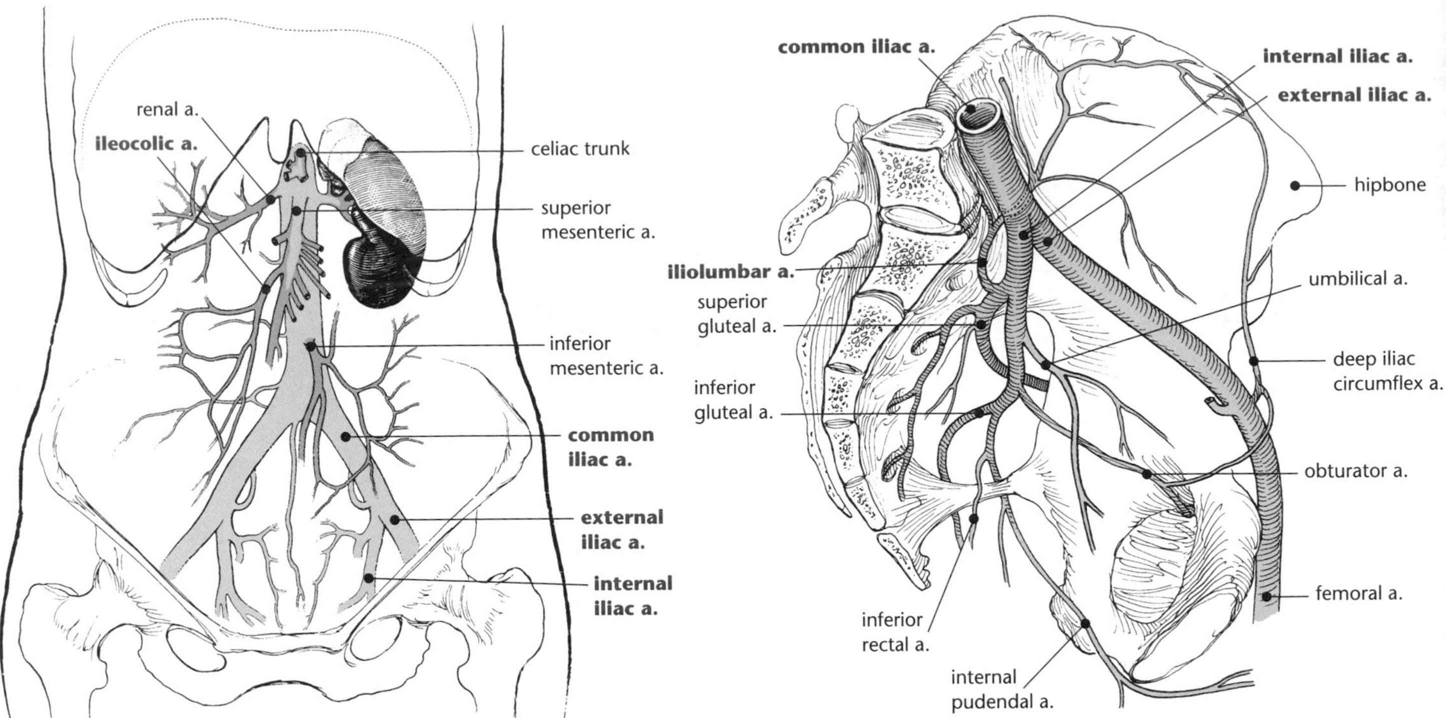

ARTERY	ORIGIN	BRANCHES	DISTRIBUTION
ileocolic a. *a. ileocolica*	superior mesenteric a.	superior (anastomoses with right colic a.), inferior (anastomoses with end of superior mesenteric a.), colic, anterior cecal, posterior cecal, appendicular, ileal	cecum, vermiform, appendix, ascending colon, distal part of ileum
iliac a., common *a. iliaca communis*	abdominal aorta about the level of L4	internal and external iliac	pelvis, genital, and gluteal regions, perineum, tower abdominal wall
iliac a., external *a. iliaca externa*	continuation of common iliac a.	inferior, epigastric, deep iliac circumflex, muscular	lower part at abdominal wall, external genitals, psoas major, cremaster, ductus deferens in male, round ligament of uterus in female
iliac a., internal hypogastric a. *a. iliaco interna*	common iliac a.	*anterior trunk:* obturator superior gluteal, inferior gluteal, umbilical, inferior vesical, uterine, vaginal middle rectal, internal pudendal: *posterior trunk:* iliolumbar, lateral sacra, superior gluteal	wall and viscera pelvis, external genitals, region of anus, medial aspect of thigh, buttock
iliac circumflex a., deep *a. circumflexa illium profounda*	external iliac a.	ascending	psoas, iliac, sartorius, and neighboring muscles; overlying skin, oblique and transverse abdominal muscles
iliac circumflex a., superficial *a. circumflexa ilium superficialis*	femoral a.	none	skin of groin, superficial lingual lymph nodes
iliolumbar a. *a. iliolumbalis*	internal iliac a.	lumbar, iliac, spinal	greater psoas muscle, quadratus, muscle of loins, gluteal and abdominal muscles; ilium, cauda equina
infraorbital a.	maxillary	orbital, anterior superior alveolar, middle superior alveolar	orbit, maxilla, maxillary sinus and teeth, lower eyelid, extrinsic eye muscles, cheek, side of nose
innominate a.		see brachiocephalic trunk	
intercostal a.'s anterior intercostal a.'s *aa. intercostales anteriores*	internal thoracic a.	muscular, cutaneous	first five or six intercostal spaces, pectoral muscles, skin of breast

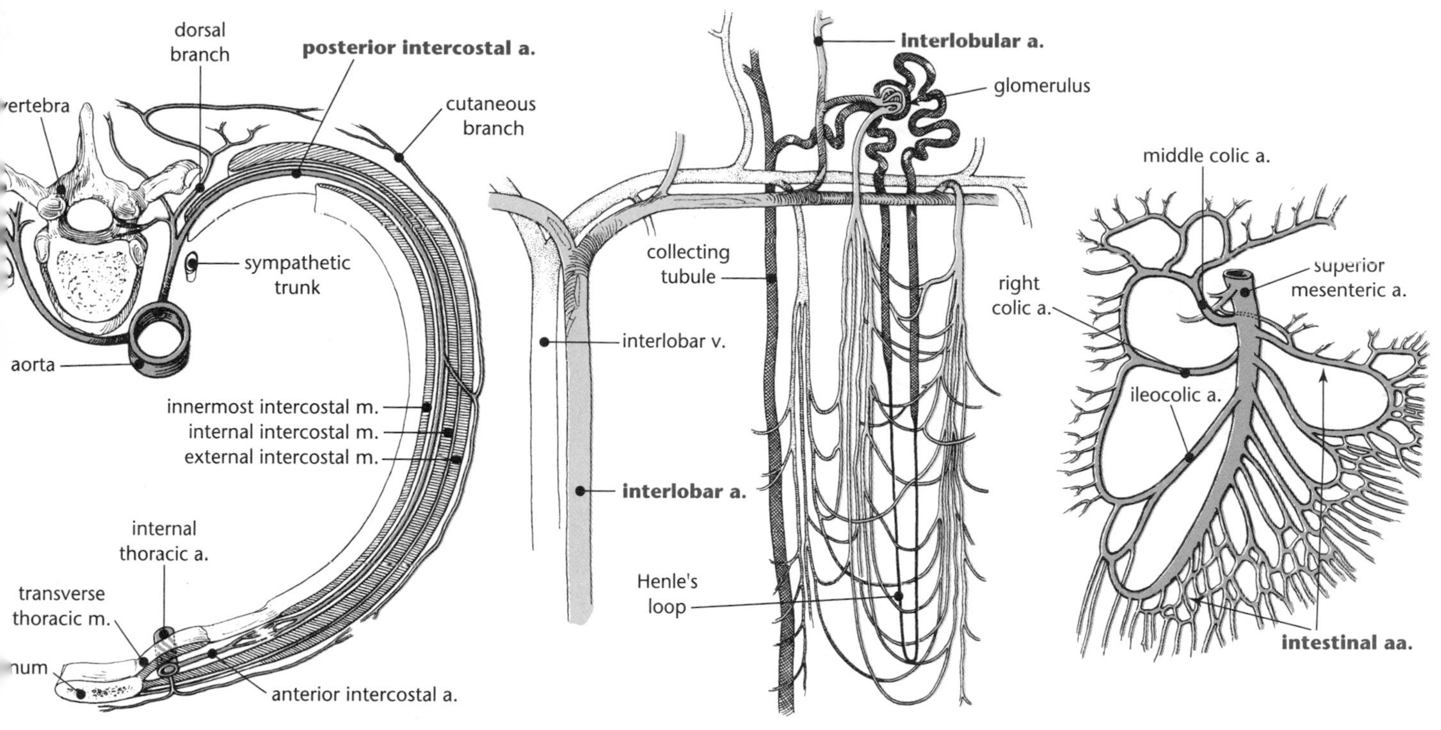

ARTERY	ORIGIN	BRANCHES	DISTRIBUTION
intercostal a., highest *a. intercostalis suprema*	costacervical trunk	first and second posterior intercostal	first and second intercostal spaces, spinal cord, back muscles
intercostal a.'s I-II, posterior *aa. intercostale's posteriores I-II*	highest intercostal a.	dorsal, spinal	upper part of thoracic wall
intercostal a.'s III-XI, posterior *aa. intercostales posteriores III-IX*	thoracic aorta	dorsal, collateral, intercostal lateral, cutaneous, muscular	lower pert of thoracic wall; mammary gland
interlobar a.'s of kidney *aa. interlobares renis*	six segmental branches of renal a.	arcuate	between pyramids of kidney
interlobular a.'s of kidney *aa. interlobulares renis*	arcuate a.'s of kidney	afferent glomeruli	renal glomeruli of kidney
interlobular a.'s of liver *aa. interlobulares hepatis*	right or left branches of proper hepatic a.	none	between lobules of liver
interosseous a., anterior volar interosseous a. *a. interossea anterior*	common interosseous a.	median, muscular, nutrient	deep muscles of front of forearm, radius, ulna
interosseous a., common a. interossen communis	ulnar a., immediately distal to tuberosity of radius	posterior and anterior interosseous	deep muscles of back of forearm, radius, ulna
interosseous a., posterior dorsal interosseous a. *a. interossea posterior*	common interosseous a.	recurrent interosseous	deep muscles of back of forearm
interosseous a.'s, palmar		see metacarpal arteries, palmar	
interosseous a., recurrent *a. interossea recurrens*	posterior interosseous a.	none	back of elbow joint
intestinal a.'s (12–15 in number) *aa. jejunales et ilei* *aa. intestinales*	superior mesenteric a.	none	jejunum, ileum
labial a., inferior *a. labialis inferior*	facial a. near angle of mouth	none	labial glands, mucous membrane, muscles of lower lip
labial a., superior *a. labialis superior*	facial a.	septal, alar	upper lip, nasal septum, ala of nose
labyrinthine a. internal auditory a. *a. labyrinthi*	basilar a. or anterior inferior cerebellar a.	vestibular, cochlear	inner ear
lacrimal a. *a. lacrimalis*	ophthalmic a. close to optic canal	lateral palpebral, zygomatic, recurrent meningeal, long posterior ciliary, muscular	lacrimal gland, conjunctiva, superior and lateral recti muscles, cheek, ciliary processes, eyelids

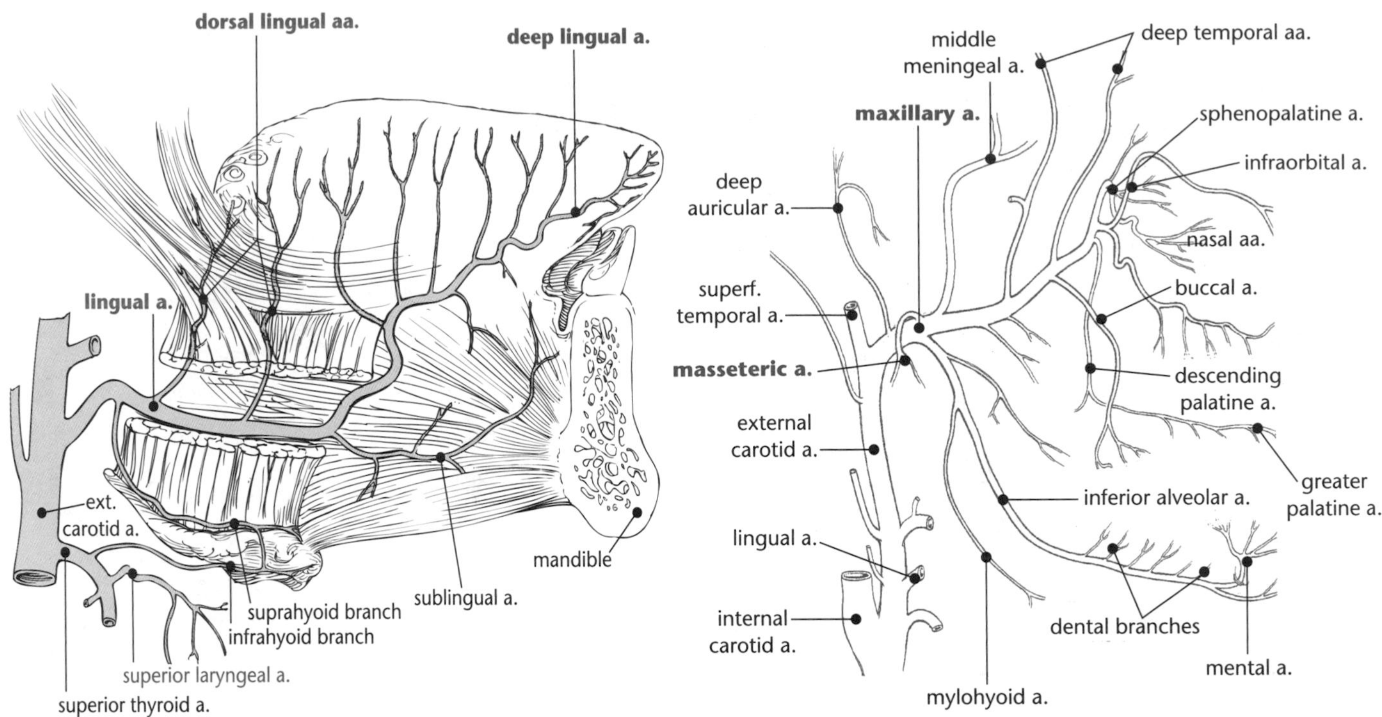

ARTERY	ORIGIN	BRANCHES	DISTRIBUTION
laryngeal a., Inferior *a. laryngea inferior*	inferior thyroid a.	none	muscles of larynx, mucous membrane of larynx
laryngeal a., superior *a. laryngea superior*	superior thyroid a. (occasionally from external carotid a.)	none	muscles, mucous membrane, and glands of larynx
lienal a.		see splenic artery	
lingual a. *a. lingualis*	external carotid a.	suprahyoid, dorsal lingual, sublingual, deep lingual	muscles and mucosa of tongue, sublingual gland, gingiva, tonsil, epiglottis
lingual a., deep ranine a. *a. profunda liguae*	lingual a. (terminal portion)	none	intrinsic lingual muscles, lingual mucosa
lingual a.'s, dorsal *a. lingualis, rami dorsales*	lingual a.	none	mucous membrane of posterior part of tongue; palatoglossal arch, tonsil, epiglottis, soft palate
lumbar a.'s (four to five in number) *aa. lumbales*	abdominal aorta	dorsal, spinal	lumbar vertebrae, hack muscles, abdominal wall
lumbar a., lowest *a. lumbalis ima*	median sacral a.	none	sacrum, iliac muscle
malleolar a., anterior lateral external malleolar a. *a. malleolaris lateralis anterior*	anterior tibial a.	none	lateral side of ankle
malleolar a., anterior medial internal malleolar a. *a. malleolaris medialis anterior*	anterior tibial a.	none	medial side of ankle
malleolar a., posterior medial internal malleolar a. *a. malleolaris medialis posterior*	posterior tibial	none	medial side of ankle
mammary a., external		see thoracic artery, lateral	
mammary a., internal		see thoracic artery, internal	
mandibular a.		see alveolar artery, inferior	
masseteric a. *a. masseterica*	maxillary a.	none	masseter muscle
maxillary a. internal maxillary a. deep facial a. *a. maxillaris*	external carotid a.	*mandibular portion:* deep auricular, anterior tympanic, inferior alveolar, middle meningeal, accessory	ear, teeth, dura mater, trigeminal ganglion,temporal, masseter, buccinator, and eye muscles, lacrimal gland, palatine

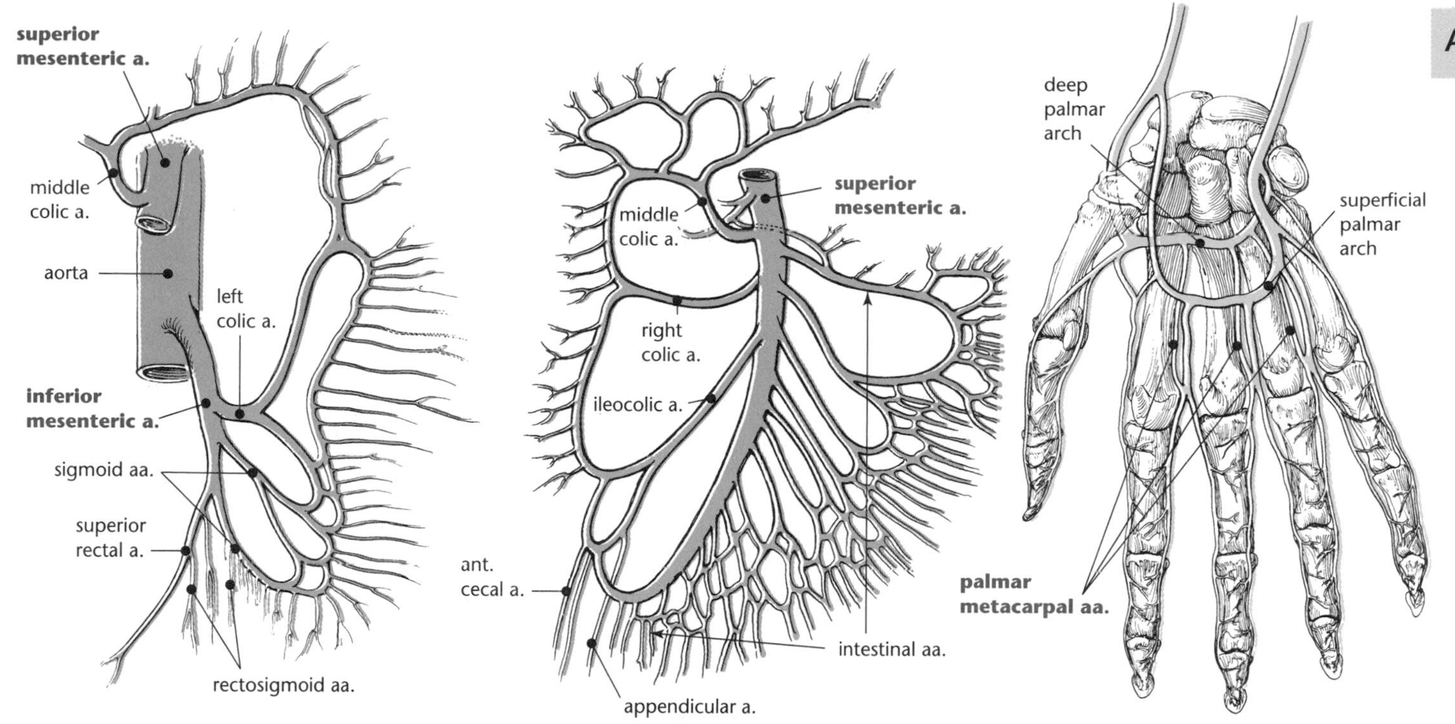

ARTERY	ORIGIN	BRANCHES	DISTRIBUTION
maxillary a. (cont'd)		meningeal; *pterygoid portion:* deep temporal, pterygoid, masseteric, buccal; *pterygopalatine portion;* posterior superior alveolar, infraorbital, descending palatine, artery of the pterygoid canal, pharyngeal, sphenopalatine	tonsil, soft palate, upper pharynx, auditory tube, nasal cavity, sinuses
maxillary a., external		see facial artery	
maxillary a., internal		see maxillary artery	
median a. *aa. mediana*	anterior interosseous a.	none	accompanies and supplies median nerve to palm
medullary a.'s *a. medullares*	vertebral a. and its branches	none	medulla oblongata
meningeal a., anterior *a. meningea anterior*	anterior ethmoidal a. or internal carotid a.	none	dora mater of anterior cranial fossa
meningeal a., middle *a. meningea media*	maxillary a.	frontal, parietal, petrosal, superior tympanic, ganglionic, temporal	cranial bones, dura mater, tensor tympani muscle, trigeminal ganglion, orbit, tympanic cavity
meningeal a., posterior *a. meningea posterior*	ascending pharyngeal a.	none	bone and dura mater of posterior cranial fossa
mesenteric a., inferior *a. mesenterica inferior*	abdominal aorta at level of L3 or L4	left colic, sigmoid, superior rectal	transverse, descending, and sigmoid colon, upper part of rectum
mesentric a., superior *a. meseterica superior*	abdominal aorta one cm below celiac trunk	inferior pancreaticoduodenal, intestinal, ileocolic, right colic, middle colic	small intestine, proximal half of colon
metacarpal a.'s dorsal (three in number) *aa. metacarpeae dorsales*	dorsal carpal branch or radial a.	dorsal digital	back of fingers
metacarpal a.'s, palmar palmar interosseous a.'s. *aa. metacarpeae palmares*	deep palmar arch	none	interosseous muscles, metacarpal bones,second, third, and fourth lumbrical muscles
metatarsal a., first dorsal *a. metatarsalis dorsalis I*	dorsal a. of foot	branch to medial side of great toe, branch to adjoining sides of the second and great toes	medial border of great toe and adjoining sides of great and second toes

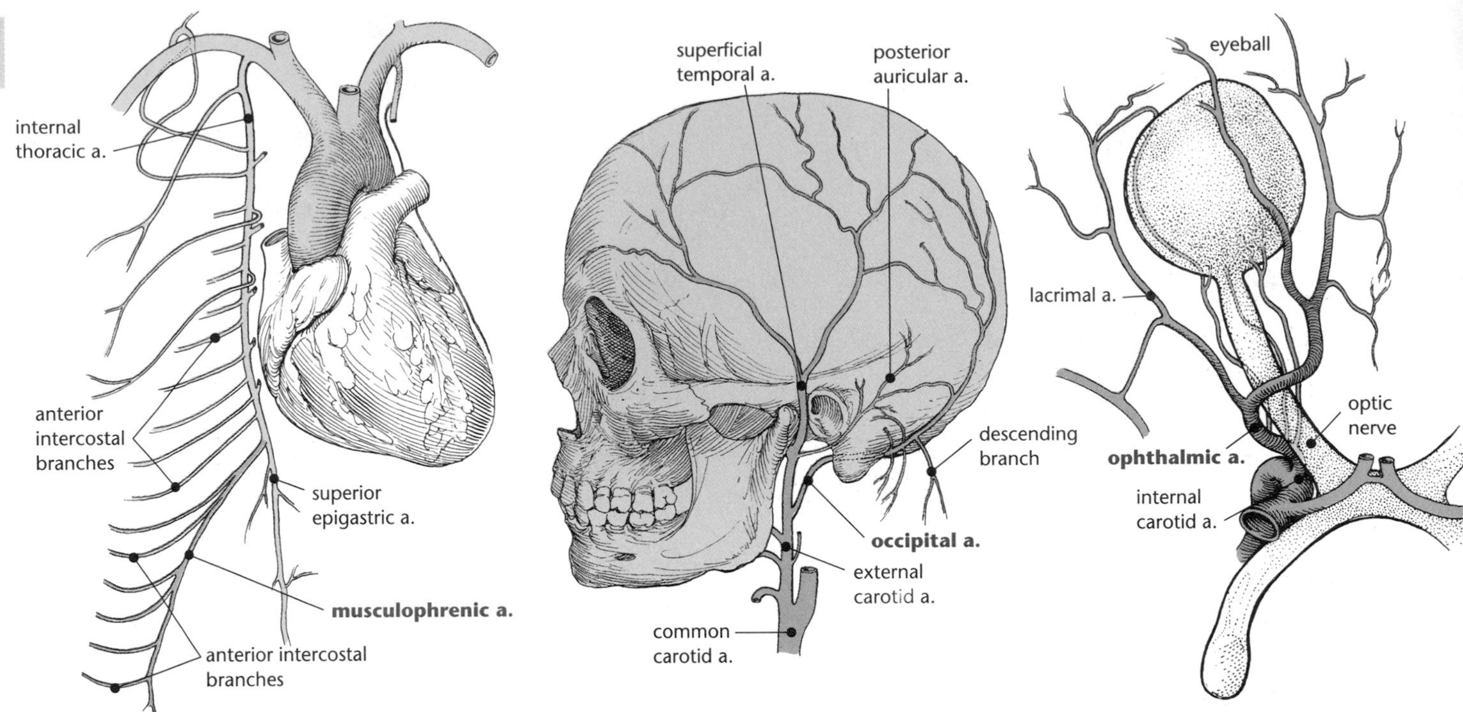

ARTERY	ORIGIN	BRANCHES	DISTRIBUTION
metatarsal a.'s, plantar (four in number) digital a.'s of foot, common *aa. metatarsales plantares*	plantar arch	plantar digital, anterior perforating	plantar surface and adjacent sides of toes
musculophrenic a. *a. musculophrenica*	internal thoracic a.	anterior intercostal	diaphragm, seventh, eighth, and ninth intercostal spaces, pericardium, abdominal muscles
mylohyoid a. *a. mylohyoideus*	inferior alveolar a.	none	mylohyoid muscle
nasal a., dorsal *a. dorsalis nasi*	ophthalmic a.	none	skin of nose, lacrimal sac
nasal a., lateral *a. nasalis lateralis*	facial a.	none	lateral nasal wall
nasal a., posterior lateral *a. nasalis posterioris lateralis*	sphenopalatine a.	none	frontal, ethmoidal, maxillary, and sphenoid sinuses
nasal a., posterior septal *a. nasalis posterioris septi*	sphenapalatine a.	none	nasal septum
nutrient a. of fibula *a. nutricia fibulae*	peroneal a.	none	substance of fibula
nutrient a.'s of humerus *aa. nutriciae humeri*	deep brachial a. about middle of arm	none	substance of humerus
nutrient a. of tibia (largest nutrient a. of bone in body) *a. nutricia tibiae*	posterior tibial a.	none	substance of tibia
obturator a. *a. obturatoria*	internal iliac a.	pubic, acetabular, obturator, anterior, posterior, vesical	bladder, ilium, pelvic muscles, hip joint
occipital a. *a. occipitalis*	external carotid a.	muscular, occipital, stern-acleidamastoid, auricular, meningeal, descending, terminal	dura mater, diploë, mastoid air cells, muscles of neck and scalp
ophthalmic a. a. ophthalmica	internal carotid a.	*orbital portion;* lacrimal, supraorbital, posterior ethmoidal, anterior ethmoidal, medial palpebral supratrochlear, dorsal nasal; *ocular portion:* central artery of the retina, short posterior ciliary, long posterior ciliary, anterior ciliary, muscular	orbit and surrounding parts; muscles and bulb of the eye

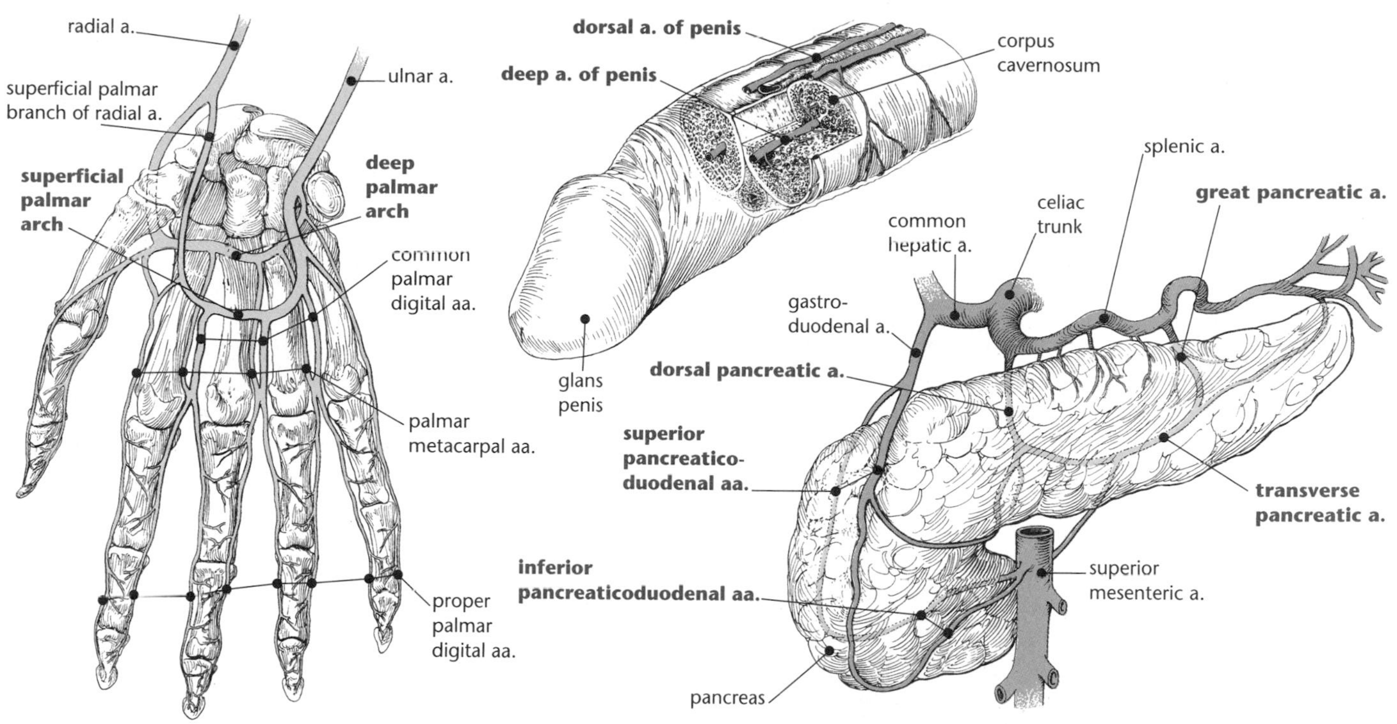

ARTERY	ORIGIN	BRANCHES	DISTRIBUTION
ovarian a.'s *aa. ovaricae*	ventral surface of abdominal aorta slightly below the renal a.'s at level of L2	ureteric, capsular, tubal; anastomoses with uterine a.	ovary, ureter, uterus, round ligament, skin of labium majus
palatine a., ascending *a. palatina ascendens*	facial a.	none	soft palate, palatine glands, auditory tube
palatine a., descending *a. palatina descendens*	maxillary a.	greater palatine lesser palatine	soft palate, hard palate, tonsil, gums, palatine glands
palatine a., greater *a. palatina major*	descending palatine a.	none	hard palate, gums, palatine glands
palatine a.'s lesser *aa. palatina minores*	descending palatine a.	none	soft palate, palatine tonsil
palmar arch, deep *arcus palmaris profundus*	radial a.	palmar metacarpal; anastomoses with deep palmar branch of ulnar	carpal extremities of metacarpal bones, interosseous muscles
palmar arch, superficial *arcus palmaris superficialis*	ulnar a.	common palmar digital	palm, fingers
palpebral a.'s, lateral *aa. palpebrales laterales*	lacrimal a.	superior, inferior	eyelids, conjunctiva
palpebral a.'s, medial *aa. palpebrales mediales*	ophthalmic a. near the pulley at the superior oblique muscle	superior, inferior	eyelids, conjunctiva, nasolacrimal duct
pancreatic a., dorsal *a. pancreatica dorsalis*	splenic a.	right, left (inferior pancreatic)	pancreas
pancreatic a., great *a. pancreatica magna*	splenic a.	none	pancreas
pancreatic a., inferior *pancreatica inferior*	dorsal pancreatic a.	none	pancreas, greater omentum
pancreaticoduodenal a., inferior duodenal a. *a. pancreaticoduodenalis inferior*	superior mesentaric a. or from its first intestinal branch	anterior, posterior	head of pancreas, descending and inferior parts of duodenum
pancreaticoduodenal a., superior *a. pancreaticoduodenalis superior*	gastroduodenal a.	ventral and dorsal pancreaticoduodenal arcade	pancreas, three parts of duodenum
penis, deep a. of a. of corpus cavernosum *a. profunda penis*	internal pudendal a.	none	corpus cavernosum of penis
penis, dorsal a. of *a. dorsalis penis*	internal pudendal a.	none	glans and prepuce of penis, integument and fibrous sheath of corpus cavernosum

ARTERY	ORIGIN	BRANCHES	DISTRIBUTION
perforating a.'s *aa. perforantes*	deep femoral a.	first, second, and third perforating	back of thigh, femur, buttock
pericardiacophrenic a. *a. pericricardiacophrenica*	internal thoracic a.	none	diaphragm, pericardium, pleura
perineal a. superficial perineal a. *a. perinealis*	internal pudendal a.	transverse perineal, posterior scrotal/labial	perineum, external genitalia, bulbocavernous and ischiocavernous muscles
peroneal a. fibular a. *a. peronea*	posterior tibial a.	muscular, nutrient (fibula), perforating, communicating, posterior lateral malleolar, lateral calcaneal	soleus and other deep calf muscles, lateral side and back of ankle and heel
pharyngeal a., ascending *a. pharyngea ascendens*	external carotid a. posterior meningeal	pharyngeal, palatine, prevertebral, inferior tympanic, of back of head and neck	wall of pharynx, soft palate, tonsil, ear, meninges, muscles
phrenic a.'s phrenic a.'s, inferior diaphragmatic a., inferior *aa. phrenicae*	abdominal aorta or celiac trunk	superior suprarenal, anterior, lateral, recurrent	diaphragm, adrenal gland
phrenic a.'s, superior *aa. phrenicae superiores*	thoracic aorta	none	diaphragm
plantar a., deep communicating a. *ramus plantaris profundus*	dorsal a. foot	first plantar metatarsal; with lateral plantar a., forms plantar arch	undersurface and adjacent sides of first and second toes
plantar a., lateral a. plantaris lateralis	posterior tibial a.	calcaneal, muscular, cutaneous; continues to form plantar arch by uniting with deep plantar branch of the dorsal artery of foot	muscles of foot, skin of toes and lateral side of foot
plantar a., medial internal plantar a. *a. plantaris medialis*	posterior tibial a.	deep, superficial	flexor muscle of toes, abductor muscle of great toe, skin of inner side of sole
plantar arch *arcus plantaris*	lateral plantar a.	perforating, plantar metatarsal	interosseous muscles, toes, sole of foot
popliteal a. *a. poplitea*	continuation of femoral a. at the adductar hiatus	muscular, sural, cutaneous, medial superior genicular, lateral superior genicular, middle genicular, medial inferior genicular, lateral inferior genicular; it divides at the distal border of the popliteus and continues as anterior and posterior tibial arteries	muscles of thigh and calf in region of knee, femur, patella, and tibia
princeps pollicis a.		see principal artery of thumb	
principal a. of thumb princeps pollicis a. *a. princeps pollicis*	radial a.	radial a. of index finger, nutrient	sides of thumb, dorsal interosseous muscles of hand, lateral side of index finger
profunda a., inferior		see collateral artery, superior ulnar	
profunda a., superior		see brachial artery, deep	
a. profunda brachii		see brachial artery, deep	
profunda femoris a.		see femoral artery, deep	
profunda linguae a.		see lingual artery, deep	
a. of pterygoid canal vidian a. *a. canalis pterygoidei*	maxillary a. or internal carotid a.	pharyngeal, tubal	sphenoid sinus, upper pharynx, auditory tube, and tympanic cavity
pudendal a.'s, external external pudic a.'s *aa. pudendae axternae*	femoral a.	anterior scrotal or anterior labial; inguinal	skin of scrotum and perineum in male; labium major and perineum in female; skin of lower abdomen
pudendal a., internal *a. pudenda interna*	internal illac a.	muscular, inferior rectal, perineal, artery of the bulb, urethral, deep artery at the penis or clitoris, dorsal artery of the penis or clitoris	muscles at perineum, anal canal, external genitalia

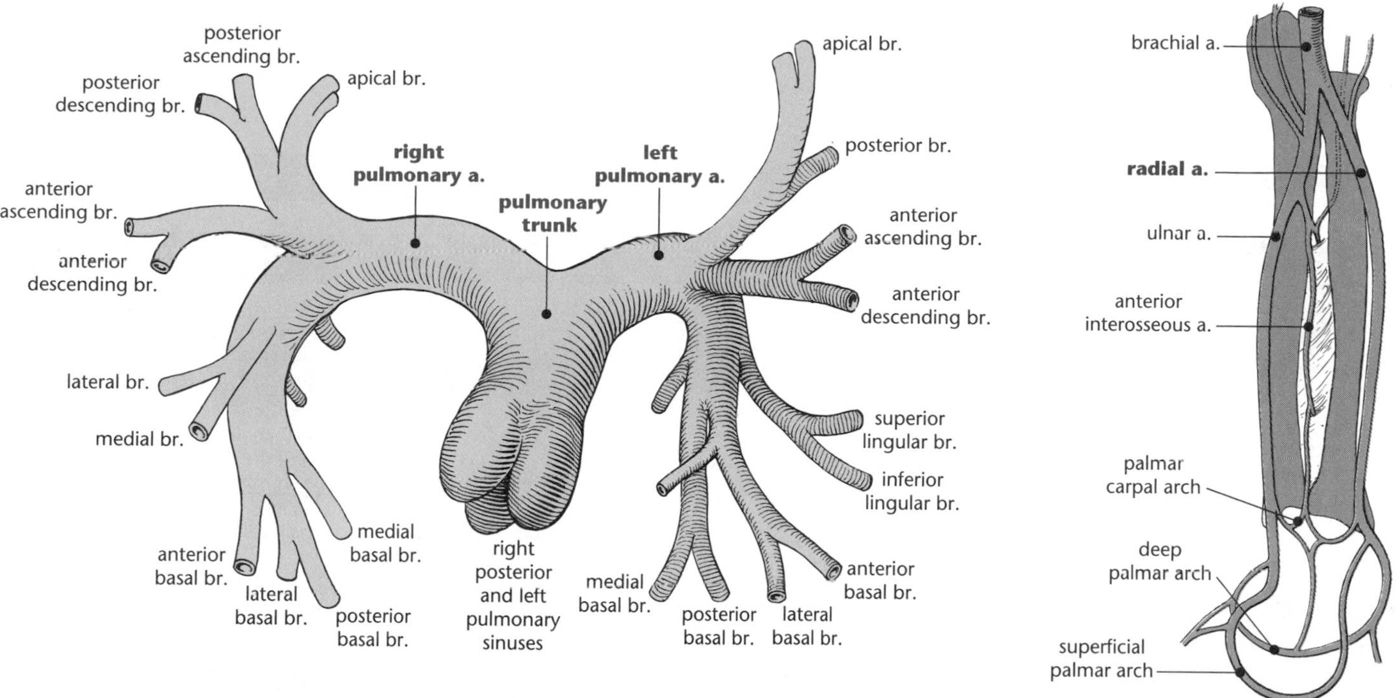

ARTERY	ORIGIN	BRANCHES	DISTRIBUTION
pulmonary a., left *a. pulmonalis sinistra*	pulmonary trunk	branches named according to the segment which they supply; e.g., apical segmental, anterior descending segmental	left lung
pulmonary a., right *a. pulmonalis dextra*	pulmonary trunk	branches named according to the segment which they supply; e.g., apical segmental, anterior descending segmental	right lung
pulmonary trunk *truncus pulmonalis*	conus of right ventricle	right and left pulmonary	lungs
radial a. *a. radialis*	brachial a.	*forearm group;* recurrent radial, muscular; *wrist group:* palmar carpal, superficial palmar, dorsal carpal; *hand group;* first dorsal metacarpal, principal a. of thumb, radial a. of index finger, deep palmar arch, palmar metacarpal, perforating, recurrent	muscles of forearm and hand, radius, skin of back of hand and palmar surface of thumb, outer aspect of index finger, intercarpal articulations
radial a. of index finger radialis indicis a. *a. radialis indicis*	radial a.	none	radial (lateral) side of index finger
radialis indicis a.		see radial artery of index finger	
ranine a.		see lingual artery, deep	
rectal a., inferior inferior hemorrhoidal a. *a. rectalis inferior*	internal pudendal a.	none	muscles and skin of anal region, rectum, external sphincter muscle
rectal a., middle middle hemorrhoidal a. *a. rectalis media*	internal iliac a.	vagina in females	rectum, prostate, seminal vesicles, vagina
rectal a., superior superior hemorrhoidal a. *a. rectalis superior*	Continuatian of inferior mesenteric a.	superior rectal artery branches; anastomoses with middle and inferior rectal arteries	rectum
recurrent a., anterior tibial *a. recurrens tibialis anterior*	anterior tibial a.	none	front and sides of knee joint, anterior tibial muscle
recurrent a., anterior ulnar *a. recurrens ulnaris, ramus anterior*	ulnar a., immediately distal to elbow joint	anterior, posterior	brachial and round pronator muscles
recurrent a., posterior tibial *a. recurrens tibialis, posterior*	anterior tibial a.	none	tibiofibular joint, knee joint, popliteus muscle

ARTERY	ORIGIN	BRANCHES	DISTRIBUTION
recurrent a., posterior ulnar *a. recurrens ulnaris, ramus posterior*	ulnar a.	none	elbow joint and neighboring muscles and skin
recurrent a., radial *a. recurrens radialis*	radial a., immediately distal to elbow	none	elbow joint, supinator, brachioradial, and brachial muscles
recurrent a., ulnar *a. recurrens ulnaris*	ulnar a.	anterior, posterior	brachial and round pronator muscles
renal a. *a. renalis*	abdominal aorta at about the level of L1	inferior suprarenal, ureteral, anterior, posterior	kidney, adrenal gland, ureter
retroduodenal a.'s *aa. retroduodenales*	gastroduodenal a., just above level of duodenum	pancreatic, duodenal	first two parts of duodenum, head of pancreas, bile duct
sacral a.'s, lateral *aa. sacrales laterales*	internal iliac a.	superior and inferior spinal branches	muscles and skin on dorsal surface of sacrum; sacral canal
sacral a., middle coccygeal a. *a. sacralis mediana*	dorsal side of aorta, slightly above its bifurcation	middle sacral artery branches; anastomose with lumbar branch of iliolumbar and lateral sacral arteries	rectum, sacrum, coccyx
scapular circumflex a. *a. circumflexa scapulae*	subscapular a.	none	subscapular, teres major, teres minor, and deltoid muscles; shoulder joint, long head of triceps
scapular a., dorsal *a. scapularis dorsalis*	thyracervical trunk, transverse cervical a. or subclavian a.	muscular	levator muscle of scapula, latissimus dorsi, trapezius, and rhomboid muscles
scapular a., transverse		see suprascapular artery	
sciatic a.		see gluteal artery, inferior	
sigmoid a.'s aa. sigmoideae	inferior mesenteric	branches of sigmoid arteries; anatomase cranially with left colic artery and caudally with superior rectal artery	caudal part of descending colon, iliac colon, sigmoid (pelvic colon)
spermatic a., external		see cremasteric artery	
spermatic a.'s internal		see testicular arteries	
sphenopalatine a. nasopalatine a. *a. sphenopalatina*	maxillary a.	posterior lateral nasal, posterior septal	frontal, maxillary, ethmoidal, and sphenoidal sinuses, nasal septum, nasapharynx
spinal a., anterior ventral spinal a. *a. spinalis anterior*	vertebral a. near termination	central	anterior side of medulla oblongata and spinal cord, filum terminale, meninges
spinal a., posterior dorsal spinal a. *a. spinalis posterior*	posterior inferior cerebellar a. or vertebral a. at side of medulla ablongata	dorsal, ventral	medulla oblongata, posterior part of spinal cord, and cauda equina, meninges, fourth ventricle
splenic a. lienal a. *a. lienalis*	celiac trunk	pancreatic, short gastric, left gastroomental, splenic, dorsal pancreatic, caudal pancreatic, great pancreatic	spleen, pancreas, stomach, greater omentum
sternocleidomastoid a. sternomastoid a. *a. sternocleidomastoidea*	occipital a. close to its commencement	none	sternocleidomastoid muscle
stylomastoid a. *a. stylomastoidea*	posterior auricular a.	mastoid, stapedial, posterior tympanic	middle ear chamber, stapes, stapedius muscle, mastoid cells, semicircular canals
subclavian a. *a. subclavia*	*right side:* brachiocephalic trunk; *left side:* arch of aorta	vertebral, thyrocervical, internal thoracic, costocervical, dorsal scapular; it becomes the axillary artery at the outer border of the first rib	neck, thoracic wall, muscles of upper arm and shoulder, spinal cord and brain
subcostal a. 12th thoracic a. *a. subcostalis*	thoracic aorta	dorsal, spinal	upper abdominal wall below twelfth rib

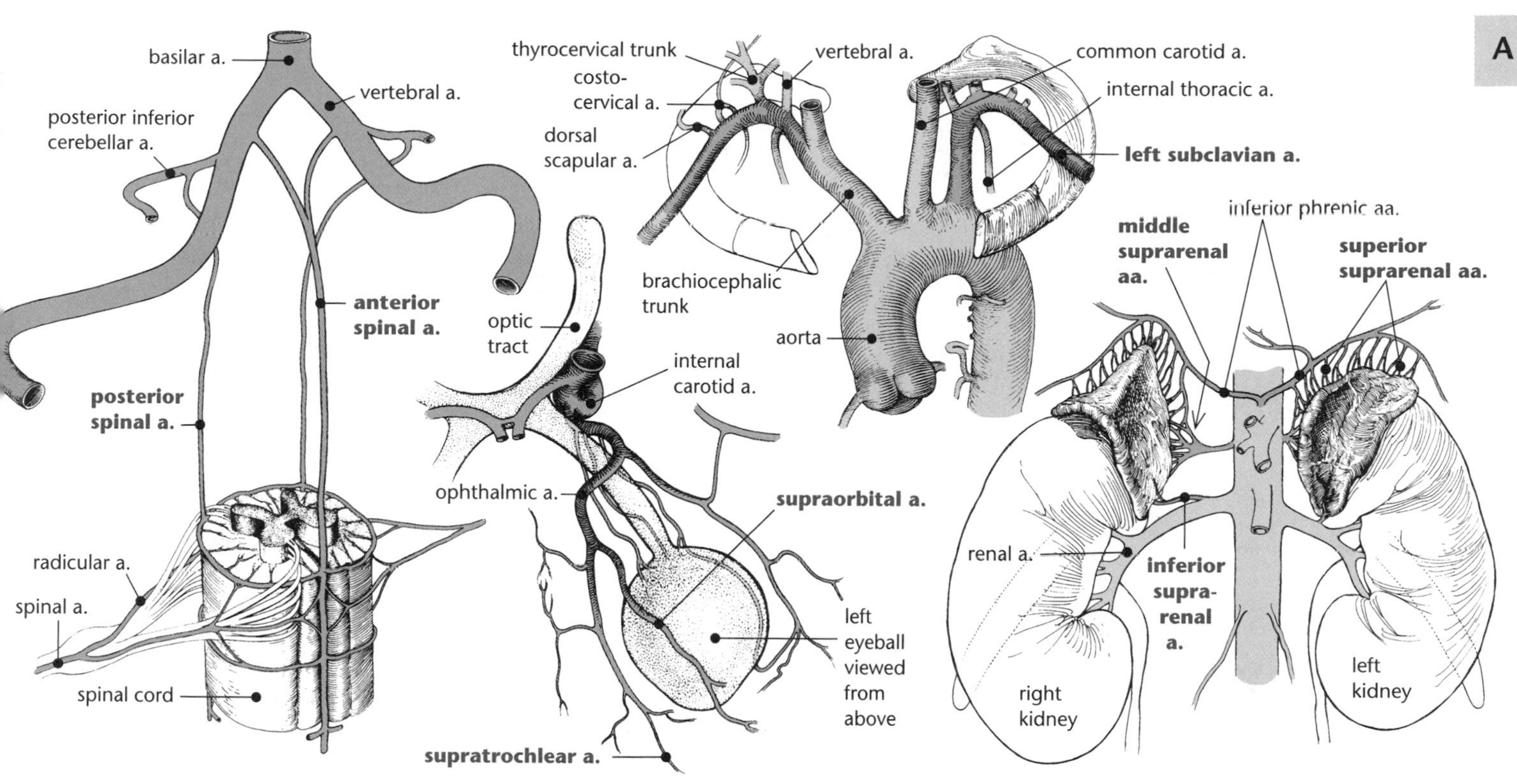

ARTERY	ORIGIN	BRANCHES	DISTRIBUTION
sublingual a. *a. sublingualis*	lingual a.	gingival, submental	sublingual gland, mylohyoid, geniohyoid, and genioglossus muscles; mucous membrane of mouth and gums
submental a. *a. submentalis*	facial a. (occasionally external maxillary a.)	superficial, deep	muscles in region of chin and lower lip, submandibular gland
subscapular a. *a. subscapularis*	axillary a.	circumflex scapular, thoracodorsal	scapular region, shoulder joint
superficial perineal a.		see perineal artery	
supraorbital a. frontal a. *a. supraorbitalis*	ophthalmic a. as it crosses the optic nerve	superficial, deep	skin, muscles, and pericranium of forehead; superior rectus muscle of eyeball, levator muscle of upper eyelid, diplöe
suprarenal a., inferior *a. suprarenalis inferior*	renal a.	none	adrenal gland
suprarenal a.'s, middle middle capsular a.'s *a. suprarenales mediae*	abdominal aorta, at level of superior mesenteric a.	anastomoses with suprarenal branches of inferior phrenic and renal arteries	adrenal gland
suprarenal a., superior *a. suprarenalis superior*	inferior phrenic a.	none	adrenal gland
suprascapular a. transverse scapular a. *a. suprascapularis*	thyroacervical trunk	acromial, suprasternal articular, nutrient, supraspinous, infraspinous	clavicle, scapula, skin of chest, skin over acromion, acromioclavicular and shoulder joints, supraspinous and intraspinous muscles
supratrochlear a. frontal a. *a. supratrachlearis* *a. frontalis*	ophthalmic a.	noise	skin, muscles, and pericranium of forehead
sural a.'s inferior muscular a.'s *aa. surales*	popliteal a. opposite the knee joint	none	gastrocnemius, soleus, and plantar muscles; neighboring skin
tarsal a., lateral tarsal a. *a. tarsea lateralis*	dorsal a. of foot	none	muscles and articulations of tarsus

ARTERY	ORIGIN	BRANCHES	DISTRIBUTION
tarsal a.'s, medial *aa. tarseae mediales*	dorsal a. of foot	none	skin and joints of medial border of foot
temporal a.'s, deep (two in number) *aa. temporales profundae*	maxillary a.	none	temporal muscle
temporal a., middle *a. temporalis media*	superficial temporal a. immediately above zygomatic arch	none	temporal muscle
temporal a., superficial *a. temporalis superficialis*	external carotid a.	transverse facial, middle temporal, zygomaticoorbital, anterior auricular, frontal, parietal, parotid	temporal, masseter, frontal, and orbicular muscles; external auditory canal, auricle, skin of face and scalp, parotid gland, temporomandibular joint
testicular a.'s spermatic a.'s, internal *aa. testiculares*	ventral surface of abdominal aorta, slightly caudal to the renal a.'s	ureteral, epididymal, cremasteric (anastomose with ductus deferens a.)	epididymis, testis, ureter, cremaster muscle
thoracic a., highest *a. thoracica suprema*	axillary a. or thoracoacromial a.	none	pectoral muscles, parietes of the thorax, anterior serratus and intercostal muscles
thoracic a., internal internal mammary a. *a. thoracica interna*	subclavian a.	pericardiacophrenic, mediastinal, thymic, sternal, anterior intercostal, perforating, musculophrenic, superior epigastric	anterior thoracic wall, diaphragm, structures in mediastinum such as pericardium and thymus gland
thoracic a., lateral long thoracic a. external mammary a. *a. thoracica lateralis*	tharacoacromial, subscapular, or axillary a.	lateral mammary (in female)	pectoral, anterior serratus, and subscapular muscles; axillary lymph nodes, mammary gland (in female)
thoracic a., twelfth		see subcostal artery	
thoracoacromial a. acromiothoracic a. *a. thoracoacromialis*	axillary a.	pectoral, acromial, clavicular, deltoid	pectoral, deltoid, and subclavius muscles; mammary gland, coracoid process, sternoclavicular joint, acromion
thoracodorsal a. *a. thoracodorsalis*	subscapular a.	none	subscapular, latissimus dorsi, anterior serratus, and intercostal muscles
thyrocervical trunk *truncus thyrocervicalis*	first portion of subclavian a.	inferior thyroid, suprascapular, transverse cervical	thyroid gland, scapular region, deep neck muscles
thyroid a., inferior *a. thyroidea inferior*	thyrocervical trunk	inferior laryngeal, tracheal, pharyngeal, esophageal, ascending cervical, muscular, glandular	larynx, trachea, esophagus, pharynx, thyroid gland, neck muscles
thyroid a., lowest *a. thyroidea ima*	arch of aorta or brachiocephalic trunk	none	thyroid gland
thyroid a., superior *a. thyroidea superior*	external carotid a.	infrahyoid, sternocleidomastoid, superior laryngeal, cricothyroid	muscles and mucosa of larynx, pharynx, esophagus; thyroid gland, muscles attached to thyroid cartilage and hyoid bone; sternocleidomastoid and neighborlng muscles and integument
tibial a., anterior *a. tibialis anterior*	popliteal a. at bifurcation	posterior tibial recurrent, fibular, anterior tibial recurrent, muscular, anterior medial malleolar, anterior lateral malleolar; continues as dorsal a. of foot at ankle joint	muscles of leg; knee joint, ankle, foot, skin of front of leg
tibial a., posterior *a. tibialis posterior*	popliteal a.	peroneal, nutrient (tibial), muscular, posterior medial malleolar, communicating, medial calcaneal, medial plantar, lateral plantar	muscles and bones of leg; ankle joint, foot
tibial recurrent a., anterior *a. recurrens tibialis anterior*	anterior tibial a.	none	anterior tibial muscle, knee joint, patella, long extensor muscle of toes
tibial recurrent a., posterior *a. recurrens tibialis* posterior	anterior tibial a.	none	popliteal muscle, knee joint, tibiofibular joint

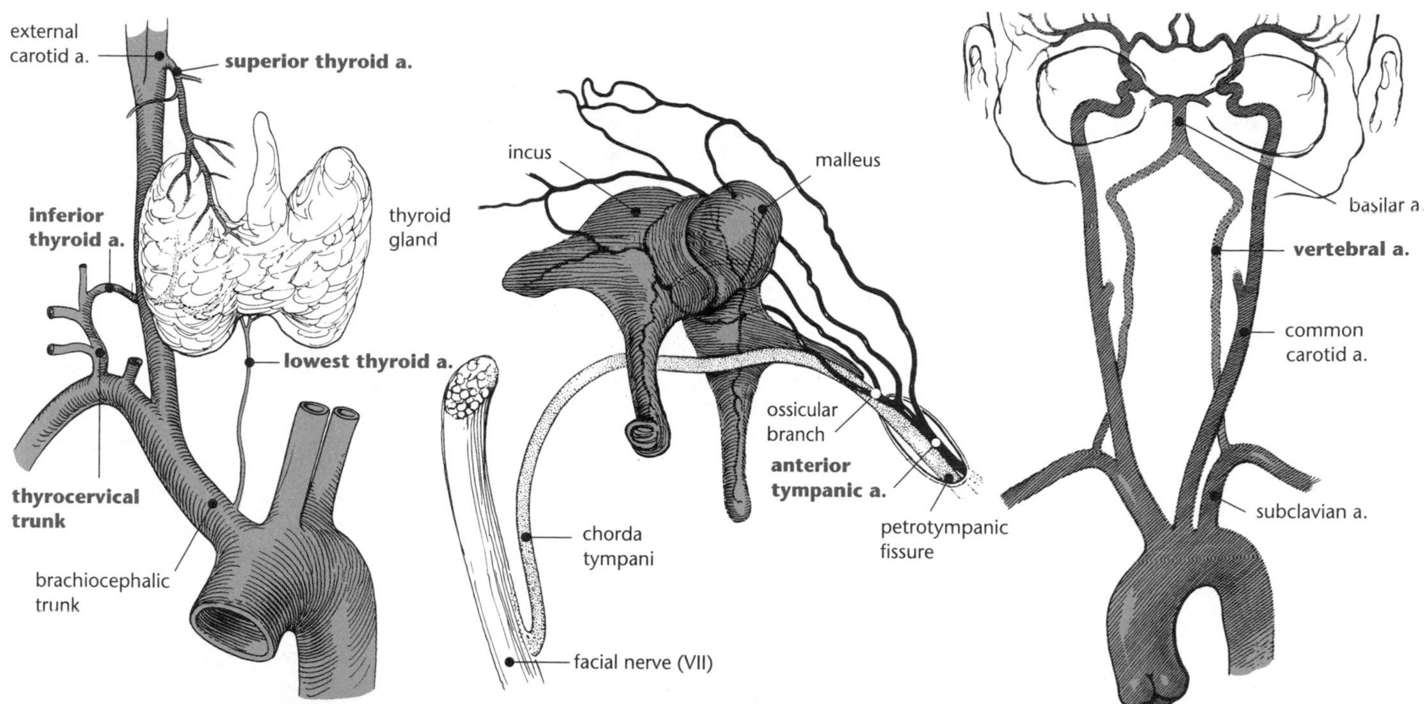

ARTERY	ORIGIN	BRANCHES	DISTRIBUTION
tympanic a., anterior tympanic a. *a. tympanica anterior*	maxillary a.	posterior, superior, ossicular	tympanic membrane, middle ear chamber, ossicles
tympanic a., inferior *a. tympanica inferior*	ascending pharyngeal a.	none	medial wall of the middle ear chamber
tympanic a., posterior *a. tympanica posterior*	stylomastoid a.	none	middle ear chamber, posterior part of tympanic membrane
tympanic a., superior *a. tympanica superior*	middle meningeal a.	none	middle ear chamber, tensor tympani muscle
ulnar a. *a. ulnaris*	brachial a., slightly distal to elbow	*forearm portion:* anterior ulnar recurrent, posterior ulnar recurrent, common interosseous, muscular; *wrist portion:* palmar carpal, dorsal carpal; *hand portion:* deep palmar, superficial palmar arch, common palmar digital	hand, wrist, forearm
umbilical a. *a. umbilicalis*	internal iliac a.	ductus deferens, superior vesical; continues as lateral umbilical ligament	urinary bladder, ureter, testes, siminal vesicles, ductus deferens
urethral a. *a. urethralis*	internal pudendal a.	none	urethra, corpus cavernosum of penis
uterine a. fallopian a. *a. uterina*	medial surface of internal iliac a.	cervical, ovarian, tubal, vaginal, ligamentous, ureteric	uterus, uterine tube, round ligament, part of vagina, ovary
vaginal a. *a. vaginalis*	internal iliac a. or uterine a.	rectal, vesical, vestibular	vagina, fundus of urinary bladder and part of rectum, vestibular bulb
vertebral a. *a. vertebralis*	subclavian a.	*cervical portion:* spinal, muscular; *cranial portion:* meningeal, posterior spinal, anterior spinal, posterior inferior cerebellar, medullary	bodies of vertebrae, deep muscles of neck, falx cerebelli, spinal cord, cerebellum, brain Stem
vesical a., inferior *a. vesicalis inferior*	Internal iliac a.	prostatic in males	fundus of bladder, prostate, seminal vesicles
vesical a.'s, superior *aa. vesicales superiores*	umbilical a.	ureteric	ureter, bladder, urachus
vidian a.		see pterygoid canal, artery of	
zygomaticoorbital a. *a. zygomaticoorbitalis*	superficial temporal a. (occasionally from the middle temporal a.)	none	orbicular muscle of eye, lateral portion of orbit

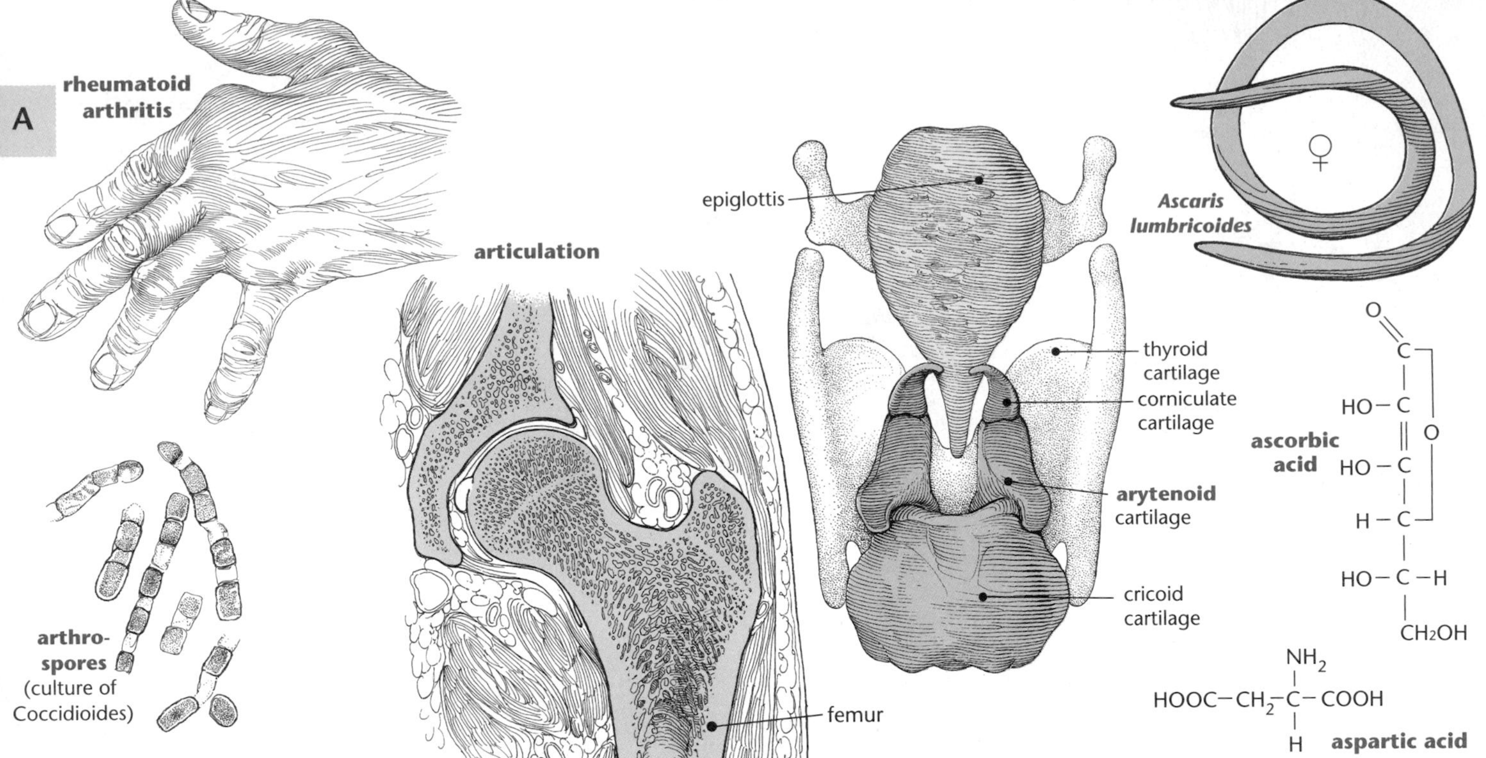

arthralgia (ar-thral´jă) Pain in a joint. Also called arthrodynia.
arthrectomy (ar-threk´to-me) Removal of a joint.
arthritic (ar-thrit´ik) Relating to or suffering from arthritis.
arthritis (ar-thrī´tis) Inflammation of the joints.
atrophic a. See rheumatoid arthritis.
chronic proliferative a. See rheumatoid arthritis.
degenerative a. See osteoarthritis.
gonococcal a. A form associated with gonorrhea, involving one or several joints, especially of the knees, ankles, and wrists; *Neisseria gonorrhoeae* can be isolated from the joint fluid.
hypertrophic a. See osteoarthritis.
juvenile a., juvenile rheumatoid a. (JRA) An uncommon, crippling disease of children involving the large joints and cervical spine with enlargement of lymph nodes, liver, and spleen. Also called Still's disease.
Lyme a. Arthritis associated with Lyme disease; affects large joints, especially the knee, causing swelling and pain in the joint. The condition may become chronic. See also Lyme disease.
pyogenic a. See suppurative arthritis.
reactive a. Arthritis occurring as a reaction to an infectious microorganism.
rheumatoid a. (RA) Chronic disease of unknown cause involving most connective tissues of the body with predilection for small joints, especially those of the fingers; marked by proliferative inflammation of the synovial membranes leading to deformity, ankylosis, and invalidism. Also called atrophic arthritis; chronic proliferative arthritis.
suppurative a. Purulent infection involving as a rule a single large joint; caused by any of several microorganisms, especially *Streptococcus hemolyticus*, *Staphylococcus aureus*, pneumococcus, and meningococcus; it usually follows injury to the affected joint. Also called pyogenic arthritis.
syphilitic a. (a) A mild chronic effusion into the knee joints (Clutton's joints) occurring during puberty in congenital syphilis. (b) Condition occurring with secondary syphilis marked by painful, stiff joints with transient swelling; inflammation of adjacent periosteum usually occurs.
tuberculous a. Arthritis caused by the tubercle bacillus; usually mono-articular, involving any joint in the body, especially the knee, hip, and spine, with destruction of contiguous bone.
arthrocentesis (ar-thro-sen-te´sis) Puncture of a joint followed by the withdrawal of fluid, usually by suction through the puncture needle.
arthrodesis (ar-thro-de´sis) Surgical fixation of a joint. Also called artificial ankylosis.
arthrodia (ar-thro´de-ă) A joint that permits a gliding motion, as between the articular processes of the vertebrae. Also called gliding joint.
arthrodial (ar-thro´de-al) Relating to arthrodia.
arthrodynia (ar-thro-din´e-ă) See arthralgia.
arthrodysplasia (ar-thro-dis-pla´zhă) Malformation of a joint or joints.
arthrogram (ar´thro-gram) X-ray image of a joint obtained in arthrography.
arthrography (ar-throg´ră-fe) **1.** Radiography of a joint after injection of a contrast medium into the joint capsule. **2.** A treatise on joints.
arthrogryposis (ar-thro-grĭ-po´sis) Permanent or persistent flexure of a joint.
a. multiplex congenita Congenital contraction of several joints of the extremities.
arthronosos (ar-thro-no´sos) Disease of the joints.
arthropathy (ar-throp´ă-the) Any disease of the joints.
diabetic a. Arthrosis occurring in diabetes as a result of disease of the trophic nerves innervating the joint.
neuropathic a. Any joint disease having a nervous origin.
tabetic a. A form of neuropathic joint disease marked by chronic, progressive degeneration and enlargement of a joint, with effusion of fluids into the synovial space. Also called Charcot's joint.
arthroplasty (ar´thro-plas-te) Surgical restoration of joint function, either by repairing damaged joint surfaces or by inserting an artificial joint.
arthropod (ar´thro-pod) Any of several invertebrate animals (phylum Arthropoda) having a segmented external covering and jointed limbs (e.g., scorpions, crabs, centipedes).
arthropyosis (ăr-thro-pi-o´sis) The production of pus within a joint. Also called arthro-empyesis.
arthroscope (ar´thro-skōp) Instrument used to view the interior of a joint and correct certain abnormalities.
arthroscopy (ar-thros´kŏ-pe) Direct visualization of the interior of a joint (e.g., of the knee joint) by means of an arthroscope.
arthrosis (ar-thro´sis) A degenerative condition of a joint.
arthrospore (ar´thro-spor) A sporelike cell produced by the fragmentation of any part of the segmented filamentous mycelium, as seen in *Coccidioides immitis*.
arthrosynovitis (ar-thro-sin-o-vi´tis) Inflammation of the synovial membrane of a joint.
arthrotomy (ar-throt´ŏ-me) Incision into a joint.
articular (ar-tik´u-lar) Relating to a joint.
articulate (ar-tik´u-lāt) **1.** Having joints. **2.** Capable of speaking in clear language. **3.** To connect.
articulation (ar-tik-u-la´shun) **1.** A joint between bones. **2.** The process of producing a speech sound.
artifact (ar´tĭ-fakt) Anything that has been artificially changed from its normal state, such as a histologic tissue that has been mechanically altered.
arytenoid (ar-ĭ-te´noid) Shaped like a ladle (e.g., a cartilage in the larynx). See arytenoid cartilage, under cartilage.
arytenoidectomy (ar-ĭ-te-noid-ek´tŏ-me) Surgical removal of an arytenoid cartilage in the larynx.
asbestos (as-bes´tos) An incombustible fibrous mineral form of magnesium and calcium silicate.
asbestosis (as-bes-to´sis) Fibrosis of the lungs caused by prolonged inhalation of asbestos particles, causing chronic shortness of breath; a pneumoconiosis.
ascariasis (as-kă-ri´ă-sis) Infestation with the large roundworm *Ascaris lumbricalis*, characterized by a larval pulmonary stage and an adult intestinal stage.
ascaridiasis (as-kar-ĭ-di´ă-sis) See ascariasis.
Ascaris (as´kă-ris) A genus of roundworms (order Nematoda) that are intestinal parasites.
A. lumbricoides A species, reddish and tapered at both ends, found in the small intestines, especially of children.
ascites (ă-si´tēz) Accumulation of free serous fluid in the abdominal cavity in clinically detectable amounts, seen sometimes as a result of cirrhosis of the liver, kidney disease, intra-abdominal cancer, and severe congestive heart failure. Also called hydroperitoneum; abdominal dropsy.
chylous a. Accumulation of a milky fluid in the peritoneal cavity. Also called chyloperitoneum.
ascitic (ă-sit´ik) Relating to ascites.
ascomycetes (as-ko-mi-se´tēs) Any of numerous fungi that contain spore-producing saclike structures (asci).
ascorbic acid (ă-skor´bik as´id) A white crystalline substance, $C_6H_8O_6$; found in citrus fruits, green leafy vegetables, and tomatoes; used in the treatment and/or prevention of scurvy. Also called vitamin C.
asepsis (a-sep´sis) Absence of disease-causing microorganisms.
aseptic (a-sep´tik) Not septic; free of contamination.
asexual (a-sek´shoo-al) Without sex.
asialia, asialism (a-si-a´le-ă, a-si-a-liz´m) Lack of saliva. Also called aptyalia.
asparaginase (as-par´ă-jin-ās) An enzyme that promotes the breakdown of asparagine to aspartic acid and ammonia; has been used to treat acute leukemia.
asparagine (as-par´ă-jēn) (Asn) A nonessential amino acid found in asparagus shoots and other plants.

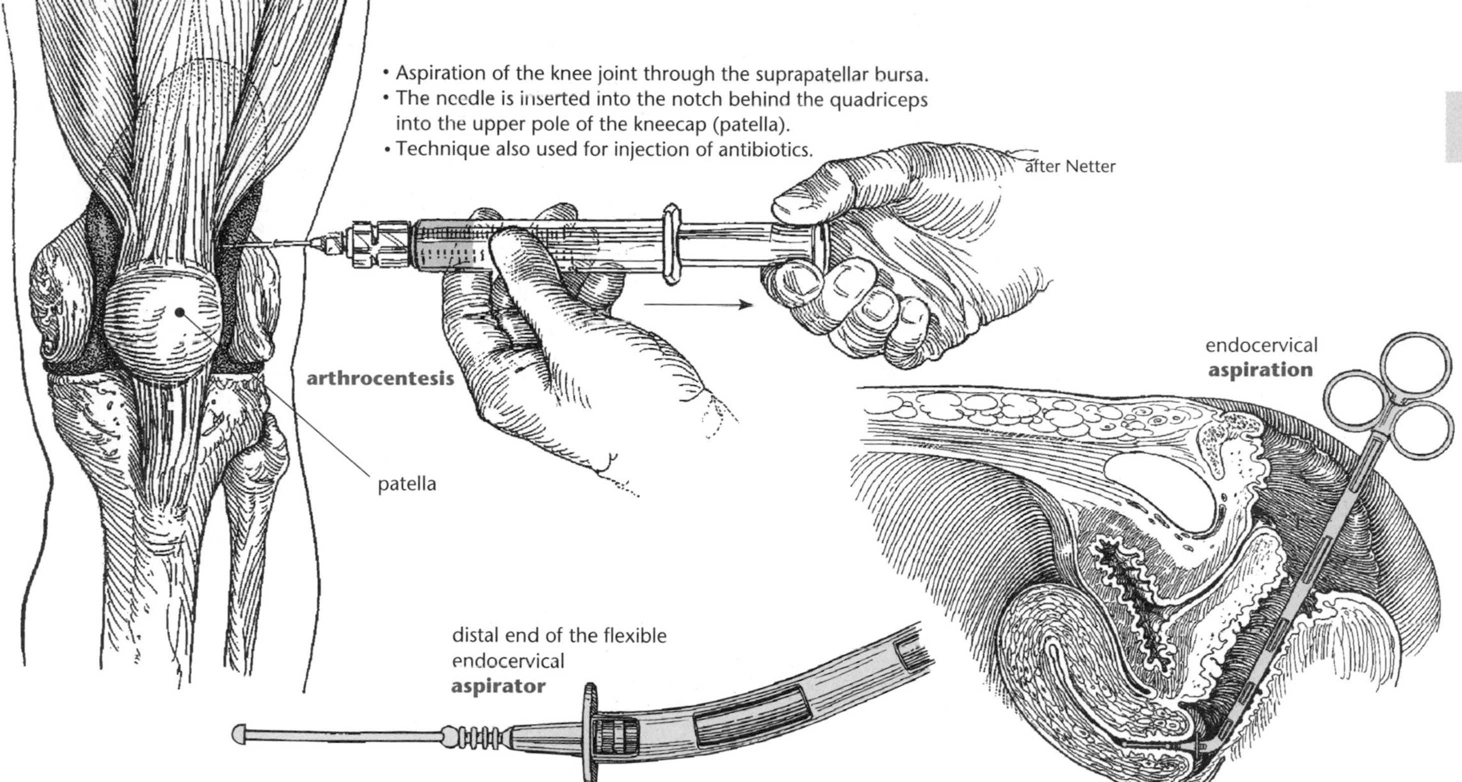
• Aspiration of the knee joint through the suprapatellar bursa.
• The needle is inserted into the notch behind the quadriceps into the upper pole of the kneecap (patella).
• Technique also used for injection of antibiotics.
after Netter
arthrocentesis
patella
endocervical
aspiration
distal end of the flexible
endocervical
aspirator

aspartame (ă-spar´tām, as´par-tām) A nutritive sweetener composed of two amino acids; approximately 180 times sweeter than sucrose (table sugar).

aspartate (as-par´tāt) A salt of aspartic acid.

a. aminotransferase (AST) Enzyme that catalyzes the reversible transfer of an amino group from L-glutamic acid to oxaloacetic acid to form α-ketoglutaric acid and L-aspartic acid. Also called aspartate transaminase; glutamic-oxaloacetic transaminase.

a. transaminase See aspartate aminotransferase.

aspartase (ăs-par´tās) An enzyme that promotes the conversion of aspartic acid to fumaric acid.

aspartate (ă-spahr´tāt) A salt of aspartic acid.

aspartate aminotransferase (ă-spahr´tāt ă-me-no-trans´fer-ās) (AST) An enzyme of the transferase class that catalyzes the reversible transfer of an amino group from L-glutamic acid to oxaloacetic acid to form α-ketoglutaric acid and L-aspartic acid; used to diagnose viral hepatitis and myocardial infarction. Also called glutamic oxaloacetic transaminase.

aspartate transaminase (ă-spahr´tāt trans-am´ĭ-nas) See aminotransferase.

aspartic acid (ă-spar´tik as´id) (Asp) A nonessential amino acid found mostly in sugar cane and sugar-beet molasses.

aspergilloma (as-per-jil-o´mă) A mass of fungus mycelium in a pulmonary cavity (intracavitary fungus ball) caused by fungi of the genus *Aspergillus*.

aspergillosis (as-per-jil-o´sis) Infection of the lungs and bronchi with *Aspergillus* fungi; usually affects debilitated patients; may also occur as an allergic reaction.

Aspergillus (as-per-jil´us) A genus of fungi (family Ascomycetes); it contains several disease-causing species.

aspermatogenic (a-sper-mă-to-jen´ik) Failing to produce spermatozoa.

asphygmia (as-fig´me-ă) Temporary absence of pulse.

asphyxia (as-fik´se-ă) Suffocation due to interference with the oxygen supply of the blood. Also called asphyxiation.

autoerotic a. Accidental cut off of air supply at the point of orgasm.

a. neonatorum Breathing failure of the newborn infant.

asphyxiant (as-fik´se-ant) Anything that causes asphyxia or suffocation

asphyxiate (as-fik´se-āt) **1.** To cause asphyxia. **2.** To undergo asphyxia; to suffocate.

asphyxiation (as-fik-se-a´shun) The causing of asphyxia.

aspirate (as´pĭ-rāt) **1.** To remove fluid from a body cavity by means of a suction device. **2.** The fluid removed.

aspiration (as-pĭ-ra´shun) **1.** Intake of foreign material into the lungs while breathing. **2.** Removal of fluid or gases by suction.

aspirator (as-pĭ-ra´tor) An instrument for removing fluids from a body cavity by suction.

aspirin (as´pĭ-rin) Common name for acetylsalicylic acid.

asporogenous (as-po-roj´ĕ-nus) Not propagating by spores.

assay (as´a) Analysis to determine the presence of a substance, its quantity, or its effects on an organism; a test; a trial.

enzyme-linked immunosorbent a. (ELISA) Blood test used to diagnose infectious diseases (e.g., AIDS and hepatitis A and B). The antigen of interest is fixed to a solid-state immunosorbent and incubated in a medium containing a test antibody raised against the antigen; then a second incubation is conducted with an enzyme-tagged detector antibody raised against the test antibody; finally, a substrate is added, which is digested by the enzyme, producing a color that can be measured by spectrophotometry.

human zona binding a. A male fertility test to determine the ability of sperm to pass through, or bind to, the zona pellucida of the ovum; two sperm samples, one from a donor and one from the patient, are exposed to different portions of surgically removed zona pellucida from ovarian tissue.

immunoradiometric a. (IRMA) A form of radioimmunoassay in which radioactively labeled antibody is added directly to the antigen being measured.

assimilate (ă-sĭm´ĭ-lāt) To consume and incorporate into the tissues.

assimilation (ă-sim-ĭ-la´shun) The process of converting food substances into tissues.

association (ă-so-se-a´shun) Relationship between persons or ideas.

astasia (as-ta´zhă) Inability to stand, in the absence of organic disorders.

asteatosis (as-te-ă-to´sis) Condition marked by deficient activity of the sebaceous glands.

a. cutis Dry-scaly skin with scanty sebaceous gland secretion.

aster (as´ter) See astrosphere.

astereognosis (ă-ster-e-og-no´sis) See tactile agnosia, under agnosia.

asterion (as-te´re-on) A craniometric point on either side of the skull at the junction of the lambdoid, occipitomastoid, and parietomastoid sutures.

asterixis (as-ter-ik´sis) A flapping movement or tremor, best seen in the outstretched hands, characteristic of certain metabolic disorders, particularly hepatic coma. Also called liver flap; flapping tremor.

asthenia (as-the´ne-ă) Loss of strength; weakness.

asthenocoria (as-the-no-kor´e-ă) Sluggish reaction of the pupil to light stimulus.

asthenopia (as-thĕ-no´pe-ă) General term denoting distress arising from the use of the eyes. See also eyestrain.

asthenospermia (as-the-no-sper´me-ă) Reduction of motility of spermatozoa.

asthma (az´mă) A reversible respiratory condition marked by airflow obstruction, causing intermittent wheezing, breathlessness, and sometimes cough with phlegm production. When the term is used alone, it usually denotes allergic asthma.

bronchial a. Recurrent acute narrowing of the large and small air passages within the lungs (bronchi and bronchioles), resulting in difficult breathing, intermittent wheezing, and coughing; due to spasm of bronchial smooth muscle, swelling of mucus membranes, and overproduction of thick, sticky mucus. Often simply called asthma.

cardiac a. An attack simulating an asthmatic episode, caused by fluid collection in the lungs secondary to failure of the left ventricle of the heart.

extrinsic a. Asthma precipitated by inhalation of such allergens as pollen, mold, animal fur, dander, feathers, or house dust.

intrinsic a. Asthma precipitated by a variety of nonspecific stimuli, including exercise (especially in cold temperatures), respiratory infections, tobacco smoke, and aspirin.

astigmatic (as-tig-mat´ik) Relating to or marked by astigmatism.

astigmatism (ă-stig´mă-tiz-m) **1.** Faulty vision caused by imperfections in the curvature of the cornea which prevent light rays from focusing at a single point on the retina; instead they are focused separately; occasionally due to defects in the curvature of the lens of the eye; may accompany myopia or hyperopia. **2.** In an electron-beam tube, a focus defect in which electrons from a single source point of a specimen come to focus at different points; the main cause of image deterioration in electron microscopy. **3.** A refractive defect of an optical system, such as a lens or mirror, that prevents sharp focusing.

astigmometer, astigmatometer (ă-stig-mom´ĕ-ter, ă-stig-mă-tom´ĕ-ter) An instrument for measuring the degree of astigmatism.

astrapophobia (as-tră-po-fo´be-ă) A morbid fear of lightning.

astringent (ă-strin´jent) **1.** Causing contraction of the tissues and arresting discharges. **2.** An agent that produces such an effect.

astroblast (as´tro-blast) An immature astrocyte.

astroblastoma (as-tro-blas-to´mă) A relatively

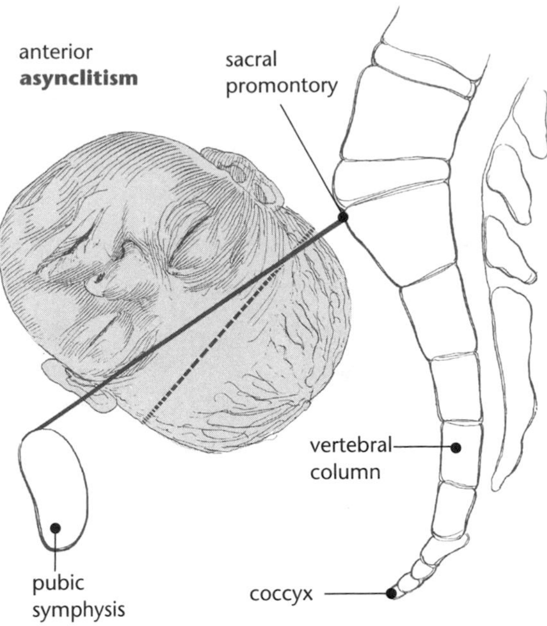

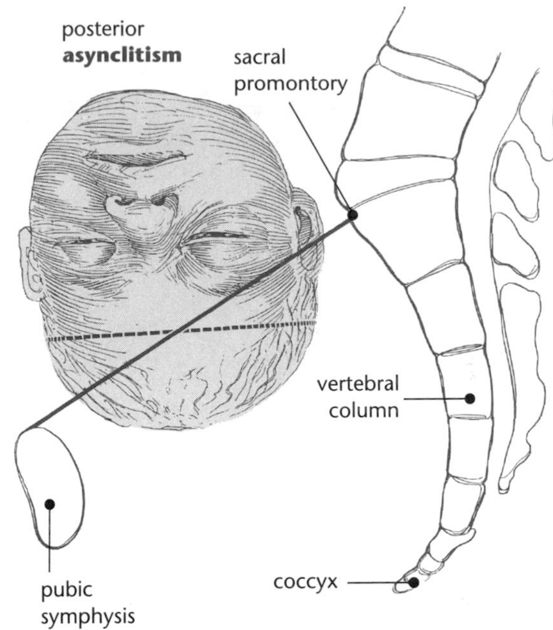

rare, rapidly growing brain tumor made up of astroblasts; two-thirds of cases occur in the cerebrum of middle-aged adults; the cerebellum is the second most frequent site.

astrocele (as´tro-sēl) See centrosphere.

astrocyte (as´tro-sīt) The largest neuroglial cell having a star-shaped cell body with numerous processes radiating outward; many of the processes end on blood vessels as perivascular feet.

astrocytoma (as-tro-si-to´mă) A non-capsulated brain tumor arising from astrocytes.

astrocytosis (as-tro-si-to´sis) An increase in the number of astrocytes; usually occurring close to degenerative lesions, abscesses, or brain tumors.

astroglia (as-trog´le-ă) A cell of non-neuronal tissue (neuroglia cell) consisting of a small body and several long straight processes.

astrokinetic (as-tro-kĭ-net´ik) Relating to the movements of the centrosome in a dividing cell.

astrosphere (as´tro-sfēr) A group of fibrillar cytoplasmic rays extending outward from the centrosome and centrosphere of a dividing cell. Also called aster; attraction sphere.

asymmetry (a-sim´ĕ-tre) Dissimilarity in corresponding parts.

asymptomatic (a-simp-to-mat´ik) Free of symptoms.

asynclitism (ă-sin´klĭ-tiz-m) In obstetrics, a situation during childbirth in which the sagittal suture of the fetal head is tilted either anteriorly or posteriorly, instead of being parallel with the pelvic planes of the mother. Formerly called obliquity.

anterior a. Deflection of the fetal head posteriorly, with the sagittal suture toward the sacral promontory of the mother, and the anterior parietal bone as the presenting part. Also called anterior parietal presentation.

posterior a. Deflection of the fetal head anteriorly; the sagittal suture lies close to the maternal symphysis, and the posterior parietal bone as the presenting part. Also called posterior parietal presentation.

asynergy (a-sin´er-je) Lack of coordination among the parts that normally work together.

asystole (ă-sis´to-le) Absence of muscular contractions of the heart.

atactilia (ă-tak-til´ē-ă) Lack of the sense of touch.

ataractic (at-ă-rak´tik) Tranquilizing; said of some drugs.

ataraxia (at-ă-rak´se-ă) Emotional tranquility.

atavism (at´ă-viz-m) The reappearance of a trait in an individual after being absent for several generations.

ataxia (ă-tak´se-ă) Lack of muscular coordination.

cerebellar a. Ataxia resulting from disease of the cerebellum.

hereditary spinal a., Friedreich's a. Hereditary disease occurring in children, marked by degeneration of the dorsal and lateral columns of the spinal cord, attended by progressive ataxia, nystagmus, and absence or diminution of deep tendon reflexes.

a. telangiectasia Hereditary progressive cerebellar ataxia associated with recurrent pulmonary infections and ocular and cutaneous telangiectases (permanent dilatation of capillaries and small arteries).

vasomotor a. Disorder of the vasomotor centers, causing spasm of the smaller blood vessels.

atelectasis (at-e-lek´ta-sis) A shrunken and airless state of the lung, or a portion of it, due to failure of expansion or resorption of air from the alveoli; it may be acute or chronic, complete or incomplete.

primary a. Failure of the lungs to expand adequately after birth; may be due to fetal hypoxia, prematurity, excessive intrapulmonary secretions, or intercurrent pneumonia; lack of surfactant, especially in premature infants, is a prime cause.

secondary a. Pulmonary collapse, especially of infants, due to respiratory distress syndrome.

ateliosis (ă-te-le-o´sis) Incomplete development. Also called infantilism.

atelognathia (at-ă-log-na´the-ă) Defective development of the lower jaw.

Atgam (at´gam) Anti-thymocyte gammaglobulin, used to suppress the immune response in organ transplantation.

atherectomy (ath-er-ek´tŏ-me) Removal of an atheroma.

rotational coronary a. Atherectomy of a hardened plaque within a coronary artery by grinding the plaque with a small diamond-studded burr.

atheroembolism (ath-er-o-em´bo-liz-m) Cholesterol and debris released from ulcerated plaques of a large artery, carried in the bloodstream and lodged in small arteries.

atherogenesis (ath-er-o-jen´ĕ-sis) The formation of atheroma in the arterial walls.

atherogenic (ath-er-o-jen´ik) Having the capacity to contribute to the formulation of atheroma.

atheroma (ath-er-o´mă) A degenerative cholesterol-containing plaque in the inner layer of an artery.

atheromatous (ath-er-o´mă-tus) Relating to atheroma.

atherosclerosis (ath-er-o-skle-ro´sis) A form of arteriosclerosis marked by deposition of lipids in the inner layer of arterial walls, resulting in the formation of elevated fatty-fibrous plaques (atheromas); the process usually begins during the first two decades of life and increases in severity with the rising age level.

athetoid (ath´ĕ-toid) Resembling athetosis.

athetosis (ath-ĕ-to´sis) Condition marked by constant, slow, involuntary writhing movements of the hands, fingers, and sometimes the feet.

athlete's foot (ăth´lēts fo͞ot) See tinea pedis.

athrepsia (ă-threp´se-ă) See marasmus.

athymia (ă-thim´e-ă) **1.** Lack of emotion. **2.** Absence of the thymus.

athyroidism (ă-thi´roid-iz-m) Condition caused by absence, or deficient functioning, of the thyroid gland. Also called athyrosis.

athyrosis (ă-thi-ro´sis) See athyroidism.

atlantoaxial (at-lan-to-ak´se-al) Relating to the atlas (first cervical vertebra) and the axis (second cervical vertebra); as the articulation of these two vertebrae.

atlanto-occipital (at-lan´to-ok-sip´ĭ-tal) Relating to the atlas (first cervical vertebra) and the occipital bone of the skull.

atlanto-odontoid (at-lan´to-o-don´toid) Relating to the atlas (first cervical vertebra) and the odontoid process of the axis (second cervical vertebra).

atlas (at´las) The first cervical vertebra articulating with the occipital bone above and the second vertebra (axis) below.

atmosphere (at´mos-fēr) **1.** The layer of gases surrounding the earth, composed of 20.94% oxygen, 0.04% carbon dioxide, 78.03% nitrogen, and 0.99% inert gases. **2.** A unit of air pressure.

atocia (ă-to´shă) Sterility in the female.

atom (at´om) A chemical unit of an element; consists of electrons moving rapidly around a dense nucleus composed of protons and neutrons; an atom is classified by the number of protons (proton or atomic number, Z) and the number of neutrons (neutron number, N) contained in its nucleus.

atomicity (ă-tom-ĭz`ĭ-te) **1.** The state of being composed of atoms. **2.** The number of replaceable atoms or groups in the molecule of a substance.

atomization (at-om-ĭ-za´shun) The process of reducing a fluid to a spray.

atomizer (at´om-īz-er) A device for delivering a liquid as a fine spray.

atonia (ă -to´ne-ă) See atony.

atonic (ă-ton´ik) Lacking normal tone or strength; said of a muscle.

atony (at´o-ne) Lack of normal tone. Also called atonia.

uterine a. Loss of muscular tone of the uterus, which may result in failure of progress of labor or postpartum hemorrhage.

atopic (a-top´ik, ă-top´ik) Displaced; not in the usual or normal place.

atopognosia, atopognosis (ă-tŏp-og-no´zhă, ă-top-og-no´sis) Loss of ability to correctly locate a

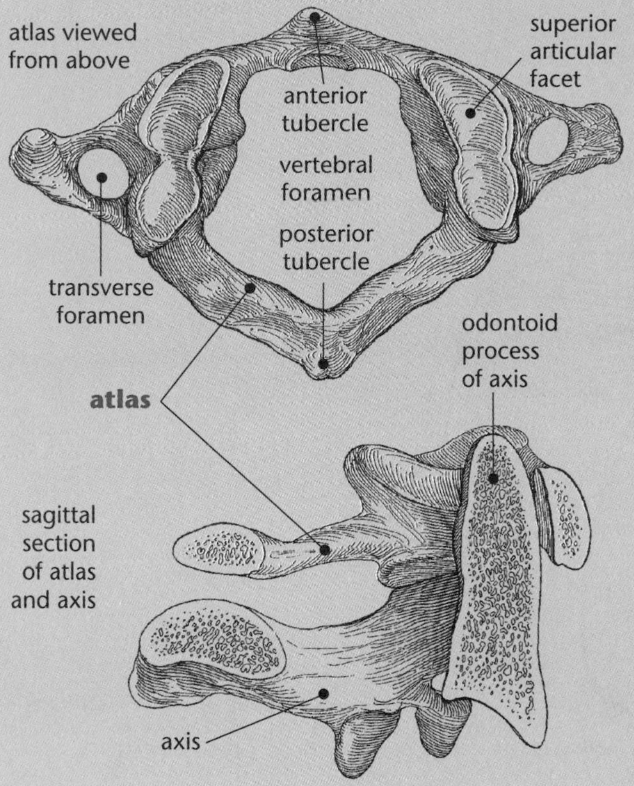

A

atlas viewed from above
superior articular facet
anterior tubercle
vertebral foramen
posterior tubercle
transverse foramen
odontoid process of axis
atlas
sagittal section of atlas and axis
axis

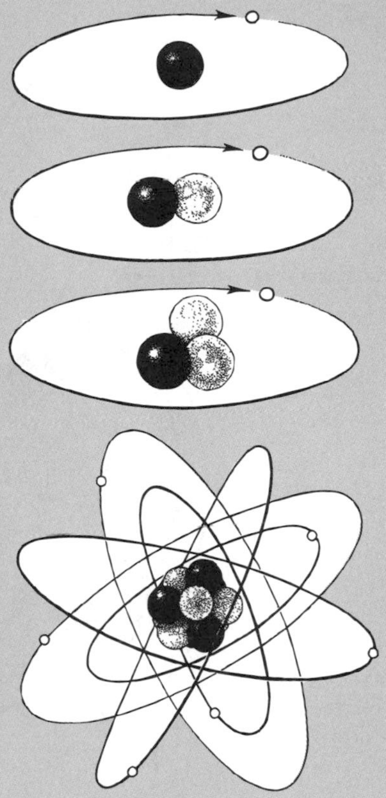

hydrogen **atom**
deuterium **atom**
tritium **atom**
carbon **atom**
6 electrons
6 protons
6 neutrons

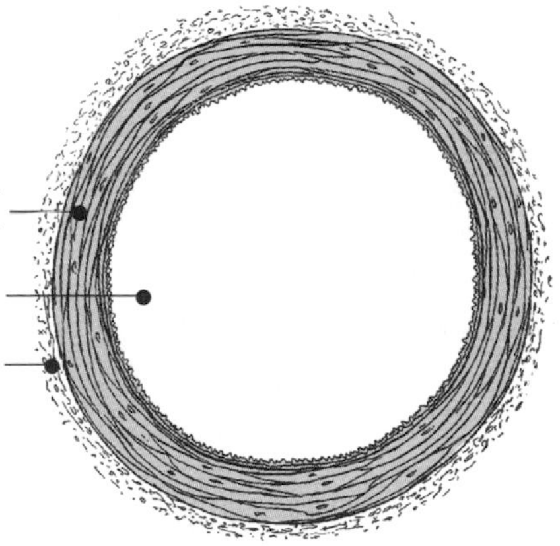

section of normal artery
muscular layer
lumen
adventitia

atherosclerosis
atheroma
muscular layer
fibrous layer
atherosclerotic narrowing of the lumen
adventitia

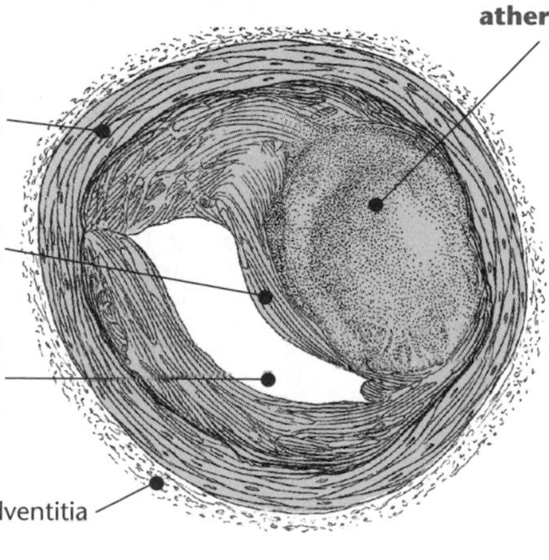

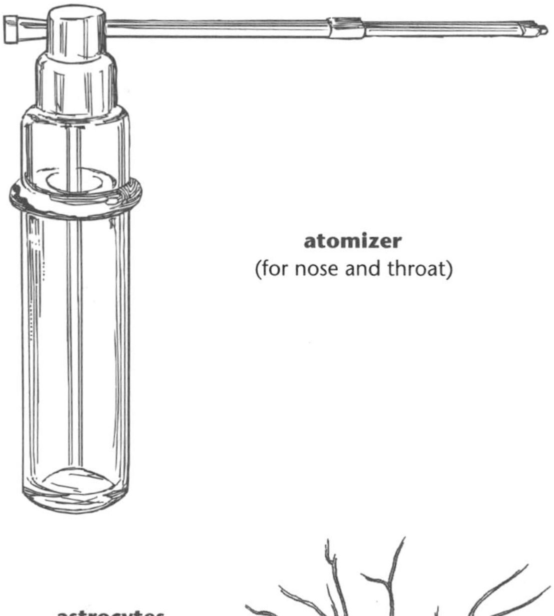

atomizer
(for nose and throat)

astrocytes
fibrous type
protoplasmic type

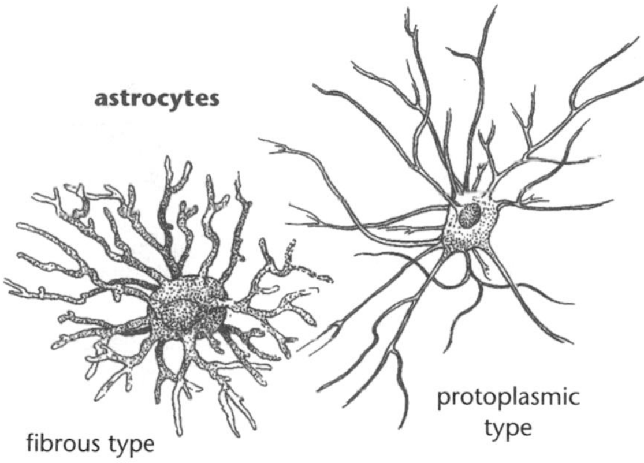

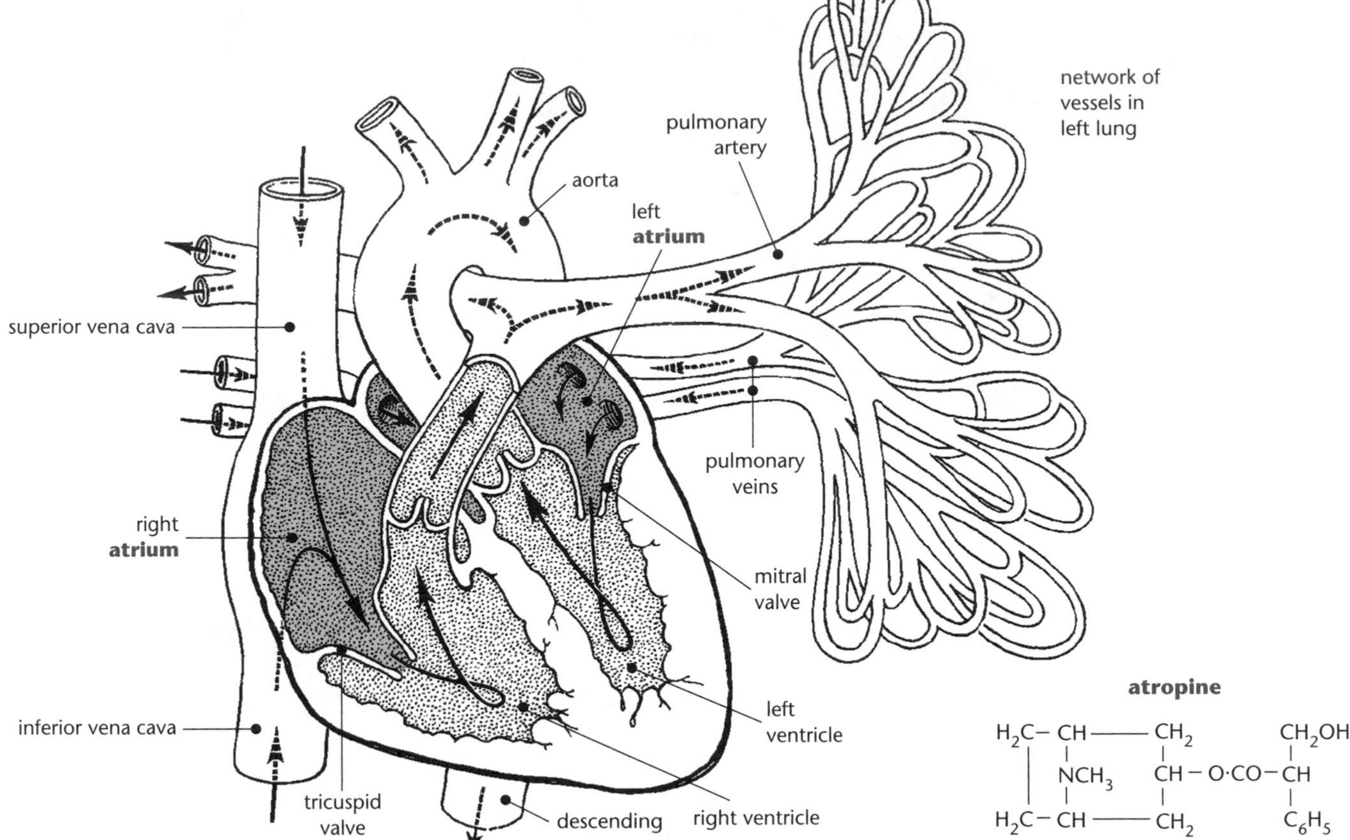

tactile stimulus.

atopy (at´ŏ-pe) Denoting an allergy characteristic of humans and tending to be inherited (e.g., hay fever, asthma).

atresia (ă-tre´zhă) Absence or closure of a normal body opening or canal.

biliary a. A condition of infants who are born without functioning bile ducts; unless they receive a liver transplant, these children usually die after several years because of resultant cirrhosis.

esophageal a. Congenital failure of the full esophageal lumen to develop.

tricuspid a. Absence of the opening between the right atrium and right ventricle.

atresic (ă-tre´zik) See atretic.

atretic (ă-tret´ik) Imperforate; lacking an opening. Also called atresic.

atretoblepharia (ă-tre-to-blĕ-far´e-ă) See symblepharon.

atrial (a´tre-al) Relating to an atrium.

atrichia (ă-trik´e-ă) Congenital or acquired absence of hair. Also called atrichosis.

atrichosis (at-rĭ-ko´sis) See atrichia.

atriomegaly (a-tre-o-meg´ă-le) Enlargement of an atrium.

atrioseptopexy (ă-tre-o-sep-to-pek´se) A heart operation to correct a defect in the interatrial septum.

atriotomy (a-tre-ot´o-me) Surgical incision of an atrium.

atrioventricular (a-tre-o-ven-trik´u-lar) (A-V) Relating to both an atrium and ventricle of the heart.

atrium (a´tre-um) **1.** One of the two (right and left) upper chambers of the heart; after birth, in the normal human the right atrium receives blood from the venae cavae and the left atrium receives blood from the pulmonary veins; the blood passes from each atrium to the respective ventricle. **2.** A shallow depression in the nasal cavity; the anterior extension of the middle meatus, located above the vestibule.

Atropa (at´ro-pă) A genus of herbs (family Solanacea).

A. belladonna A poisonous plant, commonly called nightshade, from which belladonna and atropine are derived.

atrophic (ă-trof´ik) Characterized by atrophy.

atrophied (at´ro-fēd) Wasted; shrunken.

atrophoderma (at-ro-fo-der´ma) Atrophy of the skin.

a. pigmentosum See xeroderma pigmentosum.

a. senile The characteristic dry condition of the skin in old age.

atrophy (at´ro-fe) A wasting, progressive degeneration and loss of function of any part of the body. Also called atrophia.

disuse a. Wasting of muscle tissue due to immobilization of the muscle (e.g., while in a cast).

infantile spinal muscular a. (ISMA) A rare disease of newborns inherited as an autosomal trait; it affects the motor nerve cells of the spinal cord, causing floppiness and paralysis of muscle (including those involved in breathing and feeding). Death usually occurs before the child is three years old. Cause is unknown. Also called Werdnig-Hoffmann disease; (colloquially) floppy infant.

Leber's hereditary optic a. Hereditary condition of rapid onset, affecting primarily young adult males; marked by bilateral degeneration of the optic disk, occasionally involving only the papillomacular bundle, and causing loss of central vision. Transmission is strictly on the maternal side.

peroneal muscular a. A hereditary disorder appearing during adolescence or adulthood; marked by degeneration of peripheral nerves and nerve roots, resulting in weakness and wasting of the distal muscles of the extremities, especially the legs; the wasting does not extend above the elbows or above the middle third of the thighs. Also called Charcot-Marie-Tooth disease.

Pick's a. Localized atrophy of the cerebral cortex.

progressive muscular a. See amyotrophic lateral sclerosis (ALS), under sclerosis.

spinal muscular a. (SMA) Hereditary (autosomal recessive) disease, with an early onset and a progressive course; marked by degeneration of the anterior horn cells of the spinal cord, resulting in wasting and paralysis of the muscles of the extremities and trunk.

Sudeck's a. Local bone loss (osteoporosis) usually occurring after fracture or minor injury and immobilization in a limb, especially the foot and ankle. Also called post-traumatic osteoporosis.

atropine (at´ro-pēn) An alkaloid with antimuscarinic actions obtained from *Atropa belladonna*; used to dilate the pupil, as an antispasmodic, and to inhibit gastric secretion; other effects include inhibition of salivary, bronchial, and sweat secretion, increase in heart rate, and inhibition of the urinary bladder.

atropinism (at´ro-pin-iz-m) Poisoning caused by an overdose of belladonna derivatives (atropine and scopolamine) or by accidental ingestion of plants such as jimson weed.

attachment (ă-tach´ment) **1.** A device by which something is stabilized. **2.** In dentistry, a mechanical device for the fixation of a dental prosthesis, such as a clasp, retainer, or cap.

epithelial a. A collar of epithelial cells which adheres to the tooth, at the base of the gingival sulcus, and is continuous with the free marginal gingiva.

parallel a. See precision attachment.

precision a. A device used in fixed and removable partial dentures, consisting of closely fitting male and female parts; the precise retention of the denture depends upon resistance between parallel walls of the two parts forming the attachment. Also called internal attachment; key-and-keyway attachment; parallel attachment; slotted attachment.

slotted a. See precision attachment.

attack (ă-tak´) The occurrence or establishment of a destructive process.

brain a. Popular name for stroke. See stroke.

drop a. Sudden falling without warning.

heart a. Occlusion of an artery supplying the heart, usually accompanied by pain and frequently by irritability of the myocardium and/or congestive heart failure. See also myocardial infarction; coronary thrombosis.

panic a. Intense fear, sweating, dizziness, chest pains, and trembling occurring in nonthreatening settings.

transient ischemic a. (TIA) Episode of neurologic dysfunction without permanent damage, commonly lasting from a few seconds to 10 minutes, caused by insufficient blood supply to a specific part of the brain; an episode persisting 24 hours or more is considered more likely to be a stroke.

uncinate a. See uncinate epilepsy, under epilepsy.

vagal a. See vasovagal attack.

vasovagal a. Condition characterized by slow pulse, labored breathing, and sometimes convulsions.

attenuant (ă-ten´u-ant) Any agent that dilutes a fluid, reduces the virulence of a pathogenic organism, or reduces the strength of a drug.

attenuation (ă-ten-u-a´shun) **1.** Dilution or weakening. **2.** Reduction of virulence of a pathogenic

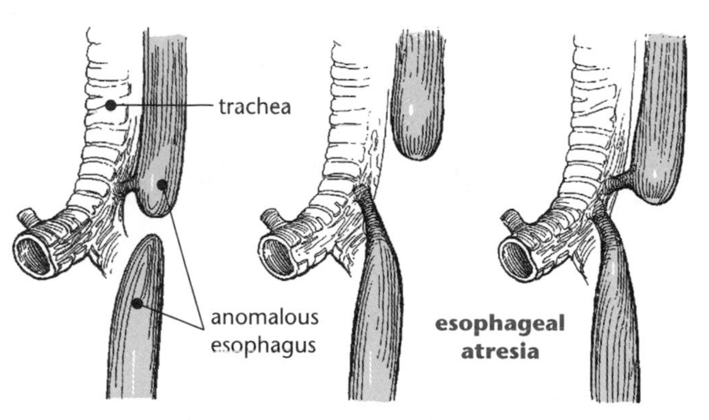

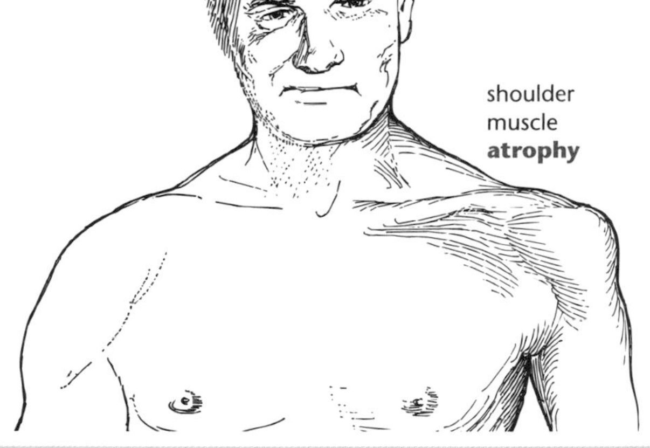

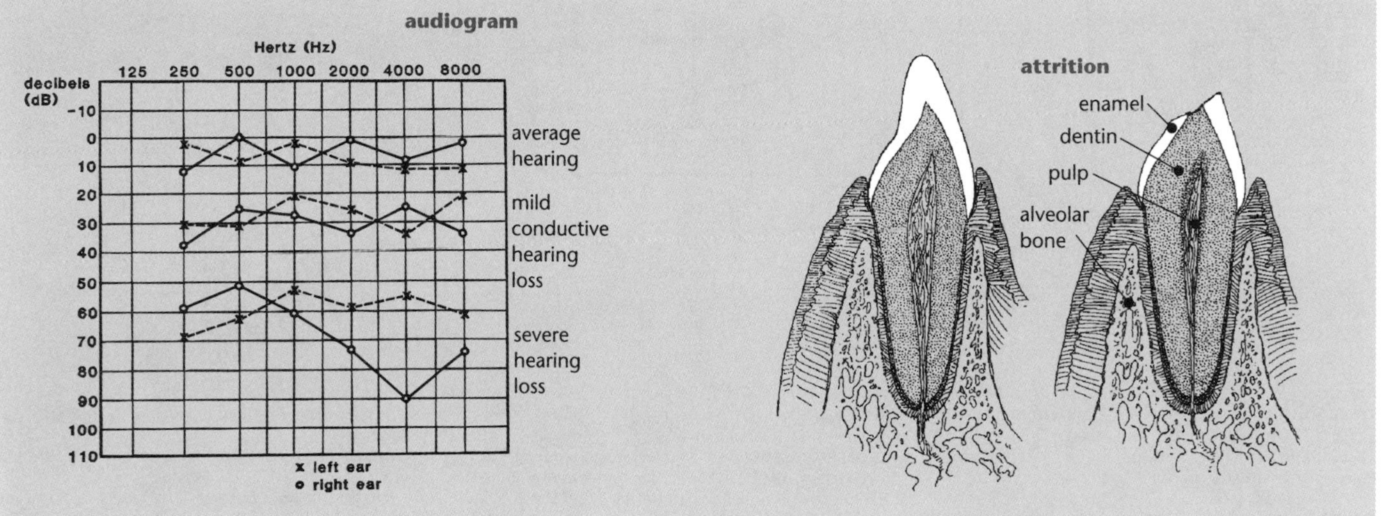

organism. **3.** Reduction of energy of a radiation beam when passed through tissue or other material

attraction (ă-trak´shun) The force acting between two bodies that draws them together.

capillary a. The force that causes a fluid to move up and along a fine, hairlike tube.

chemical a. The force causing atoms of different elements to unite.

magnetic a. The force that tends to draw iron and steel toward a magnet and resist their separation.

neurotropic a. The tendency of a regenerating axon to direct itself toward the motor end-plate.

attrition (ă-trish´un) **1.** Wearing away by friction. **2.** In dentistry, the normal wearing away of the biting surfaces of teeth due to mastication.

atypical (a-tip´ĭ-kal) Differing from the normal or usual type; not typical.

audile (aw´dil) Relating to hearing; applied to the ability to comprehend or remember most easily what has been heard, as opposed to what has been seen. COMPARE: visile.

audiogenic (aw-de-o-jen´ik) **1.** Sound producing. **2.** Caused by sound.

audiogram (aw´de-o-gram) A chart plotted from the results of hearing tests with the audiometer.

audiology (au-de-ol´ŏ-je) The study and measurement of hearing and the treatment of deafness.

audiometer (aw-de-om´ĕ-ter) Instrument for determining the acuity of hearing.

audiometry (aw-de-om´ĕ-tre) The measuring of hearing acuity with the audiometer.

auditory brainstem response a., ABR a. Measuring of hearing by eliciting responses from the auditory nerve and brainstem to repetitive acoustic stimuli. Also called brainstem evoked response audiometry.

Bekesy a. Testing of hearing with the audiometer while the patient controls the intensity of the tone.

brainstem evoked response a., BSER a. See auditory brainstem response audiometry.

AUDIT Acronym for alcohol use disorders identification test; a questionnaire used to identify at-risk drinking and alcohol abuse and dependence.

audition (aw-dish´un) **1.** The sense of hearing. **2.** The act of hearing.

auditory (aw´dĭ-tor-e) Relating to the special sense of hearing.

aura (aw´ră) The peculiar sensation that precedes an epileptic seizure, recognized by the individual.

auditory a. Noises or buzzing in the ears sometimes heard by a person prior to an epileptic attack.

olfactory a. Olfactory sensation which sometimes precedes an epileptic seizure.

visual a. Flashes of light sometimes seen by an person just before an epileptic attack.

aural (aw´ral) **1.** Relating to the ear. **2.** Relating to an aura.

auriasis (aw-ri´ă-sis) See chrysiasis.

auric (aw´rik) Relating to gold.

auricle (aw´rĭ-kl) **1.** External portion of the ear. Also called pinna. **2.** Pouchlike appendage projecting from the upper anterior portion of each atrium of the heart.

auricular (aw-rik´u-lar) **1.** Relating to the ear. **2.** Relating to an auricle of the heart.

aurotherapy (aw-ro-ther´ă-pe) See chrysotherapy.

auscultate (aws´kul-tāt) To examine the chest or abdomen by listening to sounds made by underlying organs.

auscultation (aws-kul-ta´shun) The act of auscultating.

auscultatory (aws-kul´tă-to-re) Relating to auscultation.

autacoid (aw´tă-koid) A substance (e.g., serotonin, prostaglandin) that produces a local effect on the cells adjacent to the site of production; autacoids are produced in a variety of body tissues.

autism (aw´tiz-m) A state of mind characterized by self-absorption, disregard of external reality, daydreams, and hallucinations; characteristic in schizophrenia.

early infantile a. Disorder appearing in the first three years of life marked by self-absorption, unresponsiveness to other people, ritualistic behaviors, and failure in language development.

autistic (aw-tis´tik) Relating to autism.

autoagglutination (aw-to-ă-gloo-tĭ-na´shun) The spontaneous clumping together (agglutination) of red blood cells.

autoagglutinin (aw-to-ă-gloo´tĭ-nin) A serum factor that causes the individual's own cellular elements (red blood cells, platelets, etc.) to agglutinate.

autoantibody (aw-to-an´tĭ-bod-e) Antibody that is produced in, and reacts with, an antigen in the same person or animal.

cold a. An antibody that reacts at zero to 5°C.

warm a. An antibody that reacts best at 37°C.

autoantigen (aw-to-an´tĭ-jen) An antigen that incites the production of autoantibodies.

autocatalysis (aw-to-kă-tal´ĭ-sis) A reaction that gradually accelerates due to the catalytic property of one of the products of the reaction.

autoclave (aw´to-klāv) **1.** A container used for sterilizing surgical instruments by pressured steam. **2.** To sterilize in an autoclave.

autocrine (aw´to-krin) Denoting a mode of hormone action whereby the hormone binds to receptors on the cell that produced it, affecting the function of that cell.

autodigestion (aw-to-di-jes´chun) Degeneration of tissues due to separation from blood supply; applied especially to spontaneous digestion of the walls of the stomach after death. Also called autolysis; self-digestion.

autoerotism (aw-to-er´o-tiz-m) Self-arousal and self-gratification of sexual desire.

autogamy (aw-tog´ă-me) A process of fertilization within the cell, as in certain protozoans; the nucleus divides, giving rise to two pronuclei which immediately unite.

autogenous (aw-toj´ĕ-nus) **1.** Self-producing. **2.** Having its origin within the body.

autograft (aw´to-graft) Living tissue (skin, bone, vein) that is transplanted from one site to another in the body of the same individual. Also called autotransplant; autogenous graft; autologous graft.

autohemolysin (aw-to-he-mol´ĭ-sin) An antibody that acts upon the red blood cells of the individual in whose blood it was formed.

autohemolysis (aw-to-he-mol´ĭ-sis) Destruction of the red blood cells of an individual by the action of hemolytic agents in his blood.

autohemotherapy (aw-to-he-mo-ther´ă-pe) Treatment by withdrawal and injection of the person's own blood.

autohypnosis (aw-to-hip-no´sis) Self-induced hypnosis; hypnotizing oneself. Also called self-hypnosis.

autoimmune disease (aw-to-ĭ-mūn´ dĭ-zēz´) Any disease characterized by tissue injury caused by an apparent immunologic reaction of the host with his own tissues; distinguished from autoimmune

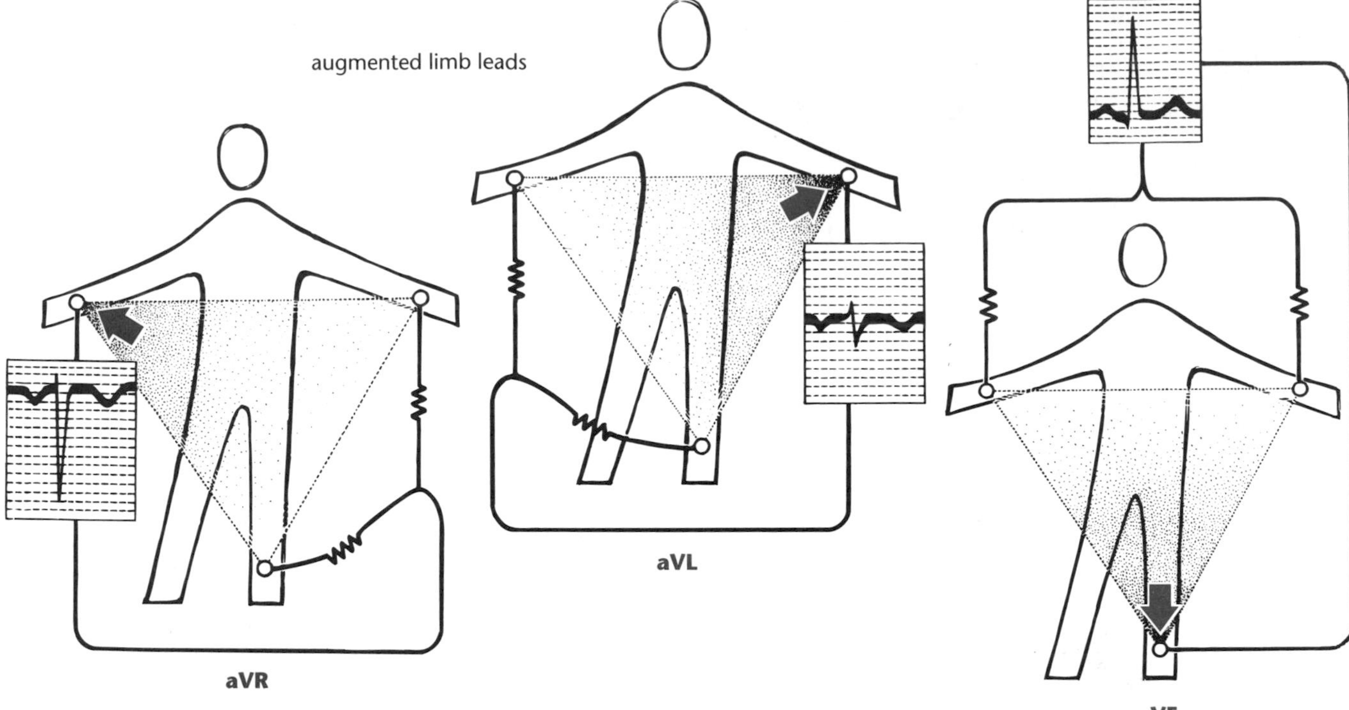

response, with which it may or may not be associated.

autoimmunize (aw-to-im´u-nīz) To immunize an individual against his own antigens.

autoinfection (aw-to-in-fek´shun) Infection with organisms already present in the body. Also called self-infection.

autoinoculation (aw-to-in-ok´u-la-shun) The spread of an infection from one site of the body to another.

autointoxication (aw-to-in-tok-sĭ-ka´shun) A condition caused by absorption of waste products or any toxin produced by the body.

autologous (aw-tol´ŏ-gus) Related to self; derived from the subject itself (e.g., a graft).

autology (aw-tol´ŏ-je) Study of one's own self.

autolysis (aw-tol´ĭ-sis) See autodigestion.

autolyze (aw´to-līz) To cause the disintegration of tissues or cells within the organism in which the autolyzing agent is produced.

automatism (aw-tom´ă-tiz-m) **1.** Involuntary or automatic action. **2.** A condition in which activity is carried out by the patient without his conscious knowledge, often inappropriate to circumstances.

autonomic (aw-to-nom´ik) Independent; self-controlling.

autopepsia (aw-to-pep´se-ă) Self-digestion, as of the gastric mucosa by its own secretion.

autopsy (aw´top-se) Examination of a dead body, usually to determine the cause of death. Also called necropsy; postmortem diagnosis; postmortem examination.

autoradiograph (aw-to-ra´de-o-graf) Image on photographic film produced by the emission of radioactive substances in tissues, showing the location and relative concentration of these substances; made by placing the structure in close contact with photographic emulsion. Also called radioautograph.

autoradiography (aw-to-ra-de-og´ră-fe) The process of making an autoradiograph.

autoregulation (aw-to-reg-u-la´shun) The intricate adaptive mechanisms that maintain a relatively constant blood flow to an organ despite changes in arterial pressure.

autosensitize (aw-to-sen´sĭ-tīz) To develop sensitivity to one's own serum or tissue.

autosome (aw´to-sōm) Any member of the 22 pairs of nonsex chromosomes.

autotopagnosia (aw-to-top-ag-no´zhă) The impaired recognition of any part of the body; may occur with lesions of the posteroinferior portion of the parietal lobe.

autotoxic (aw-to-toks´ik) Marked by autointoxication.

autotoxin (aw-to-tok´sin) Any poison acting upon the body from which it originates.

autotransfusion (aw-to-trans-fu´zhun) Transfusion of the patient's own blood.

autotransplant (aw-to-trans´plant) See autograft.

autotransplantation (aw-to-trans-plan-ta´shun) The transferring of living tissue from one part to another of the same individual.

autovaccination (aw-to-vak-sĭ-na ´shun) Vaccination with vaccine prepared from the patient's own body.

autoxidation, auto-oxidation (aw-tok-sĭ-da´shun, aw´to-oks-ĭ-da´shun) The spontaneous combination of a substance with oxygen at ordinary temperatures and without a catalyst, as in the rusting of iron.

auxotroph (awk´so-trōf) A mutant microorganism that can be cultivated only by supplementing a minimal medium with growth factors or amino acids, not required by wild-type strains.

avascular (ă-vas´ku-lar) Without blood vessels, normally or otherwise.

aVF One of three unipolar augmented limb leads. See lead.

avidity (ă-vid´ĭ-te) The binding strength between an antibody and an antigen.

avirulent (a-vir´u-lent) Not virulent; not causing disease.

avitaminosis (a-vi-tă-mĭ-no´sis) Any condition caused by deficiency of one or more vitamins in the diet.

aVL One of three unipolar augmented limb leads. See lead.

avoirdupois (av-er-dŭ-poiz´) A system of weight measurements in which 16 ounces make a pound, 1 ounce contains 16 drachms, and 1 drachm equals approximately 27.3 grains; 1 pound in this system contains 7000 troy grains or 453.6 grams; used for the British Pharmacopia prior to the introduction of metric weights.

aVR One of three unipolar augmented limb leads. See lead.

avulsion (ă-vul´shun) Pulling or tearing away; forcible separation.

axenic (a-zen´ik) Germ-free; denoting a pure culture, said of animals reared in a bacteria-free environment.

axial (ak´se-al) Relating to an axis (e.g., of the body or a body part).

axilla (ak-sil´ă) The pyramidal region at the junction of the arm and the chest; it contains the axillary vessels, lymphatics, brachial plexus, and muscles. Also called armpit.

axillary (ak´sĭ-lar-e) Relating to the axilla (armpit).

axis (ak´sis), *pl.* **ax´es** **1.** The second cervical vertebra. Also called epistropheus. **2.** Any of the imaginary lines used as points of reference, about which a body or a part may rotate. **3.** Any of various centrally located structures, such as the notochord of the embryo.

electrical a. The direction of the electromotive forces originating in the heart.

long a. A line passing lengthwise through the center of a structure.

mandibular a. A line passing through both mandibular condyles around which the mandible rotates.

optic a. (a) A line passing through the centers of the cornea and lens, or the closest approximation of this line. (b) In doubly refracting crystals, the direction in which light is not doubly refracted.

pelvic a. A hypothetical curved line passing through the center point of each of the four planes of the pelvis.

rotational a. See fulcrum line, under line.

visual a. An imaginary straight line extending from the object seen to the fovea centralis of the retina. Also called visual line.

axofugal (ak-sof´u-gal) Directed away from an axon.

axolemma (ak-so-lem´ă) The thin sheath enclosing the axon of a nerve fiber.

axon (ak´son) The long cytoplasmic process of a neuron (nerve cell). Also called neuroaxon.

axonal (ak´so-nal) Relating to an axon.

axoneme (ak´so-nēm) See axial filament, under filament.

axoplasm (ak´so-plaz-m) The cytoplasm of an axon containing mitochondria, microtubules, neurofila-ments, agranular endoplasmic reticulum, and some multivesicular bodies.

azidothymidine (az-ĭ-do-thi´mĭ-dēn) (AZT) See zidovudine.

azobilirubin (a-zo-bil´ĭ-roo´bin) A red-violet pigment resulting from the condensation of diazotized sulfanilic acid and bilirubin in the van den Bergh reaction for determination of bilirubin.

azoospermia (a-zo-o-sper´me-ă) Absence of spermatozoa in the semen, causing sterility.

azootemia (az-o-te´me-ă) An excess of urea or other nitrogenous substances in the blood.

prerenal a. Elevation of blood urea nitrogen resulting from primary alterations outside of the kidney, such as a reduction of renal blood flow due to congestive heart failure or hypotension, rather than renal disease per se.

azotification (a-zo-tĭ-fĭ-ka´shun) The action of bacteria upon nitrogenous matter in the soil. Also called nitrification.

azygos (az´ĭ-gos) A single or unpaired anatomical structure, such as the azygos vein.

azygous (az´ĭ-gus) Unpaired.

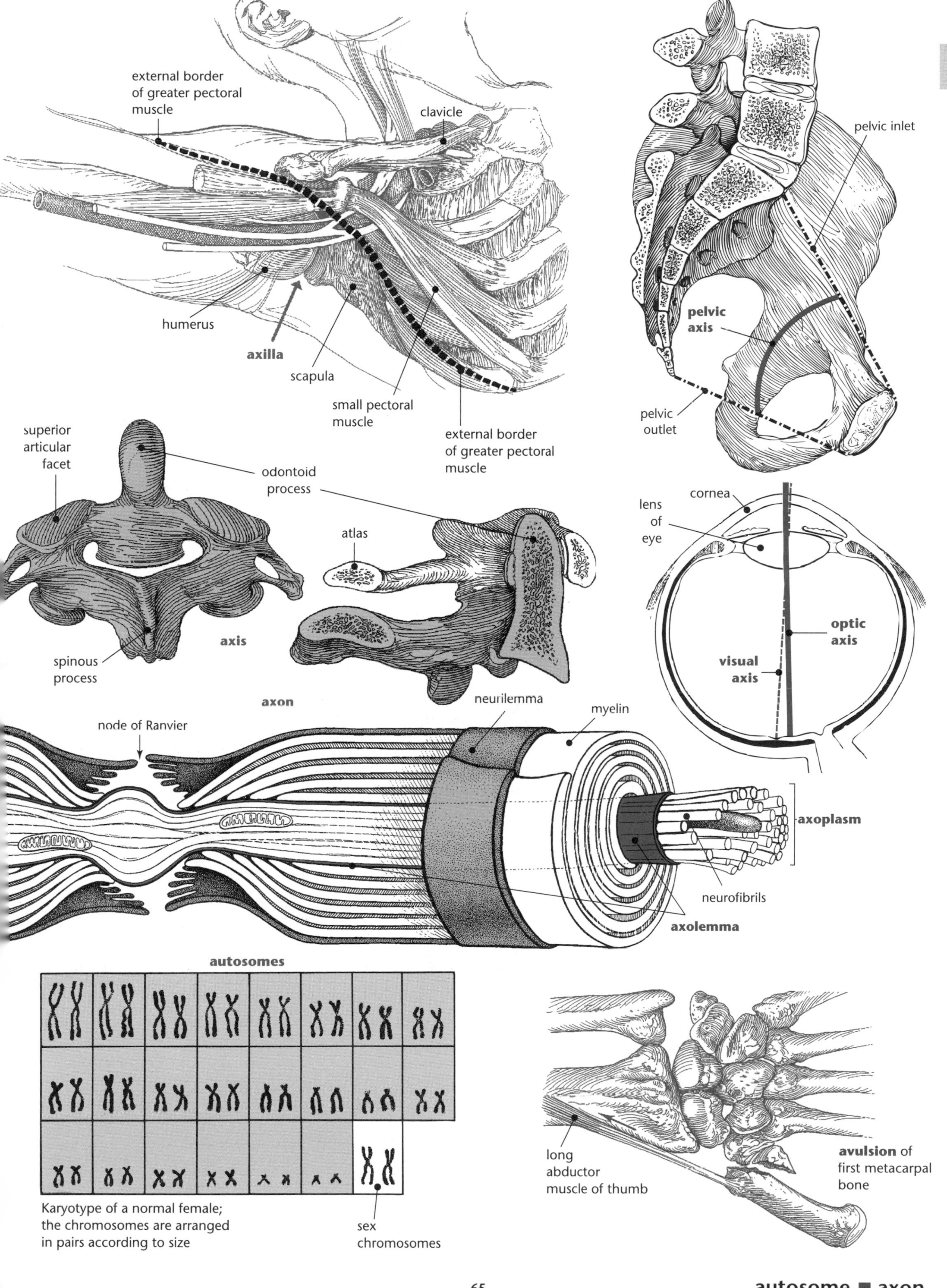

Karyotype of a normal female; the chromosomes are arranged in pairs according to size

B

B

ß (ba´tă) Beta. For terms beginning with β, see under specific term.
Babesia (bă-be´zhă) A genus of irregularly shaped protozoa (order Piroplasmida), parasites of the red blood cells, causing babesiosis in domestic and wild animals and humans.
babesiosis (bă-be-ze-o´sis) Any disease caused by a species of *Babesia* spread by ticks and afflicting many domestic animals.
Babinski's sign (bă-bin´skēz sīn) **1.** See extensor plantar reflex, under reflex. **2.** See pronation sign. **3.** Reduced contraction of the platysma muscle (at the neck) during movements of the jaw and face; occurs on the affected side in hemiplegia.
Babinski's syndrome (bă-bin´skē sin´drōm) The association of cardiac, arterial, and central nervous system disorders of late syphilis.
baby (ba´be) An infant.
blue b. An infant with a congenital heart defect in which the ductus arteriosus or foramen ovale of the heart fails to close, causing a mixing of venous and arterial blood in the left ventricle and a blood supply inadequate in oxygen; the skin usually has a bluish tint.
blueberry muffin b. The occurrence of yellowish and purple patches on the skin of a newborn; may be the result of an intrauterine viral infection transmitted from the mother through the placenta.
collodion b. A newborn infant with a thick, shiny, membranous skin that cracks and peels. The condition may disappear completely or may evolve into ichthyosis, especially lamellar ichthyosis.
test-tube b. Popular term for an infant born from an egg fertilized *in vitro* (in a Petri dish) and then implanted in the mother's uterus.
baby bottle syndrome (ba´be bŏt´l sin´drōm) See nursing bottle caries, under caries.
babygram (ba´be-gram) An x-ray film that includes the chest and abdomen of a newborn baby.
bacillary, bacillar (bas´ĭ-lar-e, bas´ĭ-lar) Relating to or caused by a bacillus.
bacillemia (bas-ĭ-le´me-ă) The presence of rod-shaped bacteria (bacilli) in the blood.
bacilli (bă-sil-i) Plural of bacillus.
bacilliform (bă-sil´ĭ-form) Shaped like a bacillus; rod-shaped.
bacilluria (bas-ĭ-lu´re-ă) The passage of urine containing rod-shaped bacteria (bacilli).
Bacillus (bă-sil´us) A genus of rod-shaped, aerobic, spore-forming, gram-positive bacteria (family Bacillaceae); some species cause disease.
B. anthracis Bacterium that causes anthrax in some animals and in humans.
B. cereus A saprophytic, spore-forming bacillus with peritrichous flagella that is responsible for a diarrheal type of food poisoning.
B. polymyxa A saprophytic, gram-negative bacillus found in soil and water; some strains produce the antibiotic polymyxin.
B. subtilis A widely distributed saprophytic, spore-forming, gram-positive bacillus found in soil and decaying organic matter; some strains produce antibiotics. Also called grass bacillus; hay bacillus.
bacillus (bă-sil´us), *pl.* **bacil´li** **1.** General term for any microorganism of the genus *Bacillus*. **2.** Term used to denote any of various rod-shaped bacteria.
Bang's b. See *Brucella abortus*, under *Brucella*.
Calmette-Guérin b. An attenuated strain of the bacterium *Mycobacterium bovis* used in the preparation of the bacille Calmette-Guérin (BCG) vaccine.
cholera b. See *Vibrio cholerae*, under *Vibrio*.
coliform bacilli A popular term denoting *Escherichia coli* and other intestinal bacteria that resemble *Escherichia*, especially in the fermentation of lactose with gas; used in reports of the degree of fecal contamination in water.
Döderlein's b. A gram-positive bacterium occurring in normal vaginal secretions; believed to be identical to *Lactobacillus acidophilus*.
Ducrey's b. See *Haemophilus ducreyi*, under *Haemophilus*.

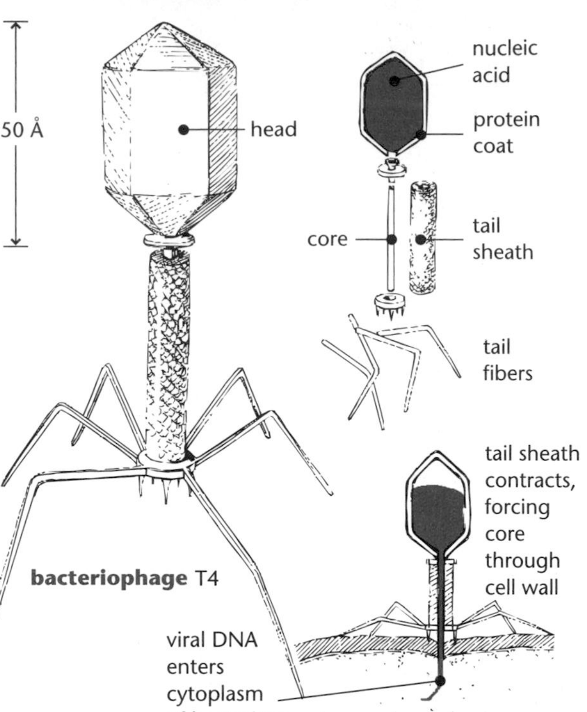

bacteriophage T4

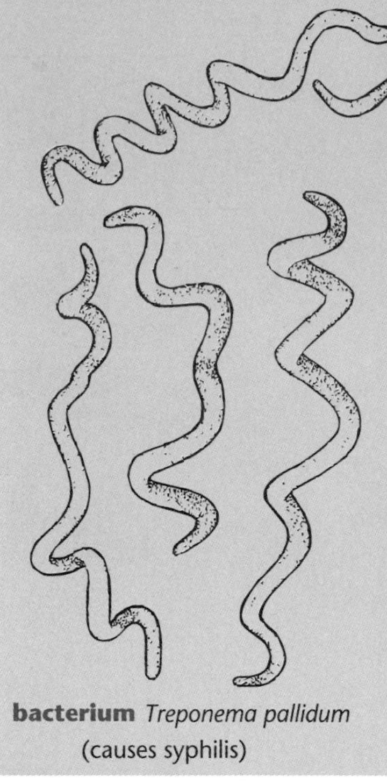
bacterium *Treponema pallidum* (causes syphilis)

Friedländer's b. See *Klebsiella pneumoniae*, under *Klebsiella*.
gas b. See *Clostridium perfringens*, under *Clostridium*.
grass b. See *Bacillus subtilis*, under *Bacillus*.
Hansen's b. See *Mycobacterium leprae*, under *Mycobacterium*.
hay b. See *Bacillus subtilis*, under *Bacillus*.
Koch's b. (a) See *Mycobacterium tuberculosis*, under *Mycobacterium*. (b) See *Vibrio cholerae*, under *Vibrio*.
Koch-Weeks b. See *Haemophilus influenzae*, under *Haemophilus*.
leprosy b. See *Mycobacterium leprae*, under *Mycobacterium*.
tubercle b. See *Mycobacterium tuberculosis* (human), under *Mycobacterium*.
Welch's b. See *Clostridium perfringens*, under *Clostridium*.
bacitracin (bas-ĭ-tra´sin) An antibiotic substance obtained from a microorganism belonging to the *Bacillus subtilis* group; used as a topical application.
back (băk) The posterior portion of the trunk.
backache (băk´āk) Pain in the back, especially in the lumbosacral or lower part of the back.
backbone (băk´bōn) **1.** See vertebral column, under column. **2.** Atoms in a polymer that are common to all its molecules. **3.** The main chain of a polypeptide.
background (băk´ground) **1.** The natural radiation of the earth and its atmosphere, and that coming from outer space. **2.** The presence of sound or radiation at a fairly constant low level.
backing (băk´ing) A metal support used in dentistry to attach a facing to a prosthesis.
backscatter (bak´skat-er) In radiology, radiation deflected more than 90° from the main beam of radiation.
bacteremia (bak-ter-e´me-ă) The presence of viable bacteria in the bloodstream.
MAC b. See *Mycobacterium avium* complex bacteremia.
***Mycobacterium avium* complex b.** Disseminated infection of the blood with a complex of bacteria that includes several strains of *Mycobacterium avium* and the closely related *Mycobacterium intracellulare*; it occurs as a common complication of advanced HIV infection, frequently as a patient's first AIDS-defining opportunistic disease, and causing a significantly increased incidence of fatigue, weight loss, fever, diarrhea, anemia, and a shortened life span. Also called MAC bacteremia.
bacteria (bak-te´re-ă) Plural of bacterium.
bacterial (bak-te´re-al) Relating to bacteria.
bactericidal (bak-ter-ĭ-si´dal) Capable of destroying bacteria.
bactericide (bak-tēr´ĭ-sīd) Any substance that destroys bacteria.
bacterid (bak´ter-id) A recurrent eruption of pus-filled blisters (pustules) localized to the palms and soles; although the primary pustule is sterile, the eruption may be aggravated by a bacterial infection; cause is unknown; previously thought to be associated with another, remote, infection. Also called pustular bacterid.
bacteriform (bak-tēr´ĭ-form) Having a bacterial form.
bacteriologic (bak-tēr-e-o-loj´ik) Relating to bacteriology.
bacteriologist (bak-ter-e-ol´ŏ-jist) A specialist in bacteriology.
bacteriology (bak-te-re-ol´o-je) The branch of microbiology concerned with the study of bacteria, especially in relation to medicine and agriculture.
bacteriolysin (bak-tēr-e-ol´ĭ-sin) An antibody that combines with the bacterial cells (antigen) that caused its formation and later destroys the cells.
bacteriolytic (bak-tēr-e-o-lit´ik) Capable of dissolving bacteria.
bacteriophage (bak-tēr´e-o-fāj) A delicate virus with considerable variation in structure that may attack and destroy bacterial cells under certain conditions; contains a DNA or RNA core (usually DNA) and a protein coat; it is the simplest replicating structure currently known to exist. Also called phage.
bacteriophagia, bacteriophagy (bak-tēr-e-o-fa´jă, bak-tēr-e-of´ă-je) The destruction of bacteria by any agent that causes disintegration.
bacteriopsonin (bak-tēr-e-op´so-nin) An opsonin or antibody that acts upon bacteria.
bacteriostasis (bak-tēr-e-os´tă-sis) The retardation of the growth and reproduction of bacteria.
bacteriostat (bak-tēr´e-o-stat) Any chemical agent that inhibits bacterial growth.
bacteriostatic (bak-tēr-e-o-stat´ik) Inhibiting the growth and reproduction of bacteria. COMPARE: bactericidal.
bacterium (bak-te´re-um), *pl.* **bacte´ria** Any of various one-celled microorganisms of the plant kingdom, existing as free-living organisms or as parasites, multiplying by subdivision, and having a large range of biochemical (including pathogenic) properties. They are classified according to their shape into: bacilli (rod-shaped), cocci (spherical), spirilla (spiral-shaped), and vibrios (comma-shaped); they are further classified on the basis of staining characteristics, colony morphology, and metabolic behavior.
enteric b. A bacterium indigenous to the intestines, usually a nonpathogenic gram-negative rod.

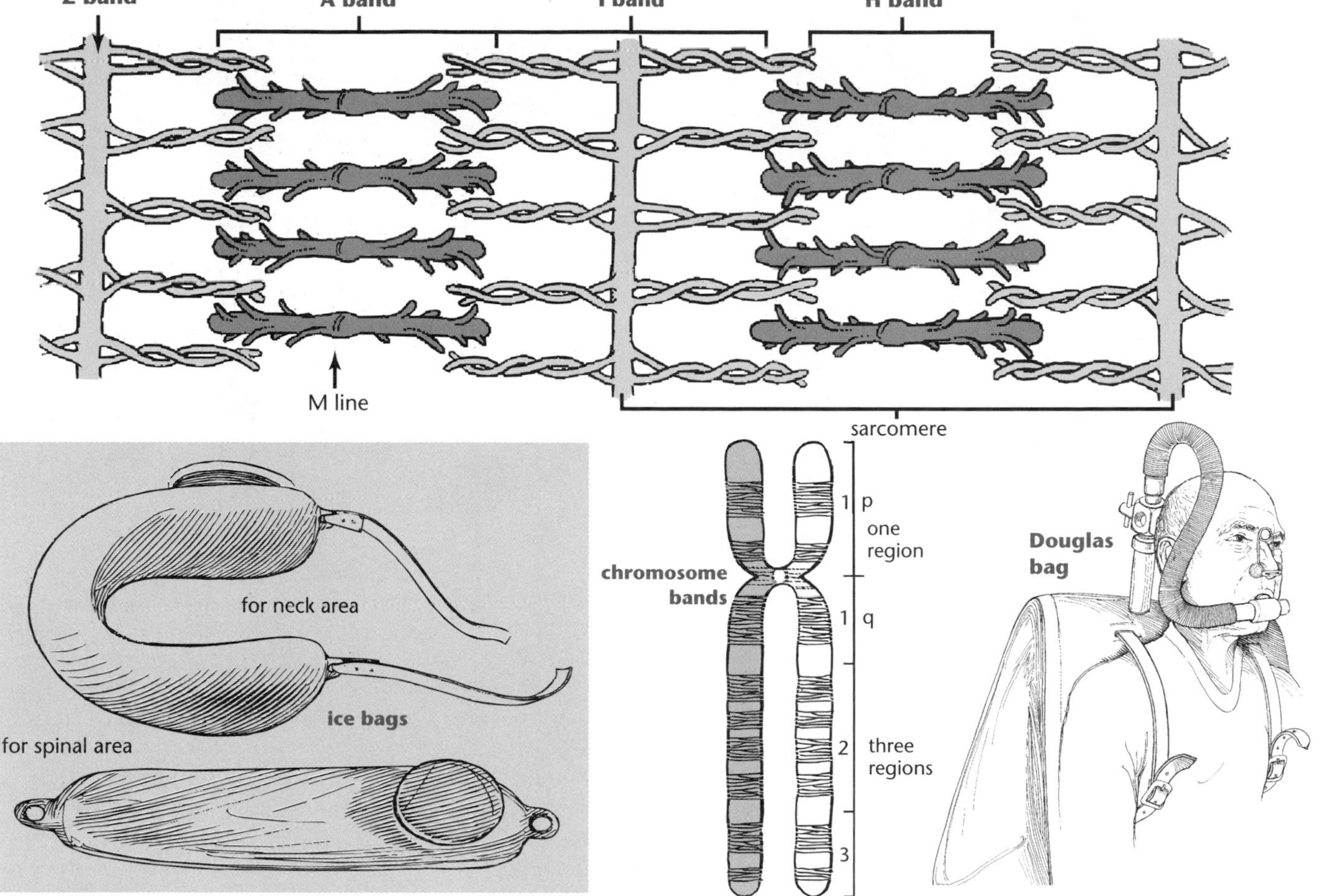

B

L-forms of bacteria Small, filterable bacterial forms with defective or absent cell walls (caused by antibiotics, specific antibodies, or lysosomal enzymes) which retain the ability to multiply.
bacteriuria (bak-te-re-u´re-ă) The presence of bacteria in the urine.
Bacteroides (bak-ter-oi´dēz) A genus of bacteria (family Bacteroidaceae) composed of gram-negative, nonmotile, anaerobic bacilli normally inhabiting the mouth, intestinal tract, and genital organs of humans; some species are pathogenic.
B. fragilis A species causing urinary tract infections; also found in puerperal infections, such as pelvic abscesses, cesarean section wound infections, and septic pelvic thrombophlebitis.
B. melaninogenicus See *Prevotella melaninogenica.*
bag (bag) **1.** A sac or pouch. **2.** Slang term for scrotum.
Ambu b. A self-reinflating bag used to produce positive pressure respiration during resuscitation.
colostomy b. A bag worn over the abdominal opening of a colostomy to collect fecal material from the intestines.
Douglas b. A device for measuring oxygen consumption of an individual, consisting of a 100-liter canvas or plastic bag with an attached mouthpiece that houses inspiratory and expiratory valves; room air is breathed in and all expired air is collected in the bag for analysis of the oxygen and carbon dioxide content.
ice b. Rubber bag into which crushed ice is put to produce local cooling; available in a variety of shapes to fit specific parts of the body.
b. of waters See amniochorion.
bagassosis (bag-a-so´sis) A chronic respiratory disorder caused by continued inhalation of the dust of bagasse (the crushed, juiceless residue of sugar cane).
balance (bal´ans) **1.** A weighing device. **2.** A state of bodily stability produced by the harmonious functional performance of its parts. **3.** In chemistry, equality of the reacting components on each side of a chemical equation.
acid-base b. The normal ratio of acid and base elements in blood plasma. Also called acid-base equilibrium.
fluid b. State of the body in relation to the intake and loss of water and electrolytes. Also called water balance.
nitrogen b. State of the body in relation to the intake and loss of nitrogen; positive nitrogen balance occurs when the amount of nitrogen excreted is smaller than the amount ingested, as during the growing age of children; negative nitrogen balance occurs when the amount of nitrogen excreted is greater than the amount ingested, as during malnutrition or febrile illnesses.
water b. See fluid balance.
balanitis (bal-ă-ni´tis) Inflammation of the glans penis.
balanoblenorrhea (bal´ă-no-blen-o-re´ă) Inflammation of the glans penis due to gonorrhea.
balanoplasty (bal´ă-no-plas-te) Any reconstructive operation upon the glans penis.
balanoposthitis (bal-ă-no-pos-thi´tis) Inflammation of the glans penis and the adjacent surface of the prepuce.
balanopreputial (bal-ă-no-pre-poo´shal) Relating to the glans penis and the prepuce.
baldness (bawld´nĕs) See alopecia.
ball (bawl) A round mass.
food b. See phytobezoar.
fungus b. A fungus mass in a body cavity.
hair b. See trichobezoar.
ballismus (bă-liz´mus) Flailing movements of one or more limbs; caused by brain damage, specifically, to the subthalamic nucleus.
balloon (bă-lo͞on´) **1.** A spherical, inflatable, nonporous sac, such as the one near the tip of a Foley catheter. **2.** To distend an organ or vessel with gas or fluid. **3.** To expand a cavity with air to facilitate its examination.
intra-aortic b. A balloon that is placed within the descending aorta and inflated intermittently in a pulsating fashion; upon activation during diastole, its pulsation increases blood pressure and organ perfusion; then, on deflation, it decreases cardiac work with each systole by decreasing afterload.
ballottement (bă-lot´ment) **1.** A method of physical examination to determine the size and mobility of an organ in the body, particularly in the presence of fluid. **2.** A method of diagnosis of pregnancy; the examining finger is inserted into the vagina and a sudden tap is given on the uterus; the fetus, if present, rises in the amniotic fluid and rebounds to its original position, striking the wall of the uterus which is felt by the examining finger.
balm (bahm) An ointment or a soothing application.
balneology (bal-ne-ol´ō-je) The branch of medical science concerned with mineral waters and their therapeutic use, especially as a bath.
balneotherapeutics, balneotherapy (bal-ne-o-ther-ă-pu´tiks, bal-ne-o-ther´ă-pe) The treatment of disease by means of baths of mineral waters.
balsam (bawl´sam) The gummy exudate of some trees and shrubs, used in pharmacologic preparations.
band (band) **1.** Any appliance or structure that encircles or binds another. **2.** Any ribbon-shaped anatomic structure.
A b. The broad, dark band produced by the thick (100 Å) myosin filaments that traverse the central part of the sarcomere. Also called anisotropic band.
absorption b.'s Areas of darkness in the spectrum indicating the regions where light was absorbed by the medium (gas, liquid or solid) through which it passed.
amniotic b.'s Abnormal strands of tissue that sometimes develop between the fetus and the sac (amniochorion) containing the fetus, believed by some to cause fetal deformities.
anisotropic b. See A band.
chromosome b. Part of a chromosome distinguishable from adjacent segments by a difference in staining intensity.
I b. A light band extending toward the center of the sarcomere from each Z line of the striated muscle fibers, composed of thin (50 Å) longitudinally oriented actin filaments. Also called isotropic band.
isotropic b. See I band.
omphalomesenteric b. An abnormal band from the intestine to the navel; a remnant of the embryonic omphalomesenteric (vitelline) duct that failed to obliterate. It occasionally results in small bowel obstruction when intestines loop around it.
orthodontic b. A thin strip of metal closely encircling the crown of a tooth in a horizontal plane.
silastic b. See Falope ring, under ring.
Z b. See Z line, under line.

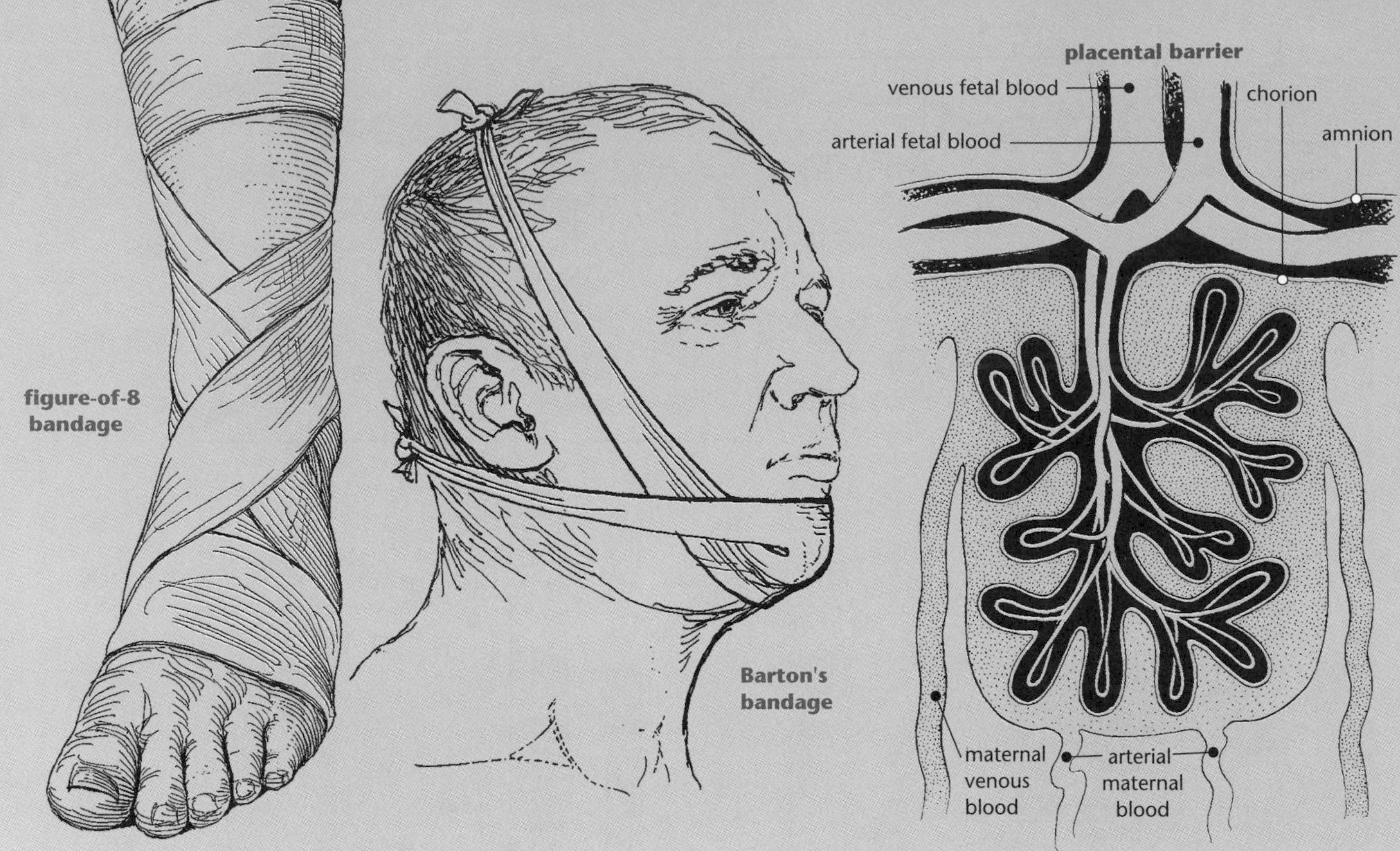

bandage (ban´dĭj) **1.** A piece of gauze or other material used to compress, check hemorrhage, prevent motion, or retain surgical dressings. **2.** To cover by wrapping with a strip of material.

Barton's b. A figure-of-eight bandage for the support of the lower jaw.

capeline b. A double-headed roller bandage for covering the head or an amputation stump.

elastic b. Bandage made of an elastic material, used to exert mild continuous pressure.

figure-of-eight b. A roller bandage applied in such a way that the turns cross like the figure 8.

Galen's b. A broad head bandage with the ends split into three sections; after the bandage is placed on the head, the anterior ends are tied behind the neck, the posterior ends on the forehead, and the middle ends under the chin.

plaster b. A bandage that is impregnated with plaster of Paris; used for immobilization.

reverse b. Bandage applied to a limb in such a way that the roller is half-twisted with each turn.

roller b. Bandage material rolled into a compact cylinder.

spica b. A figure-of-eight bandage with overlapping turns, applied to two anatomic parts of markedly different dimensions, such as the arm and thorax, thigh and pelvis, thumb and hand.

spiral b. Bandage applied spirally around a limb.

T b. A bandage shaped like the letter T, generally used to keep dressings on the perineum.

tubular b. A gauze bandage in the shape of a tube for covering small structures, such as a finger; it is put on the structure with an applicator.

Velpeau's b. A bandage used to support the arm and hold it across the chest.

bandaging (ban´dĭ-gĭng) The application of a bandage.

banding (band´ing) **1.** The act of encircling with a thin strip of flexible material. **2.** The staining of chromosomes to make characteristic cross bands visible, thus facilitating identification of chromosome pairs, allocation of phenotypic features to the specific chromosome segment, and classification of clinical syndromes.

C b., centromeric b. Banding by heating preparations in saline solution to temperatures just below boiling and staining with Giemsa stain; useful for staining material near centromeres.

chromosome b. See banding.

G b., Giemsa b. Banding by incubating preparations in saline solution and staining with Giemsa stain; it is the most commonly used technique.

NOR b., nucleolar organization region b. Banding with a silver stain, useful for staining satellites and stalks of acrocentric chromosomes.

pulmonary artery b. Surgical procedure to alleviate congestive heart failure by decreasing blood flow through the lungs and consequently reducing volume overload of the left ventricle.

Q b., quinacrine b. Banding with quinacrine fluorescent stain.

R b., reverse b. Banding by incubating preparations in buffer solution at high temperatures and staining with Giemsa stain.

bank (bank) A place for collecting and storing biological products.

blood b. A bank for blood and blood products.

eye b. A facility for obtaining and distributing corneas to eye surgeons (usually within 24 to 48 hours) for use in corneal transplants.

sperm b. A bank where sperm is preserved frozen for future use in artificial insemination. Liquid nitrogen at 196°C is used to arrest molecular movement and preserve the cells' vitality.

Banti's syndrome (ban´tēz sin´drōm) See chronic congestive splenomegaly, under splenomegaly.

bar (băr) **1.** The international unit of pressure; 1 megadyne (10^6 dyne per cm^2) atmosphere. **2.** Tissue bridging a gap between structures. **3.** A piece of metal connecting two or more parts of a removable partial denture.

Passavant's b. See Passavant's ridge, under ridge.

barbital (băr´bĭ-tawl) A colorless or white crystalline powder, $C_8H_{12}N_2O_3$; a barbituric acid derivative used as a sedative.

barbiturate (băr-bich´ŭr-āt) **1.** A salt of barbituric acid. **2.** Any derivative of barbituric acid used as a sedative.

barbituric acid (băr-bĭ-tūr´ik as´id) A crystalline substance, $CH_2(CONH)_2CO$, not itself a sedative, but from which barbiturates (sedative drugs) are derived.

bariatrician (bar-e-ă-trish´ăn) A physician who specializes in reducing the weight of obese patients.

bariatrics (bar-e-at´riks) The branch of medicine concerned with the care and treatment of overweight people.

barium (bar´e-um) A soft silvery-white metallic element; symbol Ba, atomic number 56, atomic weight 137.36.

b. sulfate A fine, white, almost insoluble powder, $BaSO_4$; used as a radiopaque contrast medium when given orally or as an enema for x-ray visualization of the gastrointestinal tract.

baroceptor (bar-o-sep´tor) See baroreceptor.

barognosis (bar-ag-no´sis) Weight perception; ability to recognize weight (e.g., when an object is placed in the hand).

baroreceptor (bar-o-re-sep´tor) A sensory nerve terminal (sense organ) that responds to changes in pressure. Also called pressoreceptor; baroceptor.

barosinusitis (bar-o-si-nu-si´tis) Inflammatory condition of paranasal sinuses caused by a sudden change in atmospheric pressure, which creates a difference between pressures within the sinuses and that of the atmosphere.

barotitis media (bar-o-ti´tis me´de-ă) Damage to the middle ear caused by the relative vacuum created in the middle ear chamber by a sudden change in atmospheric pressure (e.g., while diving or flying); usually occurs when the eustachian (auditory) tube is obstructed due to allergies or respiratory tract infection; symptoms include pain, dizziness, and hearing loss; the eardrum (tympanic membrane) may rupture. Also called aerotitis media; commonly called aviator's ear.

barotrauma (bar-o-traw´mă) Injury caused by pressure, generally to the middle ear or paranasal sinuses, due to the difference between atmospheric pressure and that within the affected cavity.

bar reader (bar rē´der) A device that provides for the placement of a bar (opaque septum) between a printed page and the viewer's eyes so as to occlude different areas of the page for each of the eyes; used principally for the diagnosis and training of simultaneous binocular vision.

barrel (bar´el) A cylinder or hollow shaft.

vaginal b. The vaginal cavity extending from the uterus to the vulva.

barren (bar´en) Popular term for a woman who is incapable of producing offspring; sterile.

barrier (bar´e-er) An impediment or obstacle.

blood-air b. The tissues in the lung, measuring about 0.2 μm in thickness, separating capillary blood from alveolar air and through which exchange of gases occurs; composed of squamous endothelium (lining the capillary), a basal membrane, and alveolar epithelium.

blood-brain b. (BBB) The tight junction

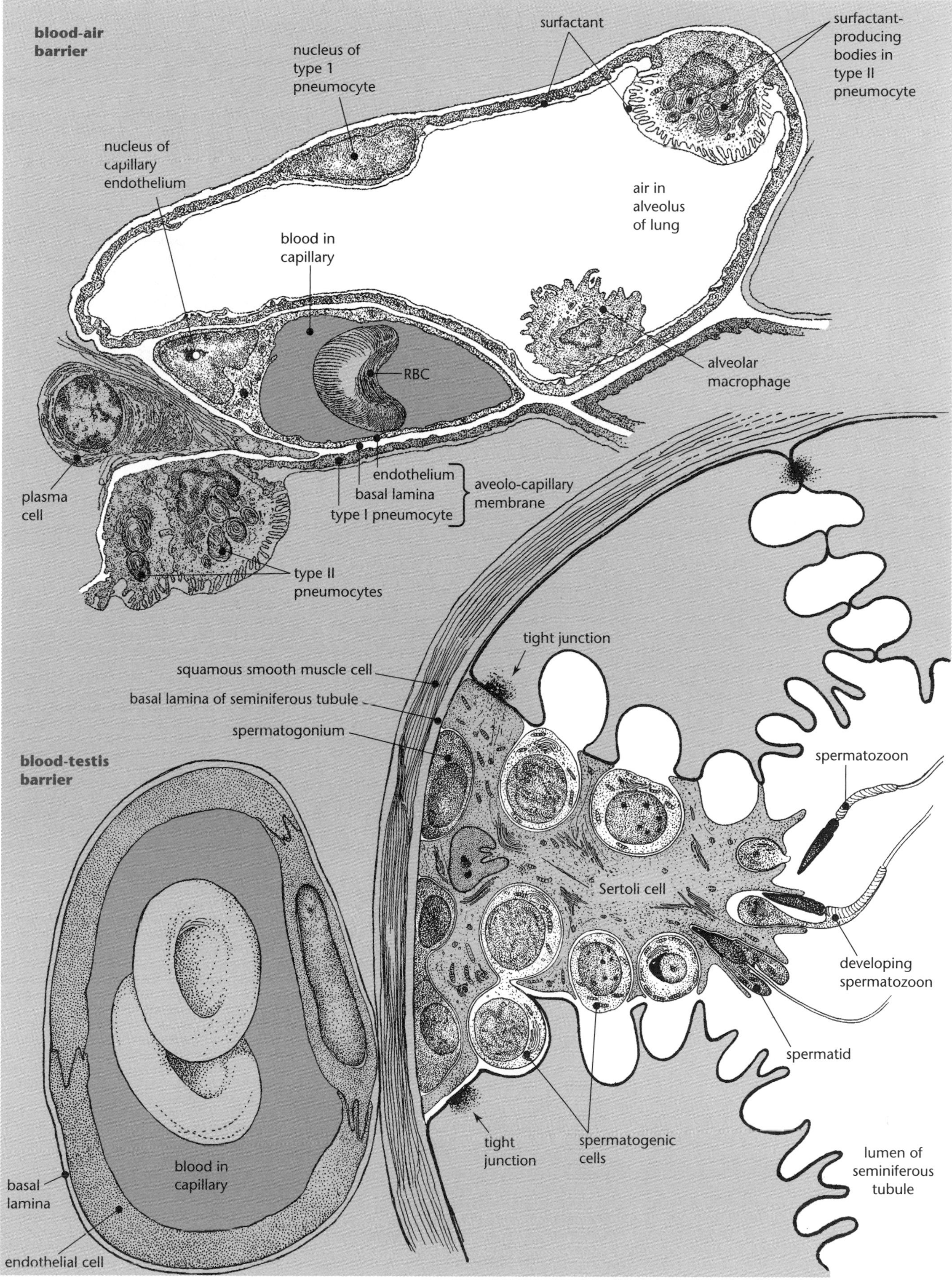
blood-air barrier
surfactant
surfactant-producing bodies in type II pneumocyte
nucleus of type 1 pneumocyte
nucleus of capillary endothelium
air in alveolus of lung
blood in capillary
RBC
alveolar macrophage
plasma cell
endothelium
basal lamina
type I pneumocyte
aveolo-capillary membrane
type II pneumocytes
tight junction
squamous smooth muscle cell
basal lamina of seminiferous tubule
spermatogonium
blood-testis barrier
spermatozoon
Sertoli cell
developing spermatozoon
spermatid
tight junction
spermatogenic cells
lumen of seminiferous tubule
blood in capillary
basal lamina
endothelial cell

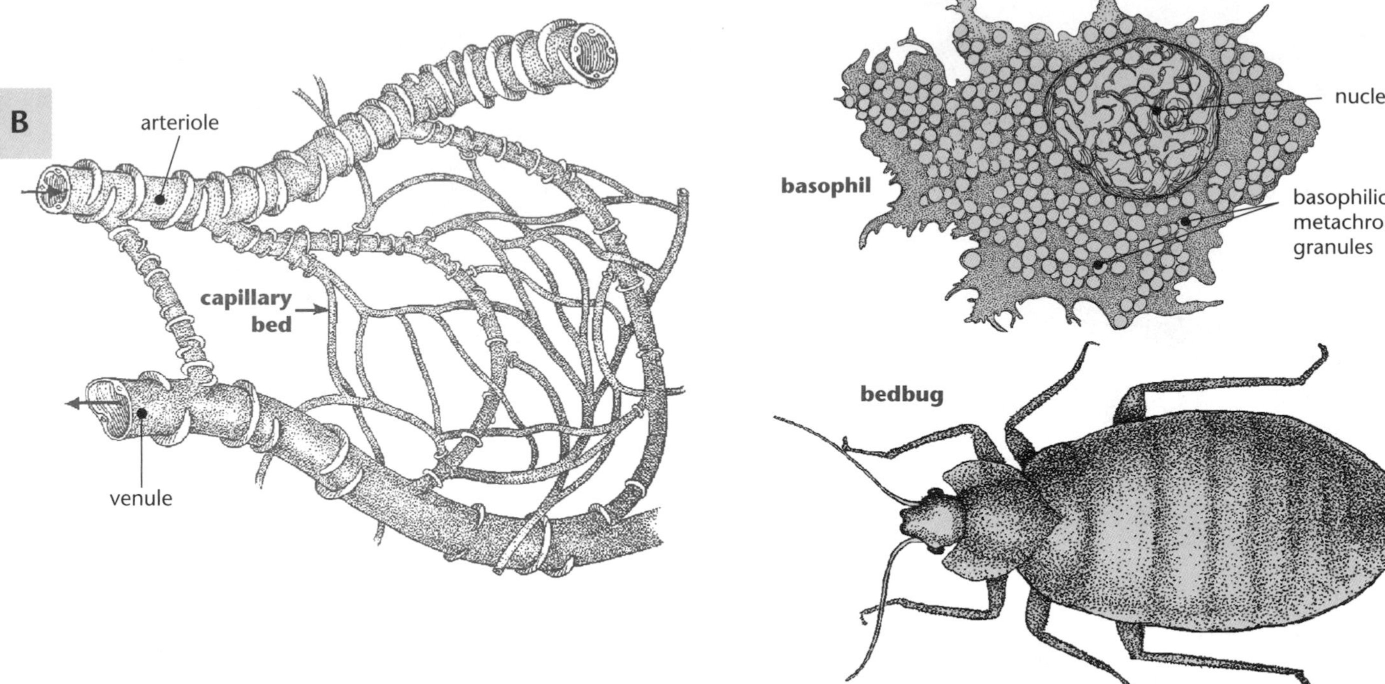

between endothelial cells of capillary walls that normally permits only a limited exchange between blood in the capillaries on the one hand and cerebrospinal fluid and extracellular fluid in the brain on the other.

blood-testis b. The tight junction barrier of the cells of Sertoli in the seminiferous tubules of the testis that restricts substances from entering the lumen of the tubules, where the spermatozoa are developing.

placental b. The semipermeable epithelial layer of the placenta separating maternal and fetal blood.

protective b. In radiology, material such as lead or concrete, used for absorbing ionizing radiation for protective purposes.

bartholinitis (bar-to-lin-i´tis) Inflammation of the greater vestibular glands (Bartholin's glands).

Bartonella bacilliformis (bar-to-nel´ă bă-sil´ĭ-for-mis) A species of gram-negative encapsulated bacteria that causes bartonellosis; transmitted to humans by the bite of sand flies.

bartonellosis (bar-to-nel-o´sis) Disease occurring mainly in Peru, caused by the bacillus *Bartonella bacilliformis*, transmitted by the bite of the sand fly; marked by a febrile stage with hemolytic anemia (Oroya fever) followed several weeks later by a nodular skin eruption (verruga peruana); occasionally one stage of the disease occurs without the other. Also called Carrión's disease. See also verruga peruana.

Bartter syndrome (bar´ter sin´drōm) An auto-somal recessive inheritance marked by juxtaglo-merular cell hyperplasia, secondary hyperaldo-steronism, hypokalemic alkalosis, and a marked increase in prostaglandin production and in plasma renin levels in the absence of hypertension.

basal (ba´sal) Relating to a base.

base (bās) **1.** The foundation or supporting part of anything. **2.** The chief ingredient of a mixture. **3.** A substance that turns litmus indicators blue and combines with an acid to form a salt. **4.** The part opposite the apex, such as the base of the heart. **5.** See Brønsted base.

acrylic resin b. A denture base made of acrylic resin.

Brønsted b. A hydrogen ion acceptor (e.g., OH^-, NH_3, HCO_3^-).

cement b. A dressing placed at the bottom of deep cavities to protect the dental pulp from thermal shock and to serve as a floor for a permanent filling.

denture b. The framework of a partial denture that rests on the ridge. Also called saddle.

record b. See baseplate.

temporary b. See baseplate.

trial b. See baseplate.

Basedow's disease (baz-ĕ-dōz dĭ-zēz´) See exophthalmic goiter, under goiter.

baseplate (bās´plāt) A temporary form corresponding to the base of a denture, used for making jaw relation plates, or for arranging artificial teeth. Also called record base; temporary base; trial base.

basial (ba´se-ăl) Relating to the basion.

basic (ba´sik) Of or relating to a base. See also basilar.

basicranial (ba-sĭ-kra´ne-al) Relating to the base of the skull.

basilar (bas´ĭ-lar) Relating to a base, such as the basilar membrane of the cochlear duct.

basilateral (ba-sĭ-lat´er-al) Relating to the base and side or sides of a structure.

basion (ba´se-on) The middle point on the anterior margin of the foramen magnum (occipital foramen).

basis (ba´sis) Latin for base.

Basle Nomina Anatomica (ba´zil no´mĭ-nă an-ă-tom´ĭ-ka) (BNA) A system of anatomic nomenclature adopted by an anatomic association; it is superseded by *Nomina Anatomica.*

basocytosis (ba-so-sī-to´sis) Abnormal increase in the number of basophils in the blood. Also called basophilic leukocytosis.

basophil (ba´so-fil) A cell, especially a white blood cell (basophilic leukocyte), containing large granules that stain readily with basic dyes.

basophilia (ba-so-fil´e-ă) **1.** Abnormal increase of basophilic leukocytes in the blood. **2.** The presence of basophilic red blood cells in the blood.

basophilic (ba-so-fil´ik) Staining easily with basic dyes.

bath (bath) **1.** The immersion of the body, or part of it, in water or any other medium. **2.** The apparatus in which the body is immersed.

colloid b. A bath containing starch, sodium bicarbonate, or any other soothing material to relieve skin irritations.

contrast b. The alternate immersion of a body part in hot and cold water (usually at half-hour intervals) to increase blood circulation to the part.

douche b. The local application of a stream of water.

sitz b. A bath in which only the hips and buttocks of the patient are immersed in a tub of water.

tepid b. A bath in water at a temperature of approximately 86°F.

water b. (a) The immersion of the body, or part of it, in water. (b) The immersion in water of a liquid-containing vessel to heat or cool the liquid.

Batten-Mayou disease (bat´ĕn-ma-yoo´ dĭ-zēz´) See cerebral sphingolipidosis, under sphingolipidosis.

battered child syndrome (bat´erd chīld sin´drōm) Multiple injuries inflicted upon a child by an older individual, usually an adult and often a parent.

Battle's sign (bat´lz sīn) Discoloration behind the ear, seen in fracture of the base of the skull.

bdellin (del´in) Any of a group of inhibitors of protein-splitting enzymes; derived from mites of the genus *Bdella.*

beaded (bēd´ed) Having the appearance of a string of beads (e.g., some bacterial colonies).

beading (be´ding) A row of small spherical masses.

b. of ribs See rachitic rosary, under rosary.

beaker (bēk´er) A wide-mouth glass cylinder with a pouring lip, used in laboratories for mixing and heating substances.

bearing down (bār´ing down) The expulsive effort of a woman during the second stage of labor.

beat (bēt) **1.** To pulsate. **2.** To strike. **3.** A pulsation, as of the heart.

apex b. The beat of the apex of the heart during ventricular systole; normally felt at the left fifth intercostal space, at the midclavicular line.

capture b. A conducted heartbeat occurring after a period of atrioventricular (A-V) dissociation.

dropped b. A nonconducted heartbeat; one that fails to appear due to an atrioventricular (A-V) block.

ectopic b. A heartbeat originating at some point in the heart other than the sinoatrial node.

escape b. An automatic heartbeat following an interval longer than the dominant cycle (i.e., after the normal beat has defaulted).

fusion b. A heartbeat arising from the simultaneous activation of either the atria or the ventricles of the heart by two impulses from different sites.

premature b. An ectopic heartbeat that depends on, and is coupled to, the preceding beat, occurring before the next dominant beat.

becquerel (bek´rel) (Bq) The SI unit of radioactivity, equal to the radioactivity of a material decaying at the rate of 1 disintegration per second.

bed (bed) **1.** A piece of furniture for resting and sleeping. **2.** In anatomy, a base or layer of tissue upon which a structure rests.

capillary b. The total mass of capillaries and their volume capacity.

Gatch b. A hinged bed in which the patient's head and knees may be elevated.

nail b. The tissue to which a fingernail or toenail is firmly attached.

bedbug (bed´bug) A blood-sucking insect, *Cimex lectularius* (family Cimicidae), about 5 mm long when fully grown, with a flat, reddish brown body and a disagreeable odor; its bite produces urticarial wheals with central hemorrhagic points; it often infests human dwellings and usually hides during the day in bed frames, torn mattresses, between

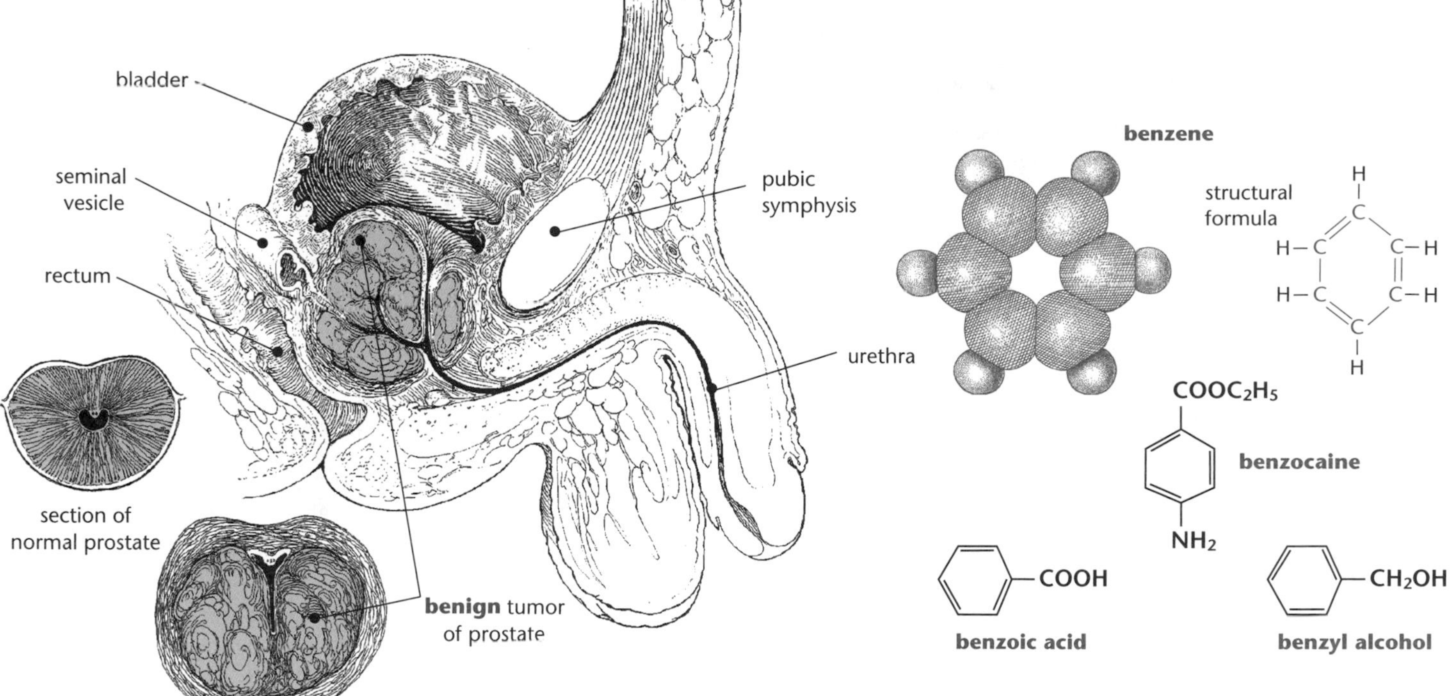

B

floorboards, and under the edges of wallpaper.

bedpan (bed´pan) A pan with a wide flat rim used for urination and defecation by a bedridden patient.

bedsore (bed´sor) See decubitus ulcer, under ulcer.

bed-wetting (bed-wet´ĭng) See nocturnal enuresis, under enuresis.

bedwing (bid´wing) Swelling of the corneal epithelium marked by irregular reflections from a multitude of droplets when seen with the slit lamp (e.g., in acute glaucoma).

bee (bē) An insect of the genus *Apis*, of which the honeybee is the most common stinging insect; it leaves its stinger and venom sac attached to the victim.

beeswax (bēz´waks) Wax secreted by the honeybee; one of the ingredients of many dental waxes.

behavior (be-hāv´yor) The manner in which a person acts or functions.

compensatory b. A behavior in which individuals suffering from anxiety disorders who are intolerant of themselves often exhibit a compensatory attitude of intolerance of others.

behavioral (be-hāv´yor-al) Relating to behavior.

behaviorism (be-hāv´yor-iz-m) A branch of psychology concerned with the observable, tangible, and objective facts of behavior, rather than with subjective phenomena such as thoughts, emotions, or impulses.

behavior modification (be-hāv´yor mod-ĭ-fĭ-ka´shun) Treatment that attempts to modify selective symptoms by techniques such as systematic desensitization and biofeedback.

Behçet syndrome, Behçet's disease (bĕ´chĕts sin´drōm, bĕ´chĕts dĭ-zēz´) Recurrent ulceration of the genitals and oral cavity with inflammation of the iris, ciliary body, and choroid and formation of a puslike fluid in the anterior chamber of the eye; pus-forming skin lesions are common and involvement of the central nervous system occurs in a variety of forms.

bejel (bej´el) See endemic syphilis, under syphilis.

bel (bel) A unit of sound intensity, being the logarithm (to the base 10) of the ratio of two levels of sound; the difference in intensity between a sound that is barely audible and one 10 times louder is 1 bel; named after Alexander Graham Bell.

belching (belch´ing) Popular term for eructation.

belladonna (bel-ă-don´ă) A poisonous plant, *Atropa belladonna*, with purple flowers and black berries. The deadly nightshade plant; its leaves and roots yield atropine, scopolamine, and other alkaloids that inhibit the action of parasympathetic nerves and are used as antispasmodics to treat gastrointestinal disorders.

belle indifference (bel an-dif-er-ahns´) See la belle indifference.

belly (bel´e) **1.** Abdomen. **2.** The prominent fleshy part of a muscle.

bellyache (bel´e-āk) Colic.

belly button (bel´e but´on) Umbilicus; navel.

Bence Jones albumin, Bence Jones protein (bens jōnz al-bu´min, bens jōnz pro-tēn) See Bence Jones protein, under protein.

bends (bendz) A manifestation of decompression sickness, consisting of severe pain in the joints and muscles, especially of the limbs and hip, which are maintained in a semiflexed position (hence the name); produced by liberation of gas bubbles in the tissues. See also decompression sickness, under sickness.

benign (be-nīn´) Denoting a condition capable of disturbing the function of an organ, without endangering the life of the individual; not malignant.

benzalkonium chloride (ben-zal-ko´ne-um klor´īd) Compound used as a local disinfectant.

benzene (ben´zēn) A thin, colorless, highly flammable liquid, C_6H_6; a coal-tar derivative, used in the manufacture of numerous chemical products. Commonly called benzol.

benzimidazole (ben-zĭ-mid´ă-zol) A compound occurring as part of the vitamin B_{12} molecule.

benzoate (ben´zo-āt) An ester or salt of benzoic acid.

benzocaine (ben´zo-kān) A surface anesthetic of the skin and mucous membranes, widely used for relief of sunburn, pruritus, and burns; an ethyl ester of aminobenzoic acid.

benzodiazepine (ben-zo-di-az´ĕ-pēn) A compound from which are derived a number of tranquilizers.

benzoic acid (ben-zo´ik as´id) A white crystalline acid occurring naturally in the resin benzoin; used in fungicides and dentifrices.

benzoin (ben´zo-in) A resin obtained as a gum from a tree, *Styrax benzoin*, sometimes used as an inhalant expectorant in the treatment of laryngitis and bronchitis.

benzyl (ben´zĭl) A hydrocarbon radical.

b. alcohol $C_6H_5CH_2OH$; a substance used as a local anesthetic.

Berger's disease (bār-zhārz´ dĭ-zēz´) See IgA nephropathy, under nephropathy.

beriberi (ber-e-ber´e) Disease resulting from a dietary deficiency of thiamine (vitamin B_1).

dry b. Chronic condition with prominent involvement of multiple peripheral nerves.

infantile b. Beriberi occurring during the first year of life, usually with prominent cardiovascular manifestations; most commonly occurs in small, breast-fed infants in the first months of life, reflecting severe thiamine deficiency in the mother.

wet b. Deficiency affecting the cardiovascular system; characterized by the heart's inability to pump sufficient blood (heart failure), which leads to congestion of blood in veins of the legs and accumulation of fluid in tissues of the legs, trunk, and sometimes the face.

berkelium (berk´le-um) A synthetic, transuranium radioactive element; symbol Bk, atomic number 97, atomic weight 247; twelve isotopes have been produced.

Bernheim syndrome (bārn´hīm sin´drōm) Right heart failure without pulmonary congestion in the presence of left ventricular enlargement.

berylliosis (ber-il-e-o´sis) Condition caused by inhalation of fumes or contact with particles of beryllium salts; marked by granulomatous growths in the lungs or skin.

beryllium (ber-il´e-um) A high melting point, corrosion-resistant metallic element; symbol Be, atomic number 4; atomic weight 9.012; used as a reflector in nuclear reactors and, in a copper alloy, for electrical contacts and nonsparking tools.

bestiality (bes-te-al´ĭ-te) Sexual activities between a human and an animal.

beta (ba´tă) **1.** The second letter of the Greek alphabet, β. **2.** The second item in a system of classification, as of chemical compounds. For terms beginning with beta, see under specific term.

beta-blocker (ba´tă blok´er) See beta-adrenergic blocking agent, under agent.

beta-fetoprotein (ba´tă fe-to-pro´tēn) A liver protein normally found in the fetus; it has been found in adults with liver disease. See also alpha-fetoprotein.

betamethasone (ba´tă-meth´ă-sōn) A potent anti-inflammatory glucocorticoid agent administered orally or as a topical application to the skin. Adverse effects of topical application include thinning of the skin; oral administration is associated with more serious adverse effects common to all steroids (e.g., enhanced susceptibility to infections, fluid retention, and high blood pressure).

beta$_2$-microglobulin (ba-tă-mi-kro-glob´u-lin) A polypeptide that is a constituent of the class I major histocompatibility antigens and other membrane proteins.

betel (be´tel) The dried leaf and nut of an East Indian plant (*Piper betle*), which are chewed for their stimulant effects. Associated with cancer of the mouth; the carcinogenic agent has not been identified.

bethanechol chloride (bĕ-than´ĕ-kol klor´īd) A parasympathomimetic drug used in the treatment of constipation, paralytic ileus, and urinary retention.

bezoar (be´zor) A hard mass found chiefly in the alimentary canal of ruminants and occasionally in humans, composed of hair and/or vegetable fibers; it

B

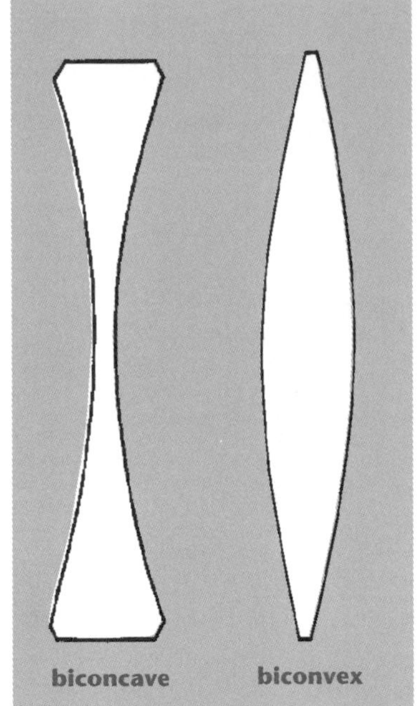

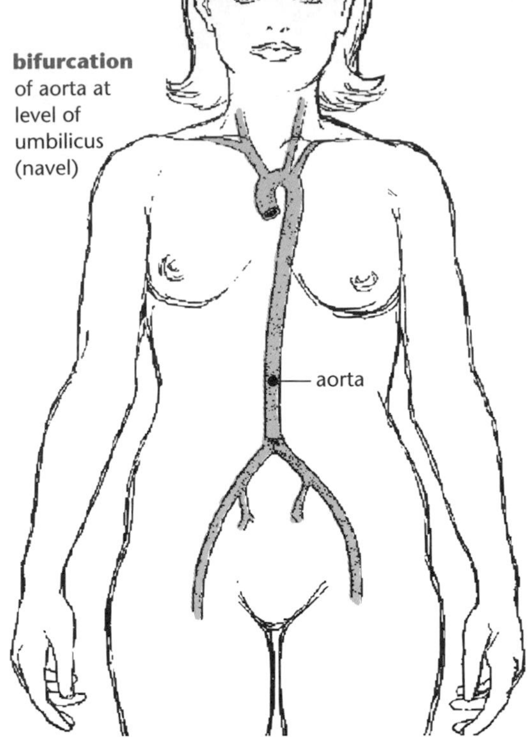

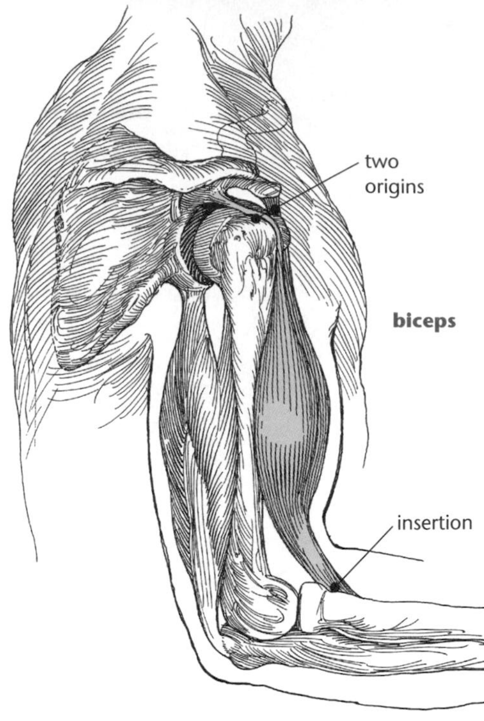

was formerly thought to have magical properties and was used as an antidote for poison.

bias (bi´as) **1.** In statistics, the distortion in the results of a study arising from systematic errors in sampling or analysis. **2.** An unvarying voltage applied to an electrode.

biauricular (bi-aw-rik´u-lar) **1.** Having two auricles. **2.** Relating to both auricles.

bibasic (bi-ba´sik) See dibasic.

bibulous (bib´u-lus) Absorbent.

bicameral (bi-kam´er-al) Composed of two chambers or cavities; said of an abscess.

bicarbonate (bi-kar´bo-nāt) A compound containing the radical group HCO_3.

standard b. The portion of bicarbonate in plasma that is derived from nonrespiratory sources; it is the bicarbonate concentration in the plasma of a whole blood sample that has been equilibrated at a 37°C temperature with a carbon dioxide pressure of 40 mm of mercury. Metabolic alkalosis and acidosis are reflected in abnormally high or low levels, respectively.

biceps (bi´seps) Denoting a muscle with two heads or points of origin.

bicipital (bi-sip´ĭ-tal) **1.** Having two heads. **2.** Of or relating to a biceps muscle.

biconcave (bi-kon-kāv´) Having a depression on both sides or surfaces.

biconvex (bi-kon-veks´) Protruding on both sides or surfaces.

bicornous, bicornuate, bicornate (bi-kor´nus, bi-kor´nu-āt, bi-kor´nāt) Having two horns or horn-shaped structures.

bicuspid (bi-kus´pid) Having two cusps or points, such as the premolars or the left atrioventricular (mitral) valve of the heart.

bifid (bi´fid) Divided into two parts, as a bifid ureter.

bifocal (bi´fo-kal) Having two focal lengths.

bifocals (bi´fo-kals) Eyeglasses in which each lens has two focal lengths, used for both distant and near vision.

bifurcate (bi-fur´kāt) To divide or separate into two parts.

bifurcation (bi-fur-ka´shun) Division or separation into two parts or branches.

bigeminal (bi-jem´ĭ-nal) Occurring in pairs.

bigeminy (bi-jem´ĭ-ne) Doubling, especially the occurrence of two pulse beats in rapid succession followed by a pause before the next two beats. Also written bigemini.

bilateral (bi-lat´er-al) Relating to or having two sides.

bile (bīl) A bitter, yellowish brown or brownish green liquid, secreted by the liver, stored in the gallbladder, and discharged into the duodenum; it aids in digestion mainly by emulsifying fats. Also called gall.

bilharziasis, bilharziosis (bil-har-zi´ă-sis, bil-har-ze-o´sis) See schistosomiasis.

biliary (bil´e-ar-e) Relating to bile and the bile ducts.

bilifuscin (bil-ĭ-fus´in) A dark green-brown pigment present in bile and bile salts.

bilious (bil´yus) **1.** See biliary. **2.** A vague popular term denoting a disturbed condition of the digestive system.

biliousness (bil´yus-nes) A vaguely defined condition marked by indigestion, excessive gas, and often constipation and headache, popularly attributed to gallbladder dysfunction.

bilirubin (bil-ĭ-roo´bin) An orange-red pigment formed from hemoglobin during destruction of erythrocytes by the reticuloendothelial system; in the presence of liver disease or excessive destruction of red blood cells, accumulation of bilirubin in the blood and tissues causes jaundice.

bilirubinemia (bil-ĭ-roo-bĭ-ne´me-ă) The presence of bilirubin in the blood, usually referring to an increased level.

bilirubinuria (bil-ĭ-roo-bĭ-nu´re-ă) The presence of the pigment bilirubin in the urine.

biliuria (bil-ĭ-u´re-ă) The presence of bile or bile salts in the urine.

biliverdin, biliverdine (bil-ĭ-ver´din) A green bile pigment formed from the oxidation of bilirubin.

bilobate (bi-lo´bāt) Composed of two lobes.

bilobular (bi-lob´u-lar) Having two lobules.

bimanual (bi-man´u-al) Performed with both hands (e.g., bimanual palpation).

bimodal (bi-mo´dal) Having two distinct modes or peaks; said of a graphic curve.

bimolecular (bi-mo-lek´u-lar) Relating to or affecting two molecules.

binary (bi´nar-e) Composed of two parts.

binaural (bi-naw´ral) Relating to both ears.

bind (bīnd) **1.** To secure, as with ligature or band. **2.** To bandage. **3.** To unite molecules. **4.** Popularly to constipate.

binder (bīnd´er) A broad abdominal bandage.

binge and purge syndrome (bĭnj and pŭrj sin´drōm) See bulimia.

binocular (bĭ-nok´u-lar, bī-nok´u-lar) **1.** Relating to both eyes. **2.** Used by both eyes at the same time, as a microscope.

binomial (bi-nōm´e-al) **1.** Composed of two names. **2.** In mathematics, an expression pertaining to two terms connected by a plus or minus sign (such as m+n or 10 –5).

binuclear, binucleate (bi-noo´kle-ar, bi-noo´kle-āt) Having two nuclei.

bioassay (bi-o-as´a) Estimation of a substance's potency by comparing its effects on living organisms or on tissue preparations with those of a standard.

bioastronautics (bi-o-as´tro-nawt´iks) The study of the effects of space travel on living organisms.

bioavailability (bi-o-ă-vāl-ă-bil´ĭ-te) The degree to which the active ingredient of a drug is absorbed by the body in the form which is physiologically active; it is an indication of both the relative amount of an administered drug that reaches the general circulation and the rate at which this occurs.

biocatalyst (bi-o-kat´ă-list) See enzyme.

biochemistry (bi-o-kem´is-tre) The chemistry of living matter or organisms. Also called biologic chemistry.

biodegradation (bi-o-deg-rah-da´shun) The process by which living organisms (e.g., soil bacteria, plants, animals) chemically decompose or break down such materials as organic wastes, pesticides, pollutant chemicals and implantable materials.

biodynamics (bi-o-di-nam´iks) The science concerned with energy as it relates to living organisms and their environment.

bioenergetics (bi-o-en-er-jet´iks) The study of energy changes produced within living tissues.

bioengineering (bi-o-en-jin-er´ing) See biomedical engineering, under engineering.

bioequivalence (bi-o-e-kwiv´ă-lens) The application of the bioavailability concept whereby it can be assumed that a drug has the same therapeutic efficacy as another drug if it achieves the same maximum concentration, the same rate of absorption, and the same total amount of absorption as a recognized standard.

bioethics (bi-o-eth´iks) The branch of ethics concerned with the moral and social implications of practices and developments in medicine and the life sciences.

biofeedback (bi-o-fēd´bak) A technique that uses electronic monitoring to give an individual immediate and continuing signals on changes in bodily functions of which he is not usually conscious, such as fluctuations in blood pressure; the subject endeavors to learn to control the function.

biogenesis (bi-o-jen´ĕ-sis) Thomas Huxley's theory that living things originate only from things already living, as opposed to spontaneous generation.

biokinetics (bi-o-kĭ-net´iks) The study of the growth changes and movements within developing organisms.

biologic, biological (bi-o-loj´ik, bi-o-loj´ĭ-kal) Relating to biology.

biologist (bi-ol´ŏ-jist) A specialist in biology.

biology (bi-ol´ŏ-je) The science concerned with the study of living organisms, their structure, function, growth, etc.

cell b. See cytology.

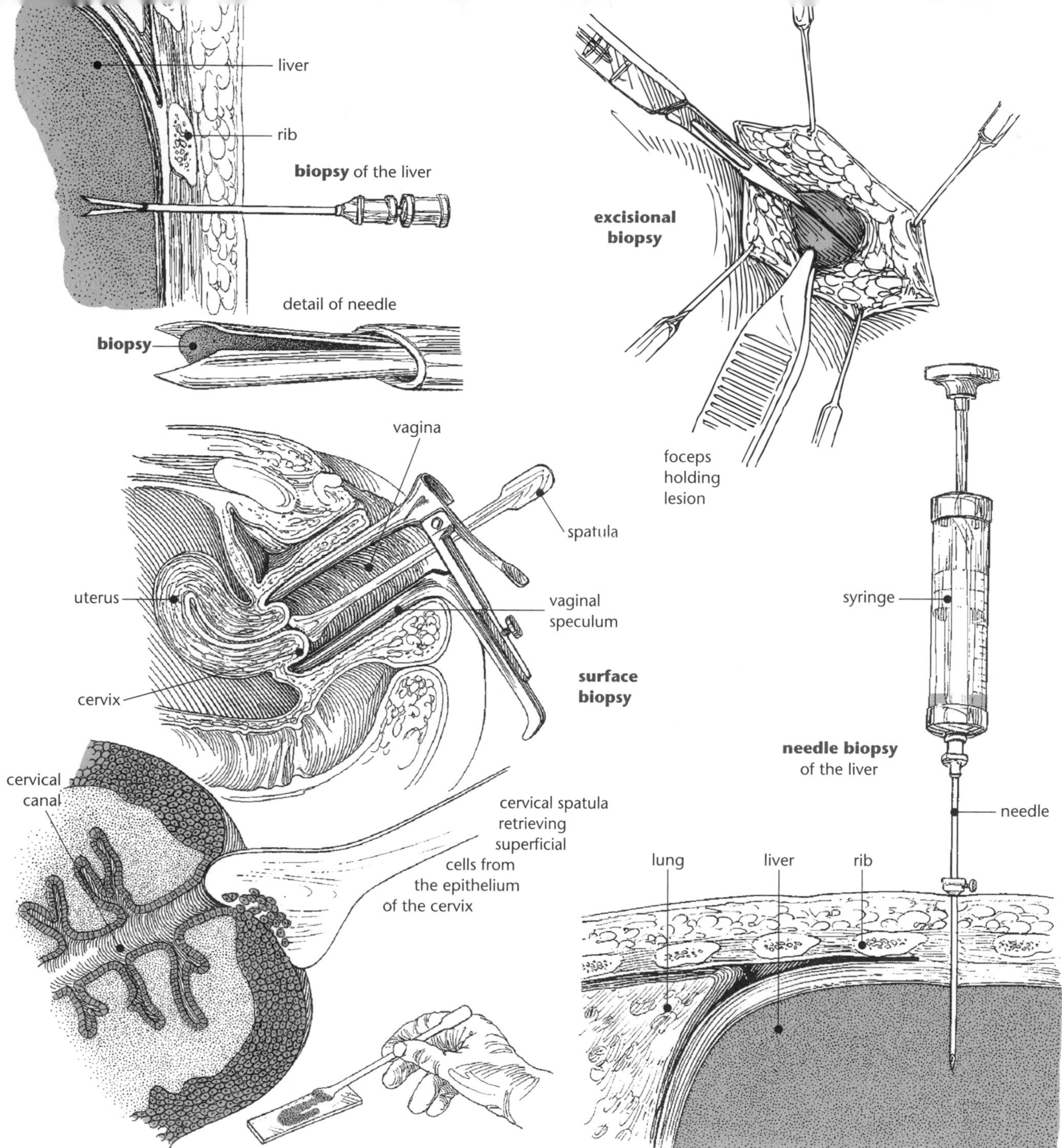

molecular b. The study of biological processes in terms of the physics and chemistry of the molecular structures involved, including chemical interactions of genetic material.

radiation b. The study of the effects of ionizing radiation on living organisms.

biomedical (bi-o-med′i-kal) Relating to the aspects of biologic sciences that pertain to clinical medicine.

biomedical engineering (bi-o-med′i-kal en-jĭ-nir′ing) See bioengineering.

biometrician (bi-o-mĕ-trish′an) A specialist in biometry.

biometry (bi-om′ĕ-tre) The statistical study of biologic information.

biomicroscope (bi-o-mi′krŏ-skōp) A microscope designed for examining living tissues in the body; one equipped with a slitlike opening through which a beam of intense light is projected into the patient's eye; used in ophthalmology to examine the structure at the front of the eye under magnification. Also called slitlamp.

biomicroscopy (bi-o-mi-kros′kŏ-pe) Examination of the eye with a biomicroscope, especially the lids, cornea, anterior chamber, and iris; interior structures of the eye (vitreous, optic nerve, retina) are usually examined by adding a self-adhering corneal contact lens.

biomolecules (bi-o-mol′ĕ-kūls) Molecules present in living matter.

bion (bi′on) Any living organism.

bionics (bi-on′iks) The application of biologic principles to the design of electronic systems.

bionosis (bi-o-no′sis) Any disease caused by living organisms.

biophysics (bi-o-fiz′iks) Application of the principles of physics to the study of biologic processes.

dental b. The relationship between the biologic behavior of the structures of the mouth and the physical action of a dental prosthesis.

radiation b. The study of the effects of radiation on living organisms.

biopolymer (bi-o-pol′ĭ-mer) A complex compound formed by a chain of simpler, similar molecules in a living organism.

biopsy (bi′op-se) (BX, Bx) The removal and examination (gross and microscopic) of tissue from the living body for the purpose of diagnosis.

aspiration b. See needle biopsy.

brush b. Removal of cells with a brush-tipped instrument; the cells of interest are entrapped in the bristles by manipulating the instrument against the suspected area of disease (e.g., within a ureter).

endoscopic b. Biopsy performed with a viewing instrument (endoscope) equipped with an attachment, either a forceps or a brush, for removing tissue or cells, respectively, from the lining of a hollow organ (e.g., the stomach, esophagus, or colon).

excisional b. The removal of an entire lesion (e.g., a lump) and a margin of surrounding normal tissue for gross and microscopic examination.

fine needle b. (FNB) Aspiration of body tissues or fluids with a suspension of cells through a fine (19 to 23 gauge) needle; may be obtained from body cavities, bone marrow, solid tumors, or organs (e.g., ovaries).

large-core needle b. (LCNB) Removal of tissues with a large-core needle; often used to obtain breast tissue from women whose mammogram shows irregularities.

needle b. Any biopsy in which biopsy material is sucked out through a needle. Also called aspiration biopsy.

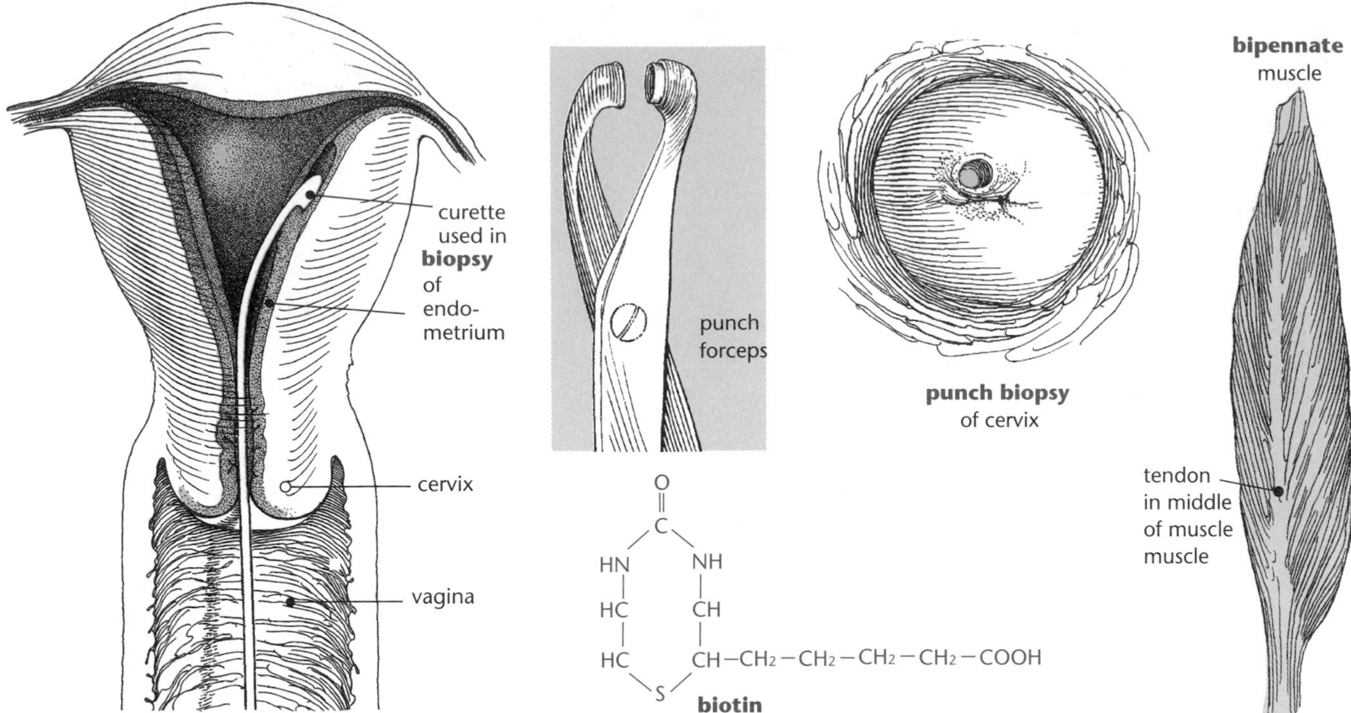

open b. Biopsy carried out during a surgical operation so that the organ may be visualized at the time of biopsy; performed when there is a need to avoid dangerously close structures, to ascertain proper sampling, or to avoid undue bleeding.

punch b. Removal of a plug of tissue by pressing down and twisting a special cutting instrument with a cylindrical sharp end. Also called trephine biopsy.

shave b. Biopsy in which a scalpel is used to cut through the base of an elevated lesion in one smooth motion.

surface b. Examination of cells scraped from a surface (e.g., from the uterine cervix).

timed endometrial b. In artificial insemination, a biopsy of the endometrium performed approximately in mid-cycle (at the time of ovulation) to determine whether the endometrium is in its secretory phase, capable of participating in implantation of the fertilized egg. Also called timed uterine-wall biopsy.

timed uterine-wall b. See timed endometrial biopsy.

trephine b. See punch biopsy.

biorhythm (bi´o-rithm) The cyclic occurrence of a biologically determined process (e.g., the sleep cycle).

biosafety (bi´o-saf-tē) The handling of all biologic materials as if they were infectious.

biosensor (bi-o-sen´sor) Any of several probes for measuring the presence or concentration of molecules, cells, and microorganisms; they translate a biochemical interaction at the probe surface into a quantifiable physical signal (e.g., a change in temperature).

biospectrometry (bi-o-spek-trom´ĕ-tre) The determination of the quantity of various substances in living tissues by means of a spectroscope. Also called clinical spectrometry.

biospectroscopy (bi-o-spek-tros´kŏ-pe) Examination of specimens of living tissue with the spectroscope. Also called clinical spectroscopy.

biostatistics (bi-o-stă-tis´tiks) The study concerned with the acquisition, analysis, and interpretation of data relating to human mortality, morbidity, natality, and demography.

biosynthesis (bi-o-sin´thĕ-sis) The formation of chemical substances by or in living organisms.

biotechnology (bi-o-tek-nol´ŏ-je) The research and development concerned with the use of organisms, cells, or cell-derived constituents to develop products that are technically, scientifically, and clinically useful. The chief focus of biotechnology is the DNA molecule and the alteration of biological function at the molecular level; its laboratory methods include transfection and cloning techniques; sequence and structure analysis algorithms; computer databases; and function, analysis, and prediction of gene and protein structure. See also genetic engineering, under engineering; recombinant DNA, under DNA; biomedical engineering, under engineering.

biotelemetry (bi-o-tel-em´ĕ-tre) The recording and measuring, without wires, of the vital processes of an organism located at a point remote from the measuring device.

biotic (bi-ot´ik) Relating to the life processes. Also called biologic.

biotin (bi´o-tin) A vitamin acting as a coenzyme, found chiefly in liver, yeast, and egg yolk. Formerly called vitamin H.

biotoxin (bi-o-tok´sin) Any toxic substance formed in the body tissues.

biotransformation (bi-o-trans-for-ma´shun) The interaction between a drug and the living organism which results in a chemical change in the drug molecule. Also called drug metabolism.

biotransport (bi-o-trans´port) The translocation of a solute through a biologic barrier without being altered.

biotype (bi´o-tīp) **1.** A group of people who have the same genotype. **2.** See biovar.

biovar (bi´o-var) A group of bacterial strains differing from other strains by identifiable physiologic characteristics.

bipara (bi-par´ă) See secundipara.

biparietal (bi-pă-ri´e-tal) Relating to both parietal bones of the skull.

biparous (bip´ă-rus) Having borne twins.

biped (bi´ped) An animal with two feet.

bipennate, bipenniform (bi-pen´āt, bi-pen´ĭ-form) Having a double feather arrangement; said of certain muscles from the arrangement of their fibers on each side of a tendon.

bipolar (bi-po´lar) **1.** Having two poles. **2.** Relating to both ends of a cell.

bipositive (bi-poz´ĭ-tiv) Having two positive charges or valences, as the calcium ion, Ca^{++}.

birefringence (bi-re-frin´jens) See double refraction, under refraction.

birth (birth) The act of being born.

live b. The complete expulsion or extraction of a fetus from the mother, regardless of the duration of pregnancy which, after such separation, breathes or shows other evidence of life (e.g., pulsation of the umbilical cord, beating of the heart, and definite movements of involuntary muscles) regardless of whether the umbilical cord has been cut or the placenta has detached.

premature b. The birth of an infant after 20 weeks of gestation but before full term is achieved.

birthmark (birth´mark) A circumscribed growth present at birth, such as a hemangioma.

biscuit (bis´kĭt bis´ket) In dentistry (in association with porcelain), the fired article before it is glazed; referred to as low, medium, or high biscuit, depending on the stage of vitrification.

bisexual (bi-sek´shoo-al) Denoting an individual who has sexual interests in both sexes. Also called ambisexual.

bis in die (bis in de´a) (b.i.d.) Latin for twice a day.

bismuth (biz´mŭth) A crystalline, brittle metallic element; symbol Bi, atomic number 83, atomic weight 209.

b. subcarbonate $(BiO)_2CO_3$; a white or pale yellow powder, used as an astringent and antacid. Also called bismuth oxycarbonate.

bisulfite (bi-sul´fīt) Any compound containing the inorganic acid group HSO_3.

bite (bīt) **1.** To grip or tear with the teeth. **2.** To pierce the skin with the teeth or a stinger. **3.** The amount of pressure produced in closing the jaws. See also interocclusal record, under record. **4.** The contact of the mandibular teeth with the maxillary teeth in any functional relation.

closed b. See small interarch distance, under distance.

open b. Condition in which some of the apposing teeth (usually the anterior teeth) fail to make contact when the jaws are fully closed. Also called apertognathia.

bitemporal (bi-tem´po-ral) Relating to both temples.

biteplate, biteplane (bīt´plat, bīt´plān) A removable dental appliance that covers the palate and has either an inclined or a flat surface at the front border; designed to offer resistance to the upper incisors when they make contact.

bivalence, bivalency (biv´ă-lens, biv´ă-len-sē) Combining power double that of a hydrogen atom; a valence of 2.

bivalent (bi-va´lent, biv´ă-lent) **1.** Having valence 2 or the combining power of two hydrogen atoms. Also called divalent. **2.** In genetics, composed of two homologous chromosomes.

biventer (bi-ven´ter) Having two bellies, said of some muscles (e.g., the digastric muscle).

blackhead (blak´hed) Popular name for a comedo.

blackout (blak´out) Temporary loss of consciousness.

black widow (blak wid´ō) One of the world's most dangerous spiders, *Latrodectus mactans*; the extremely poisonous female is about one and a half inches long with a shiny black body and a red hourglass patch on its abdomen; the male is about one-fourth the size of the female and has yellow-brown markings; name acquired from the fact that the female eats its mate after consummation of coitus.

bladder (blad´der) A distensible musculomem-

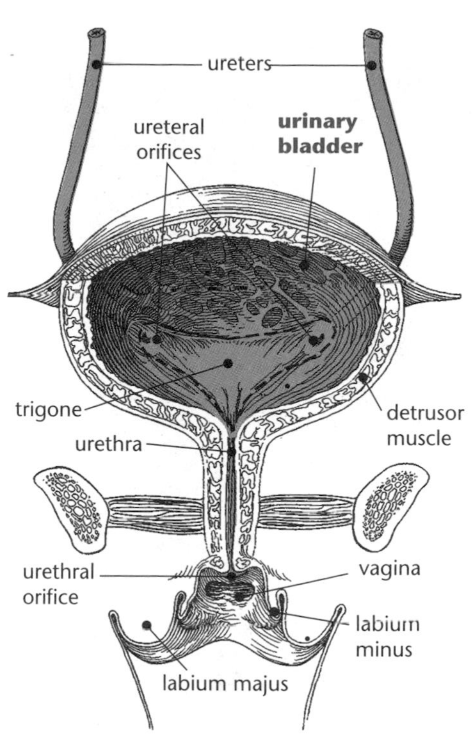

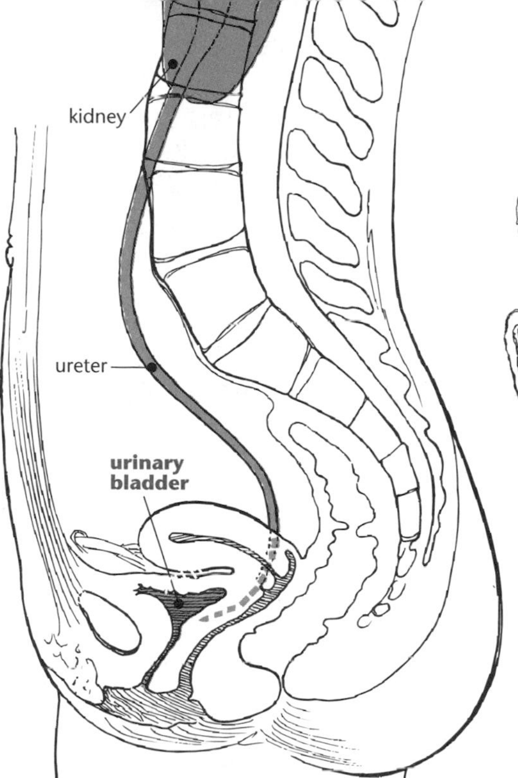

blepharochalasis

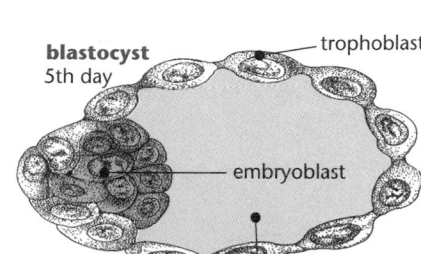

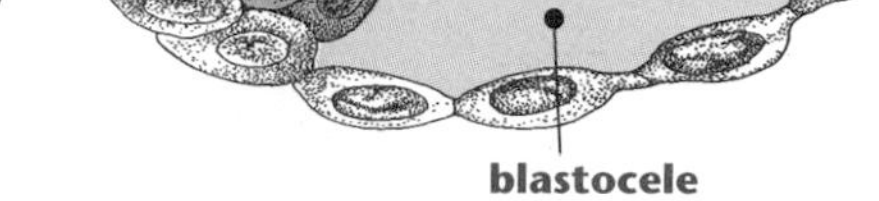

branous sac that serves as a receptacle for fluid, especially the urinary bladder.

atonic b. One that is unable to contract due to paralysis of the motor nerves that innervate it.

Christmas tree b. The characteristic appearance of a spastic bladder, caused by lesions of the upper motor nerve supply of the bladder (at the 12th thoracic or 1st lumbar level).

gall b. See gallbladder.

ileal b. See ileal conduit, under conduit.

nervous b. A constant desire to urinate, with incomplete emptying of the bladder.

neurogenic b. Any disturbance of bladder function caused by impairment of the nerve supply.

reflex neurogenic b. Condition in which the person has no awareness of filling or ability to contract the bladder voluntarily; caused by a lesion in sacral nerves 2, 3 and 4.

urinary b. The reservoir for urine; it receives urine from the kidneys via the ureters and discharges it through the urethra. Usually called bladder.

blastema (blas-te´mă) In embryology, a group of cells from which develops an organ or part.

metanephric b. A caplike cellular mass over the ampullar end of the ureteric bud and from which develop the excretory units of the kidney.

blastocele (blas´to-sēl) The fluid-filled cavity of a blastocyst.

blastocyst (blas´to-sist) The embryo at the time of its implantation into the uterine wall, consisting of a single layer of outer cells (trophoblast), a fluid-filled cavity (blastocele), and a mass of inner cells (embryoblast). Also called blastodermic vesicle.

Blastocystis (blas-to-sis´tis) A genus of yeastlike organisms parasitic in the digestive tract of mammals.

B. hominis Protozoan sometimes found in feces; it may cause diarrhea when present in large numbers; previously considered a nonpathogenic yeast.

blastogenesis (blas-to-jen´ĕ-sis) **1.** Reproduction by budding. **2.** The development of an embryo during cleavage and germ layer formation. **3.** The transformation of small lymphocytes of human blood in tissue culture into large blastlike cells capable of undergoing mitosis.

blastoma (blas-to´mă) Malignant tumor composed of embryonic, undifferentiated cells.

blastomere (blas´to-mēr) One of the cells into which the fertilized egg divides. Also called cleavage cell.

Blastomyces (blas-to-mī´sēz) A genus of pathogenic fungi (family Moniliaceae).

B. coccidioides See *Coccidioides immitis*, under *Coccidioides*.

B. dermatitidis A species that is the cause of blastomycosis.

blastomycosis (blas-to-mī-ko´sis) A chronic disease caused by inhalation of the fungus (*Blastomyces dermatitidis*), originating in the respiratory system, especially the lungs, and disseminating to the skin and sometimes to bone and other organs. Formerly called North American blastomycosis.

North American b. See blastomycosis.

South American b. See paracoccidioidomycosis.

blastopore (blas´to-pōr) A small opening into the archenteron (primitive digestive cavity) of the embryo at the gastrula stage.

blastospore (blas´to-spor) A spore developed by budding from a fungal filament or hypha.

blastula (blas´tu-lă) Early stage in the development of an embryo; a spherical structure consisting of a single layer of cells that enclose a fluid-filled cavity.

blastulation (blas-tu-la´shun) Formation of the blastocyst or blastula.

bleaching (blēch´ing) **1.** Removal of color by means of chemical agents. **2.** In dentistry, a method for returning a discolored tooth to its normal color.

bleaching agent (blēch´ing a´jent) Any chemical used for brightening discolored teeth.

bleb (bleb) A blister.

bleeder (blēd´er) **1.** A person afflicted with hemophilia or any other bleeding disease. **2.** A blood vessel from which blood escapes and which usually requires surgical intervention to arrest the bleeding.

bleeding (blēd´ing) The escape of blood.

contact b. Bleeding occurring after sexual intercourse; may be caused by cervical cancer, eversion, polyps, or infection. Also called postcoital bleeding.

dysfunctional uterine b. Bleeding from the uterus due to endocrine imbalance rather than a localized disorder.

implantation b. Slight uterine bleeding frequently occurring at the time of implantation of the fertilized ovum onto the uterine wall; caused by disruption of blood vessels at the implantation site.

intermenstrual b. See metrorrhagia.

postcoital b. See contact bleeding.

postmenopausal b. Uterine bleeding occurring after 12 months of absent menses; may be caused by disease (e.g., endometrial carcinoma).

blennadenitis (blen-ad-ĕ-ni´tis) Inflammation of the mucous glands.

blepharectomy (blef-ă-rek´to-me) Surgical removal of all or a portion of an eyelid.

blepharitis (blef-ă-ri´tis) Inflammation of the eyelids.

blepharochalasis (blef-ă-ro-kal´ă-sis) Condition of the upper eyelids marked by excessive tissue that hangs over the lid margin when the eye is open.

blepharoclonus (blef-ah-ro-klo´nus) A rhythmic spasm of the eyelids.

blepharoconjunctivitis (blef-ă-ro-kon-junk-tĭ-vi´tis) Inflammation of the eyelids and conjunctiva, especially the palpebral conjunctiva.

blepharon (blef´ă-ron) See eyelid.

blepharophimosis (blef-ă-ro-fi-mo´sis) A condition in which the aperture of the eyelids is narrow. Also called blepharostenosis.

blepharoplasty (blef´ă-ro-plas-te) Any restorative surgical procedure of the eyelids.

blepharoptosis (blef-ă-rop-to´sis) Drooping of the upper eyelid.

blepharospasm (blef´ă-ro-spaz-m) Spasmodic winking, or contraction of the muscles of the eyelid.

blepharostenosis (blef-ă-ro-sten-ō´sis) See blepharophimosis.

blepharotomy (blef-ă-rot´ŏ-me) An incision on an eyelid.

blind loop syndrome (blīnd lo͞op sin´drōm) Stagnation of intestinal contents in a blind loop or pouch in the small intestine (either present at birth or created in certain surgical procedures) resulting in increased bacterial growth with malabsorption of vitamin B_{12}, fat, and other nutrients.

blindness (blīnd´nes) Lack or loss of sight.

blue b. See tritanopia.

color b. Inability to distinguish differences between some colors.

day b. See hemeralopia.

flash b. Temporary loss of vision caused by exposure to intense light.

legal b. Loss of vision to a degree as defined by legal statute to constitute blindness; maximal correction of acuity of 20/200 or less in the better eye, and diameter of visual field of 20° or less.

letter b. A form of aphasia in which letters, though seen, relate no meaning to the mind.

night b. Impaired vision in subdued light, generally due to a deficiency of vitamin A. Also called nyctalopia.

pure word b. Inability to recognize written or printed words as conveyors of ideas.

river b. See onchocerciasis.

snow b. Temporary blindness caused by excessive exposure to sunlight reflected from snow.

blink (blĭngk) To close and open the eyelids rapidly; an involuntary act by which the tears are spread over the conjunctivas, keeping them moist.

blister (blis´ter) Common name for vesicle (2) and bulla (1).

fever b. Popular term for herpes febrilis. See under herpes.

bloat, bloating (blōt, blō´ting) Distention of the abdomen with gas.

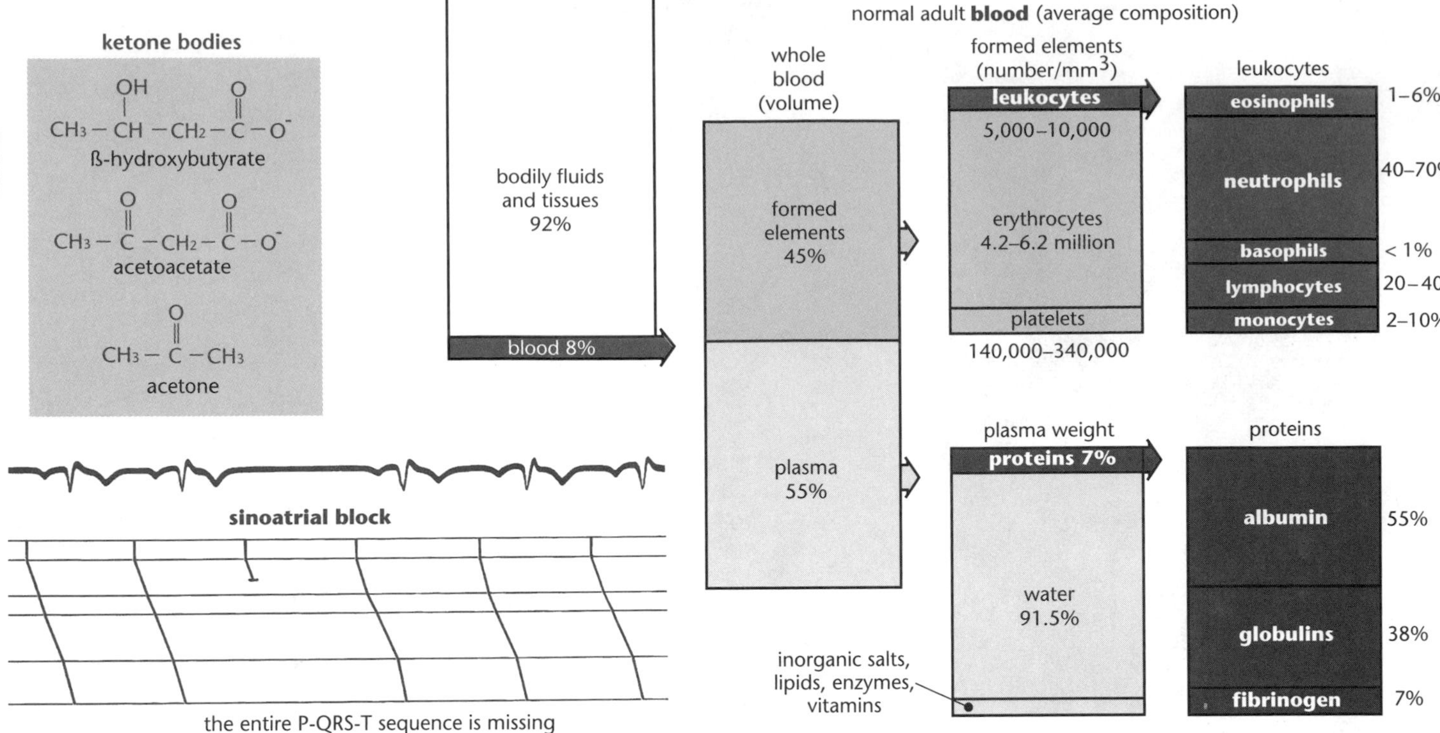

bloater (blo´ter) One who is bloated.
blue b. Informal term for describing the appearance of a patient with emphysema. The patient appears blue-purple (due to oxygen deficiency in the blood) and bloated (due to fluid collection in the tissues, chiefly caused by heart failure). COMPARE: pink puffer, under puffer.

block (blok) **1.** An obstruction to passage. **2.** An interruption of nerve impulses.
alveolar-capillary b. Impaired diffusion of gases, especially oxygen, between the capillaries and alveoli of the lungs.
anterograde b. A block in the conduction of a cardiac impulse anywhere on its normal course from the sinoatrial node to the ventricles.
arborization b. A form of intraventricular block, thought to be due to widespread blockage in the Purkinje fibers of the heart.
atrioventricular (A-V) b. Disorder of the atrioventricular bundle, causing disruption in the transmission of impulses from atria to ventricles; usually classified in three degrees: *first degree A-V b.*, conduction time of the impulses is prolonged but all impulses reach the ventricles; *second degree A-V b.*, some impulses are blocked and do not reach the ventricles so that ventricular beats are dropped; *third degree A-V b.* (complete block), no impulses can reach the ventricles. Also called heart block.
bundle-branch b. (BBB) A form of intraventricular block due to impaired conduction in one of the main branches of the atrioventricular bundle (bundle of His).
caudal b. See caudal anesthesia, under anesthesia.
epidural b. See epidural anesthesia, under anesthesia.
exit b. Interruption of the conduction of a cardiac impulse occurring at its point of exit.
heart b. See atrioventricular block.
intra-atrial b. Impaired conduction through the atria.
intraventricular b., I-V b. Delayed conduction through the ventricles.
left bundle-branch b. (LBBB) Interruption of impulse conduction within the heart, occurring in the left branch of the atrioventricular bundle (bundle of His).
lochia b. See lochiometra.
Mobitz type I b. A type of second-degree atrioventricular block in which a dropped beat occurs periodically after a series of increasingly prolonged P-R intervals. Also called Wenckebach block.
Mobitz type II b. A type of second-degree atrioventricular block in which a dropped beat occurs periodically without previously prolonged P-R intervals.
paracervical b. See paracervical block anesthesia, under anesthesia.
peri-infarction b. Delayed conduction through the myocardium at the site of an old myocardial infarct.
retrograde b. Backward conduction from the ventricles or atrioventricular (A-V) node into the atria.
saddle b. See saddle block anesthesia, under anesthesia.
sinoatrial b., S-A b., sinus b. Failure of the nervous impulse to leave the sinus node.
spinal b. See spinal anesthesia, under anesthesia.
Wenckebach b. See Mobitz type I block.

blockade (blok-ād´) **1.** Intravenous injection of harmless material, such as colloidal dyes, to render the reticuloendothelial cells temporarily functionless. **2.** Obstruction of nerve impulse transmission by a drug.
adrenergic b. Inhibition by a drug of the responses of effector cells to adrenergic sympathetic nerve impulses (sympatholytic), and to adrenaline (adrenolytic).
cholinergic b. Interruption by a drug of nerve impulse transmission at autonomic ganglionic synapses (ganglionic blockade), at myoneural junctions (myoneural blockade), and at postganglionic parasympathetic effector cells.
ganglionic b. Interruption by a drug of nerve impulse transmission at autonomic ganglionic synapses.

blocker (blok´er) See blocking agent, under agent.
calcium channel b. See calcium channel-blocking agent, under agent.
starch b.'s See glucosidase inhibitors, under inhibitor.

blood (blud) The fluid circulated by the heart through the vascular system of vertebrates; consisting of plasma (a pale yellow fluid) in which are suspended red and white blood cells and platelets; it carries oxygen and nutrients to all the body tissues and waste products to the excretory systems.
arterial b. The relatively bright red blood that has been oxygenated in the lungs and is within the left chambers of the heart and the arteries.
cord b. Blood within the umbilical cord.
occult b. Blood in the feces in amounts too small to be seen but detectable by laboratory tests.
venous b. The dark red blood within the veins; it loses oxygen and gains carbon dioxide by passing through metabolically active tissues.
whole b. Donated blood that has not been separated into its components.

bloodbank (blud bangk) See under bank.
blood banking (blud bangk'ing) See transfusion medicine, under medicine.
blood boosting (blud bo͞ost´ing) See blood doping.
blood count (blud´kount) See blood count, under count.
blood doping (blud dōp´ing) The giving of blood transfusions to athletes to enhance their perfor-mance. Also called blood boosting; blood packing.
blood group (blud gro͞op) Any of various immunologically distinct and genetically determined classes of human blood, identified clinically by characteristic agglutination reactions. For individual blood groups, see specific names.
blood grouping (blud gro͞op´ing) The classification of blood samples according to their agglutinating characteristics. Also called blood typing.
bloodletting (blud´let-ing) The removal of blood from a vein for therapeutic purposes.
blood packing (blud pak´ing) See blood doping.
bloodshot (blud´shot) The reddish appearance of an irritated part, such as the conjunctiva, due to the congested state of the blood vessels.
bloodstream (blud´strem) The blood circulating within the vascular component of the body, as opposed to blood that has been sequestered in a part (e.g., in a subdural hemangioma).
blood substitute (blud sub´stĭ-to͞ot) See blood substitute, under substitute.
blood type (blud tīp) See blood type, under type.
blood typing (blud tī´ping) See blood grouping.
blotting (blot´ing) The process of transferring electrophoretically separated particles (such as proteins and DNA fragments) onto special filters, papers, or membranes for analysis. See also Northern, Southern, and Western blot analysis, under analysis.
blue toe syndrome (blo͞o tō sin´drōm) A blue coloration of the toes leading to tissue necrosis and gangrene; caused by small emboli obstructing circulation to the skin and muscles of the digits.
blush (blush) Localized density observed in x-ray examination of blood vessels, due to increased vascularity in a tumor or to leakage of blood.
board certified (bord ser´tĭ-fīd) Denoting a physician or other health professional who is formally recognized as having passed an examination given by a specialty board after meeting certain specified criteria.
body (bod´e) **1.** The whole material structure of man or animal. **2.** The main part of anything.
acetone b.'s See ketone bodies.
alcoholic hyaline b.'s See Mallory bodies.
amygdaloid b. A motor nucleus composed of large multipolar cells that send fibers into the glossopharyngeal, vagus, and accessory nerves to

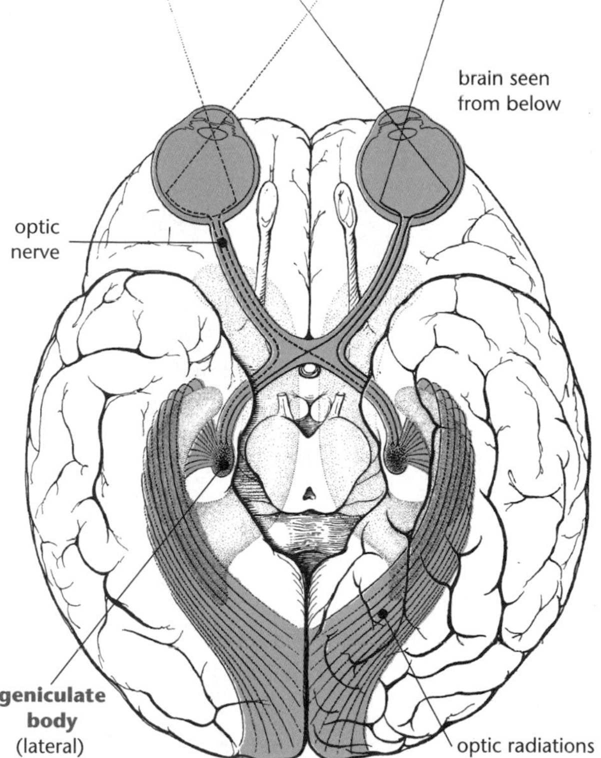

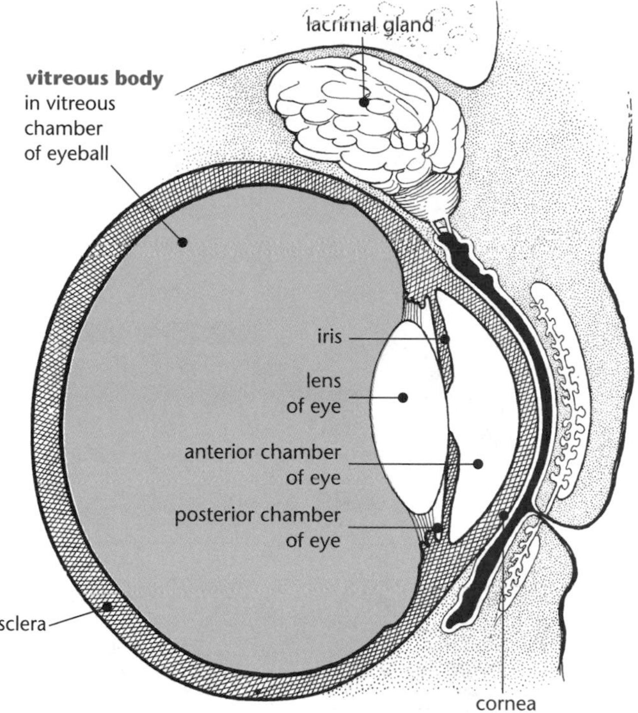

supply the pharynx and larynx.

aortic b.'s Small bilateral structures on a branch of the aorta near its arch; they contain chemoreceptors which are stimulated by decreases in blood oxygen tension.

Aschoff b.'s The specific lesions of acute rheumatic carditis occurring as nodules within the connective tissue of the myocardium; a fully developed body consists of nonspecific phagocytes, myocardial histiocytes, multinucleated cells, and fibroblastic proliferation. Also called Aschoff nodules.

Auer b.'s Elongated structures found in the cytoplasm of immature myeloid cells in acute myelocytic leukemia.

Barr chromatin b., Barr b. See sex chromatin, under chromatin.

basal b. Cylindrical thickening at the base of each cilium or flagellum; consists of nine triplets of microtubules arranged within the periphery of the cell membrane; triplets are continuous with the doublets of each cilium or flagellum. Also called basal granule.

Call-Exner b.'s Extracellular multilaminated bodies containing an accumulation of densely staining material; they are located among the granulosa cells in maturing ovarian follicles.

carotid b. A neurovascular ellipsoidal structure, 3 to 6 mm in diameter, situated on each side of the neck at the bifurcation of the common carotid artery; it is part of the visceral afferent system that helps to regulate respiration; it contains chemoreceptor endings that monitor the oxygen and carbon dioxide content of the blood circulating through the carotid body. Also called carotid glomus.

cell b. The portion of a nerve cell that surrounds and includes the nucleus, exclusive of any projections.

chromaffin b.'s See paraganglia.

ciliary b. The circular structure at the front of the eye between the outer edge of the iris and the ora serrata of the retina; it consists of six layers including the ciliary muscle (which, through the suspensory ligament, permits the lens to accommodate for near and far vision) and a layer of vessels and processes (the most vascular portion of the eye).

Councilman's b.'s Globules representing dead and shrunken hepatocytes (liver cells), formed in the liver in acute viral hepatitis. Also called Councilman's lesion.

elementary b. 1. See elementary particle, under particle. **2.** A platelet. **3.** Old term for a virion or virus particle.

foreign b. Any object or mass of material in the body that has been accidentaly or deliberately introduced from without.

geniculate b.'s Four paired oval masses located in the posteroinferior aspect of the thalamus (two lateral and two medial); the lateral are relay nuclei in the visual pathway; the medial serve as relay nuclei in the auditory pathway to the cerebral cortex.

Golgi b. See Golgi apparatus, under apparatus.

Heinz b.'s Irregularly shaped, refractile granules in red blood cells (usually located at or close to the periphery of the cell), occurring as a result of polymerization and precipitation of denatured hemoglobin molecules.

hematoxylin b.'s, hematoxyphil b.'s Relatively large, deeply staining bodies occasionally found lying free in the tissues in certain diseases, believed to be the remnants of an injured cell nucleus; the structures are so named because of their affinity for hematoxylin stain; found most commonly in systemic lupus erythematosus, especially in renal glomeruli and blood vessel walls.

herring b.'s See hyaline bodies of the pituitary.

Howell-Jolly b.'s Small, round, well defined nuclear remnants commonly found near the periphery of red blood cells following splenectomy; occasionally present in megaloblastic anemia and leukemia.

hyaline b.'s of the pituitary Cells filled with hyaline material occasionally occurring in the posterior lobe of the pituitary (hypophysis). Also called herring bodies.

inclusion b.'s Structures frequently observed in either the nucleus or the cytoplasm (occasionally in both) of cells infected with certain viruses.

juxtaglomerular b. A group of cells around the renal glomerular arterioles containing cytoplasmic granules believed to be composed of renin.

ketone b.'s Collective name for acetoacetic acid, acetone, and β-hydroxybutyrate, the end products of improper and excessive breakdown of stored fat in the liver; they accumulate in the blood and spill over in the urine in such conditions as uncontrolled or undiagnosed diabetes and in severe starvation. Also called acetone bodies; ketones.

Leishman-Donovan b.'s (L-D bodies) The ovoid, nonflagellated form of the parasite *Leishmania donovani*, usually packed in clusters within the cells of their mammalian host, causing visceral leishmaniasis (kala azar).

lipid b. See lipid droplet, under droplet.

Mallory b.'s Large accumulation of eosinophilic material in damaged liver cells; seen in certain diseases, especially those caused by alcoholism. Also called alcoholic hyaline bodies.

mamillary b. One of two small pea-shaped bodies of the hypothalamus, behind the infundibulum in the interpeduncular space; it receives fibers from the fornix and projects to the anterior thalamic nuclei.

Negri b.'s Bodies containing the rabies virus in the cytoplasm of nerve cells. Also called Negri corpuscles.

Nissl b.'s Clusters of ribosomes and endoplasmic reticulum in the cell body and dendrites of a nerve cell; they stain deeply with basic dyes.

pacchionian b.'s See arachnoid granulations, under granulation.

pampiniform b. See epoophoron.

para-aortic b.'s Small masses of chromaffin tissue (derived from neural ectoderm) found near the sympathetic ganglia along the abdominal aorta; they secrete epinephrine. Also called Zuckerkandl's bodies.

pineal b. A small gland-like structure, located on the roof of the third ventricle of the brain, overhanging the two superior quadrigeminal bodies. Also called pineal gland.

pituitary b. See hypophysis.

polar b. One of the three cells formed by the ovum during its maturation.

psammoma b.'s Minute spheres, resembling grains of sand, composed of concentrically laminated mineral deposits; found in papillary cancer.

quadrigeminal b.'s Four paired (a superior and an inferior pair) eminences forming the dorsal part of the midbrain.

residual b.'s Intracellular globules (secondary lysosomes) containing unprocessed ingested particles such as aging pigments (lipofuscin).

restiform b. See inferior cerebellar peduncle, under peduncle.

sex chromatin b. See sex chromatin, under chromatin.

trachoma b.'s Intracellular deposits found in the tarsal conjunctiva of a trachomatous eye.

vertebral b. The cylindrical ventral portion of the vertebra; adjacent vertebral bodies are joined by fibrocartilaginous disks.

vitreous b. The transparent, gelatinous mass, of a consistency slightly firmer than egg white, filling the eyeball behind the lens; composed of a delicate network (vitreous stroma) enclosing in its meshes a watery fluid (vitreous humor). Also called corpus vitreum; vitreous.

wolffian b. See mesonephros.

Zuckerkandl's b.'s See para-aortic bodies.

boil (boil) See furuncle.

bolus (bo´lus) **1.** A soft mass of food moved as a unit in the process of swallowing. **2.** A relatively large dose of a drug injected rapidly as a single unit into a vein.

bomb (bomb) An apparatus containing a radioactive

B

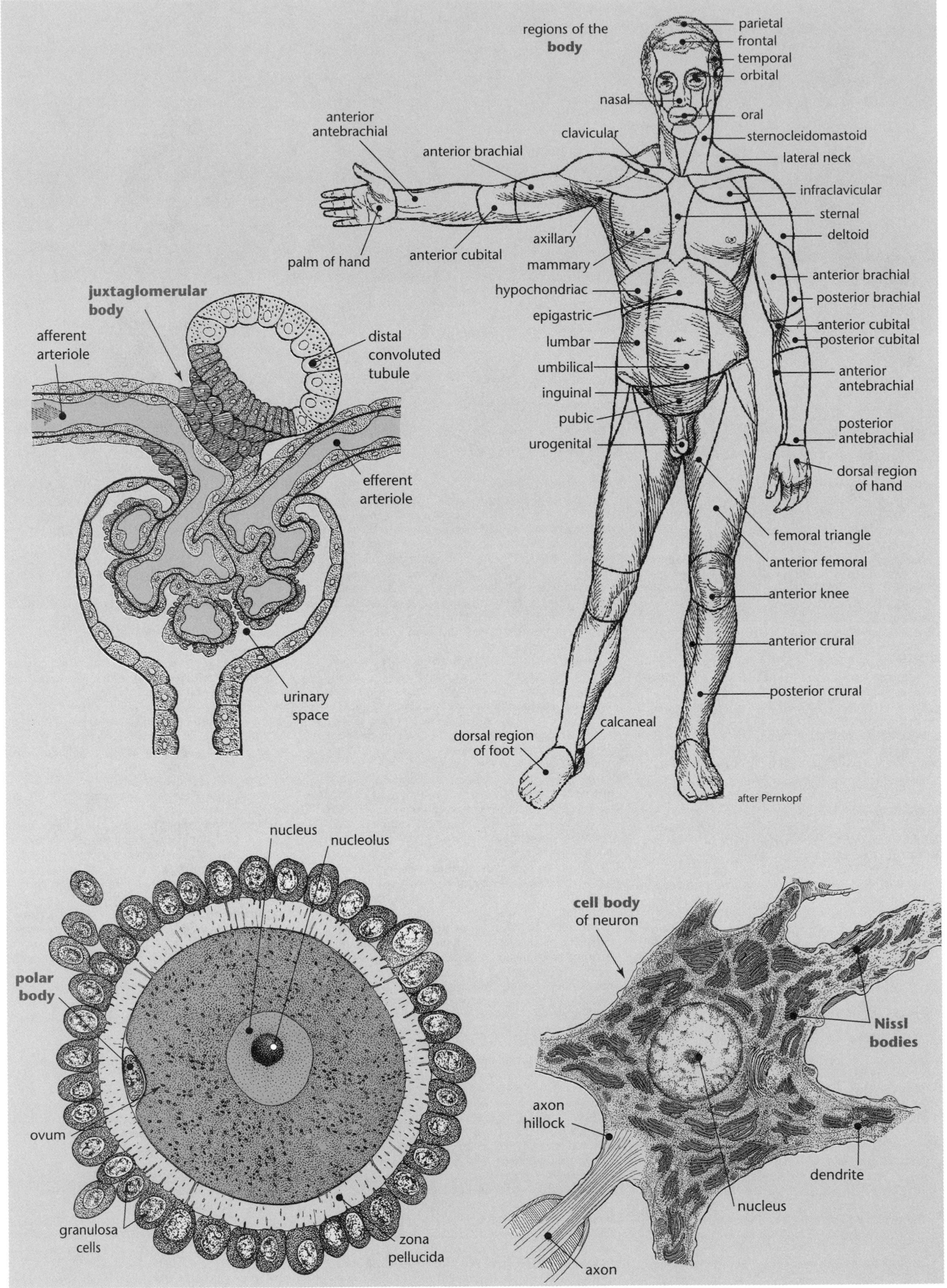
regions of the
body
parietal
frontal
temporal
orbital
nasal
oral
sternocleidomastoid
lateral neck
clavicular
anterior antebrachial
anterior brachial
infraclavicular
sternal
deltoid
axillary
mammary
palm of hand
anterior cubital
anterior brachial
posterior brachial
hypochondriac
epigastric
lumbar
umbilical
inguinal
pubic
urogenital
anterior cubital
posterior cubital
anterior antebrachial
posterior antebrachial
dorsal region of hand
femoral triangle
anterior femoral
anterior knee
anterior crural
posterior crural
calcaneal
dorsal region of foot
after Pernkopf
juxtaglomerular body
afferent arteriole
distal convoluted tubule
efferent arteriole
urinary space
nucleus
nucleolus
polar body
ovum
granulosa cells
zona pellucida
cell body of neuron
Nissl bodies
axon hillock
dendrite
nucleus
axon

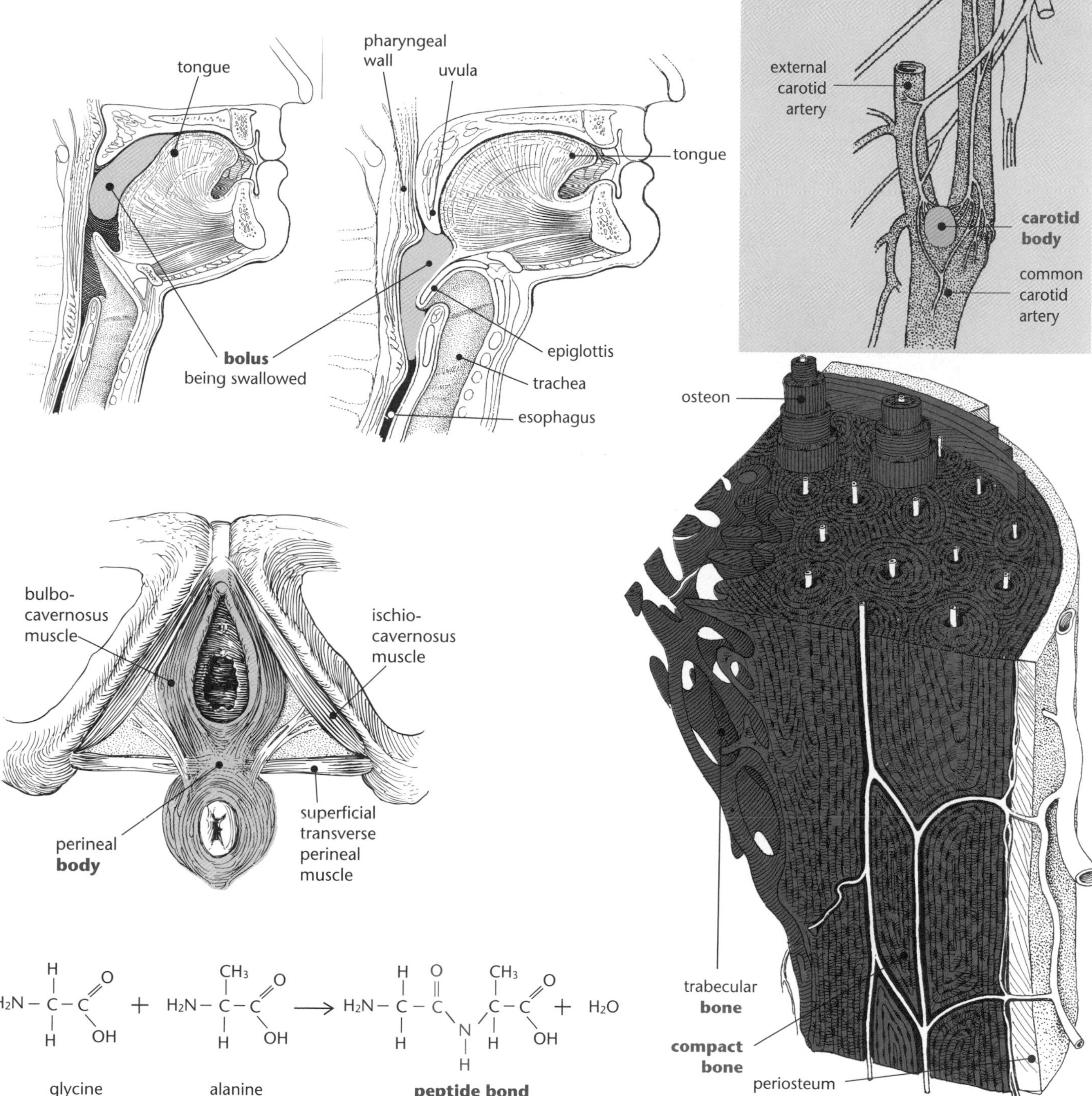

material for application of rays to a desired area of the body.

bombard (bom-bard′) To subject a specific area of the body to the action of rays.

bombesin (bom′bĕ-sin) A peptide neurotransmitter.

bond (bond) In chemistry, any of several forces holding atoms or ions together in a molecule.

covalent b. A bond resulting from the sharing of one, two, or three pairs of electrons by neighboring atoms.

electrovalent b. See ionic bond.

ionic b. A bond formed by the transfer of one or more electrons from one kind of atom to another; characteristic of salts. Also called electrovalent bond.

peptide b. A covalent bond linking two amino acids, formed when the carboxyl group of one is linked to the amino group of the other.

bone (bōn) The hard, semirigid, calcified connective tissue forming the skeleton of vertebrates. For specific bones, see table of bones.

alveolar b. The thin plate forming the walls of the tooth sockets.

ankle b. See talus, in table of bones.

breast b. See sternum, in table of bones.

brittle b.'s See osteogenesis imperfecta, under osteogenesis.

cancellous b. See spongy bone.

cheek b. See zygomatic bone, in table of bones.

collar b. See clavicle, in table of bones.

compact b. A type in which the bony substance is densely packed and the spaces and channels are narrow. Also called dense bone.

cranial b.'s The 21 bones forming the skull; the paired inferior nasal concha, lacrimal, maxilla, nasal, palatine, parietal, temporal, and zygomatic; and the unpaired ethmoid, frontal, occipital, sphenoid, and vomer.

dense b. See compact bone.

ear b.'s See auditory ossicles, under ossicle.

elbow b. See ulna, in table of bones.

b.'s of the face The bones surrounding the mouth, nose, and part of the eye sockets (orbits); i.e., the paired maxilla, zygomatic, inferior nasal concha, nasal, lacrimal, and palatine; and the unpaired mandible, ethmoid, and vomer.

flank b. See ilium, in table of bones.

flat b. Any bone of slight thickness and chiefly compact structure; generally composed of two plates arranged in a parallel direction, separated by a thin layer of spongy bone.

heel b. See calcaneus, in table of bones.

hip b. See hipbone.

innominate b. Former name for hipbone.

irregular b. Any complex bone that does not conform to the long, short, or flat shape.

jaw b. See mandible, in table of bones.

long b. Any bone having greater length than width, consisting of a tubular shaft, which contains a medullary cavity, and two expanded ends.

shin b. See tibia, in table of bones.

short b. A bone having the general appearance of a cube and a relatively large proportion of spongy bone within a layer of compact bone.

skull b.'s The 21 cranial bones plus the mandible.

spongy b. Bone having a lattice-work appearance and relatively large marrow spaces. Also called cancellous bone.

sutural b.'s See sutural bones, in table of bones.

thigh b. See femur, in table of bones.

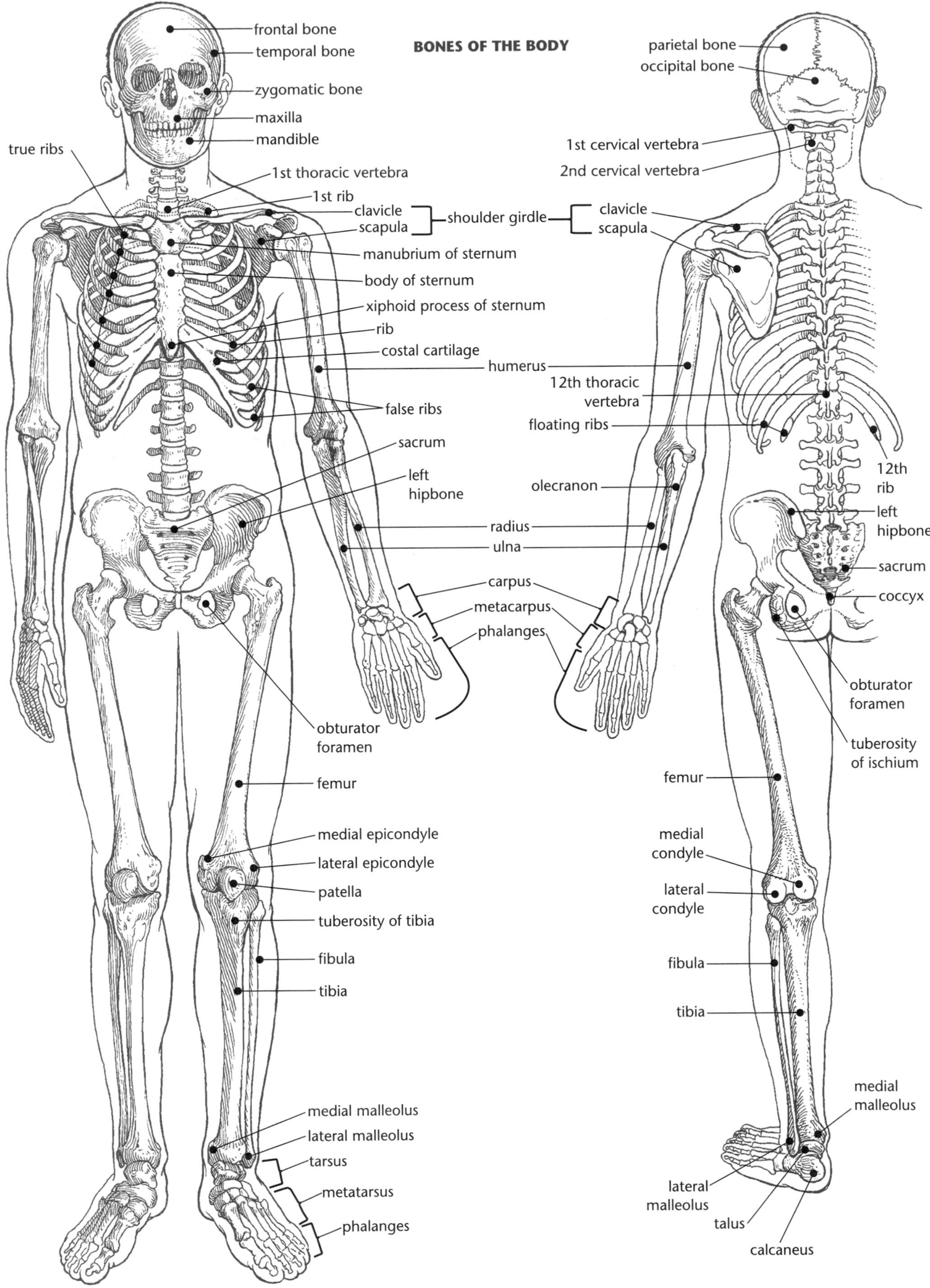
BONES OF THE BODY
frontal bone
temporal bone
zygomatic bone
maxilla
mandible
true ribs
1st thoracic vertebra
1st rib
clavicle
scapula
shoulder girdle
manubrium of sternum
body of sternum
xiphoid process of sternum
rib
costal cartilage
humerus
false ribs
sacrum
left hipbone
radius
ulna
carpus
metacarpus
phalanges
obturator foramen
femur
medial epicondyle
lateral epicondyle
patella
tuberosity of tibia
fibula
tibia
medial malleolus
lateral malleolus
tarsus
metatarsus
phalanges
parietal bone
occipital bone
1st cervical vertebra
2nd cervical vertebra
clavicle
scapula
12th thoracic vertebra
floating ribs
12th rib
olecranon
left hipbone
sacrum
coccyx
obturator foramen
tuberosity of ischium
femur
medial condyle
lateral condyle
fibula
tibia
medial malleolus
lateral malleolus
talus
calcaneus

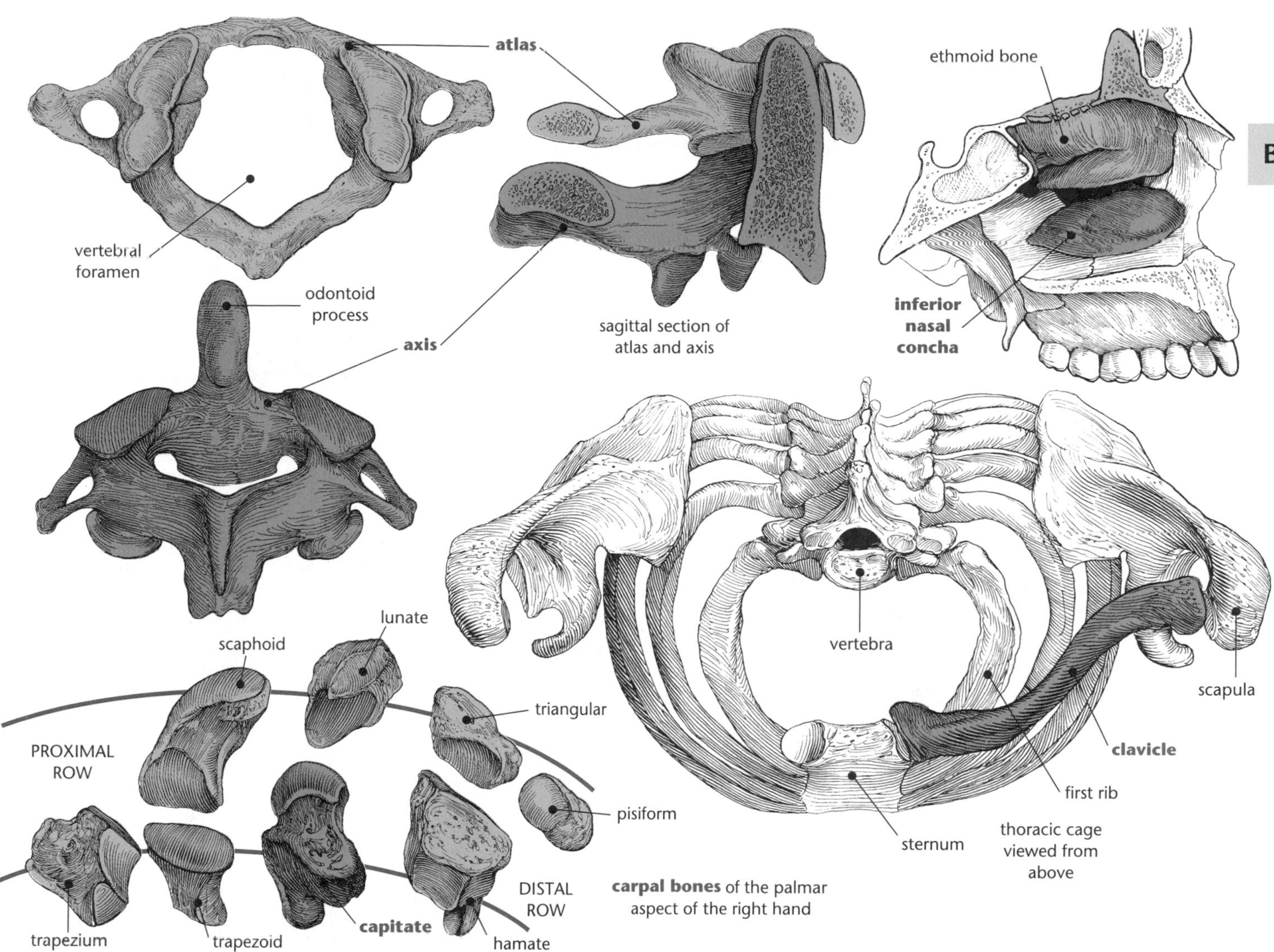

carpal bones of the palmar aspect of the right hand

B

BONE	LOCATION	DESCRIPTION	ARTICULATIONS
ankle b.		see talus	
anvil b.		see incus	
astragalus		see talus	
atlas *atlas*	neck	first cervical vertebra	occipital (above), axis (below)
axis epistropheus *axis*	neck	second cervical vertebra	atlas (above), third cervical vertebra (below)
backbones		see vertebrae	
calcaneus heel b. *calcaneus*	foot	largest of the tarsal b.'s situated at back of foot, forming heel; somewhat cuboidal	talus (above), cuboid (below)
capitate b. magnum b. *os capitatum*	wrist	largest of carpal b.'s, occupies center of wrist	second, third, and fourth metacarpal b.'s; lunate, trapezoid, scaphoid, hamate
carpal b.'s *ossa carpi*	wrist	eight in number, arranged in two rows: scaphoid, lunate, triangular (triquetral), and pisiform (proximal row); trapezium, trapezoid, capitate, and hamate (distal row)	
cheekbone		see zygomatic bone	
clavicle collar b. *clavicula*	shoulder	long curved b. placed nearly horizontally above first rib	sternum, scapula, cartilage of first rib
coccyx *os coccygis*	lower back	from three to five triangular rudimentary vertebrae with only the first not fused	sacrum
concha, inferior nasal inferior turbinate b.	skull	thin, irregular, scroll-shaped b. extending horizontally along lateral	ethmoid, maxilla, palatine

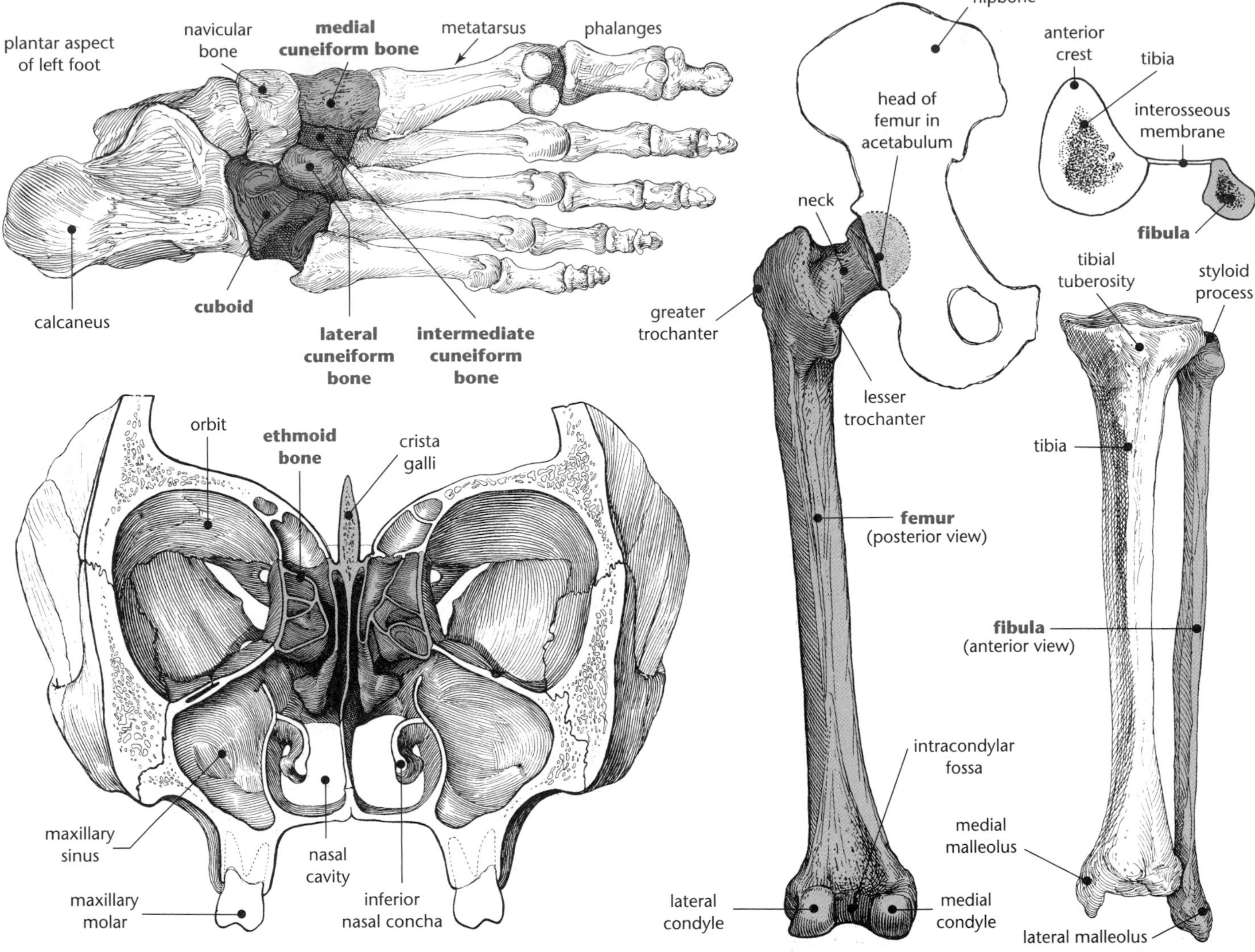

BONE	LOCATION	DESCRIPTION	ARTICULATIONS
cuboid *os cuboideum*	foot	pyramidal b. on lateral side of foot, proximal to fourth and fifth metatarsal b.'s	calcaneus, lateral cuneiform, fourth and fifth metatarsal b.'s, navicular
cuneiform b., interme-diate second cuneiform b. *os cuneiforme intermedium*	foot	wedge-shaped; smallest of the three cuneiforms, positioned between me-dial and lateral ones	navicular, medial cuneiform, lateral cuneiform, second metatarsal
cuneiform b., lateral external cuneiform b. *os cuneiforme laterale*	foot	intermediate-sized cuneiform located in center of front row of tarsal b.'s	navicular, intermediate cuneiform, cuboid; second, third, and fourth metatarsals
cuneiform b., medial internal cuneiform b. *os cuneiforme mediale*	foot	largest of the three cuneiforms, at medial side of foot between the nav-icular and base of first metatarsal	navicular, intermediate cuneiform, first and second metatarsal
elbow b.		see ulna	
epistropheus		see axis	
ethmoid b. *os ethmoidale*	skull	unpaired, T-shaped b. forming part of nasal septum and roof of cavity; curled processes form superior and middle conchae	sphenoid, frontal, both nasal, lacrimal, and palatine b's; maxillae, inferior nasal conchae, vomer
fabella *fabella*	knee	sesamoid b. in lateral head of gas-trocnemius muscle behind lateral condyle of femur	femur
femur thigh b. *femur*	thigh	longest and heaviest b. in the body, situated between hip and knee	hipbone, patella, tibia
fibula splint b. *fibula*	leg	lateral b. of leg	tibia, talus
flank b.		see ilium	

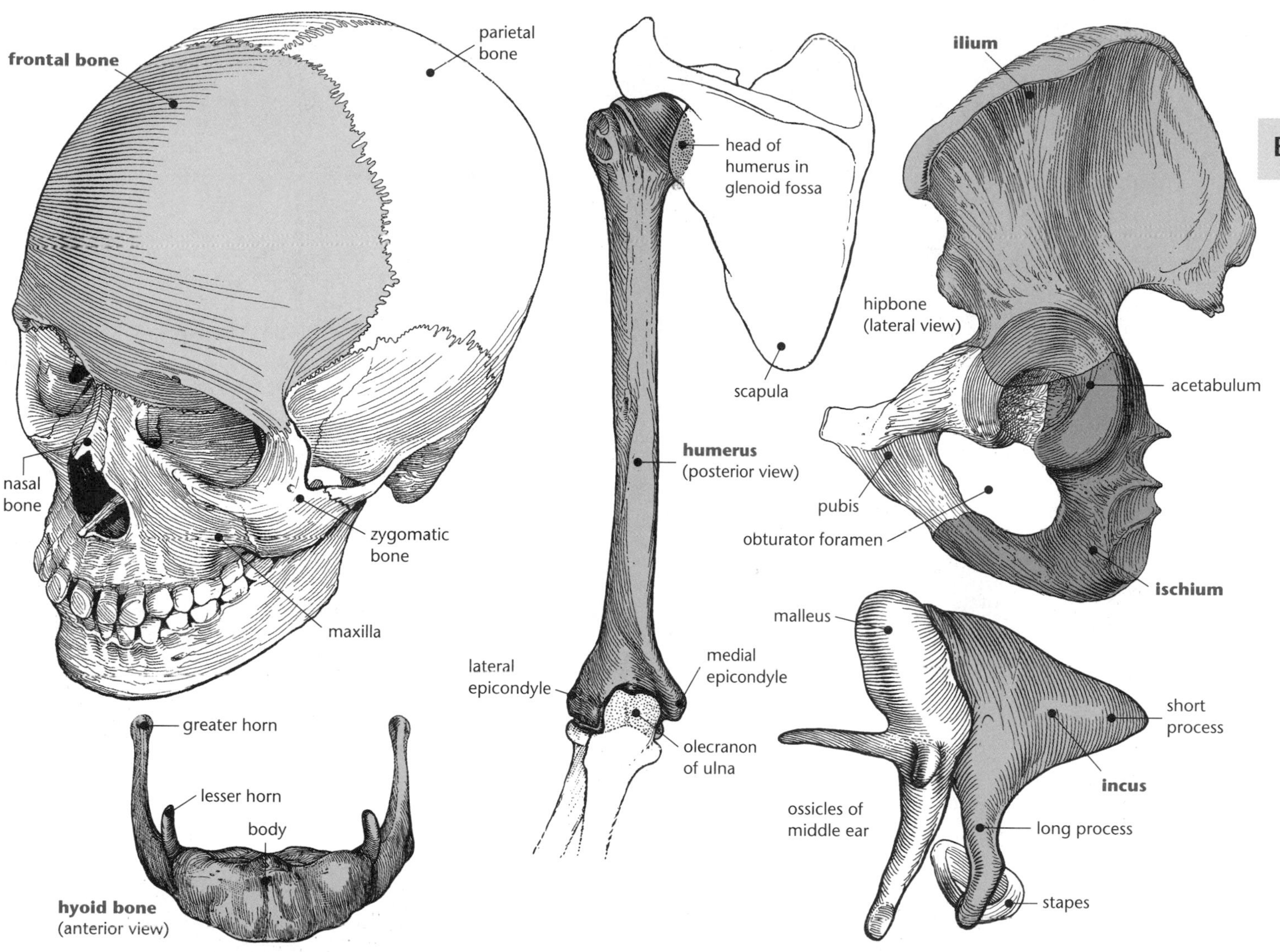

BONE	LOCATION	DESCRIPTION	ARTICULATIONS
frontal b. forehead b. *os frontale*	skull	flat b. forming anterior part of skull	ethmoid, sphenoid, maxillae, and both nasal, parietal, lacrimal, and zygomatic b.'s
greater multangular b.		see trapezium bone	
hamate b. unciform b. *os hamatum*	wrist	most medial b. of distal row of carpals; distinguished by hooklike process (hamulus) that projects from its palmar surface	lunate, triguetrum, capitate, fourth and fifth metacarpals
hammer b.		see malleus	
hipbone innominate b. *os coxae*	pelvis and hip	large, broad, irregularly shaped b. that forms greater part of pelvis; consists of three parts: ilium, ischium, and pubis	femur, sacrum, with its fellow of opposite side at pubic symphysis
humerus arm b. *humerus*	arm	longest and largest b. of upper limb, situated between shoulder and elbow	scapula, radius and ulna
hyoid b. lingual b. *os hyoideum*	neck	U-shaped b. in front of neck between mandible and larynx	suspended from tips of skull's styloid processes by ligaments
ilium flank b. *os ilium*	pelvis	broad expanded upper part of the hipbone, divisible into a body and an ala	sacrum, femur, ischium, pubis
incus anvil b. *incus*	middle ear chamber	middle b. of auditory ossicles	malleus, stapes
inferior tubinate b.		see concha, inferior nasal	
innominate b.		see hipbone	
ischium *os ischii*	pelvis	inferior and dorsal part of the hipbone, divisible into a body and a ramus	femur, ilium, pubis

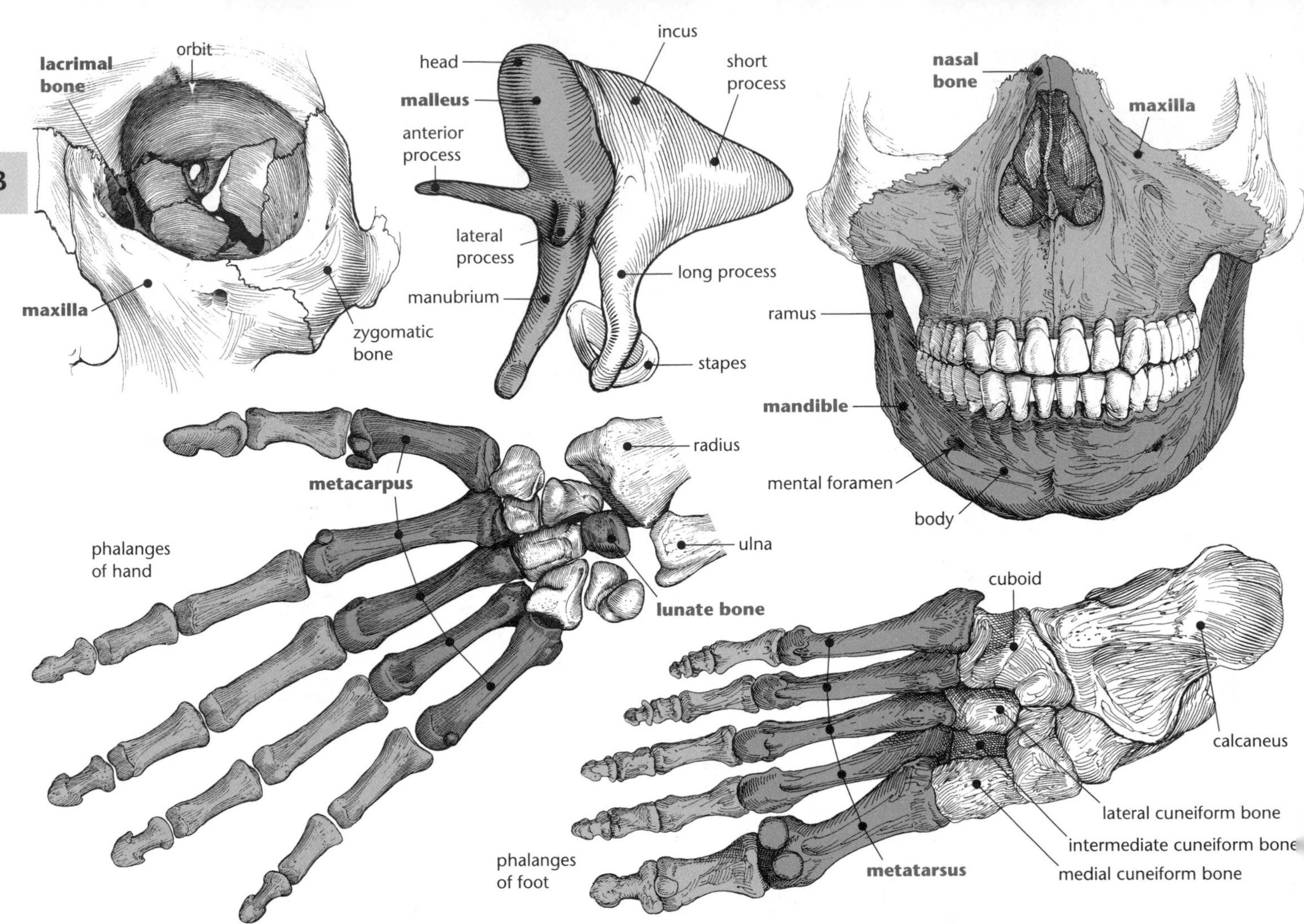

BONE	LOCATION	DESCRIPTION	ARTICULATIONS
lacrimal b. *os lacrimale*	skull	smallest and most fragile b. of the face; resembles a fingernail and is situated in anterior medial wall of orbit	ethmoid, frontal, maxilla, inferior nasal concha
lesser multangular b.		see trapezoid bone	
lunate b. semilunar b. *os lunatum*	wrist	in center of proximal row of carpus between scaphoid and triangular (triquetral) b.'s	radius, capitate, hamate, triangular, (triquetral) scaphoid
malar b.		see zygomatic bone	
malleus hammer b. *malleus*	middle ear chamber	most lateral b. of auditory ossicles, somewhat resembling a hammer and consisting of a head, neck, and three processes	tympanic membrane and incus
mandible inferior maxillary b. *mandibula*	lower portion of face	horseshoe-shaped b. containing the lower teeth; strongest b. of face	mandibular fossa of both temporal b.'s
maxilla maxillary b *maxilla*	middle portion of face	largest b. of the face except the mandible; contains the upper teeth and encloses maxillary sinus	frontal, ethmoid, nasal, zygomatic, lacrimal, vomer, inferior nasal concha, other maxilla
metacarpus metacarpal b.'s *ossa metacarpalia*	hand, between wrist and fingers	five slender b.'s of the hand proper, each consisting of a body and two extremities (head and base), and numbered from 1st to 5th starting from the thumb side	base of first metacarpal with trapezium, base of other metacarpals with each other and with distal row of carpal b.'s, heads with corresponding phalanges
metatarsus metatarsal b.'s *os metatarsalia*	foot, between distal row of tarsal b.'s and first phalanges of toes	five slender b.'s of the foot proper, each consisting of a body and two extremities (head and base), and numbered from 1st to 5th starting from the great toe side	distal tarsal b.'s, bases with each other, heads with corresponding phalanges
multangular b., greater		see trapezium bone	
multangular b., lesser		see trapezoid bone	
nasal b. *os nasale*	middle of face	one of two small oblong paired b.'s positioned side by side to form bridge of nose	frontal, ethmoid, opposite nasal, maxilla

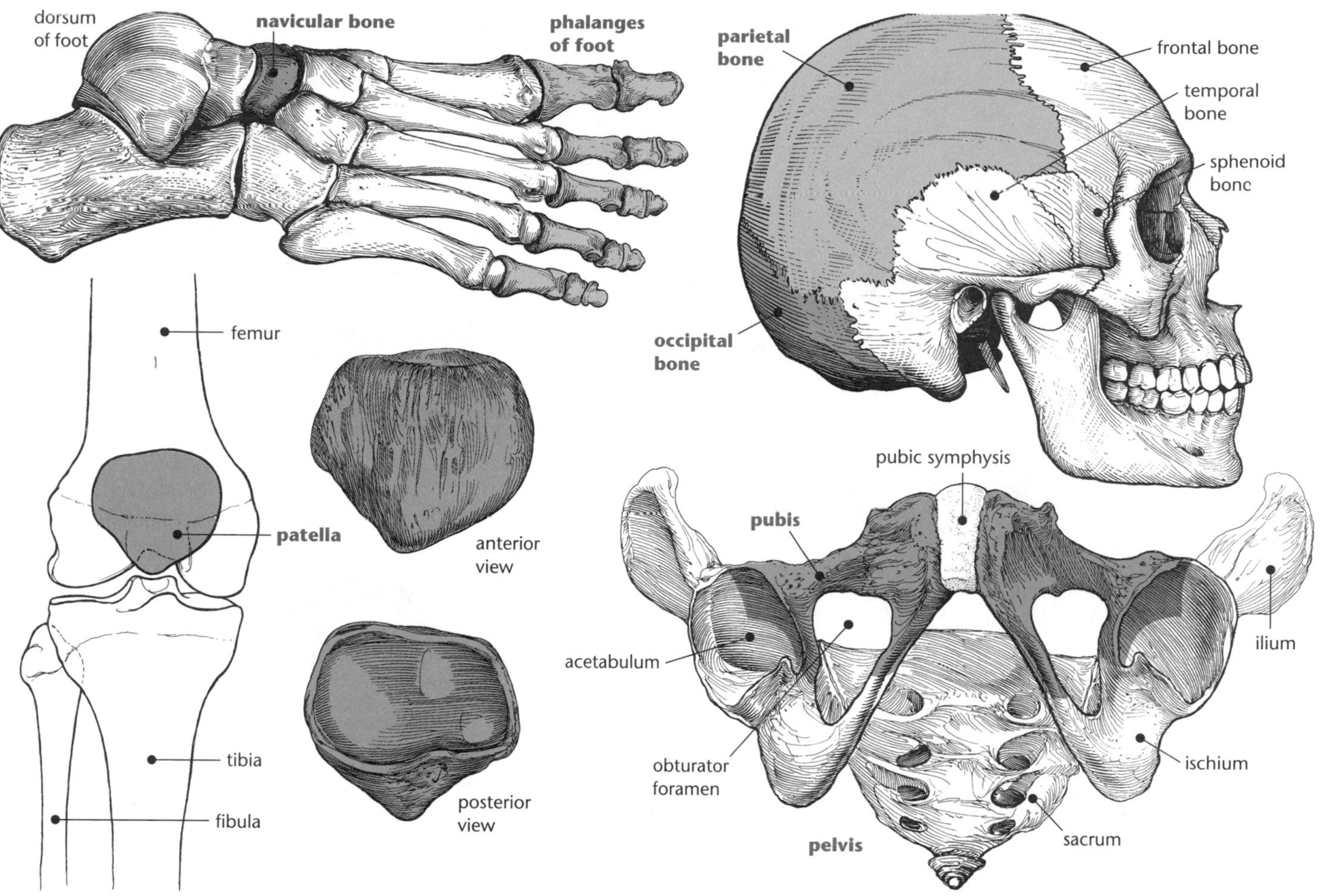

BONE	LOCATION	DESCRIPTION	ARTICULATIONS
navicular b. scaphoid b. of foot *os naviculare pedis*	foot	situated at medial side of tarsus between talus and cuneiform b.'s	talus, three cuneiforms, occasionally with cuboid
navicular b. of hand		see scaphoid bone	
occipital b. *os occipitale*	skull	unpaired saucer-shaped b. forming posterior part of base of cranium pierced by the foramen magnum	both parietals and temporals; sphenoid, atlas
palatine b. palate b. *os palatinum*	skull	one of two, somewhat L-shaped paired b.'s, the two forming the posterior part of hard palate, part of floor and lateral wall of nasal cavity, and part of floor of the orbit	sphenoid, ethmoid, maxilla, vomer, opposite palatine, inferior nasal concha
parietal b. *os parietale*	skull	paired b.'s between frontal and occipital b.'s forming sides and roof of cranium	opposite parietal, frontal, occipital, temporal, sphenoid
patella knee cap *patella*	knee	flat, rounded, triangular b. (sesamoid), situated in front of knee joint	femur
pelvis		a body ring resembling a basin, composed of two hipbones, sacrum, and coccyx	
phalanges of foot *ossa digitorum pedis*	foot	miniature long b.'s, two in great toe and three in each of other toes	proximal row of phalanges with corresponding metatarsal b.'s and middle phalanges; middle phalanges with proximal and distal phalanges; distal phalanges with middle phalanges
phalanges of hand *ossa digitorum manus*	hand	miniature long b.'s, two in thumb and three in each of other fingers	proximal row of phalanges with corresponding metacarpal b.'s and middle phalanges; middle phalanges with proximal and distal phalanges; distal phalanges with middle phalanges
pisiform b. *os pisiforme*	wrist	most medial of proximal row of carpus; smallest carpal b.	triangular (triquetral)
pubis *os pubis*	pelvis	anterior lower portion of hipbone	ilium, ischium, femur

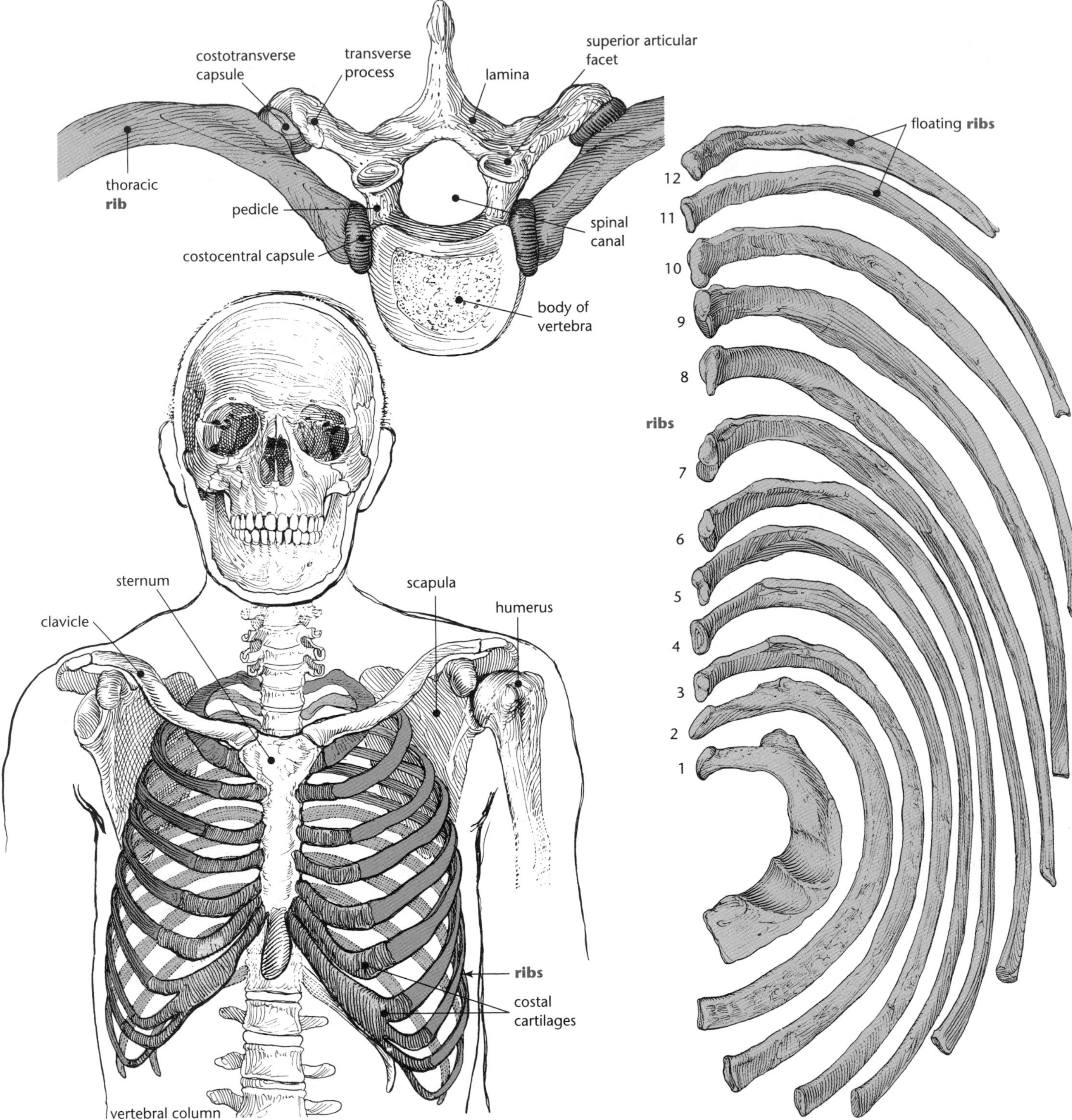

BONE	LOCATION	DESCRIPTION	ARTICULATIONS
pyramidal b.		see triangular bone	
radius *radius*	forearm between elbow and wrist	lateral b. of forearm; proximal end is small and forms small part of elbow; distal end is large and forms large part of wrist joint	humerus, ulnar, lunate, scaphoid
ribs *costae*	chest	12 pairs of thin, narrow, arch-shaped b.'s forming posterior and lateral walls of chest	all posteriorly with vertebral column; upper seven pairs anteriorly with sternum, through intervention of costal cartilages; lower five pairs anteriorly with costal cartilages; lowest two pairs free at ventral extremities (floating)

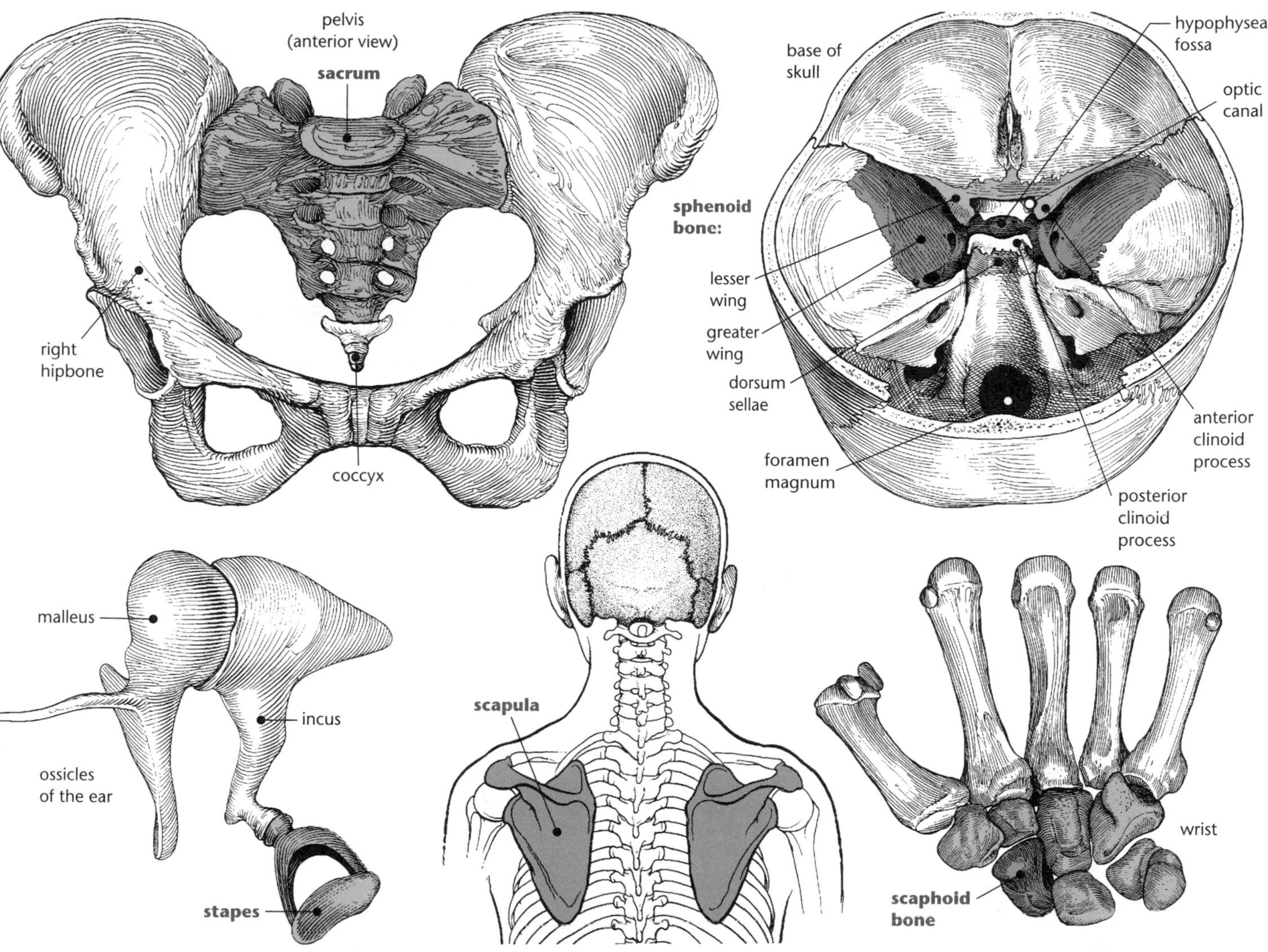

B

BONE	LOCATION	DESCRIPTION	ARTICULATIONS
sacrum *os sacrum*	lower back	large triangular b., formed by fusion of five vertebrae, and situated at dorsal part of pelvis	above with last lumbar vertebra, at each side with ilium, below with coccyx
scaphoid b. scaphoid b. of hand navicular b. of hand *os scaphoideum* *os scaphoideum manus*	wrist	largest b. of proximal row of carpus located at thumb side	radius, trapezium, trapezoid, capitate, lunate
scaphoid b. of foot		see navicular bone	
scapula shoulder blade *scapula*	shoulder	large, flat, triangular b. forming dorsal part of shoulder girdle	clavicle, humerus
semilunar b.		see lunate bone	
sesamoid b.'s *ossa sesamoidea*	extremities, usually within tendons	small rounded b.'s embedded in certain tendons; some constant ones include those in the tendons of quadriceps muscle of thigh, short flexor muscle of great toe, long peroneal muscle, anterior tibial muscle, posterior tibial muscle, and greater psoas muscle; the patella (kneecap) is the largest sesamoid b.	none
shinbone		see tibia	
sphenoid b. *os sphenoidale*	base of skull	unpaired, irregularly shaped b. forming anterior part of base of skull and portions of cranial, orbital, and nasal cavities	vomer, ethmoid, frontal, occipital, both parietals, both temporals, both zygomatics, both palatines; also articulates with tuberosity of maxilla
stapes stirrup *stapes*	middle ear chamber	most medial b. of auditory ossicles, somewhat resembling a stirrup	incus, oval window

B

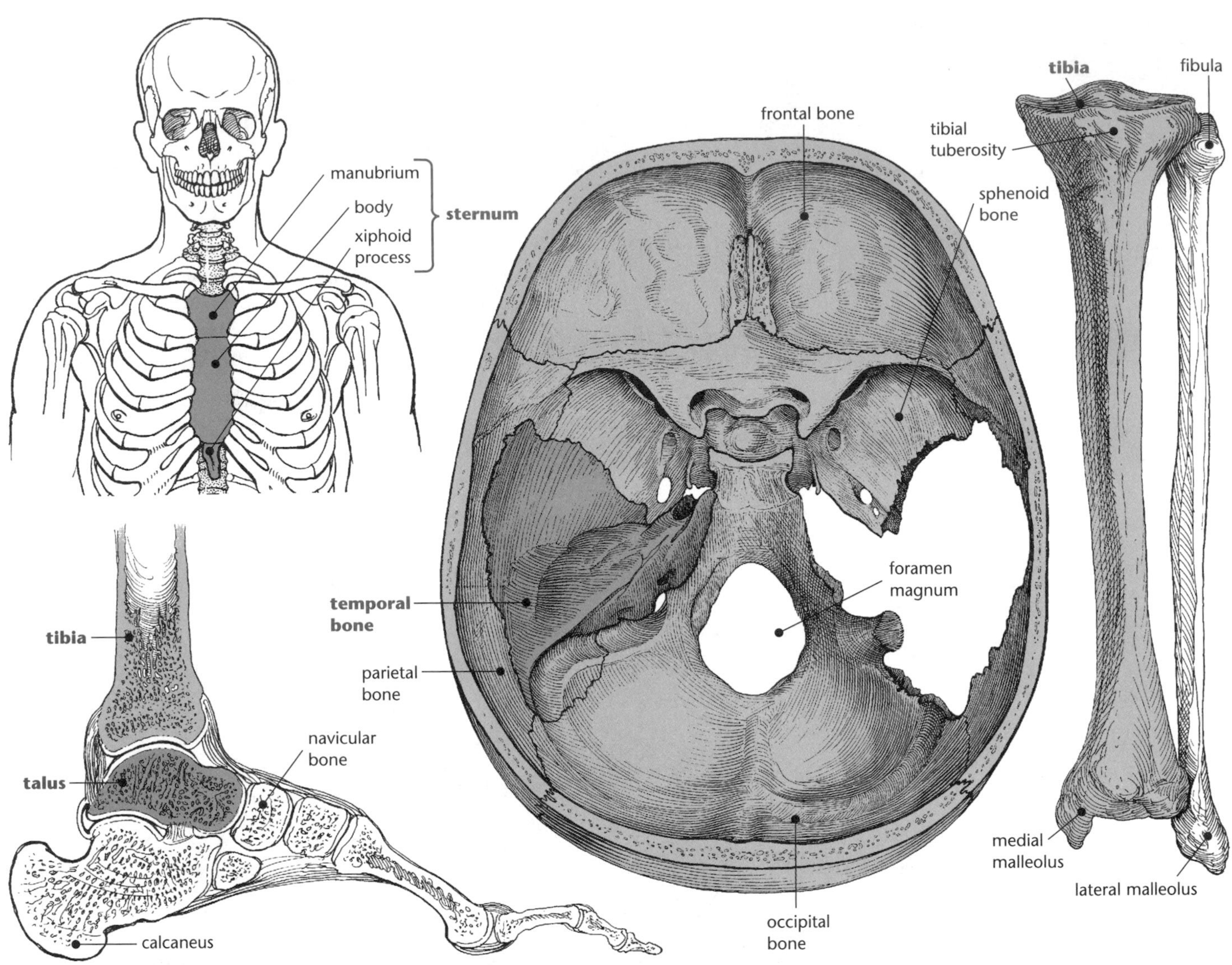

BONE	LOCATION	DESCRIPTION	ARTICULATIONS
sternum breastbone *sternum*	chest	elongated, flattened, dagger-shaped b. forming ventral wall of thorax; consists of three parts; manubrium, body, xiphoid process	both clavicles and first seven pairs of costal cartilages
stirrup b.		see stapes	
sutural b.'s wormian b.'s *ossa suturalis*	skull	irregular, isolated b.'s occasionally found along cranial sutures, especially lambdoid suture	usually occipital and parietal b.'s
talus ankle b. astragalus *talus*	ankle	second largest of the tarsal b.'s; supports tibia and rests on calcaneus	tibia, fibula, calcaneus, navicular
temporal b. *os temporale*	skull	irregularly shaped b. consisting of three parts: squamous, petrous, and tympanic, forms part of side and base of cranium	occipital, parietal, zygomatic, sphenoid, mandible
tibia shinbone tibia	leg	situated at medial side of leg between ankle and knee joint; second longest b. in the body	above with femur and fibula; below with fibula and talus
trapezium greater multangular b. *os trapezium*	wrist	most lateral of four b.'s of distal row of carpus	scaphoid, first metacarpal, trapezoid, second metacarpal
trapezoid b. *lesser multangular b.* *os trapezoideum*	wrist	smallest b. in distal row of carpus	scaphoid, second metacarpal, trapezium, capitate
triangular b. pyramidal b. triquetral b. *os triquetrum*	wrist	pyramidal shape; second from little finger side of proximal row of carpus	lunate, pisiform, hamate

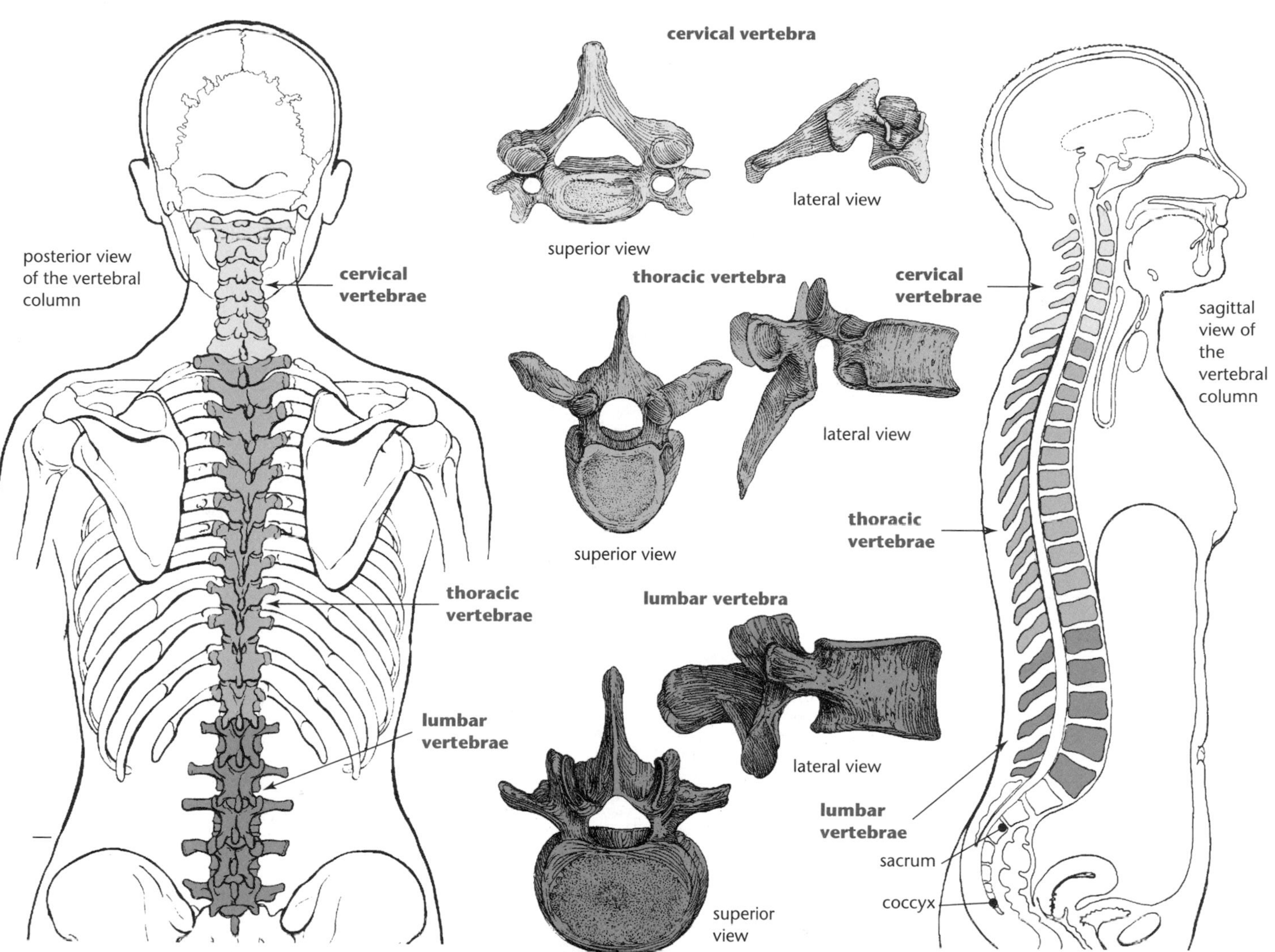

BONE	LOCATION	DESCRIPTION	ARTICULATIONS
triquetral b.		see triangular bone	
turbinate b., inferior		see choncha, inferior nasal	
turbinate b., middle			
turbinate b., superior		not a separate bone; see ethmoid bone	
ulna elbow b. *ulna*	forearm	medial b. of forearm; lies parallel with radius	humerus, radius
unciform b.		see hamate bone	
vertebrae, cervical backbones *vertebrae*	back of neck	seven segments of vertebral column; smallest of the true vertebrae; possess a foramen in each transverse process	first vertebra with skull, all others with adjoining vertebrae
vertebrae, lumbar backbones *vertebrae*	lower back	five segments of vertebral column; largest b.'s of movable part of vertebral column	with adjoining vertebrae; fifth vertebra with sacrum
vertebrae, thoracic backbones *vertebrae*	back	12 segments of vertebral column; possess facets on the sides of all the bodies and the first 10 also have facets on the transverse processes	with adjoining vertebrae, heads of ribs, tubercles of ribs (except 11th and 12th)
vomer *vomer*	skull	thin, flat b. forming posterior and inferior part of nasal septum	ethmoid, sphenoid, both maxillae, both palatine b.'s; also articulates with septal cartilage of nose
wormian b.'s		see sutural bones	
zygomatic b. malar b. cheekbone *os zygomaticum*	skull	forms prominence of cheek and lower, lateral aspects of orbit	frontal, sphenoid, temporal, maxilla

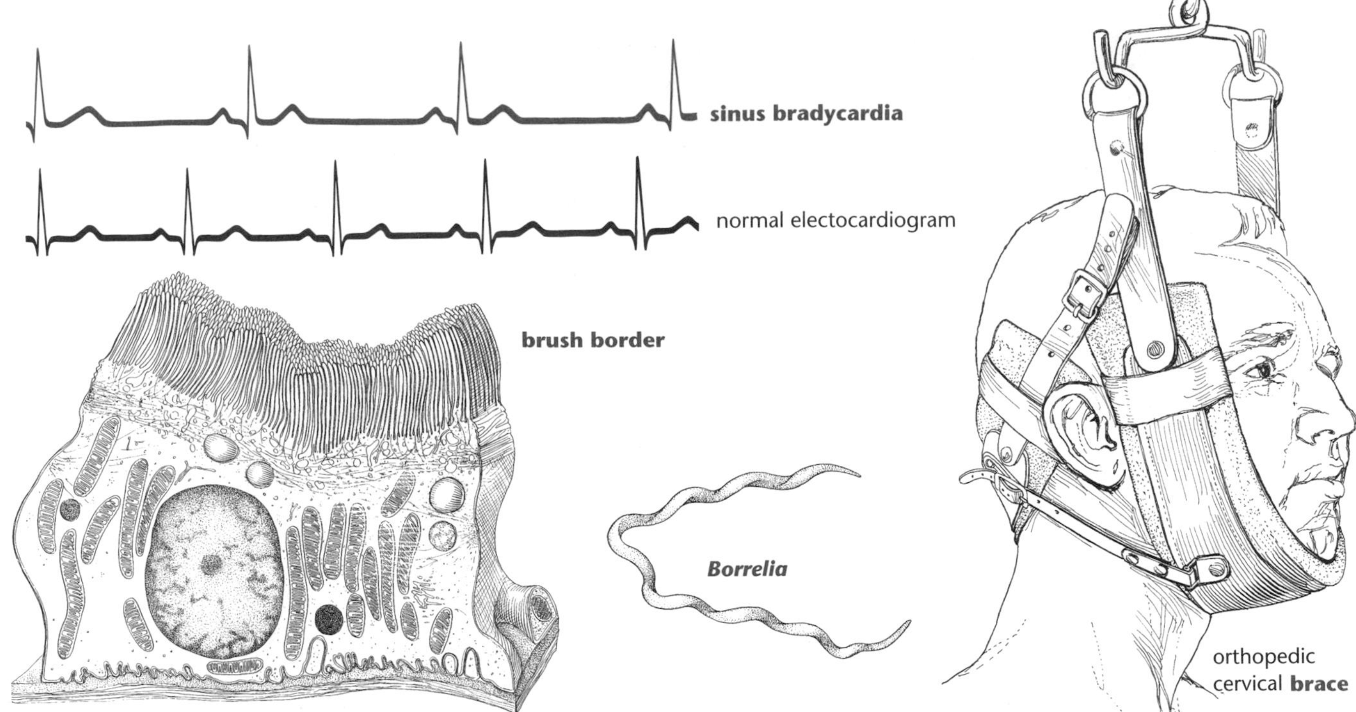

borate (bor´āt) A salt of boric acid.

borax (bor´aks) Sodium borate, $Na_2B_4O_7$; used in dentistry in the casting of fluxes and to retard the setting reaction of gypsum products.

borborygmus (bor-bo-rig´mus) Rumbling noise produced by movement of gas in the intestines.

border (bor´der) Edge or margin.

brush b. A border of many fine, closely packed microvilli, as seen on the free surface of the cuboidal cells of the proximal convoluted tubules of the kidney.

denture b. **1.** The boundary of a denture base. **2.** The area of a denture base at the junction of the polished surface with the impression (tissue) surface. Also called denture edge.

striated b. A border of many fine, closely packed microvilli on the free surface of the columnar absorptive cells of the intestine; it greatly increases the surface area of intestinal epithelium. Also called striated free border.

striated free b. See striated border.

vermilion b. The exposed reddish portion of the upper and lower lips.

Bordetella (bor-dĕ-tel´ă) A genus of gram-negative pathogenic bacteria (family Brucellaceae).

B. pertussis The causative agent of whooping cough.

boric acid (bor´ik as´id) A white or crystalline compound, H_3BO_3; used as an antiseptic.

Bornholm disease (born´hōm dĭ-zēz´) See epidemic pleurodynia, under pleurodynia.

boron (bor´on) A soft, brown nonmetallic element; symbol B, atomic number 5, atomic weight 10.82.

Borrelia (bŏ-rel´e-ă) A species of gram-negative, anaerobic, screw-shaped bacteria (family Treponemataceae). Some species are pathogenic, transmitted by the bites of arthropods.

B. burgdorferi The species causing Lyme disease in humans and borreliosis in dogs and cattle; transmitted by several species of ixodid ticks.

borreliosis (bo-rel-e-o´sis) Any disease caused by bacteria of the genus *Borrelia.*

Lyme b. See Lyme disease.

boss (bos) **1.** A round swelling. **2.** A hump on the back.

bosselation (bos-ĕ-la´shun) Condition marked by the presence of one or more round protuberances or swellings.

Bothriocephalus (both-re-o-sef´ă-lus) See *Diphyllobothrium.*

botryoid (bot´re-oid) Resembling a bunch of grapes.

bottle (bot´l) A receptacle with a narrow neck.

wash b. (a) A fluid-containing bottle with two tubes passing through its cork, arranged in such a way that blowing through one tube forces a stream of fluid through the other; used for washing chemical materials. (b) A fluid-containing bottle with a tube passing to the bottom through which gases are forced for the purpose of purifying the gases.

botulism (boch´u-liz-m) Poisoning caused by the toxin of *Clostridium botulinum* in improperly preserved food.

bougie (boo-zhe´) A flexible cylindrical instrument used in the diagnosis and treatment of strictures of tubular structures, such as the esophagus or urethra; it also serves to measure the degree of narrowing.

b. à boule See bulbous bougie.

bulbous b. A bougie with a bulb-shaped tip. Also called bougie à boule.

filiform b. A very slender bougie.

bougienage (boo-zhe-năzh) Examination or treatment (dilatation) of a tubular structure by means of a bougie or cannula.

bouillon (boo-yaw´) **1.** A clear thin broth. **2.** A culture medium prepared from beef.

Bourneville's disease (bōōrn-velz´) See tuberous sclerosis, under sclerosis.

bout (bout´) An episode.

periodic drinking b.'s A form of alcoholism in which the person overindulges in alcoholic drinks continuously for days or weeks, then recovers and abstains for several weeks or months before the next episode. Also called paroxysmal alcoholism.

bouton (boo-tan´) A swelling or thickening.

b. en chemise Abscesses of the intestinal mucosa, seen in amebic dysentery.

terminal b. See axon terminal, under terminal.

b.'s termineaux See axon terminal, under terminal.

Bovie (bo´ve) Instrument used in electrosurgical procedures. Term is also used as a verb to denote dissecting or cauterizing with the instrument.

bovine (bo´vīn) Relating to cattle.

bowel (bow´el) Popular name for intestine.

Bowen's disease (bo´enz dĭ-zēz´) Squamous cell carcinoma occurring as pink-to-brown papules at multiple sites on the skin within the epidermis.

bowleg (bo´leg) See genu varum, under genu.

brace (brās) A device for supporting a body part.

orthodontic b.'s General term for orthodontic appliances designed to move teeth into a more esthetic and/or functional position; composed of bands fitted to the teeth with attachments or brackets to hold spring wires; often the wires are supplemented by rubber bands.

brachial (bra´ke-al) Relating to the arm.

brachium (bra´ke-um), *pl.* **bra´chia** **1.** The arm, especially above the elbow. **2.** Any armlike structure.

brachybasia (brak-e-ba´zhă) The slow, shuffling gait indicative of motor nerve disease.

brachycephalic (brak-e-se-fal´ik) Characterized by brachycephalism.

brachycephalism (brak-e-sef´ă-liz-m) A deformity in which the skull has an abnormally flattened anteroposterior plane, due to premature closure of the coronal suture.

brachydactyly (brak-e-dak´tĭ-le) Abnormal shortness of fingers and toes.

brachysyndactyly (brak-e-sin-dak´tĭ-le) A combined shortness and webbing of fingers or toes.

brachytherapy (brak-e-ther´ă-pe) Local irradiation of tissues (i.e., the radiation source is placed in direct proximity to the tissues being irradiated). See also irradiation.

interstitial b. Irradiation carried out by placing removable radioactive needles or permanent isotope implants within a tumor.

intracavitary b. Irradiation by introducing into a body cavity a small sealed, or partly sealed, container (e.g., capsule, cylinder, ovoid) loaded with radioactive material.

bracket (brak´ĭt) In orthodontics, a small piece of metal fixed on the band surrounding a tooth; used to fasten the arch wire to the band.

bradycardia (brad-e-kar´de-ă) Abnormal slowness of the heartbeat, a rate usually less than 60 beats per minute.

sinus b. Bradycardia resulting from the sinus node originating impulses at a slow rate; usually due, in part at least, to vagal inhibition of the sinus node; seen often in patients with high vagal tone, in trained athletes, in hypothyroidism, and secondary to increased intracranial tension.

bradycrotic (brad-e-krot´ik) Marked by a slow pulse.

bradykinesia (brad-e-kĭn-e´zhă) Abnormal slowness of movement.

bradykinin (brad-e-ki´nin) A potent vasodilator polypeptide hormone produced by the action of kallikrein on an alpha 2-globulin.

bradypnea (brad-e-ne´ă, brad-ip´ne-ă) Abnormally slow rate of breathing, as in shock.

bradytachycardia syndrome (brad-e-tak-ĭ-kar´de-ă sin´drōm) Alternating periods of slow and rapid heart beats; usually indicates a disease of the sinoatrial node (the "pacemaker" of the heart).

braille (brāl) A system of writing and printing for the blind, consisting of raised dots representing letters and numerals; invented by Louis Braille, a French teacher of the blind.

brain (brān) The portion of the central nervous system contained within the skull; composed of the cerebrum, cerebellum, pons, and medulla oblongata. Also called encephalon.

braincase (bran´kas) The cranial part of the skull

pubic symphysis
prostate
bougienage
filiform bougie in bladder
filiform bougies passing through the urethra
penis
scrotum
rectum

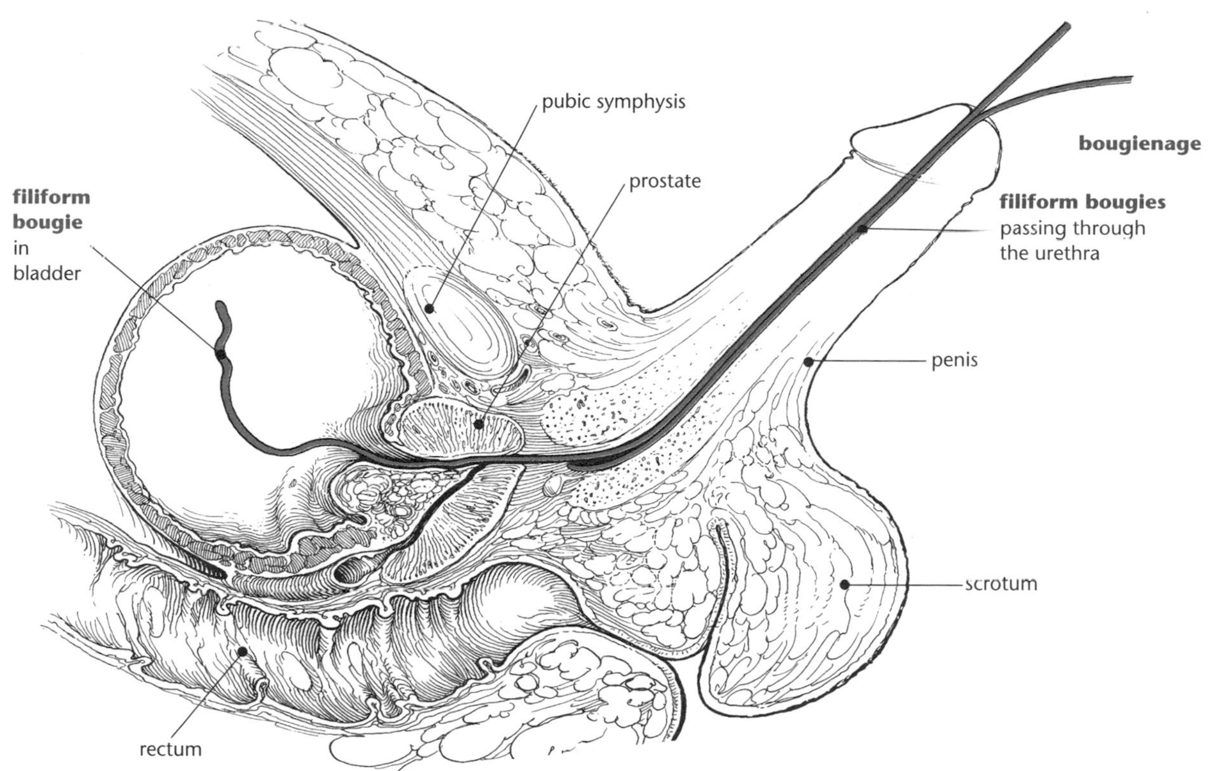

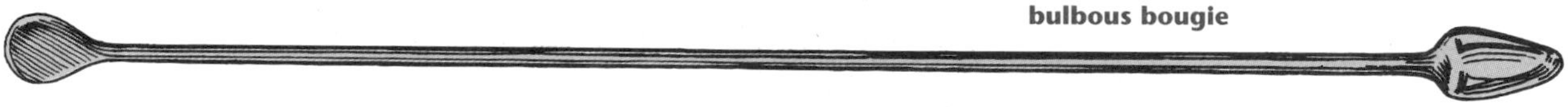

bulbous bougie

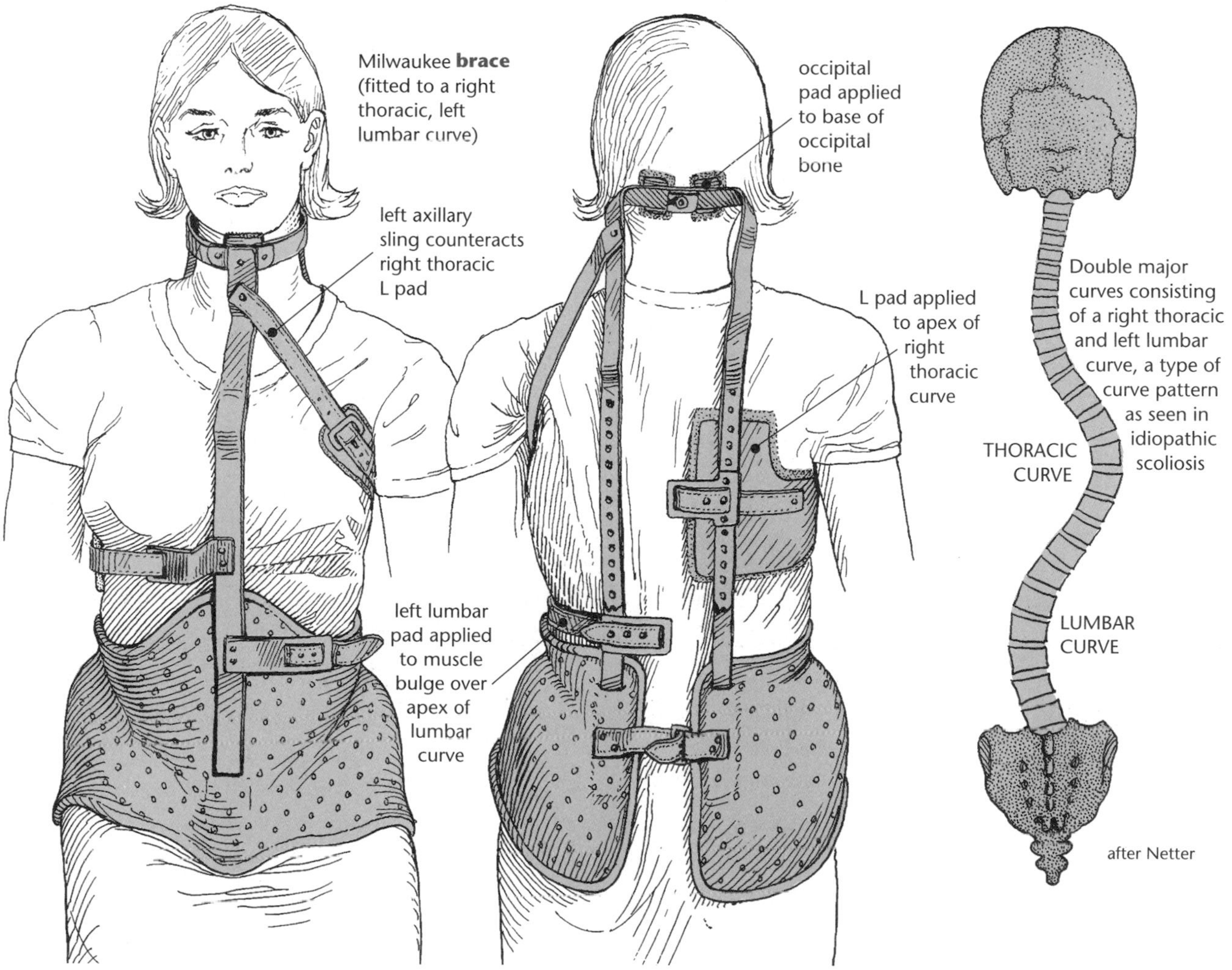

Milwaukee **brace** (fitted to a right thoracic, left lumbar curve)
left axillary sling counteracts right thoracic L pad
left lumbar pad applied to muscle bulge over apex of lumbar curve
occipital pad applied to base of occipital bone
L pad applied to apex of right thoracic curve
Double major curves consisting of a right thoracic and left lumbar curve, a type of curve pattern as seen in idiopathic scoliosis
THORACIC CURVE
LUMBAR CURVE
after Netter

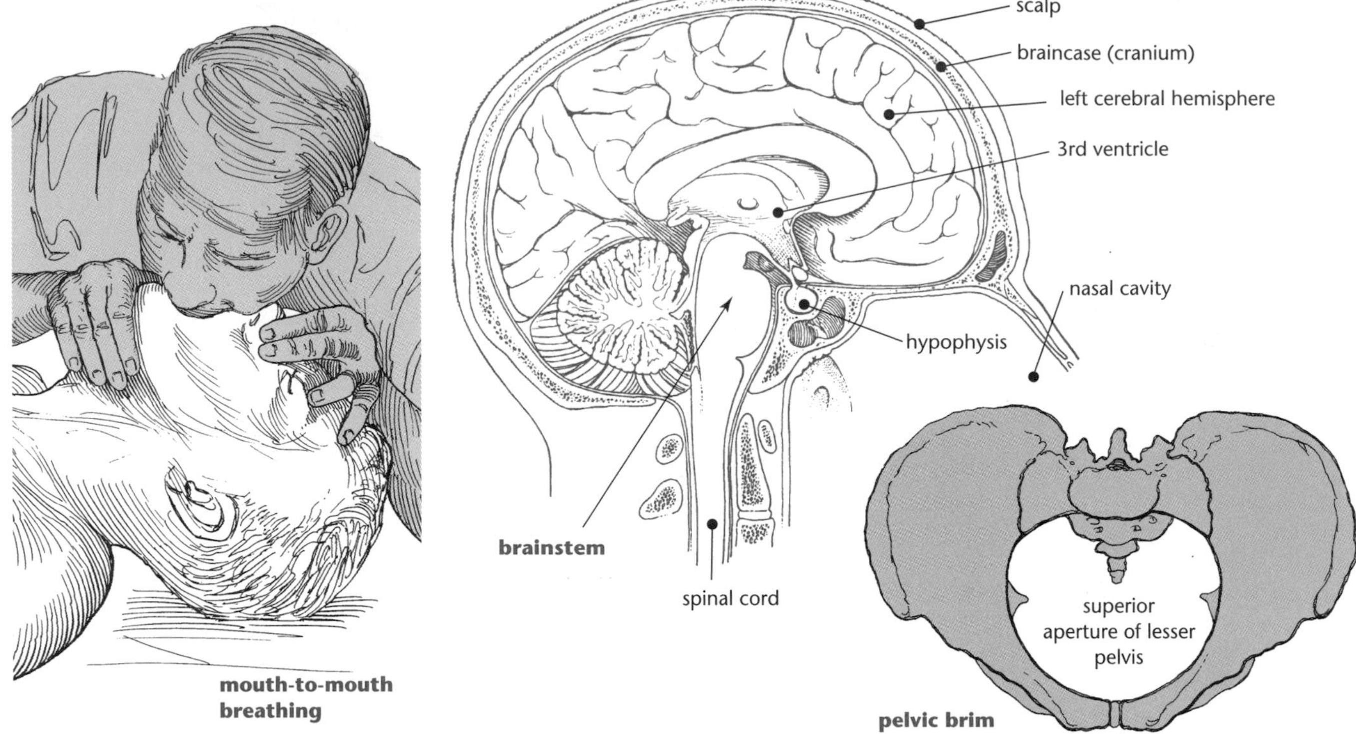

mouth-to-mouth breathing

pelvic brim

enclosing the brain; the facial bones are not included.

brainstem (brān´stem) The part of the brain connecting the forebrain (prosencephalon) and the spinal cord; it consists of the midbrain (mesencephalon), pons, and medulla oblongata.

bran (bran) A by-product of the milling of wheat to produce flour; consists mainly of the coat of the grain; used as a bulk cathartic.

branchial (brang´ke-ăl) Relating to gills.

branchiogenic, branchiogenous (brang-ke-o-jen´ik, brang-ke-oj´ĕ-nus) Originating from the embryonic branchial arches or the ridges between the branchial clefts.

brawny (brăw´ne) Dark and swollen.

breach of duty (brēch ŭv dū´tē) In medical liability claims, a physician's violation of responsibilities owed to a patient to provide medical care within accepted standards of medical practice.

breast (brest) **1.** One of the two structures attached to the fascia covering the chest muscles. In the male, breasts are rudimentary; in the female, they are the organs of lactation. The adult female breast consists of fifteen to twenty glandular lobes and their ducts (the mammary gland proper); fibrous tissue binding the glandular lobes; and fatty tissue in the spaces between the lobes; also present are blood vessels, nerves, and lymph vessels. Multiple fibrous bands pass forward to the skin and nipple, forming the Cooper's (suspensory) ligament for supporting the breast in its upright position. When distorted by a tumor, these bands cause dimpling of the skin surface. Also called mamma. See also mammary gland, under gland. **2.** The chest.

accessory b. See polymastia.

keel b. See pectus carinatum.

pigeon b. See pectus carinatum.

supernumerary b. See polymastia.

breastbone (brest´bōn) See sternum.

breath (breth) **1.** The inhaled and exhaled air in respiration. **2.** The air exhaled, as evidenced by vapor.

uremic b. The characteristic fishy or ammoniacal odor of the breath of patients with chronic kidney failure; results from the systematic accumulation of substances normally excreted in the urine.

breathing (brēth´ing) The act of taking in and expelling air from the lungs.

Biot's b. See ataxic respiration, under respiration.

bronchial b. A harsh, blowing quality of the breath heard on auscultation of the chest; often heard over a consolidated lung or over a cavity in the lung.

Cheyne-Stokes b. See Cheyne-Stokes respiration, under respiration.

continuous positive pressure b. (CPPB) See continuous positive pressure ventilation, under ventilation.

intermittent positive pressure b. (IPPB) See intermittent positive pressure ventilation, under ventilation.

mouth b. Habitual breathing through the open mouth.

mouth-to-mouth b. A stage in cardiopulmonary resuscitation (CPR) in which the rescuer places his mouth completely over the victim's mouth (and nose, if the victim is a child) and delivers two slow, independent breaths, while maintaining the victim's airway open and allowing time for the victim to exhale before delivering the second breath; each breath lasts 1.5 to 2 seconds (1–1.5 seconds for infants and children); if after the second breath normal breathing is still absent but carotid pulse is present, then breathing is again delivered, at the rate of about 12 breaths per minute (about 20 breaths/minute for infants and children). Also called mouth-to-mouth resuscitation. See also cardiopulmonary resuscita-tion (CPR), under resuscitation.

periodic b. See Cheyne-Stokes respiration, under respiration.

pursed-lip b. A technique of breathing in which air is exhaled through pursed lips in order to slow down the outflow of air from the lungs; it relieves airway discomfort in chronic obstructive pulmonary disease.

shallow b. A weak type of breathing, as seen in acute pulmonary disease.

breech (brēch) The buttocks (nates).

breed (brēd) **1.** To develop new or improved strains in animals or plants. **2.** A strain of animal or plant.

bregma (breg´mă) The point on the skull where the sagittal and coronal sutures meet.

brei (bri) A suspension of minced tissue, used especially in metabolic experimentation.

brevotoxins (brev-o-tok´sins) (BTX) Neurotoxins, produced by the alga *Ptychodiscus brevis Davis,* implicated in causing food poisoning; used in research on the nervous system.

bridge (brĭj) **1.** In dentistry, a nonremovable prosthesis consisting of one or more artificial teeth suspended between and attached to abutments (terminal natural crowns or roots). **2.** The upper part of the human nose, between the eyes.

Bright's disease (brīts dĭ-zēz´) A term applied in the past to a variety of acute and chronic renal diseases, especially those thought to represent forms of glomerulonephritis.

Brill's disease (brilz dĭ-zēz´) See Brill-Zinsser disease.

Brill-Zinsser disease (bril-zin´sĕr dĭ-zēz´) The occurrence of typhus in persons who suffered an infection of primary epidemic typhus in the past; caused by *Rickettsia prowazekii* which, according to Zinsser, remain viable in the body of the patient; recrudescence or relapse occurs years after the original infection. Also called Brill's disease; recrudescent typhus.

brim (brim) An edge.

pelvic b. The circumference of the oblique plane dividing the major and minor pelves.

British antilewisite (brit´ĭsh an-tĭ-loo´ĭ-sīt) (BAL) See dimercaprol.

brittle bones disease (brit´l bōns dĭ-zēz´) See osteogenesis imperfecta, under osteogenesis.

broach (brōch) A small instrument used in the examination or treatment of the root canal of a tooth.

Broadbent's sign (brod´bentz sīn) Pulsation observed in the left posterior axillary line, occurring synchronously with cardiac systole; a sign of adherent pericardium.

broad-spectrum (brod spek´trum) Widely effective. See also broad-spectrum antibiotic, under antibiotic.

Brock's syndrome (broks sin´drōm) See middle lobe syndrome.

bromcresol green (brom-krē´sol grēn) A slightly yellow crystalline compound, $C_{21}H_{14}Br_4O_5S$; slightly soluble in water; soluble in alcohol, ether, and ethyl alcohol; used as an indicator of pH: yellow at pH 3.8, blue-green at pH 5.4.

bromcresol purple (brom-krē´sol pur´pl) A pale yellow crystalline compound, $C_{21}H_{16}Br_2O_5S$; soluble in alcohol and dilute alkalis; used as an indicator of pH: yellow at pH 5.2, purple at pH 6.8.

bromide (bro´mīd) A binary compound of bromine and another element or organic radical; a salt of hydrobromic acid.

bromine (bro´mēn) A heavy, corrosive, reddish, volatile, nonmetallic liquid element, with a highly irritating vapor; symbol Br, atomic number 35, atomic weight 79.916.

bromocriptine (bro-mo-krip´tēn) An ergot derivative that suppresses secretion of the hormone prolactin from the adenohypophysis (anterior portion of the pituitary). Used in the treatment of conditions caused by excessive prolactin production, such as abnormal milk production (galactorrhea); formerly used for the suppression of puerperal lactation.

bromphenol blue (brōm-fe´nol bloo) An indicator of pH.

Brompton cocktail (brom´ton kŏk´tāl) A drink containing various ingredients including cocaine hydrochloride and morphine hydrochloride; given orally as a pain reliever to patients dying of cancer.

bronchi (brong´ki) Plural of bronchus.

bronchial (brong´ke-al) Relating to the bronchi.

bronchiectasis, bronchiectasia (brong-ke-ek´tă-sis, brong-ke-ek-ta´zhă) An irreversible, abnormal

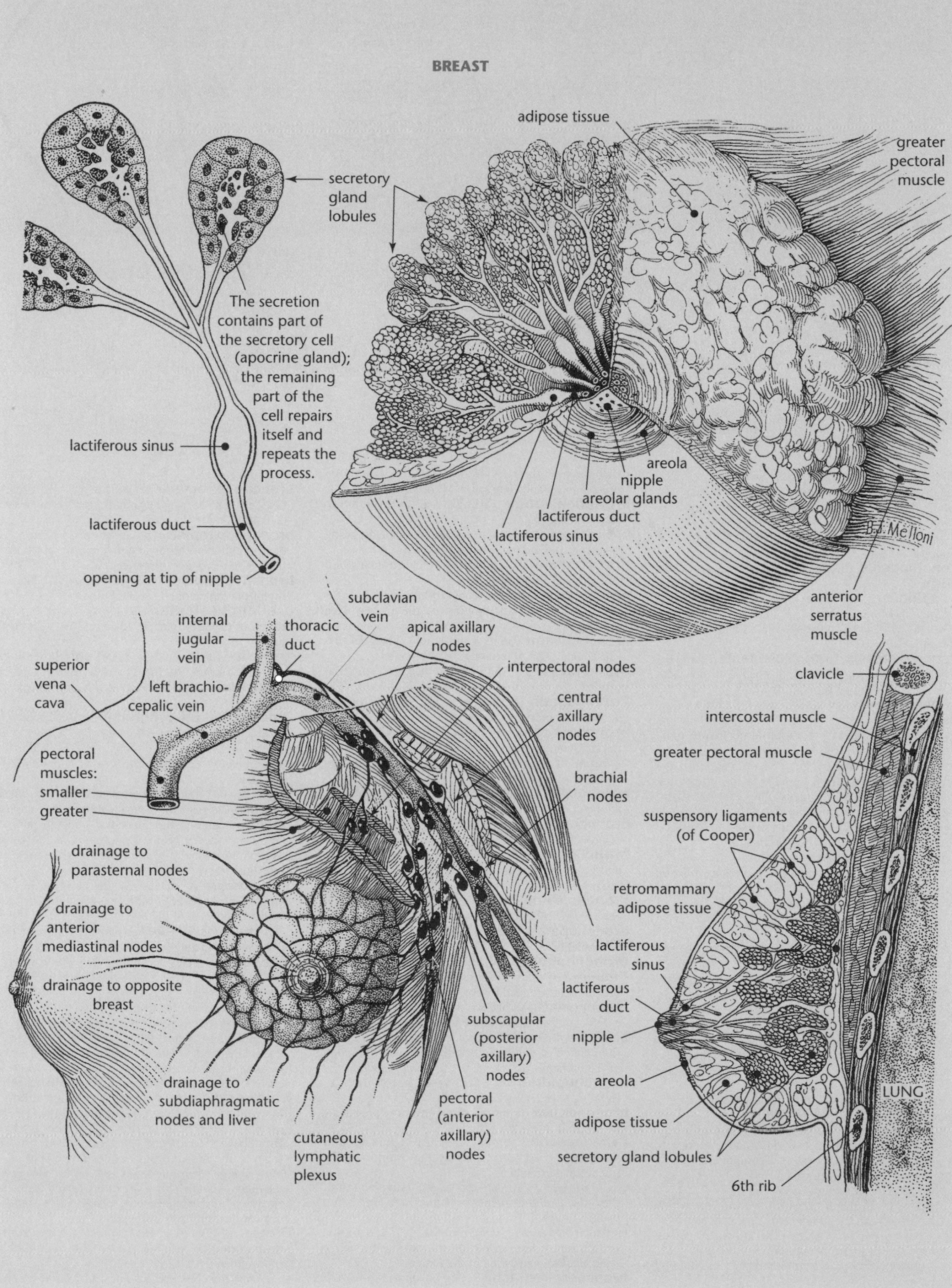
BREAST
secretory gland lobules
The secretion contains part of the secretory cell (apocrine gland); the remaining part of the cell repairs itself and repeats the process.
lactiferous sinus
lactiferous duct
opening at tip of nipple
adipose tissue
greater pectoral muscle
areola
nipple
areolar glands
lactiferous duct
lactiferous sinus
B.J. Melloni
anterior serratus muscle
subclavian vein
internal jugular vein
thoracic duct
apical axillary nodes
superior vena cava
left brachio-cepalic vein
interpectoral nodes
central axillary nodes
pectoral muscles: smaller greater
brachial nodes
drainage to parasternal nodes
drainage to anterior mediastinal nodes
drainage to opposite breast
drainage to subdiaphragmatic nodes and liver
cutaneous lymphatic plexus
subscapular (posterior axillary) nodes
pectoral (anterior axillary) nodes
clavicle
intercostal muscle
greater pectoral muscle
suspensory ligaments (of Cooper)
retromammary adipose tissue
lactiferous sinus
lactiferous duct
nipple
areola
adipose tissue
secretory gland lobules
6th rib
LUNG

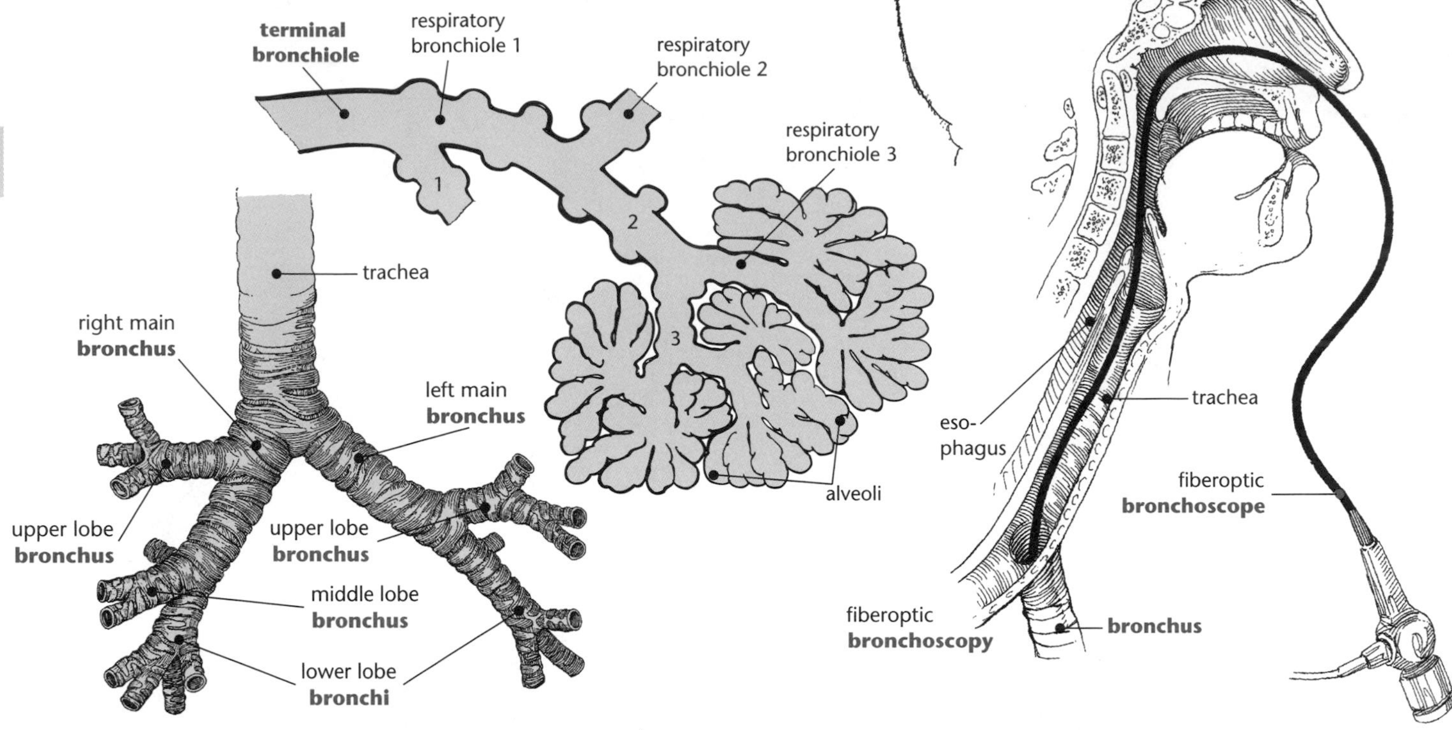

dilatation of the bronchi or bronchioles; the extent of the disorder may range from a mild involvement of a single pulmonary segment to gross distortion of the entire bronchial tree.

bronchiloquy (brong-kil'o-kwe) See bronchophony.

bronchiogenic (brong-ke-o-jen´ik) Of bronchial origin.

bronchiole (brong´ke-ōl) Any of the thin-walled extensions of a bronchus.

terminal b. The last bronchiole without alveoli in its wall.

bronchiolectasis, bronchiolectasia (brong-ke-o-lek´tă-sis, brong-ke-o-lek-ta´zhă) Chronic dilatation of the terminal bronchioles.

bronchiolitis (brong-ke-o-li´tis) Inflammation of the bronchioles.

acute b. A viral bronchiolitis occurring most commonly in children under the age of 2 years; marked by a hacking cough, difficult breathing, and wheezing resulting from damage to the bronchiole walls and formation of mucus plugs that trap air in the distal bronchioles; usually caused by a respiratory syncytial virus (RSV) but other viruses may also be responsible. Also called viral bronchiolitis.

b. fibrosa obliterans Inflammation of the bronchioles with obstruction caused by fibrous granulation tissue formed in the walls of the terminal bronchioles; it may be caused by inhalation of irritating gases or foreign bodies, or occur as a complication of pneumonia.

b. obliterans with organizing pneumonia (BOOP) A widespread inflammatory and fibrous obstruction of the bronchioles complicated by pneumonia and fibrous obstruction of the pulmonary air sacs (alveoli).

viral b. See acute bronchiolitis.

bronchiolopulmonary (brong-ke-o-lo-pul´mo-ner-e) Relating to the bronchioles and the lungs.

bronchiostenosis (brong-ke-o-stĕ-no´sis) Narrowing of the bronchi.

bronchitis (brong-ki´tis) Inflammation of the mucous membrane of the bronchi.

acute b. A form of bronchitis that is generally self-limited, lasting only a few days, with complete recovery; it usually occurs as a complication of an upper respiratory infection.

allergic b. See asthma.

chronic b. Generalized narrowing and obstruction of the airways in the lungs lasting longer than three consecutive months in at least two successive years; usually resulting from cigarette smoking or from long-term exposure to air pollutants, such as irritating fumes or dusts.

chronic obstructive b. Term used when chronic bronchitis is associated with extensive abnormalities and obstruction of the smaller airways.

bronchoalveolar (brong-ko-al-ve´o-lar) See bronchovesicular.

bronchocavernous (brong-ko-kav′er-nus) Relating to a bronchus and a pulmonary cavity.

bronchocele (brong´ko-sēl) A circumscribed dilatation of a bronchus.

bronchoconstrictor (brong-ko-kon-strik´tor) An agent that causes narrowing of the lumen of a bronchus.

bronchodilator (brong-ko-di´la´tor) An agent that causes dilatation of the lumen of a bronchus.

bronchogenic (brong-ko-jen´ik) Of bronchial origin.

bronchogram (brong´ko-gram) The radiogram obtained by bronchography.

bronchography (brong-kog´ră-fe) Rarely performed radiographic examination of the bronchi after injection of a radiopaque material; now superseded by computed tomography.

broncholith (brong´ko-lith) A bronchial calculus (stone).

broncholithiasis (brong-ko-lĭ-thi´ă-sis) Presence of bronchial calculi.

bronchomalacia (brong-ko-mă-la´shă) Degeneration of the supporting tissues of the bronchi and trachea.

bronchomotor (brong-ko-mo´tor) An agent that changes the caliber of bronchi.

bronchopathy (brong-kop´ă-the) Disease of the bronchial tubes.

bronchophony (brong-kof´ŏ-ne) Exaggerated resonance of the voice heard in auscultation over a bronchus surrounded by consolidated lung tissue.

bronchoplasty (brong'ko-plas-te) Surgical repair of a defect in the trachea or the bronchi.

bronchopneumonia (brong-ko-nōō-mo´ne-ă) Inflammation of the lungs, usually following infection of the bronchi. Also called bronchial pneumonia.

bronchopulmonary (brong-ko-pul-mo-ner´e) Relating to the bronchi and the lungs.

bronchorrhea (brong-ko-re´ă) Abnormally profuse secretion from the bronchi.

bronchoscope (brong´ko-skōp) A thin tubular instrument used for inspecting the interior of the trachea and bronchi.

bronchoscopy (brong-kos'ko-pe) Examination of the lumen of the tracheobronchial tree through a bronchoscope.

bronchospasm (brong´ko-spaz-m) Spasmodic contraction of the smooth muscles of the bronchial walls causing narrowing of the lumen.

bronchospirography (brong-ko-spi-rog'ră-fe) The measuring of the airflow in one lung only, or one lobe of a lung.

bronchospirometer (brong-ko-spi-rom´ĕ-ter) A device for measuring separately the air capacity of each lung.

bronchospirometry (brong-ko-spi-rom'ĕ-tre) The determination of the respiratory capacity of a lung by the use of a bronchospirometer.

bronchostenosis (brong-ko-stĕ-no´sis) Narrowing of the lumen of a bronchial tube.

bronchovesicular (brong-ko-vĕ-sik´u-lar) Relating to the bronchial tubes and air sacs in the lungs.

bronchus (brong'kus), *pl.* **bron´chi** Either of two main branches of the trachea leading to the bronchioles and serving to convey air to and from the lungs.

Brown-Séquard syndrome (brōōn´sa-kărz sin´drōm) Symptom complex caused by damage to one side of the spinal cord, causing paralysis and loss of discriminatory sensation on the same side of the body and loss of pain and temperature sensation on the opposite side. Also called Brown-Séquard paralysis.

Brucella (broo-sel'ă) A genus of bacteria composed of gram-negative, rod-shaped to coccoid parasitic cells; they cause primary infections of the genital organs, mammary glands, and respiratory and intestinal tracts.

B. abortus A species causing abortion in cattle and undulant fever (brucellosis) in humans. Also called Bang's bacillus.

B. melitensis A species causing undulant fever in humans and abortion in goats.

B. suis A species resembling *Brucella melitensis*; the cause of abortion in swine and brucellosis in humans.

brucellosis (broo-sĕ-lo´sis) An infectious disease caused by bacteria of the genus *Brucella* and transmitted by contact with secretions and tissues of infected animals; marked by remittent fever, general weakness, aches, and pains, sometimes becoming chronic. Also called undulant fever; Malta fever.

Brudzinski's signs (broo-jin´skēz sin´drōm) **1.** Brudzinski's neck sign: flexion of both legs and thighs upon forcible flexion of the neck. **2.** Brudzinski's contralateral leg sign: flexion of one thigh at the hip causes a similar movement of the other thigh; when one thigh and leg are flexed and the other extended, lowering of the flexed leg causes flexion of the extended one. Brudzinski's signs are seen in meningitis.

Brugia (bruj´ă) A genus of parasitic threadworms transmitted to humans and other mammals by mosquitoes.

B. malayi The species causing filarial elephantiasis in Southeast Asia.

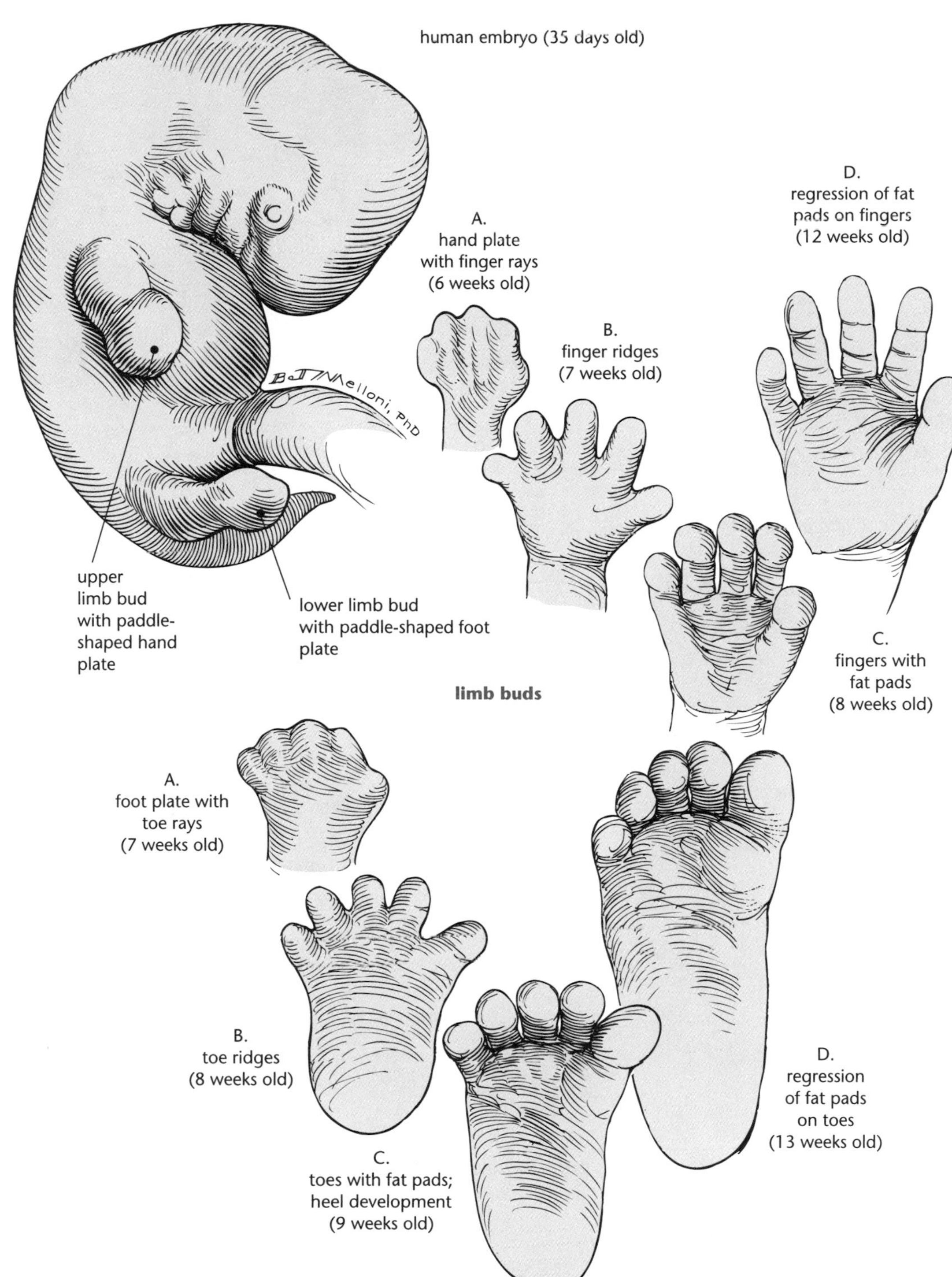

limb buds

bruise (bro͞oz) Hematoma without laceration; usually a superficial lesion but can occur in deeper structures; a contusion.

bruit (bro͞ot, bru-ē´) Sound or murmur, especially an abnormal one heard during auscultation, from the French word for noise.

abdominal b. A murmur heard on auscultation of the abdomen, generally traceable to the aorta or one of its major branches.

aneurysmal b. A blowing murmur heard over an aneurysm.

carotid b. A murmur heard over a carotid artery.

b. de canon The abnormally loud first heart sound heard intermittently in complete heart block; cannon sound.

diastolic b. Bruit occurring during the diastolic phase of the heart cycle after the second heart sound; usually connotes an abnormal valve function.

epigastric b. A murmur heard in the epigastrium during auscultation of the abdomen.

systolic b. Bruit heard during the systolic phase of the heart cycle between the first and second heart sounds.

b. de Roger See Roger's murmur, under murmur.

thyroid b. A vascular murmur heard over a hyperactive thyroid gland.

bruxism (bruk´siz-m) Forceful clenching and grinding of the teeth, especially during sleep.

bruxomania (bruk-so-ma´ne-ă) Unconscious grinding of the teeth while awake.

bubo (bu´bo) Enlargement and inflammation of a lymph node, especially in the groin or axilla.

malignant b. Bubo associated with bubonic plague.

tropical b. See lymphogranuloma venereum.

venereal b. Bubo in the groin associated with venereal disease.

bubonic (bu-bon´ik) Relating to an enlarged suppurating lymph node in the groin or axilla.

buccal (buk´al) Pertaining to the cheek.

buccolingual (buk-o-ling´gwal) **1.** Denoting the plane of a posterior tooth from its buccal surface across to its lingual surface. **2.** Relating to the cheek and the tongue.

bucco-occlusal (buk-o-ŏ-kloo´zal) Relating to the buccal and occlusal surfaces of a posterior tooth; usually denoting the line angle formed by the junction of the two surfaces.

buccopharyngeal (buk-o-fă-rin´je-al) Relating to both the mouth and the pharynx.

buccoversion (buk-o-ver´shun) Malposition of a tooth toward the cheek.

bud (bud) Any small organic part resembling a plant bud.

bronchial b. One of the outgrowths from the primordial bronchus, giving rise to the bronchial tree.

limb b. A swelling on the trunk of an embryo that gives rise to an arm or leg.

lung b.'s Two lateral outpocketings of the respiratory primordium of the foregut that give rise

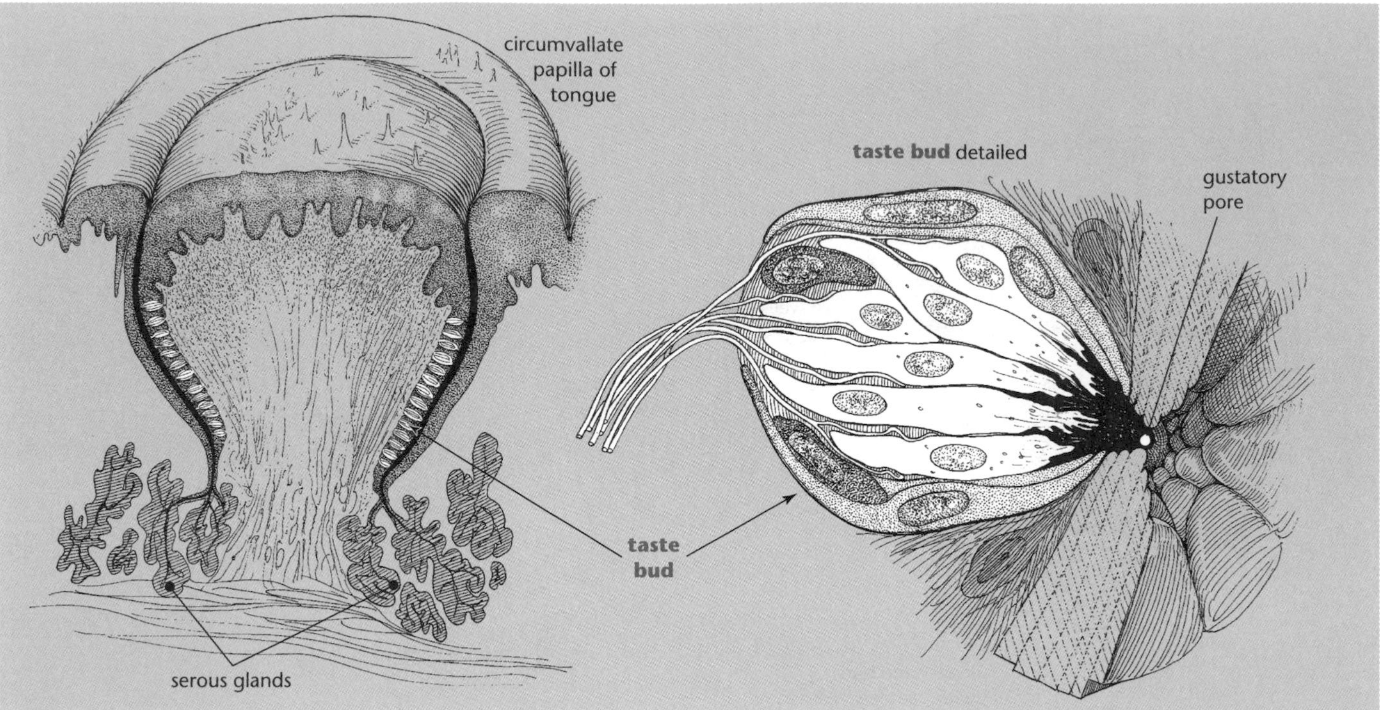

to the tracheobronchial tree.

metanephric b. An outgrowth from the mesonephric duct, giving rise to the lining of the ureter, pelvis, and calices of the kidney, and the straight collecting tubules.

taste b. One of numerous flask-shaped minute organs, located on the tongue, the under surface of the soft palate, and the posterior surface of the epiglottis; composed of modified epithelial supporting cells which surround a mass of spindle-shaped gustatory cells and the fibrils of the nerves of taste (chorda tympani and glossopharyngeal). Also called gustatory caliculus; taste bulb.

tooth b. The primordial structure from which a tooth develops.

Budd-Chiari syndrome (bud´ke-ă´re sin´drōm) See hepatic vein occlusion, under occlusion.

budding (bud´ing) See gemmation.

Buerger's disease (ber´gerz dĭ-zēz´) See thromboangiitis obliterans.

buffer (buf´er) **1.** Any substance that maintains the relative concentrations of hydrogen and hydroxyl ions in a solution by neutralizing any added acid or alkali. **2.** To add a buffer to a solution; to maintain body fluids at a relatively constant pH when acid or alkali is added to or lost from the body.

buffering (buf´er-ing) A process by which hydrogen ion concentration is maintained constant.

biologic b. Ionic shifts between intra- and extracellular spaces that protect extracellular pH.

renal b. Removal of excess acid or base by the kidney.

respiratory b. Increases or decreases in respiratory rate that act to increase or decrease CO_2 and, subsequently, H_2CO_3 and HCO_3.

bug (bug) Any of various insects of the suborder Hemiptera.

assassin b. See kissing bug.

bed b. See bedbug.

cone-nose b. See kissing bug.

kissing b. An insect (family Reduviidae) similar to the ordinary bedbug but with a cone-shaped anterior end; usually found in bedrooms where it feeds at night on the blood of its sleeping, and unsuspecting hosts; acquired its name because of its inclination to bite the lips of sleeping people. Also called cone-nose bug; assassin bug.

red b. See chigger.

bulb (bulb) **1.** Any globular structure. **2.** The medulla oblongata.

aortic b. A dilatation at the beginning of the aorta.

carotid b. See carotid sinus, under sinus.

duodenal b. See duodenal cap, under cap.

end b. One of the minute spherical bodies located at the termination of a sensory nerve fiber; present in certain parts of the skin, mucous membranes, muscles, joints, and connective tissue of internal organs.

jugular b. A dilatation of the internal jugular vein just before it joins the subclavian vein.

Krause's end b. A spherical sense organ located at the termination of some sensory nerve fibers; it responds to the sensation of cold. Also called Krause's corpuscle.

olfactory b. The expanded anterior end of the olfactory tract.

b. of penis The expanded posterior portion of the corpus spongiosum penis.

taste b. See taste bud, under bud.

bulbar (bul´bar) **1.** Relating to or resembling a bulb. **2.** Relating to the medulla oblongata.

bulbopontine (bul-bo-pon´tīn) Relating to the part of the brain composed of the pons and the portion of the medulla oblongata over it.

bulbourethral (bul-bo-u-re´thral) Relating to the bulb of the penis and the urethra.

bulimia (bu-lim´e-ă) Repeated episodes of solitary binge eating, often followed by self-induced vomiting or massive laxative use to avoid weight gain; these episodes usually alternate with periods of fasting; seen primarily in young white females. Also called binge and purge syndrome.

bulimic (bu-lim´ik) Relating to bulimia.

bulkage (bulk´ij) Any substance, such as bran, that stimulates peristalsis by increasing the bulk of the intestinal contents.

bulla (bul´ă), *pl.* **bul´lae** **1.** A blister or circumscribed elevation on the skin containing serous fluid or air, larger than 1 centimeter in diameter (e.g., as in a second degree burn). **2.** A bubble-like anatomic structure. COMPARE: vesicle.

pulmonary b. A large air-filled bulla on the surface or within the lung; seen in certain diseases.

bullous (bul´us) Relating to bullae or the nature of bullae.

bundle (bun´dl) A group of nerve or muscle fibers.

atrioventricular (A-V) b. A bundle of specialized muscular fibers located in the membranous interventricular septum of the heart; the only direct muscular connection between the atria and the ventricles; it originates at the atrioventricular (A-V) node in the floor of the right atrium, extends downward in the septum, divides into right and left branches, and ends in numerous strands (Purkinje system) in the papillary and ventricular muscles. Also called bundle of His; fasciculus atrioventricularis.

b. of His See atrioventricular bundle.

posterior longitudinal b. See medial longitudinal fasciculus, under fasciculus.

bunion (bun´yun) Painful condition of the big toe, marked by lateral angulation of the toe (hallux valgus), enlargement of the head of the metatarsal bone, and a swollen, inflamed overlying bursa; caused by poorly fitted shoes. COMPARE: hallux valgus.

bunionectomy (bun-yun-ek´to-me) Treatment of a bunion by surgical means.

buphthalmos (būf-thal´mos) A condition marked by an increase of intraocular fluid with enlargement of the eyeball and protrusion of the cornea. Also called congenital glaucoma; hydrophthalmos.

bur (ber) A rotary dental instrument with one cutting end designed in any of several shapes and a shaft at the other end which is inserted into a hand piece; used for excavating decay from a tooth, shaping cavity forms, or any surface reduction of tooth substance.

burette, buret (bu-ret´) A calibrated, uniform-bore glass tube with a stopcock at its lower end, used in the laboratory for accurate fluid dispensing.

Burkholderia (burk-hol-der´e-ă) Genus of gram-negative rod-shaped bacteria (family Pseudomonadaceae) formerly classified in the genus *Pseudomonas.*

B. mallei Species causing glanders in horses, sheep, goats, and humans. Formerly called *Pseudomonas mallei.*

B. pseudomallei Species causing melioidosis. Formerly called *Pseudomonas pseudomallei.*

burn (bern) **1.** To injure by fire, heat, or a chemical. **2.** The lesion thus produced.

brush b. Injury to the skin by friction of a rapidly moving object. Also called rope burn; mat burn.

chemical b. A burn caused by a caustic agent.

first degree b. Reddening of skin without blistering; only epidermis is affected.

flash b. A burn caused by brief exposure to radiant heat of high intensity.

mat b. See brush burn.

radiation b. A burn due to overexposure to x-rays, radium, ultraviolet rays, etc.

rope b. See brush burn.

second degree b. Blistering of skin; epidermis and dermis are involved.

thermal b. A burn produced by contact with heat.

third degree b. Destruction of full thickness of skin; may involve subcutaneous fat, muscle, and bone.

burner (ber´nĕr) The part of a lamp or stove that is lighted to produce a flame.

Bunsen b. A gas burner used in the laboratory, consisting of a metal tube with adjustable air holes at the base.

burner syndrome (ber´nĕr sin´drōm) Burning pain of the arms sometimes accompanied by

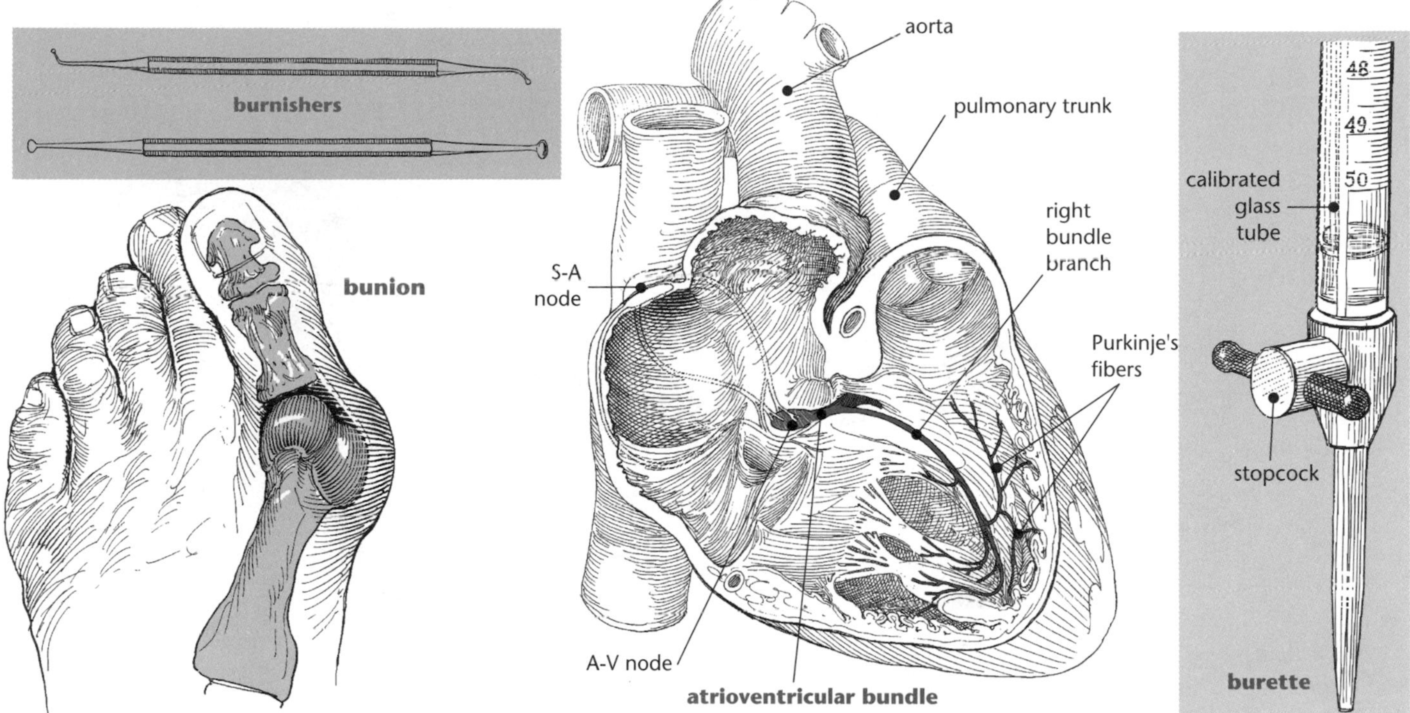

shoulder girdle weakness, experienced during contact sports; attributed to injury to the brachial plexus.

Burnett's syndrome (bur-nets sin´drōm) See milk-alkali syndrome.

burnisher (ber´nish-ĕr) A dental instrument with rounded edges for smoothing, polishing, or stretching the metallic surface of a tooth restoration.

bursa (ber´să), *pl.* **bur´sae** A closed sac lined with specialized connective tissue and containing a viscid fluid; usually present over bony prominences, between and beneath tendons, and between certain movable structures; it serves to facilitate movement by diminishing friction.

Achilles b. See bursa of calcaneal tendon.

b. of acromion A small subcutaneous bursa located at the shoulder between the upper surface of the acromion and the overlying skin.

adventitious b. An abnormal bursa developed as a result of continued irritation.

anserine b. A large bursa located at the medial side of the knee joint between the tibial (medial) collateral ligament and the tendon insertions of the semitendinous, gracilis, and sartorius muscles. Also called tibial intertendinous bursa.

b. of biceps muscle of arm See bicipitoradial bursa.

b. of biceps muscle of thigh Either of two subtendinous bursae: *lower,* a small bursa between the tendon of the biceps muscle of thigh (biceps femoris muscle) and the fibular (lateral) collateral ligament of the knee joint; *upper,* a small bursa under the tendon of origin of the long head of the biceps muscle of thigh (biceps femoris muscle) at the ischial tuberosity of the hipbone.

bicipitoradial b. A bursa interposed between the tendon of the biceps muscle of the arm (biceps brachii muscle) and the front part of the tuberosity of the radius. Also called bursa of biceps muscle of arm.

b. of big toe A bursa interposed between the lateral side of the base of the first metatarsal bone of the foot and the medial side of the adjoining shaft of the second metatarsal bone.

b. of calcaneal tendon A large bursa located at the heel, between the back of the heel bone (calcaneus) and calcaneal tendon (Achilles tendon). Also called Achilles bursa, retrocalcaneal bursa; bursa of tendo calcaneus.

b. of coracobrachial muscle An occasional bursa of the upper arm located between the tendons of the coracobrachial and subscapular muscles.

deep infrapatellar b. A bursa located below the patella (kneecap) between the lower portion of the patellar ligament and the tibia.

deep trochanteric b. See trochanteric bursa of greater gluteal muscle.

b. of Fabricius A saclike outgrowth of the cloaca in chicks, similar to the human thymus; contains lymphoid tissue and produces lymphocytes which are active in humoral immunity; it atrophies after six months. See also B lymphocytes, under lymphocyte.

b. of fibular collateral ligament A bursa interposed between the lateral part of the knee joint capsule and the fibular (lateral) collateral ligament, which it partially envelops.

gastrocnemius b. A bursa composed of two portions (lateral and medial) and located in the back of the knee, under the two heads of the gastrocnemius muscle; the medial portion is usually connected with the semimembranous bursa (of clinical importance because when distended with fluid, it is the usual cause of a popliteal cyst).

gluteofemoral b. A bursa interposed between the tendon of the greater gluteal muscle (gluteus maximus muscle) and the tendon of the lateral vastus muscle (vastus lateralis muscle).

b. of greater pectoral muscle A bursa between the tendons of insertion of the greater pectoral muscle and the latissimus dorsi muscle on the upper anterior aspect of the humerus. Also called bursa of pectoralis major muscle.

b. of greater psoas tendon See iliopectineal bursa.

iliac b. A large subtendinous bursa lying under the tendon of the iliac muscle just above the hip joint; sometimes in communication with the cavity of the hip joint.

iliopectineal b. A bursa located on the anterior surface of the hip joint capsule, between the iliofemoral and pubofemoral ligaments; it frequently communicates with the capsule of the joint. Also called bursa of greater psoas tendon; bursa of psoas major muscle.

infrapatellar b. Either of two bursae of the knee: *deep,* a bursa located just below the patella (kneecap) between the lower part of the patellar ligament and the upper part of the front of the tibia; *superficial,* a subcutaneous bursa situated between the patellar ligament and the overlying skin.

b. of infraspinous muscle A small synovial bursa interposed between the tendon of the infraspinous muscle (infraspinatus muscle) and the capsule of the shoulder joint.

interosseous cubital b. See interosseous bursa of elbow.

interosseous b. of elbow An occasional bursa interposed between the tendon of the biceps muscle of the arm (biceps brachii muscle) and the depression of the anterior ulnar between the supinator crest and tuberosity. Also called interosseous cubital bursa.

ischial b. of gluteus maximus muscle See ischiogluteal bursa.

ischiogluteal b. A large bursa separating the gluteus maximus muscle from the ischial tuberosity; chronic ischiogluteal bursitis is caused by prolonged sitting on hard surfaces and is commonly known as weaver's bottom. Also called ischial bursa of gluteus maximus muscle.

b. of lateral epicondyle A small subcutaneous bursa at the elbow occasionally found between the bony prominence of the lateral epicondyle of the humerus and the overlying skin.

b. of lateral malleolus A subcutaneous bursa at the ankle between the lateral malleolus of the fibula and the overlying skin.

b. of latissimus dorsi muscle An elongated bursa in front of the tendon of the latissimus dorsi muscle at the intertubercular sulcus of the humerus in the upper part of the arm.

b. of medial epicondyle A small subcutaneous bursa at the elbow found occasionally between the bony prominence of the medial epicondyle of the humerus and the overlying skin.

b. of medial malleolus A subcutaneous bursa at the ankle between the medial malleolus of the tibia and the overlying skin.

b. of obturator muscle The bursae of the hip: *External,* a bursa interposed between the tendon of the external obturator muscle and the hip joint capsule and femoral neck; it communicates with the synovial cavity of the hip joint. *Internal,* (a) a well-developed sciatic bursa partially encircling the tendon of the internal obturator muscle as it emerges from the lesser sciatic notch of the hipbone; (b) a narrow bursa between the tendon of the internal obturator muscle and the hip joint capsule.

olecranon b. A subcutaneous bursa located at the elbow between the skin and the tip of the olecranon process of the ulna.

omental b. See lesser sac of peritoneum, under sac.

ovarian b. A peritoneal recess between the medial surface of the ovary and the overlapping mesosalpinx.

b. of pectoralis major muscle See bursa of greater pectoral muscle.

b. of piriform muscle A small bursa under the tendons of the piriform muscle and the superior gemellus muscle at their insertion on the greater trochanter of the femur.

popliteal b. A bursa located on the posterolateral portion of the knee, under the popliteus muscle; it is often a continuation of the synovial sac of the knee.

prepatellar b. A large subcutaneous bursa situated between the lower part of the front of the patella (kneecap) and the overlying skin; chronic irritation causes prepatellar bursitis (housemaid's

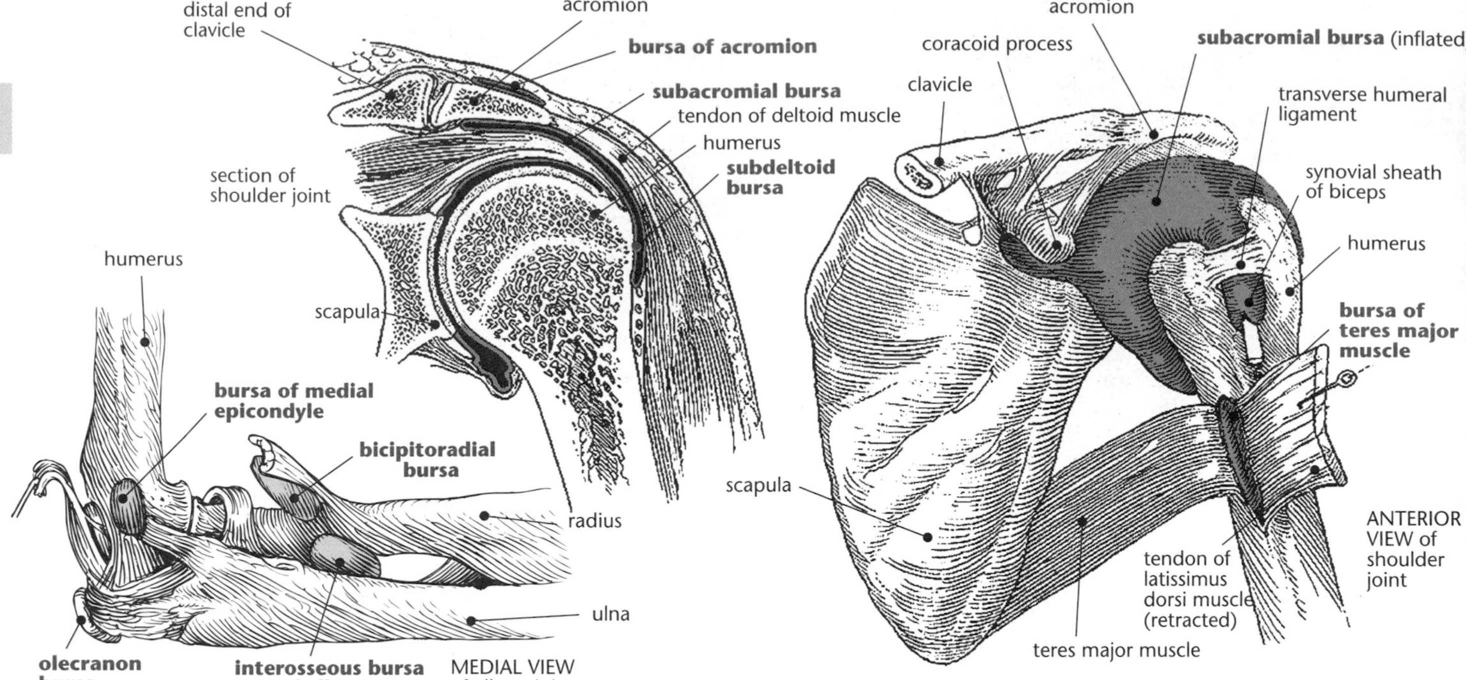

knee).

b. of psoas major muscle See iliopectineal bursa.

b. of quadrate muscle of thigh–A bursa located between the front of the quadrate muscle of thigh (quadratus femoris muscle) and the lesser trochanter of the femur. Also called bursa of quadratus femoris muscle.

b. of quadratus femoris muscle See bursa of quadrate muscle of thigh.

quadriceps b. See suprapatellar bursa.

radiohumeral b. A bursa located at the elbow, over the radiohumeral joint, between the extensor digitorum and supinator muscles.

b. of rectus muscle of thigh A small bursa between the tendon of origin of the rectus muscle of thigh (rectus femoris muscle) and the margin of the acetabulum.

retrocalcaneal b. See bursa of calcaneal tendon.

sciatic b. See bursa of obturator muscle, internal.

semimembranous b. A bursa located in the medial aspect of the knee, between the semimembranous tendon and the medial head of the gastrocnemius muscle. See also gastrocnemius bursa.

subacromial b. A large bursa located between the acromion and the capsule of the shoulder joint; usually connected with the subdeltoid bursa.

subcoracoid b. See subscapular bursa.

subdeltoid b. A bursa located between the deltoid muscle and the capsule of the shoulder joint; usually combined with the subacromial bursa.

subscapular b. A bursa between the tendon of the subscapular muscle and the glenoid border of the scapula; it communicates with the shoulder joint. Also called subcoracoid bursa.

superficial acromial b. A bursa located at the shoulder between the acromion and the skin.

b. of superior oblique muscle of eyeball A synovial sheath encircling the tendon of the superior oblique muscle of the eyeball as it passes through the cartilaginous pulley (trochlea) at the superomedial angle of the orbit. Also called synovial trochlear bursa.

suprapatellar b. An anterior extension of the synovial sac of the knee joint, between the femur and the tendon of the quadriceps muscle of the thigh (quadriceps femoris muscle). Also called quadriceps bursa; quadrate bursa; suprapatellar synovial pouch.

synovial trochlear b. See bursa of superior oblique muscle of eyeball.

b. of tendo calcaneus See bursa of calcaneal tendon.

b. of tendon of triceps muscle A bursa interposed between the tendon of the triceps muscle of the arm (triceps brachii muscle) and the olecranon process of the ulna.

b. of teres major muscle A synovial sac between the tendons of the teres major and latissimus dorsi muscles.

tibial intertendinous bursa See anserine bursa.

b. of tibial tendon Either of two bursae of the foot: *anterior,* a small bursa seen under the tendon of the anterior tibial muscle, at the medial surface of the proximal part of the first metatarsal bone; *posterior,* a small bursa interposed between the tendon of the posterior tibial muscle and the calcaneonavicular ligament on the sole of the foot.

b. of trapezius muscle A subtendinous bursa interposed between the tendinous part of the trapezius muscle and the medial end of the spine of the scapula.

trochanteric b. of gluteus maximus muscle See trochanteric bursa of greater gluteal muscle.

trochanteric b. of gluteus medius muscle See trochanteric bursa of middle gluteal muscle.

trochanteric b. of gluteus minimus muscle See trochanteric bursa of least gluteal muscle.

trochanteric b. of greater gluteal muscle A large bursa, often double, that separates the tendon of the greater gluteal muscle (gluteus maximus muscle) from the posterolateral surface of the greater trochanter of the femur, over which it glides. Also called deep trochanteric bursa; trochanteric bursa of gluteus maximus muscle.

trochanteric b. of least gluteal muscle A bursa between the tendon of the least gluteal muscle (gluteal minimus muscle) and the medial part of the anterior surface of the greater trochanter of the femur. Also called trochanteric bursa of gluteus minimus muscle.

trochanteric b. of middle gluteal muscle A bursa interposed between the tendon of the middle gluteal muscle (gluteal medius muscle) and the lateral surface of the greater trochanter of the femur. Also called trochanteric bursa of gluteus medius muscle.

b. of tuberosity of tibia A subcutaneous bursa located between the tuberosity of the tibia and the overlying skin of the knee.

bursectomy (ber-sek'to-me) Surgical removal of a bursa.

bursitis (ber-si'tis) Inflammation of a bursa.

olecranon b. Bursitis of the olecranon bursa, at the tip of the elbow. Also called miner's elbow; student's elbow.

prepatellar b. Inflammation of the bursa in front of the patella (kneecap), usually due to repeated trauma. Also called housemaid's knee.

bursocentesis (ber-so-sen-te'sis) Puncture and removal of fluid from a bursa.

bursolith (ber'so-lith) A stonelike concretion formed in a bursa.

bursotomy (ber-sot'ŏ-me) Incision into a bursa.

burst (berst) A sudden increase in activity.

respiratory b. A series of enzymatic reactions used by phagocytes to convert oxygen into substances necessary to destroy bacteria.

busulfan (bu-sul'fan) An antitumor alkylating drug used in the treatment of ovarian cancer. Its use during pregnancy is associated with fetal malformations and low birth weight.

butterfly (but'er-fli) **1.** Any material or device in the shape of a butterfly (e.g., a piece of tape for approximating the edges of a wound, or a wad of absorbent material used in gynecologic surgery). **2.** A butterfly-shaped rash on the cheeks and across the nose, characteristic of lupus erythematosus.

buttock (but'ok) One of two protuberances formed by the gluteal muscles.

button (but'n) **1.** Any knob-shaped or disk-shaped structure, lesion, or device. **2.** A collection of cells obtained after centrifuging a fluid specimen containing a small number of cells. **3.** In dentistry, the excess metal remaining from casting; located at the end of the sprue.

peritoneal b. A device for draining ascitic fluid.

terminal b. See axon terminal, under terminal.

buttonhole (but'n-hol) A small straight surgical cut into a cavity.

butyraceous (bu-ti-ra'she-us) Having the consistency of butter.

butyric acid (bu-tir'ik as'id) A saturated fatty acid of unpleasant odor occurring in rancid butter, sweat, and other substances.

butyroid (bu'ti-roid) Resembling butter.

bypass (bi'pas) A shunt; a diverted flow.

aortocoronary b. See coronary bypass.

cardiopulmonary b. Procedure in which the flow of blood is diverted from the heart and lungs; performed to permit surgery within the heart, ascending aorta, or coronary arteries; venous blood normally emptying into the right atrium is diverted from the venae cavae to an extracorporeal circuit, passed through an oxygenator where gases are exchanged, and returned to the arterial circulation.

coronary b. The suturing of a tubular graft to the aorta and a coronary artery, circumventing a clogged portion of the coronary artery, thereby restoring circulation. Also called aortocoronary bypass; coronary artery bypass graft (GABG).

byssinosis (bis-ĭ-no'sis) A form of chronic inflammatory and fibrotic disease caused by inhalation of dust in cotton, flax, and hemp mills; chief symptom is acute airway obstruction. Also called cotton-mill fever.

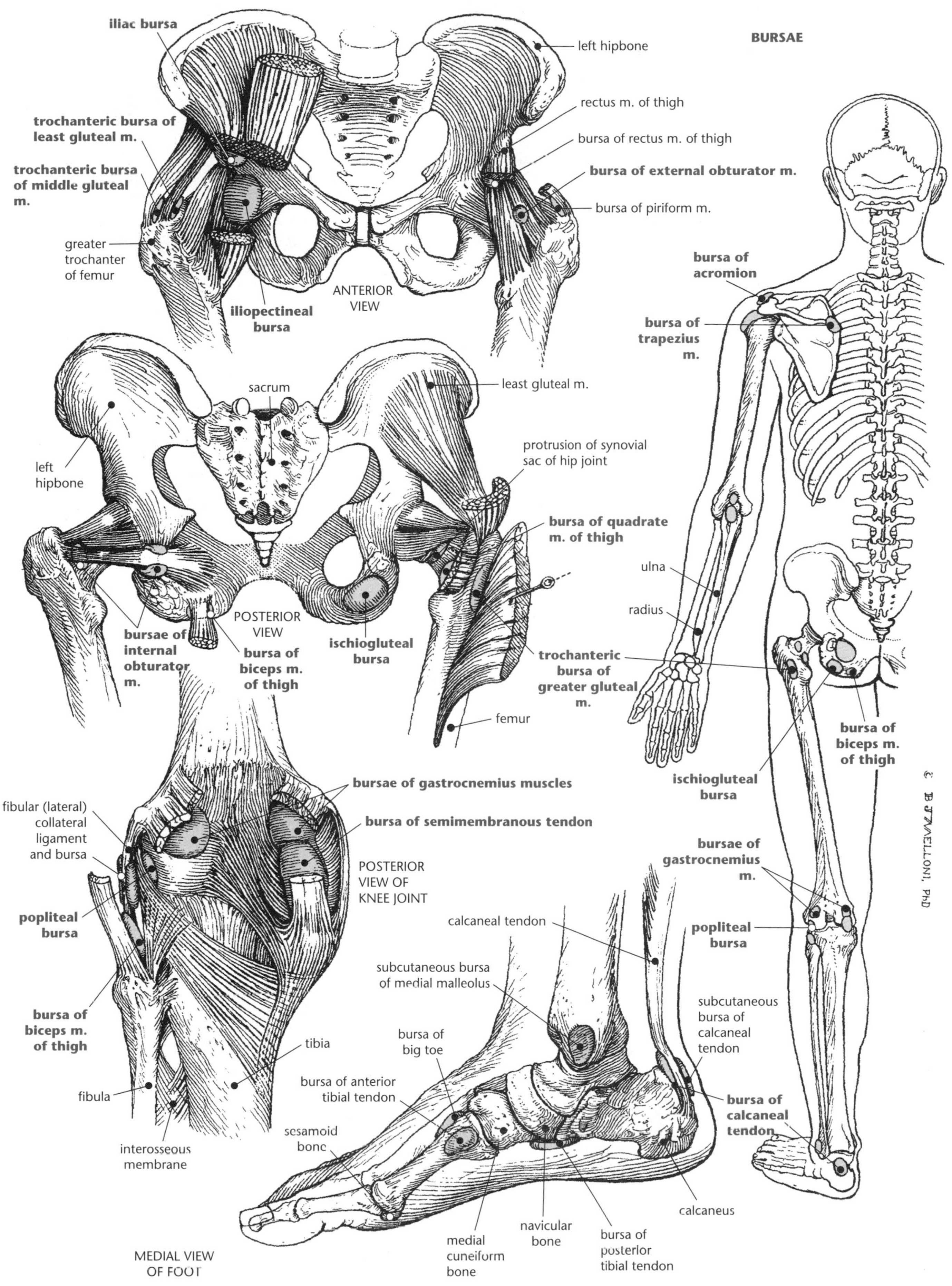
BURSAE
iliac bursa
left hipbone
rectus m. of thigh
trochanteric bursa of least gluteal m.
bursa of rectus m. of thigh
trochanteric bursa of middle gluteal m.
bursa of external obturator m.
bursa of piriform m.
greater trochanter of femur
ANTERIOR VIEW
iliopectineal bursa
bursa of acromion
bursa of trapezius m.
sacrum
least gluteal m.
left hipbone
protrusion of synovial sac of hip joint
bursa of quadrate m. of thigh
ulna
radius
POSTERIOR VIEW
bursae of internal obturator m.
bursa of biceps m. of thigh
ischiogluteal bursa
trochanteric bursa of greater gluteal m.
femur
bursa of biceps m. of thigh
ischiogluteal bursa
bursae of gastrocnemius muscles
fibular (lateral) collateral ligament and bursa
bursa of semimembranous tendon
POSTERIOR VIEW OF KNEE JOINT
popliteal bursa
bursae of gastrocnemius m.
popliteal bursa
calcaneal tendon
subcutaneous bursa of medial malleolus
subcutaneous bursa of calcaneal tendon
bursa of biceps m. of thigh
tibia
bursa of big toe
bursa of anterior tibial tendon
fibula
bursa of calcaneal tendon
interosseous membrane
sesamoid bone
calcaneus
navicular bone
medial cuneiform bone
bursa of posterior tibial tendon
MEDIAL VIEW OF FOOT
© B J Melloni, PhD

C

CA 15-3 An antigen sometimes found in the serum of patients with metastatic cancer.

CA 19-9 An antigen often found in elevated levels in the serum of patients with ovarian mucinous cystadenocarcinomas, endometrial, tubal, and endocervical cancers, and in patients with metastatic pancreatic cancer. It is part of the Lewis blood group system.

CA 125 An antigen often found in elevated levels in the serum of patients with epithelial ovarian cancer, but can also be found in a variety of benign conditions such as endometriosis.

cacao (kă-ka´o) An evergreen tropical tree, *Theobroma cacao*. Also called chocolate tree.

cachectic (kă-kek´tik) Relating to cachexia.

cachectin (kă-kek´in) Polypeptide secreted by activated macrophages (monocytes and lymphocytes), capable of causing *in vivo* hemorrhagic destruction of certain tumors. Also called tumor necrosis factor (TNF).

cachet (kă-sha´) A wafer capsule formerly used by pharmacists to enclose unpalatable drugs.

cachexia (kă-kek´se-ă) Severe malnutrition, weakness, and muscle wasting resulting from a chronic disease.

cacosmia (kak-oz´me-ă) An olfactory hallucination; a perception of unpleasant odors that do not exist.

cadaver (kă-dav´er) Corpse; a dead body.

cadaverine (kă-dav´er-in) An amine, $C_5H_{14}N_2$, found in decomposing animal tissue.

cadherin (kad-hēr´in) Any of a family of glycoproteins, present on cell membranes with a prime role in calcium-dependent cell-to-cell adhesion of normal cells.

epithelial c., E c. A major mediator of the cell-to-cell adhesion of all epithelial cells.

cadmium (kad´me-um) A soft, bluish-white metallic element; symbol Cd, atomic number 48, atomic weight 112.41; found in nature associated chiefly with zinc; used in the manufacture of storage batteries, in plating, and in alloys; inhalation may produce pulmonary edema; excessive absorption may also produce interstitial nephritis.

caduceus (kă-doo´shus) The winged staff of Mercury, with two oppositely entwined serpents; emblem of the U.S. Army Medical Corps.

café au lait (kă-făo lā) See café au lait spot, under spot.

caffeine (kă-fēn´) A bitter alkaloid compound found in coffee, tea, and cola beverages; used medicinally as a stimulant and diuretic.

caffeinism (kaf´ēn-iz-m) The chronic results of excessive consumption of beverages containing caffeine, characterized by rapid beating of the heart, irritability, and insomnia.

cage (kāj) **1.** Any enclosure used to confine. **2.** Any structure resembling a cage.

Faraday c. A cage screened from external electrical waves, used in electroencephalography.

thoracic c., rib c. The bones and musculature of the chest which enclose the thoracic organs.

caisson disease (ka´son dĭ-zēz´) See decompression sickness, under sickness.

calamine (kal´ă-mīn) **1.** A mineral, hydrous zinc silicate. **2.** A powder composed of zinc oxide (not less than 98%) with about 0.5% of ferric oxide, used in lotions and ointments to relieve itching in inflammatory skin disorders. See also calamine lotion, under lotion.

calcaneal, calcanean (kal-ka´ne-al, kal-ka´ne-an) Pertaining to the calcaneus (heel bone).

calcaneus (kal-ka´ne-us) The heel bone, articulating with the talus above and the cuboid anteriorly. See table of bones.

calcareous (kal-kar´e-us) Chalky; relating to calcium or limestone.

calcicosis (kal-sĭ-ko´sis) A lung disease (pneumoconiosis) caused by prolonged inhalation of limestone dust. Also called marble cutter's phthisis.

calcidiol (kal-sĭ-di´ol) The first product in the conversion of vitamin D_3 to the more active form, calcitriol (1, 25-dihydroxycholecalciferol); it is formed in the liver and converted to calcitriol by the kidney. Also called calcifediol; 25-hydroxy-cholecalciferol.

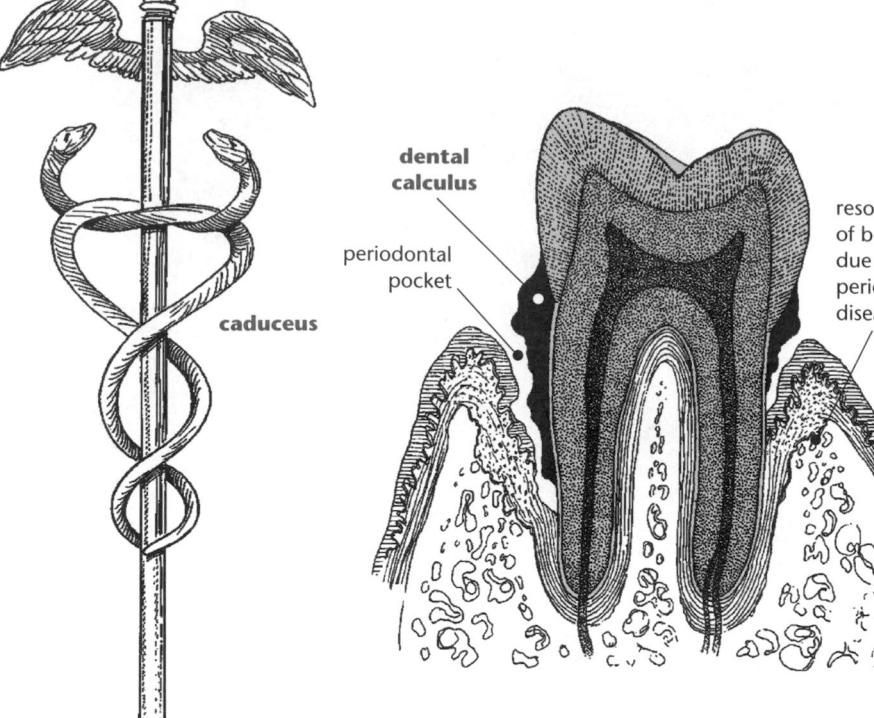

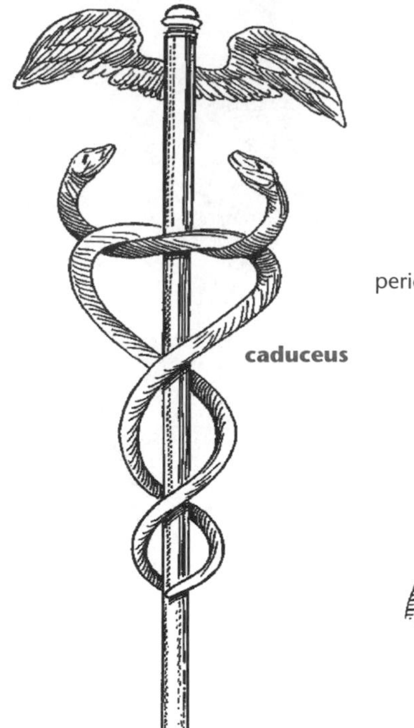

caduceus

dental calculus

periodontal pocket

resorption of bone due to periodontal disease

calcifediol (kal-sif-e-di´ol) See calcidiol.

calciferol (kal-sif´er-ol) See vitamin D_2.

calciferous (kal-sif´er-us) **1.** Containing lime. **2.** Forming any of the salts of calcium.

calcific (kal-sif´ik) Caused by or producing calcification.

calcification (kal-sĭ-f ĭ-ka´shun) **1.** Normal deposition of mineral salts in the bone and tooth tissues, thus contributing to their hardening and maturation. **2.** Pathologic hardening of organic tissue by deposits of calcium salts within its substance.

calcination (kal-sĭ-na´shun) The process of calcining.

calcine (kal´sēn) **1.** To turn a substance (e.g., gypsum) into a powder (e.g., plaster of Paris) by heating under high temperature.

calcineurin (kal-sĭ-nu´rin) Protein that binds both calcium ion (Ca^{++}) and calmodulin (a calcium regulatory protein inhibiting the latter's action).

calcinosis (kal-sĭ-no´sis) A disorder marked by the deposition of calcium salts in the skin and subcutaneous tissues, and sometimes in the tendons and muscles.

c. cutis A calcium deposit on the skin, usually occurring secondary to a preexisting skin eruption.

renal c. See nephrocalcinosis.

c. universalis Calcinosis involving widespread areas or the entire body.

calcipenia (kal-sĭ-pe´ne-ă) Condition characterized by deficiency of calcium in the tissues.

calciphilia (kal-sĭ-fil´e-ă) Condition in which the tissues tend to absorb calcium salts from the blood, thus becoming calcified.

calcitonin (kal-se-to´nin) A thyroid gland hormone which regulates calcium metabolism; it is secreted in response to a high level of blood calcium and acts to lower the level by inhibiting bone resorption. Also called thyrocalcitonin.

calcitriol (kal-sĭ-trĭ´ol) Dihydroxycholecalciferol; the active form of vitamin D.

calcium (kal´se-um) A silvery, moderately hard metallic element; symbol Ca, atomic number 20, atomic weight 40.08; together with phosphate and carbonate, it gives bone most of its structural properties; it is an essential nutrient in regulating blood coagulation, muscular contraction, conduction of nerve impulses, cell membrane function, enzyme action, and in assuring cardiac rhythmicity; several of the salts of calcium are used in medicine.

c. carbonate Chalk; an antacid and astringent; $CaCO_3$; 40% calcium by weight.

c. chloride A calcium salt used in the treatment of calcium deficiencies.

c. fluoride A compound occurring naturally in bones and teeth; CaF_2.

c. gluconate An odorless, tasteless, granular salt of calcium, 8% calcium by weight.

c. hydroxide Slaked lime, $Ca(OH)_2$, used in dentistry as a topical stimulant for production of secondary dentin to reseal the pulp cavity.

c. lactate The calcium salt of lactic acid, used as a calcium supplement.

c. oxalate A white, crystalline, insoluble calcium compound, CaC_2O_4; found as sediment in acid urine and in urinary stones.

calcium-45 A radioactive calcium isotope (^{45}Ca) having a half-life of 162.7 days; may be used as a tracer in the study of bone metabolism.

calcium channel blocker (kal´se-um chan´ĕl blok´ĕr) See calcium channel-blocking agent, under agent.

calcium pyrophosphate deposition disease (kal´se-um pi-ro-fos´fāt dĕp-o-zish´un dĭ-zēz´) (CPDD) Deposition of calcium pyrophosphate crystals in the joints, causing a gout-like arthritis.

calciuria (kal-se-u´re-ă) Urinary excretion of calcium; occasionally used as a synonym for hypercalciuria.

calcodynia (kal-ko-din´e-ă) Pain in the heel.

calculous (kal´ku-lus) Pertaining to or affected with calculus.

calculus (kal´ku-lus), *pl.* **cal´culi** An abnormal stony concretion usually composed of mineral salts and formed most frequently in the cavities of the body which serve as reservoirs for fluids. Also called stone.

articular c. Calculus formed within a joint.

biliary c. See gallstone.

dental c. A yellow to brown concretion adhering to the surface of a tooth, made up of calcium salts, microorganisms, and other debris. Also called tartar.

mulberry c. A mulberry-shaped calculus formed in the bladder, composed mainly of calcium oxalate.

renal c. See kidney stone, under stone.

salivary c. A calculus in a salivary duct or gland.

stag-horn c. A calculus with several branches occurring in the kidney pelvis.

subgingival c. A dental calculus occurring below the margin of the gum.

supragingival c. A dental calculus adherent to the exposed surface of a tooth.

urinary c. See urinary stone, under stone.

vesical c. See bladder stone, under stone.

calefacient (kal-ĕ-fa´shent) Anything that produces a localized sensation of warmth.

calf (kaf), *pl.* **cal´ves** The muscular back portion of the human leg; formed by the bellies of the gastrocnemius and soleus muscles.

caliber (kal´ĭ-ber) The diameter of a tube.

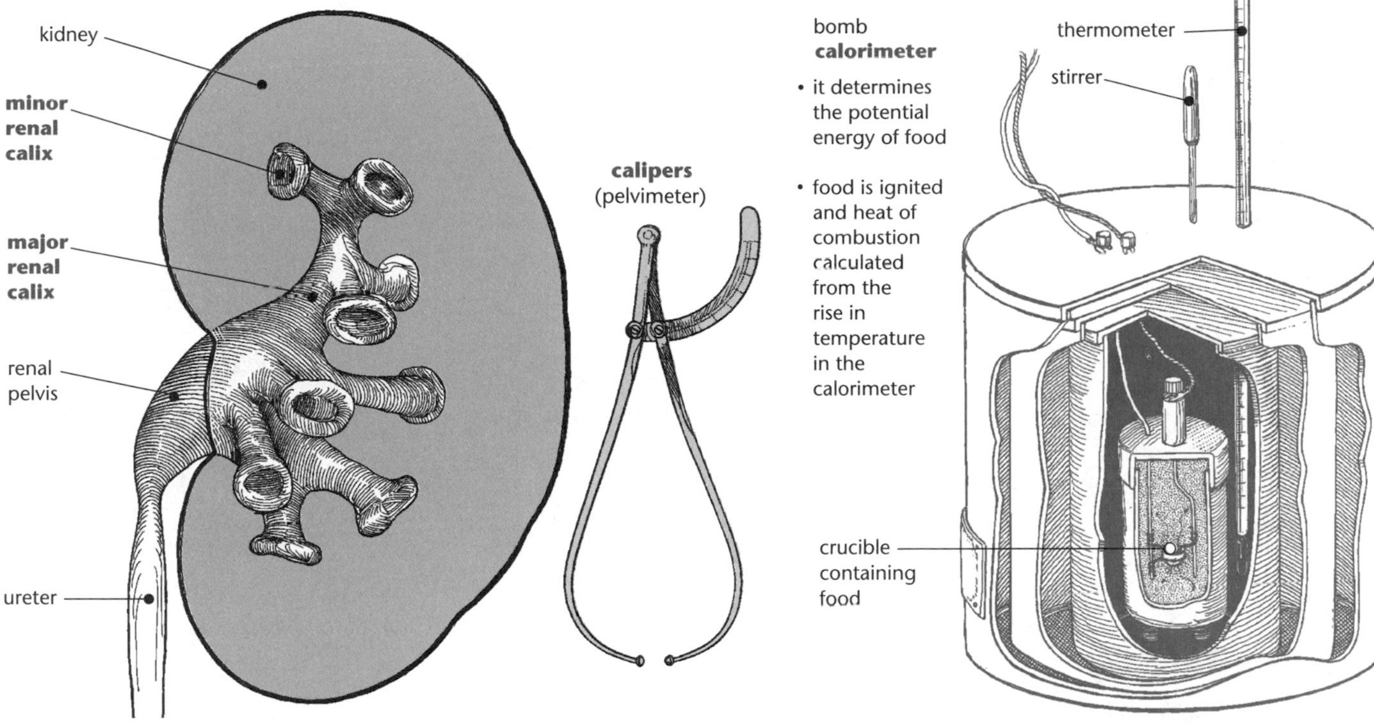

C

calibrate (kal´ĭ-brāt) **1.** To standardize systematically the graduations of a quantitative measuring apparatus. **2.** To determine the diameter of a tube.
caliceal (kal-ĭ-se´al) Relating to a calix.
calicectasis (kal-ĭ-sek´tă-sis) See caliectasis.
calices (ka´lĭ-sēz) Plural of calix.
caliculus (kă-lik´u-lus) A cup-shaped structure. Also spelled calyculus; also called calycle.
gustatory c. See taste bud, under bud.
caliectasis (kal-le-ek´tă-sis) Distention of the pelvis and calices of a kidney. Also called calicectasis; pyelocaliectasis.
californium (kal-ĭ-for´ne-um) Radioactive element; symbol Cf, atomic number 98, atomic weight 249; half-life 45 minutes.
calipers (kal´ĭ-perz) Instrument composed of two hinged legs, used for measuring diameters, such as the pelvic diameters, or intervals as on an electrocardiogram. See also pelvimeter.
calisthenics (kal-is-then´iks) **1.** A system of light gymnastic exercises to improve muscular tone and to improve physical well-being. **2.** The practice of such simple, systematic exercises.
calix (ka´liks), *pl.* **ca´lices** A cup-shaped cavity in an organ. Also written calyx.
major renal c. One of two or three cup-shaped subdivisions of the pelvis of the kidney.
minor renal c. One of several (seven to 13) cup-shaped subdivisions of the major renal calices.
Calkins' sign (kal´kins sīn) In obstetrics, the morphologic change of the uterus at delivery, from discoid to ovoid; due to a separation of the placenta from the uterine wall.
callosal (kă-lo´sal) Relating to the corpus callosum.
callosity (kă-los´ĭ-te) See callus (1).
callous (kal´ŭs) Hard and toughened; relating to a callus.
callus (kal´us) **1.** A circumscribed thickening of the skin. Also called callosity. **2.** A hard bonelike substance which is formed between and around the fragments of broken bone and eventually accomplishes repair of the fracture.
central c. Provisional callus formed within the medullary cavity of fractured bone.
definitive c. The exudate formed between the fractured surfaces of a bone, which changes into true bone.
provisional c. Callus formed between and around the fractured surfaces of a bone, keeping the ends of the bone in apposition and becoming absorbed after repair is completed.
calmodulin (kal-mod´u-lin) An intracellular calcium-binding regulatory protein that serves as a mediator of cellular responses to calcium. It is involved in a variety of cellular activities, including contraction of smooth muscle cells of the uterus during labor.
calor (ka´lor) Latin for heat.
caloric (kă-lor´ik) **1.** Relating to calories. **2.** Relating to heat.
calorie (kal´o-re) Any of several units of heat.
large c. (Cal, C) The calorie used in metabolic studies as a measurement of the energy-producing value of various foods according to the amount of heat they produce when oxidized in the body; specifically the amount of heat required to raise the temperature of one kilogram of water one degree centigrade (from 15°C to 16°C) at a pressure of one atmosphere. Also called kilocalorie (Kcal).
small c. (cal, c) The unit of heat equal to the amount of heat required to raise the temperature of one gram of water one degree centigrade at a pressure of one atmosphere. Also called gram calorie.
calorific (kal-o-rif´ik) Relating to heat generating.
calorigenic (kă-lor-ĭ-jen´ik) Producing or increasing heat.
calorimeter (kal-o-rim´ĕ-ter) An apparatus for measuring the amount of heat given off in a chemical or metabolic process.
Benedict-Roth c. See Benedict-Roth apparatus, under apparatus.
bomb c. A cylindrical apparatus for determining the potential energy of food; the food is ignited and the heat of combustion is calculated from the rise in temperature in the calorimeter.
calorimetry (kal-ŏ-rim´ĕ-tre) The measurement of the amount of heat given off by the body.
calpain (kal´pān) A calcium-sensitive, intracellular, protein-splitting enzyme (protease), thought to play a key role in degeneration of nerve tissue.
calvaria (kal-var´e-ă) The upper part of the skull.
calvarium (kal-var´e-um) Term used incorrectly for calvaria.
calx (kalks), *pl.* **cal´ces** The heel.
calyceal (kal-ĭ-se´al) See caliceal.
calycectasis (kal-ĭ-sek´tă-sis) See caliectasis.
calycle (kal´ĭ-kl) See caliculus.
calyculus (kă-lik´u-lus) See caliculus.
calyx (ka´liks), *pl.* **cal´yces** See calix.
camera (kam´er-ă, kam´ră) **1.** An apparatus used for recording images, either photographically or electronically. **2.** Any cavity of the body.
gamma c. An electronic instrument that produces images of the gamma-ray emissions from organs containing radionuclide tracers. Also called scintillation camera.
scintillation c. See gamma camera.
camphor (kam´for, kam´fer) A solid, crystalline, volatile substance obtained from an evergreen tree, *Cinnamonum camphora*, or prepared synthetically; used medicinally as an expectorant, stimulant, and diaphoretic.
camptomelic syndrome (kamp-to-me´lik sin´drōm) Flat facial features, short vertebrae, underdeveloped shoulder blades, and bowed legs, associated with abnormal development of cartilage and bone. Also called osteochondrodysplasia.
Campylobacter (kam-pĭ-lo-bak´ter) Genus of motile spiral, gram-negative bacteria (family Spirillaceae); found in the intestinal tract and reproductive organs of animals and the intestinal tract of humans.
C. jejuni See *Helicobacter jejuni*, under *Helicobacter.*
C. pylori See *Helicobacter pylori*, under *Helicobacter*.
canal (kă-nal´) A tubular structure; a channel.
adductor c. An aponeurotic canal in the middle third of the thigh; it contains the femoral artery and vein, and the saphenous nerve. Also called Hunter's canal.
Alcock's c. See pudendal canal.
alimentary c. See digestive tract, under tract.
atrioventricular c. The canal in the embryonic heart leading from the common sinoatrial chamber to the ventricle.
auditory c. (a) *External;* the auditory canal from the concha of the auricle to the tympanic membrane (eardrum); in the adult, it is approximately 25 mm in length on its superoposterior wall and 6 mm long on its anteroinferior wall. Also called external auditory meatus. (b) *Internal;* a canal through the petrous bone, about 1 cm in length, from the internal auditory foramen to the medial wall of the vestibule and cochlea: it transmits the labyrinthine blood vessels, the vestibulocochlear nerve, and the motor and sensory roots of the facial nerve. Also called internal auditory meatus.
birth c. The cavity of the uterus and vagina through which an infant passes at birth. Also called parturient canal.
carotid c. A passage through the petrous part of the temporal bone, transmitting the internal carotid artery.
central c. (a) One extending throughout the entire length of the spinal cord. (b) One extending through the middle of each osteon of compact bone.
cervical c. See canal of cervix.
c. of cervix A normally closed, flattened canal within the cervix of the uterus, approximately 2.5 cm in length, connecting the vagina to the cavity within the body of the uterus. Also called cervical canal.
external auditory c. See auditory canal.

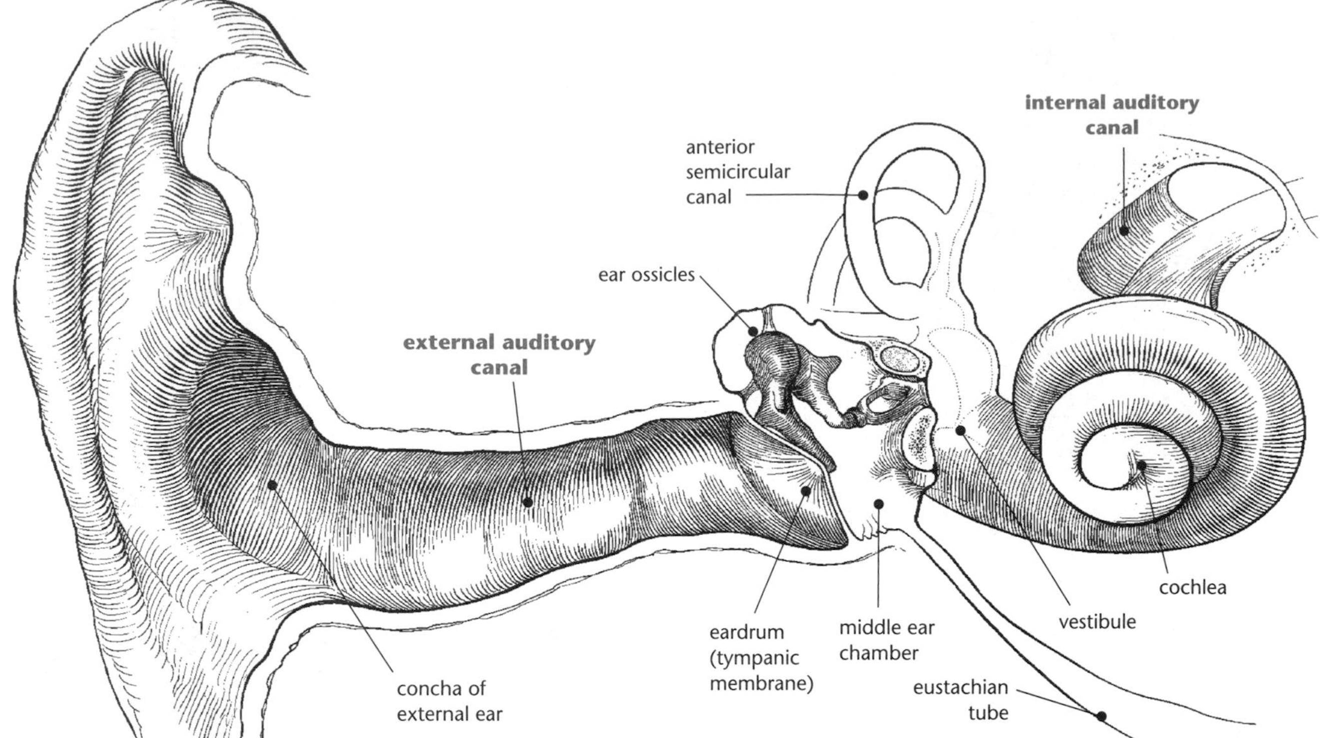

femoral c. The medial and smallest of the three compartments of the femoral sheath; it contains some lymphatic vessels and a lymph gland.

haversian c.'s See central canal (b).

Hunter's c. See adductor canal.

incisive c., incisor c. One of two canals opening on either side of the midline in the hard palate, just behind the incisor teeth; through each pass the terminal branches of the descending palatine artery and of the nasopalatine nerve.

inferior dental c. See mandibular canal.

inguinal c. An obliquely directed passage through the layers of the lower abdominal wall on either side, through which pass the spermatic cord in the male and the round ligament of the uterus in the female.

internal auditory c. See auditory canal.

mandibular c. The canal within the mandible containing the inferior alveolar vessels and nerves, from which terminal branches reach the mandibular teeth. Also called inferior dental canal.

optic c. A short canal through the sphenoid bone at the apex of the orbit which transmits the optic nerve and ophthalmic artery into the orbital cavity. Also called optic foramen.

parturient c. Birth canal.

pterygoid c. The canal that passes through the root of the pterygoid process of the sphenoid bone.

pudendal c. The fibrous tunnel within the obturator fascia that lines the lateral wall of the ischiorectal fossa; it transmits the pudendal vessels and nerves. Also called Alcock's canal.

root c., pulp c. The portion of the pulp cavity within the root of a tooth which leads from the apex to the pulp chamber and contains the pulp tissue.

Schlemm's c. See scleral venous sinus, under sinus.

semicircular c.'s The three bony canals (anterior, lateral, and posterior) in the internal ear in which the membranous semicircular ducts are located.

spinal c. See vertebral canal.

tympanic c. See scala tympani, under scala.

vertebral c. The canal formed by the vertebrae, containing the spinal cord. Also called spinal canal.

vestibular c. See scala vestibuli, under scala.

canalicular (kan-ă-lik´u-lar) Relating to a minute canal or canaliculus.

canaliculation (kan-ă-lik-u-la´shun) Formation of canals in tissues.

canaliculization (kan-ă-lik-u-lĭ-za´shun) The formation of small canals in a tissue.

canaliculus (kan-ă-lik´u-lus), *pl.* **canalic´uli** A minute channel or canal.

bile canaliculi Canaliculi between liver cells, forming a mesh.

canaliculi dentales See dental tubules, under tubule.

lacrimal c. One of two fine channels leading from the medial ends of the eyelids to the lacrimal sac.

canalis (kă-na´lis), *pl.* **cana´les** Latin for canal or channel.

Canavan's disease (kan´ă-vanz dĭ-zēz´) Spongy degeneration of the brain; an autosomal recessive inheritance usually affecting infants between three and four months of age.

cancellated (kan´sĕ-lāt-ed) Having a netlike or spongelike structure, such as the spongy bone between the cortical plates and the alveolar bone proper of the mandible.

cancellous (kan-sĕl´us) Denoting the spongy or honeycomb structure of some bone tissue; such as the ends of long bones.

cancer (kan´ser) (CA) General term for any malignant tumor.

scirrhous c. See scirrhous carcinoma, under carcinoma.

cancericidal (kan-ser-ĭ-sĭ´dal) See carcinolytic.

cancerophobia (kan-ser-o-fo´be-ă) Abnormal fear of acquiring a malignant growth.

cancerous (kan´ser-us) Relating to or of the nature of a malignant neoplasm.

cancroid (kang´kroid) Like cancer.

cancrum (kang´krum) An ulcer that spreads rapidly, occurring usually in the mucosa of the mouth or nose.

candela (kan-del´ă) (cd) The SI unit of luminous intensity equal to the luminous intensity of 5 mm^2 of platinum at its solidification point (1773.5°C). Also called new candle; international candle.

Candida (kan´dĭ-dă) A genus of yeastlike fungi.

C. albicans A species that normally inhabits the intestinal tract of humans but may cause disease under certain conditions (e.g., in debilitated individuals). Also called thrush fungus.

candidemia (kan-dĭ-de´me-ă) Presence of *Candida* organisms in the blood, usually due to systemic candidiasis.

candidiasis (kan-dĭ-di´ă-sis) Infection with microorganisms of the genus *Candida*.

candle (kan´dl) Old term for the unit of luminous intensity. See candela.

canine (ka´nīn) **1.** Relating to a dog. **2.** Relating to a cuspid (canine tooth).

canker (kang´ker) See aphthous stomatitis, under stomatitis.

cannabis (kan´ă-bis) The dried flowering tops of the *Cannabis sativa* plant, commonly known as marijuana and hashish.

cannabism (kan´ă-biz-m) Condition caused by overuse of hashish or Indian hemp; marked by hallucinations and other subjective symptoms.

cannula (kan´u-lă) A tube inserted into the body to withdraw or deliver fluid; sometimes used in conjunction with a metal rod (trocar) fitted into its lumen to puncture the wall of the cavity and then be withdrawn, leaving the cannula in place.

cannulation (kan-u-la´shun) The insertion of a cannula into a body cavity or vessel.

Cantelli's sign (kan´tel-ez sīn) See doll's eye sign.

cantharis (kan´thă-ris), *pl.* **can´tharides** Toxic preparation from the dried beetle *Lytta* (*Cantharis*) *vesicatoria*, mistakenly believed to have aphrodisiac qualities; formerly used as a counterirritant and to promote blister formation. Also called Spanish fly.

canthectomy (kan-thek´tŏ-me) Surgical excision of a canthus.

canthitis (kan-thi´tis) Inflammation of a canthus.

cantholysis (kan-thol´ĭ-sis) See canthotomy.

canthoplasty (kan´tho-plas-te) Plastic surgery of the canthus of the eye.

canthorrhaphy (kan-thor´ă-fe) Suturing of the eyelids, usually at the outer canthus, to shorten the palpebral fissure.

canthotomy (kan-thot´ŏ-me) The surgical slitting of the canthus, usually for widening the space between eyelids. Also called cantholysis.

canthus (kan´thus) The angle (nasal or temporal) formed by the junction of the upper and lower eyelids.

cap (kap) Any structure that serves as a cover.

acrosomal c. See acrosome.

contraceptive c. Any of three small contraceptive devices (cervical, vault, and vimule caps) designed to fit snugly over the uterine cervix; often used by women who cannot use a diaphragm due to anatomic changes (e.g., prolapsed uterus, cystocele).

cradle c. The grayish yellow crust formed on the scalp of an infant, caused by seborrhea. Also called milk crust.

duodenal c. The first portion of the duodenum, extending 4 to 5 cm from the pylorus. Also called duodenal bulb.

enamel c. The enamel organ covering the top of a growing tooth papilla.

knee c. See patella.

metanephric c. One of the masses of mesodermal cells adhering to the ureteral bud of an embryo and developing into the uriniferous tubules of the kidney.

capacitance (kă-pas´ĭ-tans) The quantity of electric charge that may be stored in a body.

capacitation (kă-pas-ĭ-ta´shun) The series of physiologic and biochemical events through which spermatozoa become capable of penetrating ova when coming in contact with various fluids of the uterus

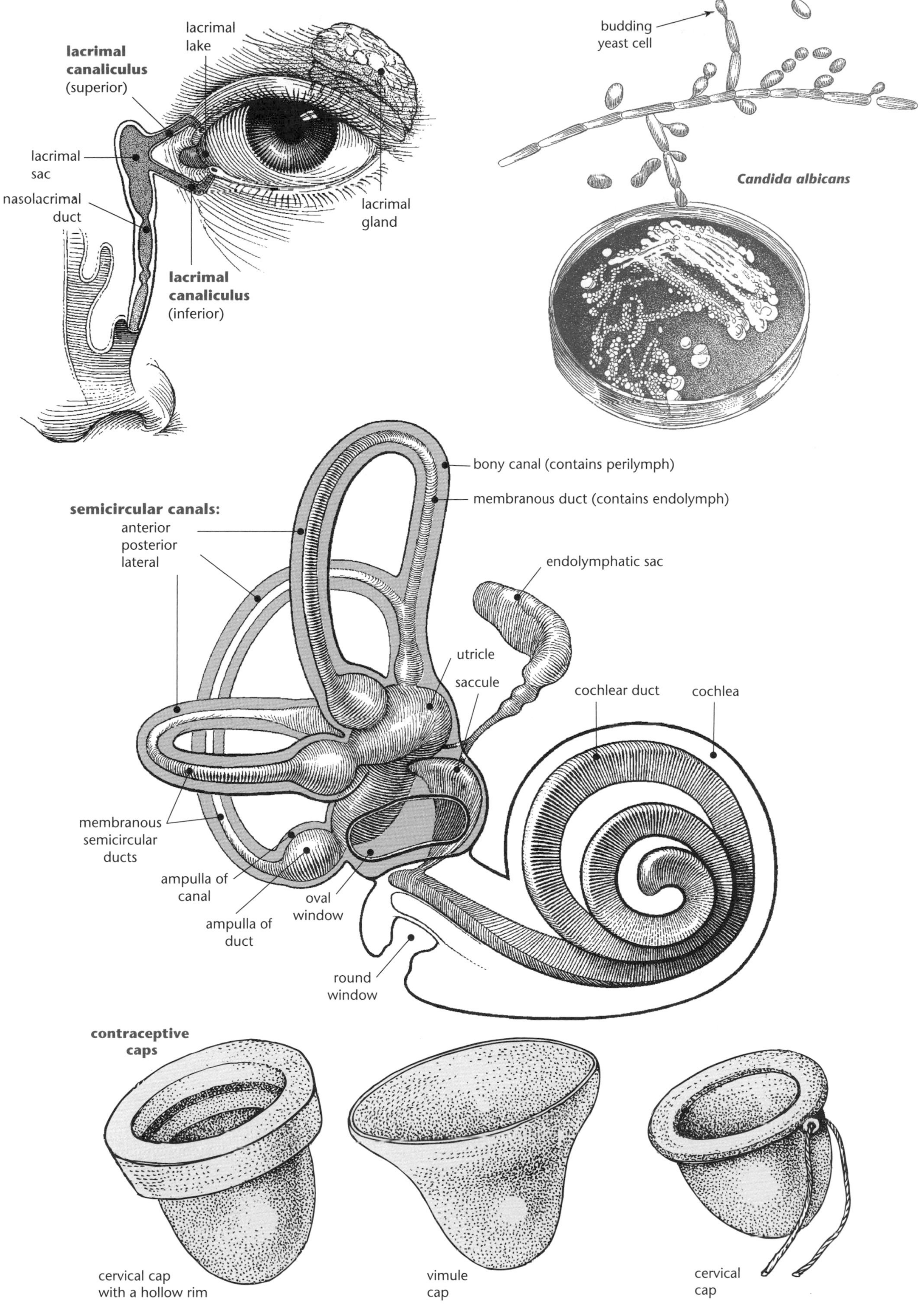
lacrimal canaliculus (superior)
lacrimal lake
lacrimal sac
nasolacrimal duct
lacrimal canaliculus (inferior)
lacrimal gland
budding yeast cell
Candida albicans
bony canal (contains perilymph)
membranous duct (contains endolymph)
semicircular canals:
anterior
posterior
lateral
endolymphatic sac
utricle
saccule
cochlear duct
cochlea
membranous semicircular ducts
ampulla of canal
ampulla of duct
oval window
round window
contraceptive caps
cervical cap with a hollow rim
vimule cap
cervical cap

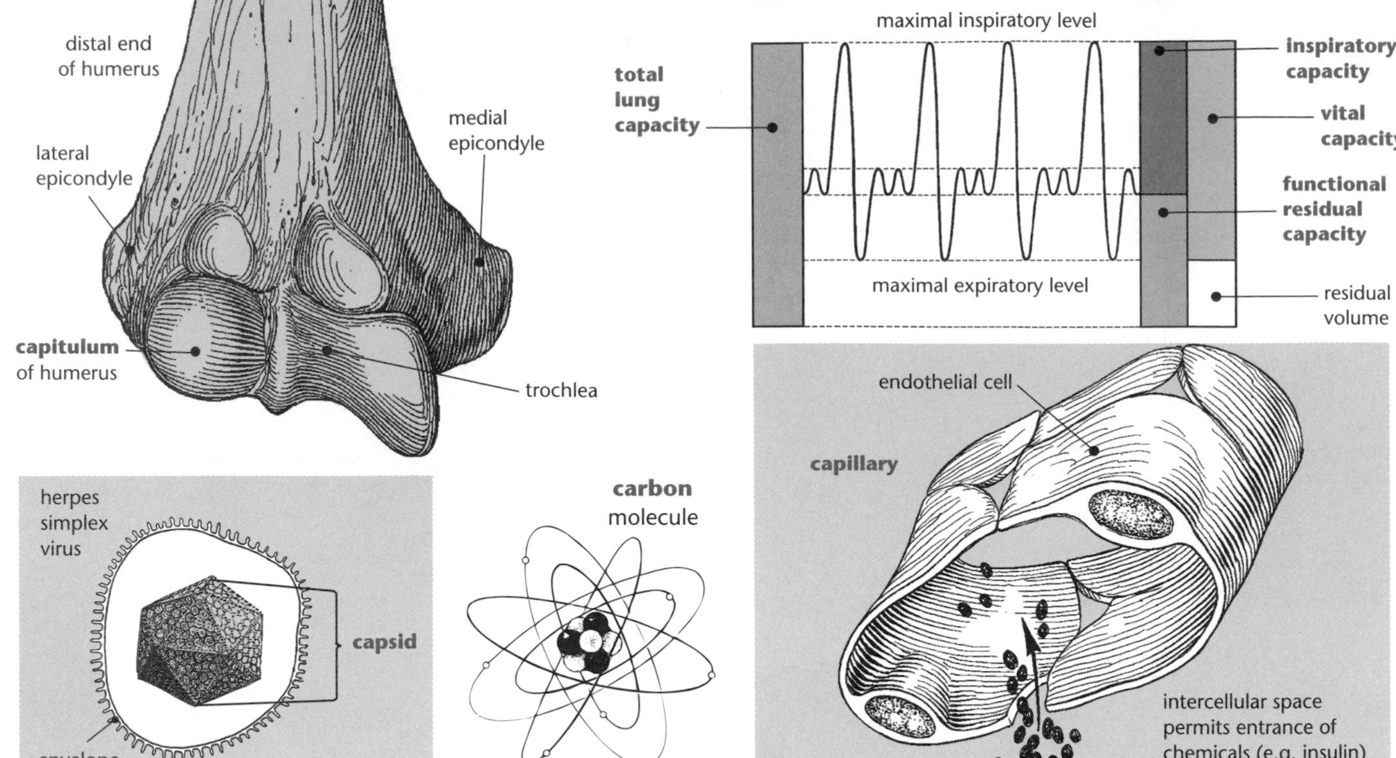

and fallopian (uterine) tube.

capacitor (kă-pas´ĭ-tor) An electric circuit element capable of temporarily holding a charge of electricity. Formerly called condenser.

capacity (kă-pas´ĭ-te) **1.** The maximum potential amount a cavity or receptacle can contain. **2.** A measure of ability.

cranial c. The cubic content of the skull.

forced vital c. (FVC) The volume of air that is forcefully and rapidly expired from full inspiration. In testing, the patient inhales maximally to full lung capacity, then exhales into an apparatus (spirometer) as forcefully, as rapidly, and as completely as possible.

functional residual c. (FRC) The volume of air remaining in the lungs at the end of exhaling during normal breathing.

heat c. The quantity of heat needed to raise the temperature of a substance 1°C.

inspiratory c. (IC) The maximum volume of air that can be inhaled into the lungs after a normal expiration.

maximum breathing c. (MBC) See maximum voluntary ventilation (MVV), under ventilation.

residual c. See residual volume, under volume.

total iron-binding c. (TIBC) A quantitative measure of the content of transferrin, the iron-binding protein, in serum.

total lung c. (TLC) The volume of air contained in the lungs at full inflation (i.e., following maximum inspiration).

vital c. (VC) The greatest volume of air that can be exhaled forcefully after a maximal inspiration.

capillariomotor (kap-ĭ-lar-e-o-mo´tor) Causing dilatation or constriction of the capillaries.

capillarity (kap-ĭ-lar´ĭ-te) The interaction between surfaces of a liquid and solid that causes the liquid to rise or fall as in capillary tubes.

capillary (kap´ĭ-lar-e) One of the minute blood vessels connecting venules and arterioles; their thin walls, which consist of a single layer of cells, permit passage of oxygen and chemicals in capillary blood into the tissues, and metabolic wastes from tissues into the capillary blood.

capitulum (kă-pit´u-lum) A small head-shaped eminence or rounded articular extremity of a bone.

Caplan's syndrome (kap´lanz sin´drōm) Large nodules surrounding blood vessels in the lungs, associated with rheumatoid arthritis and pneumoconiosis.

capping (kap´ing) **1.** Covering. **2.** In immunology, movement of cell surface antigens toward one pole (cap) of the cell surface after the antigens are cross-linked by specific antibody.

pulp c. The procedure of placing a covering over the exposed vital pulp of a tooth.

capsid (kap´sid) Protein coat of a virus.

capsule (kap´sul) **1.** A small, soluble, gelatinous container used to enclose a dose of an oral medicine. **2.** A fibrous or membranous sac surrounding a part, an organ, or a tumor. **3.** A mucopolysaccharide layer surrounding certain bacteria.

Bowman's c. See glomerular capsule.

Crosby c. An attachment at the end of a flexible tube, used to obtain a peroral biopsy of intestinal mucosa.

fibrous c. of liver (a) A thin layer of loose connective tissue enveloping the bile duct, hepatic artery, and portal vein. (b) Connective tissue surrounding the liver.

glomerular c. A double-walled membranous envelope surrounding a minute tuft of non-anastomosing capillaries (glomerulus); it is the invaginated pouchlike beginning of a renal tubule. Also called Bowman's capsule.

internal c. A broad band of white fibers located in each cerebral hemisphere, between the caudate nucleus and thalamus on the medial side and the lentiform nucleus on the lateral side; generally divided into an anterior limb, a genu, posterior limb, retrolentiform part, and sublentiform part; along with the caudate and lentiform nuclei, it forms the corpus striatum, an important unit of the extrapyramidal system.

joint c. A saclike structure enclosing the cavity of a synovial joint, composed of an outer fibrous layer and an inner synovial membrane.

c. of the lens A transparent, brittle but highly elastic membrane closely surrounding the lens of the eye.

Tennon's c. See bulbar fascia, under fascia.

capsulitis (kap-su-li´tis) Inflammation of the capsule of an organ or part.

capsuloplasty (kap´su-lo-plas-te) Surgical repair of a joint capsule, or replacement of a portion or all of the capsule.

capsulotomy (kap-su-lot´o-me) The surgical cutting of a capsule, as of the capsule of the crystalline lens in a cataract operation.

caput (kap´ut), *pl.* **cap´ita** **1.** The head. **2.** Any headlike prominence of an organ or structure.

c. succedaneum Soft swelling on the presenting part of the head of a newborn infant due to collection of fluid between the scalp and the membrane covering the skull (periosteum); results from mild trauma (e.g., when the head encounters resistance in a rigid vaginal outlet, or in a prolonged labor); typically disappears within a few days. COMPARE: cephalhematoma.

carbamide (kar´bă-mīd) An isomer of urea in anhydrous form. See urea.

carbaminohemoglobin (kar-bam-ĭ-no-he-mo-glo´bin) Carbon dioxide in combination with hemoglobin in the blood.

carbamoyl (kar´bă-moil, kar-bam´o-il) The organic group NH_2CO–. Also called carbamyl.

carbamoylglutamic acid (kar-bam-o-il-gloo-tam´ik) An intermediate in the carbamoylation of ornithine to citrulline in the urea cycle.

carbarsone (kar-bar´sōn) A crystalline odorless acid, containing 28.85% arsenic in its anhydrous state; used in the treatment of protozoan infections such as amebiasis.

carbohydrases (kar-bo-hi´drā-sēz) A general term for enzymes that promote the digestion of carbohydrates.

carbohydrates (kar-bo-hi´drāts) Any of the group of organic compounds composed of carbon, hydrogen, and oxygen, with a 2 to 1 ratio of hydrogen to oxygen (e.g., sugars, starches, cellulose).

carbolic (kar-bol´ik) Relating to phenol.

carbolic acid (kar-bol´ik ăs´id) See phenol.

carbon (kar´bon) A tetravalent organic element; symbol C, atomic number 6, atomic weight 12.011.

c. dioxide CO_2; the product of the combustion of carbon with a large supply of air. Also called carbonic acid gas.

c. monoxide CO; a colorless, odorless, poisonous gas with a strong affinity for hemoglobin; formed by the imperfect combustion of carbon with a limited supply of air.

c. tet See carbon tetrachloride.

c. tetrachloride CCl_4; a colorless oily liquid; formerly used as a local anesthetic, anthelminthic, and cleaning agent but no longer recommended because of its toxicity to the liver and kidney. Commonly called carbon tet. Also called tetrachloromethane.

carbon-12 An isotope of carbon, ^{12}C; its atomic weight, 12.000, was adopted in 1961 as the atomic weight unit (awu).

carbon-14 A radioactive carbon isotope with atomic weight 14 and a half-life of 5715 years.

carbonic acid (kar-bon´ik as´id) Carbon dioxide plus water, H_2OCO_2.

carbonize (kar-bon-īz) To convert into charcoal; to char.

carbonyl (kăr-bŏ-nīl) The organic bivalent radical = CO, characteristic of the ketones and aldehydes.

carboxyhemoglobin (kar-bok-se-he-mo-glo´bin) (HbCO) Carbon monoxide bound to the plasma pigment hemoglobin; present in the blood in carbon monoxide poisoning. Also called carbon monoxide hemoglobin.

carboxyl (kar-bok´sĭl) The characteristic mono-valent group –COOH of nearly all organic acids.

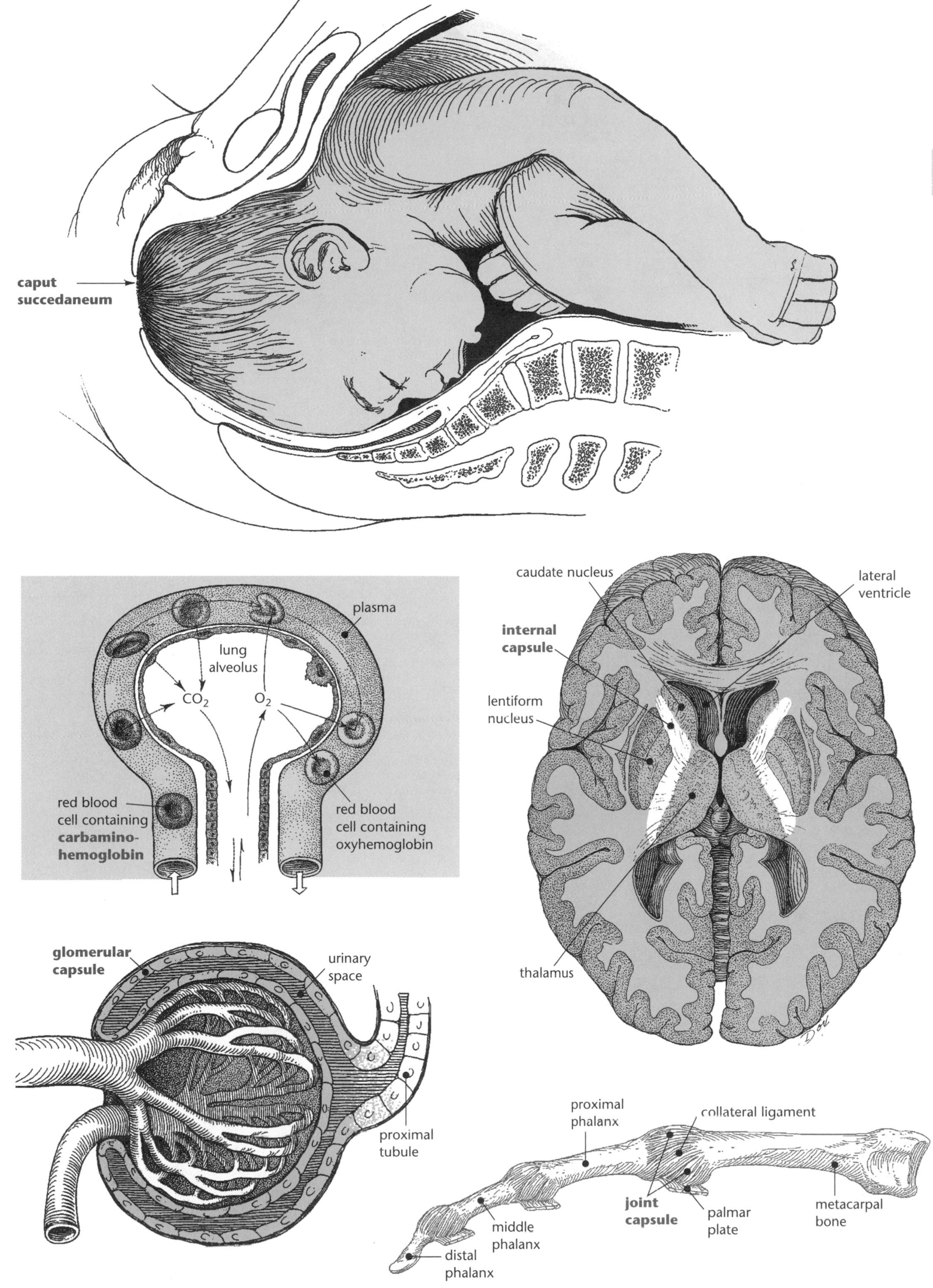
caput succedaneum
plasma
lung alveolus
CO_2
O_2
red blood cell containing carbamino-hemoglobin
red blood cell containing oxyhemoglobin
caudate nucleus
lateral ventricle
internal capsule
lentiform nucleus
thalamus
glomerular capsule
urinary space
proximal tubule
proximal phalanx
collateral ligament
joint capsule
palmar plate
metacarpal bone
middle phalanx
distal phalanx

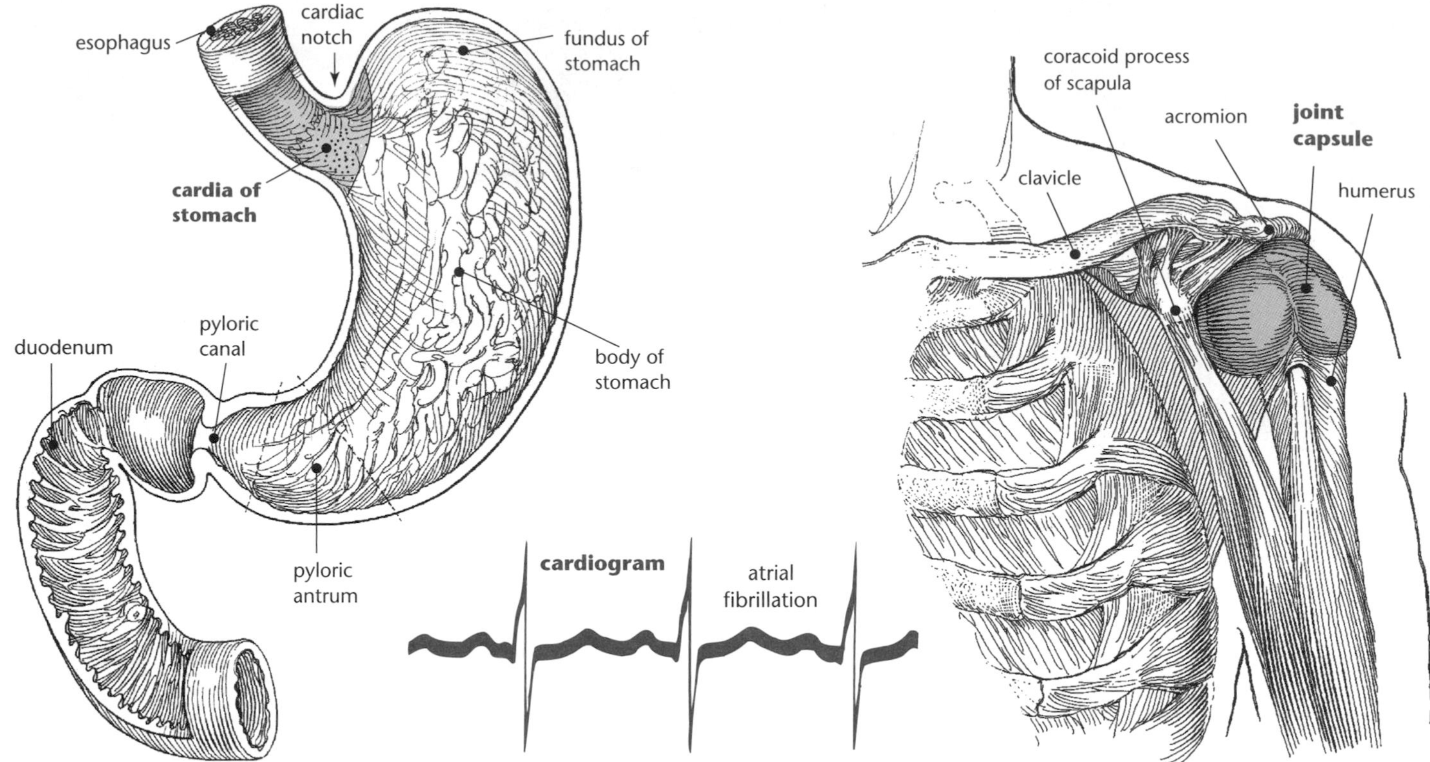

carboxylase (kar-bok´sĭ-lās) Enzyme that catalyzes the removal of carbon dioxide from the carboxyl group (COOH) of organic acids.

carboxypeptidase (kar-bok-se-pep´tĭ-dās) An enzyme of intestinal juice that acts on the peptide bond of amino acids having a free carboxyl.

c. B See protaminase.

carbuncle (kar´bung-kl) Painful infection of the skin and subcutaneous tissues with production and discharge of pus and dead tissue, similar to a boil (furuncle) but more severe, and with multiple sinus formation; usually caused by *Staphylococcus aureus*.

renal c. An abscess in the cortex of the kidney, usually resulting from the union of several smaller abscesses; it may occasionally rupture into the collecting system or it may rupture through the renal capsule, causing perirenal abscess.

carbuncular (kar-bung´ku-lar) Relating to carbuncles.

carcinogen (kar-sin´ŏ-jen) A cancer-producing agent.

carcinogenesis (kar-sĭ-no-jen´ĕ-sis) The origin, development, or production of cancer.

carcinogenic (kar-sĭ-no-jen´ik) Anything that causes cancer.

carcinoid (kar´sĭ-noid) See carcinoid tumor, under tumor.

carcinoid syndrome (kar´sĭ-noid sin´drōm) Skin flushes, diarrhea, lesions of the heart valves, and bronchial constriction; caused by release of one or more biologically active substances from a carcinoid tumor.

carcinolytic (kar-sĭ-no-lit´ik) Capable of destroying carcinomas.

carcinoma (kar-sĭ-no´mă) A malignant cellular tumor which tends to invade surrounding tissues and/or spread to other parts of the body by metastasis, causing eventual death.

alveolar cell c. See bronchiolar carcinoma.

basal cell c. (BCC) A malignant tumor derived from the basal layer of the skin or from structures derived from basal cells; it invades locally but rarely metastasizes and occurs most frequently on the face and scalp. Also called basal cell epithelioma.

bronchiolar c. A rare type of carcinoma derived either from the lining cells of the pulmonary alveoli or from the terminal bronchioles; occurring in the peripheral parts of the lung in the form of single nodules or multiple nodules that coalesce to form a diffuse mass. Also called alveolar cell carcinoma.

bronchogenic c. Carcinoma arising from a bronchus; the most common form of carcinoma of the lung.

clear cell c. of kidney See renal adenocarcinoma, under adenocarcinoma.

colloid c. See mucinous carcinoma.

embryonal c. of testis A highly malignant neoplasm of the testis appearing as a small grayish white nodule or mass, sometimes associated with hemorrhage and necrosis.

epidermoid c. See squamous cell carcinoma.

hepatocellular c. (HCC) See hepatoma.

c. *in situ* Carcinoma that is still confined to its site of origin, before it spreads to other tissues.

intraductal c. Carcinoma derived from epithelial cells of a duct, especially in the breast, which eventually fills the duct's lumen.

medullary c. A soft, fleshy, usually large tumor consisting chiefly of epithelial cells with little fibrous stroma.

mucinous c. A form of adenocarcinoma in which the degenerative process results in the formation of several areas of mucinous or hyaline material. Also called colloid carcinoma.

oat cell c. A small-celled carcinoma usually occurring in a bronchus. Also called small cell carcinoma.

papillary c. A finger-shaped carcinoma.

primary c. Carcinoma at the site of origin.

renal cell c. See renal adenocarcinoma, under adenocarcinoma.

scirrhous c. A stony-hard tumor having a great amount of fibrous tissue, usually occurring in the breast. Also called scirrhous cancer; fibrocarcinoma.

signet-ring cell c. A tumor composed of cells with a droplet of mucus in the cytoplasm, which compresses the nucleus against the cell membrane.

small cell c. See oat cell carcinoma.

spindle cell c. Carcinoma composed of elongated cells; may resemble a sarcoma.

squamous cell c. (SCC) Carcinoma derived from epithelium, often from normal epithelium, probably made susceptible by a variety of factors (e.g., chronic radiodermatitis, senile keratosis, leukoplakia or environmental agents); squamous cell carcinomas of the skin occur more frequently in persons over 40 years old. Also called epidermoid carcinoma.

transitional c. Carcinoma derived from transitional epithelium; usually occurring in the bladder, ureters, renal pelves, and nasopharynx.

villous c. Carcinoma composed of frondlike projections (villi) covered with neoplastic epithelium.

carcinomatoid (kar-sĭ-nom´ă-toid) Resembling a carcinoma.

carcinomatosis (kar-sĭ-no-mă-to´sis) Condition resulting from the spread of carcinoma to multiple sites in the body.

carcinomatous (kar-sĭ-nom´ă-tus) Having characteristics of carcinoma.

cardia (kar´de-ă) The region of the stomach near the esophageal opening.

cardiac (kăr´de-ak) **1.** Pertaining to the heart. **2.** Relating to the area of the stomach adjacent to the esophageal opening.

cardiatelia (kar-de-ă-te´le-ă) Incomplete development of the heart.

cardiectomy (kar-de-ek´tŏ-me) Surgical removal of the cardiac portion of the stomach.

cardiectopia (kar-de-ek-to´pe-ă) Development of the heart in a position other than the normal.

cardioaccelerator (kar-de-o-ak-sel´er-a-tor) An agent that hastens the heart's action.

cardiocentesis (kar-de-o-sĕn-te´sis) Surgical puncture of the heart.

cardiodynamics (kăr-de-o-di-nam´iks) The study of the movements and forces involved in the action of the heart.

cardioesophageal (kar-de-o-ĕ-sof-ă-je´al) Relating to the esophagus and adjacent part of the stomach.

cardiogenic (kar-de-o-jen´ik) Originating in the heart.

cardiogram (kar´de-o-gram) A graphic record of the activity of the heart, made with the cardiograph; the term is commonly used instead of electrocardiogram.

cardiograph (kar´de-o-graf) Instrument used to record graphically the movements of the heart.

cardiography (kar-de-og´ră-fe) The process of recording the heart movements with a cardiograph.

cardioinhibitory (kar-de-o-in-hib´ĭ-tor-e) Retarding the action of the heart.

cardiokinetic (kar-de-o-kĭ-net´ik) Having an influence on the action of the heart.

cardiolipin (kar-de-o-lip´in) A substance obtained from beef heart muscle; used as an antigen in tests for syphilis.

cardiolith (kar´de-o-lĭth) A calculus within the heart.

cardiologist (kar-de-ol´ŏ-jist) A specialist in cardiology.

cardiology (kar-de-ol´ŏ-je) The branch of medicine concerned with the diagnosis and treatment of heart disease.

cardiomegaly (kar-de-o-meg´ă-le) Enlargement of the heart. Also called megalocardia.

cardiomyoliposis (kar-de-o-mi-o-li-po´sis) Fatty degeneration of the heart muscle.

cardiomyopathy (kar-de-o-mi-op´ă-the) Disease of the muscular wall of the heart. Also called myocardiopathy.

alcoholic c. Cardiomyopathy resulting from the toxic effects of chronic alcohol consumption or from

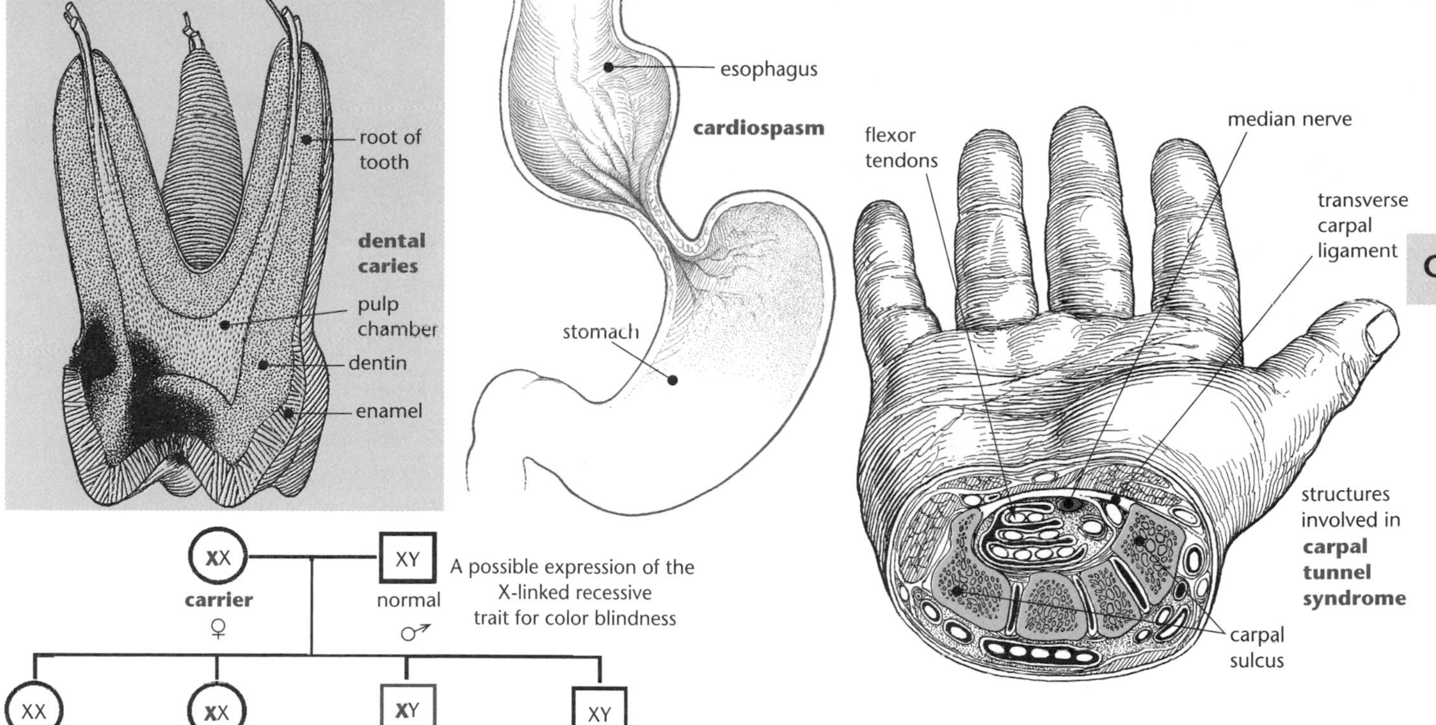

thiamine deficiency due to malnutrition (seen in alcoholics).

familial hypertrophic c. (FHCM) See hypertrophic cardiomyopathy.

hypertrophic c. (HCM) Inherited disease that is the most common cause of sudden death in the young (especially young athletes participating in strenuous sports); marked by enlargement of the heart due to hypertrophy of the left ventricle, resulting in poor diastolic relaxation, inadequate filling, and rapid emptying of the ventricle; an autosomal dominant inheritance, linked to a mutation of the beta-myosin heavy-chain gene located on chromosome 14. Also called familial hypertrophic cardiomyopathy (FHCM).

cardiomyotomy (kar-de-o-mi-ot´ŏ-me) See esophagomyotomy.

cardionatrin I (kar-de-o-na´trin) See atrial natriuretic peptide, under peptide.

cardionecrosis (kar-de-o-nĕ-kro´sis) Necrosis of the heart.

cardionephric (kar-de-o-nef´rik) See cardiorenal.

cardioneurosis (kăr-de-o-nōō-ro´sis) See cardiac neurosis, under neurosis.

cardiopathy (kar-de-op´ă-the) Any disease of the heart.

cardiopericardiopexy (kar-de-o-per-ĭ-kar´de-o-pek-se) The operative procedure of spreading sterile magnesium silicate within the pericardial sac for the purpose of creating adhesive pericarditis, thus increasing the blood supply of the heart muscle.

cardioplasty (kar´de-o-plas-te) Plastic surgery of the junction of the esophagus and stomach for the relief of spasm of the esophagus or upper end of the stomach.

cardioplegia (kar-de-o-ple´ja) Temporary interruption of the heart's activity with cold or chemical agents to allow performance of heart surgery.

cardiopulmonary (kar-de-o-pul´mo-ner-e) Relating to the heart and lungs.

cardiorenal (kar-de-o-re´nal) Relating to the heart and kidneys. Also called cardionephric; nephrocardiac.

cardiorrhexis (kar-de-o-rek´sis) Rupture of the heart wall.

cardioselectivity (kar-de-o-sĕ-lek´tiv-ĭ-tē) The quality of having a relatively greater effect on heart tissue than on other tissues.

cardiospasm (kar´de-o-spaz-m) Spasmodic constriction of the distal portion of the esophagus, at its junction with the stomach, with accompanying dilatation of the rest of the esophagus.

cardiotomy (kar-de-ot´ŏ-me) **1.** Surgical incision into the heart wall. **2.** Incision into the esophageal opening (cardia) of the stomach.

cardiotonic (kar-de-o-ton´ik) Having a favorable or tonic effect on the heart; strengthening the heart action.

cardiotoxic (kăr-de-o-tok´sik) Having a toxic effect on the heart.

cardiovascular (kar-de-o-vas´ku-lar) Relating to the heart and blood vessels.

cardioversion (kar-de-o-ver´zhun) See defibril-lation.

cardioverter (kăr´de-o-ver-ter) See defibrillator.

carditis (kar-di´tis) Inflammation of the heart.

care (kār) General term used in medicine and public health to denote the application of knowledge to the benefit of an individual person or a community.

managed medical c. Health care in which a third party payer mediates between physicians and patients. The third party may be an insurance company, corporation, or the federal government.

medical c. The application of specific training to the identification, treatment, and prevention of illness.

primary medical c. Care provided by the health professional who is approached first for treatment.

secondary medical c. Medical care by a physician at the request of the primary caregiver.

tertiary medical c. Consultative care by a specialist in a medical center (e.g., in specialized surgical procedures, critical care support).

caries (kar´ēz) Molecular death and breakdown of a bone.

contact c. Caries occurring in the proximal surface of the tooth adjacent to a restoration.

dental c. Localized, progressive decay of the teeth that starts on the surface and, if untreated, extends to the dentin and pulp with subsequent infection.

nursing bottle c.'s Caries of primary teeth associated with the use of a nursing bottle as an aid for sleeping in a child over the age of one year. Also called baby bottle syndrome.

carina (kă-ri´nă) Any ridgelike projection (e.g., central ridge formed by the bifurcation of the trachea).

cariogenesis (kar-e-o-jen´ĕ-sis) The process of caries formation.

cariogenic (kar-e-o-jen´ik) Producing caries; said of certain foods.

cariostatic (kar-e-o-stat´ik) Anything that inhibits the progress of dental caries.

carious (kar´e-us) Relating to caries.

carmine red (kar´min red) A specific stain for glycogen and mucus in which the active ingredient is carminic acid; also used for staining embryos, small animals, and large blocks of tissue.

carneous (kar´ne-us) Fleshy.

Carnivora (kar´nĭ-vor) The order of flesh-eating mammals.

carnosine (kar´no-sēn) A nitrogenous base made up of alanine and histadine, found in skeletal muscle.

Caroli's disease (kă-ro-lēz´ dĭ-zēz´) A familial disorder characterized by segmental saccular dilatation of the intrahepatic bile ducts, a marked predisposition to stone formation, inflammation of bile ducts, and lung abscesses.

carotene (kar´ŏ-tēn) A provitamin capable of conversion into vitamin A; the yellow pigment of carrots and other yellow foods.

carotenemia (kar-ŏ-tĕ-ne´me-ă) Increased carotene in the blood causing a yellowish pigmentation of the skin. Also called carotinemia; xanthemia.

carotid (kă-rot´id) **1.** Relating to the two principal arteries of the neck (carotid arteries). **2.** Denoting a carotid artery. See table of arteries.

carotid sinus syndrome (kă-rot´id sĭ´nus sin´drōm) Slow heartbeat, low blood pressure, fainting, and occasional convulsions due to overstimulation of the carotid sinus.

carotinemia (kar-o-tin-e´me-ă) See carotenemia.

carpal (kar´pal) Relating to the bones of the wrist (carpus).

carpal tunnel syndrome (kar´pal tun´el sin´drōm) A complex of symptoms caused by any condition (usually thickening of the synovia of the flexor tendons) that compresses the median nerve in the carpal tunnel of the wrist, beneath the transverse carpal ligament; marked by pain and numbness in the area of the hand innervated by the median nerve; the duration and degree of nerve compression determine the patient's complaints; in late stages there is atrophy of thenar muscles.

carpometacarpal (kar-po-met-ă-kar´pal) Relating to the wrist bones and the metacarpus (the five bones between the wrist and fingers).

carpopedal (kar-po-ped´al) Relating to the wrists and feet, as in the spasm of tetany.

carpus (kar´pus) The wrist; the eight bones of the wrist. See table of bones.

carrier (kar´e-er) **1.** An individual who, although showing no symptoms of disease, harbors infectious microorganisms and spreads the infection to others. **2.** An individual who carries a normal gene and an abnormal recessive gene which is not expressed obviously, although it may be detectable by appropriate laboratory tests. **3.** A substance in a cell that is capable of accepting an atom or a subatomic particle, thus facilitating transport of organic solutes. **4.** In dentistry, an instrument for carrying plastic amalgam to the cavity into which it is inserted.

chronic c. A person who harbors disease-producing microorganisms for some time after recovery.

passive c. One who harbors infectious micro-

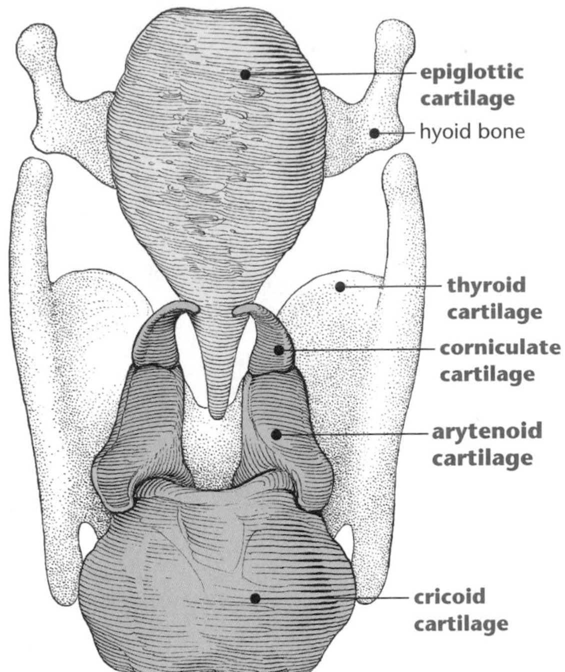

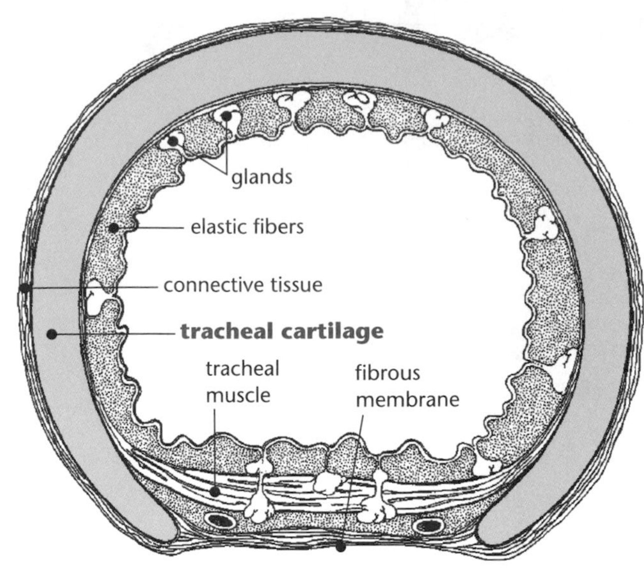

organisms without having had the disease.

Carrión's disease (kă-re-ōnz´ dĭ-zēz´) See bartonellosis.

cartilage (kar´tĭ-lij) A tough, nonvascular connective tissue making up most of the fetal skeleton and present in the adult in the articular parts of bones and certain tubular structures; there are three main varieties: hyaline cartilage (most widely distributed type), elastic cartilage, and fibrous cartilage.

accessory c.'s of nose See lesser alar cartilages.

articular c. A type of hyaline cartilage forming a thin sheet upon the joint surface of bones.

arytenoid c. One of two triangular cartilages located in the back of the larynx.

corniculate c. One of two minute cones of yellow elastic cartilage in the larynx, located at the apex of each arytenoid cartilage.

costal c. One of 24 bars of hyaline cartilage serving to prolong the ribs anteriorly and contributing to the elasticity of the chest wall.

cricoid c. The ring-shaped and lowermost of the cartilages of the larynx.

cuneiform c. One of two small rod-shaped laryngeal cartilages on either side in the aryepiglottic fold.

elastic c. Yellow fibrocartilage, a variety of cartilage containing bundles of yellow elastic fibers with little or no white fibrous tissue; found chiefly in the external ear, the auditory tube, and some laryngeal cartilages.

epiglottic c. A thin, leaflike lamina of yellow fibrocartilage located behind the root of the tongue and the body of the hyoid bone, forming the central portion of the epiglottis.

epiphyseal c. The layer of cartilage between the shaft and the epiphysis of a long bone; present during the growing years, after which the cartilage ossifies and growth in length ceases.

fibrous c. See fibrocartilage.

greater alar c.'s Two cartilaginous plates supporting the nostrils. Also called lower lateral cartilages of nose.

hyaline c. An elastic bluish-white translucent type of cartilage covered with a membrane (perichondrium) except when coating the articular ends of bones.

lateral c. One of two triangular plates of cartilage located below the inferior margin of the nasal bone. Also called upper lateral cartilage.

lesser alar c.'s Two to four cartilages located posterior to the greater alar cartilage on either side. Also called accessory cartilages of nose.

lower lateral c.'s of nose See greater alar cartilages.

c. of nasal septum A quadrilateral plate at the lower anterior part of the nasal septum; it completes the separation of the nasal cavities.

thyroid c. The largest of the cartilages of the larynx; its anterior prominence is called Adam's apple (laryngeal prominence).

tracheal c. One of 16 to 20 incomplete cartilaginous rings forming the trachea.

upper lateral c. See lateral cartilage.

cartilaginous (kar-tĭ-laj´ĭ-nus) Consisting of cartilage.

caruncle (kar´ung-kl) A small fleshy protuberance.

lacrimal c. A small pinkish protuberance at the medial junction of the eyelids.

urethral c. A small, fleshy, outgrowth at the orifice of the female urethra; may be an eversion of the urethral lining with an underlying varicose vein.

carvedilol (kar´vē-dil-ol) A nonselective beta-adrenergic blocking agent with some alpha-1 blocking activity used in the treatment of congestive heart failure; also used for hypertension.

carver (kar´ver) A dental instrument used to shape wax or amalgam.

cascade (kas-kād´) A series of sequential events (e.g., a physiologic process) that, once initiated, continues to the final state, with each event being activated by the preceding one.

cascara sagrada (kas-kār´ă să-grād´ă) The dried bark of a tree, *Rhamnus purshiana* or buckthorn; used as a laxative. Often simply called cascara.

case (kās) An instance or occurrence of disease.

index c. See proband.

caseation (ka-se-a´shun) Necrosis of tissues into a cheeselike mass.

casein (ka´sēn, ka-sēn´) The chief protein of milk.

caseinogen (ka-sēn´o-jen) The precursor of casein; a substance present in milk that, when activated by rennin, is converted into casein.

caseous (ka´se-us) Resembling cheese, as certain necrotic tissue.

cast (kast) **1.** A rigid dressing, usually made of gauze and plaster of Paris, used for immobilization of a body part. **2.** A cylindrical solid material accumulated within a tubular structure of the body.

blood c. A cast composed of a thick material containing various elements of blood, formed in kidney tubules or in bronchioles and caused by bleeding into the structures.

cellular c. A renal cast containing red and white blood cells or epithelial cells.

epithelial c. A cast containing cells from the inner lining of the tubular structure in which it was formed.

false c. See cylindroid.

fatty c. Urinary cast composed chiefly of fat globules with cholesterol esters.

granular c. A colorless renal cast composed of particles of cellular debris.

hanging c. A plaster cast applied to immobilize a fracture as well as deliver a traction force via the weight of the cast; commonly used for the treatment of the lower part of the humerus.

hyaline c. A relatively transparent urinary cast consisting mainly of precipitated protein.

mucous c. See cylindroid.

red blood cell c. See blood cast.

renal c. Urinary cast.

urinary c. A cast discharged in the urine.

walking c. A plaster cast extending from below the knee to the toes with an added attachment, such as a boot, to allow a natural gait.

waxy c. A light yellow cylinder with a tendency to split transversely, found in the urine in cases of oliguria or anuria.

white blood cell c. A urinary cast composed of white blood cells; found in interstitial nephritis.

castrate (kas´trāt) To remove the testes or the ovaries.

castration (kas-tra´shun) Removal of the testes or ovaries.

functional c. Atrophy of the gonads (testes or ovaries) by prolonged treatment with sex hormones.

catabolic (kat-ă-bol´ik) Promoting or exhibiting catabolism.

catabolism (kă-tab´o-liz-m) The breakdown of chemical compounds into more elementary principles by the body; an energy-producing metabolic process, the reverse of anabolism.

catabolite (kă-tab´o-līt) A product of catabolism.

catacrotism (kă-tak´ro-tiz-m) Anomaly of the pulse marked by one or more minor expansions of the artery following the main beat.

catalepsy (kat´ă-lep-se) A trance-like condition with rigidity of muscles allowing the body (including extremities) to assume a position for an indefinite period of time.

catalyst (kat-ă-list) A substance, usually present in small amounts, that influences the rate of a chemical reaction without being changed in the process.

negative c. Catalyst that retards a chemical reaction.

organic c. See enzyme.

positive c. A catalyst that accelerates a chemical reaction.

catalyze (kat´ă-līz) To modify the rate of a chemical reaction; to act as a catalyst.

catamnesis (kat-am-ne´sis) Seldom-used term denoting the "follow-up" medical history of a patient after an illness or discharge from the hospital.

cataphasia (kat-ă-fa´zhă) Speech disorder consisting of involuntary repetition of the same word.

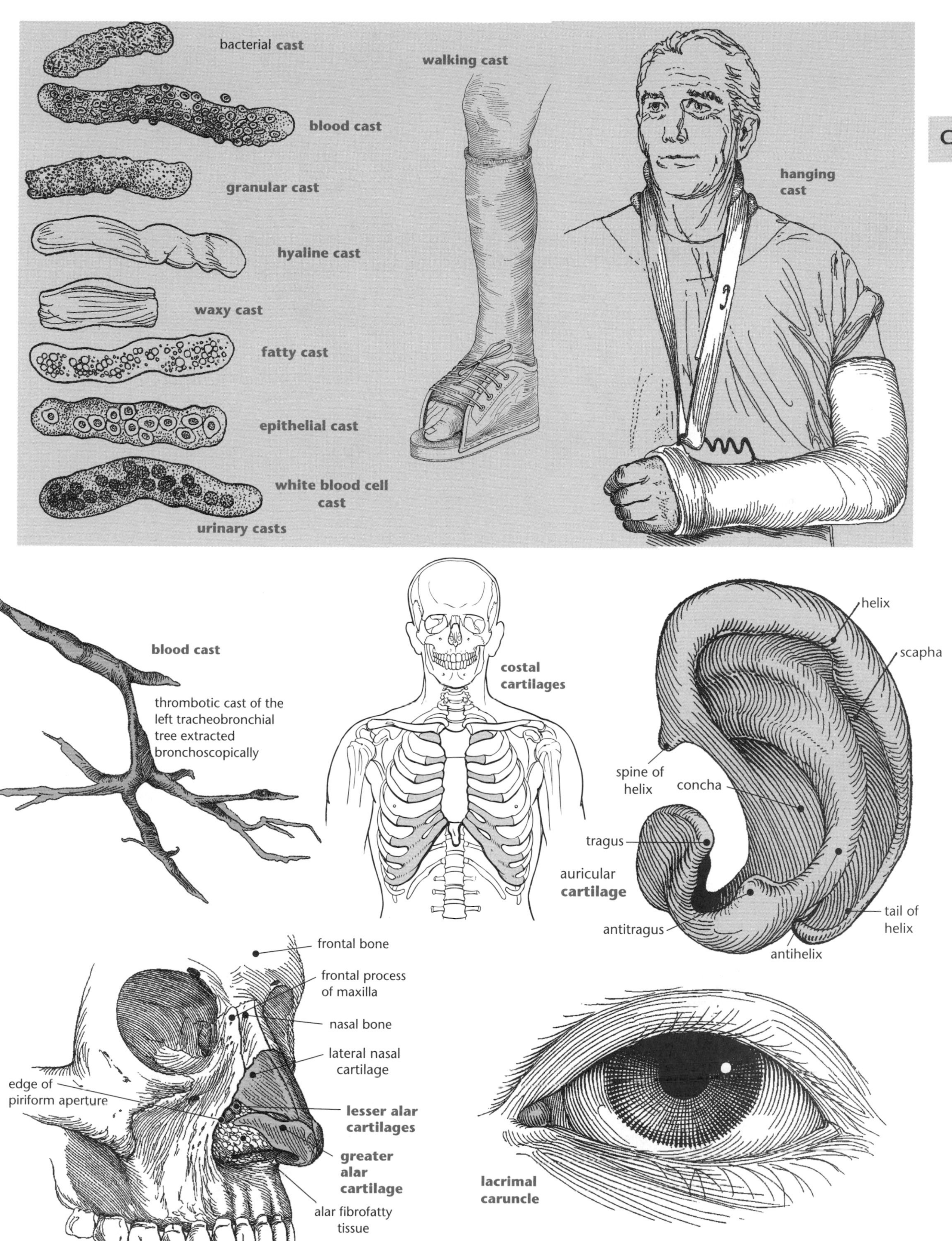
bacterial cast
blood cast
granular cast
hyaline cast
waxy cast
fatty cast
epithelial cast
white blood cell cast
urinary casts
walking cast
hanging cast
blood cast
thrombotic cast of the left tracheobronchial tree extracted bronchoscopically
costal cartilages
helix
scapha
spine of helix
concha
tragus
auricular cartilage
antitragus
tail of helix
antihelix
frontal bone
frontal process of maxilla
nasal bone
lateral nasal cartilage
edge of piriform aperture
lesser alar cartilages
greater alar cartilage
alar fibrofatty tissue
lacrimal caruncle

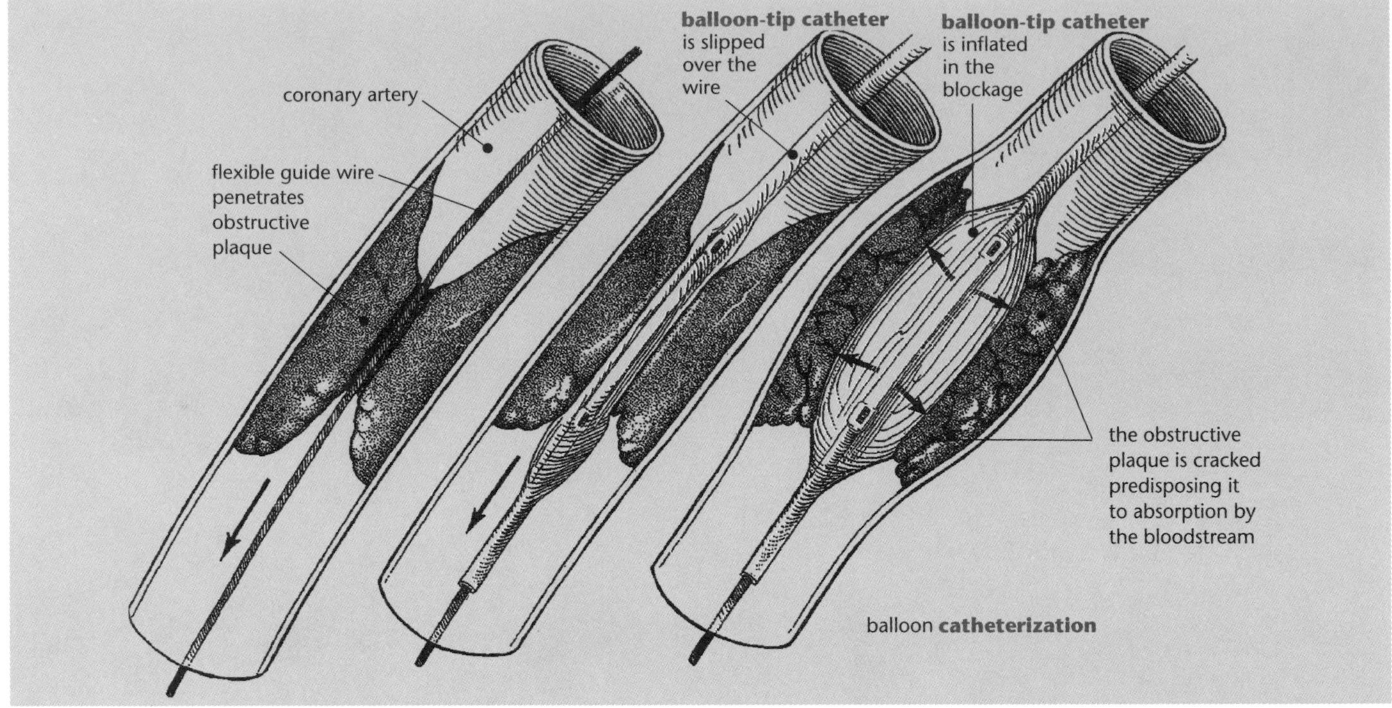

coronary artery
flexible guide wire penetrates obstructive plaque
balloon-tip catheter is slipped over the wire
balloon-tip catheter is inflated in the blockage
the obstructive plaque is cracked predisposing it to absorption by the bloodstream

balloon **catheterization**

cataplasia (kat-ă-pla´zhă) Degenerative reversion of cells or tissues to an embryonic state.

cataplexy (kat´ă-plek-se) A sudden and brief loss of muscle tone and postural reflexes, causing limpness of the body or a part, usually triggered by an emotional surge (e.g., gales of laughter, sudden elation, anger).
narcolepsy c. Transient loss of muscle tone in conjunction with intermittent attacks of uncontrollable sleep.

cataract (kat´ă-rakt) Loss of transparency of the lens of the eye and/or its capsule, resulting in partial or total blindness.
cerulean c. A nonprogressive collection of blue spots throughout the lens of the eye; appears to be congenital and is of little significance.
congenital c. Cataract present at birth due to faulty development of the fetus.
immature c. An early stage of a cataract development.
mature c. A cataract in which the entire lens substance has become opaque and can be easily separated from its capsule.
posterior subcapsular c. A type of senile cataract involving the interior aspect of the lens periphery.
radiation c. A cataract caused by continued exposure to radioactive materials.
senile c. A cataract occurring in old age.
stationary c. One that has ceased to progress.
traumatic c. Cataract caused by a foreign body injury (e.g., BB shot, rock).

catarrh (kă-tăr´) Inflammation of a mucous membrane, especially of the nose and throat, with a discharge.

catatonia (kat-ă-to´ne-ă) Marked motor anomalies usually seen in schizophrenia; may be a *withdrawn type,* characterized by generalized inhibition, mutism, stupor, and negativism; or an *excited type,* characterized by waxy flexibility or occasionally by excitement and excessive (sometimes violent) motor activity.

cat-cry syndrome (kăt-krī sin´drōm) See cri du chat syndrome.

catechol (kat´ĕ-kol) A chemical compound, 1,2-dihydroxybenzene, $C_6H_6O_2$; of interest mainly because of the importance of its aminated derivatives.

catecholamines (kat-ĕ-kol´ă-mēns) Amine compounds derived from catechol, such as epinephrine and norepinephrine, which have sympathomimetic activity and are concerned with nervous transmission, vascular tone, and many metabolic activities.

catgut (kat´gut) A tough, thin thread made from sterilized connective tissue of healthy animals; used as absorbable surgical ligatures and sutures. Also called surgical gut.

catharsis (kă-thar´sis) **1.** The promotion of vigorous bowel evacuation. **2.** Therapeutic discharge of emotional tension by recalling and talking about past events.

cathartic (kă-thar´tik) **1.** A drug that promotes evacuation of intestinal contents in a more or less fluid state by increasing motor activity of the intestine, either directly or reflexly; distinguished from a laxative which produces a milder effect. Also called purgative. **2.** Relating to a catharsis.

cathepsin (kă-thep´sin) Any intracellular protein-splitting enzyme that acts on the interior peptide bonds of a protein, causing its decomposition; cathepsins are widely distributed in animal tissues, especially the liver, kidney, and spleen.

cathepsis (kă-thep´sis) Protein hydrolysis by the action of cathepsins.

catheter (kath´ĕ-ter) A slender, usually flexible tube inserted into a body cavity to drain fluids or to introduce diagnostic or therapeutic agents.
angiographic c. A thin-walled catheter through which a contrast medium is introduced into the blood vessels of an organ for visual examination.
balloon tip c. A twin-lumen catheter with a distensible balloon at the end.
Fogarty c. A catheter having an inflatable balloon near the tip; used to remove thrombi from large veins and stones from the biliary ducts.
Foley c. An indwelling catheter equipped with a small balloon near the tip that can be inflated with air or liquid to retain the catheter in place, usually in the bladder.
indwelling c. Catheter designed to be left within a body cavity or passage for an extended period of time.
pacing c. A catheter equipped with electrodes at the tip, passed into the right atrium or ventricle to function as a heart pacer.
pigtail c. A slender catheter with a coiled end to minimize the impact of the injected substance on the vessel wall.
Swan-Ganz c. A thin, soft catheter with a balloon at the end to measure pulmonary arterial pressure; introduced into the basilic vein and carried by the bloodstream through the heart into a small artery in the lung.
two-way c. A twin-channeled catheter for irrigation.

catheterization (kath-ĕ-ter-ĭ-za´shun) Introduction of a catheter into a bodily passage.
cardiac c. Passage of a catheter into the heart by way of a blood vessel; first attempted by Forsmann on himself in 1928.
left-heart c. Introduction of a radiopaque catheter into the brachial or femoral artery and passage in a retrograde direction through the artery to the aorta and, frequently, across the aortic valve into the left ventricle.
right-heart c. Passage of a radiopaque flexible catheter into a vein, usually the basilic; the catheter is manipulated under fluoroscopic control through the venous system into the right atrium and eventually the right ventricle and pulmonary trunk.
urinary c. Insertion of a catheter into the bladder to drain urine.

catheterize (kath´ĕ-ter-īz) To introduce a catheter into a bodily canal or passage.

cathexis (kă-thek´sis) Attachment of emotional energy and significance to a person, object, or idea.

cathode (kath´ōd) (Ca, k, ka) The negatively charged electrode of an electron tube, galvanic cell (primary cell) or storage battery (secondary cells). Also called negative electrode.

cation (kat´ī-on) A positively charged ion that is characteristically attracted to the negatively charged cathode; indicated as a plus sign (e.g., H^+).

CATLINE (catalog-online) A segment of MEDLARS that contains references to books and serials catalogued at the National Library of Medicine; available at medical libraries in the MEDLARS network for immediate access to authoritative cataloging information; also used as a source of information for ordering books and journals and to provide reference and interlibrary loan services.

cat-scratch disease (kat-skrach dĭ-zēz´) Regional inflammation of lymph nodes following the scratch or bite of a cat infected with the bacterium *Bartonella henselae*. Also called cat-scratch fever.

cauda (kaw´dă), *pl.* **caudae** A tail or tapered end of a structure.
c. equina The bundle of nerves (sacral and coccygeal) in which the spinal cord ends.

caudad (kaw´dad) Directed posteriorly or toward the tail.

cauda equina syndrome (kaw´dă ē-kwī-nă sin´drōm) Dull pain and anesthesia of the buttocks, genitalia, and/or thigh with impaired bladder and bowel function; caused by compression of the spinal nerve roots.

caudal (kaw´dal) Near the tail or lower part of the body.

caudate (kaw´dāt) Possessing a tail or a tail-like appendage.

caul (kawl) The portion of fetal membranes surrounding the head of the fetus at birth when the membranes remain intact until completion of delivery.

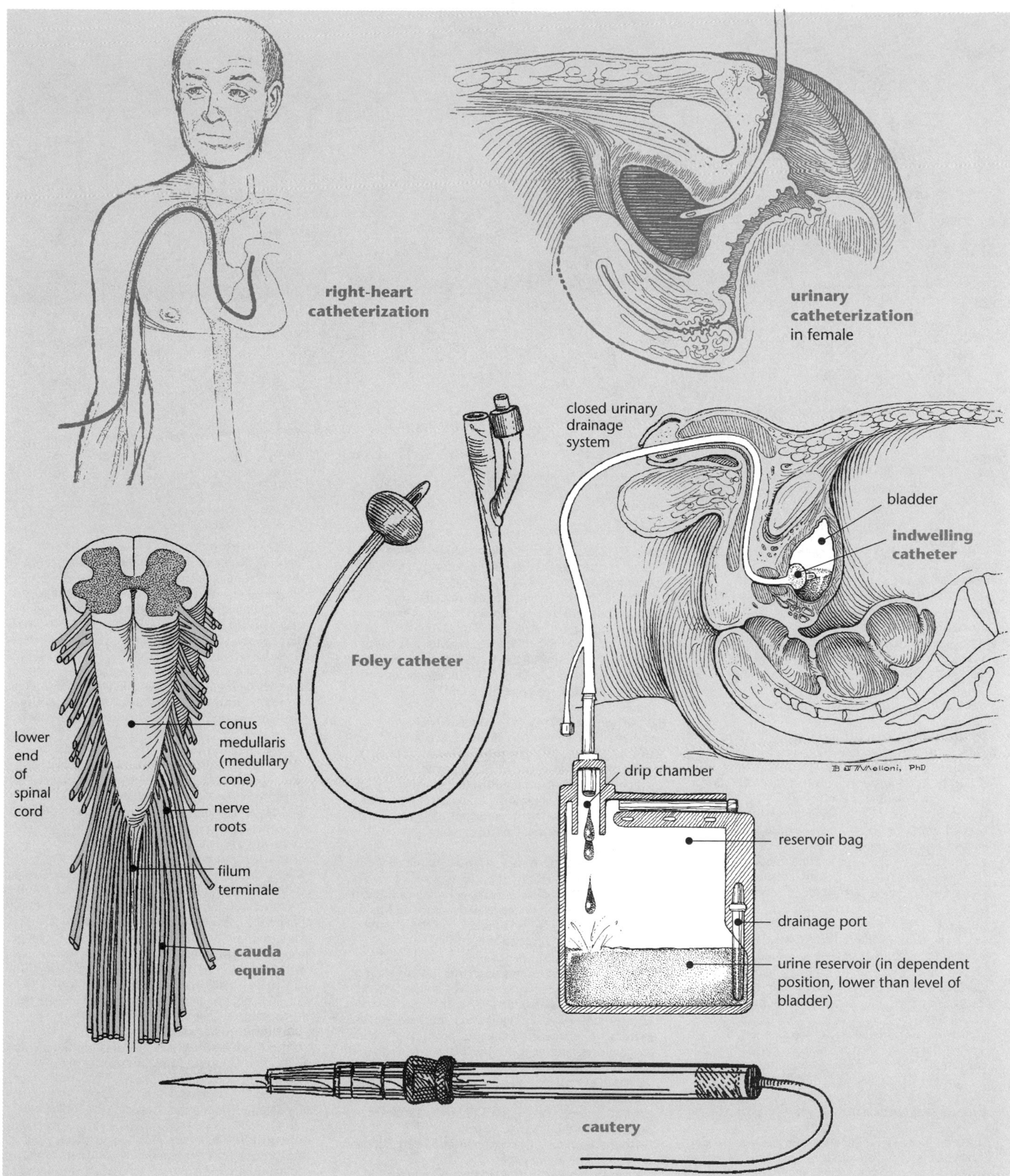

causalgia (kaw-zal´jă) A painful, burning sensation, accompanied by trophic changes in the skin and nails, due to a peripheral nerve injury, usually of the median or sciatic nerves.

caustic (kaws´tik) Corrosive; capable of burning.

cauterization (kaw-ter-ĭ-za´shun) The act of cauterizing; the application of a caustic substance or electric current for the purpose of scarring or destroying aberrant tissue.

cauterize (kaw´ter-īz) To apply a cautery.

cautery (kaw´ter-e) An agent or device used for destroying tissue by scarring or burning.

caval (kā´val) Relating to the vena cava.

caveolae (ka-ve-o´le) Minute vesicles that develop by invagination of the plasmalemma of the cell surface; they usually pinch off to form free vesicles within the cytoplasm and serve as a mechanism for cell ingestion.

cavern (kav´ern) A cavity, especially one caused by disease, as seen in tuberculous lungs.

cavernitis (kav-er-ni´tis) Inflammation of one or both columns of erectile tissue (corpus cavernosum) in the penis.

fibrous c. See Peyronie's disease.

cavernous (kav´ĕr-nus) **1.** Having cavities. **2.** Resulting from the presence of cavities.

cavernous sinus syndrome (kav´er-nus sī´nus sin´drōm) Any symptom complex that includes multiple nerve paralysis of the 3rd, 4th, and 5th cranial nerves usually due to nerve damage from a lesion of the cavernous sinus within the skull.

cavitary (kav´ĭ-tar-e) **1.** Relating to cavities. **2.** Any parasite having a body cavity and living inside the host's body.

cavitation (kav-ĭ-ta´shun) Formation of cavities, as in the lungs in pulmonary tuberculosis.

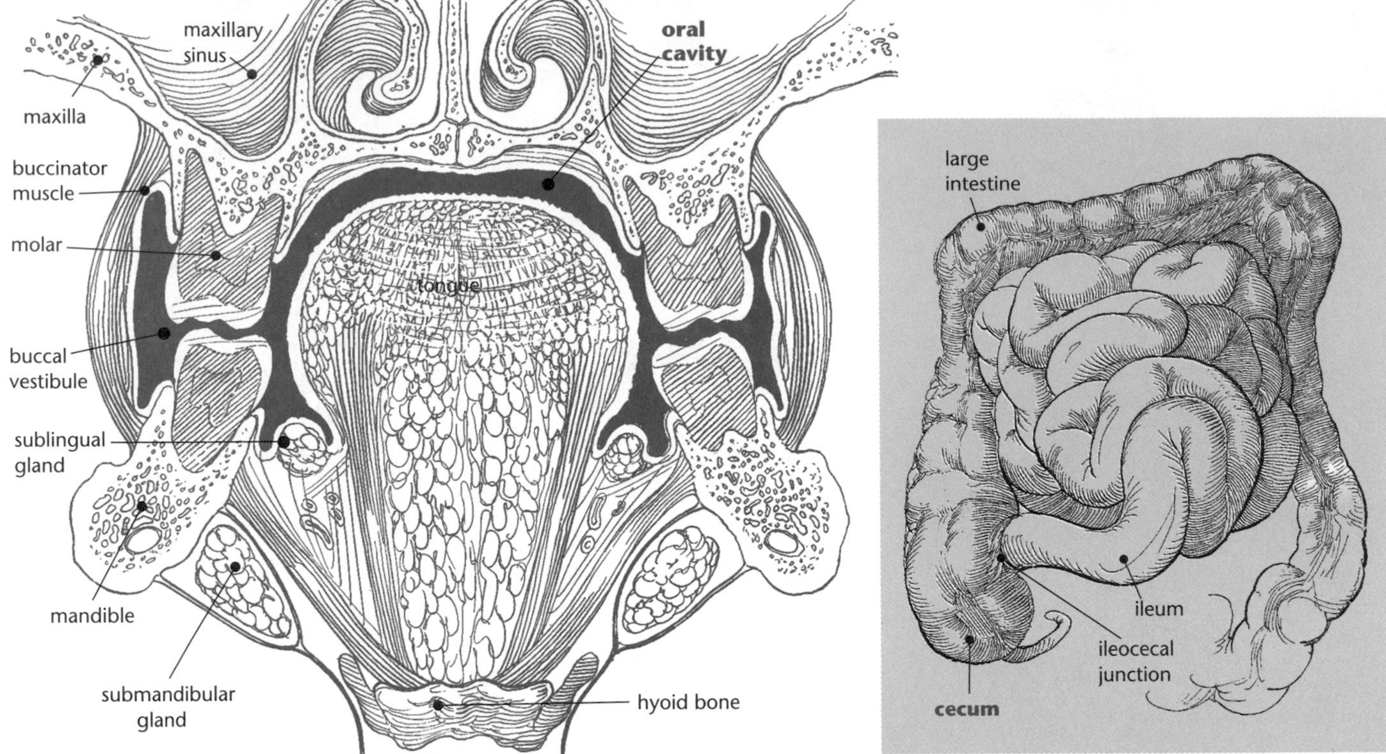

cavity (kav´ĭ-te) **1.** A hollow space within the body; a chamber. **2.** Popular term for loss of tooth structure due to decay.
abdominal c. The bodily cavity between the diaphragm above and the pelvis below.
amniotic c. The fluid-filled space within the amniochorion (membrane containing the embryo/fetus).
body c. The cavity of the body containing the organs.
buccal c. The space between the lips and the gums and teeth.
compound c. In dentistry, a cavity involving two or more surfaces of a tooth.
cranial c. The space within the skull.
distal c. In dentistry, a cavity located on the surface of a tooth away from the midline.
glenoid c. See glenoid fossa, under fossa.
medullary c. of bone The elongated cavity within the shaft of a long bone.
nasal c. An irregular space extending from the base of the cranium to the roof of the mouth and divided in two by a thin vertical septum (nasal septum).
oral c. The cavity of the mouth.
pelvic c. The short, wide, curved space within the bony framework of the minor pelvis; it contains the pelvic colon, rectum, bladder, and some of the organs of reproduction.
pericardial c. The potential cavity between the two layers of the membrane enveloping the heart (pericardium).
pleural c. The potential space between the two layers of the pleura (parietal and visceral).
prepared c. In dentistry, a dental excavation made by removal of caries and other procedures for enhancing retention of a restoration.
proximal c. In dentistry, a cavity occurring on the mesial or distal surface of a tooth.
pulp c. The central chamber of a tooth containing blood vessels, lymphatic vessels, and nerve fibers; the entire space occupied by the pulp.
tympanic c. The cavity of the middle ear, located in the temporal bone and containing the ear ossicles.
visceral c. One of the major cavities of the body: cranial, thoracic, abdominal, and pelvic.

cavogram (kā-vo-gram) A radiograph of the vena cava.

cavosurface (kăvo-sur-fis) Relating to a prepared cavity and the surface of a tooth.

cavum (kā-vum) Latin for cavity or hollow.

CD See cluster of differentiation.

cecitis (se-si´tis) See typhlitis.

cecostomy (se-kos´to-me) Surgical creation of an opening into the cecum through the abdominal wall.

cecum (se´kum) The widest, pouchlike portion of the large intestine to which the vermiform appendix is attached.

celiac (se´le-ak) Relating to the abdominal cavity.

celiac disease (se´le-ak dĭ-zēz´) Disorder characterized by intolerance to gluten (a protein present in the grains of wheat, rye, oats, and barley), abnormal structure of the small intestine, and poor absorption of food. Also called nontropical sprue; gluten-induced enteropathy. COMPARE: tropical sprue, under sprue.

celiohysterectomy (se-le-o-his-tĕ-rek´tō-me) See abdominal hysterectomy, under hysterectomy.

celioscopy (se-le-os´kŏ-pe) See laparoscopy.

celiotomy (se-le-ot´ŏ-me) See laparotomy.

cell (sel) **1.** The smallest unit of living matter capable of independent functioning, composed of protoplasm and surrounded by a semipermeable plasma membrane. **2.** Any small cavity or compartment. **3.** A receptacle.
acidophilic c. A cell whose cytoplasm or its granules have an affinity for acid dyes such as eosin.
acinar c. One of the secreting cells lining an acinus or alveolus of a compound acinous gland, such as the pancreas. Also called acinous cell.
adipose c. See fat cell.
adventitial c. See pericyte.
air c. An air-containing space (e.g., an air sinus of the skull).
alpha c. of pancreas A cell of the islet of Langerhans (islet of pancreas) marked by fine cytoplasmic granules; known to produce glucagon (hyperglycemic-glycogenolytic factor); it stains red with phloxine.
alveolar c. See type I pneumocyte, under pneumocyte.
amacrine c. A special inhibitory retinal cell, regarded as a modified nerve cell.
anaplastic c. An undifferentiated cell characteristic of carcinoma.
antigen-presenting c. (APC) A cell (formed in bone marrow) that helps to induce an immune response by capturing antigen and carrying it in a form that is recognized by T lymphocytes (in regional lymph nodes or the spleen), thereby stimulating lymphocyte activity.
antigen-sensitive c. See immunocyte.
argentaffin c. See neuroendocrine cell.
B c.'s See B lymphocytes, under lymphocyte.
B1c.'s See B1 lymphocytes, under lymphocyte.
B2c.'s See B2 lymphocytes, under lymphocyte.
balloon c. A large, degenerated cell.
band c. Any granulocytic leukocyte in which the nucleus has a simple, nonlobulated, elongated shape, resembling a band; it represents a normal stage prior to the development of a mature segmented granulocytic leukocyte (polymorphonuclear white blood cell). Also called stab cell.
basal c. A cell appearing in the deepest layer of a stratified epithelium; an early keratinocyte.
basophilic c. A cell whose cytoplasm or its granules stain strongly with basic dyes, such as aldehyde fuchsin.
beta c.'s of hypophysis The basophilic cells of the anterior pituitary (adenohypophysis); they secrete thyroid stimulating hormone (TSH), follicle stimulating hormone (FSH) and luteinizing hormones (LH).
beta c.'s of pancreas The predominant cells of the islet of Langerhans (islet of pancreas), marked by coarse cytoplasmic granules that represent a precursor of insulin; it stains blue with the Gomori stain.
Betz c.'s The large pyramidal cells of the fifth layer of the motor cortex.
bipolar c. A neuron having two processes (afferent and efferent), as those in the retina.
blast c. (a) An immature precursor cell (e.g., erythroblast, lymphoblast, neuroblast); a primitive cell, the least differentiated of a line of blood-forming elements. (b) A leukemic cell of indeterminable type.
blood c. One of the formed elements of the blood; an erythrocyte or leukocyte.
burr c. An elongated erythrocyte with multiple long, sharp, spinelike projections from the cell surface; seen in hemolytic anemias, especially those associated with uremia and carcinoma.
cartilage c. See chondrocyte.
chief c. of parathyroid gland The principal cell of the parathyroid gland; it secretes parathyroid hormone.
chief c. of stomach An enzyme-producing cell of a gastric gland in the stomach. Also called peptic cell.
chromaffin c. A cell whose cytoplasm exhibits fine brown granules when stained with a dichromate; occurring in the adrenal medulla and paraganglia of the sympathetic nervous system and some other tissues.
chromophobe c. A cell of the adenohypophysis (anterior pituitary) that has little affinity for histologic dyes.
clear c. Any cell containing non-stainable, or faintly stainable material.
cleavage c. See blastomere.
columnar c. A cell, usually epithelial, in which the height is significantly greater than the width, usually epithelial; may be a tall columnar or low columnar cell.
committed c. Any cell committed to the

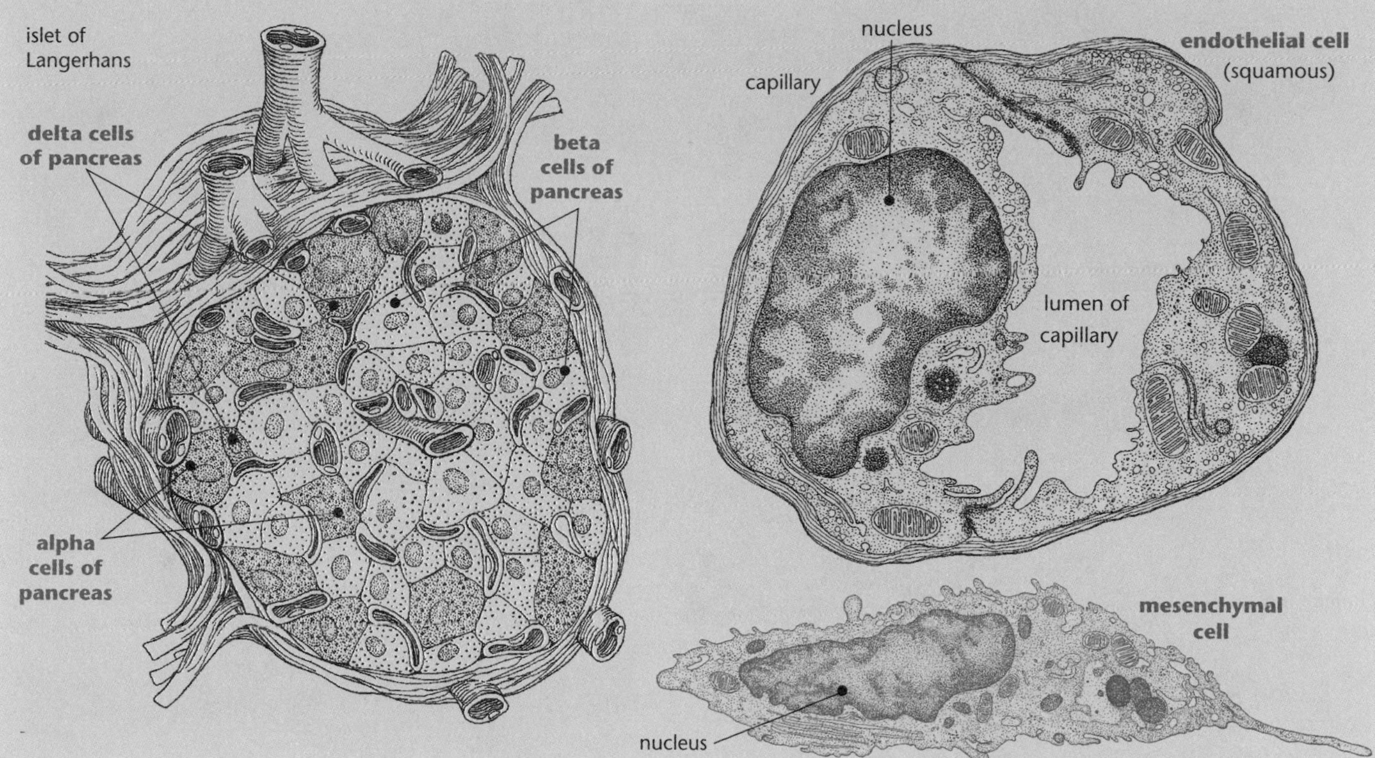

production of antibodies specific for a given antigen-determinant (e.g., primed cell, memory cell, and antibody-producing cell).

cone c. of retina One of the visual receptors sensitive to color.

cuboid c. A cell in which all diameters are approximately the same size, resembling a cube.

cytotoxic T c. See cytotoxic T lymphocyte, under lymphocyte.

daughter c. Any cell resulting from the division of a parent cell.

dentin c. See odontoblast.

dust c. See alveolar macrophage, under macrophage.

effector c. In immunology, a T lymphocyte (T cell) capable of carrying out the end function of the immunologic process (e.g., cytotoxicity, suppression).

enamel c. See ameloblast.

endothelial c. One of the thin, flat cells (squamous) forming the lining (endothelium) of the blood and lymph vessels and the inner layer of the endocardium.

epithelial c. One of a variety of cells that form epithelium.

epithelioid c. A large cell seen in certain granulomatous reactions (e.g., tuberculosis).

fat c. A very large connective tissue cell (60 to 80 µm) in which neutral fat is stored; the cytoplasm is usually compressed into a thin envelope, with the nucleus at one point in the periphery. Also called adipose cell; lipocyte.

foam c. A macrophage exhibiting a peculiar vacuolated appearance due to the presence of lipids in a multitude of small vacuoles; notably seen in xanthoma. Also called xanthoma cell.

follicular c.'s See granulosa cells.

follicular lutein c.'s See granulosa lutein cells.

fusiform c.'s of cerebral cortex Spindle-shaped cells in the sixth layer of the cerebral cortex.

ganglion c. A large nerve cell in a ganglion peripheral to the central nervous system.

Gaucher c. An abnormal cell found in spleen, liver, lymph nodes and bone marrow in Gaucher's disease; it is a round or polyhedral, pale reticuloendothelial cell 20 to 80 µm in diameter containing a gluco-cerebroside.

germ c. The ovum or spermatozoon.

germinal c.'s Cells from which other cells are derived or proliferated, especially the dividing cells in the embryonic neural tube.

ghost c. A cell in its last stages of degeneration, appearing as a shadow.

gitter c. A compound granule cell; a lipid-laden microglial cell observed near a healing cerebral infarct.

glitter c. A large leukocyte seen in the urine exhibiting brownian movement in the cytoplasm; associated with urinary tract infection.

goblet c.'s Unicellular mucous glands found in the epithelium of certain mucous membranes, especially of the respiratory and intestinal tracts.

Golgi's c.'s (a) See Golgi type I neuron, under neuron. (b) See Golgi type II neuron, under neuron.

granule c. One of many small cells in the granular layer of the cerebellar cortex.

granulosa c.'s Special epithelial cells displaying high mitotic activity; they surround the ovum in a primary follicle and, in a vesicular follicle, form the stratum granulosum, corona radiata, and cumulus oophorus; they secrete a refractile substance that forms the protective zona pellucida around the ovum and, during the early stages of follicular maturation, secrete an inhibitory substance (polypeptide) that maintains the primary oocyte in an arrested stage of meiotic prophase. Also called follicular cells.

granulosa lutein c.'s Giant glandular cells that comprise the major part of the wall of a ruptured vesicular follicle (corpus luteum) in the ovary; formed by hypertrophy of the follicular granulosa cells of the old vesicular follicle; they produce the sex steroid progesterone. Also called follicular lutein cells.

great alveolar c. See type II pneumocyte, under pneumocyte.

hair c.'s Pear-shaped epithelial cells with delicate hairlike microvilli (stereocilia) one to 100 µm in length on the free surface; they are present in neuroepithelial sensory areas of the utricle, saccule, ampullae, and the spiral organ of Corti.

HeLa c.'s The first documented, continuously cultured human malignant cells, derived from a cervical carcinoma; used in the cultivation of viruses.

helmet c. See shistocyte.

helper T c., helper c. See helper T lymphocyte, under lymphocyte.

Hürthle c. An enlarged, granular thyroid follicular epithelial cell with acidophilic cytoplasm, as seen in Hashimoto's disease.

I c. See immunocyte.

immunocompetent c. See immunocyte.

inducer c. See helper cell.

interstitial c.'s of testis See Leydig's cells.

islet c. One of the cells in the islet (island) of Langerhans of the pancreas.

juxtaglomerular c.'s A group of secretory cells forming the middle layer of the wall of the afferent arteriole just before it enters the glomerulus in the kidney; they secrete the hormone renin.

killer c.'s, K c.'s See cytotoxic T lymphocytes, under lymphocytes.

Kupffer c.'s Fixed macrophages or reticuloendothelial cells lining the capillary system of the liver (which conveys blood from the interlobular branches of the portal vein to the central vein); they are phagocytic in character and are active in freeing the bloodstream of foreign particles.

Langhans' giant c.'s (a) Multinucleated giant cells seen in tuberculosis and other granulomas; the nuclei are located, in the form of an arc, at the periphery of the cells. (b) Rounded cells with clear cytoplasm and light-staining nuclei forming the cytotrophoblast.

L.E. c. Lupus erythematosus cell; a leukocyte containing an amorphous body; this amorphous material is a phagocytosed nucleus from another cell that has been traumatized and exposed to serum antinuclear globulin; L.E. cells are formed *in vitro* in the blood of individuals with systemic lupus erythematosus, or by the action of the individual's serum on normal leukocytes.

lepra c.'s Large mononuclear phagocytes (macrophages) with foamlike cytoplasm; associated with lepromatous lesions that contain the acid-fast organisms of leprosy.

Leydig's c. Endocrine interstitial cells located between the seminiferous tubules of the testis; they secrete androgens, mainly testosterone. Also called interstitial cells of testis.

lupus erythematosus c. See L.E. cell.

lymph c. See lymphocyte.

mast c.'s Large cells with coarse cytoplasmic granules containing heparin (anticoagulant) and histamine (vasodilator) occurring in most loose connective tissue, especially along the path of blood vessels; the cells act as mediators of inflammation on contact with antigen; sometimes called tissue mast cells or histogenous mast cells to distinguish them from the hematogenous mast cells (basophilic leukocytes) circulating in the blood.

memory B c. B cell that has already encountered antigen, undergone class switching, and returned to a resting state to be reactivated by a second challenge from the antigen it recognizes; during the second challenge, the cell mounts a more sustained response. Also called immunlogic memory cell.

mesangial c. An intercapillary cell of the kidney's glomerulus located mostly near the part of the capillary facing the center of the glomerulus.

mesenchymal c. A cell present in mesenchyme and capable of differentiating into any of the special types of connective tissue or supporting tissues, smooth muscle, vascular endothelium, or blood cells.

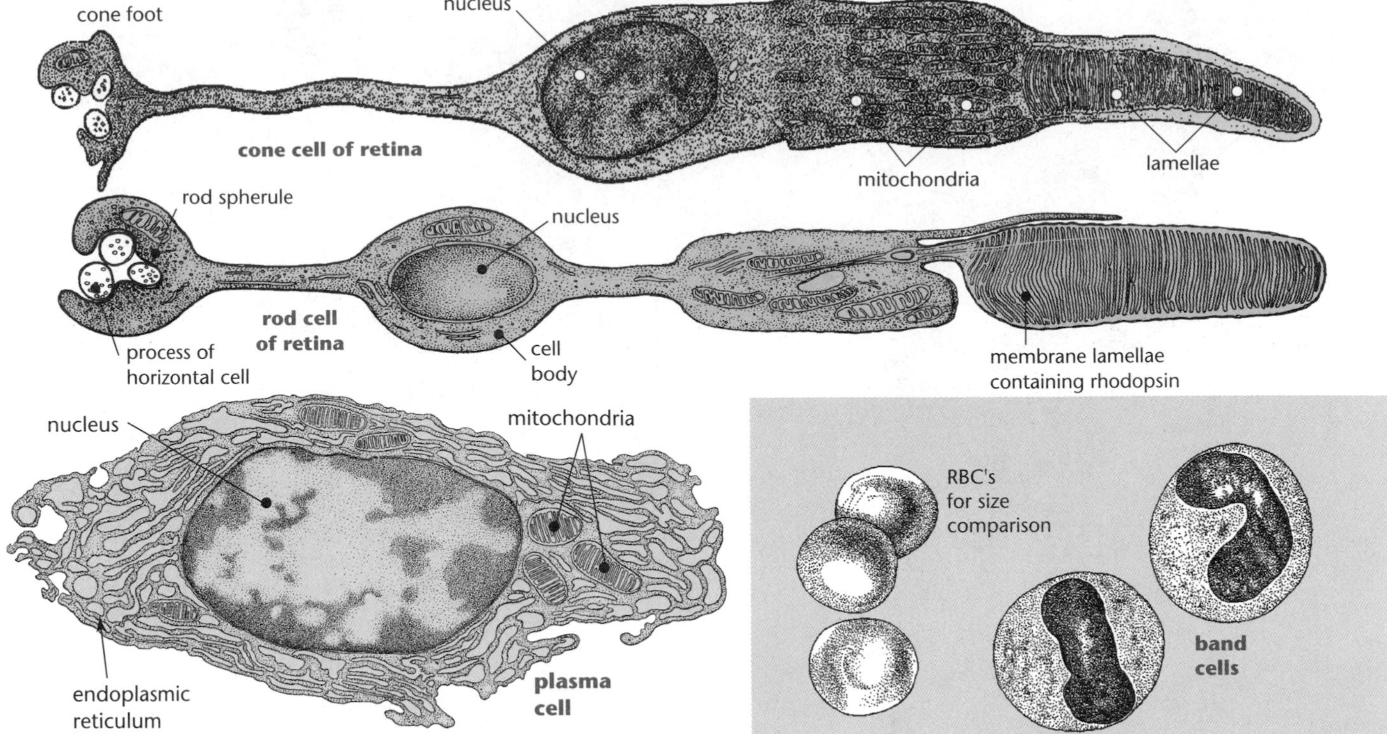

mesothelial c. One of the flat cells of the simple squamous epithelium (mesothelium) lining the pleural, pericardial, peritoneal, and scrotal cavities.

Mexican hat c. See target cell (a).

mother c. A cell that gives rise to a new generation of daughter cells by cell division. Also called parent cell.

myeloid c. Any young cell that develops into a mature granulocyte.

myoepithelial c. One of the smooth muscle cells of ectodermal origin, with processes that spiral around some of the epithelial cells of sweat, mammary, lacrimal and salivary glands; their contraction forces the secretion of the glands toward the ducts.

natural killer c., NK c. A large lymphocyte that recognizes and then kills abnormal cells (e.g., infected cells or tumor cells that lack cell-surface major-histocompatibility complex class I molecules).

nerve c. See neuron.

neuroendocrine c. A cell with an affinity for silver salts and therefore capable of being stained by them; located throughout the gastrointestinal tract.

neuroglial c. Any of the non-neuronal cells of nervous tissue including the oligodendroglia, astrocytes, microglia, and ependymal cells. Also called glial cell.

neurosecretory c. A nerve cell that elaborates a chemical substance, as those of the hypothalamus.

null c. A lymphocyte devoid of surface immunoglobulin (neither T nor B markers). Also called NUL lymphocyte.

oat c. A cell resembling an oat grain; seen in lung cancer.

olfactory c. One of the slender sensory nerve cells surmounted by sensitive hairs, present in the olfactory mucous membrane at the roof of the nose; the receptor for the sense of smell.

osteochondrogenic c. A young cell of the inner layer of periostium, capable of developing into a bone or a cartilage cell.

oxynthic c. See parietal cell.

oxyphilic c.'s (a) Parietal cells. (b) Acidophilic cells present in the parathyroid glands; they increase in number with age.

Paneth's c.'s Pyramidal-shaped cells occurring in small groups near the base of the crypts of Lieberkühn; believed to secrete digestive enzymes throughout the small intestine.

parent c. See mother cell.

parietal c. One of the cells present in the periphery of the gastric glands; it lies upon the basement membrane covered by the chief cells and secretes hydrochloric acid, which reaches the lumen of the gland through fine channels. Also called oxynthic cell.

plasma c. A cell that stores and releases antibody and is believed to be of primary importance in antibody synthesis; it has an RNA-rich cytoplasm containing an extensive system of endoplasmic reticulum studded with ribosomes; the cell is derived embryologically from a bursal equivalent tissue and is therefore a differentiated B cell; in certain diseases, such as chronic lymphocytic leukemia, there is a proliferation of this cell type.

primed c. A cell that has been primed by antigen for antibody production.

primitive reticular c.'s Cells comprising the cellular network of the stroma of bone marrow and lymphatic tissues.

Purkinje's c.'s The large nerve cells of the cerebellar cortex with flask-shaped bodies forming a single cell layer between the molecular and granular layers; their dendrites are arranged in the molecular layer in a plane transverse to the folia, and their axons penetrate the granular layer to form the only pathways out of the cerebellar cortex; they terminate in the central cerebellar nuclei.

pus c. One of the polymorphonuclear leukocytes constituting the majority of the formed elements in pus.

pyramidal c. A nerve cell of the cerebral cortex; usually triangular with an apical dendrite directed toward the surface of the cortex and several smaller dendrites at the base; the axon is given off at the base of the cell and descends to deeper layers.

red blood c. (RBC) See erythrocyte.

Reed c.'s, Reed-Sternberg c.'s Large lymphocytes usually having two nuclei containing prominent nucleoli, and with the two halves of the cell in a mirror-image form; considered the characteristic cell of Hodgkin's disease.

Renshaw c. An inhibitory interneuron in the ventral horn of the spinal cord that acts as a negative feedback monitor of motor neurons.

respiratory c. See type I pneumocyte, under pneumocyte.

reticular c.'s See primitive reticular cells.

reticuloendothelial c. Phagocytic cell of the reticuloendothelial system, similar to the leukocyte but attached to vascular and lymphatic channels rather than being circulatory.

rod c. of retina One of the visual photoreceptor cells of the retina sensitive to gray shades.

Schwann's c. A special cell that surrounds a peripheral axon forming a myelin sheath.

septal c. See type II pneumocyte, under pneumocyte.

Sertoli c.'s The elaborate nonspermatogenic sustentacular cells in the seminiferous tubules of male gonads (testes) extending from the basal lamina to the lumen; they house the developing spermatogenic cells in deep recesses and produce sex hormone-binding globulin and androgens.

Sézary c. A cell with a large convoluted nucleus and scant cytoplasm; the atypical T lymphocyte found in the Sézary syndrome.

sickle c. An abnormal crescent-shaped red blood cell; the shape is due to the presence of hemoglobin S. Also called meniscocyte.

smudge c. Any leukocyte that becomes so degenerated that the cytoplasm disappears, leaving a naked nucleus that stains poorly and exhibits no characteristic chromatin pattern; rarely found in normal blood; seen in large numbers in chronic lymphocytic leukemia.

sperm c. See spermatozoon.

squamous c. A flat, scalelike epithelial cell.

squamous alveolar c. See type I pneumocyte, under pneumocyte.

stab c. See band cell.

stellate c.'s of the cerebral cortex A star-shaped interneuron cell located in the second, third, and fourth layers of the cortex of the brain.

stem c.'s (a) Any precursor cell. (b) Cells that can produce cells that are able to differentiate into other cell types.

suppressor c.'s See suppressor T cells.

suppressor T c.'s Cells of the lymphoid system which turn off immune responses (humoral and cell-mediated) once they are started, by inhibiting the production of sensitized antibodies and antibody-forming cells; also play an active role in development of tolerance to self and heterologous antigens.

sustentacular c. One of the supporting cells of an epithelium, as seen in the spiral organ of Corti, taste bud, and olfactory epithelium.

T c.'s See T lymphocytes, under lymphocyte.

target c. (a) An abnormal erythrocyte that when stained shows a dark center surrounded by a light band encircled by a darker ring, resembling a bull's eye target; found in a variety of anemias including thalassemia and other hemoglobinopathies. Also called Mexican hat cell. (b) A cell displaying a foreign (nonself) antigen recognized by an effector T lymphocyte. (c) A cell containing specific receptors for circulating messengers such as hormones.

tart c. A granulocyte that has an engulfed nucleus of another cell that is still well preserved.

taste c. A neuroepithelial cell that perceives gustatory stimuli, situated at the center of a taste bud.

theca lutein c.'s Lutein cells within the folds of the glandular corpus luteum of the ovary and derived from the theca interna; they produce estrogens. Also called paraluteal cells.

Tiselius electrophoresis c. The cell or container

C

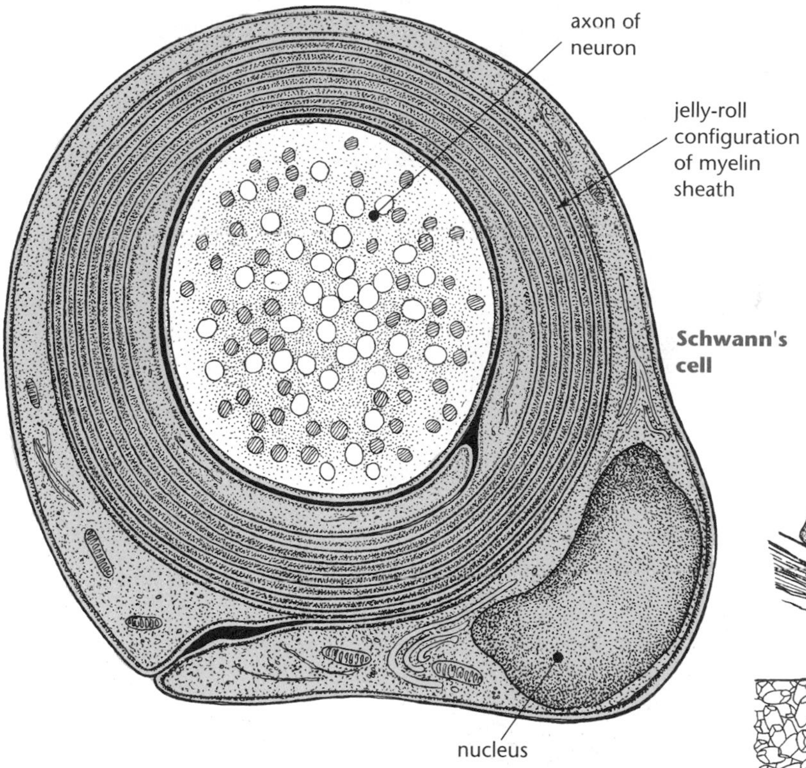

axon of
neuron
jelly-roll
configuration
of myelin
sheath
Schwann's
cell
nucleus

developing
sperm
Sertoli
cell

gelatinous
layer with
otoconia
otolithic
membrane
kinocilium
stereocilia
hair cell
(type II)
hair cell
(type I)
macula of
inner ear

BLOOD CELLS
white blood cells
neutrophil
eosinophil
basophil
granular
leukocytes
monocyte
lymphocyte
agranular
(nongranular)
leukocytes
red blood
cells
platelets

columnar cell
stereocilia
basal
cell
detail of duct of epididymis

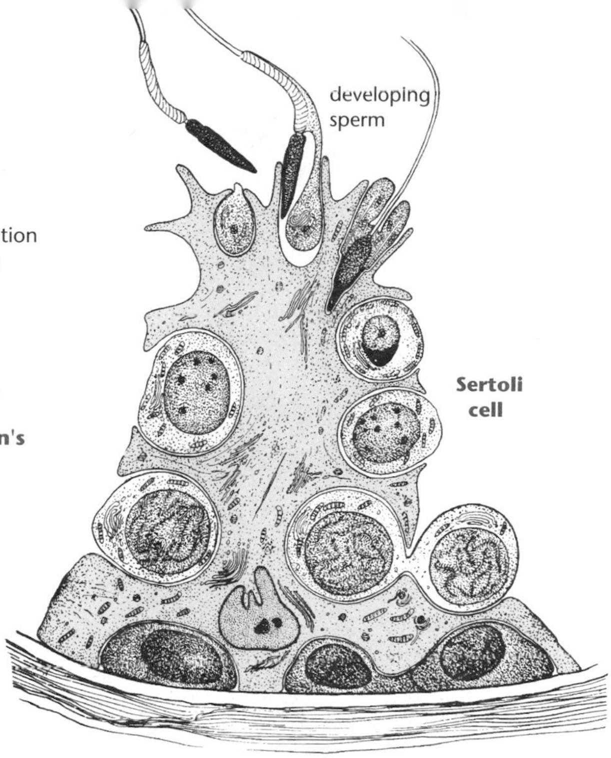

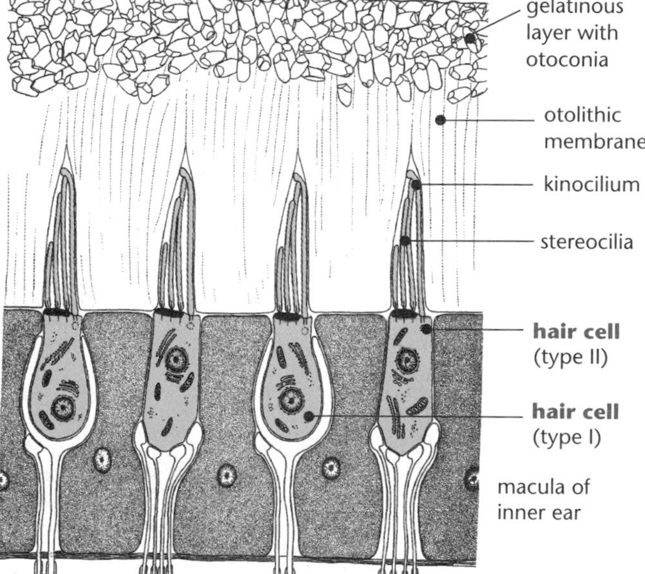

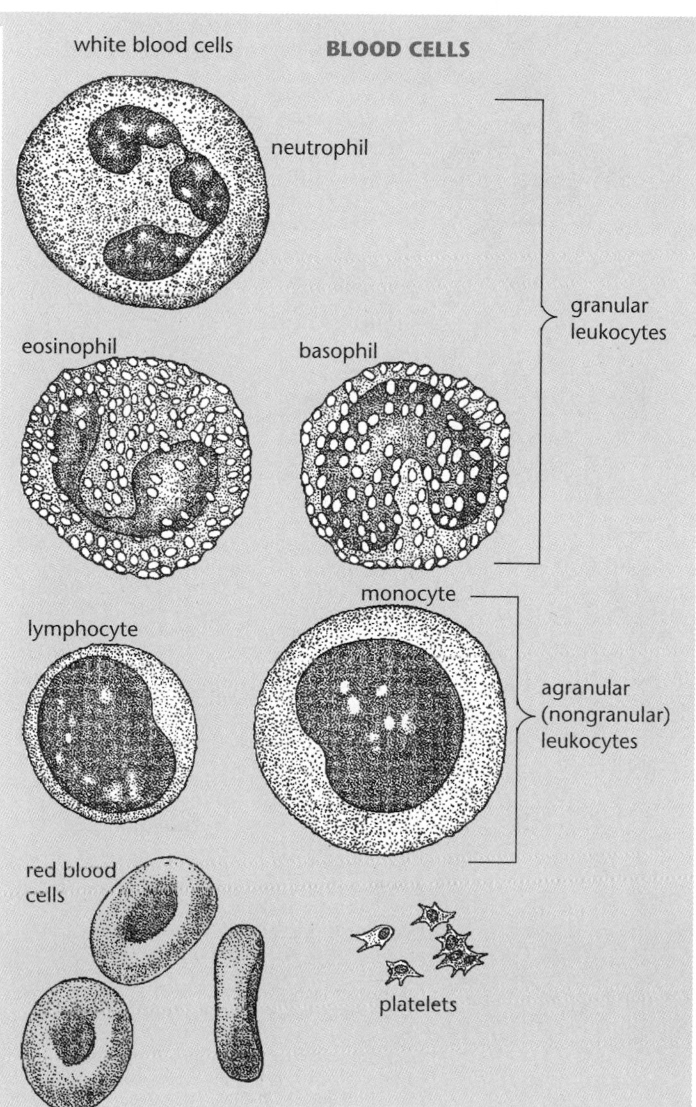

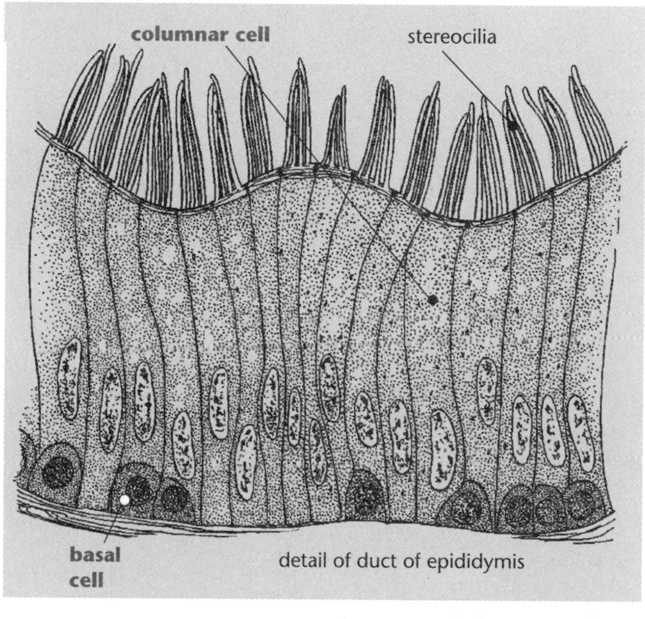

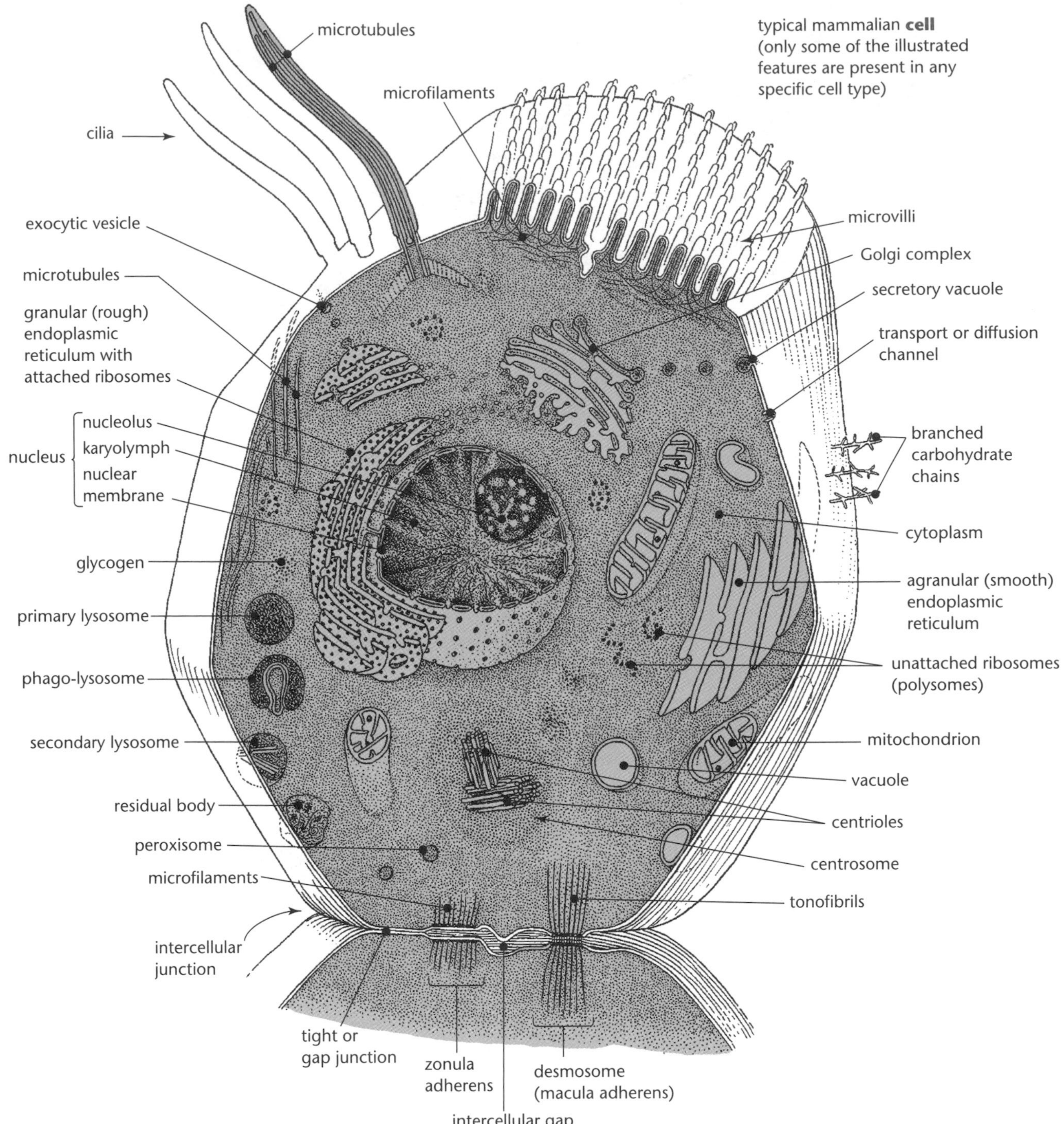

in a Tiselius apparatus containing the solution to be electrophoretically analyzed.

transitional c. (a) A monocyte. (b) Any cell thought to represent a phase of development from one form to another.

type I c. See type I pneumocyte, under pneumocyte.

type II c. See type II pneumocyte, under pneumocyte.

type 1 helper T c. See type 1 helper T lymphocyte, under lymphocyte.

type 2 helper T c. See type 2 helper T lymphocyte, under lymphocyte.

wasserhelle c.'s The water-clear cells of the parathyroid gland.

white blood c.'s (WBC) Formed elements in the blood that include granular leukocytes, lymphocytes, and monocytes.

xanthoma c. See foam cell.

cellular (sel′u-lar) Relating to, resembling, composed of, or derived from cells.

cellularity (sel-u-lar′ĭ-te) The number and quality of the cells constituting a tissue.

cellule (sel′ūl) **1.** A small cavity or compartment. **2.** A minute cell.

cellulite (sel′u-līt) Popular term for fat deposits beneath the skin.

cellulitis (sel-u-li′tis) A rapidly spreading acute inflammation of subcutaneous tissue; a complication of wound infections.

cellulose (sel′u-lōs) A carbohydrate polymer, $C_6H_{10}O_5$; the main constituent of the cell walls of plants; an important source of bulk in the diet because it is not affected by the digestive enzymes.

celom (se′lom) The body cavity of the embryo, between the two layers of the mesoderm after one unites with the ectoderm and the other with the endoderm. Also spelled coelom.

celomic (se-lom′ik) Relating to the body cavity or celom.

Celsius (sel′se-us) (C) See Celsius scale, under scale.

cement (sĕ-ment′) **1.** Cementum. **2.** Any of several materials used in dentistry, neurosurgery, and orthopedic surgery as luting and sealing agents, temporary restorations, and bases.

bone c. A luting agent for filling interstices of bone; it is widely used in the fixation of hip and knee implants.

intercellular c. Substance holding together cells, especially epithelial cells.

muscle c. See myoglia.

cementoblast (sĕ-men′to-blast) One of the cells active in the formation of cementum.

cementocyte (sĕ-men′to-sīt) Cell occupying a lacunar space in the cementum of a tooth; generally has protoplasmic processes that radiate from the cell body into the canaliculi of the cementum; derived from cementoblasts trapped within newly formed cementum.

cementoma (sĕ-men-to′mă) Periapical ossifying fibroma, an asymptomatic periapical lesion marked by proliferation of fibrous connective tissue at the

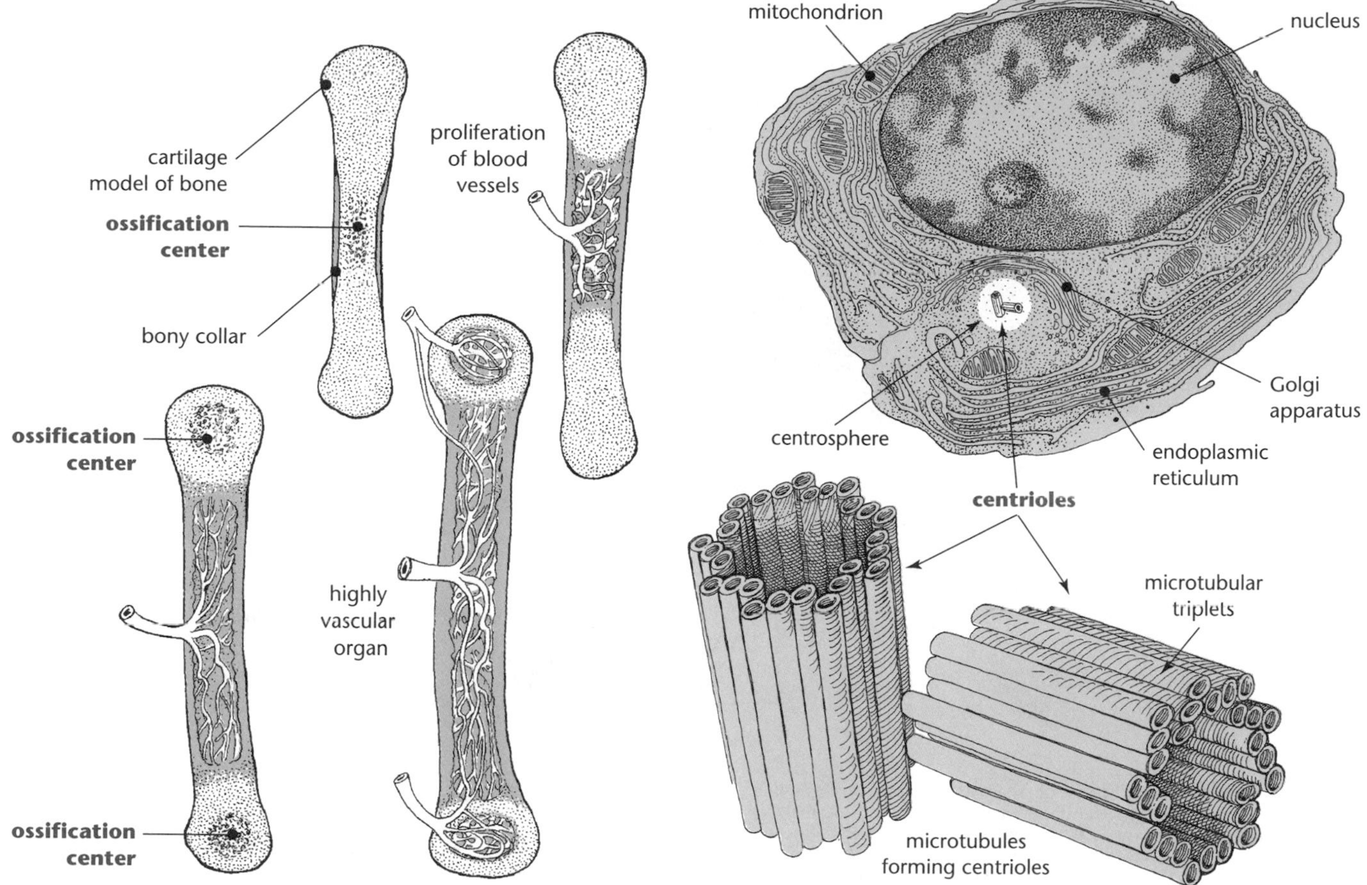

apex of a tooth; it is generally replaced by a calcified mass resembling cementum.

cementum (sĕ-men´tum) Specialized, bonelike, fibrous tissue covering the anatomic roots of human teeth; it offers attachment to the periodontal ligament; it is more resistant to resorption than bone, thus making orthodontic movement of teeth possible.

cellular c. Cementum possessing cementocytes, primarily located in the apical portion of the tooth.

center (sen´ter) **1.** The middle; the central part of an organ or structure. Also called core. **2.** A specialized region in which a process, such as ossification, begins. **3.** A collection of neurons governing a particular function. **4.** An agency designed to serve the community.

birth c., birthing c. A facility that provides prenatal, childbirth, and postnatal care and usually includes family-oriented maternity care concepts and practice.

germinal c. A light staining oval mass in the center of a secondary lymphatic nodule consisting primarily of large lymphoid cells; a site of antibody synthesis.

optical c. The point of a lens through which passing light rays suffer no angular deviation.

ossification c. Any region in which the process of bone formation first begins in a tissue.

reflex c. Any part of the nervous system where the reception of a sensory impression is automatically followed by a motor impulse.

respiratory c.'s Regions in the medulla and pons that coordinate the activity of respiration.

speech c. A unilateral area in the inferior frontal gyrus, associated with articulate speech.

vasomotor c.'s Areas of the central nervous system (in the tuber cenereum, medulla oblongata, and spinal cord) that control the constriction and dilatation of peripheral blood vessels.

vomiting c. A center in the lower part of the medulla oblongata; its stimulation may cause vomiting.

centesis (sen-te´sis) The puncturing of a cavity.

centibar (sen´tĭ-bar) A unit of atmospheric pressure; one-hundredth of a bar.

centigrade (sen´tĭ-grād) (C) **1.** Divided into or consisting of 100 gradations. **2.** See Celsius scale, under scale.

centigram (sen´tĭ-gram) (cg) One hundredth of a gram.

centiliter (sen´tĭ-le-ter) (cl) One hundredth of a liter.

centimeter (sen´tĭ-me-ter) (cm) One hundredth of a meter.

centimorgan (sen-tĭ-mor´gan) (cM) One hundredth of a morgan.

centrad (sen´trad) **1.** Toward the center. **2.** A unit of ophthalmic prism strength, equal to one hundredth of the radius of the circle; symbolized by an inverted delta (∇).

centrage (sen´trāj) Condition in which the center of the various refracting and reflecting surfaces of an optical system lie on a straight line.

central core disease (sen´tral kōr dĭ-zēz´) A congenital myopathy usually manifested before the first month of life; characterized by proximal muscle weakness, most severe in the lower limbs, resulting in delayed walking; on biopsy the central core of muscle fibers stains abnormally.

centric (sen´trik) Relating to a center.

centrifugal (sen-trif´ŭ-gal) Directed away from a center or axis; efferent.

centrifuge (sen´trĭ-fūj) **1.** An apparatus that, by means of centrifugal force, separates substances of different densities. **2.** To separate substances by rapid spinning.

centrilobular (sen-trĭ-lob´u-lar) Occurring at or near the center of a lobule.

centriole (sen´trĭ-ōl) Any of two short, cylindrical organelles (usually at right angles to each other) containing nine pairs of parallel microtubules about a central cavity, located in the centrosome and considered to play an important role in cell division; usually associated with the Golgi apparatus in a nondividing cell.

centripetal (sen-trip´ĕ-tal) Directed toward a center or axis; afferent.

centromere (sen´tro-mēr) The constricted part of the chromosome to which the spindle fibers attach during mitosis; chromosome movement occurs about this point. Also called kinetochore.

centrosome (sen´tro-sōm) Two associated centrioles, which play an important role in cell division (mitosis).

centrosphere (sen´tro-sfēr) A clear, gel-like zone of a cell that contains the centrosome.

centrum (sen´trum), *pl.* **cen´tra** The center of an anatomical structure.

cephalad (sef´ă-lad) Toward the head.

cephalalgia (sef-ă-lal´jă) See headache.

cephalhematoma (sef-al-he-mă-to´mă) Swelling with palpable edges overriding a single cranial bone without crossing suture lines, due to accumulation of blood between the bone and its covering membrane (periosteum); seen in a newborn infant who sustained a periosteal injury (e.g., with a vacuum extractor) or may occur during an uneventful delivery; may be absorbed within 3 months or, in rare occasions, persist for over 1 year. Also called cephalohematoma. COMPARE: caput succedaneum.

cephalic (sĕ-fal´ik) Relating to the head.

cephalin (sef´ă-lin) A member of a large group of lipids known as phospholipids; found in most animal tissues, especially the brain and spinal cord; important in the blood clotting process.

cephalization (sef-al-ĭ-za´shun) **1.** The gradual evolutionary concentration in the brain of important functions of the nervous system. **2.** The concentration of growth tendency at the anterior end of the embryo.

cephalocentesis (sef-ă-lo-sen-te´sis) The draining of fluid from the brain by means of a hollow needle or trocar and cannula.

cephalodynia (sef-ă-lo-din´e-ă) Headache.

cephalogyric (sef-ă-lo-ji´rik) Referring to turning movements of the head.

cephalohematoma (sef-ă-lo-he-mă-to´mă) See cephalhematoma.

cephalomegaly (sef-ă-lo-meg´ă-le) Abnormal enlargement of the head.

cephalosporin (sef-ă-lo-spōr´in) Any broad-spectrum antibiotic derived from the fungus *Cephalosporium*; the newer antibiotics are semisynthetic.

ceramide (ser´ă-mīd) General term used to designate any *N*-acyl fatty acid derivative of a sphingosine.

cercaria (ser-kar´e-ă), *pl.* **cercar´iae** A larval stage of trematode parasites. Cercariae leave their first host, usually a snail, to infest fish or vegetation, or to directly penetrate human skin.

cereal (sēr´e-al) **1.** An edible grain, the plant producing it, or the food prepared from it. **2.** Of or relating to such grain.

cerebellar (ser-ĕ-bel´ar) Relating to the cerebellum.

cerebellar syndrome (ser-ĕ-bel´ar sin´drōm) A cerebellar deficiency manifested chiefly by slurred speech, slow and clumsy movement of the limbs and staggering gait.

cerebellopontile (ser-ĕ-bel-o-pon´tēl) Relating to both the cerebellum and the pons.

cerebellorubral (ser-ĕ-bel-o-roo´bral) Relating to the cerebellum and the red nucleus.

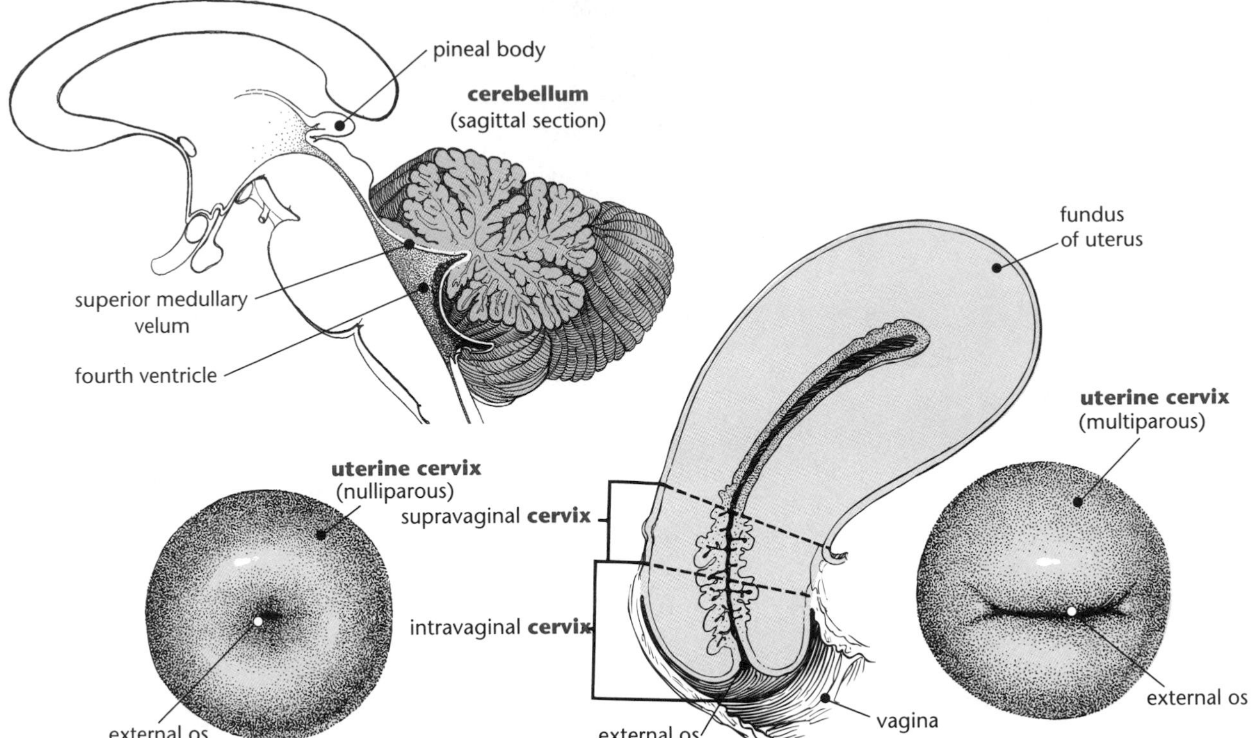

cerebellum (ser-ĕ-bel´um) The part of the central nervous system situated below and posterior to the cerebrum and above the pons and medulla oblongata; it serves to maintain equilibrium and coordination.

cerebral (sĕ-re´bral, ser´ĕ-bral) Relating to the brain.

cerebration (ser-ă-bra´shun) Conscious or unconscious mental activity.

cerebritis (ser-ĕ-brī´tis) Diffuse inflammation of the brain without suppuration.

cerebron (ser´ĕ-bron) See phrenosin.

cerebropathy (ser-ĕ-brop´ă-the) See encephalopathy.

cerebropsychosis (ser-ĕ-bro-si-ko´sis) Mental disorder caused by, or associated with, a lesion of the brain.

cerebrosclerosis (ser-ĕ-bro-sklĕ-ro´sis) Harden-ing of the brain substance.

cerebrose (ser´ĕ-brōs) A hexose (monosaccharide having six carbon atoms) present in brain tissue. Also called galactose.

cerebroside (ser´ĕ-bro-sīd) A phosphorus-free glycolipid containing a fatty acid, an unsaturated amino-alcohol, and galactose (or occasionally) glucose. Found in myelin sheaths and cell coats in nervous tissue. Also called cerebrogalactoside.

cerebrosidosis (ser-ĕ-bro-sī-do´sis) See Gaucher's disease.

cerebrospinal (ser-ĕ-bro-spi´nal) Relating to the brain and spinal cord.

cerebrotomy (ser-ĕ-brot´ŏ-me) Surgical incision of the brain substance.

cerebrovascular (ser-ĕ-bro-vas´ku-lar) Denoting the blood circulation of the brain.

cerebrum (sĕ-re´brum, ser´ĕ-brum) The brain, excluding the medulla, pons, and cerebellum.

cerium (se´re-um) A metallic element; symbol Ce, atomic number 58, atomic weight 140.115.

certifiable (ser-tĭ-fi´ă-bl) **1.** Applied to any disease required by law to be reported to health authorities whenever it occurs. **2.** Denoting a person exhibiting sufficiently severe psychotic behavior to require confinement.

certification (ser-tĭ-fĭ-ka´shun) **l.** The reporting of a contagious disease to health authorities as required by law. **2.** The process of completing the necessary legal procedures for detention and treatment in a mental hospital. **3.** The formal signing of a statement of cause of death by a medical practitioner. **4.** The formal written statement by which an agency or organization evaluates and recognizes an individual or an institution as meeting certain predetermined standards.

ceruloplasmin (sĕ-roo-lo-plaz´min) A plasma protein that carries more than 95% of the body's circulating copper; it is thought that the copper carried by ceruloplasmin goes into the cellular manufacture of cytochrome oxidase. Ceruloplasmin is deficient in Wilson's disease.

cerumen (sĕ-roo´men) The yellowish brown, waxlike secretion of the glands lining the external ear canal. Also called earwax.

ceruminolytic (sĕ-roo-mĭ-no-lit´ik) Any agent that softens or dissolves earwax in the external ear canal.

ceruminosis (sĕ-roo-mĭ-no´sis) Excessive formation of earwax.

cervical (ser´vĭ-kal) **1.** Relating to the neck. **2.** Relating to the uterine cervix.

cervical disk syndrome (ser´vĭ-kal disk sin´drōm) Pain, numbness, and muscular spasm of the neck, radiating to the shoulders, caused by irritation and compression of the cervical nerve roots by a protruding intervertebral disk.

cervical fusion syndrome (ser´vĭ-kal fu´zhun sin´drōm) See Klippel-Feil syndrome.

cervical rib syndrome (ser´vĭ-kal rib sin´drōm) Pain and tingling along the forearm and hand due to pressure upon the brachial plexus and subclavian artery by a rudimentary cervical rib, fibrous band, first thoracic rib, or tight scalene muscle.

cervicectomy (ser-vĭ-sek´tŏ-me) Amputation of the uterine cervix. Also called trachelectomy.

cervicitis (ser-vĭ-si´tis) Inflammation of the uterine cervix.

cystic c. A cervix containing multiple nabothian cysts.

cervicobrachial (ser-vĭ-ko-bra´ke-al) Relating to the neck and the arm.

cervix (ser´viks) (cx), *pl.* **cer´vices** Any constricted, necklike part of an organ or structure. The term is frequently used alone to denote the uterine cervix.

incompetent c. In pregnancy, a uterine cervix prone to dilate prematurely, usually resulting in midterm spontaneous abortion.

uterine c. The lowest portion of the uterus; its upper half, the *supravaginal cervix,* lies between the bladder and the rectouterine pouch; its lower half, the *vaginal cervix*, projects into the vagina; within the cervix is the cervical canal extending between two narrow openings: the internal os connecting with the uterine cavity, and the lower external os opening into the vagina. Popularly called neck of the womb.

cesarean (sĭ-zar´ē-ăn) **1.** See cesarean section, under section. **2.** See cesarean hysterectomy, under hysterectomy.

cesium (se´ze-um) Element of the alkali metal group, symbol Cs, atomic number 55, atomic weight 132.91.

Cestoda (ses-to´dă) A class of Platyhelminthes or flatworms, which includes the tapeworm.

cestode (ses´tōd) A tapeworm.

Chaddock's signs (chad´ŏks sīnz) Reflexes usually obtained in pyramidal tract lesions. (a) *Chaddock's toe sign:* extension of the toe on stroking the lateral malleolus and the lateral dorsum of the foot. (b) *Chaddock's wrist sign*: flexion of the wrist with fanning of the fingers upon stroking the wrist on the side of the little finger.

Chadwick's sign (chad´wiks sīnz) Bluish discoloration of the lining of the vagina and cervix; considered a probable sign of early pregnancy.

chafe (chāf) **1.** To irritate or wear away by rubbing. **2.** Irritation.

Chagas' disease (shă´găs dĭ-zēz´) Infection with the protozoan parasite *Trypanosoma cruzi*, usually transmitted by a blood-sucking arthropod when its feces contaminate skin abrasions, or by transfusion of contaminated blood; may cause encephalitis and damage to the heart and intestines. Also called American trypanosomiasis.

chain (chān) **1.** In chemistry, a group of atoms bonded together in a linear fashion. **2.** In bacteriology, a group of microorganisms attached end-to-end.

closed c. A chain formed by atoms linked together in the shape of a ring.

heavy c., H c. A large polypeptide chain of the immunoglobulin molecule, linked to light chains by disulfide bonds.

J c. A polypeptide chain present in certain immunoglobulin molecules, particularly IgM and IgA, which allows them to form polymers.

lateral c. See side chain.

light c., L c. Either of two small polypeptide chains, designated lambda and kappa, of the immunoglobulin molecule.

polypeptide c. A repeating peptide chain formed by amino acids, each of which contributes an identical group to the backbone of the chain plus a distinguishing radical as a side group.

side c. A group of atoms linked to a closed chain. Also called lateral chain.

sympathetic c. See sympathetic trunk, under trunk.

chalasia, chalasis (kă-la´zhă, kă-la´sis) The relaxation of a group of muscles, especially muscles that work together.

chalazion (kă-la´ze-on) A cyst in a tarsal (meibomian) gland that is seen merely as a lump in an otherwise normal eyelid. Also called meibomian cyst.

chalone (kal´ōn) A substance that inhibits cell division and is synthesized by mature cells of the tissue upon which it acts.

chamber (chām´ber) A closed space.

anterior c. of the eye The space between the

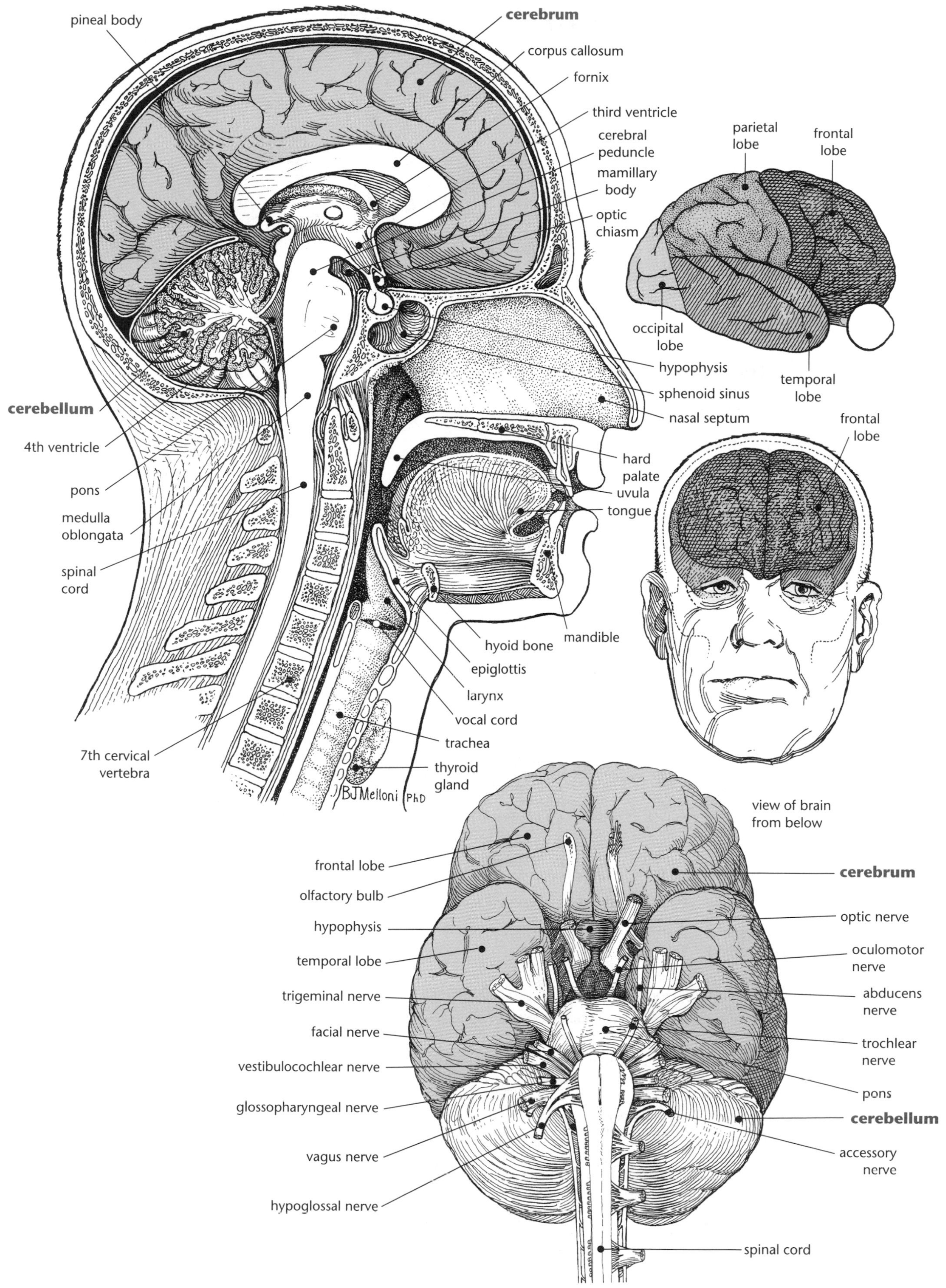
pineal body
cerebrum
corpus callosum
fornix
third ventricle
cerebral peduncle
mamillary body
optic chiasm
hypophysis
sphenoid sinus
nasal septum
hard palate
uvula
tongue
mandible
hyoid bone
epiglottis
larynx
vocal cord
trachea
thyroid gland
cerebellum
4th ventricle
pons
medulla oblongata
spinal cord
7th cervical vertebra
BJMelloni PhD
parietal lobe
frontal lobe
occipital lobe
temporal lobe
frontal lobe
view of brain from below
frontal lobe
olfactory bulb
hypophysis
temporal lobe
trigeminal nerve
facial nerve
vestibulocochlear nerve
glossopharyngeal nerve
vagus nerve
hypoglossal nerve
cerebrum
optic nerve
oculomotor nerve
abducens nerve
trochlear nerve
pons
cerebellum
accessory nerve
spinal cord

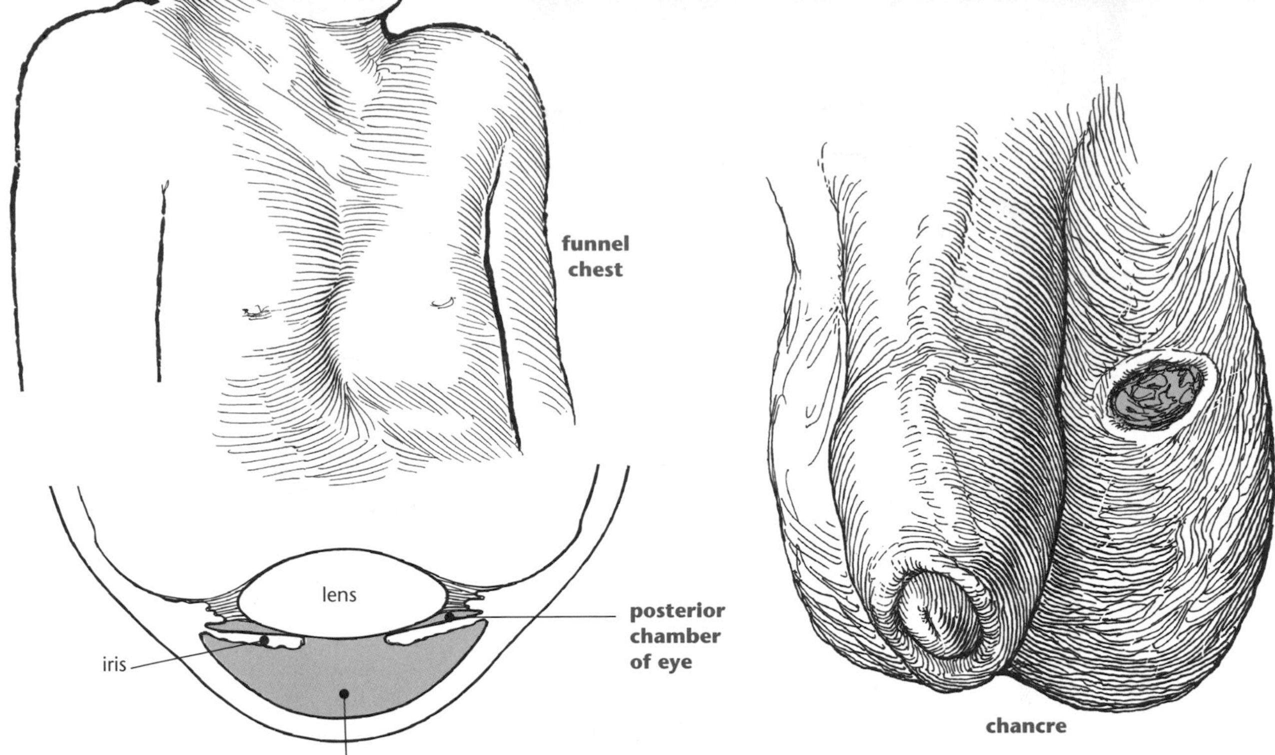

cornea and the iris; it is filled with aqueous humor.

hyperbaric c. A chamber in which the air pressure may be raised to higher than normal atmospheric pressure.

ionization c. A gas-filled enclosure fitted with electrodes between which an electric current passes when the gas is ionized by radiation.

middle ear c. See tympanic cavity, under cavity.

posterior c. of the eye The space between the iris and the lens; it is filled with aqueous humor.

pulp c. The area of the pulp cavity within the coronal portion of the tooth and into which the root canal opens.

Thoma's counting c. See Thoma-Zeiss hemocytometer, under hemocytometer.

vitreous c. The cavity of the eyeball behind the lens containing the vitreous body.

chancre (shang´ker) The first lesion of syphilis present at the site of entrance of the syphilitic infection; it appears as a hard, reddish ulcer with an eroded center covered by a yellowish secretion. Also called hard chancre; hunterian chancre; indurated chancre; true chancre; hard sore.

simple c. See chancroid.

soft c. See chancroid.

chancroid (shang´kroid) An infectious, non-syphilitic, pus-discharging, venereal ulcer caused by *Haemophilus ducreyi*. Also called soft chancre; simple chancre; soft sore.

change (chānj) A modification.

fatty c. Accumulation of fats (lipids) within cells; it occurs in all organs, most frequently in the liver in cases of cirrhosis.

fibrocystic c. of breast Benign condition of the female breast characterized by formation of cysts, overgrowth of connective tissue and intraductal epithelium, and sclerosing of gland tissue. Formerly called fibrocystic disease of breast; cystic hyperplasia of breast; chronic cystic mastitis; mammary dysplasia.

c. of life Popular term for menopause.

channel (chan´el) A passageway through which something flows.

chap (chap) **1.** To cause the skin to crack or split. **2.** A split or crack.

chaperone (shăp´ĕ-rōn) A protein that plays a role in the process of protein folding and translocation by binding to newly synthesized protein chains and preventing interactions with other proteins that might interfere with the intended pathway.

character (kar´ak-ter) **1.** A distinctive feature, attribute, or trait. **2.** The combination of a person's relatively stable personality traits and habitual modes of behavior.

charcoal (char´kōl) A black porous material obtained by burning wood with a restricted amount of air.

activated c. Medicinal charcoal, charcoal that has been treated to increase its adsorptive power, used as an antidote and to reduce hyperacidity.

Charcot-Marie-Tooth disease (shăr-kō´mă-re ´tōōth dĭ-zēz´) See peroneal muscular atrophy, under atrophy.

charley horse (char´le hors) A popular name for a cramp or stiffness of muscles, especially of the leg or arm following injury or excessive activity.

chart (chart) **1.** Information or data depicted in the form of graphs or tables. **2.** The health record of a patient. **3.** To enter information into the patient's record or to record data in graphic form.

checkbite (chek´bīt) See interocclusal record, under record.

Chediak-Higashi syndrome (cha´de-ăk he-gă´she sin´drōm) A rare hereditary condition found in infants; symptoms include decreased pigmentation of the skin, hair, and eyes, cytoplasmic inclusions of the leukocytes, and susceptibility to pyogenic infections; early death is common.

cheek (chēk) The fleshy side of the face forming the lateral wall of the oral cavity. Also called bucca; mala.

cheek biting (chēk bī´ting) Biting of the inner surface of the cheek; occasionally results in hyperkeratotic lesions and irritations of the buccal mucosa.

cheekbone (chēk´bōn) See zygomatic bone in table of bones.

cheilectomy (ki-lek´tŏ-me) **1.** Surgical removal of a portion of the lip. **2.** Cutting away of bony irregularities on the rim of a joint cavity.

cheilion (kī´lē-on) The corner or angle of the mouth.

cheilitis (kī-lī´tis) Inflammation of the lip. Also spelled chilitis.

actinic c., solar c. Inflammation of the lip characterized by a scaly crust on the vermillion border, usually due to overexposure to sunlight.

cheilognathouranoschisis (kī-lo-na-tho-u-ră-nos´kĭ-sis) Congenital malformation consisting of a cleft that extends from the palate, through the gum, to the upper lip.

cheiloplasty (kī´lo-plas-te) Plastic surgery of the lips. Also called labioplasty.

cheiloschisis (kī-los´kĭ-sis) See cleft lip, under lip.

cheilosis (kī-lo´sis) A noninflammatory condition of the lip marked by fissuring and chapping; characteristic of riboflavin deficiency.

cheiroscope (kī´ro-skōp) A binocular instrument used for antisuppression training of the eyes in strabismus.

chelate (ke´lāt) **1.** A compound containing a metal ion connected by coordinate bonds to two or more nonmetal ions in the same molecule. **2.** To effect chelation.

chelation (ke-la´shun) The coordinate bond formation between a metal ion and two or more nonmetal ions in the same molecule.

chemical (kem´ĭ-kal) **1.** Relating to chemistry. **2.** A substance produced by the interaction of elements.

chemise (shem´ēz´) A piece of linen used to secure a tampon around a catheter that has been inserted into a wound.

chemistry (kem´is-tre) The science concerned with the atomic and molecular composition of the different types of matter and the laws that govern their mutual reactions.

analytic c. The breaking up of compounds to determine and study their composition.

biologic c. See biochemistry.

inorganic c. The branch of chemistry concerned with substances not containing carbon.

organic c. The study of substances containing carbon.

physiologic c. See biochemistry.

chemobiotic (ke-mo-bi-ot´ik) Denoting a compound containing an antibiotic and another therapeutic chemical.

chemocautery (ke-mo-kaw´ter-e) The destruction of tissue by the application of a caustic substance.

chemoceptor (ke´mo-sep-tor) See chemoreceptor.

chemodectoma (ke-mo-dek-to´mă) A tumor of the chemoreceptor system, such as the carotid body, glomus jugulare, and aortic arch bodies.

chemodectomatosis (ke-mo-dek-to-ma-to´sis) Occurrence in the lungs of multiple minute tumors of the chemoreceptor type.

chemodifferentiation (ke-mo-dif-er-en-she-a´shun) Differentiation at the molecular level in the developing embryo; it precedes and controls morphologic differentiation.

chemoembolization (ke-mo-em-bŏ-liz-a´shun) Placement of a pellet containing an anticancer drug within arteries supplying blood to a malignant tumor. Pellets cut off the blood supply and deliver the drug directly to the tumor.

chemokines (ke´mo-kinz) Chemotactic hormone-like proteins (cytokines) that regulate the transit of white blood cells from blood to tissues. Each type of white blood cell has chemokine receptors that guide it to specific chemokines in the tissue.

chemokinesis (ke-mo-kĭ-ne´sis) Increased activity of cells stimulated by chemical substances.

chemoluminescence (ke-mo-loo-mĭ-nes´ens) **1.** Light produced by the transformation of chemical energy. **2.** Radiation producing chemical action.

chemolysis (ke-mol´ĭ-sis) Chemical decompo-

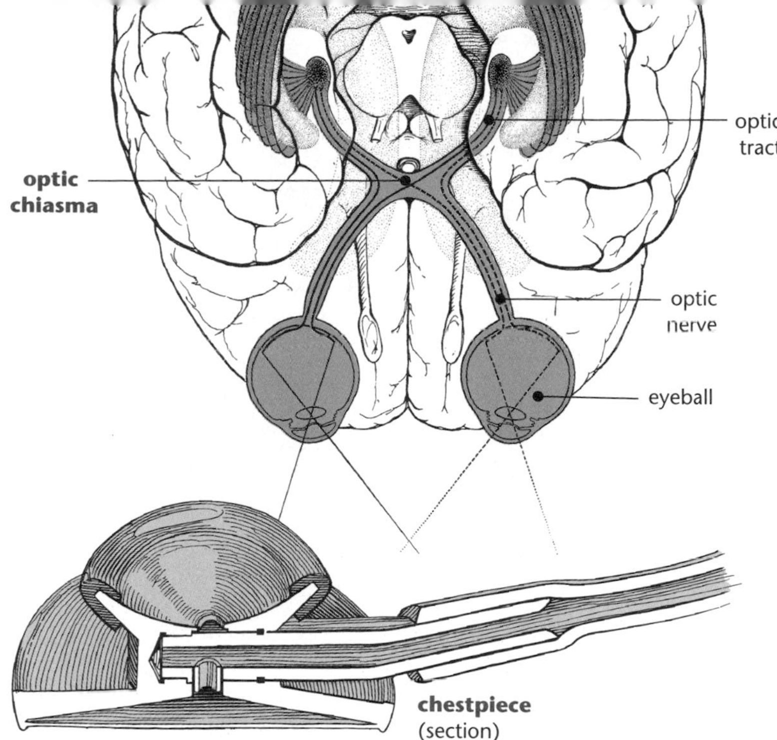

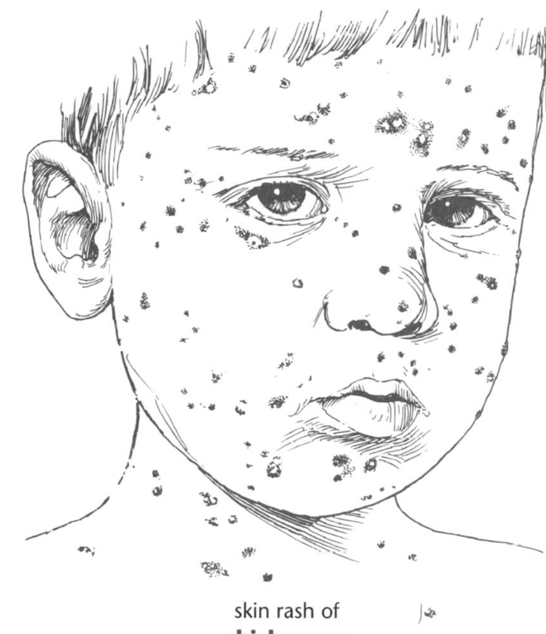

sition.

chemonucleolysis (ke-mo-noo-kle-ol´ĭ-sis) Dissolution of the center of an intervertebral disk by injecting it with an enzyme (e.g., chymopapain).

chemopallidectomy (ke-mo-pal-ĭ-dek´tŏ-me) Injection of a chemical substance in the globus pallidum in the brain; an operation performed for the relief of rigidity in parkinsonism.

chemopallidothalamectomy (ke-mo-pal-ĭ-do-thal-ă-mek´tŏ-me) Destruction of portions of brain tissue (globus pallidus and thalamus) by injection of a chemical.

chemoprophylaxis (ke-mo-pro-fĭ-lak´sis) Prevention of a specific disease by the use of a chemical.

chemoreceptor (ke-mo-re-sep´tor) An end organ (e.g., a taste bud) or sense organ (e.g., carotid body) that is sensitive to chemical stimuli. Also called chemoceptor.

chemosensitive (ke-mo-sen´sĭ-tiv) Sensitive to changes in the chemical composition of substances.

chemosis (ke-mo´sis) Eye disorder marked by swelling of the conjunctiva around the cornea.

chemosurgery (ke-mo-sur´jer-e) The use of chemical substances to destroy tissues.

chemotactic (ke-mo-tak´tic) Relating to chemotaxis.

chemotaxis (ke-mo-tak´sis) Movement of cells toward or away from a chemical substance, especially the unidirectional migration of white blood cells toward an attractant.

chemotherapeutics (ke-mo-ther-ă-pu´tiks) The branch of therapeutics dealing with the treatment of disease with chemicals.

chemotherapy (ke-mo-ther´a-pe) Treatment or prevention of disease by means of chemical substances.

chenodeoxycholic acid (ke-no-de-ok-se-kol´ik as´id) A bile that dissolves fats for intestinal absorption.

cherubism (cher´ŭ-biz-m) Uncommon hereditary disease affecting the jaws, manifested in childhood as painless bilateral swelling with upward turning of the eyes, which gives the child's face a characteristic cherubic appearance.

chest (chest) The upper part of the body between the neck and the diaphragm. Also see thorax.

barrel c. A short and round chest with ribs in a horizontal position; seen in cases of advanced emphysema.

flail c. An unstable chest wall due to multiple rib fractures causing a paradoxical motion (moving inward on inspiration and outward on expiration). Also called flapping chest wall.

funnel c. See pectus excavatum, under pectus.

keel c. See pectus carinatum, under pectus.

chestpiece (chest´pēs) The part of the stethoscope that is placed on the patient.

Chiari-Frommel syndrome (ke-ă´re-from´ĕl sin´drōm)(CFS) Prolonged milk secretion, absence of menstruation, and atrophy of the uterus after childbirth; generally associated with a benign tumor of the anterior lobe of the pituitary (adenohypophysis).

chiasma, chiasm (ki-az´mă, kī´az-m) An X-shaped crossing.

optic c. The point of crossing of the fibers of the optic nerves.

chickenpox (chik´en poks) An acute contagious disease, usually of young children, caused by the varicella-zoster virus (human herpesvirus 3); marked by a skin eruption, fever, and mild constitutional symptoms; incubation period is from 11 to 24 days. Also called varicella.

chigger (chig´er) Any of various six-legged larvae of mites, the most common being *Trombicula alfreddugesi*; the chigger usually attaches itself to parts of the body that are snugly clothed, such as the waist and ankles; itching generally begins three to six hours after it has attached. Also called red bug; harvest mite.

chigoe (chig´o) The small tropical sand flea, *Tunga penetrans*; the egg-carrying female burrows under the skin of humans, causing intense itching.

chilblains (chil´blāns) Condition resulting from prolonged exposure to extremely cold temperature, marked by inflammatory swelling of hands and feet accompanied by severe itching and burning sensations, and sometimes ulceration; usually affects individuals with a history of cold limbs in summer as well as in winter. Also called pernio. COMPARE: frostbite.

child (chīld) A young person between the periods of infancy and puberty.

battered c. A child who has been subjected to physical abuse, usually by parents, with resulting injuries.

hyperactive c. A child who shows excessive motor activity, fidgeting, talking, emotional instability, and usually short attention span (attention deficit).

childbearing (chīld´bār-ing) Pregnancy and parturition.

childbirth (chīld´birth) Parturition.

natural c. Management of parturition based on the concept that labor is easier for women who are relaxed and free of fear; this state is achieved by prenatal education, exercises, and psychologic conditioning and largely replaces anesthesia and surgical intervention. Also called physiologic childbirth.

physiologic c. See natural childbirth.

chill (chil) **1.** A moderate sensation of coldness. **2.** A feeling of coldness accompanied by shivering and fever.

Chilomastix (ki-lo-mas´tiks) A genus of protozoa parasitic in the intestines; one species, *Chilomastix mesnili*, is believed to cause diarrhea.

chimera (ki-me´ră) **1.** A person who has received genetically and immunologically different cell types, as in a graft or a bone marrow transplant. **2.** In experimental genetics, an organism developed from cells or tissues from two different species.

chimerism (ki-mēr´iz-m) The state of being a chimera.

blood c. The presence of two blood types in one individual, occurring when the blood of one dizygotic twin fetus is transferred to the other twin through a common blood vessel. Blood chimerism occurs in the second twin.

chin (chin) The central anterior prominence of the lower jaw. Also called mentum.

double c. Loose fatty flesh under the chin.

Chinese restaurant syndrome (chī-nēz´ res´ter-ant sin´drōm) Transient syndrome consisting of chest pains, throbbing of the head, and feelings of tightness of facial muscles after ingesting monosodium l-glutamate, which is generally used in Chinese food; occurs in individuals who are unusually sensitive to this additive.

chirognostic (ki-rog-nos´tik) Capable of distinguishing between right and left.

chirokinesthesia (ki-ro-kin-es-the´zhă) The subjective sensation of motions of the hand.

chiroplasty (ki´ro-plas-te) Plastic surgery of the hand.

chiropodist (ki-rop´ŏ-dist) See podiatrist.

chiropody (ki-rop´ŏ-de) See podiatry.

chiropractic (ki-ro-prak´tik) A philosophy of therapy in which disease is attributed to mild dislocations of the vertebral column, causing pressure on the nerves; the preferred method of treatment is by manipulation of the vertebrae. Also called chiropractic medicine.

chiropractor (ki-ro-prak´tor) One who practices chiropractic.

chisel (chis´el) A metal instrument with a beveled cutting edge designed after the carpenter's chisel; used in dentistry for cutting tooth enamel and in surgery for cutting bone.

chitin (kī´tin) A transparent, horny organic substance (polysaccharide), constituting the chief component of insect exoskeletons, crustacean shells; and the cell walls of certain fungi.

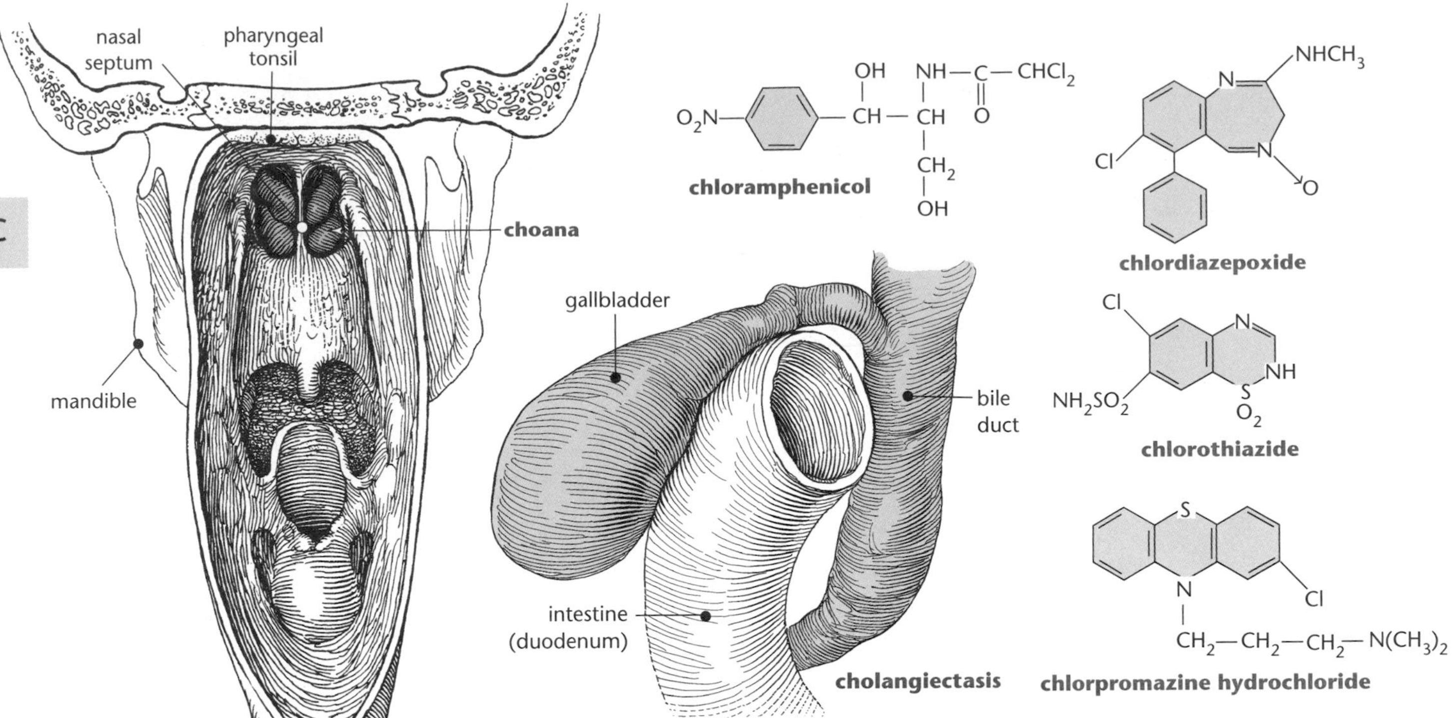

chitobiose (kī-to-bī´os) The disaccharide present in chitin.
chitosamine (kī-to´să-mēn) See glucosamine.
Chlamydia (klă-mid´e-ă) A genus of non-motile, gram-negative intracellular bacteria (family Chlamydiaceae); unlike viruses, they posses both RNA and DNA.
C. pneumoniae Species causing pneumonia and bronchitis.
C. psittaci A species causing a pulmonary infection.
C. trachomatis The cause of trachoma, inclusion conjunctivitis, lymphogranuloma venereum, urethritis, and proctitis.
chloasma (klo-az´mă) See melasma.
c. of pregnancy See melasma of pregnancy, under melasma.
chloracne (klor-ak´ne) A skin eruption, resembling acne, caused by constant contact with certain chlorinated compounds.
chloral (klor´al) A colorless oily liquid of pungent odor, CCl_3CHO; produced by the action of chlorine gas on alcohol.
c. hydrate A colorless crystalline compound, soluble in water and alcohol; used as a hypnotic and sedative.
chloralism (klor´al-iz-m) Condition caused by the constant use of chloral as an intoxicant.
chloralose (klor´ă-lōs) A crystalline substance used as a general anesthetic in laboratory animals.
chlorambucil (klor-am´bu-sil) A derivative of nitrogen mustard which retards proliferation and maturation of lymphocytes; used in the treatment of chronic lymphocytic leukemia and some lymphomas; Leukeran®.
chloramphenicol (klor-am-fen´ĭ-kol) A broad-spectrum antibiotic originally obtained from *Streptomyces venezuellae* but now produced synthetically; effective against many strains of gram-positive and gram-negative pathogenic micro-organisms; used selectively because of the occurrence (infrequently) of aplastic anemia; Chloromycetin®.
chlordane (klor´dān) A chlorinated hydrocarbon used as an insecticide; may cause human poisoning by absorption through the skin, inhalation, or ingestion.
chlordiazepoxide (klor-di-az-ĕ-pok´sīd) The nonproprietary name for Librium®, a drug widely used for treating anxiety, tension, and psychoneuroses.
chloremia (klor-e´me-ă) **1.** See chlorosis. **2.** See hyperchloremia.
chlorhydria (klor-hi´dre-ă) See hyperchlorhydria.
chloric (klor´ik) Containing chlorine.
chloride (klor´īd) Any compound of chlorine.
methyl c. The hydrochloric acid ester of methyl alcohol; a refrigerant, used in spray form as a local anesthetic. See chloromethane.
chloridimeter (klor-ĭ-dim´ĕ-ter) An apparatus for determining the amount of chlorides in fluids (e.g., blood, urine).
chloriduria (klor-ĭ-du´re-ă) The presence of chloride in the urine.
chlorinate (klor´ĭ-nāt) To combine with chlorine or a chlorine compound.
chlorinated (klor´ĭ-nāt-ed) Containing chlorine.
chlorine (klor´ēn) A greenish yellow, irritating, gaseous element; symbol Cl, atomic number 17, atomic weight 34.45; used as a disinfectant and bleaching agent.
chlorite (klor´īt) Any salt of chlorous acid.
chloroethane (klor-o-eth´ān) See ethyl chloride, under ethyl.
chloroform (klor´ŏ-form) A colorless, volatile, heavy liquid of sweetish taste, $CHCl_3$; formerly used as a general anesthetic.
chloroma (klor-o´mă) A tumor arising from myeloid tissue and containing a pale green pigment; most frequently found in the periosteum and ligamentous structures of the skull; seen usually in children and young adults.
chloromethane (klor-om-eth´āne) The hydrochloric acid ester of methyl alcohol, used in spray form as a local anesthetic. Also called methyl chloride.
chlorophyll, chlorophyl (klor´o-fil) Any of a group of green pigments in plant cells that absorb light during the food-making process of photosynthesis.
chlorophyllins (klor´o-fĭl-ins) Substances derived from chlorophyll, capable of absorbing odorous molecules and thus acting as deodorants.
chloroplast (klor´o-plast) A cytoplasmic organelle of all green plant cells; it contains chlorophyll.
chloropsia (klor-op´se-ă) A condition in which all objects appear to have a tint of green. Also called green vision.
chloroquine phosphate (klor´o-kwin fos´fāt) Quinoline diphosphate; an agent used in the treatment of malaria, hepatic amebiasis, and certain skin diseases.
chlorosis (klor-o´sis) A rarely used term for a type of iron deficiency anemia occurring in some adolescent girls; marked by a moderate reduction in red blood cells and a great reduction in hemoglobin content.
chlorothiazide (klor-o-thi´ă-zīd) A commonly prescribed diuretic and antihypertensive drug; it inhibits renal tubular reabsorption of sodium and is used in treating hypertension and edema due to congestive heart failure, liver disease, and pregnancy; Diuril®.
chlorotic (klō-rot´ik) Relating to chlorosis.
chlorpromazine hydrochloride (klōr-pro´mă-zēn hi-dro-klor´īd) A phenothiazine derivative used orally, muscularly, or intravenously to depress conditioned reflexes and the hypothalamic centers; used as a major tranquilizer, and in the management of postoperative nausea, and in radiation therapy and chemotherapy; Thorazine hydrochloride®.
chlorpropamide (klōr-pro´pă-mīd) An oral hypoglycemic agent in the sulfonylurea class; Diabinese®.
chlortetracycline (klōr-tet-ră-si´klēn) An antibiotic substance obtained from *Streptomyces aureofaciens*; active against hemolytic streptococci, staphylococci, typhoid bacilli, brucellae, and certain viruses; it has been supplanted in use by other tetracycline compounds with fewer side effects; Aureomycin®.
chloruresis (klōr-u-re´sis) The presence of chloride in the urine.
chloruretic (klor-u-ret´ik) Relating to an agent that promotes an increase of chloride excretion in the urine.
choana (ko´a-nă) The funnel-like opening of the nasal cavity into the nasopharynx on either side. Also called posterior naris.
choanal (ko´a-nal) Relating to a choana.
chokes (chōks) Popular term for a group of symptoms occurring in decompression sickness (e.g., chest pain and tightness, shallow breathing).
cholagogue (ko´lă-gog) Any agent that promotes the flow of bile.
cholangiectasis (ko-lan-je-ek´tă-sis) Dilatation of the bile duct.
cholangiocarcinoma (ko-lan-je-o-kar-sĭ-no´mă) Malignant tumor of the liver originating in the epithelium of the intrahepatic bile ducts.
cholangioenterostomy (ko-lan-je-o-en-ter-os´tŏ-me) Surgical union of the bile duct to the intestine.
cholangiography (ko-lan-je-og´ră-fe) Radiologic examination of the bile ducts after introduction of a contrast medium.
cholangiole (ko-lan´je-ōl) One of the minute terminal branches of the bile duct.
cholangiopancreatography (ko-lan-je-o-pan-kre-ă-tog´ră-fe) X-ray examination of the bile ducts and pancreas.
endoscopic retrograde c. (ERCP) Use of an endoscope to pass a catheter for injection of radiopaque medium into pancreatic and bile ducts.
cholangioscopy (ko-lan-je-os´kŏ-pe) Visual examination of the bile ducts with an endoscope.
cholangiotomy (ko-lan-je-ot´ŏ-me) Surgical incision into a bile duct.
cholangitis (ko-lan-jī tis) Inflammation of the bile

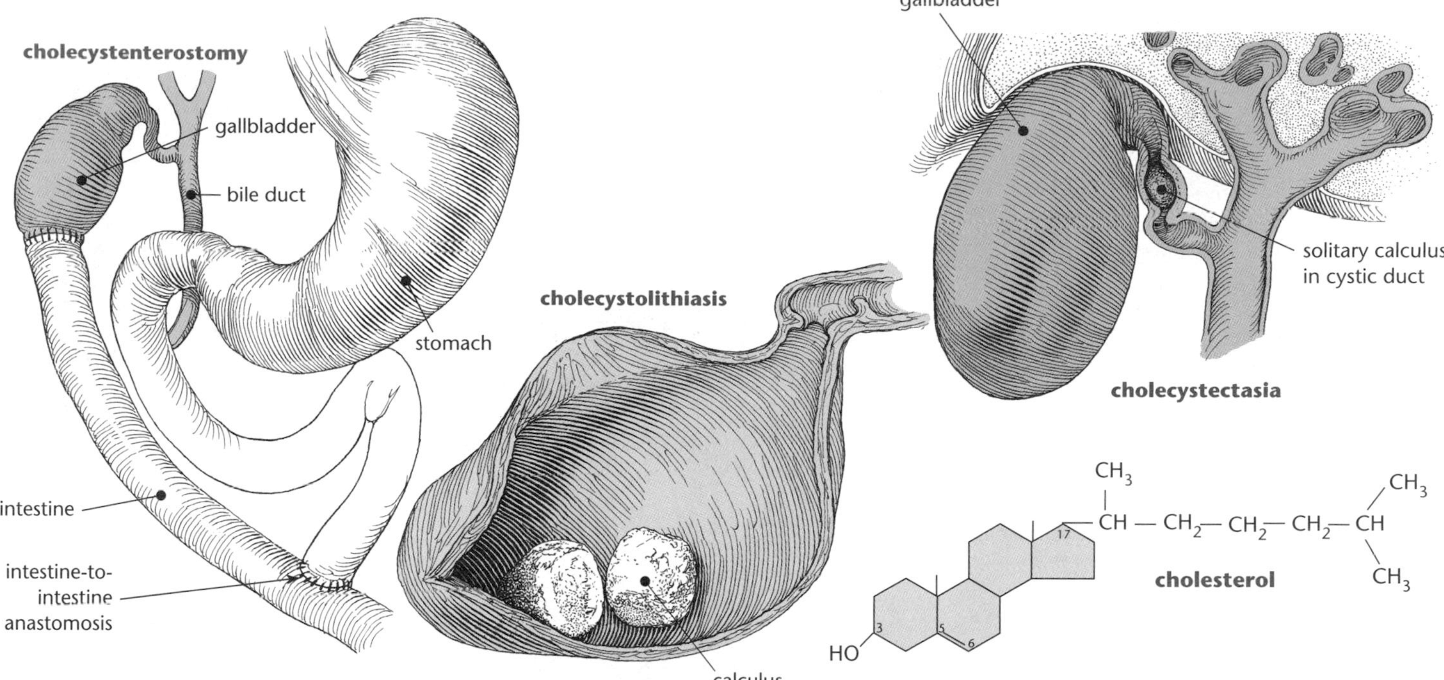

duct.

cholanopoiesis (ko-lă-no-poi-e´sis) Synthesis by the liver of cholic acid or its conjugates, or of natural bile salts.

cholecalciferol (ko-le-kal-sif´er-ol) See vitamin D_3, under vitamin.

cholechromopoiesis (ko-le-kro-mo-poi-e´sis) Synthesis of bile pigments by the liver.

cholecyst (ko´le-sist) See gallbladder.

cholecystagogue (ko-le-sis´tă-gog) An agent that stimulates gallbladder activity.

cholecystectasia (ko-le-sis-tek-ta´zhă) Dilatation of the gallbladder.

cholecystectomy (ko-le-sis-tek´tŏ-me) Surgical removal of the gallbladder.

cholecystenterostomy (ko-le-sis-ten-ter-os´tŏ-me) Surgical joining of the gallbladder and the intestine.

cholecystic (ko-le-sis´tik) Relating to the gallbladder.

cholecystis (ko-le-sis´tis) See gallbladder.

cholecystitis (ko-le-sis-ti´tis) Inflammation of the gallbladder.

cholecystoduodenostomy (ko-le-sis-to-doo-ŏ-dĕ-nos´tŏ-me) Surgical creation of a direct connection between the gallbladder and the duodenum.

cholecystogram (ko-le-sis´to-gram) An x-ray image of the gallbladder.

cholecystography (ko-le-sis-tog´ră-fe) X-ray visualization of the gallbladder after administration of a radiopaque substance, which is excreted by the liver and concentrated by the gallbladder.

cholecystojejunostomy (ko-le-sis-to-je-joo-nos´tŏ-me) Surgical establishment of a connection between the gallbladder and jejunum.

cholecystokinase (ko-le-sis-to-kī´nās) An enzyme that promotes the breakdown of cholecystokinin.

cholecystokinetic (ko-le-sis-to-kĭ-net´ik) Causing release of the gallbladder contents.

cholecystokinin (ko-le-sis-to-ki´nin) (CCK) A hormone secreted by the mucosa of the upper intestinal tract; it stimulates contraction of the gallbladder.

cholecystolithiasis (ko-le-sis-to-lĭ-thi´ă-sis) The presence of one or more stones in the gallbladder.

cholecystorraphy (ko-le-sis-tor´ă-fe) Suturing of the gallbladder.

cholecystostomy (ko-le-sis-tos´tŏ-me) Surgical formation of an opening into the gallbladder with insertion of a drainage tube through the abdominal wall.

cholecystotomy (ko-le-sis-tot´ŏ-me) Surgical incision into the gallbladder.

choledoch (ko´le-dok) The bile duct.

choledochal (ko-led´ŏ-kal) Relating to the bile duct.

choledochectomy (kol-ĕ-do-kek´tŏ-me) Surgical removal of a portion of the bile duct.

choledochitis (kol-ĕ-do-ki´tis) Inflammation of the bile duct.

choledochoduodenostomy (ko-led-o-ko-doo-o-dĕ-nos´tŏ-me) Surgical anastomosis between the bile duct and the duodenum.

choledochoenterostomy (ko-led-ŏ-ko-en-ter-os´tŏ-me) Surgical formation of a connection between the bile duct and any part of the intestine.

choledochography (ko-led-ŏ-kog´ră-fe) X-ray visualization of the bile duct after administration of a radiopaque material.

choledocholith (ko-led´ŏ-ko-lith) Stone in the bile duct.

choledocholithiasis (ko-led-ŏ-ko-lĭ-thi´ă-sis) The presence of stones in the bile duct.

choledocholithotomy (ko-led-ŏ-ko-lĭ-thot´ŏ-me) Incision into the bile duct for the removal of a stone.

choledochoplasty (ko-led-ŏ-ko-plas´te) Reparative surgery of the bile duct.

choledochorrhaphy (ko-led-ŏ-kor´ă-fe) Suturing of the bile duct.

choledochoscope (ko-led´ŏ-ko-skōp) A flexible fiberoptic instrument for inspecting the lumen of the bile duct.

choledochoscopy (ko-led-ŏ-kos´ko-pe) Visual examination of the bile duct with a choledochoscope.

choledochostomy (ko-led-ŏ-kos´tŏ-me) Surgical formation of an opening into the bile duct for drainage.

choledochotomy (ko-led-ŏ-kot´ŏ-me) Surgical incision into the bile duct.

choledochous (ko-led´ŏ-kus) Containing or conveying bile.

cholelith (ko´le-lith) See gallstone.

cholelithiasis (ko-le-lĭ-thi´ă-sis) The presence of gallstones.

cholelithotomy (ko-le-lĭ-thot´ŏ-me) Surgical removal of a gallstone.

cholemesis (ko-lem´ĕ-sis) The vomiting of bile.

cholemia (ko-le´me-ă) The presence of bile in the blood.

cholemic (ko-le´mik) Relating to the presence of bile in the blood.

choleperitonitis (ko-le-per-ĭ-tŏ-ni´tis) Inflammation caused by the presence of bile in the peritoneal cavity.

cholepoiesis (ko-le-poi-e´sis) The formation of bile.

cholera (kol´er-ă) An acute infectious disease caused by the bacterium *Vibrio cholerae*; marked by severe diarrhea, vomiting, cramps, loss of huge amounts of fluid and electrolyte, and collapse. Transmitted by contaminated drinking water.

choleresis (ko-ler´ĕ-sis) Secretion of bile by the liver, distinguished from the expulsion of bile by the gallbladder.

cholerrhagia (ko-le-ra´je-ă) Excessive secretion of bile.

cholescintigraphy (kol-e-sin-tig´ră-fe) Noninvasive scanning of the gallbladder and the cystic and bile ducts after injection of a radionuclide to determine patency of the ducts and evaluate emptying of the gallbladder.

cholestasis (ko-le-sta´sis) Suppression or arrest of the flow of bile.

cholestatic (ko-le-stat´ik) Tending to arrest the flow of bile.

cholesteatoma (ko-le-ste-ă-to´mă) A tumor-like mass in the middle ear composed of a lining of stratified squamous epithelium filled with material containing blood and cholesterol; associated with chronic middle ear infection.

cholesteremia (ko-les-ter-e´me-ă) Increased amounts of cholesterol in the blood.

cholesterol (ko-les´ter-ol) A white, waxy, crystalline organic alcohol; a universal tissue constituent, present in all animal fats and oils, in bile, brain tissue, blood, and egg yolk; it constitutes a large portion of the most common type of gallstone and is found in deposits in the vessel walls in atherosclerosis.

cholesterolosis (ko-les-ter-ol-o´sis) Focal deposits of cholesterol in the tissues, especially the gallbladder mucosa.

cholestyramine (ko-les-ti´ră-mēn) An agent that binds with dietary cholesterol and acidic drugs in the gastrointestinal tract. Used to treat hypercholesteremia.

cholic (ko´lik) Relating to the bile.

cholic acid (ko´lik as´id) A digestive acid present in bile.

choline (ko´lēn) A compound synthesized by the body and found in most animal tissues; important in fat metabolism; a precursor of acetylcholine.

cholinergic (ko-lin-er´jik) **1.** Stimulated by or capable of liberating acetylcholine; parasympathomimetic. **2.** Simulating the effects of acetylcholine.

cholinester (ko-lin-es´ter) An ester of choline.

cholinesterase (ko-lin-es´ter-ās) Any of several enzymes that promote the hydrolysis of acetylcholine.

cholinomimetic (ko-lin-o-mi-met´ik) Producing an effect similar to that of acetylcholine.

cholorrhea (kol-o-re´ă) Excessive secretion of bile.

cholylcoenzyme A (ko-lĭl-ko-en´zīm) A condensation product of choline and coenzyme A.

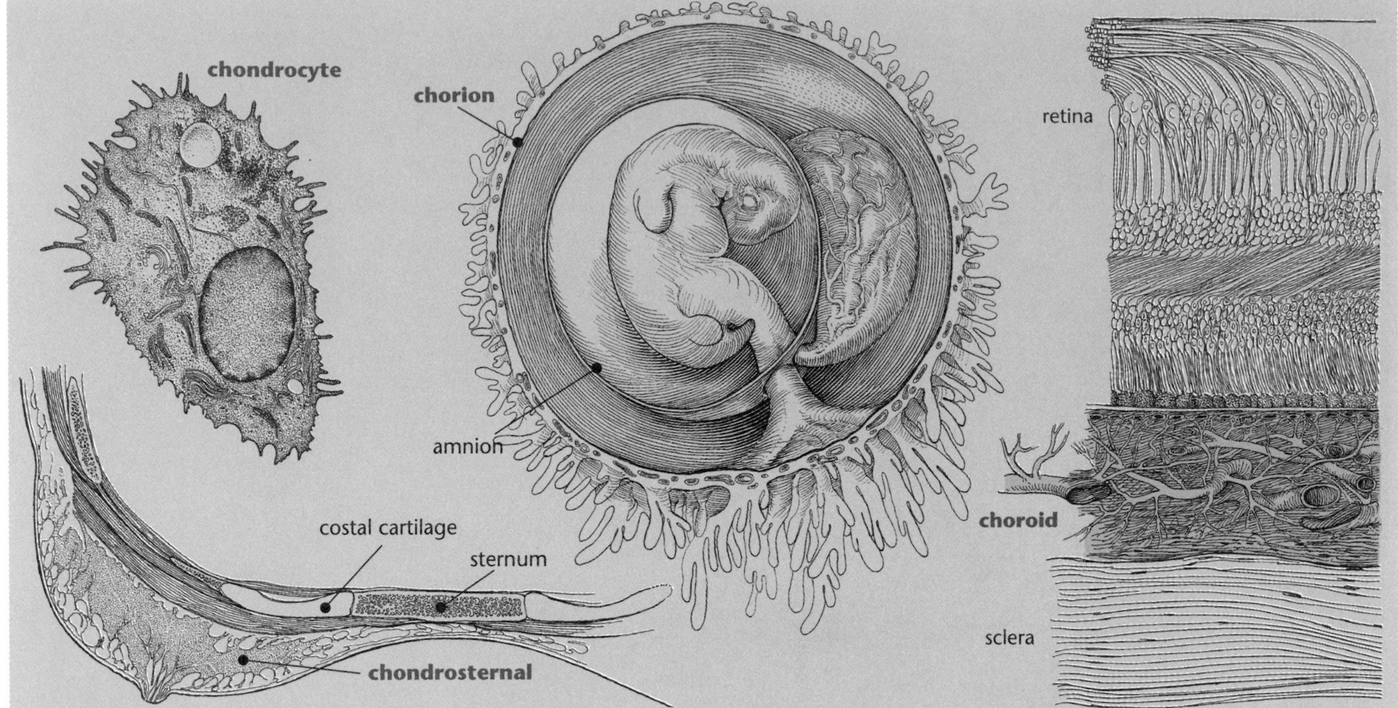

cholytaurine (ko-lil-taw´rēn) See taurocholic acid.
chondral (kon´dral) Relating to cartilage.
chondralgia (kon-dral´jă) See chondrodynia.
chondrectomy (kon-drek´tŏ-me) Removal of a cartilage.
chondrification (kon-drĭ-fĭ-ka´shun) Conversion into cartilage.
chondritis (kon-dri´tis) Inflammation of cartilage.
costal c. See costochondritis.
chondroblast (kon´dro-blast) A cartilage-pro-ducing cell.
chondroblastoma (kon-dro-blas-to´mă) A benign tumor of long bones composed of cartilage-like tissue; occurs mostly in persons under the age of 20 years.
chondrocalcinosis (kon-dro-kal-sĭ-no´sis) Calcified deposits in articular cartilage and synovial fluid of large joints, producing arthritic pain and goutlike symptoms.
chondroclast (kon´dro-klast) A giant cell concerned with the absorption of cartilage.
chondrocostal (kon-dro-kos´tal) Relating to the cartilage of the ribs.
chondrocyte (kon´dro-sīt) A cartilage cell; since the cartilage has no blood vessels, the chondrocyte receives its nutrition by diffusion from the capillaries of the perichondrium.
chondrodermatitis nodularis chronica helicis (kon-dro-der-mă-ti´tis nod-u-lar´is kron´ĭ-kă hel´ĭ-sis) The presence of painful nodules on the helix of the ear.
chondrodynia (kon-dro-din´e-ă) Pain in a cartilage. Also called chondralgia.
chondrodystrophy, chondrodystrophia (kon-dro-dis´trŏ-fe, kon-dro-dis-tro´fe-ă) Abnormal development of cartilage, especially at the epiphyses of long bones, resulting in stunted growth of the limbs and short stature (chondrodystrophic dwarfism), while the head and vertebral column develop normally. Also called chondrodysplasia.
chondrogenesis (kon-dro-jen´ĕ-sis) The forma-tion of cartilage.
chondroma (kon-dro´mă) A benign tumor com-posed of cartilage.
chondromalacia (kon-dro-mă-la´shă) Softening of an articular cartilage, most commonly seen in the kneecap (patella).
chondromatosis (kon-dro-mă-to´sis) The presence of multiple cartilaginous growths (chondromas).
chondro-osseous (kon-dro-os´e-us) Relating to cartilage and bone.
chondro-osteodystrophy (kon-dro-os´te-o-dis´tro-fe) General term for a group of disorders involving bone and cartilage (e.g., Morquio's syndrome). Also called osteochondrodystrophy.
chondropathy (kon-drop´ă-the) Any disease of cartilage.
chondrophyte (kon´dro-fīt) A cartilaginous growth at the articular surface of a bone.
chondroplasty (kon´dro-plas-te) Reparative surgery of cartilage.
chondrosamine (kon-dro´să-mēn) See galactosamine.
chondrosarcoma (kon-dro-sar-ko´mă) A malignant bone tumor derived from cartilage cells; it erodes the bone and invades adjacent soft tissues.
chondrosternal (kon-dro-ster´nal) Relating to the rib cartilages and the sternum.
chondrotome (kon´dro-tōm) A surgical knife used for cutting cartilage.
chorda (kor´dă), *pl.* **chordae** **1.** A tendon. **2.** A stringlike anatomic structure.
chordae tendineae Tendinous strands in the heart ventricles, extending from the papillary muscles to the leaflets of the atrioventricular valves.
c. tympani A branch of the facial nerve that innervates the submandibular and sublingual glands and the anterior two-thirds on the tongue.
Chordata (kor-da´tă) The phylum that includes all animals having a notochord at some developmental stage.
chordee (kor´de, kor-de´) Abnormal downward curvature of the penis due to fibrous bands on the undersurface of the corpora.
chorditis (kor-di´tis) Inflammation of a chord.
chordoma (kor-do´mă) A slow-growing malignant tumor arising from remnants of notochordal tissue; occurs along the vertebral column, especially the sacrococcygeal area and at the base of the skull.
chorea (kor-e´ă) Any of a group of disorders characterized by brief, rapid, involuntary movements of the limbs, face, trunk, and head.
acute c. See Sydenham's chorea.
chronic progressive c. See hereditary chorea.
hereditary c. A hereditary, progressive, degenerative disease of the brain beginning in adult life and causing mental deterioration; characterized by involuntary jerky movements, usually of the trunk, shoulders, and lower limbs. Also called chronic progressive chorea; Huntington's chorea.
Huntington's c. See hereditary chorea.
infectious c. See Sydenham's chorea.
senile c. Mild involuntary, usually unilateral, movements of the limbs occurring in the aged.
Sydenham's c. A symptom complex occurring in children, marked by muscle weakness, lack of coordination, and involuntary movements intensified by voluntary effort; associated with acute rheumatic fever. Also called acute chorea; St.Vitus' dance; infectious chorea.
choreic (ko-re´ik) Of or relating to chorea.
choreiform (ko-re´ĭ-form) Resembling chorea (a spasmodic nervous disorder).
choreoathetoid (kor-e-o-ath´ĕ-toid) Characterized by choreoathetosis.
choreoathetosis (kor-e-o-ath-ĕ-to´sis) Abnormal involuntary movements of the body, a combination of choreic and athetoid patterns such as twitching, writhing, contortions of the face, heel walking, and bizarre postures.
chorioadenocarcinoma (ko-re-o-ad´ĕ-no-kar-sĭ-no´mă) See invasive mole, under mole.
chorioadenoma destruens (ko-re-o-ad-ĕ-no´mă des-tru´ens) See invasive mole, under mole.
chorioamnionitis (ko-re-o-am-ne-on-i´tis) Inflammation of the fetal membranes.
chorioangioma (kor-e-o-an-je-o´mă) A rare benign tumor arising from placental capillaries, which appears as a solitary nodule in the placenta.
choriocarcinoma (ko-re-o-kar-sĭ-no´mă) **1.** Gestational choriocarcinoma; an uncommon but highly malignant tumor of the placenta derived from cells of the original placental tissues (trophoblast) most often found in the uterus after a pregnancy, frequently as a complication of a hydatidiform mole; occasionally it occurs after an abortion. Also called chorioepithelioma; chorionic epithelioma; trophoblastoma. **2.** A rare primary germ cell tumor of the ovary unrelated to gestational choriocarcinoma, associated with elevated levels of human chorionic gonadotropin (hCG).
chorioepithelioma (ko-re-o-ep-ĭ-the-le-o mă) See choriocarcinoma.
choriomeningitis (kor-e-o-men-in-ji´tis) Inflh involvement of the choroid plexuses, especially of the third and fourth ventricles.
lymphocytic c. A disease affecting rodents, especially mice, sometimes transmitted to humans; caused by an arenavirus (family Arenaviridae).
chorion (ko´re-on) The outermost membrane of the sac enclosing the fetus.
chorioepithelioma (kor-e-o-ep-ĭ-the-le-o´mă) See choriocarcinoma.
chorionic (ko-re-on´ik) Relating to the outermost of the fetal membranes (chorion).
chorioretinitis (ko-re-o-ret-i-ni´tis) Inflammation of two layers of tissue investing the eyeball, the vascular layer (choroid) and the light sensitive layer (retina). Also called Jensen's disease; retinochoroiditis.
choristoma (kor-is-to´mă) A growth composed of normal tissue occurring in abnormal locations.
choroid (kor´oid) **1.** The middle, vascular layer of

chromosomes arranged in pairs according to size

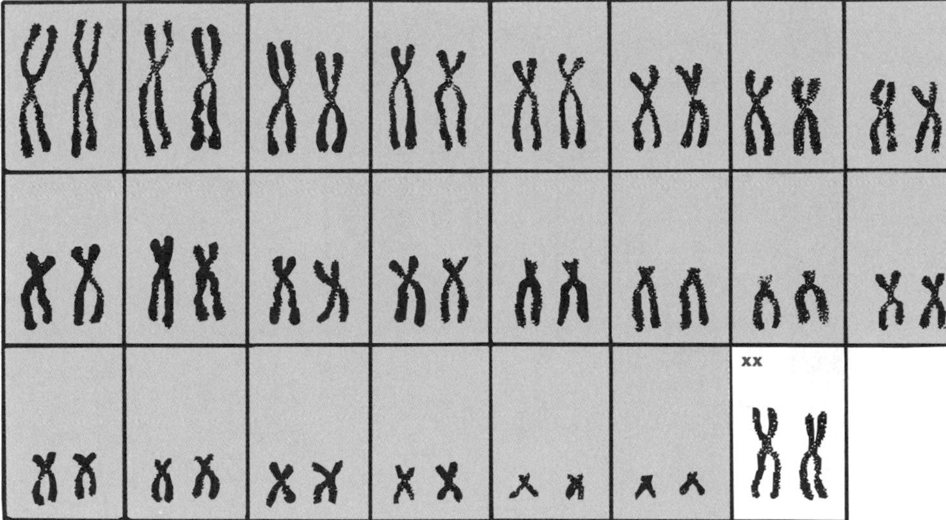

karotype of normal female

acrocentric chromosome

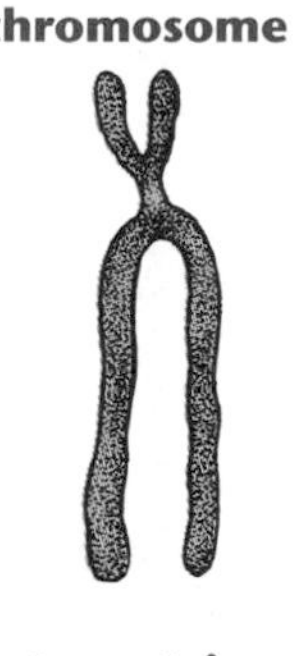

acrocentric chromosome with satellites

satellite

metacentric chromosome

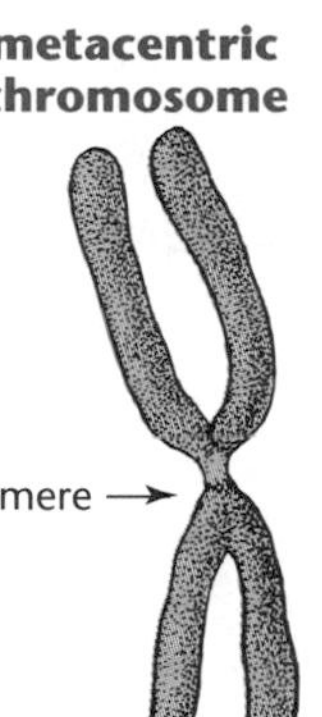

submetacentric chromosome

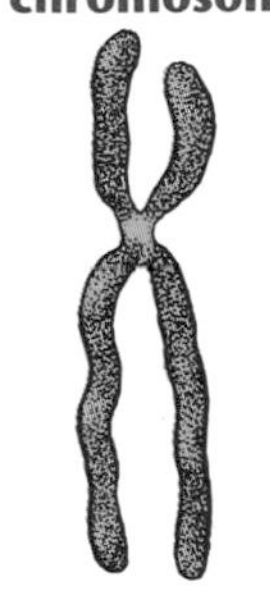

the eyeball. **2.** Resembling the outermost membrane (chorion) enclosing the fetus.

choroideremia (kor-oid-ĕr-e´me-ă) Hereditary disease marked by progressive degeneration of the vascular layer of the eye (choroid); the earliest symptom is night blindness followed by loss of peripheral vision and eventual total blindness.

choroiditis (kor-oid-i´tis) Inflammation of the vascular coat of the eye.

choroidocyclitis (kor-oi-do-sik-li´tis) Inflam-mation of the vascular coat of the eye and the ciliary body.

Christmas disease (kris´mas dĭs-zēz´) Hemo-philia B. See also factor IX.

chromaffin (kro-maf´in) Readily staining a yellow or brown color; with chromium salts; denoting certain cells present mostly in the medulla of the adrenal glands and to a lesser extent along the ganglionated sympathetic chain (paraganglia) and the abdominal aorta.

chromaffinoma (kro-maf-ĭ-no´mă) A tumor composed of chromaffin tissues.

chromaffinopathy (kro-maf-ĭ-nop´ă-the) Any disease of the chromaffin tissues.

chromate (kro´māt) A salt of chromic acid.

chromatic (kro-mat´ik) Relating to color.

chromatids (kro´mă-tids) Two daughter strands joined by a single centromere, formed by the splitting of a chromosome in the prophase stage of mitosis; eventually each chromatid becomes a chromosome.

chromatin (kro´mă-tin) The association of DNA and proteins in the cell nucleus, comprising the chromosomes and staining readily with basic dyes.

sex c. The chromatin mass in the nucleus of somatic (body) cells of the normal female; it represents a single, condensed, and inactive X chromosome. Its presence or absence in cells obtained from a smear of the inside of the cheek (buccal mucosa) has been used to determine a person's sexual genotype. Also called Barr chromatin body; Barr body; sex chromatin body.

chromatism (kro´mă-tiz´m) **1.** Abnormal pigmentation. **2.** Color distortion in an image produced by a lens. Also called chromatic aberration.

chromatogenous (kro-mă-toj´ĕ-nus) Producing pigmentation or color.

chromatogram (kro-mat´o-gram) The absorbent column containing the stratified constituents separated from a solution by chromatography.

chromatography (kro-mă-tog´ră-fe) A method of chemical analysis by means of which substances in solution are separated into constituent layers of different colors as they pass through an adsorbent (paper or powder) at different velocities.

gas c. Differential separation of complex mixtures by vaporizing and diffusing the substance along with a carrier gas through an adsorbent.

high-performance liquid c., high-pressure liquid c. (HPLC) Separation and quantitation of substances in solution by forcing the mixture through a column of sorbent and a detector; used to measure organic compounds (e.g., steroid hormones, drugs, carcinogens, toxins).

paper c. Partition chromatography in which one of the substances being separated adheres to, and forms a film on, filter paper; used in biochemistry to estimate traces of complex organic compounds. Also called paper partition chromatography.

paper partition c. See paper chromatography.

partition c. Separation of similar substances by repeated divisions between immiscible liquids.

thin-layer c. (TLC) Chromatography through a thin layer of an inert material (e.g., cellulose) supported on a glass or plastic plate.

chromatolysis (kro-mă-tol´ĭ-sis) Dissolution of the chromidial (chromophilic) substance (Nissl bodies) in the neuron following injury to the cell body or its axon.

chromatomere (kro-mă-to´mēr) A group of membrane-limited round granules containing a substance thought to have lysosomal properties.

chromatometer (kro-mă-tom´ĕ-ter) See chromometer.

chromatophilic (kro-mă-to-fil´ik) Staining easily.

chromatopsia (kro-mă-top´se-ă) Color vision, an abnormal condition in which all objects appear tinged with one particular color. Also called chromopsia.

chromatoptometry (kro-mă-top-tom´ĕ-tre) See chromometry.

chromesthesia (kro-mes-the´zhă) **1.** Condition in which colors are seen when other senses are stimulated. **2.** The perception of other sensations, such as taste or smell, when colors are seen. **3.** The color sense.

chromidium (kro-mid´e-um), *pl.* **chromid´ia** A granule in the cell cytoplasm that stains deeply with basic dyes.

chromium (kro´me-um) A steel-gray metallic element; symbol Cr, atomic number 24, atomic weight 52.01.

Chromobacterium (kro-mo-bak-tēr´e-um) A genus of gram-negative flagellated bacteria (family Rhizobiaceae); it produces a violet pigment.

chromoblast (kro´mo-blast) An embryonic pigment cell.

chromoblastomycosis (kro-mo-blas-to-mi-ko´sis) A localized skin disease caused by *Phialophora* or *Cladosporium*, principally in the tropics; the lesion is usually a slow-growing nodule that ulcerates and becomes purplish red to gray and wartlike. Also called chromomycosis.

chromocyte (kro´mo-sīt) A pigmented cell.

chromocytometer (kro-mo-sī-tom´ĕ-ter) An instrument for determining the amount of hemoglobin in red blood cells.

chromogen (kro´mo-jĕn) **1.** A substance capable of chemically changing into a pigment. **2.** A pigment-producing organelle.

chromogenesis (kro-mo-jen´ĕ-sis) The production of pigment.

chromogranin A (kro-mo-gran´in) Protein stored and released with catecholamines from the adrenal medulla.

chromometer (kro-mom´ĕ-ter) A scale used for testing color perception. Also called chromatometer.

chromometry (kro-mom´ĕ-tre) The measuring of color perception. Also called chromatoptometry.

chromomycosis (kro-mo-mi-ko´sis) See chromoblastomycosis.

chromonema (kro-mo-ne´mă), *pl.* **chromone´mata** A coiled filament that extends the entire length of a chromosome and contains the genes.

chromophil, chromophile (kro´mo-fil, kro´mo-fīl) A cell or tissue that stains readily.

chromophilia (kro-mo-fil´e-ă) The property of being readily stained; said of certain cells.

chromophilic, chromophilous (kro-mo-fil´ik, kro-mof´ĭ-lus) Staining readily.

chromophobe, chromophobic (kro´mo-fōb, kro-mo-fo´bik) Denoting a cell or tissue that resists staining.

chromophobia (kro-mo-fo´be-ă) **1.** Resistance to staining. **2.** Morbid dislike of colors.

chromophore (kro´mo-for) Color radical, a molecular group that is capable of selective absorption of light, resulting in coloration of certain substances.

chromoprotein (kro-mo-pro´tēn) A compound, such as hemoglobin, composed of a pigment and a simple protein.

chromopsia (kro-mop´se-ă) See chromatopsia.

chromoscope (kro´mo-skōp) An instrument or scale used in the study and testing of color phenomena as related to color perception.

chromosome (kro´mo-sōm) One of a group of threadlike structures contained in the nucleus of a cell; it contains DNA encoding genetic information (hereditary material from both parents); human cells normally have 46 (23 pairs) chromosomes.

acrocentric c. A chromosome with the centromere placed very close to one end so that the shorter arm is very small.

metacentric c. A chromosome with a centrally placed centromere that divides the chromosome into two arms of approximately equal length.

C

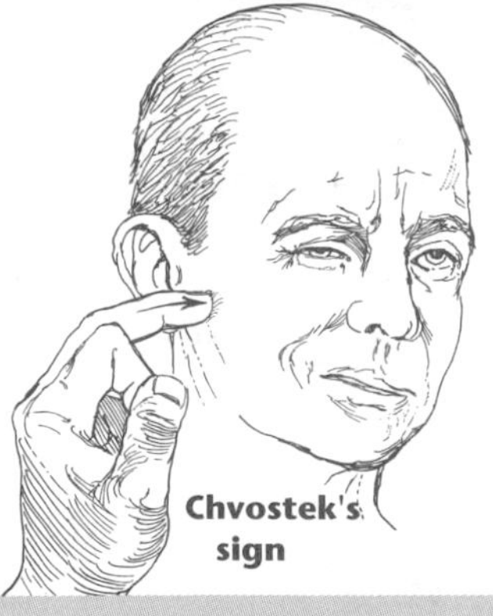

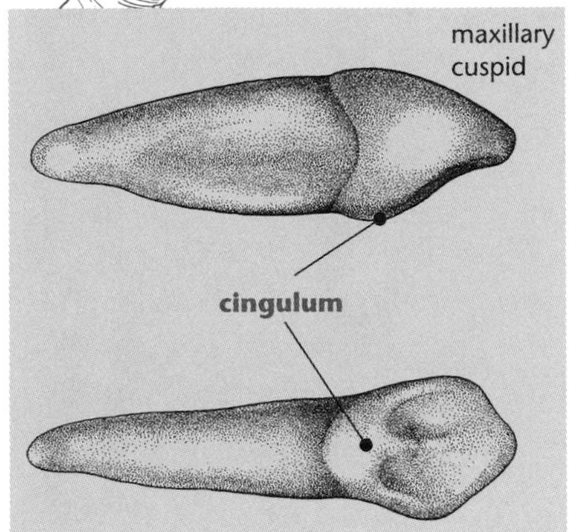

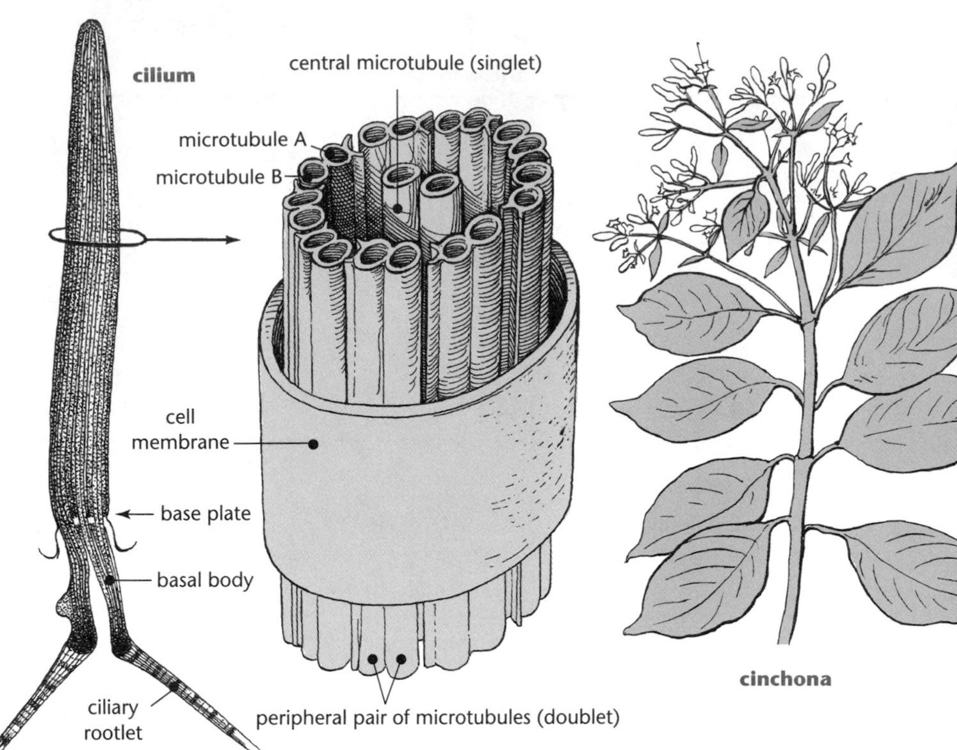

mitochondrial c. A small circular chromosome in the mitochondria of a cell (instead of the cell nucleus); it contains its own unique DNA and is the basis for maternal inheritance with a high rate of mutations; has been demonstrated in several neuromuscular disorders (e.g., Leber's hereditary optic neuropathy). See also mitochondrial DNA, under DNA.

Philadelphia (Ph^1) **c.** An abnormal minute chromosome probably derived from a small acrocentric chromosome (no. 21 or 22) by loss of a large part of the long arm; found in cultured leukocytes of many patients afflicted with chronic myelocytic leukemia.

c. satellite A small chromosomal segment separated from the main body of the chromosome by a secondary constriction; in humans, usually associated with the short arm of an acrocentric chromosome.

sex c.'s Chromosomes responsible for the determination of sex; normally females have two X chromosomes, males have one X and one Y.

submetacentric c. A chromosome with the centromere so placed that it divides the chromosome into two arms of unequal length.

telocentric c. A chromosome with a terminal centromere; such chromosomes are unstable and arise by misdivision or breakage within the centromere region.

X c. One of the sex chromosomes carried by the female in a double dose (two XX) and by the male in a single dose (one X and one Y).

Y c. One of the sex chromosomes carried by the male in a single dose (one Y and one X).

chronaxie, chronaxy (kro′nak-se, kro′nak-se) The unit of excitability of nerve or muscle tissue; the time required by an electric current (of twice the minimum strength needed to elicit a threshold response) to pass through a motor nerve and cause a contraction in the associated muscle.

chronic (kron′ik) Denoting a disease of slow progress and persisting over a long period of time; opposite of acute.

chronic granulomatous disease (kron′ik gran-u-lom′ă-tus dĭ-zēz′) (CGD) A congenital susceptibility to severe infection due to inability of polymorphonuclear leukocytes to destroy bacteria; an X-linked recessive inheritance. Also called congenital dysphagocytosis.

chronobiology (kron-o-bi-ol′ŏ-je) The study of biological rhythms in individual organisms.

chronognosis (kron-og-no′sis) Perception of the passage of time.

chronograph (kron′o-graf) Instrument for graphically recording short periods of time, such as the duration of an event or episode.

chronophotograph (kron-o-fo′to-graf) One of a series of photographs showing motion.

chronotaraxis (kron-o-tar-ak′sis) Confusion relating to the passage of time.

chronotropism (kro-not′ro-piz-m) Modification of the rate of a regular periodic movement, as of the heart beat.

chrysiasis (krĭ-si′ă-sis) Deposition of gold in the tissues following administration of gold salts. Also called auriasis.

chrysotherapy (kris-o-ther′ă-pe) The therapeutic administration of gold salts. Also called aurotherapy.

Chvostek's sign (khvos′yĕks sīn) A unilateral spasm of facial muscles elicited by a slight tap over the facial nerve; seen in tetany. Also called Weiss' sign.

chyle (kīl) A milky fluid composed of lymph and digested fat, taken up by the lymphatic capillaries (lacteals) during digestion, and transported by the thoracic duct to the left subclavian vein and by the right lymphatic duct to the junction of the right subclavian and internal jugular veins, where it becomes mixed with the circulating blood.

chylomicronemia (ki-lo-mi-kro-ne′me-ă) Increased number of microscopic particles of fat (chylomicrons) in the blood.

chylomicrons (ki-lo-mi′krons) Minute fat particles (about 1 µm in size) present in lymph; normally they are quickly cleared from the blood.

chylopericardium (ki-lo-per-ĭ-kar′de-um) A milky effusion into the pericardium due to injury or to obstruction of the thoracic duct.

chyloperitoneum ki-lo-per-ĭ-to-ne′um) See chylous ascites, under ascites.

chylopoiesis (ki-lo-poi-e′sis) The formation of chyle.

chylothorax (ki-lo-tho′raks) The collection of a milky fluid of lymphatic origin (chyle) in the pleural cavity.

chyluria (kil-u′re-ă) The presence of chyle or lymph in the urine, giving it a white, turbid appearance.

chyme (kīm) The semifluid mass of food passed from the stomach to the duodenum.

chymopoiesis (kī-mo-poi-ĕsis) The conversion of food into chyme. Also called chymification.

chymosin (ki′mo-sin) See rennin.

chymotrypsin (ki-mo-trip′sin) A digestive enzyme (proteinase) present in pancreatic juice; proposed for use in the treatment of inflammation and edema caused by trauma.

chymotrypsinogen (ki-mo-trip-sin′o-jen) Pancreatic enzyme that gives rise to chymotrypsin.

cicatrectomy (sik-ă-trek′tŏ-me) Surgical removal of a scar.

cicatrix (sik′ă-triks) A scar.

cicatrization (sik-ă-trĭ-za′shun) The formation of scar tissue.

cilia (sil′e-ă) Plural of cilium.

ciliarotomy (sil-e-ă-rot′ŏ-me) An incision through the peripheral region of the anterior surface of the iris (ciliary zone).

ciliary (sil′e-ar-e) **1.** Relating to the eyelashes or any hairlike process. **2.** Relating to certain structures of the eye.

ciliated (sil′e-āt-ed) Having hairlike processes.

cilioretinal (sil-e-o-ret′ĭ-nal) Relating to the ciliary body and the retina.

cilium (sil′e-um), *pl.* **cil′ia** **1.** A microscopic hair-like projection on a cell surface capable of vibratory or lashing movements. **2.** Eyelash.

cillosis (sil-o′sis) Twitching of the eyelids. Also called ciliosis.

cimbia (sim′be-ă) A band of white fibers across the ventral surface of the cerebral peduncle.

cimetidine (si-met′ĭ-dēn) A drug that blocks the actions of histamine on H_2 receptor sites, thus inhibiting secretion of stomach acid; effective in the treatment and prevention of peptic ulcer.

cinchona (sin-ko′nă) Any of various trees of the genus *Cinchona*, found in South America; the bark contains quinine and a number of other alkaloids.

cinchonism (sin′ko-niz-m) Toxic condition resulting from overuse of quinine or other alkaloids; marked by headache, deafness, giddiness, and ringing in the ears. Also called quininism.

cineangiocardiography (sin-ĕ-an-je-o-kar-de-og′ră-fe) The production of motion picture films showing, fluoroscopically, contrast medium passing through the heart chambers and great vessels.

cine-esophagoscopy (sin-ĕ-ĕ-sof-ă-gos′ko-pe) An image of esophageal action.

cinefluorography (sin-ĕ-floo-or-og′ră-fe) The production of motion picture film of fluoroscopic observations.

cinegastroscopy (sin-ĕ-gas-tros′ko-pe) Motion pictures of the interior of the stomach.

cinemicrography (sin-ĕ-mi-krog′ră-fe) The producing of motion picture films through a microscope.

cineradiography (sin-ĕ-ra-de-og′ră-fe) The production of motion picture films of sequential images appearing on a fluoroscopic screen. Also called cineroentgenography.

cineroentgenography (sin-ĕ-rent-gen-og′ră-fe) See cineradiography.

cineurology (sin-ĕ-u-rol′ŏ-je) Action images of the urinary tract.

cingulum (sing′gu-lum) **1.** A band of association fibers in the brain that partly encircle the corpus callosum. **2.**

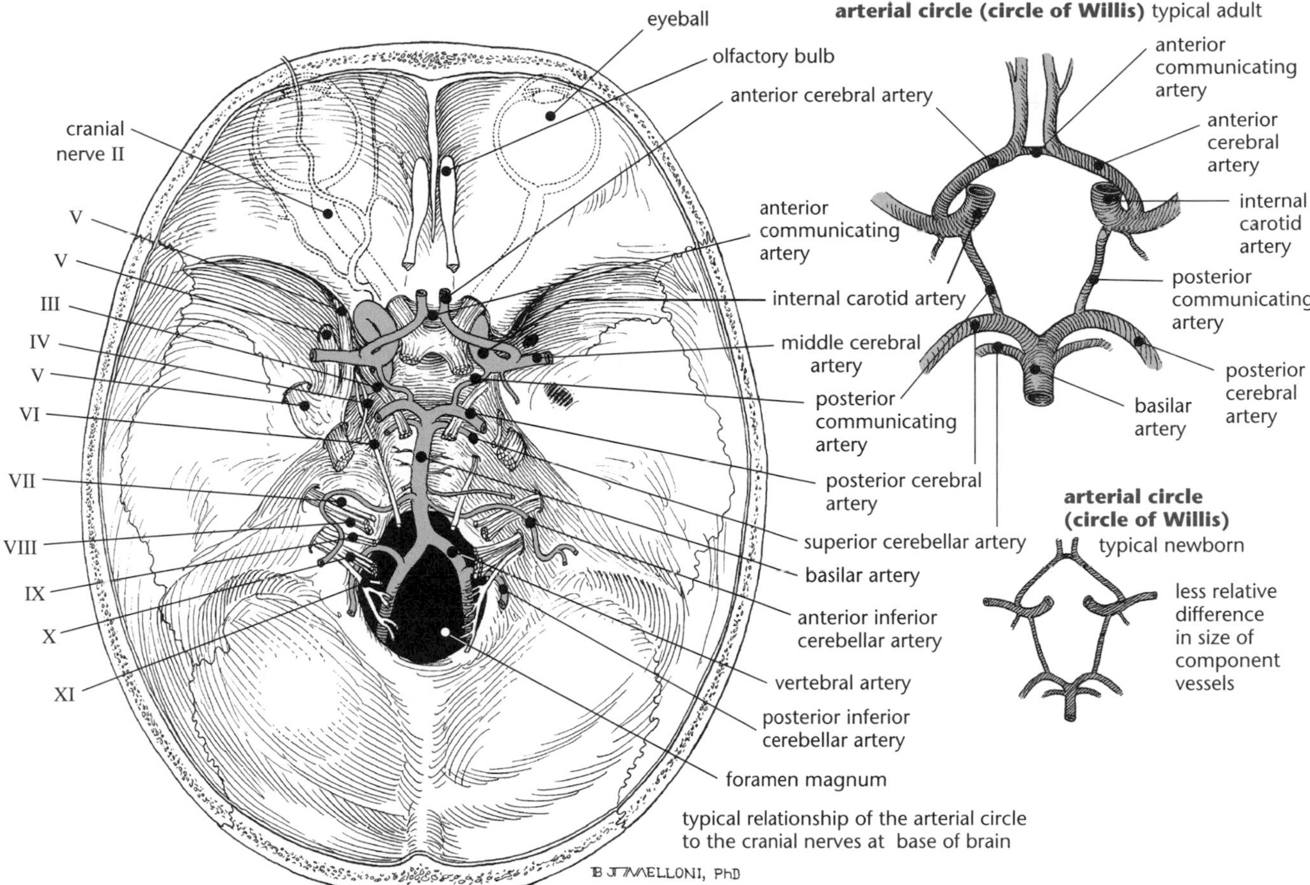

A U-shaped enamel ridge on the lingual surface of incisor teeth.

cingulotomy (sing-gu-lot′ŏ-me) Operation on the brain consisting of precise electrolytic destruction of portions of the cingulate gyrus to relieve severe chronic pain or certain intractable psychoses.

circa (sŭr′kă) (ca) Latin for approximately.

circadian (sir-ka′de-an) Denoting the rhythm of biologic phenomena that cycle approximately every 24 hours; e.g., in persons who sleep at night ACTH (and cortisol) secretion begins to rise in the early morning hours, peaks at the time of awakening, and falls to low values in the evening. Also called circadian rhythm.

circinate (sir′sĭ-nāt) Ring-shaped.

circle (sir′kl) A ring-shaped anatomic structure.

arterial c. A circle of anastomosing arteries at the base of the brain. Also called circle of Willis.

c. of Willis See arterial circle of cerebrum.

circuit (sir′kit) The path followed by an electric current.

circulation (sir-ku-la′shun) Movement through a circular course; unless otherwise specified, the term refers to blood circulation.

collateral c. Circulation of blood through small anastomosing vessels when the main course is obstructed.

coronary c. Circulation through the system of blood vessels supplying the heart muscle.

enterohepatic c. Normal circulation of substances through the liver, into the bile, through the intestines, and back to the liver.

extracorporeal c. Temporary diversion of blood circulation outside the body through a special machine (e.g., a heart-lung machine, hemodialyzer).

fetal c. The blood flow through the blood vessels of the fetus, carried to the placenta (by two arteries in the umbilical cord) and returned from the placenta to the fetus (by a vein in the umbilical cord).

lymph c. The flow of lymph through lymphatic vessels and nodes.

placental c. The flow of blood through the intervillous space of the placenta, which transfers oxygen and nutritive materials from mother to fetus and carbon dioxide and waste products from fetus to mother.

portal c. (a) Circulation of blood through capillaries in the liver from the portal to the hepatic veins. (b) In general, any blood circulation between the capillary beds of two organs.

pulmonary c. The flow of blood from the heart, through the pulmonary artery and lungs, and back to the heart through the pulmonary veins.

systemic c. General circulation, circulation throughout the whole body.

third c. See twin-twin transfusion syndrome.

circulus (sĭr′ku-lus), *pl.* **cir′culi** Latin for circle.

circumcision (sĭr-kum-sizh′un) The removal of a circular portion of the foreskin (prepuce).

circumduction (sĭr-kum-duk′shun) The circular movement of a part, as of a limb or eye.

circumflex (sĭr′kum-fleks) Denoting certain arched anatomic structures.

circumnuclear (sĭr-kum-noo′kle-ar) Surrounding a nucleus.

circumocular (sĭr-kum-ok′u-lar) Surrounding the eye.

circumoral (sĭr-kum-or′al) Around the mouth.

circumscribed (sĭr′ku,-skrībd) Confined within bounds.

circumvallate (sĭr-kum-val′āt) Any structure surrounded by a raised ring.

circumvolute (sĭr-kum-vo′lūt) Coiled or twisted around a central axis.

cirrhosis (sĭ-ro′sis) A chronic disease of the liver marked by a loss of normal lobular architecture, with nodular regeneration of parenchymal cells separated by fibrous septa, and by vascular derangement and anastomoses; these structural abnormalities interfere with liver function and circulation, and ultimately cause death.

alcoholic c. Cirrhosis characterized in its early stage by liver enlargement and fatty changes of liver cells throughout the entire organ; it slowly progresses to fat resorption, regeneration of small nodules and scarring (Laënnec's cirrhosis) with a fatal outcome; caused by long-term alcohol abuse.

biliary c. Any of several morphologically and etiologically different types of cirrhosis that have in common a long history of extra- or intra-hepatic suppression of bile flow, and an enlarged, firm, finely granular liver with a green hue; extensions of connective tissue septa into the lobular parenchyma are sparse, regenerative nodules are rare.

cardiac c. An extensive centrilobular fibrotic reaction, as in chronic passive hepatic congestion from any cause.

cryptogenic c. Cirrhosis that often has an unknown cause, but may result from chronic or recurrent viral hepatitis or from autoimmune liver disease.

Hanot's c. See primary biliary cirrhosis.

Laënnec's c. See alcoholic cirrhosis.

postnecrotic c. Cirrhosis caused by massive necrosis involving multiple lobules, with collapse of the reticular framework to form large scars alternating with large nodules of regenerated or residual liver.

primary biliary c. A type marked by fibrosis of bile ducts associated with jaundice, itching, and high levels of blood cholesterol; seen most commonly in females, usually in middle age, and thought to be an autoimmune disorder. Also called Hanot's cirrhosis.

cirrhotic (sĭ-rot′ik) Affected with cirrhosis.

cisplatin (sis′plat-in) Anticancer drug, often used to treat cancer of the testes; major adverse effects include nausea and vomiting.

cisterna (sis-ter′nă) Any dilatation or enclosed space serving as a reservoir for lymph or other body fluid.

c. cerebellomedullaris See cisterna magna.

c. chyli The triangular dilatation at the beginning of the thoracic duct, situated in front of the second lumbar vertebra; it receives two lumbar lymphatic trunks and the intestinal lymphatic trunk. Also called receptaculum chyli.

c. magna The large subarachnoid space between the medulla oblongata and the under side of the cerebellum. Also called cisterna cerebellomedullaris.

subarachnoid c. One of several intercommunicating spaces at the base of the brain formed by the separation of the arachnoid from the pia mater.

cisternal (sis-ter′nal) Relating to any fluid-containing sac or cavity in the body.

cisternography (sis-ter-nog′ră-fe) X-ray examination of the subarachnoid spaces at the base of the

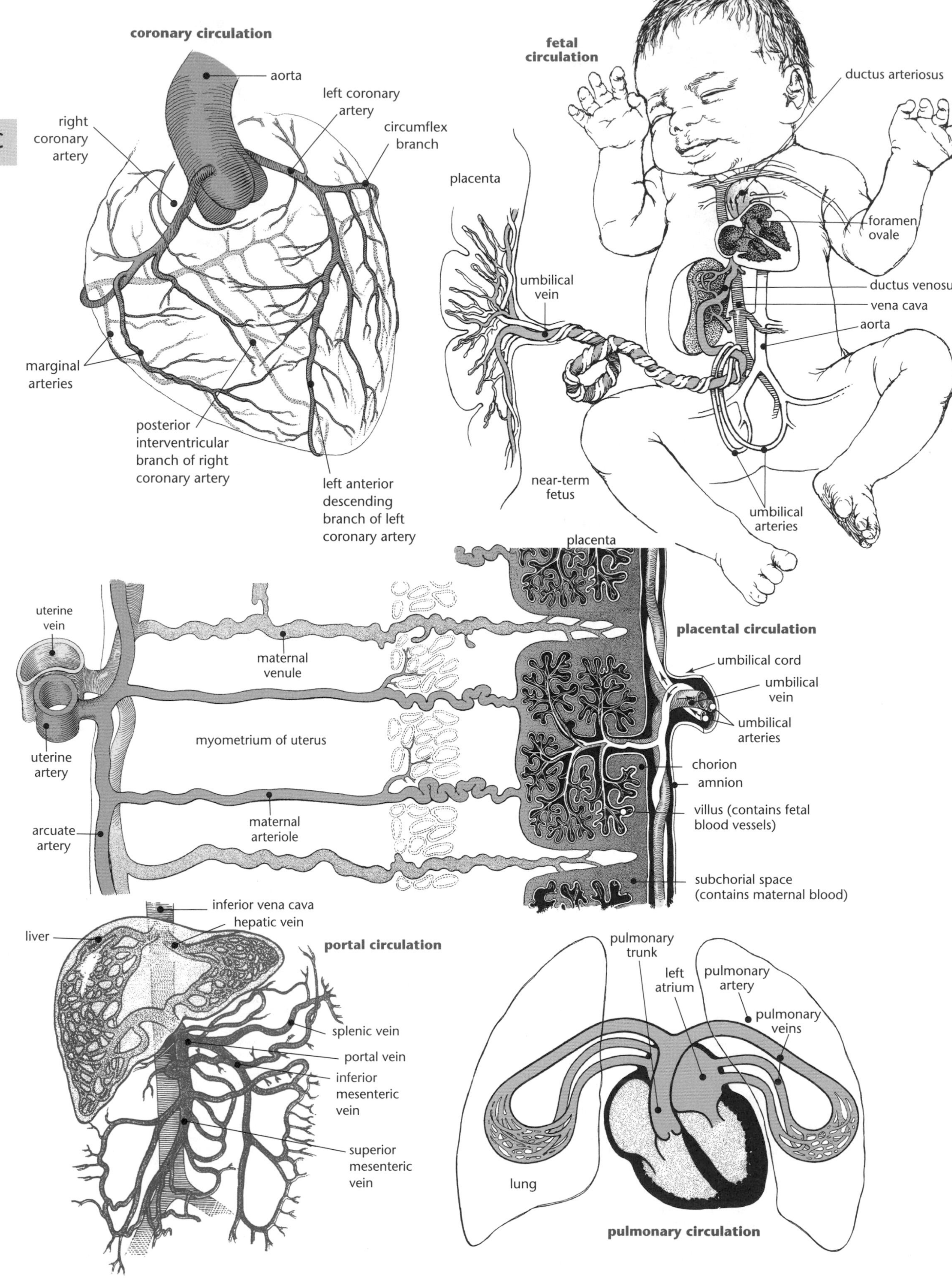
coronary circulation
aorta
left coronary artery
right coronary artery
circumflex branch
marginal arteries
posterior interventricular branch of right coronary artery
left anterior descending branch of left coronary artery
fetal circulation
ductus arteriosus
placenta
foramen ovale
umbilical vein
ductus venosus
vena cava
aorta
near-term fetus
umbilical arteries
placenta
placental circulation
uterine vein
maternal venule
umbilical cord
umbilical vein
umbilical arteries
myometrium of uterus
uterine artery
chorion
amnion
villus (contains fetal blood vessels)
arcuate artery
maternal arteriole
subchorial space (contains maternal blood)
inferior vena cava
hepatic vein
liver
portal circulation
splenic vein
portal vein
inferior mesenteric vein
superior mesenteric vein
pulmonary trunk
left atrium
pulmonary artery
pulmonary veins
lung
pulmonary circulation

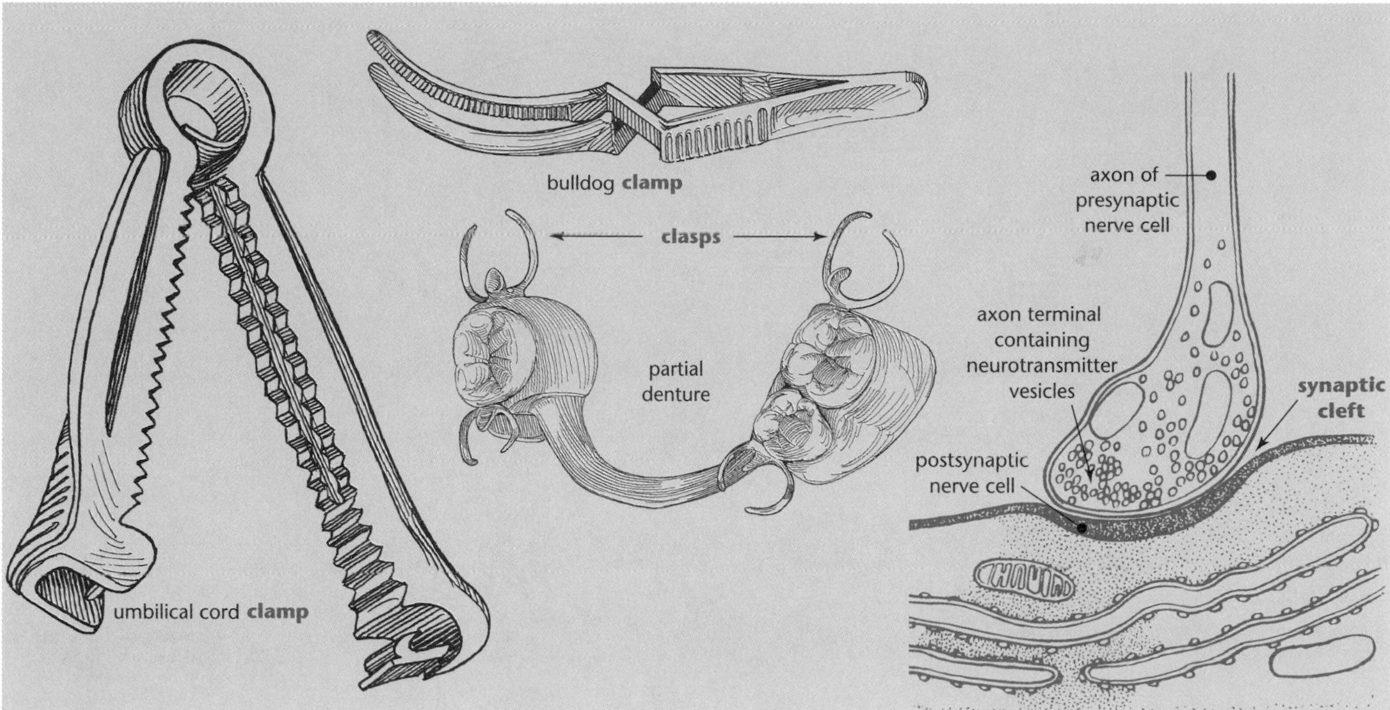

brain after infusion of a radiopaque material.

cistron (sis´tron) The smallest hereditary unit of function; the section of the DNA molecule that specifies a particular biochemical function.

citrate (sit´rāt) A salt of citric acid.

citric acid (sit´rik as´id) A colorless crystalline acid, $C_6H_8 - O_7H_2O$, present in the juice of citrus fruits.

Citrobacter (sit-ro-bak´ter) A genus of rod-shaped bacteria (family Enterobacteriaceae) causing infections in debilitated patients.

clamp (klamp) An instrument used to compress a part.

patch c. See under clamping.

clamping (klamp´ing) Compressing or isolating tissues with a clamp.

patch c. A technique for measuring ion flow across a cell membrane by electrically polarizing and maintaining that potential on an isolated portion of the membrane. Also called patch clamp.

clap (klap) Slang expression for gonorrhea.

clarificant (klar-if´ĭ-kant) Any agent that clears a turbid liquid.

clasp (klasp) In dentistry, one of the metal components of a partial denture; consists usually of two tapered retentive arms joined by a supportive body; serves to stabilize the denture.

class (klas) A biologic category ranking below a phylum and above an order.

classification (klas-ĭ-fĭ-ka´shun) A systematic grouping into categories.

Angle's c. A list of the several forms of malocclusion grouped into four main classes.

Bethesda system of c. See under system.

Breslow c. Classification of melanoma of the skin, based on the depth of invasion. It includes six levels of depth, measured in millimeters, from the epidermis through the subcutaneous fat tissue: 1.0 mm, 1.5 mm, 2 mm, 3 mm, 4 mm, and 5 mm. Also called Breslow's staging; Breslow's thickness.

Clark's c. Classification of melanoma of the skin, using five histologic depth levels of involvement. *Level I, in situ* melanoma in which all demonstrable malignant cells are in the epidermis, superficial to the basement membrane. *Level II*, tumor crosses the basement membrane and invade the papillary dermis. *Level III*, tumor fills the papillary dermis up to (but does not invade) the reticular dermis. *Level IV*, tumor invades the reticular dermis. *Level V*, tumor invades subcutaneous fat tissue. Also called Clark's level; Clark's staging.

DeBakey's c. Classification of dissecting aneurysms of the aorta: *type I*, dissection involves the ascending and descending aorta; *type II*, limited to the ascending or the transverse aorta; *type III*, involves the descending aorta only (*IIIA* to the diaphragm, *IIIB* below it).

Duke's c. Classification of the degree of spread of carcinoma of the large bowel: A, confined within the bowel; B, spread by direct continuity; no lymph node involvement; C_1, lymphatic invasion adjacent to the tumor and bowel wall; C_2, lymph node involvement at a nearby site; D, distant metastases.

Lancefield's c. The division of streptococci into several categories based on specific precipitin reactions.

New York Heart Association c. (NYHA) Functional classification of patients with cardiac disease. *Class I*, no limitation of activity; ordinary activity produces no symptoms. *Class II*, slight limitation of activity; symptoms occur on moderate exertion. *Class III*, marked limitation of activity; symptoms occur on mild exertion. *Class IV*, complete limitation of activity; symptoms occur even at rest.

clastic (klas´tik) Having a tendency to break or divide.

claudication (klaw-dĭ-ka´shun) Limping.

intermittent c. Condition marked by cramplike pains and weakness of legs induced by walking, and the disappearance of all discomfort when at rest; caused by narrowing of the arteries of the legs.

claustrophobia (klaws-tro-fo´be-ă) A morbid fear of confined spaces.

claustrum (klaws´trum) An anatomic structure resembling a barrier, such as the thin layer of gray matter on the lateral surface of the external capsule of the brain, separating the insula from the lentiform nucleus.

clava (kla´vă) See gracile tubercle, under tubercle.

clavicle (klav´ĭ-kl) Either of two long, curved bones extending from the sternum to the acromion and forming the anterior half of the shoulder girdle; its medial end articulates with the sternum and first rib; it is the only bony attachment between the upper extremity and the trunk. Also called collarbone.

clavicotomy (klav-ĭ-kot´ŏ-me) Surgical division of a clavicle.

clavus (kla´vus) Latin for corn.

clawfoot (klaw´foot) Deformity of the foot in which the longitudinal arch is extremely high and the toes are turned under. Also called pes cavus; cavus foot.

clawhand (klaw´hand) Permanent backward bending of the metacarpophalangeal joints connecting the base of the fingers to the hand, with curling of the fingers.

clearance (klēr´ans) **1.** Removal of a substance from the body by an excretory organ (e.g., the kidney). See also creatinine clearance. **2.** The space between apposed structures (e.g., teeth). **3.** In toxicology, the rate at which a toxic agent is excreted, divided by the average concentration of the agent in the plasma. It is a measure of the volume of fluid that is freed of a toxic agent per unit time, rather than the amount of toxic substance removed.

creatinine c. Rate at which the kidney removes endogenous or exogenous creatinine from blood plasma; an approximate measure of glomerular filtration rate. Normal values are 100–140 ml/minute for males and 85–125 ml/minute for females of average size (1.73 m^2 surface area), but tend to decrease above age 40.

immune c. Clearance of antigen from the blood resulting from complexing with antibodies.

inulin c. The most precise of the commonly used measures of glomerular filtration rate, since inulin is freely filtered but neither secreted nor reabsorbed by the tubules; requires infusion of inulin since this substance occurs naturally only in plants.

occlusal c. In dentistry, condition in which the upper and lower teeth pass one another horizontally without contact or interference.

osmolar c. The volume of blood that would contain the number of osmolar particles excreted by the kidney in 1 minute.

PAH c. Clearance of para-aminohippurate; an approximate measure of renal plasma flow; when combined with the extraction ratio, a more precise value is obtained.

cleavage (klēv´ij) **1.** The first stages of cell division after the egg is fertilized. **2.** The splitting up of a molecule into two or more simpler ones.

cleft (kleft) A fissure.

branchial c. In mammalian embryology, a term loosely applied to a series of bilateral ectodermal grooves along the lateral walls of the pharyngeal gut (the equivalent of gills in aquatic animals); on rare occasions, they persist in the adult form as fistulas, sinus tracts, or cysts in the neck area.

Schmidt-Lantermann c. The funnel-shaped intrusion of cytoplasm in the myelin lamellae around the axon of a nerve cell; thought to play a role in the transport of nutrients through the supporting cell.

synaptic c. The space, usually 200 to 300 Å, between the presynaptic terminal knob and the apposing postsynaptic neuron.

cleidal (klī´dăl) Relating to a clavicle. Also written clidal.

clenched fist sign (klenchd fist sīn) The gesture of a patient with angina pectoris by pressing the chest with a clenched fist.

cleoid (klē´oid) A dental carving instrument.

click (klik) A sharp sound.

ejection c. A sharp cardiac sound heard in early systole over the area of the aorta or the pulmonary artery when these vessels are dilated.

mitral c. The opening sound of the mitral (left

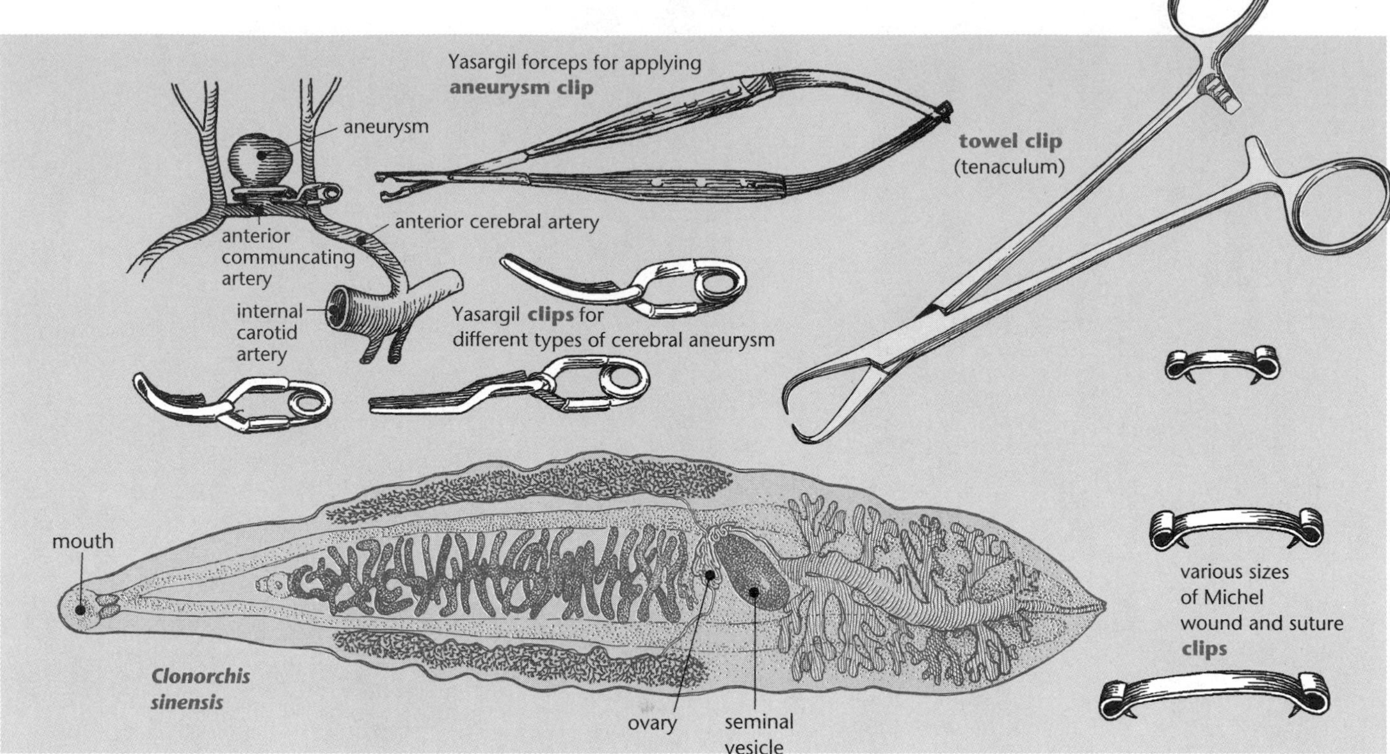

atrioventricular) valve.

systolic c. A sharp cardiac sound heard during contraction of the heart muscle (systole); often indicates prolapse of a mitral (left atrioventricular) valve.

clidal (klī´dal) See cleidal.

clidarthritis (klid-ar-thri´tis) **1.** Gouty pain in the clavicle. **2.** Inflammation of the articular portions of the clavicle.

clidocostal (klī-do-kos´tal) Pertaining to the clavicle and ribs.

clidotomy (kli-dot´o-me) Surgical division of the clavicles of a dead fetus to facilitate its delivery.

climacter (kli-mak´ter) See climacteric.

climacteric (kli-mak´ter-ik) The phase of the aging process during which a woman passes from the reproductive to the nonreproductive stage; symptoms correlate with the diminution of hormone production and ovarian function and may include hot flushes, headache, vulvar discomfort, painful sexual intercourse, and mental depression. Commonly called the change of life. The term is popularly used interchangeably with menopause.

climacterium (kli-mak-te´re-um) See climacteric.

climatology (kli-mă-tol´ŏ-je) The study of climate in relation to health and disease.

climatotherapy (kli-mă-to-ther´ă-pe) Treatment of disease by moving the patient to a suitable climate.

climax (klī´maks) **1.** The height or crisis of a disease. **2.** Orgasm.

clinic (klin´ik) **1.** An institution, building, or part of a building where treatment is given to patients not requiring hospitalization. **2.** Medical instruction given to students in which patients are examined and treated in their presence. **3.** An establishment run by medical specialists working cooperatively.

clinical (klin´ĭ-kal) **1.** Relating to the bedside observation of the course and symptoms of a disease. **2.** Relating to a clinic.

clinician (klĭn-ish´un) A practicing physician.

clinicopathologic (klin-ĭ-ko-path-ŏ-loj´ik) Relating to the signs and symptoms of a disease and the laboratory study of specimens obtained through biopsy or autopsy.

clinicopathologic conference (klin-ĭ-ko-path-ŏ-loj´ik kŏn´fĕ-rens) (CPC) A teaching conference in which the patient's case is discussed following which the pathologic data are presented.

clinocephaly (kli-no-sef´ă-le) Congenital deformity marked by flatness or concavity of the upper part of the skull. Also called saddle head.

clinodactyly (kli-no-dak´tĭ-le) Permanent curvature (lateral or medial) of one or more fingers; usually produced by a shift in alignment of the interphalangeal joint surface; seen most commonly in the little finger.

clinoid (klī´noid) Resembling a bed; said of certain anatomic structures, such as the clinoid process of the sphenoid bone.

clinoscope (klī´no-skōp) Instrument to measure cyclophoria (tendency of one eye to deviate).

clip (klip) **l.** A device used in surgical procedures to approximate cut skin edges or to stop or prevent bleeding. **2.** A clasp.

aneurysm c. Any of several noncrushing clips used in the surgical treatment of cerebral aneurysms; they usually have a spring mechanism that allows their removal, repositioning, and reapplication.

towel c. A forceps for clipping towels to the skin at the edge of the operative field. Also called towel forceps.

clithrophobia (klīth-ro-fo´be-ă) Abnormal fear of being locked in.

clitoridectomy (klit-ŏ-rĭ-dek´to-me) Surgical removal of the clitoris.

clitorimegaly (klit-ŏ-rĭ-meg´ă-le) Enlargement of the clitoris.

clitoris (klit´ŏ-ris) A structure partially enclosed between the anterior ends of the labia minora; it has a body, consisting of two corpora cavernosa that contain dense fibers enveloping erectile tissue, and a small elongated end with the glans clitoridis composed of erectile tissue. The homologue of the penis.

clitorism (klit´ŏ-rizm) **1.** Prolonged, usually painful, erection of the clitoris. **2.** Abnormally large clitoris.

clitoroplasty (klit´ŏ-ro-plas-te) Reconstructive surgery of the clitoris.

clivus (kli´vus) The internal slope at the base of the skull, from the front of the foramen magnum to the dorsum sellae, formed by the basilar portion of the occipital bone and the body of the sphenoid bone; it supports the pons and the medulla oblongata.

c. monticuli See declive cerebelli, under declive.

cloaca (klo-a´kă) **1.** The cavity into which the intestinal, urinary, and genital tracts open in certain animals. **2.** The combined intestinal and genitourinary opening in the embryo.

clomiphene citrate (klo´mĭ-fēn cĭ´trāt) A nonsteroid compound that stimulates ovulation; used to treat infertility in women who fail to produce eggs (ova); may produce multiple births.

clonal (klō-nal) Relating to a clone.

clone (klōn) **1.** A colony of genetically identical cells with a common ancestor. **2.** In molecular biology, a copy of a DNA sequence created by recombinant DNA procedures.

clonic (klon´ik) Characterized by alternate contraction and relaxation of muscles.

clonicotonic (klon-ĭ-ko-ton´ik) Characterized by rapid alternate contraction and relaxation (clonic) and continued tension (tonic); said of certain muscular spasms.

cloning (klōn´ing) **1.** The developing of a colony of cells from one cell by repeated mitosis; all cells have the same genetic constitution. **2.** The transplantation of a somatic cell nucleus into an ovum for the purpose of developing an embryo through asexual reproduction.

clonorchiosis (klo-nor-ki-o´sis) Disease, prevalent in the Far East, caused by invasion of the bile ducts by *Clonorchis sinensis*, a fluke transmitted to humans by ingestion of raw or undercooked freshwater fish infected with larvae.

Clonorchis (klo-nor´kis) A genus of flukes (family Opisthorchiidae) having both sets of sex organs in the same individual, in which self-fertilizition often occurs; some species are parasitic in the human liver.

C. sinensis A species that is the cause of clonorchiosis. Also called Chinese liver fluke.

clonus (klo´nus) A spasm in which contraction and relaxation of a muscle alternate in rapid succession.

Clostridium (klos-trid´e-um) A genus of bacteria (family Bacillaceae) characterized by gram-positive, motile (occasionally nonmotile), anaerobic, or aerotolerant rods; some species produce putrefaction of proteins.

C. bifermentans A species found in putrid meat, gaseous gangrene, and soil; some strains are pathogenic.

C. botulinum A species that produces botulinum toxin, the cause of food poisoning (botulism); there are five types (A to E), each of which elaborates an immunologically distinct form of exotoxin; the toxins of types A, B, and E cause human illness, with type A toxin being responsible for the severest and most common intoxications.

C. difficile A species that produces a toxin associated with inflammation of mucous membranes of the small intestine and colon in patients receiving antibiotic therapy.

C. histolyticum A species found in soil and feces; causes necrosis of tissue; toxic to small laboratory animals.

C. novyi A species producing a powerful exotoxin; pathogenic for humans and animals; classified into three immunologic types, A, B, and C; associated with certain liver diseases.

C. perfringens A species consisting of short encapsulated rods; the chief cause of gas gangrene; also the cause of postpartum endometritis, enteritis, and food poisoning; found in soil and milk. Formerly called *Clostridium welchii*; gas bacillus; Welch's bacillus.

C. septicum A species producing a lethal and

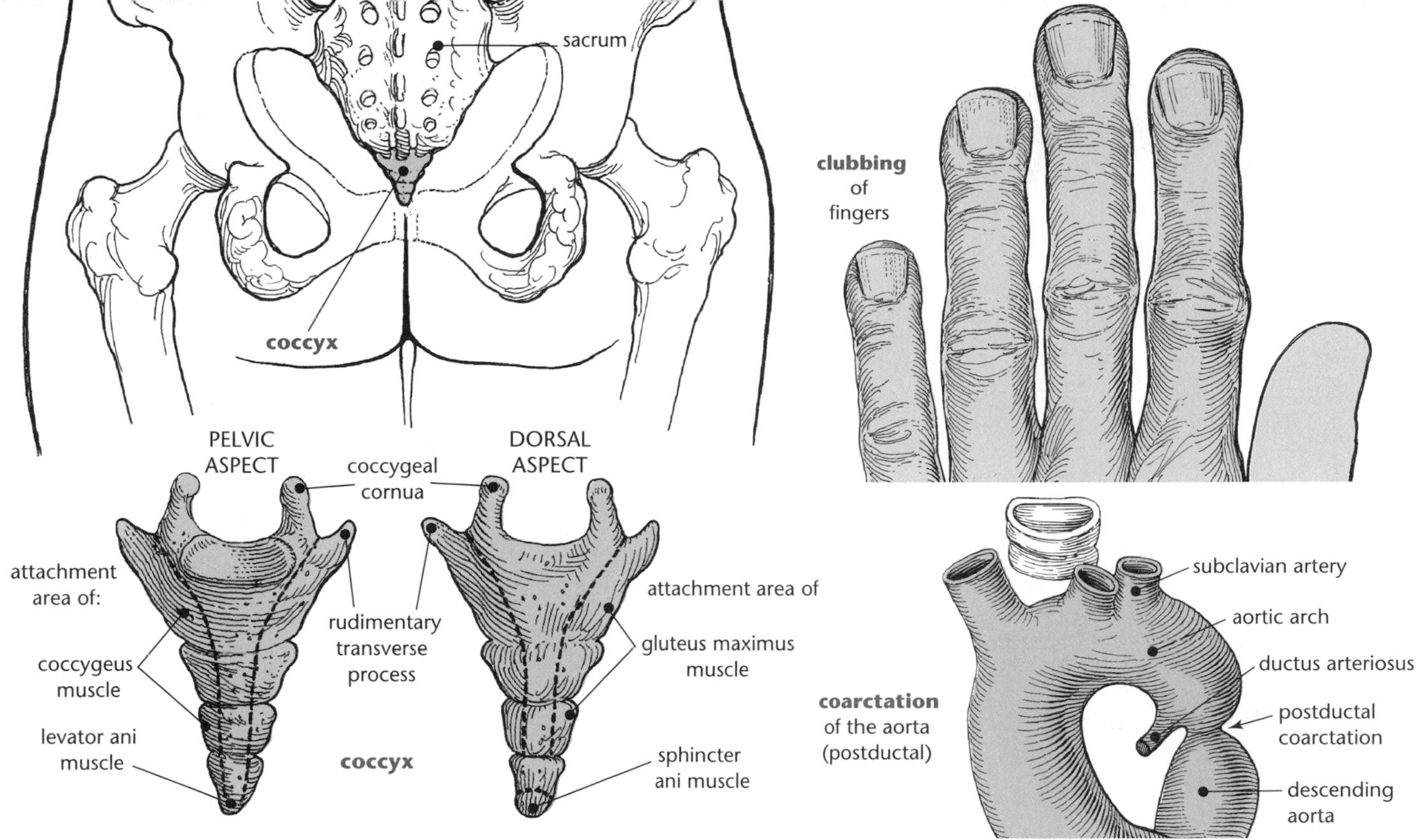

C

hemolytic exotoxin; found in wound infections.

C. tetani A species consisting of motile rods with a drumstick shape, producing an exotoxin with affinity for motor nerve centers, the cause of tetanus or lockjaw; found in soil and wounds.

C. welchii See *Clostridium perfringens*.

closure (klo´zhur) **1.** The act of closing or the state of being closed. **2.** The conclusion of a reflex pathway.

clot (klot) **1.** A thrombus. **2.** To coagulate.

blood c. A solidified elastic mass of fibrin enmeshing platelets, red blood cells, and white blood cells; produced when whole blood coagulates.

clubbing (klub´ing) Broadening and thickening of the soft tissues of the ends of fingers or toes, associated with a variety of cardiac and chronic pulmonary conditions.

clubfoot (klub´foot) See talipes equinovarus, under talipes.

clump (klump) **1.** To aggregate; to form a cluster. **2.** A mass so formed.

clumping (klump´ing) The clustering of bacteria or other cells suspended in a liquid.

cluster of differentiation (klus´ter ŭv dif-ĕ-ren´she-ā´shun) (CD) Cell surface molecules that define a particular cell line or the state of cellular differentiation and are detected by monoclonal antibodies; used to classify leukocytes into subsets. See also CD4/CD8 count, under count.

c. of d. 4 (CD4) Glycoprotein that participates in adhesion of T lymphocytes to target cells; is involved in transmitting intracellular signals during activation by antigens of the major histocompatibility complex (MHC), class II; and provides appropriate signals for B lymphocyte differentiation into immunoglobulin-secreting cells.

c. of d. 8 (CD8) Glycoprotein molecule that is a marker for T lymphocytes with suppressor and cytotoxic activity; it binds to antigens of the major histocompatibility complex (MHC), class I, on antigen-presenting cells.

clysis (klı̄´sis) Infusion of fluid into the body.

coagglutinin (ko-ă-gloo´tĭ-nin) A substance that causes agglutination of antigen only in the presence of univalent antibody; by itself it does not cause agglutination.

coagulable (ko-ag´u-lă-bl) Capable of clotting.

coagulant (ko-ag´u-lant) **1.** Causing coagulation or clotting. **2.** A substance that causes clotting.

coagulase (ko-ag´u-lās) In microbiology, an extracellular enzyme or complex that promotes plasma coagulation and is clinically associated with disease production.

coagulate (ko-ag´u-lāt) **1.** To cause the conversion of a fluid into a semisolid mass. **2.** To become such a mass.

coagulation (ko-ag-u-la´shun) **1.** Clotting; the conversion of a fluid into a jellylike solid. **2.** A clot.

disseminated intravascular c. (DIC) The presence of numerous widespread blood clots in minute blood vessels occurring as a complication of a variety of disorders; symptoms vary depending on the underlying disorder; may be acute (as in amniotic fluid embolism and major trauma) or chronic (as in cancer).

coagulative (ko-ag´u-la-tiv) Causing coagulation.

coagulin (ko-ag´u-lin) An antibody that causes coagulation of its antigen.

coagulopathy (ko-ag-u-lop´ă-the) A disease affecting the blood-clotting process.

consumption c. Condition marked by great reduction in the circulating levels of platelets and of certain coagulation factors; due to utilization of platelets in excessive blood clotting throughout the body.

coagulum (ko-ag´u-lum), *pl.* **coag´ula** A clot; a curd.

coaptation (ko-ap-ta´shŭn) The fitting together of parts, such as the ends of a broken bone.

coarct (ko´arkt) To press together; to constrict.

coarctation (ko-ark-ta´shun) A narrowing or constriction, as of a blood vessel.

coat (kōt) A membrane or a layer of tissue.

buffy c. (a) A light yellowish layer of platelets and white blood cells covering the packed red cells of centrifuged blood. (b) A layer of similar composition, plus fibrin, that covers the blood clot when coagulation is delayed so that red cells have time to settle.

cobalamin (ko-bal´ă-min) See vitamin B_{12}, under vitamin.

cobalt (ko´bawlt) A hard, brittle, steel-gray metallic element; symbol Co, atomic number 27, atomic weight 58.94; cobalt ingestion has been associated with cardiomyopathy.

cobalt-60 A radioactive isotope of cobalt, used in radiotherapy.

cobralysin (ko-bral´ĭ-sin) The substance in cobra venom that destroys red blood cells.

coca (ko´kă) A tree, *Erythroxylon coca*, with leaves that contain cocaine and other alkaloids.

cocaine (ko´kān) A crystalline narcotic alkaloid, colorless or white, extracted from coca leaves or synthesized from ergomine or its derivatives; has anesthetic, vasoconstrictive, and psychotropic properties. Popularly called coke; snow.

crack c. The potent purified form of cocaine; usually smoked, injected intravenously, or taken orally; dependence can develop in less than two weeks. Popularly called crack.

cocainize (ko´kă-nīz) To anesthetize by the administration of cocaine.

cocarboxylase (ko-kar-boks´ĭ-lās) See thiamine pyrophosphate.

cocarcinogen (ko-kar-sin´ŏ-jen) An agent that increases the activity of a carcinogen.

cocci (kok´si) Plural of coccus.

Coccidia (kok-sid´e-ă) An order of protozoans, some of which are pathogenic and parasitic in the epithelium of the small intestine.

Coccidioides (kok-sid-e-oi´dēz) A genus of zygomycetous fungi, some of which are parasitic in man.

C. immitis A species of fungi causing coccidioimycosis. Also called *Blastomyces coccidioides*.

coccidioidin (kok-sid-e-oi´din) A sterile solution prepared from *Coccidioides immitis* products. Used as a skin test for coccidioidomycosis in localities where the disease is not prevalent.

coccidioidomycosis (kok-sid-e-oi-do-mi-ko´sis) A disease caused by the fungus *Coccidioides immitis*, affecting primarily the lungs; it is frequently asymptomatic and rarely disseminated; the disease is endemic in desert areas of the United States; one form is known as desert fever; San Joaquin Valley fever.

coccidiosis (kok-sid-e-o´sis) Disease of certain vertebrates caused by any protozoans of the order Coccidia; in humans, the infection is self-limiting and accompanied by nausea and diarrhea.

coccobacillus (kok-o-bă-sil´us) An oval-shaped microorganism.

coccoid (kok´oid) Resembling a spherical bacterium (coccus).

coccus (kok´us), *pl.* **coc´ci** A bacterium of round or oval shape.

coccyalgia (kok-se-al´jă) See coccygodynia.

coccydynia (kok-se-din´e-ă) See coccygodynia.

coccygeal (kok-sij´e-al) Relating to or located in the proximity of the coccyx.

coccygectomy (kok-sĭ-jek´tŏ-me) Surgical removal of the coccyx.

coccygodynia (kok-sĭ-go-din´e-ă) Pain in the coccygeal region, frequently caused by a fall upon the buttocks. Also called coccydynia; coccyalgia.

coccyx (kok´siks), *pl.* **coc´cyges** Three or four

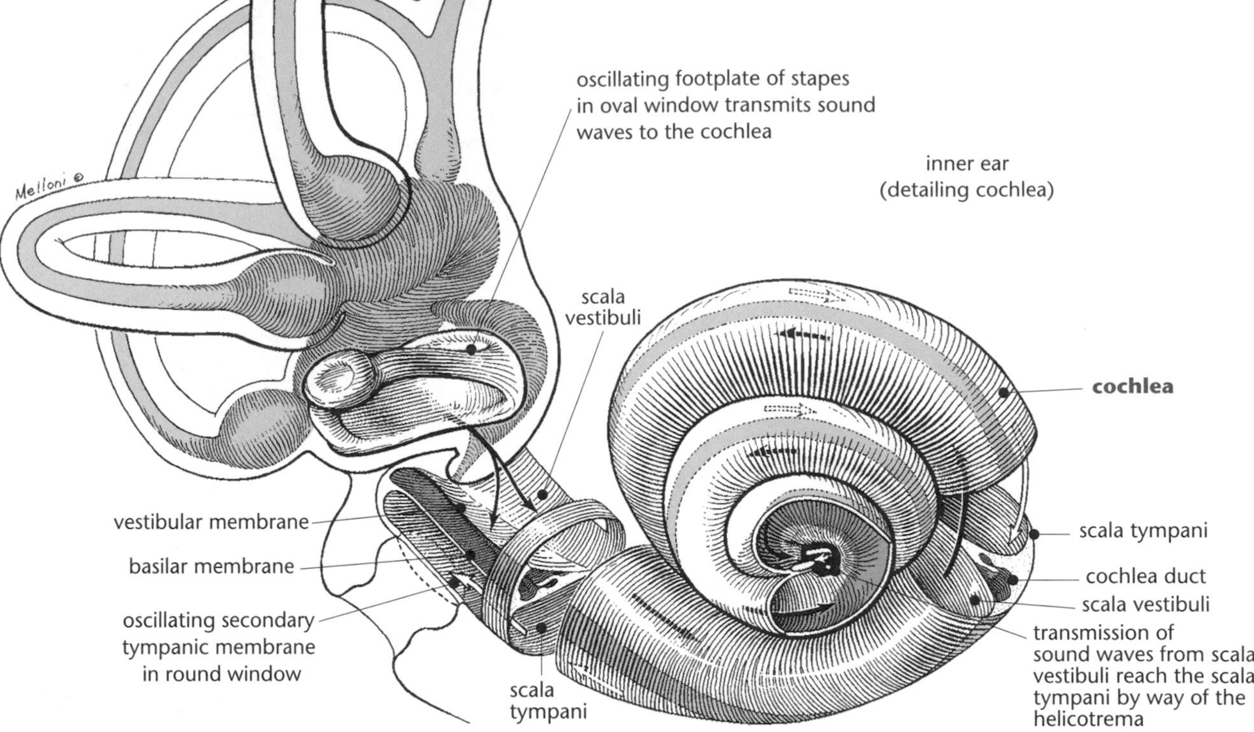

small, fused, rudimentary vertebrae that form the caudal extremity of the vertebral column.

cochlea (kok′le-ă) The spiral cavity in the inner ear; the essential organ of hearing containing the membranous cochlear duct in which the spiral organ of Corti with its nerve endings is located.

cochlear (kok′le-ar) Relating to the cochlea.

cochleare magnum (kok-le-a′re mag′num) (coch. mag.) Latin for tablespoon.

cochleovestibular (kok-le-o-ves-tib′u-lar) Relating to the cochlea and the vestibule of the ear.

cochlitis (kok-li′tis) Inflammation of the cochlea.

code (kōd) **1.** A systematic collection of rules. **2.** A system of symbols used for transmitting information.

c. blue Designation for the hospital resuscitation team or for the resuscitation procedure.

genetic c. The pattern of three adjacent nucleotides in a DNA molecule that controls protein synthesis.

c. red An emergency call designating a fire threat or alarm in an area of the hospital.

codecarboxylase (ko-de-kar-bok′sĭ-lās) A coenzyme of various amino acid decarboxylases. Also called pyridoxal phosphate.

codeine (ko′dēn) A white, crystalline narcotic alkaloid obtained from opium or morphine, used for the relief of cough and as an analgesic.

codominant (ko-dom′ĭ-nant) Of equal dominance; denoting two dissimilar alleles that are both expressed in the individual when present together in a particular locus of the chromosome.

codon (ko′don) The set of three adjacent nucleotides in DNA or RNA that codes the insertion of one specific amino acid in the synthesis of a protein chain. The term is also used for corresponding (and complementary) sequences of three nucleotides in messenger RNA into which the original DNA sequence is transcribed.

initiation c.'s Codons that act as 'start' signals, coding for synthesis of polypeptide chains.

stop c.'s See termination codons.

termination c.'s Codons that specify a stop of translation of RNA into protein. Also called stop codons.

coefficient (ko-ĕ-fish′ent) A numerical measure of the effect or change produced by variations of specified conditions, or of the ratio between two quantities.

c. of absorption **1.** The milliliters of a gas that will saturate 100 ml of liquid, at standard temperature and pressure. **2.** In radiology, the constant for radiation of a given wavelength, the value of which depends on the atomic number of the substance through which the radiation passes.

correlation c. A measure of the closeness of the relationships between variables; a value of 1 represents perfect correlation and 0 represents no relationship; the sign of the correlation coefficient is positive when the variables move in the same direction (height vs. weight) and negative when they move in opposite directions (life expectancy vs. weight).

distribution c. The constant ratio in which a substance, soluble in two immiscible solvents, distributes itself in equilibrium between the two solvents; the basis of many chromatographic separation procedures. Also called partition coefficient.

filtration c. The volume of fluid passed in unit time through a unit area of membrane per unit pressure difference.

partition c. See distribution coefficient.

permeability c. Coefficient related to the diffusion through a membrane; it is inversely proportional to the membrane thickness.

phenol c. See Rideal-Walker coefficient.

Poisseuille's viscosity c. The ratio of the shearing force per unit area between two parallel layers of a liquid in motion, to the velocity gradient between the layers; a numerical measure of the viscosity as determined by the capillary tube method; usually symbolized by h.

c. of relationship The probability that two persons with a common ancestor have a common gene that came from that ancestor.

Rideal-Walker c. The ratio of bactericidal effectiveness of a germicide compared to that of phenol as a standard; the disinfecting power of the substance is obtained by dividing the figure indicating the degree of dilution of the germicide that destroys a microorganism in a given time by that indicating the degree of dilution of phenol which destroys the same organism in the same time under the same conditions. Also called phenol coefficient.

temperature c. The fractional change in any physical property per degree rise in temperature.

coelom (se′lom) Celom.

coenzyme (ko-en′zīm) A nonprotein organic compound, produced by living cells, which plays an intimate and frequently essential role in the activation of enzymes (e.g., thiamine, riboflavin).

c. A (CoA) A widely distributed coenzyme containing adenine, ribose, pantothenic acid, and thioethanolamine; it plays an essential role in various metabolic reactions.

coeur (kŏr) French for heart.

c. en sabot The characteristic x-ray appearance of the heart in tetralogy of Fallot; it vaguely resembles a wooden shoe.

cofactor (ko′fak-tor) A substance that is essential to bring about the action of an enzyme.

cognition (kog-nish′un) **1.** The intellectual process by which knowledge is acquired, as opposed to emotional processes. **2.** The product of this process. Also called comprehension; perception.

cohesion (ko-he′zhun) The mutual attraction by which the molecules of a substance are held together.

cohort (ko′hort) In epidemiology, a group of people who share a designated characteristic and who are traced over an extended period of time.

coil (koil) Any device wound in a spiral shape.

Guglielmi detachable c. (GDC) A wire coil made of soft flexible metal (usually platinum), placed within an aneurysm to cut off blood flow and prevent rupture of the aneurysmal blood vessel.

coin-counting (koin-koun′ting) See pill-rolling tremor, under tremor.

coition (ko-ish′un) See coitus.

coitus (ko′ĭ-tus) Vaginal sexual intercourse between man and woman. Also called coition.

c. interruptus Withdrawal of the penis from the vagina just prior to ejaculation; used as a method of contraception. Also called onanism; interrupted coitus; incomplete coitus.

c. reservatus Coitus in which ejaculation is intentionally delayed or suppressed.

cola (kō′lă) See kola nut.

colchicine (kol′chĭ-sēn) An alkaloid obtained from colchicum; used in the treatment of acute gout.

cold (kōld) The common cold, a symptom complex due to a viral infection of the respiratory tract; marked by nasal discharge, sneezing, some malaise, and usually without fever.

chest c. Bronchitis.

head c. Acute rhinitis.

colectomy (ko-lek′to-me) Surgical removal of the colon, or a segment of it.

colic (kol′ik) **1.** Relating to the colon. **2.** Acute abdominal pain. **3.** A symptom complex seen in infants under three months of age, characterized by paroxysmal abdominal pain and frantic crying.

biliary c. Severe pain caused by the passage of a gallstone through the bile duct.

infantile c. Symptom complex of early infancy marked by a period of daily episodes of irritability, paroxysmal crying or screaming, and drawing up of the legs with apparent abdominal pain; episodes tend to occur in the evening and the infant does not respond to usual means of comforting.

lead c. Abdominal pain caused by lead poisoning.

renal c. Pain caused by the impaction or passage of a stone along the ureter or renal pelvis.

ureteral c. Severe pains caused by obstruction of the ureter.

coliform (ko′lĭ-form) Resembling the *Escherichia*

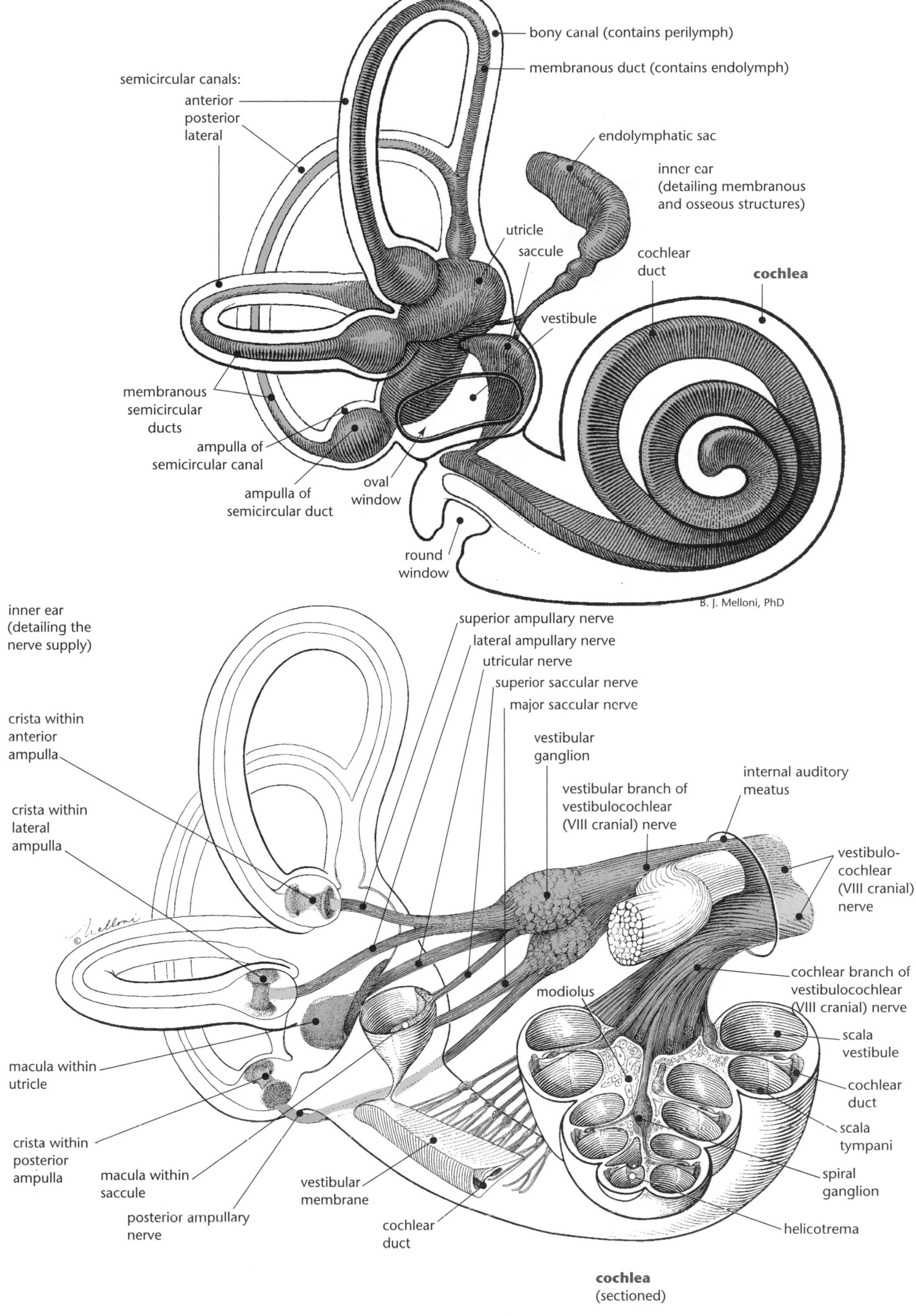
bony canal (contains perilymph)
membranous duct (contains endolymph)
semicircular canals:
anterior
posterior
lateral
endolymphatic sac
inner ear
(detailing membranous
and osseous structures)
utricle
saccule
cochlear
duct
cochlea
vestibule
membranous
semicircular
ducts
ampulla of
semicircular canal
ampulla of
semicircular duct
oval
window
round
window
B. J. Melloni, PhD
inner ear
(detailing the
nerve supply)
superior ampullary nerve
lateral ampullary nerve
utricular nerve
superior saccular nerve
major saccular nerve
crista within
anterior
ampulla
vestibular
ganglion
internal auditory
meatus
vestibular branch of
vestibulocochlear
(VIII cranial) nerve
crista within
lateral
ampulla
vestibulo-
cochlear
(VIII cranial)
nerve
cochlear branch of
vestibulocochlear
(VIII cranial) nerve
modiolus
scala
vestibule
macula within
utricle
cochlear
duct
scala
tympani
crista within
posterior
ampulla
macula within
saccule
vestibular
membrane
spiral
ganglion
posterior ampullary
nerve
cochlear
duct
helicotrema
cochlea
(sectioned)

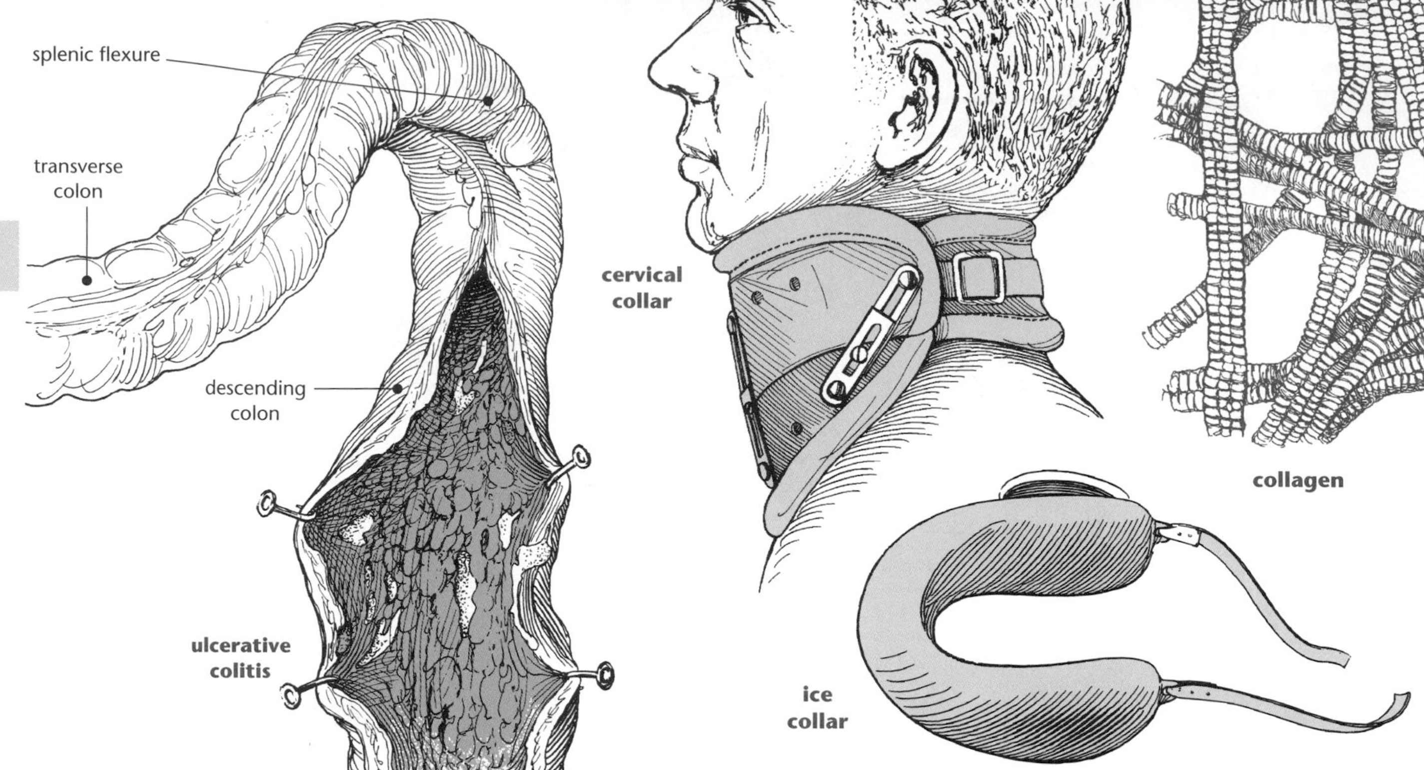

coli bacillus.
colitis (ko-li´tis) Inflammation of the colon.
granulomatous c. Disease of the colon that produces lesions involving all layers of the bowel wall, resembling the changes produced in the ileum by regional enteritis.
mucous c. See irritable colon, under colon.
pseudomembranous c. See pseudomembranous enterocolitis, under enterocolitis.
spastic c. See irritable colon, under colon.
ulcerative c. A chronic disease of unknown cause marked by ulceration of the mucosa and submucosa of the colon with bleeding and malnutrition.
collagen (kol´ă-jen) The supportive protein component of connective tissue, bone, cartilage, and skin; converted into gelatin by boiling.
collagenase (ko-laj´ĕ-nās) An enzyme that promotes the breakdown of collagen.
collagen diseases (kol´ă-jen dĭ-zēz´ĕs) A group of diseases having in common such histologic features as inflammatory damage to connective tissues and blood vessels with deposition of fibrinoid material; included in this group are such disorders as systemic lupus erythematosus, polyarteritis nodosa, dermatomyositis, scleroderma, and rheumatoid arthritis. Also called connective tissue diseases.
collagenosis (ko-laj-ĕ-no´sis) Collagen diseases.
collapse (kŏ-laps) **1.** A state of extreme prostration. **2.** The act of caving in.
collar (kol´ar) **1.** A band or device, usually one encircling the neck. **2.** An encircling anatomic structure.
cervical c. A device generally used to support, stabilize, immobilize, or hyperextend the neck in cases where a rigid cast or bracing is not indicated.
ice c. A rubber bag designed to be filled with crushed ice and placed on the neck to produce cooling, as in postoperative care of tonsillectomies.
collarbone (kol´ar-bōn) See clavicle.
collateral (ko-lat´er-al) Secondary, auxiliary, or alternative.
colliculitis (ko-lik-u-lī´tis) See verumontanitis.
colliculus (ko-lik´u-lus), *pl.* **collic´uli** A small elevation, as in the roof of the midbrain.
seminal c. An area within the prostate into which open the two ejaculatory ducts and the prostatic utricle.
colligative (kol´ĭ-ga-tiv) In physical chemistry, denotes dependence on the number of particles (molecules, atoms, or ions) present in a given space, rather than on their nature; applied to solutions.
collimation (ko-lĭ-ma´shun) The controlling of the size of x-ray beam spread by use of lead plates placed in front of the primary roentgen ray beam.
collimator (kol-ĭ-ma´tor) An apparatus, often consisting of a pair of lead plates, used to confine a beam of radiation within a specific area.
colliquation (kol-ĭ-kwa´shun) The degeneration of tissue with subsequent conversion into a liquid-like form (liquefaction).
ballooning c. Liquefaction of the cell protoplasm leading to edematous swelling and softening. Also called ballooning degeneration.
colliquative (ko-lik´wă-tiv) **1.** Denoting an excessive watery discharge. **2.** Characterized by liquefaction of tissues.
collodion (ko-lo´de-on) A colorless, flammable, syrupy solution of pyroxylin or gum cotton in ether and alcohol; used as a protective coat for cuts and surgical dressings and as a support film on copper grids in election microscopy. Also called collodium.
collodium (ko-lo´de-um) See collodion.
colloid (kol´oid) **1.** A gluelike substance, such as gelatin, consisting of a suspension of submicroscopic particles in a continuous medium. **2.** A yellowish gelatinous material present in the tissues as a result of colloid degeneration.
emulsion c. See emulsoid.
collum (kol´um) Latin for neck; denoting any necklike structure.
coloboma (kol-o-bo´mă) Any defect in which a portion of a structure, especially of the eye, is absent; it may be congenital, pathologic, or artificial.
colocolic (ko-lo-kol´ik) Denoting a surgical joining of one part of the colon to another.
colotysis (ko-lol´ĭ-sis) Freeing the colon from adhesions.
colon (kō´lon) Portion of the large intestine extending from the cecum to the rectum.
ascending c. The part of the colon extending upward on the right side of the abdomen from the cecum to the hepatic flexure. Also called right colon.
descending c. The part of the colon extending downward on the left side of the abdomen from the splenic flexure to the sigmoid colon. Also called left colon.
irritable c. (IC) A condition marked by abdominal pain, gas, constipation or diarrhea, and the passage of mucus; it usually starts in adolescence or early adult life, and the attacks frequently coincide with emotional stress. Also called irritable bowel syndrome; spastic colitis; mucous colitis; spastic colon.
lead pipe c. A term applied to the radiologic appearance of a scarred, contracted, and rigid colon, usually the consequence of advanced ulcerative colitis.
left c. See descending colon.
right c. See ascending colon.
sigmoid c. The S-shaped part of the colon in the pelvis between the descending colon and rectum.
spastic c. See irritable colon.
transverse c. The portion of the colon that crosses the abdomen from the hepatic flexure to the splenic flexure.
colonic (ko-lon´ik) Relating to the colon.
colonization (kol-ŏ-nĭ-za´shun) **1.** Innidiation; metastasis. **2.** The act of forming compact groups or colonies (e.g., the developing of colonies of the same type of microorganisms). **3.** Grouping and caring for individuals with a common disease such as leprosy.
colonorrhagia (ko-lon-o-ra´jă) See colorrhagia.
colonorrhea (ko-lon-o-re´ă) See colorrhea.
colonoscopy (ko-lon-os´kŏ-pe) Visual exami-nation of the interior of the colon with a long, flexible, fiberoptic instrument (colonoscope).
virtual c. Colonoscopy conducted with a helical CT scanner through which a sequence of two-dimensional "slices" of the abdominal area is obtained; these "slices" are then reconstructed into a three-dimensional virtual colon for viewing.
colony (kol´ŏ-ne) A visible group or growth of microorganisms on a solid medium, presumably arising from a single microorganism.
mucoid c., M-type c. A usually virulent colony marked by a well developed carbohydrate capsule which may act as a defense mechanism.
rough c., R-type c. A nonvirulent or slightly virulent colony having a granular growth, irregular margins, and flat surface.
smooth c., S-type c. A colony presenting a round, even, smooth surface; some capsule-forming species have a degree of virulence.
colopexy (ko´lo-pek-se) Shortening of an elongated gastrocolic omentum by means of sutures to support a prolapsed transverse colon; procedure is also used in the correction of a prolapsed stomach.
coloproctitis (ko-lo-prok-tī´tis) Inflammation of the colon and rectum. Also called proctocolitis; rectocolitis.
colorectal (ko-lo-rek´tal) Relating to the colon and rectum.
colorimetry (kul-or-im´ĕ-tre) **1.** The quantitative analysis of color, either in terms of hue, saturation, and brightness, or by comparison with known standards. **2.** The quantitative chemical analysis of a solution by color comparison with a standard solution.
colorrhagia (ko-lo-ra´jă) Abnormal discharge from the colon. Also called colonorrhagia
colorrhea (ko-lo-re´ă) Diarrhea thought to originate in the colon. Also called colonorrhea.
colostomy (ko-los´to-me) Surgical establishment of a permanent opening into the colon through the

The shutters of the **collimator** are wide open

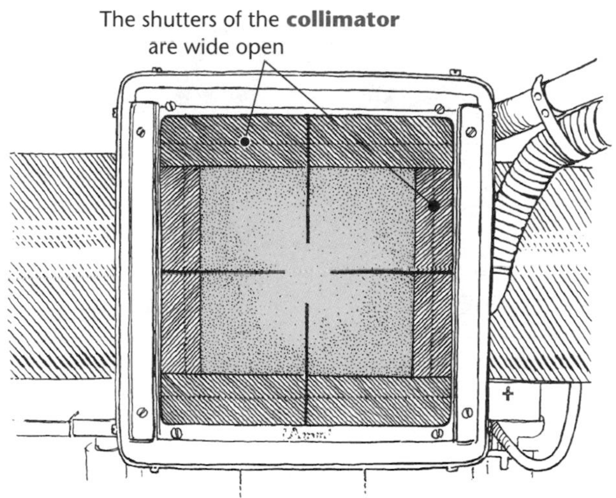

The shutters of the **collimator** are adjusted to restrict the x-ray beam to the area of diagnostic interest

B.J. MELLONI
PhD

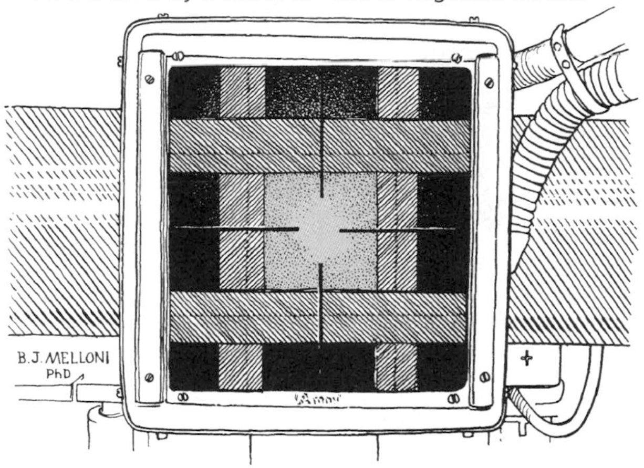

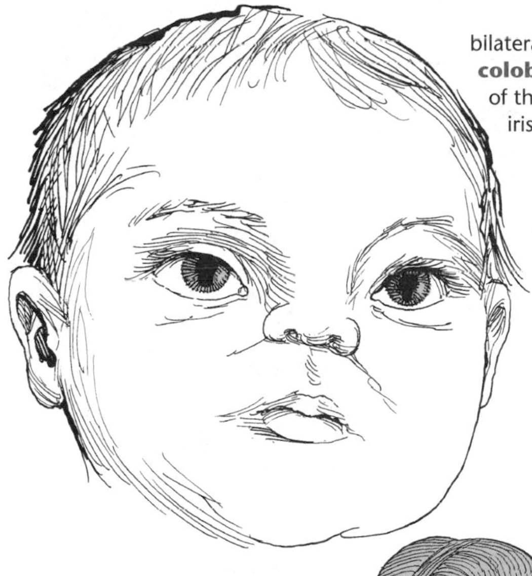

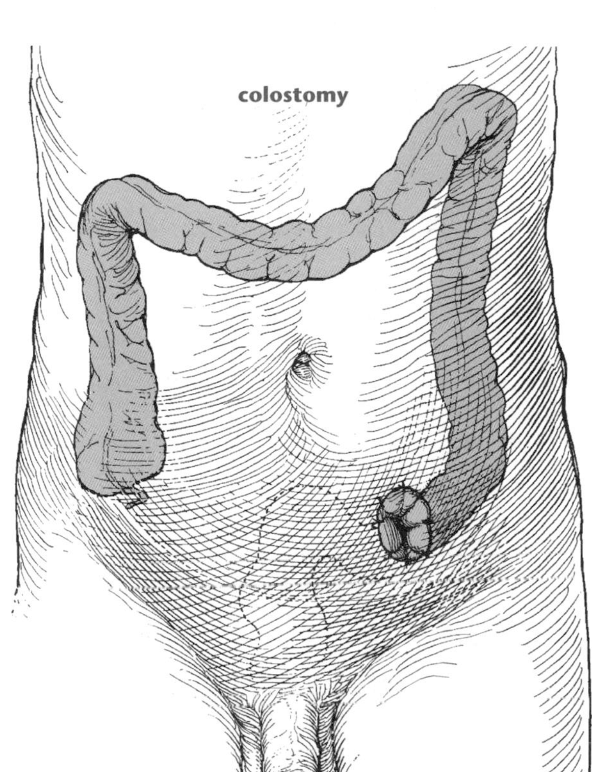

bilateral **coloboma** of the iris

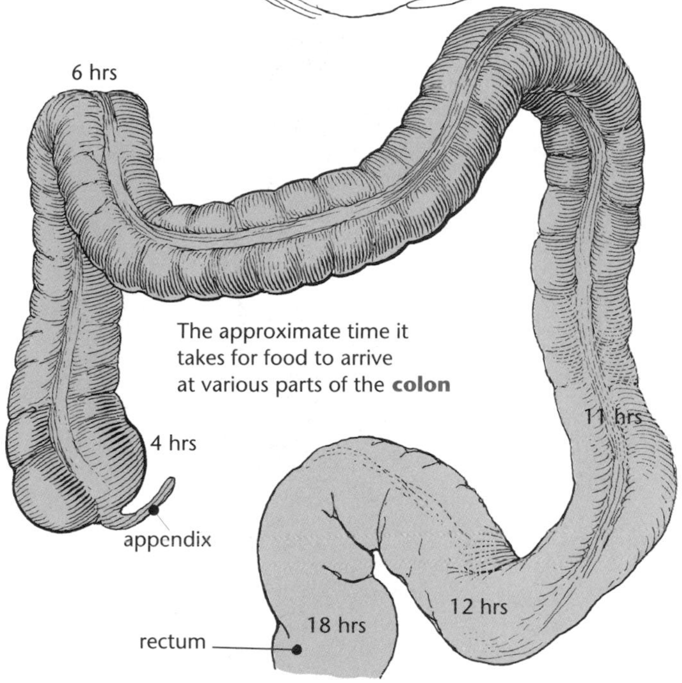

6 hrs
The approximate time it takes for food to arrive at various parts of the **colon**
11 hrs
4 hrs
appendix
12 hrs
18 hrs
rectum

colostomy

Melloni
ascending colon
transverse colon
descending colon
sigmoid colon
rectum

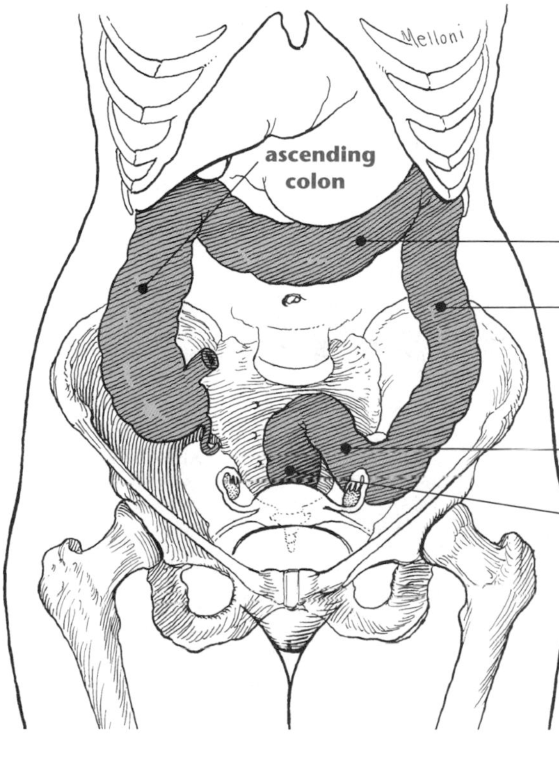

C

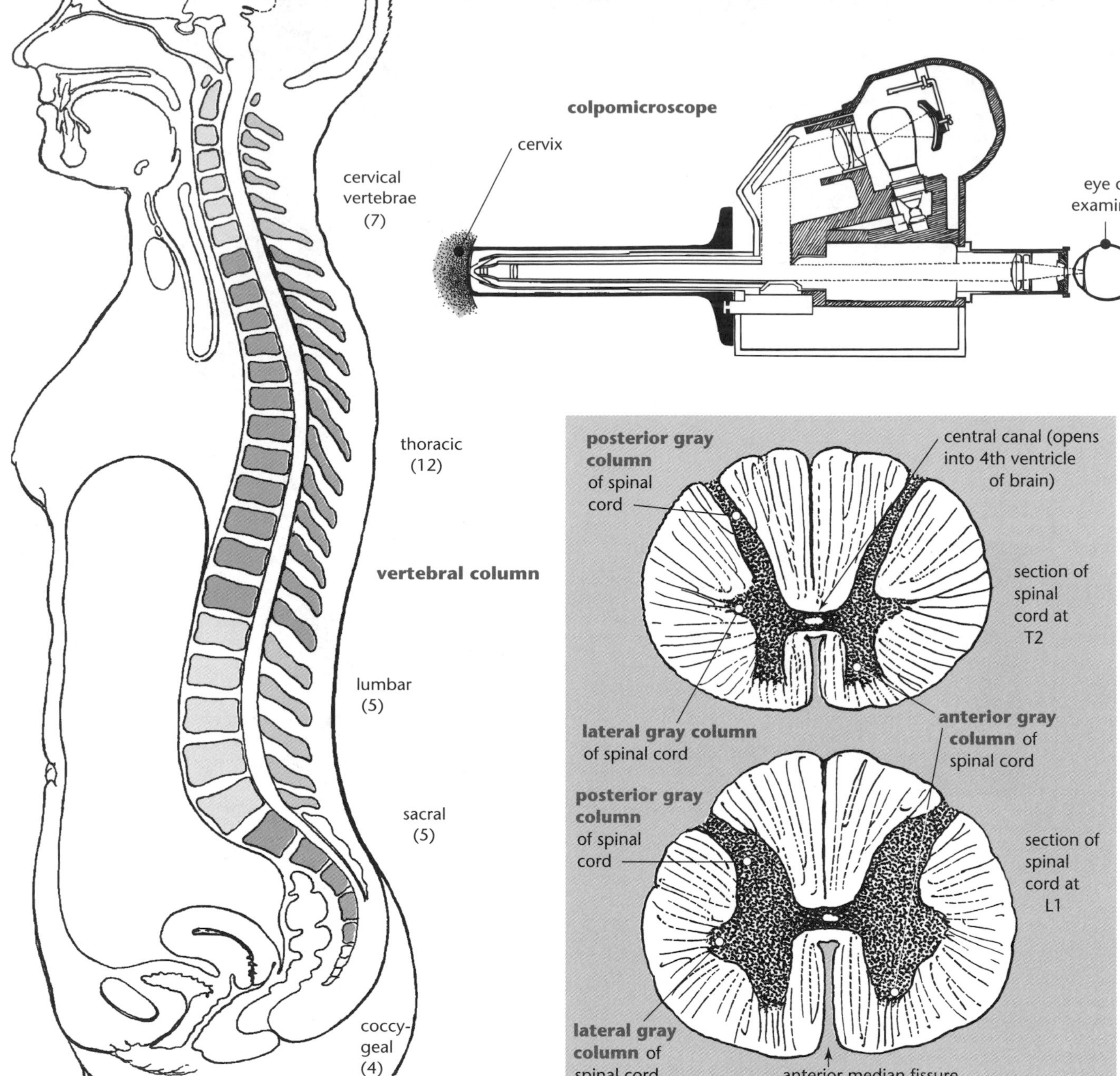

abdominal wall.

colostrorrhea (kŏ-los-tro-re´ă) A copious secretion of colostrum (first milk secreted at the end of pregnancy).

colostrum (kŏ-los´trum) A thin, sticky secretion of the breasts occurring a few days before and after childbirth. Also called foremilk.

colotomy (ko-lot´o-me) Incision of the colon.

colpatresia (kol-pă-tre´zhă) Occlusion of the vagina.

colpectomy (kol-pek´tŏ-me) Total excision of the vagina. Also called vaginectomy.

colpitis (kol-pi´tis) See vaginitis.

colpocleisis (kol-po-kli´sis) Surgical closure of the vaginal lumen.

colpodynia (kol-po-din´e-ă) See vaginodynia.

colpohysterectomy (kol-po-his-ter-ek´to-me) See vaginal hysterectomy, under hysterectomy.

colpomicroscope (kol-po-mi´kro-skōp) A high-powered microscope with a built-in light source for direct visual examination of cells and tissues of the cervix *in vivo.*

colpomicroscopy (kol-po-mi-kros´ko-pe) Examination of cells of the cervix with a colpomicroscope.

colpoperineorrhaphy (kol-po-per-ĭ-ne-or´ă-fe) Surgical repair and reinforcement of a lacerated vagina and musculature of the pelvic floor. Also called vaginoperineorrhaphy.

posterior c. Colpoperineorrhaphy performed for the correction of a large rectocele and a generalized relaxation of the pelvic floor.

colpopexy (kol´po-pek-se) Suturing a prolapsed vaginal wall in an elevated normal position. Also called vaginopexy.

colpoplasty (kol´po-plas-te) See vaginoplasty.

colpopoiesis (kol-po-poi-e´sis) Surgical construction of an artificial vagina.

colpoptosis (kol-po-to´sis) Prolapse of the vagina.

colporrhaphy (kol-por´ă-fe) **1.** Suturing of a tear in the vagina. **2.** Restructuring of the vaginal wall.

colporrhexis (kol-po-rek´sis) Laceration or tearing of the vagina.

colposcope (kol´po-skōp) A binocular microscope used for direct visualization of the cervix and to obtain biopsies from focal cervical lesions.

colposcopy (kol-pos´kŏ-pe) Visualization of cervical and vaginal tissues under magnification with a colposcope; performed after obtaining a positive Pap test or to evaluate suspicious lesions.

colpospasm (kol´po-spaz-m) See vagzinismus.

colpostenosis (kol-po-stě-no´sis) Narrowing of the vagina.

colpotomy (kol-pot´ŏ-me) Incision through the vaginal wall, usually to drain a pelvic abscess. Also called vaginotomy.

colpoxerosis (kol-po-ze-ro´sis) Abnormal dryness of the vaginal mucosa.

columbium (kol-um´be-um) An element, symbol Cb, now known as niobium.

columella (kol-u-mel´ă) **1.** A small column. **2.** The lower portion of the nasal septum.

column (kol´um) A pillar-shaped anatomic structure.

anterior gray c. The anterior (ventral) portion of the gray matter on either side of the spinal cord.

enamel c. One of the groups of fibers that make up the tooth enamel.

lateral c. The portion of gray matter of the spinal cord, extending between the anterior and posterior columns; present only in the thoracic and upper lumbar regions.

posterior gray c. The posterior (dorsal) portion of the gray matter on either side of the spinal cord.

spinal c. See vertebral column.

vertebral c. The columnar arrangement of vertebrae, from the skull through the coccyx, which encloses and supports the spinal cord. Also called spinal column; backbone; spine.

coma (ko´mă) A state in which psychologic and motor responses to stimulation are impaired. See also Glasgow coma scale, under scale.

deep c. Coma in which responses are completely lost.

diabetic c. Coma due to ketoacidosis caused by uncontrolled diabetes mellitus; symptoms leading to coma progress slowly (few days in adults, 12 to 14 hours in juveniles) and include dry mouth, thirst, and excessive urination, followed usually by nausea,

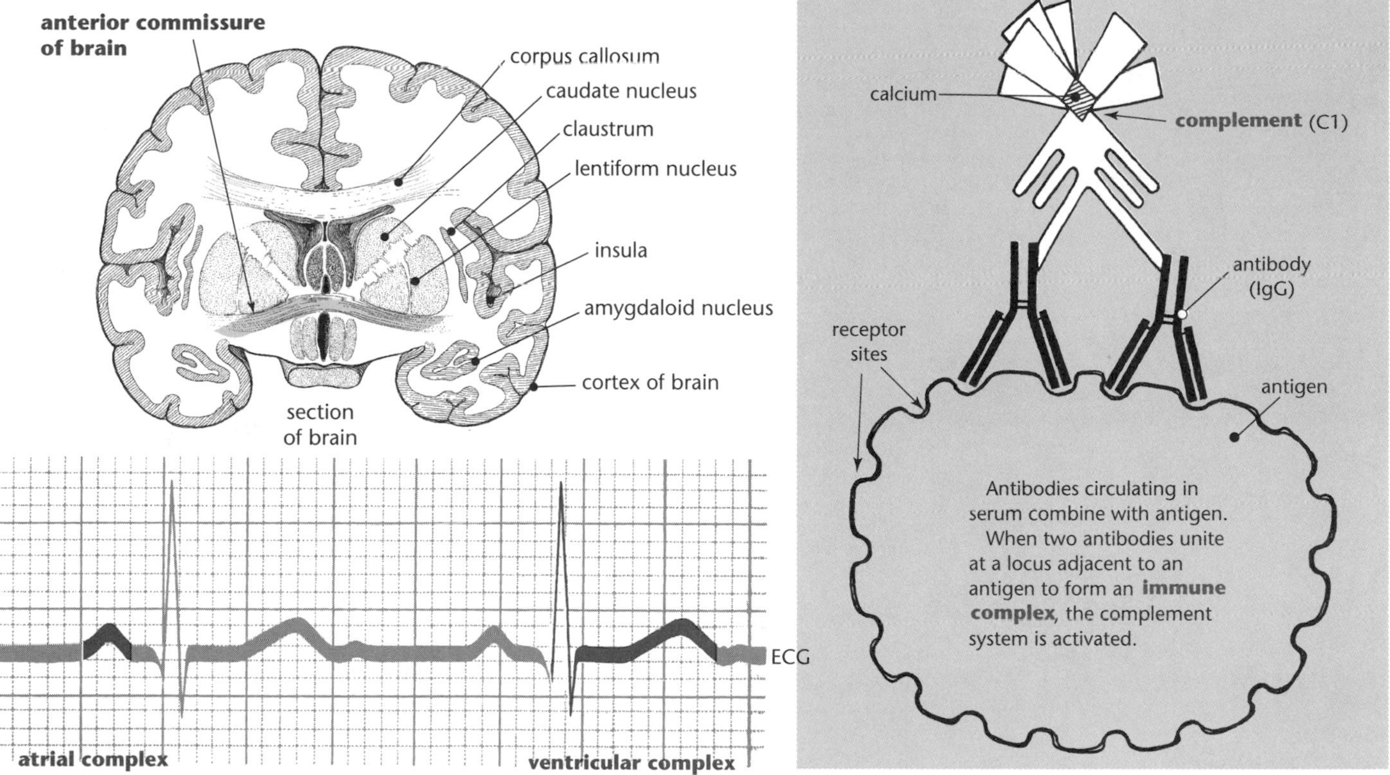

C

vomiting, and abdominal pain; those immediately preceding the coma may be labored breathing, flushed complexion, and drowsiness.

hepatic c. Coma occurring in the terminal stages of cirrhosis of the liver, hepatitis, or other liver diseases; may be preceded by mental confusion, flapping tremor, or jaundice.

hyperosmolar nonketotic c. Diabetic coma without increased ketone bodies; caused by the dehydrating effect on brain cells of the hyper-osmolarity of marked hyperglycemia.

moderately deep c. Coma in which only rudimentary responses of a reflex nature are present (e.g., corneal reflex).

comatose (ko´mă-tōs) In a condition of coma.

combustion (kom-bus´chun) Burning; oxidation or other chemical change accompanied by the production of heat and light.

heat of c. See under heat.

comedo (kom´ĕ-do), *pl.* **comedo´nes** A plug of dried sebaceous material retained in the orifice of a hair follicle. Commonly called blackhead.

comedocarcinoma (ko-me-do-kar-sĭ-no´mă) Carcinoma of the breast filling the ducts with a necrotic cheesy material that can be extruded with slight pressure.

comes (ko´mēz), *pl.* **co´mites** A companion blood vessel of another vessel or nerve.

commensal (ko-men´sal) Denoting two non-parasitic organisms that live together, one benefiting from the association while the other is neither benefited nor harmed.

comminuted (kom-ĭ-nōōt´ed) Denoting a bone broken into several fragments.

comminution (kom-ĭ-nu´shun) The process of breaking into small pieces.

commissure (kom´ĭ-shūr) **1.** Joining together; in the brain or spinal cord, bundles of nerve fibers crossing the midline from side to side. **2.** A line formed by the junction of two bones in the skull. **3.** The angle or corner of the eye, the lips, or the labia.

anterior c. of brain A bundle of white fibers crossing the midline in front of the third ventricle.

posterior c. of brain A bundle of white fibers crossing the midline posterior to the third ventricle, at its junction with the cerebral aqueduct.

commissurotomy (kom-ĭ-shūr-ot´ŏ-me) Surgical division of the bands of a commissure.

mitral c. Surgical division of the fibrous band of the mitral (left atrioventricular) valve in the heart to relieve mitral stenosis.

commitment (kŏ-mit´ment) The legal placing of a person in a mental hospital or any other protective custody.

communicable (kŏ-mu´nĭ-kă-bl) Capable of being transmitted from one person to another; applied to diseases.

communicans (kŏ-mu´nĭ-kanz) Denoting a nerve that connects two others.

compartment syndrome (kom-part´ment sin´drōm) Injury due to compression of a muscle group within its confined fascial space; may be caused by trauma, extensive exercise, or any process that causes swelling within the compartment.

compatible (kom-pat´ĭ-bl) **1.** In pharmacology, denoting two or more substances that are capable of being mixed without undergoing undesirable chemical changes or loss of therapeutic properties. **2.** Describing two samples of blood in which the serum of each does not agglutinate the red blood cells of the other; blood that causes no reaction when transfused.

compensation (kom-pen-sa´shun) **1.** The act of offsetting a functional or structural defect. **2.** A defense mechanism in which the individual, consciously or unconsciously, strives to make up for real or imagined deficiencies.

compensatory (kom-pen´să-tor-e) Serving to counterbalance or make up for a deficiency or loss.

competence (kom-pĕ-tens) **1.** The ability of an organ or part to perform a function. **2.** The ability of a group of embryonic cells to react to a given morphogenic stimulus with resulting differentiation. **3.** The state of being capable of normal adult function and rational decision making.

competition (kom-pĕ-tish´un) Process by which one substance inhibits the action of another, structurally similar, substance.

complaint (kom-plānt´) An expression of pain or discomfort.

chief c. (CC) The symptom reported by the patient as responsible for his seeking medical attention.

complement (kom´plĕ-ment) (C) A group of more than 25 proteins present in normal serum that become involved in the control of inflammation, activation of phagocytes (cells that engulf nonself particles, bacteria, and other cells), and the destructive attack on cell membranes; reaction of the complement system can be activated by the immune system.

complex (kom´pleks) **1.** A group of interrelated parts or factors. **2.** In psychiatry, a group of associated ideas (largely unconscious), having a strong emotional tone and influencing the personality. **3.** In electrocardiography, a group of deflections corresponding to a base in the cardiac cycle.

AIDS-related c. (ARC) Early symptoms of AIDS: fever, fatigue, diarrhea, weight loss, and generalized lymph node enlargement. See AIDS.

atrial c. The portion of the electrocardiogram (ECG) representing electrical activation of the atria; the P wave.

brain wave c. A combination of fast and slow electrical activities of the brain that recur often enough to be recognized as a discrete phenomenon.

castration c. Fear of injury to the genitals as punishment for forbidden sexual desires. Also called castration anxiety.

Eisenmenger's c. Congenital heart condition consisting of a ventricular septal defect with pulmonary hypertension, resulting in right-to-left shunt through the defect; it may or may not be associated with overriding aorta.

Ghon c. See primary complex.

Golgi c. See Golgi apparatus, under apparatus.

histocompatibility c. Fifty or more genes on chromosome 6 coding for cell surface proteins and involved in the immune response.

HLA c., human lymphocyte antigen c. The major histocompatibility complex in humans; consists of a group of linked gene loci on chromosome 6 coding for cell surface histocompatibility antigens; it determines tissue type and transplant compatibility.

immune c. A complex composed of antibody linked to antigen.

inferiority c. Feelings of inferiority due to real or imagined physical or social inadequacies; manifested by extreme shyness or timidity or by overcompensation through excessive ambition or aggressiveness.

juxtaglomerular c. See juxtaglomerular apparatus, under apparatus.

major histocompatibility c. (MHC) A cluster of linked loci (collectively called HLA complex in humans) located on a small region of chromosome 6; it controls production of the cell-surface proteins (histocompatibility antigens) that determine tissue type and transplant compatibility. The proteins are also involved in many aspects of immunologic recognition, such as interaction between different lymphoid cells and between lymphocytes and antigen-presenting cells.

membrane attack c. (MAC) The complex of complement components C5 through C9 that creates a hole in the membrane of cells or bacteria, allowing passage of water and small solutes.

***Mycobacterium avium* c.** (MAC) See *Mycobacterium avium* complex, under *Mycobacterium*.

Oedipus c. The natural strong attachment of a child to the parent of the opposite sex, usually occurring between three and six years of age.

oocyte-cumulus-corona c. (OCCC) The entirety of the egg and its accompanying coverings harvested from the ovary for *in vitro* fertilization.

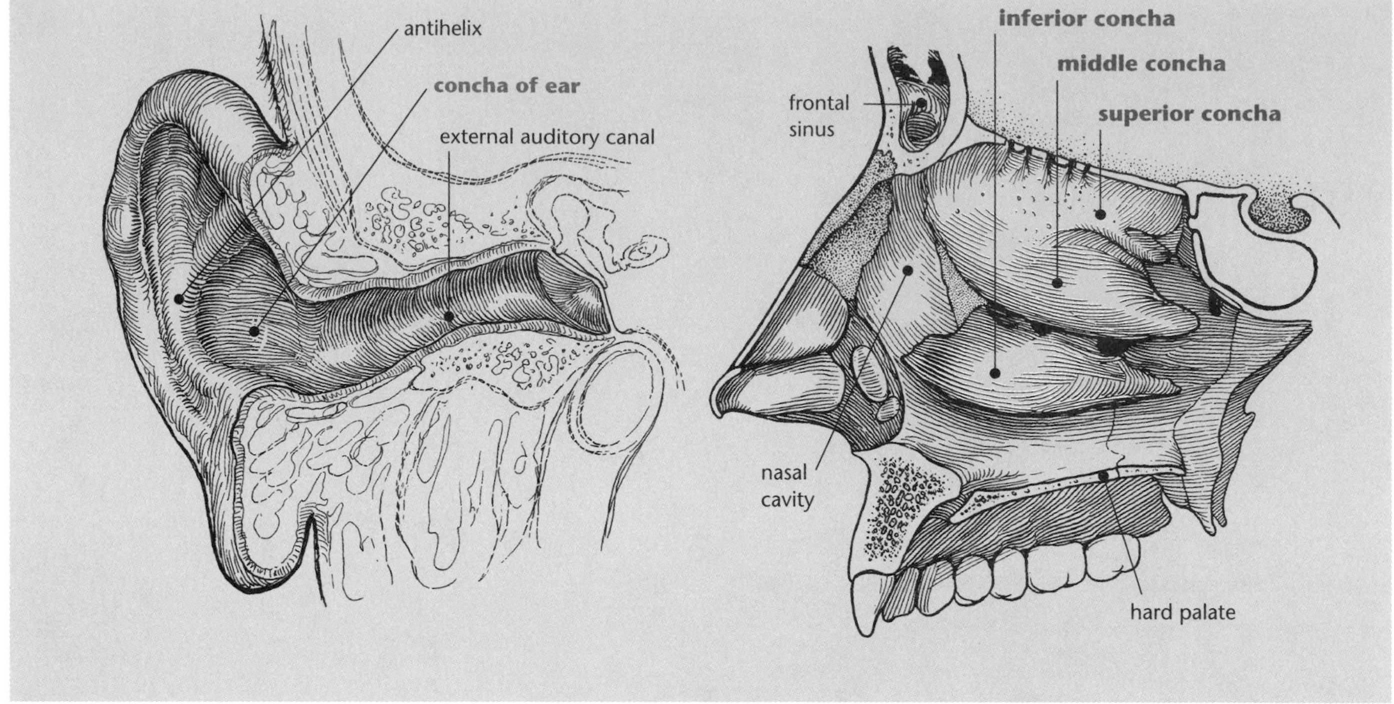

persecution c. A feeling that one's well-being is being threatened, without any basis in reality.

primary c. The combination of lung and lymph node granulomatous inflammation, occurring in primary childhood tuberculosis, in a child who has not been previously exposed to *Mycobacterium tuberculosis.* Also called Ghon complex.

QRS c. The deflection in the electrocardiogram (ECG) representing ventricular contraction of the heart.

spike and wave c. In electroencephalography (EEG), a complex consisting of a dart and dome wave, usually seen in petit mal seizures.

superiority c. Exaggerated self-assertion and aggressiveness, an overcompensation for feelings of inferiority.

ventricular c. The QRS wave in the electrocardiogram (ECG).

vitamin B c. See under vitamin.

complexion (kom-plek´shun) The appearance and general condition of the skin.

compliance (kom-pli´ans) The quality of yielding; the tendency of a hollow organ (e.g., the bladder) to distend.

lung c. Change of volume per change of pressure, an index of the mechanical properties of the lung.

component (kom-po´nent) A constituent part.

c. of complement In immunology, any of the proteins participating in the sequential activities of complement (complement cascade); each complement component takes its turn in the precise chain steps set in motion (like a domino effect) when the first protein in the complement series is activated; complement components of the classical pathway and the terminal components are named on the basis of functional activity by the symbols C1 through C9.

composition (kom-po-zish´un) **1.** The act of combining parts or elements to form a whole. **2.** In chemistry, the group of atoms that forms the molecule of a substance.

compos mentis (kom´pos men´tis) Latin term meaning of sound mind.

compound (kom´pound) **1.** A substance consisting of two or more chemical elements or parts in union. **2.** In pharmacy, a preparation containing a mixture of drugs. **3.** In dentistry, a molding or impression material that softens when heated and solidifies without chemical change when cooled. **4.** To prepare a pharmaceutical mixture.

c. A The adrenal hormone 11-dehydrocorticosterone.

acyclic c., aliphatic c. Organic compound in which the carbon atoms are linked in a linear fashion. Also called open chain compound.

aromatic c. See cyclic compound.

c. B The adrenal hormone corticosterone.

binary c. Compound whose molecule is composed of two elements or atoms of different kinds (e.g., HCl).

closed chain c. See cyclic compound.

cyclic c. Any organic compound that has atoms linked together in the form of a ring. Also called closed chain compound; ring compound.

diazo c. An organic compound containing the azo (–N=N–) group.

c. E The adrenal hormone cortisone.

endothermic c. Compound whose formation involves the absorption of heat.

exothermic c. Compound whose formation involves the emission of heat.

c. F The adrenal hormone, hydrocortisone. Also called cortisol.

heterocyclic c. See cyclic compound.

impression c. See plastic (2).

inorganic c. Any compound that does not contain carbon.

nonpolar c. Compound whose molecules have asymmetrical distribution of charge so that no positive or negative poles exist (e.g., hydrocarbons).

open chain c. See acyclic compound.

organic c. Any compound containing carbon.

ring c.'s See cyclic compound.

c. S The adrenal hormone 11-deoxycortisol.

substitution c. Compound formed when elements of a molecule are replaced by other elements or radicals.

compress (kom´pres) A pad of gauze or other soft material used as a dressing or applied to a part of the body where localized pressure is necessary.

graduated c. A compress made of several layers of cloth gradually increasing in number so that it is thickest in the center.

wet c. A compress moistened with an antiseptic solution or with hot or cold water.

compression (kom-presh´un) Pressing together.

cerebral c. Abnormal pressure on the brain (e.g., by tumor, hemorrhage, skull fracture).

digital c. Pressure applied with the fingers over a blood vessel to check bleeding.

compression syndrome (kom-presh´un sin´drōm) See crush syndrome.

compulsion (kom-pul´shun) An irresistible urge to do something contrary to the person's wishes or standards.

conation (ko-na´shun) The volitional aspect of behavior which includes impulse, drive, and purposive striving; one of three elements of behavior, the other two being cognition (thinking) and affect (feeling).

concameration (kon-kam-er-a´shun) A series of connecting cavities.

concatenate (kon-kat´e-nāt) Connected in a chainlike series.

concave (kon´kāv) Having a hollowed surface.

concavity (kon-kav´ĭ-te) A depression.

concavoconvex (kon-ka-vo-kon´veks) **1.** Concave on one side and convex on the opposite. **2.** Denoting a lens with greater concave than convex curvature.

concentration (kon-sen-tra´shun) **1.** The quantity of a specified substance in a unit amount of another substance (e.g., mg per ml). **2.** A preparation that has had its strength increased by evaporation.

maximum permissible c. (MPC) The quantity of radiation considered to be relatively safe.

molar c. (M) The portion of a constituent substance in moles divided by the volume of the mixture in liters.

concentric (kon-sen´trik) Having a common center.

conception (kon-sep´shun) **1.** The act of forming an idea. **2.** Fertilization of an ovum by a spermatozoon.

conceptus (kon-sep´tus) All the tissue products of conception from the time the sperm and ovum unite until birth; includes the placenta, fetal membranes, and the embryo/fetus.

concha (kong´kă), *pl.* **con´chae** A shell-shaped structure.

c. of ear The large shell-shaped hollow of the external ear, between the tragus and antihelix.

c. bullosa Distention of the nasal conchae, especially of the middle one; seen in some cases of chronic rhinitis.

inferior nasal c. A thin, spongy, curved bony plate forming the lower part of the lateral wall of the nasal cavity; it articulates with the ethmoid, maxilla, palatine, and lacrimal bones. Also called inferior turbinate bone.

middle nasal c. The bony middle nasal concha and its overlying mucous membrane.

sphenoidal c. A thin curved bony plate forming part of the roof of the nasal cavity. Also called sphenoturbinal bone.

superior nasal c. The upper and smaller of the two curved bony plates projecting from the inner wall of the ethmoid in the nasal cavity. Also called superior turbinate bone.

conchoidal (kong-koi´dal) Shell-like in shape.

concordant (kon-kor´dănt) In genetics, denoting a pair of twins exhibiting a certain trait. See also discordant.

concrement (kon´kre-ment) See concretion.

concrescence (kon-kres´ens) The growing together of normally separate parts, such as the roots of a tooth.

concretion (kon-kre´shun) An aggregation of solid material; a calculus.

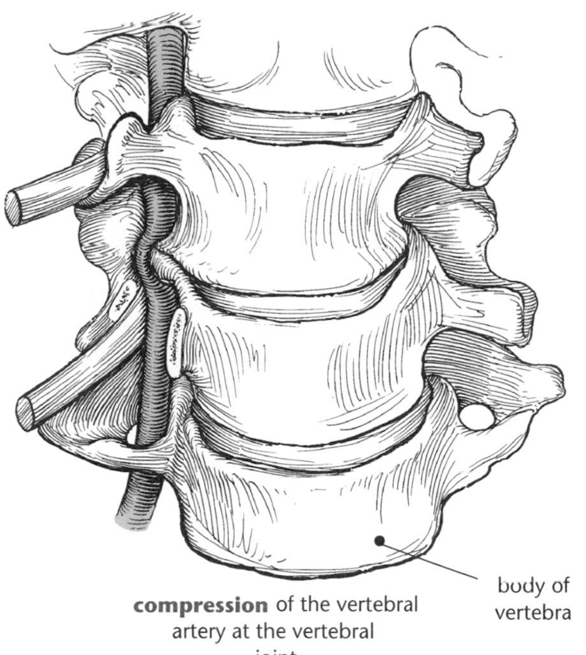

compression of the vertebral artery at the vertebral joint

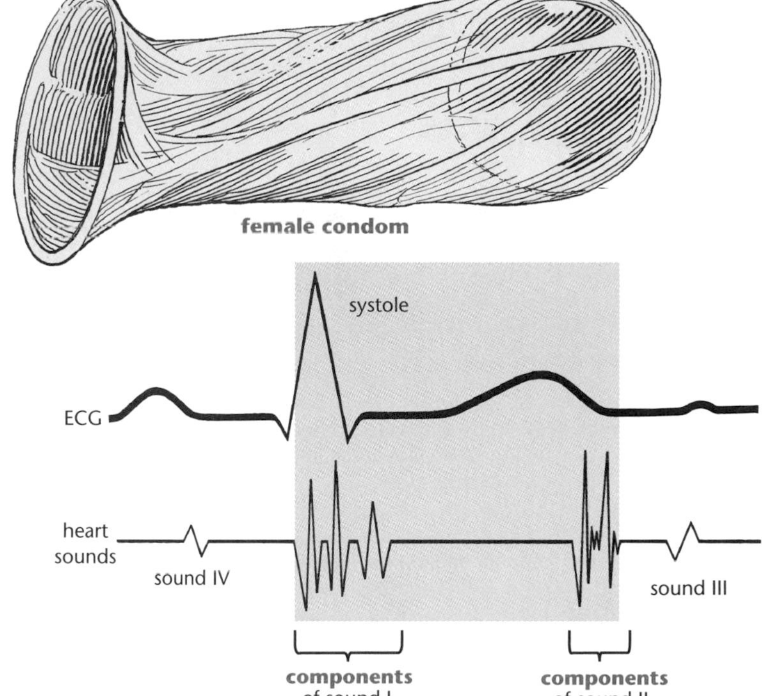

female condom

concussion (kon-kush´un) **1.** A violent jarring or shaking of a part of the body, as caused by a fall or a blow. **2.** The morbid condition resulting from such a jarring.

brain c. The immediate and temporary distur-bance of brain function as manifested by dizziness, cold perspiration, visual disturbances, and sometimes loss of consciousness.

condensation (kon-den-sa´shun) **1.** The act of making more compact. **2.** The changing of a gas to a liquid or a liquid to a solid. **3.** The representation of several ideas by a single dream-image or symbol. **4.** In dentistry, compaction.

condense (kon-dens´) To compress, such as the restorative material into the prepared cavity of a tooth.

condenser (kon-den´ser) **1.** A device for cooling a gas to a liquid, or a liquid to a solid. **2.** Dental instrument for compressing restorative material into the prepared cavity of a tooth. **3.** A simple or compound lens used to gather light rays and focus them on an object to be illuminated.

achromatic c. A condenser used in a microscope for bright field work and corrected for both spherical aberration and chromatic aberration.

dark-field c. An optical system used in microscopes, by means of which light is collected and directed upon the specimen while the remainder of the field is dark.

phase contrast c. A condenser that transmits light through rings so as to work in conjunction with a phase-altering pattern in the objective.

substage c. A lens or group of lenses converging the illuminating beam for proper passage of light through the microscope.

condition (kon-dish´un) **1.** A state, as of health. **2.** A malady. **3.** In psychology, to train an individual to respond to a specific stimulus in a particular way.

pre-existing c. In health insurance, a physical or mental condition that exists prior to the effective date of coverage of a health insurance policy or health care service contract, and for which treatment under the policy or contract may be limited or may be excluded for a set period of time.

conditioning (kon-dish´un-ing) The process of training an individual or organism to respond to a specific stimulus in a specific way, usually by simultaneous presentation of unrelated stimuli one of which evokes the desired response.

instrumental c. See operant conditioning.

operant c. The procedure whereby a stimulus, once having evoked a response that produces a reward (or removes or prevents a punishment), is thereafter more likely to evoke that response. Also called instrumental conditioning.

physical c. An improvement in strength or efficiency of muscular performance by exercise.

condom (kon´dum) A sheath, usually made of thin rubber, used to cover the penis during sexual intercourse to prevent conception or infection.

female c. Any protective sheath worn by a woman during sexual intercourse as a contraceptive sheath and as protection against minute abrasions and transmission of disease. Also called vaginal pouch.

conductance (kon-duk´tens) A measure of a material's ability to allow an electric charge to pass through it.

conduction (kon-duk´shun) The transmission of energy (heat, electricity, etc.) or nerve impulses from one point to another.

aberrant ventricular c. Abnormal pathway of a supraventricular impulse in the ventricle, caused by delayed activation of a branch of the atrio-ventricular bundle.

accelerated c. The partial or complete bypass of the normal conduction pathways by the sinus impulse, resulting in early activation of the ventricular muscle.

air c. Transmission of sound waves to the inner ear through the external auditory canal and the middle ear.

bone c. Transmission of sound waves to the inner ear through the bones of the skull.

concealed c. Partial transmission of an impulse through the A-V junction, which depolarizes only a portion of the junction, thus causing abnormal conduction of the next impulse.

delayed c. First degree atrioventricular (A-V) heart block. See under block.

intraventricular c. Conduction of the cardiac impulse through the ventricular muscle. Also called ventricular conduction.

nerve c. Transmission of an impulse through a nerve.

retrograde c. Transmission of an impulse through the cardiac muscle or the conduction system in a manner opposite to that of the normal impulse. Also called reconduction; ventriculoatrial conduction.

saltatory c. Conduction in which the nerve impulse jumps from one node of Ranvier to the next.

synaptic c. The propagation of a nerve impulse through a synapse.

ventricular c. See intraventricular conduction.

ventriculoatrial c. See retrograde conduction.

conductivity (kon-duk-tiv´ĭ-te) The ability to transmit or convey heat, electricity, sound, etc.

conductor (kon-duk´tor) **1.** Any substance capable of transmitting heat, electricity, sound, etc. **2.** A grooved probe for guiding a surgeon's knife.

conduit (kon´doo-it) A channel.

ileal c. A channel constructed from a detached segment of ileum (distal part of the small intestine) for discharging urine when the bladder has been removed; one end of the segment is attached to the ureters, the other end is attached to an opening made on the abdominal wall. Also called ileal bladder.

condylar (kon´dĭ-lar) Relating to a condyle.

condylarthrosis (kon-dĭl-ar-thro´sis) A joint in which an ovoid surface of a bone (condyle) fits into an elliptical cavity.

condyle (kon´dīl) A rounded knoblike prominence at the end of a bone by means of which it articulates with another bone.

condylectomy (kon-dil-ek´tŏ-me) Surgical removal of a condyle.

condyloma (kon-dĭ-lo´mă) A wartlike growth.

c. acuminatum A soft, pointed, warty growth, or collection of growths, usually occurring around the anus and on the external genitalia of males or females, and in the uterine cervix; caused by infection with human papillomavirus (HPV), usually types 6 and 11, chiefly transmitted through sexual contact; a squamous carcinoma association, especially in the cervix, has been reported. Also called anorectal wart; genital wart; venereal wart; moist wart; pointed wart; fig wart; verruca acuminata; papilloma venereum; pointed condyloma.

c. latum Highly infectious lesion of secondary stage of syphilis; occurs on the genitalia, around the anus, and on the inner thighs and buttocks. Also called moist papule.

condylomatous (kon-dĭ-lo´ma-tus) Relating to a condyloma.

condylotomy (kon-dĭ-lot´ŏ-me) Division of a condyle.

cone (kōn) A figure or anatomic structure tapering to a point from a circular base.

c. of light The triangular reflection of light seen on inspection of the eardrum (tympanic membrane). Also called pyramid of light.

medullary c. The tapered end of the spinal cord.

retinal c. One of about six or seven million photoreceptor cells that, with the rod cells, form the second of the 10 layers of the retina.

confabulation (kon-fab-u-la´shun) The replacement of memory lapses with detailed fabrications of imaginary experiences; may occur in organic brain disorders that affect intellectual functioning.

confectio (kon-fek´shē-ō) See confection.

confection (kon-fek´shun) A sweetened pharmaceutical preparation. Also called confectio; electuary.

configuration (kon-fig-u-ra´shun) **1.** The shape or outline of something as determined by the arrangement of its parts. **2.** The spatial grouping of atoms in a molecule.

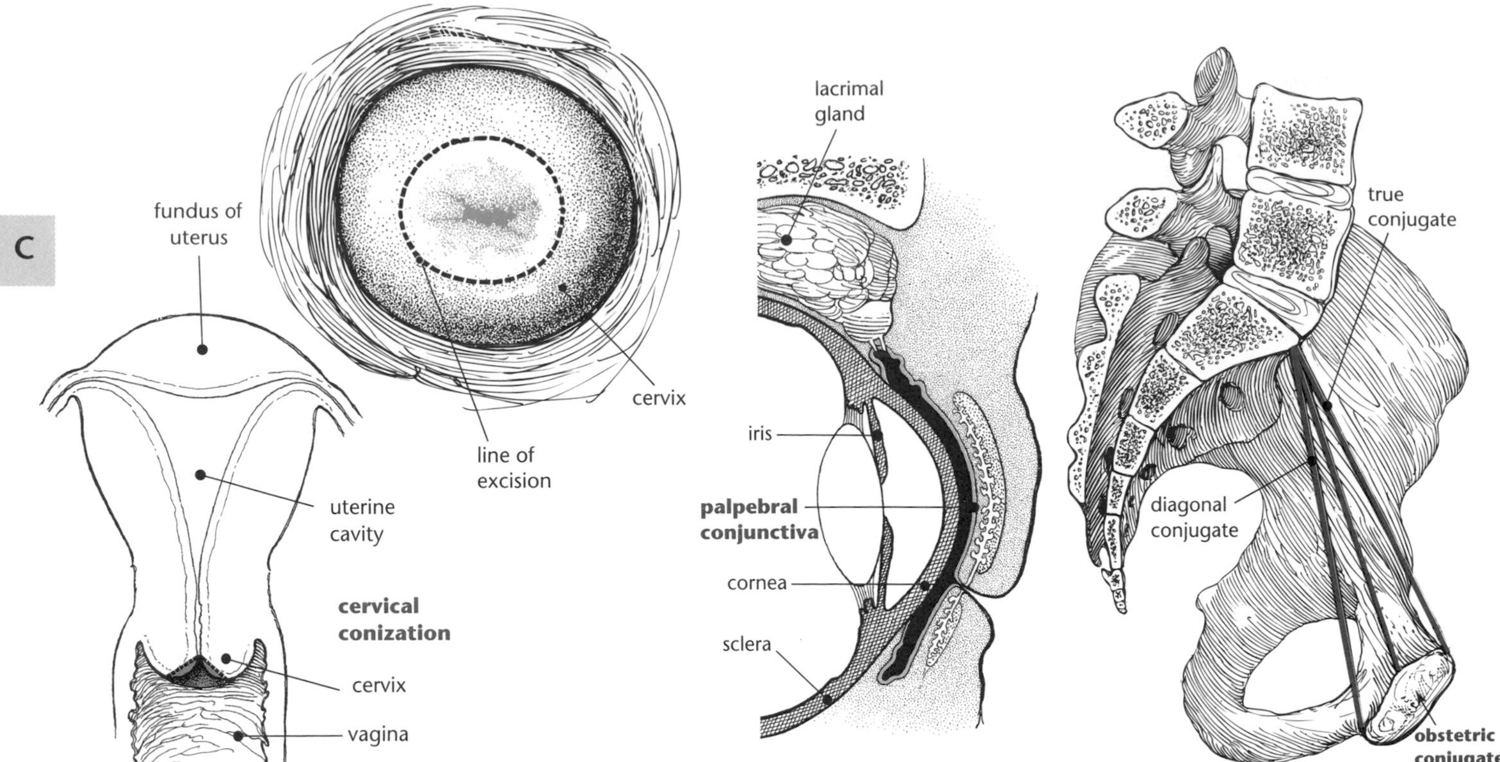

confinement (kon-fīn´ment) The period of childbirth.

conflict (kon´flikt) The struggle between two opposing emotions, thoughts, needs, or courses of action.

confluence of sinuses (kon´floo-ens ŭv sīn´nus-ez) The junction of the sinuses of the dura mater (superior sagittal, straight, occipital, and two transverse), located in a slight depression at one side of the internal protuberance of the occipital bone.

confluent (kon´floo-ent) Running together, as the skin lesions of certain diseases which are not distinct but become merged.

conformation (kon-for-ma´shun) The spatial arrangement of atoms in a molecule achieved by rotation of groups about single, covalent bonds, without breaking any covalent bonds.

conformer (kon´for-mer) A mold or shell fitted in a cavity to preserve its shape, as in the eye socket after removal of the eye prior to insertion of an artificial eye.

confusion (kon-fu´zhun) A state of perceptual disorientation, inattentiveness, and impaired ability to think clearly and with customary speed.

congener (kon´jĕ-ner) **1.** A drug that is part of a group of chemical compounds sharing the same parent compound. **2.** One of two or more muscles with the same function.

congenic (kon-jen´ik) Relating to inbred animals.

congenital (kon-jen´ĭ-tal) Present at birth.

congenital poikiloderma-juvenile cataract syndrome See Rothmund's syndrome.

congested (kon-jest´ed) Containing an abnormally large amount of blood.

congestion (kon-jest´chun) Abnormal accumula-tion of blood in a part.

hypostatic c. See venous stasis, under stasis.

passive venous c. Congestion of a part due to partial stagnation of blood in the capillaries and venules, resulting from faulty venous drainage or failure of the right ventricle of the heart.

conglutination (kon-gloo-tĭ-na´shun) **1.** Abnormal adhesion of tissues. **2.** The clumping of sensitized cells or of antigen-antibody complexes that have absorbed complement, occurring in the presence of bovine serum that contains the protein conglutinin.

conglutinin (kon-gloo´tĭ-nin) A nonantibody protein with the capability of combining with the carbohydrate portion of complement and thus capable of clumping particles covered by the complement; found in normal bovine serum.

Congo red (kong´gōred) A red azo dye, used in biologic stains and as an indicator (red in alkaline solutions and blue in acid solutions).

conidiophore (ko-nid´e-o-for) A spore-bearing specialized hyphal filament in fungi.

conidiospore (ko-nid´e-o-spōr) A fungal spore produced on a specialized conidiophore.

conidium (ko-nid´e-um), *pl.* **conid´ia** The reproductive spore of fungi produced asexually.

coniofibrosis (ko-ne-o-fi-bro´sis) Abnormal formation of fibrous tissue in the lungs, caused by prolonged exposure to dust.

coniosis (ko-ne-o´sis) Any disease caused by dust.

Conium maculatum (ko-ni´um mak´u-la-tum) A poisonous large herb, family Umbelliferae. Also called poison hemlock; spotted parsley.

conization (kon-ĭ-za´shun) Surgical removal of a conical portion of tissue.

cervical c. Removal of a lesion and surrounding tissue (tissue at risk) from the central longitudinal axis of the cervix, including the external os and a length of endocervical canal; the excised tissue may or may not have a cone shape, depending on the distribution of the lesion.

cold c. Conization performed with a knife.

laser c. Conization performed with a laser beam.

conjugase (kon´jo͞o-gās) An enzyme, present in the liver and kidney of mammals, that splits folic acid conjugates into pteroylglutamic acid and glutamic acid.

conjugate (kon´jo͞o-gāt) Paired, coupled.

diagonal c. The distance between the sacral promontory and the lower border of the pubic symphysis.

obstetric c. The distance between the sacral promontory and the inner surface of the pubic symphysis; represents the shortest anteroposterior diameter of the pelvic inlet.

true c. The anteroposterior diameter of the pelvic inlet from the sacral promontory to the upper border of the pubic symphysis. Also called conjugata vera; anteroposterior diameter of pelvic inlet.

conjugation (kon-jo͞o-ga´shun) **1.** Sexual reproduction of unicellular organisms whereby the two cells exchange genetic material. **2.** In chemistry, the combination of large molecules (e.g., proteins) with those of another substance.

conjunctiva (kon-junk´tī-vă) The thin transparent mucous membrane lining the inner surface of the eyelids (palpebral conjunctiva) and the exposed surface of the anterior sclera up to the border of the cornea (bulbar conjunctiva); the epithelial layer of the conjunctiva is continuous with the corneal epithelium.

conjunctivitis (kon-junk-tĭ-vī´tis) Inflammation of the conjunctiva resulting from bacterial, viral, or allergic agents; e.g., acute catarrhal conjunctivitis is caused by a bacterium (usually pneumococcus), epidemic keratoconjunctivitis is caused by a virus (adenovirus 8), vernal catarrh is caused by hyper-sensitivity to exogenous allergens.

acute contagious c. Bacterial conjunctivitis caused by *Haemophilus influenzae*, causing redness of the eye and a mucopurulent discharge. Also called pinkeye; acute epidemic conjunctivitis.

acute epidemic c. See acute contagious conjunctivitis.

neonatal c. See ophthalmia neonatorum, under ophthalmia.

connective tissue diseases (kŏ-nek´tiv tish´oo dĭ-zēz´ĕs) See collagen diseases.

connector (kŏ-nek´tor) In dentistry, the part of a fixed partial denture that unites its component parts (e.g., an artificial tooth).

Conn's syndrome (konz sin´drōm) See primary aldosteronism, under aldosteronism.

consanguineous (kon-san-gwin´e-us) Related by blood.

consanguinity (kon-san-gwin´ĭ-te) Kinship; blood relationship from common ancestry.

conscious (kon´shus) Being aware of one's existence, actions, and environment.

consciousness (kon´shŭs-nes) State of awareness of and responsiveness to environment.

consensual (kon-sen´shoo-al) Relating to a reflex response of one organ in response to sensory stimulation of another (e.g., the eyes).

conservative (kon-ser´vă-tiv) Applied to a cautious method of treatment.

consolidation (kon-sol-ĭ-da´shun) **1.** Solidification into a dense mass; applied especially to the inflammatory solidification of the lung in pneumonia. **2.** The mass so formed.

constant (kon´stant) (k) A quantity which, under stated conditions, does not vary with changes in the environment.

decay c. The mathematical expression for the number of atoms of radionuclide that will decay in a unit of time.

dissociation c. (K) In chemistry, the constant that depends upon the equilibrium between the dissociated and undissociated forms of a molecule in solution.

gas c. (R) The universal constant of proportionality, appearing in the equation of the general gas law, equal to the pressure of the gas times its volume divided by its temperature.

Michaelis-Menten c. (K_m) A constant expres-sing the concentration of the substrate at which half the maximum velocity of a reaction is achieved.

Plank's c. (*h*) A constant expressing the ratio of the energy possessed by a quantum of energy to its frequency; its value is approximately 6.625×10^{-27} erg-sec.

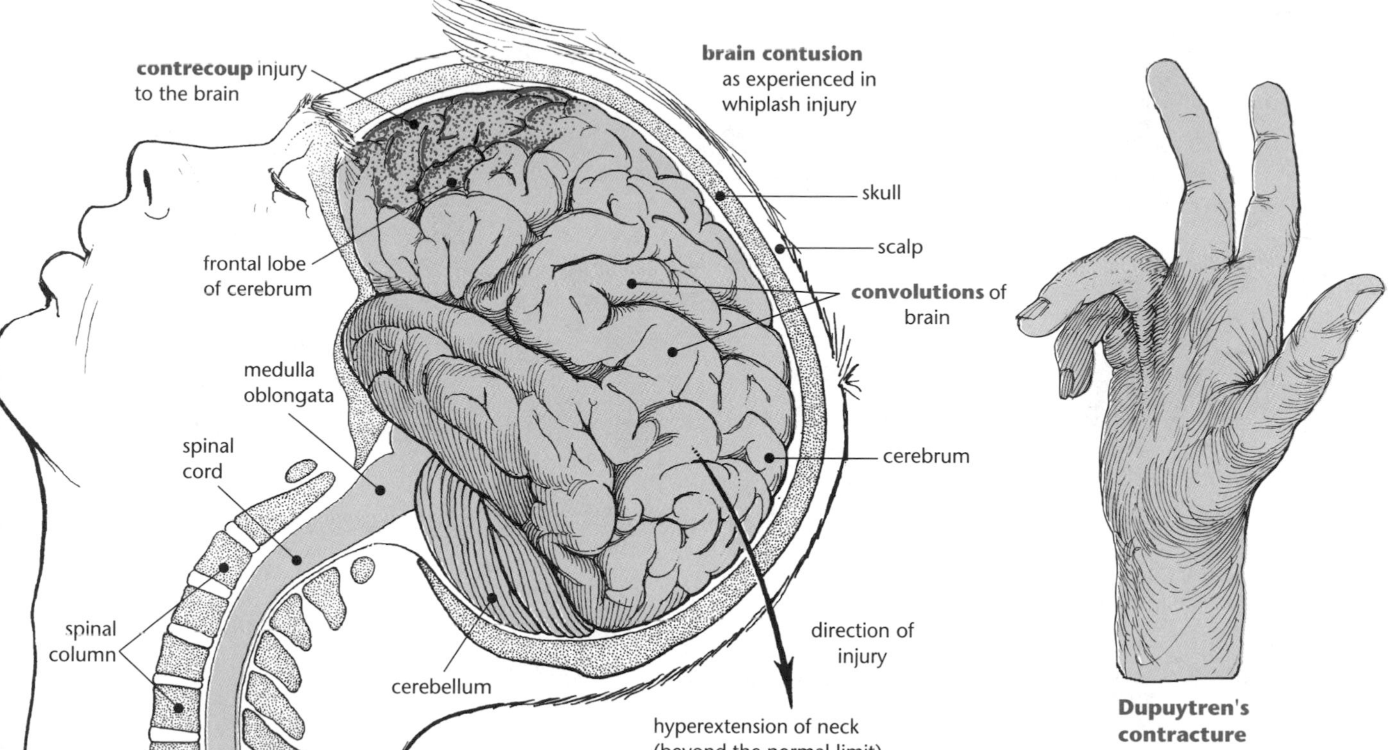

C

constellation (kon-stel-ā́shun) In psychiatry, a set of related ideas.

constipate (kon´stĭ-pāt) To slow the action of the bowels.

constipation (kon-stĭ-pā́shŭn) A decrease in the frequency of bowel movements, accompanied by a difficult prolonged effort in passing a very hard stool, followed by a sensation of incomplete evacuation.

constitution (kon-stĭ-too´shŭn) The physical make-up and state of health of the body.

constitutive (kon-stĭ´too-tiv) Produced constantly (e.g., an enzyme).

constriction (kon-strik´shun) **1.** A narrowing; a binding. **2.** A subjective sensation of being tightly bound or squeezed.

secondary c. The slender heterochromatic area of a chromosome which separates the satellite from the rest of the chromosome (the primary constriction is at the centromere).

constrictor (kon-strik´tor) Denoting a muscle that narrows a canal or opening.

consultand (kon-sul′tand) A prospective parent who seeks genetic counsel and whose genetic constitution is in question. COMPARE: proband; relative of interest.

consultant (kon-sul′tant) A physician who is called in an advisory capacity.

consultation (kon-sul-ta´shun) A conference of two or more physicians to evaluate the diagnosis and treatment of the disease in a particular patient; an evaluation or second opinion provided by a specialist.

consumption (kon-sump′shun) The act or process of expending or using up something.

oxygen c. (a) The rate at which oxygen is used by a tissue. (b) The rate at which oxygen from alveolar gas enters the bloodstream in the lungs.

contact (kon′takt) **1.** The point at which two adjacent bodies touch one another. **2.** A person who has been exposed to the virus of an infectious disease.

contact tracing (kon′takt trās′ing) Identification of persons or animals who have had an association with an infected person, animal, or contaminated environment and who, through such an association, have had the opportunity to acquire the infection; it is an accepted method of controlling sexually transmitted diseases.

contagion (kon-ta′jun) Transmission of a disease by direct or indirect contact.

contagious (kon-ta′jus) Transmissible by direct or indirect contact. Also called catching.

contagium (kon-ta′je-um) The causative agent of an infectious disease.

contaminant (kon-tam′ĭ-nant) An impurity.

contamination (kon-tam-ĭ-na´shun) **1.** The process of rendering impure or unhealthy. **2.** In an experiment, allowing the variable that is to be validated to influence the variable used for validation.

content (kon′tent) **1.** Material or substance contained. **2.** The amount of a specified substance.

contiguity (kon-tĭ-gyu′ĭ-te) The state of being adjacent in time or space; immediately preceding or following.

continence (kon′tĭ-nens) **1.** Ability to delay urination or defecation. **2.** Self-restraint, especially from sexual activity.

contour (kon´tōōr) **1.** Surface configuration. **2.** To shape into a desired form, as a denture or a broken tooth.

contraception (kon-tră-sep′shun) The prevention of conception.

contraceptive (kon-tră-sep′tiv) Any agent or device used for the prevention of conception.

barrier c. Any device for preventing the entrance of sperm into the cervical canal (e.g., male and female condoms, diaphragm, cervical cap, and spermicidal agents).

oral c. Any synthetic steroid that is similar to estrogen and progesterone (female hormones) and is taken orally at regular doses to alter the woman's hormonal balance, thereby inhibiting ovulation and preventing pregnancy. Popularly called birth control pill; the pill.

postcoital c. Oral contraceptive taken within 72 hours after sexual intercourse (coitus); usually a combination of hormones (a progestin and an estrogen). Also called morning-after pill; postcoital pill.

contract (kon-tract′) To pull together; to reduce in size or increase tension by drawing together.

contractile (kon-trak′tĭl) Able to contract.

contractility (kon-tract-til′ĭ-te) The ability to shorten or increase tension, applied to a muscle.

contraction (kon-trak′shun) (C) **1.** The shortening or increase in tension of functioning muscle. **2.** A shrinkage or reduction in size. **3.** A heartbeat.

Braxton Hicks c.'s Short, relatively painless contractions of the pregnant uterus, usually beginning at irregular intervals during early pregnancy and becoming more frequent and rhythmic as pregnancy advances, especially during the last 2 weeks of gestation, when they may be mistaken for labor pains; they occasionally occur without pregnancy (e.g., in the presence of soft tumors of the uterine wall).

hourglass c. The narrowing of the middle of a hollow organ.

isometric c. Force developed by contraction of a muscle without appreciable shortening of its length.

isotonic c. Contraction and shortening of a muscle without appreciable change in the force of the contraction.

premature c. A premature heartbeat.

contracture (kon-trak′chur) A permanent contrac-tion due to tonic spasm, muscle atrophy, or scars.

Dupuytren's c. Shortening of the palmar fascia producing permanent flexion of one or more fingers.

ischemic c. Contracture of a muscle resulting from circulatory interference, as by a tight bandage or from cold temperatures.

organic c. Contracture that is permanent, usually due to fibrosis within the muscle.

Volkmann's c. Contraction of the fingers and sometimes wrist following a severe injury or improper use of a tourniquet.

contraindication (kon-tra-in-dĭ-ka´shun) Any condition that renders undesirable the use of a medication or surgical procedure.

contralateral (kon-tră-lat´er-al) Located on the opposite side.

contrastimulant (kon-tră-stim´u-lant) **1.** Counte-racting the effects of a stimulant. **2.** Any agent producing such an effect.

contrecoup (kon-trĕ-koo′) Occurring on the opposite side, as the fracture of a portion of the skull opposite to the point of impact.

control (kon-trōl′) **1.** To verify a scientific experiment by comparing with a standard or by conducting a parallel experiment, conditions being equal except for one factor. **2.** A standard against which the results of an experiment are checked.

birth c. Limitation of the number of children conceived by the voluntary use of contraceptive measures.

contusion (kon-too´zhun) A mechanical (usually superficial) injury causing a bluish black dis-coloration; a bruise.

brain c. A localized injury to the surface of the brain, usually attended by extravasation of blood and sometimes swelling; symptoms vary according to the extent and location of the injury.

wind c. See windage.

conus (ko′nus), *pl.* **co′ni** A cone-shaped structure.

c. arteriosus The upper, anterior portion of the right ventricle of the heart, ending where the pulmonary trunk begins.

c. medullaris The tapered end of the spinal cord. Also called medullary cone.

convalescence (kon-vă-les′ens) A stage in recovery between the abatement of a disease or injury and complete health.

convection (kon-vek´shun) Heat transfer in liquids or gases by the movement of heated particles.

convergence (kon-ver′jens) **1.** The turning toward or approaching a common point from different directions (e.g., the coordinated movement of the two eyes toward a near point, or the movement of the

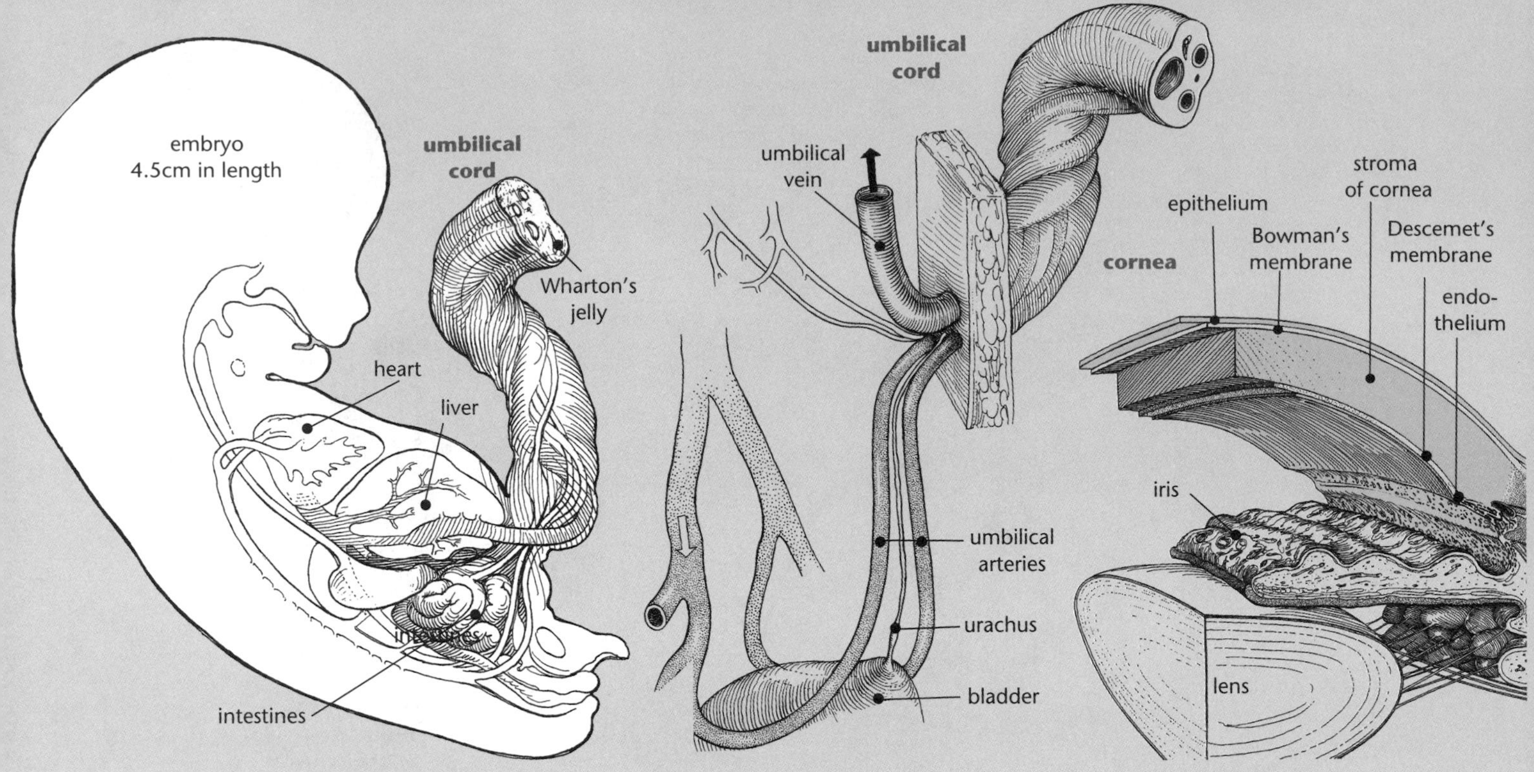

peripheral cells of the blastula toward the center during the gastrulation stage of the embryo). **2.** The connecting of several presynaptic neurons with one postsynaptic neuron.

negative c. Slight outward deviation of the visual axes (e.g., when observing a distant object).

positive c. Inward deviation of the visual axes (e.g., in convergent strabismus).

convergent (kon-ver´jent) Moving or inclined toward a common point.

conversion (kon-ver´zhun) **1.** The act of changing. **2.** In psychiatry, physical symptoms occurring as manifestation of a psychic conflict.

convertin (kon-ver´tin) See factor VII.

convex (kon-veks´) An outwardly curved surface.

convexoconcave (kon-vek-so-kon´kāv) Denoting a lens that has a greater convex than concave curvature.

convoluted (kon-vo-lo͞ot´ed) Rolled, coiled, or twisted.

convolution (kon-vo-lo͞o´shun) A twisting or infolding of an anatomic part upon itself. See also gyrus.

convulsant (kon-vul´sant) Causing convulsions.

convulsion (kon-vul´shun) A violent involuntary muscular contraction, or a series of such contractions producing jerking movements.

Cope's sign (kōps sīn) A sign of appendicitis: tenderness over the area of the appendix on extending the thigh and tenderness on compressing the femoral artery in the femoral triangle.

copolymer (ko-pol´ĭ-mer) A plastic composed of two or more chemically different monomers or base units.

copolymerization (ko-pŏ-lim-er-ĭ-zā´shun) The chemical joining of different monomers to form a compound of a high molecular weight.

copper (kop´er) A malleable, reddish brown metallic element; symbol Cu, atomic number 29, atomic weight 63.54.

coproantibodies (kop-ro-an-tĭ-bod´e) Antibodies present in the intestinal contents.

coprolalia (kop-ro-la´le-ă) The involuntary use of obscene words.

coprolith (kop´ro-lith) A mass of inspissated feces. Also called fecalith; stercolith.

coprophagia (kop-ro-fa´jă) The eating of feces. Also called scatophagy.

coproporphyrin (kop-ro-por´fĭ-rin) A porphyrin compound normally present in feces; a decomposition product of bilirubin. Also called stereoporphyrin.

copulation (kop-u-la´shun) Sexual intercourse; coitus.

cor (kōr) Latin for heart.

c. biloculare A more or less two-chambered heart due to the absence or incomplete development of the interatrial and interventricular septa.

c. bovinum An abnormally large heart as seen in the third stage of syphilis. Also called bucardia.

c. pulmonale Enlargement of the right ventricle of the heart, secondary to a disease of the lungs.

c. triloculare A three-chambered heart due to absence of either the interatrial or the interventricular septum.

coracoacromial (kor-ă-ko-ă-kro´me-al) Relating to the coracoid and acromial processes of the scapula (shoulder blade).

coracobrachial (kor-ă-ko-bra´ke-al) Relating to the coracoid process of the scapula and the arm.

coracoclavicular (kor-ă-ko-klă-vik´u-lar) Relating to the coracoid process of the scapula and the clavicle.

coracohumeral (kor-ă-ko-hu´mer-al) Relating to the coracoid process of the scapula and the humerus.

coracoid (kor´ă-koid) Shaped like a raven's beak; denoting the thick, curved process at the superior border of the scapula (shoulder blade).

cord (kord) Any flexible, stringlike structure.

medullary c.'s Columns of dense lymphoid tissue (mostly packed lymphocytes) surrounded by sinuses in the medulla of lymph nodes.

spermatic c. Cord extending from the deep inguinal ring to the testis within the scrotum; contains the deferent duct, arteries, veins, nerves, and lymph vessels held together by loose connective tissue.

spinal c. The elongated portion of the central nervous system that is enclosed by the vertebral column.

umbilical c. Cord connecting the fetus with the fetal side of the placenta; consists of a sheet of amnion encasing two arteries and one vein embedded in a loose mucoid connective tissue (Wharton's jelly); at birth it measures from 30 to 100 cm in length and 0.8 to 2.0 cm in diameter.

vocal c. See vocal fold, under fold.

cordate (kor´dāt) Heart-shaped.

cordectomy (kor-dek´tŏ-me) Surgical removal of a cord.

cordocentesis (kor-do-sen-te´sis) See percutaneous umbilical cord sampling, under sampling.

cordopexy (kor´do-pek-se) Surgical fixation of a cord.

cordotomy (kor-dot´ŏ-me) Severing of the sensory tracts of the spinal cord for the relief of intractable pain.

core (kor) **1.** The innermost or central part of something. **2.** A metal casting designed to retain in position the artificial crown of a tooth. **3.** A section of a mold used to record and maintain the relationships of parts, such as teeth or metallic restorations.

corectasis (kor-ek´tă-sis) Abnormally dilated state of the pupil.

corectopia (kor-ek-to´pe-ă) Abnormal position of the pupil to one side of the center of the iris.

corepressor (ko-re-pres´or) A small molecule, usually a product of a specific enzyme pathway, capable of combining with the inactive repressor to form an active complex which combines with the operator and prevents mRNA synthesis; a homeostatic mechanism for regulating enzyme production in repressible enzyme systems.

corestenoma (kor-e-ste-no´mă) Abnormally contracted state of the pupil.

corium (ko´re-um) See dermis.

corn (korn) A circumscribed induration and thickening of the skin.

hard c. A corn over a toe joint caused by friction and/or pressure from ill-fitting shoes.

seed c. A wart on the foot.

soft c. A thickening of the skin between two toes caused by pressure and kept soft by moisture.

cornea (kor´ne-ă) The transparent anterior part of the outer coat of the eyeball that serves as the major refracting medium; it consists of five layers; corneas donated for transplantation are now routinely preserved at eye banks.

conical c. See keratoconus.

corneal (kor´ne-al) Relating to the cornea.

corneitis (kor-ne-i´tis) See keratitis.

corneosclera (kor-ne-o-skler´ă) The cornea and sclera considered as a unit that forms the outer layer of the eyeball.

corneous (kor´ne-us) Hornlike.

corneum (kor´ne-um) The superficial layer of the skin. Also called stratum corneum.

corniculate (kor-nik´u-lāt) Having the shape of a small horn.

cornification (kor-nĭ-fĭ-ka´shun) Conversion into horny tissue or keratin.

cornu (kor´noo), *pl.* **cor´nua** **1.** A horn-shaped structure. **2.** Any structure composed of bony tissue.

corona (ko-ro´nă) Any structure resembling a crown.

c. radiata An investment of follicular cells remaining attached to the ovum when released by the ovary; a remnant of cumulus oophorus (which previously surrounded the developing oocyte within the ovary).

coronal (ko-ron´al) **1.** Relating to the crown of the head or of a tooth. **2.** Relating to the side-to-side plane of the head or any vertical plane parallel to it.

coronary (kor´ŏ-nar-e) **1.** Encircling in the manner

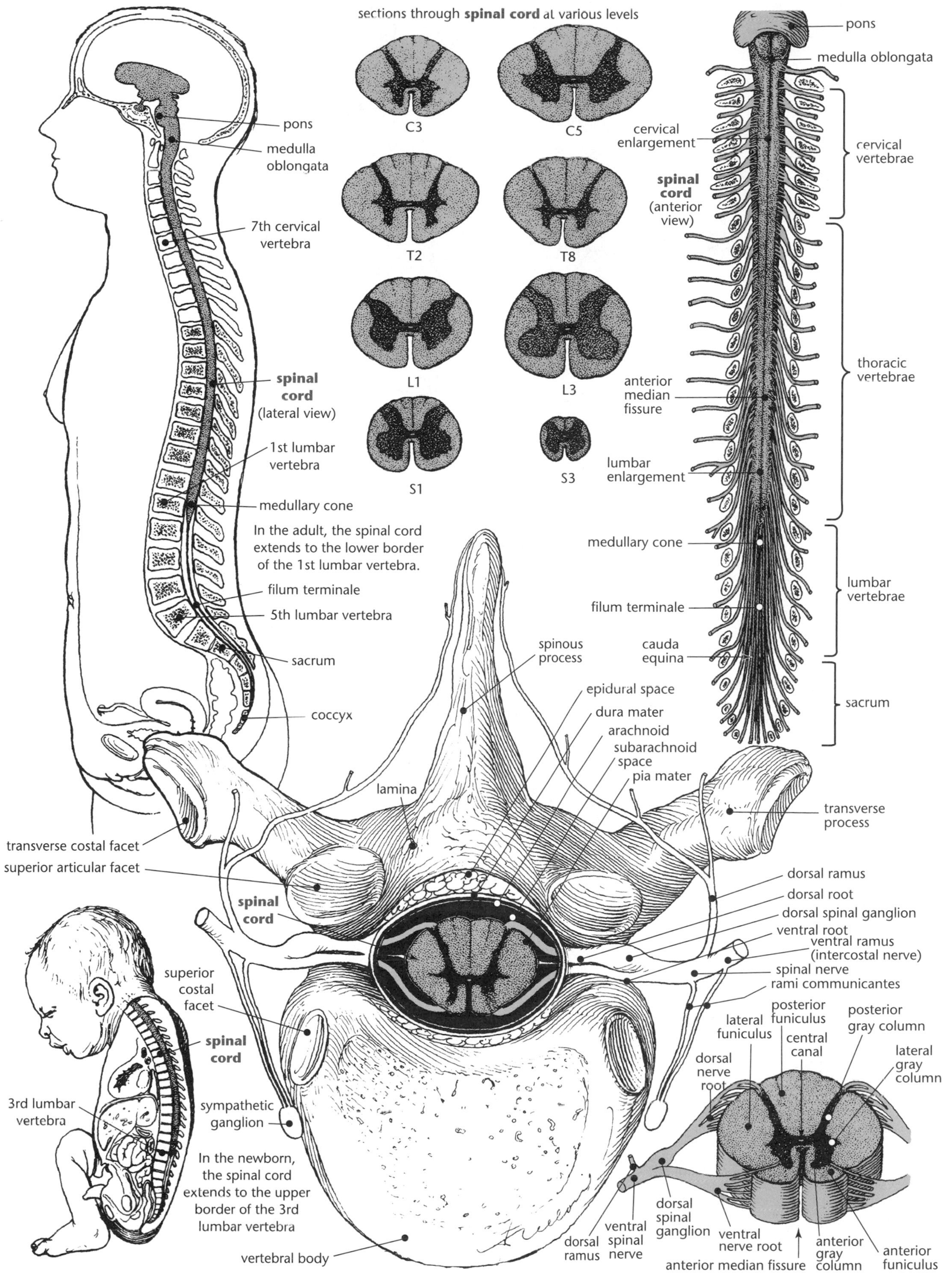
sections through spinal cord at various levels
C3
C5
T2
T8
L1
L3
S1
S3
pons
medulla oblongata
7th cervical vertebra
spinal cord (lateral view)
1st lumbar vertebra
medullary cone
In the adult, the spinal cord extends to the lower border of the 1st lumbar vertebra.
filum terminale
5th lumbar vertebra
sacrum
coccyx
pons
medulla oblongata
cervical enlargement
spinal cord (anterior view)
cervical vertebrae
thoracic vertebrae
anterior median fissure
lumbar enlargement
medullary cone
filum terminale
lumbar vertebrae
cauda equina
sacrum
spinous process
epidural space
dura mater
arachnoid
subarachnoid space
pia mater
lamina
transverse process
transverse costal facet
superior articular facet
dorsal ramus
dorsal root
dorsal spinal ganglion
ventral root
ventral ramus (intercostal nerve)
spinal nerve
rami communicantes
spinal cord
superior costal facet
spinal cord
3rd lumbar vertebra
sympathetic ganglion
In the newborn, the spinal cord extends to the upper border of the 3rd lumbar vertebra
vertebral body
lateral funiculus
posterior funiculus
central canal
posterior gray column
lateral gray column
dorsal nerve root
dorsal spinal ganglion
dorsal ramus
ventral spinal nerve
ventral nerve root
anterior median fissure
anterior gray column
anterior funiculus

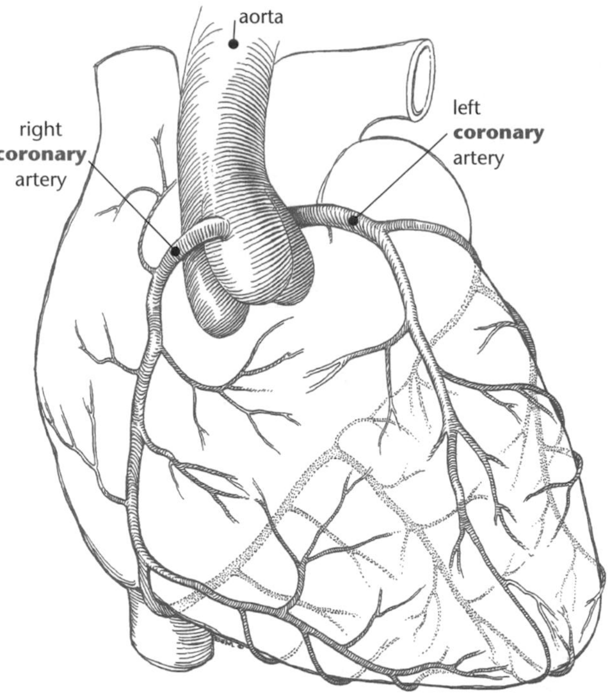

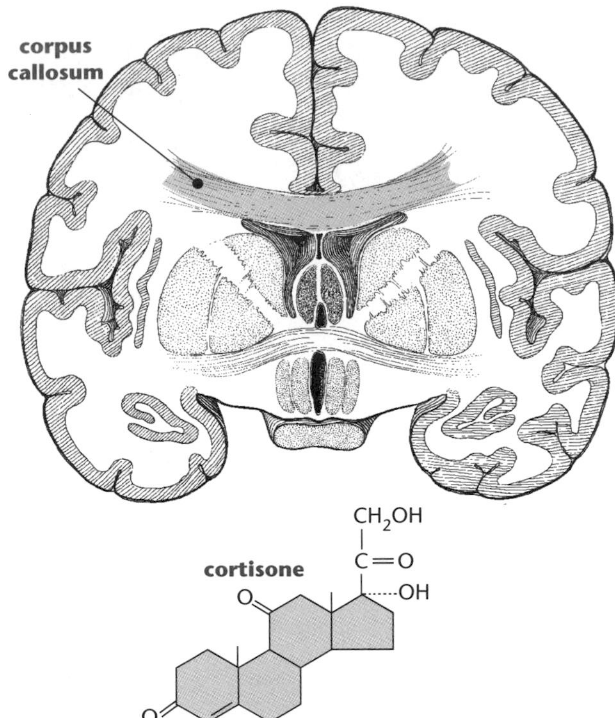

of a crown, as the vessels supplying the heart muscle. **2.** Popular term for coronary occlusion.

coronary artery disease (kor´ŏ-nar-e ar´ter-e dĭs-zēz´) (CAD) Hardening and narrowing of arteries supplying blood to the heart muscle (myocardium); usually caused by progressive plaque formation on the arterial walls.

coroner (kor´ŏ-ner) A county official empowered to investigate any death thought to be of other than natural causes, occurring within his or her jurisdiction; qualifications for the position vary with the jurisdiction. In some communities, medical examiners have replaced coroners.

coronion (ko-ro´ne-on) A craniometric point at the tip of the coronoid process of the lower jaw.

coronoid (kor´o-noid) **1.** Shaped like a crow's beak; denoting certain processes of bones, such as the coronoid process of the mandible (lower jaw). **2.** Crown-shaped.

corpora (kor´po-ră) Plural of corpus.

corporeal (kor-por´e-al) **1.** Relating to the body. **2.** Relating to a corpus.

corpulence (kor´pu-lens) Obesity.

corpus (kor´pus), *pl.* **cor´pora** Body; the main portion of a structure.

c. albicans A mass of white, collagenous scar tissue that replaces the corpus luteum when conception does not occur.

c. callosum A mass of transverse fibers connecting the two hemispheres of the brain.

c. cavernosum One of the two parallel columns of erectile tissue of the penis or of the clitoris.

c. luteum A secretory structure in the ovary formed at the site of a ruptured vesicular ovarian follicle after it has discharged its ovum; consists of a large mass of lipid-rich cells containing a yellow pigment (lutein); it secretes estrogens and progesterone, the hormones that cause thickening of the uterine lining in preparation for the implantation of the fertilized ovum; if pregnancy occurs, it continues to grow for 13 weeks before slowly regressing; if pregnancy fails to occur, the corpus luteum regresses to a mass of scar tissue (corpus albicans).

c. spongiosum The median column of erectile tissue of the penis, situated between and inferior to the corpora cavernosa and surrounding the urethra.

c. striatum The caudate and lentiform nuclei and the internal capsule considered as a whole; situated in front of and lateral to the thalamus in each hemisphere of the brain. Also called striate body.

c. vitreum See vitreous body, under body.

corpuscle (kor´pus-l) **1.** A small body or mass. **2.** A cell capable of moving freely in the body. **3.** A primary particle such as a photon or electron.

blood c. Any blood cell.

colostrum c. One of numerous large round bodies containing fat droplets, present in colostrum; thought to be modified leukocyte.

Golgi-Mazzoni c. An encapsulated sensory nerve ending found in the subcutaneous tissue of the pulp of the fingers; similar to a pacinian corpuscle, but with a thinner capsule and with axons that ramify more extensively and end in flat expansions.

ghost c. See achromocyte.

Krause's c. See Krause's end bulb, under bulb.

Meissner's c. A small, oval, encapsulated receptor organ present in the dermal papillae of the skin, particularly prevalent on the palmar and plantar surfaces; signals fine, discriminative touch sensations. Also called tactile corpuscle of Meissner.

Negri c.'s See Negri bodies, under body.

pacinian c. An encapsulated receptor organ that signals mechanical deformations as touch or vibratory sensations; characterized by an un-myelinated terminal axon covered by numerous concentric layers of connective tissue; found in subcutaneous tissue, fascial planes around joints and tendons, and in the mesentery about the pancreas; especially numerous in the palm of the hand, sole of the foot, and genital organs; it responds to deep pressure and vibrations.

phantom c. See achromocyte.

red blood c. See erythrocyte.

renal c. The invaginated pouchlike glomerular capsule (the beginning of a renal tubule) containing a central tuft of vessels (the glomerulus).

Ruffini's c.'s See Ruffini's nerve endings, under ending.

shadow c. See achromocyte.

terminal c. Any specialized encapsulated nerve ending, such as the pacinian corpuscle.

white blood c.'s See white blood cells, under cell.

correspondence (kor-ĕ-spon´dens) The state of being in harmony.

retinal c. The faculty of vision by which an object seen with the two eyes (thus forming two retinal images) is perceived as one due to the coordinate functioning of retinal receptors.

corrosive (kŏ-ro´siv) Caustic; denoting an agent that causes a gradual wearing away or disintegration of a substance by chemical alteration.

cortex (kor´teks) The external portion of an organ, such as the brain, kidney, and adrenal gland.

cortexone (kor-teks´ōn) See deoxycorticosterone.

cortical (kor´tĭ-kal) Relating to a cortex.

corticifugal (kor-tĭ-sif´u-gal) Conducting impulses away from the cerebral cortex.

corticipetal (kor-tĭ-sip´e-tal) Conducting impulses toward the cerebral cortex.

corticoid (kor´tĭ-koid) Corticosteroid.

corticopontine (kor-tĭ-ko-pon´tīn) Relating to the cerebral cortex and pons.

corticospinal (kor-tĭ-ko-spi´nal) Relating to the cerebral cortex and spinal cord.

corticosteroid (kor-tĭ-ko-ster´oid) Any of the hormones of the adrenal cortex or any synthetic substitute.

corticosterone (kor-tĭ-kos´ter-ōn) See cortisone.

corticothalamic (kor-tĭ-ko-thă-lam´ik) Relating to the cerebral cortex and thalamus.

corticotropin (kor-tĭ-ko-tro´pin) **1.** A hormone produced by the anterior lobe of the pituitary gland that stimulates the secretion of cortisone and other hormones of the adrenal cortex. **2.** A pharmaceutical preparation made synthetically or extracted from the anterior pituitary of mammals, used to stimulate the activity of the adrenal cortex. Also called adrenocorticotrophin.

cortisol (kor´tĭ-sol) See hydrocortisone.

cortisone (kor´tĭ-sōn) A hormone from the adrenal cortex active in regulating carbohydrate metabolism and the nutrition of connective tissue; its release is regulated by the action of the adrenocorticotropic hormone (ACTH) of the pituitary gland; an excess of cortisone activity is responsible for Cushing's syndrome. Also called corticosterone.

Corynebacterium (ko-rī-ne-bak-te´re-um) A genus of irregularly staining, gram-positive bacteria having a club shape and causing disease in plants and animals.

C. diphtheriae The species that causes diphtheria in humans; produces a powerful exotoxin; found in the mucous membrane of the upper respiratory tract of infected persons.

coryza (ko-rī´ză) See acute rhinitis, under rhinitis.

cosmesis (koz-me´sis) Concern for the appearance of the patient, especially in surgical operations.

cosmetic (koz-met´ik) Denoting any preparation or operative procedure intended to improve the appearance of a person.

costa (kos´tă), *pl.* **cos´tae** Latin for rib.

costal (kos´tal) Relating to a rib.

costectomy (kos-tek´tŏ-me) Surgical removal of a rib.

costocentral (kos-to-sen´tral) See costovertebral.

costochondral (kos-to-kon´dral) Relating to a rib and its cartilage.

costochondritis (kos-to-kon-drī´tis) Pain at the costochondral articulations, especially the third, fourth, and fifth joints, occasionally mistaken for pain of cardiac origin.

costoclavicular (kos-to-klă-vik´u-lar) Relating to

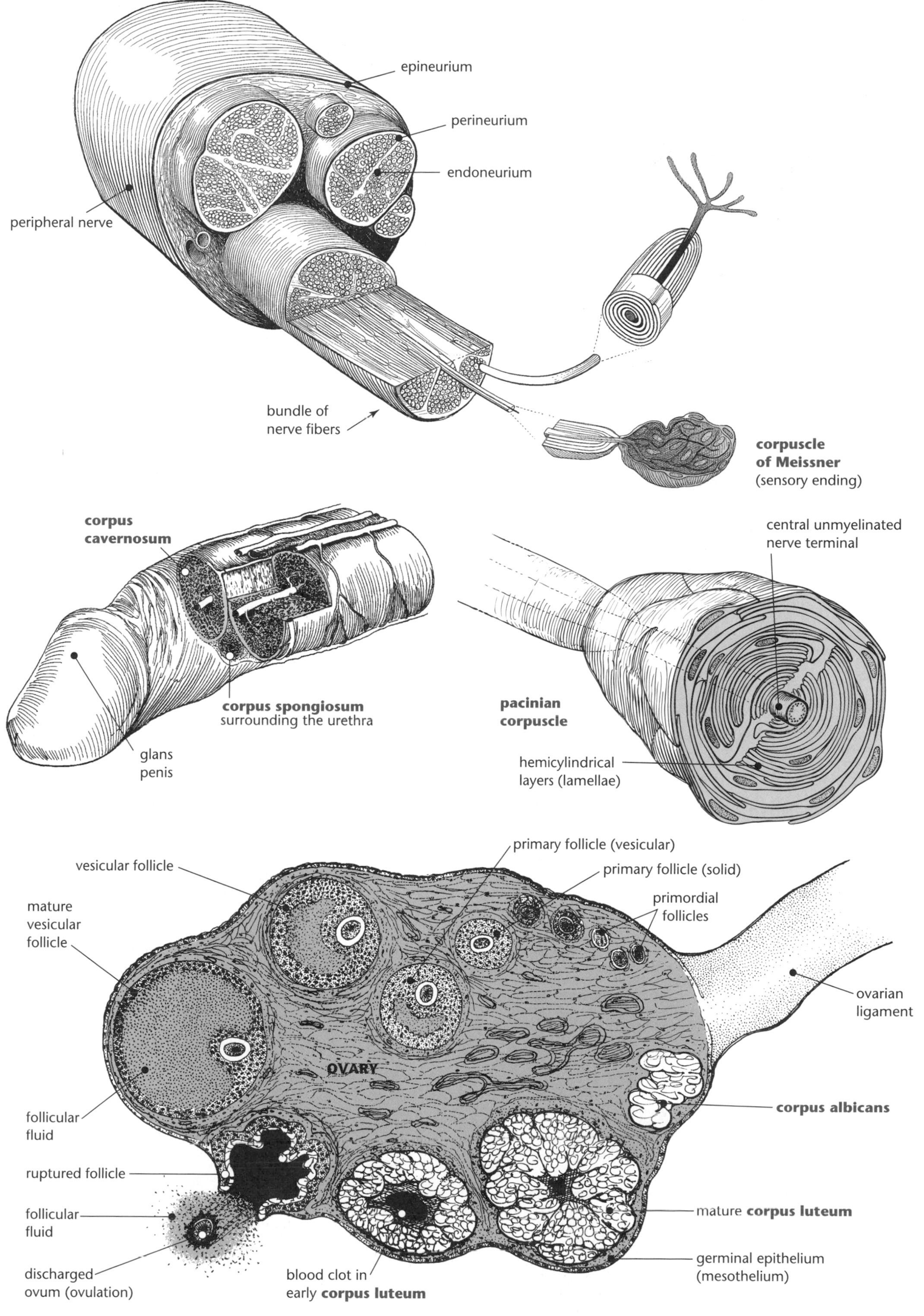
epineurium
perineurium
endoneurium
peripheral nerve
bundle of
nerve fibers
corpuscle
of Meissner
(sensory ending)
corpus
cavernosum
corpus spongiosum
surrounding the urethra
glans
penis
central unmyelinated
nerve terminal
pacinian
corpuscle
hemicylindrical
layers (lamellae)
primary follicle (vesicular)
vesicular follicle
primary follicle (solid)
primordial
follicles
mature
vesicular
follicle
ovarian
ligament
OVARY
follicular
fluid
corpus albicans
ruptured follicle
follicular
fluid
mature corpus luteum
germinal epithelium
(mesothelium)
discharged
ovum (ovulation)
blood clot in
early corpus luteum

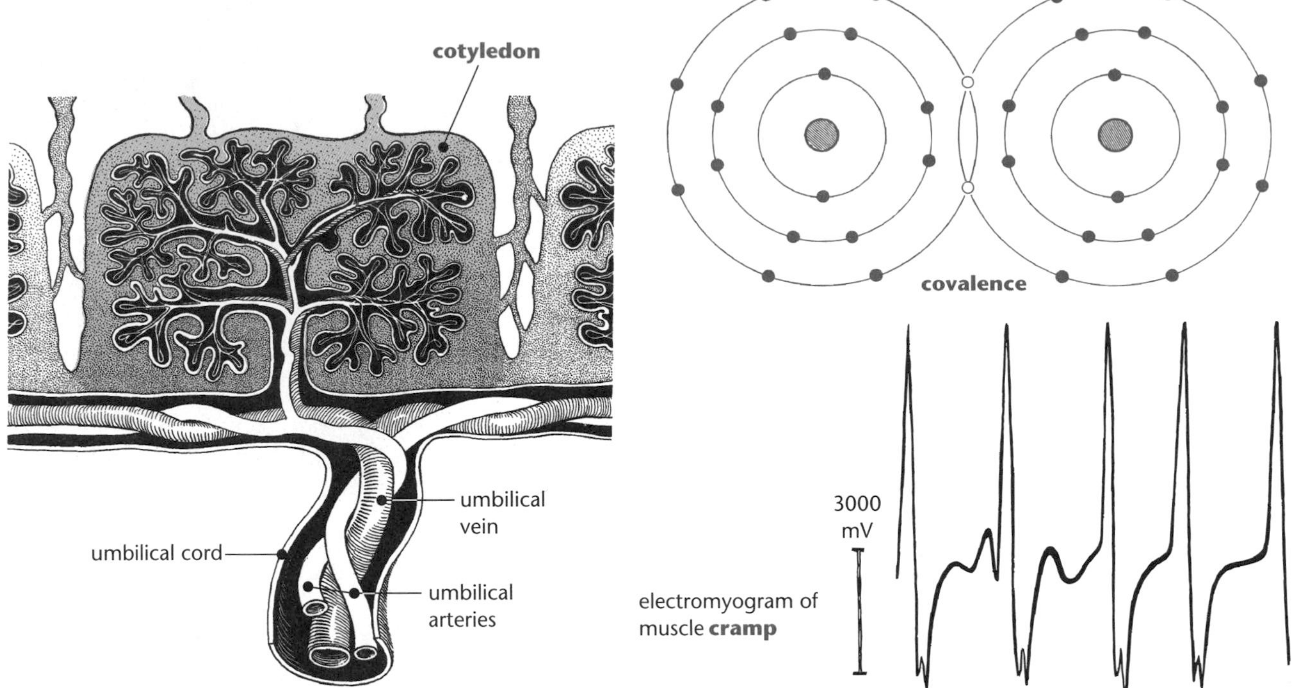

the ribs and a clavicle.

costoclavicular syndrome (kos-to-klă-vik′u-lar sin ′drōm) Vascular disorders of the upper limb due to neuromuscular compression between the clavicle and the first rib.

costophrenic (kos-to-fren′ik) Relating to the ribs and the diaphragm.

costoscapular (kos-to-skap′u-lar) Relating to the ribs and a scapula.

costosternal (kos-to-ster′nal) Relating to the ribs and the sternum.

costotome (kos′to-tōm) Instrument used for cutting through a rib.

costotomy (kos-tot′ŏ-me) Division of a rib or costal cartilage.

costovertebral (kos-to-ver′te-bral) Relating to the ribs and the thoracic vertebrae. Also called costocentral.

cotransport (ko-trans′port) The simultaneous transport of two substances across a membrane, in the same direction.

cotton (kot′n) The soft, white fiber covering the seeds of the cotton plant (genus *Gossypium).*

absorbent c. Cotton from which fatty matter and impurities have been removed.

cotyledon (kot-ĭ-le′don) One of 15 to 20 irregularly shaped subdivisions on the maternal side of the placenta (i.e., the surface attached to the uterine wall); it contains numerous villi.

cough (kawf) A forceful and sudden expulsion of air from the lungs.

whooping c. See pertussis.

coulomb (koo′lom) (Q) A unit of electrical quantity equal to the amount of charge transferred in one second by a steady current of one ampere.

counseling (kown′sel-ing) A professional service that provides an individual with a better understanding of his problems and potentialities.

genetic c. A service by individuals know-ledgeable in human genetics that provides information about inherited disorders so that people can make informed choices about family planning.

count (kount) **1.** To list one by one in order to calculate a total. **2.** The formulation of a total obtained by examining a sample.

Arneth c. The percentage of distribution of polymorphonuclear neutrophils according to the number of lobes their nuclei contain.

blood c. (a) The number of red or white blood cells in 1 mm^3 of blood. (b) The determination of these numbers.

CD4/CD8 c. The ratio of helper-inducer T lymphocytes to cytotoxic-suppressor T lymphocytes; used to monitor for signs of rejection of organ transplants and to gauge progression of HIV infection to AIDS. In healthy individuals, the ratio ranges between 1.6 and 2.2.

complete blood c. (CBC) One usually composed of a hemoglobin determination, a hematocrit, a red blood cell count, a white blood cell count, and a differential white blood cell count.

differential blood c. The percentage of various types of white blood cells in a specific volume of blood. Also called differential white blood cell count.

Schilling's blood c. A differential blood count in which the polymorphonuclear leukocytes are separated into four groups according to the number and arrangement of nuclear segments in the cells. Also called Schilling's index.

counter (koun′ter) A computer or any apparatus for counting.

Geiger c. An instrument used to detect, measure, and record the emission of radioactive particles; it consists of a negatively charged metallic cylinder in a vacuum tube containing a positively charged wire. Also called Geiger-Müller counter (GM counter).

scintillation c. Device used to detect and count radioactive particles.

counterconditioning (koun-ter-kon-dish′un-ing) In behavior therapy, establishment of a second conditioned response to nullify a previously learned response.

countercurrent (koun′ter-kur-ent) A current flowing in a direction opposite to another.

counterextension (koun-ter-eks-ten′shun) See countertraction.

counterirritant (koun-ter-ir′ĭ-tant) A substance applied locally to produce a mild superficial irritation in order to alleviate an underlying inflammation.

counterpulsation (koun-ter-pul-sa′shun) Procedure used to improve an impaired circulation (e.g., in acute myocardial infarction) by means of a pump that is synchronized to the heartbeat.

countershock (koun′ter-shok) Electric shock applied to the heart to correct a disturbance of its rhythm.

counterstain (koun′ter-stān) A second stain, usually of a contrasting color, applied to a microscopy specimen to color parts not affected by the first stain. Also called contrast stain.

countertraction (koun-ter-trak′shun) A traction or pull which is antagonistic to the action of another traction; a back-pull. Also called counterextension.

countertransference (koun-ter-trans-fer′ens) The psychoanalyst's emotional reaction to his patient; it may be conscious or unconscious.

countertransport (koun-ter-trans′port) The passage of two substances across a cell membrane, simultaneously but in opposite directions (e.g., sodium and hydrogen ions).

coup (koo) French for stroke or blow.

couple (kup′l) To copulate; said of lower animals.

coupling (kup′ling) **1.** Pairing or joining. **2.** Bigeminal rhythm; heartbeats occurring in pairs; a normal sinus beat followed by a premature heartbeat.

constant c. See fixed coupling.

fixed c. The occurrence of several premature heartbeats with a constant interval between each of them and the preceding normal heartbeat. Also called constant coupling.

variable c. The occurrence of several premature heartbeats with different intervals between each of them and the preceding normal heartbeat.

Courvoisier's sign (koor-vwah-ze-āz sīn) See Courvoisier's law, under law.

covalence (ko-va′lens) In chemistry, a bond marked by the sharing of electrons (usually in pairs) by two atoms in a chemical compound.

coverslip (kov′er-slip) See cover glass, under glass.

cowpox (kou′poks) A mild eruptive skin disease affecting the teats and udders of cattle, caused by a poxvirus. The virus can be transmitted to humans by skin contact with infected animals. See also vaccinia.

coxa (kok′să), *pl.* **cox′ae** Latin for hipbone and hip joint.

coxalgia (kok-sal′jă) Pain in the hip joint.

Coxiella burnetii (kok-se-el′ă bur-net′e) The bacterium (genus *Coxiella*) that causes Q fever.

coxodynia (kok-so-din′e-ă) Coxalgia; pain in the hip joint.

coxsackievirus (kok-sak′e-vi-rus) One of a group of viruses (genus *Enterovirus*) having pathologic effects on the brain, heart, muscle, epithelium of respiratory tract, and skin; divided into two antigenically different groups (A and B); the name is derived from the town of Coxsackie, New York, where it was discovered while an outbreak of poliomyelitis was being investigated.

C-peptide (sē-pep′tīd) See under peptide.

crack (krăk) See crack cocaine, under cocaine.

cramp (kramp) A painful muscle spasm.

heat c. Pain in the abdomen and/or legs occurring in persons working in extreme hot weather.

tailor's c. Spasm and neuralgic pain of the fingers, hand, and forearm. Also called tailor's spasm.

writer's c. Spastic pain of the muscles of the thumb and two adjoining fingers induced by excessive writing. Also called mogigraphia; graphospasm.

cranial (kra′ne-al) Relating to the skull.

craniectomy (kra-ne-ek′tŏ-me) Surgical removal of a portion of the skull.

craniocele (kra′ne-o-sēl) See encephalocele (3).

craniofacial (kra-ne-o-fa′shal) Relating to both the skull and the face.

craniology (kra-ne-ol′ŏ-je) The scientific study of the skull, especially human, in all its aspects.

craniomalacia (kra-ne-o-mă-la′shă) Thinning and

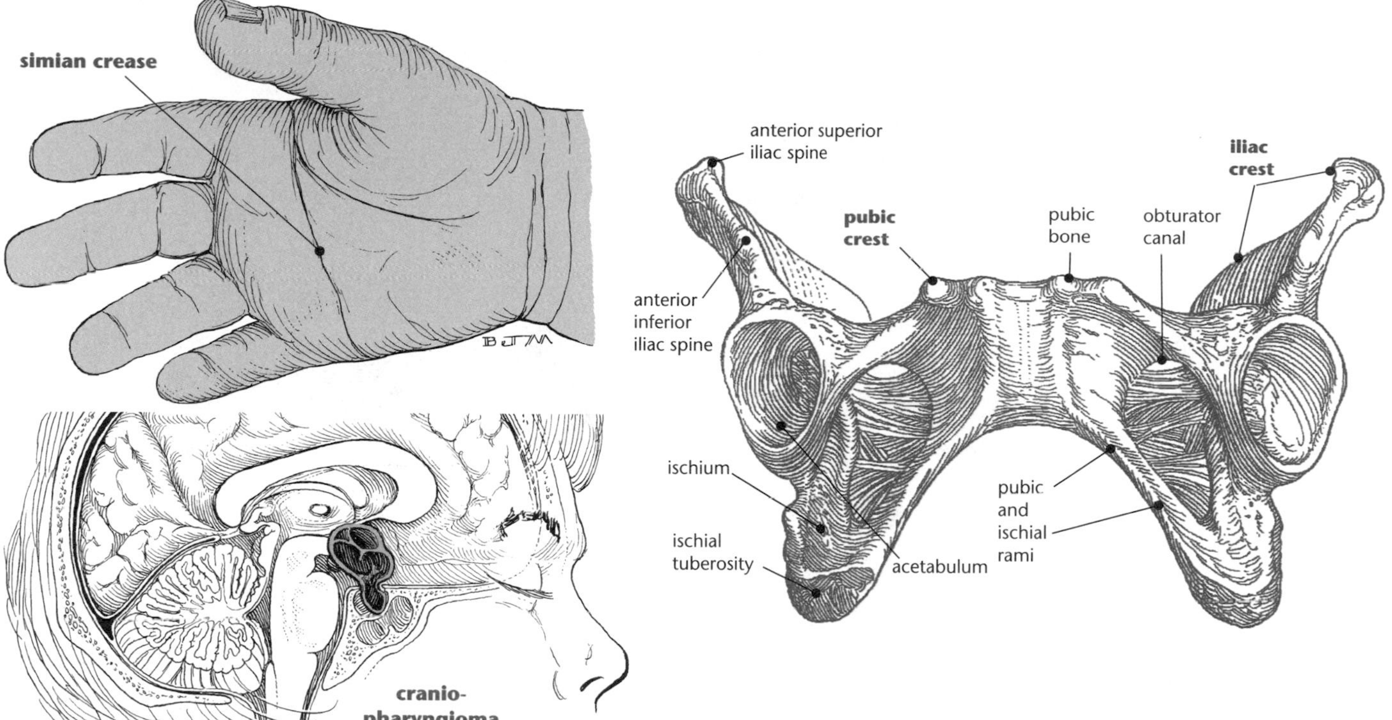

softening of the bones of the skull.

craniometer (kra-ne-om´ĕ-ter) An instrument used to measure skulls.

craniometric (kra-ne-o-met´rik) Relating to skull measurement.

craniometry (kra-ne-om´ĕ-tre) Measurement of the skull, especially human, after removal of the soft tissues.

craniopathy (kra-ne-op´ă-the) Any disease of the skull.

craniopharyngioma (kra-ne-o-fă-rin-je-o´mă) Tumor of the hypophysis arising from remnants of the embryonic adenohypophysis (Rathke's pouch); may be cystic or solid, frequently with calcium deposits. Also called Rathke's pouch tumor.

craniopuncture (kra´ne-o-punk-chur) Puncture of the skull.

craniorachischisis (kra-ne-o-ră-kis´kĭ-sis) Congenital fissure of the skull and vertebral column.

craniosacral (kra-ne-o-sa´kral) Relating to the origins of the parasympathetic nervous system.

cranioschisis (kra-ne-os´kĭ-sis) Congenital defect of the skull in which it fails to close completely, leaving a fissure.

craniosclerosis (kra-ne-o-skle-ro´sis) Abnormal thickening of the skull.

craniostenosis (kra-ne-o-ste-no´sis) Congenital malformation of the skull due to premature closure of the cranial sutures.

craniosynostosis (kra-ne-o-sin-os-to´sis) Premature closure of the sutures of the skull.

craniotabes (kra-ne-o-ta´bēz) Localized softening of an infant's skull, usually due to severe rickets.

craniotome (kra´ne-o-tōm) Instrument used in craniotomy.

craniotomy (kra-ne-ot´ŏ-me) **1.** Surgical opening into the skull. **2.** In obstetrics, puncturing of the head of a dead fetus and evacuation of the contents to facilitate its delivery.

cranium (kra´ne-um) The bones of the head in general; specifically, the bones enclosing the brain. Also called the skull.

crash cart (krash kart) A wheeled conveyance containing the necessary supplies and equipment for initiating emergency resuscitation.

crater (kra´ter) The most depressed area of an ulcer.

crateriform (kra-ter´ĭ-form) Hollowed like a bowl; in bacteriology, denoting a type of liquefaction of gelatin by bacteria in a stab culture.

crazing (kra´zing) The formation of fine cracks on the surface of a structure, such as an artificial tooth, induced by release of internal stress.

cream (krēm) **1.** The fatty constituent of milk that tends to accumulate at the surface on standing. **2.** Any of various substances resembling cream.

crease (krēs) A slight linear depression.

simian c. The single flexion crease usually present on the palms of individuals with Down syndrome. Also called simian line.

creatine (kre´ă-tin) A nitrogenous compound found mainly in muscle tissue.

c. phosphate A creatine phosphoric acid compound; a source of energy in muscle contraction. Also called phosphocreatine.

creatine phosphokinase (kre´ă-tin fos-fo-ki´nās) (CPK) An enzyme that promotes the formation of ATP (adenosine triphosphate) from phosphocreatine and ADP (adenosine diphosphate); essential to muscle contraction.

creatinine (kre-at´ĭ-nin) (Cr) A product of creatine metabolism and a normal metabolic waste; it is removed from the blood by glomerular filtration in the kidneys and excreted in the urine. Since creatinine is usually produced at a constant rate, the clearance rate and the serum level are used as an index of kidney function; normal levels in adult males range from 0.7 to 1.4 mg/dl; in adult females, from 0.6 to 1.0 mg/dl. See also creatinine clearance, under clearance.

creatinuria (kre-at-ĭ-nu´re-ă) The presence of increased amounts of creatine in the urine; usually a sign of a disorder of muscle, as in muscular dystrophy.

cremaster (kre-mas´ter) See table of muscles.

crenate, crenated (kre´nāt, kre-nāt´ed) Notched.

crenocyte (kre´no-sīt) An abnormal red blood cell with scalloped or notched edges.

crepitant (krep´ĭ-tant) Crackling.

crepitation (krep-ĭ-ta´shun) **1.** A grating sound like that produced when rubbing hair between the fingers, heard in certain diseases such as pneumonia. **2.** Noise made by friction of the two ends of a fractured bone. **3.** Sensation felt when palpating over an area in which there is subcutaneous gas.

crepitus (krep´ĭ-tus) **1.** Crepitation. **2.** A dry, crackling sound.

crescent (kres´ĕnt) Any structure shaped like a sickle.

malarial c. A gametocyte of the malarial parasite *Plasmodium falciparum*, characterized by its half-moon (crescentic) shape. Also called sickle form.

cresol (kre´sol) Any of three isomeric phenols (*ortho*-cresol, *meta*-cresol, and *para*-cresol); poisonous, colorless liquid or crystals, used as disinfectant.

CREST Acronym for a syndrome characterized by calcinosis, Raynaud's phenomenon, esophageal involvement, sclerodactyly, and telengiactasia.

crest (krest) A bony ridge.

alveolar c. The margin of the bone surrounding each tooth.

ethmoidal c. Ridge in the medial side of the maxilla; articulates with the middle concha.

ganglionic c. See neural crest.

gingival c. The edge of the free gingiva separating the gingival sulcus from the external gingiva.

iliac c. The long curved upper border of the ilium.

infundibuloventricular c. See supraventricular crest.

intertrocanteric c. Ridge between the greater and lesser trochanters of the femur, marking the junction of the neck and shaft of the bone.

nasal c. The ridge along the middle of the floor of the nasal cavity.

neural c. A band of ectodermal cells dorsolateral to the embryonic neural tube that give origin to ganglia of the cranial and spinal nerves and ganglia of the sympathetic trunk. Also called ganglionic crest.

pubic c. The rough anterior border of the pubic bone.

c. of scapular spine The border of the spine of the scapula (shoulder blade).

spiral c. The serrated edge of the osseous spiral lamina of the cochlea.

supraventricular c. The muscular ridge separating the conus arteriosus from the remaining cavity of the right ventricle of the heart. Also called infundibuloventricular crest.

cretin (kre´tin) A person afflicted with cretinism.

cretinism (kre´tin-iz-m) Condition characterized by stunted growth, apathy, distended abdomen, protruding swollen tongue, and arrested mental development, resulting from an inadequate production of thyroid hormones in early infancy.

cretinoid (kre´tin-oid) Exhibiting symptoms similar to those of cretinism.

Creutzfeldt-Jakob disease (kroits´felt-yah´kōb dĭ-zēz´) (CJD) A spongiform encephalopathy characterized by dementia accompanied by myoclonus; the dementia progresses so rapidly that deterioration is usually seen daily; the individual afflicted with the disease moves inevitably from good health to total helplessness or death within a year; caused by prions (small, proteinaceous infectious particles).

crevice (krev´is) A narrow crack.

gingival c. The space between the enamel of a tooth and the margin of the gums; in cases in which the gums have receded, between the gums and cementum.

cribriform (krib´rĭ-form) Sievelike; perforated.

cricoarytenoid (kri-ko-ăr-ĭ-te´noid) Relating to both the cricoid and arytenoid cartilages of the larynx.

cricoid (kri´koid) Ring-shaped, denoting the cartilage at the lower end of the larynx.

cricoidectomy (kri-koi-dek´to-me) Surgical removal of the cricoid cartilage.

cricothyroid (kri-ko-thi´roid) Relating to the cricoid and thyroid cartilages of the larynx.

cricotracheotomy (kri-ko-tra-ke-ot´ŏ-me) Division of the cricoid cartilage and upper trachea.

cri du chat syndrome (kre doo shă sin´drōm)

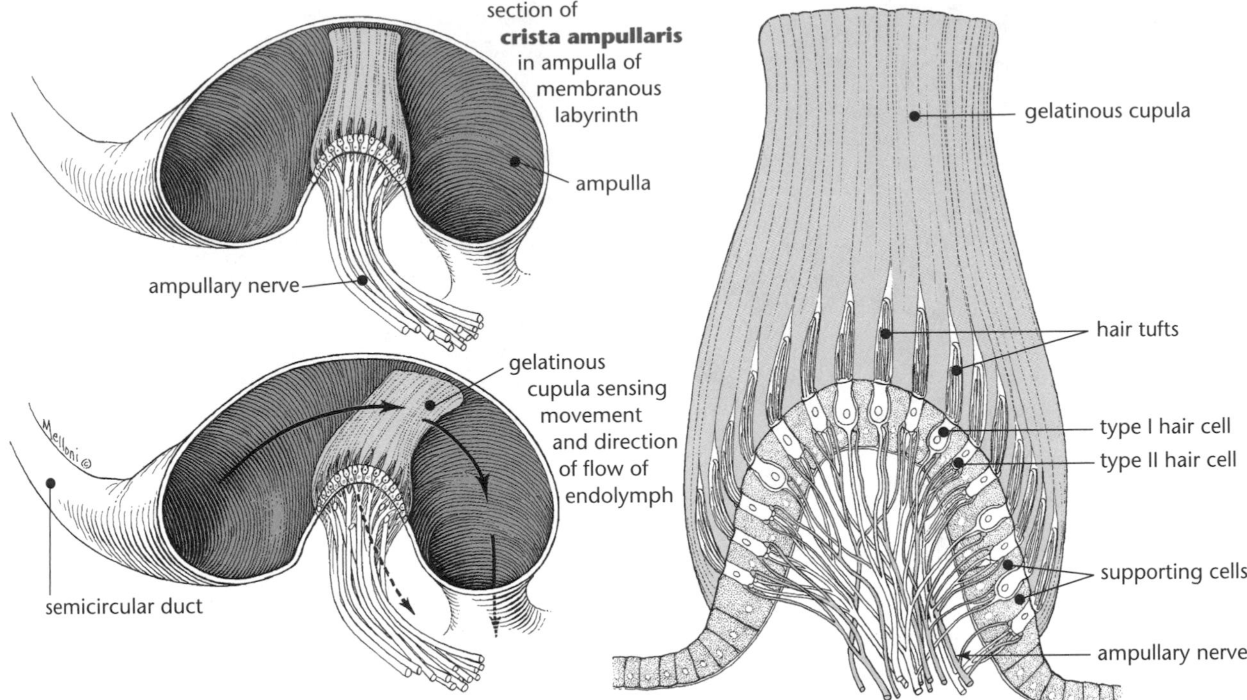

Hereditary condition marked by abnormal smallness of the head and jaw, severe mental deficiency, and a characteristic high-pitched catlike cry; caused by deletion of the short arm of chromosome 5. Also called cat-cry syndrome.

Crigler-Najjar disease (krig´ler-nă´jahr dĭ-zēz´) See Crigler-Najjar syndrome.

Crigler-Najjar syndrome (krig´ler-nă´jahr sin´drōm) An inherited disorder that may be: *type I*, a rare severe form, usually fatal soon after birth, associated with total absence of the bilirubin enzyme glucuronyltransferase; or *type II*, a mild form in which the enzyme deficiency is partial and life expectancy of the person is normal. Also called Crigler-Najjar disease.

crinogenic (krin-ō-jen´ik) Causing increased glandular secretion.

cripple (krip´l) **1.** To render disabled. **2.** One who is partially or completely disabled.

crisis (kri´sis) **1.** A sudden change, for the better or worse, in the course of a disease. **2.** A paroxysmal attack of pain or distress in an organ as seen in tabes dorsalis.

addisonian c See acute adrenocortical insufficiency, under insufficiency.

adrenal c. See acute adrenocortical insufficiency, under insufficiency.

Dietl's c. Severe abdominal pain usually caused by a kinked ureter, occurring in individuals with a floating kidney.

myasthenic c. Life-threatening exacerbation of muscle weakness and related complications in a myasthenia gravis patient.

oculogyric c. Crisis in which the eyeballs become fixed in one position (usually upward) for a length of time; occurs in encephalitis lethargica.

thyroid c. See thyrotoxic crisis.

thyrotoxic c. A sudden increase of the symptoms of thyrotoxicosis: rapid pulse, fever, nausea, diarrhea, a rise in the basal metabolic rate, and coma. Also called thyroid crisis; thyroid storm.

crista (kris´tă), *pl.* **cris´tae** A sharp upstanding ridge or crest.

c. ampullaris An elevation on the inner surface of the ampulla of each semicircular duct that contains innervated hair cells responsive to movement of the endolymph.

c. galli A perpendicular bony ridge on the upper surface of the ethmoid bone in the anterior cranial fossa; it projects above the level of the cribriform plate like a cock's comb. The anterior end of the falx cerebri is attached to it.

c. iliaca See iliac crest, under crest.

crocodile tears syndrome (krok´ŏ-dīl tirz sin´drōm) Spontaneous secretion of tears occurring simultaneously with normal salivation during eating, caused by a lesion of the facial nerve; usually follows partial recovery from facial paralysis.

Crohn's disease (krōnz dĭ-zēz´) See regional enteritis, under enteritis.

cromolyn sodium (kro´mŏ-lin so´de-um) The disodium salt of cromoglycic acid; used in the treatment of asthma and allergic rhinitis.

crossbite (kros´bīt) Condition in which the normal labiolingual or buccolingual relationship between the upper and lower teeth is reversed (the lower teeth are anterior and/or buccal to the upper teeth).

anterior c. Condition in which the upper incisors are locked lingual to the lower incisors.

crossbreed (kros´brēd) See hybrid.

cross-eye (kros´ī) See exotropia.

crossfoot(kros´fo͝ot) See talipes varus, under talipes.

crossing over (kros´ing o´ver) The exchange of material, including genes, between two paired chromosomes during meiosis.

crossmatching (kros-mach´ing) A test using cells from a recipient and serum from a donor to detect the presence of antibodies directed at recipient's cells.

croup (kro͞op) A term commonly used to denote any kind of laryngitis with laryngeal spasm in children; marked by a hoarse, barking cough (croupy cough), and difficult breathing.

croupy (kro͞op´e) Of the nature of croup.

crown (krown) The topmost part of a structure, as of the head or tooth.

anatomical c. The portion of a tooth covered by enamel.

artificial c. A restoration of the major part or of the entire coronal part of a tooth affixed to the remains of a natural tooth structure; usually made of gold, porcelain, or plastic.

clinical c. The portion of a tooth visible in the oral cavity, beyond the margin of the gums.

dowel c. A crown replacing the entire coronal part of a tooth and supported by means of a retention post extending into a filled root canal.

face c. A crown with a veneer for esthetics.

partial c. A crown that does not cover all the surfaces of a tooth; used as a retainer or single unit restoration.

crown and bridge (krown and brij) The branch of prosthodontics concerned with crown restorations and the fixed type of tooth-borne partial denture prosthesis.

crowning (krown´ing) The end of the second stage of labor in which the head of the fetus is visible, its largest diameter being encircled by the stretched vulva.

cruciate (kroo´she-āt) Shaped like a cross; overlapping or crossing.

crucible (kroo´sĭ-bl) A vessel or receptacle made of porcelain or graphite, used for melting materials at very high temperatures.

crucible former (kroo´sĭ-bl for´mer) A stand which holds a sprued wax pattern of a dental restoration; it forms the base for the casting ring.

crura (kroo´ră) Plural of crus.

crural (kroor´al) Relating to the leg or thigh.

crus (krus), *pl.* **cru´ra** **1.** Latin for leg. **2.** Any leglike structure.

common membranous c. The short duct formed by the united ends of the posterior and anterior semicircular ducts.

common osseous c. The short canal formed by the union of the posterior and anterior semicircular canals.

c. of diaphragm Either of two fibromuscular bands (right and left) that connect the diaphragm with the lumbar vertebrae; the two crura encircle the aorta.

c. of incus Either of two processes (short and long) of the incus (middle ear ossicle).

c. of penis The tapering posterior portion of the corpus cavernosum penis.

c. of stapes Either of two limbs (anterior and posterior) of the stapes (innermost ear ossicle).

crush syndrome (krush sin´drōm) Shock and renal failure following a severe crushing injury causing soft tissue trauma; acute tubular necrosis is thought to result from the myoglobin released from the damaged muscles. Also called compression syndrome.

crust (krust) **1.** A hard outer layer or covering. **2.** A scab; the dried exudate of a lesion.

Crustacea (krus-ta´she-ă) A class of predominantly aquatic animals (phylum Arthropoda) having segmented bodies covered with an exoskeleton (e.g., lobsters, crabs, shrimps, barnacles, wood lice).

crustacean (krus-ta´she-an) Relating to the class Crustacea.

crutch (kruch) A supporting device, used singly or in pairs, designed to aid those who need help in walking.

Cruveilhier-Baumgarten syndrome (kroo-vāl-ya´boum´găr-tĕn sin´drōm) Intrahepatic portal vein obstruction, usually due to cirrhosis of the liver, associated with patency of the umbilical vein, varicose paraumbilical veins, and a venous hum or thrill.

cry (kri) **1.** An inarticulate expression of distress. **2.** To utter such a sound.

epileptic c. A vocal sound sometimes made by a person at the onset of an epileptic convulsion.

cryanesthesia (kri-an-es-the´zhă) Loss of the ability to feel cold.

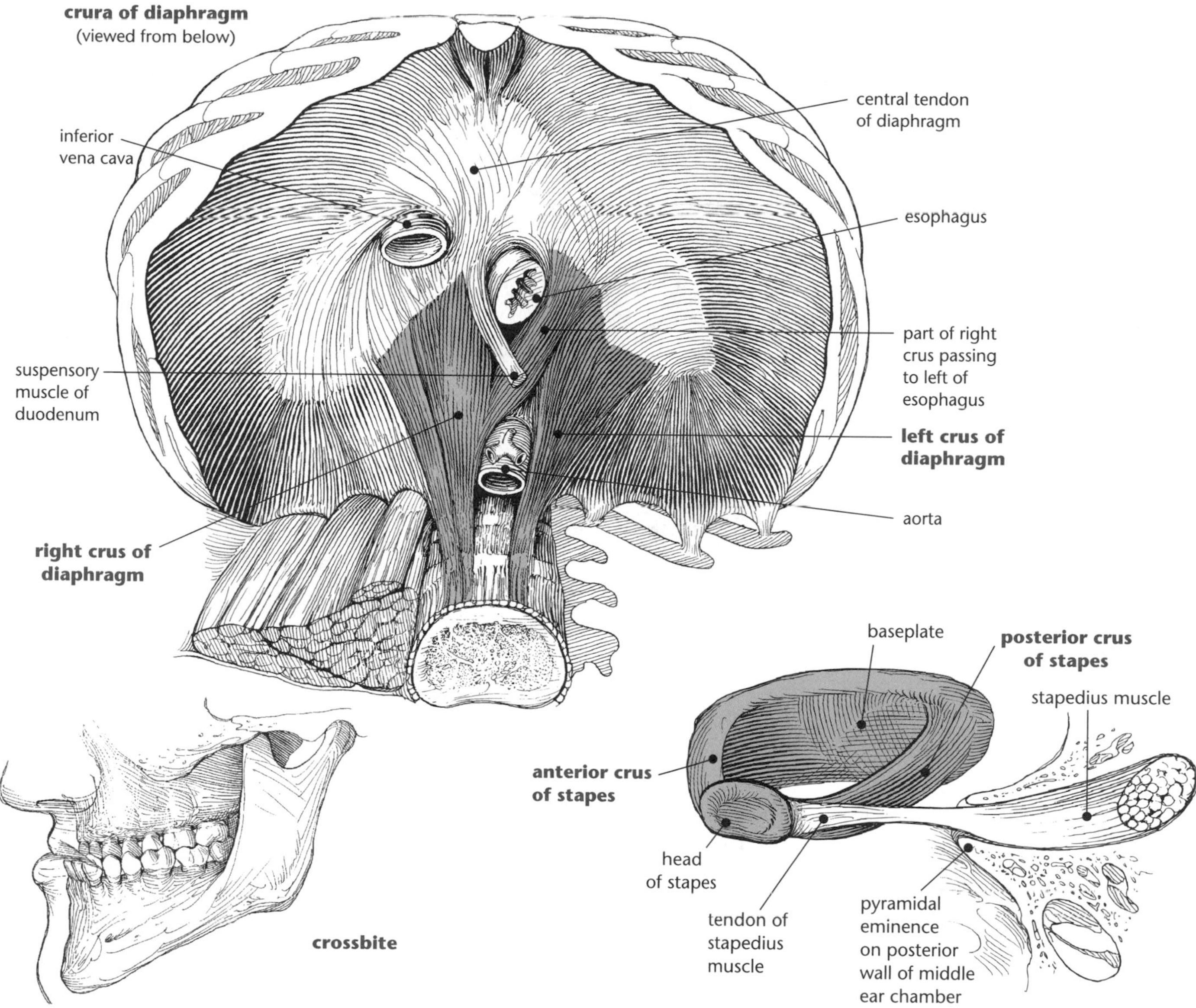

cryesthesia (kri-es-the´zhă) Abnormal sensitivity to cold temperatures.

cryobiology (kri-o-bi-ol´ŏ-je) The study of the effect of low temperatures on living organisms.

cryocautery (kri-o-kaw´ter-e) Destruction of tissue by freezing with substances such as liquid nitrogen or carbon dioxide snow.

cryoconization (kri-o-kon-ĭ-za´shun) Removal of a cone of tissue from the wall of the lower cervical canal with a freezing instrument (cryoprobe).

cryoextraction (kri-o-eks-trak´shun) Removal of a cataract with a cryoextractor.

cryoextractor (kri-o-eks-trak´tor) A copper pencil-shaped instrument with a small ball at its end that is placed in a freezing substance and used in the removal of a cataractous lens of the eye.

cryogenic (kri-o-jen´ik) Producing very low temperatures.

cryogenics (kri-o-jen´iks) The branch of physics concerned with the production and effects of very low temperatures.

cryoglobulin (kri-o-glob´u-lin) Abnormal gamma-globulin; it precipitates when exposed to low temperatures (less than 37ºC).

cryoglobulinemia (kri-o-glob-u-lĭ-ne´me-ă) The presence of abnormal quantities of cryoglobulin in the blood, which solidify within tiny blood vessels when exposed to cold temperatures and restrict blood flow to exposed parts.

cryometer (kri-om´ĕ-ter) An instrument for measuring very low temperatures.

cryopathy (kri-op´ă-the) Any condition caused by cold.

cryoprecipitate (kri-o-pre-sip´ĭ-tāt) Precipitate formed upon cooling of a solution.

cryopreservation (kri-o-prez-er-va´shun) Preservation of cells, tissues, or *in vitro* fertilized embryos by freezing (e.g., in liquid nitrogen).

cryoprobe (kri´o-prōb) A blunt surgical instrument with a tip that can be maintained at below freezing temperatures; used in cryosurgery (i.e., for destroying tissue or to cause tissue to adhere to the instrument for removal).

cryoprotein (kri-o-pro´ēn) A blood protein that precipitates from solution when cooled and redissolves upon warming.

cryoscopy (kri-os´kŏ-pe) The determination of the freezing point of a solution compared with that of distilled water; based on the principle that the freezing point is depressed according to the concentration and nature of the solute.

cryostat (kri´o-stat) Apparatus used to maintain low-temperature environments so that certain procedures (e.g., sectioning frozen tissues) may be carried out.

cryosurgery (kri-o-sur´jer-e) Surgery performed by the application of extreme cold temperatures.

cryothalamectomy (kri-o-thal-ă-mek´tŏ-me) Destruction of the thalamus by extreme cold temperatures for the treatment of Parkinson's disease.

cryotherapy (kri-o-ther´ă-pe) The therapeutic use of extremely low temperatures, as of liquid nitrogen in the treatment of chronic cervicitis.

crypt (kript) A glandular sac or pitlike depression.
- **anal c.'s** See anal sinuses, under sinus.
- **dental c.** The space filled by a developing tooth.
- **c.'s of Leiberkühn** See intestinal glands, under gland.
- **c.'s of Morgagni** See anal sinuses, under sinus.
- **tonsillar c.** One of several pits on the surface of the palatine tonsil.

cryptitis (krip-ti´tis) Inflammation of a crypt or a follicle.
- **anal c.** Inflammation of the mucous membrane of an anal crypt, especially painful during bowel movements.
- **urethral c.** Inflammation of the mucous follicles of the external orifice of the female urethra.

cryptococcin (krip-to-kok´sin) Antigen derived from the fungus *Cryptococcus neoformans*.

cryptococcosis (krip-to-kok-o´sis) A chronic disseminated disease caused by the fungus *Cryptococcus neoformans*; it causes a respiratory infection often overlooked until it spreads to other areas of the body, particularly the central nervous system where it causes meningitis.

Cryptococcus (krip-to-kok´us) A genus of yeastlike fungi (family Cryptococcaceae).
- ***C. neoformans*** Species commonly found in pigeon droppings and causing cryptococcosis in humans.

cryptogenic (krip-to-jen´ik) Of obscure origin.

cryptolith (krip´to-lith) A calculus in a crypt or pit of a structure.

cryptomenorrhea (krip-to-men-o-re´ă) Monthly occurrence of the signs of menstruation without a flow of blood, as in imperforate hymen and cervical obstruction.

cryptomerorachischisis (krip-to-me-ro-ră-kis´kĭ-sis) See spina bifida occulta, under spina.

cryptophthalmos (krip-tof-thal´mos) Congenital anomaly marked by the absence of eyelids; the skin is continuous from the forehead to the cheek over a rudimentary eye.

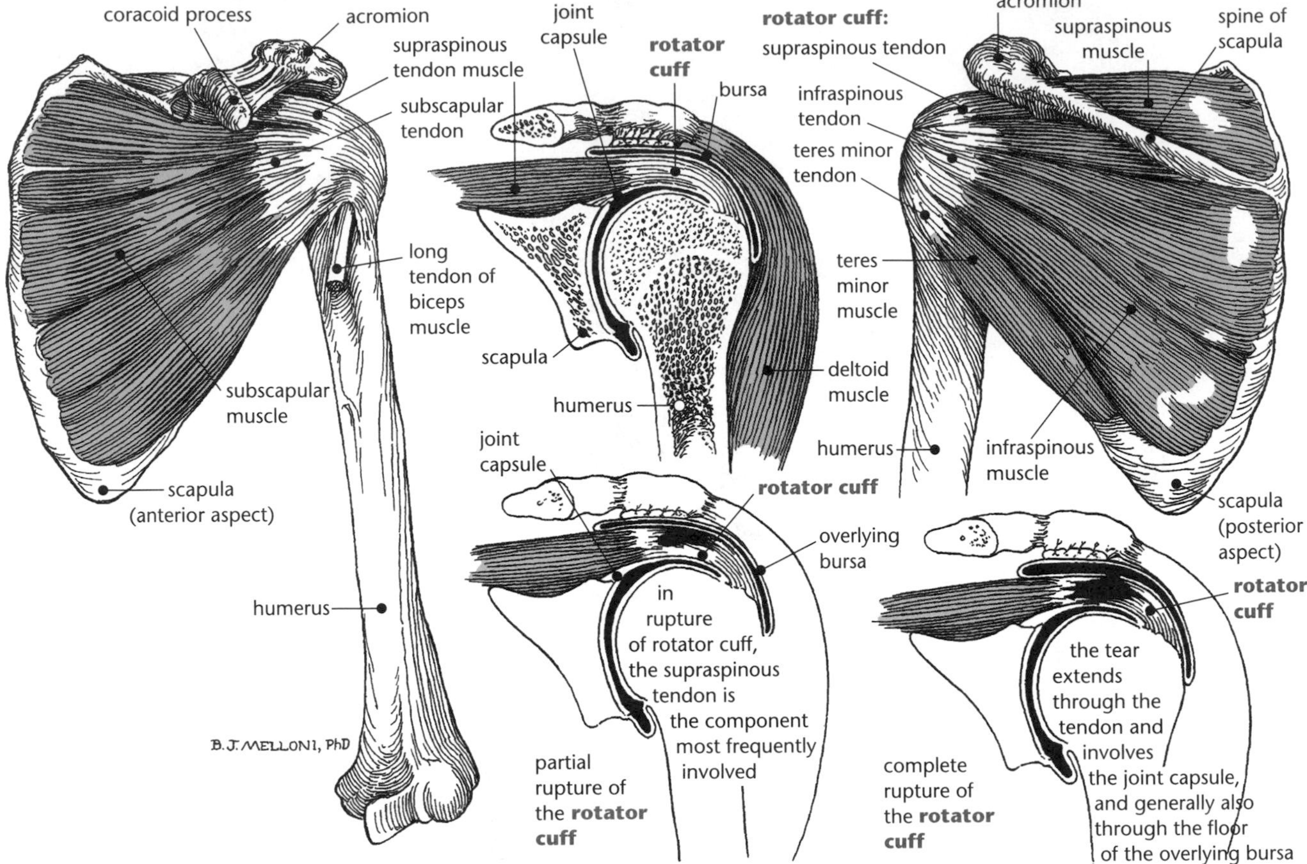

cryptorchid (krip-tor´kid) Relating to an undescended testis.

cryptorchidectomy (krip-tor-kĭ-dek´tŏ-me) Surgical removal of an undescended testis.

cryptorchidism, cryptorchism (krip-tor´kĭ-diz´m, krip-tor´kiz-m) Condition in which the descent of a testis is arrested at some point in its normal path into the scrotum; the testis may be situated anywhere between the renal and scrotal areas. Also called undescended testicle; undescended testis; retained testis.

cryptosporidiosis (krip-to-spo-rid-e-o´sis) Infection with cryptosporidia, usually characterized by diarrhea; most commonly seen in immunocompromised individuals; milder self-limited disease may be seen in immunocompetent individuals.

Cryptosporidium (krip-to-spo-rid´e-um) A genus of parasitic protozoans (family Cryptosporidae) found in the intestinal tract of many animals and humans.

cryptozoite (krip-to-zo´īt) A stage in the cycle of the malarial parasite, existing in the host's body tissues prior to entering the red blood cell.

crystal (kris´tal) **1.** A solid substance composed of atomic groupings (unit cells) having a geometric form which is characteristic for different compounds. **2.** One unit cell of such a substance.

asthma c.'s See Charcot-Leyden crystals.

Charcot-Leyden c.'s Elongated crystalline structures formed from eosinophils; found in the sputum of patients with bronchial asthma. Also called asthma crystals.

crystal violet (kris´tal vī´o-līt) A compound of one or several methyl derivatives of pararosaniline; used as a biological stain.

crystalline (kris´tă-lēn) **1.** Transparent; clear. **2.** Relating to or made of crystal or composed of crystals.

crystallization (kris-tal-ĭ-za´shun) Spontaneous grouping of the molecules of a substance into an orderly repetitive pattern; change in form to a solid phase, as when a solute precipitates from solution.

crystallography (kris-tal-og´ră-fe) The study of the structure and phenomena of crystals.

x-ray c. A technique for the three-dimensional mapping of substances (too small to be viewed even through an electron microscope) through the use of x-ray diffraction techniques.

crystalloid (kris´tă-loid) **1.** Resembling a crystal. **2.** A noncolloidal substance that, when in solution, can diffuse through a semipermeable membrane and is generally capable of being crystallized.

c. of Charcot-Böttcher A slender crystal-shaped inclusion peculiar to the Sertoli cell of the seminiferous epithelium.

crystalluria (kris-tal-u´re-ă) The presence of crystals in the urine.

cubital (ku´bĭ-tal) Relating to the forearm, the ulna, or the elbow.

cubitus (ku´bĭ-tus) The elbow.

cue (kyōō) A perceived stimulus to which a person responds.

cuff (kuf) Bandlike structure surrounding a part.

rotator c. A supportive structure covering the upper part of the shoulder joint capsule; formed by tendons of four muscles (supraspinous, infraspinous, teres minor, subscapular); provides active support for the joint in motion.

cul-de-sac (kul-de-sak´), *pl.* **culs-de-sac** A pouch or sac.

conjunctival c. See fornix of conjunctiva, under fornix.

c. of Douglas See rectouterine pouch, under pouch.

culdocentesis (kul-do-sen-te´sis) Aspiration of pus or any fluid from the rectouterine pouch through a transvaginal puncture.

culdoscope (kul do-skōp) A lighted instrument used for the visual examination of the pelvic cavity and its contents.

culdoscopy (kul-dos´kŏ-pe) Viewing of the pelvic cavity and organs with a culdoscope introduced through the posterior wall of the vagina.

Culex (ku´leks) Genus of mosquitoes (family Culicidae); some species carry and transmit disease-causing microorganisms, including those causing encephalitis.

culicide (ku-lis´ĭ-sīd) Any agent that kills mosquitoes.

culicifuge (ku-lis´ĭ-fūj) An agent that drives away mosquitoes and gnats.

Cullen's sign (kul´lenz sīn) Blue discoloration of the skin around the navel as a result of intraperitoneal hemorrhage. Also called periumbilical ecchymosis.

culture (kul´chur) **1.** The propagation of microorganisms in a nutrient medium. **2.** A colony of microorganisms grown in a nutrient medium.

pure c. A culture in which all the microorganisms are of one species.

tissue c. The growth and maintenance of tissue cells *in vitro* after removal from the body.

cum (kum) (c̄) Latin meaning with.

cumulus oophorus (ku´mu-lus o-of´ŏ-rus) The mass of granulosa cells surrounding the developing ovum in the ovarian follicle.

cuneate (ku´ne-āt) Wedge-shaped.

cuneiform (ku-ne´ĭ-form) Wedge-shaped. See table of bones.

cuneus (ku´ne-us), *pl.* **cu´nei** The posterior portion of the occipital lobe of each cerebral hemisphere.

cuniculus (ku-nik´u-lus) The burrow made in the skin by the itch mite.

cunnilingus (kun-ĭ-ling´us) Oral stimulation of the vulva or clitoris.

cunnus (kun´us) Latin for vulva.

cup (kup) A cuplike structure.

glaucomatous c. A deep depression of the optic disk, occurring in glaucoma due to increased intraocular pressure.

physiologic c. A normal depression on the surface of the optic disk.

cupola (koo´po-lă) See cupula.

cupping (kup´ing) Formation of a cup-shaped depression.

c. of optic disk Exaggerated depression at the center of the optic disk, as seen in glaucoma.

cupric (koo´prik) Relating to divalent copper.

c. sulfate Deep blue crystals used as irritant, astringent, and fungicide. Also called copper sulfate; blue vitriol.

cupula (koo´pu-lă) A dome-shaped structure. Also written cupola.

c. cristae ampullaris A gelatinous mass over the crista of the ampulla of the semicircular canal containing tufts of cilia from the underlying hair cells.

c. of pleura The domelike peak of the pleural sac covering the apex of the lung and located near the neck.

curare (koo-ră´re) An extract of alkaloids from the bark of several plants, especially *Strychnos toxifera*;

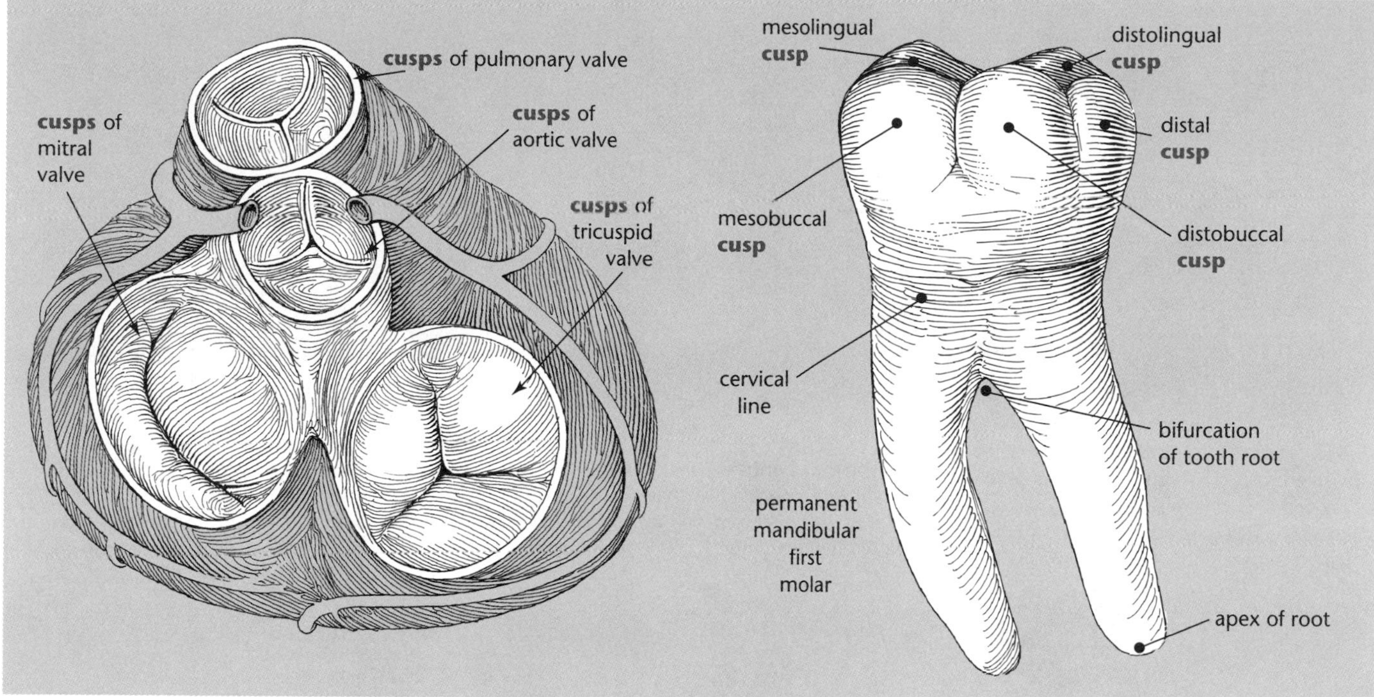

its principal active ingredient (tubocurarine) inhibits muscle contraction by interfering with the action of the neurotransmitter acetylcholine; used as a muscle relaxant.

curarization (ku-rar-i-za ´shun) Therapeutic administration of curare or related compounds.

curative (ku´ră-tiv) **1.** Serving to cure. **2.** A remedy.

curd (kerd) The coagulated part of milk.

cure (kūr) **1.** To restore to health. **2.** A method of treatment or a remedy. **3.** In dentistry, the procedure by which a plastic material (such as that of a denture base) is hardened.

curet (ku-ret´) A spoon-shaped surgical instrument used to scrape the walls of a body cavity. Also written curret.

curettage (ku-rĕ-tazh´) Surgical scraping of the interior of a cavity with a curette to remove growths or diseased tissue, or to obtain tissue for examination (biopsy).

endometrial c. Scraping of the interior lining of the uterus with a curet.

fractional c. Separate curettage of the lining of the uterus and of the cervical canal for diagnostic evaluation.

periapial c. Removal of diseased tissue sur-rounding the root of a tooth.

curette (ku-ret´) See curet.

curie (ku´re) (Ci) A unit of radioactivity equal to 3.7 x 10^{10} disintegrations per second.

curium (ku´re-um) A synthetic radioactive element; symbol Cm, atomic number 96, atomic weight 247.

current (kur´ent) A steady flow (e.g., air, electricity, or fluid).

alternating c. (AC) An electric current that reverses direction of flow at regular intervals.

direct c. (DC) An electric current that flows in one direction only.

high frequency c. An alternating electric current having a frequency of at least 10,000 cycles per second.

c. of injury The current that passes through a conductor connecting the injured and the uninjured portions of a nerve or other excitable tissue.

stabile c. A current applied with both electrodes placed in a fixed position.

curvature (kur-vă-chōōr) A bending or curving.

greater c. of stomach The left and inferior borders of the stomach.

lesser c. of stomach The right border of the stomach.

spinal c. See kyphosis; lordosis; scoliosis.

curve (kurv) **1.** A line that deviates from a straight course in a smooth, continuous, nonangular manner. **2.** A line representing plotted data on a graph.

distribution c. A curve in which the number of individuals is plotted along the ordinate and the property under investigation is plotted along the abscissa.

dose-response c., dose-effect c. Graphic representation of a curve showing the relationship between a dose of a chemical or ionizing radiation and its influence on a biological process.

dye-dilution c. A curve indicating the serial concentrations of a dye. Also called indicator-dilution curve.

frequency c. A curve representing an approximation of the rate of occurrences of a periodic event. Also called gaussian curve; probability curve.

gaussian c. See frequency curve.

indicator-dilution c. See dye-dilution curve.

Price-Jones c. A curve representing variations in the diameters of red blood cells.

probability c. See frequency curve.

c. of Spee A curve formed by the upper dental arch meeting with the lower dental arch viewed buccally from the first bicuspid to the last molar.

Starling c. A curve indicating cardiac output against atrial pressure.

strength-duration c. A curve indicating the relationship between the intensity of an electrical stimulus and the time it must flow to be effective.

stress-strain c. A curve showing the ratio of deformation to load during testing of a material under tension.

cushingoid (kōōsh´ing-oid) Having the characteristics of Cushing's syndrome or disease.

Cushing's disease (kōōsh´ingz dĭ-zēz´) Adrenocortical overactivity caused by excessive secretion of pituitary adrenocorticotropic hormone (ACTH).

Cushing's syndrome (kōōsh´ingz sin´drōm) Metabolic disorder caused by chronic excess of glucocorticoids; characterized by a round face, central obesity, prominent dorsal fat pad, florid complexion, abdominal striae, hypertension, and impaired carbohydrate tolerance among other findings.

cushion (kōōsh´un) Any anatomic structure resembling a pad.

atrioventricular canal c.'s See atrioventricular endocardial cushions.

atrioventricular endocardial c.'s A pair of apposing masses of mesenchymal tissue in the embryonic heart; they appear at the superior and inferior borders of the atrioventricular canal in a 6 mm embryo; they grow together and fuse, dividing the canal into right and left atrioventricular orifices. Also called atrioventricular canal cushions.

eustachian c. See torus tubarius, under torus.

Passavant's c. See Passavant's ridge, under ridge.

cusp (kusp) **1.** One of the triangular segments of a heart's valve. **2.** A pronounced elevation on the occlusal surface (grinding surface) of a tooth.

cuspid (kus´pid) One of the four anterior, single-cusped teeth, between the incisor and bicuspid; it is the longest and most stable tooth in the mouth. Also called canine tooth; dog tooth; eye tooth (an upper cuspid).

cuspidor (kus´pĭ-dōr) In dentistry, a bowl-shaped vessel adjacent to a dental chair, used for spitting into.

cut (kut) **1.** To incise. **2.** To dilute.

cutaneous (ku-ta´ne-ŭs) Relating to the skin.

cutdown (kut´doun) A small opening over a vein to facilitate introduction of a needle or a cannula into the vessel.

cuticle (ku´tĭ-kl) **1.** The epidermis. **2.** The thin fold of skin overlying the base of a fingernail or toenail.

cuticularization (ku-tik-u-lar-ĭ-zā´shun) The formation of skin over an abraded area.

cutis vera (ku´tis ver´ă) See dermis. Also called corium.

cuvette (ku-vet´) A glass container in which solutions are placed for photometric study.

cyanate (si´an-āt) A salt of cyanic acid.

cyanide (si´an-īd) Any of a group of compounds of hydrocyanic acid containing the radical –Cn or ion $(CN)^-$.

cyanmethemoglobin (sī-an-met-he-mo-glo´bin) Cyanide methemoglobin; a compound of cyanide and methemoglobin.

cyanocobalamin (sī-ă-no-ko-bal´ă-min) See vitamin B_{12}, under vitamin.

cyanophil (si-an´o-fil) Any cell or tissue element readily stainable with blue dyes.

cyanopsia (si-ă-nop´se-ă) A defect of vision in which all objects seem to be tinted blue.

cyanose tardive (si´ă-nōs tar´div) Term applied to the potentially cyanotic group of congenital heart diseases with an abnormal communication between systemic and pulmonary circulation; cyanosis is absent while the shunt is from left to right, but if the shunt reverses, as after exercise or late in the course of the disease, cyanosis appears. Also called delayed cyanosis.

cyanosis (si-ă-no´sis) Bluish discoloration of the skin, lips, and nail beds caused by insufficient oxygen in the blood; it appears when the reduced hemoglobin in the small vessels is 5 g per 100 ml or more.

delayed c. See cyanosis tardive.

cyanotic (si-ă-not´ik) Affected with cyanosis.

cybernetics (si-ber-net´iks) The comparative study of biologic and mechanoelectric systems of automatic control, such as the nervous system and electronic computers, for the purpose of explaining the nature of the brain.

cyclarthrodial (sĭk-lar-thro´de-al) Relating to a rotary joint.

C

CARDIAC CYCLE

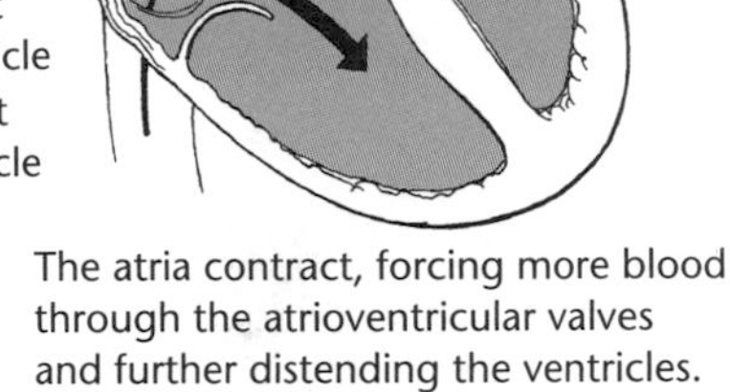

The **cardiac cycle** starts with the heart relaxed; blood streams into the atria from the venae cavae and pulmonary veins and flows through the open atrioventricular valves to the ventricles.

The atria contract, forcing more blood through the atrioventricular valves and further distending the ventricles.

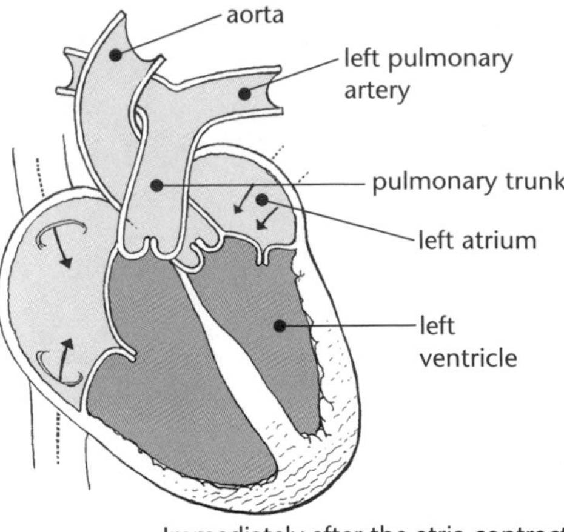

Immediately after the atria contract, the ventricles start contracting and the increase in ventricular pressure closes the atrioventricular valves.

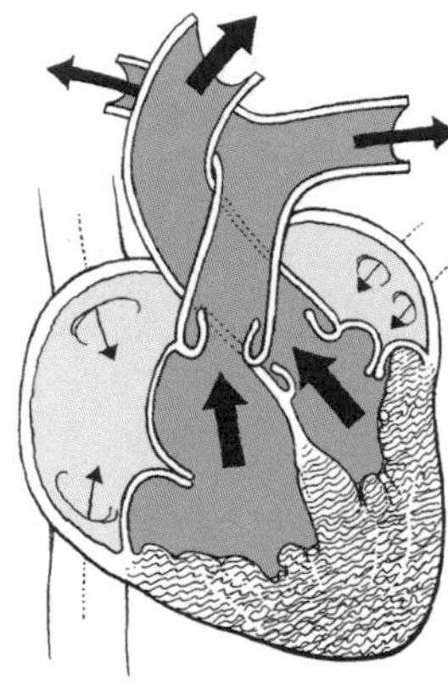

Once the ventricular pressure overcomes the residual pressure of the aorta and pulmonary trunk, it forces the semilunar valves of those vessels to open, permitting blood to be pumped out of the heart. In contracting, the ventricles force most, but not all, of the contents into the great vessels.

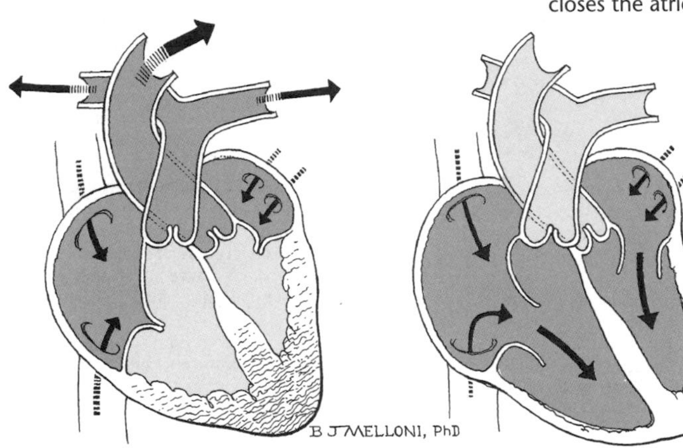

Ventricular pressure lessens when the ventricles begin to relax; pressure in the aorta and pulmonary trunk remains high and the semilunar valves close, thereby forcing blood throughout the body; at this stage of the **cardiac cycle**, all the valves are closed.

With the complete relaxation of the ventricles, the atrioventricular valves are forced open by the blood streaming in from the atria and begins a new **cardiac cycle**. This period of relaxation is the longest phase of the **cardiac cycle.**

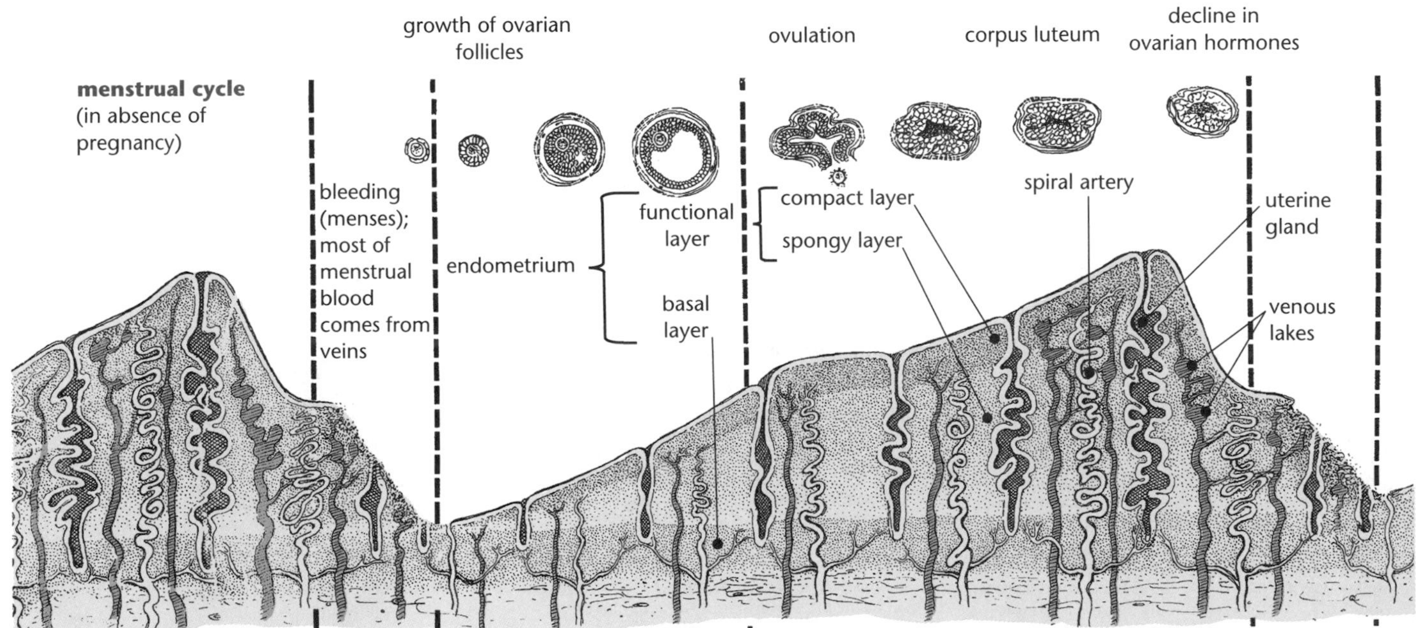

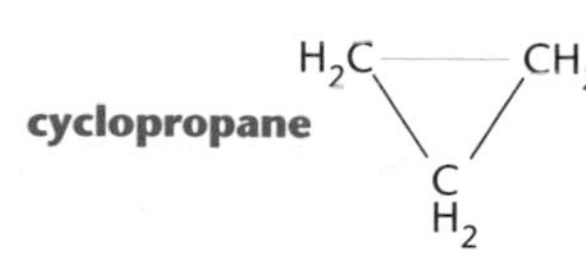

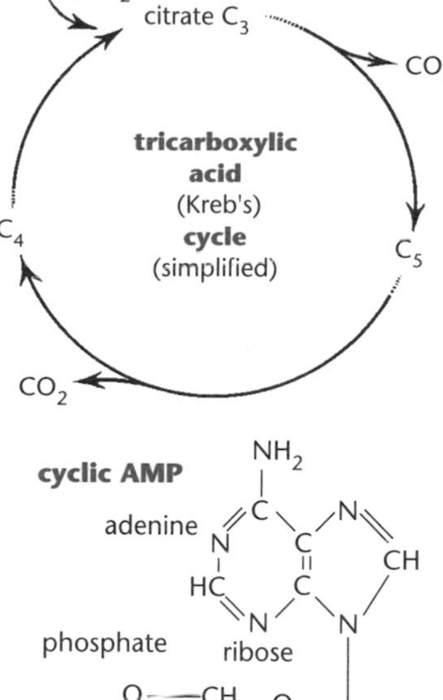

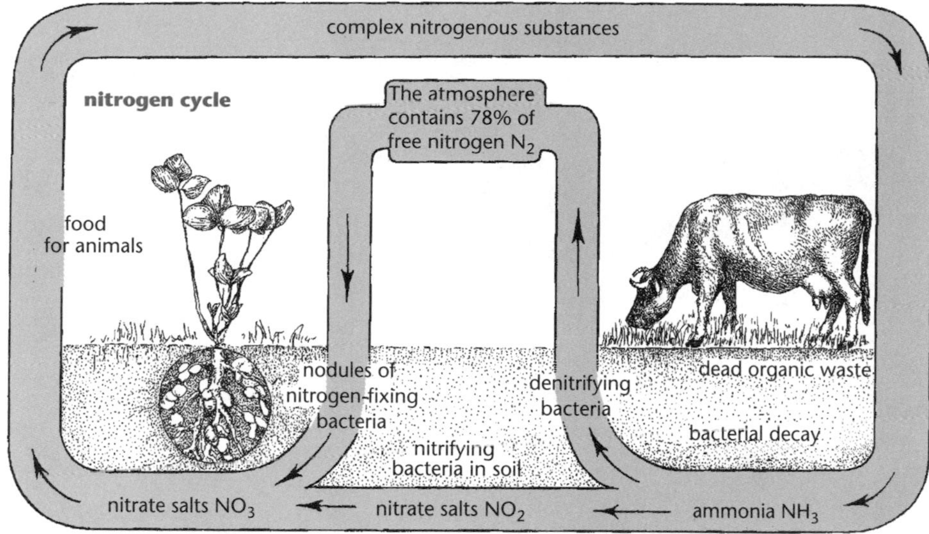

cyclarthrosis (sĭk-lar-thro´sis) A rotary joint.

cycle (si´kl) A time interval in which a regularly repeated sequence of events takes place.

anovulatory c. A sexual cycle in which no ovum is produced.

brainwave c. The complete series of changes in amplitude of a wave of the electroencephalogram before repetition occurs.

carbon c., carbon dioxide c. The natural processes through which carbon in the atmosphere, in the form of carbon dioxide, is converted into carbohydrates by photosynthesis, metabolized by living organisms, and ultimately returned to the atmosphere, again as carbon dioxide.

cardiac c. The complete round of events that occur in the heart with each heartbeat.

citric acid c. See tricarboxylic acid cycle.

endometrial c. See menstrual cycle.

exogenous c. The phase in the development of a parasite spent in the body of the invertebrate host, as of the malarial parasite in the body of a mosquito.

Krebs c. See tricarboxylic acid cycle.

life c. The entire life of an organism.

menstrual c. The sequence of normal changes taking place (about every 28 days) in the endometrium, culminating with shedding of uterine mucosa and bleeding (menstruation); they correspond to changes in the ovary (ovarian cycle) and occur in response to hormonal activity. In popular usage, the term encompasses all ovarian and uterine changes. Also called endometrial cycle.

nitrogen c. The continuous process in which nitrogen is deposited in the soil, assimilated by bacteria and plants, transferred to animals, and returned to the soil.

ovarian c. The recurrent sequence of events taking place in the ovary, including maturation and release of the ovum, in response to hormonal activity.

reproductive c. The series of physiologic changes that take place in the female reproductive organs from conception to delivery.

tricarboxylic acid c. A series of enzymatic reactions involving the complete oxidation of acetyl units, providing the main source of energy in the mammalian body and taking place mostly during respiration. Also called Krebs cycle; citric acid cycle.

urea c. The series of chemical reactions that occur in the liver, resulting in the production of urea.

cyclectomy (sĭk-lek´to-me) Surgical removal of a portion of the ciliary body.

cyclic (si´klik, sĭk´lik) Occurring periodically.

cyclic adenylic acid (si´klik ad-ĕ-nil´ik as´id) See adenosine-3´,5´-cyclic monophosphate.

cyclic AMP See adenosine-3´,5´-cyclic monophosphate.

cyclic GMP See cyclic guanosine monophosphate, under guanosine.

cyclic phosphate (si´klik fos´fāt) See adenosine-3´,5´-cyclic monophosphate.

cyclitis (si-klī´tis) Inflammation of the ciliary body.

plastic c. Severe cyclitis with exudation of a material rich in fibrin that accumulates in the anterior and posterior chambers of the eye.

purulent c. Acute cyclitis with a copious discharge of pus, usually involving the iris and choroid.

serous c. Simple cyclitis with a relatively fluid discharge.

cyclizine hydrochloride (si´klĭ-zēn hi-dro-klor´īd) An antihistamine used in preventing and relieving symptoms of motion sickness and postoperative nausea and vomiting; also relieves vertigo and other symptoms caused by vestibular disorders of the ear; Marezine®.

cyclochoroiditis (si-klo-ko-roid-i´tis) Inflammation of the ciliary body and the choroid layer of the eye.

cyclodialysis (si-klo-di-al´ĭ-sis) The surgical creation of an opening between the anterior chamber of the eye and the suprachoroidal space to reduce intraocular pressure in glaucoma.

cyclodiathermy (si-klo-di´ă-ther-me) The partial destruction of the ciliary body by the application of heat for the reduction of intraocular pressure in the treatment of glaucoma.

cycloid (si´kloid) Denoting a personality characterized by alternating states of elation and mild depression.

cyclokeratitis (si-klo-ker-ă-ti´tis) Inflammation of the ciliary body and the cornea.

cyclooxygenase (si-klo-ok´sĭ-jĕn-ās) An enzyme that promotes the first two steps in the formation of prostaglandin. Also called prostaglandin endoperoxide synthase.

cyclophoria (si-klo-for´e-ă) Tendency of one eye to deviate on its anteroposterior axis.

cyclophorometer (si-klo-for-om´ĕ-ter) Instrument used to measure cyclophoria.

cyclophosphamide (si-klo-fos´fă-mīd) A white crystalline powder used as an antitumor agent; Cytoxan®.

cycloplegia (si-klo-ple´je-ă) Paralysis of the ciliary muscle, which controls the shape of the lens of the eye during focusing.

cycloplegic (si-klo-ple´jik) **1.** Relating to cycloplegia. **2.** An agent that causes cycloplegia.

cyclopropane (si-klo-pro´pān) A colorless, inflammable, explosive gas, C_3H_6; used as a general anesthetic. Also called trimethylene.

Cyclospora (sī-klo-spor´ă) A genus of protozoan parasites found in reptiles, millipedes, and insect-eating animals; implicated in causing a form of widespread, prolonged, self-limited diarrhea.

cyclosporine (si-klo-spor´ēn) An immunosuppressive drug used in organ transplantation; it selectively inhibits T lymphocytes. Formerly called cyclosporin A.

cyclothymia (si-klo-thi´me-ă) Cyclic fluctuations of mood between elation and mild depression.

cyclotomy (si-klot´ŏ-me) Surgical incision of the ciliary muscle of the eye.

cylinder (sil´in-der) (cyl) **1.** A cylindrical lens. **2.** A rod-shaped urinary cast.

cylindroid (sil´in-droid) A ribbonlike mucous mass in the urine resembling a hyaline cast. Also called mucous cast; false cast.

cylindroma (sil-in-dro´mă) A usually benign epithelial tumor appearing as multiple nodules, especially on the scalp and face.

cylindruria (sil-in-droo´re-ă) The presence of casts in the urine.

cynophobia (si-no-fo´be-ă) Exaggerated fear of dogs.

cypridopathy (si-pri-dop´ă-the) Any venereal disease.

cypridophobia (sī-pri-do-fo´be-ă) Abnormal fear of venereal disease or of sexual intercourse.

cyst (sist) **1.** An abnormal sac within the body containing air or fluid. **2.** A bladder.

allantoic c. See urachal cyst.

Baker's c. A collection of escaped synovial fluid in the tissues outside the knee joint.

Bartholin's gland c. The most common cyst of the vulva, resulting from retention of glandular secretions due to a blocked duct.

branchial c. A cyst resulting from the nonclosure of a branchial cleft.

bursal c. A retention cyst in a bursa.

chocolate c. A cyst of the ovary containing a thick dark brown tenacious fluid; often seen in endometriosis.

corpus luteum c. A cyst in the ovary formed from corpus luteum that remains cystic with excessive fluid content instead of regressing normally; commonly associated with disturbance of or delay in menstruation.

dermoid c. A common, usually bilateral, ovarian cyst; it is lined with skin and contains displaced skin elements (i.e., sebaceous glands and hair) and often teeth and mandibular bone. Also called benign cystic teratoma; mature benign teratoma; dermoid.

dilatation c. See retention cyst.

distention c. See retention cyst.

echinococcus c. See hydatid cyst.

ependymal c. Cystic dilatation of the central

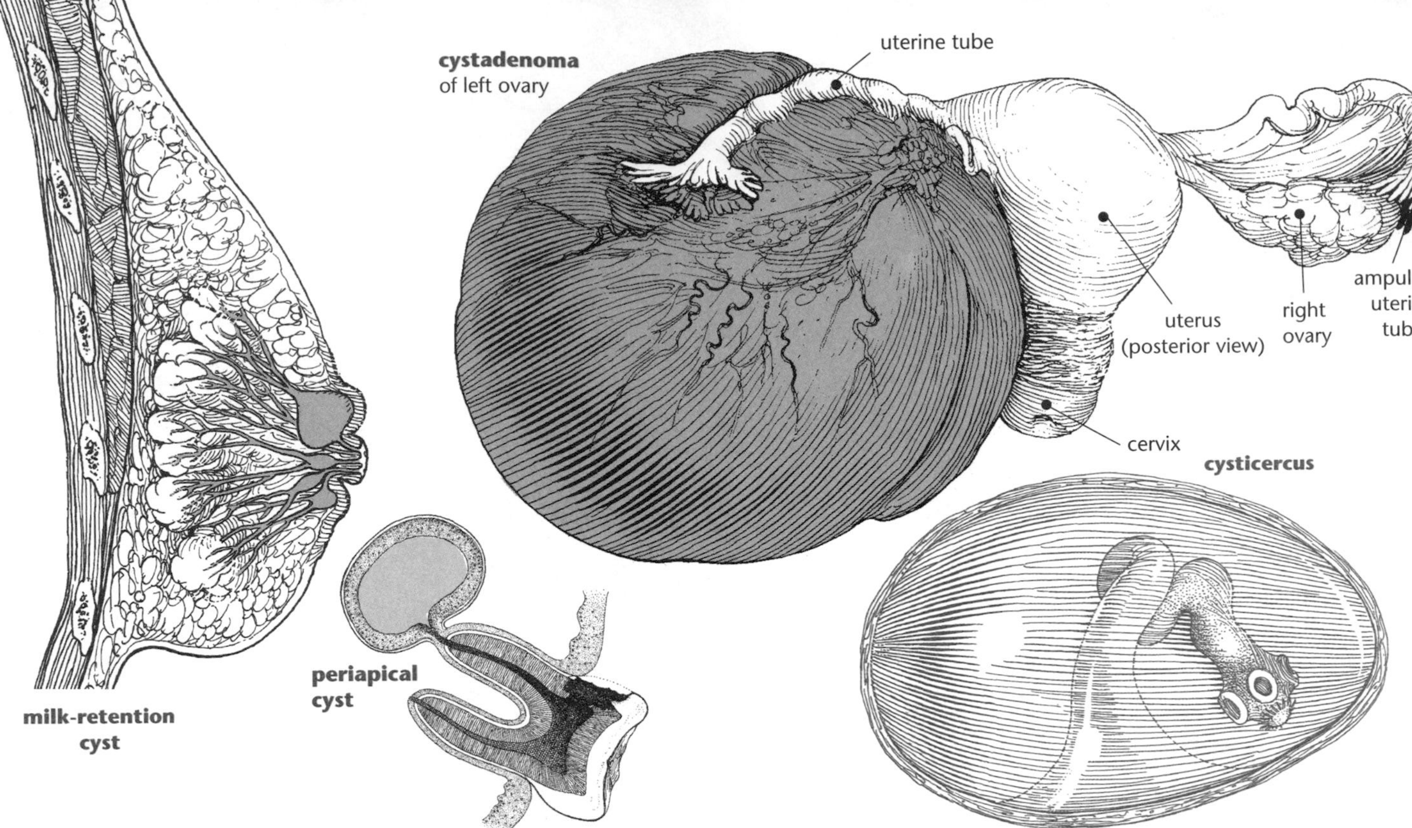

canal of the spinal cord or of the cerebral ventricles. Also called neural cyst.

hydatid c. Cyst formed, usually in the liver, by the larval stage of the tapeworm. Also called echinococcus cyst.

lacteal c. See milk-retention cyst.

meibomian c. See chalazion.

milk retention c., milk c. Retention cyst in the breast resulting from obstruction of a lactiferous duct. Also called lacteal cyst; galactocele; lactocele.

mother c. The main echinococcus cyst containing smaller daughter cysts.

mucous c. Retention cyst resulting from closure of the duct of a mucous gland.

nabothian c. Retention cyst resulting from compression of a nabothian gland in the uterine cervix. Also called nabothian follicle.

neural c. See ependymal cyst.

omphalomesenteric duct c. A cystic dilatation along the remnant of the embryonic omphalomesenteric (vitelline) duct.

ovarian c. Cystic tumor of the ovary.

periapical c. Cyst around the tip of a tooth root, usually a nonvital tooth. Also called radicular cyst; root cyst.

piliferous c. Dermoid cyst containing hair.

pilonidal c. See pilonidal sinus, under sinus.

pseudomucinous c. One containing gelatinous material.

radicular c. See periapical cyst.

retention c. Cyst resulting from obstruction or compression of the duct draining a gland. Also called dilatation cyst; distention cyst; secretory cyst.

root c. See periapical cyst.

sacrococcygeal c. See pilonidal sinus, under sinus.

sebaceous c. Cyst of the skin or scalp containing sebum and keratin; results from retention of a sebaceous gland secretion.

secretory c. See retention cyst.

serous c. Cyst containing clear serous fluid.

solitary bone c. Cyst lined with a thin layer of connective tissue and containing serous fluid; usually seen in the shaft of a long bone of a child. Also called unicameral cyst; osteocytoma.

sublingual c. See ranula.

unicameral c. Cyst contained within a single cavity. See solitary bone cyst.

urachal c. Abdominal cyst resulting from failure of a portion of the urachus to obliterate during intrauterine life. Also called allantoic cyst.

cystadenocarcinoma (sis-tad-e-no-kar-si-no´mă) A malignant tumor derived from glandular epithelium, most frequently occurring as a partially solid mass with a cystic pattern; seen chiefly in the ovaries.

cystadenoma (sis-tad-e-no´mă) Benign tumor containing large cystic masses lined with epithelium, typically found in the ovary and pancreas.

cystalgia (sis-tal´jă) Pain in the bladder.

cystathionine (sis-tă-thi´o-nēn) An intermediate in the conversion of methionine to cysteine.

cystathioninuria (sis-tă-thi-o-nē-nu´re-ă) A rare, inherited disorder of amino acid metabolism resulting in an excessive secretion of cystathionine in the urine; associated with mental retardation.

cystectasia, cystectasy (sis-tek-ta´zhă, sis-tek´tă-se) Dilatation of the bladder.

cystectomy (sis-tec´tŏ-me) **1.** Removal of a cyst. **2.** Removal of the urinary bladder.

cysteine (sis-te´ēn) (CyS) An amino acid, $C_3H_7NO_2S$, present in most proteins.

cystic (sis´tik) **1.** Relating to a cyst. **2.** Relating to the gallbladder or urinary bladder.

cystic disease of breast (sis´tik dĭ-zēz´ ŭv brĕst) See fibrocystic change of breast, under change.

cystic disease of renal medulla (sis´tik dĭ-zēz´ ŭv re´nal mĕ-dul´ă) The presence of multiple cysts in the medulla of the kidney, seen primarily in two clinical syndromes: *uremic medullary cystic disease* (nephronophthisis), an inherited disease in which medullary cysts are associated with glomerulosclerosis, interstitial fibrosis, and renal failure often appearing in childhood; *non-uremic medullary cystic disease* (sponge kidney), a relatively benign condition that may be associated with calculi or infections, usually diagnosed by intravenous pyelography.

cysticercosis (sis-tĭ-ser-ko´sis) Infestation with the larvae of the cestode *Taenia solium* (pork tapeworm).

cysticercus (sis-tĭ-ser´kus) The cystic or larval form of the tapeworm, consisting of a scolex or head enclosed in a fluid-filled sac or cyst.

cystic fibrosis of pancreas (sis´tik fi-bro´sis ŭv pan´kre-as) See under fibrosis.

cysticotomy (sis-tĭ-kot´ŏ-me) Surgical incision into the cystic duct.

cystiform (sis´tĭ-form) Resembling a cyst.

cystine (sis´tēn, sis´tĭn) A sulfur-containing amino acid present in many proteins.

cystinosis (sis-tĭ-no´sis) Failure of normal metabolism of cystine (an amino acid) due to a genetically determined enzyme deficiency; cystine accumulates and precipitates in many tissues, including the renal tubular epithelium and bone marrow; one of many causes of Fanconi syndrome.

cystinuria (sis-tĭ-nu´re-ă) **1.** The presence of cystine in the urine. **2.** A hereditary defect in renal tubular reabsorption of amino acids (cystine, lysine, arginine, and ornithine), resulting in recurrent kidney stone formation.

cystitis (sis´ti´tis) Inflammation of the urinary bladder.

interstitial c. Nonbacterial chronic cystitis causing suprapubic pain, which is relieved by voiding.

cystitomy (sis-tit´ŏ-me) **1.** Capsulotomy. **2.** Cystotomy. **3.** Cholecystotomy.

cystocele (sis´to-sēl) Hernia formed by the downward and backward displacement of the urinary bladder toward the vaginal orifice, due most commonly to weakening of its pelvic support. Also called vesicocele.

cystogram (sis´to-gram) X-ray picture of the bladder, obtained in cystography.

cystography (sis-tog´ră-fe) Radiography of the bladder after introduction of a radiopaque fluid.

cystoid (sis´toid) **1.** Resembling a cyst. **2.** A collection of soft material resembling a cyst, but without an enclosing capsule.

cystolith (sis´to-lith) A bladder stone.

cystolithectomy (sis-to-lĭ-thek´tŏ-me) Surgical removal of a bladder stone; erroneously used when referring to the removal of a gallbladder stone. Also called cystolithotomy.

cystolithiasis (sis-to-lĭ-thi´ă-sis) The presence of bladder stones.

cystolithic (sis-to-lith´ik) Relating to a bladder stone.

cystolithotomy (sis-to-lĭ-thot´ŏ-me) See cystolithectomy.

cystoma (sis-to´mă) A tumor containing cysts.

cystometer (sis-tom´ĕ-ter) A diagnostic device that measures the tone of the detrusor muscle in the wall of the urinary bladder in relation to the volume of fluid in the bladder.

cystometrogram (sis-to-met´ro-gram) A graphic record of the pressure within the urinary bladder.

cystometry (sis-tom´ĕ-tre) The continuous recording of the pressures within the urinary bladder by means of a cystometer; the procedure is used for determining the tone of the bladder when neurologic disturbance of the bladder wall is suspected.

cystoplasty (sis´to-plas-te) Surgical repair of the bladder.

cystoplegia (sis-to-ple´jĕ) Paralysis of the bladder.

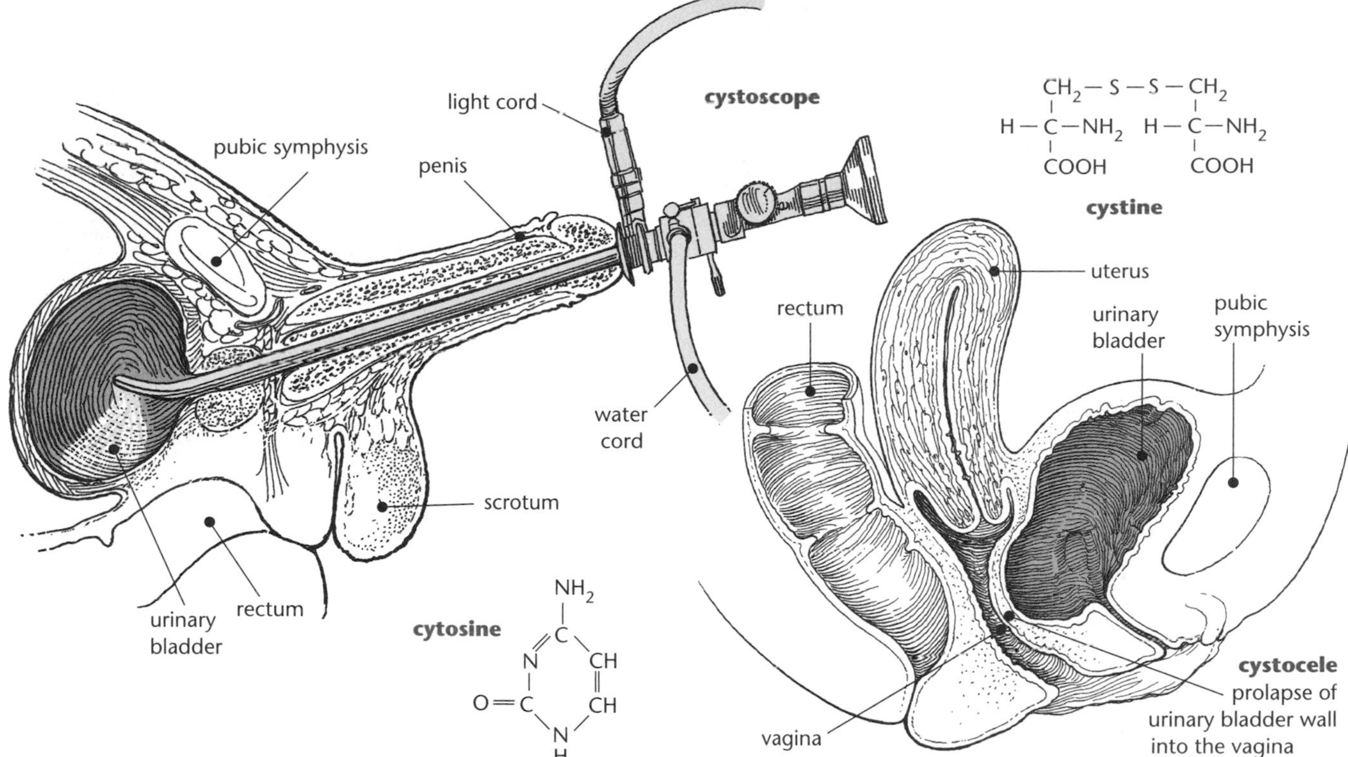

cystoptosis (sis-top-to´sis) Prolapse of the inner lining of the bladder into the urethra.
cystopyelitis (sis-to-pi-ĕ-li´tis) Inflammation of the bladder and of the pelvis of the kidney.
cystorrhagia (sis-to-ra´jă) Bleeding from the bladder.
cystorrhea (sis-to-re´ă) Discharge of mucus from the bladder. Also called vesical catarrh.
cystoscope (sis´to-skōp) A tubular instrument fitted with a light for examining the interior of the urinary bladder.
cytoscopy (sis-tos´kŏ-pe) Visual examination of the interior of the urinary bladder by means of a cystoscope.
cystospasm (sis´to-spaz-m) Spasmodic contraction of the bladder.
cystostomy (sis-tos´tŏ-me) A temporary opening made into the bladder in order to divert urine from the urethra.
cystotomy (sis-tot´ŏ-me) Surgical incision of the urinary bladder. Also called vesicotomy.
cystoureteritis (sis-to-u-re-ter-ī´tis) Inflammation of the bladder and a ureter or ureters.
cystourethritis (sis-to-u-re-thrī´tis) Inflammation of the bladder and urethra.
cystourethrocele (sis-to-u-re´thro-sēl) Prolapse of female urethra and neck of bladder.
cytarabine (si-tar´ă-bēn) See arabinosylcytosine.
cytidine (si´tĭ-dēn) A nucleoside consisting of cytosine attached through a β-glycosidic linkage to ribose.
cytoanalyzer (si-to-an´ă-li-zer) A machine used to screen smears containing cells suspected of malignancy.
cytoarchitecture (si-to-ăr-kĭ-tek´chur) The arrangement of cells in a tissue, especially of the cerebral cortex.
cytobiology (si-to-bi-ol´ŏ-je) See cytology.
cytocentrum (si-to-sen´trum) See centrosome.
cytochemistry (si´to-kem-is-tre) A branch of cell biology devoted to the chemical and physicochemical analysis of living matter.
cytochrome (si´to-krōm) A respiratory enzyme capable of undergoing alternate reduction and oxidation; chemically related to hemoglobin.
  c. oxidase The terminal enzyme in the chain of events that constitutes cellular oxygen consumption.
  c. P-450 Pigment involved in extramitochondrial transport of electrons in the liver and in mixed function oxidation reactions; important in the metabolism of many drugs; found in adrenal mitochondria and in liver microsomes; so named because the CO compound of the reduced cytochrome has an absorption maximum of 450 nanometers.
cytocide (si´to-sīd) Destructive to cells.
cytoclasis (si-tok´lă-sis) The fragmentation of cells.
cytocyst (si´to-sist) The remains of a cell enclosing a schizont (malarial parasite undergoing asexual division).
cytodendrite (si-to-den´drīt) Dendrite.
cytodiagnosis (si-to-di-ăg-no´sis) Diagnosis of disease based on the study of cells.
cytogenesis (si-to-jen´ĕ-sis) The origin of cells.
cytogenetics (si-to-je-net´iks) The combined study of heredity and the structure and function of cells.
cytokine (si´to-kīn) Any of several hormone-like proteins that act as intercellular chemical messengers to regulate many cell functions, especially the immune response; produced by various cell types (e.g., lymphocytes, monocytes, fibroblasts, macro-phages, keratinocytes).
cytology (si-tol´ŏ-je) The science concerned with the study and identification of cells. Also called cell biology; cytobiology.
  exfoliative c. Examination, for the purpose of diagnosis, of cells recovered from secretions, exudate, or washings of a tissue, such as sputum, vaginal secretion, gastric washings, etc.
cytolysin (si-tol´ĭ-sĭn) An antibody that is capable of causing the dissolution of an animal cell.
cytolysis (si-tol´ĭ-sis) The destruction of a cell.
cytomegalic (si-to-mĕ-gal´ik) Characterized by greatly enlarged cells.
cytomegalic inclusion disease (si-to-mĕ-gal´ik in-kloo´zhun dĭ-zēz´) A viral infection presenting symptoms according to the organs affected; formerly believed to affect only children, but seen now in adults with debilitating diseases; caused by a cytomegalovirus.
cytomegalovirus (si-to-meg´ă-lo-vi´rus) (CMV) One of a group of highly specific human herpes-viruses causing intranuclear inclusions and enlargement of cells of various organs; in humans, it causes cytomegalic inclusion disease. Also called human herpesvirus 5.
cytometer (si-tom´ĕ-ter) A standardized device for counting and measuring cells, particularly blood cells.
cytometry (si-tom´ĕ-tre) A method of separating and enumerating cells suspended in a fluid (e.g., blood cells).
  flow c. A high-speed procedure performed with a flow cytometer in which a laser beam rapidly scans a large number of fluorescently labeled cells suspended in a stream; the cytometer automatically sorts and counts the different types of cells as they flow individually through an aperture and cross the laser beam. The technique can analyze cell size, DNA content, viability, enzyme content, and surface characteristics; used to diagnose malignancy in difficult cases by establishing the presence of abnormal cell populations.
cytomorphology (si-to-mor-fol´ŏ-je) The study of the configuration of cells.
cytopathic (si-to-path´ik) Characterized by a diseased condition of cells.
cytopathogenic (si-to-path-o-jen´ik) Capable of producing a diseased condition in cells.
cytopathology (si-to-pă-thol´ŏ-je) The study of cells in disease.
cytopenia (si-to-pe´ne-ă) Diminution of the cellular elements in the blood.
cytophagy (si-tof´ă-je) The devouring or ingestion of cells by other cells (phagocytes).
cytoplasm (si´to-plaz-m) The protoplasm or substance of a cell surrounding the nucleus, carrying structures within which most of the life processes of the cell take place.
cytopoiesis (si-to-poi-ĕ´sis) The development of cells.
cytosine (si´to-sēn) A pyrimidine base, $C_4H_5N_3O$; a disintegration product of nucleic acid.
cytosis (si-to´sis) **1.** The presence of more than the usual number of cells. **2.** Term used with a prefix to denote certain characteristics of cells.
cytosmear (si´to-smēr) See cytologic smear, under smear.
cytosol (si´to-sol) The soluble portion of the cyto-plasm after all the particles, such as mitochondrial and endoplasmic reticular components, are removed.
cytosome (si´to-sōm) The cell body without the nucleus.
cytostatic (si-to-stat´ik) Capable of stopping cell growth.
cytostome (si´to-stōm) The opening that serves as a mouth in certain complex protozoa.
cytotaxis, cytotaxia (si-to-tak´sis, si-to-tak´se-ă) The movement of a cell toward or away from another cell in response to a specific stimulus.
cytotoxic (si-to-tok´sik) Damaging to cells. Also called cytolytic.
cytotoxin (si-to-tok´sin) An antibody that destroys or inhibits the functions of cells.
cytotrophoblast (si-to-trof´o-blast) The inner, cellular, layer of the trophoblast developed from the single-layered trophoblast at the time of implantation of the blastocyst.
cytotropic (si-to-trop´ik) Having an affinity for cells.
cytozoic (si-to-zo´ik) Living in a cell.
cytozoon (si-to-zo´on) A protozoan parasitic in a cell.

D

δ (del'tă) Delta. For terms beginning with δ, see under specific term.
dacryadenitis (dak-re-ad-ĕ-nī´tis) See dacryoadenitis.
dacryagogue (dak're-ă-gog) **1.** Promoting the flow of tears. **2.** Any agent that induces the lacrimal gland to secrete tears.
dacryoadenalgia (dak-re-o-ad-ĕ-nal´jă) Pain or discomfort in a lacrimal gland.
dacryoadenitis (dak-re-o-ad-ĕ-nī´tis) Inflammation of the lacrimal gland. Also spelled dacryadenitis.
dacryoblennorrhea (dak-re-o-blen-o-re ă) A chronic discharge of mucus from the lacrimal ducts, as in chronic dacryocystitis.
dacryocele (dak´re-o-sēl) See dacryocystocele.
dacryocyst (dak´re-o-sist) The lacrimal sac.
dacryocystalgia (dak-re-o-sis-tal´jă) Pain or discomfort in a lacrimal sac.
dacryocystectomy (dak-re-o-sis-tek´tŏ-me) Surgical removal of the lacrimal sac.
dacryocystitis (dak-re-o-sis-tī'tis) Inflammation of the lacrimal sac; most often seen in infants and in menopausal women.
dacryocystocele (dak-re-o-sis´to-sēl) Enlargement of the lacrimal sac with fluid, usually due to obstruction of the nasolacrimal duct. Also called dacryocele.
dacryocystogram (dak-re-o-sis´tŏ-gram) X-ray image of the lacrimal apparatus (tear-forming and tear-conducting structures) obtained after injection of a radiopaque substance, usually performed to locate an obstruction.
dacryocystorhinostenosis (dak-re-o-sis-to-rī-no-stĕ-no´sis) Narrowing of the nasolacrimal duct, obstructing the normal flow of tears into the nasal cavity.
dacryocystorhinostomy (dak-re-o-sis-tos´tŏ-me) The operative creation of a passage between the lacrimal sac and the nose to effect drainage of tears when the nasolacrimal duct is occluded.
dacryocystotomy (dak-re-o-sis-tot'ŏ-me) Surgical incision into the lacrimal sac.
dacryohemorrhea (dak-re-o-hem-o-re´ă) The shedding of tears mixed with blood.
dacryolith (dak´re-o-lith) A calculus in the tear-forming or tear-conducting structures. Also called tear stone.
dacryolithiasis (dak-re-o-lĭ-thī'ă-sis) The presence of calculi (dacryoliths) in the tear passages.
dacryoma (dak-re-o´mă) **1.** A cyst caused by obstruction of the lacrimal duct. **2.** A tumor of the lacrimal apparatus.
dacryon (dak´re-on) A cranial point where the lacrimal, frontal, and maxillary bones meet at the angle of the ocular orbit.
dacryops (dak're-ops) **1.** A watery condition of the eye; the constant presence of excess tear fluid on the eye due to poor drainage caused by constriction of the lacrimal punctum. **2.** Dilatation of a lacrimal duct by contained fluid.
dacryopyorrhea (dak-re-o-pi-o-re´ă) The shedding of tears containing pus.
dacryopyosis (dak-re-o-pi-o´sis) Formation or discharge of pus in the lacrimal sac or duct.
dacryorrhea (dak-re-o-re'ă) An excessive flow of tears.
dacryosolenitis (dak-re-o-so-lĕ-nī'tis) Inflammation of the lacrimal or nasal duct.
dacryostenosis (dak-re-o-stĕ-no'sis) Stricture of any lacrimal passage.
dactinomycin (dak-tĭ-no-mī'sin) An antineoplastic agent used in the treatment of Wilms' tumor in children and trophoblastic disease in women.
dactyl (dak'til) A digit; a finger or toe.
dactylalgia (dak-tĭ-lal'jă) Pain in the fingers or toes.
dactyledema (dak-til-ĕ-de'mă) Edema of a finger.
dactylitis (dak-tĭ-lī'tis) Inflammation of a digit.
dactylocampsis (dak-tĭ-lo-kamp'sis) Permanent flexion or bending of the fingers or toes.
dactylography (dak-tĭ-log´ră-fe) The study of fingerprints.
dactylogryposis (dak-tĭ-lo-grĭ-po'sis) Contraction of the fingers or toes.

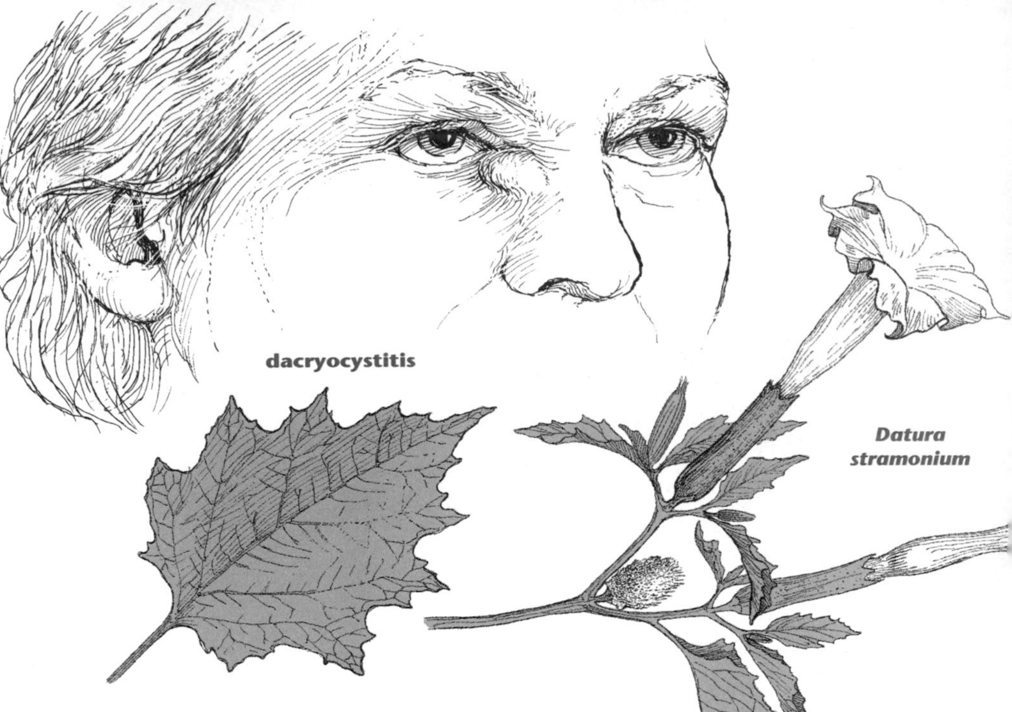

dactyloid (dak'tĭ-loid) Finger-shaped.
dactylology (dak-tĭ-lol´ŏ-je) Use of the finger alphabet as a means of communication, as by deaf-mutes.
dactylomegaly (dak-tĭ-lo-meg'ă-le) A condition in which fingers or toes are abnormally large. Also called macrodactylia.
dactyloscopy (dak-tĭ-los'kŏ-pe) The examination of fingerprints for purposes of personal identification.
dactylospasm (dak´tĭ-lo-spaz-m) Spasmodic contraction of the fingers.
dactylus (dak´tĭ-lus) A finger or a toe; usually a toe, as distinguished from digitus, a finger.
Dalrymple's sign (dal´rim-pls sīn) Abnormal wideness of the palpebral fissures, occurring in Graves' disease.
dalton (dawl'ton, dōlt'n) A unit of molecular weight equivalent to the weight of a hydrogen atom; a water molecule weighs 18 daltons and a hemoglobin molecule weighs 64,500 daltons; the terms dalton and molecular weight are used interchangeably.
dam (dam) A barrier preventing the flow of fluid; especially a thin rubber sheet used in dentistry and surgery to isolate the operative field from the access of bodily fluid. Also called rubber-dam.
  coffer d. A thin sheet of rubber stretched around the neck of a tooth to keep it dry during dental restoration.
dander (dan´der) Dry skin shed by animals (dogs, cats, etc.); the cause of allergy in certain persons.
dandruff (dan'ruf) Common name for the mild form of seborrheic dermatitis; see under dermatitis.
Dandy-Walker syndrome (dan´dē-wawk´er sin´drōm) Congenital hydrocephalus in infants due to obstruction or atresia of the median aperture of the fourth ventricle (foramen of Magendi) and the lateral aperture of the fourth ventricle (foramen of Luschka).
dapsone (dap´sōn) A compound used in the treatment of leprosy and tuberculosis.
Datura stramonium (da-too'ră stră-mo'ne-um) A species of an annual herb containing alkaloids that block the action of parasympathetic nerves; has been used as an inhalant to treat asthma. Also called jimsonweed; thorn apple.
daturine (da-too'rin) See hyoscyamine.
D&C See dilatation and curettage.
DDT Dichlorodiphenyltrichloroethane, a colorless, toxic insecticide.
D&E See dilatation and evacuation.
deacidification (de-ă-sid-ĭ-fĭ-ka'shun) The act of removing or neutralizing an acid.
deactivation (de-ak-tĭ-va´shun) The process of rendering inactive; making harmless or ineffective.
dead (ded) Lifeless.
deaf (def) Afflicted with deafness; unable to hear.
deafferentation (de-af-er-en-ta´shun) The suppression or loss of afferent nerve impulses from a portion of the body.
deaf-mute (def-myo͞ot) An individual who can neither hear nor speak.
deafmutism (def-myo͞o´tiz-m) The condition of being deaf-mute.
deafness (def´nes) Inability to hear, partial or complete.
  acoustic trauma d. See noise-induced deafness.
  conductive d. Loss of hearing caused by disease of, or injury to, the tympanic membrane or ear ossicles.
  nerve d. Former name for sensorineural deafness.
  noise-induced d. Loss of hearing caused by prolonged exposure to excessive noise.
  pure word d. Condition in which the person can hear but cannot comprehend spoken language, while comprehension of written words and ability to speak are relatively preserved; has been attributed to a lesion in or near the primary auditory cortex (Heschl's gyrus) in the temporal lobe of the brain.
  sensorineural d. Deafness caused by damage to the cochlear division of the vestibulocochlear (8th cranial) nerve, the cochlea, or the retrocochlear nerve tracts.
  sudden d. Sudden loss of hearing resulting from a systemic disease, most commonly viral infection of the inner ear or a blood clot in the labyrinthine artery.
  word d. See auditory aphasia, under aphasia.
dealbation (de-al-ba'shun) Whitening; bleaching.
dealcoholization (de-al-ko-hol-ĭ-za´shun) The removal of alcohol from a substance.
deamidate (de-am´ĭ-dāt) To remove the amido group from an organic compound. Also called desamidate; deamidize.
deaminase (de-am'ĭ-nās) An enzyme that promotes the removal of the amino group from amino compounds such as amino acids.
deaminate (de-am´ĭ-nāt) To remove, usually by hydrolysis, an amino group from an organic compound.
deamination (de-am-ĭ-na'shun) The removal of an amino group (NH_2) from an organic compound. Also called deaminization.
death (dĕth) Death as described by The Uniform Determination of Death Act passed by the US Congress (1981), which states that an individual is dead if there is (1) irreversible cessation of circulatory and respiratory functions or (2) irreversible cessation of all functions of the entire brain, including the brainstem.
  black d. The worldwide epidemic of the 14th century, believed to be pneumonic plague.
  brain d. An irreversible state persisting after a

$$H_2\overset{NH_2}{\overset{|}{C}}-CH_2-CH_2-CH_2-\overset{NH_2}{\overset{|}{CH}}-COOH \xrightarrow{\text{decarboxylase}} H_2\overset{NH_2}{\overset{|}{C}}-CH_2-CH_2-CH_2-\overset{NH_2}{\overset{|}{CH_2}}+CO_2$$

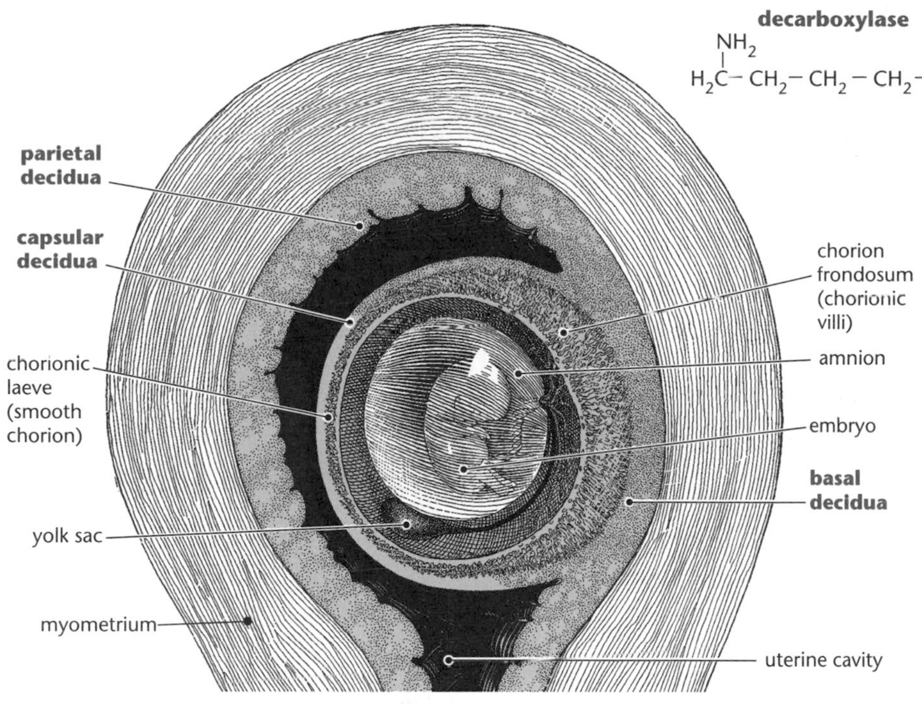

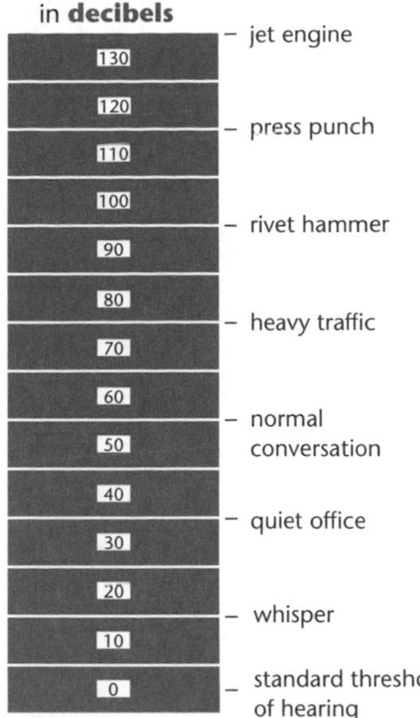

specified length of time (usually 6-24 hours) in which there is total cessation of brain function (i.e., complete unresponsiveness to all stimuli, including painful stimuli such as hard pinching), absence of brainstem reflexes (e.g., pupils are dilated and unresponsive to light), and disappearance of the electroencephalogram pattern (a "flat" electroencephalogram); heartbeat and breathing may continue only with the aid of a respirator. Two conditions are excluded: hypothermia and depression of the central nervous system by drugs. Confirmatory tests make it possible to shorten the observation period in adults; in infants and young children, a full 24-hour observation period is recommended. Also called cerebral death.

cell d. Termination of a cell's ability to carry out vital functions (i.e., metabolism, growth, reproduction, and adaptability).

cerebral d. See brain death.

clinically unexplained d. (a) Death of a patient whose prolonged, complex illness was extensively studied but a satisfactory diagnosis was not established. (b) Death of a patient whose illness was of such brief duration that there was little or no opportunity for medical observation or studies to provide a reasonable explanation.

crib d., cot d. See sudden infant death syndrome.

fetal d. Intrauterine death of a fetus. In early pregnancy, the first sign is absence of uterine enlargement; in later pregnancy, absence of fetal movement.

infant d. Death of a baby under the age of 1 year.

maternal d. The death of a woman while pregnant or within 42 days of termination of pregnancy (the puerperium), irrespective of the duration and site of pregnancy. *Direct maternal d.*, death resulting from obstetric complications of pregnancy, labor, or the puerperium; or from any intervention, incorrect treatment, or omission; or from any sequence of events derived from any of the above. *Indirect maternal d.*, death caused by a previously existing medical condition, or one developed during pregnancy and aggravated by the natural physiologic burdens of pregnancy, including the additional demands of labor and delivery.

neonatal d. Death of an infant during the first 28 days of life; usually designated *early* when it occurs during the first 7 days and *late* thereafter.

nonmaternal d. Death of a pregnant woman unrelated to the pregnant state (e.g., from an automobile accident).

perinatal d. Death occurring during the perinatal period (i.e., from completion of 20 weeks of gestation through the first 28 days after delivery).

programmed cell d. See apoptosis.

sudden cardiac d. (SCD) Unexpected cessation of cardiac contraction occurring within one hour of the onset of symptoms, usually caused by obstruction of one or more coronary arteries; other causes include constriction of the aortic valve, abnormalities of the conduction system in the heart muscle, and prolapse of the mitral (left atrioventricular) valve. In young people, it may be caused by hypertrophic cardiomyopathy (HCM) due to a genetic defect. See also hypertrophic cardiomyopathy, under cardiomyopathy.

death rattle (dĕth rat´l) The gurgling noise sometimes heard in the throat of a dying person, caused by loss of the cough reflex and accumulation of mucus.

death struggle (dĕth strug´l) The rare signs of the final moments of death; a twitching or convulsion. Also called agony; death throe; psychorrhagia.

debilitate (dĕ-bil´ĭ-tāt) To make weak or feeble; to enervate.

debility (dĕ-bil´ĭ-te) The condition of abnormal bodily weakness; lack or loss of strength.

debouch (da-bo͞osh´) To open or empty into another part of the body.

debridement (da-brēd-maw´) Removal of all devitalized tissue and debris from a traumatic or infected wound until healthy tissue is exposed.

debt (det) Deficit.

oxygen d. The extra oxygen consumed by the body, above its resting needs, to satisfy demands caused by intensive exercise.

debulking (de-bulk´ing) Operative removal of portions of a large malignant tumor to reduce its size, oxygenate the tumor tissues (oxygen is often toxic to malignant cells), and provide space to encourage proliferation of malignant cells (thus rendering the tumor more susceptible to destruction by chemotherapy; quiescent cells are not as susceptible).

decagram (dek´ă-gram) Ten grams.

decalcification (de-kal-sĭ-fĭ-ka´shun) **1.** The loss of calcium salts from bones or teeth. **2.** The removal of calcium ions from the blood to prevent or delay coagulation.

decalcify (de-kal´sĭ-fi) To remove calcium salts, especially from bones or teeth.

decalcifying (de-kal´sĭ-fi-ing) **1.** Denoting any agent or process that removes calcium salts from bones or teeth. **2.** Denoting an agent that removes calcium ion from blood to render it incoagulable.

decaliter (dek´ă-le-ter) A measure of 10 liters; 2.64 gallons; roughly 10 quarts.

decant (dĭ-kant´) To pour off the upper clear portion of a fluid without disturbing the sediment.

decapeptide (dek-ă-pep´tīd) A peptide composed of 10 amino acids.

decapitate (de-kap´ĭ-tāt) To remove the head; to behead.

decapsulation (de-kap-su-la´shun) The removal of a capsule or enveloping membrane.

decarboxylase (de-kar-bok´sĭ-lās) Any enzyme that accelerates the removal of carbon dioxide (CO_2) from the carboxyl group of a compound, especially from alpha-amino acids (e.g., lysine decarboxylase).

decarboxylation (de-kar-bok´sĭ-la´shun) Replacement of a carboxyl group from an organic compound, usually with hydrogen.

decay (de-ka´) **1.** The decomposition of organic compounds as a result of bacterial or fungal action. **2.** In physics, spontaneous, progressive decrease in the number of atoms from a radioactive substance.

deceleration (de-sel-er-a´shun) Decrease in velocity.

decerebrate (de-ser-´ĕ-brāt) **1.** To remove the portion of the brain above the lower border of the quadrigeminal bodies. **2.** An experimental animal so prepared. **3.** A person who has sustained a brain injury that renders him physiologically comparable to a decerebrate animal.

decerebration (de-ser-ĕ-bra´shun) Removal of a portion of brain in experimental animals.

decerebrize (de-ser´ĕ-brīz) To remove the brain.

decibel (des´ĭ-bel) (dB, db) A unit for measuring the ratio of two powers or intensities (electric or acoustic power); in measurement of acoustic intensities, it is equal to 10 times the common logarithm of the ratio of two levels of intensity, or to the smallest degree of loudness that is ordinarily heard by the human ear; at a distance of about four feet, an ordinary conversation produces a level of approximately 60 dB (on a scale from 1 to 130).

decidua (de-sid´u-ă) The modified, highly specialized inner lining of the pregnant uterus; i.e., the endometrium that has become thick and vascular, forming a receptive environment for implantation of the blastocyst and development of the embryo/fetus and its membranes. It is shed at childbirth except for the deepest layer. Also called decidual membrane.

basal d. The portion of decidua between the implanted chorionic vesicle and the uterine muscle (myometrium); it becomes the maternal part of the placenta.

capsular d. Endometrium that seals the implanted chorionic vesicle from the uterine cavity; it undergoes rapid regression from about the fourth month of pregnancy. Also called reflex decidua.

menstrual d. The engorged (hyperemic) endothelial mucosa of the nonpregnant uterus; shed during the menstrual period.

parietal d. The entire endometrium lining the cavity of the pregnant uterus, except the parts surrounding the implanted conceptus. Also called decidua vera; true decidua.

reflex d. See capsular decidua.

true d. See parietal decidua.

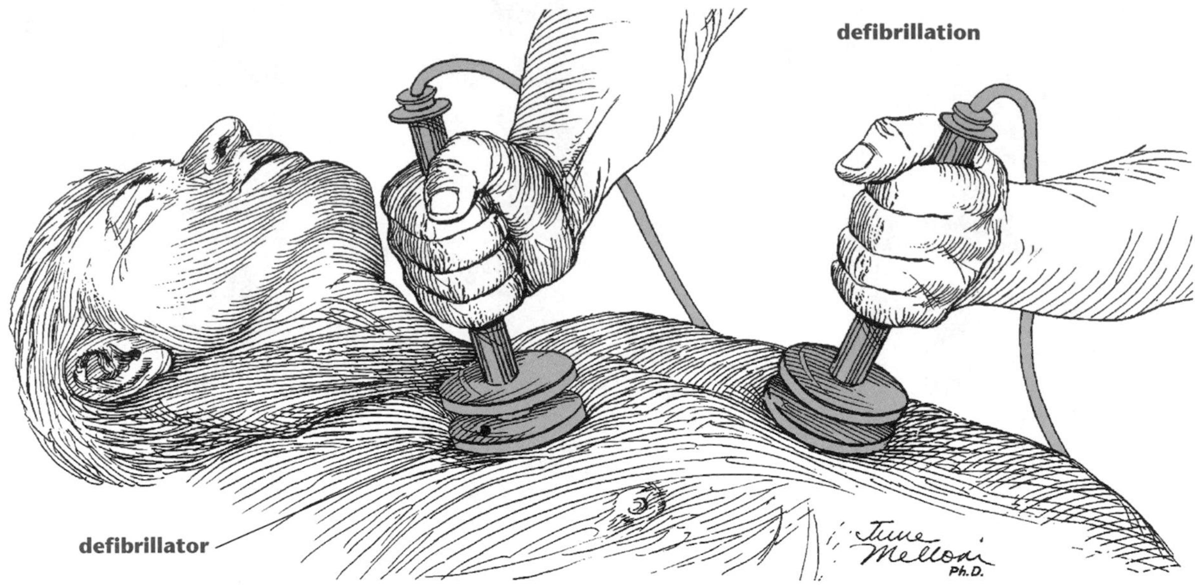

d. vera See parietal decidua.
decidual (dĕ-sid′u-al) Relating to decidua.
decidualization (de-sid-u-ă-lĭ-za′shun) The changes occurring in tissues in which the fertilized ovum implants culminating in the formation of decidua, the highly specialized endometrium; may occur also in tissues in which ectopic pregnancies take place (e.g., mucosal lining of uterine tubes, peritoneum, and ovaries).
deciduation (dĕ-sid-u-a′shun) The casting off of endometrial tissue during menstruation.
deciduoma (dĕ-sid-u-o′mă) A mass of decidual tissue in the uterus.
deciduous (dĕ-sid′u-us) Temporary; falling off at the end of a developmental stage (e.g., primary dentition).
deciliter (des′ĭ-le-ter) (dl) A measure of one-tenth (10^{-1}) of a liter.
decimeter (des′ĭ-mē-ter) (dm) A linear measure of one-tenth (10^{-1}) of a meter.
decinormal (des-ĭ-nor′mal) (0.1 N) One-tenth of normal; denoting a solution that has one-tenth of the normal strength. See also normal solution, under solution.
decipara (dĕ-sip′ă-ră) (para X) A woman who has borne 10 children.
declination (dek-lĭ-na′shun) **1.** A sloping; a bending downward. **2.** In ophthalmology, rotation of the eye about an anteroposterior axis.
decline (de-klīn′, dĭ-klīn′) **1.** The stage of abatement of symptoms of an acute disease. **2.** A period of involution. **3.** A wasting disease.
declive (de-klīv′) Latin for hill or slope.
d. cerebelli The sloping portion of the vermis of the middle lobe of the cerebellum, bounded anteriorly by the primary fissure and posteriorly by the postclival fissure.
decoction (de-kok′shun) **1.** The process of boiling down or concentrating by boiling. **2.** A medicine prepared by boiling.
decompensation (de-kom-pen-sa′shun) **1.** Failure of the heart to maintain adequate circulation in certain cardiac and circulation disorders. **2.** Failure of usual coping mechanisms resulting in personality disintegration.
decompose (de′kom-pōz) **1.** To decay. **2.** To separate a compound into its basic elements.
decomposition (de-kom-pŏ-zish′un) **1.** Organic decay; disintegration; lysis. **2.** The separation of compounds into constituents by chemical reaction.
decompression (de-kom-presh′un) The removal of pressure.
bowel d. Relief of a distended portion of the intestine by passage of a long tube connected to suction or by establishing a direct opening, such as a cecostomy.
cardiac d. Surgical incision into the pericardium for the release of accumulated fluid from the pericardial sac. Also called pericardial decompression.
cerebral d. Removal of a section of the skull, with puncture of the dura mater, to relieve intracranial pressure.
orbital d. Removal of bone from the orbit to relieve pressure behind the eyeball, as in exophthalmus.
pericardial d. See cardiac decompression.
decongestant (de-kon-jes′tant) Any agent that reduces congestion or swelling.
decongestive (de-kon-jes′tiv) Reducing congestion or swelling.
decontamination (de-kon-tam-ĭ-na′shun) **1.** Making safe by eliminating or neutralizing harmful agents (noxious chemicals, radioactive material). **2.** Removal of contamination.
decorticate (de-kor′tĭ-kāt) To surgically remove the cortex of an organ or structure.
decortication (de-kor-tĭ-ka′shun) Removal of the cortical substance (external layer) of an organ or structure, such as the brain or kidney.
decrudescence (de-kroo-des′ens) Abatement of the intensity of symptoms of disease.
decubital (de-ku′bĭ-tl) Relating to a decubitus ulcer (bedsore).
decubitus (de-ku′bĭ-tus) The act of reclining; lying down.
decussate (de-kus′āt) **1.** To cross or intersect so as to form an X. **2.** Crossed like the letter X.
decussation (de-kŭ-sa′shun) A point of crossing, especially of nerve tracts.
dedifferentiation (de-dif-er-en-she-a′shun) **1.** The reversion of specialized cellular forms to a more primitive condition. **2.** The process in which specialized tissues are the site of origin of primitive elements of the same type.
defecation (def-e-ka′shun) The discharge of feces from the bowels.
defect (de′fekt) Malformation.
atrial septal d. Defect in the septum between the atria of the heart.
birth d. See congenital malformation, under malformation.
filling d. Any abnormality in the contour of the digestive tract, as seen in an x-ray image.
ventricular septal d. (VSD) Defect in the septum between the ventricles of the heart.
defective (de-fek′tiv) Denoting a person deficient in some physical or mental attribute.
defemination (de-fem-ĭ-na′shun) The loss or decrease of feminine characteristics.
defense mechanism (de-fens′ mek′ă-niz-m) An unconscious process through which a person seeks relief from anxiety.
defensins (de-fen′sinz) See defensin peptides, under peptide.
deferent (def′er-ent) Carrying down or away.
deferentectomy (def-er-en-tek′to-me) See vasectomy.
deferentitis (def-er-en-ti′tis) Inflammation of the deferent duct. Also called vasitis; spermatitis.
deferoxamine mesylate (dĕ-fer-oks′ă-mēn mes′ĭ-lāt) Compound used in the treatment of iron poisoning, given by intramuscular injection or intravenous infusion.
defervescence (def-er-ves′ens) The lowering of fever.
defibrillation (de-fib-rĭ-la′shun) The arrest of quivering movements of cardiac muscle fibers (fibrillation).
defibrillator (de-fib-rĭ-la′tor) **1.** Anything that arrests ventricular fibrillation and restores the normal heart beat. **2.** An apparatus capable of delivering an electric shock to arrest ventricular fibrillation.
defibrination (de-fi-brĭ-na′shun) The removal of fibrin from the blood to prevent it from clotting.
deficiency (de-fish′en-se) The state of being insufficient; a lack; a shortage.
adult lactase d. Adult deficiency of the intestinal enzyme lactase, causing milk intolerance and malabsorption.
antitrypsin d. Hereditary disorder that in its severe form is frequently associated with emphysema.
glucose-6-phosphate dehydrogenase d. An X-linked genetic deficiency causing a variety of hemolytic anemias, including severe reactions upon ingestion of fava beans (favism).
hypoxanthine guanine phosphoribosyltransferase d. (HPRT) Inherited metabolic disorder occurring in two forms: *complete HPRT* (Lesch-Nyhan syndrome), characterized by excessive uric acid in the blood (hyperuricemia), self-mutilation, abnormal involuntary movements, spasticity, and mental retardation; *partial HPRT* (Kelley-Seegmiller syndrome), associated with hyperuricemia but no central nervous system involvement.
immune d. See immunodeficiency.
mental d. See mental retardation, under retardation.
pseudocholinesterase d. Hereditary disorder manifested by an excessive reaction to drugs that are usually hydrolyzed by serum pseudocholinesterase, especially some of the agents used to achieve muscular relaxation during anesthesia, such as succinylcholine.
pyruvate kinase d. Hereditary deficiency of pyruvate kinase, causing hemolytic anemia.
deficit (def′ĭ-sit) A deficiency in quantity or quality.
pulse d. The difference between the number of heartbeats (greater) and the number of beats counted at the wrist (less) due to failure of a very early ventricular contraction to propel sufficient blood to produce a palpable pulse.
definition (def-ĭ-nish′un) **1.** The power of an optical system to produce a sharp image. **2.** The maximum ability of the eye to discriminate between two points.
deflection (de-flek′shun) **1.** The act of turning aside. **2.** A wave of the electrocardiogram.
intrinsicoid d. In electrocardiography, the sudden downstroke from maximum positivity.
defloration (def-lo-ra′shun) The act of rupturing the hymen. Also called deflowering.
deflorescence (def-lo-res′ens) Disappearance of the skin eruption of any eruptive disease.
defluvium (de-floo′ve-um) Hair loss.
deformation (de-for-ma′shun) **1.** A change of form

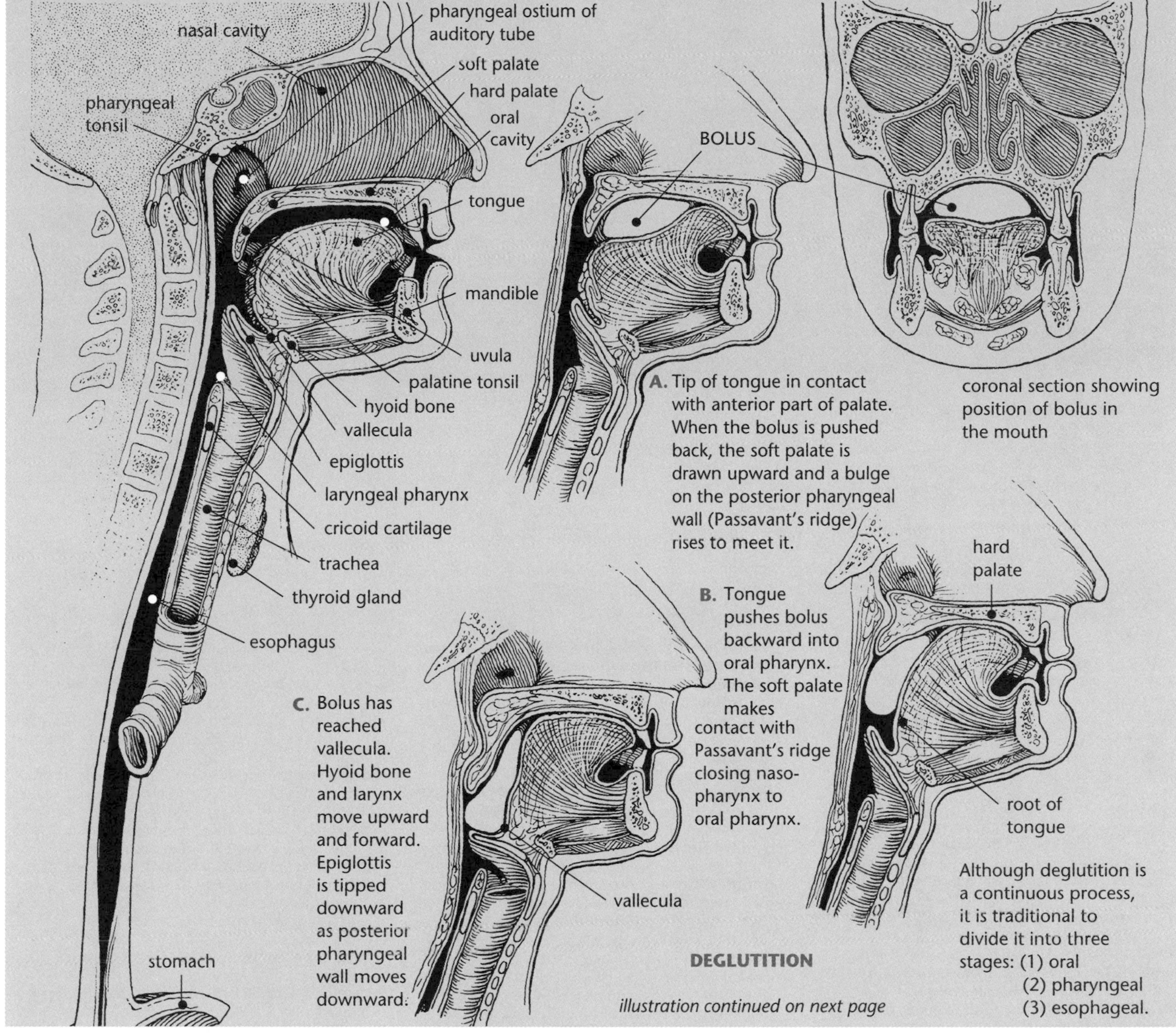
nasal cavity
pharyngeal ostium of auditory tube
soft palate
hard palate
oral cavity
pharyngeal tonsil
tongue
mandible
uvula
palatine tonsil
hyoid bone
vallecula
epiglottis
laryngeal pharynx
cricoid cartilage
trachea
thyroid gland
esophagus
stomach
BOLUS
A. Tip of tongue in contact with anterior part of palate. When the bolus is pushed back, the soft palate is drawn upward and a bulge on the posterior pharyngeal wall (Passavant's ridge) rises to meet it.
coronal section showing position of bolus in the mouth
hard palate
B. Tongue pushes bolus backward into oral pharynx. The soft palate makes contact with Passavant's ridge closing naso-pharynx to oral pharynx.
root of tongue
C. Bolus has reached vallecula. Hyoid bone and larynx move upward and forward. Epiglottis is tipped downward as posterior pharyngeal wall moves downward.
vallecula
DEGLUTITION
Although deglutition is a continuous process, it is traditional to divide it into three stages: (1) oral
(2) pharyngeal
(3) esophageal.
illustration continued on next page

from the normal. **2.** A congenital malformation. **3.** The changing of shape to adapt to a particular stress (e.g., of a red blood cell passing through the narrow lumen of a capillary).

deformity (de-for′mĭ-te) Any bodily disfigurement.

bayonet d. See Colles' fracture, under fracture.

bone d. Any deformity resulting from abnormal growth, improperly healed fractures, or softening of bone tissues.

boutonniere d. Hyperextension of the distal interphalangeal joint and flexion of the proximal joint, with splitting of the dorsal hood so that the head of the proximal phalanx protrudes through the resulting "buttonhole." Also called buttonhole deformity.

gunstock d. Displacement of the forearm to one side resulting from condylar fracture at the elbow.

lobster-claw d. A hand or foot with the middle digits fused or missing.

silver fork d. See Colles' fracture, under fracture.

swan-neck d. Hyperextension of the proximal interphalangeal joint and flexion of the distal interphalangeal joint; a frequent complication of mallet finger.

defundation (de-fun-da′shun) Surgical removal of the fundus of the uterus.

defurfuration (de-fer-fer-ā′shun) The falling off or shedding of fine scales from the skin. Also called branny desquamation.

degenerate (de-jen′er-āt) **1.** Marked by deterioration. **2.** A person who is morally degraded.

degeneration (de-jen-er-a′shun) **1.** Deterioration of physical, mental, or moral characteristics. **2.** The deterioration of tissues with corresponding functional impairment as a result of injury or disease; the process may advance to an irreversible stage and eventually cause death of the tissues (necrosis).

adipose d. See fatty degeneration.

amyloid d. Deposition of an abnormal protein-polysaccharide substance (amyloid) in the extracellular spaces of tissues.

atheromatous d. Localized accumulation of lipid material (atheroma) in the inner layers of the arterial walls.

ballooning d. Liquefaction of the cell protoplasm leading to edematous swelling and softening. Also called ballooning colliquation.

basophilic d. Blue staining of connective tissue by the hematoxylin-eosin stain in conditions such as lupus erythematosus and senile skin.

carneous d. Degeneration of a uterine leiomyoma (fibroid) usually occurring during pregnancy associated with potential preterm labor; marked by formation of soft, dark red areas of hemorrhage and necrosis; symptoms include pain, tenderness on palpation, and low-grade fever. Also called red degeneration.

colloid d. Conversion of tissues into a gumlike inspissated material.

fatty d. Any abnormal accumulation of fat within the parenchymal cells of organs or glands. Also called adipose degeneration.

fibrinoid d. The formation of a dense, homogeneous, acidophilic substance in the tissues.

hepatolenticular d. See Wilson's disease.

heredomacular d. See macular degeneration.

hyaline d. A regressive process in which cellular cytoplasm becomes glossy and homogeneous due to injury that causes coagulation and denaturation of proteins.

hydropic d. A reversible form of intracellular edema with accumulation of water within the cell.

macular d. A hereditary condition marked by progressive degeneration of the macula and loss of vision. Also called heredomacular degeneration.

mucoid medial d. See cystic medial necrosis, under necrosis.

reaction of d. The abnormal reaction of a degenerated nerve or muscle to an electric stimulus.

red d. See carneous degeneration.

secondary d. See wallerian degeneration.

senile d. The normal degeneration of tissues in old age.

vitelliform d. Autosomal dominant disease of the eye, marked by an abnormality of the retinal pigment epithelium that is visible only in the macular area as a yellow deposit resembling a "sunny side up" fried egg; may lead to loss of central vision by the second decade of life. Also called Best's disease.

wallerian d. Dissolution and resorption of the distal stump of a sectioned peripheral nerve. Also called secondary degeneration.

Zenker's d. A form of hyaline degeneration in which the cytoplasm of striated muscle cells becomes clumped, homogeneous, and waxy; occurs in patients dying of febrile illnesses, such as typhoid fever and diphtheria.

degenerative joint disease (de-jen′er-ă-tiv joint dĭ-zēz′) (DJD) See osteoarthritis.

deglutition (de-gloo-tish′un, deg-loo-tish′un) The act of swallowing.

deglutitory (de-gloo′tĭ-to-re) Relating to swallow-

after Netter

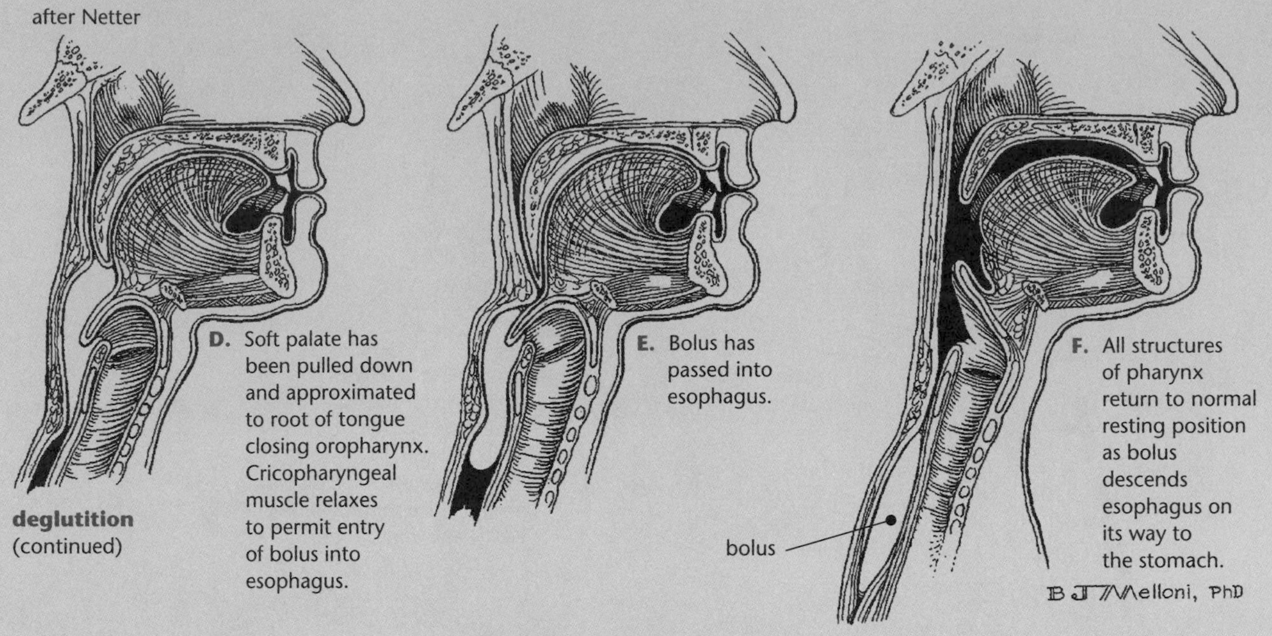

D. Soft palate has been pulled down and approximated to root of tongue closing oropharynx. Cricopharyngeal muscle relaxes to permit entry of bolus into esophagus.

E. Bolus has passed into esophagus.

F. All structures of pharynx return to normal resting position as bolus descends esophagus on its way to the stomach.

bolus

deglutition (continued)

B J Melloni, PhD

D

ing.

degranulation (de-gran-u-la´shun) The loss of granules, as in the disappearance of the neutrophilic granules in a leukocyte immediately following particle ingestion.

degree (dĭ-grē´, de-gre´) **1.** A division of a temperature scale. **2.** A unit of angular measure equal to 1/360 of the circumference of a circle. **3.** A measure of severity; extent.

degu (dăgoo) A ratlike animal from Chile possessing two anatomically separate thymus glands (cervical thymus and mediastinal thymus); used extensively by immunologists to study the thymus, which, in early life, sets up the immune defense mechanisms for the body. Also called trumpet-tailed rat.

degustation (de´gus-ta´shun) The act or sense of tasting.

dehalogenase (de-hal´ō-jen-ās) Enzyme present in the thyroid gland that promotes the removal of iodine from mono- and diiodotyrosines.

dehiscence (de-his´ens) **1.** A splitting along a line or slit. **2.** Separation of any of the suture layers of an operative wound at any stage of healing. COMPARE: evisceration (2).

uterine d. An uncommon postoperative complication of cesarean section, associated with adhesions between the abdominal wall and the uterus; symptoms include spiking temperatures, pain, and intestinal obstruction.

dehydrate (de-hi´drāt) To extract water from the body or from any substance; to make anhydrous.

dehydration (de-hi-dra´shun) Diminution of water content of the body or tissues.

dehydrocholic acid (de-hi-dro-ko´lik as´id) A synthetic bile acid that stimulates secretion of bile; used in states of deficient bile formation.

dehydroepiandrosterone (de-hi-dro-ep-ĭ-an-dros´ter-ōn) (DHEA) Steroid hormone of weak physiologic activity produced primarily by the adrenal cortex of both males and females, beginning during fetal life and usually declining at about age 25; it plays a role in the formation of testosterone and estrogen. Its role in the process of aging is being investigated.

dehydrogenase (de-hi-droj´ĕ-nās) An enzyme that catalyzes the removal of hydrogen from a substrate and the transfer of the hydrogen to an acceptor.

dehydrogenation (de-hi-dro-jĕ-na´shun) To remove hydrogen from a compound. Also called dehydrogenization.

dehypnotize (de-hip´no-tīz) To awaken from a hypnotic state.

déjà vu (da-zhă´voo´) A feeling that a new experience or situation has happened before. Also called déjà vu phenomenon.

dejection (de-jek´shun) **1.** A state of mental depression. Also called melancholy. **2.** Defecation.

Déjerine-Roussy syndrome (dĕ-zhĕ-rēn´roo-se´ sin-drōm) See thalamic syndrome.

delamination (de-lam-ĭ-na´shun) A division into layers or laminae; specifically the splitting of blastoderm into ectoderm and entoderm.

de-lead (de-led´) To remove lead from bodily tissues.

deleterious (del-ĕ-tēr´e-us) Harmful.

deletion (dĕ-le´shun) In genetics, loss of a segment of a chromosome through breakage; a chromosome aberration.

delimitation (de-lim-ĭ-ta´shun) The process of putting bounds; preventing the spread of a disease.

deliquesce (del-ĭ-kwes´) To become damp; to melt.

deliquescent (del-ĭ-kwes´ent) Denoting a solid substance that becomes liquefied by absorbing moisture from the atmosphere.

delirious (dĭ-lir´ē-us) In a state of mental confusion and excitement.

delirium (dĭ-lir´ē-um) A condition of temporary mental excitement and confusion, marked by hallucinations, delusions, anxiety, and incoherence.

d. tremens (DTs) Acute mental disturbance due to withdrawal from alcohol, marked by sweating, tremor, anxiety, precordial pain, and both visual and auditory hallucinations.

deliver (de-liv´er) **1.** To assist a woman in birth. **2.** To remove (e.g., a tumor).

delivery (de-liv´er-e) In obstetrics, the mode of actual expulsion of the infant and placenta from the uterus.

abdominal d. See cesarean section, under section.

breech d. Extraction of an infant whose pelvis or lower extremity is the presenting part.

forceps d. The use of forceps for delivery of a fetus in vertex presentation (i.e., when the top-back of the skull is foremost within the birth canal). Classified according to the level of the fetal head at the time the instrument is applied: *high forceps d.*, application of forceps to the fetal head before its engagement (i.e., before its biparietal plane has descended to a level below that of the pelvic inlet); *low forceps d.*, when the leading point of the head is at a station +2 cm or more and not on the pelvic floor; *midforceps d.*, when the leading point of the head is above station +2 cm but the head is engaged (i.e., the parietal plane of the head has descended to a level below that of the pelvic inlet).

postmortem d. Delivery of a child after death of its mother.

premature d. The birth of a fetus before 34 weeks of gestation.

delouse (dē-lous´) To rid of infestation with lice.

delta (del´tă) **1.** The fourth letter of the Greek alphabet, Δ, δ; used to denote the fourth in a series. **2.** Any triangular anatomic space. **3.** In chemistry, the capital (Δ) denotes a double bond between carbon atoms; the lower case (δ) denotes the location of a substituent on the fourth atom from the primary functional group in an organic molecule. **4.** Symbol (Δ) for change. For terms beginning with delta, see under the specific term.

delta check (del´tă chĕk) Comparison of the values of a patient's consecutive laboratory tests to detect changes.

deltoid (del´toid) Triangular; shaped like the Greek letter delta, Δ. See table of muscles.

delusion (dĭ-loo´zhun) A false belief maintained even against contradictory evidence or logical argument.

d. of grandeur Exaggerated belief in one's importance.

d. of persecution A false belief that one is being persecuted.

demarcation (de-mar-ka´shun) The marking of boundaries.

line of d. An inflamed area separating granulomatous and healthy tissue.

demasculinization (de-mas-ku-lin-ĭ-za´shun) The loss of male characteristics.

demented (de-men´ted) Afflicted with dementia or loss of reason.

dementia (dĕ-men´shă) Deterioration of intellectual function due to organic factors.

Alzheimer's d. See Alzheimer's disease.

d. praecox Obsolete term for schizophrenia.

senile d. Mental deterioration caused by atrophy of the brain due to aging.

demifacet (dem-e-fas´et) The half of a facet on the side of some thoracic vertebrae for articulation with the head of a rib. Also called costal facet.

demilune (dem´e-loon) **1.** Crescent; semilunar. **2.** The gametocyte of *Plasmodium falciparum*.

serous d. Five to10 serous cells capping the terminal end of a mucous, tubuloalveolar secretory unit of mixed salivary glands. Also called crescent of Gianuzzi.

demineralization (de-min-er-al-ĭ-za´shun) A reduction of the mineral constituent of the tissues through excessive elimination.

demipenniform (dem-e-pen´ĭ-form) Feather-shaped on one side only; said of certain muscles with a tendon on one side.

demography (de-mog´ră-fe) The study of human populations, especially their growth, geographical distribution, and vital statistics.

demonstrator (dem´on-stra-tor) A person who supplements the teachings of a professor by instructing small groups, preparing dissections, etc.

demophobia (de-mo-fo´be-ă) Morbid fear of crowds.

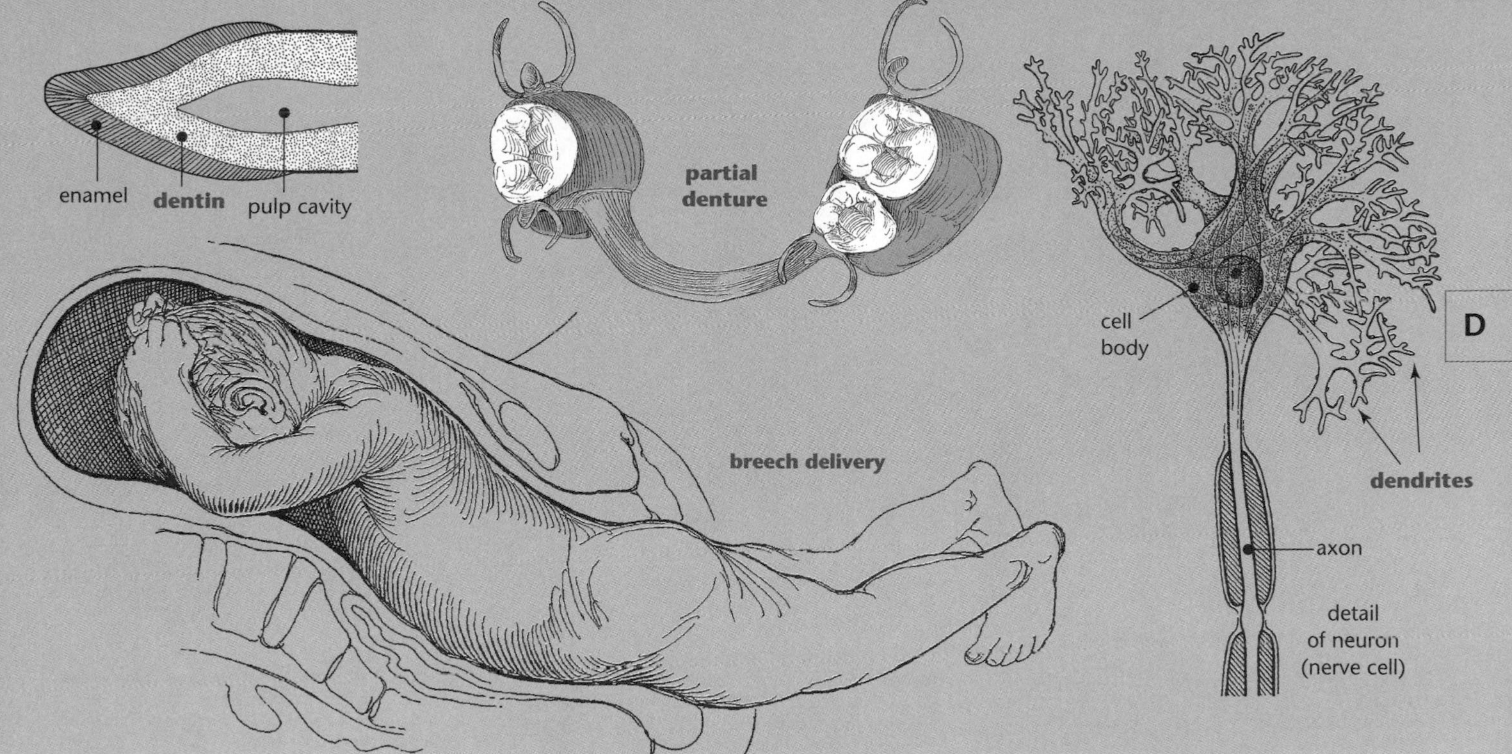

demulcent (de-mul´sent) **1.** Soothing; allaying irritation. **2.** Any gummy or oily substance having such properties.
demyelination, demyelinization (de-mi-ĕ-lin-a´shun, de-mi-ĕ-lin-ī-za´shun) Destruction or loss of myelin from the sheath of a nerve.
denarcotize (de-nar´ko-tīz) To remove or separate narcotic properties from an opiate.
denaturation (de-na-chur-a´shun) Loss of characteristic biologic activity in protein molecules due to extremes of pH or temperature.
denatured (de-na´churd) Changed in nature; adulterated.
dendriform (den´drĭ-form) Branched like a tree; tree-shaped.
dendrite (den´drīt) One of the cytoplasmic branches of nerve cells (neurons) which conducts the impulses received from the terminations of other neurons toward the cell body. Also called dendritic process.
dendritic (den-drit´ik) Relating to or resembling dendrites or protoplasmic processes of the nerve cells.
dendroid (den´droid) Branched; treelike.
denervate (de-ner´vāt) To remove or sever the nerve supply to a bodily part.
dengue (deng´gă) Epidemic disease of tropical and subtropical regions caused by a dengue virus (genus *Flavivirus*) and transmitted by *Aedes* mosquitoes; marked by severe headache, intense pain of the back and joints, high fever, and a spotty rash; after three or four days, all symptoms subside only to reappear 24 hours later with a characteristic skin eruption. Also called breakbone fever; dandy fever.
denial (dĕ-ni´al) An unconscious psychological defense mechanism, in which consciously intolerable thoughts, wishes, feelings, or needs are rejected or blocked out.
denidation (den-ī-da´shun) Disintegration and expulsion of the superficial uterine mucosa.
denitrify (de-ni´trĭ-fi) To remove nitrogen from a compound.
de novo (de no´vo) Newly; anew.
dens (dens), *pl.* **den´tes** **1.** Latin for tooth. **2.** A toothlike structure, such as the odontoid process of the axis (second vertebra).
densimeter (den-sim´ĕ-ter) An instrument for determining the density of a fluid.
densitometer (den-sĭ-tom´ĕ-ter) **1.** Device for determining the density of a liquid. **2.** Device for determining the degree of bacterial growth in a medium. **3.** Device for determining the optical density of a material (e.g., x-ray film) by way of a photocell that measures light transmission through given areas of the film.
densitometry (den-sĭ tom´ĕ-tre) Technique for measuring variations in density of a substance.
density (den´sĭ-te) **1.** The state of compactness; the amount of matter per unit volume expressed in grams per cubic centimeter. **2.** The measure of the degree of resistance to the speed of a transmission.
bone d. In clinical practice, the amount of mineral per square centimeter of bone; usually measured by photon absorptiometry or by x-ray computed tomography. Actual bone density is expressed in grams per milliliter.
count d. See photon density.
optical d. The light-absorbing quality of a translucent substance.
photon d. In radioisotope scanning, the number of counted events per square centimeter or per square inch of imaged area. Also called count density.
vapor d. The ratio of the weight of a vapor or gas to an equal volume of hydrogen.
dental (den´tal) Relating to teeth.
dentalgia (den-tal´jă) Toothache.
dentate (den´tāt) Notched; having toothlike projections.
denticle (den´tĭ-kl) See pulp stone, under stone.
denticulate (den-tik´u-lāt) Having toothlike projections.
dentiform (den´tĭ-form) Shaped like a tooth.
dentifrice (den´tĭ-fris) A compound, such as a paste or powder, used in conjunction with a toothbrush for cleaning the teeth.
dentigerous (den-tij´er-us) Containing teeth, as certain cysts.
dentin (den´tin) The hard tissue forming the main substance of teeth; it surrounds the tooth pulp and is covered by enamel on the crown and by cementum on the roots.
primary d. Dentin formed before the eruption of a tooth.
secondary d. Highly irregular dentin formed after tooth eruption due to irritation from caries or injuries, or the normal wearing down of the teeth.
dentinal (den´tĭ-nal) Relating to dentin.
dentine (den´tēn) Dentin.
dentinogenesis (den-ti-no-jen´ĕ-sis) The development of dentin.
dentinoma (den-tĭ-no´mă) An extremely rare encapsulated tumor composed of connective tissue and masses of dentin.
dentinum (den-ti´num) Latin for dentin.
dentist (den´tist) One who is trained and licensed to practice dentistry.
dentistry (den´tis-tre) The science and art concerned with the diagnosis, prevention, and treatment of diseases of the oral cavity and associated tissues, especially the restoration or replacement of defective teeth. Also called odontology.
cosmetic d. Any procedure or treatment for improving the appearance of teeth.
forensic d. Application of dental science to legal investigations or problems (e.g., dental identification of dead bodies, analysis of bite marks, evaluation of alleged dental malpractice). Also called legal dentistry; dental jurisprudence; forensic odontology.
legal d. See forensic dentistry.
pediatric d. See pedodontics.
dentition (den-tish´un) The arrangement of the natural teeth in the dental arch.
deciduous d. Set of 20 teeth erupting between 6 and 26 months of age and replaced by the permanent dentition. Also called primary dentition.
delayed d. Eruption of the first deciduous teeth after 13 months of age or of the first permanent teeth after 7 years of age. Also called retarded dentition.
permanent d. Set of 32 teeth that begin to erupt when a child is about 6 years old.
primary d. See deciduous dentition.
retarded d. See delayed denition
transitional d. Dentition containing deciduous and permanent teeth.
dentulous (den´tu-lus) Possessing natural deciduous or permanent teeth.
denture (den´chur) An artifical substitute for missing natural teeth and surrounding tissues.
complete d. A dental prosthesis that replaces all the natural teeth and associated structures in a jaw.
fixed partial d. A partial denture that is supported by the teeth or roots and cannot be readily removed. Also called fixed bridge.
immediate d. A denture made before the anterior teeth are extracted and inserted immediately after extraction for cosmetic reasons.
partial d. A dental prosthesis replacing one or more teeth and held in place by remaining teeth and underlying tissues; may be removable or fixed.
denucleated (de-noo´kle-āt-ed) Deprived of a nucleus.
denudation (den-u-da´shun) To make bare; to divest of covering.
deodorant (de-o´dor-ant) An agent that counteracts undesirable odors.
deossification (de-os-ĭ-fĭ-ka´shun) Removal of the mineral elements of bone.
deoxycholic acid (de-ok-se-ko´lik as´id) A digestive bile acid formed in the small intestine by the action of intestinal bacteria on cholic acid.
deoxycorticosterone (de-ok´se-kor-tĭ-kos´ter-ōn, de-ok´se-kor-tĭ-ko-ster´ōn) (DOC) A steroid hormone formed in the adrenal cortex; a precursor of corticosterone. Also called deoxycortone.
d. acetate (DOCA, DCA) A salt-retaining steroid.
deoxycortone (de-ok-se-kōr´tōn) See deoxycorticosterone.

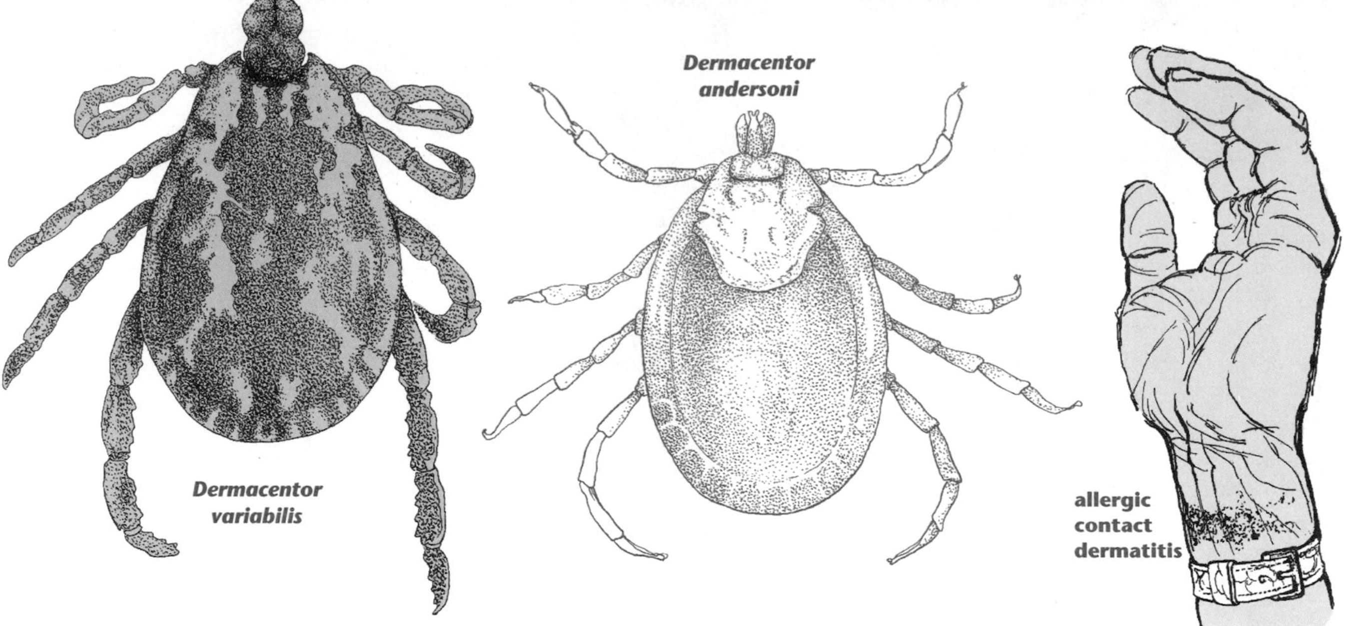

deoxygenate (de-ok-sĭ-jen´āt) To deprive of oxygen.

deoxyribonuclease (de-ok-se-ri-bo-noo´kle-ās) (DNAase) An enzyme that breaks down deoxyribonucleic acid (DNA) to nucleotides.

deoxyribonucleic acid (de-ok-se-ri-bo-noo-kle´ik as´id) (DNA) The molecular basis of heredity. See DNA.

deoxyribonucleoprotein (de-ok-se-ri-bo-noo-kle-o-pro´tēn) A nucleoprotein that yields deoxyribonucleic acid (DNA) on hydrolysis.

deoxyribonucleoside (de-ok-se-ri-bo-noo´kle-o-sīd) A compound consisting of a purine or pyrimidine base combined with deoxyribose (a DNA sugar).

deoxyribonucleotide (de-ok-se-ri-bo-noo´kle-o-tīd) A substance composed of a purine or pyrimidine base bonded to deoxyribose (a DNA sugar), which in turn is bound to a phosphate group.

deoxyribose (de-ok-se-ri´bōs) The pentose sugar constituent of deoxyribonucleic acid (DNA).

deoxysugar (de-ok-se-shōōg´ar) Any of several sugars containing fewer oxygen atoms than carbon atoms in the molecule, resulting in one or more carbons lacking an attached hydroxyl group.

depancreatize (de-pan-kre´ă-tīz) To remove the pancreas.

dependence (de-pen´dens) A psychologic and/or physical need for a substance, person, or object.

alcohol d. See alcoholism.

drug d. General term for a condition in which the user of a drug has a compelling desire to continue taking the drug either to experience its effects or to avoid the discomfort that occurs when it is not taken. Dependence may be *psychological,* an emotional drive to continue taking a drug, which the user believes is necessary to maintain a sense of optimal well-being; or *physical,* an adaptive state of the body resulting from the continued drug use. Formerly called drug addiction; drug habituation.

substance d. See drug dependence.

Dependovirus (de-pen-do-vi´rus) A genus of viruses (family Parvoviridae) that require the presence of adenovirus to replicate. Also called adeno-associated virus; adenosatellite virus.

depersonalization (de-per-son-al-ĭ-za´shun) A condition in which a person loses his sense of personal identity or feels his body to be unreal.

dephosphorylation (de-fos-for-ĭ-la´shun) The removal of a phosphate group from a compound through the action of an enzyme.

depigmentation (de-pig-men-ta´shun) Partial or complete loss of pigment.

depilate (dep´ĭ-lāt) To remove hair, usually from the surface of the body.

depilation (dep-ĭ-la´shun) The removal of hair.

depilatory (de-pil´ă-tor-e) **1.** An agent that removes or destroys hair from the body. **2.** Capable of removing hair.

deplete (de-plēt´) To exhaust; to empty.

depletion (de-ple´shun) **1.** The process of emptying. **2.** Excessive loss of body constituents that are necessary for normal functioning. **3.** The condition resulting from such process.

deplumation (de-ploo-ma´shun) Abnormal loss of the eyelashes.

depolarization (de-pōl-ar-ĭ-za´shun) The elimination or neutralization of polarity.

deportation (de-por-ta´shun) The act of carrying away.

trophoblastic d. See trophoblastic embolization, under embolization.

deposit (de-poz´it) Sediment.

depot (de´po) An organ or tissue in which drugs or biologic substances are deposited and stored by the body.

depravity (de-prav´ĭ-te) **1.** Moral deterioration or corruption. **2.** A perverse act.

depressant (de-pres´ant) Serving to reduce functional activity.

depressed (de-prest´) **1.** Sunk below level of surrounding parts. **2.** Below normal functional level. **3.** Dejected.

depression (de-presh´un) **1.** Emotional dejection; morbid sadness accompanied by loss of interest in surroundings and lack of energy. **2.** Area lower than the surrounding level.

anaclitic d. Impairment of an infant's development (physical, intellectual, and social) which sometimes follows a sudden separation from its mother or mother substitute.

endogenous d. Depressive disorder occurring without predominant psychosocial causative factors, thus presumed to be somatic in origin; symptoms include a depressed mood with disturbances of sleep, appetite, sexual interest, and motor regulation.

major d. Disorder that, every day for at least 2 weeks, includes at least four of the following symptoms: (a) decreased or increased appetite with corresponding change in weight; (b) insomnia (especially very early awakening) or sleeping for excessively long periods; (c) motor retardation, or agitation; (d) loss of interest and pleasure in surroundings and decreased sexual drive; (e) feelings of excessive guilt, self reproach, or worthlessness; (f) decreased ability to make decisions; (g) fatigue; (h) recurrent suicidal thinking or attempts.

postpartum d. A temporary mood disturbance experienced by some women, usually 3 to 10 days after delivery; characterized by crying, irritability, anxiety, forgetfulness, and mood swings from sadness to elation. Commonly called baby blues; postnatal blues; three-day blues.

reactive d. Depression caused by an external predominant factor and relieved by the removal of that factor.

depressomotor (de-pres-o-mo´tor) **1.** Serving to retard motor activity. **2.** Anything that causes such an effect.

depressor (de-pres´or) **1.** Anything that depresses or reduces functional activity, such as certain nerves, muscles, or chemicals. **2.** An instrument or device used to push structures out of the way during an examination or operation.

tongue d. A broad wooden blade used to push the tongue against the floor of the mouth during examination of the throat.

deprivation (dep-rĭ-va´shun) Loss or absence of stimuli, nurture, organs, powers, or attributes that are needed.

sensory d. A diminution of sensory stimuli.

depth (depth) A dimension downward or inward.

anesthetic d. The depth of depression of the central nervous system caused by an anesthetic drug; an indication of the potency of the anesthetic.

d. of focus The variation of the distance between an object and a lens or optical system without causing objectionable blurring.

depulization (de-pyoo-li-ză´shun) Destruction of fleas, especially those carrying the plague bacillus. The term is generally used with reference to antiplague measures.

depurant (dep´yoo-rant) **1.** Anything that purifies. **2.** An agent that promotes the excretion of waste matter.

derangement (de-rānj´ment) **1.** Mental disorder. **2.** Disarrangement of the regular order; disorder.

derivation (der-ĭ-vă´shun) **1.** The source from which something originates. **2.** The diversion of fluids from one part of the body to another.

derivative (de-riv´ă-tiv) **1.** In chemistry, a compound obtained from another and containing some of the elements of the original substance. **2.** Resulting from derivation.

dermabrasion (der-mă-bra´zhun) Operative procedure used to remove acne or chicken pox scars, tattoos, and superficial foreign bodies acquired during road or industrial accidents; the most popular method consists of freezing the skin, followed by mechanical removal of the epidermis and upper dermis with a high-speed rotary steel brush. Also called mechanical abrasion; planing.

Dermacentor (der-mă-sen´tor) A genus of ticks (family Ixodidae).

D. andersoni The wood tick, a transmitter of Rocky Mountain spotted fever and tularemia and the cause of tick paralysis.

D. variabillis The American dog tick, the transmitter of spotted fever and tularemia.

dermal (der´măl) Relating to the skin.

dermalaxia (der-mă-lak´se-ă) Softening of the skin.

dermametropathism (der-mă-mĕ-trop´ă-thiz-m) A method of diagnosing certain skin disorders by observing the markings when a blunt instrument is drawn across the skin.

dermatitis (der-ma-ti´tis), *pl.* **dermatitides** Inflammation of the skin.

allergic contact d. Localized dermatitis characterized by a sharply demarcated area of redness and itchiness, often with an eruption of blisters;

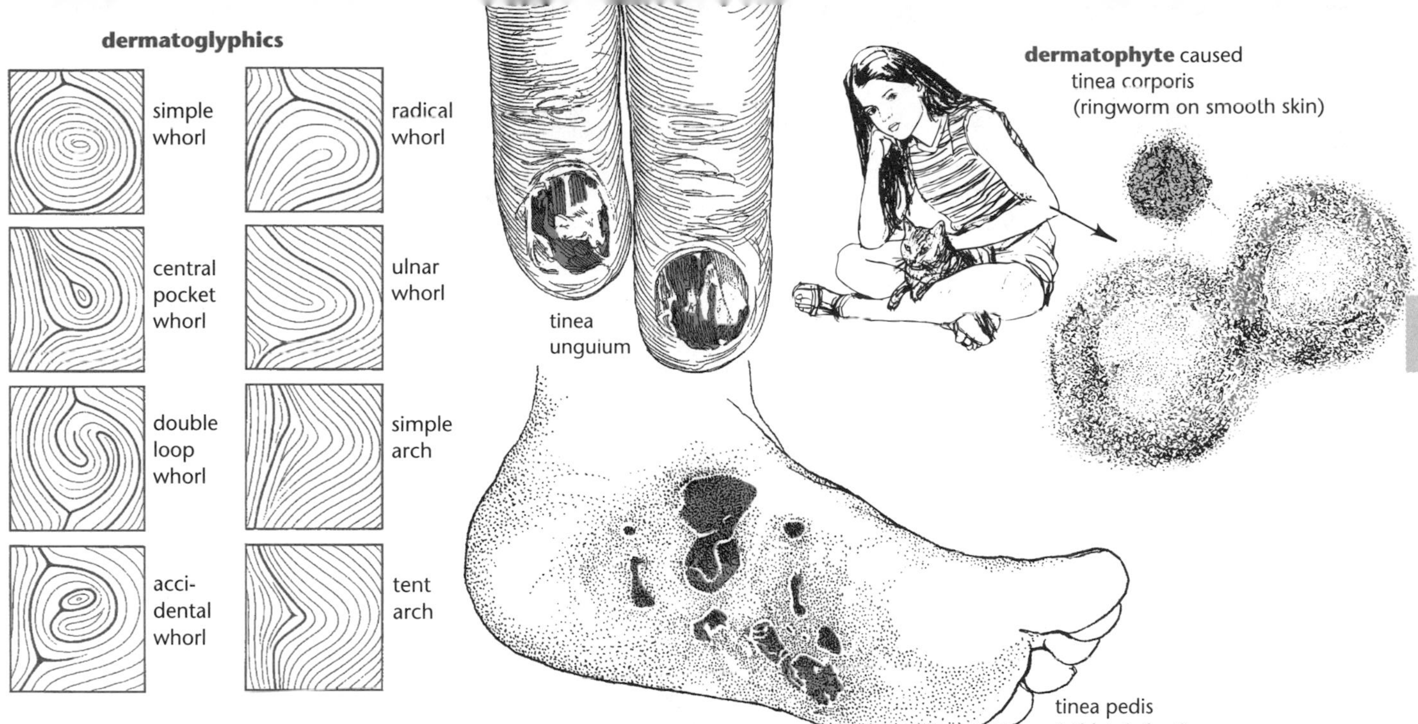

results from contact with any of a variety of natural or manufactured substances (allergens) to which the skin has already been exposed and sensitized; occurs as a delayed cutaneous hypersensitivity reaction to the substance. Common allergens include cosmetics, deodorants, depilatories, hair products, topical medications, clothing, and jewelry; industrial products include epoxy resins, formaldehyde, dyes, metals and acrylic monomers.

atopic d. Dermatitis usually seen in people susceptible to asthma and hay fever; lesions occur predominantly in front of the elbows and behind the knee. Also called atopic eczema.

chemical d. Dermatitis produced by contact with chemicals.

contact d. Cutaneous reaction caused by direct contact with a substance to which the person is hypersensitive. Also called contact allergy.

d. exfoliativa infantum, d. exfoliativa neonatorum A pustular dermatitis with abundant flaking and red coloration of the skin accompanied by fever, malaise, and occasionally gastrointestinal symptoms; it affects young infants and is frequently fatal.

exfoliative d. Generalized exfoliation, redness, and severe scaling of the skin with constitutional symptoms.

d. herpetiformis (DH) Chronic disorder marked by an eruption of itchy burning clusters of vesicles and papules occurring mostly on the forearms and abdomen. Also called Duhring's disease; hydroa herpetiforme.

d. medicamentosa See drug eruption, under eruption.

rhus d. A delayed hypersensitivity reaction marked by an eruption of weeping, crusting vesicles; caused by contact with urushiol from species of the genus *Rhus* (poison ivy, poison oak, or poison sumac).

seborrheic d. A condition of unknown cause with a predilection for the scalp but also seen on the eyebrows, behind the ears, the chest, back, and pubic area; characterized by varying degrees of redness, scaling, and sometimes itching. Commonly known in its mild form as dandruff; seborrhea.

solar d. Dermatitis produced in persons allergic to the sun's rays.

stasis d. Dermatitis occurring usually on the lower legs in association with varicose veins.

Dermatobia (der-mă-to´be-ă) A genus of flies (family Oestridae) that includes the parasitic botflies.

dermatocele (der-mă-to´sēl) A localized loose condition of the skin.

dermatoconiosis (der-mă-to-ko-nī-o´sis) Occupational dermatitis caused by irritation of the skin by dust.

dermatofibroma (dĕr-mă-to-fi-bro´mă) A benign skin tumor believed to be a capillary hemangioma that has become indurated, cellular, and fibrous. Also called sclerosing hemangioma; histiocytoma.

dermatofibrosarcoma protuberans (der-mă-to-fi-bro-sar-ko´mă pro-too´ber-ans) A skin tumor composed of several small nodules covered with dark reddish blue skin; it tends to recur after removal.

dermatoglyphics (der-mă-to-glif´iks) **1.** The variety of pattern configurations of epidermal ridges on the volar aspect of the hands and feet; the ridge configuration may be altered in some disorders. **2.** The study of skin patterns, especially of the palms of the hands and soles of the feet.

dermatograph (der´mă-to-graf) The linear wheal made in dermatographism.

dermatographism (der-mă-tog´ră-fiz-m) Formation of wheals after stroking the skin with a pencil or blunt instrument. Also called dermatography; skin writing.

dermatography (der-mă-tog´ră-fe) See dermatographism.

dermatoid (der´mă-toid) Resembling skin.

dermatologist (der-mă-tol´o-jist) A specialist in disorders of the skin and related systemic diseases. Popularly called skin specialist.

dermatology (der-mă-tol´o-je) The medical specialty concerned with the diagnosis and treatment of diseases of the skin and its appendages.

dermatome (der´mă-tōm) **1.** Surgical instrument used in cutting thin slices of skin for grafting. **2.** In embryology, the dorsolateral wall of a somite from which the skin is derived. **3.** A skin area supplied by sensory fibers of a single spinal nerve.

dermatomegaly (der-mă-to-meg´ă-le) Congenital defect consisting of an excessive amount of skin which hangs in folds; cutis laxa.

dermatomycosis (der-mă-to-mi-ko´sis) Any cutaneous fungal infection.

dermatomyositis (der-mă-to-mi-o-si´tis) Disorder of skin and muscle characterized by a blue-violet rash on the face (especially around the eyes) and on the back of the hands and fingers, with muscle weakness especially on the shoulder and pelvic areas; two varieties are known, affecting children or adults; the adult form is sometimes associated with an occult internal cancer.

dermatonosology (der-mă-to-no-sol´o-je) The classification of skin diseases. Also called dermonosology.

dermatopathology (der-mă-to-pă-thol´o-je) The study of skin diseases.

dermatopathy (der-mă top´ă-the) Any disease of the skin.

Dermatophagoides (der-ma-tof a-goi´des) Genus of mites; some species, especially *Dermatophagoides farinae* and *Dermatophagoides pteronyssinus,* provide the principal source of allergic material of house dust.

dermatophyte (der´mă-to-fīt) Any fungus capable of invading the keratinized tissue of skin, hair, and nails and causing such conditions as athlete's foot, nail infections, tinea corporis, and scalp ringworm.

dermatophytid (der-mă-tof´ĭ-tid) Secondary skin eruption, usually on the fingers and hands, following sensitization of fungi. Often called id. See also id reaction, under reaction.

dermatophytosis (der-mă-to-fi-to´sis) Any superficial fungal infection caused by a dermatophyte.

dermatoplasty (der´mă-to-plas-te) Skin grafting to correct defects or replace loss of skin.

dermatosis (der-mă-to´sis), *pl.* **dermato ´ses** Any skin eruption.

dermatoses of pregnancy Skin eruptions that are unique to the pregnant state (e.g., pruritis gravidarum, pruritis urticarial papules and plaques of pregnancy [PUPPP], herpes gestationis).

dermatoskeleton (der-mă-to-skel´ĕ-ton) See exoskeleton (2).

dermatotherapy (der-mă-to-ther´ă-pe) The treatment of skin diseases.

dermatotropic (der-mă-to-trop´ik) Acting selectively on the skin. Also called dermotropic.

dermatrophia, dermatrophy (der-mă-tro´fe-ă, der-măt´ro-fe) Thinning or atrophy of the skin.

dermis (der´mis) The connective tissue layer of the skin just below the epidermis; composed of a thin superficial layer and a deep dense layer with reticular fibers; it contains blood vessels, lymph channels, nerves, sebaceous glands, hair follicles, and sweat glands. Also called corium; true skin; cutis vera.

dermoblast (der´mo-blast) One of the mesodermal cells that develops into the dermis.

dermographia (der-mo-graf´e-ă) See dermatographism.

dermographism (der-mog´ră-fiz-m) See dermatographism.

dermoid (der´moid) **1.** Resembling skin. **2.** See dermoid cyst, under cyst.

dermonosology (der-mo-no-sol´o-je) See dermatonosology.

dermoskeleton (der-mo-skel´ĕ-ton) See exoskeleton (2).

dermostosis (der-mo-sto´sis) Bony formations on the skin.

dermotoxin (der-mo-tok´sin) A substance that causes pathologic changes in the skin.

dermotropic (der-mo-trop´ik) See dermatotropic.

dermovascular (der-mo-vas´ku lar) Relating to the blood supply of the skin.

desaturation (de-sach-ŭ-ra´shun) The chemical process of transforming a saturated compound into an unsaturated one.

descemetitis (des-ĕ-mĕ-ti´tis) Inflammation of the

descensus testis

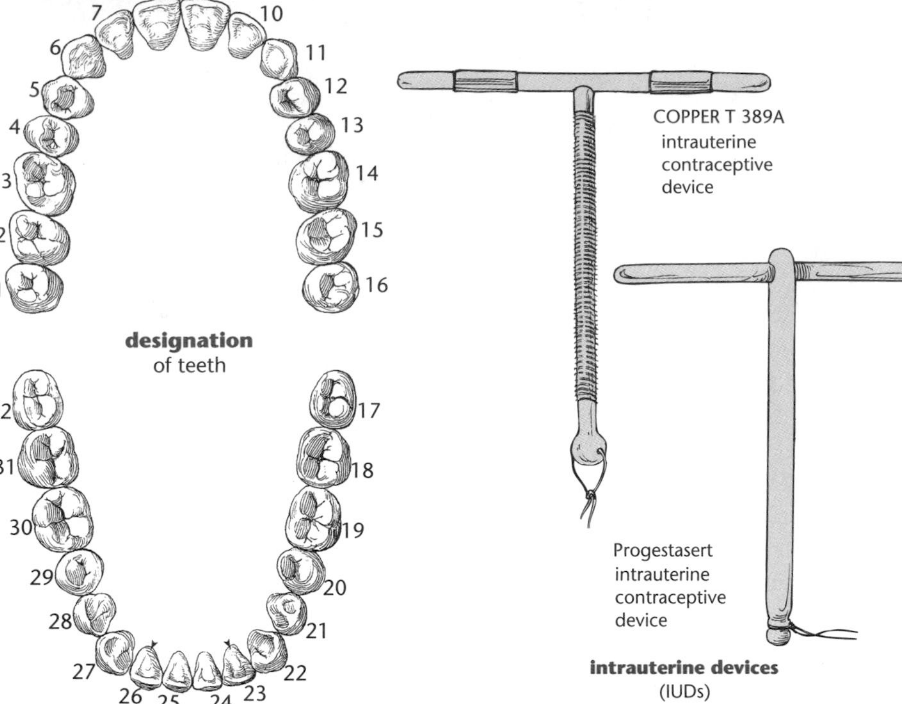

designation of teeth

intrauterine devices (IUDs)

posterior limiting (Descemet's) membrane of the cornea.

descensus (de-sen´sus) Falling; descent.

d. testis Descent of the testis from the abdomen into the scrotum shortly before the end of intrauterine life.

d. uteri See prolapse of uterus, under prolapse.

desensitization (de-sen-sĭ-tĭ-za´shun) **1.** Reduction of immediate hypersensitivity reactions by injection of graded doses of the offending substance (allergen). Also called immunotherapy; hyposensitization. **2.** A method of treating an emotional disorder (e.g., behavior therapy).

desensitize (de-sen´sĭ-tīz) **1.** To subject a person to desensitization. **2.** To reduce or eliminate sensation.

desiccant (des´ĭ-kant) **1.** An agent possessing a high affinity for water, used to absorb moisture; a drying agent. **2.** Promoting dryness. Also called exsicant.

desiccate (des´ĭ-kāt) To dry. See also electrodesiccation.

desiccator (des´ĭ-ka-tor) A closed vessel containing a dehydrating agent (calcium chloride, sulfuric acid, etc.) in which a substance or an apparatus is placed for drying and to be kept free from moisture.

designation (dez-ĭg-nā´shun) Distinguishing name.

desmin (dez´min) A 52-kd protein, the chief intermediate filament of striated (skeletal and cardiac) muscle; it maintains the structural and functional integrity of muscle fibrils and serves as a cytoskeletal protein linking Z bands to the plasma membrane of the muscle cell.

desmitis (des-mi´tis) Inflammation of a ligament.

desmoid (dez´moid) A nodule resulting from the proliferation of fibrous tissue of muscle sheaths, especially of the abdominal wall; usually occurring in women following pregnancy. Also called desmoid tumor.

desmoplasia (dez-mo-pla´zhă) Disproportionate formation of fibrous tissue.

desmoplastic (dez-mo-plas´tik) **1.** Causing adhesions. **2.** Causing fibrosis in the vascular stroma of a tumor.

desmopressin acetate (dez-mo-pres´in as´ĕ-tāt) A synthetic analog of vasopressin used as an antidiuretic.

desmorphology (des-mor-fol´ŏ-je) See teratology.

desmosome (dez´mo-sōm) Two apposed, small, ellipsoidal plates, about 0.5 μm in diameter, along the interfaces between the plasma membrane of adjacent cells; it serves as a site of adhesion; visible only by electron microscopy. Also called macula adherens.

half-d. A plate on one cell without a companion plate butting up against it, as found at the basal plasma membrane in some epithelia. Also called hemidesmosome.

despumation (des-pu-ma´shun) The removal of impurities or scum from the surface of a liquid.

desquamate (des´kwă-māt) To cast off or shed the outer layer of a surface, as the scaling off of the epidermis.

desquamation (des-kwa-ma´shun) The shedding or peeling of the superficial layer of the skin (epidermis) in flakes or scales.

branny d. See defurfuration.

detachment (de-tach´ment) **1.** The state of being separated (e.g., the separation of the retina from its normally attached choroid). **2.** In psychiatry, the condition of being free from emotional or social involvement.

deterioration (de-tir-ē-ŏ-rā´shun) Any worsening condition or progressive impairment.

determinant (de-ter´mĭ-nant) The determining factor that establishes the characteristics of an entity.

antigenic d. The exact site on the surface of an antigen molecule or a hapten (smaller molecule) to which attaches a specific antibody produced by the host's immune system; a single antigen molecule may have several determinants recognized separately and specifically by the host's immune system. Also called epitope.

determination (de-ter-mĭ-na´shun) The estimation of the extent, quality, or character of anything.

determinism (de-ter-min-iz-m) The doctrine that any event is the inevitable consequence of prior influences and hence can be completely explained by its antecedents.

De Toni-Fanconi syndrome (dĕ to´ne-fan-ko´ne sin´drōm) Multiple defects of renal tubular function manifested by aminoaciduria, phosphaturia, glycosuria, a variable degree of renal tubular acidosis, and abnormal softening of bone tissue.

detoxicate (de-tok´sĭ-kāt) To remove the effects or counteract the toxic properties of a poison.

detoxication (de-tok-sĭ-ka´shun) **1.** The process of neutralizing the toxic properties of a substance. **2.** The recovery from the toxic effects of a substance.

detrusor (de-troo´sor) Denoting a muscle that effects an expulsion or pushing out of something (e.g., the detrusor muscle of the bladder).

detubation (de-tu-ba´shun) Removal of a tube from the body (e.g., of a tracheostomy tube).

detumescence (de-too-mes´ens) The return to the flaccid state or to the normal size of a swollen organ or part.

d. of penis The return of the penis to the flaccid state from an erection.

deuteranopia (doo-ter-ă-no´pe-ă) A form of color blindness in which red, orange, yellow, and green cannot be differentiated when their brightnesses and saturations are equal; similarly, blue, violet, and blue-purple appear to differ only in brightness and saturation, but not in hue; a sex-linked hereditary defect, occurring in about one percent of males and only rarely in females.

deuterium (doo-te´re-um) (D) See hydrogen-2.

d. oxide (D_2O) See heavy water, under water.

deuteron (doo´ter-on) (d) A subatomic particle consisting of a proton and a neutron; the nucleus of deuterium (heavy hydrogen). Also called deuton; diplon.

deuton (doo´ton) See deuteron.

deutoplasm (doo´to-plaz-m) The nonliving material in the cytoplasm, especially reserve food substance or yolk in the ovum.

Deutschländer's disease (doich´len-ĕrz dĭs-zēz´) See fatigue fracture, under fracture.

devascularization (de-vas-ku-lar-ĭ-za´shun) Removal of blood vessels from a part.

deviance (de´ve-ans) See deviation (2).

deviation (de-ve-a´shun) **1.** A turning aside. **2.** Departure from a norm, rule, or accepted course of behavior.

axis d. Deflection of the electrical axis of the heart to the right or to the left. Also called axis shift.

parallel conjugate d. (a) The normal joint and equal movement of the two eyes in the same direction when shifted from one object to another. (b) Pathologic failure of both eyes to turn to one side simultaneously; the person compensates by rotating or tilting the head.

primary d. In strabismus, deviation of the defective eye measured with the normal eye fixed on an object.

secondary d. In strabismus, deviation of the normal eye when the defective eye is made to fixate on an object.

skew d. Movement of both eyes in different directions.

standard d. (SD) In statistics, a measure of dispersion or variation in a distribution.

device (de-vīs´) Something made or constructed for a particular purpose.

contraceptive d. Any device used to prevent conception, including intrauterine devices and barrier type contraceptives (e.g., male and female condoms, diaphragm, cervical cap, spermicidal agents). See also method.

intrauterine d. (IUD) A metal or plastic loop or spiral inserted into the uterus to prevent conception. Also called intrauterine contraceptive device.

intrauterine contraceptive device See intrauterine device.

ventricular assist d. (VAD) A device used to increase the function of one or both ventricles of the heart; consists of one or two pumps (either implanted or externally placed) with afferent and efferent conduits attached to provide pulsative blood flow.

Classification of DIABETES MELLITUS and other categories of glucose intolerance

	CLASS	FORMER TERMINOLOGY	CLINICAL CHARACTERISTICS
DIABETES MELLITUS (DM)	Type 1 diabetes type I diabetes	juvenile diabetes juvenile-onset diabetes juvenile-onset-type diabetes JOD ketosis-prone diabetes brittle diabetes insulin-dependent diabetes	Persons in this subclass are dependent on injected insulin to prevent ketosis, acidosis, and hyperglycemia; in the preponderance of cases, onset is in youth, but type 1 diabetes may occur at any age; characterized by insulinopenia.
	Type 2 diabetes type II diabetes	adult-onset diabetes maturity-onset diabetes non-insulin-dependent diabetes	Persons in this subclass are not insulin-dependent or ketosis-prone, although they may use insulin for correction of symptomatic or persistent hyperglycemia and they can develop ketosis under special circumstances; serum insulin levels may be normal, elevated or depressed; in the preponderance of cases, onset is after 40, but type 2 diabetes is known to occur at all ages; about 60–90% of type 2 diabetic subjects are obese and constitute a subtype of type 2 diabetes; in these individuals, glucose intolerance is often improved by weight loss; hyperinsulinemia and insulin resistance characterize some individuals in this subtype.
	Other types, including diabetes mellitus associated with certain conditions and syndromes: 1) pancreatic disease 2) hormonal 3) drug or chemical induced 4) insulin receptor abnormalities 5) certain genetic syndromes 6) other types	secondary diabetes	In addition to the presence of the specific conditions or syndrome, diabetes mellitus is also present.
IMPAIRED GLUCOSE TOLERANCE (IGT)	Nonobese IGT Obese IGT IGT associated with certain syndromes, which may be 1) pancreatic disease 2) hormonal 3) drug or chemical induced 4) insulin receptor abnormalties 5) genetic syndromes	asymptomatic diabetes chemical diabetes subclinical diabetes borderline diabetes latent diabetes	Mild glucose intolerance of subjects in this class may be attributable to normal variation of glucose tolerance within a population; in some subjects, impaired glucose tolerance (IGT) may represent a stage in the development of type 2 or type 1 diabetes mellitus, although the majority of persons with IGT remain in this class for many years or return to normal glucose tolerance.
GESTATIONAL DIABETES (GDM)	Gestational diabetes	same	Glucose intolerance that has its onset or recognition during pregnancy thus, diabetics who become pregnant are not included in this class; associated with increased perinatal complications and with increased risk for progression to diabetes within 5–10 years after parturition; usually requires treatment with insulin; necessitates reclassification after pregnancy terminates. Adapted from the National Diabetes Association

Devic's disease (dĕ-vēks′ dĭ-zēz′) See neuromyelitis optica.
devitalization (de-vi-tal-ĭ-za′shun) In dentistry, the destruction of the pulp of a tooth.
devitalized (de-vi′tal-īzd) Without vitality; dead.
devolution (dev-o-loo′shun) **1.** Degeneration; catabolism. **2.** The opposite of evolution.
dexter (deks′ter) (D) Latin for right.
dextrad (deks′trad) Toward the right.
dextral (deks′tral) **1.** Relating to the right side. **2.** Right-handed.
dextran (deks′tran) Any of various large polymers of glucose, used in solution as a plasma substitute.
dextrin (deks′trin) A soluble carbohydrate formed by the hydrolysis of starch, the first stage in the formation of glucose; commercial dextrin is a white or yellow powder; used in solution as an adhesive.
dextrin 6-glucosyltransferase (deks′trin gloo-kō-sil-trans′fer-ās) A bacterial enzyme that promotes the synthesis of dextrans from dextrins. Also called dextran dextrinase.
dextroamphetamine sulfate (deks-tro-am-fet′ă-men sul′fāt) A sympathomimetic agent; a stimulant to the central nervous system and appetite depressant; Dexedrine®.
dextrocardia (deks-tro-kar′de-ă) **1.** Abnormal location of the heart on the right side of the chest. **2.** Condition in which the major portion of the heart is displaced to the right side (e.g., when the right lung collapses).
dextrocular (deks-tro-ok′u-lar) Relating to the right eye.
dextromethorphan hydrobromide (deks-tro-meth-ōr′fan hi-dro-bro′mīd) Pharmaceutical preparation taken orally as a cough suppressant.
dextroposition (deks-tro-po-zish′un) Abnormal right-sided location of an organ normally located in the left side.
d. of heart Condition either congenital or acquired (as in collapse of the right lung), in which the major portion of the heart lies on the right side.
dextrorotatory (deks-tro-ro′tar-e) Turning the plane of polarization to the right; bending rays of light clockwise; said of some crystals and solutions.
dextrose (deks′trōs) See glucose.
dextrothyroxin sodium (deks tro-thi-rok′sin so′de-um) *d*-Thyroxine, a thyroid hormone analog used to reduce the cholesterol content in the tissues.
dextroversion (deks-tro-ver′shun) Displacement or turning toward the right.
diabetes (di-ă-be′tēz) General term for diseases characterized by excessive excretion of urine; when used alone the term refers to diabetes mellitus.
d. 1 See type 1 diabetes mellitus.
d. 2 See type 2 diabetes mellitus.
adult-onset d. See type 2 diabetes mellitus.
alloxan d. The production of diabetes mellitus in

D

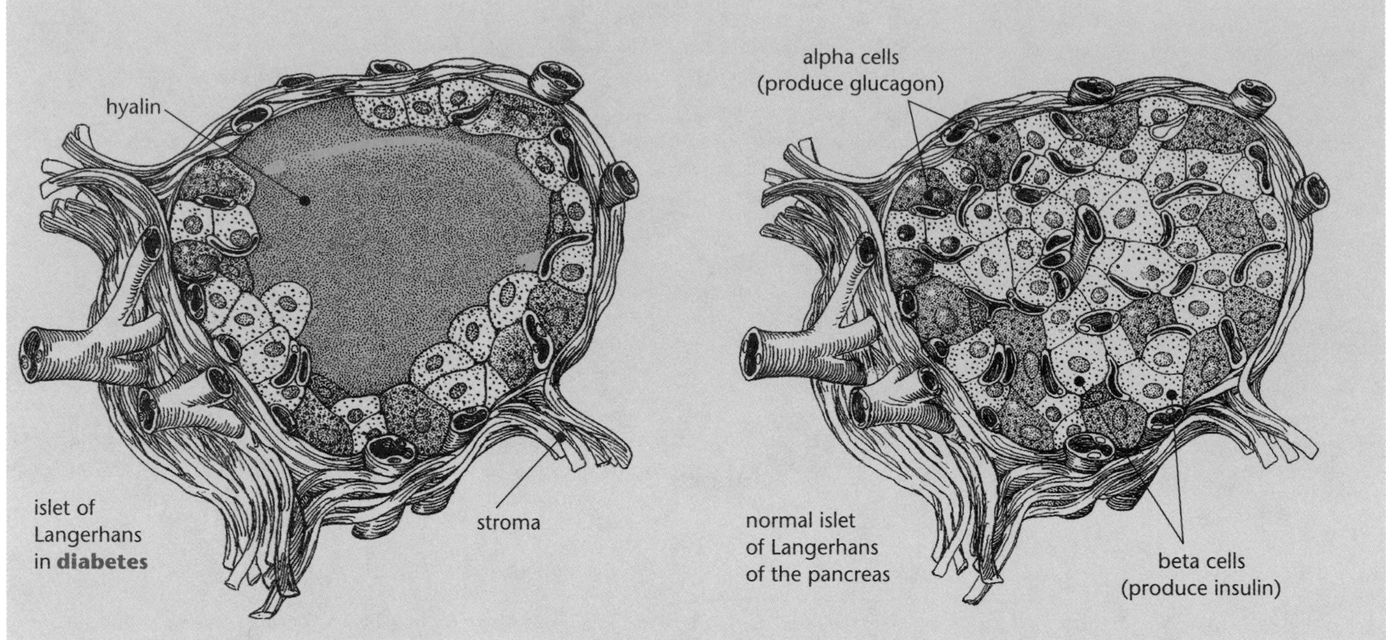

experimental animals by the administration of alloxan, an agent that damages the insulin-producing cells of the pancreas.

brittle d. See labile diabetes.

bronzed d. Diabetes associated with hemochromatosis. See also hemochromatosis.

gestational d. mellitus (GDM) Glucose intolerance detected by a glucose tolerance test during pregnancy in the absence of clinical evidence usually associated with overt carbohydrate intolerance; although limited to pregnancy, patients who develop gestational diabetes are at increased risk of developing diabetes mellitus subsequently in the nonpregnant state. Also called pregnancy-induced glucose intolerance.

d. insipidus A comparatively rare form of diabetes characterized by excessive thirst and the passage of large amounts of dilute urine (of low specific gravity), due to an inadequate production of antidiuretic hormone (vasopressin) by the posterior lobe of the pituitary; normally, the antidiuretic hormone curtails the amount of water the kidney releases in the urine. Compare with nephrogenic diabetes insipidus.

insulin-dependent d. mellitus (IDDM) See type 1 diabetes mellitus.

juvenile d., juvenile-onset d. Former terms for type 1 diabetes mellitus.

labile d. Diabetes mellitus that is difficult to control, with unpredictable and frequent episodes of hyper- and hypoglycemia. Formerly called brittle diabetes.

latent d. mellitus See impaired glucose tolerance, under tolerance.

maturity-onset d. mellitus See type 2 diabetes mellitus.

maturity-onset d. of youth (MODY) A subtype of type 2 diabetes mellitus characterized by a gradual onset during late adolescence or early adulthood.

d. mellitus (DM) A chronic systemic disease of disordered metabolism of carbohydrate, protein, and fat; its primary feature is inappropriately high levels of glucose in the blood (hyperglycemia), from which the term *mellitus* (Latin for "honeyed") was derived. The condition has been classified into two major categories (type 1 diabetes mellitus and type 2 diabetes mellitus); in the former there is insulin deficiency and in the latter there is diminished insulin effectiveness. Longstanding diabetes mellitus is associated with increased risk of coronary artery disease, peripheral vascular disease and hypertension, retinopathy, nephropathy, and neuropathy. Poor diabetic control correlates with more complications. Pregnancy in diabetic women whose condition is poorly controlled may have deleterious effects in both mother and child. Maternal effects can include: the likelihood of preeclampsia-eclampsia, increased risk of acquiring bacterial infections, birth canal injuries (due to abnormally large size of the fetus), cesarean delivery (with increased risk of complications), and large volume of amniotic fluid (with attending cardiorespiratory symptoms).

nephrogenic d. insipidus A rare familial form of diabetes insipidus due to severely diminished ability of the kidney tubules to reabsorb water; it does not respond to the administration of antidiuretic hormone. Also called vasopressin-resistant diabetes.

noninsulin-dependent d. mellitus (NIDDM) See type 2 diabetes mellitus.

preclinical d. mellitus See impaired glucose tolerance, under tolerance.

steroidogenic d. Abnormal glucose tolerance, or overt diabetes mellitus, induced by adrenocortical steroid hormones (e.g., cortisone) or therapeutic analogs (e.g., prednisone). The condition may be temporary or may become permanent.

subclinical d. mellitus See impaired glucose tolerance, under tolerance.

type 1 d. mellitus An often severe type of diabetes mellitus characterized by a sudden onset of insulin deficiency, with a tendency to develop ketoacidosis; may occur at any age, but is most common in childhood and adolescence (peak age of onset is 11-15 years); the disorder is due to destruction of the beta cells of the islets of Langerhans in the pancreas, possibly by a viral infection and autoimmune reactions; symptoms and signs include elevated blood glucose levels (hyperglycemia) excessive urination (polyuria), chronic excessive thirst (polydipsia), excessive eating (polyphagia), weight loss, and irritability; affected persons must have injections of insulin to survive. Also called diabetes 1. Formerly called juvenile diabetes, juvenile-onset diabetes; insulin dependent diabetes mellitus (IDDM); diabetes mellitus type I.

type 2 d. mellitus A form of diabetes mellitus characterized by a gradual onset that may occur at any age but is most common in adults over the age of 40 years, especially those with a tendency to obesity (peak age of onset is 50-60 years); may be due to a tissue insensitivity to insulin, or to a delayed insulin release from the pancreas in response to glucose intake; a genetic predisposition is noted when it occurs in young people. Also called diabetes 2. Formerly called adult-onset diabetes mellitus; maturity-onset diabetes mellitus; non-insulin dependent diabetes mellitus (NIDDM); diabetes mellitus type II.

vasopressin-resistant d. See nephrogenic diabetes insipidus.

diabetic (di-ă-bet′ik) Relating to diabetes.

diabetogenic (di-ă-bet-o-jen′ik) Causing diabetes.

diabetologist (di-ă-bĕ-tol′o-jist) A specialist in the study and treatment of diabetes.

diabetology (di-ah-be-tol′o-je) The field of medicine concerned with the study and treatment of diabetes.

diacetylmorphine (di-ă-se-til-mor′fēn) See heroin.

diacylglycerol (di-a-sil-glis′er-ol) (DAG) A diester of glycerol (trihydric sugar alcohol); it acts as a second messenger in calcium-mediated responses to hormones by activating protein kinase C (an enzyme).

diadochokinesia, diadochokinesis (di-ad-ŏ-ko-ki-ne′zhă, di-ad-ŏ-ko-ki-ne′sis) The normal ability of alternating opposite muscular actions (e.g., extension and flexion of a limb).

diagnose (di′ag-nōs) To identify the nature of a disease; to make a diagnosis.

diagnosis (di-ag-no′sis) The determination of the nature of a disease.

antenatal d. See prenatal diagnosis.

clinical d. A diagnosis based on the signs and symptoms of a disease.

differential d. The determination of which of two or more diseases with similar symptoms is the one with which the patient is afflicted; consideration or listing of diseases possibly responsible for a patient's illness, based on information available at the time, e.g., symptoms, signs, physical findings, and laboratory data.

d. by exclusion A diagnosis made by excluding all but one of the disease processes thought to be possible causes of the symptoms being considered.

laboratory d. A diagnosis made by a chemical, microscopic, bacteriologic, or biopsy study of secretions, discharges, blood, or tissue.

pathologic d. 1. A diagnosis (sometimes a postmortem diagnosis) made from a study of the lesions present. **2.** A diagnosis of the pathologic conditions present, determined by a study and comparison of the symptoms.

physical d. A diagnosis based on information obtained through physical examination of the patient, using the techniques of inspection, palpation, percussion, and auscultation.

postmortem d. See autopsy.

prenatal d. Diagnosis of disorders made by examining fetal cells obtained either by amniocentesis (from amniotic fluid), chorionic villous sampling (from placenta), or fetal blood sampling (from umbilical cord). Also called antenatal diagnosis.

diagnostician (di-ag-nos-tish′un) One who is experienced in determining the nature of diseases; formerly used to apply to physicians with extensive training and experience in medicine, comparable to internists of today.

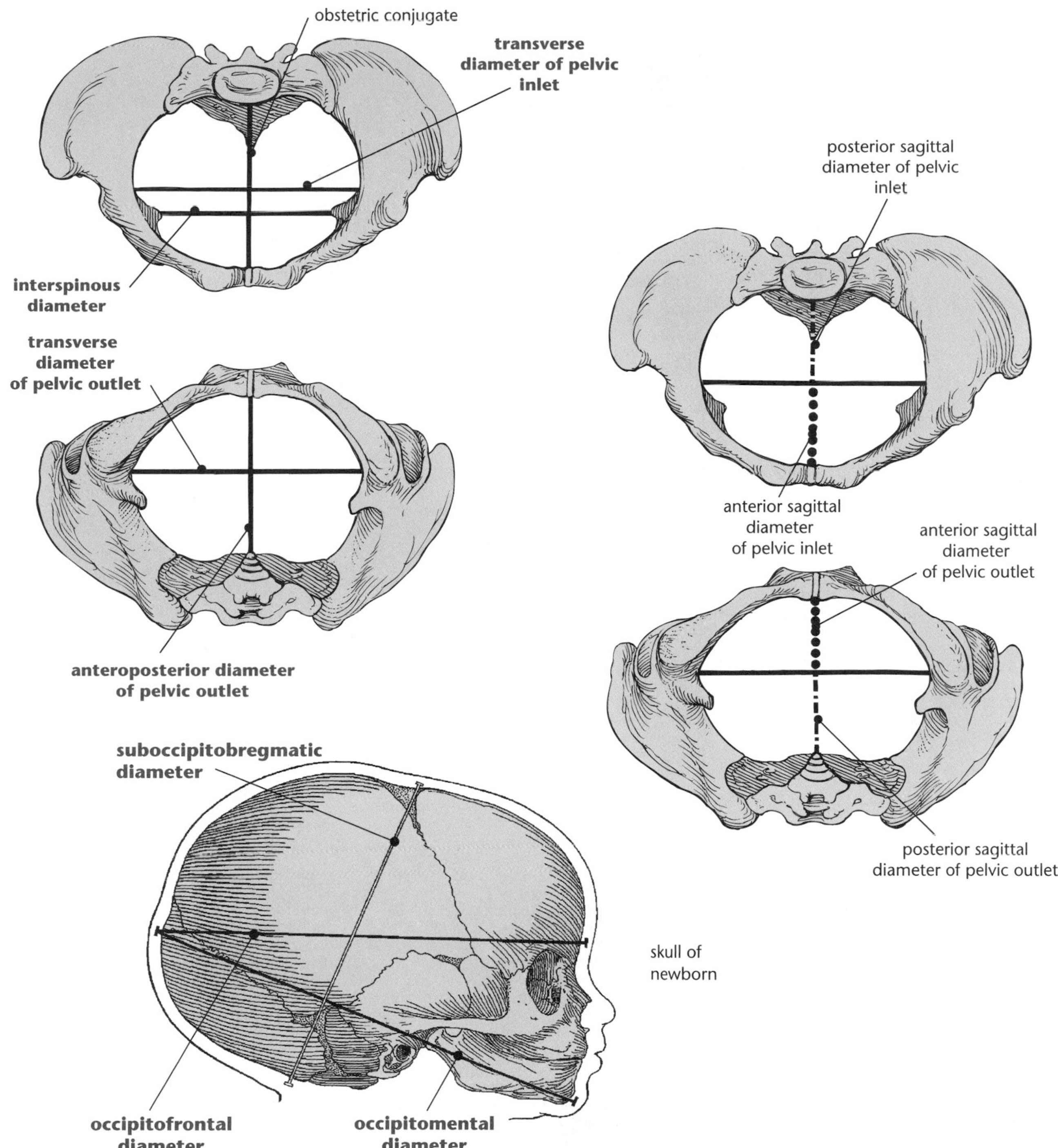

diagram (di´ă-gram) A simple graphic representation.

Venn d. In statistics, a diagram employing circles or ellipses to represent the extent to which two or more quantities or concepts are mutually inclusive or exclusive.

diakinesis (di-ă-ki-ne´sis) The terminal part of the prophase stage in meiosis during which the spireme threads break up into shorter and thicker chromosomes, and the nucleolus and nuclear membrane disappear.

dialysance (di-al´ĭ-sans) The amount of blood (measured in milliliters) completely cleared of a substance by a dialyzing membrane in a period of time, usually one minute.

dialysate (di-al´ĭ-sāt) Fluid used in dialysis.

dialysis (di-al´ĭ-sis) The separation of smaller molecules (crystalloids) from larger molecules (colloids) in a solution by selective diffusion through a semipermeable membrane.

chronic ambulatory peritoneal d. (CAPD) A treatment modality in which the patient exchanges the dialyzing fluid three to five times daily through a permanently placed catheter.

chronic cycling peritoneal d. (CCPD) See continuous cycling peritoneal dialysis.

continuous cycler-assisted peritoneal d. See continuous cycling peritoneal dialysis.

continuous cycling peritoneal d. (CCPD) Peritoneal dialysis in which automated equipment (cycles) is set each night at bedtime to make several exchanges of fluid while the patient sleeps. Also called continuous cycler-assisted peritoneal dialysis; chronic cycling peritoneal dialysis.

peritoneal d. Dialysis in which sterile dialyzing fluid is introduced into the abdominal cavity; the peritoneum acts as the semipermeable membrane.

dialysis disequilibrium syndrome Nausea, vomiting, hypertension, and central nervous system signs occasionally occurring within hours after starting hemodialysis for kidney failure; thought to be due to removal of metabolites (especially urea) from the extracellular fluid and blood at a much greater rate than from the brain cells, with subsequent cerebral edema.

dialyze (di´ă-līz) To perform dialysis.

dialyzer (di´ă-līz-er) A semipermeable membrane used in dialysis as a filter.

diameter (di-am´e-ter) **1.** A straight line passing through the center of any circular anatomic structure or space; frequently used to specify certain dimensions of the female pelvis and fetal head. **2.** The distance along such a line. **3.** The thickness or width of any structure or opening.

anteroposterior d. of midpelvis The distance between the pubic symphysis and sacrum at the junction of the fourth and fifth vertebrae; it is on the midplane or plane of least pelvic dimensions.

anteroposterior d. of pelvic inlet See diagonal conjugate and true conjugate, under conjugate.

anteroposterior d. of pelvic outlet The distance between the lower rim of the pubic symphysis and the sacrococcygeal junction.

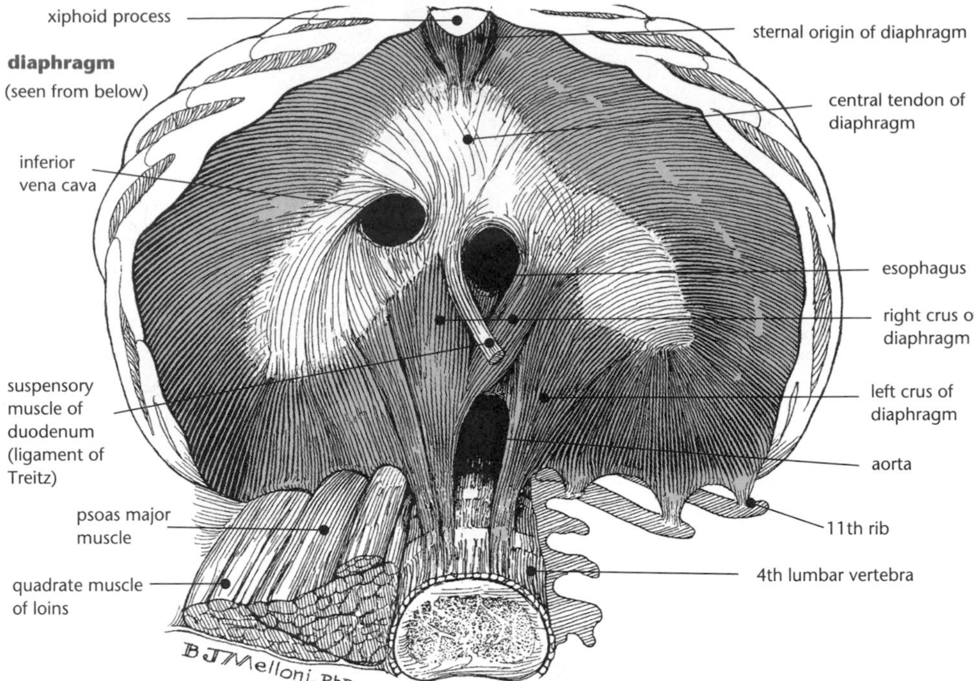

Sometimes the tip of the coccyx is used for the posterior point.

biischial d. of pelvic outlet See transverse diameter of pelvic outlet.

biparietal d. The greatest transverse diameter of a skull; it extends from one parietal bone to the other; in the fetus at term it usually measures 9.25 cm.

bispinous d. See interspinous diameter.

bitemporal d. The distance between the two temporal sutures of the fetal skull at term, usually around 8.0 cm.

bituberous d. See transverse diameter of pelvic outlet.

interspinous d. The transverse diameter of the midpelvis between the two ischial spines; usually the smallest diameter of the pelvis. Also called bispinous diameter; transverse diameter of midpelvis.

intertuberous d. See transverse diameter of pelvic outlet.

oblique d.'s of pelvis (a) Of the inlet: two diameters, each measured from one sacroiliac joint to the opposite junction of the ischial and pubic rami (iliopubic eminence). (b) Of the outlet: the distance from the midpoint of the sacrotuberous ligament to the opposite junction of the ischial and pubic rami (iliopubic eminence).

occipitofrontal d. The diameter of a skull from the frontal bone between the eyebrows (glabella) to the prominent portion of the occipital bone (external occipital protuberance).

occipitomental d. The distance of a skull from the chin to the most prominent portion of the occipital bone (external occipital protuberance).

suboccipitobregmatic d. The diameter of a fetal skull at term from the middle of the large fontanel to the under surface of the occipital bone, just where it joins the neck.

transverse d. of midpelvis See interspinous diameter.

transverse d. of pelvic inlet The greatest distance between opposite sides of the pelvic brim (i.e., between the iliopectineal lines on either side).

transverse d. of pelvic outlet The distance between the two ischial tuberosities. Also called bituberous diameter; intertuberous diameter; biischial diameter.

diamine (di-ă-mēn) An organic compound containing two amino groups (e.g., $NH_2CH_2CH_2NH_2$, ethylene diamine).

diapause (di´ă-pawz) A period of biological dormancy, such as the suspension of growth and decreased metabolism in insects during a specific stage in their life cycle.

diapedesis (di-ă-pĕ-de´sis) **1.** The passage of blood or any of its corpuscles through the pores of blood vessels. **2.** The process by which phagocytic cells leave the blood stream and accumulate at extravascular sites of tissue injury.

diaphoresis (di-ă-fo-rē´sis) Sweating.

diaphoretic (di-ă-fo-ret´ik) An agent that causes sweating, especially profuse sweating.

diaphragm (dī´ă-fram) **1.** The musculomembranous structure which separates the thoracic and abdominal cavities. **2.** Any dividing membrane. **3.** A device with a variable aperture that controls the amount of light illuminating a specimen on a light microscope. **4.** The adjustable grid of lead strips used for minimizing radiation exposure to patients when taking x-ray pictures.

contraceptive d. A flexible ring covered with rubber or other plastic material, fitted over the cervix of the uterus to prevent pregnancy.

pelvic d. The part of the pelvic floor formed by the paired levator ani and coccygeus muscles and their fasciae.

urogenital d. A deep musculomembranous structure extending between the ischiopubic rami; composed of the sphincter urethrae and deep transverse perineal muscles.

diaphysis (di-af´ĭ-sis) The shaft of a long bone.

diaphysitis (di-ă-fiz-ī´tis) Inflammation of the body or shaft of a long bone.

diaplacental (di-ă-plă-sen´tal) Passing through the placenta.

diapophysis (di-ă-pof´ĭ-sis) The upper articular surface of a transverse vertebral process.

diarrhea (di-ă-re´ă) An increase in the looseness or fluidity and frequency of bowel movements beyond what is normal for the person.

nocturnal d. Diarrhea occurring primarily at night: seen in diabetes mellitus.

traveler's d. Diarrhea affecting travelers usually during the first week of a trip and lasting 1 to 3 days.

diarthric (di-ar´thrik) Relating to two joints.

diarthrosis (di-ar-thro´sis) A joint that permits relatively free movement. Also called diarthrodial; synovial joint.

diaschisis (di-as´kĭ-sis) A sudden functional disorder caused by a focal disturbance of the brain.

diastalsis (di-ă-stal´sis) The type of peristalsis of the small intestine in which a wave of inhibition precedes the wave of contraction.

diastase (di´ă-stās) A mixture of amylolytic or starch-splitting enzymes that convert starch into dextrin and maltose; present in some germinating grains such as malt.

diastasis (di-as´tă-sis) Separation of two bones normally joined together without existence of a true joint, as in separation of the epiphysis from the shaft of a long bone.

d. recti Separation of the abdominal rectus muscles from the midline, usually seen after pregnancy or abdominal surgery.

diastema (di-ă-ste´mă) Excessive space between two adjacent teeth.

diastole (di-as´to-le) Rhythmic relaxation of the muscles of the heart chambers during which time they fill with blood.

diastolic (di-ă-stol´ik) Relating to a diastole.

diataxia (dia-ă-tak´se-ă) Loss of muscular co-ordination on both sides of the body.

diathermy (di´ă-ther-me) Local generation of heat in the body tissues by a high frequency electric current.

medical d. Production of sufficient heat to warm the tissues without destroying them.

shortwave d. Heating of tissues by means of an oscillating current of high frequency; used in physiotherapy to relieve pain.

surgical d. High frequency diathermy used for the destruction of diseased tissues (electrocoagulation), cauterization, etc.

diathesis (di-ath´ĕ-sis) An inherited predisposition to a disease or abnormality; a constitutional susceptibility.

cystic d. A predisposition to the formation of cysts in an organ.

gouty d. A predisposition to gout.

hemorrhagic d. A predisposition to spontaneous bleeding.

diatom (di´ă-tom) A microscopic, unicellular alga with a hard silica-containing cell wall.

diatomaceous (di-ă-to-ma´shus) Consisting of the siliceous skeletons or shells of the unicellular diatoms.

diatomic (di-ă-tom´ik) Consisting of two atoms.

diazepam (di-az´ĕ-pam) A benzodiazepine derivative, $C_{16}H_{13}ClN_2O$; used primarily as an antianxiety agent and as an adjunct in the treatment of muscular spasms; also used to treat alcohol withdrawal; Valium®.

diazotize (di-az´o-tīz) To treat an amine with nitrous acid.

diazoxide (di-az-ok´sīd) A nondiuretic thiazide derivative used intravenously to acutely lower blood pressure in the treatment of hypertensive crises; Hyperstat®.

dibasic (di-băsik) Having two replaceable hydrogen atoms; denoting a compound with two hydrogen atoms replaceable by a monovalent metal. Also called bibasic.

dibenzopyridine (di-ben-zo-pir´ĭ-dēn) See acridine.

Dibothriocephalus (di-both-re-o-sef´ă-lus) See *Diphyllobothrium*.

dicentric (di-sen´trik) Having two centromeres, as in certain abnormal chromosomes.

dichloride (di-klor´īd) A chemical compound

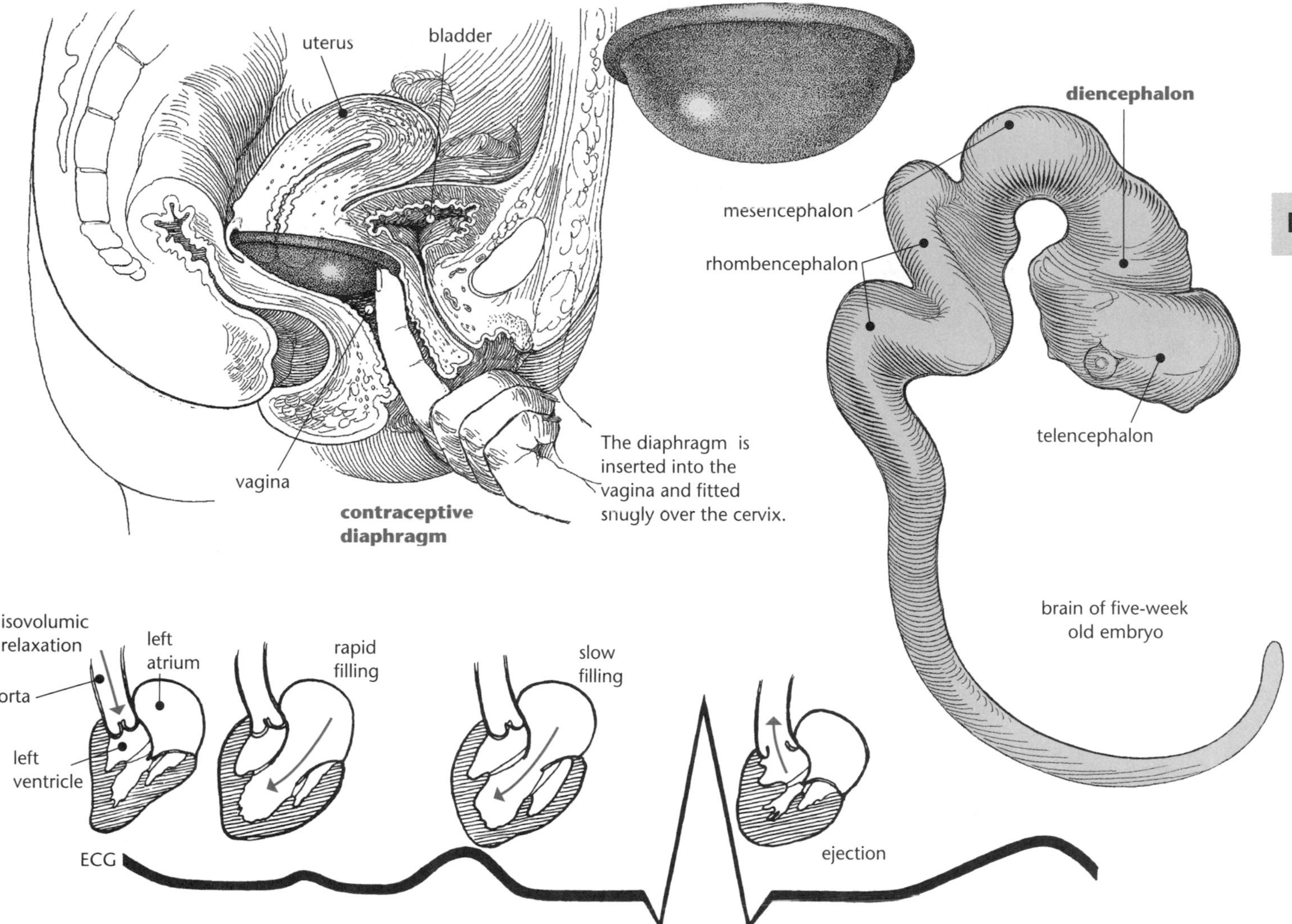

containing two chloride atoms per molecule.

dichotomy (di-kot´ŏ-me) Division or cutting into two parts.

dichromate (di-kro´māt) A chemical compound containing the radical $Cr_2O_7^=$. Also called bichromate.

dichromatic (di-kro-mat´ik) **1.** Having two colors. **2.** Relating to dichromatism.

dichromatism (di-kro´mă-tiz-m) A defect in color perception; the spectrum is seen as composed of only two colors separated by an achromatic or colorless band. Also called dichromatopsia.

dichromatopsia (di-kro-mă-top´se-ă) See dichromatism.

dichromism (di-kro´miz-m) The property of exhibiting two colors, as in certain crystals when seen from different directions, or certain solutions in varying degrees of concentration.

dichromophil, dichromophile (di-kro´mo-fil, di-kro´mo-fīl) Denoting tissues that take both acid and basic stains but in different areas.

dicrotic (di-krot´ik) Double beat, denoting a pulse with two beats for each heartbeat.

dictyoma (dik-te-o´mă) Tumor of the retina.

dicumarol (di-koo´mă-rol) A coumarin derivative that inhibits the formation of prothrombin in the liver; a long-acting anticoagulant agent. Also called bishydroxycoumarin.

didactic (di-dak´tik) Intended to instruct by means of lectures or textbooks rather than by clinical demonstrations with patients.

didactylism (di-dak´til-iz-m) Having two fingers on a hand or two toes on a foot.

didymus (did´ĭ-mus) A testis; from the Greek word *didymos*, meaning twin.

die (di) A specialized model made from an impression, such as the positive reproduction of a prepared tooth; usually made of metal or super-hard dental stone.

diencephalon (di-en-sef´ă-lon) The portion of the embryonic brain between the mesencephalon and the telencephalon from which develop the thalamus, metathalamus, epithalamus, subthalamus, and hypothalamus; it encloses the third ventricle; together with the telencephalon it makes up the prosencephalon.

diener (de´ner) A laboratory assistant.

diet (di´et) **1.** Body nourishment. **2.** Regulated nourishment, especially as prescribed for medical reasons. **3.** To follow a specific dietary plan, especially for reduction of body weight by limitation of caloric intake.

adequate d. See balanced diet.

balanced d. A diet containing the essential ingredients in proper proportion for adequate nutrition. Also called adequate diet.

bland d.'s Regular diets modified to be free from roughage or spicy, irritating foods; progressive regimen (bland 1, 2, 3, or 4), generally used in treatment of upper gastrointestinal disturbances. Also called Sippy diet.

cholesterol-lowering d. See low saturated fat diet.

clear liquid d. Diet used postoperatively for individuals unable to tolerate full liquids or solid food.

diabetic d.'s Any of nine balanced diets recommended by the American Diabetes Association for diabetic individuals; they are relatively free of sugar and high carbohydrate foods and have caloric levels from 1200 to 3500, commonly divided in fifths (i.e., three meals and two snacks) per day.

elimination d. A diet omitting foods suspected of causing allergic reactions; usually eliminated are eggs, milk, and wheat, less frequently, nuts, chocolate, and fish.

full liquid d. A diet composed of foods which are in liquid form at body temperature; it basically serves as a pre- or postoperative diet, and as a transition to a more liberal soft regimen.

Giordano-Giovannetti d. A low protein diet that helps to relieve gastrointestinal symptoms of patients with chronic renal failure. Also called Giovannetti diet.

Giovannetti d. See Giordano-Giovannetti diet.

gluten-free d. Diet in which all wheat products are eliminated; used in the treatment of celiac disease.

high-fiber d. Diet that is relatively high in dietary fiber (i.e., fiber found in fruit, vegetables, and whole grains).

high potassium d.'s Diets for individuals undergoing vigorous diuretic therapy; they provide approximately 100 mEq of potassium per day.

Kempner rice-fruit d. Diet consisting chiefly of rice and fruits with addition of minerals and vitamins and restriction of salt; recommended to patients with hypertension or chronic kidney disease.

low calcium d. A daily diet of from100 to200 mg of calcium; used in the treatment of hyperparathyroidism and urinary calcium stones, or as a test

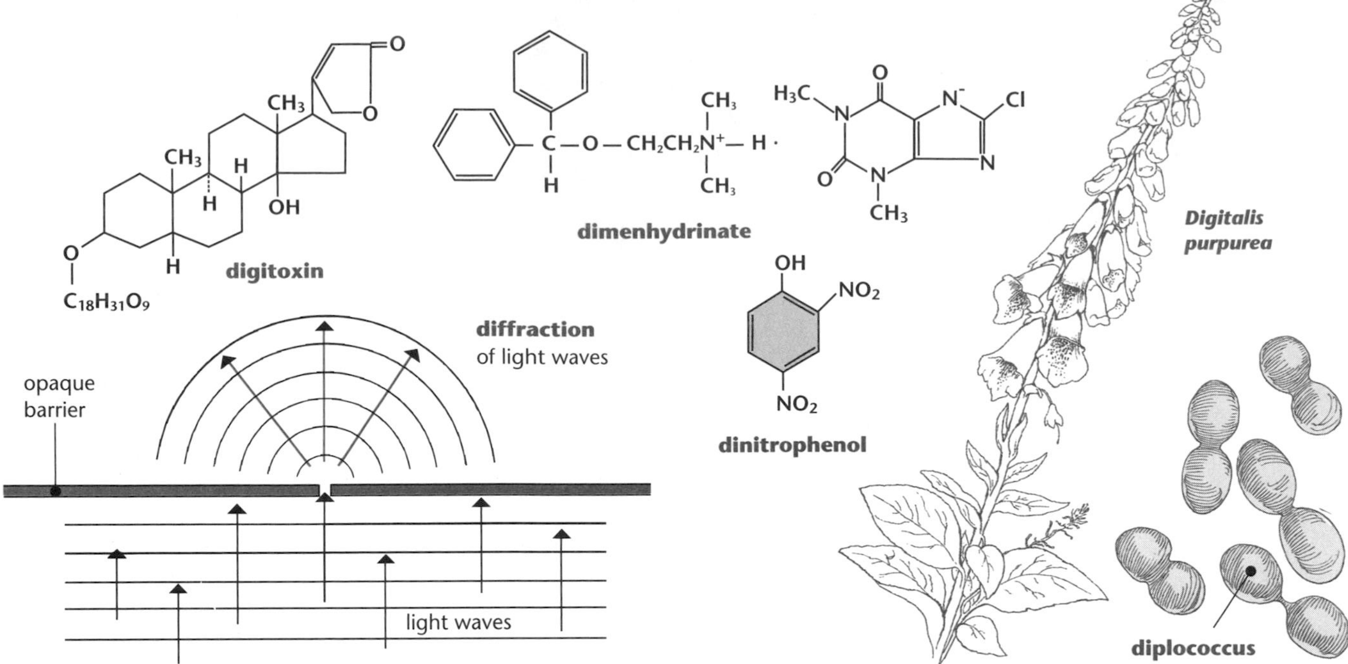

diet to determine urinary calcium excretion; diets of 250 mg of calcium may be used to treat hypercalciuria.

low cholesterol d. See low saturated fat diet.

low fat d. A diet containing minimal amounts of fats (40-50 g per day); may include lean meat, fish, skimmed milk, cottage cheese, and cereal products; the caloric level may be varied through changes in protein and carbohydrate levels.

low residue d. A diet low in cellulose content, as in fruits, vegetables, and unrefined cereals; vegetables are pureed to change the consistency of the cellulose.

low saturated fat d. A diet high in polyunsaturated fatty acids of vegetable origin, with restrictions on foods high in cholesterol and saturated fatty acids, such as eggs, butter, and meat. Also called cholesterol-lowering diet; low cholesterol diet.

low sodium d.'s Diets providing low levels of sodium for the treatment of congestive heart failure, and other conditions associated with edema; four levels of low sodium diets are commonly used: 250 mg, 500 mg, 1000 mg, and 2000 mg of sodium (a regular diet without added salt provides about 4 g of sodium). Also called salt-free diet.

Ornish reversal d. Diet for reversing coronary artery disease; consists of 10% calories from fat, 70 to 75% from carbohydrate, and 15 to 20% from protein.

reduction d.'s Diets for weight reduction, with caloric levels of 800, 1000, 1200, 1500, and 1800, that are adequate in protein and restricted in carbohydrate and fat.

regular d. One adequate to meet recommended daily allowances of the National Research Council; it contains approximately 80 to 100 g of protein, 4 g of sodium, 83 mEq of potassium, and 2000 cal.

renal d.'s Diets low in protein, sodium, and potassium; used in the treatment of renal failure. COMPARE: Giordano-Giovannetti diet.

salt-free d. See low sodium diet.

Sippy d. See bland diet.

soft d. A regular diet modified to include foods that are easily digested, excluding those high in indigestible cellulose and gas-forming fruits and vegetables; it contains approximately 75 g of protein, 4 g of sodium, 72 mEq of potassium, and 2000 cal.

dietetic (di-ĕ-tet´ik) **1.** Of or relating to diet. **2.** Specially prepared or processed food for regulated diets.

dietetics (di-ĕ-tet´iks) The study of diet in relation to health and disease.

diethylstilbestrol (di-eth-il-stil-bes´trol) (DES) A synthetic compound with estrogenic properties; formerly used to treat threatened miscarriage, a practice now abandoned because of the drug's carcinogenic tendency in the daughters of women who took it while pregnant. Also called stilbestrol.

dietitian (di-ĕ-tish´an) A specialist in dietetics.

dietogenetics (di-ĕ-to-jĕ-net´iks) The study of the relationship between the genetic constitution of an individual, his diet, and various food requirements.

dietotherapy (di-ĕ-to-ther´ă-pe) The treatment of disease by a regulated selection of food.

difference (dif´er-ens) **1.** A specific variation. **2.** The amount by which one quantity varies from another.

arteriovenous oxygen d. The difference in the oxygen content of the arterial blood entering and the venous blood leaving a specified area or organ.

differential (dif-er-en´shal) Relating to a difference.

differentiation (dif-er-en-she-a´shun) **1.** In biology, the process of developing into specialized organs; said of embryonic tissues. **2.** See differential diagnosis, under diagnosis.

diffraction (dĭ-frak´shun) The interaction of solid matter with any waveform (i.e., light, sound, or electronic waves), especially the tendency of light rays to bend or deflect from a straight line when passing by the edge of an opaque barrier.

diffuse (dĭ-fūs´) **1.** Spread out; not circumscribed, localized, or limited. **2.** To move by diffusion.

diffusion (dĭ-fū´zhun) **1.** The process of uniformly spreading out or scattering; the passage of the molecules of one substance between the molecules of another to form a mixture of the two substances. **2.** Dialysis.

digastric (di-gas´trik) Having two bellies, as in the digastric muscle.

Digenea (di-je´nē-ă) A subclass of flatworms or flukes (class Trematoda), parasitic in man and other mammals.

DiGeorge's syndrome (dĭ-jor´jez sin´drōm) A multiorgan congenital disorder resulting from damage to the third and fourth pharyngeal pouches during early embryonic development (before the eighth week of pregnancy); characterized by a reduced development or total absence of the thymus and parathyroid glands, frequently accompanied by anomalies of other structures formed at the same embryonic age, including defects of the heart and great vessels, stricture of the esophagus, widely separated eyes, and low-set ears. Also called thymic hypoplasia syndrome.

digest (dī-jest´, dĭ-jest´) **1.** To break up food into simpler, assimilable compounds by the muscular and chemical action of the digestive tract. **2.** To absorb mentally.

digestant (dī-jes´tant, dĭ-jes´tant) An agent that aids the process of digestion.

digestion (dī-jes´chun, dĭ-jes´chun) The process taking place in the alimentary canal whereby the nutritive components of food are converted into simpler chemical substances that can be absorbed by the intestines.

digestive (dī-jes´tiv, dĭ-jes´tiv) Relating to digestion.

digit (dij´it) A finger or toe.

clubbed d.'s See clubbing.

digital (dij´ĭ-tal) Relating to a digit or digits, especially a finger.

Digitalis (dij-ĭ-tal´is) Genus of perennial flowering plants; two species, *D. lanata* and *D. purpurea* (purple foxglove), are the main sources of steroid glycosides, used in the treatment of heart disease.

digitalization (dij-ĭ-tal-ĭ-za´shun) The treatment of an individual with digitalis or a related cardiac glycoside, to achieve a desired therapeutic effect.

digitate (dij´ĭ-tāt) Having fingerlike processes.

digitation (dij-ĭ-ta´shun) A finger-like process.

digitoxin (dij-ĭ-tok´sin) A glycoside obtained from *Digitalis purpurea*; used in the treatment of congestive heart failure.

digitus (dij´ĭ-tus), *pl.* **dig´iti** Latin for finger.

digoxin (di-jok´sin) A glycoside obtained from the leaves of *Digitalis lanata*; used in the treatment of congestive heart failure.

DiGuglielmo syndrome (de goo-glĭ-el´mō sin´drōm) See erythroleukemia.

dihydrate (di-hi´drāt) A compound having two molecules of water.

dihydroergotamine (di-hi-dro-er-got´ă-mēn) (DHE 45) A crystalline compound produced by the hydrogenation of ergotamine; used in the treatment of migraine headache.

dihydrostreptomycin (di-hi-dro-strep-to-mi´sin) Compound made by the hydrogenation of streptomycin; has antibiotic properties.

dihydrotachysterol (di-hi-dro-tak-is´tĕ-rol) (AT 10) A synthetic sterol that produces effects similar to those of vitamin D.

dihydrotestosterone (di-hi-dro-tes-tos´ter-ōn) (DHT) A potent androgenic hormone, secreted by both the ovary and adrenal (suprarenal) glands but primarily formed in peripheral tissues (e.g., hair follicles) by the action of the enzyme 5a reductase upon testosterone; believed to play a significant role in somatic virilization during embryonic development.

diiodotyrosine (di-i-o-do-ti´ro-sēn) (T_2, DIT) A precursor of the thyroid hormone thyroxine.

diisopropyl flurophosphate (di-i-so-pro´pĭl floor-o-fos´făt) (DFP) See isofluorphate.

dilatation (dil-ă-ta´shun) The condition of being enlarged, occurring normally, artificially, or as a result of disease; said of a tubular structure, a cavity, or an opening.

gastric d. Acute distention of the stomach with fluid and air; commonly seen following surgery or

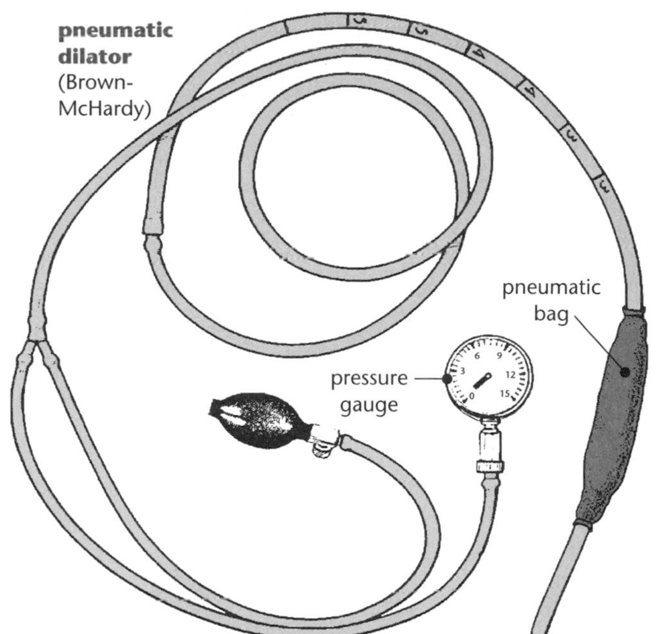

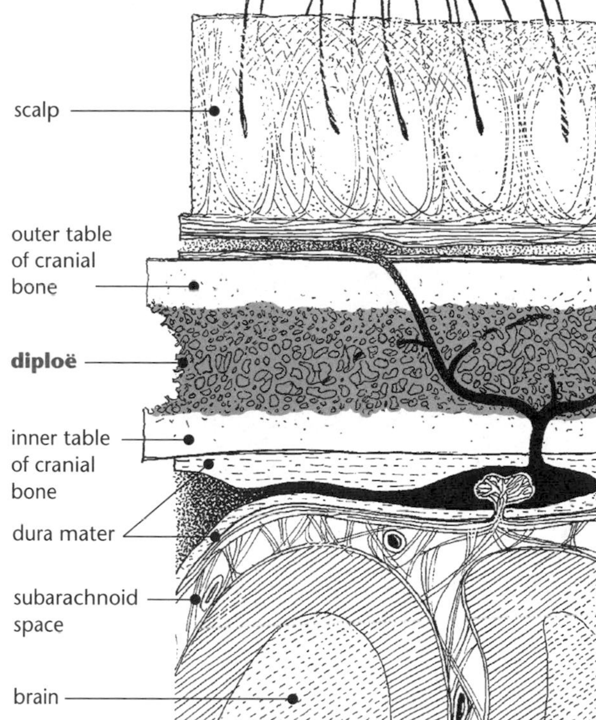

trauma.

post-stenotic d. Enlargement of a blood vessel distal and adjacent to an abnormally constricted area of the vessel or a valve.

dilatation and curettage (dil-ă-ta´shun ku-rĕ-tazh´) (D&C) Dilatation of the uterine cervix and scraping of the lining of the uterus (endometrium) with a curette.

dilatation and evacuation (dil-a-ta´shun e-vak-u-a´shun) (D&E) Abortion performed after 16 weeks of pregnancy; consists of wide cervical dilatation followed by mechanical destruction and removal of fetal parts and removal of the placenta with a large-bore vacuum curette.

dilatation and extraction (dil-a-ta´shun eks-trak´-shun) (D&X) See dilatation and evacuation.

dilate (di-lāt´) To enlarge; to stretch.

dilator (di-la´tor) Instrument for enlarging a passage or cavity.

dildo, dildoe (dil´dō) An object having the approximate size and shape of an erect penis; used to produce sexual pleasure by vaginal insertion.

diltiazem (dil-tī´ă-zem) A calcium channel blocking agent used in the treatment of hypertension and angina pectoris; especially useful in Prinzmetal's angina.

diluent (dil´u-ent) A substance that reduces the concentration of a solution.

dilution (di-loo´shun) **1.** The process of reducing the concentration of a solution or substance. **2.** A weakened solution or substance; an attenuated mixture.

dimenhydrinate (di-men-hī´drĭ-nāt) Drug used in preventing and treating motion sickness; Dramamine®.

dimension (dĭ-men´shun) Any measurable distance.

vertical d. In prosthodontics, the distance between two points on the face, one above and one below the mouth, usually in the midline; it may be measured when the opposing occlusal surfaces are in maximum contact (occlusal vertical dimension) or in rest position, when the jaws are not in contact (rest vertical dimension).

dimer (dī´mer) Chemical compound formed by combining two identical simpler molecules.

dimercaprol (di-mer-kap´rol) A compound used as an antidote for lewisite and other arsenic poisoning. Also called British antilewisite (BAL).

dimethyl sulfoxide (di-meth´il sul´fok´sīd) (DMSO) An industrial solvent occasionally used in medicine as a skin penetrant to facilitate absorption of medications from the skin.

dimorphism (di-mor´fiz-m) The property of occurring in two forms.

dinitrophenol (di-ni-tro-fe´nol) (DNP) A drug that causes an increase in rate of metabolism by interruption of the coupling of oxidation and phosphorylation; not used clinically because of its toxicity.

dinucleotide (di-noo´kle-o-tīd) One of the compounds into which nucleic acid splits on hydrolysis; it may split into two mononucleotides.

diopter (di-op´ter) (D) The unit used to designate the refractive power of a lens or an optical system.

dioptometer (di-op-tom´ĕ-ter) An instrument for measuring refraction and accommodation of the eye. Also called dioptrometer.

dioptric (di-op´trik) **1.** Relating to the unit of refractive power of lenses. **2.** Refractive.

dioptrics (di-op´triks) The science of the refraction of light.

dioptrometer (di-op-trom´ĕ-ter) See dioptometer.

diotic (di-ŏtik) In audiology, denoting an arrangement in which each ear receives the same signal.

dioxide (di-ok´sīd) An oxide containing two atoms of oxygen per molecule.

dioxin (di-oks´in) A hydrocarbon; a pesticide contaminant thought to produce cancer and birth defects.

dipeptidase (di-pep´tĭ-dās) One of the protein-splitting enzymes that causes the breakdown of a dipeptide into its two constituent amino acids.

dipeptide (di-pep´tīd) Two amino acids linked by a peptide bond.

dipeptidyl carboxypeptidase (di-pep-tĭ-dil kar-bok-se-pep´tĭ-dās) See peptidyl-dipeptidase A.

diphenhydramine hydrochloride (di-fen-hi´dră-mēn hi-dro-klo´rīd) An antihistamine used in the prevention and treatment of motion sickness, postoperative nausea, nausea and vomiting of pregnancy, and some allergies; Benadryl®.

diphenylhydantoin (di-fe-nil-hi-dan´toin) An anticonvulsant agent, used primarily to treat epilepsy; Dilantin®.

2,3-diphosphoglycerate (di-fos-fo-glis´er-āt) (DPG) A chemical present in the red blood cells that binds to hemoglobin and has a great effect on its oxygen affinity; in its absence, hemoglobin unloads less oxygen in passing through tissue capillaries.

diphosphopyridine nucleotide (di-fos-fo-pir´ĭ-dēn noo´kle-o-tīd) (DPN) Old term for nicotinamide adenine dinucleotide (NAD).

diphtheria (dif-ther´e-ă) An acute contagious disease caused by a bacillus, *Corynebacterium diphtheriae*; marked by inflammation of the upper respiratory tract, fibrin formation (false membrane) of the mucous membranes, and elaboration of soluble exotoxin that acts on the heart and cranial or peripheral nerve cells.

diphtheroid (dif´thĕ-roid) **1.** Resembling diphtheria. **2.** A bacterium resembling the organism that causes diphtheria.

diphyllobothriasis (di-fil-o-both-ri´ă-sis) Infestation with *Diphyllobothrium latum* (broadfish tapeworm), caused by ingestion of inadequately cooked infected fish.

Diphyllobothrium (di-fil-o-both´re-um) A genus of tapeworms (family Diphyllobothriidae). Formerly called *Bothriocephalus; Dibothriocephalus.*

D. latum Intestinal parasite transmitted to man by ingestion of undercooked infected freshwater fish. Also called fish tapeworm.

diplacusis (dip-lă-koo´sis) Condition in which one sound is heard differently by the two ears, resulting in the perception of two sounds instead of one.

diplegia (di-ple´ge-ă) Paralysis of corresponding parts on both sides of the body. Also called bilateral paralysis.

congenital facial d. See Möbius' syndrome.

diplobacteria (dip-lo-bak-tēr´e-ă) Bacteria linked in pairs.

Diplococcus (dip-lo-kok´us) Former name for a genus of bacteria.

D. pneumoniae See *Streptococcus pneumoniae*, under *Streptococcus.*

diplococcus (dip-lo-kok´us), *pl.* **diplococ´ci** Any of various spherical or ovoid bacteria joined together in pairs.

diploë (dip´lo-e) The spongy (cancellous) bone with a limited marrow cavity between the two tables (layers) of the cranial bones.

diploid (dip´loid) Having two sets of chromosomes, the total number of chromosomes being twice that of a gamete.

diplomate (dip´lo-māt) A board-certified physician.

diplon (dip´lon) See deuteron.

diplopia (dĭ-plo´pe-ă) The condition of seeing one object as two. Also called double vision.

diplotene (dip´lo-tēn) In meiosis, the fourth of five stages of prophase in which the intimately paired homologous chromosomes begin to separate, forming a characteristic chiasma or X appearance; at this stage, blocks of genes are exchanged between homologous chromosomes.

dipsesis (dip-se´sis) Abnormally excessive thirst. Also called dipsosis.

dipsomania (dip-so-ma´ne-ă) An insatiable, uncontrollable desire for alcoholic drinks.

dipsosis (dip-so´sis) See dipsesis.

dipstick (dip´stik) A cellulose strip impregnated with any of various chemicals that undergo a color change when in contact with certain substances (e.g., glucose and protein); used to detect the presence of these substances in a sample of urine.

dipyridamole (di-pi-rid´ă-mōl) A crystalline compound used to reduce platelet aggregation and as a dilator of coronary blood vessels.

director (di-rek´tor) **1.** The head of a service of an organized group. **2.** A grooved instrument for guiding

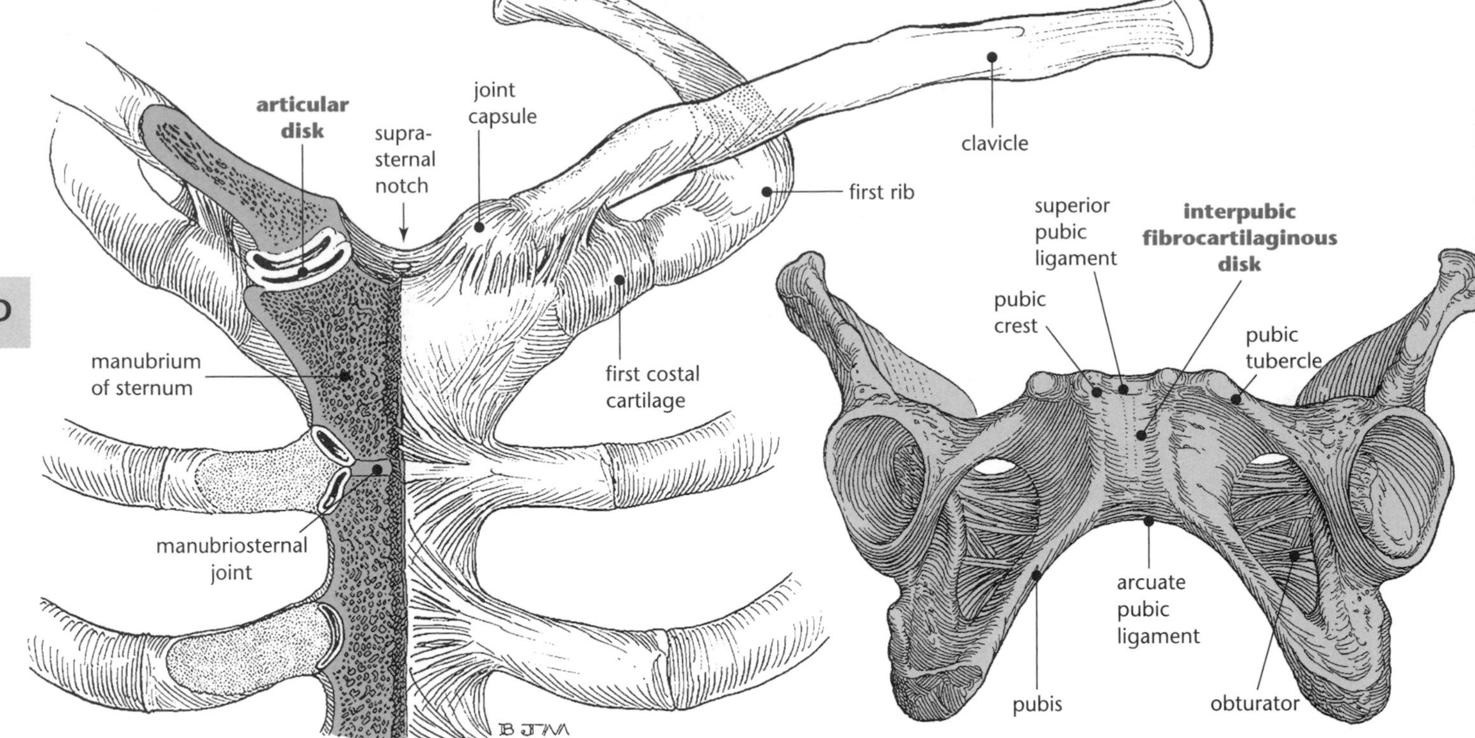

and limiting the motion of a surgical knife.

medical d. A physician employed by a hospital or clinic to serve in a medical and administrative capacity as head of the medical staff; may also serve as liaison for the medical staff with the administration and governing board.

dirigation (dir-i-ga´shun) The process of developing voluntary control over usually involuntary body functions.

dirigomotor (dir-i-go-mo´tor) Anything that controls muscular activity.

dirt-eating (durt et´ing) See geophagia.

Dirofilaria (di-ro-fĭ-lar´e-ă) A genus of filaria (family Onchocercidae, superfamily Filarioidea) known to infest mammals; rarely found in humans.

D. immitis The heartworm, a parasite in the pulmonary arteries of dogs.

disability (dis-ă-bil´ĭ-te) **1.** A legal loss of function and earning power. **2.** Incapacity. **3.** Any handicap.

learning d. (LD) A complex of symptoms that involves impairment of some or all of the following functions: learning, language, perception, memory, and concentration; neurologic examination usually yields minor abnormalities, if any; diagnosis rests on psychological assessment of cognitive function.

disaccharidase (di-sak´ă-ri-dās) Any enzyme that promotes the hydrolysis of a disaccharide.

disaccharide (di-sak´ă-rīd) A class of sugars, including sucrose, lactose, and maltose, that yield two monosaccharides on hydrolysis.

disarticulation (dis-ar-tik-u-la´shun) Amputation of a limb by separating the bones at the joint.

disc (disk) See disk.

discectomy (dis-kek´tŏ-me) Surgical removal of an intervertebral disk.

discharge (dis-charj) **1.** Material that is released as an excretion or a secretion. **2.** To pour forth; to emit. **3.** The activation of a nerve cell.

discission (dĭ-sizh´un) Surgical procedure in which the capsule of the lens of the eye is either punctured or cut.

discogenic (dis-ko-jen´ik) Referring to a disorder originating in an intervertebral disk.

discography (dis-kog´ră-fe) See diskography.

discoid (dis´koid) **1.** Having the shape of a disk. **2.** A dental disk-shaped carving and excavating instrument.

disconjugate (dis-kon´jōō-gāt) Not moving or functioning together. The opposite of conjugate.

discopathy (di-kop´ă-the) See diskopathy.

discordant (dis-kor´dant) In genetics, denoting a pair of twins in which only one member exhibits a certain trait. See also concordant.

discrete (dis-krēt´) Denoting certain lesions of the skin that are separate, not joined or confluent.

discutient (dis-ku´shent) Denoting an agent that causes the dispersal of a tumor or any pathologic accumulation.

disease (dĭ-zēz´) Any abnormal condition, affecting either the whole body or any of its parts, which impairs normal functioning. The following are classes of diseases. For individual diseases, see specific names.

communicable d. Any disease transmissible by infection or contagion directly or through a carrier of the pathogen.

congenital d. A disease present at birth.

contagious d. A disease transmissible by direct or indirect contact.

deficiency d. A disease due to a prolonged lack of vitamins, minerals, or any other essential dietary component.

endemic d. A disease present in a specific locality more or less continuously.

functional d. See functional disorder, under disorder.

hereditary d. A disease transmitted genetically from parent to offspring.

infectious d. A disease caused by the presence of a pathologic microorganism.

mental d. See mental disorder, under disorder.

occupational d. A disease caused by the environment of a particular occupation.

organic d. Disease involving structural changes in the body.

periodic d. Any disease that recurs regularly.

sexually transmitted d.'s (STDs) Disorders spread by intimate contact (including sexual intercourse, kissing, cunnilingus, anilingus, fellatio, mouth-breast contact, and anal intercourse); many can be acquired transplacentally by the fetus or through contact with maternal secretions by the newborn; causative microorganisms include herpesvirus 1 and 2, cytomegalovirus, *Chlamydia*, group B *Streptococcus*, molluscum contagiosum virus, *Sarcoptes scabiei*, hepatitis viruses, and human immunodeficiency virus (HIV). Also called venereal diseases.

social d. Obsolete term for sexually transmitted disease.

systemic d. A disease affecting several organs or the entire body.

venereal d. (VD) See sexually transmitted diseases.

disengagement (dis-en-gāj´ment) In obstetrics, the emergence of the presenting part of the fetus through the vulva.

disequilibrium (dis-e-kwĭ-lib´re-um) Lack of balance or stability.

disimpaction (dis-im-pak´shun) **1.** Separation of an impacted bone fracture. **2.** The breaking up of a fecal impaction.

disinfectant (dis-in-fek´tant) Any agent that kills disease-causing microorganisms; generally used on inanimate objects.

disinfection (dis-in-fek´shun) Destruction of infectious agents on a surface by chemical or physical means.

terminal d. Elimination of the infectious agent from personal clothing and possessions in the immediate environment of the patient.

disintegration (dis-in-tĕ-gra´shun) **1.** Breakdown or separation of component parts. **2.** Disorganization of mental processes.

disk (disk) Any platelike structure. Also written disc.

articular d. A circular fibrocartilaginous pad present in some synovial joints and attached to the joint capsule; eg., the articular disk of the temporomandibular joint, which separates the cavity of the capsule into two separate compartments, thus reducing friction between the articulating surfaces of the bones.

dental d. A small disk of paper or plastic, coated with cuttle-fish bone, emery, garnet, or sand; used in dentistry to cut, smooth, or polish teeth and dental restorations.

epiphyseal d. See epiphyseal plate, under plate.

herniated d. Posterior rupture of the inner portion of an intervertebral disk, causing pressure on the nerve roots with resulting pain; occurring most commonly in the lower back. Also called slipped disk; ruptured disk; prolapsed disk.

intercalated d. The double membrane separating cells of cardiac muscle fibers.

interpubic fibrocartilaginous d. The fibrocartilaginous disk uniting the articular surfaces of the pubic bones at the symphysis.

intervertebral d. The fibrocartilaginous tissue between the bodies of adjacent vertebrae, consisting of a jellylike center surrounded by a fibrous ring.

optic d. The portion of the optic nerve in the eyeball formed by retinal nerve fibers converging to a central area; it appears as an elevated pinkish white oval or circular disk; it is the blind spot in the visual field.

prolapsed d. See herniated disk.

ruptured d. See herniated disk.

slipped d. See herniated disk.

tactile d. The saucer-shaped termination of specialized sensory nerve fibers in contact with a modified cell in the deep layers of the epidermis. Also called meniscus tactus.

temporomandibular articular d. The articular disk of the temporomandibular joint; it separates the joint cavity into two compartments. Also called

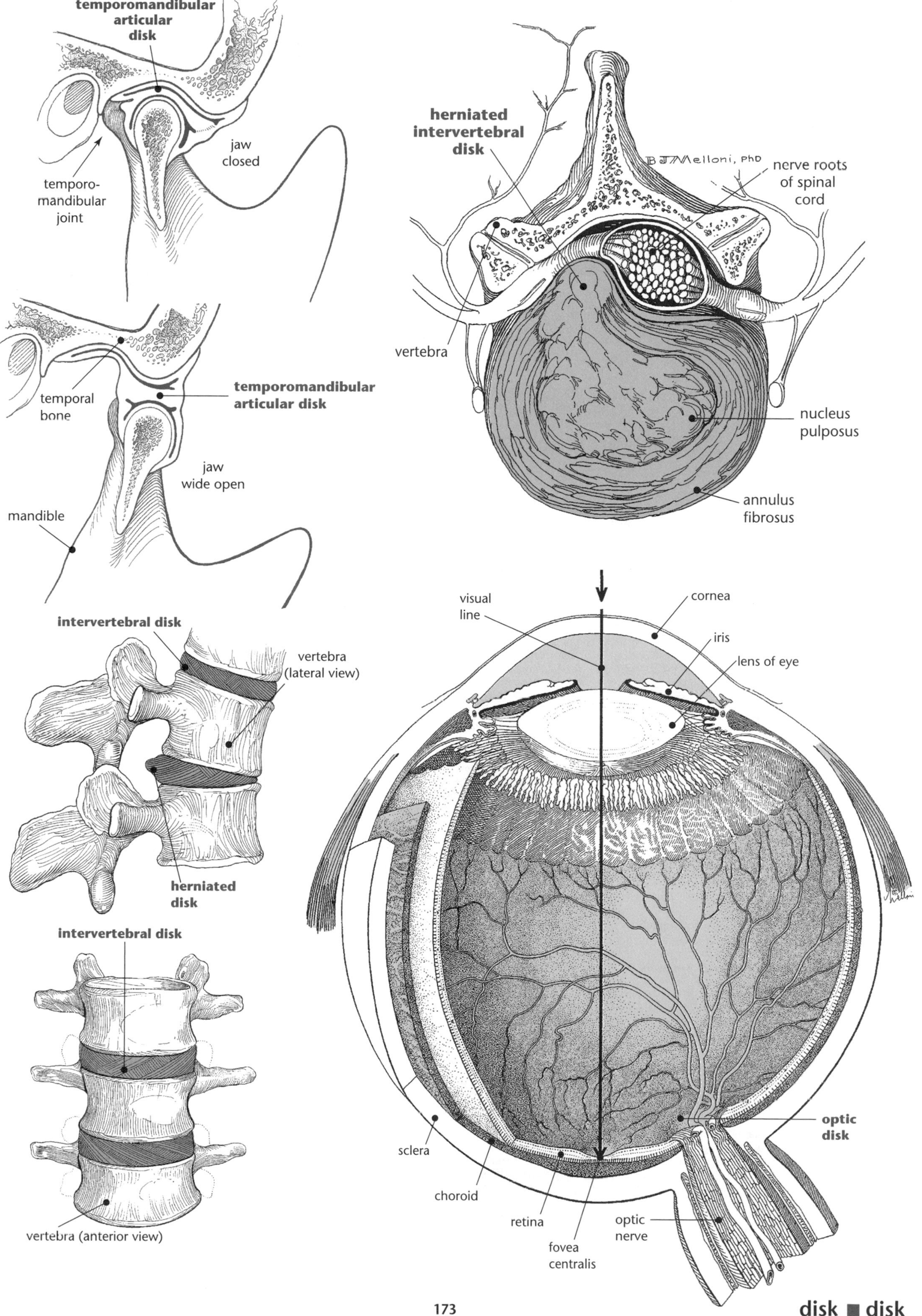

temporomandibular articular disk
temporo-mandibular joint
jaw closed
temporal bone
temporomandibular articular disk
jaw wide open
mandible
herniated intervertebral disk
B J Melloni, PhD
nerve roots of spinal cord
vertebra
nucleus pulposus
annulus fibrosus
intervertebral disk
vertebra (lateral view)
herniated disk
intervertebral disk
vertebra (anterior view)
visual line
cornea
iris
lens of eye
optic disk
sclera
choroid
retina
fovea centralis
optic nerve

D

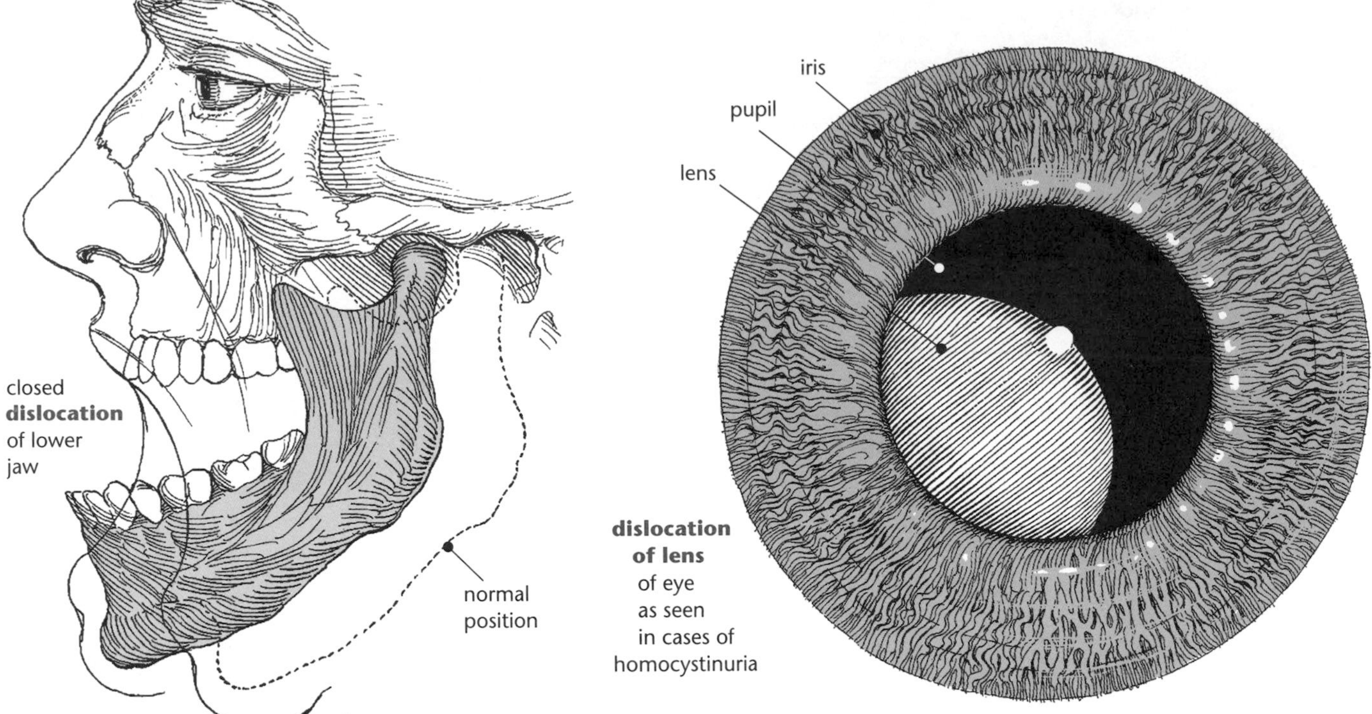

temporomandibular meniscus.

diskectomy (dis-kek′tŏ-me) The surgical removal, in part or whole, of an intervertebral disk.

diskitis (dis-kī′tis) Inflammation of a disk, especially of one between the vertebrae.

diskography (dis-kog′ră-fe) Radiographic visualization of intervertebral disk space after injection of a radiopaque substance. Also written discography.

diskopathy (dis-kop′ă-the) Any disease of an intervertebral disk. Also written discopathy.

disk syndrome (disk sin′drōm) Pain in the lower back, radiating to the thigh with occasional loss of ankle and knee reflexes, resulting from compression of spinal nerve roots by an intervertebral disk.

dislocate (dis′lo-kāt) To shift from the usual or normal position, especially to displace a bone from its socket.

dislocation (dis-lo-ka′shun) **1.** Displacement of a limb or organ from the normal position. See also ectopia. **2.** Specifically, a displacement of a bone from its socket or joint.

d. of lens See ectopia lentis, under ectopia.

dismutase (dis′mu-tās) An enzyme that promotes the reaction of two identical molecules to produce two molecules in different oxidation states.

disorder (dis-or′der) A disturbance of function or health.

affective d.'s A group of disorders characterized chiefly by a disturbance of mood, not due to any other physical or mental disorder.

antisocial personality d. Disorder beginning before the age of 15, marked by a life pattern of repeated conflict with society and its rules, lack of remorse or shame, and inability to sustain meaningful interpersonal relationships; in childhood, it is characterized by truancy, lying, running away from home, vandalism, etc.; in adulthood, features include disregard for others and others' property, irresponsibility, an inconsistent work record, and a tendency to blame others or give plausible rationalizations for deviant behavior. Formerly called psychopathic personality; psychopathy.

attention-deficit hyperactivity d. (ADHD) Disorder with onset before seven years of age, characterized by age-inappropriate short attention span and impulsiveness, poor modulation of emotions and behavior, and difficulty screening out extraneous stimuli; symptoms are especially noticeable in group settings; may or may not have hyperactivity as a prominent component; some difficulties often persist into adulthood. Formerly called minimal brain dysfunction; hyperkinetic reaction of childhood; learning disability; hyperactive child.

autosomal dominant d. Disorder occurring when only one abnormal gene is present and the corresponding gene (allele) on the homologous chromosome is normal. Also called autosomal dominant disease.

autosomal recessive d. Disorder that is apparent only when both corresponding genes (alleles) in homologous chromosomes are abnormal. Also called autosomal recessive disease.

bipolar d. Disorder marked by alternating moods of elation and depression. Formerly called manic-depressive psychosis; manic-depressive illness; manic-depressive disorder.

borderline personality d. Behavioral pattern marked by impulsiveness, intense interpersonal relationships, and instability in mood and emotion.

character d. Deeply ingrained, maladaptive patterns of behavior unaccompanied by subjective feelings of anxiety or guilt.

conversion d. Condition in which unconscious or repressed emotional conflict finds expression as aberrant body functioning (e.g., blindness, deafness, paralysis, pain). Also called hysteria; conversion hysteria; hysterical neurosis; conversion reaction.

functional d. Mental disorder not caused by organic disease.

generalized anxiety d. Generalized persistent anxiety of at least one month's duration without the specific symptoms of phobias, panic attacks, or obsessions or compulsions; symptoms include motor tension, autonomic hyperactivity, apprehensive expectation, vigilance, and scanning.

genetic d. Disorder in which the genetic component expresses itself in a predictable manner without much influence from the environment.

immunoproliferative d. Proliferation of cells of the lymphoreticular system associated with autoallergic disturbances or gamma-globulin abnormalities.

manic-depressive d. See bipolar disorder.

mendelian d. Pathologic condition determined at a single chromosomal gene locus, whether autosomal or on a sex chromosome, and transmitted in a dominant or recessive way.

mental d. Any psychiatric disorder listed in the Standard Nomenclature of Diseases and Operations of the American Medical Association, or in the Diagnostic and Statistical Manual for Mental Disorders of the American Psychiatric Association. Also called mental illness.

myeloproliferative d. Any of a group of disorders characterized primarily by excessive proliferation of blood cells in the bone marrow (e.g., polycythemia vera, chronic myelogenous leukemia).

neuropsychologic d. Impairment of mental function due to a lesion in the brain; it may have a sudden onset and a short duration (acute) or it may be prolonged (chronic).

obsessive-compulsive d. (OCD) Anxiety disorder characterized by obsessions (recurrent ideas, thoughts, or impulses) and compulsions (repetitive behaviors designed to produce or prevent some future situation or event), which are severe enough to interfere with personal or social functioning.

paranoid personality d. A pervasive suspiciousness of others in a variety of contexts; the motives of others are interpreted as malevolent and directed specifically to cause harm to the individual.

personality d. General term used to denote any long-standing maladaptive pattern of behavior; distinguished from neurotic and psychotic symptoms.

posttraumatic stress d. (PTSD) Anxiety disorder resulting from having experienced an overwhelming stress or trauma (e.g., rape or assault), characterized by recurrent nightmares, flashbacks, intrusive recollections, general detachment, excessive startle response, and abnormal response to stimuli that recall the traumatic event. Also called post-traumatic neurosis; posttraumatic stress syndrome.

psychophysiologic d., psychosomatic d. Disturbances of visceral functioning secondary to long-continued emotional attitudes or stress.

schizoid personality d. Personality disorder in which there is a deficit in the capacity to form social relationships as shown by withdrawal, aloofness, and lack of humor.

seasonal affective d. (SAD) An affective disorder characterized by recurrent episodes of major depression occurring in fall and winter with remission through spring and summer.

sleep d. Any disturbance of sleep (e.g., somnambulism).

disorganization (dis-or-gan-i-za′shun) Destruction or breakdown of tissues with resulting loss of function.

disorientation (dis-or-e-en-ta′shun) Loss of the sense of direction or location.

dispensary (dis-pen′să-re) **1.** An office in any institution (hospital, school, etc.) from which medical supplies and medicines are distributed. **2.** An outpatient department of a hospital.

dispensatory (dis-pen′să-tor-e) A book describing the sources, preparation, contents, and uses of medicines.

dispense (dis-pens′) To prepare and distribute medicines to the sick.

disperse (dis-pers′) To scatter.

dispersion (dis-per′zhun) **1.** The process of dispersing or the state of being dispersed. **2.** A suspension of solid, liquid, or gaseous particles of colloidal size in another medium.

coarse d. A suspension of relatively large

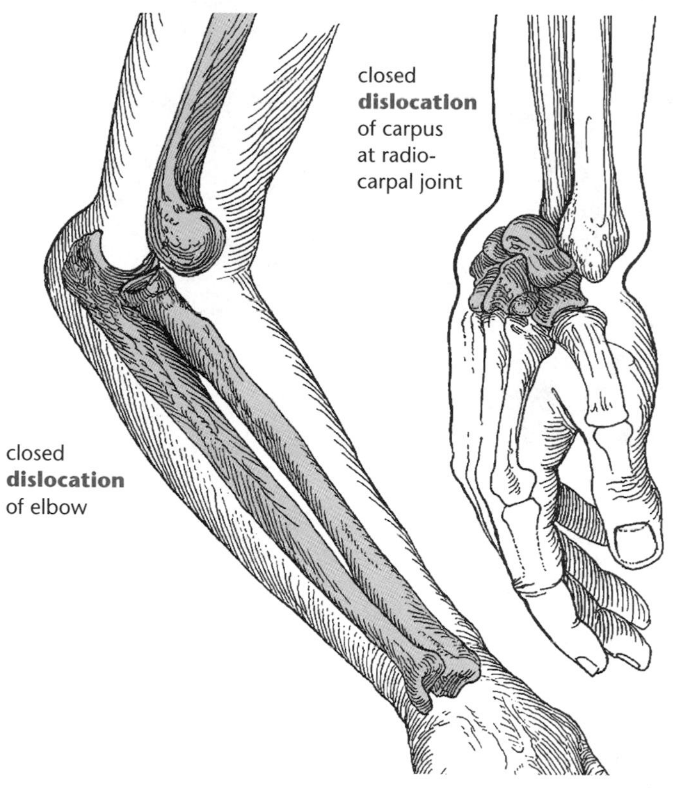

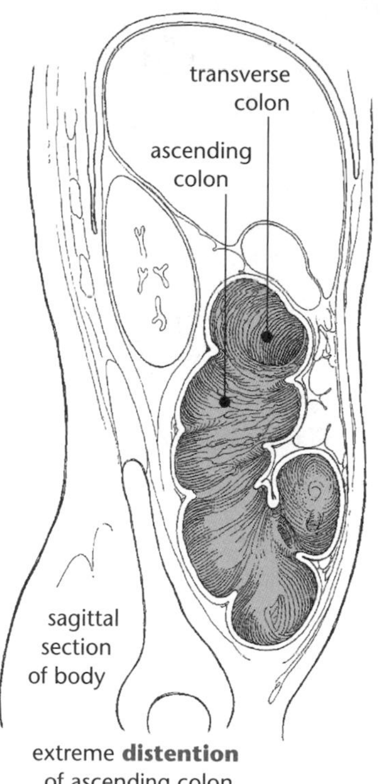

extreme **distention** of ascending colon

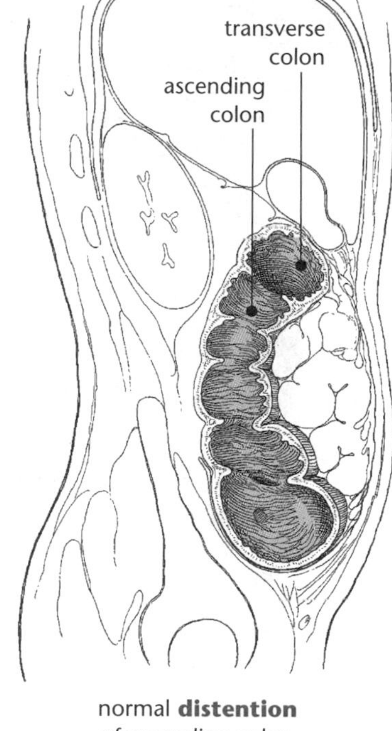

normal **distention** of ascending colon

D

particles in a liquid.

molecular d. One in which the dispersed particles are individual molecules; a true solution.

displacement (dis-plās′ment) **1.** The condition of being moved from a normal position. **2.** In chemistry, a reaction in which an atom, molecule, or radical group is removed from a compound and replaced with another. **3.** The weight of a fluid expelled by a floating body or by another fluid of greater density. **4.** An unconscious defense mechanism in which an emotion, such as anger, is unconsciously directed to an object or person other than the direct cause of frustration; e.g., an angry individual beating the wall with his fist.

dissect (dĭ-sekt′, dī-sekt′) To cut apart, especially in the study of anatomy.

dissection (dĭ-sek′shun, dī-sek′shun) **1.** The act of dissecting. **2.** A tissue that has been dissected.

disseminated (dĭ-sem′ĭ-nāt-ed) Widely distributed throughout an organ, tissue, or the body; scattered; dispersed.

dissimulation (di-sim-u-lā′shun) The act of feigning health by a sick person.

dissociation (di-so-she-a′shun, di-so-se-a′shun) **1.** Separation. **2.** Change of a complex chemical compound into a simple one.

albuminocytologic d. Increase in the protein content of the cerebrospinal fluid without increase in cell count.

atrioventricular d. Independent action of the atria and ventricles of the heart.

complete A-V d. Complete atrioventricular block; independent contraction of atria and ventricles caused by failure of impulses to reach the ventricles.

electromechanical d. Continuing transmission of impulses within the heart without resulting contractions of the heart muscle (e.g., in cardiac rupture).

incomplete A-V d. Atrioventricular dissociation interrupted by ventricular captures.

interference d. Atrioventricular dissociation occasionally interrupted by ventricular captures.

dissolve (dĭ-zolv′) **1.** To cause a substance to change from a solid to a dispersed state by placing it in contact with a solvent fluid. **2.** To melt; to reduce to a liquid state.

distad (dis′tad) Toward the periphery.

distal (dis′tal) **1.** Farthest from a point of reference. **2.** In dentistry, the location most distant from the median line of the jaw.

distance (dis′tans) The space between two points.

interocclusal d. The distance or space between the occlusal surfaces of the mandibular and maxillary teeth when the mandible is in the physiologic rest position. Also called freeway space.

map d. The distance between two gene loci in a chromosome; measured in centimorgans.

reduced interarch d. See overclosure.

small interarch d. A small space between the upper (maxillary) and lower (mandibular) dental arches. Also called closed bite.

distemper (dis-tem′per) Infectious viral disease of certain mammals, especially young dogs, often causing paralysis and death.

distensibility (dis-ten-sĭ-bil′ĭ-te) The ability to stretch.

distention, distension (dis-ten′shun) The state of being stretched or distended.

distill (dis-til′) To subject a liquid mixture to vaporization and subsequent condensation with collection of components by differential cooling.

distillation (dis-tĭ-la′shun) The vaporization of a liquid mixture by heat followed by separation of its components by condensation of the vapor.

distobuccal (dis-to-buk′al) Relating to the distal and buccal surfaces of a posterior tooth; usually denoting the line angle formed by the junction of the two surfaces.

distobucco-occlusal (dis-to-buk-o-ŏ-kloo′zal) Relating to the distal, buccal, and occlusal surfaces of a posterior tooth; usually denoting the point angle formed by the junction of the three surfaces.

distolabioincisal (dis-to-la′be-o-in-sī′zal) Relating to the distal, labial, and incisal surfaces of an anterior tooth; usually denoting the point angle formed by the junction of the three surfaces.

distolingual (dis-to-ling′gwal) Relating to the distal and lingual surfaces of a tooth; usually denoting the line angle formed by the junction of the two surfaces.

distolinguoincisal (dis-to-ling-gwo-in-si′zal) Relating to the distal, lingual, and incisal surfaces of an anterior tooth; usually denoting the point angle formed by the junction of the three surfaces.

distomiasis (dis-to-mi′ă-sis) Condition caused by the presence of flukes in the organs or tissues.

disto-occlusal (dis-to-ŏ-kloo′zal) Relating to the distal and occlusal surfaces of a posterior tooth; usually denoting the line angle formed by the junction of the two surfaces.

distortion (dis-tor′shun) **1.** A deformed image caused by irregularities in a lens. **2.** A mechanism aiding in the disguising or repression of unacceptable thoughts.

distraction (dis-trak′shun) **1.** Mental or emotional disturbance. **2.** Separation of joint surfaces without fracture or dislocation. **3.** In orthodontics, unusually large distance of structures, such as teeth, from the median plane.

distress (dis-tres′) Physical or mental anguish or pain.

fetal d. Metabolic derangements in the fetus affecting the functions of vital organs to the point of temporary or permanent injury or death.

distribution (dis-trĭ-bu′shun) **1.** The arrangement of blood vessels and nerves in the body. **2.** The areas of the body supplied by the terminal branches of such structures.

disulfiram (di-sul′fĭ-ram) A counterdrug that produces an aversion to alcohol; Antabuse®.

diuresis (di-u-re′sis) Discharge of increased amounts of urine.

alcohol d. Production of unusually large quantities of urine after consumption of alcoholic beverages.

osmotic d. Diuresis due to concentration in the kidney tubules of substances that limit the reabsorption of water.

solute d. Diuresis caused by increased concentration of solute in the blood or resulting from excretion of increased amounts of solute in the urine.

water d. Diuresis caused by diminution of antidiuretic hormone, resulting in excretion of increased amounts of urine without a marked change in the excretion of solute.

diuretic (di-u-ret′ik) An agent that increases the volume flow of urine.

diurnal (di-ŭr′nal) Relating to the daylight hours. Opposite of nocturnal.

divalent (di-va′lent) See bivalent (1).

divergence (di-ver′jens) **1.** The act or state of spreading apart from a common point. **2.** The spreading of branches of a presynaptic neuron to form synapses and cause activity with a number of postsynaptic neurons.

diverticular (di-ver-tik′u-lar) Of or relating to a diverticulum.

diverticular disease of colon Condition occurring most commonly in people over 40 years of age; marked by formation of outpouchings of the mucous lining of the colon, which protrude through defects in the muscular wall of the bowel at points of blood vessel entry; may be asymptomatic or may cause intermittent cramping pain and bleeding; occasionally may undergo inflammatory changes and infection. Also called diverticulosis. See also diverticulitis.

diverticulectomy (di-ver-tik-u-lek′tŏ-me) Surgical removal of a diverticulum or of diverticula.

diverticulitis (di-ver-tik-u-li′tis) Inflammation and infection of intestinal diverticula causing a cramping pain, usually in the lower left side of the abdomen, associated with nausea and fever.

diverticulosis (di-ver-tik-u-lo′sis) See diverticular

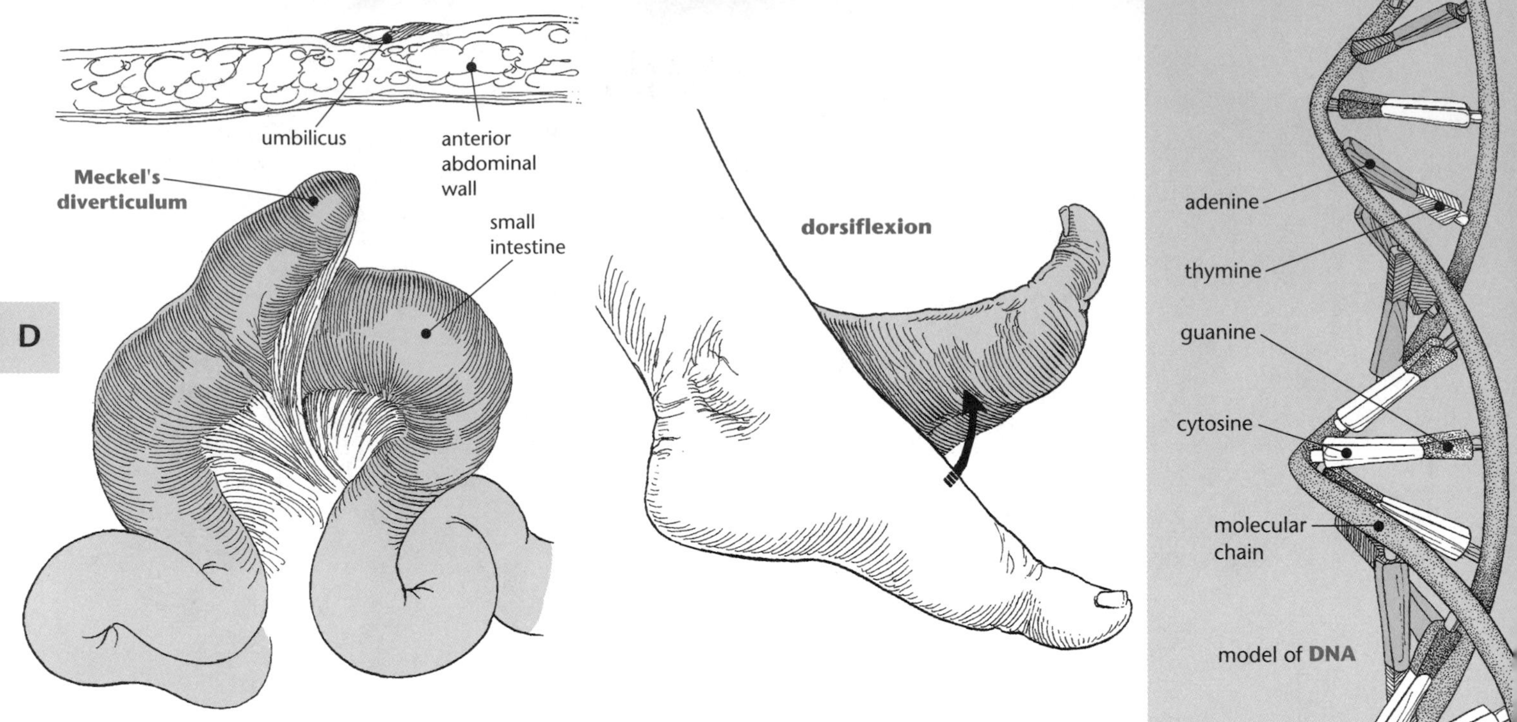

disease of colon.

diverticulum (di-ver-tik´u-lum), *pl.* **divertic´ula** A saccular dilatation protruding from the wall of a tubular organ.

esophageal d. Diverticulum through a weak spot in the esophageal wall.

hypopharyngeal d. See pharyngoesophageal diverticulum.

intestinal d. A herniation of the mucous membrane through a defect in the muscular layer of the intestinal wall.

Meckel's d. A congenital sacculation or appendage of the ileum.

pharyngoesophageal d. A diverticulum between the inferior pharyngeal constrictor muscle and the cricopharyngeal muscle. Also called hypopharyngeal diverticulum; Zenker's diverticulum.

traction d. One formed by the pulling force of adhesions, occurring mainly in the esophagus.

urethral d. An outpouching of the urethral lumen; in the female, it may vary in size from 3 mm to 8 cm in diameter; when large, the diverticulum may be buried along the entire length of the urethra.

vesicourachal d. A diverticulum of the bladder into the urachus resulting from persistent patency of part of the allantoic duct which prenatally extends from the bladder to the umbilical cord.

Zenker's d. See hypopharyngeal diverticulum.

division (dĭ-vizh´on) Separation.

meiotic d. See meiosis.

mitotic d. See mitosis.

divulse (dĭ-vuls´) To separate by tearing.

divulsion (dĭ-vul´shun) Removal by tearing or pulling apart.

dizygotic (di-zi-got´ik) (DZ) Relating to fraternal (nonidentical) twins (i.e., twins derived from two separate ova).

dizygous (di-zi´gus) Dizygotic.

dizziness (diz´e-nes) An abnormal sensation of unsteadiness characterized by a feeling of movement within the head, without actual motion.

DNA Deoxyribonucleic acid, the molecular basis of heredity, present in chromosomes; it is the largest biologically active molecule presently known and is responsible for the replication of the key substances of life, proteins and nucleic acid; it consists of two long chains of alternate sugar (with attached base) and phosphate groups twisted into a double helix.

antisense DNA See antisense strand, under strand.

genomic DNA The chromosomal DNA sequence (segment) of a gene, including the DNA sequence of coding and noncoding regions. Also applies to DNA that has been isolated directly from cells or chromosomes or cloned copies of all or part of such DNA.

mitochondrial DNA The unique DNA packed in the circular chromosome of mitochondria; it is present in numerous copies in each cell and is maternally transmitted to the offspring due to the abundance of mitochondria in the ovum (the sperm mitochondria are in the sperm's tail, which does not penetrate the ovum during fertilization).

recombinant DNA Biologically active DNA that has been formed by the *in vitro* joining of segments of DNA from different species.

Z DNA A form of DNA that is twisted in the opposite direction from the usual DNA spiral; while its detailed function is not fully known, Z DNA may play a role in controlling gene expression.

doctor (dok´tor) **1.** A person holding a doctorate degree awarded by a college or university in any specialized field, such as anatomy. **2.** A person trained in and licensed to practice the healing arts, as a physician, dentist, or veterinarian. **3.** To treat medically.

dolichocephalic (dol-ĭ-ko-se-fal´ik) Having a disproportionately long head; denoting a skull with a cephalic index of below 80. Also called dolichocephalous.

dolichocephalous (dol-ĭ-ko-sef´ă-lus) See dolichocephalic.

dolichopelvic (dol-ĭ-ko-pel´vik) Having a long narrow pelvis.

doll's eye sign (dŏlz ī sīn) Phenomenon occurring in healthy newborn infants; when the head is turned to one side, the eyes tend not to move with it. Also called Cantelli's sign.

domain (do-mān´) One of the regions of a peptide molecule having a coherent structure or functional significance that distinguishes it from other regions of the same molecule.

dominance (dom´ĭ-nans) The state of being dominant.

cerebral d. The dominance in function of one cerebral hemisphere over the other, with control of speech, analytical processing, and mathematics usually controlled by the left hemisphere and spatial concepts and language related to visual images by the right hemisphere.

dominant (dom´ĭ-nant) **1.** Exerting a controlling influence. **2.** In genetics, a characteristic that is apparent even when the gene for it is carried by only one of a pair of homologous chromosomes (i.e., inherited from only one parent).

donor (do´nor) **1.** One who contributes tissue (e.g., blood for transfusion, organs for transplant, spermatozoa for artificial insemination). **2.** In chemistry, a substance that donates part of itself to another substance (the receptor).

methyl d.'s Compounds that, in living tissue, can supply methyl groups for transfer to other compounds.

dopa, DOPA (do´pă) 3,4-Dihydroxyphenylalanine, a crystalline amino acid; a precursor of norepinephrine, epinephrine, and melanin.

dopamine (do´pă-mēn) The precursor of the hormone norepinephrine; found primarily in the adrenal medulla, brain (in high concentrations), sympathetic ganglia, and carotid body (where it acts as a neurotransmitter).

dopaminergic (do-pă-mēn-er´jik) Relating to the action of dopamine; applied to nerve cells and cell receptors.

dope (dōp) A narcotic or habit-forming drug taken for pleasure or to maintain an addiction.

doping (dōp´ing) Popular term for the practice of taking any substance with the intent of stimulating physical and psychological strength; usually applied to athletes.

Doppler (dŏp´ler) Instrument that emits an ultrasonic beam, which changes in frequency as it reflects (echoes) from moving structures (e.g., blood flow within blood vessels or the heart); useful to diagnose vascular and heart disease.

dornase (dor´nās) See streptodornase.

pancreatic d. A deoxyribonuclease preparation made from beef pancreas, used as an inhalation to reduce the tenacity of thick secretions.

dorsal (dor´sal) **1.** Relating to the back of the body or the posterior part of an anatomic structure. **2.** The upper (as opposed to the plantar) surface of the foot.

dorsiflexion (dor-sĭ-flek´shun) Flexion or turning upward, as of the foot or toes.

dorsolumbar (dor-so-lum´bar) Relating to the back of the body in the region of the lower thoracic and upper lumbar vertebrae.

dorsum (dor´sum) The back or the upper or posterior surface.

d. sellae The portion of the sphenoid bone that forms the posterior boundary of the sella turcica.

dosage (do´sij) **1.** The determination of the proper amount of a dose. **2.** In genetics, the number of copies of a particular gene present in a chromosome.

dose (dōs) (D) A specified quantity of medication to be taken or administered at one time or at stated intervals.

absorbed d. The amount of ionizing radiation absorbed by the tissues at one time.

booster d. A supplementary dose given sometime after the initial dose to maintain immunity.

curative d. The amount of a substance required to cure a disease or correct a deficiency.

daily d. The total amount of a medicine taken within 24 hours.

divided d. Fractional portions of a medicine administered at short intervals so that the full dose is given within a definite period.

erythema d. The minimal safe amount of radiation required to produce redness of the skin

artificial crown
collar
dowel
packed root canal
hematoma

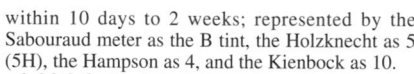

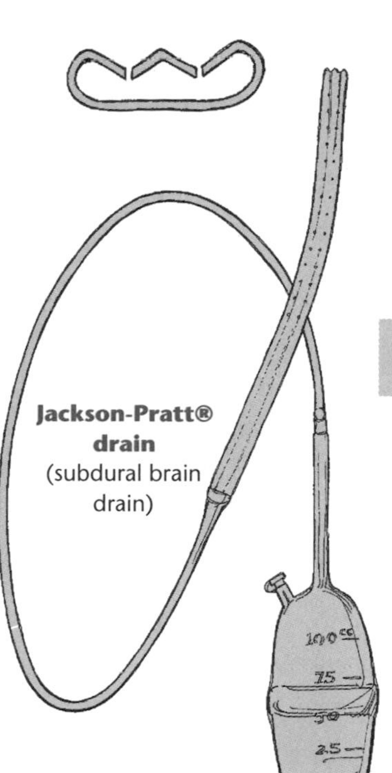

within 10 days to 2 weeks; represented by the Sabouraud meter as the B tint, the Holzknecht as 5 (5H), the Hampson as 4, and the Kienbock as 10.

initial d. A relatively large dose administered at the beginning of a treatment. Also called loading dose.

loading d. See initial dose.

maintenance d. The amount of a medicine administered to keep the patient under the influence of the drug after larger previous amounts.

maximal permissible d. (MPD) The greatest amount of radiation to which a person may be exposed without causing harmful effects.

minimal infective d. (MID) The smallest amount of infectious material that produces disease.

minimal lethal d. (MLD, mld) The smallest amount of a toxin required to kill an experimental animal.

minimal reacting d. (MRD, mrd) The smallest amount of a toxic substance required to cause a reliable level of reaction in a susceptible test animal.

sensitizing d. The first dose of an allergen administered to an experimental animal, which renders the animal susceptible to a hypersensitivity reaction upon a subsequent exposure to the same allergen.

skin d. (SD) The quantity of radiation received on the skin surface.

dosimetrist (do-sim′ĕ-trist) A person who plans and calculates the proper radiation dose necessary for treatment in radiation therapy.

dosimetry (do-sim′ĕ-tre) Determination of correct dosage.

dot (dot) A small mark or spot.

Maurer's d.'s Red-staining granules sometimes seen in the cytoplasm of red blood cells infected with the malarial parasite *Plasmodium falciparum*.

Schuffner's d.'s The characteristic small dark granules seen in red blood cells infected with malarial parasites (particularly *Plasmodium vivax*), giving the cells a dotted or stippled appearance. Also called Schuffner's granules.

dotage (do′taj) The mental weakness common in old age.

doublet (dub′let) **1.** A combination of two similar structures, such as a combination of two joined microtubules in a cilium or flagellum. **2.** A pair of lenses mounted together to form a single lens system.

douche (do͞osh) A stream of liquid, vapor, or gas directed into a cavity of the body, particularly the rinsing of the vagina with a liquid.

dovetail (dŭv′tāl) In dentistry, a fanned-out prepared cavity resembling the tail of a dove, made deliberately to prevent displacement of the restoration.

dowel (dow′l) A pin, usually made of metal, fitted into the root canal of a natural tooth to give support to an artificial crown.

down-regulation (doun-reg-u-la′shun) The rapid development of a resistant-to-treatment or tolerant state resulting from repeated administration of a pharmaceutically or physiologically active agent.

Down syndrome (doun sin′drōm) Congenital defect caused by a chromosomal abnormality; the affected person has three chromosomes (trisomy) instead of the normal two for the pair designated Number 21; marked by various degrees of mental retardation and characteristic physical features such as short flattened skull, epicanthal folds, thickened tongue, broad hands and feet, and other anomalies. Also called mongolism; trisomy 21.

doxorubicin (dok-so-ro͞o′bĭ-sin) An anticancer drug.

dracunculiasis (drā-kung-ku-li′ă-sis) Infection with *Dracunculus medinensis* acquired by drinking contaminated water. Also called guinea worm infection.

Dracunculus (dră-kung′ku-lus) A genus of nematode worms that have a crustacean as an intermediate host.

D. medinensis A skin-infecting worm. Ingested larvae penetrate the stomach or intestinal wall, where they mature and mate; the female develops over a period of one year, then migrates to the skin. Also called guinea worm; Medina worm; serpent worm.

drain (drān) **1.** To draw off the fluid from a bodily cavity, especially to provide for its exit as soon as it is formed. **2.** To discharge. **3.** A device (tube or wick) used to remove fluid from a wound.

cigarette d. A cigarette-shaped gauze wick enclosed in a thin-walled rubber tube.

Jackson-Pratt® d. A flexible silicon rubber suction drain with small intraluminal ridges which prevent collapse of its lumen and with a radiopaque marker incorporated in the side; used to drain the subdural space after removal of a subdural hematoma. Also called subdural brain drain.

Penrose d. Cigarette drain.

stab d. A drain passed through a puncture wound some distance from the operative incision.

subdural brain d. See Jackson-Pratt® drain.

sump d. A drain composed of two tubes, the larger one containing a slender tube which is attached to a suction pump.

drainage (drān′ij) **1.** The continuous withdrawal of fluids from a cavity or wound. **2.** The material withdrawn or discharged.

capillary d. Drainage effected by means of a wick of gauze, strands of hair, or other material.

closed d. Drainage of chest cavity carried out with protection against the entrance of outside air into the cavity.

open d. Drainage of chest through an opening in the chest wall without sealing off the outside air.

postural d. A gravitational method of draining accumulated secretions in the airways of the lungs; the patient lies on an inclined surface with head downward in alternating positions (on the back, side, and abdomen).

tidal d. Drainage of a paralyzed urinary bladder by an irrigation apparatus.

dram (dram) **1.** An avoirdupois unit of weight equal to 27.34 grains or 0.062 ounce. **2.** An apothecary unit of weight equal to 60 grains or 1/8 ounce.

drawer sign (draw′er sīn) A sign elicited from a patient lying on his back with his knee flexed at 90 degrees while the examiner grasps the upper part of the patient's leg with both hands and pulls the head of the tibia; a forward movement indicates rupture of the anterior cruciate ligament; if the tibia can be pushed under the femoral condyle, the posterior cruciate ligament is ruptured. Also called Rocher's sign.

drawsheet (draw′shēt) A narrow sheet stretched crosswise under a patient in bed; used as an aid in moving or turning the patient.

dream (drēm) A series of images experienced during sleep, usually with a definite sense of reality.

wet d. See nocturnal emission, under emission.

dress (dres) To apply a dressing.

dressing (dres′ing) **1.** Material or preparation applied to a wound or lesion to prevent infection or absorb discharges. **2.** The application of such materials.

occlusive d. Dressing that covers and seals a wound completely.

pressure d. A dressing consisting of gauze and abundant resilient material held in place with elastic bandage; thus pressure is applied on the wound to prevent accumulation of fluids.

Dressler's syndrome (dres′lĕrz sin′drōm) See postmyocardial infarction syndrome.

dribble (drĭb′l) **1.** To drool. **2.** To flow in drops (e.g., leakage of urine in urinary incontinence).

drift (drift) Unobtrusive and cumulative changes over time in the genetic composition of a population.

drill (dril) A cutting instrument for boring holes in bones or teeth by rotary motion.

drip (drip) **1.** To fall in drops. **2.** A liquid that falls in drops. **3.** Colloquial expression referring to a discharge.

intravenous d. The continuous intravenous injection of a substance a drop at a time.

postnasal d. Excessive discharge of mucus from the posterior nares.

dromic (drŏmik) Denoting nerve impulses conducted in a normal direction.

dromotropic (drom-o-trop′ik) Affecting

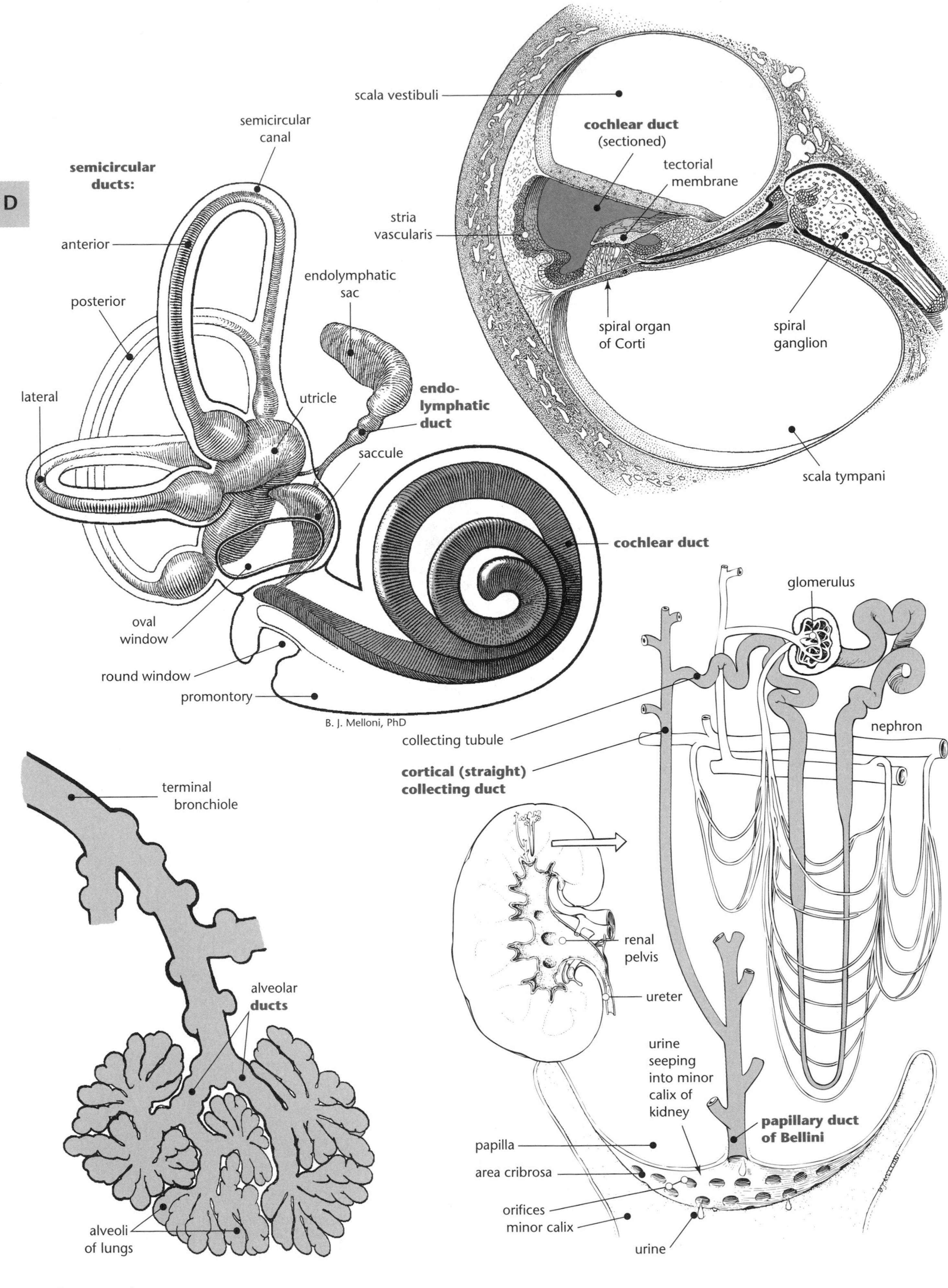
scala vestibuli
semicircular canal
semicircular ducts:
cochlear duct (sectioned)
tectorial membrane
anterior
stria vascularis
endolymphatic sac
posterior
spiral organ of Corti
spiral ganglion
lateral
utricle
endo-lymphatic duct
saccule
scala tympani
cochlear duct
glomerulus
oval window
round window
promontory
B. J. Melloni, PhD
collecting tubule
nephron
cortical (straight) collecting duct
terminal bronchiole
renal pelvis
alveolar ducts
ureter
urine seeping into minor calix of kidney
papillary duct of Bellini
papilla
area cribrosa
orifices
minor calix
alveoli of lungs
urine

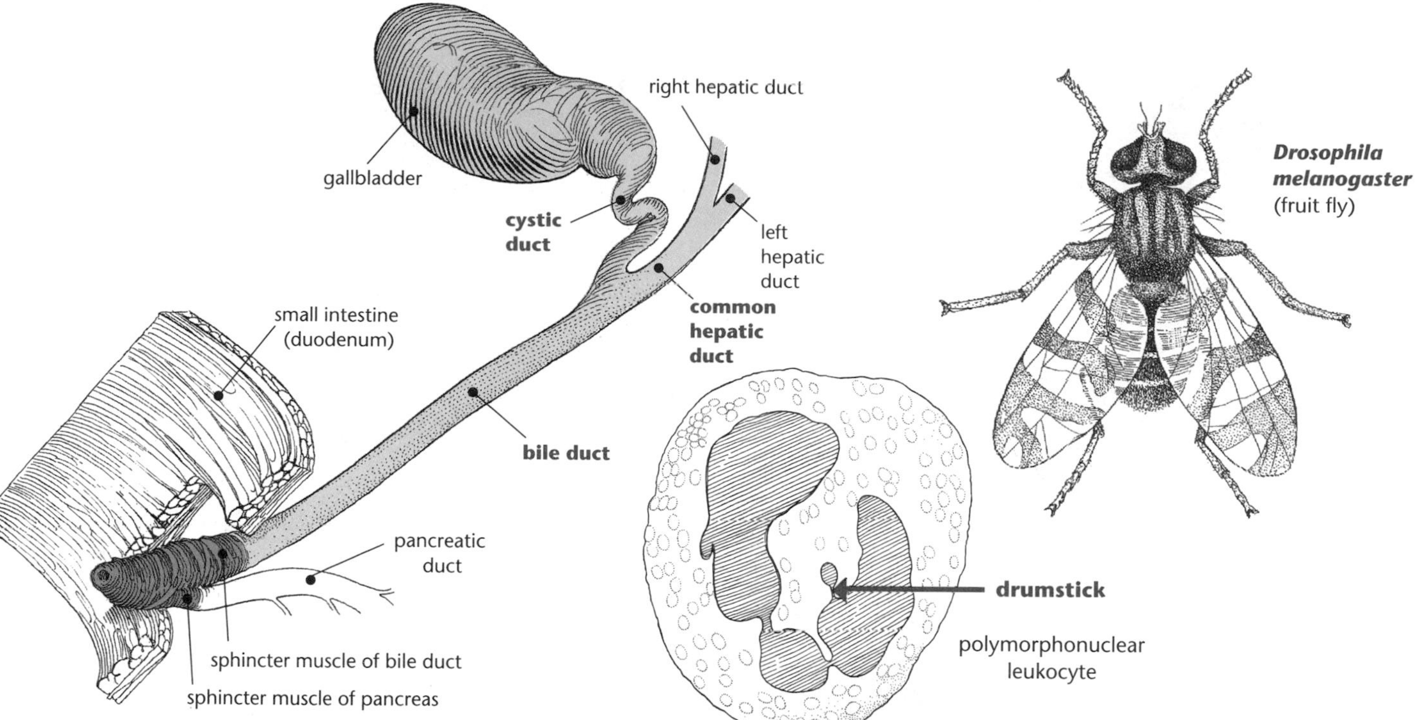

conductivity of nerves.

drop (drŏp) **1.** The smallest possible quantity of a liquid heavy enough to fall in a pear-shaped globule. **2.** To fall in drops or to let fall in drops.

foot d. See footdrop.

hanging d. A drop of a fluid on the undersurface of the object glass examined under the microscope.

toe d. See footdrop.

wrist d. See wristdrop.

droplet (drŏp´let) A very small drop.

lipid d. A spherical body of lipid occurring freely in the cytoplasm of cells; it is not ordinarily membrane bound and is generally surrounded by mitochondria. Also called lipid body; lipid inclusion.

drops (drŏps) Popular name for any liquid medicine administered with a dropper.

eye d. See ophthalmic solution, under solution.

knockout d. Popular name for chloral alcoholate; made by mixing chloral hydrate with any alcoholic drink and given with criminal intent to produce rapid unconsciousness.

dropsy (drŏp´se) Old term for describing generalized fluid-retaining states.

abdominal d. See ascites.

Drosophila (dro-sof´ĭ-lă) A genus of flies containing about 900 species, including the fruit fly (*D. melanogaster*), which is used extensively in genetic studies.

drowsiness (drou´ze-nes) A state of impaired consciousness and marked desire to sleep.

drug (drug) Any chemical substance capable of affecting living processes.

d.'s of abuse A group of substances most frequently taken for the effects they produce on the brain and spinal cord; usually they are the psychoactive drugs (alcohol, sedative-hypnotics, opiates and opioids, stimulants, and hallucinogenics).

backdrop d. A drug of pharmacologic equivalence to another.

crude d. Any medicinal material before refining.

designer d.'s A group of highly potent drugs of abuse produced in clandestine laboratories; they are either analogs of narcotic analgesics and stimulants (e.g., meperidine, fentanyl, and amphetamines) or are variants of phencyclidine (PCP); they are manufactured in such a way that their chemical structures do not fall within the federal laws controlling manufacture and distribution of drugs listed under the Controlled Substances Act.

ethical d. See prescription drug.

generic d. A drug whose name is not protected by a trademark; it may be manufactured by any pharmaceutical company.

nonprescription d. A pharmaceutical that does not require a prescription to be purchased. Commonly called over-the-counter drug.

nonsteroidal anti-inflammatory d. (NSAID) Any of a group of drugs that reduce inflammation, fever, and pain and do not contain such steroids as hydrocortisone or prednisone. Examples include aspirin, ibuprofen, and acetaminophen.

orphan d. See orphan product, under product.

over-the-counter d. See nonprescription drug.

prescription d. One that requires the approval of a licensed health professional to be purchased. Also called ethical drug.

psychedelic d. See hallucinogen.

psychotropic d. Any drug that influences psychic functions, behavior, or experiences, such as chlorpromazine (Thorazine®).

recreational d. See street drug.

stimulant d. Any drug that increases the excitability of the central nervous system (CNS), either as its principal action or as a side or adverse effect.

street d. A drug taken for self-gratification rather than for medical reasons. Also called recreational drug.

sulfa d.'s See sulfonamides.

drug-fast (drug´ fast) Relating to microorganisms that resist the action of a chemical.

drug holidays (drug hŏl´ĭ-dāz) Periods of time during which a chronically medicated patient abstains from taking the medication to allow return of normal function or to maintain sensitivity to the drug.

drug misuse (drug mis-yo͞os´) **1.** The occasional nonmedical use of a drug. **2.** The inappropriate medical use of drugs (i.e., for conditions for which they are not suited). **3.** The appropriate medical use of a drug but in inappropriate dosages. Also see drug abuse, under abuse.

drumstick (drum´stĭk) A minute protrusion from the nucleus of a polymorphonuclear leukocyte, present in about two percent of these cells when two X chromosomes are present, as in normal females (XX) or in patients with Klinefelter's syndrome who have an extra sex chromosome (XXY).

drunkenness (drung´ken-nĭs) Intoxication, usually with alcohol.

drusen (droo´zen) Small, circular, yellow or white hyaline or colloid nodules occurring in the innermost layer of the vascular coat of the eye (choroid); usually they do not interfere with vision.

dry eye syndrome (drī ī sin´drōm) See keratoconjunctivitis sicca, under keratoconjunctivitis.

Dubin-Johnson syndrome (doo´bin-jon´son sin´drōm) Congenital familial defect in the excretory function of the liver resulting in mild jaundice, the presence of large amounts of bilirubin in the blood, and frequently a dark pigment in the liver cells. Also called chronic idiopathic jaundice.

Duchenne-Aran disease (du-shen´ar-an´ dĭ-zēz´) See amyotrophic lateral sclerosis, under sclerosis.

duct (dukt) A tube or channel, usually for conveying the product of a gland to another part of the body.

accessory pancreatic d. The smaller of the two pancreatic ducts that enter the duodenum. Also called duct of Santorini.

Bartholin's d. See major sublingual duct.

Bellini's d. See papillary duct of Bellini.

bile d. Duct formed by union of the common hepatic duct and cystic duct; it conveys bile to the duodenum.

cochlear d. A spirally arranged membranous tube within the cochlea of the inner ear.

collecting d.'s The ducts (within the renal cortex and medulla) conveying fluid from the nephron to the pelvis of the kidney. *Cortical collecting d.*, receives fluid from the connecting tubule of the nephron; *medullary collecting d.*, receives fluid from a number of cortical collecting ducts; *papillary d. of Bellini*, receives fluid from several medullary collecting ducts and empties it into the pelvis of the kidney. Formerly called collecting tubules.

common hepatic d. Duct formed by the union of the right and left hepatic ducts.

cystic d. Duct leading from the gallbladder to the bile duct.

deferent d. The duct that conveys sperm from the epididymis to the ejaculatory duct. Also called vas deferens; ductus deferens; spermatic duct.

ejaculatory d. Duct formed by the union of the deferent duct (vas deferens) and the excretory duct of the seminal vesicle; it opens into the prostatic urethra.

endolymphatic d. A duct in the labyrinth of the inner ear that connects the endolymphatic sac with the utricle and saccule.

excretory d. of the seminal vesicle The duct that drains the seminal vesicle and leads to the ejaculatory duct.

lactiferous d. One of about eighteen ducts that drain milk from the lobes of the mammary gland and open at the nipple. Also called milk duct.

major sublinqual d. Duct that drains the sublingual salivary gland and opens at the sublingual papilla in the floor of the mouth. Also called Bartholin's duct.

mesonephric d. Either of the two embryonic ducts that develop in the male into the deferent duct; in the female it disappears. Also called wolffian duct.

milk d. See lactiferous duct.

mullerian d. See paramesonephric duct.

nasolacrimal d. A duct conveying tears from the lacrimal sac to the nasal cavity.

omphalomesenteric d. See yolk stalk, under stalk.

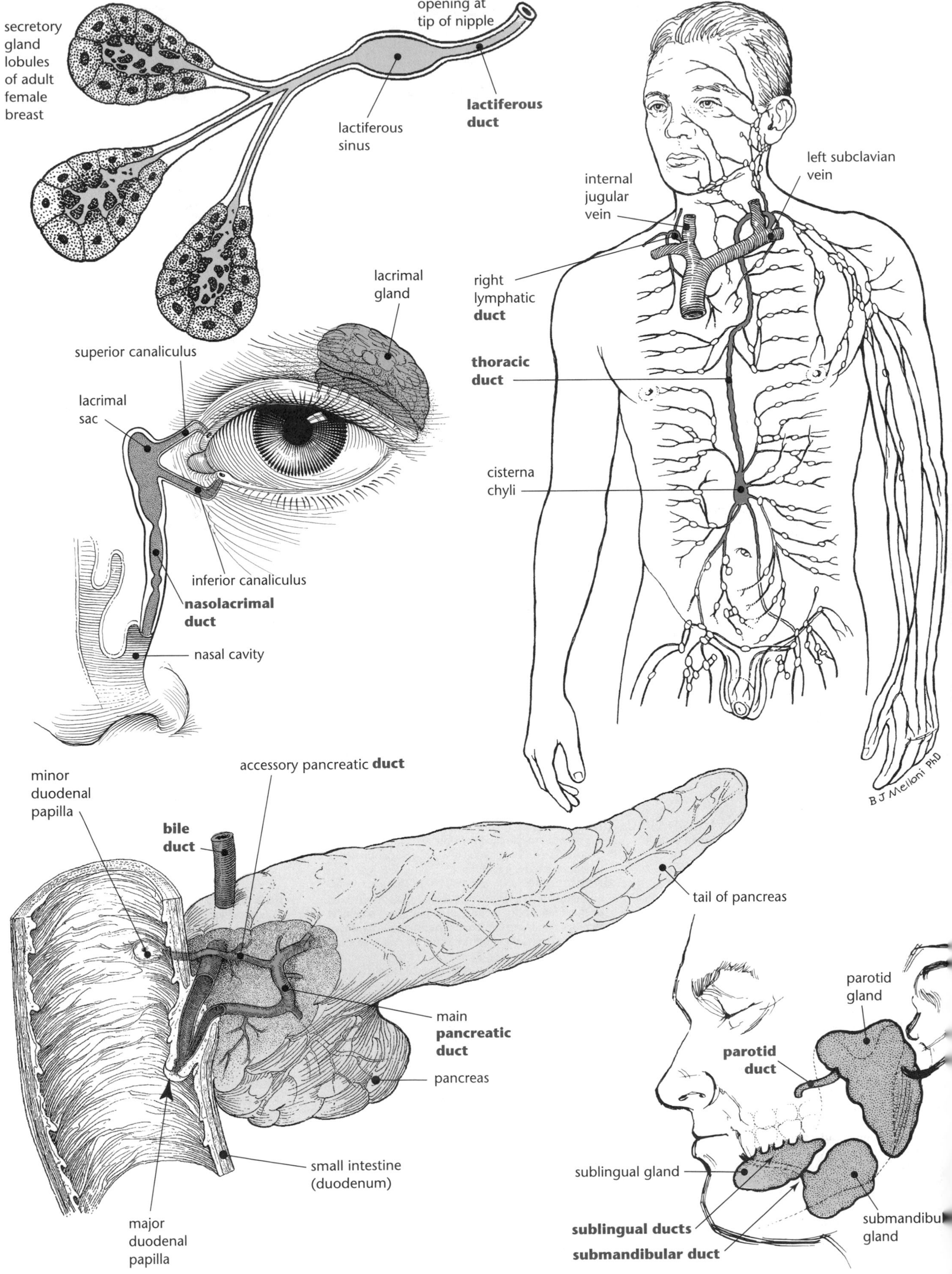
secretory gland lobules of adult female breast
opening at tip of nipple
lactiferous sinus
lactiferous duct
internal jugular vein
left subclavian vein
right lymphatic duct
thoracic duct
cisterna chyli
lacrimal gland
superior canaliculus
lacrimal sac
inferior canaliculus
nasolacrimal duct
nasal cavity
B J Melloni PhD
minor duodenal papilla
accessory pancreatic duct
bile duct
tail of pancreas
main pancreatic duct
pancreas
small intestine (duodenum)
major duodenal papilla
parotid gland
parotid duct
sublingual gland
sublingual ducts
submandibular duct
submandibu
gland

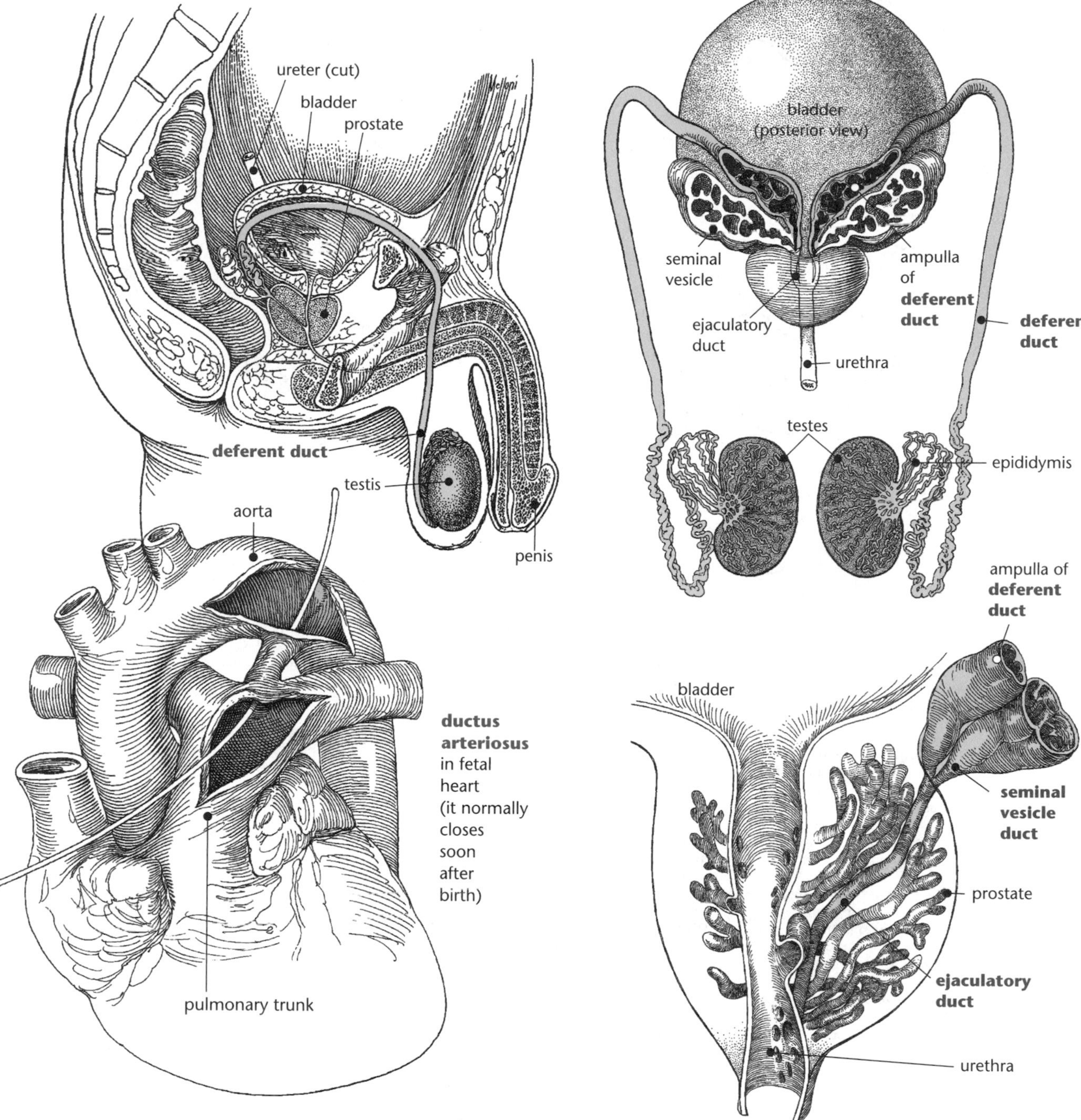

pancreatic d. The main excretory duct of the pancreas; it opens into the duodenum.

papillary d. of Bellini One of numerous ducts in the inner part of the renal medulla, formed by the junctions of several medullary collecting ducts. Also called Bellini's duct.

paramesonephric d. Either of the two embryonic ducts that develop, in the female, into the uterine tubes, vagina, and uterus; it disappears in the male. Also called mullerian duct.

paraurethral d. One of several ducts of the paraurethral (Skene's) glands. Also called Schüler's duct.

parotid d. The duct that conveys saliva from the parotid gland to the mouth at the level of the upper second molar.

perilymphatic d. A minute canal connecting the perilymphatic space of the cochlea with the subarachnoid space.

d. of Santorini See accessory pancreatic duct.

Schüler's d. See paraurethral duct.

semicircular d. One of three membranous tubes within the semicircular canal of the internal ear; it contributes to balance and orientation.

spermatic d. See deferent duct.

sublingual d.'s A group of 8 to 20 excretory channels conveying saliva from the sublingual gland to the floor of the mouth; most are small channels that open on the summit of the sublingual fold; those from the anterior part of the gland occasionally join to form a larger channel that opens at or near the sublingual papilla adjacent to the frenulum of the tongue.

submandibular d. A duct about 5 cm long that drains the submandibular gland and opens at the tip of the sublingual papilla on the floor of the mouth adjacent to the frenulum of the tongue. Also called Wharton's duct.

sudoriferous d. The duct leading from the body of a sweat gland to the surface of the skin. Also called sweat duct.

sweat d. See sudoriferous duct.

thoracic d. The largest lymphatic channel in the body; it conveys lymph into the left subclavian vein.

thyroglossal d. An embryonic duct extending along the midline of the neck; its lower part gives rise to the isthmus of the thyroid gland; normally the remainder disappears but occasionally it persists in the adult and forms a cyst or a fistula.

utriculosaccular d. A duct located in the inner ear extending from the utricle and joining the endolymphatic duct.

venous d. In the fetus, the continuation of the umbilical vein through the liver to the inferior vena cava; it obliterates after birth, becoming the ligamentum venosum.

vitelline d. See yolk stalk, under stalk.

Wharton's d. See submandibular duct.

wolffian d. See mesonephric duct.

ductile (duk´til) Capable of being drawn out into a wire or molded into a new shape.

duction (duk´shun) The movement of an eye by the extrinsic muscles.

ductus (duk´tus), *pl.* **duc´tus** Latin for duct, a tubular structure.

d. arteriosus A fetal communicating channel between the left pulmonary artery, at its base, and the beginning of the descending aorta; it normally obliterates a few days after birth, remaining in the adult as a fibrous structure (ligamentum arteriosum).

d. deferens See deferent duct, under duct.

patent d. arteriosus (PDA) A ductus arteriosus that remains open (patent), with blood flowing abnormally from the aorta to the pulmonary artery.

Duhring's disease (doo´ringz dĭ-zēz´) See dermatitis herpetiformis, under dermatitis.

dull (dul) **1.** Not sharp; said of an instrument, pain, or sound. **2.** Lacking mental alertness.

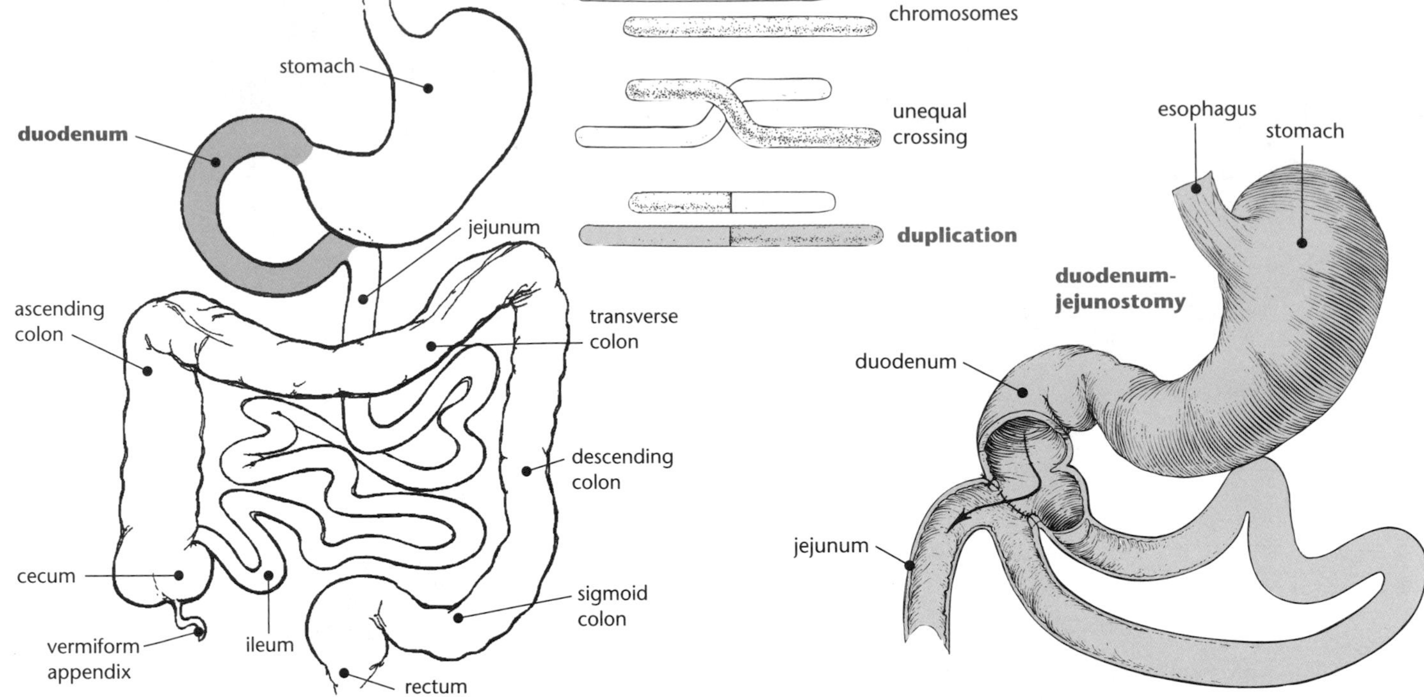

dullness, dulness (dul′nĭs) The quality of sound elicited by percussion over a solid part or organ, characterized by very little resonance.
shifting d. Dull sound produced by percussion, usually of the abdominal cavity, that shifts location as the patient is moved; indicative of the presence of free fluid.
dumping syndrome (dump′ing sin′drōm) Symptoms occurring within 30 minutes after the end of a meal, including nausea, warmth, sweating, palpitation, pallor, headache, diarrhea, pain in the upper abdomen, and weakness; caused by excessively rapid emptying of the stomach, usually following loss of the pylorus in stomach resection. Also called postgastrectomy syndrome.
duodenal (doo′o-dē-nal) Relating to the duodenum.
duodenectomy (doo-o-dĕ-nek′tŏ-me) Surgical removal of the duodenal portion of the small intestine, total or partial.
duodenitis (doo-o-de-nī-tis) Inflammation of the duodenal portion of the small intestine.
duodenocholecystostomy (doo-o-de-no-ko-le-sis-tos′tŏ-me) Surgical formation of a passage between the gallbladder and the duodenum.
duodenocholedochotomy (doo-o-de-no-ko-led-o-kot′ŏ-me) Surgical incision into the bile duct and the adjoining portion of the duodenum.
duodenoenterostomy (doo-o-de-no-en-ter-os′tŏ-me) Surgical formation of a passage between the duodenum and another part of the small intestine.
duodenojejunostomy (doo-o-de-no-jĕ-joo-nos′tŏ-me) Surgical formation of a passage between the duodenum and the jejunum.
duodenolysis (doo-o-de-nol′ĭ-sis) The operation of freeing the duodenum from adhesions.
duodenorrhaphy (doo-o-de-nor′ă-fe) Suturing of the duodenum.
duodenoscopy (doo-o-de-nos′kŏ-pe) Visual observation of the interior of the duodenum by means of an endoscope.
duodenostomy (doo-o-de-nos′tŏ-me) Surgical formation of an orifice or passage into the duodenum.
duodenotomy (doo-o-de-not′ŏ-me) Surgical incision into the duodenum.
duodenum (du-o-de′num) The first portion of the small intestine, extending from the lower end of the stomach to the jejunum and shaped like a horseshoe around the head of the pancreas; the term comes from the Latin *duodeni* (twelve) because it measures about 12 fingerbreadths (25-30 cm) in length.
duplication (doo-plĭ-ka′shun) In genetics, a chromosome aberration consisting of the presence of an extra piece of chromosome, usually originated by unequal exchange of fragments between homologous chromosomes; the other chromosome has a segment missing (deletion).
dura (doo′ră) See dura mater.
dural (doo′ral) Relating to the dura mater.
dura mater (doo′ră ma′ter) A tough, fibrous, whitish membrane; the outermost of the three membranes covering the brain and spinal cord. Also called dura.
dwarf (dwarf) An abnormally small person. Also called nanus; person of short stature.
dwarfism (dwarf′iz-m) In a broad sense, failure to achieve full growth potential; may be induced by ecological factors (e.g., dietary intake, systemic disease), by genetic factors, or by endocrine factors; lack of height is only one of the resulting features.
achondroplastic d. A form caused by congenital abnormality in the process of ossification of cartilage; affected individuals have a relatively elongated trunk, short extremities, and a large head.
pituitary d. Dwarfism accompanied by sexual infantilism and decreased function of the thyroid and adrenal glands; caused by lesions of the anterior portion of the pituitary gland early in childhood.
primordial d. Inadequate term designating a condition characterized by insufficient growth with normal functional development.
D&X Dilatation and extraction. See dilatation and evacuation.
dyad (di′ad) **1.** A pair. **2.** A bivalent element or radical. **3.** One pair of chromosomes after the disjunction of a tetrad at the first meiotic division.
dye (dī) Any coloring substance.
dynamics (di-nam′iks) **1.** The science of the relationship between motion and the forces causing it. **2.** The emotional forces determining patterns of behavior.
dynamograph (di-nam-′o-graf) See ergograph.
dynamometer (di-nă-mom′ĕ-ter) See ergometer.
dyne (dīn) A unit of force equal to the force required to give a body of 1 g an acceleration of 1 cm per second squared.
dysacusis, dysacusia (dis-ă-koo′sis, dis-ă-koo′ze-ă) **1.** Defect of hearing marked by inability to discriminate between sounds; distinguished from lack of sensitivity to sound. **2.** Pain in the ear caused by sound.
dysarthria (dis-ar′thre-ă) Impairment of ability to produce clear speech caused by muscular dysfunction secondary to central or peripheral nervous system disease.
dysarthrosis (dis-ar-thro′sis) **1.** Malformation of a joint. **2.** Impairment of articulation. **3.** A false joint.
dysautonomia (dis-aw-to-no′me-ă) Dysfunction of the autonomic nervous system.
familial d. Congenital nerve disorder affecting infants and children; characterized by indifference to pain, inability to shed tears, emotional instability, drooling, excessive sweating, and poor motor control. Also called Riley-Day syndrome.
dysbarism (dis′bar-iz-m) General term denoting physiologic changes resulting from changes in barometric pressure, such as the effects of rapid decompression.
dysbasia (dis-ba′zhă) Difficult or distorted walking; it may be organically or psychically determined.
dyscephaly (dis-sef′ă-le) Malformation of the head and face.
dyschezia (dis-ke′zhă) Difficult or painful defecation.
dyschiria (dis-ki′re-ă) Disorder in which the individual is unable to tell which side of his body has been touched.
dyschondrogenesis (dis-kon-dro-jen′ĕ-sis) Defective development of cartilage.
dyschondroplasia (dis-kon-dro-pla′zhă) See enchondromatosis.
dyschromia (dis-kro′me-ă) Any abnormality in the pigmentation (color) of the skin or hair.
dyscoria (dis-kor′e-ă) Irregularly shaped pupil.
dyscrasia (dis-kra′zhă) A general morbid condition of the body.
bleeding d. A pathologic condition due to abnormal hemostasis (e.g., hemophilia).
plasma cell d.'s A group of disorders (e.g., multiple myeloma, primary amyloidosis) characterized by proliferation of a single clone of immunoglobulin-secreting cells and increased levels of a single homogeneous immunoglobulin in serum or urine. Also called monoclonal gammopathy.
dysdiadochokinesia (dis-di-ad-ŏ-ko-ki-ne′zhă) Inability to make alternating movements in rapid succession, such as extending and flexing a limb.
dysentery (dis′en-ter-e) Disease marked by frequent watery stools containing blood and mucus, attended by abdominal pain, dehydration, and sometimes fever.
amebic d. Dysentery due to infection with *Entamoeba histolytica*, which may cause ulceration of the colon; symptoms vary from slight abdominal discomfort and diarrhea alternating with constipation to profuse bleeding and discharge of mucus and pus.
bacillary d. Dysentery caused by bacteria of the genus *Shigella*.
dyserethism (dis-er′e-thiz-m) A slow response to stimuli.
dysergia (dis-er′jă) Motor incoordination.
dysesthesia (dis-es-the′zha) Painful or disagreeable sensation produced by ordinary stimuli.
dysfunction (dis-funk′shun) Abnormal or impaired functioning of an organ or bodily system.
erectile d. (ED) Term suggested as more precise than impotence for describing the inability to attain

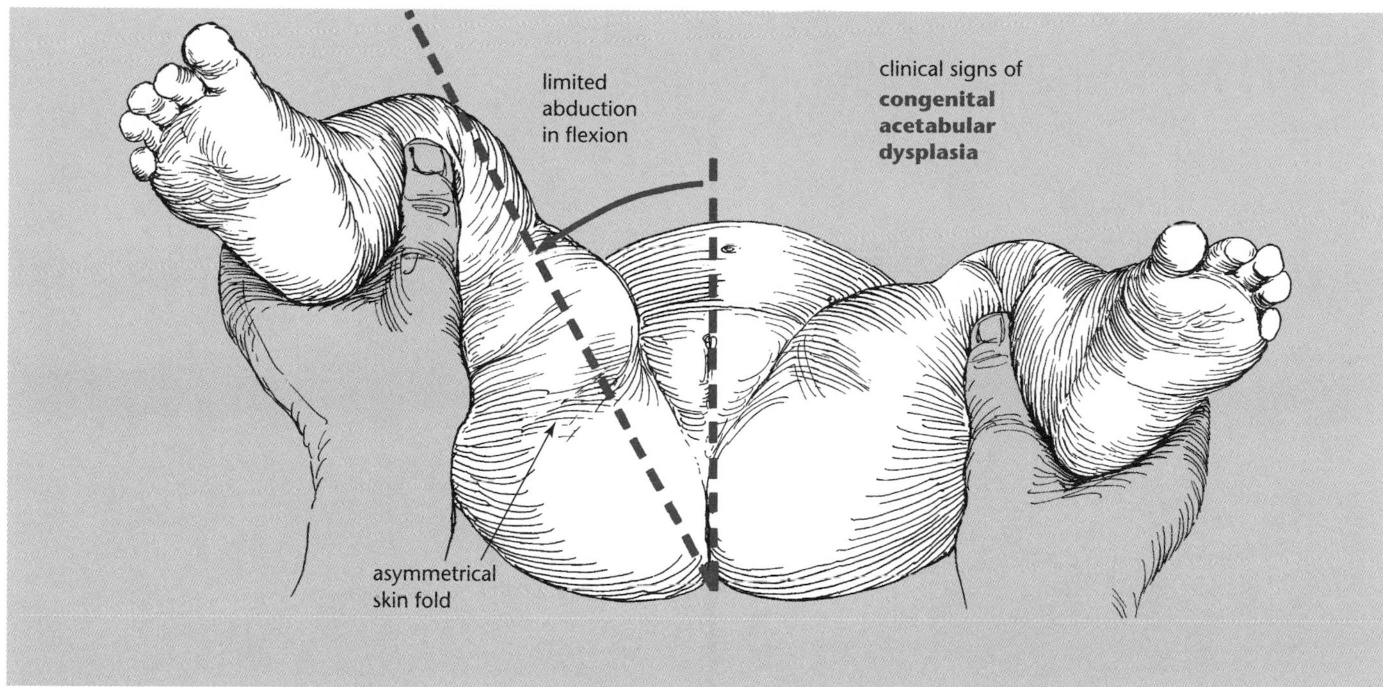

and/or maintain erection of the penis sufficient for satisfactory sexual intercourse; it is considered part of the overall multifaceted process of male sexual function; causes may be organic (from the nervous or vascular systems) or psychological, but they most commonly appear to derive from problems in all three areas acting in concert; assessment and treatment of the dysfunction may require a multidisciplinary approach. Also called impotence.

minimal brain d. (MBD) See attention-deficit hyperactivity disorder, under disorder.

dysgammaglobulinemia (dis-gam-ă-glob-u-lin-e´me-ă) Disorders or abnormalities of gamma globulins in the blood serum.

dysgenic (dis-jen´ik) Relating to dysgenesis.

dysgenesis (dis-jen´ĕ-sis) The study of the factors causing defective or deficient embryonic development.

gonadal d. Defective development of ovaries or testes.

seminiferous tubule d. Underdevelopment of male genital organs, overdevelopment of breasts, reduced sperm production, and reduced androgen secretion; characteristics constantly present in the Klinefelter's syndrome.

dysgerminoma (dis-jer-mĭ-no´mă) A rare malignant ovarian tumor composed of undifferentiated germinal epithelium; the counterpart of seminoma of the testis. Also called ovarian seminoma.

dysgeusia (dis-goo´zha) A general term describing any distortion of taste perception.

dysgnathia (dis-na´the-ă) Any abnormality of the maxilla or mandible.

dysgnosia (dis-no´zha) Any disorder of the intellect.

dysgraphia (dis-graf´e-ă) Difficulty in writing, usually due to ataxia, tremor, or motor neurosis.

dyshemopoiesis (dis-he-mo-poi-e´sis) Defective or imperfect blood formation.

dyshidrosis, dysidrosis (dis-hi-dro´sis, dis-id-ro´sis) **1.** An abnormality of sweat production. **2.** A recurrent eruption of blisters primarily on the hands and feet, accompanied by intense itching. Also called pompholyx.

trichophytic d. Tinea pedis.

dyskeratoma (dis-ker-ă-to´mă) Skin tumor containing cells that display abnormal keratinization.

warty d. A benign skin tumor with a central keratin plug, occurring on the scalp, face, or neck.

dyskinesia (dis-ki-ne´zhă) Any abnormality of voluntary movements.

dyslalia (dis-la´le-ă) Impairment of speech due to defective speech organs.

dyslexia (dis-lek´se-ă) Difficulty in reading due to impaired ability to identify and understand written symbols, and a tendency to reverse certain letters and words.

dyslogia (dis-lo´je-ă) Impairment of the thought processes and speech.

dysmegalopsia (dis-meg-ă-lop´se-ă) Abnormal visual perception in which objects appear larger than they are.

dysmelia (dis-me´le-ă) Congenital absence of a portion of one or more limbs.

dysmenorrhea (dis-men-o-re´ă) Painful menstrual periods. Popularly called menstrual cramps; cramps.

functional d. See primary dysmenorrhea.

primary d. Dysmenorrhea occurring in the absence of organic disease. Also called functional dysmenorrhea.

secondary d. Dysmenorrhea caused by inflammation, tumor, infection, or anatomic factors.

dysmetria (dis-me´tre-ă) Inability to stop a muscular movement at a desired point.

dysmorphism (dis-mor´fiz-m) Abnormality of shape.

dysontogenesis (dis-on-to-jen´e-sis) Abnormal development.

dysosmia (dis-oz´me-ă) A general term describing any distortion of smell perception.

dysostosis (dis-os-to´sis) Defective bone formation.

cleidocranial d. Autosomal dominant inheritance marked by partial or complete absence of the collarbones (clavicles) and delay in ossification of the skull, often with underdeveloped facial bones, and defective teeth.

craniofacial d. An autosomal dominant inheritance characterized by a wide skull, widely separated eyes, undersized upper jaw, beaked nose, and exophthalmos. Also called Crouzon's disease.

mandibulofacial d. Hereditary abnormalities of the palpebral fissures, mandible and zygomatic bones, and lower lids, with malposition and malocclusion of teeth, low-set malformed ears, and high or cleft palate; called Franceschetti's syndrome when complete, and Treacher Collins' syndrome when partial.

d. multiplex See Hurler's syndrome.

dyspareunia (dis-pă-roo´ne-ă) Painful intercourse.

dyspepsia (dis-pep´se-ă) Indigestion.

dysphagia (dis-fa´je-ă) Difficulty in swallowing.

d. lusoria Dysphagia due to compression of the esophagus by a congenital abnormality of a blood vessel, usually the right subclavian artery when it abnormally comes off the thoracic aorta.

sideropenic d. See Plummer-Vinson syndrome.

dysphasia (dis-fa´zha) Loss of ability to produce or comprehend spoken or written language, or both, due to disease of the brain.

dysphonia (dis-fo´ne-ă) A disturbance or impairment of voice.

abductor spasmodic d. Difficulty in speaking caused by forceful, involuntary separation of the vocal folds, which produces breathy speech interruptions.

adductor spasmodic d. Difficulty in speaking caused by forceful, involuntary approximation of the vocal folds, which interrupts the air stream and produces a strained, hoarse, choppy voice.

dysphoria (dis-for´e-ă) An emotional state characterized by depression, restlessness, and malaise, usually accompanied by poor self-esteem.

dysplasia (dis-pla´zhă) **1.** In pathology, abnormality of cell growth in which some cells in a tissue have some of the characteristics of malignancy but not enough for a diagnosis of an early cancer; unlike cancer (which is irreversible), dysplastic tissue may sometimes reverse spontaneously to normal. **2.** In embryology, abnormal or altered development of a body part.

cervical d. Dysplasia involving the superficial layer (epithelium) of the uterine cervix; it is considered a precancerous lesion. Depending on the thickness of the involved epithelium, it is designated mild (CIN I), moderate (CIN II), or severe (CIN III/ carcinoma *in situ*). The human papilloma virus (HPV) has been implicated as a causative agent, especially types 16, 18, and 31. Also called cervical intraepithelial neoplasia (CIN).

chondroectodermal d. An inherited disorder marked by short extremities with normal trunk, polydactyly, and abnormal development of teeth and nails; frequently associated with congenital heart defects. Also called Ellis-van Creveld syndrome.

congenital acetabular d. Congenital dislocation of the hip; a complete or partial displacement of the femoral head out of the acetabulum; not related to trauma or to other musculoskeletal disease.

dentin d. Hereditary abnormality of dentin formation marked by disarrangement of dentin tubules by masses of collagenous matrix, poorly developed tooth roots, and absence of pulp canals and chambers.

ectodermal d. General term denoting abnormal development of tissues derived from ectoderm.

fibromuscular d. Nonatherosclerotic disease of arteries, especially the renal arteries, causing constriction of the vessels.

fibrous d. of bone Condition in which the marrow of one or more bones is replaced by fibrous tissue.

hereditary renal-retinal d. Inherited disorder marked by retinitis pigmentosa, diabetes insipidus,

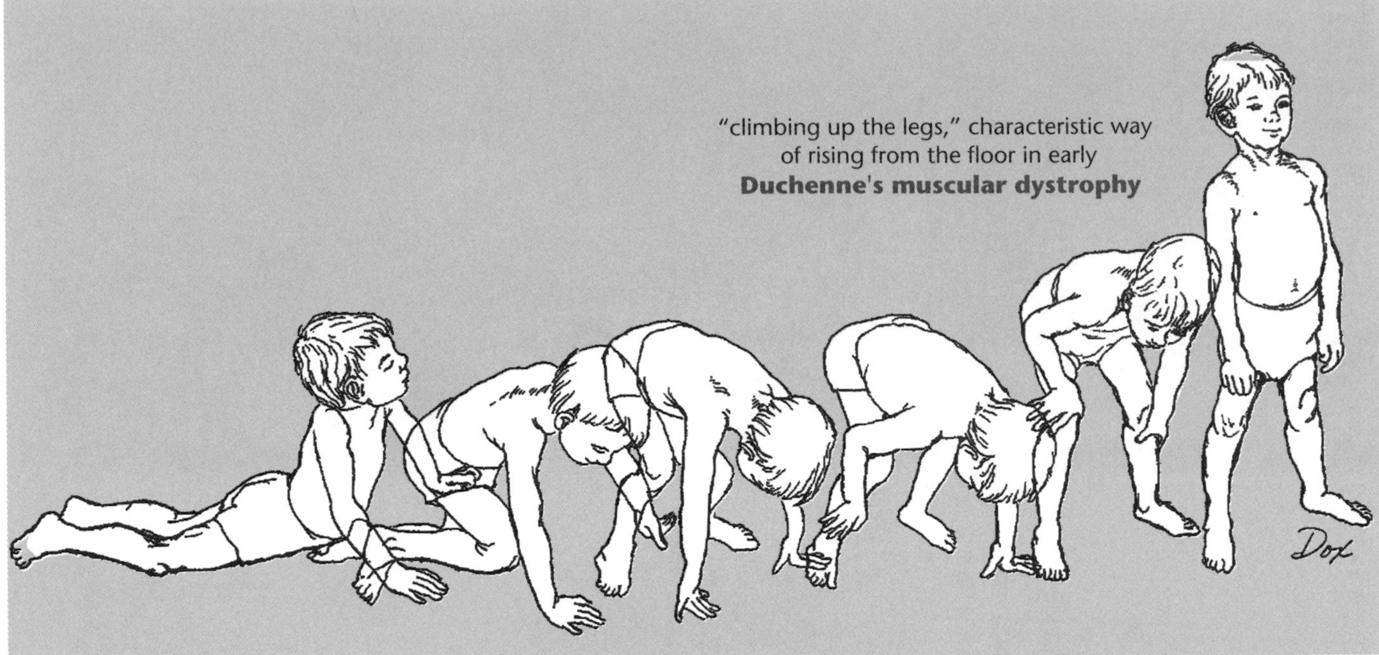
"climbing up the legs," characteristic way
of rising from the floor in early
Duchenne's muscular dystrophy
Dox

and progressive uremia.

mammary d. See fibrocystic change of breast, under change.

polyostotic fibrous d. The occurrence of fibrous dysplasia in several bones, usually on one side of the body.

vulvar d. Dysplasia of the vulva characterized as multicentric mucosal lesions; graded as mild (VIN I), moderate (VIN II), or severe (VIN III), depending on the degree of involvement; it is associated with the presence of human papilloma virus (HPV), especially types 16 and 18 (in 80-90% of cases). Also called vulvar intraepithelial neoplasia (VIN). See also Bowen's disease.

dysplastic (dis-plas´tik) Relating to or marked by abnormality of development.

dyspnea (disp´ne-ă) Difficult or labored breathing usually associated with serious disease of the heart or lungs.

cardiac d. Dyspnea originating from a heart condition.

exertional d. Excessive shortness of breath brought about by physical effort.

paroxysmal nocturnal d. (PND) Acute dyspnea occurring suddenly at night, caused by pulmonary congestion and edema.

dyspneic (disp-ne´ik) Relating to dyspnea.

dyspraxia (dis-prak´se-ă) Impaired ability to perform learned movements, usually due to a brain lesion.

dysproteinemia (dis-pro-tēn-e ´me-ă) Abnormality in blood proteins.

dysrhythmia (dis-rith´me-ă) A disturbance of the heart rhythm.

dyssomnia (dis-som´ne-ă) Any of a group of sleep disorders included in the International Classification of Sleep Disorders, designated as *intrinsic* (e.g., narcolepsy, sleep apnea, restless leg syndrome), *extrinsic* (e.g., altitude insomnia, drug-or-alcohol-dependent sleep disorders), and *circadian rhythm* sleep disorder (e.g., shift-work sleep disorder, jet-lag syndrome).

dysstasia (dis-sta´zhă) Difficulty in standing.

dyssynergia, dyssynergy (dis-sin-er´je-ă, dis-sin-er´je) Disturbance of muscular coordination.

detrusor-sphincter d. Disturbance of the normal coordination between bladder muscles during voiding efforts in which spasm of the urinary sphincter occurs simultaneously with detrusor muscle contraction.

dysthymia (dis-thi´me-ă) Chronic mild depression.

dystocia (dis-to´se-ă) Difficult labor.

fetal d. Difficult labor due to abnormalities of position or size of the fetus.

maternal d. Difficult labor due to uterine inertia, tumors, or deformities of the birth canal.

dystonia (dis-to´ne-ă) Abnormal tonicity of musculature.

cervical d. Asymmetric muscle spasms of the neck, causing turning or tilting movements and sustained abnormal postures of the head; may be accompanied by moderate head tremor and musculoskeletal pain. Also called spasmodic torticollis.

dystopia (dis-to´pe-ă) Malposition.

dystopic (dis-top´ik) Out of place.

dystrophin (dis´trŏ-fin) Protein present in normal muscle, bound to the membrane of the muscle; it helps to maintain the integrity of the muscle fiber; in its absence, the muscle fiber degenerates. Dystrophin is absent in people afflicted with Duchenne's muscular dystrophy.

dystrophy (dis´tro-fe) Disorder caused by faulty nutrition or by lesions of the pituitary gland and/or brain.

adiposogenital d. Condition caused by lesions of the pituitary and hypothalamus, marked by increased body fat, especially about the abdomen, hips, and thighs, with underdeveloped genital organs and hair loss; usually manifested during puberty and often mistaken for obesity. Also called Fröhlich's syndrome.

Becker's muscular d. (BMD) Genetic disorder similar to Duchenne's muscular dystrophy but much milder, occurring later in childhood and progressing at a much slower rate; some patients may remain ambulatory for many years; caused by mutations in the structural gene for the protein dystrophin; an X-linked recessive inheritance.

cerebrooculorenal d. See oculocerebrorenal syndrome.

childhood muscular d. See Duchenne's muscular dystrophy.

Duchenne's muscular d. (DMD) Genetic disorder occurring as an X-linked recessive inheritance and affecting males almost exclusively; characterized by dystrophin deficiency and progressive muscle weakness starting in the pelvic girdle and spreading rapidly, a swaying gait, frequent falls, and difficulty arising from the floor (the child usually "climbs up his legs"); deposits of fibrofatty tissue replace muscle fibers and may occupy a greater volume than the normal muscle (pseudohypertrophy); may also involve the heart muscle; manifestations of the disorder begin between three and five years of age and it is usually fatal by the third decade. The defective gene is in the short arm of the X chromosome. Also called childhood muscular dystrophy; pseudohypertrophic muscular dystrophy; Duchenne's paralysis.

Fuch's endothelial d. An eye disorder secondary to spontaneous loss of endothelium of the central cornea; characterized by formation of epithelial blisters, reduced vision, and pain.

muscular d. (MD) Any of several genetic disorders that are characterized primarily by progressive deterioration of muscle fibers.

myotonic d. Genetic disorder, occurring as an autosomal dominant inheritance (genetic defect on chromosome 19); it typically becomes evident in the second to third decades of life with varying degrees of muscular involvement and severity; symptoms include stiffness and eventual atrophy of muscles, especially of the face and neck, associated with slurred speech and cataracts. Also called myotonia atrophica.

pseudohypertrophic muscular d. See Duchenne's muscular dystrophy.

reflex sympathetic d. (RSD) Disturbance of the sympathetic nervous system affecting an extremity, marked by intense burning pain, redness or pallor, skin changes, and rapid demineralization of bone; frequently follows an injury (e.g., bone fracture, injury to nerves or blood vessels). Also called shoulder-hand syndrome; sympathetic reflex dystrophy.

dysuria (dis-u´re-ă) Difficulty or pain in urination.

E

ear (ēr) The compound organ of hearing and equilibrium; it is sensitive to sound waves, to the effects of gravity, and to motion; consists of the *external e.*, which includes the auricle (pinna) and the external auditory canal; the *middle e.*, which consists of the tympanic chamber and the movable ossicles within; and the *inner e.*, which includes the semicircular canals, vestibule, and cochlea.
aviator's e. See barotitis media.
cauliflower e. Boxer's ear, a thickened deformed ear caused by injury to the tissues due to repeated blows.
darwinian e. An ear in which the upper border of the auricle is flat with a sharp edge.
dog e. Redundant skin left at one end of a sutured incision due to mismatching of cut edges during suturing of the wound.
glue e. Colloquialism for otitis media with thick fluid in the middle ear chamber, causing marked conductive hearing loss.
swimmer's e. Infection of the auditory canal (otitis externa) associated with swimming; may be fungal or bacterial in nature.
earache (ēr′āk) Pain in the ear. Also called otalgia.
eardrum (ēr′drum) See tympanic membrane, under membrane.
earth (erth) **1.** Soil. **2.** An amorphous pulverizable mineral. **3.** A metallic oxide characterized by a high melting point (e.g., alumina).
alkaline e. Any oxide of the elements in the family to which calcium and magnesium belong.
diatomaceous e. Purified siliceous earth composed mainly of shell wall remains of minute aquatic unicellular diatoms; used as an inert filler in many dental materials and as a mild abrasive and polishing agent. Also called infusorial earth.
infusorial e. Diatomaceous earth.
rare e. Any of those rare elements with atomic numbers from 57 to 71 that closely resemble one another chemically.
earth-eating (erth-e′ting) See geophagia.
earwax (ēr′waks) See cerumen.
Eaton-Lambert syndrome (e′ton-lam′bert sin′drōm) Syndrome usually associated with tumor, especially small carcinoma of the lung; marked by progressive muscular weakness and pain in the limbs with peculiarly slow movements and curare sensitivity; electromyography is diagnostic.
ebonation (e-bo-na′shun) The removal of loose bone chips after an injury.
ebullism (eb′u-liz-m) Formation of water vapor in the tissues due to extreme reduction in barometric pressure occurring at altitudes above 60,000 feet.
ebur (e′bur) Resembling ivory.
eburnation (e-bur-na′shun) The transformation of bone into a dense ivory-like substance.
eccentric (ek-sen′trik) **1.** Situated away from the center. **2.** Deviating from the established norm. **3.** One who deviates markedly from normal or conventional conduct or speech; abnormal in emotional reactions and in general behavior, with no intellectual defect; an erratic person.
eccentrochondroplasia (ek-sen-tro-kon-dro-pla′zhă) Abnormal ossification, especially in long bones, in which osseous tissue is formed from areas other than the epiphysial cartilage.
ecchondroma (ek-kon-dro′mă) A benign cartilaginous tumor; an outgrowth of normally situated cartilage projecting through the shaft of a bone. Also called ecchondrosis.
ecchondrosis (ek-kon-dro′sis) See ecchondroma.
ecchymoma (ek-ĭ-mo′mă) A slight blood-containing swelling due to a bruise.
ecchymosis (ek-ĭ-mo′sis), *pl.* **ecchymo′ses** A bruise; a "black and blue spot" on the skin caused by escape of blood within the skin from injured vessels.
e. of eyelid Injury popularly called black eye.
periumbilical e. See Cullen's sign.
ecchymotic (ek-ĭ-mot′ik) Relating to an ecchymosis.
eccrine (ek′rin) See exocrine.
eccrinology (ek-ri-nol′o-je) The study of secretions and excretions.
eccrisis (ek′rĭ-sis) **1.** The excretion of waste products. **2.** Any waste product.

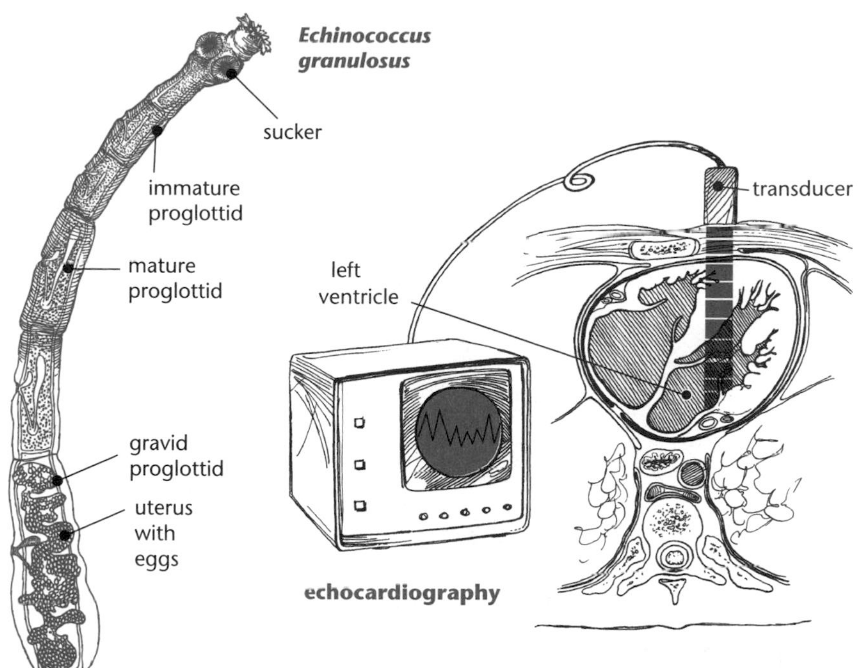

eccritic (ek-rit′ik) Anything that promotes excretion of waste products.
eccyesis (ek-si-e′sis) See ectopic pregnancy, under pregnancy.
ecdemic (ek-dem′ik) Indicating a disease brought into an area from without; not endemic.
ecdysis (ek-dĭ-sis) Desquamation or shedding of an outer covering. Also called molting.
echidnase (e-kid′nās) Enzyme present in the venom of vipers that causes swelling and inflammation in the snake-bitten victim.
echinococcosis (e-ki-no-kok-o′sis) Infection caused by the larval form of *Echinococcus granulosus* or *Echinococcus multilocularis*, producing expanding cysts in the liver or lungs; anaphylactic reaction may occur from rupture of cyst fluid into the pleural or peritoneal cavity. Also called hydatid disease.
Echinococcus granulosus (e-ki-no-kok′us gran-u-lo′sus) A species of tapeworm occurring in the adult form in dog's intestines; the larval forms occur in humans, forming hydatid cysts in the liver and other tissues.
Echinodermata (e-ki-no-der′mă-tă) A phylum of radially symmetrical invertebrates often having a body covered with spines; includes starfishes, sea urchins, sea lilies.
echinosis (ek-ĭ-no′sis) Abnormal irregular appearance of red blood cells; having lost their smooth surface, they resemble the shell of a sea urchin.
Echinostoma (ek-ĭ-nos′to-mă) Genus of flukes with a characteristic collar of spines, distributed widely in Southeast Asia; some species infect humans, causing diarrhea.
echinulate (e-kin′u-lāt) Having small spines; applied in bacteriology to cultures that spread out in pointed outgrowths.
echo (ek′o) Repetition of a sound; reflection of a sound wave to its point of origin.
echocardiogram (ek-o-kar′de-o-gram) Graphic display obtained from the application of ultrasonic procedures.
echocardiography (ek-o-kar-de-og′ră-fe) The use of an ultrasonic apparatus that sends sound impulses toward the walls of the heart, which in turn bounce or echo the sounds back; the patterns produced are graphically displayed for interpretation; used for determining the movement patterns of the heart and its valves, chamber size, wall thickness, and the presence of pericardial fluid.
cross-sectional e. See two-dimensional echocardiography.
Doppler e. Measurement of blood flow within the heart using a motion-mode (M-mode) and two-dimensional echocardiogram while simultaneously recording the audible Doppler signals (e.g., direction, velocity, intensity, amplitude) reflected from the moving column of red blood cells.
transesophageal e. (TEE) Technique in which a small transducer, attached to the end of an endoscope, is introduced into the esophagus to obtain images of the posterior aspect of the heart and thoracic aorta. Particularly useful to detect vegetations on the mitral valve in bacterial endocarditis.
two-dimensional e. Technique in which the ultrasound beam rapidly moves through an arc, producing a cross-sectional or fan-shaped image of heart structures. Also called cross-sectional echocardiography.
echoencephalography (ek-o-en-sef-ă-log′ră-fe) A method of examing the brain by recording the reflection of high frequency (ultrasonic) sound waves; it is used to obtain a safe, rapid, and painless estimate of the position of the midline of the third ventricle; useful in evaluating patients with suspected subdural or epidural hemorrhage or other conditions which might cause a brain shift.
echography (ĕ-kog′ră-fe) See ultrasonography.
echolalia (ek-o-la′le-ă) Involuntary echolike and meaningless repetition of another's words or phrases.
echopathy (ĕ-kop′ă-the) A syndrome characterized by the senseless imitation of speech (echolalia) or gestures and postures (echopraxia) of others; may occur during the catatonic phase of schizophrenia.
echophony, echophonia (ĕ-kof′ō-nē, ek-o-fo′ne-ă) The echo of the voice sometimes heard in auscultation of the chest.
echopraxia (ek-o-prak′se-ă) The involuntary and meaningless imitation of movements made by another.
echovirus (ek′o-vi-rus) Virus of the genus *Enterovirus* (family Picornaviridae) associated with aseptic meningitis and gastroenteritis in humans; the term is an acronym of enteric cytopathogenic human orphan virus.
eclampsia (ĕ-klamp′se-ă) Acute disorder of pregnant and puerperal women, representing a progression of preeclampsia; marked by seizures occurring most commonly before delivery, usually after the 20th week of gestation; postpartum episodes occur chiefly in the first 48 hours after delivery, but may occur as late as 6 weeks. Seizure-induced complications may include pulmonary edema and retinal detachment. Fever is an unfavorable prognostic sign.
puerperal e. Eclampsia occurring within six weeks after delivery.
eclamptic (ĕ-klamp′tik) Relating to eclampsia.
eclamptogenic, eclamptogenous (ĕ-klamp-to-jen′ik, ĕ-klamp-to-jen′us) Causing eclampsia.
E. coli (e ko′lī) Abbreviation for *Escherichia coli.*

E

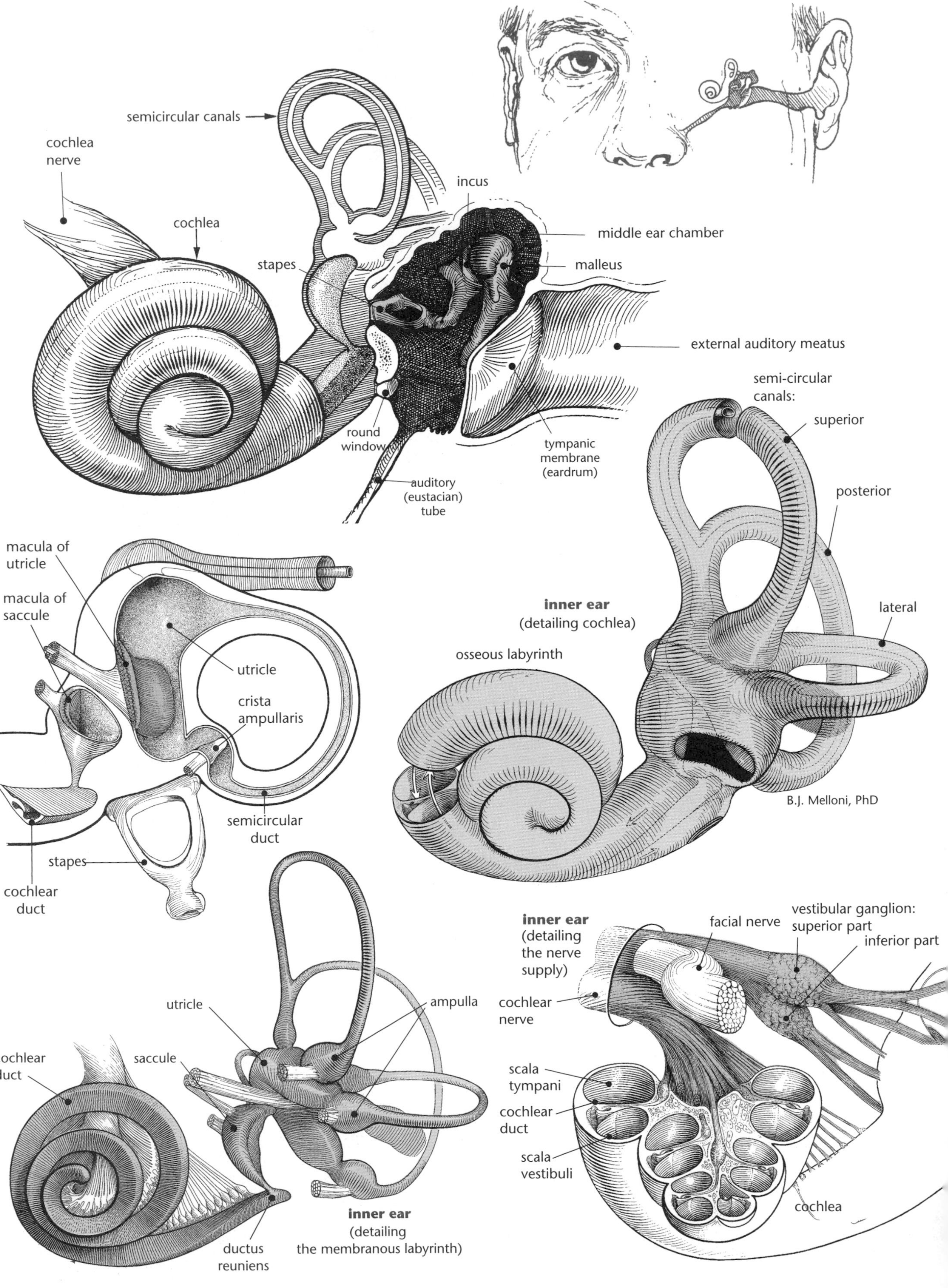

semicircular canals
cochlea
nerve
cochlea
stapes
incus
middle ear chamber
malleus
external auditory meatus
round
window
auditory
(eustacian)
tube
tympanic
membrane
(eardrum)
semi-circular
canals:
superior
posterior
lateral
macula of
utricle
macula of
saccule
utricle
crista
ampullaris
semicircular
duct
stapes
cochlear
duct
inner ear
(detailing cochlea)
osseous labyrinth
B.J. Melloni, PhD
utricle
ampulla
cochlear
duct
saccule
ductus
reuniens
inner ear
(detailing
the membranous labyrinth)
inner ear
(detailing
the nerve
supply)
facial nerve
vestibular ganglion:
superior part
inferior part
cochlear
nerve
scala
tympani
cochlear
duct
scala
vestibuli
cochlea

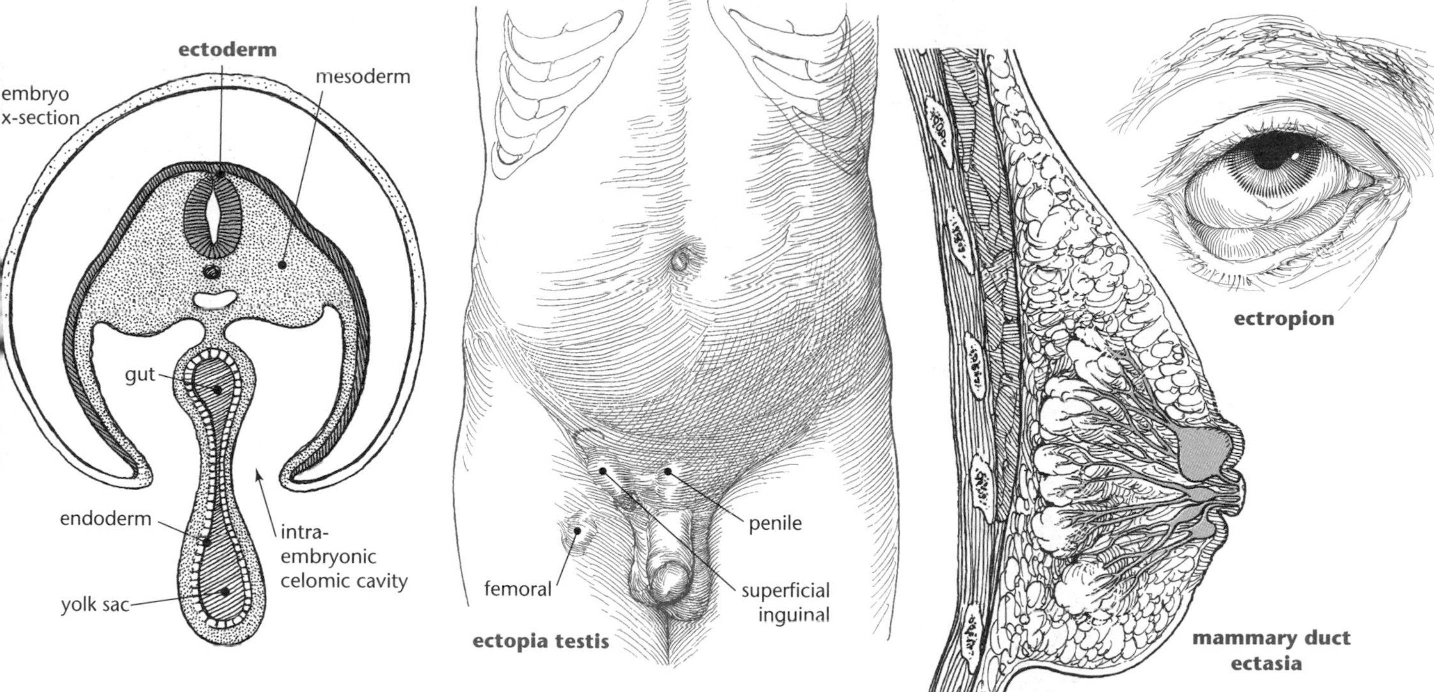

E

See under *Escherichia.*
ecology (e-kol'o-jē) The science of the relationship between organisms and their evironment.
economy (ĭ-kon'ŏ-me) The functional arrangement of organs and structures within the body.
ecosystem (ek-o-sis'tem) An ecological system; a community of organisms, together with its physical environment, considered as an entity.
ecotaxis (ek'o-tak-sis) Migration of lymphocytes from the thymus and bone marrow to other tissues that provide an appropriate microenvironment.
ecstasy, MDMA (ek'sta-se) Popular name for 3,4-methylenedioxymethamphetamine, a hallucinogenic drug of abuse; it produces euphoria followed by depression and difficulty in concentration.
ectasia, ectasis (ek-ta'zha, ek'tă-sis) Dilatation of a hollow organ or a tubular structure.
mammary duct e. A breast condition affecting multiparous women 50–60 years of age; characterized by thickening (inspissation) of secretions within major excretory ducts, duct dilatation, and periductal inflammation; the condition may superficially resemble cancer of the breast.
ectatic (ek-tat'ik) Relating to ectasia.
ectethmoid (ek-teth'moid) See ethmoidal labyrinth, under labyrinth.
ecthyma (ek-thi'mă) A pustular eruption, usually seated upon a shallow ulcer, that evolves into a firm crust or scab; caused by staphylococci or streptococci; scarring is a characteristic sequela.
contagious e. See orf.
ectiris (ek-tī'ris) The anterior or outer layer (endothelium) of the iris.
ectoantigen, exoantigen (ek-to-an'tĭ-jen, ek-so-an'tĭ-jen) Any molecule inciting antibody production that is separate or separable from its source.
ectoblast (ek'to-blast) See ectoderm.
ectocardia (ek-to-kar'de-ă) Abnormal position of the heart.
ectocervical (ek-to-ser'vĭ-kal) Relating to the vaginal portion of the uterine cervix.
ectochoroidea (ek-to-ko-roi'de-ă) See suprachoroid.
ectocornea (ek-to-kor'ne-ă) The anterior or outer epithelium of the cornea.
ectocrine (ek'to-krin) **1.** A substance, synthesized or resulting from the decomposition of organisms, that affects plant life. **2.** See ectohormone.
ectocyst (ek'to-sist) The outer layer of a hydatid cyst.
ectoderm (ek'to-derm) The outermost of the three germ layers of the embryo; it gives rise to the nervous system and to the epidermis and its derivatives, such as hair and the lens of the eye.
ectodermal, ectodermic (ek-to-der'mal, ek-to-der'mik) Relating to the ectoderm.
ectodermatosis (ek-to-der-mă-to'sis) See ectodermosis.
ectodermosis (ek-to-der-mo'sis) A disorder arising from the maldevelopment of any organ or tissue derived from the ectoderm. Also called ectodermatosis.
ectogenous (ek-toj'ĕ-nus) Originating outside the body.
ectohormone (ek-to-hor'mōn) A substance that is secreted by an organism (mostly an invertebrate) into its immediate environment and modifies the functional activity of some distant organism; a parahormonal mediator of ecological importance.
ectomere (ek'to-mēr) Any cells, formed by division of the fertilized egg, that participate in the formation of the ectoderm.
ectomorph (ek'to-morf) A person with a constitutional body type in which tissues derived from the ectoderm predominate; morphologically, the body is lean and the limbs predominate over the trunk.
ectomorphic (ek-to-mor'fik) Having the characteristics of an ectomorph.
ectopagia (ek-top'ă-je-ă) The lateral fusion of conjoined twins.
ectoparasite (ek-to-par'ă-sīt) A parasite that lives on the surface of the body of its host.
ectopia (ek-to'pe-ă) **1.** Congenital displacement of a body part. Also called ectopy. **2.** In cardiology, a state in which heartbeats originate at some point in the heart other than the sinoatrial node.
e. lentis Partial or complete displacement of the lens of the eye; may be *hereditary*, a usually bilateral dislocation occurring as part of a syndrome or disorder (e.g., Marfan's syndrome, homocystinuria); or *traumatic*, a dislocation following a contusion injury (e.g., a blow to the eye with a fist). Also called dislocation of lens.
e. testis A condition in which a testicle has strayed from the path of normal descent into the scrotum; it may be due to an abnormal connection of the distal end of the gubernaculum testis, a connection which leads the gonad to an abnormal position.
ectopic (ek-top'ik) **1.** Located in, or arising from, a place other than normal (e.g., heartbeats arising from other than the S-A node). **2.** Popular term for ectopic pregnancy. See under pregnancy.
ectopic ACTH syndrome (ek-top'ik a-c-t-h sin'drōm) Secretion of ACTH by nonendocrine tumors producing hypokalemic alkalosis and weakness.
ectoplacental (ek-to-plă-sen'tal) Outside or surrounding the placenta.
ectoplasm (ek'to-plaz-m) Clear, thin cytoplasm at the periphery of a cell; it is more gelled than the rest of the cytoplasm in the cell; the clarity is due to the exclusion of all organelles except filaments.
ectopy (ek'to-pe) See ectopia.
ectostosis (ek-to-sto'sis) Formation of bone beneath the perichondrium or the periostium.
ectothrix (ek'to-thriks) Denoting a type of fungal infection in which the hyphae grow both within and on the surface of the hair shaft. COMPARE: endothrix.
ectotoxin (ek-to-tok'sin) See exotoxin.
ectozoon (ek-to-zo'on) Any parasitic animal living on the surface of the host.
ectrodactyly (ek-tro-dak'tĭ-le) Congenital absence of a digit or of digits.
ectrogeny (ek-troj'ĕ-ne) Congenital absence of a part.
ectromelia (ek-tro-me'le-ă) **1.** Congenital absence of one or more limbs. **2.** A viral disease of mice causing, among other symptoms, gangrene and loss of feet; it effects a high mortality in laboratory mouse colonies. Also called mousepox.
ectropion (ek-tro'pe-on) Eversion or outward turning of the margin of an eyelid.
ectrosyndactyly (ek-tro-sin-dak'tĭ-le) A congenital absence of one or more digits and the fusion of the others.
eczema (ek'zĕ-mă) General term for a group of acute or chronic inflammatory skin disorders characterized by redness, thickening, oozing, and the formation of papules, vesicles, and crusts; often accompanied by itching and burning.
allergic e. Eczema occurring as an allergic reaction.
atopic e. See atopic dermatitis, under dermatitis.
e. herpeticum A generalized widespread infection of the skin caused by the herpes simplex virus.
e. madidans A moist eruption. Also called weeping eczema.
e. marginatum See tinea cruris, under tinea.
nummular e. Eruption of coin-sized and coin-shaped patches of vesicular dermatitis, usually affecting the extensor surfaces of the hands, arms, and legs.
pustular e. Eczema in which the lesions become covered with pus crusts; a secondary infection usually caused by staphylococci.
e. rubrum Eczema presenting excoriated, oozing lesions.
stasis e. Eczema of the legs, frequently with ulceration, caused by impaired circulation.
e. vesiculosum An eruption of vesicles.
weeping e. See eczema madidans.
winter e. Dry scales on the skin resulting from rapid evaporation of moisture from the skin surface.
eczematous (ek-zem'ă-tus) Affected with or of the nature of eczema.

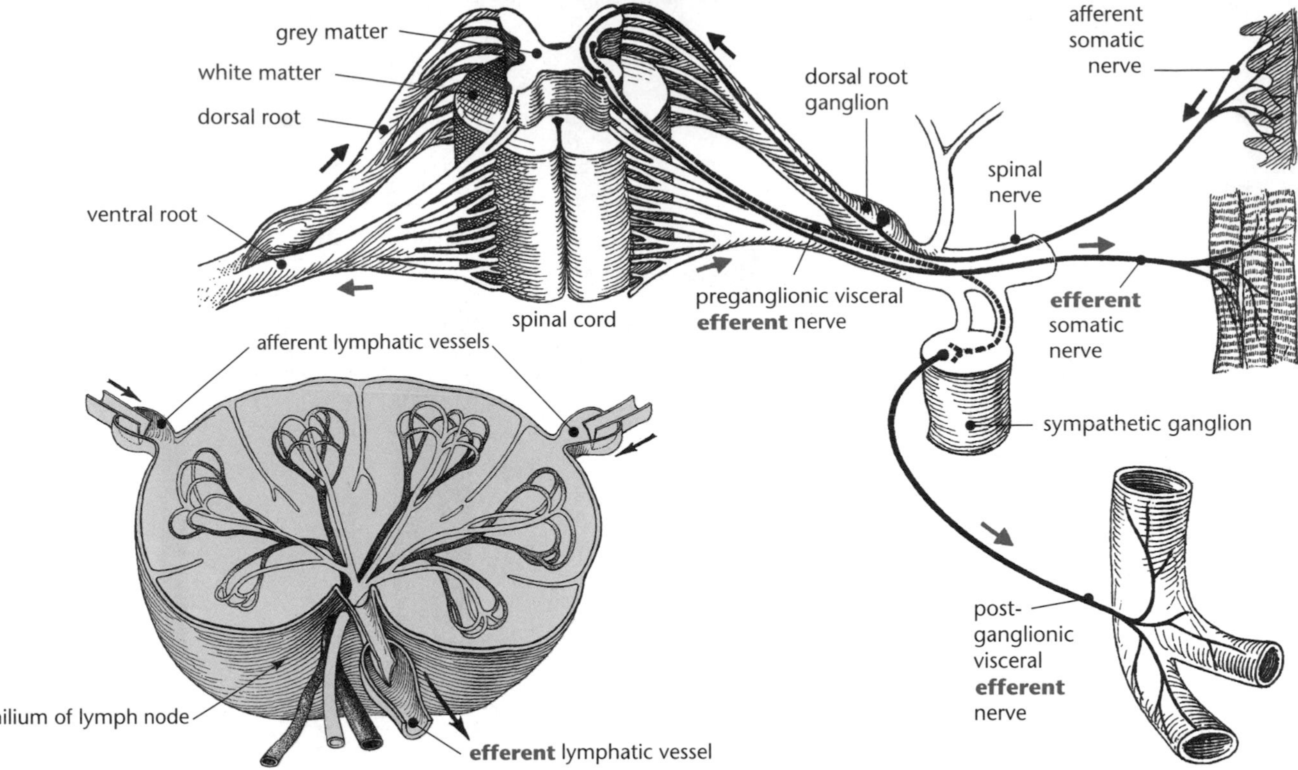

edema (ĕ-de´mă) Swelling of any part of the body due to collection of fluid in the intercellular spaces of tissues.

angioneurotic e. Recurrent local edema due to increased vascular permeability of allergic or nervous origin; affecting most commonly the eyelids, lips, tongue, lungs, larynx, or extremities and occurring in persons having a variety of allergies. Also called giant urticaria.

Berlin's e. Edema of the macular area of the retina, giving it a white appearance, caused by a severe blow to the eyeball. Also called concussion edema.

brawny e. See nonpitting edema.

cardiac e. Edema caused by heart disease with resulting increase in venous pressures.

cerebral e. Edema of the brain caused by tumors, infarction, generalized edema due to heart or kidney disease, or certain toxic conditions.

concussion e. See Berlin's edema.

dependent e. Swelling of the limbs, especially the legs due to accumulation of fluid.

hereditary angioneurotic e. (HANE) A condition inherited as an autosomal dominant trait, characterized by recurrent attacks of angioedema with involvement of the gastrointestinal tract and the larynx; due to deficiency of C1 esterase inhibitor or to an inactive form of the inhibitor.

high altitude pulmonary e. (HAPE) An acute form of altitude sickness causing edema of the lungs.

menstrual e. Increase in weight and retention of water during or just before menstruation.

e. neonatorum A generalized, usually fatal, edema in the newborn.

nutritional e. Swelling caused by prolonged dietary deficiency; usually due at least in part to hypoproteinemia.

nonpitting e. Edema that does not produce indentations by pressure; usually seen in metabolic abnormalities. Also called brawny edema.

pitting e. Condition in which pressure on an edematous area causes indentations that remain for a time after the pressure is released.

pulmonary e. Escape of fluid into the air sacs and interstitial tissue of the lungs; causes include left ventricular failure, mitral stenosis, and chemicals that are pulmonary toxins.

edematous (ĕ-dem´ă-tus) Characterized or affected by edema.

edentulous (e-den´tu-lus) Toothless.

edge (ej) **1.** A rim, margin, border, or ridge. **2.** The sharpened side of a blade.

cutting e. **1.** The beveled, knifelike working angle of a dental hand instrument. **2.** The incisal edge of an anterior tooth.

e. strength In dentistry, the ability of a fine margin to resist fracture.

eduction (e-duk´shun) The process of coming out, as emerging from general anesthesia.

effect (ĕ-fekt´) A result; something brought about by a force or an agent.

Bohr e. The effect of carbon dioxide (CO_2) on the oxygen affinity of blood, i.e., CO_2 in the tissues facilitates the removal of oxygen from hemoglobin, resulting in a greater availability of oxygen to the tissues.

Compton e. A change in wavelength of a bombarding photon with the displacement of an orbital electron.

cumulative e. The sudden pronounced effect resulting after several ineffective doses. Also called cumulative action.

Doppler e. The apparent change in frequency of sound or light waves when the observer and the source are in relative motion; the frequency increases when they approach one another and decreases when they move away. Also called Doppler phenomenon.

Hawthorne e. The changes observed in people included in a research project when they know they are being studied.

inotropic e. The increased force of cardiac muscular contractions occurring during pregnancy to compensate for the need for an increased cardiac output, which is typical of the pregnant state.

Pasteur e. The slowing down of fermentation by oxygen, first observed by Pasteur.

side e. An effect other than that for which a drug or therapy is administered, especially an undesirable secondary effect.

toxic e. A drug-produced harmful effect on some biologic mechanism.

effector (ĕ-fek´tor) An end organ that, upon receiving a nerve impulse, distributes it, activating either secretion of a gland or contraction of a muscle.

allosteric e. Any small molecule that modifies enzyme activity by binding at sites other than the catalytically active sites.

efferent (ef´er-ent) Conveying a nerve impulse away from a central organ or area.

effervesce (ef-er-ves´) To emit gas bubbles to the surface, as in a carbonated liquid.

effervescent (ef-er-ves´ent) **1.** Bubbling; giving off gas. **2.** Producing effervescence.

efficacy (ef´ĭ-kă-se) The ability to produce a desired effect; effectiveness.

efficiency (ĕ-fish´en-se) The ability to accomplish a desired effect or produce results with a minimum of unnecessary effort; competency.

visual e. A rating used in determining compensation for ocular injuries based on measurable functions of central acuity, field vision, and ocular motility.

effloresce (ef-lōr-es´) **1.** To lose water upon exposure to a dry atmosphere, thus becoming a powder. **2.** To become covered with a powdery substance.

efflorescent (ef-lōr-es´ent) Tending to effloresce.

effluvium (ĕ-floo´ve-um) Shedding of hair.

effuse (ĕ-fus´) Spread out widely and thinly on a surface; denoting the surface character of a bacterial culture.

effusion (ĕ-fu´zhun) **1.** The escape of fluid into a body cavity. **2.** The fluid effused.

pleural e. Fluid filling the membranous sac covering the lung and lining of the chest.

egg (eg) **1.** The female reproductive cell of birds and reptiles. **2.** See ovum. Also called oocyte.

fertilized e. See zygote.

ego (e´go) The awareness of the existence of the self as different from others; in psychoanalytic theory, one of the three parts of the psychic apparatus that mediates between the other two parts (id and superego) and reality.

egocentric (e´go-sen´trik) Marked by constant or extreme preoccupation with one's own interests.

ego-dystonic (e´go-dis-ton´ik) Denoting those aspects of the personality that are alien or unacceptable to the self.

egomania (e´go-man´ne-ă) Pathologic preoccupation with one's self.

egophony (e-gof´o-ne) A form of bronchophony; the bleating nasal quality of voice heard over an area of compressed lung above a pleural effusion or an area of consolidation; transmission of the spoken voice is altered so that long e (ē) sounds like long a (ā).

ego-syntonic (e´go-sin-ton´ik) Denoting those aspects of the personality that are acceptable to the self.

Ehlers-Danlos syndrome (a´lerz-dan-los´ sin´drōm) Inherited disorder marked by hyperelasticity of the skin, fragility of cutaneous blood vessels, overextension of joints, and the formation of pigmented nodules (raisin tumors) at the site of skin injury.

Ehrlichia (ār-lik´e-ă) A genus of nonmotile gram-negative bacteria (order Rickettsiales) causing disease in dogs and humans.

ehrlichiosis (ār-lik-e-o´sis) Infection with *Ehrlichia canis* causing symptoms similar to those of Rocky Mountain spotted fever, but without a rash; transmitted from dogs by ticks.

eicosanoid (i-ko´să-noid) A 20-carbon unsaturated

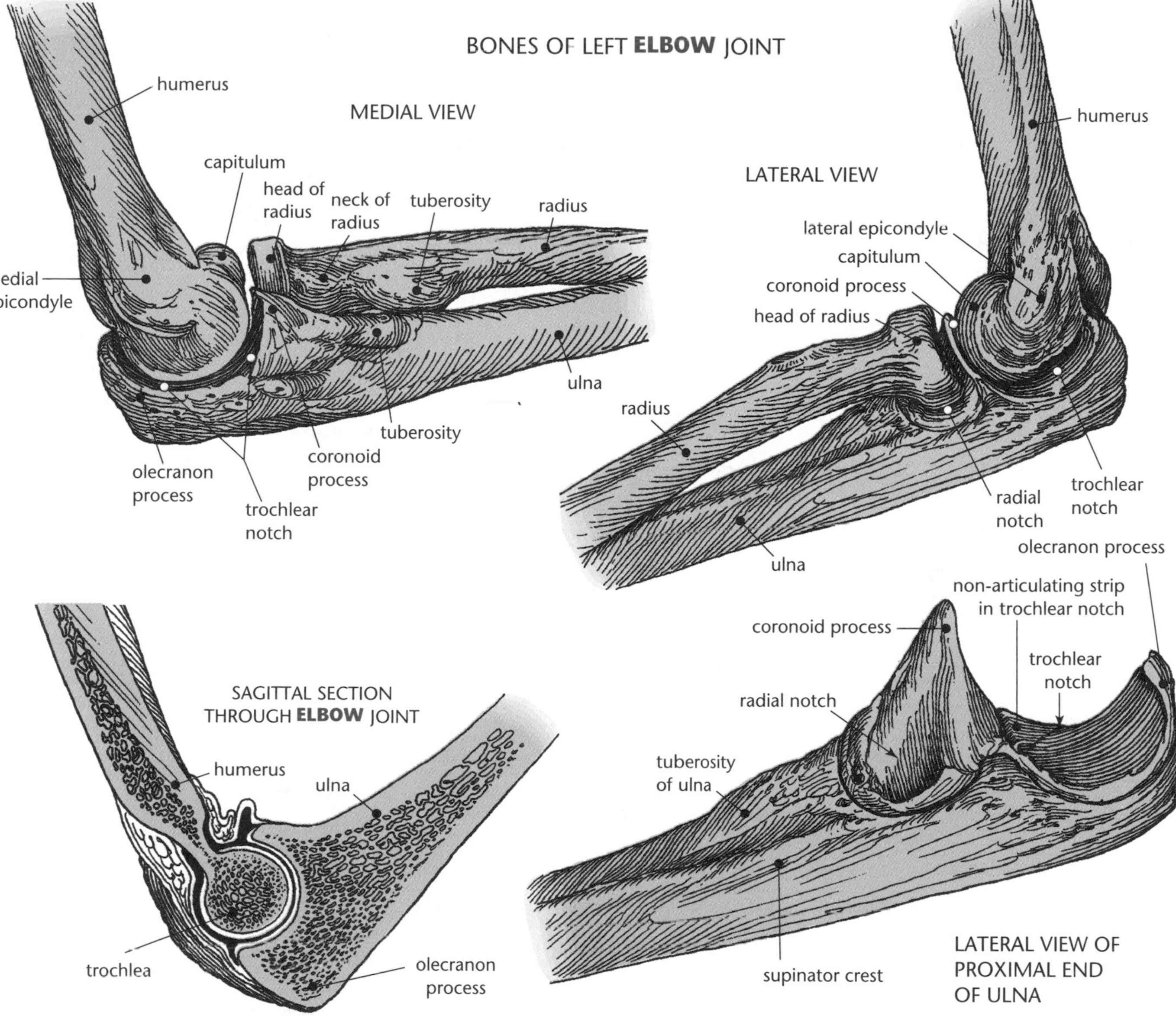

fatty acid derived from arachidonic acid (e.g., prostaglandins and leukotrienes).

eikonometer (i-ko-nom´ĕ-ter) Any instrument used to measure the difference in size of the images seen by the two eyes; an examination for aniseikonia.

einsteinium (īn-stī´ne-um) A synthetic radioactive element; symbol Es, atomic number 99, atomic weight 254.

Eisenmenger's syndrome (i´sen-meng-erz sin´drōm) Strictly defined, a ventricular septal defect, overriding aorta, right ventricular hypertrophy, and a normal or dilated pulmonary artery; because these terms have been frequently used to describe cases with right to left shunt without all of the above components, they are not regarded as useful terms by cardiologists.

ejaculate (e-jak´u-lāt) **1.** To discharge abruptly, especially semen. **2.** The semen discharged. Also called ejaculum.

ejaculation (e-jak-u-la´shun) Emission of the semen.

inhibited e. A rare condition in which erection is normal (or prolonged) but ejaculation does not occur.

premature e. Emission of the semen prior to or immediately upon engaging in sexual intercourse.

retrograde e. Condition in which the ejaculate is forced backward into the bladder due to failure of the sphincter muscle of the bladder to close at orgasm; may result from neurological disease, a surgical operation upon the neck of the bladder and prostatic urethra, transurethral resection of the prostate (TURP), or certain antihypertensive medications.

ejaculatory (e-jak´u-lă-to-re) Of or relating to ejaculation.

ejaculum (e-jak´u-lum) See ejaculate.

ejector (e-jek´tōr) Anything that removes any material forcefully.

saliva e. A device containing a perforated suction tube used to remove fluids from the mouth.

elastance (e-las´tans) A measure of a structure's ability to return to its initial or original form following deformation; e.g., the measure of the ability of a hollow organ, such as the bladder, to revert toward its original dimensions upon removal of the distending force (urine).

elastic (e-las´tik) **1.** Capable of being stretched, bent, or deformed in any way, and then return to original form. **2.** A rubber band used in orthodontics to apply force to the teeth.

intermaxillary e. A rubber band placed between orthodontic appliances of upper and lower jaws to cause tooth movement as the jaw opens and closes.

intramaxillary e. A rubber band placed within an orthodontic appliance.

elastica (e-las´tĭ-kă) A general term for elastic tissue, such as the elastic layer in the wall of an artery.

elasticin (e-las´tĭ-sin) See elastin.

elasticity (e-las-tis´ĭ-te) The quality of being elastic.

modulus of e. A measure of elasticity or stiffness of a material determined by dividing the stress by the corresponding strain value.

elastin (e-las´tin) A yellow scleroprotein present in elastic fibers that allows them to stretch about one and one-half times their original length.

elastomer (e-las´to-mĕr) Any of various polymers that can be stretched like rubber, and that will relax to their original dimensions when unstressed.

elastometer (e-las-tom´ĕ-ter) A device for measuring the elasticity of bodily tissues.

elastosis (e-las-to´sis) Degeneration of the elastic tissues.

e. dystrophica See angioid streaks, under streak.

e. perforans serpiginosa Circinate group of asymptomatic keratotic papules, marked by thickened epidermis around a central keratin plug overlying an accumulation of elastic tissue.

senile e. A dermatosis marked by degeneration of elastic tissue in the skin of the elderly or in those afflicted with chronic actinic effect.

elbow (el´bo) The joint between the arm and the forearm.

bend of the e. See cubital fossa, under fossa.

miner's e. See olecranon bursitis, under bursitis.

nursemaid's e. Popular term for partial dislocation (subluxation) of the head of the radius in which the radial head slips under the annular ligament at the elbow joint, with the ligament remaining intact; a common injury of infants and young children as a result of being suddenly pulled or lifted by the arm or hand. Also called pulled elbow.

point of the e. See olecranon.

pulled e. See nursemaid's elbow.

student's e. See olecranon bursitis, under bursitis.

tennis e. See lateral epicondylitis, under epicondylitis.

tip of the e. See olecranon.

electroanalysis (e-lek-tro-ă-nal´ĭ-sis) Quantitative separation of metals by means of an electric current.

electrocardiogram (ECG)

R R P T U P T voltage variations Q S Q S time

E

EEG surface **electrodes**

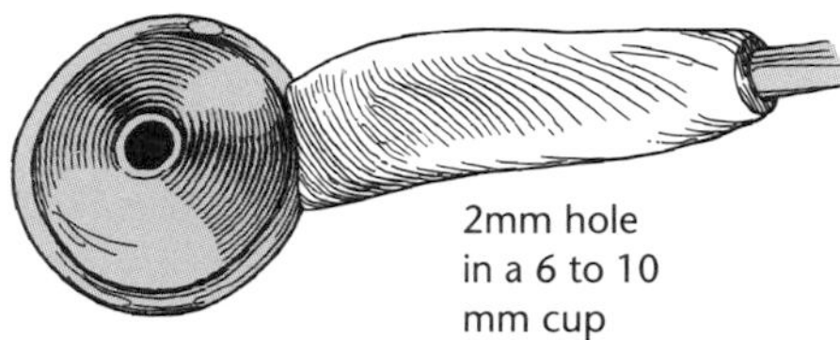

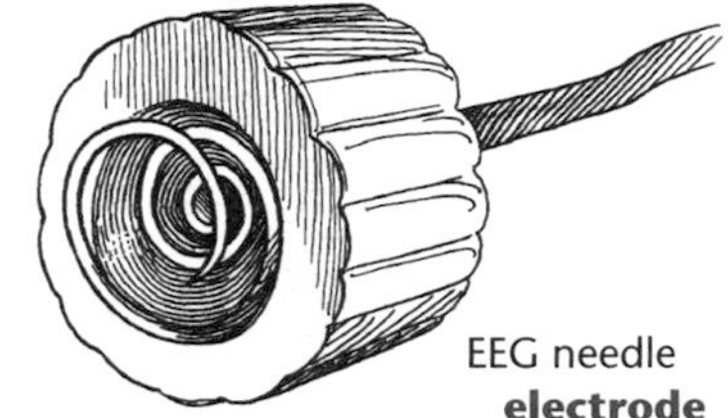

EEG needle **electrode**

frontal-central L R

central-occipital L R

frontal-temporal L R

temporal-occipital L R

electroencephalograms (EEGs)

electroanesthesia (e-lek-tro-an-es-the´zhă) Anesthesia induced by an electric current.

electrocardiogram (e-lek-tro-kar´de-o-gram) (ECG, EKG) A graphic record of the electric current produced by the contraction of the heart, obtained with an electrocardiograph; the voltage variations, resulting from the depolarization and repolarization of the heart muscle and producing electric fields, are plotted against time on paper tape.

electrocardiograph (e-lek-tro-kar´de-o-graf) An instrument for recording the electric currents produced by heart muscle in the process of contraction; a galvanometer which records voltage variations.

electrocardiography (e-lek-tro-kar-de-og´ră-fe) A method of recording the electric current generated by the activity of the heart muscle by means of an electrocardiograph.

fetal e. Electrocardiography of a fetus while in the uterus.

electrocardioscope (e-lek-tro-kar´de-o-skōp) An oscilloscope for the continuous monitoring of the electrocardiogram (ECG).

electrocauterization (e-lek-tro-kaw-ter-i-za´shun) Cauterization by means of an electrically heated platinum wire.

electrocautery (e-lek-tro-kaw´ter-e) An instrument for cauterizing tissue in which a platinum wire is heated by a current of electricity.

electrochemistry (e-lek-tro-kem´is-tre) The science of chemical reactions produced by electricity; study of the electrical aspects of chemical reactions.

electrocoagulation (e-lek-tro-ko-ag-u-la´shun) The hardening of diseased tissues induced by high frequency currents; a form of surgical diathermy.

electrocontractility (e-lek-tro-kon-trak-til´ĭ-te) The capability of muscle tissue to contract in response to an electric stimulation.

electroconvulsant (e-lek-tro-kon-vul´ant) Denoting a type of therapy for emotional disorders in which an electric current is passed through the head of the patient to produce convulsions; see also electroshock therapy, under therapy.

electrocorticogram (e-lek-tro-kor´tĭ-ko-gram) A record of electrical activity emanating from the cerebral cortex; obtained by placing electrodes in direct contact with the cortex.

electrocute (e-lek´tro-kūt) To cause death by passing a high voltage electric current through the body.

electrode (e-lek´trōd) A conductor of electricity through which current enters or leaves a medium.

central terminal e. In electrocardiography, one in which the wire connections from the two arms and left leg are fastened together and connected to the electrocardiograph to form the indifferent electrode.

exploring e. In electrocardiography, electrode that is placed on the chest near the heart region and paired with an indifferent electrode.

glass e. An electrode made of a thin-walled glass bulb containing a platinum wire, a standard buffer solution, and quinhydrone; used in determining hydrogen ion (pH) concentrations.

hydrogen e. An electrode considered the ultimate standard of reference in all hydrogen ion (pH) determinations; made by partly immersing platinum black in platinum and allowing it to absorb hydrogen to saturation.

indifferent e. In electrocardiography, an electrode having multiple terminals.

negative e. See cathode.

positive e. See anode.

electrodesiccation (e-lek-tro-des-ĭ-ka´shun) Destruction of tissue by dehydration using monopolar electric current through a needle electrode.

electrodialysis (e-lek-tro-di-al´ĭ-sis) Dialysis by the application of an electric field across the semipermeable dialysis membrane, used especially to separate electrolytes.

electroejaculation (e-lek-tro-e-jak-u-la´shun) In reproductive medicine, the application of an electrical stimulus to an area near the prostate gland to cause an involuntary ejaculation of a semen sample for *in vitro* fertilization; used in certain types of male infertility (e.g., in spinal cord injury).

electroencephalogram (e-lek-tro-en-sef´ă-lo-gram) (EEG) A graphic record of the electric activity of the brain obtained with an electroencephalograph.

depth e. An electroencephalogram obtained by placing electrodes directly on subcortical structures.

low voltage e. An electroencephalogram in which no activity larger than 20 μV can be recorded between any two points on the scalp.

electroencephalograph (e-lek-tro-en-sef´ă-lo-graf) An instrument used to record the electric currents produced in the brain.

electroencephalography (e-lek-tro-en-sef-ă-log´ră-fe) The recording of the electric currents generated by the activity of the brain, especially the cerebral cortex, by means of an electroencephalo-graph.

electroexcision (e-lek-tro-ek-siz'zhun) Surgical removal of tissue by electrical means.

electrogastrograph (e-lek-tro-gas´tro-graf) An instrument for recording the bioelectrical potentials associated with gastrointestinal activity.

electrogram (e-lek´tro-gram) Any electrically produced graph or tracing, such as an electrocardiogram or electroencephalogram.

His bundle e. (HBE) An electrogram usually made by placing a catheter electrode near the tricuspid (right atrioventricular) valve; mainly used to determine the site, extent, and mechanism of arrhythmias.

electrography (e-lek-trog´ră-fe) The production of electrograms.

electrolarynx (e-lek-tro-lar´inks) A vibrating mechanism that makes it possible for a person to speak intelligibly after his larynx has been surgically removed.

electrolysis (e-lek-trol´ĭ-sis) **1.** Chemical decomposition of a compound in solution by passage of an electric current. **2.** Destruction of hair follicles by electric means to remove unwanted hair.

electrolyte (e-lek´tro-līt) Any substance that, when in solution, dissociates into ions, thus becoming capable of transmitting an electric current.

electrolytic (e-lek-tro-lit´ik) **1.** Relating to or produced by electrolysis. **2.** Relating to an electrolyte.

electrolyze (e-lek´tro-līz) To cause a chemical decomposition by means of an electric current.

electromyogram (e-lek-tro-mi´o-gram) (EMG) A graphic record obtained by electromyography of the somatic electric currents associated with muscle activity.

electromyography (e-lek-tro-mi-og´ră-fe) The recording of the electric currents generated by muscular activity.

electron (ĕ-lek´tron) An elementary, subatomic particle of nature; it has a negative charge of 1 and a mass of 9.1×10^{-28} g.

valence e. An electron in an atom capable of participating in the formation of chemical bonds with other atoms.

electronarcosis (e-lek-tro-nar-ko´sis) The passing of an electric current through the brain via scalp electrodes to produce narcosis or unconsciousness.

electronegative (e-lek-tro-neg´ă-tiv) **1.** Possessing a negative electric charge. **2.** Referring to those elements whose unchanged atoms have a tendency to attract electrons and become anions (e.g., oxygen and chlorine).

electron gun (e-lek´tron gun) An electrode, as in a cathode-ray tube, that emits a controlled beam of accelerated electrons.

electronic (e-lek-tron´ik) **1.** Relating to electrons. **2.** Relating to electronics.

electronics (e-lek-tron´iks) The study of electronic phenomena.

electron-volt (e-lek´tron vōlt) (eV) The energy imparted to an electron by a potential of one volt; equal to 1.6×10^{-12} erg.

electronystagmography (e-lek-tro-nis-tag-mog´ră-fe) (ENG) The electronic recording of eye movements in nystagmus.

number of **electrons** in some atoms

element	symbol	atomic number	Shell						
			K	L	M	N	O	P	Q
hydrogen	H	1	1						
lithium	Li	3	2	1					
carbon	C	6	2	4					
nitrogen	N	7	2	5					
oxygen	O	8	2	6					
sodium	Na	11	2	8	1				
chlorine	Cl	17	2	8	7				
potassium	K	19	2	8	8	1			
calcium	Ca	20	2	8	8	2			
mercury	Hg	80	2	8	18	32	18	2	
radium	Ra	88	2	8	18	32	18	18	2

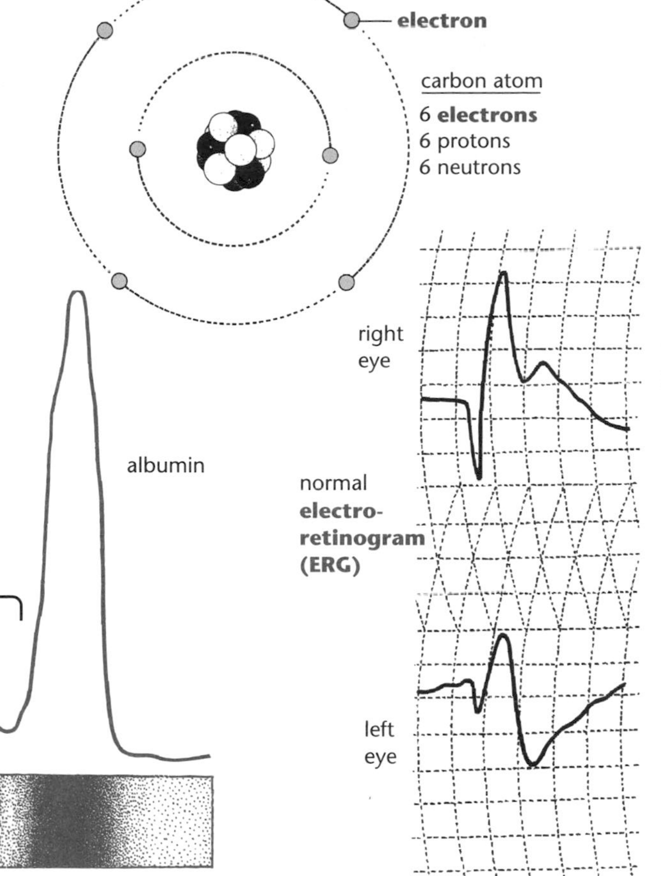

paper electrophoresis

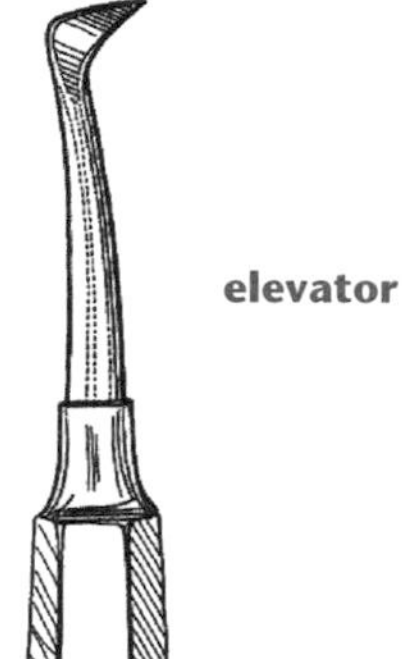

electro-oculogram (e-lek-tro-ok´u-lo-gram) (EOG) A record of eye positions made by an electro-oculograph.

electro-oculography (e-lek-tro-ok-u-log´ră-fe) The production of records of eye position (electro-oculograms) by recording, during eye movement, the difference in electrical potential between two electrodes placed on the skin at either side of the eye.

electrophoresis (e-lek-tro-fŏ-re´sis) The movement of charged particles in an electric field toward either the anode or the cathode; used as a means of separating substances in a medium.

paper e. The migration of charged particles along a strip of filter paper, saturated with a few drops of an electrolyte, when a potential gradient is placed across the paper.

thin-layer e. (TLE) The movement of charged particles through a thin layer of an inert material such as cellulose.

electrophysiology (e-lek-tro-fiz-e-ol´ŏ-je) The study of electrical phenomena related to physiologic processes.

electroplate (e-lek´tro-plāt) To plate or coat with a thin layer of metal by electrolysis or electrodeposition; in dentistry, impressions are plated to form metalized working dies.

electropositive (e-lek-tro-poz´ĭ-tiv) Having a positive electric charge; denoting an element whose atoms tend to release electrons to form a chemical bond (e.g., sodium, potassium, calcium).

electroresection (e-lek-tro-re-sek´shun) Removal of tissue with an electrical cutting loop.

electroretinogram (e-lek-tro-ret´ĭ-no-gram) (ERG) The electrical potential of the retina recorded by a galvanometer from the surface of the eyeball and originated by a pulse of light; it depicts the integrity of the neuroepithelium of the retina.

electroscope (e-lek´tro-skōp) An instrument for detecting the presence of electric charges.

electroshock (e-lek´tro-shok) See electroconvulsive therapy, under therapy.

electrostethograph (e-lek-tro-steth´o-graf) An electrical instrument for recording the respiratory and cardiac sounds of the chest.

electrotherapy, electrotherapeutics (e-lek-tro-ther´ă-pe, e-lek-tro-ther-ă-pu´tiks) The treatment of disease by means of electricity.

electrothermal (e-lek-tro-ther´mal) Relating to electricity and heat; especially, the production of heat electrically.

element (el´ĕ-ment) **1.** A substance made up of atoms having the same number of protons in each nucleus. **2.** An irreducible substance or indivisible constituent of a composite entity.

electronegative e. An element having more than four valence electrons and tending to gain electrons in a chemical combination.

electropositive e. An element having fewer than four valence electrons and tending to release electrons in a chemical combination.

radioactive e. An element that spontaneously transforms into another element with emission of radioactivity.

trace e.'s Elements present in the body in minute amounts; important in metabolism or to form essential compounds.

eleotherapy (el-e-o-ther´ă-pe) See oleotherapy.

elephantiasis (el-ĕ-fan-ti´ă-sis) Thickening and inflammation of the skin and subcutaneous tissues, especially of the legs and genitalia, due to a long-term obstruction of the lymphatic circulation from any cause.

filarial e. Elephantiasis caused by infection of the lymphatic system by the threadlike worms *Wuchereria bancrofti* or *Brugia malayi*. Also called lymphatic filariasis.

elephant man disease (el´ĕ-fant man dĭ-zēz´) **1.** See Proteus syndrome. **2.** See neurofibromatosis (II).

elevator (el´ĕ-va-tor) **1.** An instrument used as a lever to pry up a depressed bone fragment. **2.** An instrument for extracting teeth and roots that cannot be grasped with a forceps.

eliminant (e-lim´ĭ-nănt) An agent that promotes the excretion or removal of waste.

elimination (e-lim-ĭ-na´shun) The expulsion of waste material from the body.

ELISA Acronym for enzyme-linked immunosorbent assay. See under assay.

elixir (ĕ-lik´ser) A clear, sweetened solution of alcohol and water, used as a vehicle for medicine taken orally.

ellipsoid (ĕ-lip´soid) Having an oval shape; applied especially to certain anatomic structures such as the oval masses of cells surrounding the second part of the penicillate artery of the spleen, and the outer portion of the inner rod segment of the retina.

elliptocytosis (ĕ-lip-to-si-to´sis) Inherited disorder in which a large number of red blood cells (25 to 90%) have an oval or elliptical shape. Also called ovalocytosis.

Ellis-van Creveld syndrome (el´is-van kre´veld sin´drōm) See chondroectodermal dysplasia, under dysplasia.

elongation (e-long-ga´shun) **1.** The act of increasing in length, or the condition of being lengthened. **2.** A measure of the ability of a metal to increase in length before breaking; indicates the ductility of a metal.

eluate (el´u-āt) The material separated by elution.

eluent (e-loo´ent) The liquid used in elution.

elution (e-loo´shun) Separation of substances by washing.

elutriation (e-loo-tre-a´shun) The process of purifying, separating, or removing by washing, decanting, and settling.

emaciation (e-mă-she-a´shun) Excessive wasting of the body; extreme leanness.

emaculation (e-mă-ku-la´shun) The removal of blemishes from the skin.

emanation (em-ă-na´shun) **1.** The act of giving off; exhalation. **2.** The gaseous product of disintegration of a radioactive substance.

emancipation (e-man-sĭ-pa´shun) In embryology, the gradual separation or segregation of different areas of the embryo into fields of specialized developmental potentialities.

emasculation (e-mas-ku-la´shun) See castration.

embalm (em-bahm´) To treat a dead body with preservatives to prevent its decay.

embed (em-bed´) To surround a tissue specimen with a firm substance, such as wax, to facilitate the cutting of thin slices.

embolectomy (em-bo-lek´tŏ-me) Surgical removal of an embolus.

emboli (em´bo-li) Plural of embolus.

embolic (em-bol´ik) Of or relating to an embolus or to embolism.

emboliform (em-bol´ĭ-form) Resembling an embolus or a wedge.

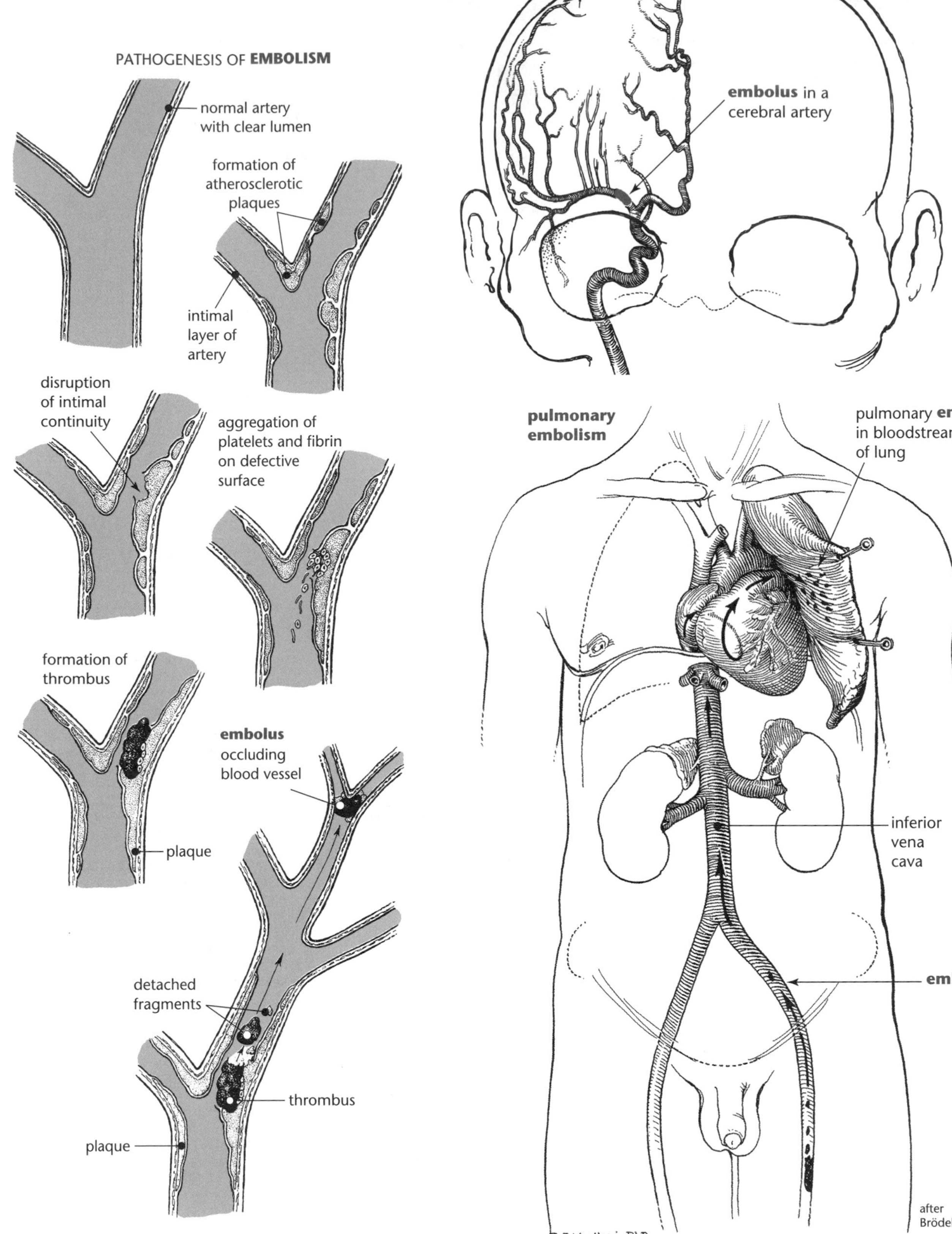

embolism (em´bo-liz-m) The sudden obstruction of a blood vessel by a clot or any foreign material (embolus) formed or introduced elsewhere in the circulatory system and carried to that point by the bloodstream.

air e. The presence of air bubbles in the blood vessels. Also called gas embolism.

amniotic fluid e. (AFE) A rare complication of childbirth in which amniotic fluid enters the blood circulation of the woman in labor through ruptured uterine veins, causing hemorrhage, shock, pulmonary embolism and, frequently, maternal death; principal predisposing factors include tumultuous uterine contractions and premature detachment of the placenta.

crossed e. See paradoxical embolism.

fat e. The presence of fat globules in the blood. Also called oil embolism.

gas e. See air embolism.

oil e. See fat embolism.

paradoxical e. The presence in an artery of an embolus that originated in a vein, having passed to the arterial circulation through a septal defect in the heart. Also called crossed embolism.

pulmonary e. (PE) The plugging of pulmonary arteries with fragments of a thrombus, most frequently from the leg after an operation.

septic pulmonary e. The lodging in a pulmonary artery of an infected thrombus that has become detached from its site of origin.

embolization (em-bo-lĭ-za´shun) **1.** The process by which natural or artificial substances in the circulation impede or obstruct blood or lymph flow. **2.** The deliberate occlusion of a blood vessel with any of a variety of materials (e.g., gelatin, sponge, coil, balloon) to stop uncontrollable internal bleeding or to cut off blood flow to a difficult to remove vascular tumor (thereby reducing its size); may be performed during a surgical operation or transcutaneously

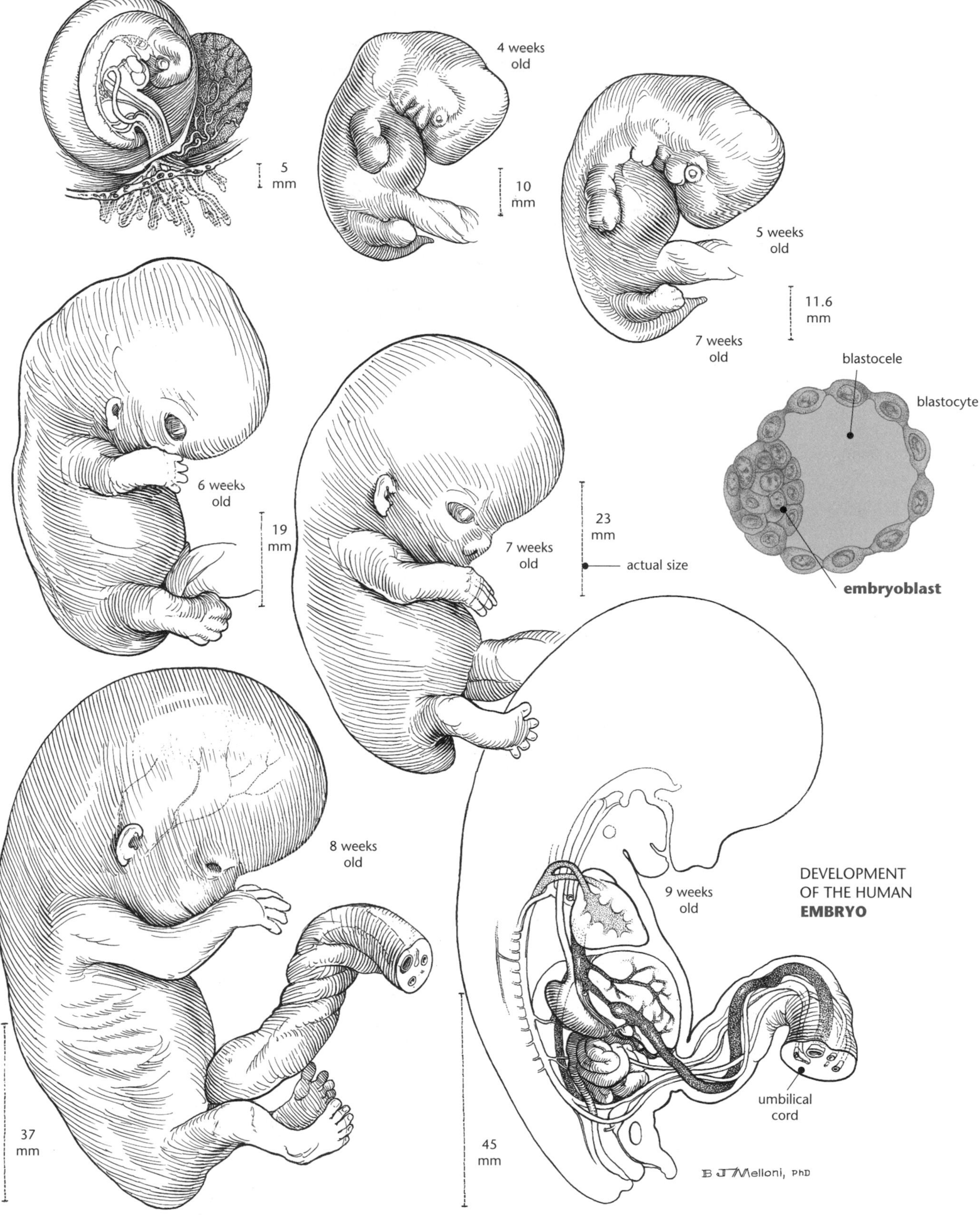

through a catheter. Also called embolotherapy.

percutaneous transcatheter e. See embolization (2).

trophoblastic e. Condition occurring as a complication of a molar pregnancy, marked by deposition of variable amounts of trophoblast in small pulmonary vessels (the trophoblast is carried in the blood circulation to the lungs), causing respiratory complications that may include (when volume of deposits is large) acute pulmonary embolism. Also called trophoblastic deportation.

embololalia (em-bŏ-lo-la´le-ă) The involuntary insertion of meaningless words in a sentence.

embolotherapy (em-bŏ-lo-ther´ă-pe) See embolization (2).

embolus (em´bo-lus) A plug within a vessel (a blood clot or other substance such as air, fat, or a tumor) that is carried in the blood stream from another site until it lodges and becomes an obstruction to circulation.

pantaloon e. See saddle embolus.

saddle e. Embolism that straddles the bifurcation of an artery (e.g., the aorta) and occludes both branches (the common iliac arteries). Also called pantaloon embolus.

embrasure (em-bra´zhur) The space produced by the diverging surfaces of adjacent teeth; it may be labial, buccal, lingual, incisal, occlusal, or gingival.

embrocation (em-bro-ka´shun) **1.** The rubbing of the body with liquid medication. **2.** The liquid used.

embryo (em´bre-o) An organism in the earliest stage of development; in man, from the time of conception to the end of the second month in the uterus.

embryoblast (em´bre-o-blast) An aggregation of cells that stick together and collect at the embryonic pole of the blastocyst and that give rise to the tissues of the embryo. Also called inner cell mass.

embryogenesis (em-bre-o-jen´ĕ-sis) The development of the embryo from the fertilized egg.

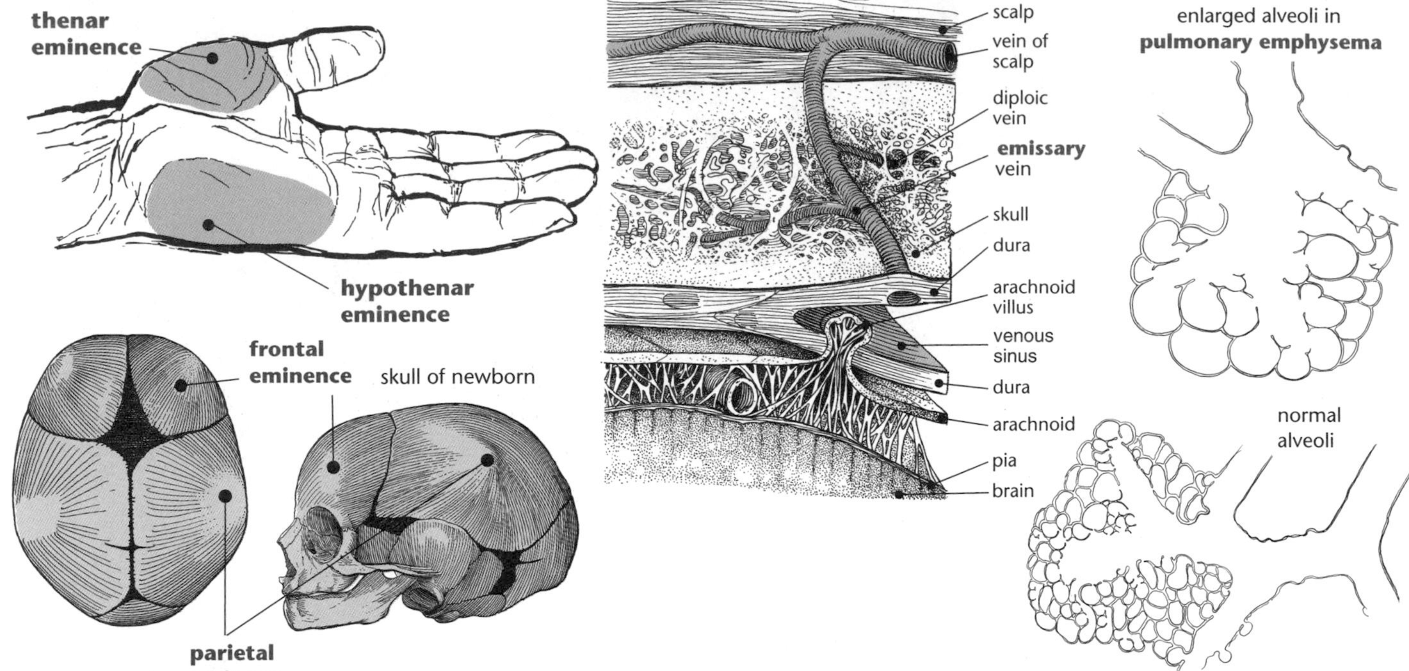

embryogenic, embryogenetic (em-bre-o-jen′ik, em-bre-o-jĕ-net′ik) Producing an embryo; relating to the origin of an embryo.

embryogeny (em-bre-oj′ĕ-ne) The origin of the embryo.

embryologist (em-bre-ol′ŏ-jist) A scientist who specializes in embryology.

embryology (em-bre-ol′ŏ-je) The science concerned with the formation and development of living organisms from the fertilization of the ovum until birth; the study of the development of the embryo. Also called developmental anatomy.

embryoma (em-bre-o′mă) See embryonal tumor, under tumor.

e. of kidney See Wilm's tumor, under tumor.

embryomorphous (em-bre-o-mor′fus) Similar to the structure of the embryo.

embryonic (em-bre-on′ik) **1.** Relating to an embryo. **2.** Undeveloped; rudimentary.

embryonization (em-bre-o-nī-za′shun) Reversion of any tissue to a primitive or embryonic stage.

embryopathy (em-bre-op′ă-the) A morbid condition in the embryo or fetus resulting from interference with normal development.

embryophore (em′bre-o-for) A membrane around the embryo of a tapeworm forming the inner layer of the egg shell.

embryotomy (em-bre-ot′ŏ-me) Any mutilating operation on the fetus to facilitate its removal through the birth canal,when delivery is not otherwise possible.

embryotoxon (em-bre-o-tok′son) A congenital opacity in the deep layers of the peripheral part of the cornea.

embryotroph (em′bre-o-trōf) **1.** The nutriment supplied to the embryo. **2.** The fluid adjacent to the blastodermic vesicle of deciduate placental mammals during implantation.

emedullate (e-med′u-lāt) To extract bone marrow.

emergency (e-mer′jen-se) A serious situation, developing suddenly and unexpectedly, and requiring immediate medical attention.

emergent (e-mer′jent) **1.** Developing suddenly and unexpectedly, and requiring prompt action. **2.** Coming out; leaving a body cavity or other part.

emery (em′er-e) A fine-grained abrasive composed of an extremely hard mineral; aluminum oxide combined with iron, magnesia, or silica.

emesis (em′ĕ-sis) Vomiting.

emetic (ĕ-met′ik) **1.** Causing vomiting. **2.** An agent that causes vomiting.

emetine (em′ĕ-tēn) A bitter-tasting alkaloid, $C_{29}H_{40}N_2O_4$; used parenterally as an amebicide.

emetocathartic (em-ĕ-to-kă-thar′tik) **1.** Both emetic and cathartic. **2.** Any agent that induces vomiting and bowel evacuation.

emigration (em-ĭ-gra′shun) A process of active motility, whereby motile white blood cells escape from small blood vessels to the surrounding tissues through the intercellular junctions of the vessel walls; monocytes, basophils, eosinophils, neutrophils, and lymphocytes are cells with the ability to emigrate.

eminence (em′ĭ-nens) A circumscribed, elevated area or prominence, especially of a bone.

frontal e. The rounded elevation on the skull on either side just above the eye.

hypothenar e. The prominence on the ulnar side (medial part) of the palm produced by the short muscles of the little finger; one of three muscle divisions of the hand.

parietal e. The prominence on either side of the skull just above the superior temporal line.

thenar e. The elevation on the radial side (lateral part) of the palm of the hand produced by the short muscles of the thumb; one of three muscle divisions of the hand.

emiocytosis (e-me-o-si-to′sis) See exocytosis.

emissary (em′ĭ-sar-e) Providing an outlet for a fluid, such as the veins that connect the venous sinuses within the skull with the veins of the scalp.

emission (e-mish′un) A discharge.

nocturnal e. Ejaculation of semen during sleep. Popularly called wet dream.

emmenagogue (e-men′ă-gog) **1.** Increasing or producing menstrual flow. **2.** Any agent producing such an effect.

emmenia (e-me′ne-ă) Menses.

emmetropia (em-ĕ-tro′pe-ă) The normal condition of the refractive system of the eye in which the light rays entering the eyeball focus exactly on the retina.

emollient (e-mol′e-ent) **1.** Soothing. **2.** An agent that softens and soothes the skin or mucous membranes.

emotion (e-mo′shŭn) Any strong feeling (joy, anger, fear).

emotional (e-mo′shun-al) **1.** Relating to an emotion. **2.** Easily affected with emotions.

empathic (em-path′ik) Relating to or marked by empathy.

empathy (em′pă-the) The intimate understanding of, and identification with, the feelings of another person.

emphysema (em-fĭ-se′mă) A swelling due to the abnormal presence of air in tissues or cavities of the body. The term usually refers to a condition of the lungs.

bullous e. Emphysema characterized by the presence of confluent air spaces in the lungs measuring over 1 cm in diameter; usually associated with generalized pulmonary emphysema.

centrilobular e. Emphysema in which the alveoli occupying the central area of each acinus become dilated and destroyed; generally more prominent in the upper lobes, but extending to all lung areas; commonly seen in chronic bronchitis.

compensatory e., compensating e. Dilatation of a portion of a lung when another portion is unable to function properly.

irregular e. A form in which the alveoli of the affected acinus are not uniformly involved; scar formation occurs almost invariably.

mediastinal e. The presence of air in the mediastinal tissue.

panlobular e. Emphysema marked by enlarged lungs with loss of vascular lung markings in areas of radiologic hyperlucency in the lower lobes; seen in individuals with homozygous α-1-antitrypsin deficiency.

paraseptal e. Emphysema with blebs and bullae that are largely localized subpleurally.

pulmonary e. Lung disease characterized by enlargement of the alveoli (air spaces distal to the terminal bronchioles) with loss of elastic fibers and rupture of their walls.

subcutaneous e. The presence of air or gas in the subcutaneous tissues.

empirical, empiric (em-pir′ĭ-kal, em-pir′ik) Based upon practical experience.

empiricism (em-pir′ĭ-siz-m) The view that experience serves as a guide to medical practice or to the therapeutic use of any remedy; reliance on experience as the only source of knowledge.

empyema (em-pi-e′mă) Pus in a body cavity, especially the pleural cavity.

e. of gallbladder Empyema occurring as a progression from acute gallbladder inflammation to persistent cystic duct obstruction, acummulation of bile, and invasion of stagnant bile by pus-forming microorganisms.

empyocele (em′pi-o-sēl) Accumulation of pus in the scrotum. Also called suppurating hydrocele.

emulsify (e-mul′sĭ-fi) To convert into an emulsion.

emulsion (e-mul′shun) A preparation composed of two liquids that do not mix, one being dispersed in the other in the form of small globules.

emulsive (e-mul′siv) A substance that can be emulsified or by which a fat or resin can be emulsified.

emulsoid (e-mul′soid) A dispersion in which the dispersed particles are relatively liquid and absorb some of the liquid in which they are dispersed. Also called emulsion colloid.

enamel (ĕ-nam′el) The hard, vitreous substance that covers the anatomic crown of a tooth.

mottled e. Defective structure of enamel due to excessive ingestion of fluoride during tooth formation; the affected teeth may have white, yellow, or brown spots which sometimes are pitted.

enamelogenesis (e-nam-el-o-jen′ĕ-sis) See

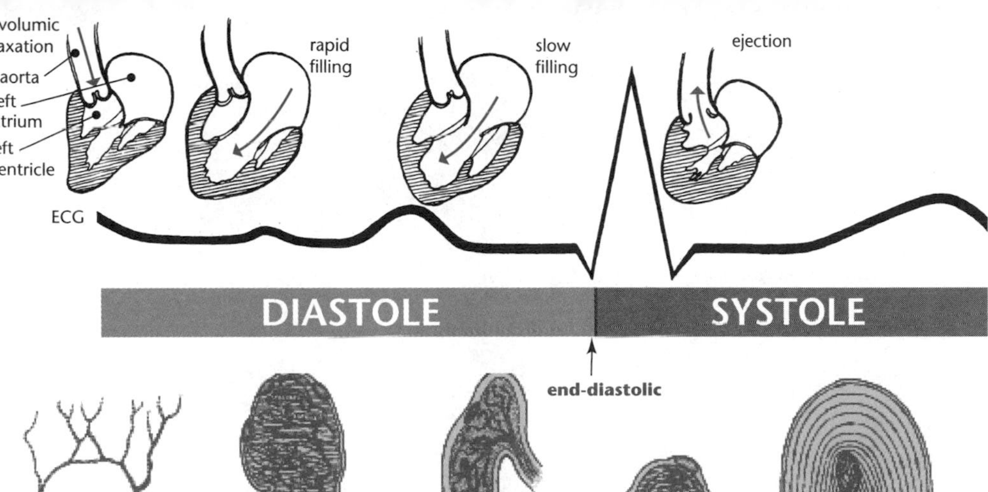

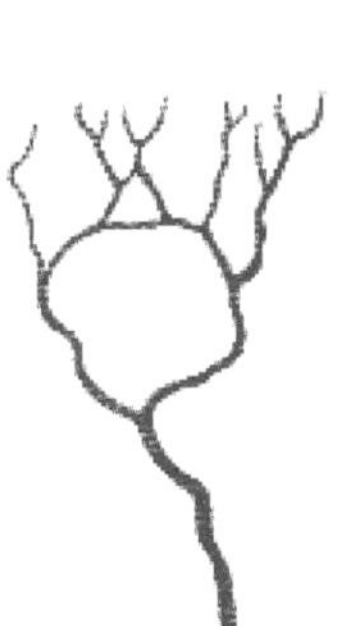
free nerve endings (pain)

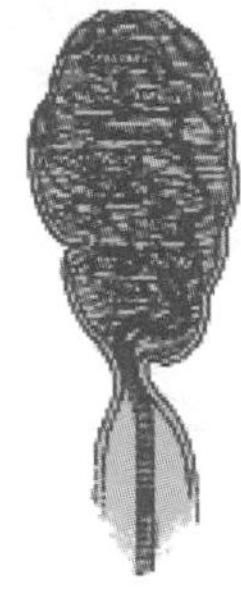
Meissner's corpuscle (touch)

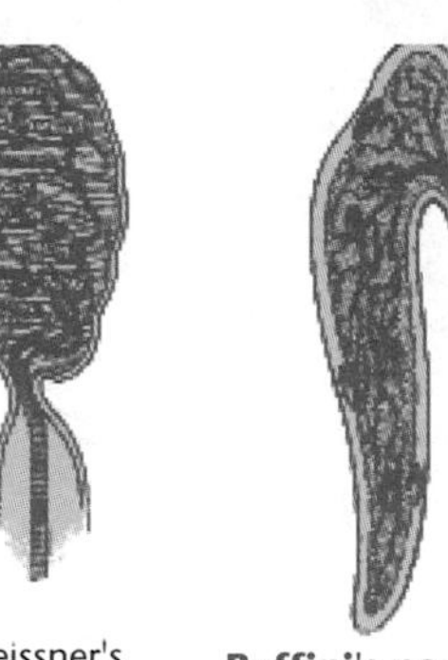
Ruffini's nerve endings (warmth)

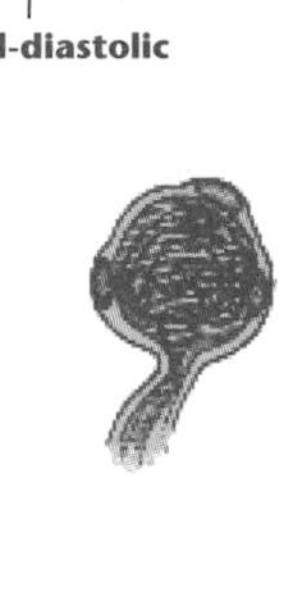
Krause's end-bulb (cold)

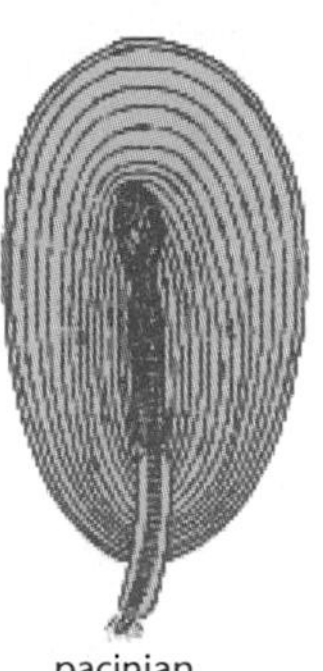
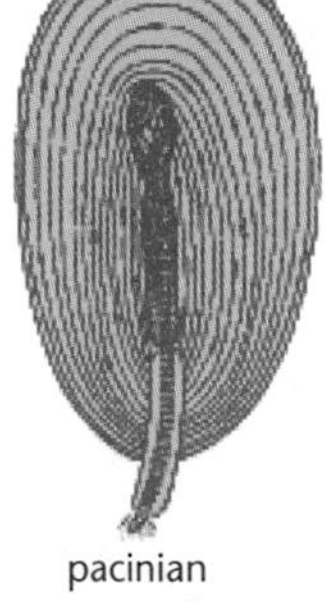
pacinian corpuscle (pressure)

endo-mysium of extrafusal muscle fibers
neuromuscular spindle
intrafusal muscle fibers:
nuclear chain type
nuclear bag type
flower-spray nerve ending (secondary sensory)
annulospiral nerve ending (primary sensory)
external capsule
internal capsule

amelogenesis.

e. imperfecta See amelogenesis imperfecta, under amelogenesis.

enameloma (e-nam-el-o´mă) Spherical nodule of enamel attached to a tooth, usually on the root. Also called enamel pearl.

enanthem, enanthema (e-nan´them, en-an-the´mă) Eruption on a mucous membrane, especially one accompanying an eruptive fever.

enantiomer (en-an´te-o-mer) One of a pair of molecules that are mirror images of each other; although they have the same chemical properties, certain of the physical and essentially all the physiologic properties are different.

enantiomerism (en-an-te-om´er-iz-m) In chemistry, isomerism in which the molecules in the configuration are related to one another like an object and its mirror image, thus not superimposable.

enantiomorph (en-an´te-o-morf) A crystal that is similar in form, but with the mirror image of another.

enantiopathy (en-an-te-o´pă-the) **1.** Treating with antidotes or substances that produce effects opposite to those of the morbid state being treated. **2.** The mutual antagonism of two morbid states.

enarthrodial (en-ar-thro´de-al) Relating to a ball and socket joint (enarthrosis).

enarthrosis (en-ar-thro´sis) A joint that permits extensive movement in almost any direction, as seen in the hip and shoulder. Also called ball and socket joint.

en block (ăn blok´) As a whole.

encanthis (en-kan´this) **1.** A small tumor at the inner canthus of the eye. **2.** Inflammation of the lacrimal caruncle (the pink fleshy mound at the medial canthus).

encapsulated (en-kap´su-lāt-ed) Encased in a capsule.

encephalemia (en-sef-ă-le´me-ă) Congestion of the brain.

encephalic (en-sĕ-fal´ik) **1.** Relating to the brain. **2.** In the skull.

encephalitic (en-sef-ă-lit´ik) Relating to inflammation of the brain.

encephalitis (en-sef-ă-li´tis) Inflammation of the brain, classified when possible by reference to the etiologic agent or pathogenic mechanism; headache, nausea, vomiting, fever, and lethargy are common initial symptoms.

acute necrotizing e. Encephalitis with tissue destruction affecting chiefly the temporal lobes; usually caused by herpes simplex virus.

e. periaxialis diffusa A rapidly progressive disease occurring chiefly in children; marked by widespread demyelinization of the cerebral cortex, with convulsions, mental symptoms, motor and sensory disturbances, and gradual loss of sight; death usually occurs within three years after onset.

encephalocele (en-sef´ă-lo-sēl) **1.** The cranial cavity. **2.** The ventricles of the brain. **3.** Protrusion of brain tissue through a congenital defect of the skull. Also called craniocele.

encephalodynia (en-sef-ă-lo-din´e-ă) Headache.

encephalogram (en-sef´ă-lo-gram) An x-ray picture of the head.

encephalography (en-sef-ă-log´ră-fe) Roentgenography of the brain. COMPARE: echoencephalography.

encephalolith (en-sef´ă-lo-lith) A cerebral calculus; a calculus in the brain.

encephalomalacia (en-sef-ă-lo-mă-la´shă) Softening of the brain.

encephalomeningitis (en-sef-ă-lo-men-in-ji´tis) See meningoencephalitis.

encephalomyelitis (en-sef-ă-lo-mi-ĕ-li´tis) Acute inflammation of the brain and spinal cord. Also called myeloencephalitis.

benign myalgic e. See epidemic neuromyasthenia, under neuromyasthenia.

encephalomyelocele (en-sef-ă-lo-mi´ĕ-lo-sēl) Congenital bone defect of the occipital area with herniation of the meninges, medulla, and spinal cord.

encephalomyelopathy (en-sef-ă-lo-mi-ĕl-op´ă-the) Any disease of the brain and spinal cord.

encephalomyeloradiculopathy (en-sef-ă-lo-mi-ĕ-lo-ră-dik-u-lop´ă-thē) Disease involving the brain, spinal cord, and roots of spinal nerves.

encephalon (en-sef´a-lon) See brain.

encephalopathy (en-sef-ă-lop´ă-the) Any disease of the brain. Also called cerebropathy.

bovine spongiform e. (BSE) Disease of cattle marked by spongy changes in the gray matter of the brainstem; thought to be caused by a prion. Also called mad-cow disease.

hepatic e. Metabolic disorder of the nervous system marked by flapping tremor (asterixis), musty odor of the breath, and disturbances of consciousness that may progress to deep coma; associated with advanced disease of the liver or with passage of toxic substances from the portal to the systemic circulation via a portocaval shunt.

hypertensive e. A form associated with severe arterial hypertension; marked by headache, nausea, vomiting, papilledema, convulsions, and coma.

lead e. Inflammation of the brain, vomiting, stupor, convulsions, and coma caused by ingestion or absorption of lead compounds.

encephalopsychosis (en-sef-ă-lo-si-ko´sis) Any psychosis caused by physical damage to the brain.

enchondroma (en-kon-dro´mă) A benign tumor composed of cartilaginous tissue and occurring within a bone.

enchondromatosis (en-kon-dro-ma-to´sis) A nonhereditary condition marked by the presence of multiple enchondromas in a long bone, resulting in shortening of the limb. Also called Ollier's disease; dyschondroplasia.

enchondrosarcoma (en-kon-dro-sar-ko´mă) A malignant bone tumor arising from a preexistent benign cartilaginous tumor within the bone (enchondroma).

enclave (en´klāv) A mass of tissue totally enclosed within another.

enclitic (en-klit´ĭk) Denoting the relation of the planes of the fetal head to those of the pelvis of the mother.

encoding (en-kōd´ing) Modification of stimuli received through the senses; first stage in the memory process.

encyesis (en-si-e´sis) A normal pregnancy in the uterus.

encysted (en-sist´ed) Enclosed in a cyst or a membranous sac.

Endamoeba (end-ă-mē´bă) A genus of amebae not parasitic in man; the term is sometimes used incorrectly for *Entamoeba*.

endarterectomy (end-ar-ter-ek´tŏ-me) Surgical removal of atheromas with the lining of an artery.

endarterial (end-ar-ter´e-al) Within an artery; relating to the intima or inner layer of the arterial wall.

endarteritis (end-ar-ter-i´tis) Inflammation of the inner layer of an artery. Also called endoarteritis.

endarterium (end-ar-ter´e-um) The intima or inner layer of the arterial wall.

endaural (end-aw´ral) **1.** Within the ear. **2.** Through the ear canal.

end-bulb (end´bulb) See end bulb, under bulb.

Krause's e-b. See Krause's end bulb, under bulb.

end-diastolic (end-di-ă-stol´ik) **1.** Occurring at the termination of diastole, just before the next systole (e.g., end-diastolic pressure). **2.** Interrupting the final stage of diastole, barely premature (e.g., end-diastolic extrasystole).

endemic (en-dem´ik) Relating to any disease prevalent continually in a particular locality.

endergonic (end-er-gon´ik) Indicating a chemical reaction that is accompanied by an absorption of free energy, regardless of the form of energy involved.

endermic, endermatic (en-der´mik, en-der-mat´ik) Through the skin, as the action of certain medicines when absorbed through the skin.

end-feet (end-´fēt) See axon terminal, under terminal.

ending (end´ing) A termination, as of a nerve.

annulospiral nerve e. A coiled nerve ending around the nuclear region of a muscle fiber; sensitive to stretch.

flower-spray nerve e.'s Intricate series of nerve

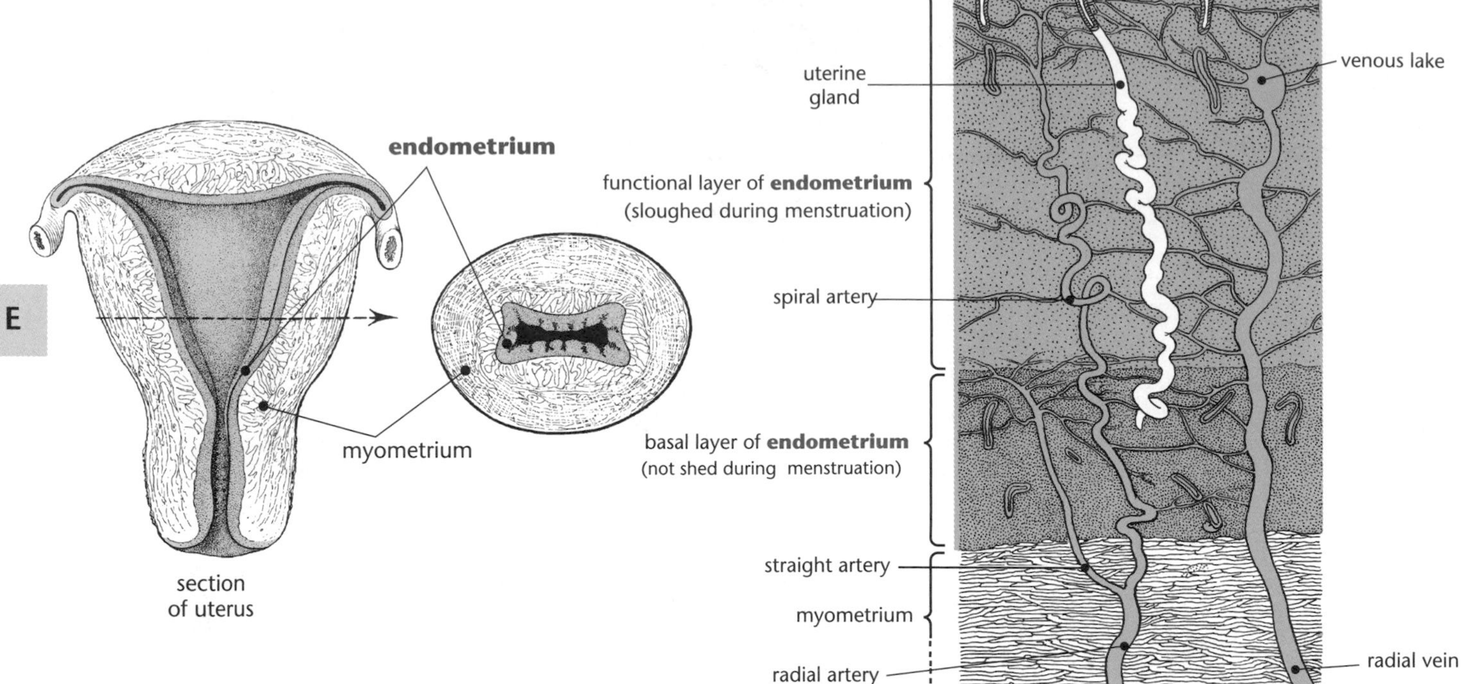

branches on the contractile part of the intrafusal muscle fibers; sensitive to increased tension.

free nerve e.'s Network of nerve endings found throughout the body, in skin, mucous membranes, and deep tissues; their fibers are both myelinated and non-myelinated.

gamma-efferent nerve e.'s The terminal part of motor fibers that innervate the intrafusal muscle fibers near their ends.

nerve e. Any one of the specialized terminations of sensory or motor nerve fibers.

Ruffini's nerve e.'s Sensory nerve endings that serve as joint receptors, mechanoreceptors, receptors for position sense, and skin receptors; characterized by whorls of fine fibers that end as numerous knobs. Also called Ruffini's corpuscles.

endoarteritis (en-do-ar-ter-i´tis) See endarteritis.

endoauscultation (en-do-aws-kul-ta´shun) Auscultation of the heart or stomach by passing a stethoscopic tube or electronic amplifier into the esophagus or heart.

endobronchial (en-do-brong´ke-al) Within the bronchial tubes. Also called intrabronchial.

endocardial (en-do-kar´de-al) **1.** Relating to the endocardium. **2.** In the heart.

endocardiography (en-do-kar-de-og´ră-fe) Recording of the electric currents traversing the heart muscle, prior to a heartbeat, with the exploring electrode within the heart chambers.

endocarditis (en-do-kar-dī´tis) Inflammation of the lining membrane of the heart chambers.

abacterial thrombotic e. See nonbacterial thrombotic endocarditis.

atypical verrucous e. See Libman-Sacks endocarditis.

bacterial e. Endocarditis due to bacteria or other microorganisms, causing deformity of the valve leaflets; it may be acute, usually caused by pyogenic organisms such as staphylococci, or subacute (chronic), usually due to *Streptococcus viridans* or *Streptococcus faecalis*.

Libman-Sacks e. A nonbacterial endocarditis associated with systemic lupus erythematosus (SLE). Also called atypical verrucous endocarditis.

Löffler's e. An uncommon condition characterized by fibrosis and large thrombi of the heart wall, frequently associated with eosinophilia and congestive heart failure. Also called Löffler's disease.

marantic e. See nonbacterial thrombotic endocarditis.

nonbacterial thrombotic e. Endocarditis associated with verrucous lesions and clots, occurring in the last stages of many chronic infections and wasting diseases. Also called abacterial thrombotic endocarditis; marantic endocarditis; terminal endocarditis.

rheumatic e. Endocarditis with special involvement of the valves associated with rheumatic fever.

subacute infective e. Endocarditis with insidious onset of symptoms, caused by an organism of moderate to low virulence; symptoms include nondescript malaise, low grade fever without chills, weight loss, and flulike symptoms.

terminal e. See nonbacterial thrombotic endocarditis.

vegetative e., verrucous e. A type associated with the formation of fibrinous clots on the ulcerated valves.

endocardium (en-do-kar´de-um) The serous membrane that lines the chambers of the heart.

endoceliac (en-do-se´le-ak) In any of the cavities of the body. Also called intracelial.

endocervical (en-do-ser´vĭ-kal) Within the uterine cervix. Also called intracervical.

endocervicitis (en-do-ser-vĭ-si´tis) Inflammation of the mucous membrane of the uterine cervix.

endochondral (en-do-kon´dral) Within cartilage. Also called intracartilaginous.

endocranial (en-do-kra´ne-al) **1.** Within the skull. **2.** Relating to the skull.

endocrine (en´do-krĭn) Secreting internally; denoting a gland whose secretions are discharged into the blood or lymph.

endocrinology (en-do-krĭ-nol´ŏ-je) The branch of science dealing with endocrine glands and their secretions.

endocrinopathy (en-do-krĭ-nop´ă-the) Any disease of the endocrine glands.

endocrinotherapy (en-do-krĭ-no-ther´ă-pe) Treatment of disease with extracts of endocrine glands.

endocrinous (en-do-krin´us) Relating to any internal secretion.

endocytosis (en-do-si-to´sis) The uptake of particles by a cell through invagination of its plasma membrane.

endoderm (en´do-derm) The innermost of the three germ layers of the embryo; it gives rise to the lining of the gastrointestinal tract from pharynx to rectum and to neighboring glands such as the liver, pancreas, thyroid, etc. Also called entoderm.

endodontics (en-do-don´tiks) The branch of dentistry concerned with the diagnosis and treatment of diseases of the tooth pulp and/or infection of the root canal and periapical areas.

endodontist (en-do-don´tist) A specialist in endodontics.

endoenzyme (en-do-en´zīm) An enzyme that is retained by and acts within the cell that produced it.

endogenous (en-doj´ĕ-nus) Originating within the body.

endointoxication (en-do-in-tok-sĭ-ka´shun) Poisoning by a toxin produced within the organism.

endolaryngeal (en-do-lă-rin´je-al) Within the larynx.

endolith (en´do-lith) See pulp stone, under stone.

endolymph (en´do-limf) The fluid contained in the membranous labyrinth of the inner ear; an isotonic solution that is of high potassium and low sodium concentration.

endometrial (en-do-me´tre-al) Relating to the endometrium.

endometrioma (en-do-me-tre-o´mă) A mass of ectopic endometrium in endometriosis.

endometriosis (en-do-me-tre-o´sis) An abnormal condition in which the uterine mucous membrane invades other tissues in the pelvic cavity; the uterus and ovaries are the most common sites; other areas include the intestines, umbilicus, bladder, and ureters.

e. interna See adenomyosis.

endometritis (en-do-me-trī´tis) Inflammation of the inner lining of the uterus.

endometrium (en-do-me´tre-um) The mucosal layer lining the cavity of the uterus; its structure changes with age and with the menstrual cycle.

endomitosis (en-do-mi-to´sis) See endopolyploidy.

endomorph (en´do-morf) A person having a body build characterized by prominence of the abdomen and other parts developed from the embryonic endodermal layer.

endomysium (en-do-mis´e-um) The microscopic sheath of delicate connective tissue that surrounds and separates individual muscle fibers.

endoneurium (en-do-nu´re-um) The delicate connective tissue sheath surrounding and separating individual nerve fibers.

endonuclease (en-do-nu´kle-ās) A nuclease (phosphodiesterase) that cleaves polynucleotides into poly- or oligonucleotide fragments of varying size.

restrictive e. One of many endonucleases isolated from bacteria that act as molecular scissors to cut DNA molecules at specific locations; used extensively as a laboratory tool. Also called restrictive enzyme; commonly called chemical knife.

endoparasite (en-do-par´ă-sīt) A parasite that lives within the body of its host.

endopeptidase (en-do-pep´tĭ-dās) A proteolytic enzyme that is capable of hydrolyzing a peptide linkage at points within the chain, not near the ends (e.g., pepsin, trypsin, and ribonuclease).

endophlebitis (en-do-fle-bi´tis) Inflammation of the inner layer of a vein.

endophthalmitis (en-dof-thal-mi´tis) Inflammation of the internal structures of the eye.

endoplasm (en´do-plaz-m) The inner portion of the

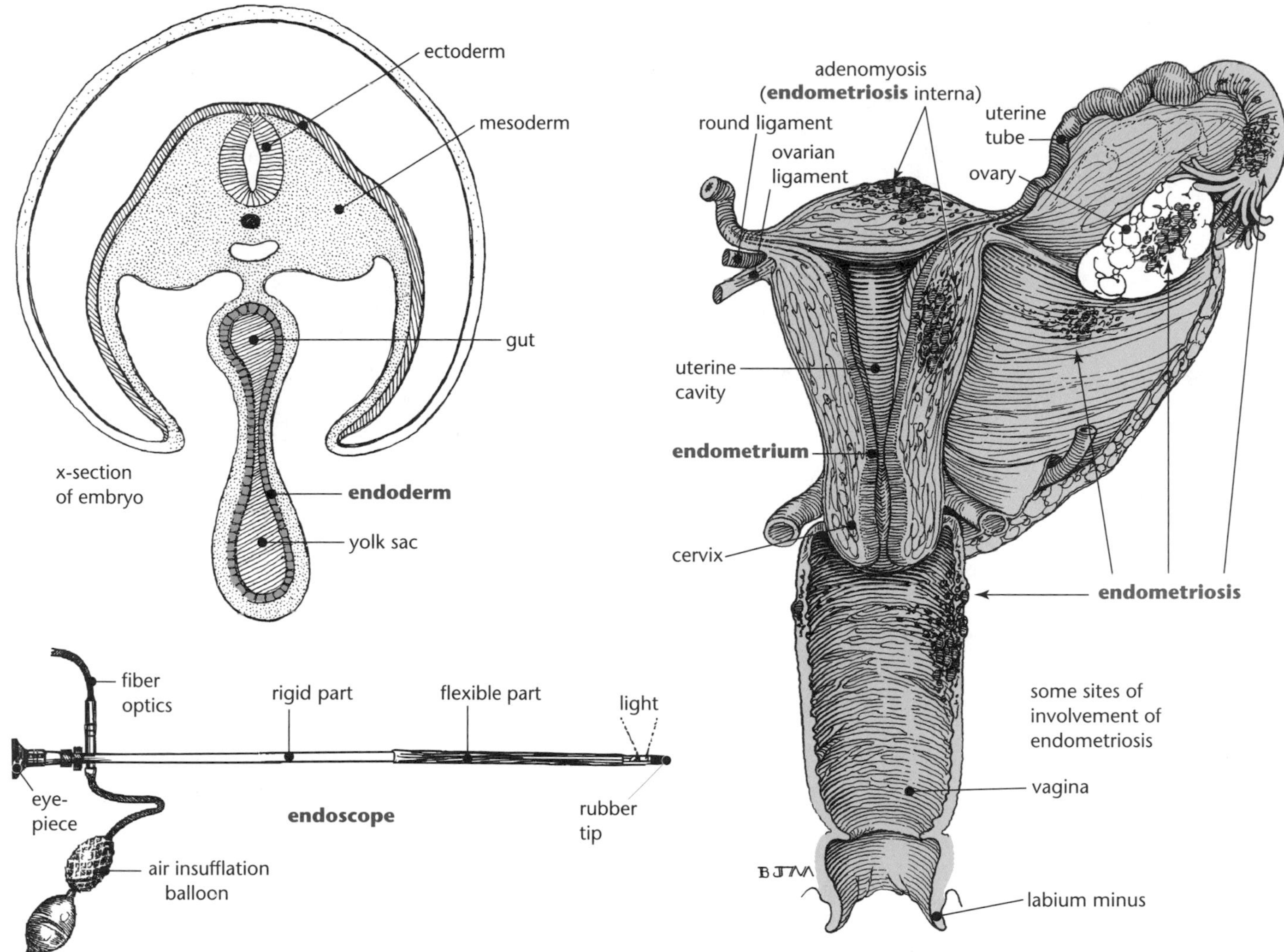

cytoplasm; it is less viscous than the ectoplasm and contains most of the cell's solid structures.

endopolyploidy (en-do-pol-e-ploi´de) The reproduction of nuclear elements without accompanying spindle formation or cytoplasmic division, resulting in a polyploid nucleus. Also called endomitosis.

end-organ (end-or´gan) See end organ, under organ.

endorphin (en-dor´fin) One of a group of low-molecular weight peptides normally found in the brain and other parts of the body; capable of producing effects similar to those of opiates.

endosalpinx (en-do-sal´pinks) The mucous membrane that lines the interior of a uterine (fallopian) tube.

endoscope (en´do-skōp) An instrument used to examine the interior of a hollow organ or a cavity (e.g., gastroscope, proctoscope, and cystoscope).

endoscopy (en-dos´kŏ-pe) Inspection of the interior of a canal or any air or food passage by means of an endoscope.

endoskeleton (en-do-skel´ĕ-ton) The internal supporting bony skeleton of vertebrates.

endosmosis (en-dos-mo´sis) The passage of a fluid through a membrane into a cavity or a cell containing fluid of a lesser density; osmosis in a direction toward the interior of a cell or a cavity.

endosonography (en-do-so-nog´ră-fe) See endoscopic ultrasonography, under ultrasonography.

endosonoscopy (en-do-so-nos´ko-pe) Ultrasonic scanning with transducers, used as miniature probes introduced into hollow or tubular structures (e.g., gastrointestinal tract, bladder).

endospore (en´do-spor) **1.** A small, resistant, asexual spore, such as that formed within the vegetative cells of some bacteria, particularly those belonging to the genera *Bacillus* and *Clostridium*. **2.** The innermost layer of the wall of a spore.

endosteitis, endostitis (en-dos-te-i´tis, en-dos-ti´tis) Inflammation of the tissue lining the medullary cavity of a bone (endosteum).

endosteoma (en-dos-te-o´mă) A benign tumor in the medullary cavity of a bone.

endosteum (en-dos´te-um) The membrane lining bone cavities.

endothelin (en-do-thēl´in) Peptide derived from the inner lining of blood vessels that induces constriction of the smooth muscle of the vessels.

endothelioma (en-do-the-le-o´mă) Any tumor, benign or malignant, derived from the endothelial tissue of blood vessels, lymphatic vessels, or serous membranes.

endothelium (en-do-the´le-um) A thin layer of cells lining serous cavities, blood vessels, and lymph vessels.

endothermic (en-do-ther´mik) Denoting a chemical reaction that produces heat absorption.

endothrix (en´do-thriks) Within the hair shaft; denoting a type of fungal infection in which the hyphae grow only within the hair shaft, where they form long, parallel rows of arthrospores. COMPARE: ectothrix.

endotoxemia (en-do-tok-se´me-ă) Presence of endotoxins in the blood, which may cause shock.

endotoxin (en-do-tok´sin) A toxin produced and retained by bacterial cells and released only by destruction or death of the cells. Also called intracellular toxin.

endotracheal (en-do-tra´ke-al) Within the trachea.

endplate, end-plate (end´plāt) The terminal part of a motor nerve fiber that transmits nerve impulses to muscle.

end-product (end prod´ukt) A chemical product that represents the final sequence of metabolic reactions.

end-stage renal disease (end-stāj re´nal dĭ-zez´) (ESRD) Failure of kidney function to a degree that the kidneys can no longer support life; may result from a variety of diseases but in the United States diabetes mellitus and hypertension together are responsible for the greatest number of cases. By HCFA (Health Care Financing Administration) regulation, a serum creatinine level of 8.0 mg/dl or greater, or a creatinine clearance of 10 ml/min or less, qualifies an individual to receive renal replacement therapy without further justification. If symptoms are severe, individuals may require dialysis at lesser levels of serum creatinine or higher levels of creatinine clearance.

enema (en´ĕ-mă) **1.** Infusion of a fluid into the rectum for cleansing or other therapeutic purposes. **2.** The liquid so infused.

barium e. Instillation of the radiopaque medium barium sulfate in solution prior to x-ray examination of the bowel.

high e. Enema instilled high into the colon, usually with the aid of a tube. Also called entero-clysis.

energetics (en-er-jet´iks) The physics of energy and its changes.

energy (en´er-je) (W) The exertion of power to effect physical change; the capacity for doing work, associated with material bodies or existing independent of matter.

e. of activation The amount of energy needed by molecules to initiate a reaction.

binding e. The energy released in binding a group of protons and neutrons into an atomic nucleus.

chemical e. Energy emanating from a chemical reaction or absorbed in the formation of a chemical compound.

conservation of e. The principle that the total amount of energy remains constant, none being lost or created in the conversion of one type of force into another.

free e. A thermodynamic function, symbolized as ΔG, that expresses the maximum amount of work that can be obtained from a chemical reaction. Also called Gibbs free-energy function.

nuclear e. The energy given off by a nuclear reaction, especially by fission, fusion, or radioactive deterioration; the energy stored in the formation of an atomic nucleus.

potential e. The energy that a particle has by virtue of its position relative to a reference position and which is not being exerted at the time.

enervation (en-er-va´shun) Lack of energy and vigor; lassitude.

engagement (en-gāj´ment) In obstetrics, a cardinal movement of labor during which the biparietal plane

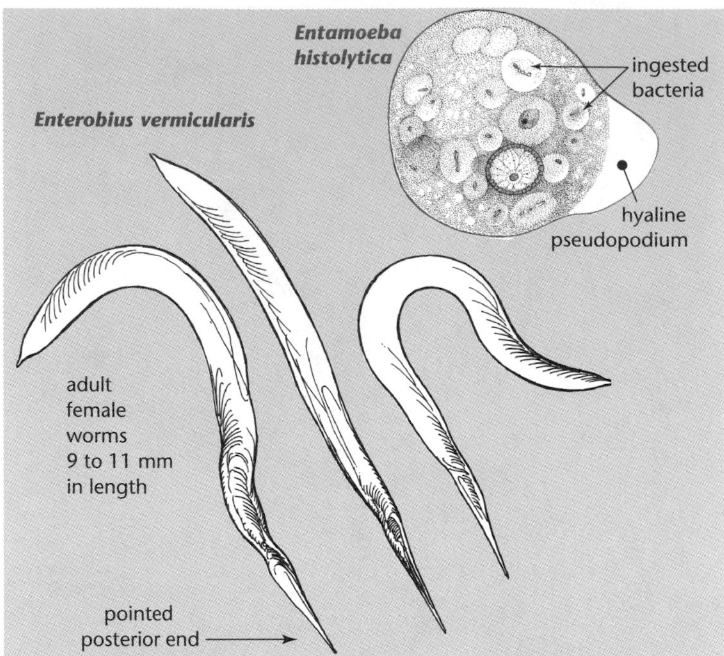

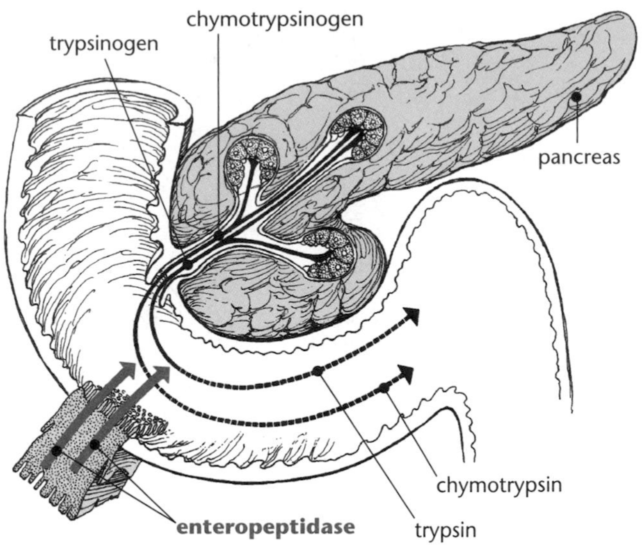

of the fetal head descends to a level below the plane of the pelvic inlet.

engineering (en-jin-er´ing) The practical application of the principles of mathematics and the physical sciences.

biomedical e. Application of engineering in solving biologic and medical problems; includes development of prostheses (e.g., artificial limbs and heart valves) and electrical devices (e.g., pacemakers). Also called bioengineering.

genetic e. Direct alteration of the genetic material of a living organism to study genetic processes, to modify heredity, to produce hormones or proteins, and potentially to correct genetic defects. See also recombinant DNA, under DNA.

engorged (en-gōrjd´) Congested or filled to excess; distended with blood or other fluid.

enhancement (en-hans´ment) **1.** Augmentation. **2.** In immunology, prolongation of a process by suppressing opposing factors (e.g., prolongation of graft survival by therapy with antibodies directed toward the graft allogens). **3.** Improvement of the definition of an x-ray or computer image.

acoustic e. In ultrasonography, overamplification of echoes returning from behind fluid-filled structures.

contrast e. Increase in definition obtained by using a material that accentuates vascular structures, such as iodinated substances for computed tomography (CT) scans and gadolinium for magnetic resonance imaging (MRI) scans.

ring e. In computed tomography, a bright circle seen on an image made after injection of a contrast medium; indicates localization of the contrast on the periphery of an abscess.

enkephalin (en-kef´ă-lin) A pentapeptide present in many parts of the brain and in nerve endings elsewhere in the body; believed to be a neurotransmitter.

enol (e´nol) An organic compound containing a hydroxyl group (alcohol) attached to a doubly bonded (ethylenic) carbon atom; the name is derived from ethyl*ene* alcoh*ol*.

enophthalmos (en-of-thal´mos) Backward displacement of the eyeball causing it to recede within the orbit.

enostosis (en-os-to´sis) A bony growth within a bone.

ensiform (en´sĭ-form) Shaped like a sword.

entactin (ent-ak´tin) An adhesive glycoprotein that binds to laminin (another adhesive glycoprotein) in the basal lamina of the renal glomerulus. See also laminin.

Entamoeba (en-tă-me´bă) A genus of protozoan parasites.

E. coli A nonpathogenic species found in the intestine.

E. gingivalis A species occurring in the mouth.

E. histolytica A species that infects human intestines, causing amebic dysentery; it may also invade the liver.

enteral (en´ter-al) Within the intestine.

enterectomy (en-ter-ek´tŏ-me) Surgical removal of a segment of the intestine.

enteric (en-ter´ik) Relating to the intestines.

enteritis (en-ter-ĭ´is) Inflammation of the intestines.

regional e. A chronic recurrent disease, mainly of young adults, marked by inflammation and ulceration of segments of the small intestine and colon; causing abdominal pain, diarrhea, fever, and weight loss; cause is unknown. Also called regional ileitis; terminal ileitis; Crohn's disease.

enteroanastomosis (en-ter-o-ă-nas-to-mo´sis) See enteroenterostomy.

Enterobacter (en-ter-o-bak´ter) Genus of gram-negative, rod-shaped, gas-producing bacteria found in soil, sewage, feces, and dairy products; several species cause opportunistic diseases; of these, *E. cloacae* accounts for the majority of hospital-acquired infections of the lungs, urinary tract, and blood.

Enterobacteriaceae (en-ter-o-bak-te-re-a´se-e) A family of gram-negative rod-shaped bacteria (order Eubacteriales); many of its members cause hospital-acquired infections (e.g., *Escherichia, Enterobacter, Klebsiella, Providencia*).

enterobiasis (en-ter-o-bĭ´ă-sis) Intestinal infection with nematode worms.

Enterobius (en-ter-o´be-us) A genus of nematode worms (family Oxyuridae).

E. vermicularis The pinworm; a short roundworm infecting the large intestine.

enterocele (en´ter-o-sēl) Herniation through the rectouterine pouch; may protrude anteriorly into the rectovaginal septum (forming a bulge on the posterior vaginal wall), posteriorly into the anal canal (simulating a prolapsed rectum), or in both directions as a "saddle hernia" (through the vagina and through the anal canal). It is almost always associated with other musculofascial weakness (e.g., cystocele, rectocele, uterine prolapse). Also called posterior vaginal hernia; cul-de-sac hernia; Douglas' pouch hernia.

enterocleisis (en-ter-o-kli´sis) Occlusion of the intestinal tract.

omentum e. The operative use of omentum to close an opening in the intestine.

enteroclysis (en-ter-ok´lĭ-sis) See high enema, under enema.

Enterococcus (en-ter-o-kok´ŭs) A genus of gram-positive, round bacteria previously classified as members of the genus *Streptococcus*; some species cause infections in humans, especially in elderly or debilitated patients.

E. faecalis A species isolated from the human intestinal tract; it is a cause of subacute bacterial endocarditis. Formerly called *Streptococcus faecalis.*

E. faecium A species normally inhabiting the human intestinal tract; has been found in intra-abdominal abscesses and in infectious complications of liver and gallbladder surgery. Formerly called *Streptococcus faecium.*

enterococcus (en-ter-o-kok´us) Any streptococcus that inhabits the intestinal tract.

enterocolitis (en-ter-o-ko-li´tis) Inflammation of the mucous membrane of the small intestine and colon.

pseudomembranous e. An acute form with formation and passage in the feces of membrane-like material; often occurring after prolonged antibiotic therapy.

enterocolostomy (en-ter-o-ko-los´tŏ-me) Operative creation of an opening between the small intestine and any part of the colon.

enterocyst (en´ter-o-sist) A cyst of the intestinal wall.

enteroenterostomy (en-ter-o-en-ter-os´tŏ-me) Operative connection of any two noncontinuous segments of intestine. Also called enteroanastomosis; intestinal anastomosis.

enterogastrone (en-ter-o-gas´trōn) One of the gastrointestinal hormones released during digestion; it is secreted by the upper intestinal mucosa when a significant amount of gastric contents reaches the upper intestine, and inhibits secretion and movements of the stomach.

enterokinase (en-ter-o-ki´nās) See enteropeptidase.

enterokinetic (en-ter-o-kĭ-net´ik) Stimulating contraction of the gastrointestinal tract.

enterolith (en´ter-o-lith) Any concretion or calculus in the intestine.

enterology (en-ter-ol´o-je) The branch of medicine concerned with the intestinal tract.

enteron (en´ter-on) The intestinal tract, especially the small intestine.

enteroparesis (en-ter-o-par-e´sis) Weakness and relaxation of the intestinal walls.

enteropathogenic (en-ter-o-path-o-jen´ik) Causing intestinal disease.

enteropathy (en-ter-op´ă-the) Any disease of the intestines.

gluten-induced e. See celiac disease.

enteropeptidase (en-ter-o-pep´tĭ-dās) An enzyme secreted by the duodenal mucosa that converts

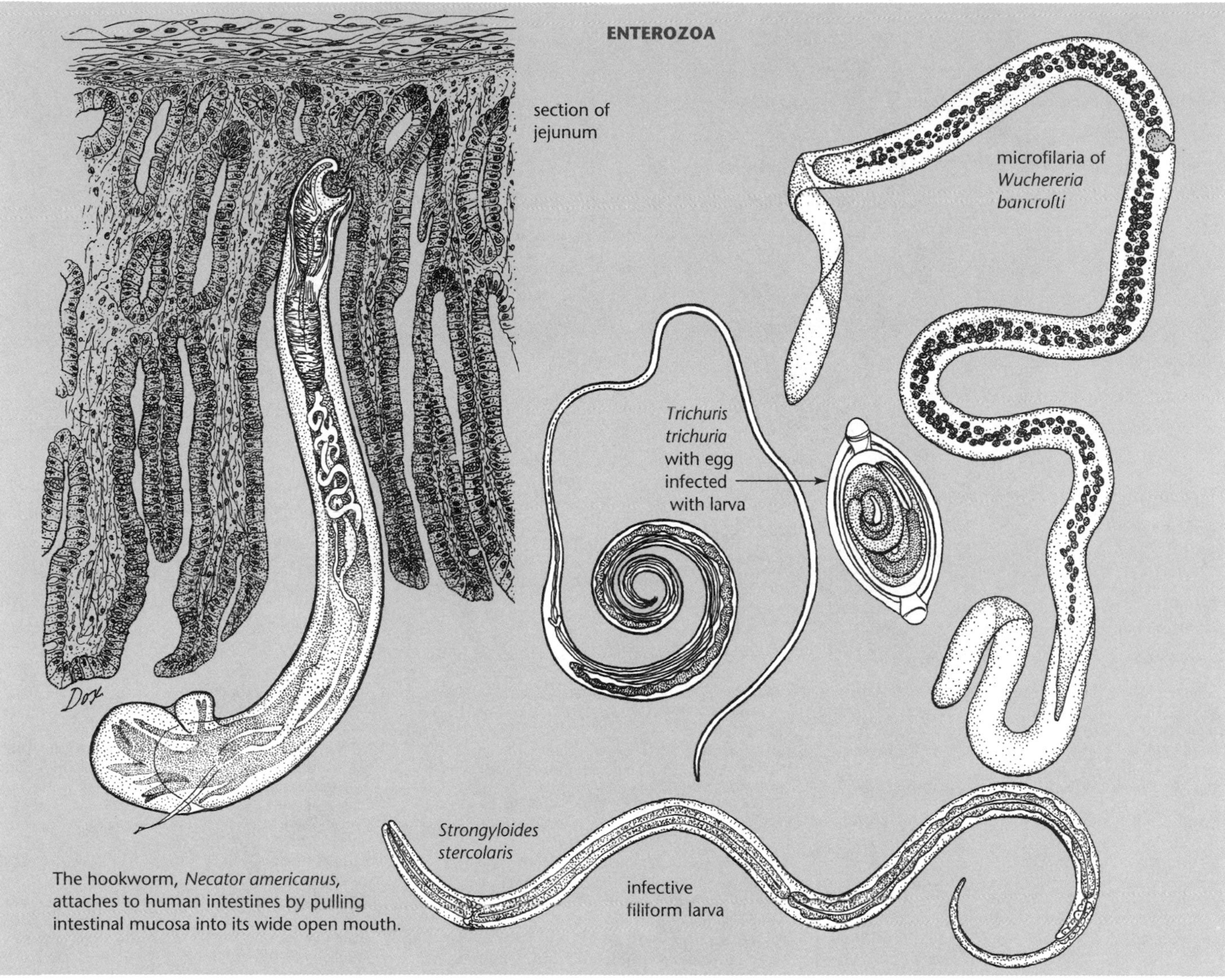

trypsinogen (pancreatic secretion) to trypsin (protein-splitting enzyme). Also called enterokinase.

enteropexy (en′ter-o-pek-se) Fixation of a portion of the intestine to the abdominal wall.

enteroptosis, enteroptosia, (en-tĕr-o-to′sis, en-tĕr-o-to′sē-ă) Downward displacement of the intestines in the abdominal cavity, as observed sometimes in obese individuals.

enterospasm (en′ter-o-spaz-m) Intestinal spasm or colic.

enterostenosis (en-ter-o-stĕ-no′sis) Narrowing or stricture of the intestinal lumen.

enterostomy (en-ter-os′tŏ-me) The establishment of an opening into the intestine, temporary or permanent, through the abdominal wall.

enterotomy (en-ter-ot′ŏ-me) Incision into the intestine.

enterotoxin (en-ter-o-tok′sin) A cytotoxin specific for the cells of the mucous membrane of the intestine.

Enterovirus (en′ter-o-vi-rus) A genus of viruses (family Picornaviridae) that infect the intestinal tract primarily but multiply also in muscles, nerves, and other tissues; includes viruses causing poliomyelitis, meningitis, gastroenteritis, and viral hepatitis, type A.

enterozoon (en-ter-o-zo′on) An intestinal parasite.

enthesitis (en-thĕ-si′tis) Irritation of the attachments of muscle or tendons to bone.

entoderm (en′to-derm) See endoderm.

entomology (en-to-mol′o-je) The study of insects.

entomophobia (en-to-mo-fo′be-ă) Abnormal fear of insects.

entopic (en-top′ik) Occurring or located in the normal site; opposed to ectopic.

entoptic (en-top′tik) Located within the eyeball.

entozoon (en-to-zo′on), *pl.* **entozo′a** A parasitic animal living in any of the internal organs of its host.

entropion (en-tro′pe-on) Inversion or inward displacement of the margin of an eyelid.

entropy (en′tro-pe) **1.** That fraction of energy not available during a chemical reaction for the performance of work, because it has gone to increasing the random motion of the atoms or molecules in a system. **2.** A measure of the ability of a system to undergo spontaneous change.

enucleate (e-noo′kle-āt) **1.** To remove whole, as in shelling out a nut. **2.** To destroy or remove the nucleus.

enucleation (e-noo-kle-a′shun) The surgical removal of a tumor or of an organ, such as the eyeball, in its entirety, without rupture.

enuresis (en-u-re′sis) Involuntary release of urine.

nocturnal e. Involuntary and repeated release of urine while asleep, occurring in children beyond the age of toilet training; may be of nervous or emotional origin, or may be caused by infection or inflammation of the urinary tract. Commonly called bed-wetting.

environment (en-vī′ron-ment) The collection of physical or external conditions affecting the growth and development of organisms.

enzootic (en-zo-ot′ik) Indicating a disease of animals that is indigenous to a specific locality, analogous to an endemic disease among humans.

enzymatic (en-zĭ-mat′ik) Relating to an enzyme.

enzyme (en′zīm) A protein secreted by the body that acts as a catalyst by promoting or accelerating a chemical change in other substances while remaining unchanged in the process.

autolytic e. An enzyme capable of causing autolysis or digestion of the cell in which it was formed.

branching e. See α-glucan-branching glycosyltransferase.

digestive e. An enzyme that promotes the hydrolysis of protein, carbohydrate, and fat in the digestive tract prior to absorption.

extracellular e. Any enzyme that performs its functions outside of the cell in which it originates (e.g., a digestive enzyme).

induced e. An enzyme produced by the addition of its specific substrate to cells that normally do not metabolize that substrate.

proteolytic e. See protease.

restrictive e. Enzyme that acts as molecular scissors by cutting DNA molecules at specific locations.

transferring e. See transferase.

enzymic (en-zim′ik) Enzymatic.

enzymology (en-zi-mol′ŏ-je) The branch of science concerned with the study of enzymes, their structure and function.

enzymolysis (en-zi-mol′ĭ-sis) The chemical decomposition brought about by an enzyme.

eosin (e′o-sin) A crystalline product of coal tar, used in solution to stain cells for microscopic study; it imparts a reddish color to the specimen.

eosinoblast (e-o-sin′o-blast) A young granular white blood cell (myeloblast) that develops into an eosinophil.

eosinopenia (e-o-sin-o-pe′ne-ă) Deficiency of eosinophilic leukocytes in the blood.

eosinophil (e-o-sin′o-fil) A cell, especially a white blood cell (eosinophilic leukocyte), that stains easily with eosin dye.

eosinophilia (e-o-sin-o-fil′e-ă) The presence of an

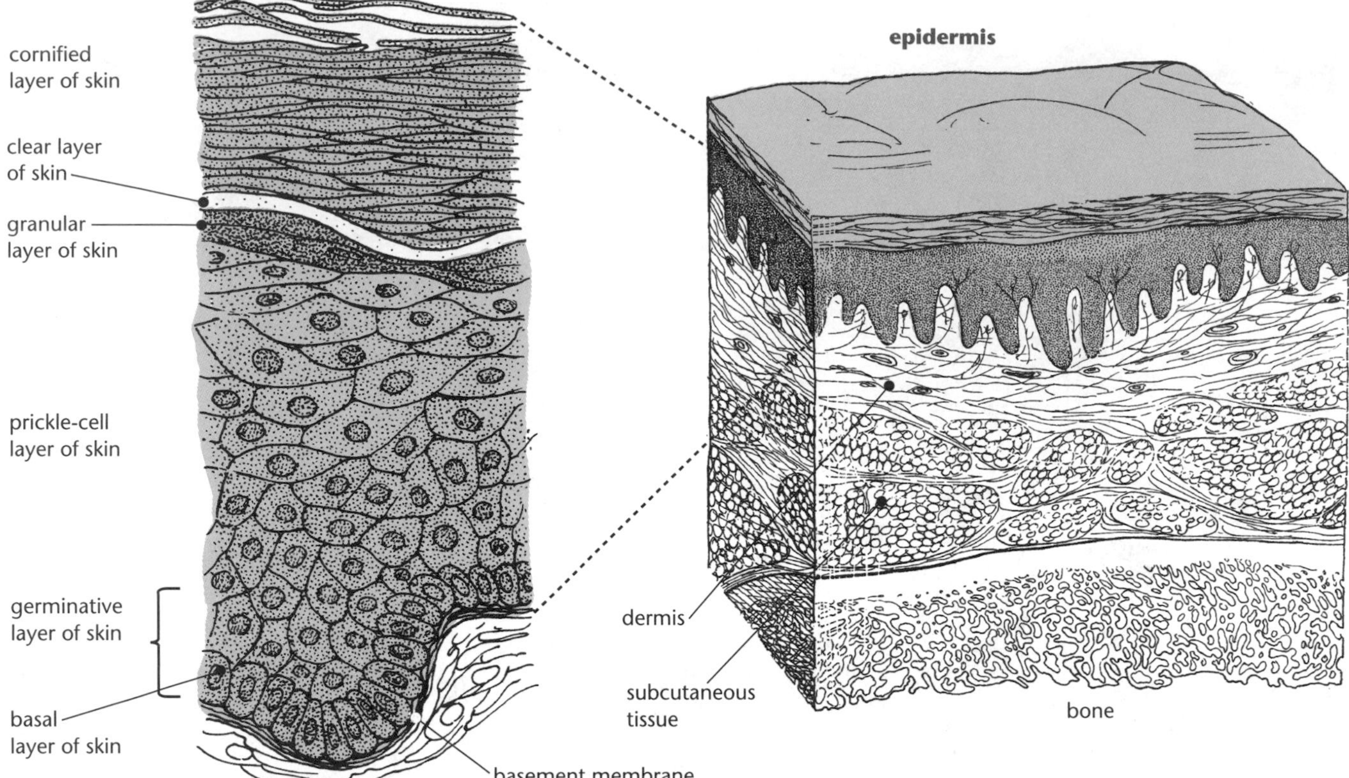

abnormally large number of eosinophils in the blood. Also called eosinophilic leukocytosis.

simple pulmonary e. Disorder marked by transient infiltrates of the lungs, low fever, and increased number of eosinophils in peripheral blood; usually lasting less than a month. Also called Löffler's syndrome.

eosinophilic (e-o-sin-o-fil´ik) Easily stained with eosin dyes. Also called oxyphilic.

ependyma (ĕ-pen´dĭ-mă) The lining membrane of the cerebral ventricles and the central canal of the spinal cord.

ependymoma (ĕ-pen-dĭ-mo´mă) A brain tumor derived from cells of the membrane lining the ventricles (ependyma); occurring most frequently in children and young adults and constituting approximately 1 to 3% of all intracranial tumors.

ephedrine (ĕ-fed´rin, ef´ĕ-drin) A sympathomimetic amine obtained from species of *Ephedra* or produced synthetically; it dilates the bronchi and is used in the prevention and treatment of bronchial asthma; it acts, in part, by releasing catecholamines from their storage vesicles.

ephelis (ĕ-fe´lis) See freckle.

epicanthus (ep-ĭ-kan´thus) A semilunar skin fold of the upper eyelid extending from its medial surface downward to cover the medial corner (inner canthus) of the eye; it is normal in individuals of certain races; may also occur in others as a congenital anomaly, as in Down syndrome. Also called epicanthal fold.

epicardia (ep-ĭ-kar´de-ă) The portion of the esophagus from the diaphragm to the stomach.

epicardium (ep-ĭ-kar´de-um) The visceral or inner layer of the pericardium that is in contact with the heart.

epicondyle (ep-ĭ-kon´dīl) The bony prominence situated above or upon a smooth articular eminence of a long bone.

lateral e. 1. Of the femur, a prominence situated above the lateral condyle; it gives attachment to the fibular collateral ligament of the knee joint. **2.** Of the humerus, a small tuberculated eminence situated at the lower end of the bone; it gives attachment to the radial collateral ligament of the elbow joint, and to a tendon common to the origin of the supinator and some of the extensor muscles.

medial e. 1. Of the femur, a large convex eminence located above the medial condyle to which the tibial collateral ligament of the knee joint is attached. **2.** Of the humerus, a large projection situated above and medial to the condyle; it gives attachment to the ulnar collateral ligament of the elbow joint, to the pronator teres, and to a common tendon of origin of most of the forearm's flexor muscles.

epicondylitis (ep-ĭ-kon-dĭ-li´tis) Inflammation of tissues surrounding a bony prominence (epicondyle) at a joint.

lateral humeral e. Pain and tenderness of the tendons near the lateral epicondyle of the humerus; a syndrome affecting the midportion of the upper extremity, usually due to repetitive rotatory motions of the forearm (believed to cause microscopic tears and subsequent chronic tendinitis). Also called tennis elbow.

epicranium (ep-ĭ-kra´ne-um) The scalp; the structures (muscle, aponeurosis, and skin) covering the skull.

epicrisis (ep-ĭ-kri´sis) A crisis occurring after the first crisis of a disease; a secondary crisis.

epicritic (ep-ĭ-krit´ik) Denoting sensory nerve fibers in the skin and oral mucosa that perceive slight variations of touch and temperature.

epidemic (ep-ĭ-dem´ik) **1.** The outbreak and rapid spread of a disease in one community, affecting many people at the same time during a specified time period. **2.** Relating to epidemics.

epidemiography (ep-ĭ-de-me-og´ră-fe) A treatise of one or several epidemic diseases.

epidemiologist (ep-ĭ-de-me-ol´o-jist) A person who specializes in epidemiology.

epidemiology (ep-ĭ-de-me-ol´o-je) The scientific study of epidemics and epidemic diseases, especially of the factors that influence the incidence, distribution, and control of infectious diseases; the study of disease occurrence in human populations.

epidermal (ep-ĭ-der´mal) Relating to the epidermis.

epidermatoplasty (ep-ĭ-der-mat´o-plas-te) Skin grafting.

epidermis (ep-ĭ-der´mis) The outer, thinner layer of the skin, consisting of layers of stratified squamous epithelium; it is devoid of blood vessels and contains a limited distribution of nerve endings. See also skin.

epidermoid (ep-ĭ-der´moid) **1.** Resembling epidermis. **2.** A tumor containing aberrant epidermal cells.

epidermodysplasia verruciformis (ep-ĭ-der-mo-dis-pla´shă ve-roo´sĭ-form-is) Development of numerous flat warts, especially on the hands and feet, some of which tend to become cancerous.

epidermolysis (ep-ĭ-der-mol´ĭ-sis) A loose state of the superficial layer of the skin, often tending to form blisters.

Epidermophyton (ep-ĭ-der-mof´ĭ-ton) A genus of fungi causing skin disorders.

epididymectomy (ep-ĭ-did-ĭ-mek´tŏ-me) Surgical removal of the epididymis.

epididymis (ep-ĭ-did´ĭ-mis), *pl.* **epidid´ymides** A tortuous, cordlike structure connected to the posterior surface of the testis serving for maturation and transport of spermatozoa; consists of a head, a body, and a tail that is continuous with the deferent duct.

epididymitis (ep-ĭ-did-ĭ-mi´tis) Inflammation of the epididymis.

epididymo-orchitis (ep-ĭ-did-ĭ-mo-or-ki´tis) Inflammation of both the epididymis and the testis.

epididymotomy (ep-ĭ-did-ĭ-mot´ŏ-me) Surgical incision into the epididymis, usually for relief of tension and pain in epididymitis.

epididymovasostomy (ep-ĭ-did-ĭ-mo-vaz-os´tŏ-me) The surgical joining of the epididymis and the deferent duct, usually for the purpose of bypassing an obstruction in the deferent duct.

epidural (ep-ĭ-doo´ral) Outside or upon the dura mater.

epigastrium (ep-ĭ-gas´tre-um) The upper central area of the abdomen; pit of the stomach.

epigenesis (ep-ĭ-jen´ĕ-sis) The concept that an organism develops by the new formation of structures, as opposed to the old theory of preformation, i.e., that an organism develops by the growth of structures already existing in miniature in the egg.

epiglottis (ep-ĭ-glot´is) The leaf-shaped cartilage that covers the aperture of the larynx during the act of swallowing to prevent food from entering the trachea.

epiglottitis (ep-ĭ-glŏ-ti´tis) Inflammation of the epiglottis; it may cause respiratory obstruction, especially in children.

acute e. Condition usually seen in children and necessitating emergency treatment (e.g., tracheal intubation); characterized by sudden onset of fever, difficult swallowing, drooling, muffled voice, and a shrill respiratory sound; almost always caused by *Haemophilus influenzae type B; Streptococcus pneumoniae* has also been implicated.

epilation (ep-ĭ-la´shun) The removal of hairs with their roots.

epilemma (ep-ĭ-lem´ă) See endoneurium.

epilepsy (ep´ĭ-lep-se) A chronic disorder, or group of disorders, characterized by recurrent, unpredictable seizures occurring spontaneously without consistent provoking factors; the seizures reflect a temporary physiologic dysfunction of the brain in which nerve cells (neurons) in the cerebral cortex

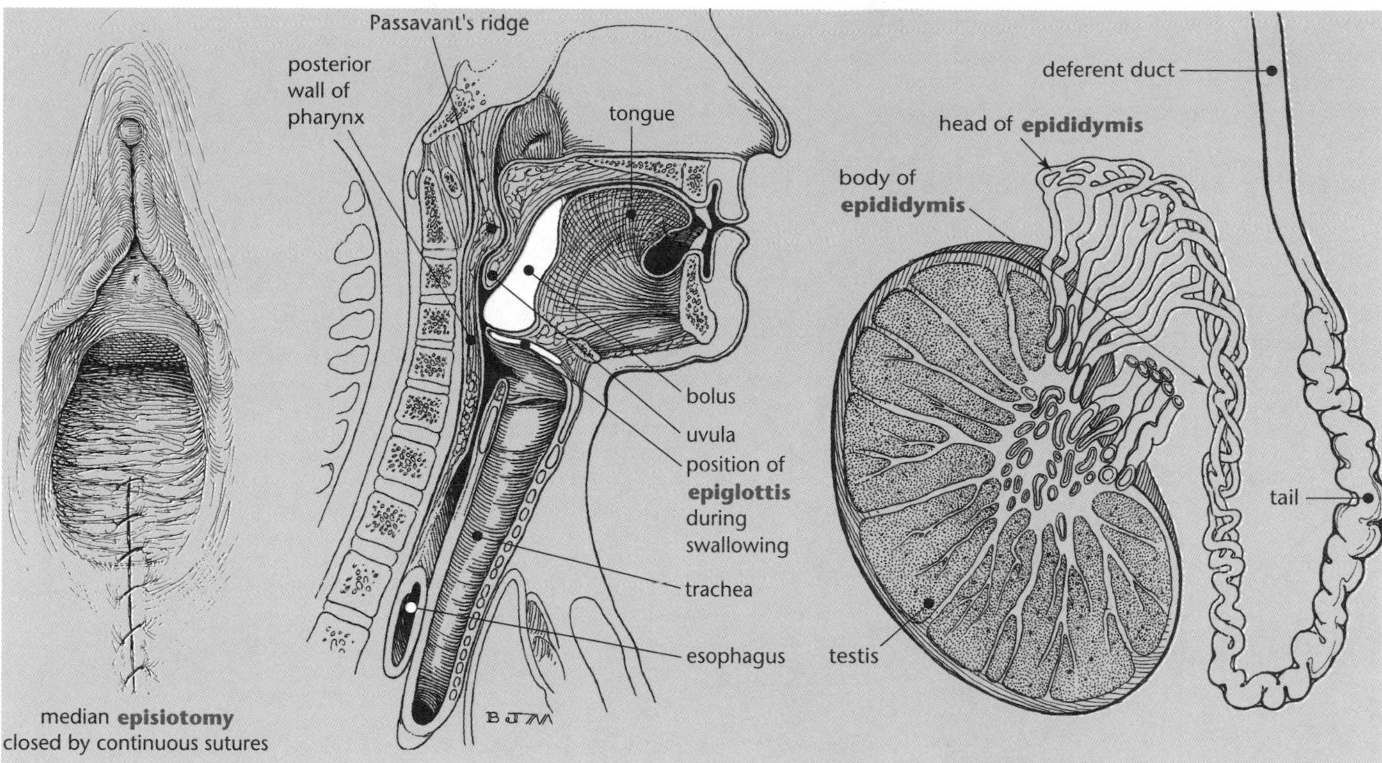

produce excessive electrical discharges.

childhood absence e. Brief or mild seizures, lasting from 5 to 30 seconds, characterized by sudden cessation of activity and a blank stare. Typically begins at age six or seven years. Also called petit mal epilepsy.

focal e. Epilepsy characterized by minor seizures restricted to isolated areas of the body, arising in a localized area of a cerebral hemisphere. Also called partial epilepsy; local epilepsy.

generalized e. Epilepsy characterized by seizures that result from involvement of both cerebral hemispheres; may range from minor (absence seizures) to major (tonic-clonic seizures).

generalized tonic-clonic e. Epilepsy marked by loss of consciousness and stiffness of the entire body, i.e., sustained (tonic) muscular contractions, followed by jerking (clonic) movements. Also called grand mal epilepsy; major epilepsy; grand mal; falling sickness. See also status epilepticus.

grand mal e. See generalized tonic-clonic epilepsy.

jacksonian e. Focal epilepsy in which the seizure arises in a localized area of the motor cortex and spreads to adjacent areas, manifested by a twitching beginning at the periphery of a structure and progressing to involve the entire musculature of one side.

juvenile absence e. Absence and generalized epilepsy beginning at the age of puberty.

local e. See focal epilepsy.

major e. See generalized tonic-clonic epilepsy.

nocturnal e. Epilepsy in which the attacks occur mainly at night, while the person sleeps.

partial e. See focal epilepsy.

petit mal e. See childhood absence epilepsy.

posttraumatic e. Epilepsy caused by brain damage incurred in a head injury; most frequently seen in penetrating brain injuries and in depressed skull fractures with injury to underlying brain; it also occurs in closed head trauma.

psychomotor e. Obsolete term. See temporal lobe epilepsy.

sleep e. See narcolepsy.

temporal lobe e. A type of focal epilepsy in which the seizure arises from all or part of the temporal lobe, often producing auditory, olfactory, or gustatory hallucinations, as well as bizarre activity and behavior; it often arises after injury to the temporal lobe. Formerly called psychomotor epilepsy.

uncinate e. A type of temporal lobe epilepsy in which the seizure arises from the anteromedial aspect of the temporal lobe, causing impairment of consciousness and a dreamy state with hallucinations of smell and taste; usually caused by a medial temporal lesion.

epileptic (ep-ĭ-lep′tik) **1.** Relating to epilepsy. **2.** One who is afflicted with epilepsy.

epileptoid (ep-ĭ-lep′toid) Resembling epilepsy; said of certain convulsions.

epimandibular (ep-ĭ-man-dib′u-lar) On the lower jaw.

epimenorrhea (ep-ĭ-men-o-re′ă) Menstruation occurring at excessively short intervals.

epimerase (ĕ-pim′ĕ-rās) One of a group of enzymes that promote epimeric changes.

epimers (ep′ĭ-merz) Two sugars that differ from one another only in the configuration around a single carbon atom (e.g., glucose and galactose).

epimicroscope (ep-ĭ-mi′kro-skōp) Opaque microscope, a microscope with a condenser around the objective; used for observing opaque or translucent specimens.

epimorphosis (ep-ĭ-mor-fo′sis) Regeneration of a cut part of an organism.

epimysium (ep-ĭ-mis′e-um) A sheath of connective tissue surrounding individual muscles.

epinephrine (ep-ĭ-nef′rin) **1.** Hormone produced by the medulla of the adrenal gland; it stimulates the sympathetic nervous system. **2.** A crystalline compound, $C_9H_{13}NO_3$, extracted from the adrenal glands of some mammals or produced synthetically; it produces cardiac stimulation, constriction or dilatation of blood vessels, and bronchial relaxation; used as a heart stimulant and in the treatment of bronchial asthma and acute allergic disorders, and as a local vasoconstrictor. Also called adrenaline.

epineural (ep-ĭ-noo′ral) Located upon a neural arch.

epineurial (ep-ĭ-noo′re-al) Relating to the connective tissue surrounding a nerve trunk.

epineurium (ep-ĭ-noor′e-um) The outermost connective tissue of a peripheral nerve.

epipharynx (ep-ĭ-far′inks) Nasopharynx.

epiphenomenon (ep-ĭ-fĕ-nom′ĕ-non) A symptom occurring during the course of a disease but not necessarily associated with it.

epiphora (ĕ-pif′o-ră) Persistent overflow of tears onto the cheek, due to obstruction of the tear-conducting passages, eversion of the margin of the lower lid, or excessive secretion of tears.

epiphysiodesis, epiphyseodesis (ep-ĭ-fiz-e-od′ĕ-sis) An operation creating a permanent premature closure of an epiphysial plate, resulting in cessation of bone growth.

epiphysiolysis (ep-ĭ-fiz-e-ol′ĭ-sis) The separation of an epiphysis from the shaft of the bone.

epiphysis (ĕ-pif′ĭ-sis), *pl.* **epiph′yses** The end of a long bone, developed separately, and initially separated from the shaft by cartilage.

epiphysitis (ĕ-pif-ĭ-si′tis) Inflammation of an epiphysis.

traumatic tibial e. A knee injury most commonly seen in adolescents active in sports; produced when the powerful vastus muscle complex, which inserts into a small area of the tibial tuberosity, exerts a sufficiently forceful contraction to separate a small portion of bone in an area of developmental bone formation; symptoms include a "knee knob" or protrusion below the knee cap (patella), tenderness elicited by pressure, and pain when the knee is extended against resistance. Also called Osgood-Schlatter disease; Osgood-Schlatter syndrome.

epiplocele (ĕ-pip′lo-sēl) A hernia of the omentum.

epiploectomy (ĕ-pip-lo-ek′tŏ-me) Surgical removal of the omentum.

epiploic (ep-ĭ-plo′ik) Relating to the omentum.

epiplopexy (ĕ-pip′lo-pek-se) See omentopexy.

episclera (ep-ĭ-skler′ă) The loose connective tissue that constitutes the external surface of the sclera and contains a large number of small blood vessels.

episcleritis (ep-ĭ-sklĕ-ri′tis) Inflammation of the connective tissue of the eye between the sclera and the conjunctiva.

episioperineoplasty (ĕ-piz-e-o-per-ĭ-ne′o-plas-te) Reparative surgery of the vulva and perineum.

episioperineorrhaphy (ĕ-piz-e-o-per-ĭ-ne-or′ă-fe) Suturing of a lacerated vulva and perineum.

episioplasty (ĕ-piz-e-o-plas′te) Surgical repair of a defect of the vulva.

episiorrhaphy (ĕ-piz′e-or′ă-fe) Suturing of a lacerated vulva.

episiotomy (ĕ-piz-e-ot′o-me) Incision of the perineum during childbirth, performed to prevent vaginal, vulvar, or perineal tear by controlled enlargement of the vaginal orifice, to shorten the second stage of labor, and to prevent undue pressure on the fetal skull during delivery. The two most commonly used incisions are the mediolateral and median (midline). Also called perineotomy.

episome (ep′ĭ-sōm) A class of genetic elements of bacteria that may exist either as autonomous entities, replicating in the host independent of the bacterial chromosome, or as segments of the bacterial chromosome, replicating with it.

simple squamous **epithelium**

simple cuboidal **epithelium**

stratified squamous **epithelium**

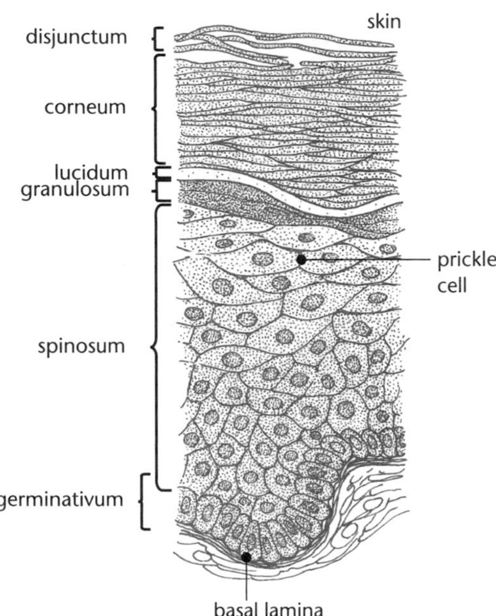

simple columnar **epithelium**

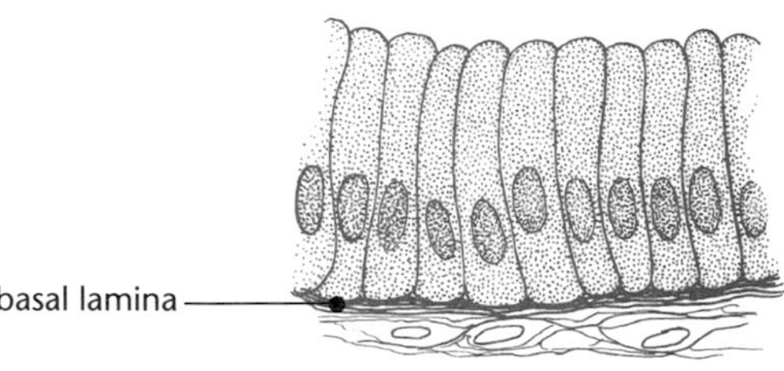

ciliated pseudostratified columnar **epithelium**

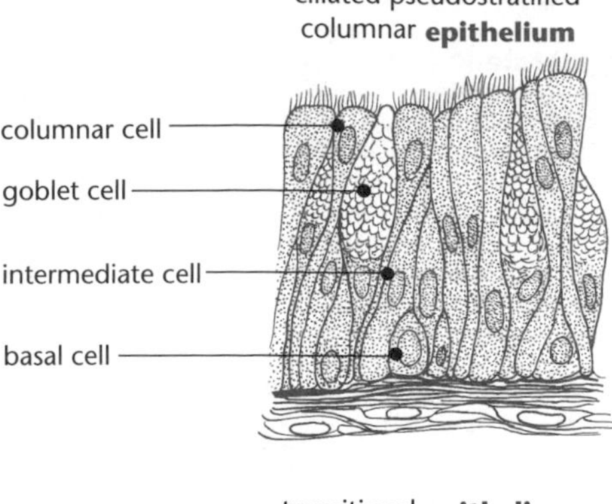

transitional **epithelium**

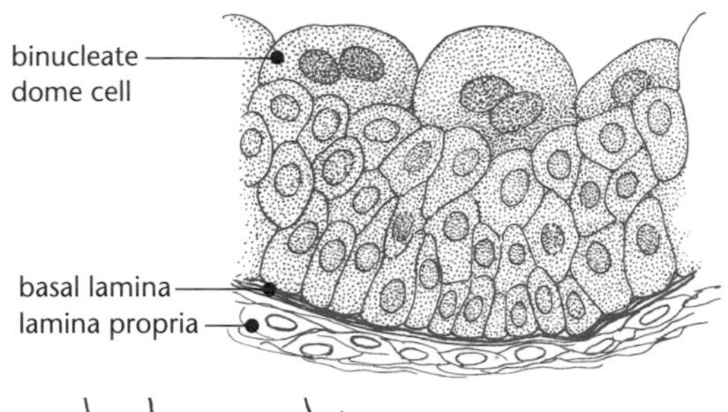

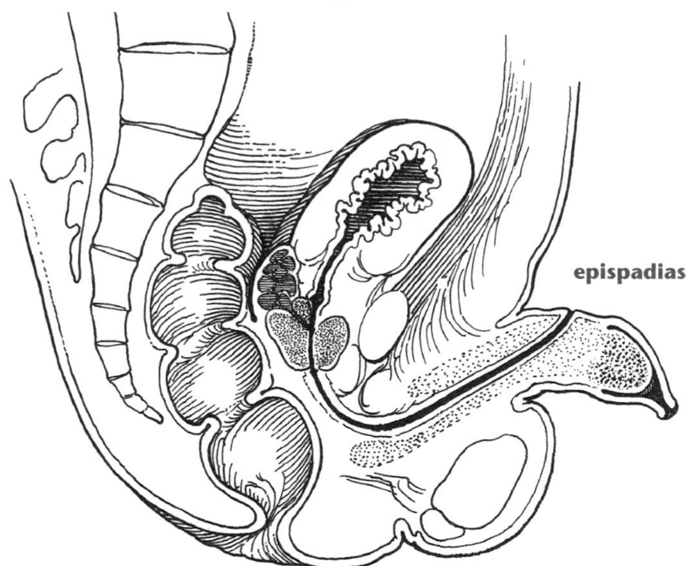

epispadias

epispadias (ep-ĭ-spa′de-ăs) A rare congenital defect in the male in which the urethra opens on the dorsal surface of the penis; also a similar defect in the female in which a fissure is present in the upper wall of the urethra.
epispastic (ep-ĭ-spas′tik) Anything that causes blistering.
epispinal (ep-ĭ-spi′nal) On the vertebral column, spinal cord, or any spinelike structure.
episplenitis (ep-ĭ-splĕ-ni′tis) Inflammation of the capsule of the spleen.
epistasis (ĕ-pis′tă-sis) **1.** The film formed on the surface of a liquid. **2.** The nonreciprocal interaction of nonallelic genes in which one suppresses the action of another.
epistaxis (ep-ĭ-stak′sis) Nosebleed.
episternal (ep-ĭ-ster′nal) Situated over or on the sternum.
epithalamus (ep-ĭ-thal′ă-mus) A small area of the diencephalon consisting of the trigonum habenulae, the pineal body, and the posterior commissure.
epithelial (ep-ĭ-the′le-al) Relating to or composed of epithelium.
epithelialization (ep-ĭ-the-le-al-ĭ-za′shun) The final stage in the healing of a surface injury in which epithelium is formed over the denuded area. Also called epithelization.
epithelioid (ep-ĭ-the′le-oid) Resembling epithelium.
epithelioma (ep-ĭ-the-le-o′mă) A malignant tumor consisting of epithelial cells and arising mainly in the skin and mucous membrane.
basal cell e. See basal cell carcinoma, under carcinoma.
Malherbe's calcifying e. See pilomatricoma.
epithelium (ep-ĭ-the′le-um) The nonvascular cellular layer that covers the internal and external surfaces of the body.
acetowhite e. Epithelium that turns white upon application of acetic acid. Acetic acid coagulates proteins of the cell nucleus and cytoplasm, making the proteins opaque and white.
germinal e. Specialized peritoneal mesothelium (low cuboidal) that forms a continuous covering over the ovary; it was once thought to give rise to primordial germ cells (oogonia).
epithelization (ep-ĭ-the-lĭ-za′shun) See epithelialization.
epitope (ep′ĭ-tōp) See antigenic determinant, under determinant.
epityphlitis (ep-ĭ-tif-li′tis) See paratyphlitis.
epizoic (ep-ĭ-zo′ik) Living as a parasite on the surface of the host's body.
epizoon (ep-ĭ-zo′on), *pl.* **epizo′a** An animal parasite living on the exterior of the host's body.
eponychia (ep-o-nik′e-ă) Infection at the groove of the nail.
eponychium (ep-o-nik′e-um) **1.** The fold of skin overlying the root of the nail; its free, cornified margin forms the cuticle. **2.** The horny epidermis at the site of the future nail in the embryo.
eponym (ep′o-nim) The name of a disease, structure, or surgical procedure that includes the name of a person (e.g., Pott's disease).
eponymic (ep-o-nim′ik) Named after a particular person.
epoophoron (ep-o-of′ŏ-ron) The vestiges of the mesonephros (wolffian body) consisting of rudimentary tubules located in the mesosalpinx between the ovary and the uterine tube. Also called pampiniform body; organ of Rosenmüller.
epoxy (ĕ-pok′se) In chemistry, an oxygen atom bound to two linked carbon atoms.
epulis (ĕ-pu′lis) A tumor of the gums.
e. gravidarum Tumor of the gums occurring during pregnancy. Also called epulis of pregnancy.
equation (e-kwa′zhun) A mathematical or chemical representation as a linear array of symbols expressing the quality of two things, separated into left and right sides by an equal sign.
Arrhenius' e. An equation relating chemical reaction rate with temperature.
Bohr's e. The equation for calculating the volume of the dead space gas in the respiratory tract by measuring the expired air and subtracting it from the alveolar gas volumes.
Einthoven's e. See Einthoven's law, under law.
Hasselbalch's e. See Henderson-Hasselbalch

equivalent measures and weights

US Customary Unit (Avoirdupois)	US Equivalents	Metric Equivalents
LENGTH		
inch	0.083 foot	2.54 centimeters
foot	1/3 yard or 12 inches	0.3048 meters
yard	3 feet or 36 inches	0.9144 meters
CAPACITY		
fluid ounce	8 fluid ounces	29.573 milliliters
pint	16 fluid ounces	0.473 liter
quart	2 pints	0.946 liter
gallon	4 quarts	3.785 liters
WEIGHT		
grain	0.036 dram	64.798 milligrams
dram	27.344 grains	1.772 grams
ounce	16 drams	28.350 grams
pound	16 ounces	453.592 grams
Apothecary Weight Unit	**US Customary Equivalents**	**Metric Equivalents**
scram	20 grains	1.296 grams
dram	60 grains	3.888 grams
ounce	480 grains	31.103 grams

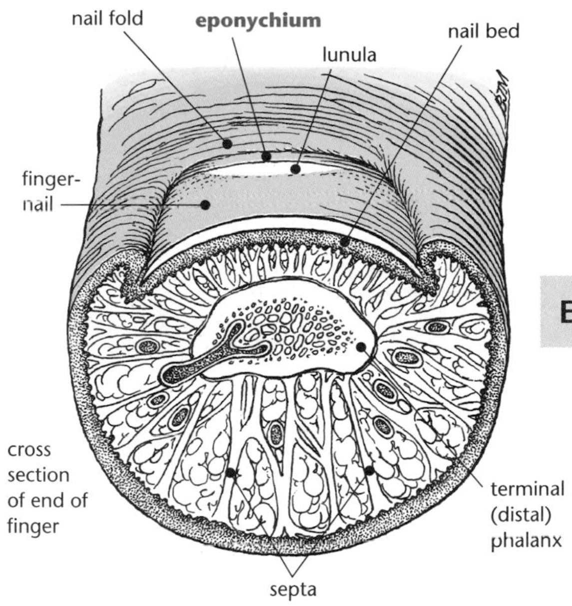

E

equation.

Henderson-Hasselbalch e. An equation for determining the pH of a buffer solution such as blood plasma; pH = pK + log ([HCO_3^-/ CO_2]). Also called Hasselbalch's equation.

equator bulbi oculi (e-kwa´tor bul´bi ok´u-li) Equator of the eyeball; an imaginary circle around the eyeball at the same distance from both poles.

equicaloric (e-kwĭ-kă-lor´ik) Having the same heat value.

equilibration (e-kwil-ĭ-bra´shun) **1.** The act of bringing about or maintaining equilibrium. **2.** In dentistry, the equalization of pressure.

equilibrium (e-kwĭ-lib´re-um) **1.** Condition in which all acting forces cancel each other, resulting in a stable unchanging system. **2.** In chemistry, a stable condition created by two reactions occurring at equal speed in opposite directions. **3.** Mental or emotional stability. **4.** A state of bodily balance.

acid-base e. See acid-base balance, under balance.

Donnan e. The condition that exists when two solutions are separated by a semipermeable membrane (i.e., permeable only to some of the ions of the solutions); the unequal distribution of ions between the two solutions causes an electrical potential between the two sides of the membrane.

equimolar (e-kwĭ-mo´lar) Containing the same number of moles or having equal molarity.

equimolecular (e-kwĭ-mo-lek´u-lar) Denoting solutions that contain an equal number of molecules.

equinus (e-kwi´nus) Talipes equinus.

equivalence, equivalency (e-kwiv´ă-lens, e-kwiv´ă-len-se) **1.** In chemistry, the relative combining powers of a set of atoms or radicals. **2.** Valence.

equivalent (e-kwiv´ă-lent) **1.** Equal in any way (substance, value, force, etc.). **2.** Having similar or equal effects.

chemical e. See gram equivalent.

gram e. (a) The weight (usually in grams) of a substance that can combine with, or displace, a unit weight of hydrogen from a compound or its equivalent of another substance. (b) The atomic or molecular weight in grams of an atom or group of atoms involved in a chemical reaction divided by the number of electrons donated, taken up, or shared by the atom or group of atoms in the course of that reaction. (c) The weight of a substance contained in 1 liter of 1 normal solution. Also called chemical equivalent; equivalent weight; combining weight.

nitrogen e. The nitrogen content of protein.

erbium (er´be-um) A soft, malleable, silvery rare earth element; symbol Er, atomic number 68, atomic weight 167.27.

erectile (ĕ-rek´til) Capable of becoming turgid; applied to vascular tissue.

erection (ĕ-rek´shun) **1.** The state of erectile tissue when filled with blood. **2.** An erect penis.

erector (ĕ-rek´or) Something that raises or makes erect; denoting specifically certain muscles that hold up or cause the erection of a body part.

erethism (er´ĕ-thiz-m) An exaggerated degree of irritability or excitability, either general or in any part of the body, accompanied by mental changes such as instability, memory loss, lack of attention, decrease in intellect, and shyness; may be associated with inorganic mercury poisoning.

erg (erg) A unit of energy equal to the force capable of moving a 1-gram weight a distance of 1 centimeter.

ergastoplasm (er-gas´to-plaz-m) See granular endoplasmic reticulum, under reticulum.

ergocalciferol (er-go-kal-sif´er-ol) See vitamin D_2, under vitamin.

ergodynamograph (er-go-di-nam´o-graf) An instrument used to record the degree of muscular force and the amount of work accompanied by muscular contraction.

ergograph (er´go-graf) An instrument for recording the work capacity of a muscle.

ergometer (er-gom´ĕ-ter) An apparatus for measuring the force of muscular contraction under controlled conditions. Also called dynamometer.

ergonomics (er-go-nom´iks) The study of activities and behavior of people working with mechanical and electronic equipment, taking into account the anatomic, physiologic, and psychologic attributes of the people working in the given environment. Also called human factor engineering.

ergonomist (er-gon-o´mist) A specialist in ergonomics.

ergosterol (er-gos´tĕ-rol) A crystalline sterol present in plant and animal tissues, which, under ultraviolet irradiation, is converted to vitamin D_2; derived from yeast and other fungi.

ergot (er´got) Any fungus of the genus *Claviceps* that attacks cereal plants; it has blood vessel-constricting and muscle-contracting properties and yields drugs of clinical usefulness.

ergotamine (er-got´ă-min) An alkaloid derived from ergot that stimulates smooth muscle, especially of the blood vessels and uterus.

ergotism (er´got-iz-m) Poisoning by ergot-infected grain such as rye or from excessive use of medicinal ergot; constriction of the arterioles leads to pain and necrosis of the extremities. Also called ergot poisoning.

erg-second (erg-sek´und) A unit of work or energy multiplied by time; equal to the amount of energy required to move a weight of one gram a distance of one centimeter in one second.

erogenous (ĕ-roj´ĕ-nus) Producing sexual desire. Also called erotogenic.

erosion (e-ro´zhun) **1.** A gradual wearing away. **2.** In dentistry, the progressive loss of tooth substance by a chemical process without the aid of bacteria, producing a hard, polished, smooth depression on the surface of the tooth.

erotic (ĕ-rot´ik) Relating to sexual arousal.

eroticism, erotism (ĕ-rot´ĭ-siz-m, er´o-tiz-m) **1.** Erotic character. **2.** A state of sexual excitement.

erotogenic (ĕ-rot-o-jen´ik) See erogenous.

erratic (ĕ-rat´ik) **1.** Denoting symptoms that do not follow a usual pattern. **2.** Unconventional.

error (er´or) **1.** Any defect, as in structure or function. **2.** A false result in a study or experiment.

alpha e. See type I error.

beta e. See type II error.

inborn e. of metabolism Inherited disorders caused by a gene-determined defect; each involves a single enzyme; manifestations may be the result of accumulation of the substance upon which the enzyme acts (substrate), a deficiency of the product of the enzyme, or the result of forcing metabolism through an auxiliary path.

interobserver e. Differences in interpretation by two or more researchers recording observations of the same phenomenon.

intraobserver e. Differences in interpretation by one researcher recording observations of the same phenomenon at different times.

random e. The variation in a measurement that has no apparent relation to any other measurement; regarded as due to chance.

refractive e. Defect in the refractive system of the eye that prevents light rays from being brought to a focus on the retina.

systematic e. Error that has an identifiable source (e.g., faulty instruments).

type I e. Rejection of a true null hypothesis. Also called alpha error.

type II e. Acceptance of a false null hypothesis (the hypothesis states that results observed in a study, experiment, or test do not differ from those that might be expected by the operation of chance alone). Also called beta error.

erubescence (er-o͞o-bes´ens) A flushing or reddening of the skin; a blush.

eructation (ĕ-ruk-ta´shun) The act of belching.

erupt (e-rupt´) To break or pierce through; said of a tooth.

eruption (e-rup´shun) **1.** The act of breaking out, as in the appearance of lesions on the skin. **2.** Redness

E

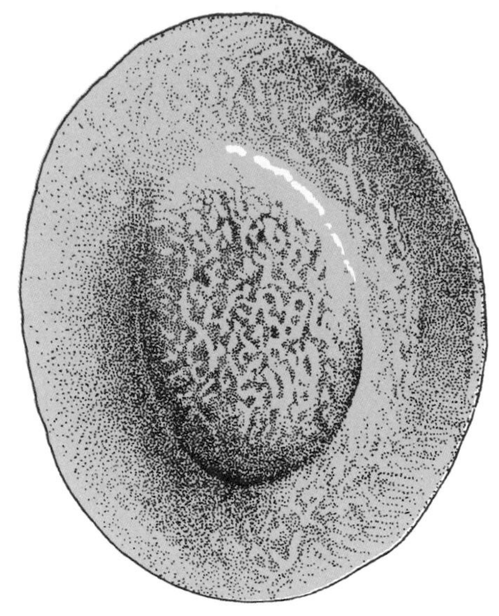

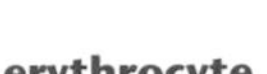

erythrocyte

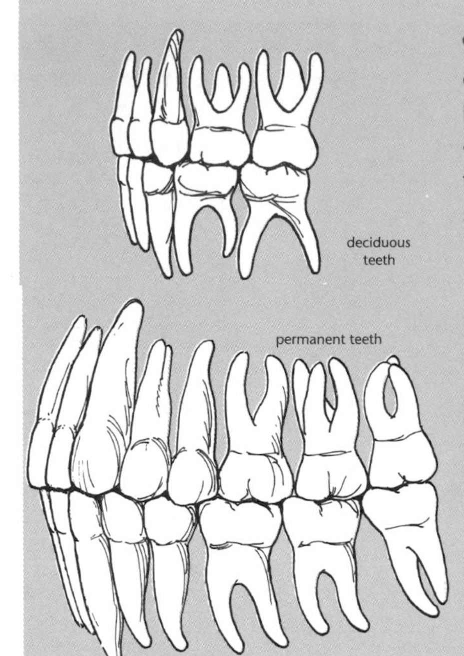

eruption of deciduous teeth	
central incisors	6–8 months
lateral incisors	7–9 months
cuspids	16–18 months
first molars	12–14 months
second molars	20–24 months

eruption of permanent teeth	
central incisors	6–8 years
lateral incisors	7–9 years
cuspids	9–12 years
first bicuspids	10–12 years
second bicuspids	10–12 years
first molars	6–7 years
second molars	11–13 years
third molars	17–21 years

or blemishing of the skin or mucosa as a manifestation of disease. **3.** Cutting a tooth; the passage of a tooth through the gum.

creeping e. See cutaneous larva migrans, under larva migrans.

drug e. Skin rash caused by a drug taken internally, generally the result of allergic sensitization. Also called dermatitis medicamentosa.

erysipelas (er-ĭ-sip´ĕ-las) An acute contagious disease caused by *Streptococcus pyogenes*, marked by a circumscribed red eruption on the skin, chills, and fever.

erysipeloid (er-ĭ-sip´ĕ-loid) Infection of the hands with the bacillus *Erysipelothrix rhysiopathiae*, marked by red lesions and occurring in persons handling infected fish or meat.

Erysipelothrix (er-ĭ-sip´ĕ-lo-thriks) A genus of bacteria (family Corynebacteriaceae) containing gram-positive, rod-shaped organisms that have a tendency to form long filaments; parasitic on mammals, birds, and fish.

erysipelotoxin (er-ĭ-sip-ĕ-lo-tok´sin) A toxin produced by *Streptococcus pyogenes*, species of bacteria causing erysipelas.

erythema (er-ĭ-the´mă) Redness of the skin.

e. chronicum migrans Annular erythema beginning several weeks after the bite of a tick and spreading peripherally with a central clearing; the first lesion of Lyme disease.

e. infectiosum Mild viral infection, most commonly seen in school-aged children, marked by a lacelike skin rash; caused by human parvovirus B19. Also called fifth disease; slapped cheek disease.

e. marginatum A type of erythema multiforme in which the lesions have a disc shape with elevated edges.

e. migrans An oval or round, slowly spreading ring around a central tick bite; often associated with Lyme disease.

e. multiforme An acute inflammatory skin disease, marked by the symmetrical eruption of macules, papules, or vesicles of various shapes presenting a multiform appearance; may be an allergic reaction; severe cases may have a fatal termination; in mild cases (Hebra's disease) the eruption usually recurs.

e. multiforme bullosum A blister-like eruption on the lips, tongue, and mucous membrane of the mouth.

e. multiforme exudativum A rare severe form of erythema multiforme characterized chiefly by eruptive, ulcerative lesions of the skin, oral mucosa, and eyes; frequently the genitalia, lungs, and joints are affected. Also called Stevens-Johnson syndrome.

e. nodosum Inflammation of subcutaneous fat (panniculitis) occurring as a hypersensitivity reaction, characterized by bright red, painful nodules on the shins and frequently on the anterior thighs and extensor surfaces of the forearms. Also called nodal fever.

e. toxicum A diffuse eruption of the skin due to an allergic reaction to a toxic substance.

erythermalgia (er-ĭ-ther-mal´jă) See erythromelalgia.

erythralgia (er-ĭ-thral´jă) A state of painful redness of the skin.

erythrasma (er-ĭ-thraz´mă) A contagious skin disease caused by the bacterium *Corynebacterium minutissimum*; marked by an eruption of reddish brown patches in the armpits and groin which glow under Wood's light.

erythredema (ĕ-rith-rĕ-de´mă) See acrodynia.

erythremia (er-ĭ-thre´me-ă) See polycythemia vera.

erythrityl tetranitrate (ĕ-rith´rĭ-tĭl tet-ră-ni´trāt) A compound used in the treatment of angina pectoris.

erythroblast (ĕ-rith´ro-blast) A young red blood cell in its immature, nucleated stage.

acidophilic e. See orthochromatic normoblast, under normoblast.

basophilic e. See basophilic normoblast, under normoblast.

orthochromatic e. See orthochromatic normoblast, under normoblast.

polychromatophilic e. See polychromatic normoblast, under normoblast.

erythroblastemia (ĕ-rith-ro-blas-te´me-ă) The presence of nucleated red blood cells (erythroblasts) in the peripheral blood; may be seen in a variety of pathologic conditions.

erythroblastopenia (ĕ-rith-ro-blas-to-pe´ne-ă) Deficiency in bone marrow of erythroblasts (red blood cells in an early stage of development).

erythroblastosis (ĕ-rith-ro-blas-to´sis) Excessive number of immature red blood cells (erythroblasts) in the circulating blood.

e. fetalis See hemolytic disease of the newborn.

erythrochromia (ĕ-rith-ro-kro´me-ă) A red coloration.

erythroclasis (er-ĭ-throk´lă-sis) Fragmentation of red blood cells.

erythrocuprein (ĕ-rith-ro-koo´prēn) A copper-containing protein present in human red blood cells.

erythrocyanosis (ĕ-rith-ro-si-ă-no´sis) Swollen and reddish condition of the limbs upon exposure to cold, but not freezing, temperatures.

erythrocyte (ĕ-rith´ro-sīt) A mature red blood cell or corpuscle that transports oxygen to the tissue by means of the hemoglobin it contains; normally it is a yellowish, non-nucleated, biconcave disk, measuring approximately from 7.2 to 8.6 m in diameter; the thickness at the center is slightly less than 1 µm and at the rim approximately 2 µm; in a normal human adult, 2,500,000 erythrocytes are formed every second; their life span is about 120 days.

crenated e. An erythrocyte possessing a scalloped border.

erythrocythemia (ĕ-rith-ro-si-the´me-ă) See polycythemia.

erythrocytic (ĕ-rith-ro-sit´ik) Relating to a red blood cell.

e. ghost The remaining membranous sac of a red blood cell after the loss of hemoglobin.

erythrocytolysin (ĕ-rith-ro-si-tol´ĭ-sin) A substance capable of causing dissolution of red blood cells.

erythrocytolysis (ĕ-rith-ro-si-tol´ĭ-sis) See hemolysis.

erythrocytometer (ĕ-rith-ro-si-tom´ĕ-ter) See hemo-cytometer.

erythrocytopenia (ĕ-rith-ro-si-to-pe´ne-ă) See erythropenia.

erythrocytorrhexis (ĕ-rith-ro-si-to-rek´sis) Partial escape of protoplasm from red blood cells, causing changes in the cells' shape. Also called erythrorrhexis.

erythrocytosis (ĕ-rith-ro-si-to´sis) Excessive formation of red blood cells.

erythrocyturia (ĕ-rith-ro-si-tu´re-ă) Red blood cells in the urine.

erythroderma (ĕ-rith-ro-der´mă) A nondescriptive term denoting abnormal redness of the skin, especially over large areas of the body.

erythrodontia (ĕ-rith-ro-don´shă) Reddish discoloration of the teeth.

erythrogenesis imperfecta (ĕ-rith-ro-gen´ĕ-sis im-per-fek´tă) See congenital hypoplastic anemia, under anemia.

erythrogenic (ĕ-rith-ro-jen´ik) **1.** Causing a rash. **2.** Producing red blood cells (seldom used term).

erythrogonium (ĕ-rith-ro-go´ne-um), *pl.* **erythrogo´nia** Denoting tissues from which red blood cells develop.

erythroid (er´ĭ-throid) Reddish.

erythrokinetics (ĕ-rith-ro-ki-net´iks) The maintenance of a steady number of circulating red blood cells in the normal individual by the balance achieved between the amount removed from and the amount delivered to the peripheral blood per unit of time.

erythroleukemia (ĕ-rith-ro-loo-ke´me-ă) Disorder of the red cell-forming process (erythropoiesis); marked chiefly by abnormal proliferation of erythroid and myeloid precursors in bone marrow, bizarre red blood cell morphology, anemia, hemorrhagic disorders, and enlargement of the spleen and liver. Also called DiGuglielmo's syndrome; erythremic

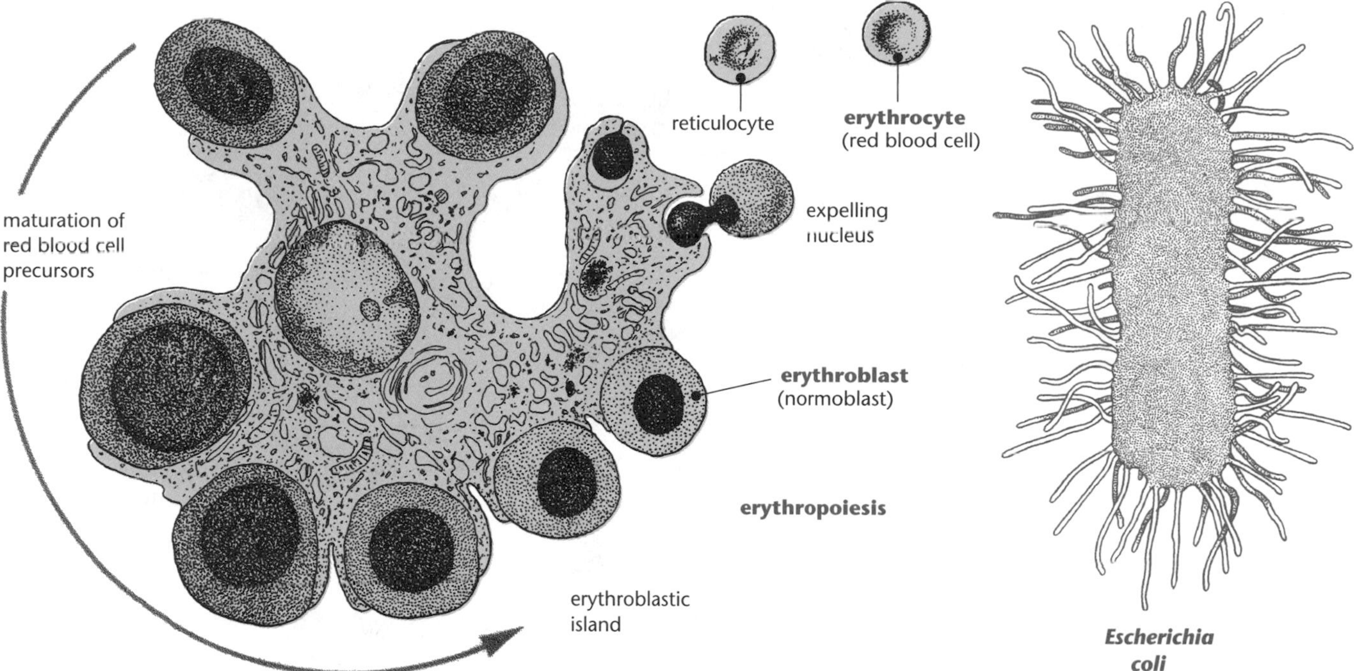

Escherichia coli

myelosis.

erythrolysin (er-ĭ-throl´ĭ-sin) See hemolysis.

erythromelalgia (ĕ-rith-ro-mel-al´jă) A circulatory disorder causing a burning sensation of the hands and/or feet, sometimes involving the whole extremity and lasting minutes or hours; usually of unknown cause but may be associated with other conditions (e.g., connective tissue disorders).

erythromelia (ĕ-rith-ro-me´le-ă) Diffuse atrophy of the skin.

erythromycin (ĕ-rith-ro-mi´sin) An antibiotic substance obtained from a strain of *Streptomyces erythreus*; Ilotycin®.

erythron (er´ĭ-thron) The total mass of erythropoietic cells and circulating erythrocytes, viewed as a functional, though dispersed, organ.

erythrophagia (ĕ-rith-ro-fa´jă) See erythrophagocytosis.

erythroneocytosis (ĕ-rith-ro-neo-si-to´sis) Presence in the peripheral blood of regenerative forms of red blood cells.

erythropenia (ĕ-rith-ro-pe´ne-ă) Deficiency of red blood cells. Also called erythrocytopenia.

erythrophagia (ĕ-rith-ro-fā´jă) See erythrophagocytosis.

erythrophagocytosis (ĕ-rith-ro-fag-o-si-to´sis) The ingestion and digestion of red blood cells by other cells, such as monocytes and polymorphonuclear leukocytes. Also called erythrophagia.

erythropoiesis (ĕ-rith-ro-poi-e´sis) The formation of red blood cells.

ineffective e. Condition in which red blood cells are produced normally but do not last to maturity.

erythropoietic (ĕ-rith-ro-poi-et´ik) Relating to the origin of red blood cells.

erythropoietin (ĕ-rith-ro-poi´ĕ-tin) Erythropoiesis-stimulating factor (ESF); a hormone produced principally in the kidney which stimulates red blood cell production. Also called erythropoietic factor; hematopoietin.

erythroprosopalgia (ĕ-rith-ro-pros-o-pal´jă) Burning pain and redness of the face, believed to indicate organic disease of the nervous system.

erythropsia (er-ĭ-throp´se-ă) The subjective sensation that all objects are covered with a red tint. Also called red vision.

erythropyknosis (ĕ-rith-ro-pik-no´sis) Degeneration of red blood cells, which become dark and shrunken (brassy bodies); occurs in malaria.

erythrorrhexis (ĕ-rith-ro-rek´sis) See erythrocytorrhexis.

erythruria (er-ĭ-throo´re-ă) Passing of urine of a red color.

escape (es-kāp´) The emergence of a lower, suppressed, cardiac pacemaker to initiate ventricular contraction when the normal, higher pacemaker defaults, or when atrioventricular (A-V) conduction fails.

nodal e. Escape with the A-V node as pacemaker.

ventricular e. Escape with an ectopic ventricular focus as pacemaker.

eschar (es´kar) A scab or slough.

escharotic (es-kă-rot´ik) Caustic.

Escherichia (esh-ĕ-rik´e-ă) A genus of bacteria (family Enterobacteriaceae) containing short, gram-negative rods; the motile species are covered with flagella; they ferment glucose and lactose with acid and gas formation, are present in feces, and may cause disease in man.

E. coli A motile species normally present in the intestines of humans; some strains may cause bloody diarrhea, kidney failure, and death.

enterohemorrhagic *E. coli* (EHEC) Strain producing a toxin resembling that of *Shigella* organisms; invades the lining of the colon, causing necrosis and acute bloody diarrhea.

enteroinvasive *E. coli* (EIEC) Strain that penetrates the intestinal mucosa and reproduces in the epithelial cells of the colon; causes severe diarrhea similar to that of shigellosis.

enteropathogenic *E. coli* (EPEC) Strain that adheres to the lining of the small intestine, causing intestinal illness, which is especially severe in newborn infants and young children.

enterotoxigenic *E. coli* (ETEC) Strain that attaches primarily to the lining of the duodenum; its toxins cause wasting diarrhea, especially among children in tropical regions; responsible for most cases of traveler's diarrhea.

escutcheon (es-kuch´an) A shield-shaped surface (e.g., the pattern of pubic hair).

eserine (es´er-in) See physostigmine.

e. salicylate See physostigmine salicylate, under physostigmine.

esodic (ĕ-sod´ik) See afferent.

esophagalgia (ĕ-sof-ă-gal´jă) Pain in the esophagus. Also called esophagodynia.

esophageal (ĕ-sof-ă je´al) Relating to the esophagus.

esophagectasis, esophagectasia (ĕ-sof-ă-jek-ta´sis, ĕ-sof-ă-jek-ta´shă) Abnormal dilatation of the esophagus.

esophagectomy (ĕ-sof-ă-jek´tŏ-me) Surgical removal of a portion of the esophagus.

esophagitis (ĕ-sof-ă-ji´tis) Inflammation of the esophagus.

candidal e. Esophagitis caused by infection with Candida organisms; predisposing factors include deficiency of the immune system (e.g., in AIDS), diabetes, malignancy, and corrosive injuries; symptoms include painful, difficult swallowing and oral thrush.

herpes e. Esophagitis caused by herpes I or II, varicella-zoster virus, or cytomegalovirus, which produce painful, difficult swallowing, fever, and bleeding.

pill-related e. Esophagitis with a tendency to form strictures caused by habitual lying down after swallowing pills with small sips of fluid or by swallowing pills with insufficient fluid to sweep them into the stomach.

peptic e. See reflux esophagitis.

reflux e. Inflammation of the distal esophagus caused by reflux of gastric or duodenal contents through an incompetent lower esophageal sphincter; frequently associated with a hiatal hernia. Also called peptic esophagitis.

esophagocardioplasty (ĕ-sof-ă-go-kar´de-o-plas-te) A reparative operation on the esophagus and the cardiac area of the stomach.

esophagocele (ĕ-sof´ă-go-sēl) Protrusion of the mucous membrane of the esophagus through a defect in its muscular layer.

esophagodynia (ĕ-sof-ă-go-din´e-ă) See esophagalgia.

esophagoenterostomy (ĕ-sof-ă-go-en-ter-os´tŏ-me) Surgical connection of the esophagus and intestine after excision of the stomach.

esophagogastrectomy (ĕ-sof-ă-go-gas-trek´tŏ-me) Surgical removal of a portion of the lower esophagus and proximal stomach, usually performed for eradicating neoplasms.

esophagogastroduodenoscopy (ĕ-sof-ă-go-gas-tro-doo-od-ĕ-nos´kŏ-pe) (EGD) Visual inspection of the lining of the esophagus, stomach, and upper duodenum using a flexible fiberoptic or video endoscope.

esophagogastrostomy (ĕ-sof-ă-go-gas-tros´kŏ-pe) The surgical formation of an artificial opening between the esophagus and the stomach.

esophagojejunostomy (ĕ-sof-ă-go-je-joo-nos´tŏ-me) Surgical union between the esophagus and jejunum.

esophagomalacia (ĕ-sof-ă-go-mă-la´shă) Softening of the walls of the esophagus.

esophagomyotomy (ĕ-sof-ă-go-mi-ot´ŏ-me) Operation for the relief of sustained muscular contraction (achalasia) at the junction of the esophagus and stomach; consists of a longitudinal cut through the sphincter muscle down to, but not including, the mucosa. Also called cardiomyotomy.

esophagoplasty (ĕ-sof´ă-go-plas-te) Surgical repair of a defect of the esophagus.

esophagoplication (ĕ-sof-ă-go-pli-ka´shun) Surgical reduction of a pouch or dilatation in the

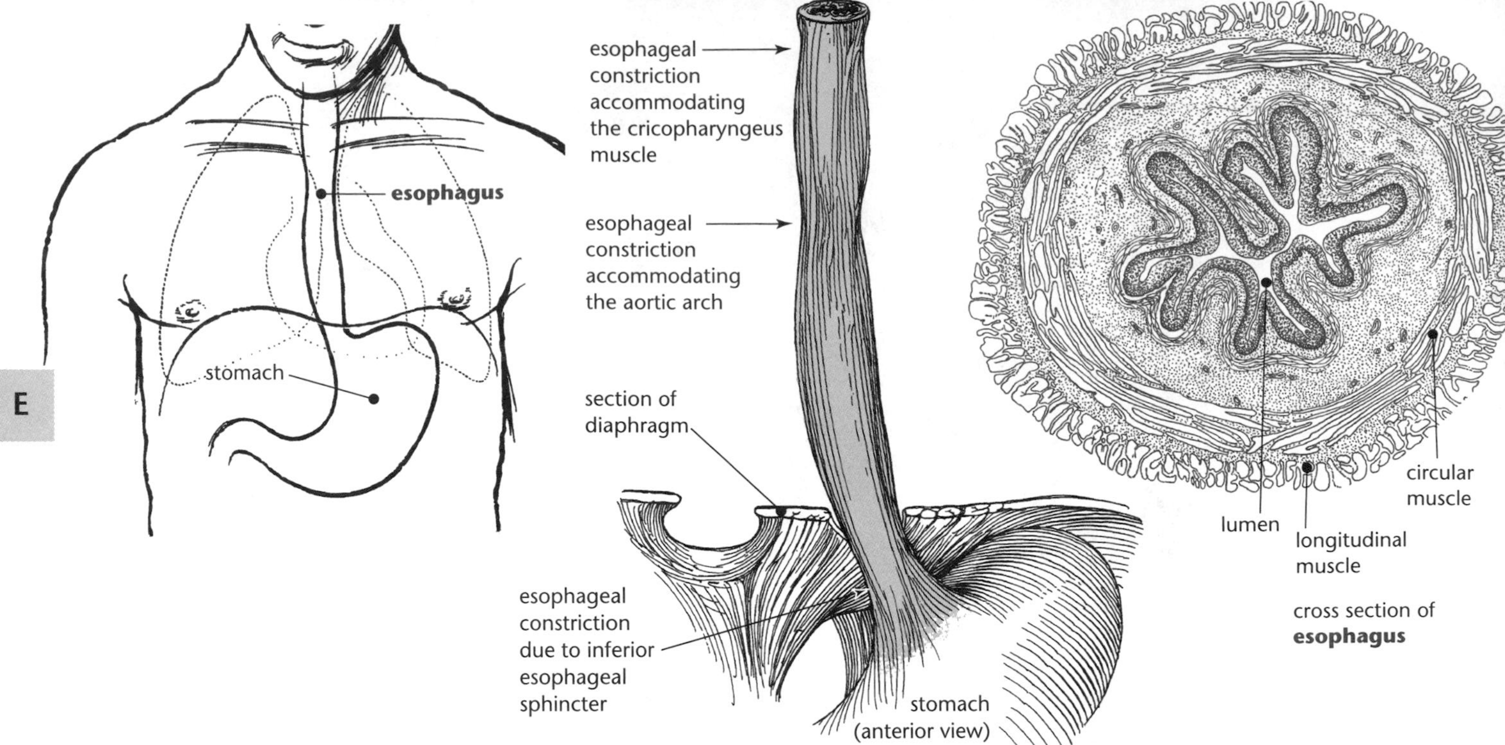

esophagus by making longitudinal folds on its walls.

esophagoscope (ĕ-sof′ă-go-skōp) An instrument for inspecting the interior of the esophagus.

esophagoscopy (ĕ-sof-ă-gos′ko-pe) Examination of the interior of the esophagus with an esophagoscope.

esophagostenosis (ĕ-sof-ă-go-stĕ-no′sis) Stricture or narrowing of the esophagus.

esophagostomy (ĕ-sof-ă-gos′tŏ-me) External opening made surgically into the esophagus.

esophagotomy (ĕ-sof-ă-got′ŏ-me) Incision through the esophagus.

esophagram (ĕ-sof′ă-gram) A roentgenogram of the esophagus.

esophagus (ĕ-sof′ă-gus) The musculomembranous tube extending downward from the pharynx to the cardia of the stomach.

esophoria (es-o-fo′re-ă) Tendency of the eyes to turn inward, manifested when fusion is prevented by covering one eye.

esophoric (es-o-for′ik) Relating to esophoria or the tendency of the eyes to deviate inward.

esotropia (es-o-tro′pe-ă) Inward deviation of the eyes. Also called cross-eyes; convergent strabismus.

esotropic (es-o-trop′ik) Relating to convergent strabismus or the inward turning of one eye.

essence (es′ens) **1.** The intrinsic properties or qualities of a thing. **2.** The fluid extract of a substance that retains its fundamental properties (e.g., the alcoholic solution of a volatile oil).

essential (ĕ-sen′shal) **1.** Necessary. **2.** Having no apparent external cause; said of a disease.

ester (es′ter) Any of a group of organic compounds formed by the condensation of an alcohol and carboxylic acid.

esterase (es′ter-ās) Any enzyme that promotes the hydrolysis of an ester.

esthesia (es-the′zha) The perception of sense impressions.

esthesiogenesis (es-the-ze-o-jen′ĕ-sis) The origin or production of a reaction in a sensory zone.

esthesiography (es-the-ze-og′ră-fe) **1.** Delineating on the skin the areas of tactile and other forms of sensibility. **2.** A description of the mechanism of sensation.

estival (es′tĭ-val) Occurring in the summer.

estivoautumnal (es-tĭ-vo-aw-tum′nal) Occurring in summer and autumn.

estradiol (es-tră-dī′ol) Estrogenic hormone essential for the development and functioning of female reproductive organs; a synthetic preparation is used in estrogen replacement therapy.

ethinyl e. Semisynthetic derivative of estradiol used as an ingredient of oral contraceptives and in estrogen replacement therapy.

estriol (es′tre-ol) A relatively weak estrogenic hormone; a major metabolic product of the hormones estradiol and estrone.

estrogen (es′tro-jen) General term for the female sex hormones, responsible for stimulating the development and maintenance of female secondary sex characteristics; formed in the ovary, placenta, testis, adrenal cortex, and some plants; therapeutic uses (with natural or synthetic preparations) include the relief of menopausal symptoms and amelioration of cancer of the prostate gland.

estrone (es′trōn) An estrogenic hormone found in the ovary and in the urine of pregnant mammals.

ethanol (eth′ă-nol) See alcohol (2).

ethchlorvynol (eth-klōr′vĭ-nol) A hypnotic and anticonvulsant drug, generally used for inducing sleep in simple insomnia and as a daytime sedative; Placidyl®.

ether (e′thĕr) **1.** Any of a group of organic compounds in which two hydrocarbon groups are linked by an oxygen atom. **2.** Term used for the anesthetic diethyl ether.

diethyl e. An inflammable, volatile liquid, $C_4H_{10}O$, obtained from the distillation of ethyl alcohol and sulfuric acid; used as an anesthetic. Also called ethyl ether.

ethyl e. See diethyl ether, under ether.

hydrochloric e. See ethyl chloride, under ethyl.

ethereal (e-the′re-al) **1.** Relating to ether. **2.** Evanescent.

etherification (e-ther-ĭ-fĭ-ka′shun) The conversion of an alcohol into ether.

etherify (e-ther′ĭ-fī) To convert into ether.

etherize (e′ther-iz) To produce anesthesia with ether.

ethical (eth′ĭ-kal) **1.** Relating to ethics. **2.** Being in accord with professionally accepted codes.

ethics (eth′iks) Standards of behavior governing an individual or a profession.

ethmoid (eth′moid) Resembling a sieve (e.g., the ethmoid bone).

ethmoidectomy (eth-moid-ek′tŏ-me) Surgical removal of the ethmoid cells or of part of the ethmoid bone.

ethmoiditis (eth-moi-di′tis) Inflammation of the ethmoid sinus.

ethmosphenoid (eth-mo-sfe′noid) Relating to both the ethmoid and the sphenoid bones.

ethnopsychiatry (eth-no-si-kī′ă-tre) The study of varied cultural patterns and their influence on emotional maturation.

ethyl (eth′ĭl) The univalent hydrocarbon radical C_2H_5—.

e. alcohol See alcohol (2).

e. chloride A gas at ordinary temperatures, a volatile liquid when compressed; used to produce local anesthesia by superficial freezing. Also called chloroethane.

ethylcellulose (eth-ĭl-sel′u-lōs) An ethyl ether of cellulose, used as a tablet binder; Ethocel®.

ethylene (eth′ĭ-lēn) A colorless, flammable gas, CH_2CH_2, somewhat lighter than air; formerly used as an inhalation anesthetic.

e. dibromide (EDB) Chemical widely used as a fumigant of fruits, soil and grain; identified as a carcinogen.

ethylenediaminetetraacetic acid (eth-ĭ-lēn-di-ă-mēn-tet-ră-ă-se′tik as′id) (EDTA) A heavy-metal antagonist (chelating agent) that forms complexes (chelates) with divalent and trivalent metals; used in the treatment of lead poisoning.

ethynodiol diacetate (ĕ-thi-no-dī′ol di-as′ĕ-tāt) A progestin used in combination with an estrogen in oral contraceptives.

etiocholanolone (e-te-o-ko-lan′o-lōn) A metabolite of adrenocortical and testicular hormones excreted in the urine.

etiologic (e-te-o-loj′ik) Relating to the causes of disease.

etiology (e-te-ol′ŏ-je) The study of causes, specifically the cause of a disease.

Eubacterium (u-bak-te′re-um) A genus of anaerobic bacteria (family Propionibacteriaceae) containing gram-positive rods; some species may be pathogenic.

eubiotics (u-bi-ot′iks) The science of hygienic living.

eucaryote (u-kar′e-ōt) See eukaryote.

eucholia (u-ko′le-ă) The normal state of the bile.

euchromatin (u-kro′mă-tin) Chromatin that shows the staining characteristics of the chromosome arms and the majority of the chromosome complement and stains lightly during interphase. COMPARE: heterochromatin.

eugenics (u-jen′iks) The branch of science concerned with the study of the hereditary improvement of man by genetic control.

eugenol (u′jĕn-ol) Eugenic acid, a light yellow oily liquid obtained from oil of cloves; used in dentistry as an antiseptic and local anesthetic.

euglobulin (u-glob′u-lin) A simple protein insoluble in pure water, but soluble in saline solutions.

euglycemia (u-gli-se′me-ă) Normal level of sugar in the blood. Also called normoglycemia.

euglycemic (u-glī-se′mik) Relating to eugly-cemia. Also called normoglycemic.

eugonic (u-gon′ik) Growing rapidly on an artificial medium; applied to certain bacterial cultures.

eukaryosis (u-kar-e-o′sis) The state of having a true nucleus, as in the higher types of cells.

eukaryote (u-kar′e-ōt) An organism with cells that

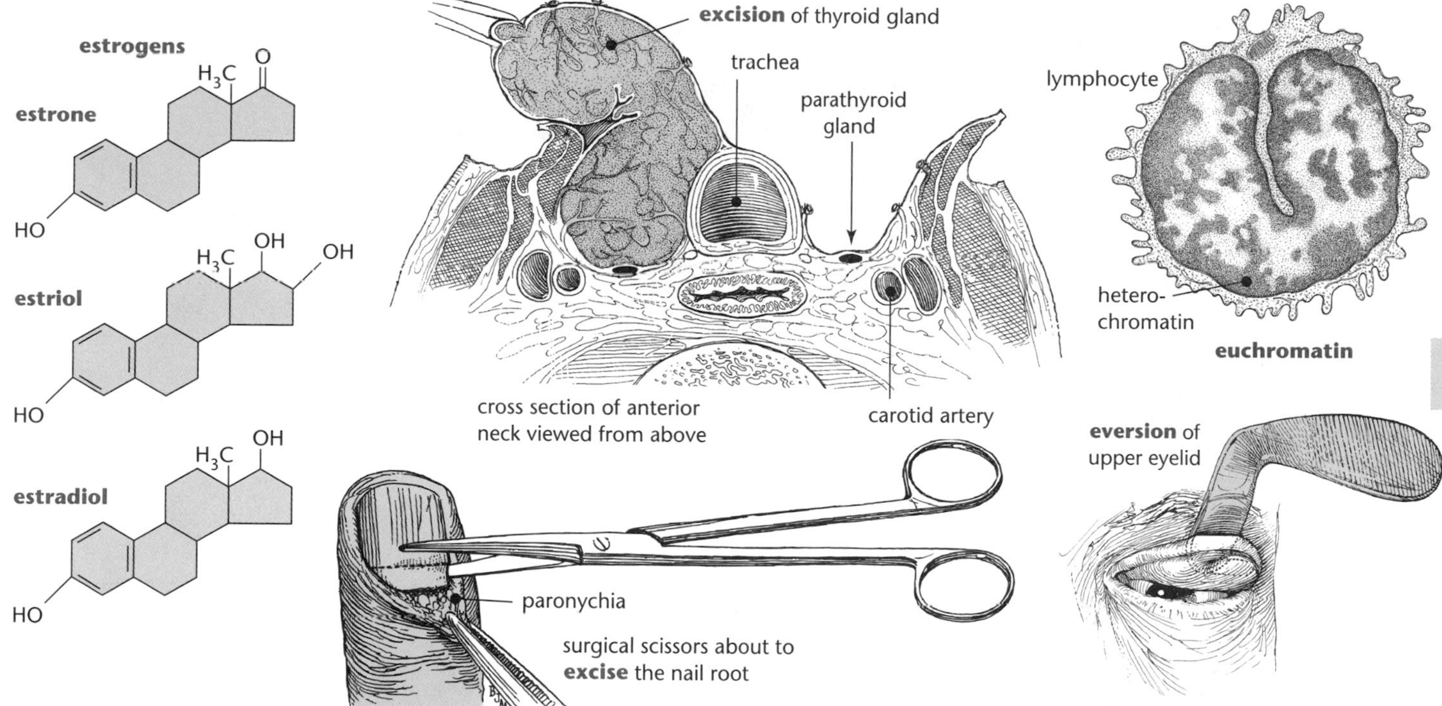

E

have a well-defined nucleus (with nuclear membrane, membrane-bound organelles, and ribosomes) and a mitotic cycle. Also written eucaryote.

eunuch (u´nuk) A castrated male, or one whose testes have never developed.

eunuchoid (u´nŭ-koid) Having the characteristics of a eunuch.

eunuchoidism (u´nŭ-koi-diz-m) Condition in which the testes fail to function.

euosmia (u-os´me-ă) **1.** A pleasant odor. **2.** A normal state of the sense of smell.

eupepsia (u-pep´se-ă) Good digestion.

euphoria (u-for´e-ă) **1.** A feeling of well-being. **2.** An exaggerated feeling of happiness.

euplasia (u-pla´zhă) The normal state of cells or tissues.

euplastic (u-plas´tik) Able to heal readily.

euploidy (u-ploi´de) In genetics, the condition of having the normal full complement of chromosomes; i.e., the chromosome number of a cell is an exact multiple of the haploid number normal for the species from which it originated.

eupnea (ūp-ne´ă) Normal, easy breathing.

europium (u-ro´pe-um) A rare earth element; symbol Eu, atomic number 63, atomic weight 151.96.

eustachitis (u-stă-ki´tis) Inflammation of the mucous membrane of the auditory (eustachian) tube.

euthanasia (u-thă-na´zhă) **1.** The act of inducing a painless, easy death, as in persons with a painful terminal illness. **2.** Painless death.

active e. Deliberate actions, such as disconnecting life-support systems or giving a lethal overdose of a drug, that serve to cause or hasten death. Also called mercy killing; positive euthanasia.

negative e. See passive euthanasia.

positive e. See active euthanasia.

passive e. The withholding of therapy or measures that prolong life, allowing nature to take its course; the patient is kept as comfortable and as painfree as possible. Also called negative euthanasia; nonintervention.

euthyroidism (u-thi´roid-iz-m) A normal condition of the thyroid gland.

eutonic (u´ton-ik) See normotonic.

eutrophia (u-tro´fe-ă) A state of normal nourishment and development.

evacuant (e-vak´u-ant) **1.** Promoting a bowel movement. **2.** An agent having such an effect.

evacuate (e-vak´u-āt) **1.** To empty the bowels. **2.** To create a vacuum or very low pressure by removing air or any gas from a closed vessel.

evacuation (e-vak-u-a´shun) **1.** Emptying of the bowels. **2.** The waste material discharged from the bowels. **3.** The creation of a vacuum.

evagination (e-vaj-ĭ-na´shun) Protrusion of a part or organ.

evaluation (e-val-u-a´shun) Examination and judgment of the significance of something.

clinical e. Evaluation based on direct observation of a patient.

evanescent (ev-ă-nes´ent) Of short life or duration.

Evans blue (ev´anz bloo) A diazo dye injected intravenously to determine blood or plasma volume by the method of dilution (the dye adheres to plasma proteins).

evaporation (e-vap-o-ra´shun) The change of a liquid into a vapor.

eventration (e-ven-tra´shun) **1.** Protrusion of the intestines through an opening in the abdominal wall. **2.** Removal of the abdominal organs.

eversion (e-ver´zhun) Turning outward, as of a foot, or inside out, as of an eyelid.

evert (e-vert´) To turn outward.

evisceration (e-vis-er-a´shun) **1.** Removal of internal organs. **2.** A critical postoperative complication involving an abdominal wall incision in which all layers of the wound separate, allowing intestinal protrusion through the opening. Also called burst abdomen. COMPARE: dehiscence.

e. of the eye Surgical removal of the contents of the eyeball, leaving the sclera intact.

e. of the orbit Removal of all the contents of the orbit. Also called exenteration.

evolution (ev-o-loo´shun) A continuous and gradual process of change from one state or form to another.

evulsion (e-vul´shun) A pulling out or forcible extraction.

Ewart's sign (u´arts sīn) An area of dullness over the area of the left lung, at the lower angle of the left shoulder blade (scapula), due to compression from a large pericardial effusion. Also called Pins' sign.

exacerbation (eg-zas-er-ba´shun) Increase in the severity of a disease or any of its symptoms.

examination (eg-zam-ĭ-na´shun) Any inspection or investigation for the purpose of diagnosis.

cytologic e. The microscopic examination of cells for the detection of cancer or for the evaluation of hormonal effect; the cells may be obtained by collecting a bodily secretion, such as sputum, urine or vaginal fluid, by scraping a tissue, such as the cervix, or by needle aspiration. Also called Papanicolaou examination.

Papanicolaou e. See cytologic examination.

postmortem e. See autopsy.

examiner (eg-zam´ĭn-er) A person who conducts examinations.

medical e. (a) An appointed medical officer with training and/or expertise in forensic pathology who investigates sudden, violent, or unexplained deaths, or any other category of death as defined by law. In many jurisdictions, medical examiners have replaced elected coroners. (b) A physician employed by public or private enterprise whose duties are defined by the employer (e.g., examination of applicants for work-men's compensation, or of prospective purchasers of life insurance).

exanthema, exanthem (eg-zan-the´mă, eg-zan´them) **1.** Any disease accompanied by a skin eruption. **2.** A skin eruption.

e. subitum An acute febrile disease occurring within the first 3 years of life, most commonly between 6 and 18 months; after 2 to 4 days of fever, the temperature falls and a macular or maculopapular rash appears; caused by human herpesvirus 6 (HH6). Also called roseola infantum.

exanthematous (eg-zan-them´ă-tus) Relating to exanthema.

excavation (eks-kă-va´shun) **1.** A natural body cavity or recess. **2.** A cavity resulting from a pathologic process.

atrophic e. An exaggerated depression of the optic disk caused by atrophy of the optic nerve.

glaucomatous e. See glaucomatous cup, under cup.

physiologic e. See physiologic cup, under cup.

excavator (eks´kă-va-tor) **1.** A spoonlike instrument used to scrape out pathologic tissue. **2.** A dental instrument used to remove carious material from a cavity.

exchange (eks-chanj´) The substitution of one thing for another.

plasma e. Removal of plasma and replacement with any of various fluids (e.g., saline or dextran solutions, albumin preparations, fresh frozen plasma, plasma protein fractions); used in the treatment of autoimmune diseases and diseases of excess plasma factors.

excipient (ek-sip´e-ent) A more or less inert substance used as a diluent or vehicle for a drug.

excise (ek-sīz´) To remove surgically.

excision (ek-sizh´un) The surgical removal of a part or organ.

loop e. See loop electrosurgical excision procedure (LEEP), under procedure.

microscopically controlled e. See Mohs' technique, under technique.

excitability (ek-sīt-ă-bil´ĭ-te) The state of being capable of quick response to a stimulus; the property of muscle tissue by virtue of which it reacts to stimulation by propagation of the impulse.

excitation (ek-si-ta´shun) **1.** Stimulation. **2.** In physics, an increase of energy.

excitement (ek-sīt´ment) The state of being agitated.

excitoglandular (ek-si-to-glan´du-lar) Increasing

exotoxins produced by some bacteria pathogenic to man

TOXIN	DISEASE	SPECIES	ACTION
tetanospasmin	tetanus	*Clostridium tetani*	spastic hemolytic cardiotoxin
diphtheritic toxin	diphtheria	*Corynebacterium diphtheriae*	necrotizing
α-toxin	pyogenic infection	*Staphylococcus aureus*	necrotizing, hemolytic, leukocidic
whooping cough toxin	whooping cough	*Bordetella pertussis*	necrotizing
neurotoxin	dysentery	*Shigella dysenteriae*	hemorrhagic paralytic
neurotoxin	botulism	*Clostridium botulinum*	paralytic

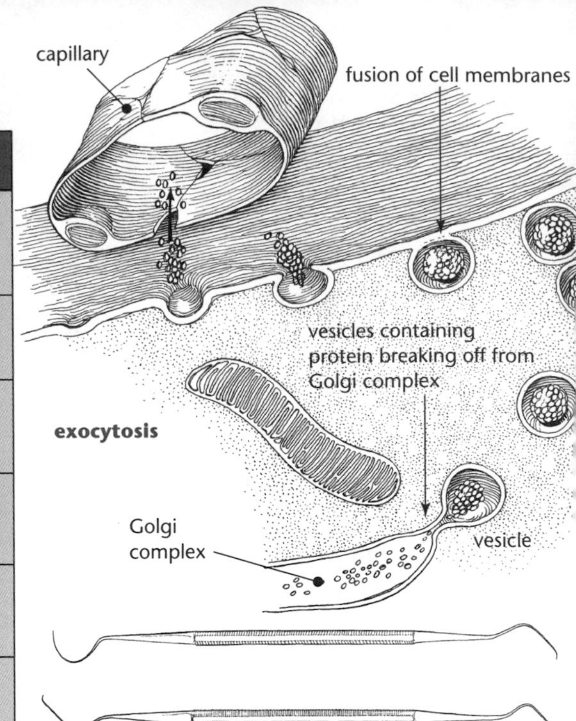

exocytosis

dental **explorers**

E

the activity of a gland.

excoriate (eks-ko͞r'e-āt) To scratch or abrade the skin.

excoriation (eks-kōr-e-a'shun) A scratch mark.

neurotic e. Self-inflicted skin lesions by emotionally disturbed persons, usually by the forcible use of fingernails.

excrement (eks'krĕ-ment) Feces.

excrescence (eks-kres'ens) Any abnormal outgrowth from the surface.

excreta (eks-kre'tă) Discharged natural wastes from the body (e.g., urine, feces).

excrete (eks-krēt') To discharge waste material from the body.

excretion (eks-kre'shun) **1.** Process by which the waste products of metabolism or undigested food residues are eliminated from the body. **2.** The product of such a process.

excretory (eks'kre-tor-e) Relating to or used during excretion.

excursion (eks-ker'shun) An oscillating or alternating motion from an axis or a mean position.

exenteration (ek-sen-ter-a'shun) Surgical removal of all the contents of a body cavity. See also evisceration.

exercise (ek'ser-sīz) Physical activity performed to develop or maintain fitness; it may require bodily exertion (active exercise) or effortless motion (passive exercise).

compulsive e. Athletic activity that has become essential for the emotional well-being of the individual.

Kegel's e. Repetitive contraction and relaxation of pelvic floor muscles for treatment of urinary stress incontinence.

exergonic (ek-sĕr-gon'ik) Indicating a chemical reaction that is accompanied by a release of free energy, regardless of the form of energy involved.

exflagellation (eks-flaj-ĕ-la'shun) The development of microgametes (male gametes) from microgametocytes (mother cells), as in malaria.

exfoliation (eks-fo-le-a'shun) **1.** The shedding, peeling, or scaling of skin. Also called desquama-tion. **2.** In dentistry, the casting off of deciduous teeth.

exhalation (eks-hă-la'shun) **1.** The act of breathing out. **2.** Exhaled gas or vapor.

exhale (eks'hāl) **1.** To breathe out. **2.** To emit gas or vapor.

exhaustion (eg-zaws'chun) **1.** Extreme fatigue. **2.** Removal of contents. **3.** Removal of the active ingredients of a drug.

heat e. Condition marked by prostration and weakness caused by prolonged exposure to hot temperatures.

exhibitionism (eg-zĭ-bish'un-iz-m) A morbid compulsion to expose the genitalia.

exhumation (eg-zu-ma'shun) The process of taking a body out of a place of burial.

exocrine (ek'so-krin) **1.** Denoting a gland that discharges its secretion through a duct. **2.** Denoting the secretion of such a gland.

exocytosis (ek-so-si-to'sis) Secretion of a substance from a cell (e.g., to secrete insulin from a beta cell of the pancreas, the intracellular sac containing insulin granules migrates to the periphery of the cell and fuses with the cell's plasma membrane upon contact; then the site of fusion ruptures and insulin passes out of the cell and into the bloodstream). Also called emiocytosis.

exodontics (ek-so-don'tiks) The branch of dentistry concerned with the extraction of teeth.

exoenzyme (ek-so-en'zīm) See extracellular enzyme, under enzyme.

exogenous (ek-soj'ĕ-nus) Originating outside the body.

exomphalos (eks-om'fă-los) See omphalocele.

exon (ek'son) A region of DNA that codes for a section of the processed messenger RNA (mRNA) which, in turn, is translated into protein. Also called coding sequence.

exonuclease (ek-so-noo'kle-ās) A nuclease (enzyme) that digests or cleaves DNA from the ends of strands (polynucleotide chains).

exopathy (ek-sop'ă-the) Any disease originating from causes outside the body.

exophoria (ek-so-for'e-ă) Tendency of the eyes to turn outward, manifested when fusion is prevented by covering the eye.

exophthalmic (ek-sof-thal'mik) Relating to or afflicted with exophthalmos.

exophthalmometer (ek-sof-thal-mom'ĕ-ter) An instrument used to measure the degree of protrusion of the eyeball. Also called proptometer.

exophthalmos (ek-sof-thal'mos) Abnormal protrusion of the eyeball.

malignant e. Severe, usually bilateral, protrusion of the eyeballs; occurring mostly in middle age; it may be unresponsive to treatment and can lead to blindness.

exophytic (ek-so-fit'ik) Tending to grow outward, such as a tumor that arises at or near the surface of an organ or tissue and grows outward.

exoskeleton (ek-so-skel'ĕ-ton) **1.** The external, supportive covering of certain invertebrates. **2.** Structures, such as hair, nails, feathers, scales, etc., developed from the ectoderm or mesoderm in vertebrates. Also called dermatoskeleton; dermoskeleton.

exospore (ek'so-spōr) A spore produced by budding, as a fungal spore.

exosporium (ek-so-spor'e-um) The outer covering of a spore.

exostosis (ek-sos-to'sis), *pl.* **exosto'ses** A bony growth on the surface of a bone.

hereditary multiple e. The presence of multiple exostoses in the long bones of children due to a hereditary defect of ossification in cartilage, resulting in severe skeletal deformity and stunting of growth. Also called diaphyseal aclasis.

solitary osteocartilaginous e. See osteochondroma.

exoteric (ek-so-ter'ik) Belonging to factors outside the organism.

exothermic, exothermal (ek-so-ther'mik, ek-so-ther'mal) **1.** Releasing heat, as in certain chemical reactions. **2.** Relating to the external warmth of the body.

exotoxin (ek-so-tok'sin) A toxin produced and released by bacterial cells as a normal physiologic process. Also called extracellular toxin.

exotropia (ek-so-tro'pe-ă) Outward deviation of the eyes. Also called divergent strabismus; walleye.

expansiveness (ek-span'siv-nes) An exaggerated sense of importance.

expectorant (ek-spek'tŏ-rant) **1.** Promoting the expulsion of mucus or other material from the air passages. **2.** A medicine so acting.

expectoration (ek-spek-tŏ-ra'shun) Mucus or other secretions coughed up from the air passages. Also called sputum.

experiment (ek-sper'ĭ-ment) A test.

blind e. See blind trial, under trial.

control e. Experiment to check the results of other experiments by keeping the same conditions except for one particular factor.

double-blind e. See double blind trial, under trial.

expiration (ek-spĭ-ra'shun) **1.** The act of breathing out. **2.** The act of dying.

expiratory (ek-spi'ră-tor-e) Relating to expiration.

expire (ek-spīr') **1.** To exhale; to breathe out. **2.** To die.

explant (eks-plant') In tissue culture, to transfer living tissue from the body to another medium.

exploration (eks-plo-ra'shun) A surgical, digital, or instrumental examination of tissue as an aid in diagnosis; a diagnostic search or investigation.

explorer (ek-splor'er) A sharp, curved dental probe used to examine teeth.

exponent (ek-spo'nent) **1.** A number or symbol written as a superscript, denoting the number of times a factor is to be involved in a repeated multiplication. **2.** One who defines or advocates.

express (ek-spres') **1.** To squeeze out. **2.** To show; to give form.

expression (ek-spresh'un) The act of expressing.

differential gene e. Gene expression that responds to signals such as those from hormones.

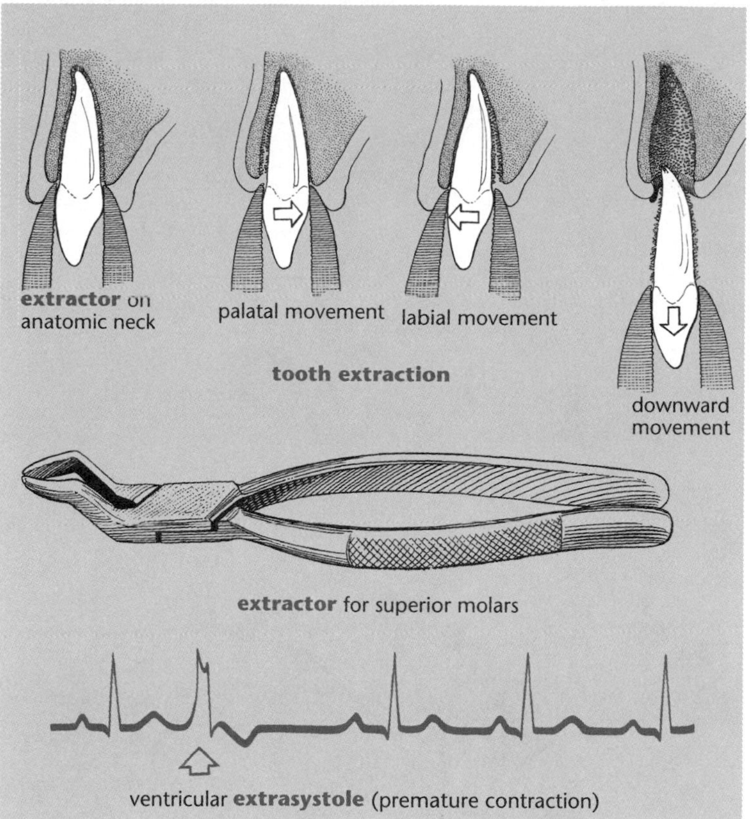

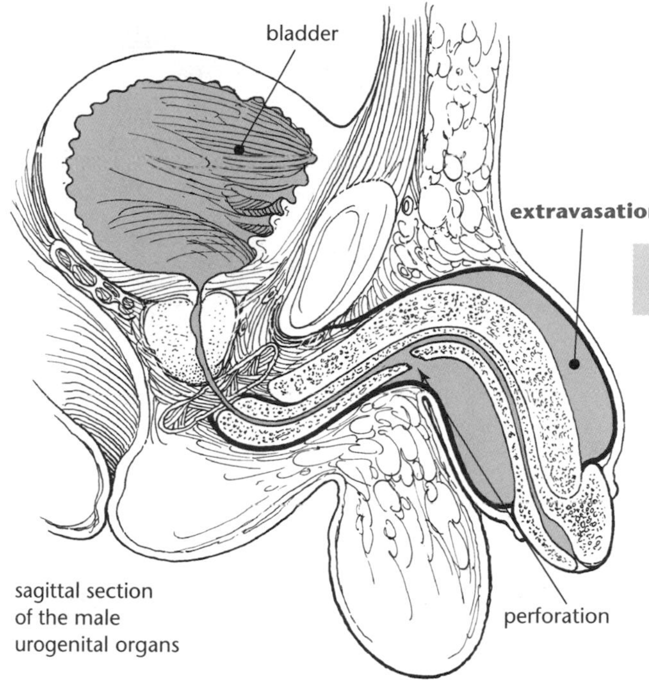

gene e. The detectable effect of a gene; manifestation of a heritable trait in an individual carrying the gene for that trait.

expressivity (eks-pres-siv´ĭ-te) In clinical genetics, the extent to which a genetic trait or defect is manifested.

variable e. A manifestation of a trait that may range from mild to severe; the trait is never completely unexpressed; a frequent characteristic of autosomal dominant traits.

exsanguinate (ek-sang´gwĭ-nāt) To drain blood; to make bloodless.

exsiccant (ek-sik´ant) **1.** Drying; dehydrating; absorbing. **2.** A dusting or drying powder.

exsiccate (ek´sĭ-kāt) To dry; to remove moisture.

exsiccation (ek-sĭ-ka´shun) The process of removing moisture.

exstrophy (ek´stro-fe) Congenital turning inside out of an organ.

e. of bladder Malformation in which the interior of the posterior wall of the bladder becomes visible through an opening in the abdominal wall and the anterior bladder wall.

exsufflation (ek-sŭ-fla´shun) Forcible expiration; forced expulsion of the breath by a mechanical apparatus.

extension (ek-sten´shun) The act of straightening a limb or the condition of being straightened.

extensor (ek-sten´sor) A muscle that, by contracting, straightens a limb.

exteriorize (ek-stēr´e-ŏ-rīz) To direct a patient's interests toward others, outside the self.

extern (eks´tern) A nonresident medical student or recent graduate who assists in the care of hospitalized patients.

external (ek-ster´nal) Situated on the outside; on the surface.

exteroceptor (ek-stĕr-o-sep´tor) A sensory nerve ending in the skin or mucous membrane which is affected primarily by the external environment (e.g., Meissner's corpuscle for touch, Krause's end bulb for cold, Ruffini's nerve endings for warmth, Golgi-Mazzoni corpuscle for pressure, and free nerve endings for pain).

extinction (ek-stink´shun) **1.** In physiology, relating to the point at which a nerve, after responding to a stimulus, becomes completely inexcitable. **2.** In psychology, the process by which a stimulus-response bond is broken.

extirpation (eks-tir-pa´shun) Complete removal of a part or of a pathologic growth.

extorsion (ek-stor´shun) The act of rotating outward.

extra-articular (eks-tră-ar-tik´u-lar) Outside a joint.

extracapsular (eks-tră-kap´su-lar) Located or occurring outside a capsule (e.g., a fracture occurring outside a joint capsule).

extracellular (eks-tră-sel´u-lar) Occurring outside a cell.

extracorporeal (eks-tra-kor-po´re-al) Outside the body.

extracorpuscular (eks-tră-kor-pus´ku-lar) Outside the blood corpuscles.

extracranial (eks-tră-kra´ne-al) Outside the skull.

extraction (eks-trak´shun) **1.** The act of drawing out or removing. **2.** The process of preparing an extract.

breech e. Extraction of the infant from the birth canal by its buttocks or lower limbs.

tooth e. Removal of a tooth.

extractor (eks-trak´tor) An instrument used in drawing out a body part; especially forceps for extracting teeth.

vacuum e. Any device used to apply traction to the fetal head during delivery, attached by suction to the scalp after the head has passed through the pelvic inlet (i.e., after engagement). Also called vacuum forceps.

extradural (eks-tră-doo´răl) Located outside the dura mater.

extrahepatic (eks-tră-hĕ-pat´ik) Located outside the liver.

extramedullary (eks-tră-med´u-lar-e) Located outside any medulla.

extraneous (ek-stra´ne-us) Originating outside the organism, or not belonging to it.

extraocular (eks-tră-ok´u-lar) External to the eye.

extraperitoneal (eks-tră-per-ĭ-to-ne´al) Located outside the peritoneal cavity.

extrapolate (ek-strap´o-lāt) To estimate a value or values beyond the observable range from a known trend of variables; broadly, to estimate or infer from known values.

extrapulmonary (eks-tră-pul´mo-nar-e) Located outside of the lungs.

extrapyramidal (eks-tră-pĭ-ram´ĭ-dal) Outside of pyramidal tracts; said of descending nerve tracts that are not part of the pyramids of the medulla.

extrapyramidal disease (eks-tră-pĭ-ram´ĭ-dal dĭ-zēz´) Any disease affecting the extrapyramidal areas of the brain.

extrasensory (eks-tră-sen´sōr-e) Not perceptible by the senses, as some forms of perception such as telepathy or clairvoyance. Also called supernatural.

extrasystole (eks-tră-sis´to-le) A premature contraction of the heart originating at a site other than the usual (ectopic); it may arise from the atrium, the atrioventricular (A-V) node, or the ventricle; the term is loosely applied to all premature contractions, but more correctly limited to interpolated premature contractions.

atrial e. Extrasystole due to irritability of the atria; the early contractions emanate from an impulse in the atria outside the sinoatrial (S-A) node.

atrioventricular nodal e. Extrasystole emanating from the atrioventricular (A-V) node and leading to a simultaneous or near simultaneous contraction of atria and ventricles. Also called nodal extrasystole; A-V nodal extrasystole.

A-V nodal e. See atrioventricular nodal extrasystole.

interpolated e. A ventricular extrasystole which, instead of being followed by a compensatory pause, is sandwiched between two consecutive sinus cycles.

nodal e. See atrioventricular nodal extrasystole.

supraventricular e. An extrasystole emanating from a center above the ventricles, i.e., atrium or atrioventricular (A-V) node.

ventricular e. A premature contraction of the ventricles.

extrauterine (eks-tră-u´ter-in) Located outside the uterus.

extravasate (eks-trav´ă-sāt) **1.** To escape from a vessel into the tissues. **2.** The material that has escaped.

extravasation (ek-strav-ă-sa´shun) Escape of fluid from a vessel into the surrounding tissues.

extravascular (eks-tră-vas´ku-lar) Outside the blood vessels or lymphatics.

extraversion (eks-tra-ver´zhun) See extroversion.

extravert (eks´tră-vert) See extrovert.

extremity (eks-trem´ĭ-te) A limb; an arm or a leg.

extrinsic (ek-strin´zik) Originating outside of a part where it is found or on which it acts.

extroversion, extraversion (eks-tro-ver´zhun, eks-tra-ver´zhun) **1.** A turning inside out, as of the uterus. **2.** A personality trait in which a person's interests lie mainly in the environment and others rather than in himself.

extrovert (eks´tro-vert) A person whose interests lie outside of himself, or who is outwardly directed.

extrude (eks-trood´) **1.** To push out, or reposition distally. **2.** In dentistry, to move a tooth into a more occlusal position with the teeth of the opposing jaw.

extrusion (ek-stroo´zhun) The process of forcing out of a normal position.

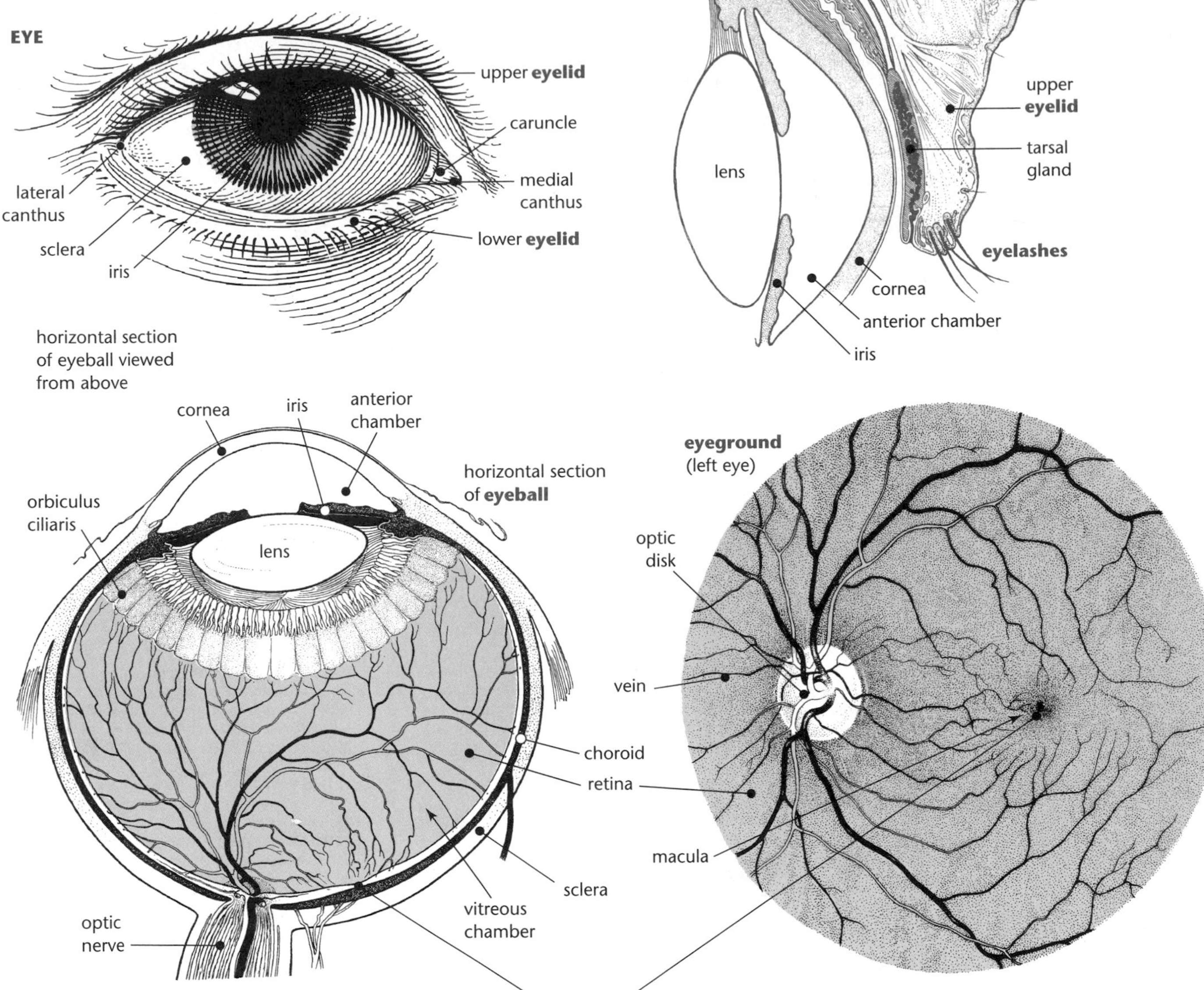

E

extubation (eks-tu-ba´shun) The removal of a tube, specifically, the removal of an intubation tube from the larynx.
exuberant (eg-zoo´ber-ant) Denoting excessive growth, as of tissue or granulation.
exudate (eks´u-dāt) Material gradually discharged and deposited in the tissues or a cavity, usually as a result of inflammation.
exudation (eks-u-da´shun) The oozing of fluids through the tissues into a cavity or to the surface, usually as a result of inflammation.
exudative (eks-u´dă-tiv) Relating to the process of exudation.
exude (ĕg-zo͞od´) To ooze; to pass out gradually through the tissues or through an opening.
eye (i) The organ of vision; in humans, it is a nearly spherical body consisting of three concentric coats; the outermost, fibrous, protective coat, made up of an opaque, white, posterior portion (five-sixths) called the sclera and an anterior transparent part called the cornea; the middle, vascular, nutritive coat, made up (from behind forward) of choroid, ciliary body, and iris; and the innermost, nervous coat called the retina; within, it contains the anterior and posterior chambers, filled with a clear fluid (aqueous humor), the crystalline lens, and the gelatinous vitreous body.
dancing e.'s See opsoclonus.
fixating e. In strabismus, the eye that is directed toward the object of regard.
lazy e. See amblyopia.
pink e. See acute contagious conjunctivitis, under conjunctivitis.
shipyard e. See epidemic keratoconjunctivitis, under keratoconjunctivitis.
white of the e. The visible portion of the sclera.
eyeball (i´bawl) The globe of the eye.
eyebrow (i´brow) **1.** The row of hairs growing between the upper eyelid and the forehead. **2.** The bony ridge over the eye. Also called supercilium.
eyeglasses (i´glas-es) A pair of ophthalmic lenses mounted on a frame, used as an aid to vision. Also called spectacles; glasses.
eyeground (i´ground) The inner surface of the eye seen through the pupil on ophthalmoscopic examination. Also called ocular fundus.
eyelash (i´lash) One of the short hairs growing on the margin of the eyelid. Also called cilium.
eyelid (i´lid) One of two folds (upper and lower) that cover and protect the anterior portion of the eyeball.
eyepiece (i´pēs) The lens or system of lenses closest to the eye in an optical instrument such as a microscope, that further magnifies the image formed by the objective lens.
eyestrain (i´strān) Fatigue or discomfort associated with the use of the eyes, due to uncorrected errors of refraction, imbalance of the eye muscles, or prolonged use of the eyes.
eyewash (i´wosh) The medicated irrigating solution used in bathing the eyes.

F

fabella (fă-bel´ă) Latin meaning little bean; in anatomy, the small sesamoid bone sometimes found in the tendon of the lateral origin of the gastrocnemius muscle.

fabrication (fab-rĭ-ka´shun) See confabulation.

face (fās) The front of the head from the forehead to the chin and from car to ear.

hippocratic f. See hippocratic facies, under facies.

masklike f. See Parkinson's facies, under facies.

moon f. The rounded face observed in individuals with Cushing's disease or in hypercorticoidism.

face-bow (fās´bo) Instrument used to record the relationship of the jaws to the temporomandibular joint.

face-lift (fās´lift) See rhytidectomy.

facet (fas´ĕt) An extremely smooth surface on a bone.

articular f. A small planar or rounded smooth surface on a bone which articulates with another structure.

costal f. See demifacet.

facetectomy (fas-ĕ-tek´tŏ-me) Surgical removal of the facet of a vertebra.

facial (fa´shal) **1.** Relating to the face. **2.** The application of cosmetic creams in conjunction with gentle massage of the face.

facies (fa´she-ēz), *pl.* **fa´cies** The outward appearance and expression of the face.

adenoid f. The open-mouthed expression of children with adenoid growths.

hippocratic f. A pinched expression of the face with sunken eyes, hollow cheeks and temples, relaxed lips, and leaden complexion, observed in a person dying after an exhausting illness. Also called hippocratic face.

Parkinson's f. Lack of facial expression due to Parkinson's disease. Also called masklike face.

facilitation (fă-sil-ĭ-ta´shun) Reinforcement of the activity of nervous tissue by the introduction of external impulses; an important protective reflex of the spinal cord (e.g., the reflex withdrawal from pain).

facing (fās´ing) Plastic or porcelain material used to cover the labial or buccal surface of a dental crown.

faciobrachial (fa-she-o-bra´ke-ăl) Relating to the face and the arms.

faciocervical (fa-she-o-ser´vĭ-kal) Relating to the face and neck.

facioplegia (fa-she-o-ple´jă) See facial nerve palsy, under palsy.

factitious (fak-tish´ŭs) Artificial; contrived.

factor (fak´tor) (F) **1.** An agent or element that contributes to an action, process, or result. **2.** A gene. **3.** An essential element in a diet, such as a vitamin.

ABO f.'s See ABO blood group.

angiogenesis f. Substance, secreted by macrophages, that stimulates growth of new blood vessels (e.g., in cancers and in healing wounds).

antiberiberi f. See thiamine.

antihemophilic f. A See factor VIII.

antihemophilic f. B See factor IX.

antiheparin f. A glycoprotein released from platelets, following platelet aggregation, which shortens the thrombin clotting time in the presence of heparin. Also called platelet factor 4.

antinuclear f. (ANF) See antinuclear antibody, under antibody.

atrial natriuretic f. (ANF) See atrial natriuretic peptide, under peptide.

branching f. See α-glucan-branching glycosyltransferase.

chemotactic f.'s Soluble substances produced by the reaction of antigen with sensitized leukocytes; they induce migration of neutrophils and monocytes from blood vessels into tissues to ingest and destroy potentially dangerous agents, such as bacteria.

Christmas f. See factor IX.

citrovorum f. See folinic acid.

clotting f.'s, coagulation f.'s Various plasma and tissue components involved in blood clotting.

colony-stimulating f. A glycoprotein that regulates the production and growth of blood cells and promotes restoration of the blood-forming function (e.g., after bone marrow suppression in chemotherapy).

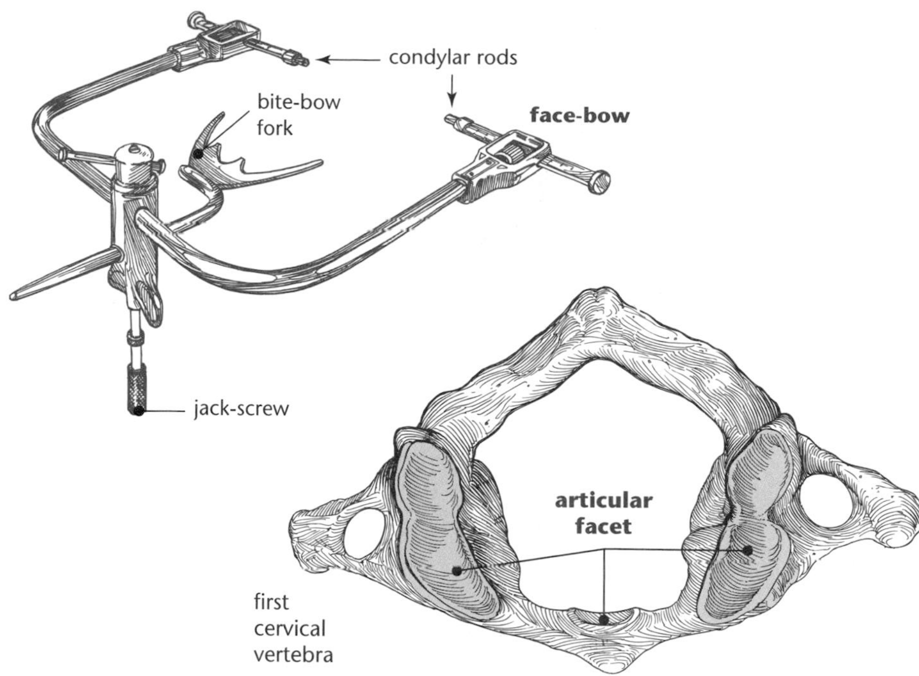

coronary risk f. Any of several factors that make the likelihood of suffering a coronary occlusion greater than average (e.g., high blood pressure, diabetes mellitus, elevated blood lipids, smoking, and heredity).

corticotropin-releasing f. (CRF) See corticotropin-releasing hormone, under hormone.

coupling f.'s Proteins restoring phosphorylating ability to mitochondria that have lost this ability or that have become uncoupled.

endothelial relaxing f. A product of activated macrophages that acts as a neurotransmitter; capable of destroying tumor cells, intracellular bacteria and parasites.

endothelium-derived relaxing f. (EDRF) A substance released from endothelial cells of blood vessels in response to the binding of vasodilators to receptors on the cells; it relaxes vascular smooth muscle. Now known to be nitric oxide.

epidermal growth f. (EGF) Protein substance isolated from submaxillary glands of male mice that, when injected into newborn mice, causes rapid eyelid opening, eruption of teeth, and epidermal growth. Large doses may inhibit these processes.

f. I See fibrinogen.

f. II See prothrombin.

f. III See thromboplastin.

f. IV Calcium ions, the presence of which is necessary for many steps of the blood coagulation process.

f. V See accelerator globulin, under globulin.

f. VII A substance that acts as an accelerator in the extrinsic pathway of prothrombin activation; it is not consumed during the clotting of blood and is consequently found in the serum following normal coagulation. Deficiency is associated with hemorrhagic disease of the newborn and purpura in the adult. Also called convertin; cothromboplastin; proconvertin; serum prothrombin conversion accelerator (SPCA); stable factor.

f. VIII The antihemophilic globulin present in plasma, essential in the first phase of blood clotting. Deficiency causes the hereditary disease, hemophilia A. Also called antihemophilic globulin; antihemophilic factor A; antihemolytic factor.

f. IX A factor essential in the first phase of blood clotting. Deficiency is inherited, causing hemophilia B (Christmas disease). Also called Christmas factor; plasma thromboplastin component (PTC); antihemophilic factor B.

f. X A procoagulant in normal plasma; a factor required for conversion of the plasma protein prothrombin to the enzyme thrombin. Deficiency may be congenital, but it also occurs in hemorrhagic disease of the newborn, liver disease, and deficiency of vitamin K.

f. XI A factor essential in the first phase of blood clotting. Deficiency is most commonly congenital, producing a mild bleeding tendency.

f. XII A stable factor present in normal blood and serum; it initiates the process of blood coagulation when the plasma contacts collagen or a foreign surface; it may be bypassed when absent so that hemostasis occurs normally despite a prolonged coagulation time. Deficiency is caused by an autosomal recessive gene and does not cause a bleeding tendency.

f. XIII A transpeptidase present in normal plasma which cross-links subunits of fibrin monomer to form insoluble fibrin polymer; thrombin catalyzes the conversion of factor XIII into its active form.

fibroblast growth f. (FGF) A growth factor that plays a role in wound healing and may cause growth of new blood vessels when produced by tumor cells. It also facilitates entry of herpes simplex virus (HSV-1) into vertebrate cells that normally have FGF receptors on their membranes.

follicle-stimulating hormone-releasing f. (FRF; FSH-RF) See follicle-stimulating hormone-releasing hormone, under hormone.

granulocyte colony-stimulating f. (G-CSF) A glycoprotein that regulates the production of red and white blood cells; it causes committed cell lines to proliferate and mature.

granulocyte-macrophage colony-stimulating f. (GM-CSF) Glycoprotein secreted by T lymphocytes, monocytes, fibroblasts, and endothelial cells; it binds to specific receptors in stem cells, causing the cells to differentiate into granulocytes and macrophages.

growth f.'s Polypeptides that exert positive and negative effects on the cell cycle; they are produced by a variety of cell types and bind to specific receptors on the cell membrane to trigger intracellular biochemical signals, thus regulating cell proliferation and differentiation; a growth factor may act on the cell that produced it or on a neighboring cell.

growth hormone-releasing f. (GRF, GH-RF) See growth hormone-releasing hormone, under hormone.

insulin-like growth f.'s (IGF) Serum peptides resembling insulin in structure and biologic activities; formed primarily in the liver and ovary; they are important as mediators of growth hormone. Two forms have been isolated: *IGF-I* (somatomedin C), active in embryonic development; and *IGF-II*, active postnatally. Also called somatomedins.

intrinsic f. (IF) A mucoprotein produced by the parietal cells of gastric glands essential for absorption of vitamin B_{12} in the ileum. Deficiency causes

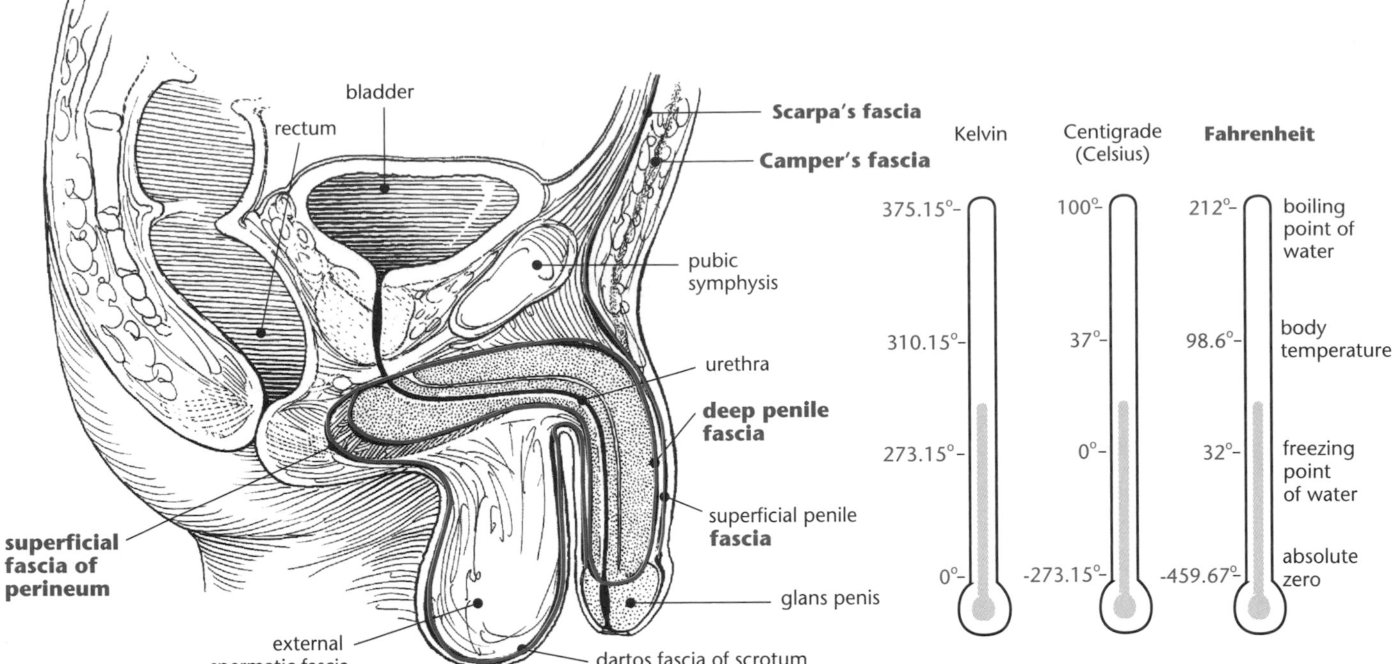

pernicious anemia.

labile f. See factor V.

lopotropic f. See choline.

luteinizing hormone-releasing f. (LRF) See luteinizing hormone-releasing hormone, under hormone.

macrophage-activating f. (MAF) A group of soluble substances (products of lymphocytes) that participate in inducing immunologic responses. Interferon-gamma (INF-γ) is a major type.

macrophage colony-stimulating f. (M-CSF) Glycoprotein secreted by monocytes, endothelial cells, and fibroblasts; it stimulates committed cell lines to proliferate and mature into macrophages.

multi-colony-stimulating f. (multi-CSF) See interleukin 3.

ovarian cancer activating f. See lysophosphatidic acid.

pellagra-preventing f. (P-PF) See nicotinic acid.

platelet f. 1 (PF-1) Plasma factor V absorbed on the surface of the platelet.

platelet f. 2 (PF-2) Fibrinogen activator on the surface of the platelet.

platelet f. 3 (PF-3**)** A lipoprotein of the platelet membrane that reacts with factors VIII and IX to activate factor X; it then participates with factor V and with activated factor X to convert prothrombin to thrombin.

platelet f. 4 (PFA) See antiheparin factor.

platelet-aggregating f., platelet-activating f. (PAF) Substance released from basophilic leukocytes that induces aggregation of platelets and is involved in immune responses.

platelet derived growth f. (PDGF) A heat-stable polypeptide within the alpha-granules of circulating blood platelets; stimulates fibroblast proliferation and thus helps repair injured cells; normally released only when blood clots; incriminated as a possible link to neoplasia if unregulated.

releasing f. (RF) A substance of hypothalamic origin capable of accelerating the rate of excretion of a given hormone by the anterior pituitary gland.

rheumatoid f. (RF) Antibody found in the serum of many individuals with rheumatoid arthritis (70%) and some other conditions; it produces agglutination when added to a suspension of particles coated with pooled human gamma globulin.

risk f. In epidemiology, an attribute or exposure that is associated with increased probability, but not necessarily the cause, of a specified outcome (e.g., developing a disease or dying from it).

secretor f. An inherited factor that permits the secretion of water-soluble forms of A- and B-group antigens into saliva and other body fluids.

spreading f. See hyaluronidase.

stable f. See factor VII.

sun-protection f. (SPF) The increased amount of ultraviolet radiation required to produce redness of the skin in the presence of a sunscreen.

testis-determining f. (TDF) A factor encoded by a gene on the Y chromosome that incites the undifferentiated gonad to develop as a testis.

thyrotropin-releasing f. (TRF) See thyrotropin-releasing hormone, under hormone.

transfer f. (TF) (a) A genetic particle in bacterial cells that is transferred from one bacterial cell to another. (b) A substance, free of nucleic acid and antibody, capable of transferring antigen specific cell-mediated immunity from donor to recipient.

transforming growth f. (TGF) One of two polypeptide growth factors that act to stimulate or inhibit growth of a variety of cells.

transforming growth f.-alpha (TGF-α) A polypeptide similar to epidermal growth factor that acts as an angiogenic factor *in vivo* and stimulates epidermal cell growth in culture.

transforming growth f.-beta (TGF-β) A polypeptide cytokine that stimulates fibroblasts in wound healing; also has antiproliferative activity, which inhibits some immune responses.

tumor-angiogenesis f. (TAF) A diffusible factor which is mitogenic to capillary endothelium and stimulates rapid formation of new vessels; secreted by malignant tumors and not found in normal tissue with the exception of the placenta; it has a molecular weight of approximately 100,000 and contains 25% ribonucleic acid.

tumor necrosis f. (NTF) See cachectin.

vascular endothelial growth f. (VEGF) An angiogenic protein that is thought to stimulate proliferation only of the endothelial cells of blood vessels; it is associated with tumor spread and with recurrence of the tumor after its removal.

vascular permeability f. (VPA) A protein that renders minute blood vessels hyperpermeable to plasma and plasma proteins. Thought to be an initial step in the growth of new blood vessels (angiogenesis) in tumors.

von Willebrand's f. (VWF) A large glycoprotein polymer that has binding sites for factor VIII.

facultative (fak´ŭl-ta-tiv) **1.** Relating to a mental faculty. **2.** Capable of adapting to varying environmental conditions; said of certain parasites. Opposite of obligate.

faculty (fak´ŭl-te) **1.** An inherent ability. **2.** Any of the powers of the human mind.

fagopyrism (făg-op´ĭ-riz-m) Skin irritation and edema caused by excessive ingestion of buckwheat (*Fagopyrum esculentum*).

Fahrenheit (far´ĕn-hīt) (F) Denoting a temperature scale that records the freezing point of water at 32° and the boiling point at 212° under normal atmospheric pressure.

failure (fāl´yer) **1.** The condition of being insufficient. **2.** A cessation of normal functioning.

backward heart f. The theory of backward heart failure maintains that congestive heart failure results in engorgement of the veins and raises pressure proximal to the failing heart chambers.

cardiac f. See heart failure.

congestive heart f. Abnormal circulatory congestion resulting from heart failure.

forward heart f. The theory of forward heart failure maintains that congestive heart failure results from inadequate cardiac output, resulting in inadequate kidney blood flow and retention of sodium and water.

heart f. Failure of the heart to function effectively as a pump so that it cannot deliver an adequate supply of oxygenated blood to the tissues. Also called myocardial failure; cardiac insufficiency.

high output f. Condition in which the cardiac output, although at normal levels or higher, is inadequate to meet the demands of the body; seen in states such as marked anemia, Paget's disease, and arteriovenous fistulas.

left ventricular f. Heart failure manifested by congestion of the lungs.

low output f. Subnormal cardiac output seen in heart failure, usually due to coronary, hypertensive, or valvular disease.

myocardial f. See heart failure.

pacemaker f. Failure of an artificial pacemaker to stimulate the heart muscle.

power f. See pump failure.

pump f. Failure of the heart as a mechanical pump rather than disturbance of the electrical impulse (arrhythmia). Also called power failure.

renal f. Loss or diminution of kidney function with consequent increase of urea and creatinine; may be acute (ARF) or chronic (CRF).

respiratory f. The failure of the pulmonary system to maintain normal gas tensions of oxygen, carbon dioxide, or both in the arterial circulation.

right ventricular f. Heart failure manifested by distention of the neck veins, edema, and enlargement of the liver.

faint (fānt) **1.** To lose consciousness. **2.** Syncope, generally due to abrupt, usually brief, failure of normal circulation of blood to the brain. **3.** Weak; feeble; lacking strength.

fainting (fān´ting) Temporary unconsciousness caused by diminished blood supply to the brain.

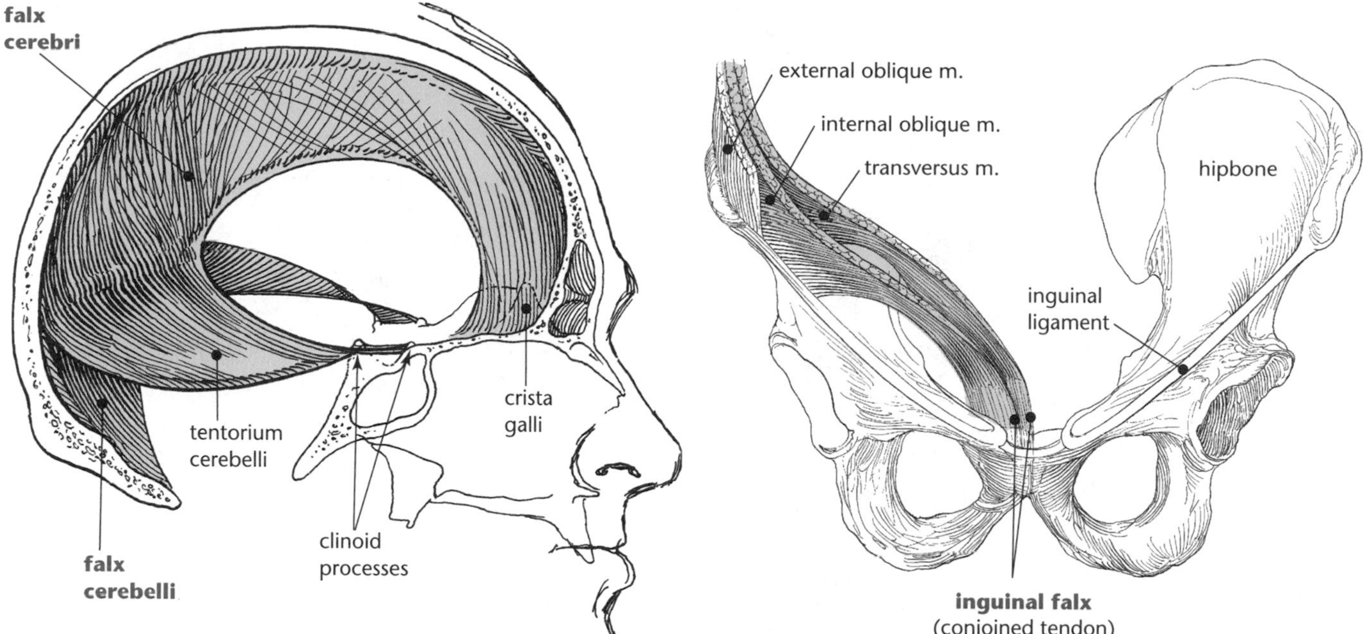

falces (fal´sez) Plural of falx.

falciform, falcate (fal´sĭ-form, fal´kāt) Sickle-shaped.

falling of the womb (fōl´ing ŭv thĕ wo͞om) See prolapse of uterus, under prolapse.

falloscopy (fal-os-ko´pe) Transvaginal inspection of the lumen of the entire length of a fallopian (uterine) tube with a fine fiberoptic endoscope.

Fallot's tetralogy (fă-lōz te-tral´ŏ-je) See tetralogy of Fallot, under tetralogy.

false-negative (fawls´ neg´ă-tiv) Denoting a test result that wrongly indicates that a person does not have the attribute or disease for which the test is conducted.

false-positive (fawls´ pos´ĭ-tiv) Denoting a test result that wrongly indicates that a person has the attribute or disease for which the test is conducted.

falx (falks) A sickle-shaped structure.

f. cerebelli The fold of cranial dura mater separating the lateral lobes of the cerebellum.

f. cerebri The fold of cranial dura mater between the cerebral hemispheres.

inguinal f. The united tendons of the abdominal transverse and the internal oblique muscles which insert into the crest of the pubic bone and the pectineal line. Also called conjoined tendon.

familial (fă-mil´e-ăl) Denoting any trait that is more common among relatives of an affected person than in the general population; could be due to genetic or environmental causes, or both.

family (fam´ĭ-le) **1.** A group of individuals composed of parents and their offspring. **2.** In biologic classification, a category ranking above a genus and below an order.

CEPH f.'s In genetics, a reference group of 40 Caucasian families from whom cell lines have been collected and distributed to researchers collaborating with the *Centre d'Etrude du Polymorphism Humain* for the mapping of the human genome.

Fanconi syndrome (fahn-ko´ne sin´drōm) A functional disturbance of the proximal kidney tubules resulting in generalized glucosuria, aminoaciduria, phosphaturia, and renal tubular acidosis; it may be inherited (e.g., in cystinosis), or acquired as a consequence of numerous causes including drugs, heavy metal poisoning, or disease (e.g., amyloidosis).

farad (far´ăd) (F) A unit of electrical capacity, equal to the capacity of a condenser having a charge of 1 coulomb under an electromotive force of 1 volt.

faraday (far´ă-da) The amount of electricity required to dissolve or deposit 1 gram equivalent weight of a substance in electrolysis, approximately 9.6494×10^4 coulombs.

faradic (fă-rad´ik) Relating to induced electricity.

farcy (far´se) The cutaneous form of glanders, characterized by ulceration of the skin at the site of inoculation of the bacillus followed by involvement of the lymphatic system.

farinaceous (far-i-nā´shus) Of the nature of or containing starch.

farsightedness (far-sīt´ed-nes) See hyperopia.

fascia (fash´e-ă), *pl.* **fas´ciae** A sheet of connective tissue that covers the body under the skin, and envelops the muscles and various organs.

f. of abdominal wall A thick subcutaneous fascia composed of a superficial fatty layer (Camper's fascia) and a deeper membranous layer (Scarpa's fascia); it is continuous with the superficial fascia of the perineum and the superficial fascia of the thigh; in the male, it is continuous with the fascia in the penis and scrotum; in the female, with the fascia in the labia majora.

Buck's f. See deep penile fascia.

bulbar f. Connective tissue sheath enveloping the eyeball with the exception of the cornea; attached to the sclera at the sclerocorneal junction. Also called Tenon's capsule.

Camper's f. Superficial fatty layer of the subcutaneous fascia of the lower part of the anterior abdominal wall.

f. of clitoris The dense fibrous tissue that encases the two corpora cavernosa of the clitoris.

Colles' f. See superficial fascia of perineum. See also Scarpa's fascia.

cremasteric f. The part of the fascia of the cremasteric muscle that invests the spermatic cord.

cribriform f. The part of the superficial fascia of the thigh that covers the sephanous opening.

deep f. The gray, dense, membranous sheet investing the trunk, neck, limbs, and part of the head; it also covers and holds the muscles and other structures in their proper positions, separating them or joining them for independent or integrated function, respectively.

deep penile f. A fascial sheath of the penis surrounds the corpora cavernosa and the corpus spongiosum. Also called Buck's fascia.

f. lata The broad fascia investing the muscles of the thigh.

nuchal f. Fascia of dorsal region of neck.

palmar f. See palmar aponeurosis, under aponeurosis.

plantar f. See plantar aponeurosis, under aponeurosis.

Scarpa's f. The deep membranous layer of the subcutaneous fascia of the abdomen; it is continuous with the deep layer of the superficial fascia of the perineum (Colles' fascia).

subcutaneous f. The connective tissue between the skin and the deep fascia, composed of an inner layer and an outer layer that normally contains an accumulation of fat. Also called superficial fascia.

subserous f. The layer of connective tissue beneath the lining of the body cavities and attaching it to the deep fascia; it also covers and supports the viscera. Also called tela subserosa.

superficial f. See subcutaneous fascia.

superficial f. of perineum The subcutaneous tissue of the urogenital region, composed of two layers: (a) A superficial fatty layer that is continuous superiorly with Camper's fascia (the superficial fatty layer of the lower abdomen). (b) A deep membranous layer continuous superiorly with Scarpa's fascia (the deep layer of the superficial abdominal fascia); also called Colles' fascia.

transversalis f. The fascial lining of the abdominal cavity between the deep or inner surface of the abdominal musculature and the peritoneum.

triangular f. See reflex inguinal ligament, under ligament.

fascial (fash´e-al) Relating to a fascia.

fascicle (fas´ĭ-kl) A small bundle of fibers, as of nerve or muscle fibers.

fascicular (fă-sik´u-lar) Pertaining to a fascicle or arranged in bundles.

fasciculation (fă-sik-u-la´shun) **1.** The formation of small bundles of fibers (fasciculi). **2.** Involuntary contraction or twitching of a group of muscle fibers; a coarser form of muscular contraction than fibrillation.

fasciculus (fă-sik´u-lus), *pl.* **fasciculi** A small bundle of muscle or nerve fibers.

inferior longitudinal f. A bundle of association fibers running through the occipital and temporal lobes of the cerebrum.

medial longitudinal f. A bundle of fibers running under the fourth ventricle from the midbrain to the spinal cord. Also called posterior longitudinal bundle.

proper fasciculi Ascending and descending association fibers surrounding the gray columns of the spinal cord.

fasciitis (fas-e-i´tis) Inflammation of fascia.

group A streptococcal necrotizing f. Destruction of muscle tissue by group A streptococcus (GAS); occurs as complication of a wound infection with GAS, usually after injury or surgery.

necrotizing f. A serious, rapidly spreading bacterial infection of superficial fascia with extensive necrosis; usually caused by group A streptococcus (GAS); may occur after trauma, surgery, or inadequate care of abscesses.

Fasciola (fă-si´o-lă) A genus of flukes; family Fasciolidae.

F. hepatica The liver fluke of sheep and cattle; a

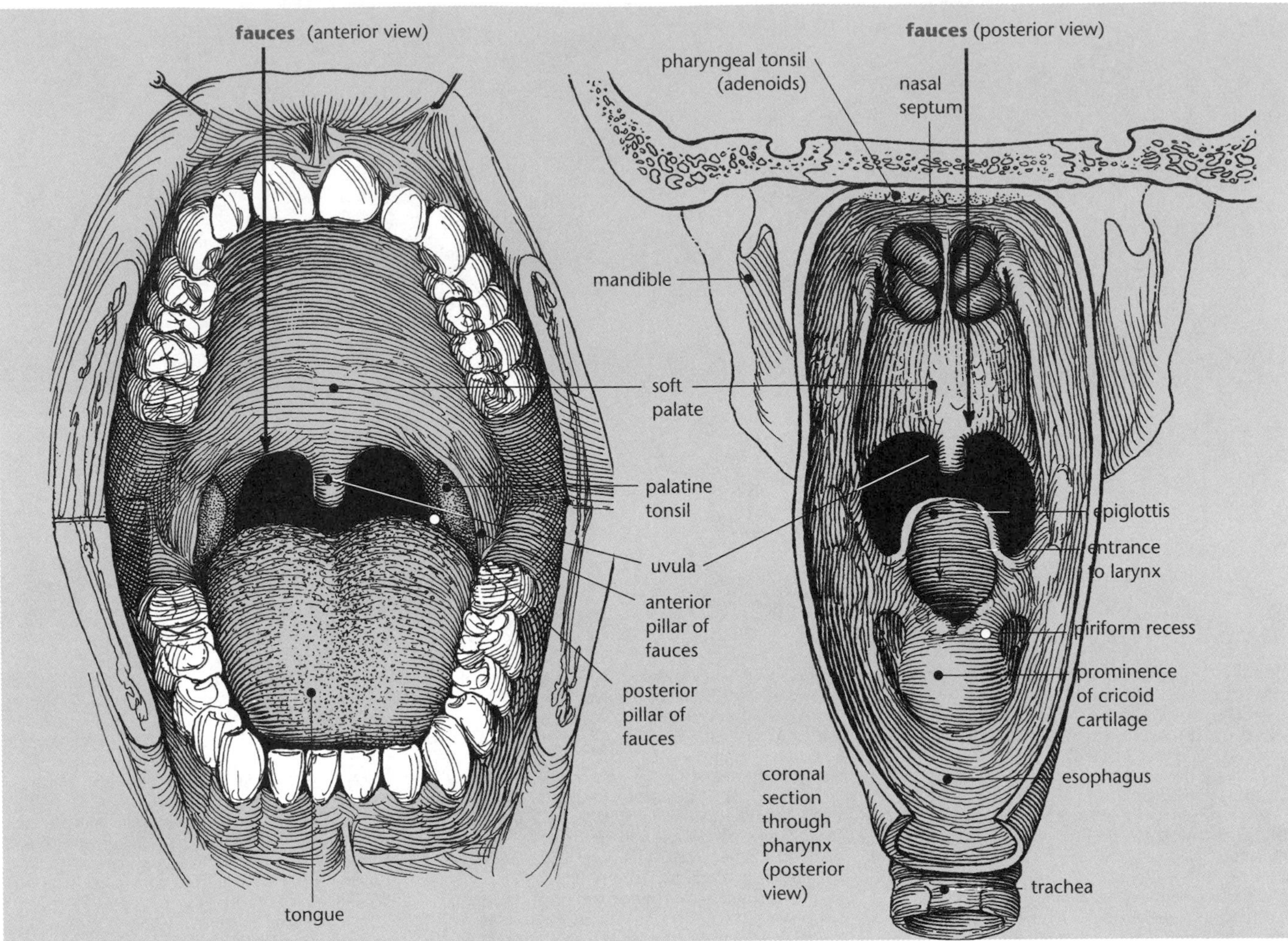

species occasionally transmitted to man through the ingestion of uncooked infected liver.

fascioliasis (fas-e-o-li´ă-sis) Infection with flukes of the genus *Fasciola.*

Fasciolopsis (fas-e-o-lop´sis) A genus of intestinal flukes; family Fasciolidae.

fascioplasty (fash´e-o-plas-te) Reparative surgery on a fascia.

fasciorrhaphy (fash-e-or´ă-fe) Suture of a fascia or an aponeurosis. Also called aponeurorrhaphy.

fasciotomy (fash-e-ot´ŏ-me) Surgical incision through a fascia.

fast (fast) Resistant to change.

fastigium (fas-tij´e-ŭm) **1.** The peak or highest point of the roof of the fourth ventricle of the brain. **2.** The height of a fever or any acute state.

fat (fat) **1.** Any of several organic compounds that yield fatty acids and glycerol upon saponification. **2.** A mixture of such compounds comprising most of the cell contents of adipose tissue; occurring also in lesser amounts in other animal cells and some plant cells.

brown f. A lobulated brown mass of tissue composed of cells containing numerous fat globules, found primarily in the interscapular region of the human newborn, hibernating animals, and other mammals. Also called interscapular gland.

saturated f. See saturated fatty acid, under acid.

unsaturated f. See unsaturated fatty acid, under acid.

fatal (fā´tal) Causing death.

fatality (fă-tăl´ĭ-tē) Anything resulting in death.

fatigability (fat-ĭ-gă-bil´ĭ-tē) Condition of becoming easily tired.

fatigue (fă-tēg´) A feeling of exhaustion with decreased efficiency resulting from physical or mental exertion.

battle f. A severe anxiety state seen in front-line soldiers, characterized by loss of effectiveness, poor judgment, physical complaints, and/or feeling of imminent death.

fat-pad (fat´pad) A circumscribed mass of adipose tissue.

fatty acid (fat´e as´id) See fatty acids, under acid.

fauces (faw´sēz) The passage from the oral cavity to the oral pharynx, including the lumen and its boundaries; the aperture by which the mouth communicates with the pharynx.

anterior pillar of the f. Palatoglossal fold that rises archlike on each side of the posterior limit of the oral cavity.

posterior pillar of the f. Palatopharyngeal fold just posterior to the palatine tonsil.

faveolus (fa-ve´o-lus) A small depression.

favism (fa´vis-m) Acute hemolytic anemia caused by ingestion of the fava bean (*Vicia faba*) or inhalation of the pollen of its flower; occurs in people with inherited deficiency of the enzyme glucose-6-phosphate dehydrogenase (G6PD); the defect renders red blood cells susceptible to destruction by chemicals in the bean.

favus (fa´vus) A chronic fungus infection, usually of the scalp, caused by *Trichophyton schoenleini.* Also called tinea capitis.

fear (fēr) A feeling of apprehension or alarm in response to an external source of danger.

morbid f. See phobia.

features (fe´churz) The outward appearance of the face or any of its parts.

febrifacient (fĕb-rĭ-fa´shent) **1.** Any substance that produces a fever. **2.** Causing fever.

febrile (fĕb´ril) Having fever.

fecal (fe´kal) Relating to feces.

fecalith (fe´kă-lith) An intestinal fecal concretion. Also called coprolith; stercolith.

fecaluria (fe-kăl-u´re-ă) The passage of fecal matter with the urine in persons with a connecting channel (fistula) between the rectum and the bladder.

feces (fe´sēz) The waste matter discharged from the bowel.

feculent (fek´u-lent) Fecal; foul.

fecundability (fe-kun-dă-bil´ĭ-te) The probability of achieving pregnancy within one menstrual cycle.

fecundate (fe´kun-dāt) To fertilize; to impregnate.

fecundation (fe-kun-da´shun) Fertilization; impreg-nation.

fecundity (fĕ-kun´dĭ-te) The probability of producing a live birth within a single menstrual cycle.

feeble (fē´bl) Infirm; weak; lacking vitality.

feedback (fēd´bak) **1.** The process whereby a portion of a system's output, as of an amplifier, is returned to the input; return of information from the output to the control system so as to modify the nature of the control. **2.** The portion of the output so returned. **3.** The feeling created by another person's reactions to oneself.

negative f. A signal or information returning from the output to the control system which results in reduced output.

positive f. A signal or information returning to the control system from the output which results in increased output.

feeding (fēd´ing) The giving or taking of nourishment.

bolus f. Tube feeding in which a set amount of nutrients is administered at intermittent periods throughout the day.

intravenous f. Introduction of liquid nutrient preparations directly into the blood circulation through a vein.

nasogastric f. Administration of liquid food through a lubricated tube passed (nasally or orally) into the stomach. Also called enteral tube alimentation.

feeling (fēl´ing) **1.** A sensation perceived by the sense of touch. **2.** Emotional or affective state or process. **3.** A vague belief.

fellatio (fĕ-la´she-o) Oral penile stimulation.

felon (fel´on) Acute staphylococcal infection of the distal fat pad at the tip of a finger or toe, causing localized swelling and intense throbbing pain. Also called whitlow.

fertilization

The penetration of sperm through the corona radiata and the zona pellucida is accomplished by the release of acrosomal enzymes (acid phosphatase and acrosomase) by many sperms.

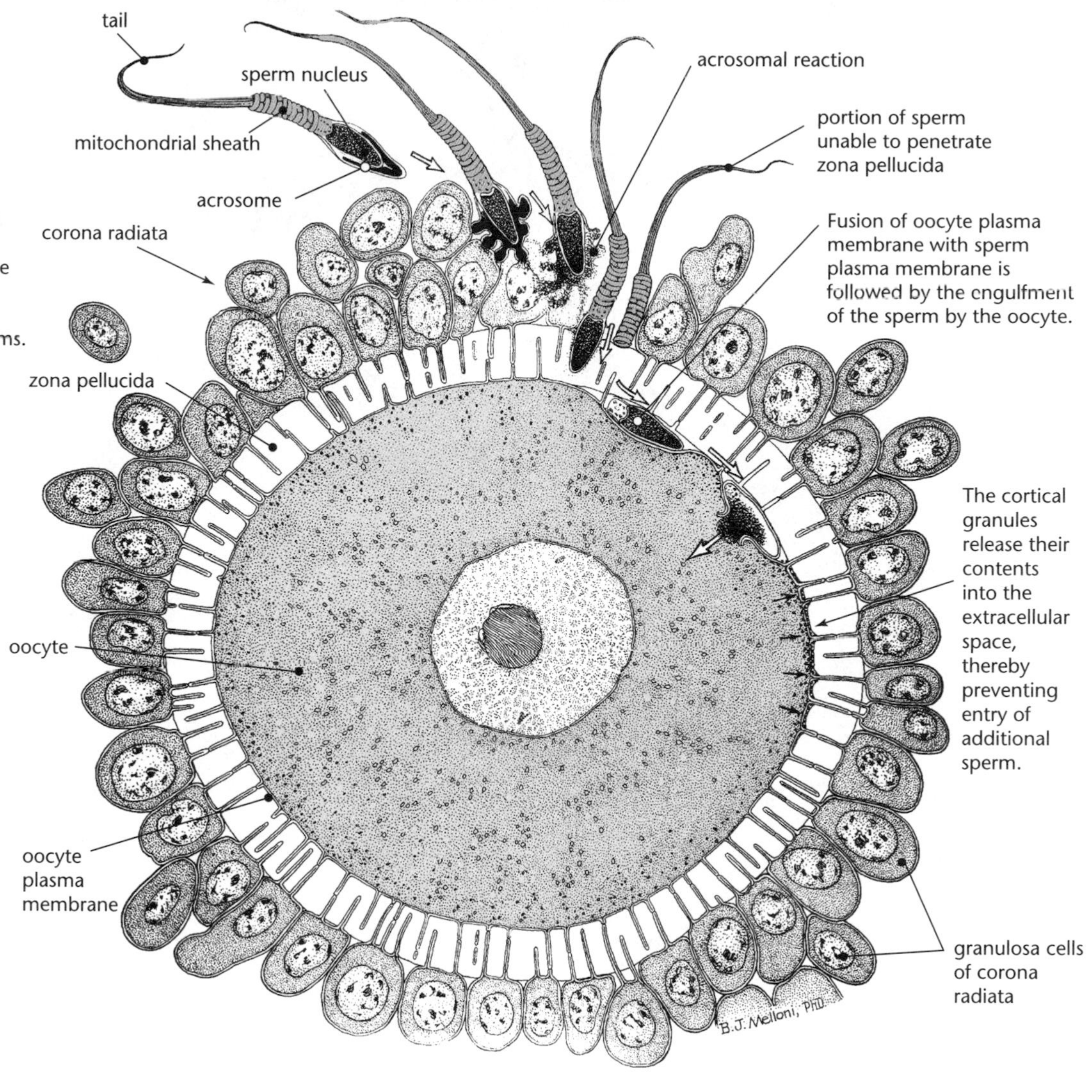

tail
sperm nucleus
mitochondrial sheath
acrosome
corona radiata
zona pellucida
oocyte
oocyte plasma membrane
acrosomal reaction
portion of sperm unable to penetrate zona pellucida
Fusion of oocyte plasma membrane with sperm plasma membrane is followed by the engulfment of the sperm by the oocyte.
The cortical granules release their contents into the extracellular space, thereby preventing entry of additional sperm.
granulosa cells of corona radiata
B.J. Melloni, PhD

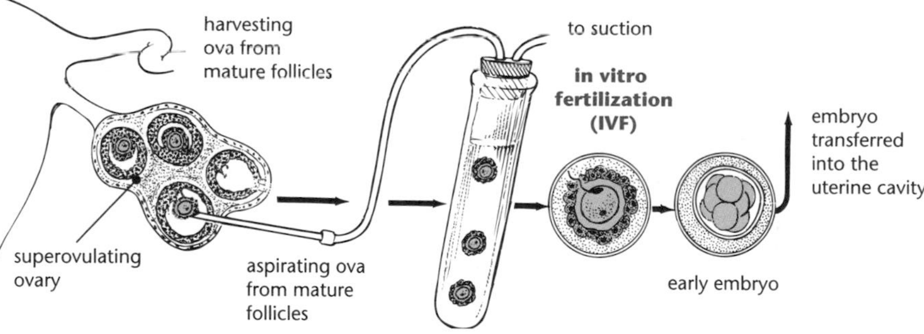

Felty's syndrome (fel´tēz sin´drōm) Rheumatoid arthritis, leukopenia, and enlargement of the spleen.

female (fe´māl) Relating to the sex that bears young or produces ova or eggs.

feminism (fem´ĭ-niz-m) The possession of female characteristics by the male.

feminization (fem-ĭ-nĭ-za´shun) The development of female characteristics by the male.

femoral (fem´or-ăl) Relating to the femur or to the thigh.

femur (fe´mur) The thighbone; the longest and largest bone in the body; see table of bones.

fenestra (fĕ-nes´tră), *pl.* **fenes´trae** A window-like opening.

f. cochleae See round window, under window.

f. vestibuli See oval window, under window.

fenestrated (fen´ĕs-trāt-ed) Pierced with one or more small window-like openings.

fenestration (fen-ĕs-tra´shun) **1.** The act of perforating. **2.** See fenestration operation, under operation.

ferment (fĕr-ment´) To undergo or to cause fermentation.

fermentable (fĕr-ment´ă-bl) Capable of undergoing fermentation.

fermentation (fĕr-mĕn-ta´shun) A chemical decomposition induced in a carbohydrate by an enzyme.

fermentative (fĕr-ment-ă-tiv) Having the ability to cause fermentation.

fermium (fĕr´me-ŭm) Radioactive element; symbol Fm, atomic number 100, atomic weight 253.

ferning (fern´ing) The typical palm-leaf or "arborization" pattern observed in a dry specimen of endocervical mucus or amniotic fluid; used as an adjunctive test to confirm amniochorion rupture during pregnancy. Ferning is a normal physiologic phenomenon in a specimen obtained at midmenstrual cycle (i.e., from days 7 to 18, peaking on day 14). Also called cervical mucus arborization.

ferric (fer´ik) Relating to or containing iron; especially a salt containing iron in its highest valence (3).

ferritin (fer´ĭ-tin) A protein rich in iron (up to 23%) formed by the union of ferric iron with apoferritin; occurs mainly in the liver, spleen, and intestinal mucosa.

ferroporphyrin (fer-o-pōr´fĭ-rin) A derivative of ferrous porphyrin in which a central iron atom is linked to the nitrogen atoms of the porphyrin.

ferroprotein (fer-o-pro´tēn) A protein containing iron in a prosthetic group.

ferroprotoporphyrin (fer-o-pro-to-por´fĭ-rin) See heme.

ferrous (fer´ŭs) Relating to or containing iron; especially a salt containing iron in its lowest valence (2).

f. fumarate A reddish orange compound used to treat iron deficiency.

f. sulfate Compound used in treating uncomplicated iron deficiency anemia. Also called green vitriol.

ferruginous (fĕ-roo´jĭ-nus) Containing iron. Also called chalybeate.

ferrum (fer´ŭm) Latin for iron.

fertile (fer´til) Capable of reproducing.

fertility (fer-til´ĭ-te) The capacity to conceive and bear offspring.

fertilization (fer-tĭ-lĭ-za´shun) The union of a spermatozoon with an ovum.

direct ovum f. See subzonal insemination, under insemination.

***in vitro* f.** (IVF) Fertilization that occurs outside the body, in a glass Petri dish.

fervescence (fĕr-ves´ĕns) An increase of fever.

fester (fes´tĕr) To form pus.

festinant (fes´tĭ-nant) Accelerating; rapid.

festination (fes-tĭ-na´shŭn) The involuntary acceleration of walking that occurs when the center of

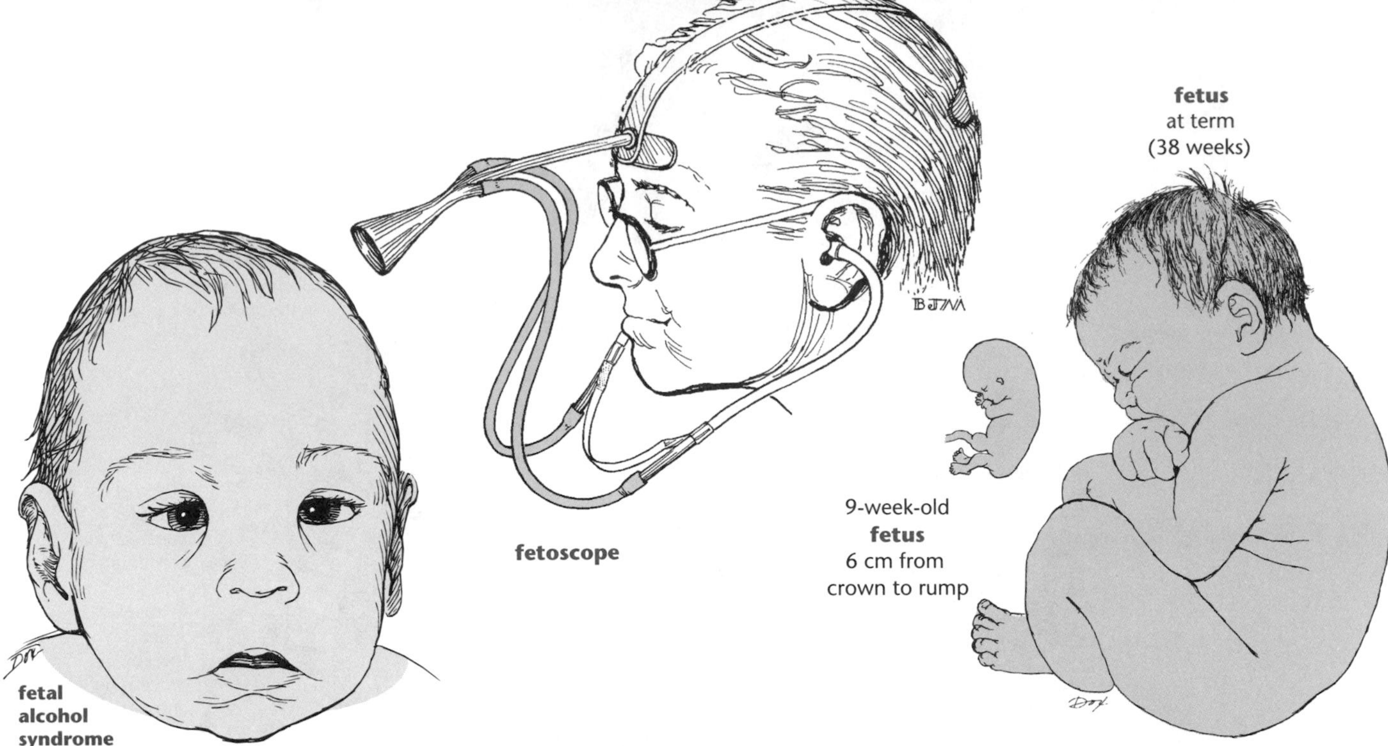

F

gravity is displaced, as seen in Parkinson's disease and some other nervous diseases. Also called festinating gait.

festooning (fes-tōōn´ing) The process of cutting, carving, or grinding material to accommodate the contours of natural tissue, as in the cutting of a round copper band to fit around a prepared tooth and rest snugly on the gingiva prior to taking an impression.

fetal (fe´tal) Relating to a fetus.

fetal alcohol syndrome (fe´tal al´kŏ-hol sin´drōm) Congenital mental and growth retardation, heart defects, and defective facial features caused by alcohol consumption by the child's mother during early pregnancy.

fetal loss (fe´tal los) See spontaneous abortion, under abortion.

feticide (fe´tĭ-sīd) Intentional destruction of the fetus in the uterus.

fetid (fe´tid) Having a disagreeable odor.

fetish (fĕt´ish) An object to which excessive attention or reverence is attached; often a source of sexual stimulation or gratification.

fetishism (fĕt´ish-iz-m) Excessive emotional attachment to an inanimate object or body part that serves as a substitute for a human sexual object.

fetography (fe-tog´ră-fe) Roentgenography of the fetus *in utero*.

fetology (fe-tol´ŏ-je) The study of the fetus and its diseases.

fetometry (fe-tom´ĕ-tre) Estimation of the size of the fetal head prior to delivery.

fetoplacental (fe-to-plă-sen´tal) Relating to the fetus and placenta.

α-fetoprotein (al´fă fe-to-pro´tēn) (AFP) See alpha-fetoprotein.

fetor (fe´tor) An offensive odor.

f. hepaticus An unpleasant odor of the breath of individuals with severe liver disorders.

f. oris Halitosis.

fetoscope (fe´to-skōp) **1.** Instrument for listening to the fetal heart sounds through the maternal abdomen. **2.** A fiberoptic endoscope for direct viewing of the fetus in the uterus.

fetus (fe´tus) The developing offspring in the uterus, from the end of the seventh week of gestation to birth; during the first eight weeks of development, it is called embryo.

fever (fe´ver) **1.** A rise in body temperature above the normal range (an early morning temperature of 99.0°F (32.2°C) or greater, or an evening temperature of 100°F (37.8°C) or greater. **2.** Condition in which the body temperature is above the normal. Also called pyrexia.

blackwater f. See malarial hemoglobinuria, under hemoglobinuria.

breakbone f. See dengue.

canicola f. Disease caused by the bacterium *Leptospira canicola*; transmitted to man by contact with infected dog urine.

carbuncular f. See anthrax.

cat-scratch f. See cat-scratch disease.

childbed f. See puerperal fever.

Colorado tick f. Viral disease similar to Rocky Mountain spotted fever but without the rash; marked chiefly by fever and low levels of white blood cells (leukopenia); transmitted to humans by the tick *Dermacentor andersoni*.

cotton-mill f. See byssinosis.

dandy f. See dengue.

deer-fly f. See tularemia.

desert f. See coccidioidomycosis.

drug f. Fever occurring as an adverse reaction to a drug; usually disappears when the drug intake is discontinued.

familial Mediterranean f. (FMF) Recurrent attacks of abdominal pain, inflamed peritoneum, fever, and sometimes a rash; the condition is asymptomatic between attacks.

Fort Bragg f. See pretibial fever.

glandular f. See infectious mononucleosis, under mononucleosis.

Haverhill f. Disorder caused by infection with *Streptobacillus moniliformis*; marked by fever, rash, and arthritis (usually of the large joints and spine), lasting two to three weeks. Although the same organism causes rat-bite fever, Haverhill fever is not transmitted by the bite of an infected rat.

hay f. Seasonal inflammation of the mucous membranes of the nose characterized by watery nasal discharge, and itching of the eyes and nose; caused by an allergic reaction to pollens; not actually associated with a rise in body temperature. Also called seasonal allergic rhinitis.

hemorrhagic f. Disease of viral origin marked primarily by fever, capillary hemorrhages, and shock.

icterohemorrhagic f. See Weil's disease.

island f. See tsutsugamushi disease.

Japanese river f. See tsutsugamushi disease.

jungle yellow f. A form of yellow fever transmitted by forest mosquitoes rather than by *Aedes aegypti* (the domestic mosquito).

Lassa f. A highly contagious, often fatal, disease marked by fever, chills, muscle aches, rashes, nausea, severe sore throat, bleeding gums, and oral ulcerations; caused by the Lassa virus (genus *Arenavirus*, family Arenaviridae); transmitted by a rat (*Mastomys natalensis*).

malignant tertian f. See falciparum malaria, under malaria.

Malta f. See brucellosis.

Mediterranean f. **1.** Old term for brucellosis. **2.** See familial Mediterranean fever.

mill f. See byssinosis.

mountain f. Altitude sickness; see under sickness.

nodal f. See erythema nodosum.

Oroya f. See bartonellosis.

paratyphoid f. An infectious disease with symptoms resembling those of typhoid fever, but milder; caused by strains of *Salmonella*.

pharyngoconjunctival f. Fever, pharyngitis, and acute follicular conjunctivitis caused by a virus, usually type 3 adenovirus; conjunctivitis is the chief complaint; it primarily affects children, who acquire it from swimming pools.

phlebotomus f. An influenza-like febrile disease of short duration caused by a virus of the Bunyaviridae family; transmitted mostly by the bloodsucking sandfly *Phlebotomus papatasii*. Also called sandfly fever.

pretibial f. A mild condition first seen among military personnel at Fort Bragg, North Carolina; marked by mild fever, enlargement of the spleen, and a rash on the anterior surface of the legs; caused by a strain of the bacterium *Leptospira interrogans*. Also called Fort Bragg fever.

puerperal f. Fever occurring after childbirth; may be due to infection. Popularly called childbed fever.

Q f. A bacterial disease resembling influenza, caused by *Coxiella burnetii*; marked by headache, fever, and constitutional symptoms; sometimes associated with inflammation of the lungs; usually acquired by inhalation of the agent.

quartan f. See malariae malaria, under malaria.

quotidian f. See quotidian malaria, under malaria.

rabbit f. See tularemia.

rat-bite f. Disease marked by inflammation of the lymph nodes and lymph vessels, joint pains, and a rash on the legs due to infection with *Spirillion minor* or *Streptobacillus moniliformis*; transmitted by the bite of an infected rat or any rodent. Also called rat-bite disease; sodoku.

recurrent f. See relapsing fever.

relapsing f. Acute infectious bacterial disease marked by recurrent periods of fever, each lasting about six days; caused by species of the genus *Borrelia*; transmitted by the bite of a louse or a soft tick. Also called recurrent fever.

rheumatic f. (RF) Acute, recurrent inflammatory disease occurring one to five weeks after a throat infection with a group A streptococcus; diagnosis depends on the presence of two of the following five major criteria (Jones criteria): skin rash, typically in a bathing suit distribution (erythema marginatum); inflammation of large joints; abnormal involuntary movements (Sydenham's chorea); subcutaneous

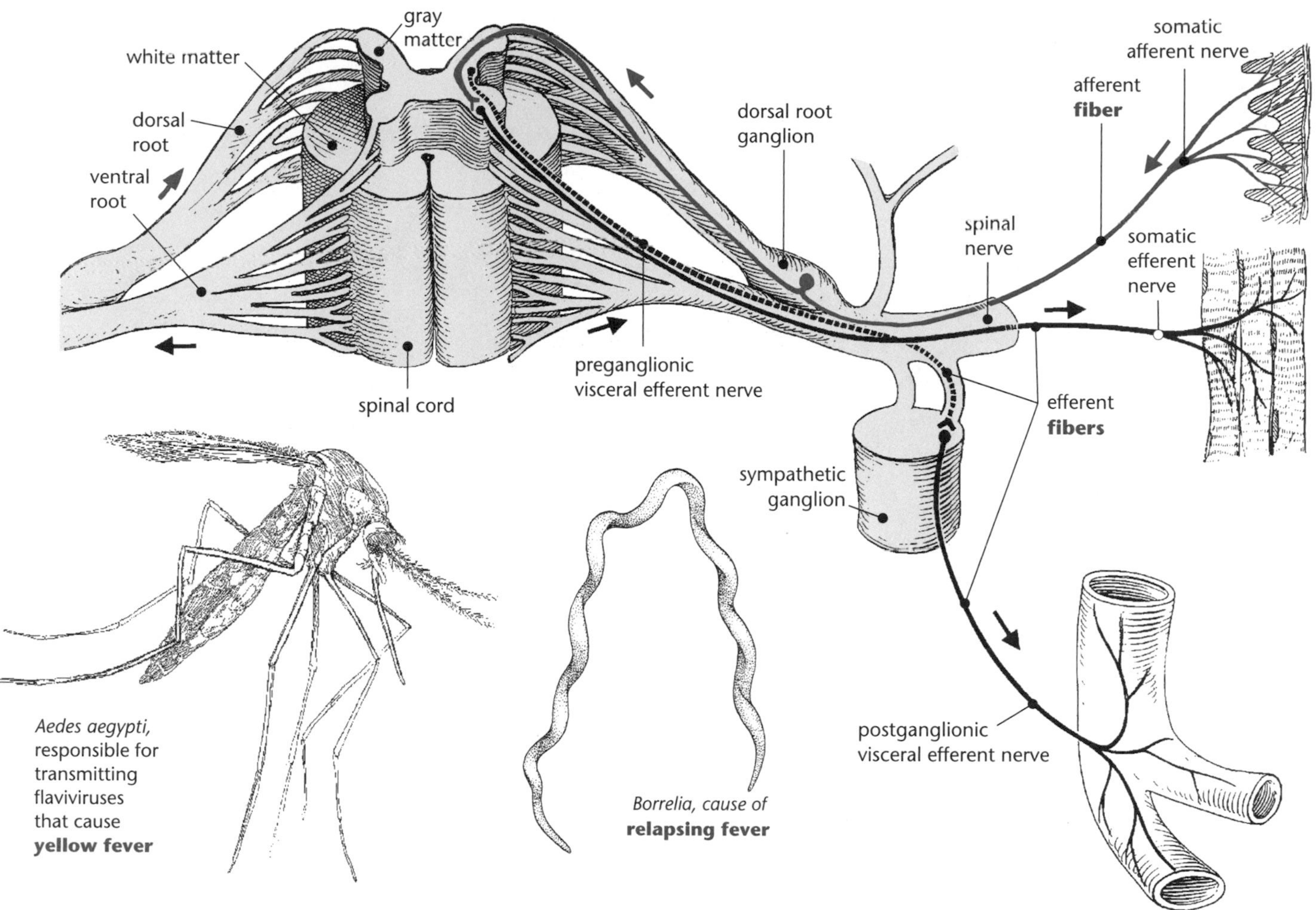

Aedes aegypti, responsible for transmitting flaviviruses that cause **yellow fever**

Borrelia, cause of **relapsing fever**

nodules; and inflammation of the heart wall (carditis) with involvement of the heart valves.

Rocky Mountain spotted f. (RMSF) Acute infectious bacterial disease marked by fever, bone and muscle pain, headache, prostration, and a generalized rash; caused by *Rickettsia rickettsii*, transmitted by several varieties of hard ticks.

sandfly f. See phlebotomus fever.

San Joaquin Valley f. See coccidioidomycosis.

scarlet f. Streptococcal infection, usually of the throat, marked by sore throat, fever, a characteristic "sandpaper" rash over the trunk and extremities (which erupts one to three days after onset of throat symptoms), and a red "strawberry" tongue. Also called scarlatina.

tertian f. See vivax malaria, under malaria.

tick f. 1. Any infectious disease transmitted by infected ticks.

trench f. A relapsing type of fever caused by *Rochalimaea quintana*; transmitted by deposits of body lice feces into broken skin.

tsutsugamushi f. See tsutsugamushi disease.

typhoid f. Acute infectious disease caused by *Salmonella typhi*, characterized mainly by fever, skin rash on the abdomen and chest, intestinal distention with gas, and enlargement of the liver and spleen; infection is acquired by eating or drinking contaminated food or water; may be transmitted by a person who is a symptomless carrier of the organism.

undulant f. See brucellosis.

uveoparotid f. See uveoparotitis.

West Nile f. Acute illness marked by fever, headache, a papular rash, inflammation of lymph nodes, and reduced number of white blood cells; caused by the mosquito-borne West Nile virus (family Flaviviridae).

yellow f. Acute infectious disease caused by a virus of the family Flaviviridae, transmitted by a mosquito (*Aedes aegipti*); characterized by fever, degeneration of the liver (producing jaundice), and intestinal disturbances.

fiber (fi´ber) Any slender, threadlike structure.

A f.'s Myelinated fibers of somatic nerves having a conduction rate of up to 120 m/sec.

accelerator f.'s Nerve fibers of the sympathetic nervous system that, when stimulated, increase the force and rapidity of the heartbeat. Also called augmentor fibers.

adrenergic f.'s Nerve fibers that release norepinephrine or epinephrine at their synapse (e.g., postganglionic sympathetic nerve fibers).

afferent f.'s Nerve fibers conveying impulses to a nerve center in the brain or spinal cord.

alpha f.'s Large-caliber myelinated motor or proprioceptive nerve fibers conducting impulses at rates near 100 m/sec.

association f.'s Nerve fibers that connect different areas of the cerebral cortex in the same hemisphere or different segments of the spinal cord in the same side.

augmentor f.'s See accelerator fibers.

B f.'s Small fibers of the autonomic nervous system having a conduction rate of 3 to 15 m/sec.

beta f.'s Motor nerve fibers having a conduction speed rate of about 40 m/sec.

C f.'s Unmyelinated nerve fibers of the autonomic nervous system having a conduction rate below 4 m/sec.

cholinergic f.'s Nerve fibers that release acetylcholine at the synapse.

collagen f.'s, collagenous f.'s The flexible fibers making up the principal constituent of connective tissue. Also called white fibers.

depressor f.'s Sensory (afferent) nerve fibers that, when stimulated, diminish vascular tone and lower blood pressure.

dietary f. The fiber of plant tissue that is resistant to hydrolysis by digestive enzymes.

efferent f.'s Nerve fibers that convey impulses from a nerve center in the brain or spinal cord outward to organs and tissues.

elastic f.'s Fibers of elastic properties forming a network in the substance of some connective tissue. Also called yellow fibers.

extrafusal f., EF f. Any skeletal muscle fiber excluding the intrafusal fibers in muscle (neuromuscular) spindles.

gamma f.'s Myelinated nerve fibers having a conduction rate of less than 20 m/sec.

gray f.'s See unmyelinated fibers.

inhibitory f.'s Nerve fibers that slow down the action of an organ.

intrafusal f., IF f. One of 6 to 14 fine, small, specialized muscle fibers composing a muscle (neuromuscular) spindle; innervated by both motor and sensory nerve endings.

myelinated f.'s Nerve fibers possessing a myelin sheath.

nerve f. One of the slender units of a nerve trunk; the axon of a nerve cell.

nonmyelinated f.'s Unmyelinated fibers.

pressor f.'s Sensory nerve fibers which, upon stimulation, cause narrowing of blood vessels and rise of blood pressure.

projection f.'s Nerve fibers that connect the cerebral cortex with other areas of the brain.

Purkinje's f.'s Specialized fibers formed of modified heart muscle cells located beneath the endocardium; concerned with the conduction of stimuli from the atria to the ventricles.

Sharpey's f.'s Thick perforating collagenous or fibroelastic bundles that attach periosteum to bone; they are continuations of the periosteal fibers and pierce the bone obliquely or at right angles to its long axis.

skeletal muscle f.'s Long, parallel muscle fibers with cross-sectional dimensions of about 10 to 100 mm; marked by transverse striations and nuclei located just under the cell membrane (sarcolemma).

smooth muscle f.'s Narrow and tapering muscle fibers without transverse striations.

spindle f. See mitotic spindle, under spindle.

unmyelinated f.'s A group of small axons lacking a myelin sheath but associated with a longitudinal chain of Schwann cells that extend cytoplasm between the individual axons. Also called gray fibers; nonmyelinated fibers.

white f.'s See collagen fibers.

yellow f.'s See elastic fibers.

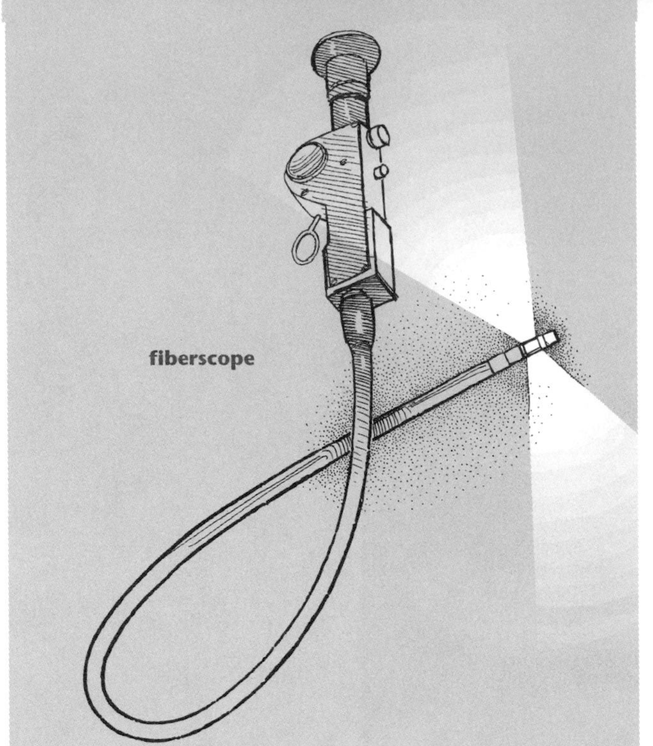

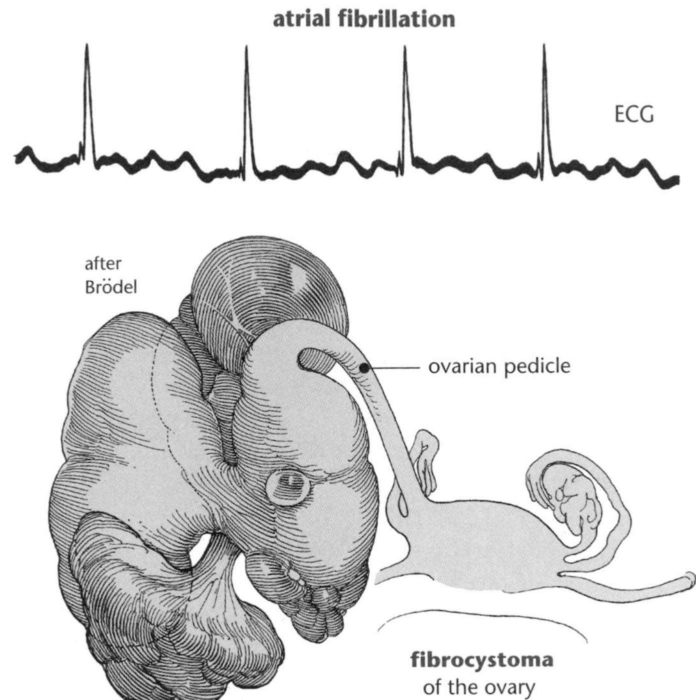

fibrocystoma of the ovary

F

fiberoptics (fi-ber-op´tiks) The transmission of images along a bundle of fine, parallel, flexible rods of plastic or glass.
fiberscope (fī´ber-skōp) A viewing instrument with very fine, flexible glass rods for light transmission (fiberoptics).
fibril (fi´bril) A minute, slender fiber or filament.
Ebner's f.'s Slender collagen fibers in the cementum and dentin of a tooth.
fibrillar, fibrillary (fī´brĭ-lar, fī´bri-lar-ē) **1.** Relating to a fibril. **2.** Relating to twitching of small skeletal or smooth muscles.
fibrillate (fī´brĭ-lāt) **1.** To be in a state of fibrillation. **2.** To become fibrillar. **3.** Composed of fibrils.
fibrillation (fi-brĭ-la´shun) **1.** The rapid contractions or quivering of muscular fibrils. **2.** The formation of fibrils.
atrial f. The replacement of the normal rhythmic contractions of the cardiac atria by rapid irregular quivers.
ventricular f. Rapid, irregular twitchings that replace the normal contractions of the muscular walls of the ventricles.
fibrilliform (fi´bril-ĭ-form) Having the general configuration of a fibril.
fibrillin (fi´bril-in) One of the protein components of connective tissue; it is markedly reduced in certain disorders (e.g., Marfan's syndrome).
fibrillogenesis (fi-bril-o-jen´ĕ-sis) The normal development of minute fibrils in collagenous fibers of connective tissue.
fibrin (fi´brin) A fibrous, insoluble protein derived from fibrinogen through the action of thrombin; the basic component of a blood clot.
fibrination (fi´brin-a-shun) **1.** The formation of a fibrin. **2.** The formation of an abnormally large amount of fibrin; denoting the condition of the blood in certain inflammatory diseases. Also called fibrinosis.
fibrinogen (fi-brin´o-jen) A protein, present in dissolved form in blood plasma, that is converted into a network of delicate filaments (fibrin) by the action of the enzyme thrombin; the blood cells become entangled in the fibrin network, thus producing coagulation. Also called factor I.
fibrinogenopenia (fi-brin-o-jen-o-pe´ne-ă) Deficiency in the concentration of fibrinogen in the blood.
fibrinoid (fi´brin-oid) **1.** Resembling fibrin. **2.** An acidophilic, homogeneous, refractile material.
fibrinolysin (fi-brĭ-nol´ĭ-sin) An enzyme that dissolves fibrin in clotted blood.
fibrinolysis (fi-brĭ-nol´ĭ-sis) The destruction of fibrin in clotted blood by enzyme action, resulting in the dissolution of a clot.
fibrinopeptide A (fi-brĭ-no-pep´tīd a) A peptide thought to be the product of fibrinolysis. Elevated levels are found in the blood after a stroke.
fibrinopurulent (fi-brĭ-no-pu´roo-lent) Relating to a discharge that contains pus and a large amount of fibrin.
fibrinosis (fi-brĭ-no´sis) See fibrination (2).
fibrinous (fi´brin-ŭs) Relating to or composed of fibrin.
fibroadenoma (fi-bro-ad-ĕ-no´mă) A benign tumor derived from glandular epithelium.
fibroadipose (fi-bro-ad-ĕ-no´mă) Containing both fibrous and fatty elements. Also called fibrofatty.
fibroblast (fi´bro-blast) An elongated, flattened, spindle-shaped cell with cytoplasmic processes at each end, having a flat, oval nucleus showing a finely granular chromatin with one or two nucleoli; one of the most common cell types found in growing connective tissue.
fibrocarcinoma (fi-bro-kar-sĭ-no´mă) See scirrhous carcinoma, under carcinoma.
fibrocartilage (fi-bro-kăr´tĭ-laj) A type of cartilage containing collagenic fibers.
fibrochondritis (fi-bro-kon-dri´tis) Inflammation of fibrocartilage.
fibrochondroma (fi-bro-kon-dro´mă) A benign tumor composed primarily of cartilage and an abundant amount of fibrous tissue.
fibrocyst (fi´bro-sist) A lesion consisting of a cyst within a fibrous network.
fibrocystic (fi-bro-sis´tik) Marked by the presence of fibrocysts.
fibrocystic disease of breast (fi-bro-sis´tik dĭ´zēz´ ŭv brest) See fibrocystic change of breast, under change.
fibrocystic disease of pancreas (fi-bro-sis´tik dĭ- zēz´ ŭv pan´kre-ăs) See cystic fibrosis of pancreas.
fibrocystoma (fi-bro-sis-to´mă) A benign tumor characterized by cysts within a conspicuous fibrous stroma.
fibrocyte (fi´bro-sīt) A resting or quiescent fibroblast.
fibroelastic (fi-bro-e-las´tik) Made up of collagen and elastic fibers.
fibroelastosis (fi-bro-e-las-to´sis) Overgrowth of fibroelastic tissue.
endocardial f. See endomyocardial fibroelastosis.
endomyocardial f. Congenital heart disease characterized by fibroelastic thickening of the mural endocardium, especially of the left ventricle; the rest of the chambers and the valves may also be involved. Also called endocardial sclerosis.
fibroenchondroma (fi-bro-en-kon-dro´mă) A benign tumor located within a bone and composed of mature cartilage and abundant fibrous tissue.
fibroepithelioma (fi-bro-ep-ĭ-the-le-o´mă) A skin tumor composed of fibrous tissue and basal cells of the epidermis; it may be transformed into a basal cell carcinoma. Also called premalignant fibroepitheli-oma.
fibrofatty (fi-bro-fat´e) See fibroadipose.
fibroid (fī´broid) **1.** Resembling or containing fibers. **2.** Colloquial clinical term for certain types of leiomyoma (a benign tumor), especially those occurring in the uterus.
fibrolipoma (fi-bro-lĭ-po´mă) A tumor composed predominantly of fat cells but containing abundant fibrous tissue. Also called lipoma fibrosum.
fibroma (fi-bro´ma) A benign tumor derived from fibrous connective tissue.
ameloblastic f. A benign tumor composed of ameloblasts (epithelial cells of a developing tooth) and dense connective tissue; occurs in the lower jaw (mandible) during childhood.
concentric f. A benign growth that occupies the entire inner wall of the uterus.
f. molluscum gravidarum The occurrence of numerous, small fibrous tumors of the skin, colorless or pigmented, appearing during pregnancy and disappearing at its termination.
fibromatosis (fi-bro-mă-to´sis) **1.** Condition marked by the development of multiple fibromas. **2.** Abnormal overdevelopment of fibrous tissue.
retroperitoneal f. See sclerosing retroperitonitis, under retroperitonitis.
fibromuscular (fi-bro-mus´ku-lar) Denoting tissues that are both fibrous and muscular.
fibromyoma (fi-bro-mi-o´mă) See leiomyoma.
fibromyositis (fi-bro-mi-o-si´tis) Chronic inflammation of a muscle with overgrowth of its connective tissue.
fibronectin (fi-bro-nek´tin) An adhesive glycoprotein present in plasma, where it participates in the phagocytosis of bacteria and other cells, or on the cell surface, where it mediates cellular adhesive interactions.
fibroplasia (fi-bro-pla´shă) Abnormal production of fibrous tissue.
retrolental f. See retinopathy of prematurity, under retinopathy.
fibroplastic (fi-bro-plas´tik) Producing fibrous tissue.
fibrosarcoma (fi-bro-sar-ko´mă) A malignant tumor composed of fibrous connective tissue.
ameloblastic f. Fibrosarcoma derived from tooth-forming tissues and containing a large number of epithelial cells of developing teeth (ameloblasts).
fibrosis (fi-bro´sis) The formation of fibrous tissue, denoting especially an abnormal degenerative

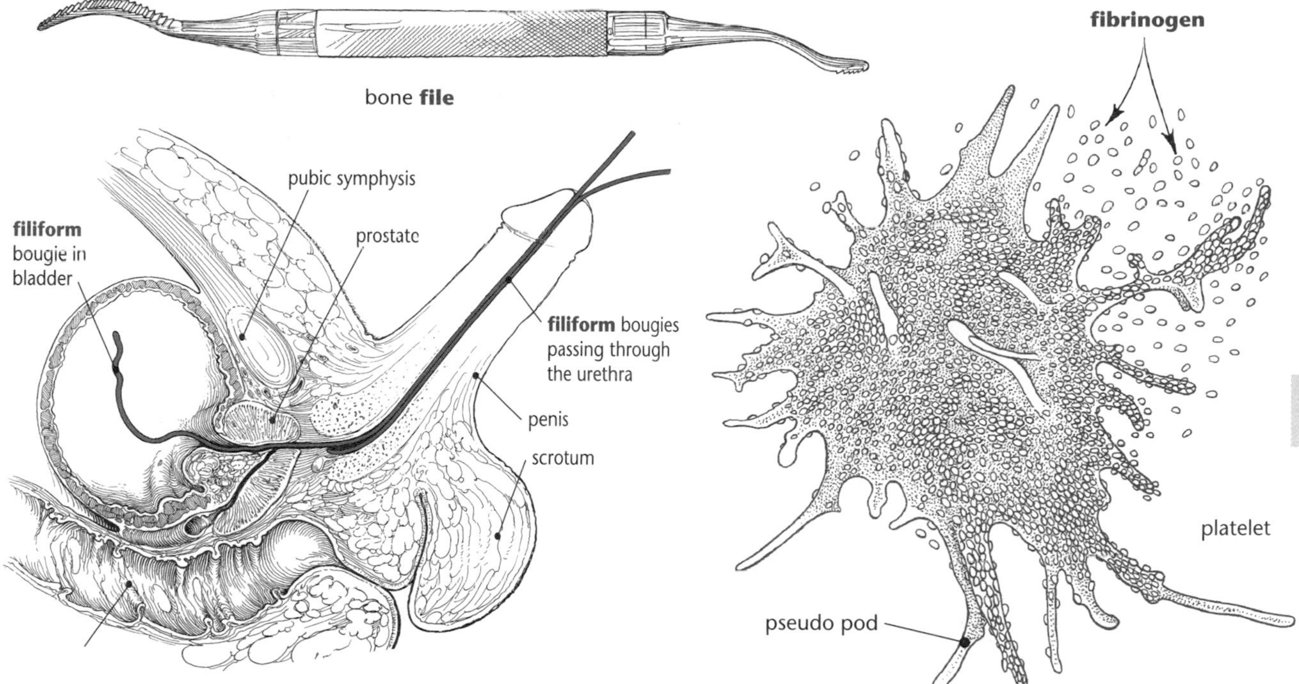

process.

cystic f. (CF) Autosomal recessive disorder marked by dysfunction of any of the exocrine glands, resulting in abnormally increased concentration of sodium and potassium in sweat and overproduction of viscid mucus, which causes obstruction of the structures involved (e.g., pancreatic and bile ducts, intestines, bronchi); it affects mainly infants and children; common forms include meconium ileus in the newborn and chronic pulmonary disease and pancreatic insufficiency in older children. Also called cystic fibrosis of pancreas; fibrocystic disease of pancreas; mucoviscidosis.

cystic f. of pancreas See cystic fibrosis.

endomyocardial f. Thickening of the ventricular myocardium.

idiopathic retroperitoneal f. See sclerosing retroperitonitis, under retroperitonitis.

perimuscular f. Fibrosis involving the renal arteries. Also called subadventitial fibrosis.

retroperitoneal f. See sclerosing retroperitonitis, under retroperitonitis.

subadventitial f. See perimuscular fibrosis.

fibrositis (fi-bro-si'tis) Inflammatory hyperplasia of fibrous or connective tissue of the muscles.

fibrous (fi-brus) Composed of, or resembling connective tissue fibers.

fibula (fib'u-lă) The lateral and smaller of the two bones of the leg, between the knee and ankle. See table of bones.

fibular (fib'u-lar) Relating to the fibula.

fibulocalcaneal (fib-u-lo-kal-ka'ne-ăl) Relating to the fibula and the calcaneus.

field (fēld) A limited area.

auditory f. The area within which a definite sound is heard.

magnetic f. The area of space about a magnet in which its magnetic force is perceptible.

visual f. (F) The area of physical space visible to the eye in a fixed position.

figure (fig'yur) Shape; form.

mitotic f. The appearance of a cell undergoing mitosis.

filament (fil'ă-ment) A fine threadlike structure.

acrosomal f. A stiff filament extruded by the acrosomal cap at the head of the spermatozoon, when it contacts the surface of a targeted ovum.

actin f. The smaller of the two contractile elements in muscle fibers, measuring about 50 Å in width; in skeletal and cardiac muscles, one end is attached to the Z line, a transverse septum that gives the muscle a characteristic striated appearance; the other free end interdigitates with the myosin filament in the contraction and relaxation of muscle.

axial f. The central filament of the tail of a spermatozoon, consisting of a central pair of fibrils within a symmetrical set of nine doublet fibrils, enveloped by an outer ring of nine larger dense fibers. Also called axoneme.

myosin f. The thicker of the two contractile elements in all muscle fibers; in skeletal and cardiac muscles, it measures about 100 Å in width, and traverses the central portion of each sarcomere, producing a dense A band; when interdigitating with the free ends of actin filaments, it is responsible for the contraction and relaxation of muscle.

root f.'s See radicular fila, under filum.

spermatic f. The short naked fragment at the terminal part of the tail of a spermatozoon. Also called end piece.

filamentous (fil-ă-men'tus) Threadlike in bacteriology, denoting a colony made up of long, interwoven, threadlike structures.

filaria (fĭ-lar'e-ă), *pl.* **filar'iae** Common name for threadworms of the family Onchocercidae.

filariasis (fil-ă-ri'ă-sis) Any disease caused by the presence of parasitic threadworms in the body.

lymphatic f. See filarial elephantiasis, under elephantiasis.

filaricide (fĭ-lar'ĭ-sīd) Any agent that destroys parasitic nematode worms.

filariform (fĭ-lar'ĭ-form) Hairlike, as filariae.

Filarioidea (fĭ-lar-e-oi'de-ă) A superfamily of true nematode worms that infest humans and other vertebrates.

file (fīl) A device used for cutting, smoothing, or grinding.

filial (fil'ē-ăl) Relating to a son or daughter.

filiform (fil'ĭ-form) **1.** Thread-shaped. **2.** An extremely slender bougie. **3.** In bacteriology, denoting an even, hairlike growth along the line of inoculation in streak or stab cultures.

fillet (fil'et) **1.** A thin strip of bandage or tape used for making traction. **2.** A band of fibers. Also called lemniscus.

filling (fil'ing) Any substance used to fill a space, cavity, or container (e.g., amalgam placed into a tooth cavity to restore the missing portion of the tooth).

acrylic resin f. A material used for restorations in teeth when esthetic properties are needed.

combination f. A tooth restoration composed of two or more layers of different materials.

compound f. A restoration that involves more than one surface of a tooth.

direct f. A restoration prepared directly in the tooth cavity.

indirect f. A restoration constructed from an accurate impression of the tooth and then cemented into the tooth cavity.

overhanging f. A restoration with excessive material at the junction of the filling and the tooth.

permanent f. A filling intended to be functional for as long a period as possible.

root canal f. Material placed in the root canal of a tooth to eliminate the space once occupied by the dental pulp.

silicate f. A restoration of lost tooth structure made with silicate cement, essentially acid-soluble glass.

temporary f. An interim filling.

treatment f. A temporary filling for allaying the sensitivity of dentin prior to placing the final restorative material.

zinc oxide-eugenol f. A temporary filling material, often referred to as ZOE.

film (film) **1.** A thin adherent coating on the surface of teeth, consisting chiefly of a mucinous mixture of saliva, microorganisms, and blood and tissue elements. **2.** A thin cellulose sheet coated with a light-sensitive emulsion used in taking photographs.

bite wing f. Dental x-ray film with an appendage that is held between the occlusal surfaces of the teeth.

film badge (film baj) A small device containing x-ray sensitive film, worn by individuals who are exposed to ionizing radiation, to record the amount of radiation to which they have been exposed; exposure is determined by measuring the degree of darkening of the film.

film fault (film fōlt) A defect in an x-ray film due either to physical or chemical causes or to electrical errors in its production.

fogged f. f. Hazy appearance of a roentgenogram; may be caused by exposure of film to light or stray radiation, subjection to unusual temperatures or chemical actions, or use of outdated film.

film holder (film hōld'er) A light-tight film container used in extraoral roentgenography.

filopodium (fi-lo-po'de-ŭm), *pl.* **filopo'dia** A slender process used for locomotion by certain free-living amebae.

filter (fil'ter) **1.** Any device used to separate particles from a liquid or gas. **2.** A device or screen that permits the passage of rays of certain wavelengths only. **3.** To pass a substance or rays through such devices.

Berkefeld f. A filter made of diatomaceous earth through which bacteria do not pass; available in three grades of porosity: W, fine; N, normal; V, coarse.

Greenfield f. A springed device consisting of six thin struts inserted into the vena cava to prevent blood clots in the legs from reaching the circulation of the lungs.

vena cava f. Any device anchored within the vena cava to prevent passage of blood clots into the pulmonary circulation.

filterable, filtrable (fil'ter-ă-bl, fil'tră-bl) **1.**

F

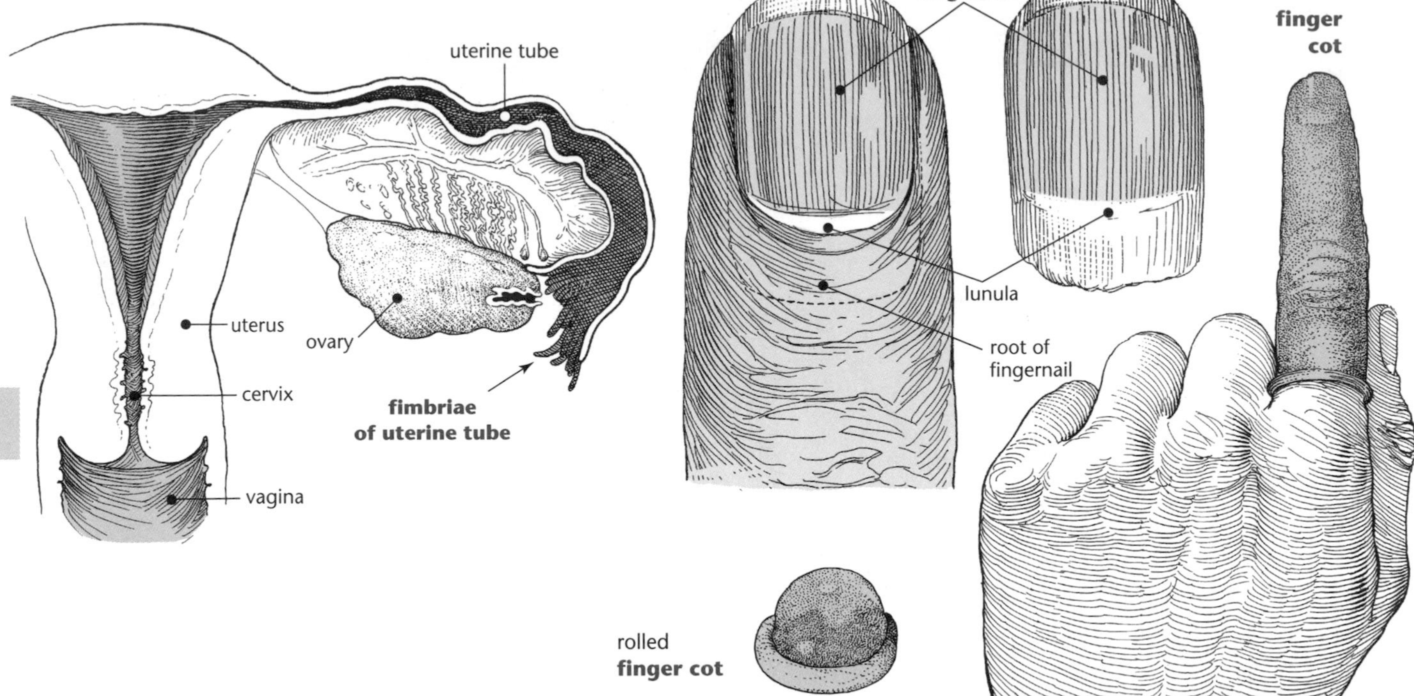

Capable of passing through a filter. **2.** Applied to viruses, minute enough to be able to pass through a fine filter.

filtrate (fil´trāt) Liquid that has passed through a filter.

filtration (fil-tra´shun) The process of passing a fluid through a filter employing differential pressure.

filum (fī´lum), *pl.* **fi´la** A filamentous or threadlike structure or part.

radicular fila Filaments into which the roots of all nerves divide before entering or leaving the spinal cord and brainstem. Also called root filaments; nerve rootlets.

f. of spinal dura mater The thin sheath covering the filum terminale and attached to the periosteum of the coccyx; it is an extension of the dura mater covering the spinal cord.

f. terminale, terminal f. The slender fibrous prolongation of the spinal cord extending from the level of the second lumbar vertebra to the coccyx; it anchors the spinal cord to the coccyx.

fimbria (fim´bre-ă), *pl.* **fimbriae** **1.** Any fringelike structure. **2.** See pilus (2).

f. hippocampi A narrow band of white fibers along the medial border of the hippocampus.

ovarian f. The longest and most deeply grooved fimbria of the fallopian (uterine) tube that runs along the lateral border of the mesosalpinx to attach to the tubal extremity of the ovary.

fimbriae of uterine tube The numerous irregular fringelike processes at the end of the distal part of the uterine tube.

fimbriate, fimbriated (fim´bre-āt, fim´bre-āt-ed) **1.** Fringed; having fimbriae. **2.** In bacteriology, denoting a colony with slender fringelike projections.

fimbrioplasty (fim-bre-o-plas´te) A corrective operation on the fringed processes of the uterine tube.

finger (fing´ger) One of five digits of the hand.

baseball f. See mallet finger.

drop f. See mallet finger.

clubbed f. See clubbing.

drumstick f. See clubbing.

fifth f. The little finger.

first f. The thumb.

fourth f. The ring finger, the thumb being considered the first.

hammer f. See mallet finger.

hippocratic f. See clubbing.

index f. The second digit, the thumb being considered the first; the finger next to the thumb. Also called forefinger.

mallet f. A finger marked by constant flexion of the distal phalanx; it cannot be actively extended due to detachment of the extensor tendon. Also called baseball finger; drop finger; hammer finger.

middle f. The third finger.

ring f. The fourth finger.

second f. The index finger.

snapping f. See trigger finger.

third f. The middle finger.

trigger f. A finger that locks in a flexed position; it can be extended only with difficulty associated with a snapping or clicking noise; it is due to narrowing of the flexor sheath at the level of the metacarpal neck. Also called snapping finger.

webbed f.'s Congenital abnormality in which two or more fingers are united in various degrees by a fold of skin.

fingeragnosia (fing-ger-ag-no´zhă) Loss of ability to recognize the individual fingers of the hand.

finger cot (fing´ger kŏt) A protective rubber covering for the finger; used in digital examinations.

fingernail (fing´ger-nāl) A horny plate on the dorsal surface of the tip of each finger. See also nail.

fingerprint fing´ger-print) An impression of the configuration of the ridges on the skin surface of the distal phalanx of a finger; usually used as a means of identification; the patterns are sometimes of clinical significance.

Galton's system of classification of f.'s The arch-loop-whorl system of classifying variations in the dermatographic patterns.

fingerprinting (fing-ger-print´ing) The act of making fingerprints.

DNA f. See DNA typing, under typing.

first aid (furst ād) Emergency assistance given to the injured or sick before the availability of professional medical care.

fission (fish´ŭn) **1.** Division of a cell; form of asexual reproduction. **2.** The splitting of an atom in two parts.

fissiparous (fĭ-sip´ă-rus) Reproducing by fission.

fissura (fis-u´ră), *pl.* **fissu´rae** Fissure; cleft.

fissuration (fish-u-ra´shun) **1.** The condition of being fissured. **2.** The formation of a fissure.

fissure (fish´ur) A cleft, groove, or slit.

anal f. A painful, difficult to heal slit in the mucous membrane of the anus.

anterior median f. The deep groove in the midline of the anterior aspect of the spinal cord.

auricular f. A groove, between the tympanic and the squamous and mastoid parts of the temporal bone, in which the auricular branch of the vagus nerve is located.

calcarine f. See calcarine sulcus, under sulcus.

central f. See central cerebral sulcus, under sulcus.

cerebral f.'s See cerebral sulci, under sulcus.

dentate f. See hippocampal fissure.

enamel f. A deep groove on the surface of a tooth resulting from imperfect fusion of adjoining dental lobes.

hippocampal f. A fissure located between the hippocampal convolution and the fascia dentata of the brain. Also called dentate fissure.

horizontal f. of cerebellum A deep cleft encircling the circumference of the cerebellar hemispheres. Also called horizontal sulcus of cerebellum.

inferior orbital f. A groove between the greater wing of the sphenoid and the orbital plate of the maxilla.

lateral f. of cerebrum See lateral cerebral sulcus, under sulcus.

longitudinal f. of cerebrum The deep median groove that divides the cerebrum into right and left hemispheres.

f.'s of lungs Fissures separating the lobes of the lungs.

primary f. Fissure that separates the cranial from the middle lobe of the cerebellum; it forms the anterior border of the declive of the vermis.

postclival f. A fissure between the declive and the folium vermis of the middle lobe of the cerebellum.

f. of Rolando See central cerebral sulcus, under sulcus.

superior orbital f. A cleft between the greater and lesser wings of the sphenoid bone. Also called sphenoidal fissure.

f. of Sylvius See lateral cerebral sulcus, under sulcus.

transverse f. of cerebellum A cleft between the corpus callosum and the fornix above and the diencephalon below.

fistula (fis´tu-lă) An abnormal passage between two internal organs, or from an organ to the surface of the body; usually designated according to the organs with which it communicates.

anal f. A fistula opening near the anus; it may or may not open into the rectum.

arteriovenous f. An abnormal communication (congenital or traumatic) between an artery and a vein.

branchial f. A congenital defect consisting of a narrow canal on the lateral aspect of the neck in front of the sternocleidomastoid muscle, resulting from incomplete closure of a branchial cleft.

bronchoesophageal f. Passage between a bronchus and the esophagus.

bronchopleural f. A fistula connecting a bronchus and a collection of pus in the pleural cavity.

carotid-cavernous f. Arteriovenous connection formed by rupture of the intracavernous portion of the carotid artery.

colovesical f. A fistula between the colon and the bladder. Also called vesicocolonic fistula.

Eck f. A communication formed by the

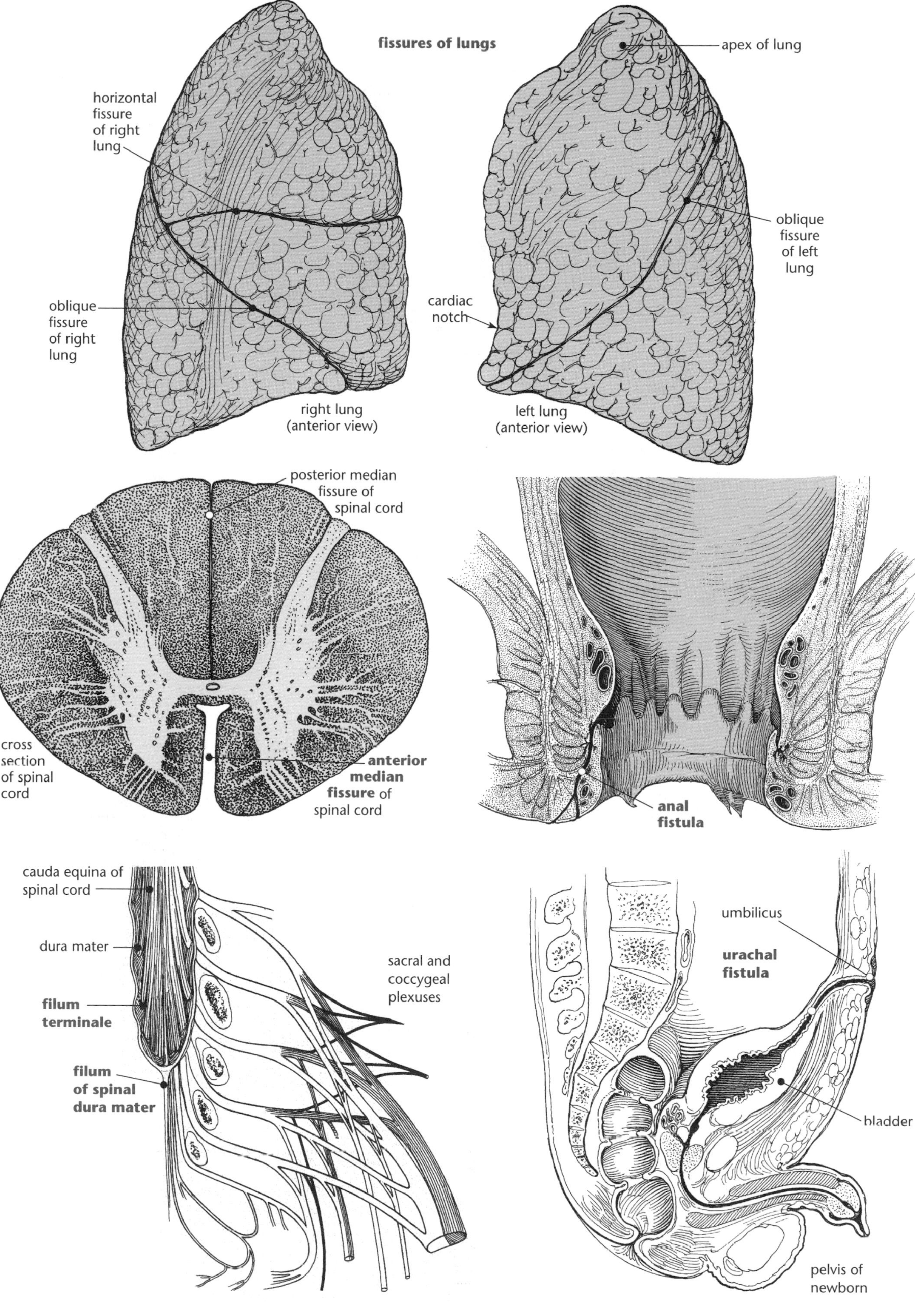

fissures of lungs
horizontal fissure of right lung
oblique fissure of right lung
right lung (anterior view)
apex of lung
oblique fissure of left lung
cardiac notch
left lung (anterior view)
posterior median fissure of spinal cord
cross section of spinal cord
anterior median fissure of spinal cord
anal fistula
cauda equina of spinal cord
dura mater
filum terminale
filum of spinal dura mater
sacral and coccygeal plexuses
umbilicus
urachal fistula
bladder
pelvis of newborn

F

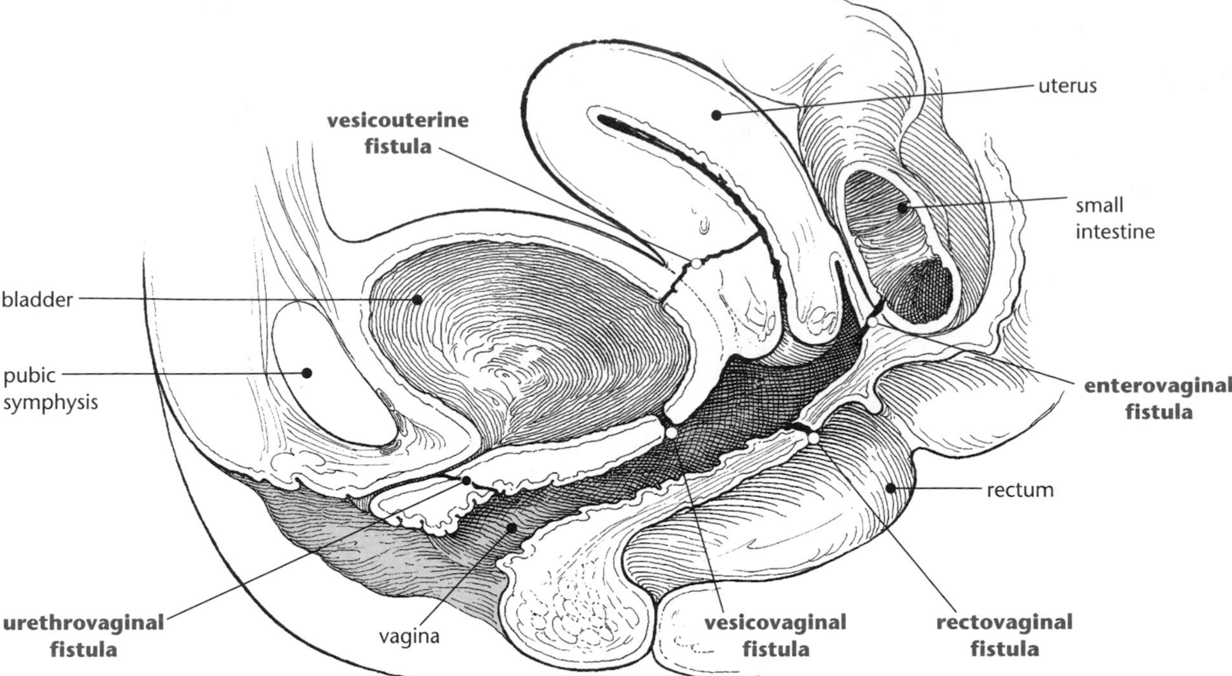

experimental anastomosing of the vena cava and portal vein with subsequent ligation of the portal vein, for the purpose of shutting off the liver of an experimental animal from its portal circulation.

enterovaginal f. A fistula between the small intestine and the vagina, usually associated with intestinal disease, especially diverticulitis.

gastrocolic f. A fistula between the stomach and the colon.

internal f. Abnormal passage between two internal organs.

pilonidal f. See pilonidal sinus, under sinus.

rectovaginal f. A fistula between the rectum and the vagina, caused by direct surgical damage, disease of the rectum, or obstetrical injury.

Thiry's f. Artificial fistula made for collecting the intestinal juice of an experimental animal; consisting of an isolated segment of intestine, having one end closed and the other attached to the skin of the abdomen.

Thiry-Vella f. Experimental fistula created by suturing to the skin of the abdomen the two ends of an isolated segment of intestine. Also called Vella's fistula.

tracheoesophageal f. Congenital fistula between the trachea and esophagus.

urachal f. Congenital abnormality that occurs when the lumen of the embryonic allantois (which extends from the navel to the bladder) persists over the entire length, allowing urine to drain from the navel. Also called patent urachus.

urethrovaginal f. A fistula between the urethra and the vagina; may be due to obstetrical injury or may be congenital.

Vella's f. See Thiry-Vella fistula.

vesicocolonic f. See colovesical fistula.

vesicouterine f. A fistula between the bladder and the uterus, usually caused by cancer of the cervix or by surgical injury to the bladder.

vesicovaginal f. A fistula between the bladder and the vagina, often the result of traumatic delivery; almost invariably causes urinary incontinence.

fistulation (fis-tu-la´shun) Formation of a fistula. Also called fistulization.

fistulatome (fis´tu-lă-tōm) A thin-bladed long knife used for slitting a fistula. Also called syringotome.

fistulatomy (fis-tu-lot´ŏ-me) See fistulotomy.

fistulectomy (fis-tu-lek´tŏ-me) Surgical repair of a fistula by the removal of its walls.

fistulization (fis-tu-lī-zā´shun) See fistulation.

fistulotomy (fis-tu-lot´ŏ-me) Surgical incision of a fistula. Also called fistulatomy; syringotomy.

fistulous (fis´tu-lus) Relating to or having fistulas.

fitness, physical (fit´nes) A state of well being that enables a person to perform his daily work without undue fatigue.

Fitz-Hugh-Curtis syndrome (fitz´hu-kĕr´tis sin´drōm) See perihepatitis.

fixation (fik-sā´shun) **1.** The act of fastening in a stationary position. **2.** In ophthalmology, the act of directing the eye toward an object, causing its image to fall on the fovea. **3.** In histology, the preservation of tissue elements with minimal alteration of the normal state. **4.** In chemistry, the conversion of a gaseous compound into solid or liquid form. **5.** In psychiatry, the arrest of one or more aspects of psychosocial development at an immature stage.

bifoveal f. Fixation in which the images of the object of regard center simultaneously on the foveae of both eyes, as occurs in normal vision. Also called binocular fixation.

binocular f. Bifoveal fixation.

complement f. (CF) Fixation that occurs when an antigen is allowed to combine with its specific antibody in the presence of complement; used in the detection of antibodies in serum.

external f. The holding together of a broken bone by means of a plaster cast encircling the injured part or a plaster splint until successful healing occurs.

internal f. The use of devices such as metallic pins, screws, wires, or plates, applied directly to the bony fragments to hold them in apposition and alignment.

fixation disparity (fik-sā´shun dis-par´ĭ-te) Condition in which the images of the object of regard do not fall on corresponding retinal points, due to a slight over- or under-convergence of the eyes.

fixative (fik´să-tiv) A substance used to preserve histologic specimens.

FK-506 See tacrolimus.

flaccid (flăk´sid) Flabby; limp.

flagellantism (flaj´ĕ-lan-tiz-m) Erotic stimulation derived from whipping, or being whipped by, a sexual partner.

flagellate (flaj´ĕ-lāt) A protozoon having one or more flagella.

flagellosis (flaj-ĕ-lo´sis) Infection with flagellated protozoa.

flagellum (flă-jel´ŭm), *pl.* **flagel´la** A hairlike protoplasmic structure, present in some microorganisms; it is usually several microns in length and composed of two tightly entwined filaments, each about 100 Å in diameter; it grows out from the basal body in the cytoplasm of the cell and is used for locomotion.

flange (flanj) **1.** A protruding rim or edge. **2.** In dentistry, the part of the denture base which extends from the cervical ends of the teeth to the border of the denture.

buccal f. The portion of the flange of a denture which occupies the vestibule of the mouth adjoining the cheek.

denture f. The nearly vertical extension from the body of a denture into any of the oral vestibules.

labial f. The portion of the flange of a denture which occupies the vestibule of the mouth adjoining the lips.

lingual f. The portion of the flange of a mandibular denture which occupies the space adjacent to the tongue.

flank (flank) The side of the body between the bottom of the ribs and the iliac crest. Also called latus.

flap (flap) **1.** A flat piece of tissue cut away from the underlying parts but attached at one end; used to cover a defect in a neighboring part or the sawn end of a bone after amputation. **2.** A characteristic flapping movement of the hands in certain disorders.

bone f. In neurosurgery, a section of the skull attached to muscles and/or other structures which serve as a hinge.

liver f. See asterixis.

pedicle f. A piece of detached tissue (including skin and subcutaneous tissues) in which the attached end or base contains an adequate blood supply.

sliding f. A flap used to either lengthen or shorten a localized area of tissue.

flare (flār) Diffuse redness of the skin surrounding an injured point.

flash (flash) **1.** A sudden, brief, intense burst of light or heat. **2.** In dentistry, excess material squeezed out of the sections of a mold.

hot f. See hot flush, under flush.

flashback (flash´băk) The spontaneous and unpredictable reversion of perceptual distortions resulting from having previously taken psychedelic drugs; it can last from several seconds to half an hour.

flask (flask) **1.** A bottle with a narrow neck, used in the laboratory. **2.** A metal case or tube used in investing procedures.

casting f. See refractory flask.

crown f. A small dental flask.

dental f. A metal case in which a sectional gypsum mold is made for the purpose of shaping and curing resinous structures, such as dentures or other resinous restorations.

Dewar f. A glass vessel, often silvered, with two walls; used for maintaining materials at constant temperature or, more usually, at low temperature. Also called vacuum flask.

Erlenmeyer f. A flask with a conical body, broad base, and a narrow neck.

Florence f. A globular long-necked bottle of thin glass used for holding water or other liquid in laboratory work.

refractory f. A metal tube in which a refractory mold is made for casting metal dental restorations or

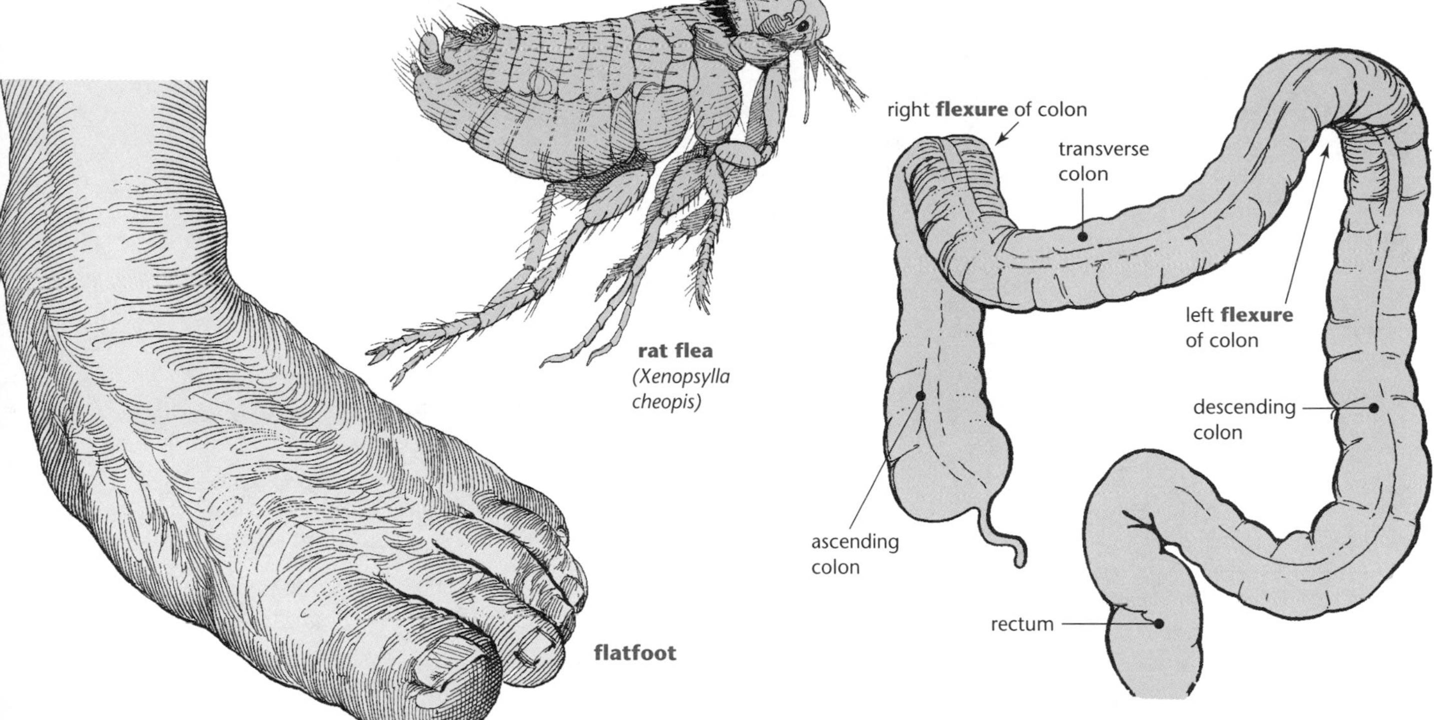

appliances. Also called casting flask; casting ring.

vacuum f. See Dewar flask.

volumetric f. A flask calibrated to contain or to deliver a definite amount of liquid.

flasking (flask´ing) In dentistry, the investing of the cast and a wax denture prior to molding the denture-base material into the form of the denture.

flatfoot (flat´fo͝ot) Condition marked by varying degrees of diminution or depression of the longitudinal arch of the foot, resulting in impairment of its weight-bearing capability; it may be congenital or acquired. Also called pes planus; splay foot.

flatulence (flat´u-lens) Excessive quantities of gas in the stomach and intestines, causing distention.

flatulent (flat´u-lent) Relating to flatulence.

flatus (fla´tus) Intestinal gas expelled through the rectum.

flatworm (flat´werm) Any member of the phylum Platyhelminthes (e.g., tapeworms and flukes).

flavin (fla´vin) Any of various nitrogenous yellow pigments present in numerous plant and animal tissues.

f. adenine dinucleotide (FAD) A nucleotide containing riboflavin which participates as a coenzyme in oxidation-reduction reactions.

f. mononucleotide (FMN) A cofactor containing riboflavin in cellular oxidation-reduction systems.

Flavivirus (fla´vĭ-vi-vus) A genus of arthropod-borne viruses (family Flaviviridae) that cause diseases such as yellow fever, dengue, and encephalitis. Formerly classified as arbovirus, group B.

Flavobacterium (fla-vo-bak-tēr´e-ŭm) A genus of bacteria; gram-negative rods that, when motile, move by means of flagella located around the mouth opening; they characteristically produce yellow, orange, red, or yellow-brown pigments; some species are pathogenic.

flavoenzyme (fla-vo-en´zīm) Any enzyme having a flavin nucleotide as coenzyme.

flavor (fla´vor) **1.** The distinctive taste of any substance. **2.** Inert substance added to a pharmaceutical preparation to give it a pleasing taste.

flea (fle) A blood-sucking insect of the genus *Pulex*.

rat f. A general term for *Pulex fasciatus*, *Pulex pallidus*, *Typhlopsylla musculi*, and *Xenopsylla cheopis*; parasitic on the rat and a vector for bubonic plague.

sand f. See chigoe.

flesh (flesh) **1.** Muscular tissue and other soft tissues of the body excluding the viscera. **2.** The meat of animals. **3.** Excess tissue; stoutness.

goose f. Popular term for cutis anserina, the temporary rough appearance of the skin caused by contraction of the arrectores pilorum muscles (erectors of the hair) as a reaction to cold, fear, or other stimuli. Also called goose bumps.

proud f. Excessive granulation on the surface of a wound or ulcer.

flex (fleks) To bend or approximate two parts which are united by a joint.

fleximeter (flek-sim´ĕ-ter) Instrument for measuring the degree of flexion possible in a joint.

flexion (flek´shun) **1.** The act of bending a limb at a joint so that its proximal and distal parts are brought together; the bending forward of the spine. **2.** The condition of being bent.

palmar f. Flexion at the wrist, causing the hand to be bent toward the anterior surface of the forearm.

plantar f. Flexion at the ankle joint, causing the foot to be bent downward.

flexor (flek´sor) A muscle that flexes a joint. See table of muscles.

flexura (flek-shoo´ră) Latin for a bend.

flexure (flek´shur) A bend.

caudal f. The bend at the caudal end of the embryo. Also called sacral flexure.

cephalic f. The bend at the cephalic region of the embryo. Also called cranial flexure.

cervical f. The bend at the junction of the embryonic brain and spinal cord.

cranial f. See cephalic flexure.

hepatic f. The bend between the ascending and transverse colon, near the liver.

pontine f. A concave flexure dividing the rhombencephalon portion of the embryonic brain into anterior and posterior halves.

sacral f. See caudal flexure.

splenic f. The bend between the transverse and descending colon, near the spleen. See also splenic flexure syndrome.

flitting flies (flĭt´ing flīs) See floaters.

floaters (flō´terz) Opaque deposits in the normally transparent vitreous body; may be congenital or due to degenerative changes of the retina or the vitreous body. Also called muscae volitantes; flitting flies.

floating (flōt´ing) Unattached; unduly movable.

floccillation (flok-sĭ-la´shun) Aimless plucking at the bedclothes, occurring in delirious patients. Also called carphologia; crocidismus.

flocculation (flok-u-la´shun) The formation of flaky masses or precipitation in a solution being tested.

flocculent (flok´u-lent) **1.** A fluid containing irregularly shaped fluffy particles. **2.** In bacteriology, denoting a liquid culture containing small adherent masses of bacteria.

flocculus (flok´u-lus) Latin for small tuft; in anatomy, the small lobule of the posterior lobe of the cerebellum, which adjoins the middle cerebellar peduncle and is continuous with the nodule of the vermis.

flood (flŭd) Colloquial term for profuse bleeding from the uterus, e.g., after childbirth (postpartum hemorrhage) or during menstruation (menorrhagia).

flora (flo´ră) Plant life.

intestinal f. The bacteria in the intestinal contents.

florid (flor´id) **1.** Denoting a flushed appearance, as of the skin. **2.** Having a bright red color, as of a lesion.

floss (flŏs) **1.** To use thread (dental floss) or ribbon (dental tape) to remove particles from spaces between teeth. **2.** Dental floss.

flow (flo) **1.** To move freely. **2.** Popular term for the menstrual discharge.

effective renal plasma f. (ERPF) The amount of plasma passing through the kidneys as measured by clearance of *p*-aminohippurate.

gene f. The gradual diffusion of genes from one population to another by migration and mating rather than by mutation.

flowers (flou´ĕrz) In chemistry, a powdery mineral substance produced by condensation or sublimation.

f. of zinc See zinc oxide.

flowmeter (flo´me-ter) Device used to measure the flow of liquids in vessels.

floxuridine (floks-ūr´ĭ-dēn) (5-FUDR) 5-Fluoro-2´-deoxyuridine; a derivative of fluorouracil; used in the treatment of gastrointestinal cancer.

flu (floo) A general term given to many brief illnesses presumed to be caused by viruses, mostly the influenza virus; symptoms usually include sudden onset of fever, shivering, headache, muscular aches, and malaise; fever generally lasts three to four days.

fluctuant (fluk´choo-ănt) Having a yielding feel to palpation, suggesting a liquid center.

fluctuate (fluk´choo-āt) **1.** To vary irregularly or change from time to time. **2.** To undulate or move in waves.

fluctuation (fluk-choo-a´shun) **1.** A variation. **2.** A wavelike motion produced when a body cavity filled with fluid is palpated.

fluid (floo´id) **1.** Any nonsolid substance, either liquid or gas. **2.** Flowing.

allantoic f. The fluid within the allantoic cavity.

amniotic f. The fluid within the amnion in which the fetus floats.

cerebrospinal f. (CSF) The fluid filling the ventricles of the brain and the subarachnoid spaces of the brain and spinal cord.

extracellular f. (ECF) The body fluid outside of the cells, composed of interstitial fluid, blood, plasma, and lymph; approximately 20% of body weight.

follicular f. An albuminous fluid secreted by the granulosa (follicular) cells in a developing ovarian follicle; it creates intercellular spaces which eventually give rise to a follicular cavity, the antrum. Also

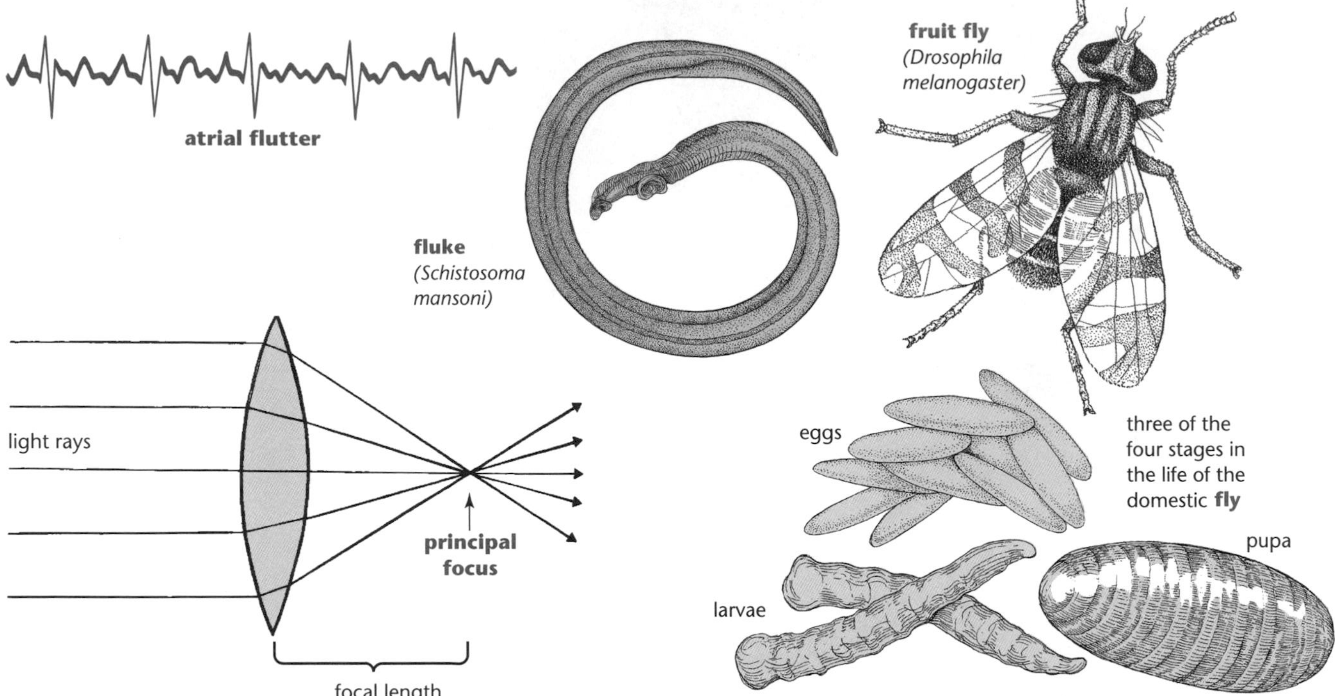

called liquor folliculi.

infranatant f. The clear liquid that settles on the bottom of a container after separation from an insoluble liquid or solid through the action of gravity or a centrifugal force.

interstitial f. Fluid lying in the spaces between cells; comprises the major part of extracellular fluid.

intracellular f. The fluid within the tissue cells, constituting about 40% of the body weight.

intraocular f. The fluid within the anterior and posterior chambers of the eye.

seminal f. See semen.

supernatant f. The clear fluid that settles on top of the contents of a vessel after separating from an insoluble liquid or solid through normal gravity or a centrifugal force.

fluidextract (floo-id-ek´strakt) An alcohol solution of a vegetable drug in which one milliliter of the solution contains the active ingredients of one gram of the standard solution it represents.

fluidglycerate (floo-id-glis´ĕr-āt) A pharmaceutical preparation containing approximately 50% by volume of glycerin and one gram of the active principle of the specific drug in each milliliter.

fluidram (floo-ĭd-ram´) A measure of capacity equal to 1/8 of a fluid ounce; a teaspoonful.

fluke (flo͞ok) Common name for species of the class Trematoda (flatworms), especially the parasitic variety.

blood f. Fluke of the genus *Schistosoma*, parasitic in the mesenteric-portal bloodstream and the vesical and venous plexuses.

Chinese liver f. A fluke parasitic in the bile ducts. Also called *Clonorchis sinensis*.

large intestinal f. A large fluke parasitic in the intestines. Also called *Fasciolopsis buski*.

liver f. See *Fasciola hepatica*, under *Fasciola*.

lung f. A fluke parasitic in the lungs. Also called *Paragonimus westermani*.

flumina pilorum (floo´mĭ-nă pī-lor´ŭm) The lined pattern along which hairs grow on the head and throughout the body. Also called hair streams.

fluocinolone acetonide (floo-ŏ-sin´ŏ-lon as´ĕ-tō-nīd) A fluorinated corticosteroid used topically in the treatment of certain dermatoses.

fluorescein (flo͞o-res´ēn) A material used, because of its fluorescence, as a marker, as in immunofluorescent studies and in circulatory studies, particularly of the eye.

sodium f. An orange-red powder used in solution to detect lesions of the cornea.

fluorescence (flo͞o-res´ĕns) The ability of certain substances to emit light, to become self-luminous, while exposed to direct light rays from another source, especially ultraviolet rays.

fluoridation (floor-ĭ-da´shun) The addition of fluoride (fluorine compound) to the public water supply to prevent tooth decay.

fluoride (floor´īd) A compound containing fluorine.

fluorine (floor´ēn) A gaseous chemical element of the halogen group; symbol F, atomic number 9, atomic weight 19.

fluorometer (floor-om´ĕ-ter) A device for detecting and measuring fluorescence.

fluoroquinolones (floor-o-kwin´o-lōnz) A class of antibiotics effective against a wide variety of microorganisms.

fluoroscope (floor´-o-skōp) A type of x-ray apparatus in which x rays going through part of the body strike upon a fluorescent screen of calcium tungstate, rendering an image on the screen of varying densities of the body.

fluoroscopic (flo͝or-o-skop´ik) Relating to fluoroscopy.

fluoroscopy (flo͝or-os´kŏ-pe) Direct examination of the inner parts of the body by use of the fluoroscope.

fluorosis (flo͝or-o´sis) Abnormal condition caused by an excessive intake of floride, manifested mainly by mottling of the enamel of the teeth.

fluorouracil (floor-o-ūr´ă-sil) (5-FU) 5-Fluorouracil; an antineoplastic drug, $C_4H_3FN_2O_2$, used in the treatment of gastrointestinal cancer and topically for the treatment of multiple premalignant actinic keratoses.

fluoxetine (floo-ok´sĕ-tēn) An antidepressant compound that prevents serotonic reuptake; Prozac®.

flush (flush) **1.** To wash with a brief gush of water. **2.** Sudden redness of the skin, especially of the face and neck.

carcinoid f. Periodic cutaneous flushing, especially of the head and neck, often precipitated by stress, ingestion of food or alcohol, or palpation of the liver; associated with a carcinoid tumor.

histamine f. Flush associated with the release of histamine.

hot f. Sudden feeling of intense heat in the face, neck, and chest, followed by sweating and sometimes palpitations; occurs about 5 to 10 times per day lasting from a few seconds to several minutes; experienced by about 50% of women during the natural menopause and by those who have had both ovaries removed (surgical menopause). Also called hot flash.

flutamide (floo´tă-mīd) Anticancer drug that blocks androgen from binding to its receptor in peripheral tissues; used to treat prostatic cancer.

flutter (flut´ĕr) Rapid vibrations or pulsations.

atrial f. Extremely rapid but rhythmic contractions of the cardiac atria, usually at a rate of 240 to 300 per minute, often producing "sawtooth" waves in the electrocardiogram. Also called auricular flutter.

auricular f. See atrial flutter.

diaphragmatic f. Rapid contractions of all or part of the diaphragm.

ventricular f. Rapid contractions of the ventricles producing electrocardiographic complexes that have a regular undulating pattern without distinct QRS and T waves.

flutter-fibrillation (flut´ĕr-fib-rĭ-la´shun) An electrocardiographic pattern of atrial activity showing both flutter and fibrillation.

flux (fluks) **1.** Excessive discharge of any body secretion. **2.** Denoting the movement of ions or molecules through a membrane. **3.** In dentistry, a substance that increases fluidity of molten metal, thereby promoting fusion; also used to remove oxides from metal surfaces during soldering of dental prostheses.

fly (flī) Any of numerous winged insects of the order Diptera; many are vectors of disease.

black f. A dark, two-winged insect of the genus *Simulium*, vector of *Onchocerca volvulus*, the parasite causing onchocerciasis. Also called buffalo gnat.

flesh f. A fly whose larvae (maggots) develop in putrefying or living tissues.

fruit f. *Drosophila melanogaster*, a fly used extensively in genetic studies.

mangrove f. Fly of the genus *Chrysops*; vector of *Loa loa*, the eye worm causing loiasis.

sand f. See sandfly.

Spanish f. See cantharis.

tsetse f. See *Glossina*.

foam (fōm) **1.** Collection of numerous small bubbles on the surface of a liquid. **2.** To produce such bubbles.

focal (fo´kal) Relating to a focus; localized.

focal glomerulonephritis (fo´kăl glo-mer-u-lo-nĕ-frī´tis) See under glomerulonephritis.

focal length (fo´kăl lĕngth) (f) The distance from a point where the image of a distant object is formed (focal point) to a point in or near the lens.

focal plane (fo´kal plān) The plane at right angles to the optical axis at the focal point.

focal point (fo´kal point) The point where the light rays coming from a distant object converge after passing through a lens, coming to a focus and forming an image.

foci (fo´si) Plural of focus.

focimeter (fo-sim´ĕ-ter) Instrument used to determine the vergence power of a lens or system of lenses.

focus (fo´kus), *pl.* **foci** **1.** The point in an optical system where light rays meet. **2.** To adjust a lens system to produce a distinct, clear image. **3.** The principal site of a disease.

conjugate foci Two points in an optical system so interrelated that rays originating at one point are

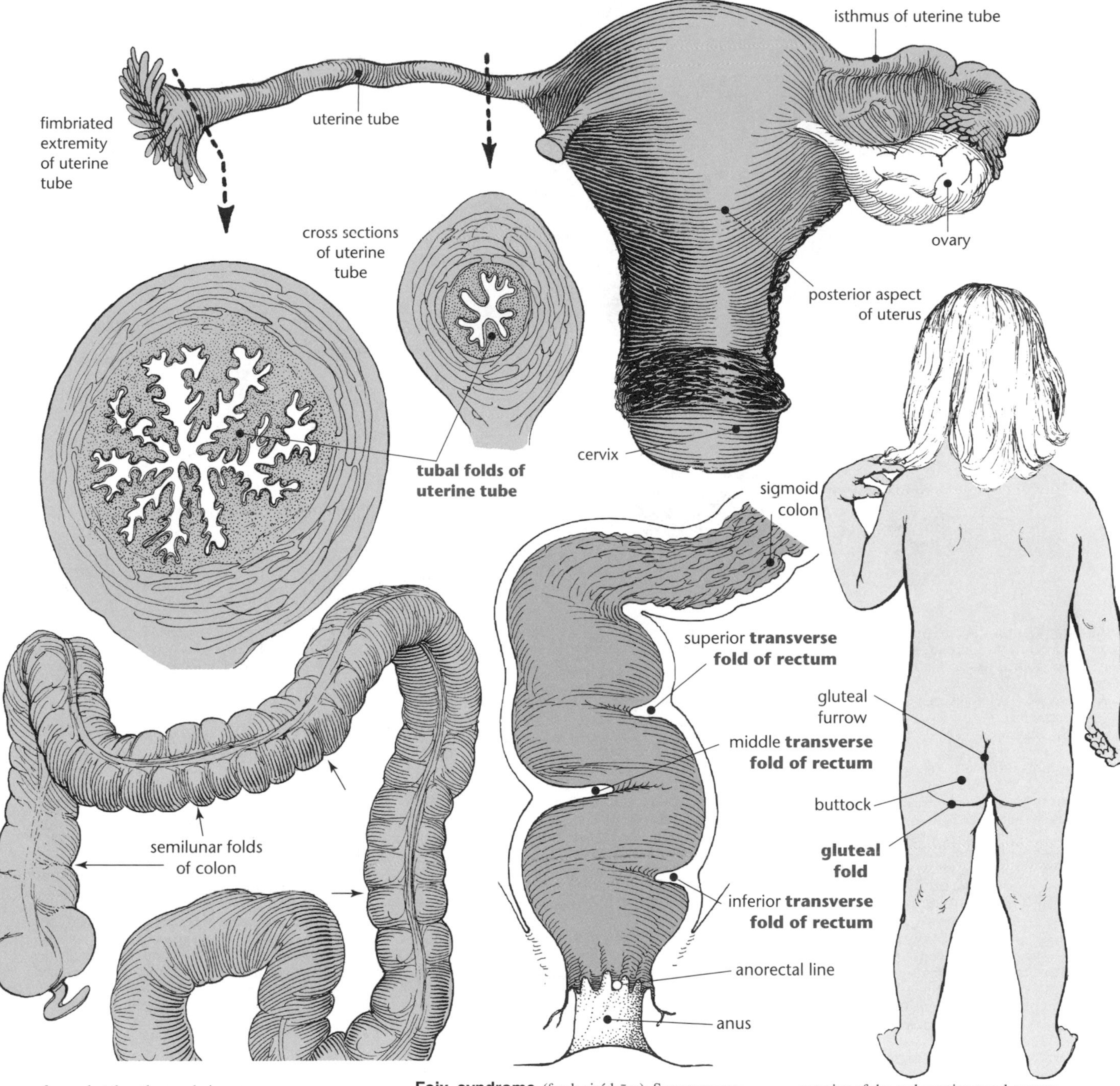

focused at the other, and vice versa.

Ghon's f. Ghon's primary lesion; see under lesion.

principal f. The real or virtual axial meeting point of rays passing into a lens parallel to its optical axis.

real f. The point at which convergent light rays meet forming a real image.

virtual f. The point at which the backward extensions of diverging light rays intersect, forming a virtual image.

fog (fog) **1.** Hazy or dense appearance of a roentgenogram caused by stray radiation, accidental exposure to light, subjection to unusual temperatures or chemical actions, or the use of outdated film. **2.** To subject a film to such conditions.

fogging (fog´ing) In ophthalmology, the deliberate undercorrection of myopia (nearsightedness) or overcorrection of hyperopia (farsightedness); a procedure used to prevent unconscious accommodation of the eye during the testing for astigmatism.

foil (foil) An extremely thin, pliable sheet of metal.

gold f. A foil of pure gold used in dentistry to restore carious or fractured teeth.

platinum f. A foil of pure platinum used in dentistry, because of its high fusing point, as a matrix for soldering procedures and to provide the internal forms of porcelain restorations.

Foix syndrome (fwah sin´drōm) See cavernous sinus syndrome.

folate (fo´lāt) A salt of folic acid.

fold (fōld) The doubling of a part upon itself.

axillary f. One of the musculocutaneous ridges (anterior and posterior) bounding the armpit.

circular f. See plica circularis.

Douglas f.'s See rectouterine folds.

glosso-epiglottic f.'s Three folds of mucous membrane (one median, two lateral) reflected from the base of the tongue onto the epiglottis.

gluteal f. A fold marking the posterior upper limit of the thigh and the lower limit of the buttock.

lacrimal f. A fold of mucous membrane in the nasal cavity at the lower end of the nasolacrimal duct; it keeps air from entering the lacrimal sac when the nose is blown.

medial umbilical f. The fold of peritoneum that covers the obliterated umbilical artery as it ascends from the pelvis toward the umbilicus.

median umbilical f. The fold of peritoneum that covers the median umbilical ligament extending from the apex of the urinary bladder to the umbilicus. Also called urachal fold.

nasojugal f. A fold indicating the confluence of the orbicularis oculi and the quadratus labii muscles.

neural f.'s Folds of ectoderm forming the margins of the embryonic neural groove.

rectouterine f.'s Folds of peritoneum that extend from the uterine cervix on either side of the rectum, to the posterior wall of the pelvis. Also called Douglas' folds.

rectovaginal f. A fold of peritoneum extending from the front of the rectum to the back of the posterior fornix of the vagina; it forms the floor of the deep rectovaginal pouch. Also called posterior ligament of uterus.

rectovesical f. The peritoneal fold that bounds the rectovesical pouch in the male.

salpingopharyngeal f. One of the vertical ridges of mucous membrane extending from the lower portion of the elevation of the auditory tube along the wall of the pharynx on either side.

sublingual f. The fold formed by the mucous membrane of the floor of the mouth, elevated by the sublingual gland and containing its excretory ducts.

transverse f.'s of rectum The three or four crescentric transverse folds in the rectum. Also called rectal valves.

tubal f.'s of uterine tube A series of major plicated folds of mucous membrane projecting into the lumen of the fallopian (uterine) tube; especially well developed in the ampulla of the tube.

urachal f. See median umbilical fold.

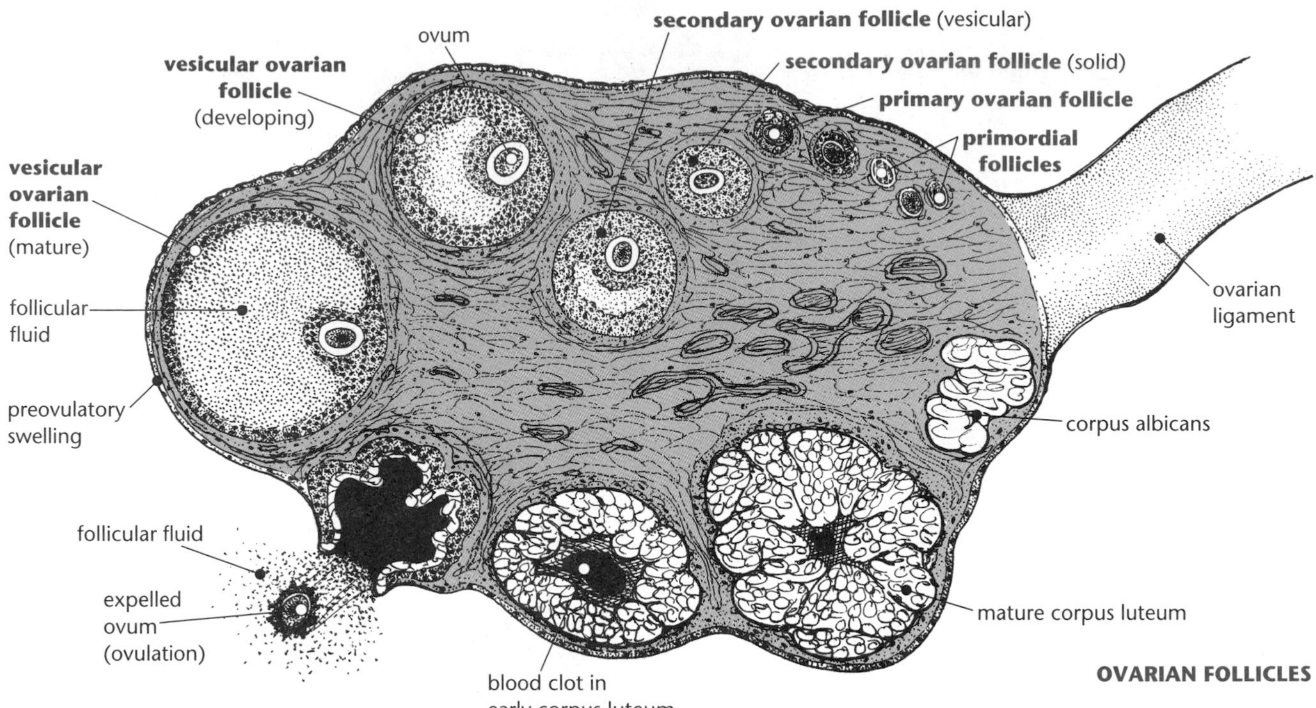

OVARIAN FOLLICLES

uterovesical f. A fold of peritoneum extending from the front of the uterus to the upper surface of the urinary bladder. Also called anterior ligament of uterus.

Vater's f. A fold located above the greater papilla of the duodenum.

vocal f. The true vocal cord; it contains the vocal ligament.

foliaceous, foliate (fo-le-ā'shun, fo'le-āt) Resembling a leaf.

folic acid (fo'lik as'id) A constituent of the vitamin B complex; extracted from liver and green leaves, and produced synthetically; deficiency may occur in malnourished individuals, alcoholics, and in malabsorption states and result in a megaloblastic anemia. Also called pteroylmonoglutamic acid.

folic acid antagonist (fo'lik as'id an-tag'ŏ-nist) One of a group of compounds that neutralize the action of folic acid; used in the treatment of neoplastic disorders, especially of the hematopoietic system.

folie (fo-le') French for madness or psychosis.

f. à deux Psychosis affecting two closely associated persons in which they share the same delusions. Also called communicated insanity; double insanity.

f. gémellaire Psychosis occurring simultaneously in twins who are not necessarily closely associated at the time.

folinic acid (fo-lin'ik as'id) A reduced form of folic acid. Also called leucovorin.

folium (fo'le-ŭm), *pl.* **folia** A broad thin anatomic structure.

folia of the cerebellum (fo'le-ă ŭv thĕ ser-ĕ-bel'ŭm) The numerous long parallel infoldings of the cerebellar cortex.

follicle (fol'lĕ-kl) **1.** A somewhat spherical mass of cells usually containing a cavity. **2.** A small crypt, such as the depression in the skin from which the hair emerges. **3.** A small circumscribed body.

atretic ovarian f. A follicle that degenerates before reaching maturity.

dental f. The fibrous layer of mesenchyme surrounding a developing tooth. Also called dental sac.

graafian f. See vesicular ovarian follicle.

hair f. A saclike invagination of the epidermis from which the root of a hair develops.

lymph f. A small mass of lymphoid tissue, as seen in the mucosa of the gut. Also called lymphatic nodule.

lymphoid f. A collection of proliferating pale-staining cells in lymphoid tissue, as in the cortex of lymph nodes.

nabothian f. A cyst resulting from obstruction of a mucous gland of the uterine cervix. Also called nabothian cyst.

ovarian f. The ovum together with its surrounding cells, at any stage of development, located in the cortex of the ovary.

primary ovarian f. A developing follicle in the ovary before the appearance of a fluid-filled antrum; it is composed of a growing primary oocyte and a single or several layers of cuboidal follicular cells surrounded by a sheath of stroma (theca); it usually develops during adolescence.

primordial f. An immature ovarian follicle consisting of the original primordial germ cell, the oogonium, and a thin single layer of squamous (flattened) follicular cells; at birth there are about 400,000 primordial follicles in each ovary; most undergo atresia.

sebaceous f. Oil gland of the skin; it opens into a hair follicle.

solid secondary ovarian f. A follicle in the ovary in which follicular fluid is gradually accumulating between the follicular (granulosa) cells; it first appears during puberty.

thyroid f. The minute components of the thyroid gland in which the thyroid hormone is stored.

vesicular ovarian f. A large mature follicle in the ovary in which the ovum (oocyte) attains full size (about four times that of the primordial germ cell); at this stage of development, the follicle migrates toward the surface of the ovary, causing a preovulatory swelling. Also called graafian follicle.

follicular (fo-lik'u-lar) **1.** Having or resembling a follicle or follicles. **2.** Growing out of follicles.

folliculitis (fo-lik-u-li'tis) Inflammation of hair follicles.

f. barbae Tinea barbae.

folliculoma (fo-lik-u-lo'mă) **1.** See granulosa cell tumor, under tumor. **2.** Cystic enlargement of a vesicular ovarian (graafian) follicle.

folliculosis (fo-lik-u-lo'sis) Abnormally increased development of lymph follicles.

conjunctival f. A chronic condition, frequently found in children, marked by the presence of multiple tiny lymphatic nodules in the conjunctiva of the lower lids.

folliculus (fo-lik'u-lus), *pl.* **follic'uli** Follicle.

fomentation (fo-mĕn-ta'shun) The therapeutic application of warmth and moisture.

fomes (fo'mēz), *pl.* **fo'mites** Anything (clothing, toys, etc.) capable of transmitting the microorganisms causing a contagious disease.

fontanel, fontanelle (fon-tă-nel') Any of the normally six unossified spaces in the fetal and infant skull, covered by a fibrous membrane. Commonly called soft spot.

anterior f. A diamond-shaped fontanel located at the junction of the frontal, sagittal, and coronal sutures. Also called frontal fontanel; bregmatic fontanel.

anterolateral f. See sphenoidal fontanel.

bregmatic f. See anterior fontanel.

frontal f. See anterior fontanel.

mastoid f. The fontanel on either side at the junction of the mastoid angle of the parietal bone with the mastoid portion of the temporal bone and the occipital bone. Also called posterolateral fontanel.

occipital f. See posterior fontanel.

posterior f. A triangular fontanel at the union of the lambdoid and sagittal sutures. Also called occipital fontanel.

posterolateral f. See mastoid fontanel.

sphenoidal f. An irregularly shaped fontanel located on either side at the junction of the frontal bone with the sphenoidal angle of the parietal bone, the squamous portion of the temporal bone and the greater wing of the sphenoid bone. Also called anterolateral fontanel.

fonticulus (fon-tik'u-lus), *pl.* **fontic'uli** See fontanel.

food (fo͞od) Nourishment, usually of plant or animal origin. Also called aliment.

conventional f. Common food not subjected to unusual processing.

engineered f. Food made from vegetable or synthetic substances. Also called fabricated food.

enriched f. Food to which vitamins (thiamine, niacin, riboflavin) and iron have been added within specified limits. Also called fortified food.

fabricated f. See engineered food.

formulated f. Imitation of common food, such as an imitation dairy product, or new types of food; blended cereal grains, legumes, roots or tubers, and sources of proteins and calories frequently serve as bases.

fortified f. See enriched food.

food analog (fo͞od an'ă-log) Engineered food product designed to look like a traditional food item such as chicken or bacon.

foot (fo͝ot) The distal end of the lower extremity. Also called pes.

athlete's f. See tinea pedis, under tinea.

ball of the f. The anterior padded portion of the sole of the foot.

cavus f. See clawfoot.

claw f. See clawfoot.

club f. See talipes equinovarus, under talipes.

contracted f. See talipes cavus, under talipes.

drop f. See footdrop.

flat f. See flatfoot.

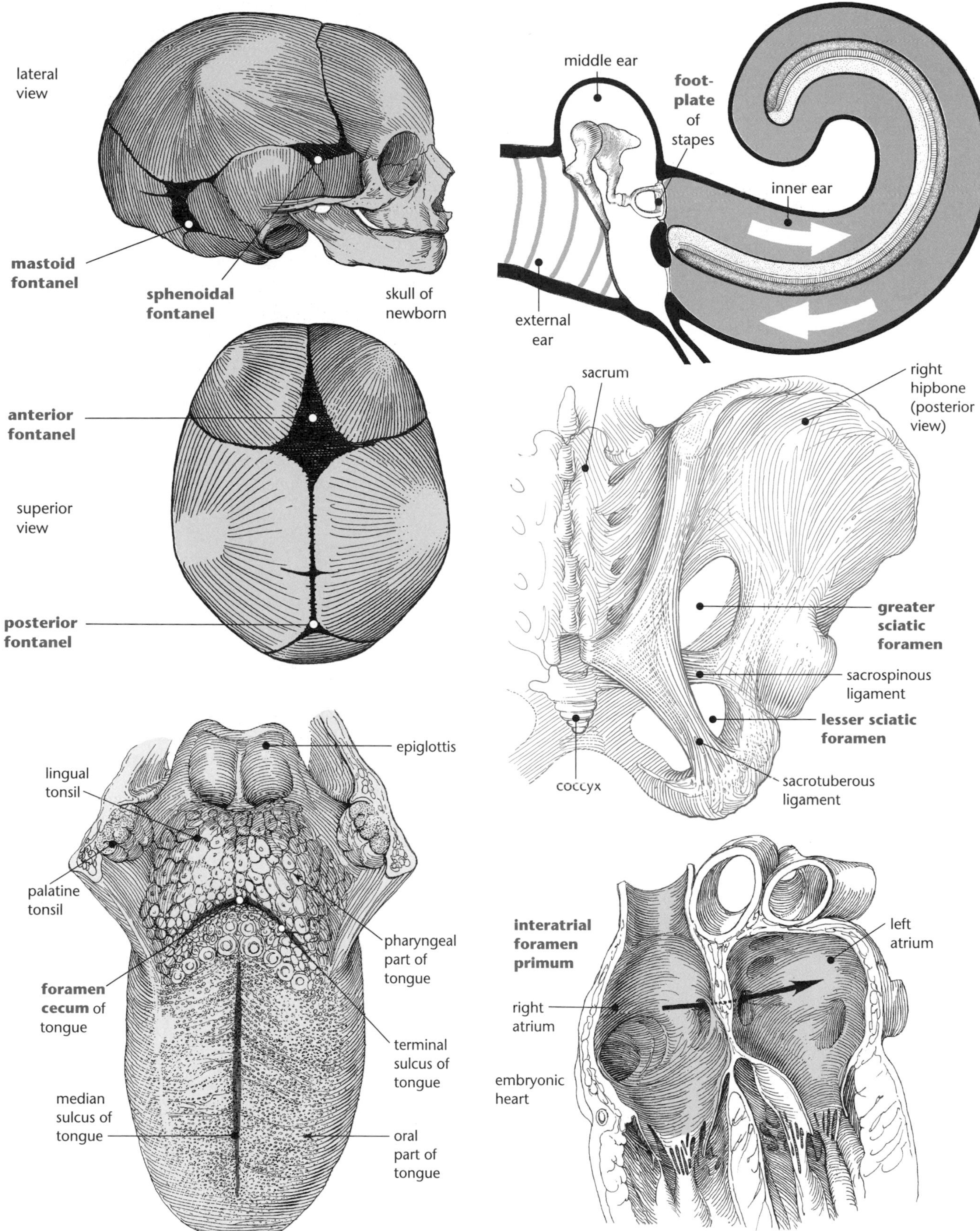

immersion f. A nonfreezing injury to the feet caused by prolonged exposure to cold (not freezing) water or mud; usually includes three clinical stages: *ischemic immersion f.*, initially the feet become cold, numb, swollen, and whitish or purplish; *hyperemic immersion f.*, a few (2 to 3) days after removal from cold, feet become hot, red, painful, blistered, and (in severe cases) bleed and become gangrenous; *posthyperemic immersion f.*, abnormal sensations frequently occur, which may last for years. Also called trench foot.

Madura f. Former name for mycetoma.

splay f. See flatfoot.

trench f. See immersion foot.

foot and mouth disease (fo͝ot ănd mouth dĭ-zēz′) A highly infectious disease of cattle, swine, and sheep; when it occurs in man (rarely), it is characterized by fever and a vesicular eruption of the palms, soles, and the oropharyngeal mucosa.

footcandle (fo͝ot′kan-dl) A unit of illumination on a surface one foot distant from a uniform point source of light of one candela, equal to one lumen per square foot; replaced in the International System of Units by the candela.

footdrop (fo͝ot′drop) Paralysis or weakness of the dorsiflexor muscles of the foot and ankle causing the foot to fall and the toes to drag on the ground during walking. Also called toe drop.

footplate (fo͝ot′plāt) The base of the stapes (smallest ossicle) of the middle ear chamber which is attached

THE **FORAMINA** AT BASE OF CRANIUM AND STRUCTURES TRANSMITTED THROUGH THEM

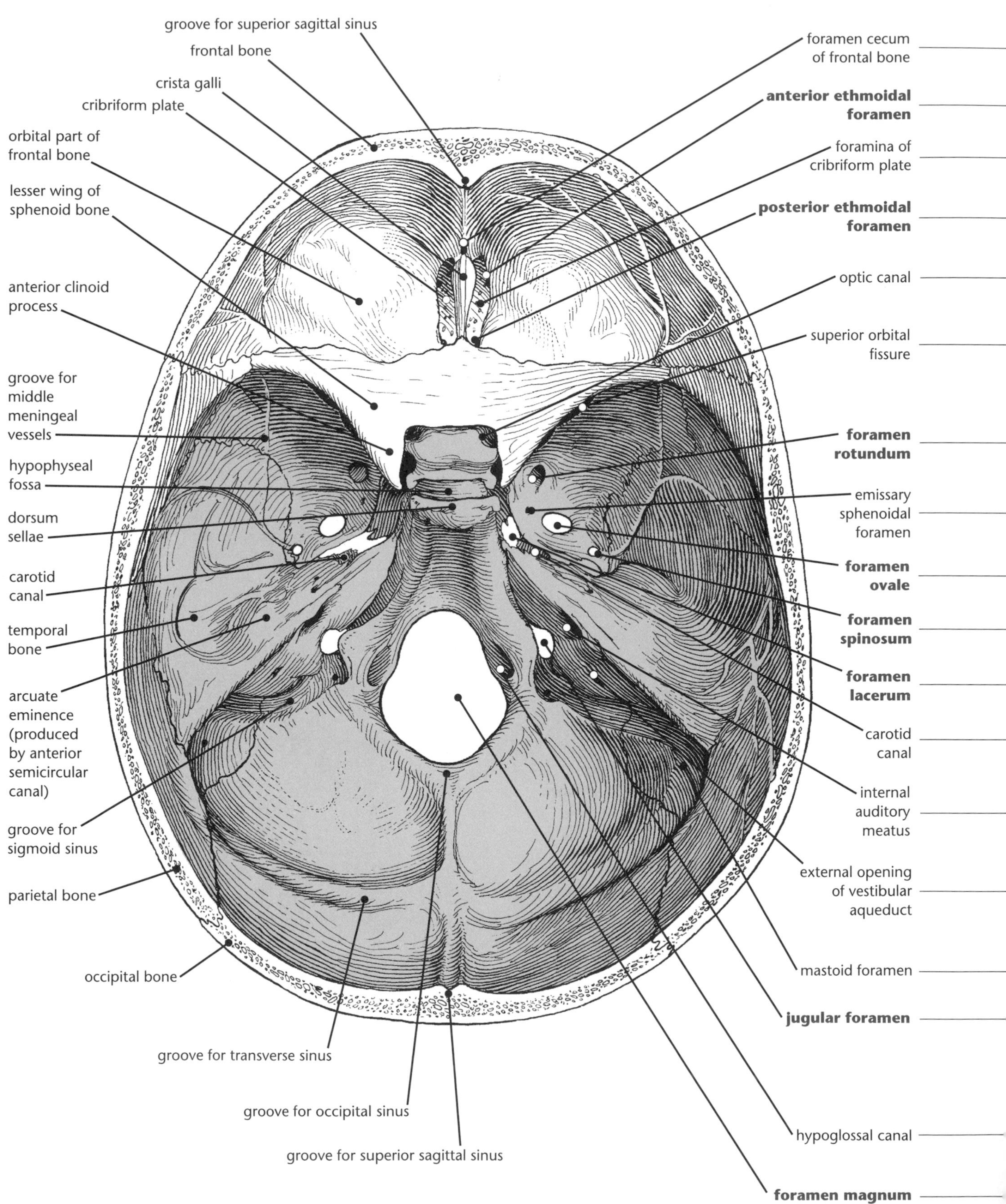
groove for superior sagittal sinus
frontal bone
crista galli
cribriform plate
orbital part of frontal bone
lesser wing of sphenoid bone
anterior clinoid process
groove for middle meningeal vessels
hypophyseal fossa
dorsum sellae
carotid canal
temporal bone
arcuate eminence (produced by anterior semicircular canal)
groove for sigmoid sinus
parietal bone
occipital bone
groove for transverse sinus
groove for occipital sinus
groove for superior sagittal sinus
foramen cecum of frontal bone
anterior ethmoidal foramen
foramina of cribriform plate
posterior ethmoidal foramen
optic canal
superior orbital fissure
foramen rotundum
emissary sphenoidal foramen
foramen ovale
foramen spinosum
foramen lacerum
carotid canal
internal auditory meatus
external opening of vestibular aqueduct
mastoid foramen
jugular foramen
hypoglossal canal
foramen magnum

STRUCTURES TRANSMITTED

emissary veins to superior sagittal sinus

anterior ethmoidal artery, vein and more

olfactory nerve

posterior ethmoidal artery, vein and nerve

optic (2nd cranial) nerve, opthalmic artery, meninges

oculomotor (3rd cranial) nerve, trochlear (4th cranial) nerve, terminal branches of opthalmic nerve, abducent (6th cranial) nerve, opthalmic veins)

maxillary nerve

emissary vein from cavernous sinus

mandibular nerve, accessory meningeal artery, lesser petrosal nerve (inconstant)

middle meningeal artery and vein, meningeal branch of mandibular nerve

internal carotid artery and accompanying sympathetic and venous plexus

internal carotid artery

facial (7th cranial) nerve, vestibulocochlear (8th cranial) nerve, nervus intermedius, labyrinthine vessels

endolymphatic duct

emissary vein from sigmoid sinus

glossopharyngeal (9th cranial) nerve, vagus (10th cranial) nerve, accessory (11th cranial nerve), sigmoid sinus, inferior petrosal sinus, posterior meningeal artery

hypoglossal (12th cranial) nerve, meningeal branch of ascending pharyngeal artery

medulla oblongata, spinal roots of accessory (11th cranial) nerve, meningeal branches of vertebral arteries, meninges

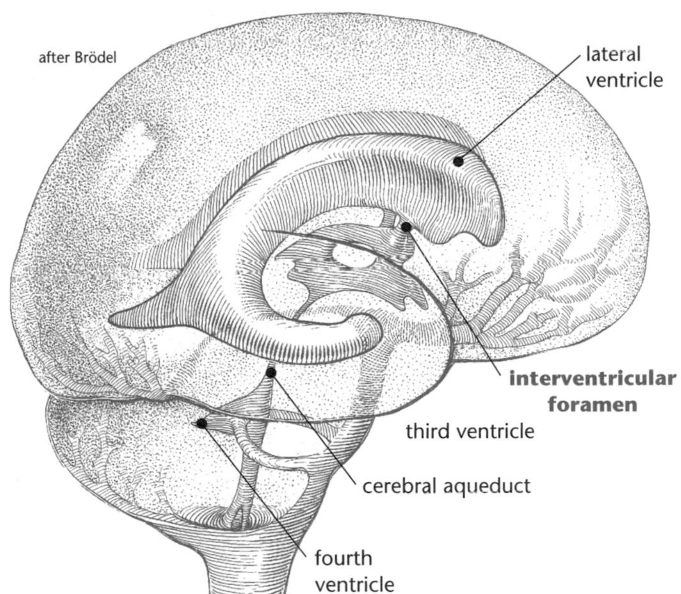

F

to the oval window by the annular ligament.

foramen (fo-ra´men), *pl.* **fora″mina** A natural opening through a bone or a membranous structure; a short passage.

apical dental f. The opening at the tip of the root of a tooth through which pass the vessels and nerves supplying the pulp.

carotid f. The inferior opening of the carotid canal giving passage to the internal carotid artery.

f. cecum The pit on the dorsal surface of the tongue representing the remains of the upper portion of the embryonic thyroglossal duct.

epiploic f. The opening connecting the two sacs of the peritoneum, namely the greater sac and the lesser sac (omental bursa). Also called Winslow's foramen.

ethmoidal f. One of two openings (anterior and posterior) in the orbit, giving passage to vessels and nerves.

great f. See foramen ovale.

greater sciatic f. A large opening bounded by the sacrum, the greater sciatic notch of the hipbone, and the sacrotuberous and sacrospinous ligaments.

incisal f. The relatively large opening in the midline of the hard palate just behind the central incisors; the opening of the nasopalatine canal.

inferior dental f. See mandibular foramen.

infraorbital f. The external opening of the infraorbital canal, on the anterior aspect of the maxilla.

interatrial f. primum **1.** The temporary opening of the embryonic heart between the right and left atria. Also called ostium primum. **2.** The abnormal persistence of such an opening in the adult heart.

interatrial f. secundum A secondary opening appearing in the embryonic heart between the right and left atria, just prior to the closure of the interatrial foramen primum. Also called ostium secundum.

interventricular f. An oval opening between the third and lateral ventricles of the brain. Also called foramen of Monro.

intervertebral f. One of several openings into the spinal canal formed by adjoining vertebrae.

jugular f. Opening located between the lateral portion of the occipital bone and the petrous portion of the temporal bone.

f. lacerum The opening between the apex of the petrous portion of the temporal bone and the body of the sphenoid bone; during life, it is closed with fibrous tissue, giving passage only to the small nerve of the pterygoid canal and a small meningeal branch of the ascending pharyngeal artery. Also called lacerated foramen.

lesser sciatic f. An opening bounded by the lesser sciatic notch and the sacrotuberous and sacrospinous ligaments.

f. of Luschka See lateral aperture of the fourth ventricle, under aperture.

f. of Magendi See median aperture of the fourth ventricle, under aperture.

f. magnum The large opening at the base of the skull through which passes the spinal cord. Also called great foramen.

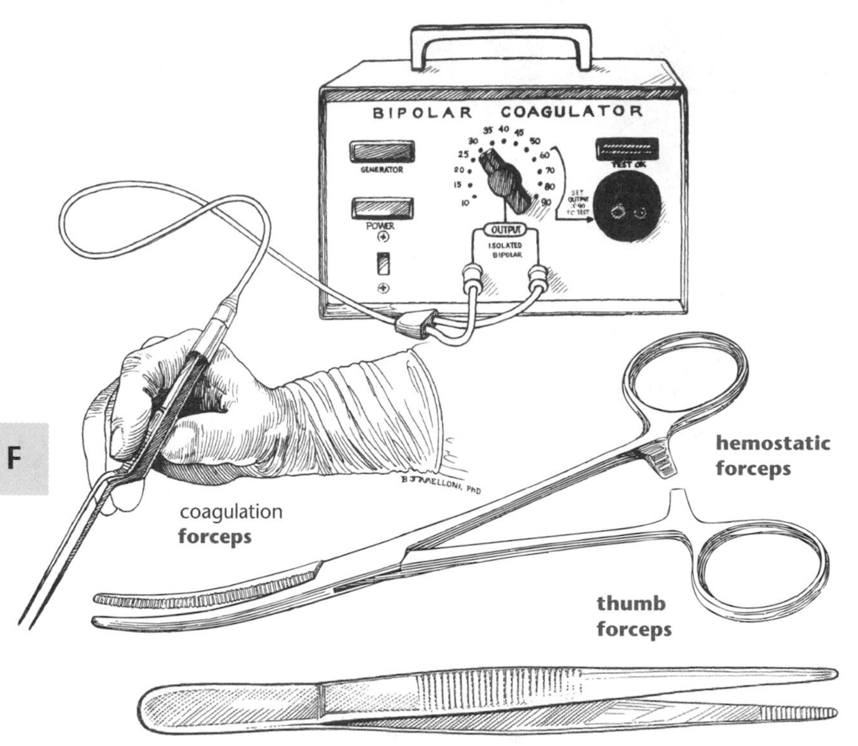

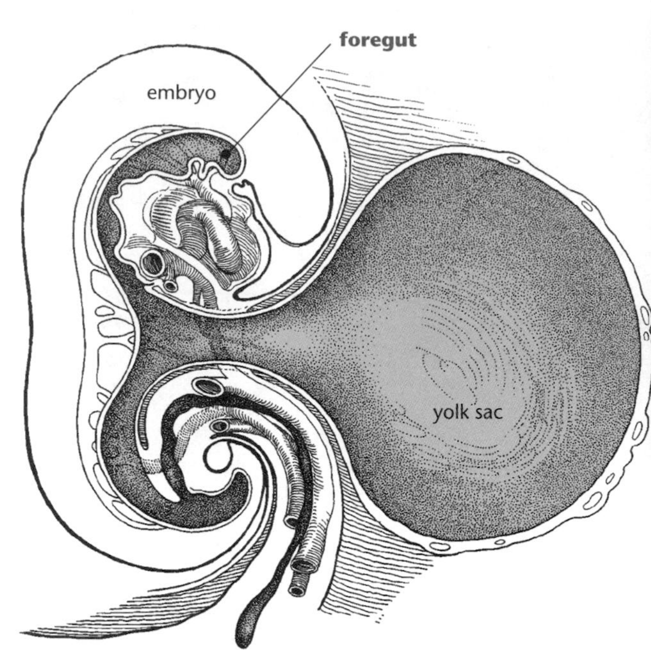

mandibular f. An opening located in the medial aspect of each ramus of the mandible. Also called inferior dental foramen.

mental f. One of two lateral openings on the body of the lower jaw, usually beneath the second bicuspid tooth. Also called mental canal.

f. of Monro See interventricular foramen.

obturator f. The large opening in the hipbone bounded by the pubis and ischium; it is almost completely closed by the obturator membrane except for a small gap (obturator canal) through which the obturator nerve and vessels pass as they leave the pelvis to enter the thigh.

optic f. See optic canal, under canal.

f. ovale (a) The oval opening between the atria of the fetal heart. (b) A large opening in the great wing of the sphenoid bone, through which pass the third portion of the trigeminal nerve and the small meningeal artery.

f. quadratum See foramen of the vena cava.

palatine foramina Anterior and posterior openings on either side of the hard palate.

f. rotundum An opening located in the great wing of the sphenoid bone, through which passes the maxillary nerve.

f. spinosum An opening located in the great wing of the sphenoid bone, transmitting the middle meningeal artery.

stylomastoid f. An opening on the petrous portion of the temporal bone, between the styloid and mastoid processes; it affords passage to the facial nerve and the stylomastoid artery.

supraorbital f. A canal or groove in the supraorbital margin of the frontal bone that gives passage to the supraorbital nerve and vessels. Also called supraorbital notch.

f. of the vena cava Opening in the diaphragm giving passage to the inferior vena cava. Also called foramen quadratum.

vertebral f. The space between the arch and the body of a vertebra.

Winslow's f. See epiploic foramen.

foramina (fo-ram´ĭ-na) Plural of foramen.

Forbes-Albright syndrome (forbz-awl´brīt sin´drōm) Combination of a profuse secretion of milk and absence of the menses, unassociated with recent pregnancy or with acromegaly; believed to be due to oversecretion of the hormone prolactin stimulated by certain pituitary tumors.

force (fōrs) (F) Strength; capacity to produce work or motion, or cause physical change.

electromotive f. (EMF) Force causing the flow of electricity from one point to another, giving rise to an electric current.

f. of mastication Force applied by the muscles during the act of chewing. Also called masticatory force.

masticatory f. See force of mastication.

van der Waals' f.'s The nondescript, attractive forces between atoms or molecules other than electrostatic (ionic), covalent (sharing of electrons), or hydrogen bonding (sharing a proton).

forceps (for´seps) An instrument resembling a pair of tongs, used for grasping, compressing, manipulating, or extracting tissue or specific structures.

alligator f. A long, slender forceps with small jaws, the lower of which is stationary.

Allis f. Forceps with serrated jaws for grasping tissues.

bone f. A strong forceps used for grasping or cutting bone.

bulldog f. A forceps for clamping cut blood vessels.

capsule f. Forceps used for extracting the lens in a cataract operation.

chalazion f. A thumb forceps with a flattened plate at the end of one arm and a ring on the other.

dental extracting f. Forceps used for grasping teeth in order to luxate and extract them from the alveolus.

hemostatic f. A forceps with a catch for locking the blades, used for grasping the cut end of a blood vessel to control hemorrhage.

mosquito f. A very small hemostatic forceps.

needle f. Forceps used for grasping a needle during surgical procedures. Also called needle holder.

obstetrical f. Forceps used for grasping and making traction on the fetal head in a difficult labor.

thumb f. Forceps used by compression with thumb and forefinger for grasping soft tissue; used especially during suturing.

forearm (for´arm) The part of the upper extremity between the elbow and wrist. Also called antebrachium.

forebrain (for´brān) See prosencephalon.

forefinger (for´fĭng-ger) See index finger, under finger.

foregut (for´gut) The cephalic portion of the primitive digestive tract in the embryo. Also called headgut.

foremilk (for´milk) Popular name for colostrum.

forensic (fo-ren´zik) Relating to or used in legal proceedings.

foreplay (for´plā) Sexual stimulation leading to sexual intercourse.

foreskin (for´skin) See prepuce.

forewaters (for´wah-terz) In obstetrics, the part of the amniotic sac that pouches into the cervix in front of the fetal head or presenting part.

form (form) Shape; mold.

accolé f. See appliqué form.

appliqué f. A ring of young species of the malarial parasite *Plasmodium falciparum* that parasitize the marginal portion of red blood cells. Also called accolé form.

convenience f. In dentistry, a form modified beyond the basic to allow access of instrumentation for the preparation of a cavity or the insertion of the restorative material.

L-f. See L-phase variant, under variant.

resistance f. In dentistry, the shape given to the prepared cavity of a tooth to enable the restoration to withstand the stress of mastication.

retention f. In dentistry, the provision made in the prepared cavity of a tooth to prevent displacement of the restoration by lateral forces as well as the stress of mastication.

sickle f. See malarial crescent, under crescent.

formaldehyde (for-mal´dĕ-hīd) A colorless, pungent, gaseous aldehyde, CH_2O, used in solution as a disinfectant and preservative.

formalin (for´mă-lin) A 37% aqueous solution of formaldehyde. Also called formol.

formation (for-ma´shun) **1.** The process of giving form or producing. **2.** Something that is formed.

personality f. The development or structure of the components of the personality.

reaction f. The development of conscious atti-tudes that are the opposite of unacceptable impulses the person harbors consciously or unconsciously.

reticular f. A collection of intermingled fibers and gray matter in the pons, the anterolateral portion of the medulla oblongata, and the cervical spinal cord. Also called reticular substance.

rouleaux f. The arrangement of red blood cells in groups resembling stacks of coins.

forme fruste (form froost), *pl.* **formes frustes** French expression for a partial or atypical form of a disease.

formic (for´mik) Relating to ants.

f. acid A colorless caustic liquid, HCOOH, used in solution as an astringent and counterirritant; it occurs naturally in ants and other insects.

formication (for-mĭ-ka´shun) A paresthesia in which there is an abnormal tactile sensation of ants or other small insects crawling over the skin.

formiminoglutamic acid (for-mim-ĭ-no-gloo-tam´ik as´id) (FIGlu) An intermediate metabolite of histidine which can appear in the urine of folic acid-deficient individuals.

formol (for´mol) See formalin.

formula (for´mu-lă) **1.** A symbolic representation of the composition of a chemical substance. **2.** An established group of symbols that express a concept. **3.** A recipe of ingredients in fixed proportion; e.g., a

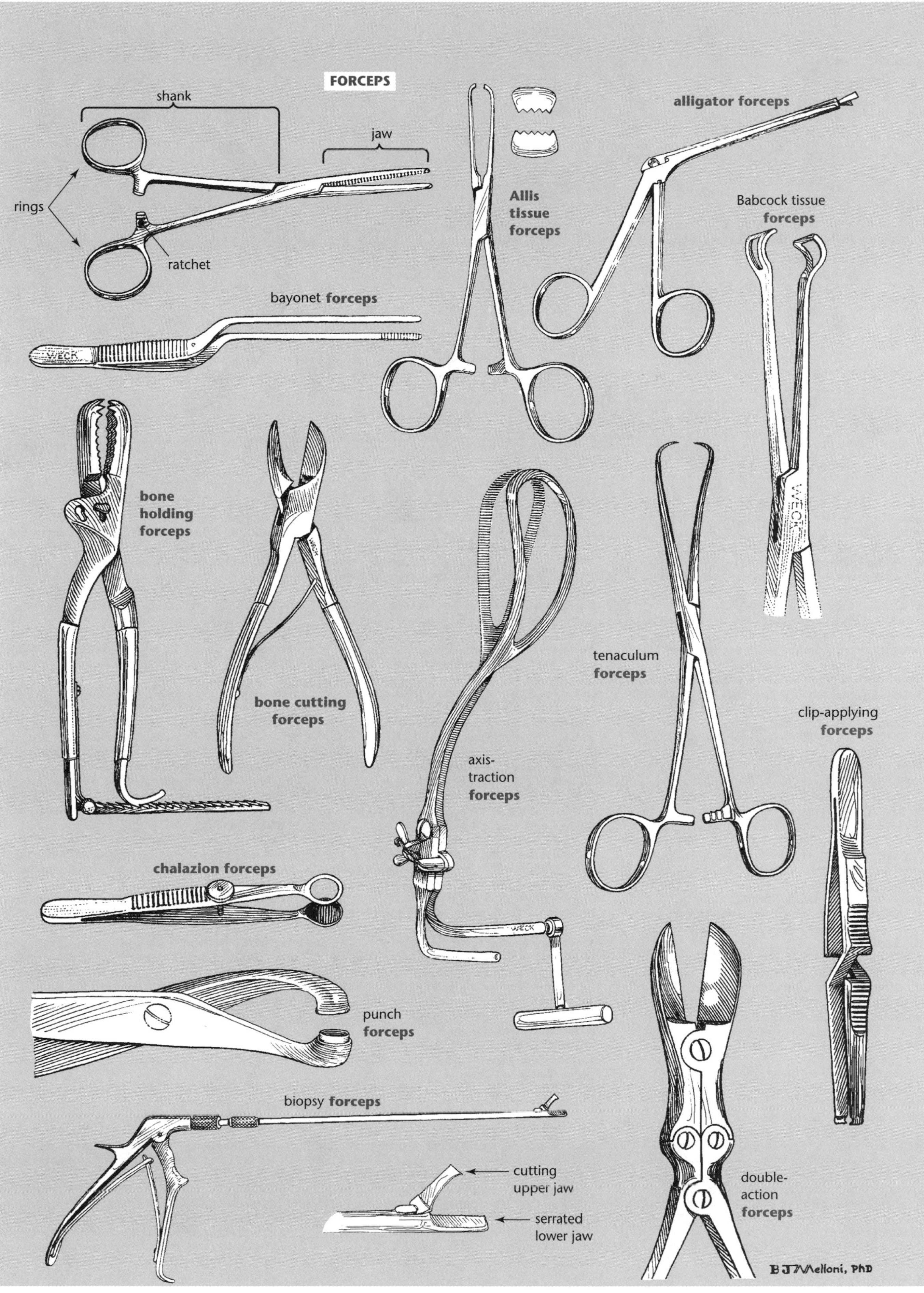
FORCEPS
shank
jaw
rings
ratchet
bayonet forceps
Allis tissue forceps
alligator forceps
Babcock tissue forceps
bone holding forceps
bone cutting forceps
tenaculum forceps
clip-applying forceps
axis-traction forceps
chalazion forceps
punch forceps
biopsy forceps
cutting upper jaw
serrated lower jaw
double-action forceps
BJ Melloni, PhD

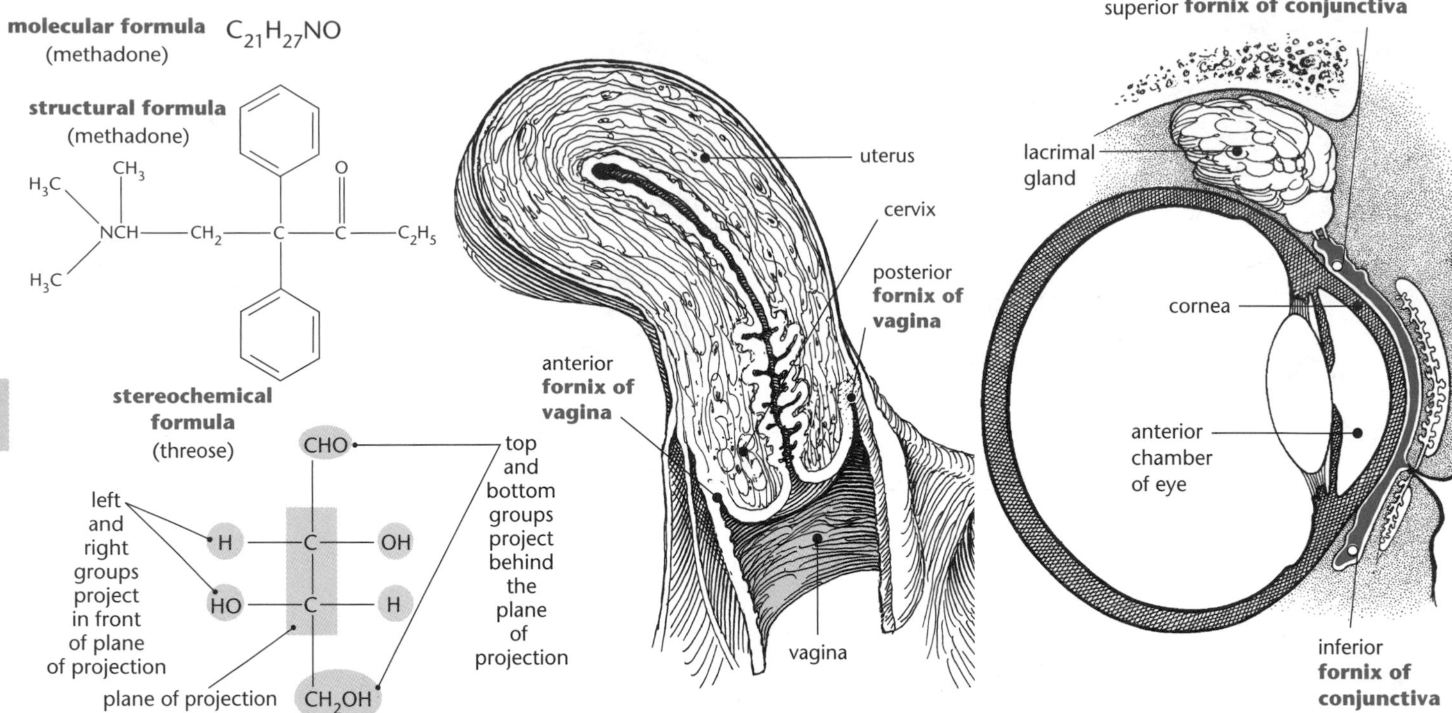

milk mixture for feeding an infant. **4.** A prescription containing directions for the preparation of a medicine.

Arneth f. A formula that expresses the approximate ratio of polymorphonuclear neutrophils in normal individuals, based on the number of lobes in the nuclei, as follows: 1 lobe, 5%; 2 lobes, 35%; 3 lobes, 41%; 4 lobes, 17%; 5 lobes, 2%.

Bazett's f. A formula for correcting the observed electrocardiogram Q – T interval for cardiac rate: corrected Q – T equals Q – T seconds divided by the square root of R – R seconds.

Bernhardt's f. A formula for determining the ideal weight, in kilograms, for an adult: the height in centimeters multiplied by the chest circumference in centimeters divided by 240.

DuBois f. A formula for determining the body's surface area from the height (in cm) and weight (in kg) of an individual: $A = H^{0.725} \times W^{0.425} \times$ constant 71.84.

Fischer's projection f. A two-dimensional representation of three-dimensional molecules in which the carbon chain is depicted vertically.

Gorlin f. A formula for calculating the area of the orifice of a cardiac valve, based on the flow across the valve and the mean pressures in the chambers on either side of the valves.

graphic f. See structural formula.

molecular f. A chemical formula depicting the number of atoms of each element in the molecules of a substance.

spatial f. See stereochemical formula.

stereochemical f. A formula depicting a spatial representation of the relative positions of the linked atoms, and the numbers of atoms of each element present in a molecule of a substance.

structural f. A graphic chemical formula showing the linkage of the atoms and groups of atoms, as well as their kind and number.

formulary (for´mu-lar-e) A collection of formulas for the preparation of medicines.

formyl (for´mĭl) The radical HCO– of formic acid.

fornix (for´niks), *pl.* **fornices** Any arched structure, or the space created by such a structure.

f. of cerebrum A harp-shaped, bilateral structure in the brain, composed of two posterior pillars (crura of the fornix), the body, and two anterior pillars (columns of the fornix); it is situated under the corpus callosum and is made up of white fibers arising from the hippocampus and terminating mainly in the mamillary bodies.

f. of conjunctiva The space formed by the reflection of the conjunctiva from the upper eyelid to the eyeball (superior fornix) and from the eyeball to the lower eyelid (inferior fornix).

f. of vagina The space between the vaginal wall and the uterine cervix.

fossa (fos´ă), *pl.* **fossae** A pit or depression.

acetabular f. A circular, nonarticular depression on the floor of the acetabulum; it lodges a mass of fat.

amygdaloid f. The hollow between the anterior and posterior pillars of the fauces containing the pharyngeal tonsil.

axillary f. The armpit; axilla.

coronoid f. The depression on the anterior aspect of the lower end of the humerus where the coronoid process of the ulna rests during full flexion of the forearm.

cranial f. One of three depressions (anterior, middle, and posterior) on the internal aspect of the base of the skull lodging the cerebrum and cerebellum.

cubital f. The depression in front of the elbow. Also called bend of the elbow; antecubital space.

glenoid f. The depression in the head of the scapula for articulation with the head of the humerus forming the shoulder joint.

greater supraclavicular f. The triangular depression on each side of the neck above the clavicle, bounded by the lateral border of the sternocleidomastoid muscle, the clavicle, and the omohyoid muscle.

hyaloid f. The concavity on the anterior aspect of the vitreous body in which the lens of the eye lies. Also called lenticular fossa.

hypophysial f. A pit on the sphenoid bone lodging the pituitary gland. Also called pituitary fossa.

lacrimal f. One located in the medial wall of the orbit, formed by the frontal process of the maxilla and the lacrimal bone; it houses the lacrimal sac.

lenticular f. See hyaloid fossa.

lesser supraclavicular f. The space between the two heads of origin of the sternocleidomastoid muscle. Also called Zang's space.

mandibular f. One of two depressions on the temporal bone that receives the condyle of the lower jaw.

olecranon f. A depression on the back of the lower end of the humerus in which the olecranon process of the ulna rests when the elbow is extended.

f. ovalis (a) A depression on the septal wall of the right atrium representing the site of the foramen ovale of the fetal heart. (b) The saphenous opening in the upper thigh, below and lateral to the pubic tubercle, giving passage to the great saphenous vein.

pituitary f. See hypophysial fossa.

popliteal f. The diamond-shaped space at the back of the knee.

pterygoid f. The fossa between the lateral and medial pterygoid plates of the sphenoid bone.

radial f. A depression on the anterior aspect of the humerus, the site of articulation with the radius.

submandibular f. See submandibular fovea, under fovea.

tonsillar f. The depression between the palatoglossal and palatopharyngeal arches occupied by the palatine tonsil.

fossette (fos-et´) A small deep ulcer of the cornea.

fossula (fos´u-lă), *pl.* **fossulae** **1.** A small depression. **2.** One of several small depressions on the surface of the cerebrum.

fossulate (fos´u-lāt) Containing many small depressions.

Foster Kennedy's syndrome (fōs´tĕr kĕn´ĕ-dē sin´drōm) See Kennedy's syndrome.

foundation (foun-da´shun) A base, especially one that provides support to a structure.

denture f. The portion of the oral structures that supports a denture.

fourchette (fo͞or-shet´) See frenulum of labia minora, under frenulum.

fovea (fo´ve-ă), *pl.* **foveae** A small depression.

central f. An area approximately 1.5 mm in diameter in the macula lutea of the retina; it is the area of greatest visual acuity.

submandibular f. A pit on the inner surface of the lower jaw on each side which lodges the submandibular gland. Also called submandibular fossa.

foveate, foveated (fo´ve-āt, fo´ve-ā-ted) Pitted; having small depressions.

foveation (fo-ve-ā´shun) The formation of a pit (e.g., the pitted scar of smallpox).

foveola (fo-ve´o-lă) A minute depression, fovea, or pit.

f. of coccyx A small depression or dimple often present in the skin over the tip of the coccyx.

gastric f. One of the numerous small pits in the gastric mucosa at the bottom of which open the gastric glands.

granular foveolae of Pacchioni See granular foveolae.

granular foveolae Small depressions on the inner surface of the skull, on each side of the sagittal sulcus; they accommodate the arachnoid granulations (pacchionian bodies). Also called granular foveolae of Pacchioni.

foveolate (fo-ve´o-lāt) Having minute depressions or pits on the surface.

Fox-Fordyce disease (foks-for´dīs dĭ-zēz´) An uncommon disease of the apocrine glands affecting mainly women from puberty to menopause; characterized by numerous small, follicular, closely aggregated, flesh-colored, intensely pruritic papules

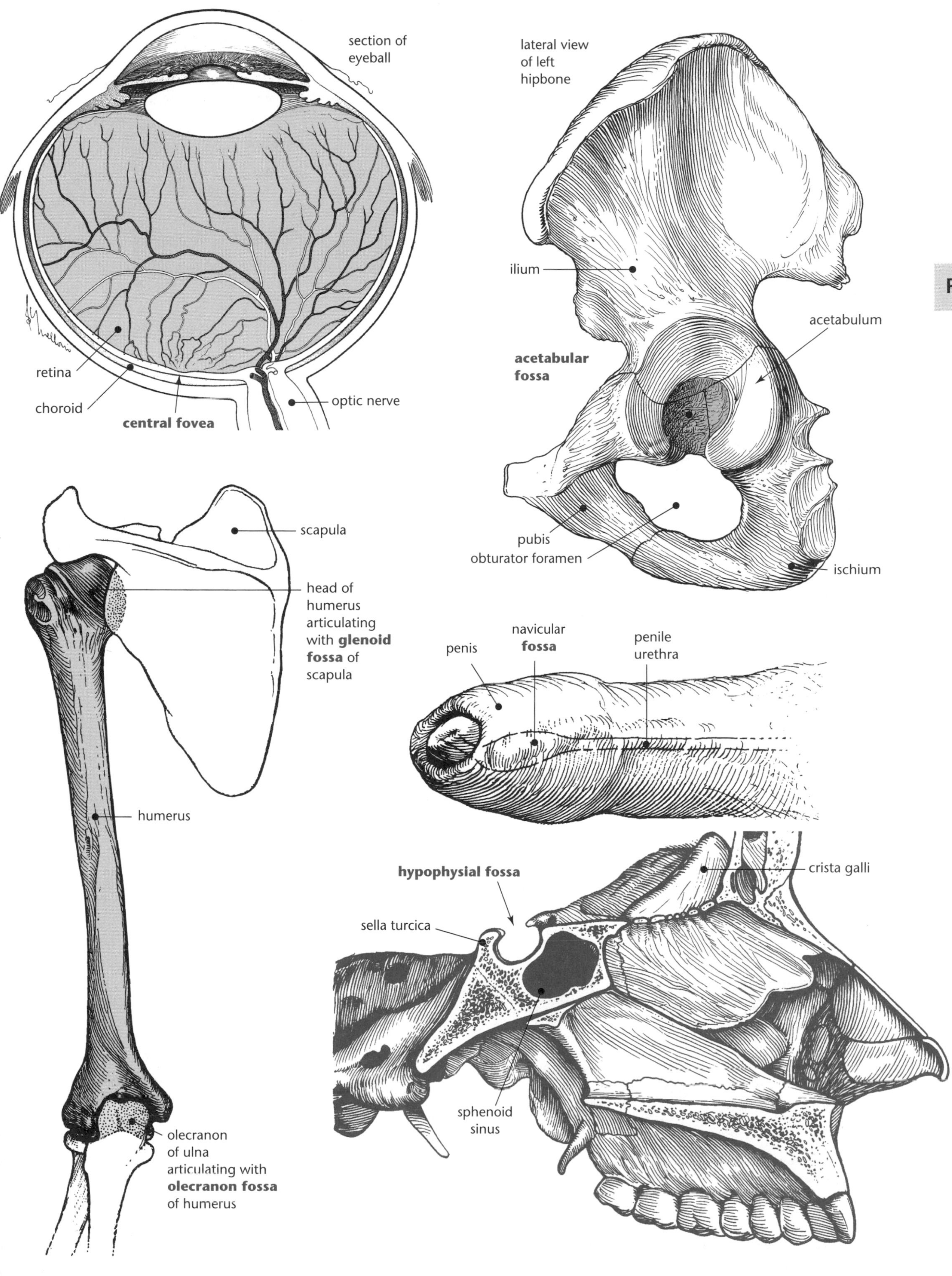
section of
eyeball
retina
choroid
central fovea
optic nerve
lateral view
of left
hipbone
ilium
acetabulum
acetabular
fossa
pubis
obturator foramen
ischium
scapula
head of
humerus
articulating
with glenoid
fossa of
scapula
humerus
olecranon
of ulna
articulating with
olecranon fossa
of humerus
penis
navicular
fossa
penile
urethra
hypophysial fossa
crista galli
sella turcica
sphenoid
sinus

F

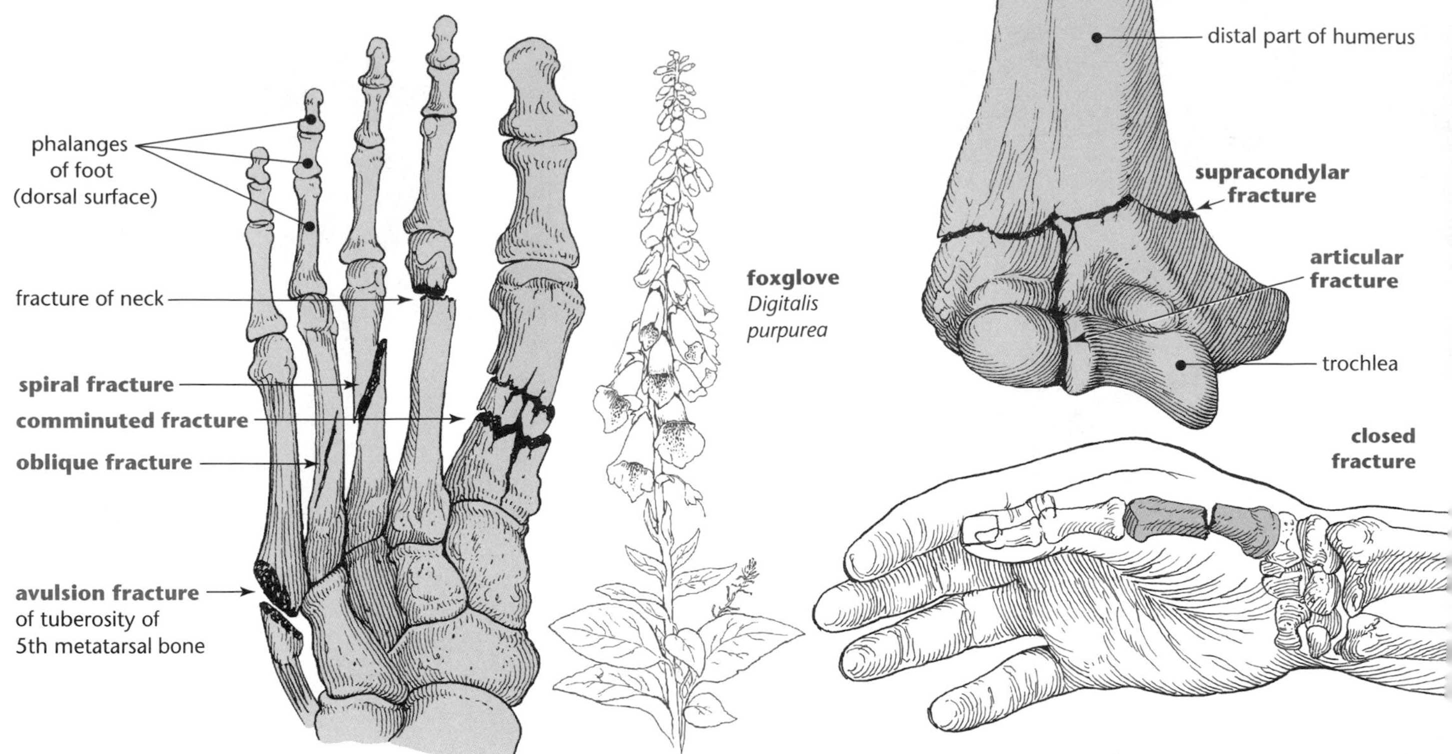

in the armpits and on the breasts, pubic area, and perineum; thought to be due to poral closure of the glands.

foxglove (foks´glov) Any of various plants of the genus *Digitalis* from which the drug digitalis is prepared.

fraction (frak´shun) **1.** A quotient of two quantities. **2.** In chemistry, a component of a substance separated by crystallization or distillation.

blood plasma f. The separated components of plasma.

ejection f. A measure of the ability of the left ventricle of the heart to expel blood.

filtration f. (FF) The fraction of plasma entering the kidney that filters into the renal tubules; glomerular filtration rate/renal plasma flow.

fractionation (frak-shun-a´shun) The breaking up of a total therapeutic dose of radiation into small fractions of low intensity given over a period of time, usually at daily or alternate daily intervals.

fracture (frak´chur) (fx) The breaking of a bone or cartilage.

articular f. A fracture involving the joint surface of a bone.

avulsion f. A breaking off of a small portion of bone at the site of attachment of a tendon or ligament.

basal skull f. A fracture occurring on the floor of the skull.

bimalleolar f. See Pott's fracture.

blowout f. A fracture of the floor of the orbit caused by a blow to the eye.

capillary f. A hairline fracture.

closed f. A fracture in which the skin is not broken. Also called simple fracture.

Colles' f. Fracture of the lower end of the radius bone. Popularly called bayonet deformity; silver fork deformity.

comminuted f. Fracture in which the bone is splintered into several pieces.

compound f. Former name for open fracture.

depressed skull f. A fracture with inward displacement of the skull.

de Quervain's f. A fracture-dislocation of the wrist; specifically, fracture of the scaphoid (navicular) bone, with dislocation of the lunate bone.

Dupuytren's f. Fracture of the lower extremity of the fibula or lateral malleolus, with dislocation of the ankle joint.

extracapsular f. A fracture near but outside of the joint capsule.

fatigue f. Fracture of a metatarsal shaft, usually the second or third, associated with prolonged weightbearing activities as in walking for long periods (e.g., during basic military training), ballet dancing, and athletics; believed to be due to muscle fatigue, when the muscle action is no longer optimal and allows increased loading of the bone. Also called march fracture; stress fracture; Deutschländer's disease.

fissured f. See linear fracture.

greenstick f. An incomplete fracture in which one side of the bone is only bent.

impacted f. A fracture in which one fragment is embedded in the substance of the other and fixed in that position.

incomplete f. A fracture in which the line of fracture does not include the whole bone.

intracapsular f. A fracture within a joint capsule.

linear f. A fracture running parallel with the long axis of the bone. Also called fissured fracture.

longitudinal f. A fracture in which the direction of the fracture line is along the axis of the bone.

march f. See fatigue fracture.

oblique f. A fracture running obliquely to the axis of the bone.

occult f. Condition in which originally there is no evidence of a fracture, but after three or four weeks an x-ray image shows new bone formation.

open f. A fracture that is accompanied by an open wound through which the broken bone may protrude. Formerly called compound fracture.

periosteal f. A fracture occurring beneath the periosteum, without displacement.

Pott's f. A fracture-dislocation of the ankle joint; specifically, fracture of the medial malleollus of the tibia, with fracture of the lower extremity of the fibula (lateral malleolus) and dislocation of the ankle joint. Also called bimalleolar fracture.

simple f. See closed fracture.

spiral f. Fracture of a long bone in which the fracture line runs in a spiral direction around the shaft of the bone; caused by a twisting force.

sprain f. Avulsion fracture.

stellate f. A fracture with several break lines radiating from a central point.

strain f. The breaking off by sudden force of a piece of bone attached to a tendon or ligament.

stress f. See fatigue fracture.

supracondylar f. A fracture in the distal end of the humerus.

transcervical f. A fracture through the neck of the femur.

transcondylar f. A fracture through the condyles of the humerus.

transverse f. A fracture in which the break line runs perpendicular to the axis of the bone.

fracture-dislocation (frak´chur- dis-lo-ka´shun) Dislocation and fracture of a bone near its articulation.

fragile X syndrome (fră-jil ĕks sĭn´drōm) Inherited defect of the X chromosome causing mental retardation and large testicles, ears, and chin in males, and mild retardation in females.

fragility (fră-jil´ĭ-te) Brittleness; tendency to break or disintegrate.

capillary f. Increased susceptibility of capillary walls to rupture.

erythrocyte f. Fragility of red blood cells due to mechanical trauma or when the saline content of the blood is altered.

fragment (frag´ment) A small detached piece from a larger entity.

Fab f.'s The two fragments of the immunoglobulin molecule, each containing an antigen-binding site, derived by the enzymatic action of papain.

Fc f. The crystallizable fragment of the immunoglobulin molecule, derived by the enzymatic action of pepsin.

frambesia (fram-be´zhă) See yaws.

frame (frām) A structure designed to immobilize or give support to a part.

Balkan f. An overhead bar supported from the floor or bedposts to suspend a fractured limb. Also called Balkan splint.

Foster f. A reversible bed similar to a Stryker frame.

Stryker f. A device that supports the patient and allows turning without individual motion of parts.

framework (frām´work) **1.** Stroma. **2.** In dentistry, the skeletal portion of a partial denture around which and to which the remaining portions of the prosthesis are attached.

frameshift (frām´shift) See frameshift mutation, under mutation.

Franceschetti's syndrome See mandibulofacial dysostosis, under dysostosis.

Francisella tularensis (fran-sĭ-sel´ă too-lă-ren´sis) A gram-negative, aerobic bacterium that causes tularemia in humans; transmitted from wild animals by bloodsucking insects or by drinking contaminated water. Formerly called *Pasteurella tularensis.*

francium (fran´se-ŭm) An unstable radioactive metallic element; symbol Fr, atomic number 87, with mass number 223; the heaviest member of the alkali family of elements: the most stable of its isotopes has a half-life of 21 minutes.

frank (frahngk) Clinically evident.

freckle (frek´kl) A brownish spot on the skin. Also called ephelis.

freeze-drying (frēz-drī´ing) A method of tissue preparation in which the tissue specimen is instantly frozen and then dehydrated in a high vacuum.

freeze-etching (frēz-ech´ing) A method of tissue preparation in which the tissue specimen is instantly

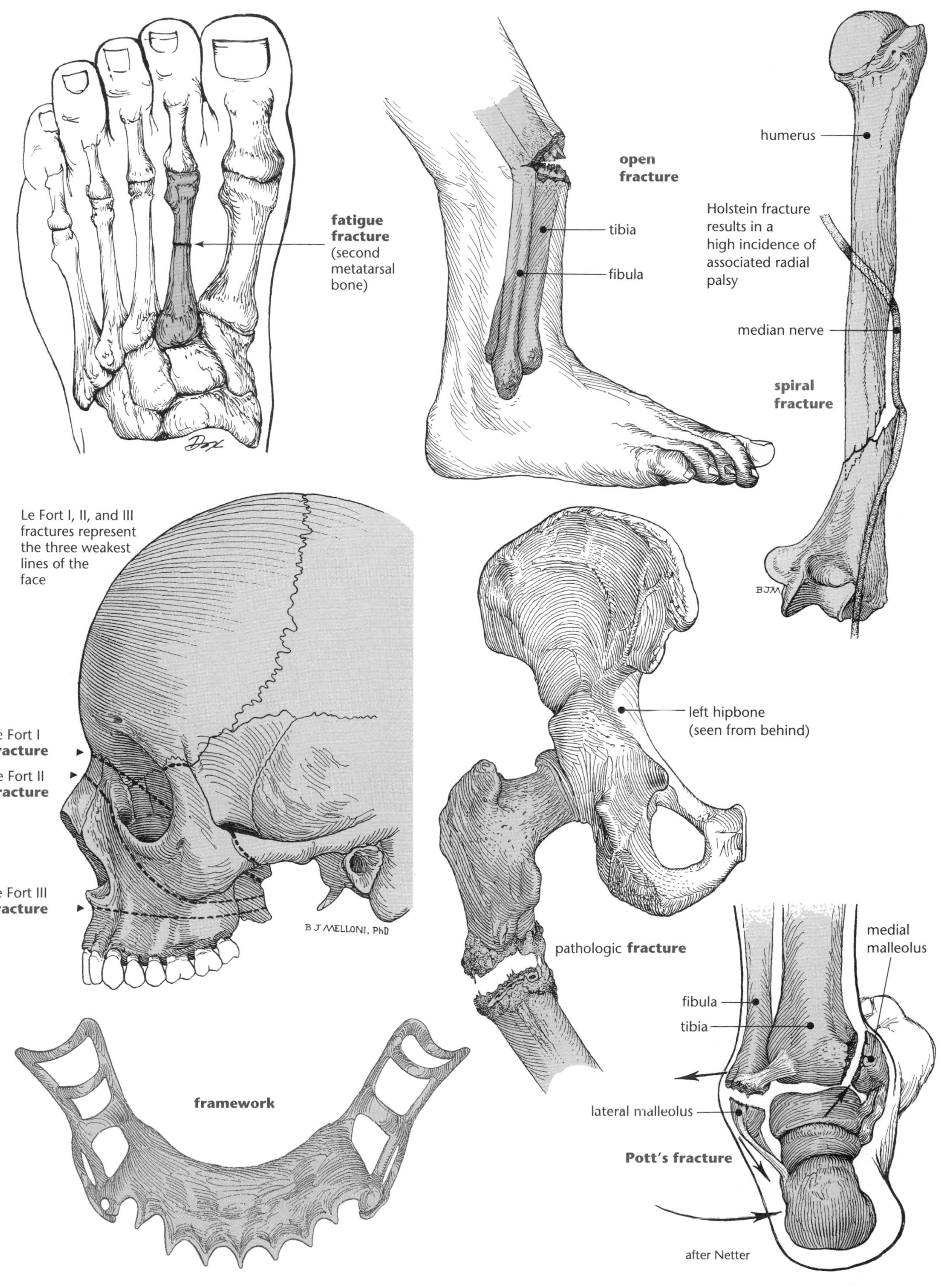
fatigue fracture (second metatarsal bone)
open fracture
tibia
fibula
humerus
Holstein fracture results in a high incidence of associated radial palsy
median nerve
spiral fracture
BJM
Le Fort I, II, and III fractures represent the three weakest lines of the face
Le Fort I fracture
Le Fort II fracture
Le Fort III fracture
BJ MELLONI, PhD
left hipbone (seen from behind)
pathologic fracture
medial malleolus
fibula
tibia
lateral malleolus
Pott's fracture
after Netter
framework

F

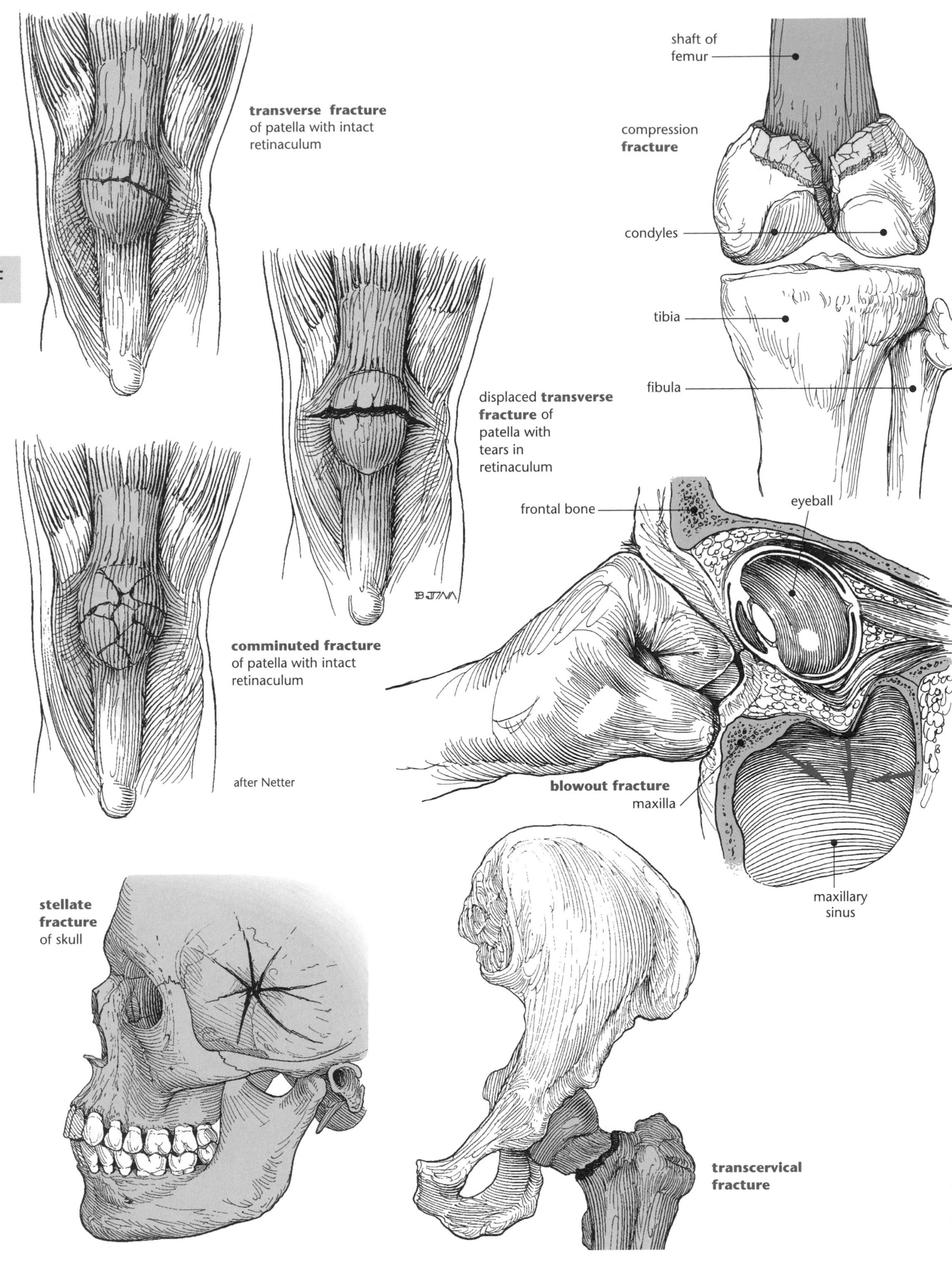
transverse fracture
of patella with intact
retinaculum
displaced transverse
fracture of
patella with
tears in
retinaculum
comminuted fracture
of patella with intact
retinaculum
after Netter
shaft of
femur
compression
fracture
condyles
tibia
fibula
frontal bone
eyeball
blowout fracture
maxilla
maxillary
sinus
stellate
fracture
of skull
transcervical
fracture

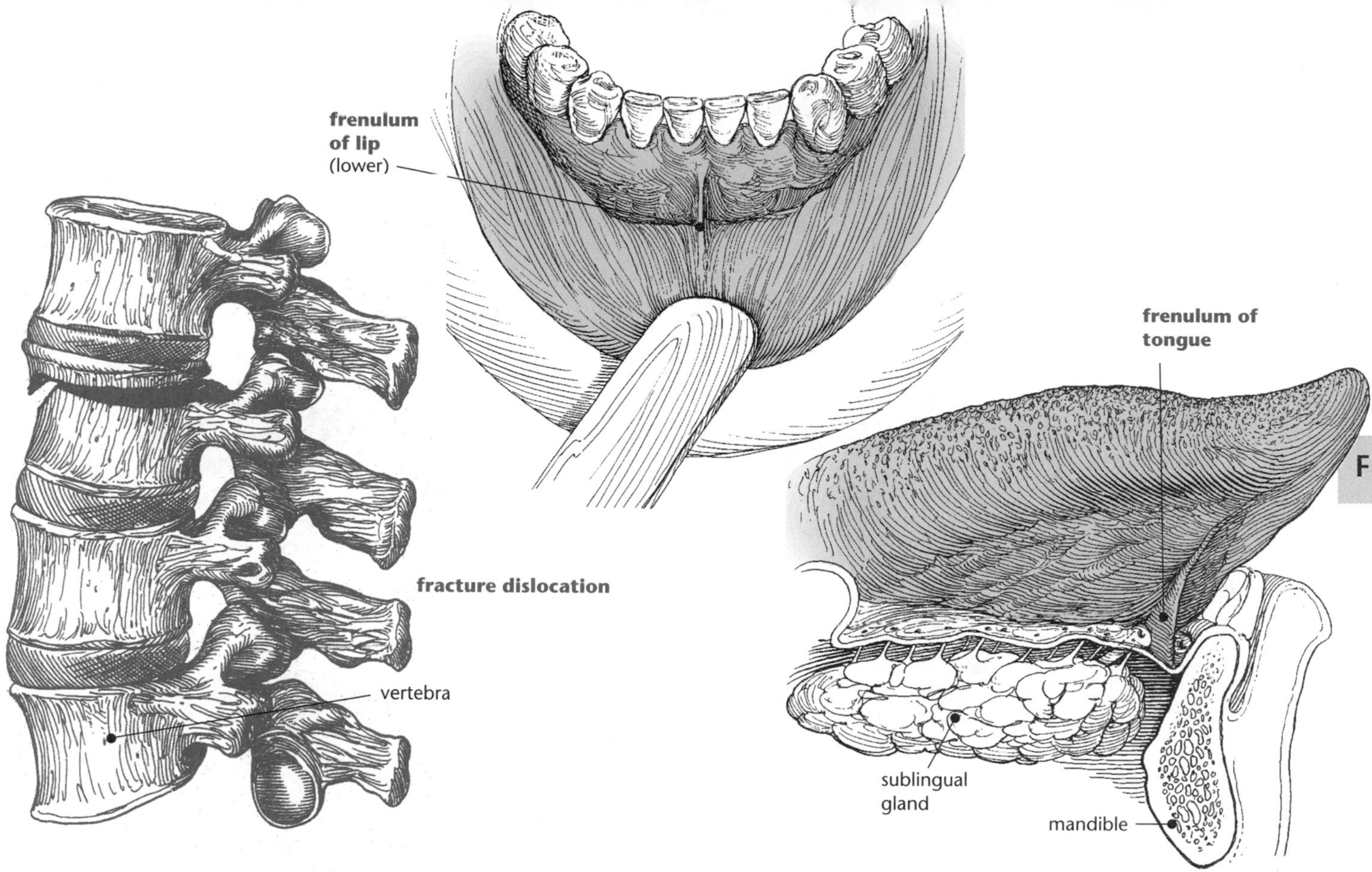

frozen (–190°C), fragments are splinted away, and then the ice is sublimed away in a vacuum to a depth of about 100 Å; it produces an etching effect especially suitable for the study of the inner surface of plasma membranes.

freezing (frēz´ing) Hardening from exposure to low temperatures.

gastric f. Freezing the secretory cells of the stomach to reduce the secretion of gastric acid; used in the treatment of peptic ulcer.

fremitus (frem´ĭ-tus) A vibration usually produced in the chest and felt on palpation.

pleural f. Vibration produced by the rubbing together of the roughened surfaces of the pleural membranes, as in pleurisy.

tactile f. Vibration felt by the hand when placed on the chest of a person speaking.

vocal f. Vibration in the chest produced by the spoken voice.

frenectomy (fre-nek´tŏ-me) The surgical removal of a frenum.

frenotomy (fre-not´ŏ-me) The dividing of the frenulum of the tongue for the relief of tongue-tie.

frenulum (fren´u-lum), *pl.* **fren´ula** A small fold of mucous membrane that extends from a fixed to a movable part and limits the motion of the movable part. Also called frenum.

f. of clitoris A fold connecting the undersurface of the clitoris with the labia minora.

f. of ileocecal valve The prolongation of the two semilunar lips of the ileocecal "valve" that coalesce and project into the lumen of the large intestine as a narrow membranous ridge; it is at the junction of the ileum and the large intestine. Also called frenulum of Morgagni.

f. of labia minora The posterior union of the two labia minora. Also called fourchette; frenulum of pudendal lips.

f. of lips Either one of the folds extending from the gums to the midline of the upper or lower lips. Also called frenulum labii.

f. of Morgagni See frenulum of ileocecal valve.

f. of prepuce A fold that unites the foreskin (prepuce) to the undersurface of the glans penis.

f. of pudendal lips See frenulum of labia minora.

f. of tongue A fold extending from the midline of the undersurface of the tongue to the floor of the mouth. Also called frenulum linguae.

frenum (fre´num), *pl.* **frena** See frenulum.

frequency (fre´kwen-se) The number of regular recurrences of a given event.

critical flicker fusion f., critical fusion f. The minimal number of intermittent or discontinuous visual stimuli per second that gives rise to a continuous visual sensation obliterating the flicker.

dominant f. The particular frequency appearing most frequently in an electroencephalogram (EEG).

urinary f. Urination at intervals that are shorter than usual for a given person, without increase in daily output of urine. It is normal in pregnancy.

friable (frī´ă-bl) Crumbly; easily torn or damaged.

fricative (frik´ă-tiv) In phonetics, a sound produced by the forcing of breath through a narrow orifice, as the sounds of the letters f, v, s, z.

frigid (frij´id) **1.** Very cold. **2.** Abnormally lacking the desire for sexual intercourse; said chiefly of women. **3.** Unable to achieve orgasm during sexual intercourse.

frigidity (frĭ-jid´ĭ-te) A psychologically based inability to respond adequately to a sexual relationship; said chiefly of women.

fringe (frĭnj) See fimbria.

fringing (frĭnj´ing) Bulbous deformation of the calyx of the kidney and tortuous elongation of the stem sometimes seen in the early stages of tuberculosis of the kidney.

Fröhlich's syndrome (frer´liks sin´drōm) See adiposogenital dystrophy, under dystrophy.

Froin's syndrome (frwahnz sin´drōm) Clear yellow color of the lumbar spinal fluid with increased protein content and rapid coagulation, indicating that the communication between the lumbar region and the cerebral ventricles has been cut off; seen in certain organic nervous diseases.

frons (fronz) Latin for forehead.

frontal (frŭn´tal) Relating to the forehead.

frostbite (frost´bīt) Local condition of varying degrees of severity caused by freezing of tissues upon exposure to extreme cold temperatures; may lead to gangrene; the fingers, toes, ears, and nose are usually affected. COMPARE: chilblains.

frost (frost) A covering resembling minute ice crystals.

uremic f. Tiny flakes of urea sometimes seen on the skin of patients with uremia.

fructans (frook´tans) Polysaccharides of fructose with a high molecular weight.

fructokinase (frook-to-kĭ´nās) A liver enzyme that promotes the reaction of ATP (adenosine triphosphate) and d-fructose to form fructose 6-phosphate.

fructolysis (frook-ro-lī´sis) The conversion of fructose to lactate.

fructosan (frook´to-san) A polyfructose, such as inulin, present in certain tubers. Also called levan; levulin; levulan.

fructose (frook´tōs) The sweetest of the simple sugars (monosaccharides) present in honey and fruits; in the body it is formed as one of the two products of sucrose hydrolysis; used intravenously as a nutrient replenisher. Also called fruit sugar; levulose.

fructosemia (frook-to-se´me-ă) The presence of fructose in the blood; seen in hereditary fructose intolerance.

fructosuria (frook-to-su´re-ă) The presence of fructose in the urine due to a disorder of metabolism in which blood fructose levels are excessive and fructose appears in the urine.

frusemide (frus´ĕ-mīd) See furosemide.

frustration (frŭs-tra´shun) In psychology, the denial of gratification by reality.

fuchsin (fyo͝ok´sin) Rosaniline monohydrochloride; a bright red dye used in histology and bacteriology.

fugue (fyo͞og) A dissociation consisting of physical flight from a disturbing environment and, when the usual mental state returns, the individual has no recollection of his actions during this period.

fulgurant (ful´gu-rant) Sudden, flashing, like lightning; usually said of pain.

fulguration (ful-gu-ra´shun) Destruction of tissue surface by means of a high frequency electric current to coagulate surface bleeding.

fulminating, fulminant (ful-mĭ-nā´ting, ful´mĭ-nant) Of sudden, violent onset and rapid course.

fumagillin (fyo͞o-mă-jil´in) A crystalline antibiotic used as an amebicide.

fumigation (fyo͞o-mĭ-ga´shun) Disinfection by exposure to the fumes of a germicide.

fuming (fyo͞om´ing) Releasing a visible vapor.

function (funk´shun) **1.** The natural or special type of activity that is proper for an organ or part. **2.** To perform such an action. **3.** The general properties of any substance.

Gibbs free energy f. See free energy, under energy.

fundal (fun´dal) Relating to a fundus.

fundiform (fun´dĭ-form) Sling-shaped.

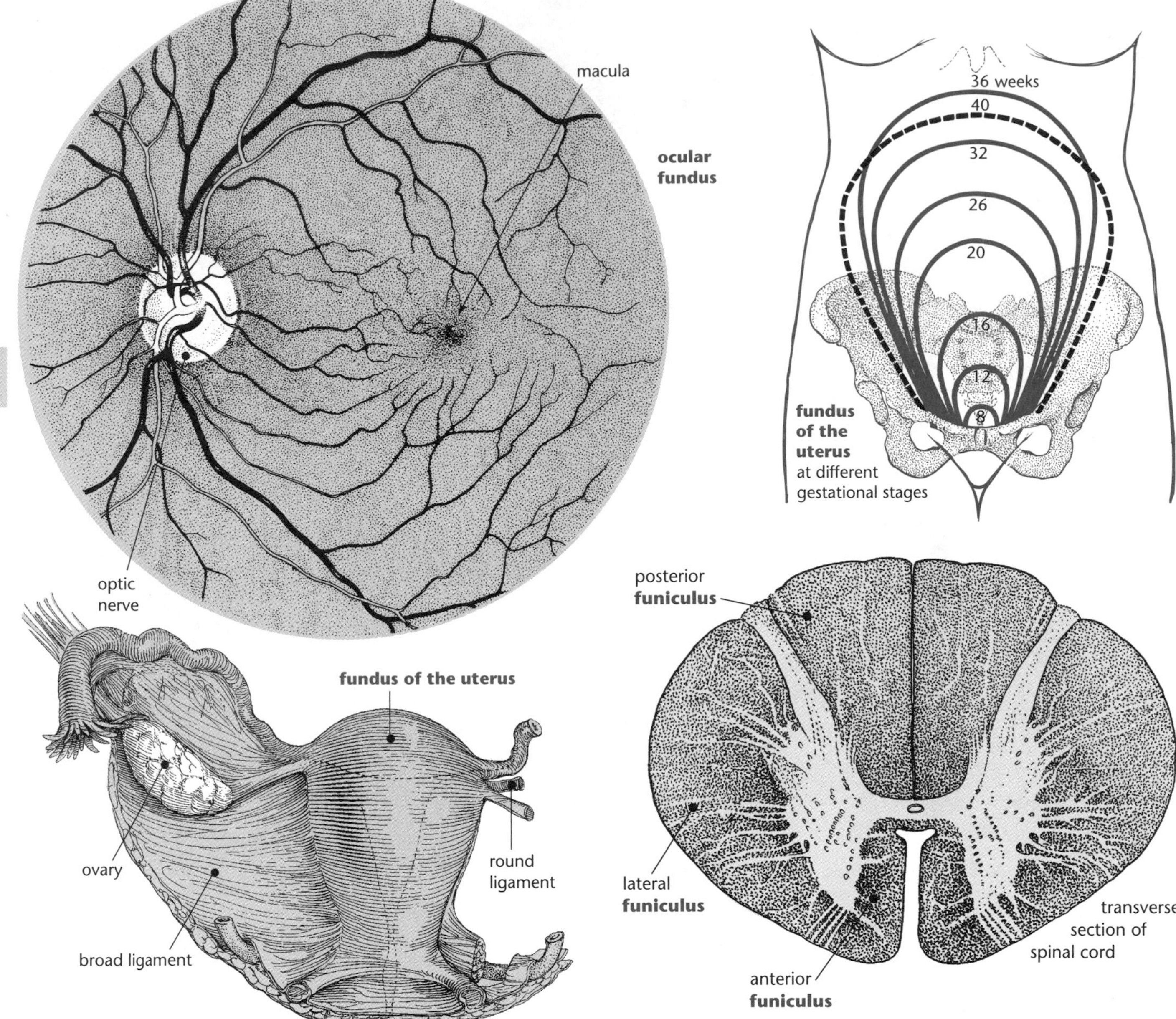

fundoplication (fun-do-plī-ka´shun) Suturing of the fundus of the stomach, as in the treatment of hiatal hernia.

fundus (fun´dus), *pl.* **fun´di** The portion of a hollow organ farthest from, above, or opposite its opening.

f. of the stomach The dome-shaped part of the stomach above its junction with the esophagus.

f. of the uterus The rounded portion of the uterus above the openings of the uterine tubes.

ocular f. The posterior portion of the interior of the eye. See also eyeground.

funduscopy (fun-dus´kŏ-pe) See ophthalmoscopy.

fungal (fun´gal) Relating to a fungus.

fungate (fun´gāt) To grow rapidly or to assume a funguslike form.

fungemia (fŭn-je´me-ă) The presence of viable fungi in the blood.

Fungi (fun´jī) A kingdom of organisms that includes saprophytic and parasitic plants, unable to manufacture their own food because they lack photosynthetic pigments.

fungi (fun´jī) Plural of fungus.

fungicide (fun´jĭ-sīd) Any substance that destroys fungus.

fungiform (fun´jĭ-form) Having the shape of a fungus.

fungistat (fun´jĭ-stat) An agent that inhibits the growth of fungi.

fungoid (fun´goid) Resembling a fungus.

fungous (fun´gus) Relating to a fungus.

fungus (fun´gus), *pl.* **fun´gi** General term for a large group of spore-bearing organisms characterized by lack of chlorophyll, asexual reproduction, and parasitic qualities.

thrush f. See *Candida albicans,* under *Candida.*

funic (fu´nik) Relating to the umbilical cord.

funicle (fu´nĭ-kl) A small cordlike structure.

funicular (fu-nik´u-lar) **1.** Having a cordlike appearance. **2.** Relating to the umbilical cord.

funiculitis (fu-nik-u-lī´tis) **1.** Inflammation of the spermatic cord. **2.** Inflammation of the portion of a spinal nerve located within the intervertebral canal.

funiculus (fu-nik´u-lus), *pl.* **funic´uli** **1.** One of the three main divisions or columns of white matter on either side of the spinal cord, called anterior, lateral, and posterior. **2.** The spermatic cord from the testis to the deep inguinal ring. **3.** The umbilical cord.

funiform (fu´nĭ-form) Cordlike.

funis (fu´nis) **1.** The umbilical cord. **2.** A cordlike structure.

funnel (fun´el) A conical vessel with a tube extending from its apex.

Buchner f. A porcelain funnel consisting of an upper cylindrical portion and a lower conical part, separated by a perforated plate upon which filter paper can be fitted.

fura-2 (fu´ră) A biofluorescent indicator that binds calcium; used to measure concentration of free calcium ion.

furfur (fur´fŭr) An epidermal scale.

furfuraceous (fur-fyu-rā´shus) Scaly; denoting a type of desquamation.

furosemide (fu-ro´sĕ-mīd) A powerful diuretic used orally or intravenously. Also called frusemide; Lasix®.

furrow (fur´o) A groove.

digital f. One of the grooves on the palmar surface of the fingers.

gluteal f. The groove between the buttocks.

palpebral f. The groove of the upper eyelid extending from the inner to the outer canthi.

furuncle (fu´rung-kl) An abscess or pyogenic infection of a sweat gland or hair follicle, usually caused by *Staphylococcus aureus.* Also called boil.

furuncular (fu-rung´ku-lar) Relating to a furuncle (boil).

furunculoid (fu-rung´ku-loid) Like a furuncle (boil).

furunculosis (fu-rung-ku-lo´sis) A condition marked by the presence of numerous furuncles (boils).

fuscin (fu´sin) The brown pigment of the retina.

fusiform (fu´zĭ-form) Tapering at both ends.

fusion (fu´zhun) **1.** The process of melting. **2.** Joining together by surgery (e.g., two parts of a joint). **3.** The integration into one perfect image of the images seen simultaneously by the two eyes. **4.** The abnormal union of two adjacent anatomic parts.

renal f. Abnormal fusion of the kidneys; named according to either the shape or the location (e.g., horseshoe kidney, cake or lump kidney, sigmoid kidney).

spinal f. The surgical fusion of two or more vertebrae to eliminate motion between them.

fusospirochetal (fu-so-spi-ro-ke´tal) Relating to the associated fusiform and spirochetal organisms.

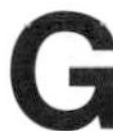

G

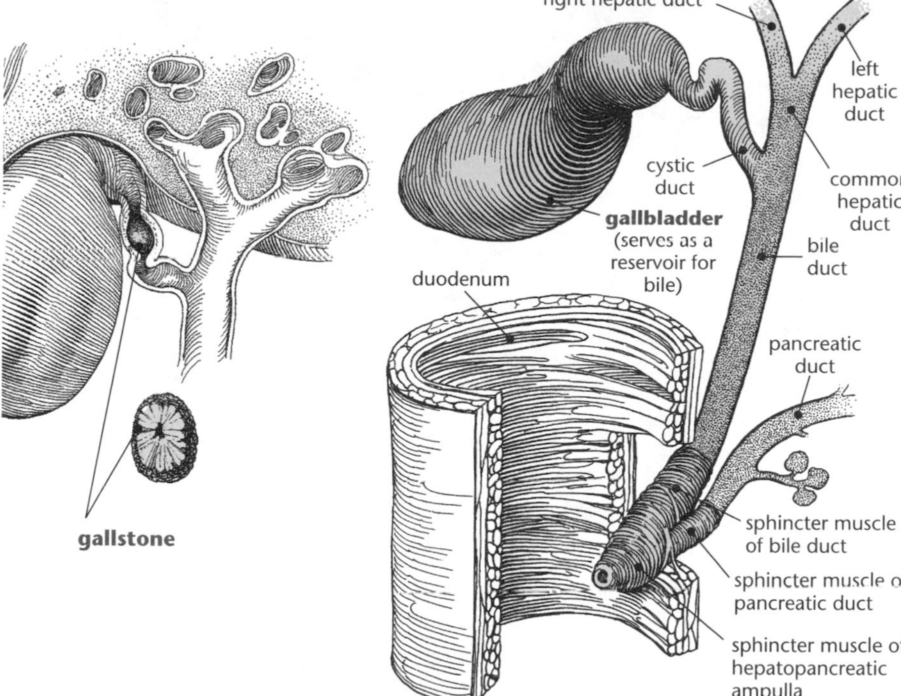

γ (gam´ă) Gamma. For terms beginning with γ, see under specific term.

gadolinium (gad-o-lin´e-um) Rare element; symbol Gd, atomic number 64, atomic weight 157.25; used to improve definition of tissue in magnetic resonance imaging (MRI).

gag (gag) **1.** To retch; to cause to retch. **2.** An instrument placed between the upper and lower jaws to keep the mouth open during operations on the tongue or throat.

gain (gan) **1.** To build up an increase; to acquire. **2.** The ratio of increase of output current, voltage, or power over input; the amplification factor of an electronic circuit.

primary g. The alleviation of anxiety provided by a neurotic illness or symptom.

secondary g. The additional indirect satisfaction or advantage (e.g., manipulating other people or receiving monetary reward) derived from a neurotic illness or symptom.

Gaisböck's syndrome (gīs´bekz sin´drōm) Hypertension and polycythemia without splenomegaly, occurring in middle-aged white males; the polycythemia is relative, with normal red blood cell mass but decreased plasma volume; cause in unknown.

gait (gāt) A manner of walking or running.

antalgic g. A self-protective limp due to pain.

ataxic g. An unsteady, irregular gait.

cerebellar g. A staggering gait with a tendency to fall, indicative of cerebellar disease; "drunken gait".

festinating g. See festination.

high steppage g. A gait in which the foot is raised high and brought down suddenly, the whole sole striking the ground in a flapping fashion.

tabetic g. A slapping gait characteristic of tabes dorsalis.

waddling g. Gait characterized by exaggerated hip elevation and lateral trunk movement, typical of muscular dystrophy and other disorders of muscle.

galactacrasia (gal-ak-tă-kra´shă) Abnormal composition of human milk.

galactagogue (gă-lak´tă gog) An agent that promotes the flow of milk.

galactan (gă-lak´tan) Any of several carbohydrates that yield galactose on hydrolysis.

galactic (gă-lak´tik) Relating to milk; inducing the flow of milk.

galactoblast (gă-lak´to-blast) See colostrum corpuscle, under corpuscle.

galactocele (gă-lak´to-sēl) See milk-retention cyst, under cyst.

galactokinase (gă-lak-to-ki´nās) An enzyme that, in the presence of ATP (adenosine triphosphate), promotes the phosphorylation of galactose to galactose 1-phosphate.

galactophore (gă-lak´to-for) A milk duct.

galactophorous (gal-ak-tof´o-rus) Conveying milk.

galactophygous (gal-ak-tof´ĭ-gus) Diminishing or arresting the flow of milk. Also called lactifugal.

galactopoiesis (gă-lak-to-poi-e´sis) Milk production.

galactopoietic (gă-lak-to-poi-et´ik) **1.** Relating to the secretion of milk. **2.** Any agent that promotes the secretion of milk.

galactorrhea (gă-lak-to-re´ă) Excessive discharge of milk from the breasts after the child has been weaned, or unrelated to a recent pregnancy.

galactosamine (gă-lak-to´să-mēn) A crystalline amino sugar derived from of galactose. Also called chondrosamine.

galactose (gă-lak´tōs) A white crystalline simple sugar, $C_6H_{12}O_6$, not found free in food; it is produced in the body by the digestion of lactose (milk sugar) and then converted into glucose for energy. Commonly called brain sugar.

galactosemia (gă-lak-to-se´me-ă) Defect in metabolism of galactose, a nutrient of milk, in which the conversion of galactose to glucose is deficient; the disorder usually becomes evident soon after birth by feeding problems, mental and physical retardation, enlargement of the liver and spleen, and elevated blood and urine galactose levels; can be treated effectively by excluding milk from the diet.

galactosis (gal-ak-to´sis) The formation of milk.

galactosuria (gă-lak-to-su´re-ă) Presence of galactose in the urine.

galactotherapy (gă-lak-to-ther´ă-pe) Treatment with a milk diet.

galactozymase (gă-lak-to-zi´mās) A starch-hydrolyzing enzyme present in milk.

galea (ga´le-ă) **1.** A helmet-shaped structure. **2.** A form of head bandage.

g. aponeurotica See epicranial aponeurosis, under aponeurosis.

galeatomy (ga-le-at´o-me) Surgical cutting of the epicranial aponeurosis (galea aponeurotica).

galectin-3 (ga-lek´tin thre) Protein thought to have a role in tumor development and inflammation.

galena (ga-lēn´ă) See lead sulfide, under lead.

galenical (gă-len´ĭ-kal) A medication prepared by extracting the active constituents of a plant.

galeophobia (ga-le-o-fo´be-ă) Morbid fear of cats.

gall (gawl) **1.** Bile. **2.** An erosion or sore.

gallamine triethiodide (gal´ă-mēn tri-ĕ-thi´o-dīd) Compound used as a skeletal muscle relaxant.

gallbladder (gawl´blad-er) A pear-shaped sac which stores bile and is situated under the liver.

Courvoisier's g. A gallbladder distended by obstruction of the biliary ducts.

hourglass g. Congenital abnormality of the gallbladder in which a septum divides it into two functioning halves.

porcelain g. Extensive calcification within the gallbladder wall occurring in chronic inflammation of the organ (chronic cholecystitis).

strawberry g. Gallbladder with a red and congested mucosa, dotted with yellowish deposits of cholesterol.

gallium (gal´e-um) A rare metallic element; symbol Ga, atomic number 31, atomic weight 69.72; liquid near room temperature.

gallium-67 (^{67}Ga) A radionuclide used to detect inflammatory or metastatic lesions.

gallium-68 (^{68}Ga) A positron-emitting isotope of gallium, used in bone scanning to detect metastatic bone lesions; has a 68-minute half-life.

gallon (gal´on) A U.S. measure of liquid volume or capacity equal to 4 quarts or 231 cubic inches; it is the equivalent of 3.785 liters.

gallop (gal´op) A triple or quadruple cadence of heart sounds resembling the canter of a horse, heard on auscultation, due to the addition of a third and/or fourth heart sound. Also called cantering or gallop rhythm.

atrial g. Presystolic gallop sound related to atrial contraction, occurring in late diastole and designated as a fourth heart sound. Also called presystolic gallop.

presystolic g. Atrial gallop.

protodiastolic g. See ventricular gallop.

summation g. Atrial and ventricular gallop sounds occurring simultaneously.

ventricular g. Third heart sound occurring in early diastole (0.14 to 0.16 seconds after the second heart sound). Also called protodiastolic gallop.

gallstone (gawl´stōn) A stone formed in the gallbladder or a bile duct, thought to be due to a defect in composition of the bile.

ball-valve g. A single stone that frequently moves within the gallbladder, causing intermittent obstruction of the bile duct and pain.

cholesterol g. A gray-yellow crystalline transluscent stone occurring singly, spherical (when small), or egg-shaped (when large) and reaching a size up to 6 cm in diameter.

mixed g. The most common type of gallstone, typically multiple, multifaceted, and 1 to 3 cm in diameter; composed of varying proportions of cholesterol, calcium carbonate, phosphates, and bilirubin.

pigmented g. A small, jet-black stone occurring in great numbers; composed of the bile pigment bilirubin.

silent g. Gallstone that does not produce symptoms.

Galton's delta (gawl´tonz del´tă) The middle triangular pattern of the lines of a fingerprint.

galvanic (gal-van´ik) **1.** Relating to chemically produced direct current electricity. **2.** Having the effect of an electric shock.

galvanism (gal´vă-niz-m) **1.** Direct current electricity, especially when produced by chemical action. **2.** Treatment with direct current electricity. Also called galvanotherapy.

galvanization (gal-vă-nī-za´shun) The application of a direct electric current.

galvanize (gal´vă-nīz) To stimulate with an electric current.

galvanocautery (gal-vă-no-kaw´ter-e) Cautery with a wire that has been heated with a galvanic current.

galvanocontractility (gal-vă-no-kon-trak-til´ĭ-te) The ability of a muscle to contract under direct current.

galvanofaradization (gal-vă-no-far-ă-di-za´shun) The simultaneous application of continuous and interrupted electric currents.

galvanometer (gal-vă-nom´ĕ-ter) An instrument for measuring the strength of a current of electricity.

Einthoven's string g. See string galvanometer.

string g. A galvanometer designed to record the electrical potentials produced in the heart; the forerunner of the electrocardiograph. Also called Einthoven's string galvanometer.

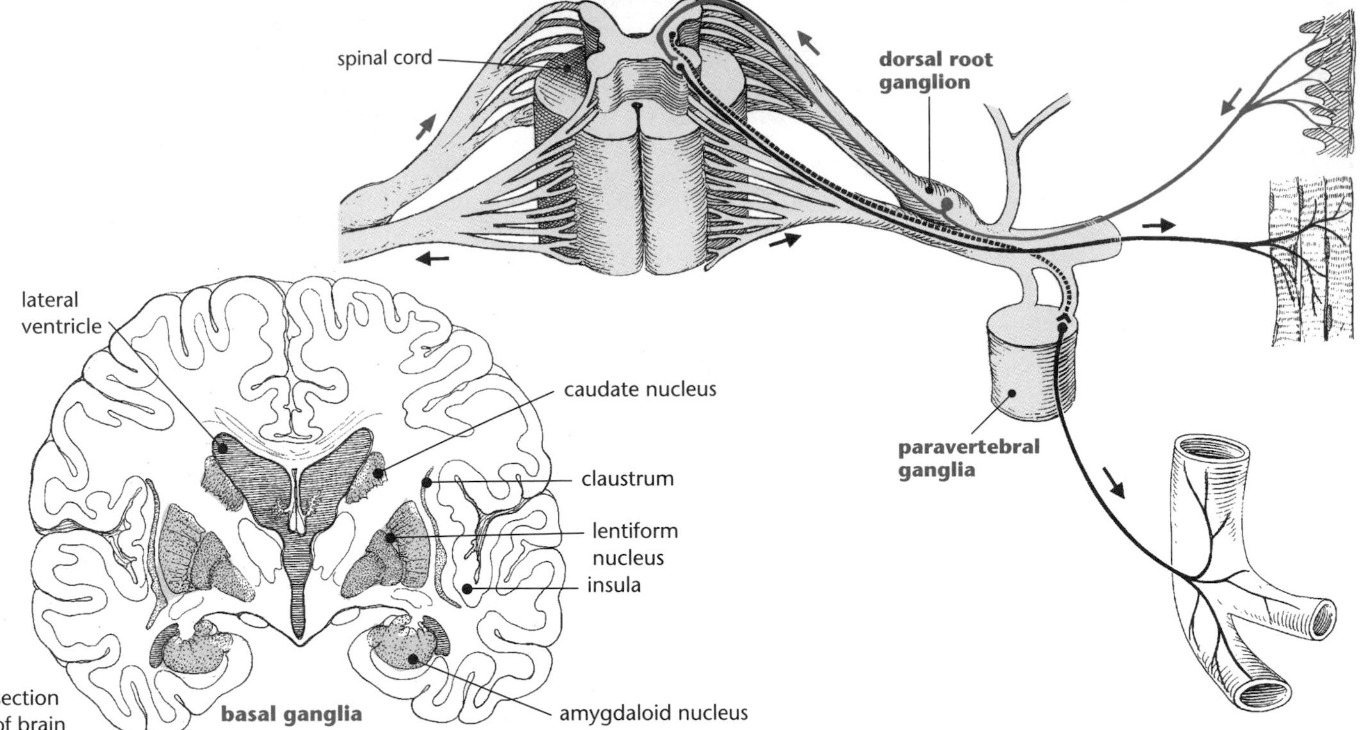

galvanopalpation (gal-vă-no-pal-pa´shun) The testing of cutaneous nerve responses by means of a weak electric current.

galvanoscope (gal´vă-no-skōp) Instrument used for detecting the presence and direction of electric currents.

galvanosurgery gal-vă-no-ser´jer-ē) Surgical procedure using a direct electric current.

galvanotherapy (gal-vă-no-ther´ă-pē) See galvanism (2).

galvanotonus (gal-vă-not´o-nus) Tonic muscular response to stimulation with an electric current.

gamete (gam´et) One of two sex cells (ovum or spermatozoon) that combines with another in true conjugation to form a zygote, from which a new organism develops; it contains only one chromosome of each chromosome pair.

gametocide (gă-me´to-sīd) Any agent destructive to gametes.

gametocyte (gă-me´to-sīt) A cell from which gametes are produced by division; a spermatocyte or an oocyte.

gametogenesis (gam-e-to-jen´ĕ-sis) The production of gametes (ova or spermatozoa).

gametogony, gametogonia (gam-e-tog´ŏ-ne, gam-e-to-go´ne-ă) Stage in the sexual cycle of protozoa in which gametocytes are formed.

gamma (gam´ă) **1.** The third letter of the Greek alphabet, γ; used to indicate the third in a series. **2.** In chemical nomenclature, used to indicate the third carbon of an aliphatic chain and the location opposite the alpha position in the benzene ring.

gamma-aminobutyric acid (gam´ă ă-me-no-bu-tir´ik as´id) (GABA, Abu) γ-aminobutyric acid; an amino acid neurotransmitter present in brain tissue that inhibits nerve impulses.

gammagram (gam´ă-gram) A graphic record of the γ-rays emitted by a substance or tissue.

gammopathy (gam-op´ă-the) General term for any disorder characterized by an abnormal proliferation of antibody-forming cells and the presence of abnormally high levels of immunoglobulins (or any of their constituents) in the plasma and/or the urine; most of these disorders are malignant (e.g., multiple myeloma and heavy chain disease).

benign monoclonal g. (BMG) See monoclonal gammopathy of undetermined significance.

monoclonal g. See plasma cell dyscrasias, under dyscrasia.

monoclonal g. of undetermined significance (MGUS) Condition marked by elevated levels of M protein in the serum but without symptoms of any immunoglobulin-producing disease; usually follows a benign course but in some cases (about 18%) a plasma cell dyscrasia develops. Also called benign monoclonal gammopathy.

polyclonal g. Gammopathy that involves two or more classes and types of immunoglobulin.

gamogenesis (gam-o-jen´ĕ-sis) Sexual reproduction.

ganciclovir (gan-si´klo-vir) Agent used in the treatment of cytomegalovirus (CMV) infections.

ganglia (gang´gle-ă) Plural of ganglion.

gangliate (gang´gle-āt), **gang´liated** See ganglionated.

gangliectomy (gang-gle-ek´tŏ-me) Surgical removal of a ganglion.

gangliform (gang´glĭ-form) Resembling a ganglion.

ganglioblast (gang´gle-o-blast) An embryonic cell from which ganglion cells develop.

glioma (gang-gle-o´mă) See ganglioneuroma.

ganglion (gang´gle-on), *pl.* **gang´lia, gang´lions** **1.** A collection of nerve cell bodies located outside of the brain and spinal cord. **2.** A cystic swelling resembling a tumor, occurring on a tendon sheath or joint capsule.

Arnold's g. See otic ganglion.

autonomic g. Any ganglion of the sympathetic and parasympathetic nervous systems.

basal ganglia Ganglia located within the white matter of each cerebral hemisphere; they serve as important links along various motor pathways of the central nervous system; they include the caudate, lentiform, and amygdaloid nuclei and the claustrum.

cardiac g. One of several ganglia in the cardiac plexus located between the arch of the aorta and the bifurcation of the pulmonary trunk.

celiac g. One of two large sympathetic ganglia in the upper part of the abdomen on either side of the aorta near the origin of the celiac artery. Also called solar ganglion.

cervical g. One of three (superior, middle, and inferior) sympathetic ganglia in the neck.

cervicothoracic g. A ganglion of the sympathetic trunk containing two components, the inferior cervical and the first thoracic ganglia, which are often fused. Also called stellate ganglion.

ciliary g. A parasympathetic ganglion lying behind the orbit between the optic nerve and the lateral rectus muscle.

coccygeal g. An unpaired ganglion of the sympathetic trunk located on the anterior aspect of the tip of the coccyx. Also called ganglion impar.

dorsal root g. A ganglion located on the dorsal root of each spinal nerve containing the cell bodies of the sensory neurons of the nerve. Also called spinal ganglion; posterior root ganglion.

ganglia of glossopharyngeal nerve The two sensory ganglia (superior and inferior) situated on the glossopharyngeal nerve as it passes through the jugular foramen.

ganglia of sympathetic trunk See paravertebral ganglia.

gasserian g. See trigeminal ganglion.

geniculate g. A ganglion of the facial nerve.

g. impar See coccygeal ganglion.

otic g. A parasympathetic ganglion located just below the foramen ovale medial to the mandibular nerve; its preganglionic fibers are derived from the glossopharyngeal nerve and its postganglionic fibers innervate the parotid gland. Also called Arnold's ganglion.

parasympathetic ganglia Aggregations of nerve cell bodies of the parasympathetic nervous system; the ciliary, pterygopalatine, otic, and submandibular ganglia of the head and several others located near the organs of the thorax, abdomen, and pelvis.

paravertebral ganglia Sympathetic ganglia located at intervals on each sympathetic trunk along the side of the vertebral column; generally there are 3 cervical, 12 thoracic, 4 lumbar, and 4 sacral. Also called ganglia of sympathetic trunk.

posterior root g. See spinal ganglion.

prevertebral ganglia The sympathetic ganglia situated in front of the vertebral column and forming the plexuses of the thorax and abdomen; distinguished from the paravertebral ganglia, which lie along each side of the vertebral column.

pterygopalatine g. The largest of the four parasympathetic ganglia associated with cranial nerves of the head; it is located in the pterygopalatine fossa just posterior to the middle nasal concha; it sends postganglionic parasympathetic fibers to the lacrimal glands, nose, oral cavity, and the upper-most part of the pharynx. Also called sphenopalatine ganglion.

g. of Scarpa See vestibular ganglion.

semilunar g. See trigeminal ganglion.

solar g. See celiac ganglion.

sphenopalatine g. See pterygopalatine ganglion.

spinal g. See dorsal root ganglion.

spiral g. of cochlea The ganglion of bipolar nerve cell bodies located within the modiolus of the inner ear; it sends fibers peripherally to the spiral organ of Corti and centrally to the cochlear nuclei of the brainstem.

stellate g. See cervicothoracic ganglion.

submandibular g. One of the four parasympathetic ganglia associated with cranial nerves of the head; it is located just above the deep part of the submandibular gland; its preganglionic fibers are derived from the facial nerve and its postganglionic fibers innervate the submandibular and sublingual

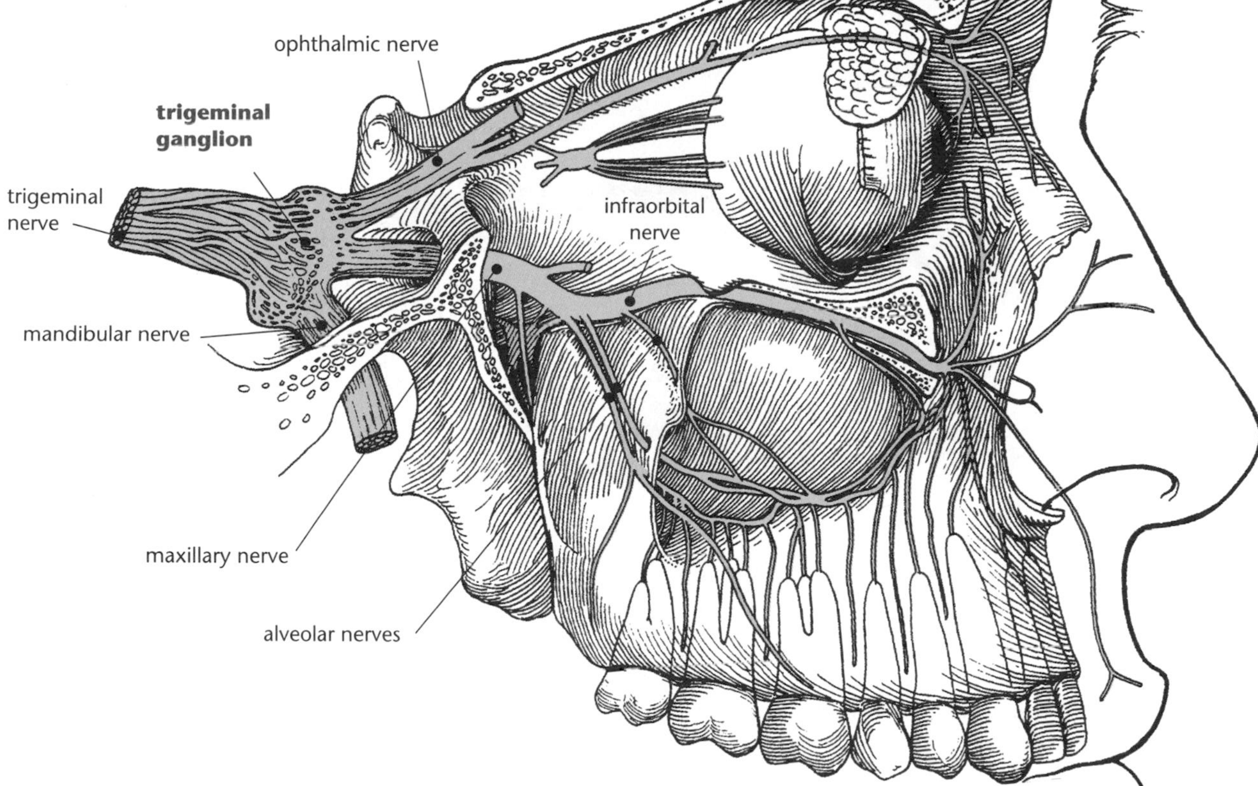

glands.

thoracic g. A ganglion on the thoracic portion of the sympathetic trunk.

trigeminal g. The large flattened ganglion on the sensory root of the trigeminal nerve, located on the anterior aspect of the petrous portion of the temporal bone. Also called semilunar ganglion; gasserian ganglion.

ganglia of vagus nerve Two ganglia of the vagus nerve: *inferior,* situated on the nerve a short distance below the jugular foramen, in front of the transverse processes of the first and second cervical vertebrae; and *superior,* situated on the nerve as it passes through the jugular foramen at the base of the skull.

vestibular g. A collection of bipolar nerve cell bodies forming a swelling of the vestibulocochlear nerve in the internal auditory meatus; it is subdivided into superior and inferior parts. Also called ganglion of Scarpa.

ganglionated (gang´gle-ŏ-nāt-ed) Having ganglia. Also called gangliated; gangliate.

ganglionectomy (gang-gle-ŏ-nek´tŏ-me) Surgical removal of a ganglion.

stellate g. See stellectomy.

ganglioneuroma (gang-gle-o-nōō-ro´mă) A small, encapsulated, benign, slow-growing tumor, composed of mature ganglion cells and nerve fibers. Also called ganglioma; neurocytoma.

ganglionic (gang-gle-on´ik) Of or relating to a ganglion, generally a nerve ganglion.

ganglionitis (gang-gle-ŏ-nī´tis) Inflammation of any ganglion.

ganglioplegic (gang-gle-ŏ-ple´jik) Denoting a compound that blocks transmission of impulses (usually for a short period of time) through an autonomic ganglion.

ganglioside (gang-gle-ŏ-sīd) A class of sphingoglycolipids present in neural tissue containing *N*-acetylneuraminic acid (NANA).

gangliosidosis (gang-gle-o-si-do´sis) Any disease involving an accumulation of specific gangliosides in the nervous system. Also called ganglioside lipidosis.

gangosa (gan-go´să) Ulceration of the soft and hard palate, nasopharynx, and nose; a sequel to yaws. Also called rhinopharyngitis mutilans.

gangrene (gang´grēn) Decay of body tissues, due to inadequate blood (nutritive) supply; a form of necrosis combined with putrefaction.

cold g. See dry gangrene

diabetic g. Gangrene due to arteriosclerosis accompanying diabetes.

dry g. Gangrene not preceded by inflammation. Also called cold gangrene; necrotic gangrene; mummification.

gas g. Gangrene occurring in extensively traumatized and soil-contaminated wounds infected with toxigenic anaerobic *Clostridium*; characterized by the presence of gas in the affected tissue.

moist g. A soft and moist gangrene due to the action of putrefactive bacteria.

necrotic g. See dry gangrene.

gangrenous (gang´grĕ-nus) Affected with gangrene.

gap (gap) An interval or an opening.

air-bone g. The lag between hearing acuity by air conduction and by bone conduction.

anion g. The difference between the measured cations and the measured anions in plasma. A simplified formula is: anion gap = (Na) – (HCO_3 + Cl). The normal range is 8 to 16 mEq/liter. Used in the evaluation of acid-base disorders.

auscultatory g. A silent interval sometimes noticed during determination of blood pressure. Also called silent gap.

silent g. See auscultatory gap.

velopharyngeal g. The space behind the palate between the nose and throat.

Gardner's syndrome (gahrd´nerz sin´drōm) Hereditary syndrome of multiple polyps (over 500) of the rectum and colon, associated with cysts and tumors of skin and bone; transmitted by an autosomal dominant trait; carcinoma of the colon develops in more than 50% of patients by age 40, and colectomy is usually recommended as a prophylactic procedure.

Gardnerella (gard-ner-el´ă) A genus of anaerobic nonmotile bacteria.

G. vaginalis A species that is the major cause of vaginosis, transmitted by sexual contact.

gargle (gar´gl) **1.** To rinse the throat and mouth by forcing exhaled air through a liquid held in the mouth while the head is tilted back. **2.** A medicated solution used for rinsing the throat and mouth.

gas (gas), *pl.* **gas´es 1.** An airlike state of matter distinguished from the solid and liquid states by freely moving molecules capable of great expansion and contraction with changes in pressure and temperature; a vapor. **2.** Gaseous anesthesia.

alveolar g. Air remaining in the lungs after a normal expiration in which the O_2 and CO_2 tensions are in equilibrium with those of the arterial blood. Also called alveolar air.

inert g. 1. Any of the gases, helium, neon, argon, krypton, xenon, and radon (nitron), which are present in the atmosphere and exhibit no chemical affinity. **2.** Totally unreactive gas, except under extreme conditions.

laughing g. See nitrous oxide.

marsh g. See methane.

mustard g. Dichlorodiethyl sulfide, an oily, volatile substance used in chemical warfare during World War I as a gaseous blistering agent; inhalation of the poison gas may result in chemical bronchopneumonia; progenitor of the so-called nitrogen mustards used in cancer chemotherapy.

tear g. Any gaseous agent, such as chloroacetophenone (CAP), that irritates the eyes, producing blinding tears.

water g. An industrial fuel gas produced by passing steam over red-hot coal or coke; consists mainly of hydrogen, hydrocarbons, and carbon monoxide.

gaseous (gash´us) Relating to or of the nature of a gas.

gasiform (gas´ĭ-form) Gaseous.

gasogenic (gas-o-jen´ik) Gas-producing.

gasometer (gas-om´ĕ-ter) A calibrated apparatus for measuring the volume of gases; generally used for measuring respiration gases.

gasometry (gas-om´ĕ-tre) The scientific measurement of gases; the determination of the relative proportion of gases in a mixture.

gastrectomy (gas-trek´tŏ-me) Surgical removal of part or all of the stomach. Also called gastric resection.

gastric (gas´trik) Relating to the stomach.

gastrin (gas´trin) One of the gastrointestinal hormones released during digestion; it is secreted by the mucosa of the pyloric region of the stomach upon contact with food; it increases the secretion of hydrochloric acid and, to a lesser degree, of pepsinogen.

gastrinoma (gas-trĭ-no´mă) A gastrin-producing tumor, usually of the pancreas, associated with the Zollinger-Ellison syndrome.

gastritis (gas-tri´tis) Inflammation of the stomach lining (mucosa).

antral g. See type B gastritis.

atrophic g. Chronic form of gastritis with degeneration of the rugal folds (rugae).

erosive g. Gastritis with erosions of the stomach lining, may be asymptomatic or associated with nausea, discomfort of the upper abdomen, and slow oozing of blood into the intestines; or may induce vomiting of blood; may be caused by irritation (e.g., by aspirin or alcohol consumption) or by severe stress (e.g., head injuries, burns, surgery, or liver failure). Also called hemorrhagic gastritis.

fundal g. See type A gastritis.

hypertrophic g. Gastritis marked chiefly by abnormally large rugal folds due to an increased number of cells (hyperplasia) of the stomach lining; may involve the superficial cells (e.g., in Ménétrièr's

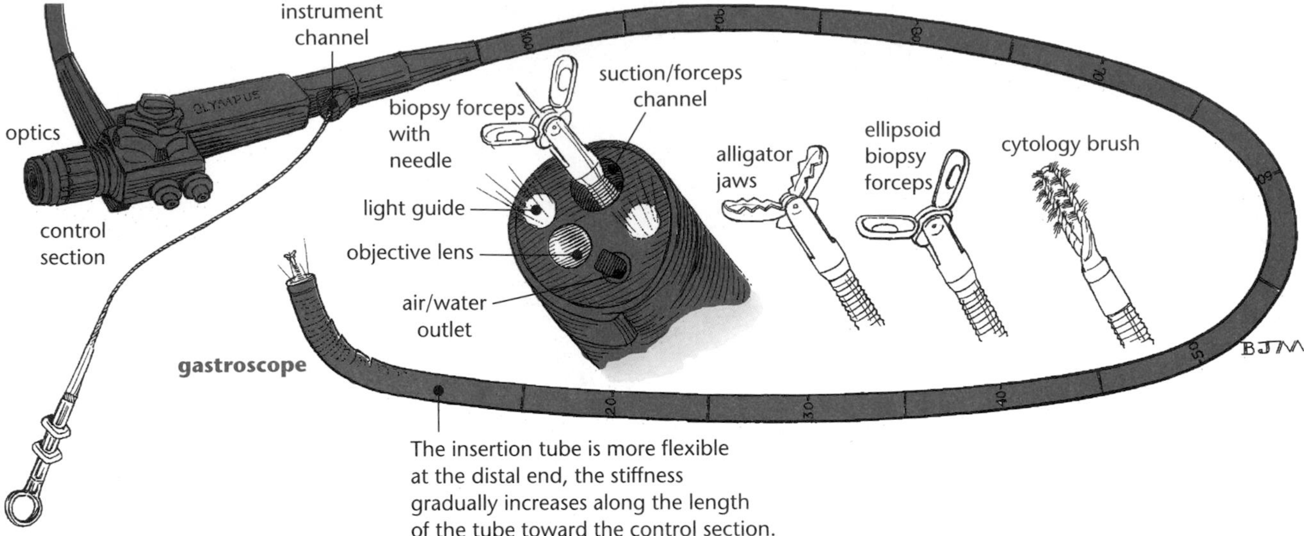

disease), or the chief mucosal cells (e.g., in hypersecretory gastropathy), or may be secondary to excessive gastrin secretion by a tumor (as in the Zollinger-Ellison syndrome).

interstitial g. Gastritis involving the muscular layer of the stomach wall as well as the mucosa.

phlegmonous g. Severe inflammation with purulent infiltration of the stomach wall.

pseudomembranous g. Inflammation of the stomach marked by the formation of a false membrane.

type A g. Chronic gastritis generally involving the uppermost region (fundus) and body of the stomach; it is usually asymptomatic and most commonly seen in elderly people; may be associated with pernicious anemia, Hashimoto's thyroiditis, and Addison's disease; long-standing disease has an increased risk of becoming cancerous. Also called fundal gastritis.

type B g. A common form of chronic gastritis primarily affecting the lower portion (antrum) of the stomach; believed to be caused by infection with a bacterium (*Helicobacter pylori*); occurs in all age groups and may be asymptomatic or cause upset stomach, burning pain, and belching. Also called antral gastritis.

gastroanastomosis (gas-tro-ă-nas-to-mo´sis) Surgical connection of the pyloric and cardiac ends of the stomach. Also called gastrogastrostomy.

gastroblenorrhea gas-tro-blen-o-re´ă) Excessive secretion of mucus by the stomach.

gastrocele (gas´tro-sēl) A hernia of a portion of the stomach.

gastrocnemius (gas-tro-ne´me-us) See table of muscles.

gastrocolic (gas-tro-kol´ik) Relating to the stomach and colon.

gastrocolitis (gas-tro-ko-li´tis) Inflammation of the stomach and colon.

gastrocoloptosis (gas-tro-ko-lo-to´sis) Downward displacement of the stomach and colon.

gastrocolostomy (gas-tro-ko-los´tŏ-me) The surgical construction of a passage between the stomach and colon.

Gastrodiscoides hominis (gas-tro-dis-koi´dēz hom´ĭ-nis) A species of trematode worms parasitic in the intestines of swine and humans.

gastroduodenal (gas-tro-doo-o-de´nal) Relating to both the stomach and the duodenum.

gastroduodenoscopy (gas-tro-doo-o-dĕ-nos´kŏ-pe) Visualization of the interior of the stomach and duodenum with the aid of a gastroscope.

gastroduodenostomy (gas-tro-doo-o-dĕ-nos´tŏ-me) Surgical creation of an artificial passage between the stomach and duodenum.

gastroenteric (gas-tro-en-ter´ik) See gastrointestinal.

gastroenteritis (gas-tro-en-ter-i´tis) Inflammation of the mucous membrane of the stomach and intestines.

gastroenteroanastomosis (gas-tro-en-ter-o-ă-nas-to-mo´sis) A surgical connection between the stomach and any noncontinuous portion of the intestine.

gastroenterologist (gas-tro-en-ter-ol´ŏ-jist) A specialist in diseases of the stomach and intestines.

gastroenterology (gas-tro-en-ter-ol´ŏ-je) The branch of medicine concerned with disorders of the stomach and intestines and also with the esophagus, the liver, and the gallbladder.

gastroenteropathy (gas-tro-en-ter-op´ă-the) Any disease of the alimentary canal.

gastroenteroptosis (gas-tro-en-ter-o-to´sis) The downward displacement, or prolapse, of the stomach and a portion of the intestine.

gastroenterostomy (gas-tro-en-ter-os´tŏ-me) Surgical creation of a passage between the stomach and the intestine.

gastroenterotomy (gas-tro-en-ter-ot´ŏ-me) Surgical incision into the stomach and intestine.

gastroepiploic (gas-tro-ep-ĭ-plo´ik) Relating to the stomach and greater omentum.

gastroesophageal (gas-tro-ĕ-sof-ă-je´al) Relating to the stomach and the esophagus.

gastroesophageal reflux disease (gas-tro-ĕ-sof-ă-je´ăl re´fluks dĭ-zēz´) (GERD) Any condition resulting from the backflow of stomach or duodenal contents through an incompetent lower esophageal sphincter; symptoms include heartburn and regurgitation.

gastroesophagitis (gas-tro-ĕ-sof-ă-ji´tis) Inflammation of the stomach and esophagus.

gastroesophagostomy (gas-tro-ĕ-sof-ă-gos´tŏ-me) Surgical creation of a new opening or connection between the stomach and esophagus.

gastrogastrostomy (gas-tro-gas-tros´tŏ-me) See gastroanastomosis.

gastrogavage (gas-tro-gă-vahzh´) Feeding by way of a gastrostomy (surgical opening through the stomach wall).

gastrogenic (gas-tro-jen´ik) Originating in the stomach.

gastrograph (gas´tro-graf) An instrument for recording the motions of the stomach.

gastrohepatic (gas-tro-hĕ-pat´ik) Relating to the stomach and the liver.

gastrohydrorrhea (gas-tro-hi-dro-rē´ă) Secretion by the stomach of a large quantity of a watery fluid.

gastrointestinal (gas-tro-in-tes´tĭ-năl) (GI) Relating to the stomach and intestines. Also called gastroenteric.

gastrojejunocolic (gas-tro-jĕ-joo-no-kol´ik) Relating to the stomach, jejunum, and colon (e.g., a fistula penetrating the three structures).

gastrojejunostomy (gas-tro-jĕ-joo-nos´tŏ-me) Surgical creation of an opening or connection between the stomach and jejunum.

gastrolith (gas´tro-lith) A calculus in the stomach; a gastric calculus.

gastrolithiasis (gas-tro-lĭ-thi´ă-sis) The presence of one or more calculi in the stomach.

gastrology (gas-trol´ŏ-je) The scientific study of the stomach and its diseases; the term gastroenterology is more commonly used.

gastromalacia (gas-tro-mă-la´shă) Softening of the stomach wall.

gastromegaly (gas-tro-meg´ă-le) Abnormal enlargement of the stomach.

gastropathy (gas-trop´ă-the) Any disease of the stomach.

hypersecretory g. Thickening of the stomach lining with excessive acid secretion (not associated with a gastrin-secreting tumor); ulceration frequently occurs.

gastropexy (gas´tro-pek-se) Surgical attachment of the stomach to the abdominal wall.

gastrophrenic (gas-tro-fren´ik) Relating to the stomach and the diaphragm.

gastroplasty (gas´tro-plas-te) Surgical correction of any defect of the stomach.

gastroplication (gas-tro-plĭ-ka´shun) A surgical procedure to reduce the size of the stomach, usually by suturing a fold along its length.

gastroptosis, gastroptosia (gas-trop-to´sis, gas-trop-to´siă) Downward displacement of the stomach.

gastropyloric (gas-tro-pi-lor´ik) Relating to the stomach as a whole and to the pylorus.

gastrorrhagia (gas-tro-ra´jă) Copious bleeding from the stomach.

gastrorrhaphy (gas-tror´ă-fe) Suture of the stomach.

gastrorrhexis (gas-tro-rek´sis) A rupture of the stomach.

gastroschisis (gas-tros´kĭ-sis) In newborn infants, a full-thickness defect of the abdominal wall located just to the right of the intact umbilical cord; consists of an opening 2 to 4 cm in diameter through which protrudes an exposed loop of intestine (without a protective covering sac).

gastrosplenic (gas-tro-splen´ik) Relating to the stomach and spleen.

gastrostaxis (gas-tro-stak´sis) Chronic slight bleeding from the mucosal lining of the stomach; occurs in certain types of chronic gastritis.

gastroscope (gas´tro-skōp) An instrument for

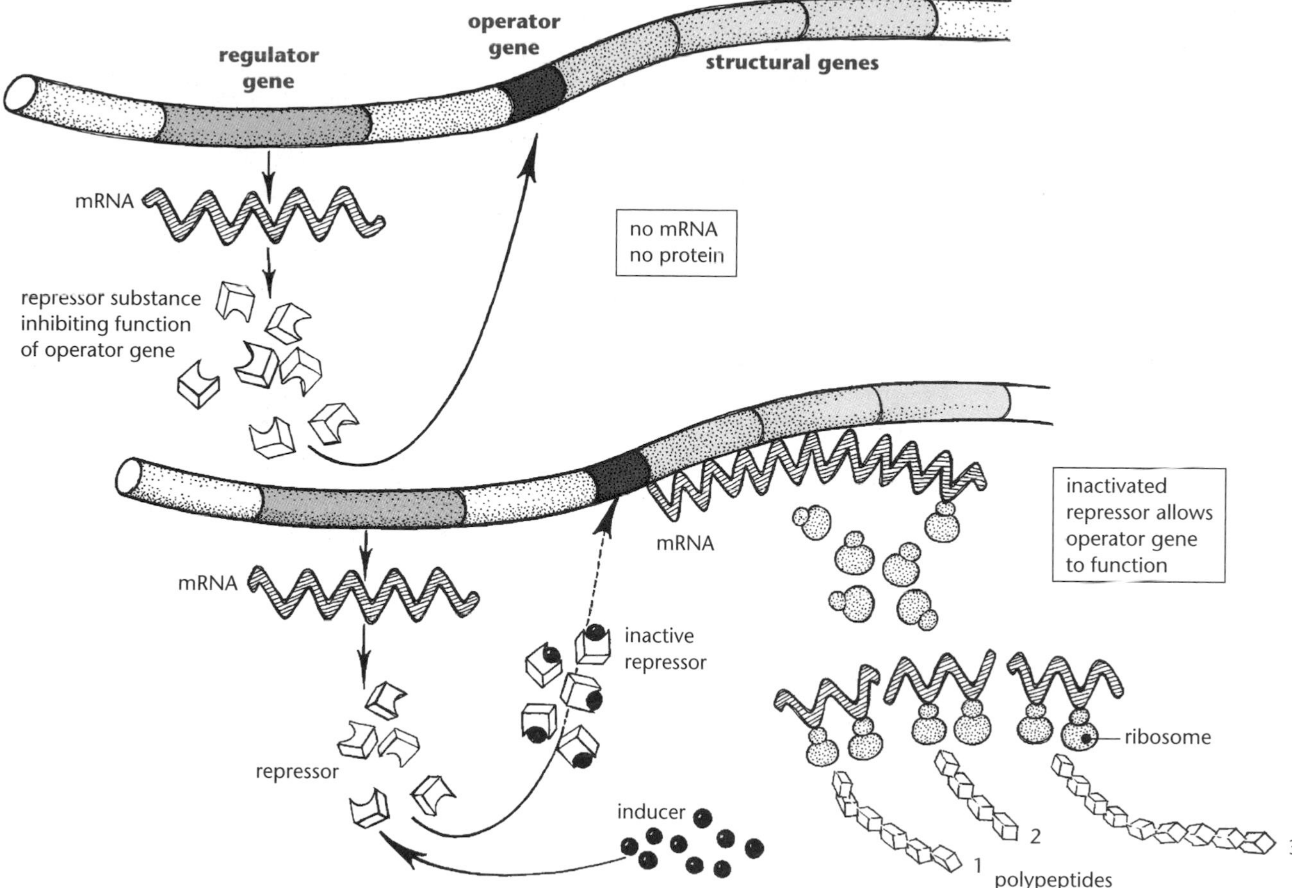

viewing the interior of the stomach.

gastroscopy (gas-tros´kŏ-pe) Examination of the interior of the stomach with the gastroscope.

gastrospasm (gas´tro-spaz-m) Spasmodic contraction of the stomach.

gastrostenosis (gas-tro-stĕ-no´sis) Constriction of the stomach.

gastrostomy (gas-tros´tŏ-me) Surgical construction of a passage into the stomach.

percutaneous endoscopic g. Inspection of the stomach interior with an endoscope introduced through a puncture of the abdominal wall and stomach.

gastrotomy (gas-trot´ŏ-me) Surgical incision into the stomach.

gastrotropic (gas-tro-trop´ik) Having an effect on the stomach.

gastrula (gas´troo-lă) An embryo at the stage of development following the blastula when the gastrulation movements occur.

gastrulation (gas-troo-la´shun) The formation of a gastrula; in embryology, the process by which a third germ layer of cells (mesoderm) migrates between the bilaminar disk making it trilaminar (ectoderm, mesoderm, and endoderm); it occurs during the third week of embryonic development.

gatekeeper (gāt´kēp-er) The health professional who performs gatekeeping.

gatekeeping (gāt-kēp´ing) In health care, the process by which a primary care physician directly provides care to a patient and determines the need for specialty referrals.

gather (gath´er) To come to a head; said of a boil when maturing.

gathering (gath´er-ing) Colloquial term for the maturing of a boil or abscess when it fills with pus.

gating (gāt´ing) **1.** Control of passage of substances through a protein channel in the cell membrane by opening or closing the opening (gate) into the channel; the mechanism may be electrical (e.g., alteration in membrane potential) or chemical (e.g., binding a ligand). **2.** Activity in a special nerve fiber to control impulse transmission through a synapse.

Gaucher's disease (go-shāz´ dĭ-zēz´) A disease characterized by the deposit of glucocerebroside, a glycolipid, in reticuloendothelial cells; manifestations include bone lesions and enlargement of the spleen, liver, and lymph nodes. Also called cerebrosidosis.

gauge (gāj) A measuring instrument.

bite g. See gnathodynamometer.

Boley g. A caliper-type gauge used in dentistry to obtain measurements necessary for dental prosthesis.

catheter g. A metal plate with perforations of different sizes used to determine the size of catheters.

Gaultheria (gawl-the´re-ă) A genus of plants including the species *Gaultheria procumbens*, commonly known as wintergreen and teaberry; it yields a volatile oil rich in methyl salicylate.

gaunt (gawnt) **1.** Very slim and bony. **2.** Emaciated.

gauntlet (gawnt´let) A glovelike bandage protecting the hand and fingers.

gauze (gawz) A thin, open weave surgical dressing or bandage.

absorbent g. A bleached cotton gauze of varied thread counts and weight.

petrolatum g. Absorbent gauze impregnated with white petrolatum.

gavage (gă-vahzh´) The passage of nutritive material into the stomach by means of a nasogastric tube.

gel (jel) **1.** The semisolid state of a coagulated colloid. **2.** To become a gel.

gelate (jel´āt) See gel.

gelatin (jel´ă-tin) A colorless, transparent protein derived from the collagen of tissue by boiling in water; used for nutritional purposes and also as a packaging agent for pharmaceuticals.

zinc g. Jelly containing zinc oxide, gelatin, glycerin, and water; used between layers of bandage as a protective dressing.

gelatinize (jĕ-lat´ĭ-nīz) **1.** To convert to gelatin. **2.** To become gelatinous.

gelatinoid (jĕ-lat´ĭ-noid) Like gelatin.

gelatinous (jĕ-lat´ĭ-nus) Pertaining to or containing gelatin.

gelation (jĕ-la´shun) The transformation of a colloid suspended in solution into a gel.

gelose (jĕ´lōs) In general, any amorphous polysaccharide, such as agar, obtained from red algae and capable of forming a jelly.

gelosis (jĕ-lō´sis) A hard mass in the tissues, especially in a muscle.

gelsolin (jel-sol´in) Enzyme present in nerve cells that, when activated by increased intracellular calcium levels, acts on the cell membrane receptors to block further calcium influx into the cell.

gemellology (jem-el-ol´ŏ-je) The study of twins and twinning.

geminate (jem´ĭ-nāt) Occurring in pairs.

gemma (jem´ă) **1.** Any budlike structure, such as a tastebud. **2.** Any outgrowth or bud that becomes a new organism.

gemmation (je-ma´shun) Asexual reproduction in which a new organism develops as an outgrowth of the parent. Also called budding.

gemmule (jem´yūl) **1.** A bud that develops into a new organism. **2.** One of several spherical enlargements sometimes present on the protoplasmic processes (dendrites) of a nerve cell.

gender (jen´der) (g) Sex category.

gene (jēn) The hereditary unit occupying a fixed position (locus) on the chromosome; capable of reproducing itself at each cell division and of governing the formation of proteins. In molecular terms, it is a segment of the DNA molecule containing the code for a specific function.

allelic g. See allele.

autosomal g. A gene present on any chromosome other than a sex (X or Y) chromosome.

codominant g. In clinical genetics, two or more alleles of a gene that express a recognizable effect on a heterozygous individual.

dominant g. A gene that produces a recognizable effect in the organism whether paired with an identical or a dissimilar gene.

g. expression See under expression.

g. flow See under flow.

holandric g. See Y-linked gene.

housekeeping g.'s Genes present in all or most cells because their products are required for basic functions.

g. library See under library.

g. map See chromosome map, under map.

operator g. One of the regular genes whose function is to activate messenger-RNA production; it is part of the feedback system for determining the rate of enzyme production.

g. pool See under pool.

g. product See under product.

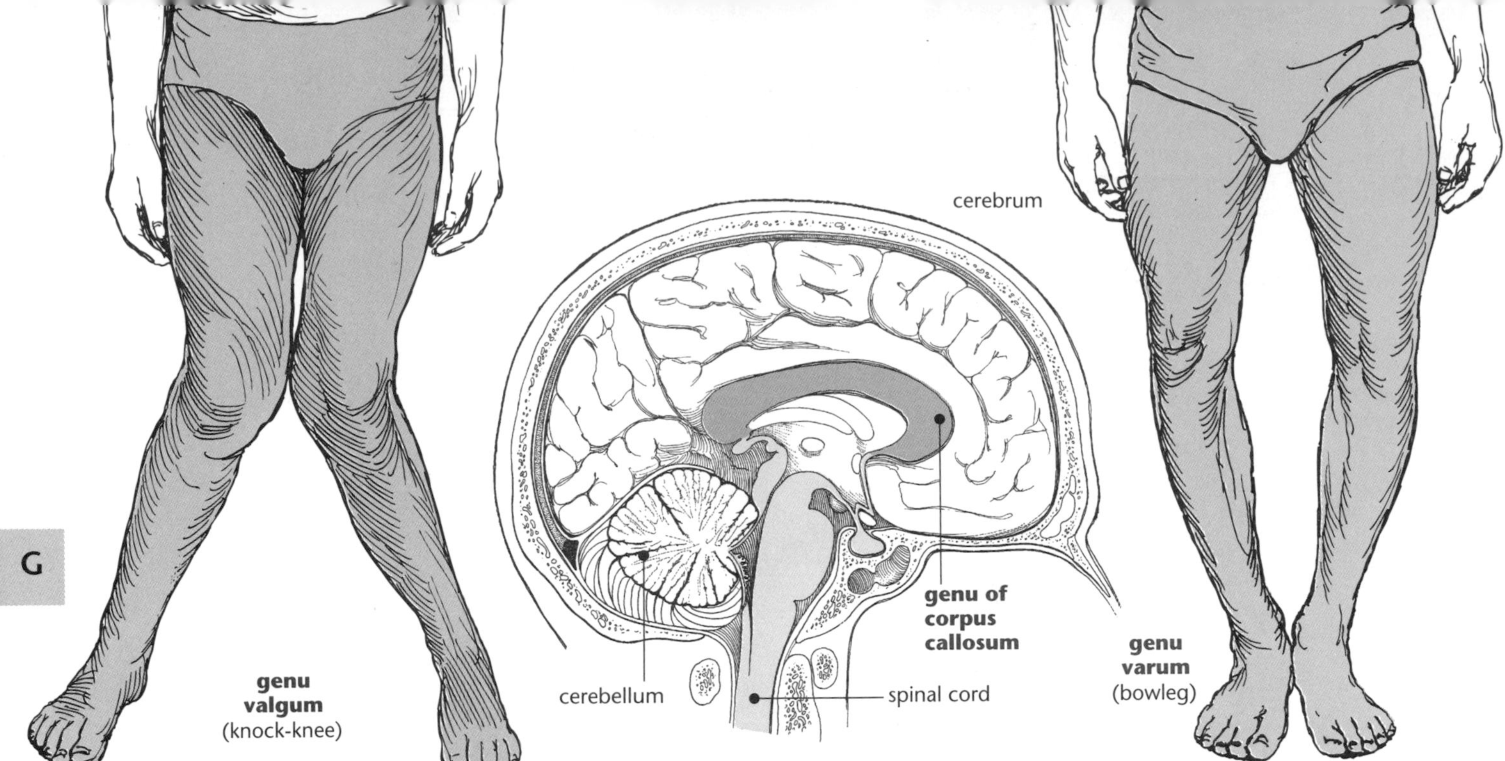

recessive g. A gene that is expressed only when homozygous (i.e., the individual inherits it from both parents); it does not produce a detectable effect in the organism when occurring in combination with a dominant gene (i.e., the individual inherits it only from one parent).

regulator g. A gene that controls the rate of protein synthesis; it controls the production of a repressor protein that acts on the operator gene.

sex-linked g. See X-linked gene and Y-linked gene.

structural g. A gene that specifies the formation of a particular polypeptide chain.

X-linked g. A gene located on an X (female) chromosome.

Y-linked g. A gene located on a Y (male) chromosome.

gene dosage (jēn do´saj) The number of times a specific gene is present in the nucleus of a cell.

genera (jen´er-ă) Plural of genus.

generalist (jen´er-al-ist) A physician who treats a broad range of diseases; a family or general physician, or an internist who does not subspecialize.

generalize (jen´er-al-īz) To become general; said of a primary local lesion that has become widespread or systemic.

generation (jen-er-a´shun) A stage in the succession of descent of the offspring of plants or animals.

filial g. Offspring resulting from a genetically specified mating: first filial generation (F_1), offspring of the first experimental crossing of animals or plants (parental generation with which the experiment starts is P_1); second filial generation (F_2), offspring resulting from intercrossing or self-fertilization of F_1 individuals; third, fourth, etc. filial generation (F_3, F_4, etc.), offspring of continued crossing of heterozygotes with continuation of F_2 ratios.

generative (jen´er-ă-tiv) Relating to reproduction.

generator (jen´er-a-tor) **1.** A machine for producing electrical energy from some other form of energy. **2.** A device that generates vapor, gas, or aerosol from a liquid or solid.

aerosol g. A device for generating airborne suspensions of small particles, usually for inhalation therapy.

asynchronous pulse g. A cardiac pacemaker in which the rate of discharge does not depend on the natural cardiac activity. Also called fixed rate pulse generator.

atrial synchronous pulse g. A ventricular stimulating pacemaker whose rate of discharge is determined by the atrial rate. Also called atrial triggered pulse generator.

atrial triggered pulse g. See atrial synchronous pulse generator.

demand pulse g. See ventricular inhibited pulse generator.

fixed rate pulse g. See asynchronous pulse generator.

pulse g. A generator serving as the source for an artificial pacemaker assembly; it generates and discharges electrical impulses to stimulate the heart.

radionuclide g. A receptacle containing a large quantity of a certain radionuclide that decays down to a secondary radionuclide of shorter half-life; the shorter form affords a continuing supply of relatively short-lived radionuclides for laboratory use. Also called "radioactive cow."

standby pulse g. See ventricular inhibited pulse generator.

ventricular inhibited pulse g. A generator that suppresses its electrical output in response to natural ventricular activity but which, in the absence of such cardiac activity, functions as an asynchronous pulse. Also called demand pulse generator; standby pulse generator.

ventricular synchronous pulse g. A pulse generator that delivers its output synchronously with naturally occurring ventricular activity but which, in the absence of such activity, functions as an asynchronous pulse. Also called ventricular triggered pulse generator.

ventricular triggered pulse g. See ventricular synchronous pulse generator.

generic (jĕ-ner´ik) **1.** Relating to a genus. **2.** See generic name, under name.

genesial, genesic (jĕ-ne´zhal, jĕ-nes´ik) **1.** Pertaining to origin. **2.** Pertaining to generation.

genesiology (jĕ-ne-ze-ol´ŏ-je) The study of generation and reproduction.

genesis (jĕn´ĕ-sis) Creation; origin.

genetic (jĕ-net´ik) **1.** Relating to the study of heredity. **2.** Determined by genes.

geneticist (jĕ-net´ĭ-sist) A scientist who specializes in genetics.

genetics (je-net´iks) The science of heredity; especially the study of the origin of the characteristics of the individual and hereditary transmission.

medical g. The branch of human genetics concerned with the relationship between heredity and disease.

genetotrophic (jĕ-net-o-trof´ik) Denoting inherited nutritional factors, applied especially to certain hereditary deficiency disorders.

genial (jĕ-ni´ăl) Relating to the chin.

genic (jen´ik) Relating to genes.

geniculate, geniculated (jĕ-nik´u-lāt, jĕ-nik´u-lā-tĕd) Shaped like a flexed knee.

geniculum (jĕ-nik´u-lŭm), *pl.* **genic´ula** A sharp kneelike bend in a small structure.

g. of facial canal The bend in the facial canal that houses the geniculum of the facial nerve.

g. of facial nerve (a) A bend of the horizontal portion of the facial nerve at the lateral end of the internal acoustic meatus, above the promontory of the middle ear. (b) A loop of facial nerve fibers curving around the abducens nucleus on the floor of the 4th ventricle of the brain.

genioglossus (je-ne-o-glos´us) See table of muscles.

geniohyoid (je-ne-o-hi´oid) See table of muscles.

genioplasty (je´ne-o-plas-te) Reparative or plastic surgery of the chin. Also called genyplasty.

genital (jen´ĭ-tal) Relating to reproduction.

genitalia (jen-ĭ-ta´e-ă) The genitals.

genitality (jen-ĭ-tal´ĭ-te) In psychoanalysis, a general term denoting the genital constituents of sexuality.

genitals (jen´ĭ-tals) The organs of reproduction.

genitourinary (jen-ĭ-to-u´rĭ-nar-e) (GU) Relating to the organs of reproduction and the urinary tract. Also called urogenital.

genodermatosis (jen-o-der-mă-to´sis) A genetically determined disorder of the skin.

genome (je´nōm) A complete set of chromosomes (with their genes) from one parent; the total genetic endowment.

genomic (je-no´mic) Relating to a genome.

genotype (jen´o-tīp) The genetic or hereditary constitution of an individual.

genotypical (jen-o-tĭp´ĭ-kal) Relating to a genotype.

gentamicin sulfate (jen-tă-mi´sin sul´fāt) A broad spectrum aminoglycoside antibiotic that inhibits the growth of bacteria; Garamycin®.

gentian violet (jen´shun vi´ŏ-lit) A compound composed of one or several methyl derivatives of pararosaniline; used as a biological stain, a bactericide in the treatment of minor lesions of the oral mucosa, and a fungicide in the treatment of candidiasis. Also called crystal violet.

genu (je´nu) **1.** The knee. **2.** Any structure resembling a flexed knee.

g. of corpus callosum The anterior extremity of the corpus callosum.

g. recurvatum The backward bending of the knee joint.

g. valgum A deformity of the leg at the level of the knee, usually bilateral, marked by a lateral angulation of the tibia. Also called knock-knee.

g. varum A deformity, usually bilateral, in which the leg has an outward curvature at the level of the knee. Also called bowleg.

genual (je´nu-al) Relating to the knee.

genus (je´nus), *pl.* **ge´nera** The biologic classification ranking below a family and above a species; a category denoting resemblances in general features

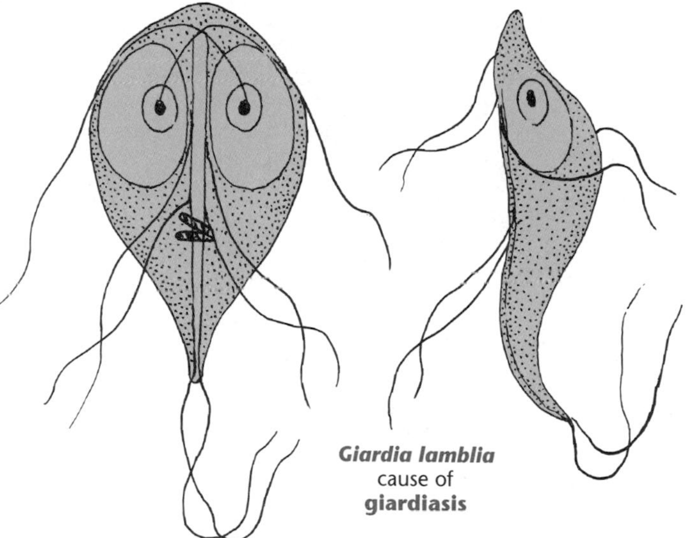

Giardia lamblia cause of **giardiasis**

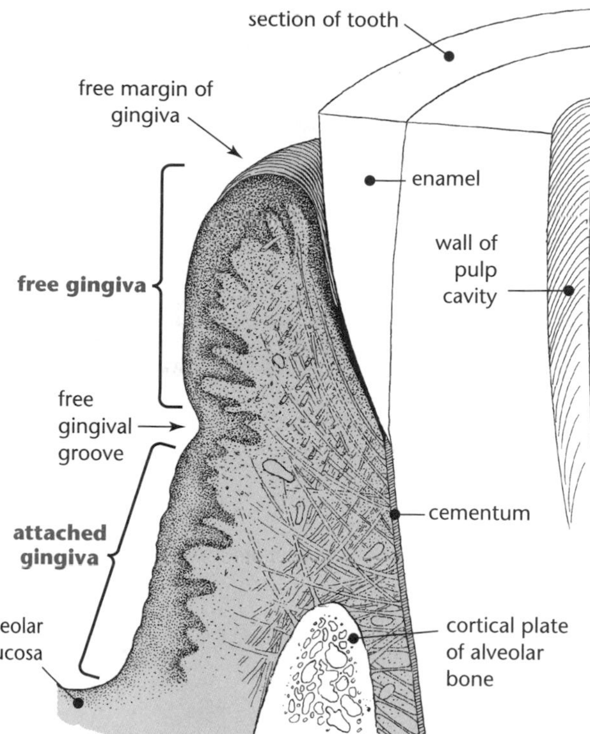

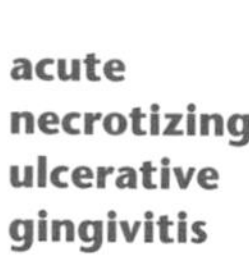
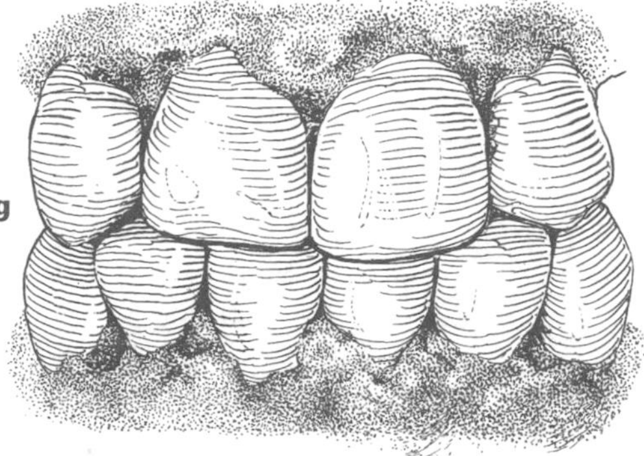

acute necrotizing ulcerative gingivitis

but differences in details.

genyplasty (jen-e-plas´te) See genioplasty.

geophagia (je-o-fa´ja) The habit of eating clay or dirt; a form of pica.

geotrichosis (je-o-tri-ko´sis) Condition caused by infection with the fungus *Geotrichum*.

Geotrichum (je-ot´rĭ-kum) A genus of yeastlike fungi, one species of which infects the lungs and bronchi of humans.

geriatric (jer-e-at´rik) Relating to old age.

geriatrician (jer-e-ă-trish´an) A physician who specializes in the treatment of diseases related to old age.

geriatrics (jer-e-at´riks) See geriatric medicine, under medicine.

germ (jerm) **1.** A pathogenic microbe. **2.** An embryonic structure capable of developing into a new organism; a primordium.

wheat g. The vitamin-rich embryonic or germinating portion of the wheat kernel; used as a cereal or dietary supplement.

germanium (jer-ma´ne-um) A metallic element; symbol Ge, atomic number 32, atomic weight 72.6.

germicidal (jer-mĭ-si´dal) Destructive to disease-causing microorganisms.

germicide (jer´mĭ-sīd) An agent that kills germs.

germinal (jer´mĭ-nal) **1.** Pertaining to germination. **2.** Pertaining to the nature of a germ.

germinoma (jer-mĭ-no-mă) Any tumor arising from germinal tissue (e.g., of the ovaries or testes).

geroderma (jer-o-der´mă) Atrophy of the skin.

gerodontics, gerodontology (jer-o-don´tiks, jer-o-don-tol´ŏ-je) The diagnosis and treatment of dental disorders of the aged.

geromarasmus (jer-o-mă-raz´mus) The atrophy of old age.

gerontal (jer-on´tal) Relating to old age.

gerontology (jer-on-tol´ŏ-je) The study of medical and social problems associated with aging.

gerontopia (jer-on-to´pe-ă) See senopia.

gerontotherapeutics (jer-on-to-ther-ă-pu´tiks) Treatment of diseases of the aged.

gerontoxon (jer-on-to-tok´son) See arcus senilis, under arcus.

gestagen (jes´tă-jen) A general term denoting hormones that produce progestational changes in the uterus.

gestalt (gĕ-shtawlt´) A unified system of physical, psychological, or symbolic phenomena having properties that cannot be derived solely from its components.

gestation (jes-ta´shun) See pregnancy.

gestational trophoblastic disease (GTD) Any of a group of pregnancy-related tumors or tumor-like conditions that have a progressive potential of becoming cancerous; characterized by proliferation of trophoblastic tissue; the lesions include invasive mole, hydatidiform mole, choriocarcinoma, and placental-site tumors. Also called gestational trophoblastic neoplasia (GTN).

Gianotti-Crosti syndrome (jē-ă-not´e-kros´te sin´drōm) Cutaneous manifestation of hepatitis B virus infection marked by an eruption of papules, especially on the arms and sides of the face, associated with mild fever and malaise; it generally disappears without treatment within 30 to 60 days. Also called papular acrodermatitis of childhood.

giantism (ji´ant-izm) Gigantism.

Giardia (je-ahr´de-ă) A genus of flagellate protozoa some of which are parasitic in the intestinal tract of humans and domestic animals.

G. lamblia A species with a broad rounded anterior end and a tapered pointed posterior; it has four pairs of flagella, two nuclei, a convex dorsal surface, and a concave ventral surface that forms a functional sucking disk in the anterior half of the body; a common cause of diarrhea and intestinal symptoms.

giardiasis (je-ahr-di´ă-sis) Infection with *Giardia lamblia*, transmitted via the fecal-oral route.

gibberish (jib´er-ĭsh) Incoherent, rapid talk.

gibbous (gib´us) Humpbacked.

gibbus (gib´us) A hump or kyphos.

GIFT Acronym for gamete intra-fallopian transfer; the placing of sperm and unfertilized ova together in a uterine (fallopian) tube to enhance the possibility of fertilization.

gigantism (ji-gan´tizm) An abnormal condition of excessive growth in height, greatly exceeding the average for the person's race.

gigavolt (jig´ă-vōlt) A billion volts.

gilbert (gil´bert) The electromagnetic unit of electromotive force.

Gilbert's syndrome (gil´bertz sin´drōm) See familial nonhemolytic jaundice, under jaundice.

Gilles de la Tourette's syndrome (zhēl-dĕ-lă-too-rets´ sin´drōm) A rare form of generalized tic usually beginning in childhood, between 2 and 15 years of age; marked by uncontrolled continuous gestures, facial twitching, foul language, and repetition of sentences spoken by other persons. Also called Gilles de la Tourette's disease; Tourette's disease; Tourette's syndrome.

gingiva (jin´jĭ-vă), *pl.* **gin´givae** (G) The gum; the fibrous tissue, covered by mucous membrane, that envelops the alveolar process and surrounds the neck of the tooth.

attached g. The portion of gingiva attached to the tooth and alveolar bone beyond the gingival groove.

buccal g. The portion of gingiva facing the cheek.

free g. The unattached margin of gingiva closely surrounding the tooth.

labial g. The portion of gingiva facing the lips.

lingual g. The portion of gingiva facing the tongue.

gingival (jin´jĭ-val) Pertaining to the gums.

gingivectomy (jin-jĭ-vek´tŏ-me) Surgical removal of diseased gum tissue.

gingivitis (jin-jĭ-vi´tis) Inflammation of the gums.

acute necrotizing ulcerative g. A bacterial (fusospirochetal) infection, usually of sudden onset, characterized by tender, bleeding gums with ulcer formation (especially between the teeth), a gray exudate, and fetid breath; most commonly occurring in individuals with poor oral hygiene. Also called trench mouth; Vincent's infection; Vincent's angina.

gingivoplasty (jin´jĭ-vo-plas-te) Surgical contouring of the gingiva.

gingivosis (jin-jĭ-vo´sis) A noninflammatory desquamative condition of the gums.

gingivostomatitis (jin-jĭ-vo-sto-mă-ti´tis) Inflammation of the gums and oral mucosa.

ginglymus (jing´glĭ-mus) See hinge joint, under joint.

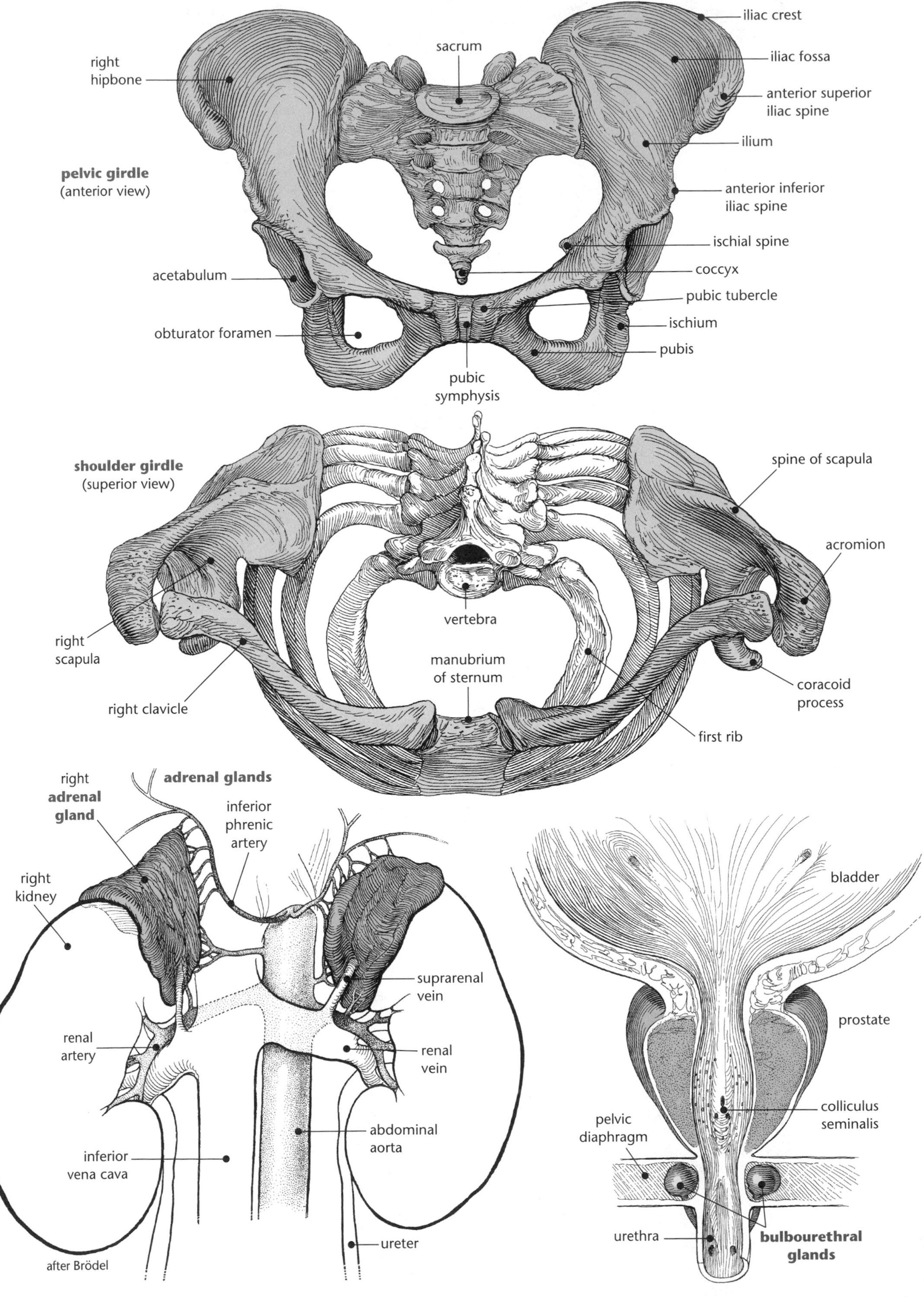
pelvic girdle
(anterior view)
right
hipbone
sacrum
iliac crest
iliac fossa
anterior superior
iliac spine
ilium
anterior inferior
iliac spine
ischial spine
coccyx
acetabulum
pubic tubercle
ischium
obturator foramen
pubis
pubic
symphysis
shoulder girdle
(superior view)
spine of scapula
acromion
vertebra
right
scapula
manubrium
of sternum
coracoid
process
right clavicle
first rib
right
adrenal
gland
adrenal glands
inferior
phrenic
artery
right
kidney
suprarenal
vein
renal
artery
renal
vein
abdominal
aorta
inferior
vena cava
ureter
after Brödel
bladder
prostate
colliculus
seminalis
pelvic
diaphragm
urethra
bulbourethral
glands

G

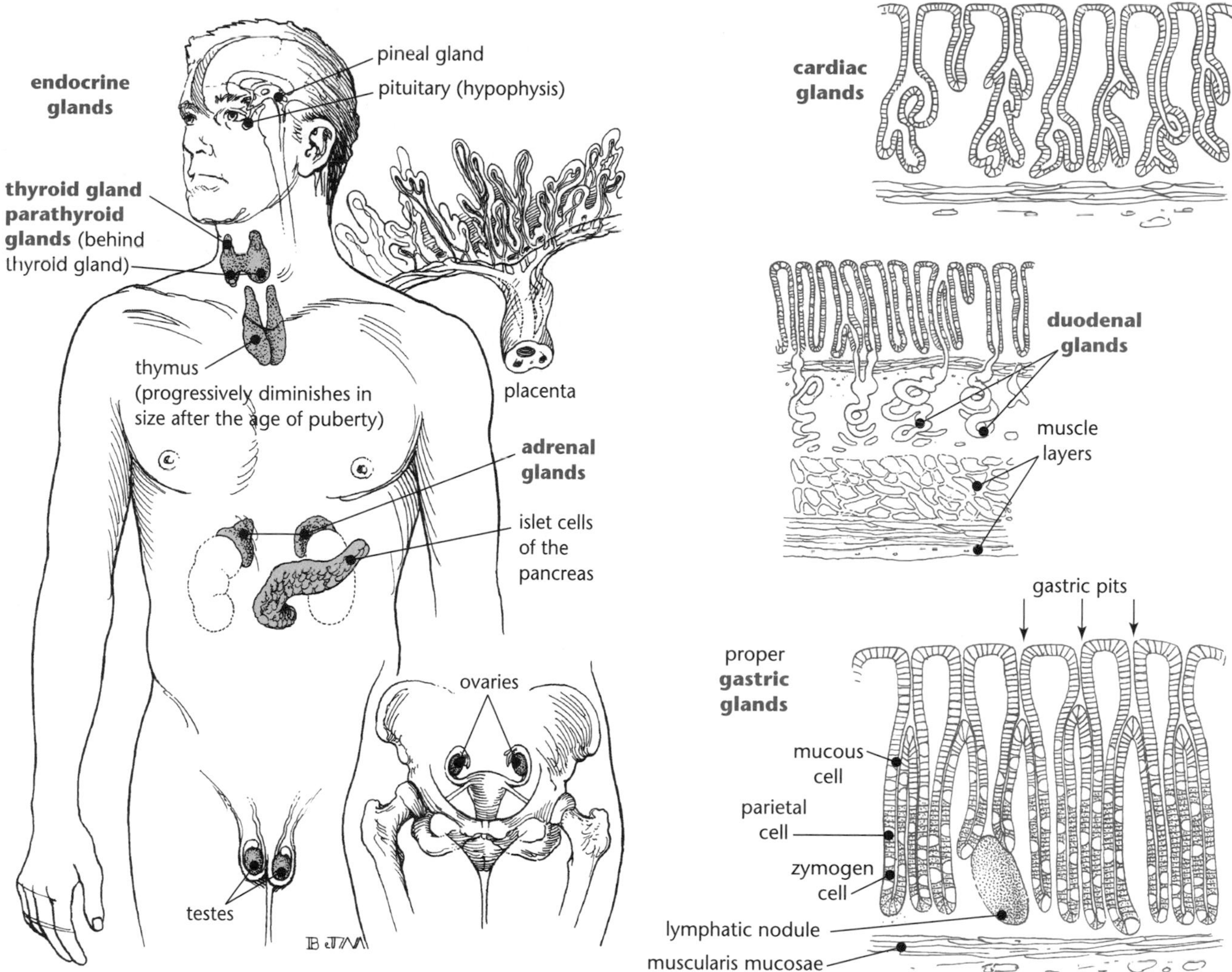

girdle (ger´dl) **1.** An encircling band. **2.** Any encircling structure or region.
pectoral g. See shoulder girdle.
pelvic g. The bony ring formed by the sacrum and the two hipbones.
shoulder g. A girdle formed by the collarbones (clavicles), shoulder blades (scapulae), and the upper part of the breastbone (sternum). Also called pectoral girdle.
girth (gurth) Circumference; the distance around anything, particularly the abdomen.
glabella (glă-bel´ă) The smooth area of the frontal bone, between the eyebrows.
glabrous (gla´brus) Hairless; smooth and bare.
gladiolus (glă-di´o-lus) The body or main portion of the breastbone (sternum).
gland (gland) (gl) A secreting organ.
accessory g. A small detached mass of glandular tissue located near a gland or similar structure.
accessory adrenal g.'s Adrenocortical bodies occurring in areolar tissue around principal glands, or in the spermatic cord, epididymis, and broad ligament of uterus.
acinous g. A gland made up of one or several saclike structures.
adrenal g. A flattened, somewhat triangular endocrine gland resting upon the upper end of each kidney; it produces steroid hormones (aldosterone, androgens, glucocorticoids, progestins, and estrogens), epinephrine, and norepinephrine. Also called suprarenal gland; adrenal body.
apocrine g. A gland producing a secretion which contains part of the secreting cells.
areolar g.'s A group of small sebaceous glands in the skin of the areola appearing as small nodules, which provide lubrication for the nipple; they enlarge markedly during the third trimester of pregnancy. Also called Montgomery glands; Montgomery follicles.
Bartholin's g. See greater vestibular gland.
Brunner's g.'s See duodenal glands.
bulbourethral g.'s Two pea-shaped glands in the urogenital diaphragm, dorsal and lateral to the membranous portion of the male urethra; during sexual stimulation, the glands secrete a mucuslike substance into the urethra that serves as a lubricant for the epithelium. Also called Cowper's glands.
cardiac g.'s The tubular, branched, slightly coiled, mucus-producing glands located in the transition zone between the esophagus and stomach; they also secrete electrolytes.
compound g. A gland composed of numerous small sacs (acini) whose excretory ducts combine to form larger ones.
Cowper's g.'s See bulbourethral glands.
ductless g. See endocrine gland.
duodenal g.'s Small, branched, compound tubular glands in the submucous layer of the first part of the duodenum; they secrete an alkaline mucoid substance into the crypts of Lieberkühn (intestinal glands) or directly to the surface between the duodenal villi. Also called Brunner's glands.
endocrine g. A gland without an excretory duct; its secretion (hormone) is released directly into the bloodstream.
endo-exocrine g. A gland (e.g., pancreas) that produces both internal and external secretions.
excretory g. Any gland that separates waste material from the blood.
exocrine g. A gland that discharges its secretion through a duct onto the internal or external surface of the body; it may be simple or compound.
gastric g.'s Numerous, straight, sometimes branched, tubular glands in the mucosa of the fundus and body of the stomach (they are absent in the cardiac and pyloric regions); they contain the cells that produce digestive enzymes. Also called peptic glands.
greater vestibular g. One of two small mucus-secreting glands on either side of the vaginal orifice, in the groove between the hymen and the labium minus; its major function is lubrication of the introitus. Also called Bartholin's gland; vulvovaginal gland.
holocrine g. A gland whose secretion is composed of the disintegrated secreting cell in addition to its accumulated secretion.
interscapular g. See brown fat, under fat.
intestinal g.'s Simple tubular glands in the mucous membrane of the intestines, concerned with the secretion of digestive enzymes and some hormones. Also called crypts of Lieberkühn.
lacrimal g. A gland that secretes tears; located in the upper lateral portion of the orbit.
Littre's g.'s See urethral glands of male urethra.
mammary g. A compound milk-producing gland that forms the major part of the female breast during the childbearing age and reaches functional maturity after pregnancy; consists of 15 to 20 lobes, each composed of many lobules; every lobe has a separate duct opening at the apex of the nipple. In the male, the gland is rudimentary. See also breast.
meibomian g. See tarsal gland.
mixed g. Gland in which some secretory units contain both serous and mucous cells (e.g., submandibular gland).
Montgomery g.'s See areolar glands.
parathyroid g.'s The smallest of the endocrine glands, situated between the dorsal borders of the thyroid gland and its capsule; usually four in number, each the approximate size of an apple seed, they produce parathyroid hormone (parathormone) which regulates the calcium and phosphate metabolism of the body.
paraurethral g. See urethral glands of female urethra.
parotid g. Salivary gland located below and in

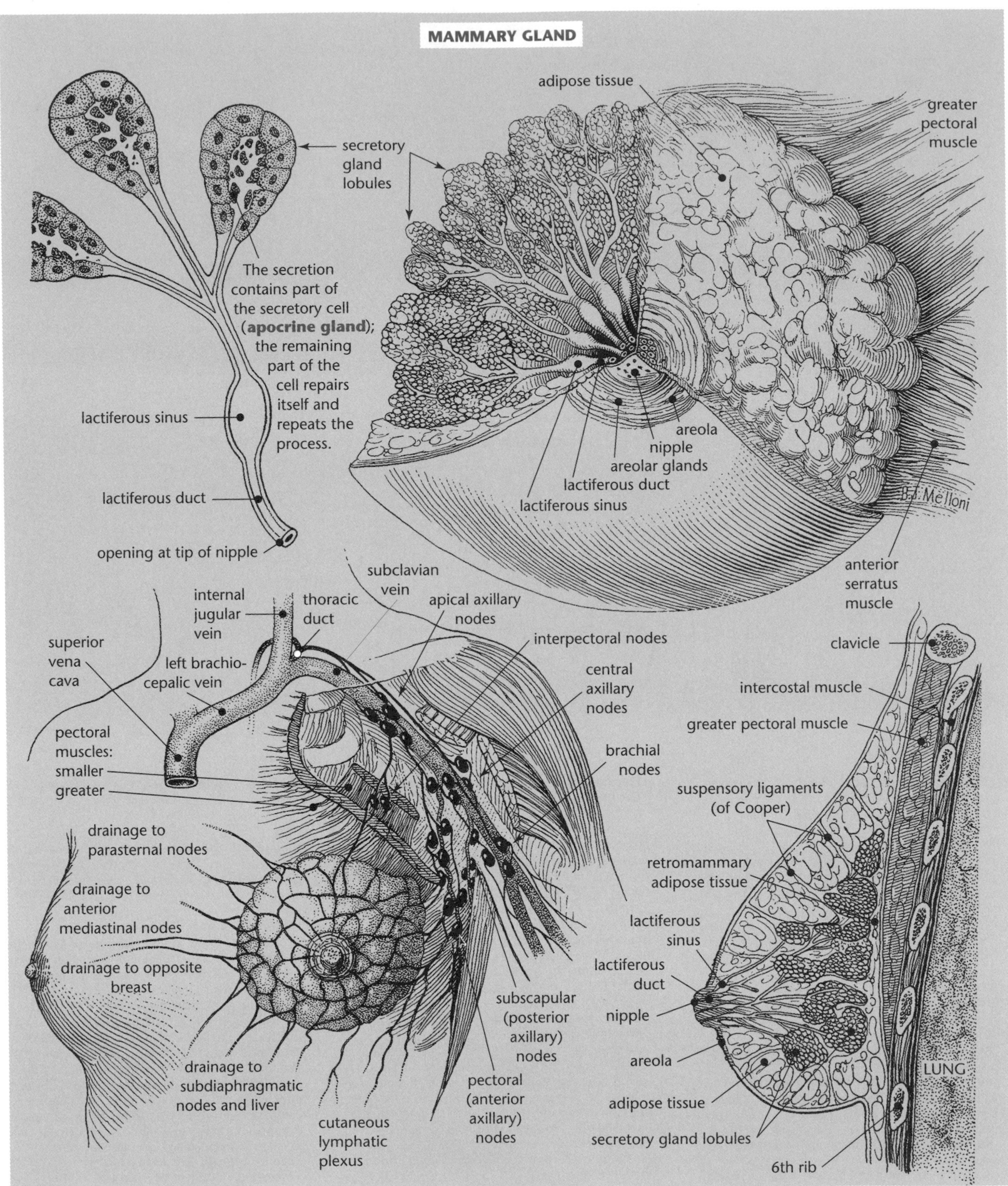

front of each ear.

pineal g. See pineal body, under body.

pituitary g. See hypophysis.

pyloric g. One of the simple, coiled, mucus-producing tubular glands of the pyloric part of the stomach.

racemose g. An acinous gland, like the parotid, whose acini are arranged like grapes on a stem.

sebaceous g. A simple branched holocrine gland in the dermis that secretes an oily substance (sebum) and usually opens into the distal part of the hair follicle; some open directly onto the skin surface (e.g., on the vermilion border of the lips).

seromucous g. See mixed gland.

simple g. A gland consisting of a single system of secretory passages opening into anonbranching duct; divided into tubular, tubuloalveolar, and alveolar types.

Skene's g. See urethral glands of female urethra.

sublingual g. One of two salivary glands in the floor of the mouth with a series of ducts (10 to 30) opening into the mouth at the side of the tongue's frenulum; most of the secretory units are mucus secreting with serous demilunes.

submandibular g. One of two predominately serous salivary glands in the upper neck; the main duct opens into the mouth beneath the tongue.

suprarenal g. See adrenal gland.

sweat g.'s Coiled tubular glands, located deep in the skin, that secrete a watery solution rich in sodium and chloride (sweat). Also called sudoriferous glands.

tarsal g. One of numerous sebaceous glands in the eyelids. Also called meibomian gland.

thymus g. See thymus.

thyroid g. The largest endocrine gland in man,

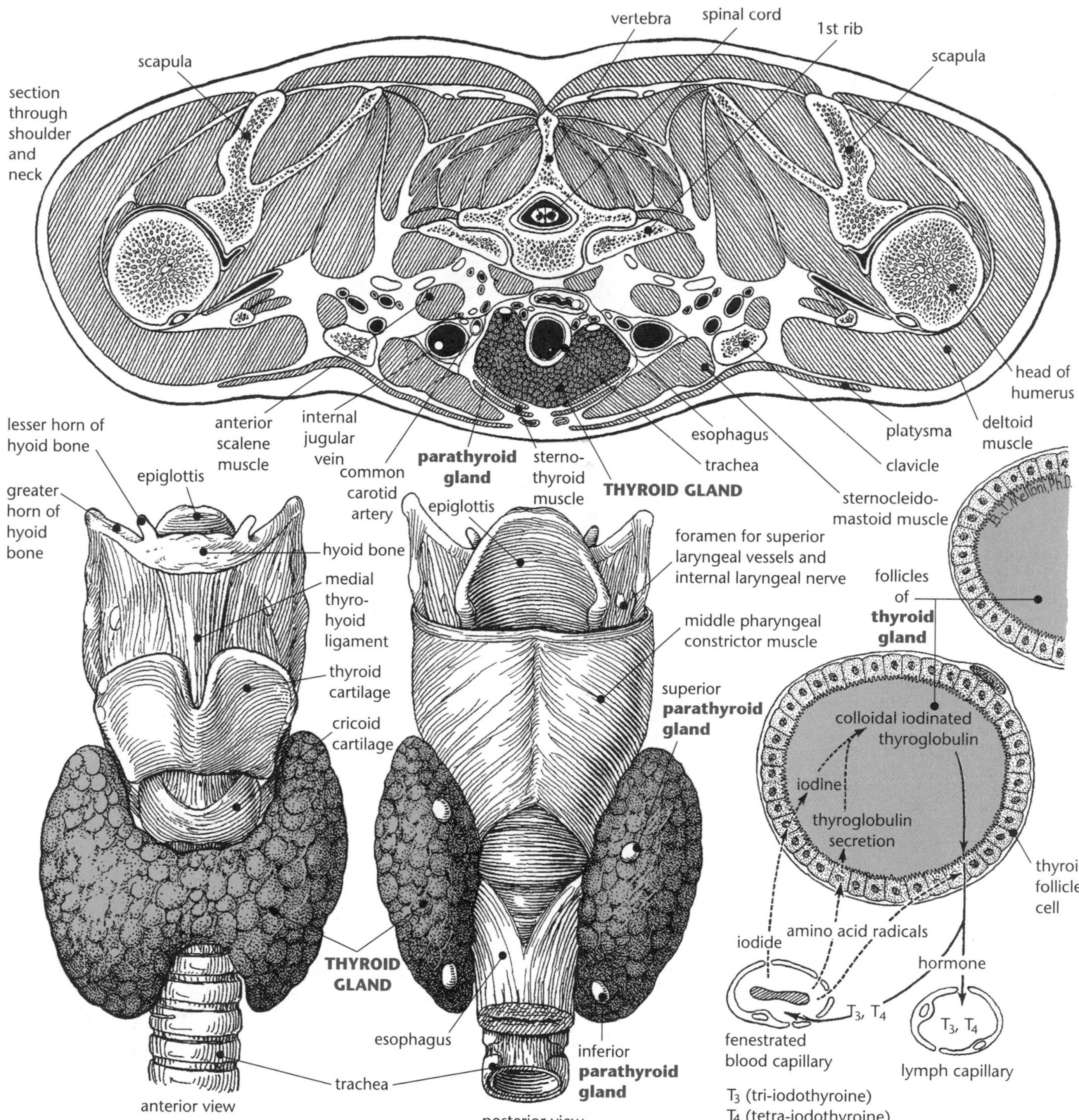

situated in front of the lower part of the neck, and consisting of right and left lobes, on either side of the trachea, joined by a connecting isthmus; it secretes the iodine-rich hormones thyroxin and triiodothyronine which are concerned with regulating the rate of metabolism; also thought to secrete thyrocalcitonin.

tubular g. A gland composed of one or more tubules closed at one end.

urethral g.'s of female urethra Numerous small glands in the mucous membrane of the urethra; some empty directly onto the urethral surface, others are grouped along the side and drain through a common duct.

urethral g.'s of male urethra Numerous small glands in the mucous membrane of the penile urethra. Also called Littre's glands.

uterine g.'s The numerous tubular glands extending through the whole thickness of the endometrium and opening into the cavity of the uterus; they secrete a fluid that keeps the interior of the uterus moist.

vulvovaginal g.'s See greater vestibular glands.

glanders (glan´derz) An infectious disease of horses, mules, and donkeys caused by the gram-negative bacillus *Pseudomonas mallei*; marked by fever and ulcers of the respiratory tract or skin; occasionally transmitted to humans. The cutaneous form is called farcy.

glandilemma (glan-dĭ-lem´ă) The enveloping membrane or capsule of a gland.

glandula (glan´du-lă) A small gland.

glandular (glan´du-lar) Relating to a gland.

glandule (glan´dūl) A small gland.

glans (glanz), *pl.* **glan´des** A small glandlike structure.

g. clitoridis, g. of clitoris A small rounded tip of the body of the clitoris.

g. penis The caplike extension of the corpus spongiosum at the tip of the penis.

Glanzmann's disease (glahnz´manz dĭ-zēz´) See thrombasthenia.

glass (glas) Any of a class of transparent or translucent brittle materials composed of silica with oxides of several bases, and considered physically as supercooled liquids instead of true solids.

cover g. A thin piece of glass used to cover an object examined under the microscope.

crown g. Glass having a low dispersion and usually a low index of refraction; a compound of lime, potash, alumina, and silica; used in ophthalmic lenses.

flint g. A heavy, brilliant optical glass having a high dispersion and usually a high index of refraction.

optical g. Glass carefully manufactured to obtain controlled index of refraction and dispersion, purity, transparency, homogeneity, and workability; the two most common types are crown and flint.

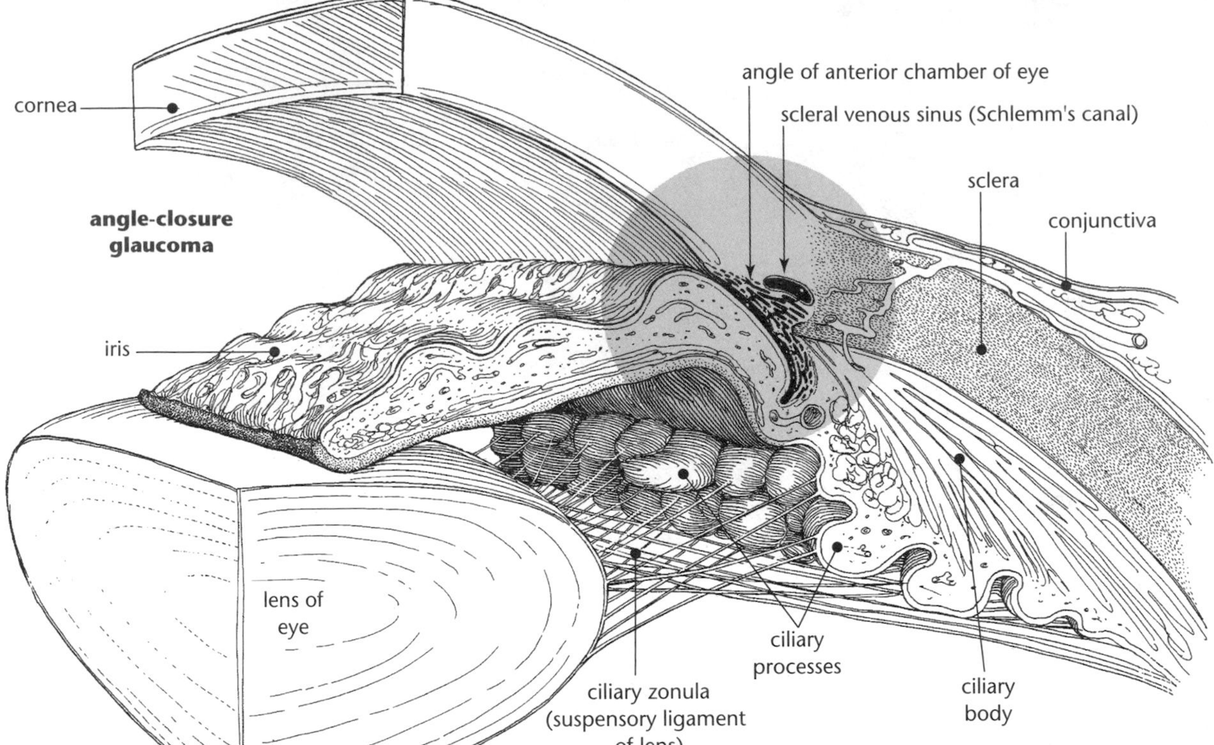

G

quartz g. Crystal made by fusing pure quartz sand; it transmits ultraviolet rays.

Wood's g. A glass containing nickel oxide; used for diagnostic purposes, as in ringworm of the scalp where infected hairs are fluorescent when viewed under light filtered through this glass; also used in conjunction with certain dyes, such as fluorescin, for visualizing abrasions of the cornea.

glasses (glas´ĕz) Eyeglasses.

glaucoma (glaw-ko´mă) An abnormal increase in intraocular pressure.

acute g. See angle-closure glaucoma.

angle-closure g. Glaucoma of sudden onset occurring when the outermost part of the iris is pushed against the inner periphery of the cornea, closing the anterior chamber angle and preventing the outflow of aqueous humor from the anterior chamber of the eye; may be precipitated by drugs used to dilate the pupil, or may result from hemorrhage or swelling of the iris or of the ciliary body. Also called acute glaucoma; narrow-angle glaucoma.

congenital g. See buphthalmos.

narrow-angle g. See angle-closure glaucoma.

open-angle g. A chronic, slowly progressive, bilateral glaucoma due to some defect in the trabecular meshwork of the anterior chamber angle resulting in failure of aqueous humor to drain properly.

phacolytic g. Glaucoma occurring as a complication of cataract; fluid from the liquified cortex of the lens seeps into the anterior chamber of the eye, causing swelling of the uvea which obstructs the outflow system and prevents adequate escape of the aqueous humor from the anterior chamber.

secondary g. Increased ocular pressure occurring as a manifestation of another, preexisting, intraocular disease.

glenohumeral (glĕ-no-hu´mer-ăl) Relating to the glenoid fossa and the humerus.

glenoid (gle´noid) Resembling a socket; applied to articular depressions forming the shoulder joint (glenoid fossa) and the articulation of the jaw (glenoid or mandibular fossa).

glia (gli´ă) The non-neuronal tissue of the brain and spinal cord. Also called neuroglia.

gliacyte (gli´ă-sīt) A cell of the non-nervous components of nervous tissue (neuroglia).

gliadin (gli´ă-din) Any of various simple proteins obtained from wheat and rye glutens. Also called glutin.

glial (gli´al) Relating to the non-nervous elements of nervous tissue.

glide (glīd) An effortless movement.

mandibular g. The side-to-side, protrusive, and intermediate movement of the mandible that occurs when the occlusal surfaces of teeth are in contact.

glioblastoma (gli-o-blas-to´mă) General term for malignant tumors containing neuroglial cells (gliacytes).

g. multiforme The most malignant and rapidly growing tumor of the cerebral hemispheres, composed of undifferentiated cells. Now called grade IV astrocytoma.

glioma (gli-o´mă) Any tumor derived from the various types of cells that make up brain tissue (e.g., astrocytoma, choroid plexus papilloma, ependymoma, oligodendroglioma).

gliomatosis (gli-o-mă-to´sis) Presence of gliomas within the brain substance.

gliomatous (gli-o´mă-tus) Relating to or of the nature of a glioma.

gliosis (gli-o´sis) Overgrowth of the non-nervous cellular elements of the brain and spinal cord.

globi (glo´bi) **1.** Plural of globus. **2.** Brown granular masses sometimes seen in the granulomatous lesions of leprosy.

globin (glo´bin) A simple protein constituent of the blood pigment hemoglobin.

globule (glob´yūl) A minute spherical body, especially a small drop of liquid.

Morgagni's g.'s Minute opaque spheres of fluid beneath the capsule and lens fibers, sometimes seen in cases of cataract. Also called Morgagni's spheres.

globulin (glob´u-lin) Any of a class of simple proteins that are insoluble in water, soluble in saline solutions, and coagulable by heat; found in blood and cerebrospinal fluid; human serum globulin is divided into alpha, beta, and gamma fractions on the basis of electrophoretic mobility.

accelerator g. (AcG, ac-g) A blood-coagulating factor of plasma that speeds the conversion of prothrombin to thrombin in the presence of thromboplastin and ionized calcium. Also called factor V.

antihemophilic g. (AHG) **1.** See factor VIII. **2.** A sterile preparation of normal human plasma which shortens the clotting time of hemophilic blood; used as an antihemophilic.

antilymphocyte g. (ALG) See antilymphocyte serum, under serum.

gamma g., γ-g. Serum proteins that constitute the majority of immunoglobulins and antibodies; used in the prevention of numerous diseases, including measles and certain types of hepatitis.

immune serum g. A sterile preparation containing a number of antibodies normally present in adult human blood; used as an immunizing agent.

thyroxine-binding g. (TBG) An alpha globulin with a strong affinity for the hormone thyroxine, thus acting as a carrier of thyroxine in the blood; significant changes in levels of TBG may alter measured T_4 levels.

globulinuria (glob-u-lĭ-nu´re-ă) The presence of globulin in the urine.

globus (glo´bus) A globe or ball.

g. hystericus A hysterical sensation of having a lump or ball in the throat.

g. pallidus The inner gray portion of the lentiform nucleus in the brain.

glomangioma (glo-man-je-o´mă) Painful, small benign tumor of a glomus body, mainly occurring under the nails of the fingers and toes.

glomerular (glo-mer´u-lar) Relating to a glomerulus.

glomerulitis (glo-mer´u-li´tis) Inflammation of the glomeruli of the kidney.

glomerulonephritis (glo-mer-u-lo-nĕ-fri´tis) (GN) Kidney disease that is marked by alteration in the structure of the glomeruli; it may be acute, subacute, or chronic.

acute crescentic g. See rapidly progressive glomerulonephritis.

acute proliferative g. Disorder occurring primarily in children and sometimes in young adults, most often following streptococcal infections; classical symptoms include fluid retention, periorbital edema, diminished urinary output, dark tea-colored urine, and elevation of the blood pressure; hematuria, red blood cell casts, and proteinuria are characteristic. Also called acute nephritis; proliferative glomerulonephritis.

chronic g. Glomerulonephritis of insidious onset or occurring as a sequel to acute glomerulonephritis; marked by kidney failure, hypertension, and proteinuria; kidneys become symmetrically shrunken and granular. Also called chronic nephritis.

diffuse g. Glomerulonephritis involving most of the renal glomeruli.

focal g. Glomerular damage restricted to some but not all glomeruli; may be a mild condition or a manifestation of a more serious progressive disease (e.g., lupus erythematosus, polyarteritis nodosa.

focal embolic g. A complication of subacute bacterial endocarditis.

global g. Complete involvement of the affected glomerulus, as opposed to segmental involvement.

hypocomplementemic g. See membranoproliferative glomerulonephritis.

immune complex g. Glomerulonephritis in which deposition of immune complexes in the renal glomerulus activates potent mediators of inflammation (such as complement proteins) and a variety of other cells, ultimately causing damage to the glomerulus and renal failure.

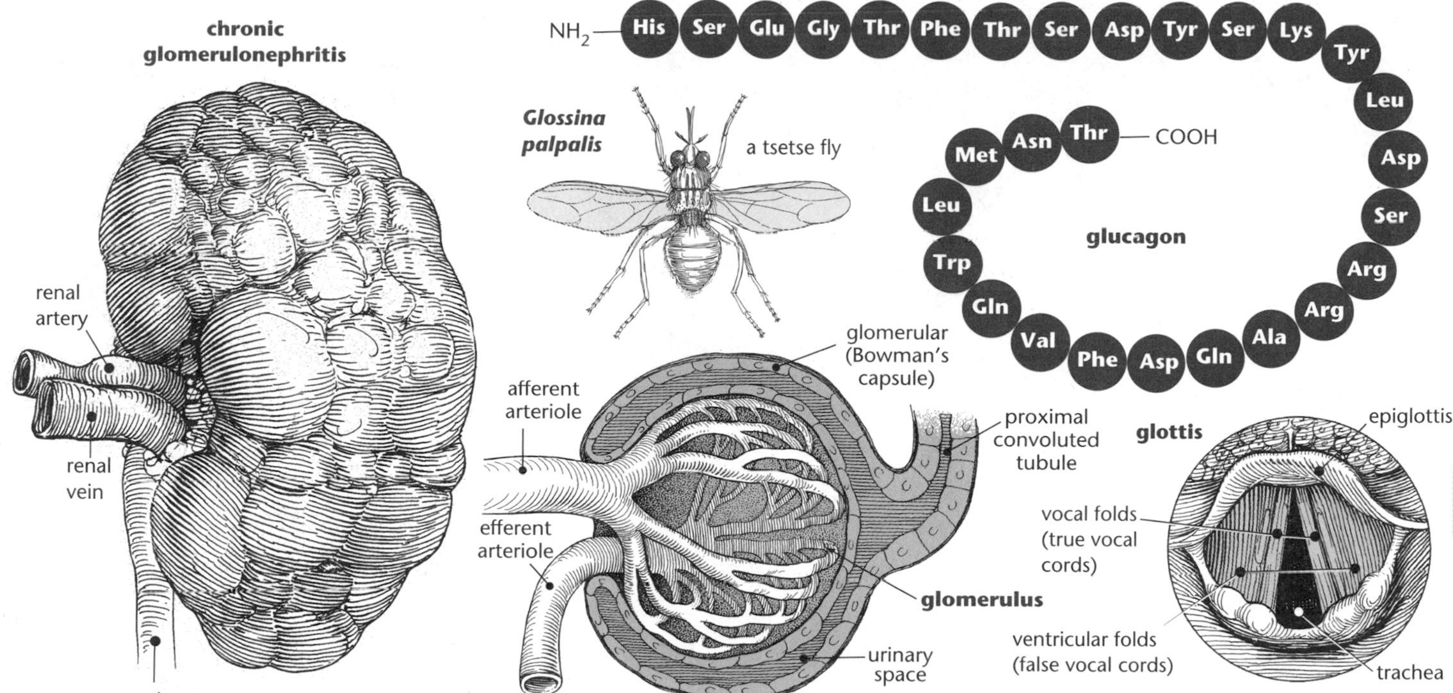

lobular g. See membranoproliferative glomerulonephritis.

membranoproliferative g. (MPGN) Disease of children and young adults, marked by proliferation of glomerular cells combined with capillary wall thickening; symptoms suggest either acute glomerulonephritis or a nephrotic syndrome with microscopic blood in the urine (hematuria); some types involve the immune system, with complement depression ranging from intermittent to persistent. Also called hypocomplementemic glomerulonephritis; mesangiocapillary glomerulonephritis; lobular glomerulonephritis.

membranous g. (MGN) A type marked by thickening of the basement membrane in the glomerular capillaries, causing proteinuria and generalized edema, and often associated with the nephrotic syndrome; a characteristic spiking appearance is found in the basement membrane on microscopy.

mesangiocapillary g. See membranoproliferative glomerulonephritis.

mesangioproliferative g. Changes in mesangial cells and proliferation (focal and diffuse) in a variety of glomerulonephritides including lupus nephritis and IgA nephropathy.

poststreptococcal g. Acute glomerulonephritis.

proliferative g. See acute proliferative glomerulonephritis.

rapidly progressive g. A form having an insidious beginning, without a previous episode of streptococcal infection, or possibly an unresolved poststreptococcal nephritis with renal insufficiency leading to death within a few months; characterized by marked crescent formation. Also called acute crescentic glomerulonephritis.

segmental g. Glomerulonephritis affecting only portions of the glomeruli.

subacute g. A term used variously to describe rapidly progressive glomerulonephritis or a type with nephrotic syndrome and a prolonged course.

glomerulopathy (glo-mer-u-lop´ă-the) Any disease of the filtering units (glomeruli) of the kidney.

glomerulosclerosis (glo-mer-u-lo-sklĕ ro´sis) Fibrosis and degeneration of the structures within the filtering units (glomeruli) of the kidney.

diabetic g. Glomerulosclerosis in which scarring occurs in a nodular pattern at the periphery of the glomeruli; occurs as a complication of diabetes mellitus, predominantly the insulin-dependent type; associated with excretion of protein in the urine, swelling of soft tissues, and high blood pressure.

focal segmental g. A form of progressive renal disease beginning in juxtamedullary capillaries and extending in a centrifugal pattern; usually presents in children or adolescents as a nephrotic syndrome.

glomerulus (glo-mer´u-lus), *pl.* **glomer´uli** **1.** A small cluster of nerves or capillaries; when used alone the term refers to a tuft of capillaries at the beginning of each uriniferous tubule in the kidney (malpighian tuft). **2.** The coiled secretory portion of a sweat gland.

glomus (glo´mus) A minute globular body composed of anastomoses between arterioles and venules and having a rich nerve supply.

carotid g. See carotid body, under body.

intravagal g. A collection of chemoreceptor cells on the auricular branch of the vagus nerve; a tumor of this glomus may cause loss of hearing.

jugular g. A glomus in the adventitia of the jugular bulb.

glossa (glos´ă) Latin for tongue.

glossal (glos´al) Relating to the tongue.

glossalgia (glos-al´jă) A painful tongue. Also called glossodynia.

glossectomy (glos-ek-tŏ-me) Amputation of the tongue or of a portion of it.

Glossina (glo-si´nă) A genus of bloodsucking flies, the tsetse flies, which transmit the microorganisms causing African sleeping sickness in humans and domestic animals.

glossitis (glos-i´tis) Inflammation of the tongue. Also called glottitis.

glossodynia (glos-o-din´e-ă) See glossalgia.

glossograph (glos´o-graf) Instrument used to record the movements of the tongue in speaking.

glossolalia (glos-o-la´le-ă) Meaningless speech; unintelligible and rapid chatter.

glossolysis (glos-ol´i-sis) See glossoplegia.

glossopharyngeal (glos-o-fă-rin´je-al) Relating to the tongue and pharynx.

glossoplasty (glos´o-plas-te) Reparative surgery of the tongue.

glossoplegia (glos´o-ple´jă) Paralysis of the tongue. Also called glossolysis.

glossoptosis (glos-op-to´sis) Downward displacement of the tongue.

glossorrhaphy (glos-or´ă-fe) Suture of the tongue.

glossospasm (glos´o-spaz-m) Spasmodic contraction of the tongue.

glossotomy (glos-ot´ŏ-me) Any surgical incision on the tongue.

glossotrichia (glos-o-trik´e-ă) See black tongue, under tongue.

glottic (glot´ik) Relating to either the tongue or the glottis.

glottis (glot´is) The vocal apparatus located in the larynx, consisting of the vocal cords and the opening between them.

glottitis (glo-ti´tis), *pl.* **glot´tides** Inflammation of the glottis.

glucagon (gloo´kă-gon) A polypeptide hormone, normally produced by α-cells of the islets of Langerhans in the pancreas when the blood sugar level gets too low; it aids in the breakdown of glycogen in the liver, thus elevating the blood sugar concentration.

glucan (gloo´kan) A polyglucose (e.g., starch amylose, glycogen amylose).

α-glucan-branching glycosyltransferase (gloo´kan-branch´ing gli-ko-sĭl-trans´fer-ās) An enzyme in muscle that cleaves α-1,4 linkages in glycogen or starch, transferring the fragments into α-1,6 linkages and creating branches in the polysaccharide molecules. Also called branching enzyme.

α-1,4-glucan 4-glucanohydrolase (gloo´kan gloo-kan-o-hi´dro-lās) Alpha-1,4-glucan 4-glucanohydrolase; an enzyme that, through a reaction with water, breaks down amylose (a straight chain polysaccharide) to form glucose and maltose; present in plants and obtained in crystalline form from pancreatic juice and saliva. Formerly called α-amylase.

α-1,4-glucan maltohydrolase (gloo´kan mawl-to-hi´dro-lās) Alpha-1,4-glucan maltohydrolase; an enzyme that, through a reaction with water, splits amylopectin (a branched polysaccharide) to form maltose; present in soybeans, wheat, barley, and other similar plants. Formerly called β-amylase.

glucocorticoid (gloo-ko-kor´tĭ-koid) Any steroid hormone of the adrenal cortex (or synthetic steroid) concerned with gluconeogenesis from amino acids and catabolism of protein; this class of compounds has other activities including anti-inflammatory activity and ability to suppress the synthesis of ACTH and MSH; cortisol is the major naturally occurring hormone of this type in humans.

glucogenic (gloo-ko-jen´ik) Producing glucose.

glucokinase (gloo-ko-ki´nās) A specific phosphorylation enzyme for glucose, present in the liver and muscle; it catalyzes the conversion of glucose to glucose 6-phosphate, in which one molecule of adenosine triphosphate (ATP) is used.

glucokinetic (gloo-ko-ki-net´ik) Mobilizing glucose in the body, as in the maintenance of sugar level.

gluconeogenesis (gloo-ko-ne-o-jen´ĕ-sis) Formation of glucose from noncarbohydrate sources, such as protein and fat.

glucosamine (gloo-kos´să-mēn) An amino sugar present in mucopolysaccharides. Also called chitosamine.

glucosan (gloo´ko-san) Any anhydride of glucose; a polysaccharide yielding glucose on hydrolysis (e.g., cellulose, glycogen, starch, dextrin).

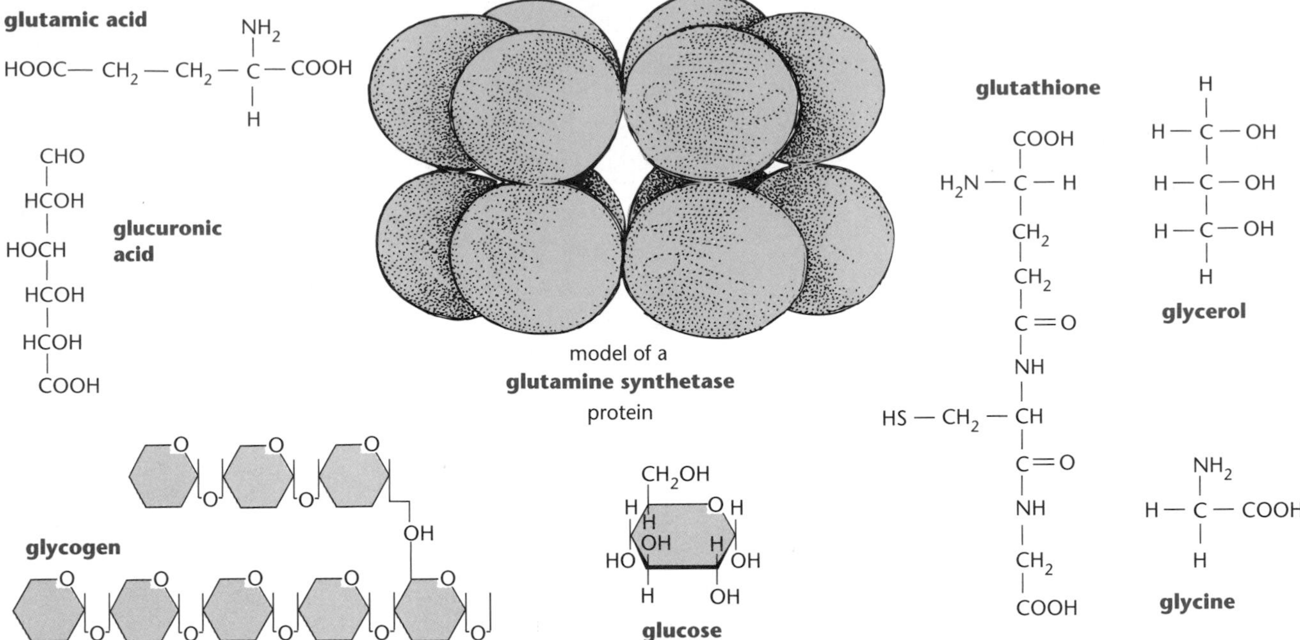

glucose (gloo´kōs) A dextrorotatory monosaccharide or simple sugar, $C_6H_{12}O_6 \cdot H_2O$, occurring as an odorless, sweet, crystalline powder; present in animal and plant tissue and obtained synthetically from starch; used in medicine as an intravenous nutrient. Also called blood sugar; grape sugar; dextrose.

glucose 6-phosphatase (gloo´kōs siks-fos´fă-tās) (G6P) A microsomal enzyme catalyzing the hydrolysis of glucose 6-phosphate to glucose and inorganic phosphate; present in liver, kidney, intestinal mucosa, and endometrium; it enables the liver to regulate blood sugar (glucose) concen-tration. Inherited deficiency of this enzyme causes glycogen storage disease (type 1 glycogenosis).

glucose 6-phosphate dehydrogenase (gloo ´kōs siks-fos´fă-tās de-hi´dro-jĕn-ās) (G6PD) Enzyme that promotes the oxidation of glucose 6-phosphate to 6-phosphogluconolactone.

glucoside (gloo´ko-sīd) One of a variety of substances in nature containing glucose combined by an ether linkage.

glucosuria (gloo-ko-su´re-ă) Presence of glucose in the urine.

glucuronic acid (gloo-ku-ron´ik as´id) The uronic acid of glucose, $HOOC(CHOH)_4CHO$; it inactivates various substances (e.g., benzoic acid, phenol, and the female sex hormones); the glucuronides so formed are excreted in the urine.

β-glucuronidase (gloo-ku-ron´ĭ-dās) An enzyme catalyzing the hydrolysis of various β-D-glucuronides, liberating free glucuronic acid; active in the liver, spleen, endometrium, breasts, adrenal glands, and testes.

glucuronide (gloo-ku-ron´īd) A glycoside of glucuronic acid.

glue-sniffing (gloo snĭf´ing) The intentional inhalation of fumes from plastic cements, resulting in central nervous system stimulation followed by depression.

glutamic acid (gloo-tam´ik as´id) (Glu) An amino acid present in protein; involved in ammonia production in the kidney.

glutamic-oxaloacetic transaminase (gloo-tam´ik ok-să-lo-ă-se´tik trans-am´ĭ-nās) (GOT) See aspartate aminotransferase (AST).

glutamic-pyruvic transaminase (gloo-tam´ik pi-roo´vik trans-am´ĭ-nās) (GPT) See alanine aminotransferase (ALT).

glutamine (gloo´tă-mēn) (Gln) An amino acid found as a constituent of proteins and in free form in blood; it yields glutamic acid and ammonia on hydrolysis.

g. synthetase An enzyme that catalyzes the amination of glutamic acid to glutamine which occurs concurrently with the hydrolysis of ATP to ADP and orthophosphate (P_1).

glutaraldehyde (gloo-tă-ral´dĕ-hīd) A tissue fixative that causes a fine precipitation of protein, thus permitting sections to be cut without appreciable distortion of structure; universally used as a prefixer in electron microscopy, generally followed by fixation with osmium tetroxide.

glutathione (gloo-tă-thi´ōn) A crystalline tripeptide of glycine, cystine, and glutamic acid that is present in blood and other tissues; it activates certain proteins and takes part in oxidation-reduction processes; the reduced form is abbreviated GSH; in the oxidized form two molecules are linked together and abbreviated GSSG.

gluteal (gloo´te-ăl) Relating to the buttocks.

gluten (gloo´tĕn) A mixture of insoluble plant proteins present in grains such as wheat, rye, oats, and barley; used as an adhesive and as a flour substitute.

glutethimide (gloo-teth´ĭ-mīd) A compound that is a depressant of the central nervous system; used as a hypnotic; Doriden®.

gluteus (gloo´te-us), *pl.* **glu´tei** Any of the three buttock muscles. See table of muscles.

glutin (gloo´tin) See gliadin.

glutinous (gloo´tĭ-nus) Sticky.

glutitis (gloo-ti´tis) Inflammation of the muscles of the buttock.

glycemia (gli-se´me-ă) The presence of sugar (glucose) in the blood.

glyceraldehyde (glis-ĕr-al´dĕ-hīd) Compound formed by the oxidation of glycerol. Also called glyceric aldehyde.

glyceridase (glis´ĕr-ĭ-dās) General term for any of several enzymes that promote the hydrolysis of glycerol esters.

glyceride (glis´ĕr-īd) An ester of glycerol.

glycerin (glis´ĕr-in) A clear, syrupy sweet liquid, $C_3H_8O_3$, used as a sweetener, a lubricant, and a solvent for drugs. See also glycerol.

glycerol (glis´ĕr-ol) A sweet, syrupy trihydric alcohol, occurring in combination as glycerides and produced by the fermentation of sugar; pharmaceutical preparations are known as glycerin.

glyceryl (glis´ĕr-il) The trivalent radical, $C_3H_5^{\equiv}$ of glycerol.

g. guaiacolate Guaifenesin.

g. trinitrate Nitroglycerin.

glycine (gli´sēn) (Gly) The principal amino acid present in sugarcane, $C_2H_5NO_2$; the simplest of the amino acids and one of the first to be isolated from proteins. Also called aminoacetic acid.

glycinuria (gli-si-nū´rē-ă) The presence of glycine in the urine.

glycocalix (gli-ko-kal´iks) A carbohydrate-rich outer fuzz coating on the free surface of certain epithelial cells; it is rich in mucoid components. Also spelled glycocalyx.

glycocholic acid (gli-ko-ko´lik) The principal acid of the bile.

glycogen (gli´ko-jĕn) The form in which carbohydrate is stored in the body, especially in the liver and muscles; a highly branched glucosan of high molecular weight; it is broken down as needed to glucose molecules.

glycogenase (gli-ko-jen´ās) The enzyme that promotes the breakdown of glycogen to glucose.

glycogenesis (gli-ko-jen´ĕ-sis) The formation of glycogen from glucose or other monosaccharides.

glycogenolysis (gli-ko-jĕ-nol´ĭ-sis) The breakdown of glycogen to simpler products.

glycogenosis (gli-ko-jĕ-no´sis) Abnormal accumulation of glycogen in the tissues. Also called glycogen storage disease.

generalized g. See type II glycogenosis.

glucose 6-phosphatase hepatorenal g. See type I glycogenosis.

myophosphorylase deficiency g. See type V glycogenosis.

type I g. Disorder thought to be caused by deficiency of the enzyme glucose 6-phosphatase, resulting in excessive accumulation of glycogen in the liver and kidneys. Also called von Gierke's disease; glucose 6-phosphatase hepatorenal glycogenosis.

type II g. Disease of infancy caused by deficiency of an enzyme, lysomal α-1,4,-glucosidase, resulting in accumulation of glycogen in the heart muscles, liver, and nervous system; newborn infants have marked cardiac enlargement and congestive heart failure usually leading to death within two years of age. Also called generalized glycogenosis; Pompe's disease.

type V g. Disease caused by deficiency of muscle glycogen phosphorylase (enzyme that catalyzes the splitting of glycogen to glucose), resulting in accumulation of glycogen in the muscles. Also called McArdle's disease; myophosphorylase deficiency glycogenosis.

glycogen storage disease (gli´ko-jĕn stōr´ij dĭ-zēz´) See glycogenosis.

glycogeusia (gli-ko-joo´se-ă) A subjective sweet taste in the mouth.

glycol (gli´kol) One of a group of alcohols containing two hydroxyl groups.

glycolysis (gli-kol´ĭ-sis) The energy-producing process in the body, especially in muscles, in which sugar is broken down into lactic acid; since oxygen is not consumed, it is frequently termed anaerobic glycolysis.

glycolytic (gli-ko-lit´ik) Causing the hydrolysis of

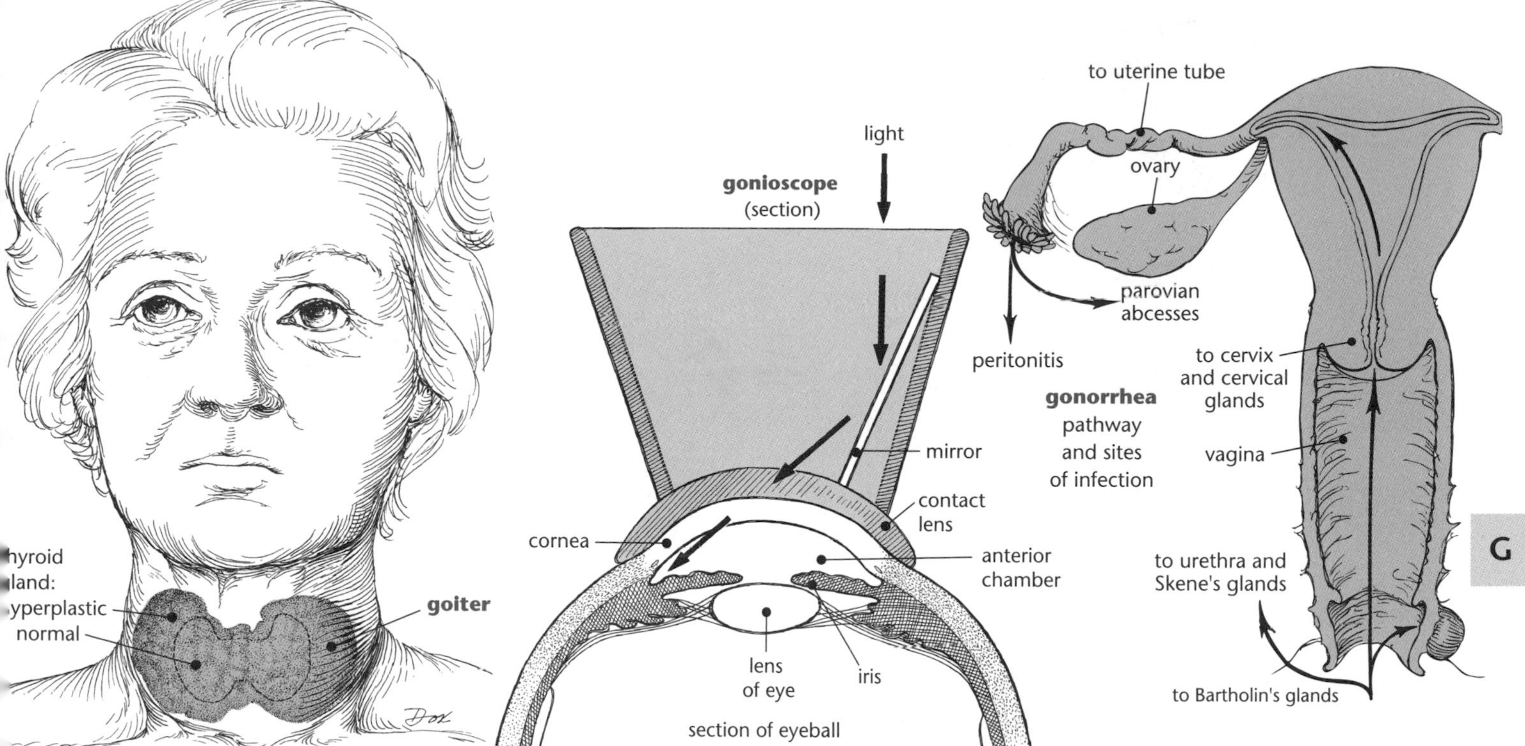

G

sugar.

glyconeogenesis (gli-ko-ne-o-jen´ĕ-sis) The new formation of sugar; the formation of glucose or glycogen from substances other than carbohydrates, such as protein or fat.

glycoprotein (gli-ko-pro´tēn) Any of several protein-carbohydrate compounds (conjugated proteins); they include the mucins, the mucoids, and the chondroproteins.

glycoside (gli´ko-sīd) Any of a group of compounds containing a carbohydrate and a noncarbohydrate residue in the same molecule; on hydrolysis they produce sugars and related compounds; found in animal tissues and in many drugs and spices.

glycosphingolipid (gli-ko-sfing-o-lip´id) A ceramide linked to one or more sugars by the terminal OH group.

glycostatic (gli-ko-stat´ik) Tending to maintain a constant glycogen level in the tissues.

glycosuria (gli-ko-su´re-ă) Excretion of sugar in the urine in excess of the normal amount; frequently a sign of diabetes mellitus.

renal g. Glycosuria occurring with normal blood sugar levels due to failure of the renal tubules to reabsorb filtered glucose to the normal degree.

glycyrrhiza (glis-ĭ-ri´ză) The dried roots of *Glycyrrhiza glabra*; used in pharmaceutical preparations. Also called licorice; licorice root.

glycyrrhizic acid (glis-ĭ-ri´zik as´id) A glycoside present in glycyrrhiza which in large amounts produces aldosteronelike effects in the kidney, causing retention of sodium and water and excessive excretion of potassium. Also called glycyrrhizin.

glycyrrhizin (glis-ĭ-ri´zin) See glycyrrhizic acid.

gnat (nat) One of several minute, winged, biting insects; a midge.

buffalo g. See black fly, under fly.

gnathalgia (nath-al´jă) See gnathodynia.

gnathic (nath´ik) Relating to the jaw.

gnathion (nath´e-on) The lowest point of the midline of the mandible; a craniometric point.

gnathitis (nath-i´tis) Inflammation of the jaw.

gnathodynamometer (nath-o-di-nă-mom´ĕ-ter) Instrument used in dentistry to measure the biting force of the jaw. Also called bite gauge; occlusometer.

gnathodynia (nath-o-din´e-ă) Pain in the jaw. Also called gnathalgia.

gnathoplasty (nath´o-plas-te) Plastic or reparative surgery of the jaw.

gnathostatics (nath-o-stat´iks) In orthodontic diagnosis, a technique based on relationships between the teeth and certain skull landmarks.

Gnathostoma (nath-os´to-mă) Genus of parasitic, pathogenic roundworms (family Gnathostomatidae). Formerly called *Chiranthus*.

G. spinigerum Parasites, frequently aquired by humans by ingestion of the larvae in undercooked fish, causing migratory swelling of the subcutaneous tissues or abscesses in the intestinal wall; the wandering larvae may also invade the eyes and brain.

gnathostomiasis (nath-o-sto-mi´ă-sis) Infection with *Gnathostoma spinigerum.*

gnosia (no´se-ă) The ability to recognize the nature and significance of objects, based on the reception of sensory stimuli (auditory, visual, or tactile).

gnotobiote (no-to-bi´ōt) A laboratory animal that is germ-free, or is contaminated with only known microorganisms.

gnotobiotic (no-to-bi-ot´ik) Having the characteristics of a gnotobiote.

goiter (goi´ter) Enlargement of the thyroid gland causing a visible swelling in front of the neck.

adenomatous g. Goiter due to the presence of a benign tumor of glandular tissue (adenoma).

colloid g. A soft goiter in which the follicles of the gland are distended and filled with colloid.

cystic g. An enlarged thyroid gland containing one or more cysts.

exophthalmic g. Goiter associated with protrusion of the eyeballs, as seen in Graves' disease.

parenchymatous g. Uniform enlargement of the thyroid gland due to excessive proliferation of its follicles and epithelium.

toxic g. A goiter with excessive secretions, causing signs and symptoms of hyperthyroidism.

goitrogen (goi´tro-jen) Any agent causing goiter.

gold (gōld) A soft, deep yellow, corrosion-resistant element; one of the least destructible, and most chemically inert metals known; symbol Au, atomic number 79, atomic weight 196.9.

white g. A gold alloy with a high palladium content.

gold-198 (^{198}Au) A radioactive isotope of gold; used in colloidal suspension for treating some forms of cancer.

gomphosis (gom-fo´sis) A type of fibrous articulation in which a bony process fits into a socket, as of a tooth and its socket.

gonad (go´nad) A sexual gland.

female g. Ovary.

male g. Testis.

gonadectomy (go-nă-dek´tŏ-me) The surgical removal of an ovary or a testis.

gonadoblastoma (gon-ă-do-blas-to´mă) A benign combined germ-cell and gonadal stromal growth.

gonadogenesis (gon-ă-do-jen´ĕ-sis) The development of the embryonic gonads.

gonadotropic (gon-ă-do-trop´ik) Influencing the gonads, as the hormones of the anterior pituitary gland that stimulate the ovaries and testes.

gonadotropin (gon-ă-do-tro´pin) A hormone that stimulates either the ovaries or the testes.

chorionic g. See human chorionic gonadotropin.

human chorionic g. (hCG) A polypeptide hormone produced by cells that enter into formation of the early placenta; its secretion begins soon after implantation of the fertilized ovum, with concentration peaking at 60 to 95 days; also produced by abnormal chorionic epithelial tissue such as hydatidiform moles, chorioadenoma destruens, and choriocarcinoma; used in diagnostic tests.

gonalgia (go-nal´jă) Pain in the knee.

gonecystolith (gon-ĕ-sis´to-lith) A concretion of calculus in a seminal vesicle.

goniometer (go-ne-om´ĕ-ter) **1.** An instrument for measuring angles. **2.** A device for testing labyrinthine disease.

gonion (go´ne-on) The most posterior, inferior, and lateral point of the external mandibular angle.

goniopuncture (go-ne-o-punk´chur) Operation for congenital glaucoma in which a puncture is made in the trabecular meshwork (at the angle of the anterior chamber) through the corneoscleral junction of the opposite side.

gonioscope (go´ne-o-skōp) A combination of a contact lens and mirror which allows the observer to look directly into the angle of the anterior chamber of the eye.

gonioscopy (go-ne-os´kŏ-pe) Examination of the angle of the anterior chamber of the eye by means of a gonioscope.

goniosynechia (go-ne-o-sĭ-nek´e-ă) Adhesion of the iris to the inner surface of the cornea at the angle of the anterior chamber; seen in angle-closure glaucoma.

goniotomy (go-ne-ot´ŏ-me) Operation for the management of congenital glaucoma in which a cut is made through one-third of the trabecular meshwork of the eye to drain the aqueous humor into Schlemm's canal (scleral venous sinus).

gonococcal (gon-o-kok´al) Relating to gonococci.

gonococcemia (gon-o-kok-se´me-ă) The presence of gonococci in the blood.

gonococcus (gon-o-kok´us), *pl.* **gonococ´ci** (GC) The bacterium that causes gonorrhea, *Neisseria gonorrhoeae*.

gonocyte (gon´o-sīt) A primitive reproductive cell.

gonorrhea (gon-o-re´ă) Contagious disease marked by inflammation of the mucous membrane of the genital tract, purulent discharge, and painful, frequent urination; if untreated, it may cause complications (e.g., epididymitis, prostatitis, tenosynovitis, arthritis, endocarditis) and may lead to sterility in females and urethral stricture in males; caused by *Neisseria*

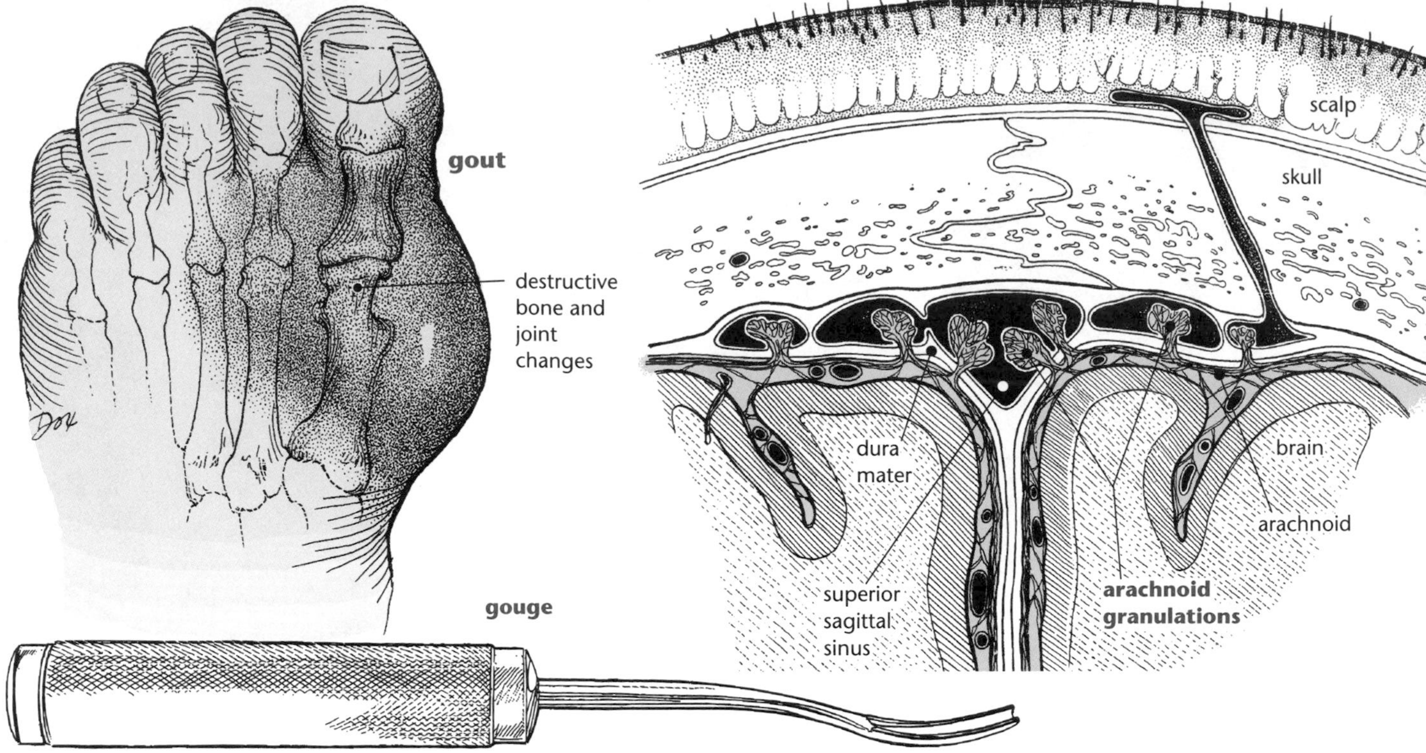

G

gonorrhoeae, transmitted chiefly by sexual intercourse; incubation period: 2 to 5 days.

oral g. See gonococcal pharyngitis, under pharyngitis.

pharyngeal g. See gonococcal pharyngitis, under pharyngitis.

rectal g. Gonorrhea of the rectum; may be asymptomatic or cause a purulent discharge, swelling, and pain.

gonorrheal (gon-o-re´al) Relating to gonorrhea.

gonycampsis (gon-ĭ-kamp´sis) Any abnormal curvature of the knee.

Goodpasture's syndrome (good´pas-chŭrz sin ´drōm) Glomerulonephritis associated with diffuse pulmonary hemorrhage; caused by an antigen directed against the basement membrane of glomerulus capillaries and pulmonary alveoli. Also called hemorrhagic pulmonary-renal syndrome.

gouge (gouj) **1.** A strong chisel with a troughlike blade, usually used for cutting and removing bone. **2.** To cut or scoop out in large amounts.

goundou (goon´doo) An endemic disease of West Africa marked by egg-shaped swelling of the maxillary bone, on either side of the nose; associated with yaws.

gout (gout) A metabolic disorder marked by an excess of uric acid in the blood, by painful inflammation of joints, especially of the big toes, and by deposits of sodium biurate in the cartilages of the affected joints and in the kidney.

saturnine g. Gout accompanying lead poisoning.

secondary g. Gout occurring as a result of increased nucleoprotein metabolism and uric acid production.

tophaceous g. Gout marked by the presence of tophi (deposits of sodium urate) about the joints and cartilaginous areas.

gouty (gou´te) Relating to gout.

G protein (jepro´tēn) See under protein.

gradient (gra´de-ent) Rate of change of temperature, pressure, distance, time, or any such variable value.

density g. A solution with a continuous concentration increase of the solute from top to bottom of the container.

mitral g. The difference in diastolic pressure between the left atrium and left ventricle.

systolic g. The difference in pressure during systole between two communicating chambers of the heart.

ventricular g. In electrocardiography, the algebraic sum of the areas within the QRS complex and the T wave of the electrocardiogram.

grading (grād´ing) A histologic method of providing an estimate of the gravity of a cancerous tumor, based on the degree of cell differentiation and the number of cell divisions within the tumor.

graduate (graj´o͞o-āt) A laboratory vessel marked off in units of fluid volume.

Graefe's sign, von Graefe's sign (gra´fez sīn) Immobility or lagging of the upper eyelid on downward movement of the eye. Also called lid lag.

graft (graft) **1.** Any tissue transplanted into a body part. **2.** To insert such a tissue.

accordion g. See mesh graft.

allogeneic g. See allograft.

autogenous g. See autograft.

autologous g. See autograft.

corneal g. See keratoplasty.

coronary artery bypass g. (CABG) See coronary bypass, under bypass.

cutis g. A piece of skin from which the epidermis and subcutaneous tissue have been removed.

delayed g. Grafting postponed until infection has been eliminated.

full thickness g. Skin graft consisting of superficial and deep layers of the skin (i.e., epidermis and dermis).

isogeneic g. See isograft.

isologous g. See isograft.

isoplastic g. See isograft.

mesh g. A graft that has been passed under a special cutting machine to create a mesh pattern; the perforations allow expansion of the graft from about 1 1/2 to 9 times its original size; useful for covering irregularly shaped wounds. Also called accordion graft.

partial-thickness g. See split-thickness graft.

pedicle g. A stalk of skin and subcutaneous tissue left attached at the donor site until its free end has taken at the recipient site. Also called double end or island graft.

pinch g.'s Circular bits of skin a few millimeters in diameter.

postage stamp g. Multiple, small, thick-split skin graft. Also called checkerboard graft.

prosthetic g. A graft composed of synthetic material; often used in bypass operations of large caliber arteries.

reversed autogenous saphenous vein g. A segment of the patient's own saphenous vein turned inside out prior to insertion to prevent the vein's valves from obstructing the blood flow; used in bypass operations of small caliber vessels, such as coronary arteries.

skin g. A piece of skin completely removed from one area of the body (or from another person) and placed in a new bed of blood supply in a denuded area of the body.

split-skin g. See split-thickness graft.

split-thickness g. (a) A skin graft consisting of the epidermis and part of the thickness of the dermis. (b) A graft of a mucous membrane that does not include all the layers of the membrane. Also called partial-thickness graft; split-skin graft.

syngeneic g. See isograft.

tendon g. A piece of tendon used to repair a defect.

xenogeneic g. See xenograft.

grafting (graft´ing) Transplantation of tissue from one part of the body to another or from one body to another.

graft-versus-host disease (graft-ver´sus-hōst dĭ-zēz´) Disease resulting from an immune reaction of transplanted lymphocytes (e.g., in a bone marrow graft) against antigens of the recipient (host).

grain (grān) **1.** A minute hard particle. **2.** Unit of mass or weight equivalent to 0.065 gram.

gram (gram) (g) Metric unit of mass or weight, equal to 0.001 kilogram.

gramicidin (gram-ĭ-si´din) An antibioic compound used in combination with other drugs of the same class, and in the form of eye drops or ointments, for the topical treatment of bacterial infection of the eyes and skin.

gram-meter (gram-me´ter) A unit of energy equal to the force required to raise a weight of 1 gram to a height of 1 meter.

gram-negative (gram-neg´ă-tiv) Denoting a microorganism that fails to retain the violet dye used in Gram's stain.

gram-positive (gram-poz´ĭ-tiv) Denoting a microorganism that retains the violet dye used in Gram's stain.

grandiose (gran´de-ōs) In psychiatry, an exaggerated feeling of self importance; having delusions of great fame or power.

grand mal (grahn mahl) See generalized tonic-clonic epilepsy, under epilepsy.

granular (gran´u-lar) **1.** Composed of or resembling granules or grains. **2.** Particles with a strong affinity for stains.

granulation (gran-u-la´shun) **1.** The act or process of dividing substances into small particles or granules; the state of being granular. **2.** The formation of small, rounded, fleshy masses on the surface of a healing wound; also, one of these fleshy masses. **3.** A granular mass in or on the surface of an organ or membrane, such as a mass of lymphoid tissue on the conjunctiva of the eyelids. **4.** The formation of crystals by prolonged agitation of a supersaturated solution of a salt.

arachnoid g.'s Small masses of arachnoid projecting into the venous sinuses and on the outer surface of the dura mater, causing pits on the inner surface of the cranium; they usually appear at the

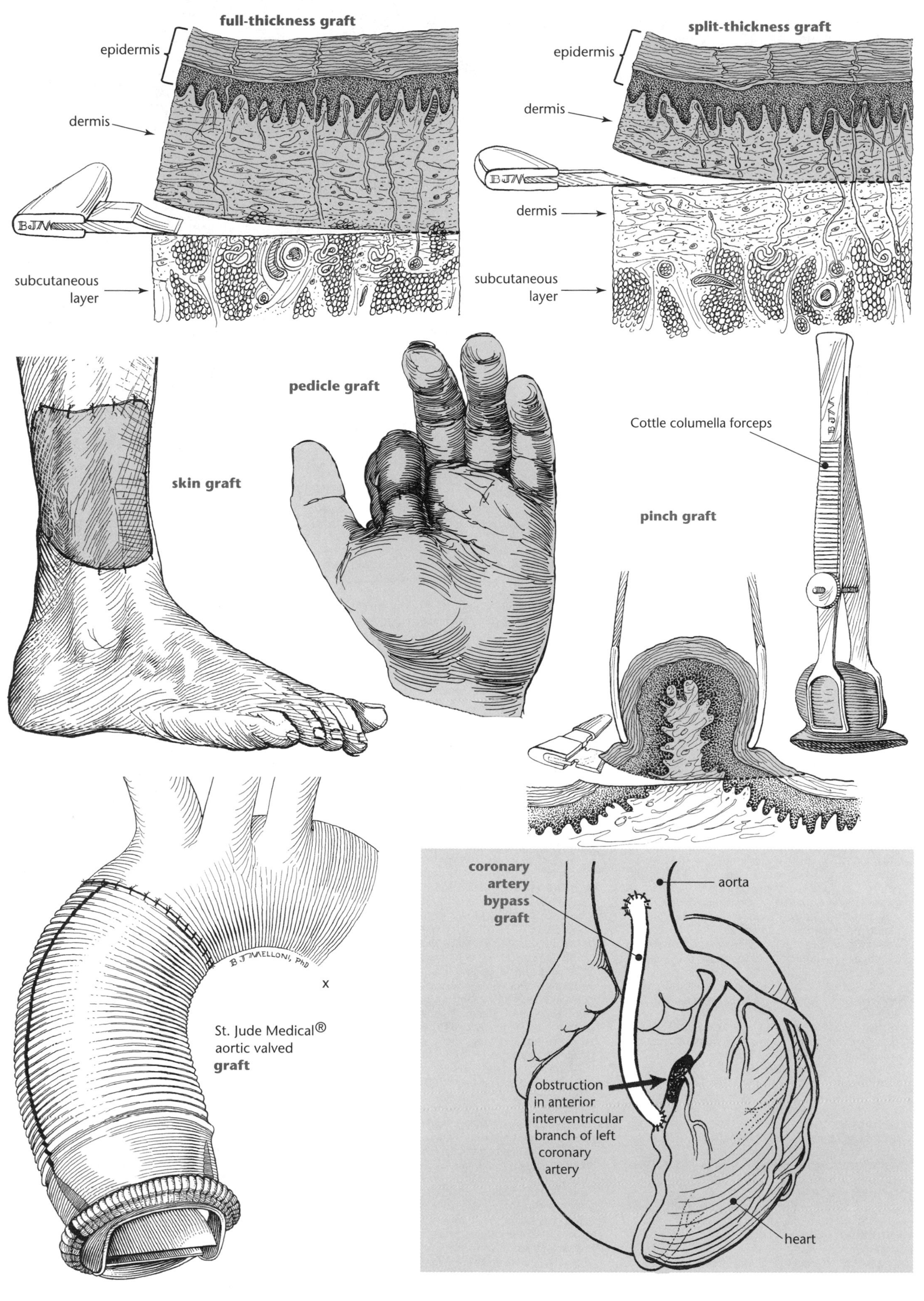
full-thickness graft
epidermis
dermis
subcutaneous
layer
split-thickness graft
epidermis
dermis
dermis
subcutaneous
layer
G
skin graft
pedicle graft
Cottle columella forceps
pinch graft
coronary
artery
bypass
graft
aorta
obstruction
in anterior
interventricular
branch of left
coronary
artery
heart
St. Jude Medical®
aortic valved
graft

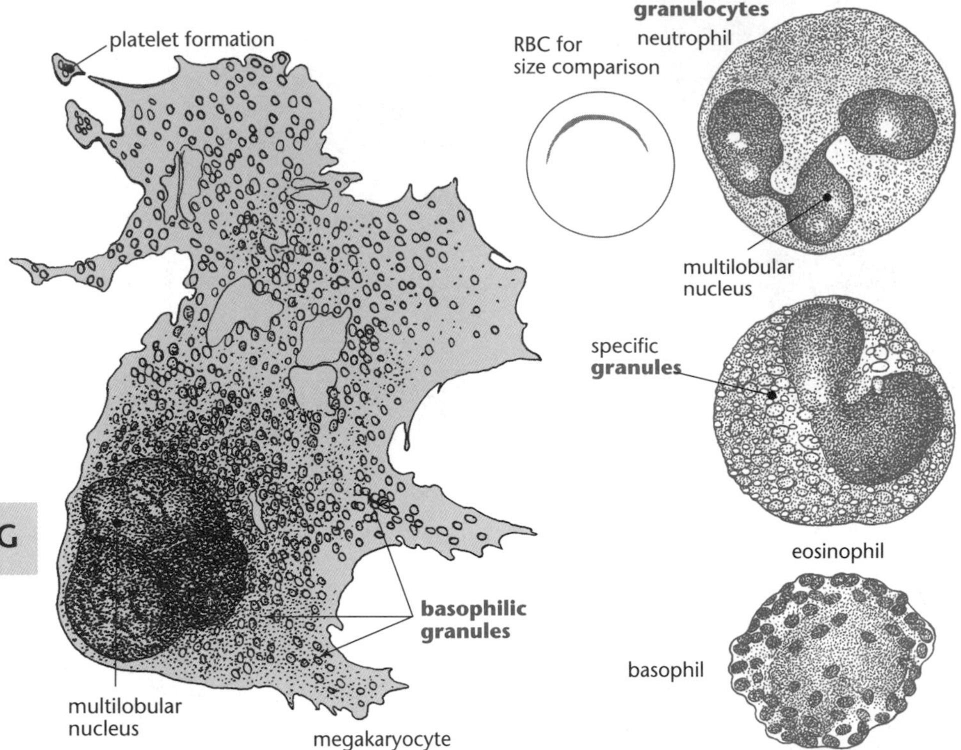

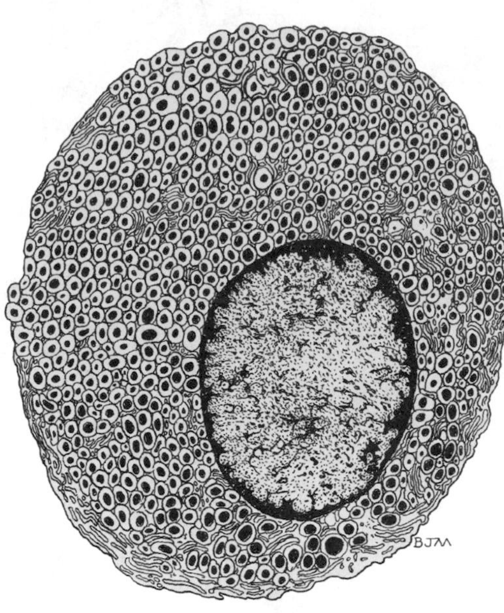

age of seven years and increase in size and number as age advances. Also called pacchionian bodies; pacchionian granulations.

pacchionian g.'s See arachnoid granulations.

granule (gran´ul) **1.** A grain or small particle; a minute discrete mass. **2.** A small pill, usually sugar coated.

acidophilic g. A granule staining readily with acid dyes such as eosin.

azurophilic g., azure g. A granule that stains readily with azure dye.

basal g. See basal body, under body.

basophilic g. A granule staining readily with basic dyes such as azure A.

brain sand g.'s Sandlike matter composed of calcium carbonate, present in the pineal body and near the choroid plexus. Also called acervulus; brain sand.

chromophobe g. A granule that does not stain or stains poorly.

Crooke's g.'s Masses of basophilic material in the basophilic cells of the anterior lobe of the pituitary gland; seen in Cushing's disease or after the administration of ACTH.

lamellated g. See keratinosome.

matrix g.'s Highly electron-dense intramitochondrial granules, about 500 Å in diameter; thought to be the binding sites for calcium ions.

membrane-coating g. See keratinosome.

osmophilic g. A granule that flourishes in the medium of high osmotic pressure.

secretory g.'s Temporarily stored intracellular membrane-bound particles, formed in the granular endoplamic reticulum and the Golgi complex.

zymogen g. One of several granules present in enzyme-secreting cells such as those in salivary glands.

granuloblast (gran´u-lo-blast) See myeloblast.

granulocyte (gran´yu-lo-sīt) A mature granular white blood cell (leukocyte) that develops in the bone marrow from a myeloblast; depending on the specific granules, it may be a neutrophilic (polymorphonuclear) granulocyte, an eosinophilic granulocyte, or a basophilic granulocyte.

granulocytopenia (gran-u-lo-si-to-pe´ne-ă) Deficiency of granular leukocytes (granulocytes) in the blood. Also called granulopenia.

granulocytopoiesis (gran-u-lo-si-to-poi-e´sis) See granulopoiesis.

granulocytosis (gran-u-lo-si-to´sis) The presence of an excessive number of granulocytes in the blood or in the tissues.

granuloma (gran-u-lo´mă) A tumor composed of granulation tissue.

dental g. A mass of chronic inflammatory tissue, usually asymptomatic, occurring at the root of a tooth. Also called periapical granuloma.

eosinophilic g. See unifocal Langerhans-cell histiocytosis, under histiocytosis.

giant-cell g. A tumor-like mass protruding from the gums (gingiva) believed to be of inflammatory origin.

g. inguinale A chronic sexually transmitted disease marked by granulomatous ulcerations in the inguinal region and the genitalia; caused by *Calymmatobacterium granulomatis*.

periapical g. See dental granuloma.

pyogenic g., g. pyogenicum A red, small, benign overgrowth of granulation tissue on the skin or oral mucosa arising as a result of trauma.

swimming pool g. A chronic warty growth, which may ulcerate, arising on abrasions, resulting from infection with *Mycobacterium marinum* in swimming pools, aquariums, or any body of water.

granulomatosis (gran-u-lo-mă-to´sis) Any disorder marked by the presence of multiple granulomas.

lipoid g., lipid g. See xanthomatosis.

lipophagic intestinal g. See Whipple's disease.

Wegener's g. A rare, often fatal, disease marked by ulceration of the upper respiratory tract progressing to involvement of the lungs, acute necrotizing arteritis, and glomerulonephritis.

granulomatous (gran-u-lom´ă-tus) Resembling a granuloma.

granulopenia (gran-u-lo-pe´ne-ă) See granulocytopenia.

granuloplastic (gran-u-lo-plas´tik) Capable of forming granules.

granulopoiesis (gran-u-lo-poi-e´sis) The formation of granulocytes. Also called granulocytopoeisis.

granulosis, granulosity (gran-u-lo´sis, gran-u-los´ĭ-te) A mass of minute granules.

graph (graf) Any pictorial device that displays a relationship of varying values.

graphology (graf-ol´ŏ-je) The analysis of handwriting to assess the character of the writer.

graphospasm (graf-o-spaz-m) See writer's cramp, under cramp.

GRAS (gras) Acronym for generally regarded as safe, denoting any safe food additive.

grave (grāv) Indicating symptoms of an extremely serious or dangerous character. Also called critical.

gravel (grav´ĕl) Numerous minute concretions, usually of uric acid, calcium oxalate, or phosphates, formed in the kidney and bladder.

Graves' disease (grāvz dĭ-zēz´) Disorder resulting from excessive production of thyroid hormone; symptoms include generalized enlargement of the thyroid gland, bulging eyeballs, muscular tremors, rapid pulse rate, and weight loss.

gravid (grav´id) Pregnant.

gravida (grav´ĭ-dă) A pregnant woman. A Roman numeral designates the number of pregnancies (e.g., gravida I is a woman in her first pregnancy, gravida II in her second).

gravidity (gră-vid´ĭ-te) **1.** The pregnant state. **2.** The total number of pregnancies a woman has had, including a current pregnancy.

gravimeter (gră-vim´ĕ-ter) See hydrometer.

gravimetric (grav-ĭ-met´rik) Determined by weight.

gravity (grav´ĭ-te) (G) The gravitational force.

specific g. (sp. gr.) The ratio of the mass of any substance (usually liquid) compared to the mass of an equal volume of another substance (usually distilled water at 4°C).

Grey Turner's sign (gra tur´nerz sīn) See Turner's sign.

grid (grid) **1.** A frame of parallel horizontal and vertical lines forming squares of uniform size, used as a reference for plotting curves. **2.** In radiology, an instrument composed of alternate strips of lead and radiolucent material, placed in apposition to a film to absorb secondary or scattered radiation.

Wetzel g. A chart for evaluating the growth and physical fitness of young and adolescent children.

grief (grēf) A state of intense mental anguish normally resulting from the loss of a valued object or person.

grinding (grīnd´ing) In dentisty, the shaping of a tooth with abrasive tools.

selective g. The grinding of selective spots on the occlusal surfaces of teeth marked with articulating paper to equalize occlusal stress.

grinding-in (grīnd´ing-in) In dentistry, the act of correcting occlusal errors in natural and artificial teeth. Also called equilibrating.

grip, grippe (grip) See influenza.

devil's g. See epidemic pleurodynia, under pleurodynia.

griseofulvin (gris-e-o-ful´vin) A fungistatic antibiotic derived from a species of *Penicillium*; used systemically in the treatment of superficial fungal infections; Fulvicin-U/F®.

gristle (gris´l) Cartilage.

groin (groin) The inguinal region; the region around the crease formed at the junction of the thigh and trunk.

Grönblad-Strandberg syndrome (grern´blahd strahnd´berg sin´drōm) An elastic tissue degeneration that involves the retina, gastrointestinal tract, and especially the skin.

groove (grōōv) A narrow, elongated depression.

carotid g. The groove through the sphenoid bone in which the internal carotid artery lies in its course through the cavernous sinus.

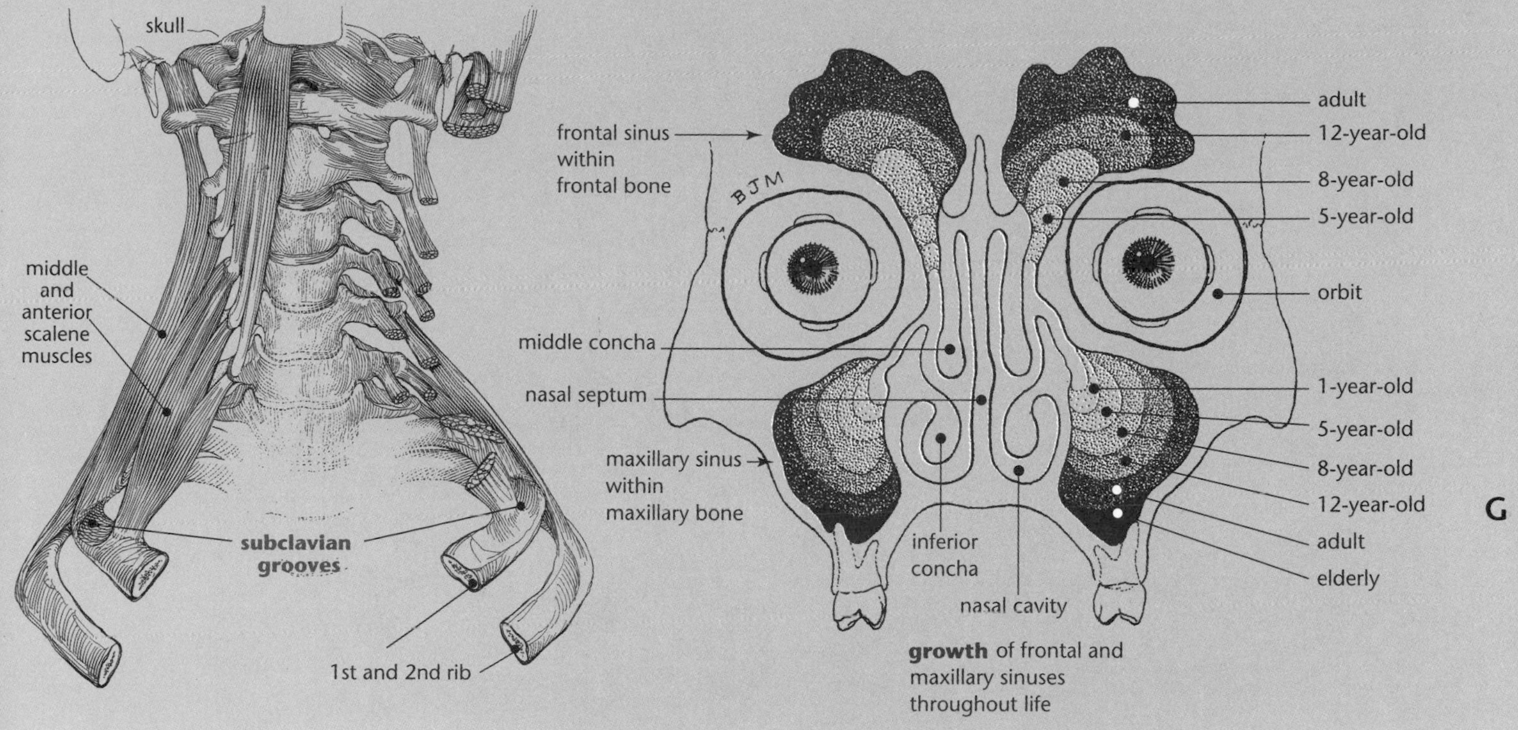

growth of frontal and maxillary sinuses throughout life

G

costal g. A groove in the lower border of the rib, housing the intercostal vessels and nerve.

developmental g. A groove on the enamel of a tooth, marking the fusion of the lobes of the crown during tooth development.

neural g. The transitory median dorsal groove in the thickened ectoderm (neural plate) of young embryos; the closure of the groove forms a closed tubular structure with a long caudal portion, the future spinal cord, and a broader cephalic portion, which becomes the brain.

subclavian g. A shallow groove on the first rib between the anterior and middle scalene muscles through which the subclavian artery and the inferior trunk of the brachial plexus pass.

group (grōōp) **1.** A collection of related objects. **2.** In chemistry, a radical.

characteristic g. A distinctive group of atoms that make one substance different from others.

diagnosis-related g. (DRG) A classification of patients into diagnostic categories to serve as a basis for payment of hospital charges by Medicare or other third party payment plans.

family g. See kindred.

HACEK g. A group of bacteria that require an enhanced carbon dioxide atmosphere to thrive and which have an ability to infect human heart valves; they include *Haemophilus* species, *Actinobacillus actinomycetemcomitans, Cardiobacterium hominis, Eikenella corrodens,* and *Kingella kingae.*

Lancefield g.'s See Lancefield's classification, under classification.

symptom g. 1. See syndrome. **2.** A complex in the electrocardiogram. See complex.

growth (grōth) **1.** The progressive development of an organism or any of its parts. **2.** A tumor.

appositional g. Growth through the addition of layers, typical of rigid structures. Also called growth by accretion.

differential g. The various growth rates of related tissues, as in embryonic structures, with resulting change in proportions.

interstitial g. Growth through formation of new tissue throughout the structure, as occurs in soft tissues.

psychological g. Growth toward self-actualization or personal maturity.

zero population g. (ZPG) The state of a total population that neither increases nor decreases, occurring when the number of births and immigrants equals the number of deaths and emigrants.

grub (grub) The maggot-like larva of certain insects.

gruel (grōō´ĕl) Thin porridge; any semifluid food made of cereal boiled in water.

grunt (grunt) A deep, guttural sound in the chest; a frequent sign of chest pain implying an acute pneumonic process with pleural involvement; also seen in pulmonary edema and in the respiratory distress syndrome of the neonatal period.

expiratory g. A laryngeal sound sometimes heard during surgical manipulation of the subdiaphragmatic areas.

gryposis (grĭ-po´sis) Any abnormal curvature.

guaiacol (gwi´ă-kol) A colorless, oily liquid, $C_7H_8O_2$, obtained from creosote or made synthetically from pyrocatechin; used chiefly as an expectorant, intestinal disinfectant, and local anesthetic.

guaifenesin (gwi-fen´ĕ-sin) Compound used to reduce the viscosity of mucus in the bronchial tree.

guanethidine sulfate (gwan-eth´ĭ-dēn sul´fāt) A potent antihypertensive drug, thought to interfere with the release of norepinephrine at the sympathetic neuroeffector junction; Ismelin Sulfate®.

guanidine (gwan´ĭ-dēn) A strong base obtained from the oxidation of guanine; the amidine of aminocarbamic acid, CH_5N_3, considered by some to be one of the factors responsible for part of the uremic syndrome in renal failure.

guanidinemia (gwăn-ĭ-dĭ-ne´me-ă) The presence of guanidine in the blood.

guanidinosuccinic acid (gwăn-ĭ-de-no-sŭk-sin´ik as´id) A metabolic by-product found in the body in excessive amounts in renal failure and implicated in the clotting abnormality and the neuropathy of the chronic uremic syndrome.

guanine (gwăn´ēn) A crystalline purine base.

guanosine (gwăn´o-sin) 9-β-D-Ribosylguanine; guanine combined with D-ribose.

cyclic g. monophosphate (cGMP) A nucleotide that serves as a second messenger; it plays a role complementary to that of cyclic AMP in regulating intracellular processes, one nucleotide promoting those that the other inhibits; when the cyclic GMP level goes up, the cyclic AMP level goes down and vice versa.

g. monophosphate (GMP) See guanylic acid.

guanylate cyclase (gwă´nĭ-lāt si´klās) Enzyme responsible for forming cyclic guanosine monophosphate (cGMP) and pyrophosphate (PP).

guanylic acid (gwă-nil´ik as´id) A major constituent of ribonucleic acid (RNA). Also called guanosine monophosphate (GMP).

guarding (gahrd´ing) Spasm of muscles at the site of injury or disease occurring as the body's protection against further injury.

abdominal g. A sign of acute peritonitis marked by involuntary rigid contraction of the abdominal rectus muscles, occurring when the examiner gently depresses the abdomen with both hands; the muscles contract, remaining taut, rigid, and boardlike throughout deep respiration.

gubernaculum (goo-ber-nak´u-lum) A guiding cord connecting two structures.

g. dentis The connective tissue band connecting the permanent tooth follicle to the gingiva.

g. testis A ligamentous cord extending from the lower end of the fetal testis through the inguinal canal to the floor of the developing scrotum; it guides the descent of the testis from the abdomen into the scrotum.

guide (gid) A device that directs the course of something by preceding it (e.g., a guide wire) or by confining its motion (e.g., by means of grooves).

mold g. A guide for specifying the shape of artificial teeth.

Guillain-Barré syndrome (ge-yă bă-ra´ sin´drom) (GBS) Disorder of motor nerves occurring after a viral infection, trauma, or surgery; marked by inflammatory changes of peripheral nerves (near the spinal cord), which cause bilateral weakness, most commonly beginning in the lower extremities and progressing rapidly to paralysis; patients usually recover completely when respiratory and vasomotor failure do not occur; thought to be an autoimmune reaction. Also called idiopathic polyneuritis.

guillotine (gil´ŏ-tēn) A surgical cutting instrument with a knifeblade that slides in the grooves of a guide.

guinea pig (gin´ē pig) Any of several small tropical American burrowing rodents of the genus *Cavia*, used extensively for experimental work.

gullet (gul´ĭt) The pharynx and the esophagus; the passage leading from the mouth to the stomach.

gum (gum) **1.** The dried viscous sap exuded by certain trees and plants; it is water-soluble, noncrystalline, and brittle. **2.** The gingiva.

g. arabic A gummy exudate of various African trees of the genus *Acacia*; used in the preparation of medicinal drugs. Also called acacia.

gumboil (gum´boil) Colloquial term for a chronic alveolar abscess that drains itself by perforating the gum. See also alveolar abscess, under abscess.

gumma (gum´ă), *pl.* **gum´mas, gum´mata** A soft, gummy, infectious tumor that occurs, irregularly, during the third stage of syphilis.

gummatous (gum´ă-tus) Relating to or of the nature of a gumma.

Gunn's syndrome (gunz sin´drōm) See jaw-winking syndrome.

Günther's disease (gēn´therz dĭ-zēz´) See congenital erythropoietic porphyria, under porphyria.

gurney (gur´ne) A wheeled stretcher or cot for transporting patients, usually within a hospital.

gustation (gus-tā´shun) **1.** The sense of taste. **2.** The act of tasting.

gustatory (gus´tă-tor-ē) Of or relating to the sense

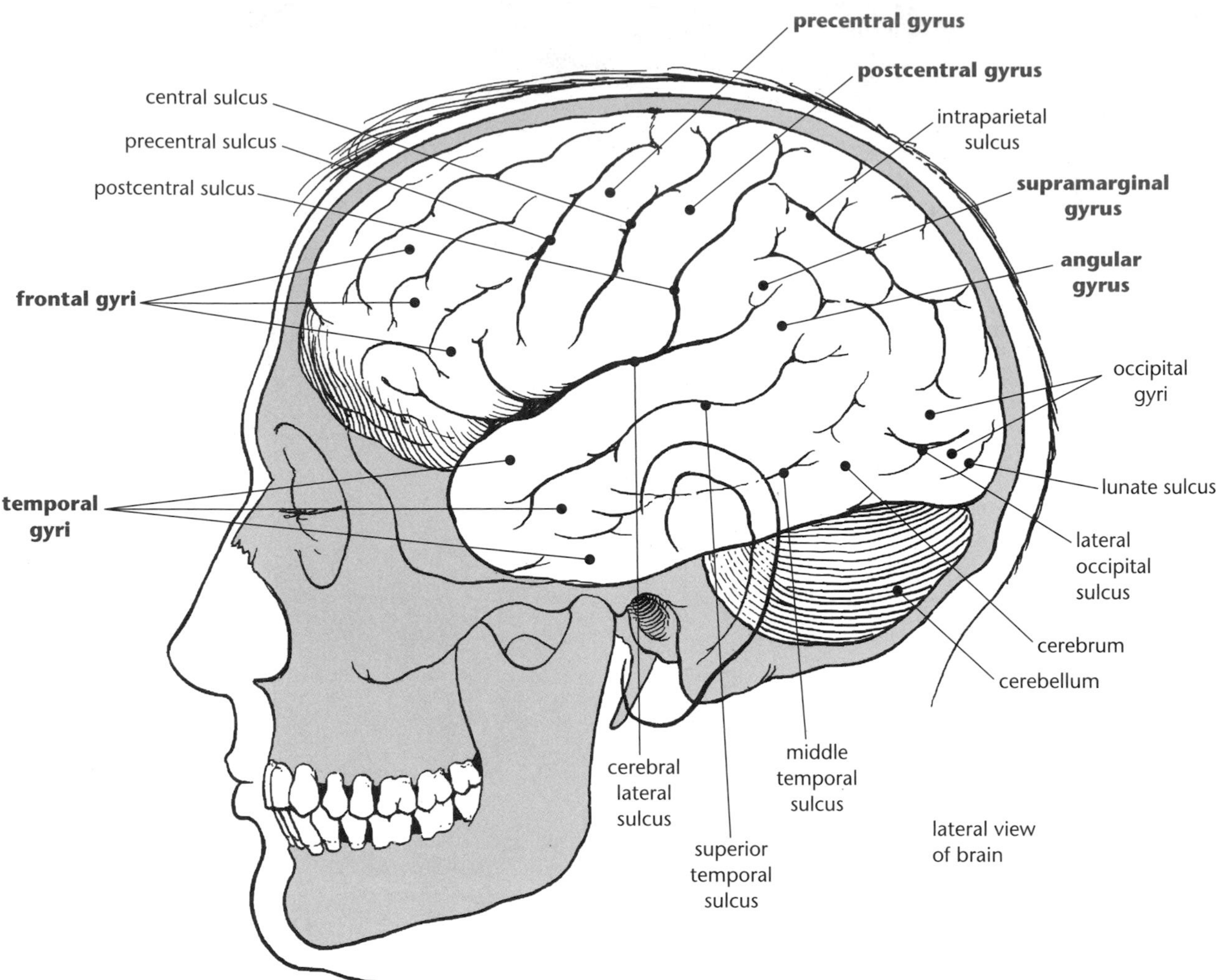

of taste.

gut (gut) **1.** The intestine. **2.** The digestive tube of the embryo.

surgical g. See catgut.

gutta (gut´ă) (gt) Latin for a drop.

gutta-percha (gut´ă -per´chă) A milky latex sap of several tropical trees (family Sapotaceae); used in the manufacture of splints and as a thin waterproof sheet to protect wounds; in dentistry, used for temporary scaling of dressings in cavities and for filling of root canals.

guttate (gŭt´āt) Resembling a drop; said of certain skin lesions.

guttatim (gŭ-ta´tim) Latin for drop by drop.

gutter (gut´er) Groove; recess.

paracolic g. The recess between the abdominal wall and the lateral side of the ascending or the descending colon.

guttur (gut´ur) Latin for throat.

guttural (gut´ur-ăl) Relating to the throat.

gymnophobia (jim-no-fo´be-ă) Morbid fear of the sight of the naked body.

gynandrism (jĭ-nan´driz-m) Female pseudohermaphroditism. See pseudohermaphroditism.

gynandroid (jĭ-nan´droid) A female pseudohermaphrodite.

gynandromorphous (jĭ-nan-dro-mor´fus) Having both male and female characteristics.

gynatresia (jin-ă-tre´zhă) Occlusion of a part of the female genital tract, usually the vagina.

gynecoid (jin´ĕ-koid) Resembling a female.

gynecologic (gi-nĕ-kŏ-loj´ik) Pertaining to gynecology.

gynecologist (gi-nĕ-kol´ŏ-jist) A specialist in gynecology.

gynecology (gi-nĕ-kol´ŏ-je) (GYN) The medical-surgical specialty concerned with disorders of the female, including the genital tract and organs, endocrinology and reproductive physiology.

gynecomania (jin-ĕ-ko-ma´ne-ă) Insatiable sexual desire for women.

gynecomastia (jin-ĕ-ko-mas´te-ă) Excessive development of the male breast.

gynecoplasty (jin-ĕ-ko-plas´te) Reparative surgery of the female genitalia.

gynephobia (jin-ĕ-ko-fo´be-ă) Morbid fear of or aversion to women.

gynopathy (jin-op´ă-the) Any disease characteristic of women.

gypsum (jip´sum) The dehydrate of calcium sulfate, $CaSO_4 \cdot 2H_2O$, from which plaster of Paris and dental stone are derived.

gyration (ji-ra´shun) **1.** Revolution about a stationary point. **2.** An arrangement or group of gyri in the brain.

gyri (ji´ri) Plural of gyrus.

gyrus (ji´rus) A convolution on the surface of the brain, between two furrows (sulci).

angular g. A convolution arching over the upturned end of the superior temporal sulcus.

cingulate g. A long curved convolution lying above and in front of the corpus callosum; it is continuous posteriorly with the isthmus.

dentate g. A narrow crenated strip of cortex between the fimbria hippocampi and the hippocampal gyrus; it is continued posteriorly, under the splenium of the corpus callosum, as the delicate fasciolar gyrus.

fasciolar g. The transitional band between the dentate gyrus and the supracallosal gyrus (indusium griseum); located near the splenium of the corpus callosum.

frontal gyri The three (superior, middle, and inferior) gyri of the frontal lobe.

hippocampal g. See parahippocampal gyrus.

lingual g. A median occipitotemporal gyrus between the calcarine and collateral sulci.

parahippocampal g. A convolution that lies between the collateral sulcus and the hippocampal sulcus, on the inferior surface of each cerebral hemisphere; posteriorly, it is continuous above the cingulate gyrus through the isthmus and below the lingual gyrus. Also called hippocampal gyrus.

paraterminal g. See subcallosal gyrus.

postcentral g. The anterior convolution of the parietal lobe, bounded in front by the central (rolandic) sulcus and posteriorly by the interparietal sulcus.

precentral g. The posterior convolution of the frontal lobe bounded posteriorly by the central (rolandic) sulcus and anteriorly by the precentral sulcus.

subcallosal g. A thin sheet of gray matter which covers the undersurface of the rostrum of the corpus callosum. Also called paraterminal gyrus.

supracallosal g. A thin sheet of gray matter which covers the superior surface of the corpus callosum of the brain. Also called indusium griseum.

supramarginal g. A convolution that arches over the upturned end of the lateral sulcus.

temporal gyri The three convolutions (superior, middle, inferior) on the lateral side of the temporal lobe, inferior to the lateral sulcus.

transverse temporal gyri Two or three convolutions lying transversely on the superior temporal gyrus, mostly in the lateral sulcus.

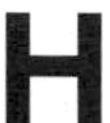

H

habena (hă-be′nă) **1.** A restricting band or frenum. **2.** A restraining bandage.

habenula (hă-ben′u-lă) The dorsal pedicle of the pineal gland.

habit (hab′it) **1.** A constant tendency to perform an act, acquired by frequent repetition of the act. **2.** Colloquial term for addiction.

habituation (ha-bich-oo-a′shun) **1.** The process of forming a habit. **2.** The method by which the nervous system gradually reduces response to a repeated stimulus.

drug h. See drug dependence, under dependence.

habitus (hab′ĭ-tus) Physical and constitutional characteristics of a person, especially as related to susceptibility to some disease.

HACEK Acronym for *Haemophilus, Actinobacillus, Cardiobacterium, Eikenella, Kingella.* See under group.

Haemodipsus ventricosus (he-mo-dip′sŭs ven-tri-ko′sus) The rabbit louse; it transmits the causative agent of tularemia (*Fracisella tularensis*) to humans.

Haemophilus (he-mof′ĭ-lus) A genus of gram-negative, rod-shaped bacteria that require blood components for growth; some cause disease in humans. Also spelled *Hemophilus.*

H. aegyptius A species that causes subacute catarrhal conjunctivitis in warm climates.

H. ducreyi A species that is the causative agent of chancroid (soft chancre). Also called Ducrey's bacillus.

H. influenzae The influenza bacillus; a species found in the respiratory tract; causes acute respiratory infections, acute conjunctivitis, and purulent meningitis in children (rarely in adults). Formerly called Koch-Weeks bacillus; Pfeiffer's bacillus; Weeks' bacillus.

H. parahaemolyticus A species found in the upper respiratory tract; frequently associated with pharyngitis.

hafnium (haf′ne-um) Chemical element; symbol Hf, atomic number 72, atomic weight 178.5.

hagiotherapy (hag-e-o-ther′ă-pē) Treatment of disease by placing the patient in contact with religious relics, or by participating in religious observances.

hair (har) Pilus; a long threadlike skin appendage covering almost the entire surface of the human body except the palms of the hands, the soles of the feet, the dorsal surface of the distal phalanges, the umbilicus, the glans penis, the inner surface of the prepuce of the penis, the clitoris, and the major and minor labia; consists of a portion implanted in the skin (root), in a flasklike pit in the skin (hair follicle), and a portion projecting from the surface (shaft). Hair on the normal scalp grows approximately half an inch per month.

auditory h.'s Hairlike stereocilia emanating from the hair cells of the cochlear receptor of the inner ear; each cell is capped with 50 to 100 stereocilia.

burrowing h. Hair that continues to grow but fails to emerge from the flesh, generally forming a small cicumscribed, superficial elevation of the skin (papule), which may become infected; most commonly occurs on the neck. COMPARE: ingrown hair.

embryonic h. See lanugo.

gustatory h. See taste hair.

ingrown h. Hair that emerges from the skin but then curves and reenters it, generally causing a papule; commonly seen in closely shaved hair. COMPARE: burrowing hair.

lanugo h. See lanugo.

primary h. See lanugo.

secondary h. See vellus.

sensory h.'s Hairlike structures on the surface of sensory epithelial cells.

taste h. One of the short hairlike processes projecting into the lumen of a taste bud; each hair is composed of groups of fine microvilli. Also called gustatory hair.

terminal h. Coarse hair that replaces secondary hair (vellus) in various areas of the body during adult years, including eyebrows, axillary, scalp, and pubic hairs, hairs in the nose and ears and on the face and chest in the male.

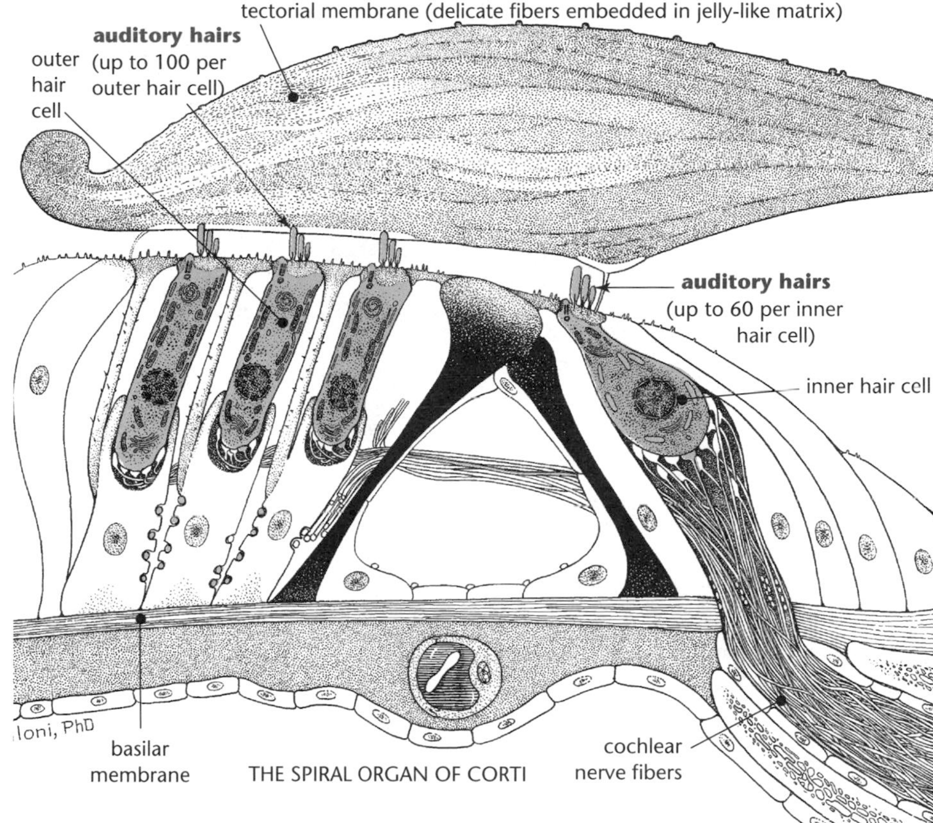

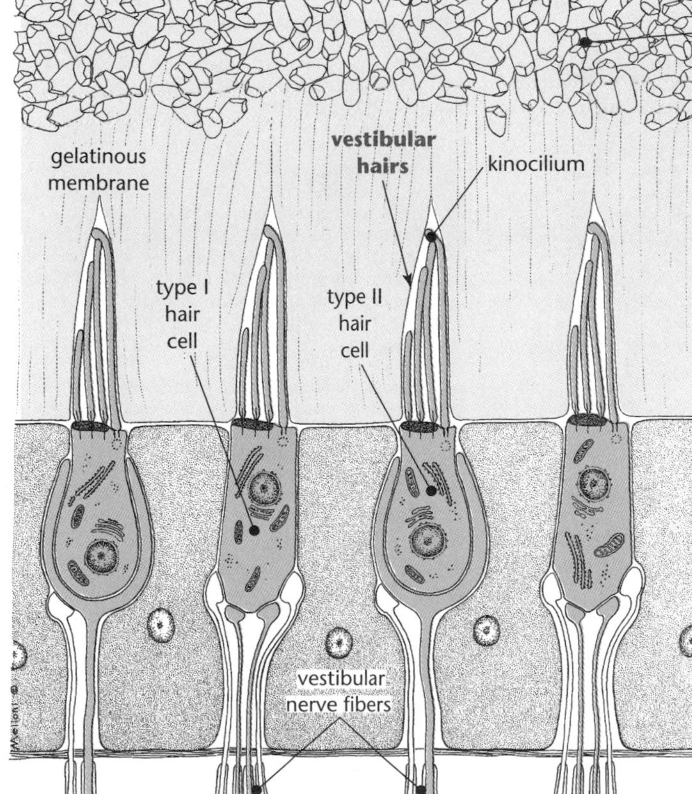

vellus h. See vellus.

vestibular h.'s Sensory hairs (stereocilia) emerging from type I and II hair cells of the vestibular receptors (cristae and maculae) of the inner ear; the apical ends of both types of hair cells bear a tuft of 40 or more stereocilia and a single kinocilium (motile cilium).

hair streams (har strēmz) See flumina pilorum.

halazone (hal′ă-zōn) An antibacterial substance used in the sterilization of water supplies.

100
75
50
25
Percent of activity
64 mc
32 mc
16 mc
8 mc
4 mc
2 mc
1 mc
1 9 17 25 33 41 49
Days
half-life decay curve of radioactive iodine (^{131}I)

varus of metatarsal bone
hallux valgus
flat, wide transverse arch
thickened metatarsal head
lateral shift of sesamoids

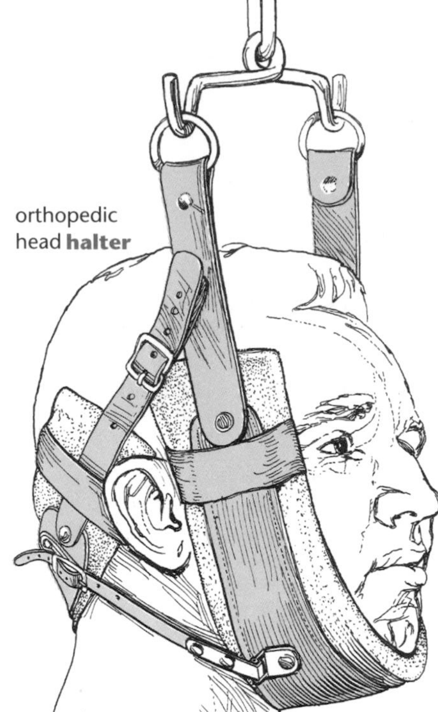

half-life (haf´līf) (HL) The time required for half of the radioactivity originally associated with a radioactive substance to disintegrate (radioactive decay).

biologic h-l. ($T_{1/2}$) **1.** The time required for a radioactive isotope within the body to lose half of its activity; this depends on both the natural half-life of the isotope and the rate of excretion from the body. **2.** The time it takes for the body to eliminate 50% of a drug.

halide (hal´īd) A salt of a halogen (bromide, chlorine, fluorine, or iodine).

halitosis (hal-ĭ-to´sis) Unpleasant breath; some causes are poor mouth hygiene, infection in the oronasopharyngeal structures, and lung abscess.

halitus (hal´ĭ-tus) **1.** Latin for breath. **2.** An exhalation.

hallucal (hal´u-kal) Relating to the big toe.

hallucination (hă-loo-sĭ-na´shun) Perception of objects or events that do not exist.

hypnagogic h. Vivid sensory, dreamlike experiences occurring during the period between wakefulness and sleep.

hallucinatory (hă-loo´sĭ-nă-tor´e) **1.** Characterized by hallucination. **2.** Capable of inducing hallucination.

hallucinogen (hă-loo´sĭ-no-jen) Any agent that induces hallucinations.

hallucinosis (hă-loo-sĭ-no´sis) Psychotic condition in which a person experiences hallucinations while conscious.

hallux (hal´uks), *pl.* **hal´luces** The big toe; the first digit of the foot.

h. dolorosa A painful condition usually associated with flatfoot, in which walking causes severe discomfort in the metatarsophalangeal joint of the big toe.

h. malleus Big toe that is congenitally bent downward.

h. rigidus Stiff toe; painful flexion of the big toe due to stiffness in the metatarsophalangeal joint.

h. valgus Abnormal angulation of the big toe toward the other toes of the same foot; the condition is generally attributed to narrow or pointed shoes; predisposing congenital and familial factors may exist. COMPARE: bunion.

h. varus Abnormal angulation of the big toe away from the other toes of the same foot.

halo (ha´lo) **1.** A circular configuration around a focus. **2.** Colored rings seen around lights or bright objects by patients afflicted with any process involving edema of the cornea (e.g., glaucoma).

halo sign A radiologic sign of a dead or dying fetus; the subcutaneous layer of fat over the fetal head appears elevated.

halogen (hal´ŏ-jen) Any of a group of chemically related nonmetallic elements that form similar saltlike compounds in combination with sodium; they include bromine, chlorine, fluorine, iodine, and the radioactive element astatine.

haloid (hal´oid) Resembling a halogen.

halophil, halophile (hal´o-fil, hal´o-fīl) A microorganism that thrives in a salty environment.

halothane (hal´o-thān) A liquid hydrocarbon used as a general anesthetic; associated with liver damage in susceptible individuals; Fluothane®.

halter (hawl´ter) A device for securing the head, particularly for traction.

ham (ham) **1.** The buttock and back part of the thigh. **2.** See popliteal fossa, under fossa.

hamartoblastoma (ham-ar-to-blas-to´mă) Malignant tumor believed to be derived from a hamartoma.

hamartoma (ham-ar-to´mă) Tumorlike, nonmalignant growth composed of cellular elements normally present in that site, but poorly developed.

Hamman-Rich syndrome (ham´an-rich sin´drōm) Progressive interstitial fibrosis of both lungs leading to pulmonary insufficiency, right-sided heart failure, and death; the cause is unknown.

Hamman's sign (ham´anz sīn) A rasping sound, synchronous with the heart beat, occurring in pneumomediastinum.

hammertoe (ham´er-tō) A deformed toe in which the second and third phalanges are bent downward.

hamster (ham´ster) Any of several ratlike Eurasian rodents (family Cricetidae) extensively used in experimental work.

hamstring (ham´string) See hamstring tendon, under tendon.

hamular (ham´u-lar) Shaped like a hook.

hamulus (ham´u-lus) Any hook-shaped process, as at the end of a bone.

lacrimal h. The hooklike process of the lacrimal bone articulating with the maxilla and forming the upper aperture of the bony nasal duct.

pterygoid h. The hooklike process of the sphenoid bone.

h. of spiral lamina The hooklike termination of the spiral lamina of the cochlea.

hand (hand) The terminal part of the upper extremity below the forearm.

accoucheur's h. The characteristic position of the hand produced by spasm in tetany.

claw h. See clawhand.

opera glass h. Deformity of the hand marked by shortening of the fingers and transverse folding of the skin caused by absorption of the phalanges, seen in chronic absorptive arthritis. Also called main en lorgnette.

spade h. The characteristic coarse, thick, square hand of acromegaly or myxedema.

trident h. A hand in which the fingers are short and thick and nearly equal in length, with a deflection (at the second phalangeal joint) of the index and middle fingers toward the radial side and the ring and little fingers toward the ulnar side, causing the fingers to spread out; characteristic hand of achondroplasia.

hand-foot-and-mouth disease (hand-fo͝ot-and mouth dĭ-zēz´) Contagious disease of children characterized by painful ulcerative stomatitis of the tongue, soft palate, and oral mucosa, associated with a vesicular eruption on hands and feet; caused by coxsackieviruses A5, A10, and A16.

handpiece (hand´pēs) In dentistry, the part of a mechanized, hand-held device that holds rotary instruments such as burs and mandrels during operative procedures; it is connected to a dental engine.

high-speed h. One that operates at rotational speeds in excess of 12,000 revolutions per minute.

ultra-high-speed h. One that operates at rotational speeds of 100,000 to 300,000 revolutions per minute.

ultrasonic h. One that vibrates at a frequency of 29,000 cycles per second (above audible range).

water-turbine h. One with a turbine powered by water under great pressure.

Hand-Schüller-Christian disease (hand-shēl´er-kris´chan dĭ-zēz´) See multifocal Langerhans-cell histiocytosis, under histiocytosis.

hangnail (hang´nāl) A partly detached piece of skin at the base or side of the nail.

Hansen's disease (han´senz dĭ-zēz´) See leprosy.

hapalonychia (hap-ă-lo-nik´e-ă) A state or condition characterized by soft fingernails or toenails; it can be normal or acquired as a result of malnutrition or debility.

haplodont (hap´lo-dont) Having peglike, even-surfaced molar teeth.

haploid (hap´loid) Referring to the reduced number of chromosomes in the gametes (i.e., spermatozoon and ovum) relative to that in the zygotes or in the body cells (diploid); the haploid number is half the diploid number.

haplopia (hap-lo´pe-ă) Single, normal vision, distinguished from double vision or diplopia.

haplosis (hap-lo´sis) The meiotic reduction of the diploid number of chromosomes to the haploid number.

haplotype (hap´lo-tīp) Closely linked alleles on a single chromosome that are usually inherited as a unit.

hapten, haptene (hap´tĕn, hap´tēn) Any incom-

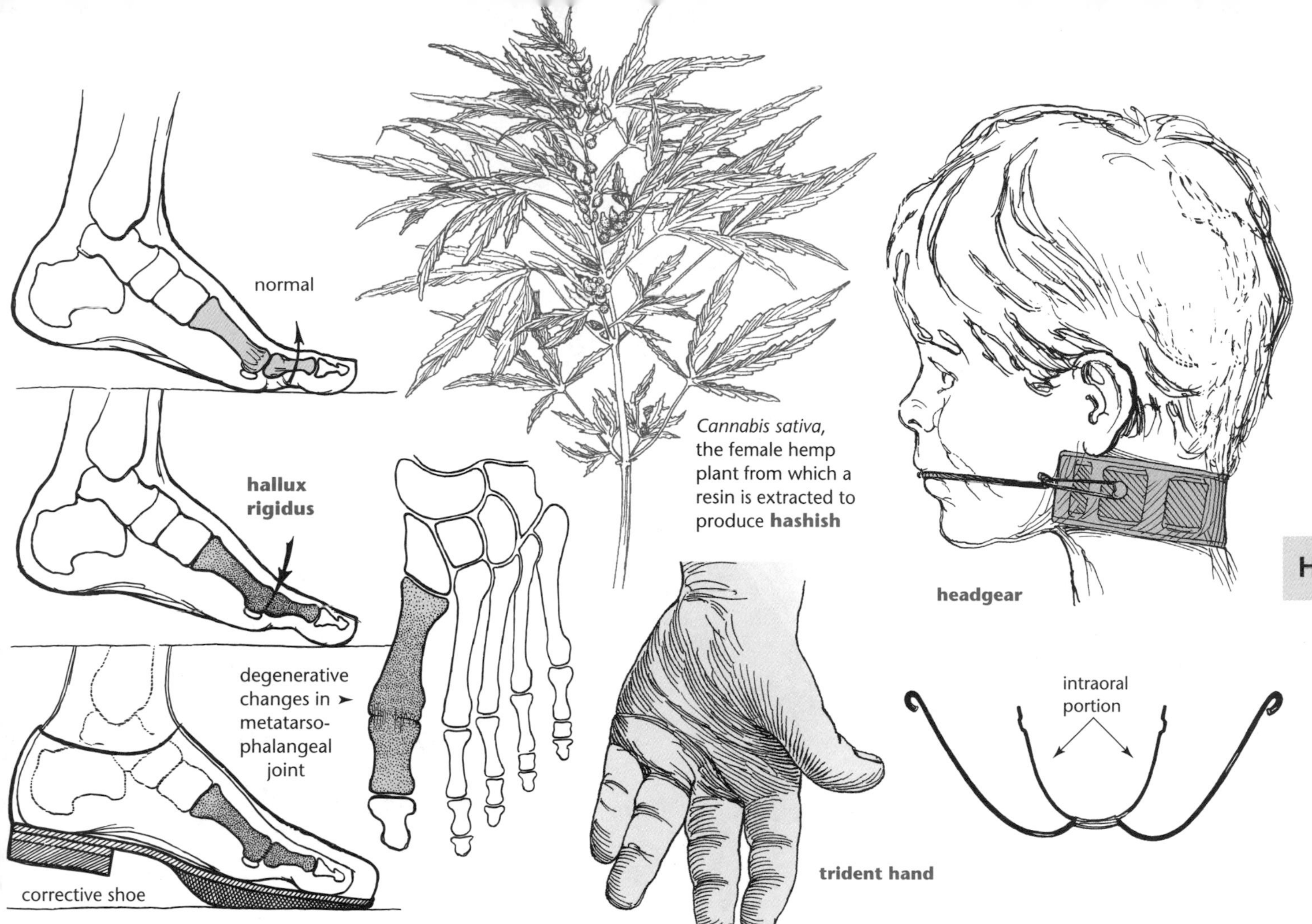

Cannabis sativa, the female hemp plant from which a resin is extracted to produce **hashish**

H

plete antigen that combines specifically with antibody but that does not incite the production of antibody unless attached to a high molecular weight carrier.

haptoglobin (hap-to-glo´bin) A protein present in human blood serum having the ability to combine with hemoglobin; a low level of haptoglobin indicates recent hemolysis.

haptometer (hap-tom´ĕ-ter) Instrument used to determine sensitivity to touch.

haptophore (hap´to-for) The atom group in the molecule of an antigen or antibody by means of which it becomes attached to a cell or to its corresponding antibody or antigen, respectively.

hardness (hard´nis) The ability of a material to resist scratching, abrasion, or attrition.

harelip (hār´lip) See cleft lip, under lip.

harmony (har´mo-ne) Agreement.

occlusal h. A contact between upper and lower teeth that is devoid of defects.

harpoon (har-po͞on´) An instrument with a barbed head used to remove small pieces of tissue for microscopic examination.

Hartnup disease (hahrt´nup dĭ-zēz´) A hereditary disorder of amino acid transport, marked by a pellagra-like skin rash upon exposure to sunlight, temporary muscular incoordination, and excretion of excessive amounts of amino acid in the urine. Also called H disease.

hasamiyami (has-ă-mē-yar´me) A fever occurring in Japan in the autumn, caused by a bacterium (*Leptospira autumnalis*).

Hashimoto's disease See Hashimoto's thyroiditis, under thyroiditis.

hashish (ha-shēsh) An intoxicating extract made from the dried flowers of the hemp plant, *Cannabis sativa*. Also written hasheesh.

hatchet (hach´it) An angled cutting hand instrument used in dentistry to remove enamel and dentin.

haunch (hawnch) The region of the upper thigh, buttock, and hip.

haustra (haws´tră) Plural of haustrum.

haustral (haws´tral) Relating to the pouches or sacculations of the colon.

haustration (haws-tra´shun) Increase in size of the sacculations of the large intestine.

haustrum (haws´trum), *pl.* **haus´tra** One of the sacculations of the colon.

haversian (ha-ver´zhăn) Term applied to the various osseous structures described by Clopton Havers.

H disease (āch dĭ-zēz´) See Hartnup disease.

head (hed) **1.** The upper or anterior vertebrate extremity, containing the brain and organs of special senses. **2.** The proximal end of a bone, closest to a point of reference. **3.** The end of a muscle that is attached to the less movable of two structures of its attachment. **4.** Slang expression denoting one who frequently uses narcotics.

headache (hed´āk) Pain in the head. Also called cephalalgia.

blind h. See migraine.

cluster h. A recurrent unilateral headache in the orbitotemporal area; usually of brief duration, often severe, generally occurring in regular intervals of six-week cycles; usually accompanied by stuffiness of the nose and tearing of the eye on the same side as the pain; can be precipitated by the use of histamine, alcohol, or nitroglycerin; more prevalent among males who smoke heavily. Also called histaminic headache; Horton's headache.

histaminic h. See cluster headache.

Horton's h. See cluster headache.

migraine h. See migraine.

organic h. Headache caused by disease of the brain or its membranes.

sick h. See migraine.

tension h. Headache caused by sustained contraction of skeletal muscle about the scalp, face, and especially the neck.

vascular h. See migraine.

headgear (hed´gēr) **1.** In orthodontics, an apparatus encircling the head or neck which provides anchorage for the attachment of an intraoral appliance. **2.** In radiology, a protective device to guard the head from injury by radiation.

heal (hēl) **1.** To close naturally, said of an incision, wound, or ulcer. **2.** To restore to health; to cure.

healer (hē´ler) One who heals or cures, especially a physician.

healing (hēl´ing) **1.** The process of return to normal health. **2.** Denoting an agent that promotes such a process.

h. by first intention The immediate healing of a wound without suppuration or granulation. Also called primary adhesion; primary union.

h. by second intention Healing by the union of two granulating surfaces after some suppuration has taken place. Also called secondary adhesion; secondary union.

h. by third intention Filling of a wound with granulations followed by formation of scar tissue.

health (helth) **1.** The state of an organism with respect to its physical, mental, and social well being. **2.** The state of an organism functioning optimally without disorders of any nature.

public h. The organized programs, services, and institutions involved with the prevention and control of disease of the population as a whole on the international, national, state, or municipal level.

health maintenance organization (HMO) (helth mān´tĕ-nans or-gă-ni-za´shun) A prepaid health plan that provides members comprehensive services from a limited group of physicians, hospitals, and other providers of health care.

healthy (hel´thē) Pertaining to good health.

hear (hēr) To perceive sound.

hearing (hēr´ing) The capacity to perceive sound.

color h. A subjective color sensation produced by certain sound waves. Also called pseudochromesthesia.

monaural h. Hearing with only one ear.

hearing aid (hēr´ing ād) A small device that amplifies sound; used to compensate for a hearing loss.

hearing loss (hēr´ing los) Reduced auditory sensitivity.

sensorineural hearing l. Loss of hearing due to dysfunction of the end organ or nerve fibers or both.

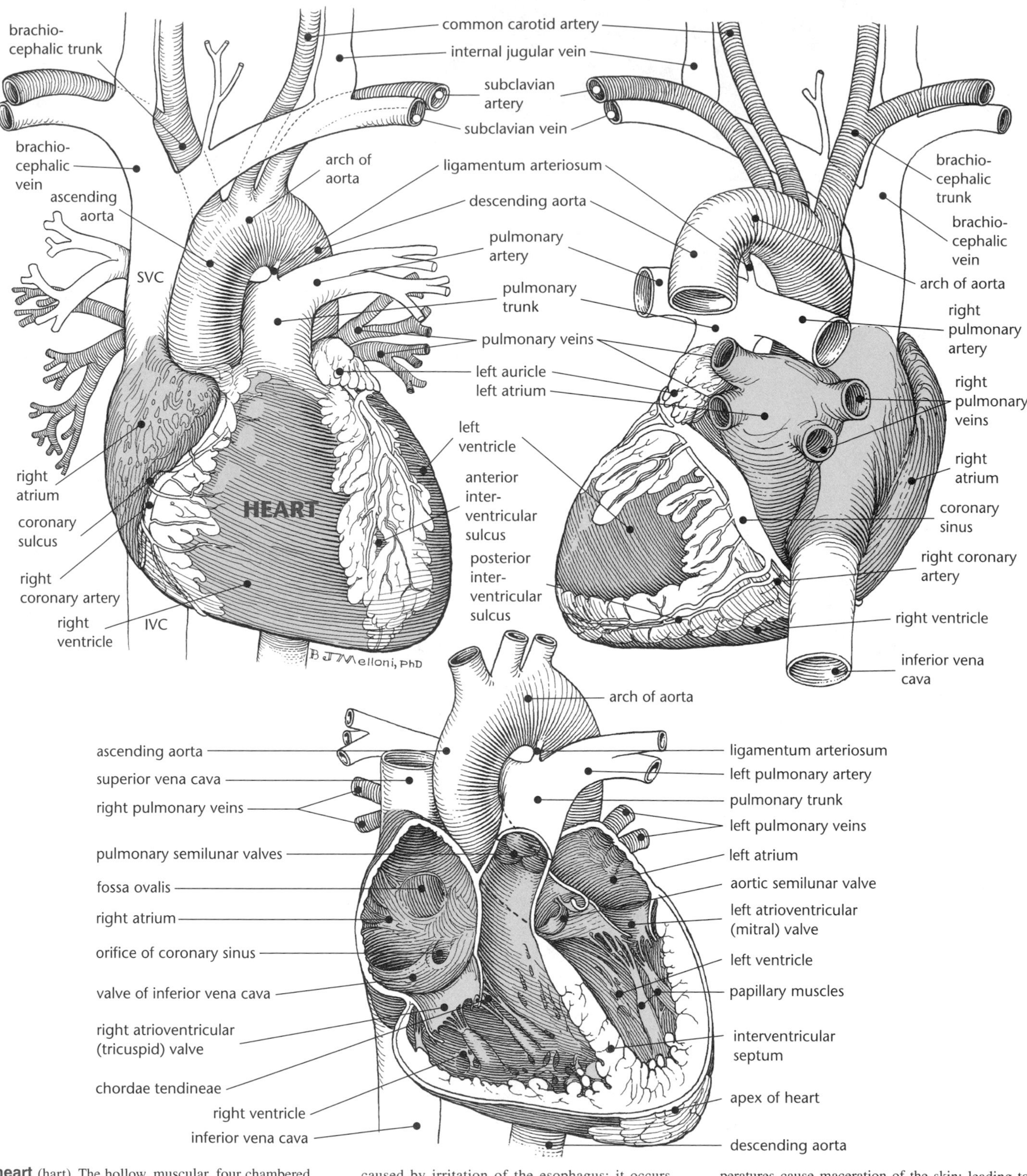

heart (hart) The hollow, muscular, four chambered organ that maintains the circulation of the blood by receiving it from the veins and pumping it into the arteries; it lies between the lungs and is enclosed in the pericardium. Also called cor.

artificial h. A device that partially or completely replaces the function of the natural heart.

dextroposition of h. See under dextroposition.

h. failure See under failure.

left h. The left atrium and left ventricle considered together.

right h. The right atrium and right ventricle considered together.

heartbeat (hart´bēt) One complete cycle of dilatation and contraction of the heart.

heartburn (hart´bern) Burning sensation in the lower chest and upper central area of the abdomen, caused by irritation of the esophagus; it occurs because of reflux of stomach contents due to an incompetent esophageal sphincter. Also called pyrosis.

heartworm (hart´werm) A parasitic nematode worm (*Dirofilaria immitis*) that usually lodges in the right chambers of the heart of dogs; very rarely seen in humans.

heat (hēt) **1.** A state characterized by elevation of temperature. **2.** A form of energy in transit from a body of higher temperature to another of lower temperature.

h. of combustion The quantity of heat released in the complete oxidation of one mole of a substance at constant pressure.

prickly h. A common, noncontagious skin disorder of hot, humid climates; elevated temperatures cause maceration of the skin; leading to blockage of sweat pores, retention of sweat, and formation of tiny vesicular papules that itch and burn. Also called miliaria rubra; heat rash.

saddle h. See clinocephaly.

heatlabile (hēt´lā´bl) Susceptible to being destroyed by a rise in temperature.

heavy-chain disease (hev´ē-chān dĭ-zēz´) Any of a group of malignant diseases characterized by overproduction of a specific immunoglobulin fragment that is detected in the blood or urine, and proliferation of lymphoid tissue; varieties include alpha-chain disease, gamma-chain disease, and mu-chain disease.

hebephrenia (he-bĕ-fre´ne-ă) A type of schizophrenia, usually developing after the onset of puberty, characterized by shallow, inappropriate emotions,

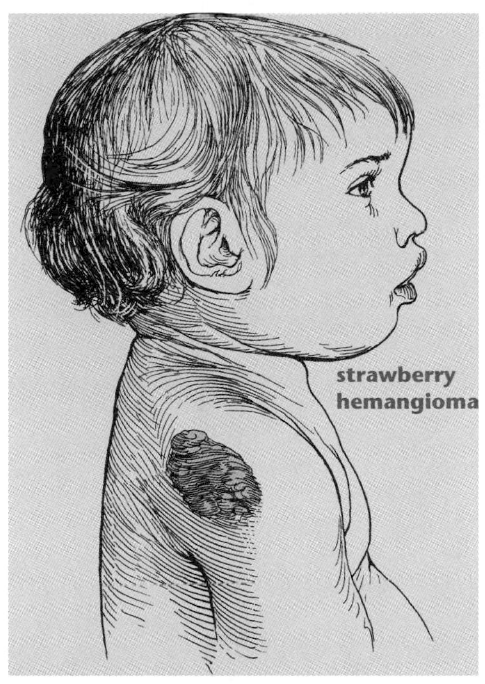

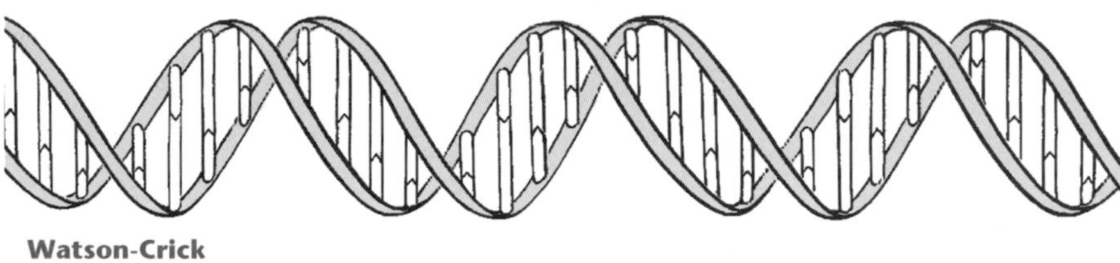

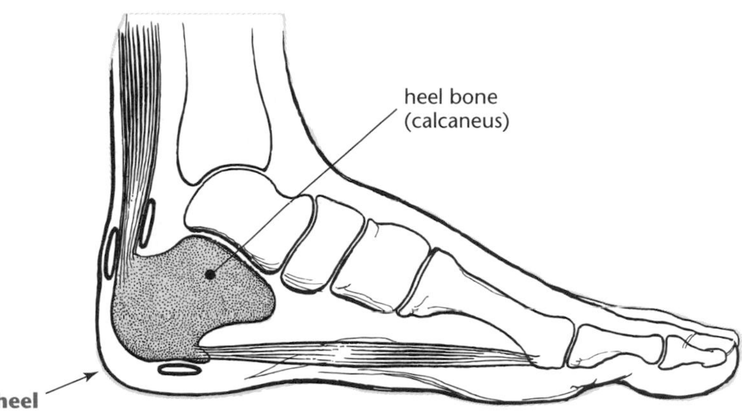

unpredictable childish behavior and mannerisms, and delusions.

hectic (hek´tik) **1.** Relating to the daily fever characteristic of certain diseases such as tuberculosis. **2.** Feverish; flushed.

hectogram (hek´tŏ-gram) One hundred grams, the equivalent of 1543.7 grains or 3.527 avoirdupois ounces.

hectoliter (hek-to-le´ter) One hundred liters, the equivalent of 105.7 quarts.

hedonic (he-don´ik) Relating to pleasure.

hedonics (he-don´iks) The study of pleasurable and unpleasurable feelings as they relate to behavior.

hedonism (hēd´n-ĭz-m) A constant pursuit of or devotion to pleasure and avoidance of pain; exhibited in some forms of character disorder.

heel (hēl) The rounded posterior portion of the foot.

heel bone (hēl bōn) Calcaneus. See table of bones.

Hegar's sign (ha´garz sīn) A compressibility and softening of the lower uterine segment (cervical isthmus) detected by bimanual examination; a reasonably reliable sign of pregnancy.

helicine (hel´ĭ-sēn) Relating to a spiral or helix.

Helicobacter (hel-ĭ-ko-bak´ter) Genus of motile, spiral, gram-negative bacteria found in the intestinal tract and reproductive organs of animals and the intestinal tract of humans. Some species cause disease.

H. jejuni Species that is the major cause of enterocolitis ranging from self-limited mild intestinal disturbances to severe recurrent diarrhea with inflammatory changes resembling those of ulcerative colitis or Crohn's disease. Formerly called *Campylobacter jejuni.*

H. pylori A species causing active chronic inflammation of the stomach (type B gastritis); found in 90% of patients with duodenal ulcers; may be responsible for most gastric and duodenal ulcers and associated with cancer of the stomach. Formerly called *Campylobacter pylori.*

helicoid (hel´ĭ-koid) Spiral.

helicotrema (hel-ĭ-ko-tre´mă) The passage at the apex of the cochlea of the inner ear through which the scala vestibuli and scala tympani communicate with one another.

heliopathy (he-le-op´ă-thē) Injury from exposure to sunlight.

heliotaxis (he-le-o-tak´sis) The tendency of a microorganism to move toward (positive heliotaxis) or away from (negative heliotaxis) a light source.

helium (he´le-um) A gaseous element; symbol He, atomic number 2, atomic weight 4.003; present in small amounts in the atmosphere.

helix (he´liks) **1.** The folded skin and cartilage forming the margin of the outer ear (auricle). **2.** A coiled curve or structure.

alpha-h. The right-handed helical form of many proteins.

DNA h. See Watson-Crick helix.

double h. See Watson-Crick helix.

twin h. See Watson-Crick helix.

Watson-Crick h. A three-dimensional model of the DNA molecule; it consists of a double helix resembling a ladder that has been twisted into a spiral; the sides of the ladder are formed by the deoxyribose-phosphate units and are held together by rungs composed of pairs of bases (adenine and thymine or cytosine and guanine) joined together by hydrogen bonds. Also called DNA helix; double helix; twin helix.

HELLP syndrome A form of severe preeclampsia marked by hemolysis, elevated liver function, and low platelets.

helminth (hel´minth) **1.** A parasitic intestinal worm, especially the nematode or trematode. **2.** A wormlike parasite.

helminthemesis (hel-min-them´ĕ-sis) The vomiting of parasitic worms.

helminthiasis (hel-min-thi´ă-sis) The condition of having intestinal worms.

helminthic (hel-min´thik) Relating to worms, especially parasitic intestinal worms.

helminthoid (hel-min´thoid) Resembling a worm.

helminthology (hel-min-thol´ŏ-je) The study of worms, especially the parasitic intestinal worms. Also called scolecology.

heloma (he-lo´mă) A corn or callosity.

helosis (he-lo´sis) The condition of having horny thickening of the skin, usually on a toe.

helotomy (he-lot´ŏ-me) The surgical removal of corns or of calluses.

hemabarometer (he-mă-bar-om´e-ter) A device for determining the specific gravity of the blood.

hemacytometer (he-mă-si-tom´ĕ-ter) See hemocytometer.

hemacytozoon (he-mă-si-to-zō´on) See hemocytozoon.

hemadsorption (he-mad-zorp´shun) Phenomenon in which a substance adheres to the surface of a red blood cell.

hemagglutinin (he-mă-gloo´tĭ-nin) A protein in blood serum that causes clumping of red blood cells; also present in the surface projections of some viruses.

hemagogue, hemagog (he´mă-gog) Any agent that promotes the flow of blood, particularly during menstruation.

hemal (he´mal) **1.** Relating to the blood. **2.** Relating to the part of the body in front of the spinal column; ventral.

hemangiectasia, hemangiectasis (he-man-je-ek-ta´shă, he-man-je-ek´tă-sis) Dilatation of blood vessels.

hemangioblast (he-man´je-o-blast) An embryonic cell derived from the mesoderm; it develops into cells that give rise to endothelium of blood vessels, to reticuloendothelial elements, and to all types of blood-forming cells.

hemangioblastoma (he-man-je-o-blas-to´mă) A brain tumor composed of angioblasts. Also called angioblastoma.

hemangioendothelioblastoma (he-man-je-o-en-do-the-le-o-blas-to´mă) A tumor of vascular origin in which the endothelial cells seem to be predominantly immature types.

hemangioendothelioma (he-man-je-o-en-do-the-le-o´mă) A tumor derived from blood vessels, composed chiefly of masses of endothelial cells.

hemangioma (he-man-je-o´mă) A benign tumor made up of blood vessels.

capillary h. A congenital tumor composed of minute, closely packed, thin-walled blood vessels that, for the most part, are of the caliber of capillaries; it varies from bright red to blue and may occur in any tissue or organ; the most common sites are the skin, subcutaneous tissues, and mucous membranes of the oral cavity and lips.

cavernous h. A tumor containing large blood filled spaces. Also called cavernous angioma.

port-wine h. See nevus flammeus, under nevus.

sclerosing h. See dermatofibroma.

senile h. A bright red capillary hemangioma varying in size from pinhead to several centimeters in diameter; may be flat or slightly raised; seen in young adults and, most frequently, in elderly individuals. Also called cherry angioma.

strawberry h. A bright red raised tumor; present at birth as a pinhead-sized flat lesion that quickly increases in size and becomes elevated and rough; approximately 90% of these hemangiomas disappear without treatment by the ages of 5 to 7. Also called nevus vasculosus.

hemangiomatosis (he-man-je-o-mă-to´sis) The presence of numerous hemangiomas.

hemangiopericytoma (he-man-je-o-per-ĭ-si-to´mă) Malignant tumor composed of numerous tiny blood channels encased in masses of connective tissue cells (pericytes). Also called perithelioma.

hemangiosarcoma (he-man-je-o-sar-ko´mă) A rare malignant tumor composed chiefly of anaplastic cells derived from blood vessels.

hemarthrosis (he-mar´thro´sis) Blood in a joint space, resulting usually in pain, tenderness, and swelling.

hematemesis (he-mă-tem´ĕ-sis) Vomiting of blood.

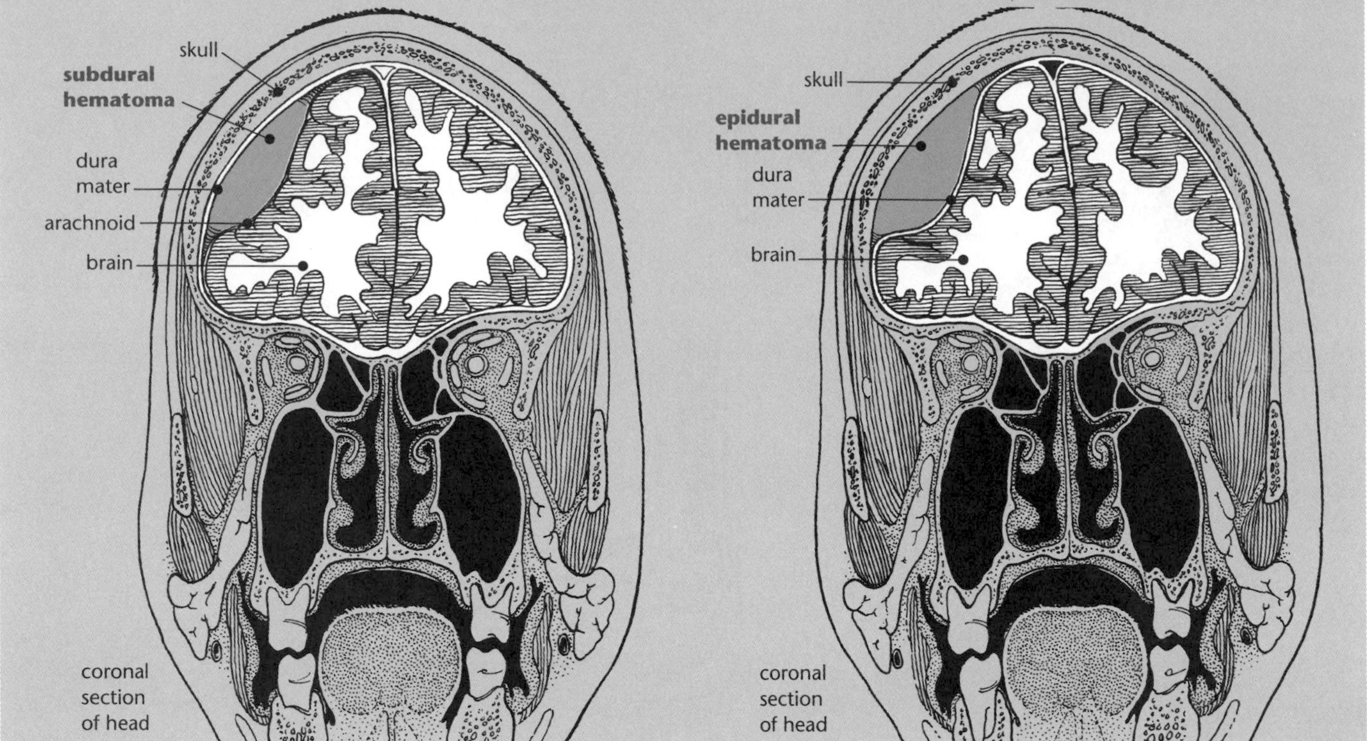

H

hematherm (he´mă-therm) Denoting a warm-blooded animal.
hemathermal (he-mă-ther´mal) Warm-blooded; said of humans and certain animals. Also called hemathermous.
hemathermous (he-mă-ther´mus) See hemathermal.
hematic (he-mat´ik) **1.** Relating to blood. **2.** See hematinic.
hematin (he´mă-tin) The hydroxide of heme.
hematinic (he-mă-tin´ik) Any agent that improves the condition of the blood.
hematoblast (he-mat´o-blast) A primitive blood cell from which develop erythroblasts, lymphoblasts, myeloblasts, and other immature blood cells.
hematocele (he-mat´o-sēl) A swelling caused by the effusion and collection of blood into a cavity of the body, especially under the serous covering of the testis.
hematochezia (hem-ă-to-ke´ze-ă) The passage of bloody stools.
hematocolpometra (hem-ă-to-kol-po-me´tră) Accumulation of blood in the uterus and vagina resulting from an imperforate hymen or any other obstruction.
hematocolpos (hem-ă-to-kol´pos) Distention of the vagina with accumulated menstrual blood usually due to an imperforate hymen.
hematocrit (he-mat´o-krit) (Hct) **1.** The volume percentage of red blood cells in whole blood; in the normal male it constitutes about 45 to 50% of the whole blood volume; in the normal female it constitutes approximately 40 to 45%. Also called packed cell volume. **2.** A small centrifuge used to separate the cellular elements of blood from the plasma.
hematocyanin (he-mă-to-si´ă-nin) See hemocyanin.
hematocystis (he-mă-to-sis´tis) Effusion of blood into the urinary bladder.
hematocyte (he´mă-to-sīt) See hemocyte.
hematocytometer (he-mă-to-si-tom´ĕ-ter) Hemocytometer.
hematocytozoon (he-mă-to-si-to-zō´on) See hemocytozoon.
hematocyturia (he-mă-to-si-tu´re-ă) The presence of red blood cells in the urine. Also called true hematuria.
hematogenesis (he-mă-to-jen´ĕ-sis) See hemopoiesis.
hematogenic, hematogenous (he-mă-to-jen´ik, he-mă-toj´ĕ-nus) Derived from or circulated by the blood.
hematoid (he´mă-toid) Resembling blood.
hematoidin (he-mă-toid´in) Pigment derived from the breakdown of hemoglobin; formed in the tissues as a result of hemorrhage.
hematologist (he-mă-tol´ŏ-jist) A specialist in hematology.
hematology (he-mă-tol´ŏ-je) The medical specialty concerned with the diagnosis and treatment of disorders of blood and blood-forming tissues.
hematolysis (he-mă-tol´ĭ-sis) See hemolysis.
hematoma (he-mă-to´mă) A localized mass of blood outside of the blood vessels, usually found in a partly clotted state.
epidural h. Hematoma between the dura mater and skull.
hepatic h. Hematoma formed just within the capsule of the liver due to liver damage by pre-eclampsia and eclampsia; causes upper abdominal pain and tenderness.
pelvic h. Any hematoma formed in or around structures of the pelvis; designated vulvar, paravaginal, broad ligament, and retroperitoneal hematomas according to their location.
umbilical cord h. Hematoma formed in the umbilical cord, usually caused by rupture of a varicosed umbilical vein; may also develop after umbilical vessel venipuncture (directed by ultrasound) to obtain a fetal blood sample.
subdural h. Hematoma between the dura mater and arachnoid (membranes) of the brain.
hematometra (he-mă-to-me´tra) Distention of the uterus with accumulated blood. Also called hemometra.
hematometry (he-mă-tom´ĕ-tre) Examination of blood to determine any or all of the following: the total number, types, and proportions of blood cells; the number or proportion of other formed elements; and the percentage of hemoglobin. Also called hemometry.
hematomyelia (he-mă-to-mi-e´le-ă) Effusion of blood into the spinal cord.
hematopathology (he-mă-to-pă-thol´ŏ-je) The branch of medicine concerned with diseases of the blood and blood-forming tissues.
hematopathy (he-mă-top´ă-the) See hemopathy.
hematopenia (he-mă-to-pe´ne-ă) Blood deficiency.
hematopoiesis (he-mă-to-poi-e´sis) See hemopoiesis.
hematopoietin (he-mă-to-poi´ĕ-tin) See erythropoietin.
hematoporphyrin (he-mă-to-por´fĭ-rin) A dark red substance formed by the decomposition of hemoglobin. Also called hemoporphyrin.
hematosalpinx (he-mă-to-sal´pinks) Distention of a uterine tube with a collection of blood. Also called hemosalpinx.
hematosepsis (he-mă-to-sep´sis) See septicemia.
hematospermia (he-mă-to-sper´me-ă) Blood in the seminal fluid. Also called hemospermia.
hematostaxis (he-mă-to-stak´sis) Spontaneous bleeding caused by a blood disease.
hematotrachelos (he-mă-to-tră-ke´los) Distention of the uterine cervix, as with accumulated menstrual blood due to an imperforate hymen.
hematoxylin (he-mă-tok´sĭ-lin) A crystalline compound, extracted from the tropical American tree, logwood; used as a stain in histology and bacteriology; it imparts a bluish tint to the specimen.
hematozoon (he-mă-to-zō´on), *pl.* **hematozo´a** Any parasitic protozoan or microorganism that lives in the circulating blood of its host.
hematuria (he-mă-tu´re-ă) Discharge of red blood cells in the urine.
heme (hēm) The nonprotein, iron-containing porphyrin molecule that forms the oxygen-binding element of hemoglobin. Also called ferroprotoporphyrin. Formerly called hematin.
hemeralopia (hem´er-ă-lo´pe-ă) Defective vision in daylight, with good vision in dim light. Also called day blindness; night sight.
hemialgia (hem-e-al´ja) Pain on one side of the body only.
hemiamblyopia (hem-e-am-ble-o´pe-ă) See hemianopsia.
hemianacusia (hem-e-an-ă-koo´ze-ă) Loss of hearing in one ear.
hemianalgesia (hem-e-an-al-je´zhă) Loss of sensibility to pain on one side of the body.
hemianesthesia (hem-e-an-es-the´zhă) Loss of sensibility to touch on one side of the body.
alternate h. Hemianesthesia affecting one side of the head and the other side of the body and extremities. Also called crossed hemianesthesia.
crossed h. See alternate hemianesthesia.
hemianopia (hem-e-ă-no´pe-ă) Loss of vision in one half the visual field of one or both eyes. Also called hemiamblyopia; hemianopsia.
bitemporal h. Bilateral hemianopsia affecting the temporal halves of the visual fields of both eyes.
congruous h. Bilateral hemianopsia affecting the nasal half of one visual field and the temporal half of the other, the defects in the two visual fields being identical in size, shape, and location, resulting in a single defect of the binocular field.
crossed h. Bilateral hemianopsia affecting the upper half of one visual field and the lower half of the other.
heteronymous h. Bilateral hemianopsia affecting either both temporal halves or both nasal halves of the visual fields.
homonymous h. Bilateral hemianopsia affecting

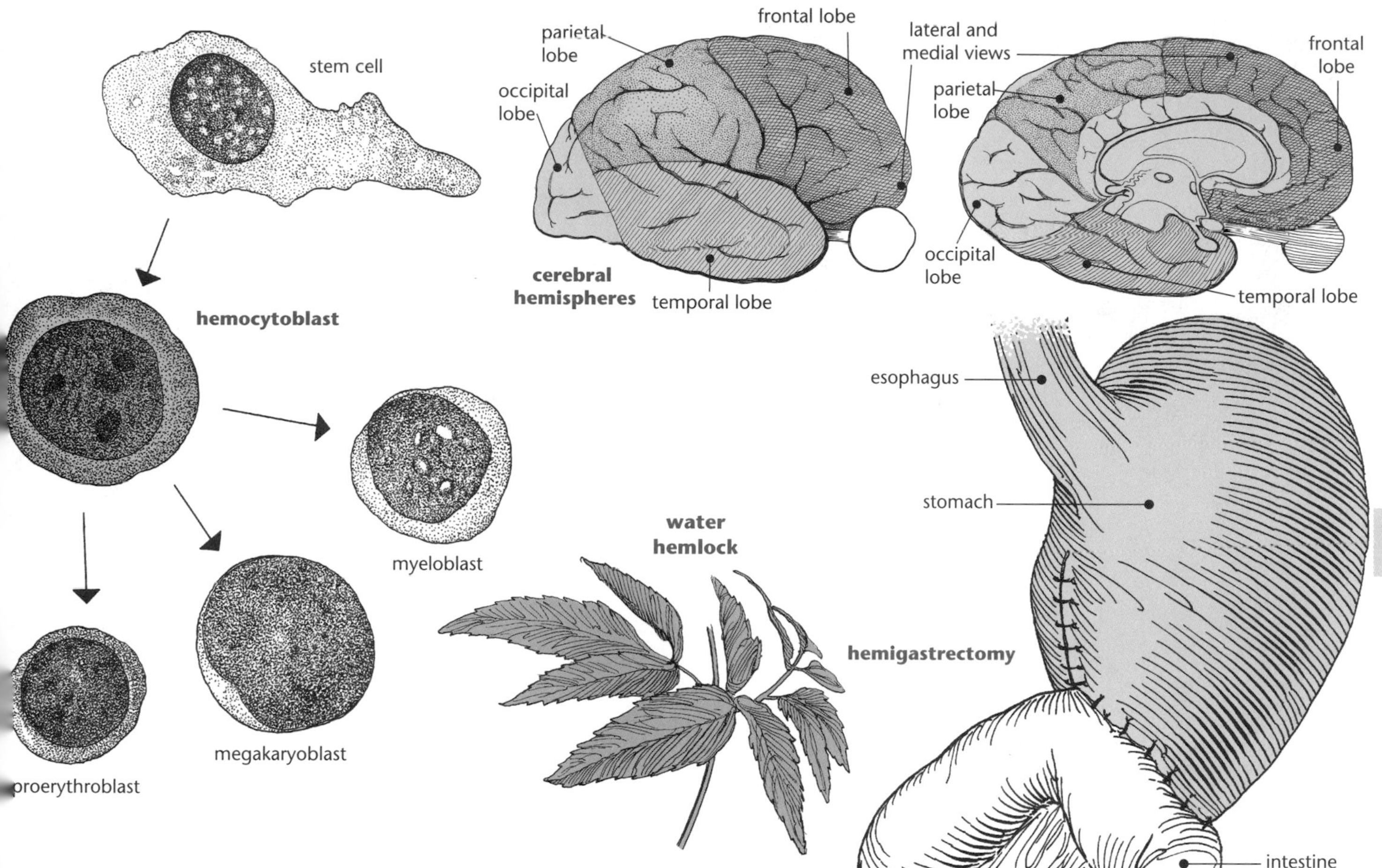

the nasal half of one visual field and the temporal half of the other.

incomplete h. Hemianopsia not affecting the entire half of the visual field.

quadrantic h. See quadrantanopsia.

hemianopsia (hem-e-an-op′se-ă) See hemianopia.

hemianosmia (hem-e-an-oz′me-ă) Loss of the sense of smell on one side only.

hemiatrophy (hem-e-at′ro-fe) Atrophy confined to one side of an organ or bodily region, as of the face or tongue.

facial h. Atrophy, usually progressive, affecting the tissues of one side of the face. Also called Romberg's disease; facial trophoneurosis.

hemiballismus (hem-e-bă-liz′mus) Violent, involuntary movements of the extremities involving one side of the body, due to a lesion in the contralateral subthalamic body.

hemiblock (hem′e-blok) Blocking of the heart impulse in either of the two main divisions of the bundle of His (atrioventricular bundle).

hemic (he′mik, hem′ik) Relating to the blood.

hemicentrum (hem-e-sen′trum) Either lateral half of the body of a vertebra.

hemichorea (hem-e-kor′e-ă) Chorea in which the uncontrollable and irregular movements of the muscles are largely confined to one side of the body.

hemicolectomy (hem-e-ko-lek′tŏ-me) Removal of part of the colon.

hemicrania (hem-e-kra′ne-ă) Pain on one side of the head.

hemidiaphoresis (hem-e-di-ă-for-e′sis) Sweating on one side of the body.

hemigastrectomy (hem-e-gas-trek′tŏ-me) Excision of one half of the stomach, usually of the pyloric end.

hemihypertrophy (hem-e-hi-pĕr-tro′fe) Congenital overgrowth of one side of the body.

hemikaryon (hem-ĭ-kar′e-on) A cell nucleus containing the haploid number of chromosomes.

hemilaminectomy (hem-e-lam-ĭ-nek′tŏ-me) The surgical removal of a portion of the vertebral lamina in order to gain exposure to an underlying nerve root or intervertebral disk; often used to denote unilateral laminectomy.

hemimelia (hem-e-me′le-ă) A congenital defect marked by absence of all or part of the distal portion of a limb or limbs.

hemin (he′min) A crystalline compound, $C_{34}H_{32}N_4O_4FeCl$; the chloride of heme. Also called Teichmann's crystals.

heminephrectomy (hem-e-nĕ-frek′tŏ-me) Surgical excision of part of a kidney.

hemiparesis (hem-e-pa-re′sis) Muscular weakness or mild paralysis of one side of the body.

hemiplegia (hem-e-ple′jă) Paralysis of one side of the body.

alternate h. Millard-Gubler syndrome.

hemiplegic (hem-e-ple′jik) One whose body is paralyzed on one side.

Hemiptera (he-mip′ter-ă) A large order of insects that includes the common bedbug.

hemisphere (hem′is-fēr) Half of a symmetrical, spherical object.

cerebral h. A lateral half of the cerebrum.

hemithorax (hem-e-thor′aks) One side of the chest.

hemizygosity (hem-e-zi-gos′ĭ-te) The state of having only one of a pair of genes.

hemizygote (hem-e-zi′gōt) An individual or cell having only one of a pair of genes.

hemizygous, hemizygotic (hem-e-zi′gus, hem-e-zi-got′ik) Having unpaired genes; said of the male with respect to the X chromosome.

hemlock (hem′lok) Any of several poisonous plants (genus *Conium*) capable of producing motor paralysis. Commonly called poison hemlock.

water h. Probably the most poisonous plant in the United States; the poison is found principally in the roots, which are often mistaken for parsnips.

hemoagglutinin (he-mo-ă-gloo′tĭ-nin) An antibody in serum that causes agglutination of red blood cells (erythrocytes).

hemobilia (he-mo-bil′e-ă) Bleeding into the biliary passages.

hemochromatosis (hem-o-kro-mă-to′sis) A disorder of iron metabolism resulting in accumulation of excess iron in the tissues of many organs, especially the skin, liver, and pancreas, leading to fibrosis and functional insufficiency of those organs that are severely involved; the heart and other muscles and endocrine glands are also affected; deposition of iron in the skin causes a bronzed pigmentation; deposits in the pancreas lead to a form of diabetes (bronzed diabetes). Also called iron storage disease.

hemochrome (he′mo-krōm) See hemochromogen.

hemochromogen (he-mo-kro′mo-jen) A substance formed by the union of heme with a nitrogenous compound, such as a protein or base. Also called hemochrome.

hemochromometer (he-mo-kro-mom′ĕ-ter) An apparatus for estimating the percentage of hemoglobin in the blood by comparing the solution of blood with a standard solution of an appropriate compound, such as ammonium picrocarminate.

hemoclasis (he-mok′lă-sis) Hemolysis or destruction of red blood cells.

hemoconcentration (he-mo-kon-sen-tra′shun) Increase in the concentration or proportion of formed elements in the circulating blood, usually resulting from the loss of plasma from the bloodstream.

hemocyanin (he-mo-si′ă-nin) An oxygen-carrying blue respiratory pigment (chromoprotein) occurring in the blood of lower sea animals (e.g., mollusks) in which copper is an essential component. Also called hematocyanin.

hemocyte (he′mo-sīt) Any cell or formed element of the blood; a blood corpuscle; a blood cell. Also called hematocyte.

hemocytoblast (he-mo-si′to-blast) A primitive cell derived from the hemohistioblast; the name given to the cell from which granulocytes, red cell precursors, and megakaryocytes are derived.

hemocytometer (he-mo-si-tom′ĕ-ter) An instrument used for estimating the blood cell count in a measured volume of blood. Also called hemacytometer; erythrocytometer.

Thoma-Zeiss h. An apparatus used to count blood cells. Also called Thoma's counting chamber.

hemocytotripsis (he-mo-si-to-trip′sis) The destruction of blood cells by mechanical means (e.g., compression between hard surfaces).

hemocytozoon (he-mo-si-to-zō′on) An animal parasite of blood cells. Also called hemacytozoon; hematocytozoon.

hemodialysis (he-mo-di-al′ĭ-sis) Removal of waste

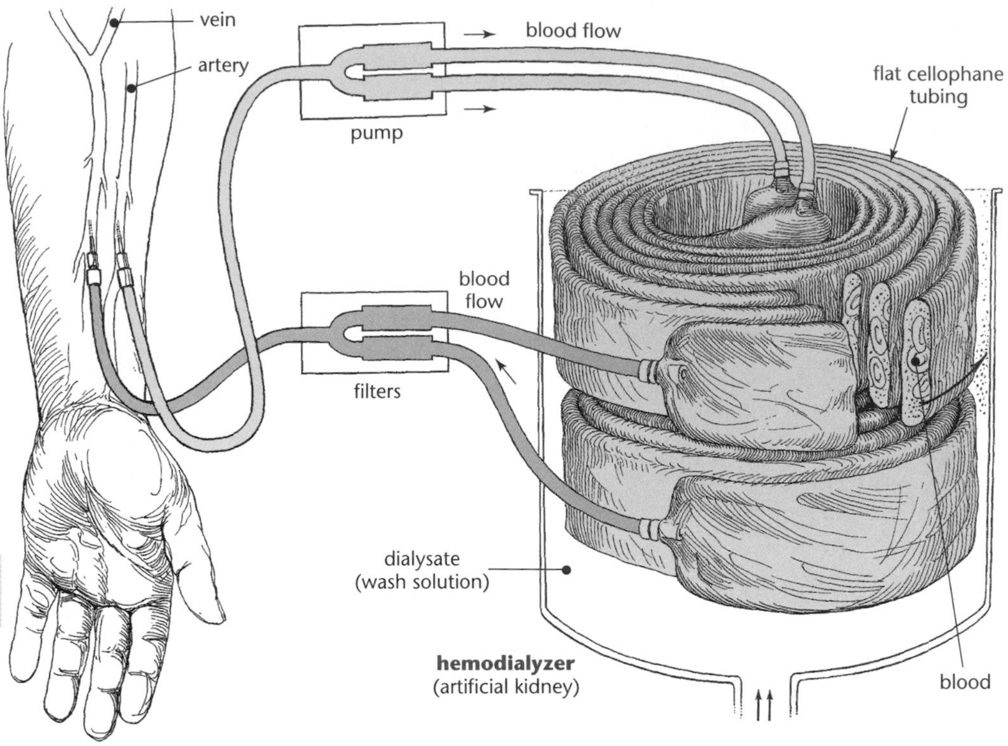

hemodialyzer
(artificial kidney)

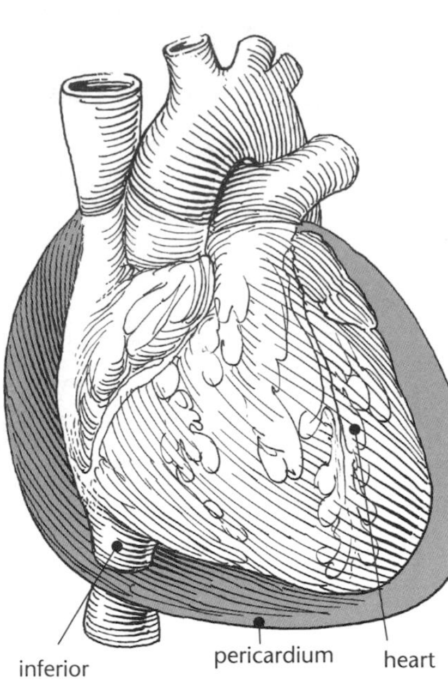

hemopericardium

materials or poisons from the blood by means of a hemodialyzer (artificial kidney).

hemodialyzer (he-mo-dī´ă-līz-er) An apparatus for removing waste products from the blood and correcting electrolyte and volume disturbances in acute or chronic kidney failure and in certain types of poisoning or drug overdose; toxic elements are removed by passing the blood through a semipermeable membrane lying in a bathing solution, then returning it to the body. Commonly called artificial kidney; kidney machine.

hemodilution (he-mo-di-lu´shun) Increase in the plasma content of the blood with resulting decrease in the concentration of red blood cells.

hemodynamic (he-mo-di-nam´ik) Relating to blood circulation.

hemodynamics (he-mo-di-nam´iks) The science of the forces connected with the circulation of the blood.

hemofiltration (he-mo-fil-tra´shun) A technique used for purifying the blood by filtering out components of the blood smaller than albumin and replacing a similar quantity of a balanced electrolyte solution; by this process, unwanted solutes such as urea, creatinine and other nitrogenous wastes are removed from the body.

hemoflagellates (he-mo-flaj´ĕ-lāts) Flagellated blood parasites.

hemofuscin (he-mo-fūs´in) A brown pigment derived from hemoglobin; sometimes found in urine along with hemosiderin; an indication of increased red blood cell destruction.

hemogenesis (he-mo-jen´ĕ-sis) See hemopoiesis.

hemoglobin (he-mo-glo-bin) (Hb) The oxygen-bearing protein of red blood cells; it is bright red when saturated with oxygen and purplish when it is not carrying oxygen.

h. A (Hb A) The predominant form of hemoglobin of human adults.

h. A_2 (Hb A_2) Hemoglobin making up about 1.5 to 3% of the total hemoglobin concentration. An elevated proportion is usually indicative of beta-thalassemia.

h. A1c See glycated hemoglobin.

h. C (Hb C) An abnormal hemoglobin characterized by an amino acid substitution (lysine for glutamic acid at position 6 of the beta chain); it reduces the normal plasticity of red blood cells. When present, target cells are seen. When homozygous, it is associated with chronic hemolytic anemia.

carbon monoxide h. See carboxyhemoglobin.

h. F (Hb F) Hemoglobin of a normal fetus; the major hemoglobin component during intrauterine life. Also called fetal hemoglobin.

fetal h. See hemoglobin F.

glycated h. A fraction of hemoglobin A to which glucose binds; high concentrations occur in patients with elevated blood sugar levels. Also called hemoglobin A1c; glycosylated hemoglobin.

glycosylated h. See glycated hemoglobin.

h. H (Hb H) An abnormal hemoglobin composed of four beta chains with a marked affinity for oxygen. It is associated with a variant of alpha-thalassemia.

oxygenated h. See oxyhemoglobin.

reduced h. Hemoglobin present in venous blood, after it has released its oxygen in the tissues.

h. S (Hb S) Abnormal hemoglobin characterized by an amino acid substitution (valine for glutamic acid at position 6 of the beta chain); associated with sickle cell anemia. Also called sickle cell hemoglobin.

sickle cell h. See hemoglobin S.

hemoglobinemia (he-mo-glo-bin-e´me-ă) The presence of free hemoglobin in plasma, resulting from mechanical injury to the red blood cells within the vessels.

hemoglobinometer (he-mo-glo-bin-om´ĕ-ter) An apparatus for estimating the amount of hemoglobin in the blood. Also called hemometer.

hemoglobinopathy (he-mo-glo-bin-op´ă-the) A hematologic disorder in which the type of hemoglobin within an individual's red blood cells differs qualitatively or quantitatively from that contained in normal red blood cells.

hemoglobinuria (he-mo-glo-bĭ-nu´re-ă) The presence of free hemoglobin in the urine, an indication of recent injury or destruction of red blood cells of at least moderate severity.

malarial h. Uncommon condition caused by infection with the malarial parasite *Plasmodium falciparum*. Also called blackwater fever.

march h. Episodes of hemoglobinuria caused by prolonged, intense physical activity (e.g., in marathon running).

paroxysmal nocturnal h. (PNH) Chronic disorder marked primarily by hemolytic anemia, hemoglobinuria (chiefly at night), yellow discoloration of the skin and mucous membranes, and enlargement of the spleen and liver. Also called Marchiafava-Micheli syndrome.

hemogram (he´mo-gram) A record of the number, proportion, and morphologic features of the cellular elements of blood.

hemohistioblast (he-mo-his´te-o-blast) An undifferentiated mesenchymal cell of the reticuloendothelial system from which all blood cells are derived; it is probably similar in morphology to other blood blasts. Also called stem cell.

hemolith (he´mo-lith) A concretion in the wall of a blood vessel.

hemolysin (he-mol´ĭ-sin) **1.** An anti-red blood cell antibody that activates complement (C´) to cause destruction (lysis) of red blood cells. Formerly called amboceptor. **2.** Any substance produced by a living agent and capable of destroying red blood cells by liberating their hemoglobin.

immune h. Hemolysin made by injecting an animal with red blood cells or whole blood from another species.

hemolysinogen (he-mo-li-sin´ŏ-jen) Antigenic substance in red blood cells that stimulates the formation of hemolysin.

hemolysis (he-mol´ĭ-sis) Destruction of red blood cells and liberation of hemoglobin. Also called erythrocytolysis; hematolysis.

hemolytic (he-mo-lit´ik) Causing disintegration of red blood cells.

hemolytic disease of newborn (he-mo-lit´ik dĭ-zēz´ ŭv noo´born) A condition resulting from an incompatibility of fetal and maternal red blood cell groups in which fetal red blood cells (antigens) are destroyed by the transplacental passage of maternal antibodies of the IgG type. Although most often caused by Rh factor incompatibility, it occurs with other less common blood groups, such as Kell and Duffy. ABO blood group incompatibility may also cause a milder form of this disease, and is usually manifest in the neonatal period. Also called erythroblastosis fetalis; hemolytic anemia of newborn.

hemolytic-uremic syndrome (he-mo-lit´ik-u-re´mik sin´drōm) A syndrome usually occurring in children, characterized by hemolytic anemia with abnormally shaped erythrocytes, thrombocytopenia, and uremia; minor respiratory or gastrointestinal infection often precedes onset.

hemolyze (he´mo-līz) To disintegrate red blood cells, causing liberation of hemoglobin from the cells.

hemomanometer (he-mo-mă-nom´ĕ-ter) An instrument for determining blood pressure. Also called hematomanometer.

hemomediastinum (he-mo-me-di-as-ti´num) Effusion of blood into the mediastinum. Also called hematomediastinum.

hemometer (he-mom´ĕ-ter) **1.** See hemoglobinometer. **2.** Term occasionally used for hemocytometer.

hemometra (he-mo-me´tră) See hematometra.

hemometry (he-mom´ĕ-tre) See hematometry.

hemopathy (he-mop´ă-the) Any disorder of the blood or blood-forming tissues. Also called hematopathy.

hemoperfusion (he-mo-per-fu´zhun) Passage of the blood over a sorbent (e.g., activated charcoal) in order to remove a toxic substance.

hemopericardium (he-mo-per-ĭ-kar´de-um)

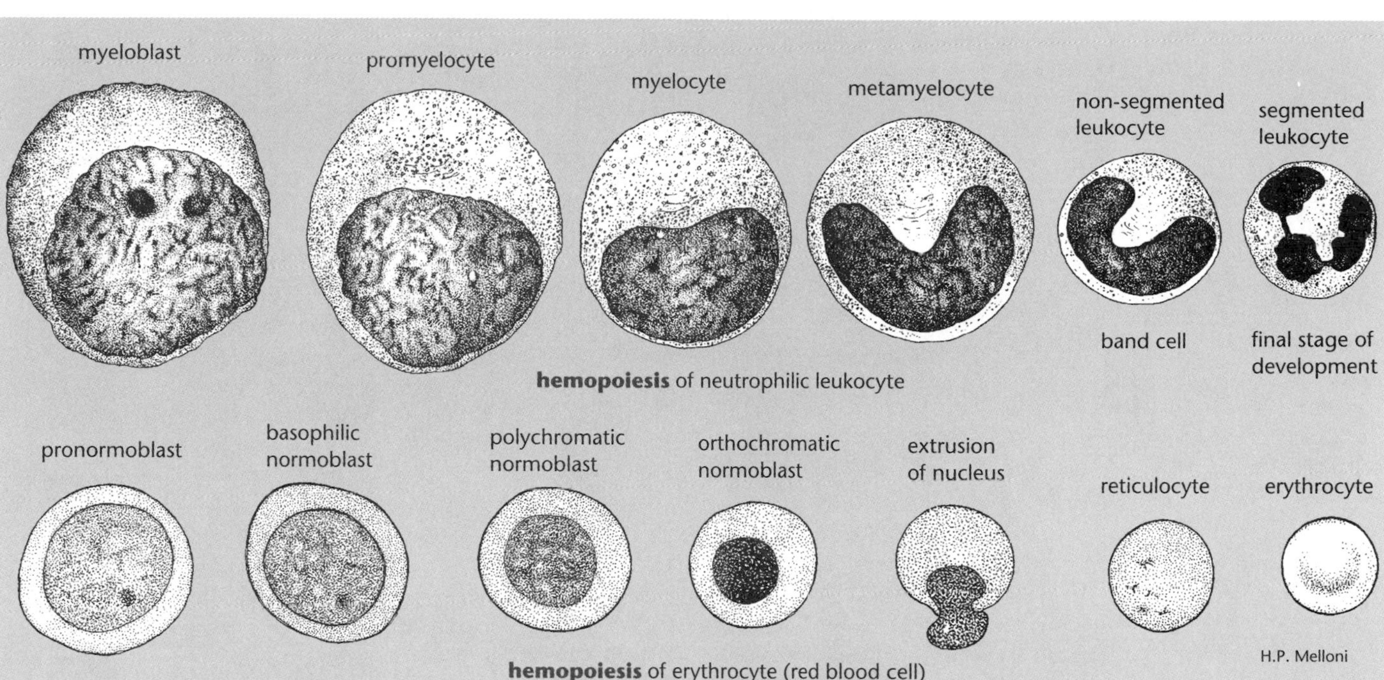

Accumulation of blood in the pericardial sac.

hemoperitoneum (he-mo-per-ĭ-to-ne´um) Escape of blood into the peritoneal cavity.

hemopexin (he-mo-pek´sin) A serum protein in human plasma, containing 20% carbohydrates; important in binding heme and porphyrins.

hemophagocyte (he-mo-fag´o-sīt) A phagocytic cell that engulfs and destroys red blood cells.

hemophagocytosis (he-mo-fag-o-si-to´sis) The process of engulfment of red blood cells by phagocytic cells.

hemophil, hemophile (he´mo-fil, he´mo-fīl) Denoting microorganisms that thrive in media containing blood.

hemophilia (he-mo-fil´e-ă) Inherited hemorrhagic disease caused by deficiency of factor VIII (antihemophilic factor). Occurs in two main forms, hemophilia A and hemophilia B.

h. A Hemophilia transmitted as an X-linked recessive inheritance; marked by prolonged clotting time, easy bruising, and bleeding into joints and muscles; caused by a reduced amount or activity of factor VIII, a component of the blood-clotting process. The defective gene is transmitted from an affected male to his grandsons through his daughters, who (except in rare occasions) are asymptomatic. Also called classic hemophilia. See also factor VIII, under factor.

h. B Disorder of the blood clotting process caused by hereditary deficiency of factor IX (plasma thromboplastin component); transmitted as an X-linked recessive inheritance. Also called Christmas disease.

classic h. See hemophilia A.

hemophiliac (he-mo-fil´e-ak) An individual afflicted with hemophilia. Popularly called bleeder.

hemophilic (he-mo-fil´ik) Relating to hemophilia.

Hemophilus (he-mof´ĭ-lus) See *Haemophilus*.

hemophobia (he-mo-fo´be-ă) An abnormal fear of the sight of blood.

hemophthalmia (he-mof-thal´me-ă) Bleeding into the eyeball.

hemopneumopericardium (he-mo-noo-mo-per-ĭ-kar´de-um) The presence of blood and air in the membrane enveloping the heart. Also called pneumohemopericardium.

hemopneumothorax (he-mo-noo-mo-thor´aks) Accumulation of air and blood in the pleural cavity.

hemopoiesis (he-mo-poi-e´sis) The formation of blood cells. Also called hematopoiesis; hematogenesis; hemogenesis.

hemopoietic (he-mo-poi-et´ik) Relating to the formation of blood cells.

hemoporphyrin (he-mo-por´fĭ-rin) See hematoporphyrin.

hemoprecipitin (he-mo-pre-sip´ĭ-tin) An antibody that combines with and precipitates soluble antigenic material from erythrocytes; a precipitin specific for blood.

hemoprotein (he-mo-pro´tēn) A conjugated compound consisting of a protein linked to heme.

hemopsonin (he-mop-so´nin) An antibody that combines with red blood cells and renders them susceptible in phagocytosis.

hemoptysis (he-mop´tĭ-sis) Spitting of blood from lesions in the larynx, trachea, or lower respiratory tract.

hemopyelectasia (he-mo-pi-ĕ-lek´tă-sis) Dilatation of the kidney pelvis with blood and urine.

hemorheology (he-mo-re-ol´ŏ-je) The science of the relation of pressures, flow, volumes, and resistances in blood vessels.

hemorrhage (hem´ŏ-rij) Bleeding, especially profuse.

accidental h. See abruptio placentae.

antepartum h. Excessive bleeding occurring at the onset of labor, as seen in premature separation of a placenta previa.

cerebral h. Bleeding from blood vessels within the brain, usually in the area of the internal capsule.

fetomaternal h. The leakage of red blood cells from the fetal to the maternal circulation.

internal h. Bleeding into an organ or a body cavity.

postpartum h. Excessive bleeding (in excess of 500 ml) following a vaginal delivery; designated *early* when it occurs within 24 hours after delivery, and *late* when it occurs between 24 hours and 6 weeks after delivery.

secondary h. Bleeding that occurs at an interval after an injury or operation.

subgaleal h. Hemorrhage under the scalp of a newborn infant caused by trauma to the head as it is forced against the uterine cervix during birth.

third-trimester h. Hemorrhage occurring during late pregnancy; may be due to nonobstetric conditions (including invasive carcinoma of the cervix), or to obstetric causes (e.g., premature separation of the placenta, placenta previa, or extrusion of the cervical plug).

vitreous h. Bleeding into the vitreous body (within the eyeball); may be caused by rupture of adjacent vessels by trauma (e.g., contusion, concussion, penetrating injuries) or acute vitreous collapse; or by systemic disease (e.g., diabetes, hypertension, leukemia).

hemorrhagic (hem-ŏ-raj´ik) Relating to or characterized by bleeding or hemorrhage.

hemorrhagic disease of newborn (hem-ŏ-raj´ik dĭ-zēz´ ŭv noo´born) Deficiency of vitamin K-dependent clotting factors (II, VII, IX, X), causing bleeding in an infant in the first days of life; sites of bleeding usually include the gastrointestinal tract, umbilical stump, circumcision site, and nose.

hemorrhagic pulmonary-renal syndrome (hem-ŏ-raj´ik pool´mo-nar-e-re´nal sin´drōm) See Goodpasture's syndrome.

hemorrhagin (hem-ŏ-ra´jin) Any of a group of toxins that destroy the endothelial cells in capillaries, causing numerous hemorrhages in the tissues; found in certain poisonous substances (e.g., rattlesnake venom, seeds of the castor oil plant).

hemorrheology (he-mo-re-ol´o-je) The study of the effects of blood flow in blood vessels and the formed elements of blood.

hemorrhoidal (hem-ŏ-roi´dal) **1.** Relating to hemorrhoids. **2.** Denoting blood vessels supplying the area of the rectum and anus.

hemorrhoidectomy (hem-ŏ-roid-ek´tŏ-me) Surgical removal of hemorrhoids.

hemorrhoids (hem´ŏ-roids) A dilated (varicose) condition of veins at or within the anus; may become strangulated, ulcerated, or fissured; generally associated with recurrent constipation, pregnancy (due to pressure against the veins) or, occasionally, portal hypertension. Also called piles.

external h. Varicosities of the inferior hemorrhoidal veins situated external to the rectoanal line and covered by skin.

internal h. Varicose enlargement of the superior hemorrhoidal veins situated above the rectoanal line and covered with mucous membrane, causing, at the early stages, intermittent bleeding during or following defecation; the condition may develop in various degrees: the hemorrhoids do not protrude through the anal canal (1st degree); protrusion occurs through the anal canal during defecation, receding spontaneously afterward (2nd degree); protrusion becomes more pronounced, occurring on any extra exertion and receding only by manual reduction (3rd degree); the hemorrhoids are permanently prolapsed (4th degree).

hemosalpinx (he-mo-sal´pinks) See hematosalpinx.

hemosiderin (he-mo-sid´er-in) A granular iron-containing yellow pigment formed during decomposition of hemoglobin; deposits are formed in a variety of tissues when there has been red blood cell breakdown.

hemosiderosis (he-mo-sid-er-o´sis) Deposition of hemosiderin (a yellow substance containing iron) in the tissues.

idiopathic pulmonary h. Recurrent hemorrhage of the lungs; cause unknown.

hemospermia (he-mo-sper´me-ă) See hemato-

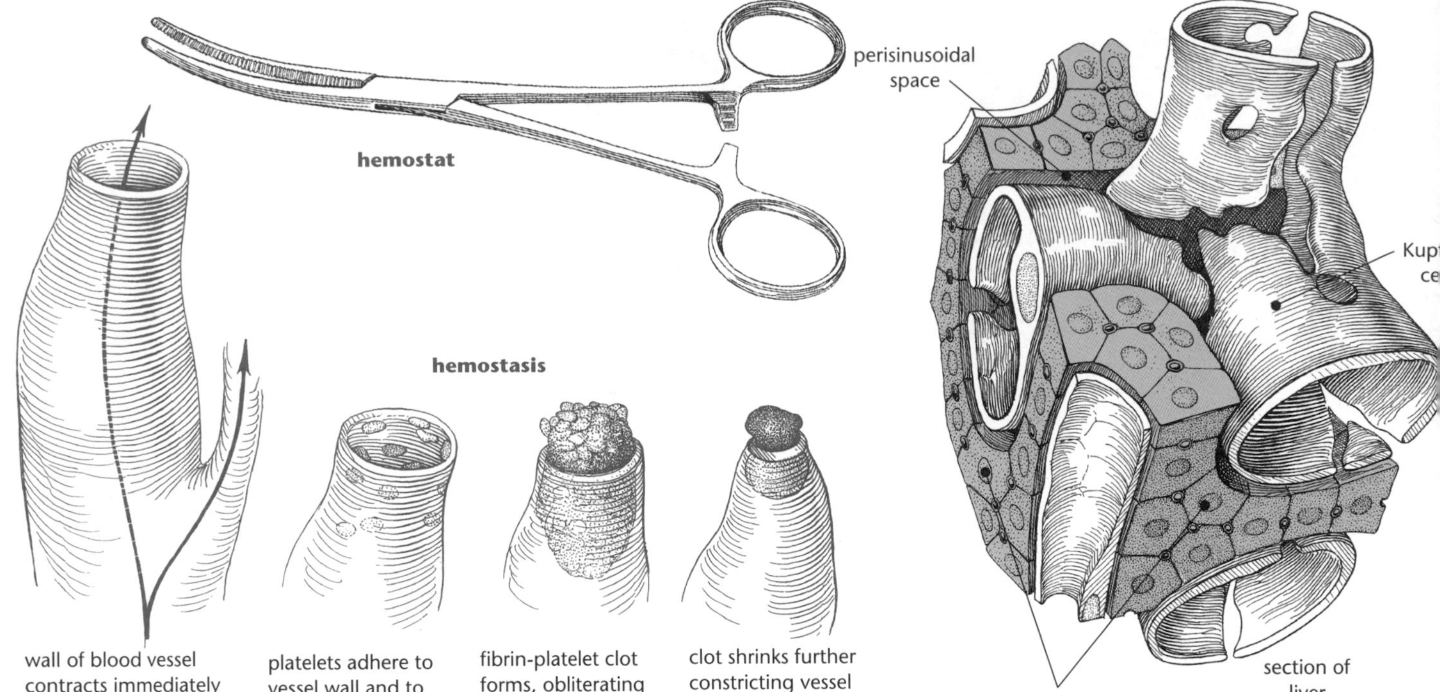
hemostat
hemostasis
wall of blood vessel contracts immediately after vessel is cut
platelets adhere to vessel wall and to one another
fibrin-platelet clot forms, obliterating lumen of vessel
clot shrinks further constricting vessel wall
perisinusoidal space
section of liver
hepatocytes

spermia.

hemostasis (he-mo-sta´sis) **1.** The arrest of bleeding. Also called hemostasia. **2.** The arrest of the flow of blood through a part or vessel.

hemostat (he´mo-stat) An instrument or an agent that stops bleeding.

hemostatic (he-mo-stat´ik) **1.** Arresting hemorrhage. **2.** Any agent that checks bleeding.

hemostyptic (he-mo-stip´tik) A chemical hemostatic; any chemical agent that stops bleeding by astringent properties.

hemothorax (he-mo-thor´aks) Accumulation of blood in the pleural cavity.

hemotoxic (he-mo-tok´sik) Injurious to blood cells.

hemotoxin (he-mo-tok´sin) Any toxin that is capable of destroying red blood cells.

hemotympanum (he-mo-tim´pă-num) Collection of blood in the middle ear.

hemozoon (he-mo-zō´on) Hematozoon.

henry (hen´re) (H) Unit of electric inductance; may be self-inductance of one circuit (when an increase of current at the rate of 1 amp/sec causes an electromotive force of 1 volt) or mutual inductance of two circuits (when the current of one circuit changing at the rate of 1 amp/sec produces an electromotive force of 1 volt in the other circuit).

hepar (he´par) Latin for liver.

heparin (hep´ă-rin) A mucopolysaccharide acid composed of D-glucuronic acid and D-glucosamine; found especially in liver and lung tissue; it has the ability to keep blood from clotting; used chiefly in the prevention and treatment of thrombosis.

heparinize (hep´ă-rĭ-nīz) To administer or apply heparin in order to delay the clotting time of blood.

hepatalgia (hep-ă-tal´jă) Pain in the liver. Also called hepatodynia.

hepatectomy (hep-ă-tek´tŏ-me) Surgical removal of a portion of the liver.

hepatic (hĕ-pat´ik) Relating to the liver.

hepatitis (hep-ă-tī´tis) Inflammation of the liver.

h. A Hepatitis caused by hepatitis A virus (HAV), transmitted through fecal contamination of food and water (fecal-oral route), with a 15- to 45-day incubation period; may occur sporadically or in epidemics; does not produce a chronic disease or a carrier state; passive immunization can be induced by administration of immune globulin. Formerly called infectious hepatitis.

anicteric h. Hepatitis in which hyperbilirubinemia is mild, serum transaminase levels are elevated, and liver biopsy resembles icteric forms.

h. B Hepatitis caused by hepatitis B virus (HBV), present in body fluids (e.g., saliva, semen, and vaginal fluid), spread by transfusion of infected blood, the use of contaminated needles, needle-prick accidents, the sexual route, or from mother to child (vertical transmission); incubation period is 4 to 26 weeks (typically 6–8 weeks); may produce an asymptomatic carrier state and play a significant role in development of cancer of the liver (hepatocellular carcinoma). Formerly called serum hepatitis.

h. C Hepatitis caused by hepatitis C virus (HCV), transmitted via transfusion of infected blood or blood products, the use of contaminated needles, needle-prick accidents, the sexual route, and from mother to newborn (predominantly with HIV coinfection); manner of transmission is unknown in many instances; often causes chronic hepatitis leading to cirrhosis; incubation period is 8 to 12 weeks. Formerly called transfusion-associated non-A, non-B hepatitis.

cholestatic h. Hepatitis in which the signs of bile duct obstruction are more prominent than those of liver cell necrosis; may be seen occasionally in viral hepatitis or may be drug induced. Must be differentiated from extrahepatic bile obstruction.

chronic h. Condition in which there is biochemical or serologic evidence of continuing inflammatory liver disease for more than six months, producing symptoms and without steady improvement.

chronic active h. Progressive destruction of the liver architecture characterized by piecemeal necrosis and formation of intralobular septa leading eventually to cirrhosis and liver failure; usually associated with hepatitis B and C viruses (HBV and HCV); nonviral causes include metabolic disorders and drug-induced hepatitis. Also called chronic aggressive hepatitis.

chronic aggressive h. See chronic active hepatitis.

chronic persistent h. (CPH) A usually benign, self-limited condition, considered a delayed recovery from an acute infection with hepatitis viruses A, B, or C or combined B and D viruses, and lasting up to several years; symptoms are usually minor and liver function tests show only mild abnormalities. The patients may be carriers of the viruses, often asymptomatic.

h. D Hepatitis caused by hepatitis D virus (HDV), developed only in the presence of hepatitis B virus (HBV); may occur when transfused blood contains both viruses (coinfection), or as an additional infection of a chronic HBV carrier (superinfection); incubation period is 30 to 120 days 9 (typically 60 days). Also called delta hepatitis; delta agent hepatitis.

delta h., delta agent h. See hepatitis D.

drug-induced h., toxic h. Acute hepatitis produced by ingesting a drug (e.g., phenytoin or salicylates), or from occupational exposure to a chemical (e.g., polypropylene chloride).

h. E Self-limited hepatitis (with a high mortality rate in pregnant women) caused by hepatitis E virus (HEV), transmitted through fecally contaminated food and water (fecal-oral route); may occur in waterborne epidemics; incubation period is 14 to 60 days (typically 40 days); it does not produce a chronic state. Formerly called non-A, non-B hepatitis.

fulminant h. A rapidly progressive form of hepatitis with necrosis of large areas of the liver; usually fatal within two weeks.

infectious h. (IF) See hepatitis A.

neonatal h. General term for a variety of disorders of newborn infants, involving injury to liver cells and tissues and causing hyperbilirubinemia and jaundice; cause is unknown; may be associated with hepatitis B.

non-A, non-B, non-C (NANBNC) **h.** See hepatitis C and E.

serum h. (SH) See hepatitis B.

viral h. Hepatitis caused by a virus. Unless otherwise specified, the term refers to infection of the liver by a group of viruses (A, B, C, D, and E viruses) that have an affinity for the liver and produce similar patterns of clinical and morphologic acute hepatitis, but vary in their potential to induce chronic or fulminant hepatitis or the carrier state of the disease.

hepatization (hep-ă-tī-za´shun) The conversion of loose tissue into a mass resembling liver, as the consolidation of lung tissue in pneumonia.

hepatocyte (hĕ-pat´ŏ-sīt) A parenchymal liver cell.

hepatoduodenostomy (hĕ-pat-o-doo-od-ĕ-nos´tŏ-me) Surgical creation of a passage between the hepatic duct and the duodenum.

hepatodynia (hĕ-pat-o-din´e-ă) See hepatalgia.

hepatogenic (hĕ-pat-o-jen´ik) Formed by or originating in the liver. Also called hepatogenous.

hepatogram (hĕ-pat´o-gram) A radioisotopic scan of the liver.

hepatography (hep-ă-tog´ră-fe) **1.** The making of a roentgenogram of the liver. **2.** A treatise on the liver.

hepatolienography (hĕ-pat-o-li-ĕ-nog´ră-fe) **1.** See hepatosplenography. **2.** A treatise on the liver and spleen.

hepatolith (hĕ-pat´o-lith) A calculus in the liver; a biliary calculus.

hepatolithiasis (hĕ-pat-o-lĭ-thī´ă-sis) Stones in the liver.

hepatologist (hep-ă-tol´ŏ-jist) A specialist on diseases of the liver.

hepatology (hep-ă-tol´ŏ-je) Study of the liver and its diseases.

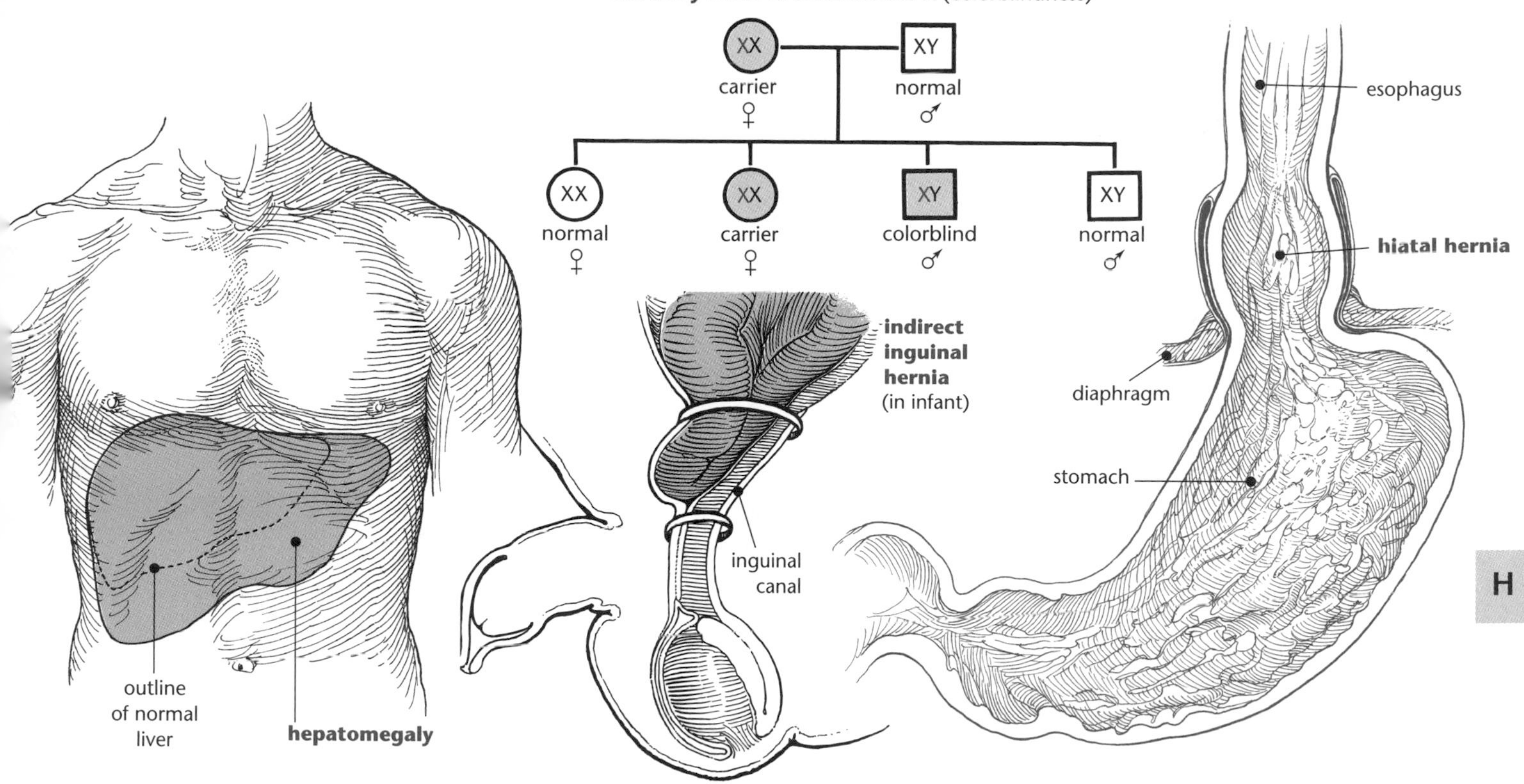

hepatolysin (hep-ă-tol′ĭ-sin) An agent destructive to the parenchymal cells of the liver.

hepatoma (hep-ă-to′mă) Malignant tumor of the liver originating in the parenchymal cells; commonly arises in the presence of chronic hepatitis. Also called hepatocellular carcinoma.

hepatomegaly (hĕ-pat-o-meg′ă-le) Enlargement of the liver.

hepatonecrosis (hĕ-pat-o-nĕ-kro′sis) Death of liver tissue.

hepatopathy (hep-ă-top′ă-the) Any disease of the liver.

hepatorenal (hĕ-pat-o-re′nal) Relating to the liver and kidney.

hepatorenal syndrome (hĕ-pat-o-re′nal sin′drōm) Renal failure occurring in the presence of severe disease of the liver or biliary tract, characterized initially by abnormally low urinary output (oliguria), marked sodium retention, and a rise in blood urea nitrogen usually out of proportion to the increase in serum creatinine.

hepatorrhaphy (hep-ă-tor′ă-fe) The surgical suturing of the liver.

hepatoscan (hĕ-pat′o-skan) The scanning of the liver after intravenous injection of a radioactive substance that is taken up by the hepatic reticuloendothelial system.

hepatosplenography (he-pat-o-splĕ-nog′ră-fe) Roentgenography of the liver and spleen after introduction of a radiopaque medium.

hepatosplenomegaly (hĕ-pat-o-sple-no-meg′ă-le) Enlargement of the liver and the spleen.

hepatotoxic (hĕ-pat-o-tok′sik) Relating to substances that damage the liver.

hepatotoxin (hĕ-pat-o-tok′sin) Any agent that destroys the liver cells.

heptapeptide (hep-tă-pep′tīd) Peptide containing seven amino acids.

herbivorous (her-biv′ŏ-rus) Feeding on plants.

hereditary (he-red′ĭ-tar-e) Genetically transmitted from parent to child. COMPARE: heritable.

heredity (he-red′ĭ-te) **1.** The genetic transmission of a specific trait from parent to offspring. **2.** The totality of physical and mental traits and potentialities so transmitted to the offspring.

autosomal h. The transmission of a trait by a gene situated on an autosome.

sex-linked h. The transmission of a trait by a gene situated on a sex chromosome.

heredoataxia (her-ĕ-do-ă-tak′se-ă) See Friedreich's ataxia, under ataxia.

heredodegeneration (her-ĕ-do-de-jen-er-a′shŭn) The genetic retrogressive change in cells and tissues.

heredopathia atactica polyneuritiformis (her-ĕ-do-path′e-ă ă-tak′tĭ-ka pol-e-nōō-ri′tĭ-for-mis) See Refsum's disease.

heritable (her′ĭ-tă-bl) Capable of being inherited, such as a trait, provided that it is present in the germ cell of a parent. COMPARE: hereditary.

hermaphrodism (her-maf′ro-diz-m) See hermaphroditism.

hermaphrodite (her-maf′ro-dīt) An individual who has genital tissues of both sexes.

hermaphroditism (her-maf′ro-dī-tiz-m) The presence in the same individual of both ovarian and testicular tissues. Also called hermaphrodism; intersexuality.

hermetic (her-met′ik) Completely sealed against the escape or entry of air.

hernia (her′ne-ă) Protrusion of part of an organ through an abnormal opening in the wall that normally contains it.

abdominal h. Hernia protruding through or into any part of the abdominal wall.

concealed h. Hernia not found on inspection or palpation.

congenital diaphragmatic h. Protrusion of abdominal organs into the chest cavity through a developmental defect in the diaphragm, usually a large posterolateral opening (foramen of Bochdalek) or through an enlarged foramen of Morgagni, behind the breastbone. Also called diaphragmatic hernia.

Cooper's h. Femoral hernia with two sacs, one in the femoral canal and the other passing through a defect in the superficial fascia and appearing immediately beneath the skin.

cul-de-sac h. See enterocele.

diaphragmatic h. See congenital diaphragmatic hernia.

dorsal h. See lumbar hernia.

Douglas' pouch h. See enterocele.

epigastric h. Hernia through the linea alba above the navel.

fascial h. See fatty hernia.

fatty h. Hernia in which a mass of adipose tissue protrudes through a gap or tear in a fibrous layer of tissue (fascia or aponeurosis). Also called pannicular hernia; fascial hernia.

femoral h. Protrusion of a sac-enclosed loop of intestine through the femoral ring and into the femoral canal. May be one of two types: *incomplete femoral h.*, if it remains in the canal as far as the saphenous opening; or *complete femoral h.*, if it passes through the opening and into the loose tissues of the groin; seen most frequently in women, especially those who have borne several children.

gastroesophageal h. See hiatal hernia.

hiatal h., hiatus h. (HH) Displacement of the upper part of the stomach into the thorax through the esophageal opening (hiatus) of the diaphragm. See also paraesophageal hernia; sliding hiatal hernia.

incarcerated h. See irreducible hernia.

incisional h. Hernia through a surgical incision, occurring almost exclusively in the abdominal wall. Also called ventral hernia.

inguinal h. Hernia in the groin area. *Direct inguinal h.*, when the herniation passes through the inguinal triangle and enters the inguinal canal; sometimes it emerges from the superficial inguinal ring and lies over the body of the pubic bone. *Indirect inguinal h.*, when the hernial sac enters the inguinal canal through the deep inguinal ring; it may descend farther and emerge from the canal through the superficial inguinal ring. *Complete inguinal h.*, when the sac descends into the scrotum.

internal h. Any hernia occurring in a large abdominal fossa, fovea, or foramen (i.e., paraduodenal, mesenteric, or omental hernia, or one into the epiploic foramen).

irreducible h. Hernia which, as a result of adhesions or for any other reason, cannot be reduced without surgical intervention. Also called incarcerated hernia.

lumbar h. A hernia in the lower back, between the last rib and iliac crest, frequenlty described by patients a "a lump in the flank". Also called dorsal hernia.

pannicular h. See fatty hernia.

paraesophageal h. A type of diaphragmatic hernia in which the stomach, or a portion of it, passes into the thorax immediately adjacent to, and to the left of, the esophagogastric junction.

posterior vaginal h. See enterocele.

rectovaginal h. See enterocele.

reducible h. Hernia that can be reduced (i.e., its contents can be returned to their original position by manipulation).

sciatic h. A herniation of intestine through the great sacrosciatic foramen.

scrotal h. See inguinal hernia.

sliding hiatal h., sliding esophageal hiatal h. Hernia in which the junction of the stomach and esophagus moves from time to time or permanently into the thorax through the diaphragm.

strangulated h. An irreducible hernia with cut off blood supply so that the herniated intestine has

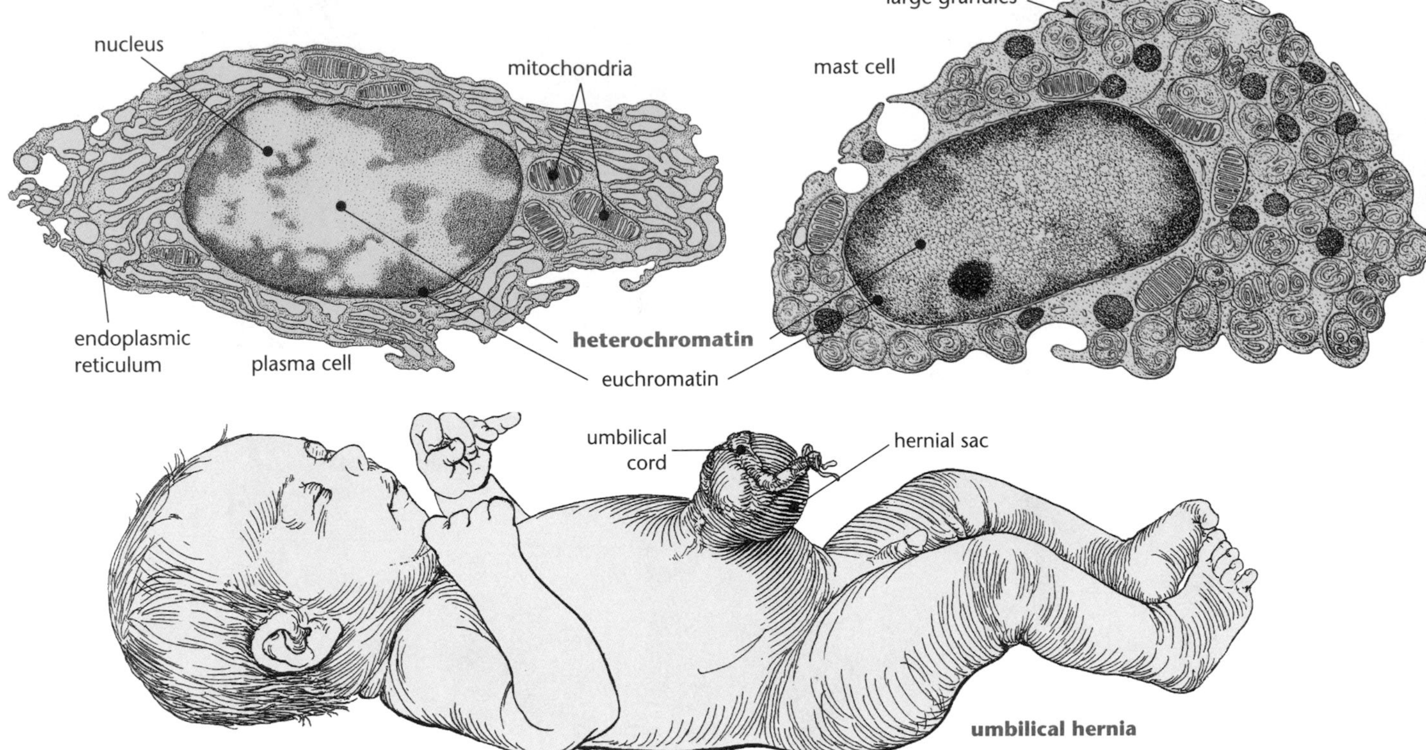

become, or is likely to become, gangrenous.

umbilical h. Hernia in which part of the intestine protrudes through the umbilical ring; it usually results from a fascial and muscular defect with failure of the umbilical ring to close.

ventral h. See incisional hernia.

herniated (her′ne-āt-ed) Pertaining to any structure protruding through a defect or abnormal opening.

herniation (her-ne-a′shun) The process of forming an abnormal protrusion.

foraminal h. Protrusion of the cerebellar tonsils through the foramen magnum. Also called tonsillar herniation.

tonsillar h. See foraminal herniation.

herniorrhaphy (her-ne-or′ă-fe) Surgical repair of a hernia.

heroin (her′o-in) A highly addictive narcotic prepared from morphine by acetylation; a white, odorless, bitterish crystalline compound, $C_2H_{23}O_5N$. Also called diacetylmorphine.

herpangina (her-pan-ji′nă) An infection of the throat usually caused by a coxsackie virus (coxsackie A); marked by intense swelling of the area, sudden onset of fever, loss of appetite, difficulty in swallowing (dysphagia), and sometimes abdominal pain, nausea, and vomiting; vesiculopapular lesions about 1 to 2 mm in diameter are present around the tonsils.

herpes (her′pēz) Inflammatory eruption of a cluster of deep-seated vesicles caused by a herpesvirus.

corneal h. See herpetic keratitis, under keratitis.

h. febrilis Herpes simplex caused by human herpesvirus 1 (HHV-1), transmitted primarily by oral secretions; characterized by recurrent blisters and ulcers usually on the lips (herpes labialis), nostrils, and/or lining membrane of the oral cavity. Also called cold sore; fever blister.

genital h., h. genitalis Sexually transmitted herpes simplex of the genital organs, usually caused by human herpesvirus 2 (HHV-2); blisters appear from 2 to 12 days after contact with a person who has active lesions. Infection may be transmitted to the newborn from the mother. See also neonatal herpes.

h. gestationis An eruption of reddish plaques and vesicles, usually in the arm and legs, occurring during the second or third trimester of pregnancy; despite its name, the condition is not caused by a herpesvirus; cause is unknown.

h. gladiatorum Infection with human herpesvirus 1 (HHV-1), causing lesions of the eyes, scalp, and skin of the face, neck, trunk, or limbs, accompanied by fever, chills, sore throat, and inflammation of lymph nodes; seen primarily in wrestlers and rugby players.

h. labialis See herpes febrilis.

neonatal h. Infection of the newborn with human herpesvirus 2 (HHV-2); a potentially fatal infection acquired during one of three periods: intrauterine through the placenta; during birth as an ascending infection through ruptured membranes (80%), or by delivery through infected cervix and vagina; or after birth.

h. simplex An acute eruption of painful blisters caused by human herpesvirus 1 and 2 (HHV-1, HHV-2); once established, the infection remains in the body and recurs at intervals with complete healing of the eruption between episodes; reappearance may be precipitated by emotional stress, febrile disease, local trauma, or menstruation.

h. simplex 2 Genital herpes.

h. zoster A painful, itchy eruption of vesicles, usually on one side of the body along the course of one or more cutaneous nerves; caused by human herpesvirus 3 (HHV-3), which infects ganglia of the sensory (posterior) roots of spinal nerves, or of the fifth cranial nerve. The condition is considered a reactivation of the virus, which remains latent in the ganglia following the primary infection (chickenpox); may be precipitated by physical or emotional stress or by malignancies (e.g., lymphoma, Hodgkin's disease). Also called shingles.

venereal h. Genital herpes.

Herpesviridae (her-pēz-vi′rĭ-de) A family of viruses (120 to 200 nanometers in diameter) that share the following features: they contain double-stranded DNA, replicate in the cell nucleus, accumulate between inner and outer layers of nuclear membrane and in the cisterna of endoplasmic reticulum, are transported to the cell surface through modified endoplasmic reticulum, and may remain latent in their host for several years or the lifetime of the host. See also herpes and herpesvirus.

herpesvirus (her-pēz-vi′rus) Any virus belonging to the family Herpesviridae. See also herpes and Herpesviridae.

human h. 1 (HHV-1) Herpes simplex 1; the virus causing herpes simplex 1, responsible for most cases of nongenital herpes. The organism enters the cell through the fibroblast growth factor receptor on the cell membrane.

human h. 2 (HHV-2) Herpes simplex 2; the herpesvirus infecting primarily the genital organs of both male and female (including the cervix and vagina), and the anal and perianal areas of homosexual men. The organism has been recovered from the urethra and prostate of asymptomatic men.

human h. 3 (HHV-3) Herpes varicella-zoster virus; the organism causing two clinical forms of infection: acute HHV-3 (varicella, commonly called chickenpox) and chronic HHV-3 (herpes zoster, commonly called shingles). Also called varicella-zoster virus.

human h. 4 (HHV-4) A herpesvirus with specificity for B cells (B lymphocytes); the cause of infectious mononucleosis, transmitted by saliva; associated with malignancies such as Burkitt's lymphoma, anaplastic nasopharyngeal cancer, and B-cell lymphomas in immunosuppressed patients (e.g., organ transplants and AIDS). Also called Epstein-Barr virus (EBV).

human h. 5 (HHV-5) See cytomegalovirus.

human h. 6 (HHV-6) A herpesvirus with affinity for B cells (B lymphocytes), occurring frequently as a coinfection with human immunodeficiency virus (HIV). An initial (primary) infection with HHV-6 is a frequent cause of exanthem subitum, an acute febrile illness in infants and young children usually associated with a variety of clinical manifestations; it is also associated with syndromes resembling infectious mononucleosis.

human h. 7 (HHV-7) A herpesvirus isolated from activated, CD4-positive T lymphocytes obtained from the blood of healthy people.

herpetiform (her-pet′ĭ-form) Resembling herpes.

hertz (hertz) (Hz) Unit of frequency of a periodic process equivalent to one cycle per second.

heterecious (het-er-e′shus) Having more than one host, i.e., spending different stages of its life cycle on two or more unrelated hosts (e.g., tapeworms).

heterochromatin (het-er-o-kro′mă-tin) Chromatin that stains darkly throughout the cell cycle, even during interphase. COMPARE: euchromatin.

heterochromia (het-er-o-kro′me-ă) Difference in color of a part or parts that are normally alike in color, as of the two irides.

heteroerotic (het-er-o-er-ot′ik) Relating to sexual feelings that are directed toward another person, as opposed to autoerotic.

heterogametic (het-er-o-gă-met′ik) Having gametes (sex cells) of different types with respect to the sex chromosomes, as in human males.

heterogamy (het-er-og′ă-me) **1.** The union of two gametes of different size, structure, and function. **2.** Alternation of two kinds of generations, one that reproduces bisexually and another in which the

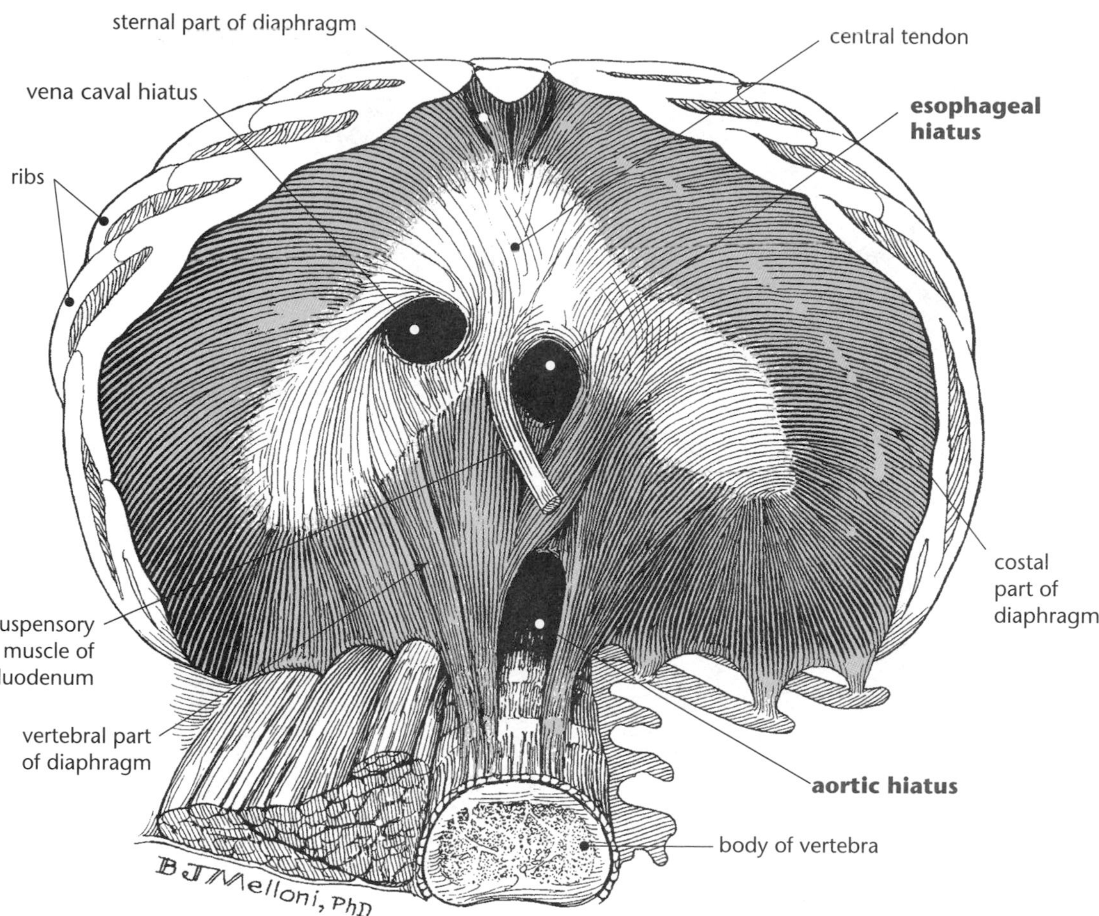

female reproduces without fecundation by the male (parthenogenetic), as in some aphids.

heterogeneity (het-ĕr-o-jĕ-ne´ĭ-te) The quality of certain genetic disorders that consist of two or more fundamentally distinct entities; formerly thought to represent single entities.

heterogeneous, heterogenous (het-er-o-je´ne-us, het-er-oj´ĕ-nus) Composed of dissimilar elements or characteristics; not homogeneous.

heterogenetic, heterogenic (het-er-o-jĕ-net´ik, het-er-o-jen´ik) Derived from a different species.

heterolalia (het-er-o-la´le-ă) The involuntary uttering of meaningless words instead of those intended. Also called heterophasia.

heterologous (het-er-ol´ŏ-gus) **1.** Composed of tissues not normal to the anatomic area. **2.** See xenogeneic.

heterolysis (het-er-ol´ĭ-sis) Dissolution or digestion of cells of one species by a lytic agent from a different species.

heteromeric (het-er-o-mer´ik) **1.** Possessing different chemical composition. **2.** Denoting spinal nerve cells that have processes crossing the midline to the opposite side of the spinal cord.

heteromorphism (het-er-o-mor´fiz-m) In cytogenetics, a difference in shape or size between homologous chromosomes.

heteronymous (het-er-on´ĭ-mus) **1.** Relating to different sides of the two visual fields (e.g., the right side of one field and the left side of the other, both nasal fields or both temporal fields). **2.** Having different but correlated names.

heterophasia (het-er-o-fa´zhă) See heterolalia.

heterophonia (het-er-o-fon´ne-ă) **1.** The change of voice in the male at puberty. **2.** Any abnormality in the voice.

heterophoria (het-er-o-for´e-ă) The tendency of the optic axes to deviate toward or away from each other.

heterophthalmus (het-er-of-thal´mus) A difference in appearance of the two eyes, as in the coloration of the irides.

Heterophyes (het-er-of´e-ēz) A genus of small parasitic flukes.

heterophyiasis (het-er-o-fi-i´ă-sis) Infection with a heterophyid fluke.

heterophyid (het-er-o-fi´ĭd) A fluke of the genus *Heterophyes*.

heteroplasia (het-er-o-pla´zhă) **1.** The presence of tissue elements in an abnormal location (e.g., the growth of bone where normally there should be fibrous connective tissue). **2.** The malposition of a part that is otherwise normal (e.g., the presence of a ureter at the lower pole of a kidney).

heteroplasty (het´er-o-plas-te) **1.** Surgical grafting of tissue donated from another individual. **2.** The replacement of tissue with synthetic material.

heteroploidy (het´er-o-ploi-de) The state of an individual or cell with a chromosome number other than the normal diploid number.

heteropsia (het-er-op´se-ă) Unequal vision in the two eyes.

heterosexuality (het-er-o-sek-shoo-al´ĭ-te) The state of having one's sexual interests directed toward a member of the opposite sex, as opposed to homosexuality.

heterotaxia, heterotaxis (het-er-o-tak´se-ă, het-er-o-tak´sis) Abnormal arrangement of bodily organs or parts; anomalous structural arrangement.

heterotaxic (het-er-o-tak´sik) Occurring in an abnormal place.

heterotransplant (het-er-o-trans´plant) See xenograft.

heterotropia (het-er-o-tro´pe-ă) See strabismus.

heterotypic (het-er-o-tip´ik) Not typical.

heterozygosity (het-er-o-zi-gos´ĭ-te) The state of having one or more pairs of dissimilar alleles.

heterozygote (het-er-o-zi´gōt) A zygote produced by the union of two gametes of different genetic composition.

heterozygous (het-er-o-zi´gus) Having differing alleles at a given locus on a pair of homologous chromosomes.

hexacanth (hek´să-kanth) The motile, six-hooked, first-stage larva of a tapeworm. Also called oncosphere.

hexachlorophene (hek-să-klo´ro-fēn) A bactericidal agent, $(C_6HCl_3OH)_2CH_2$ used as a local antiseptic.

hexadecanoic acid (hek-să-dek-ă-no´ik as´id) See palmitic acid.

hexapeptide (hek-să-pep´tīd) A peptide containing six amino acids.

hexenmilch (hek´sen-milkh) German for witch's milk; a milky fluid sometimes secreted by the breasts of newborn infants.

hexokinase (hek-so-ki´nās) An enzyme (present in yeast, muscle, and other tissues) that promotes the phosphorylation of glucose and other hexoses to form hexose-6-phosphate.

hexosamine (hek-sōs´ă-min) A primary amine derivative of a hexose resulting when NH_2 replaces OH (e.g., glucosamine).

hexosan (hek´so-san) Any of several polysaccharides that yield a hexose on hydrolysis.

hexose (hek´sōs) A monosaccharide having six carbon atoms in the molecule (e.g., glucose and fructose).

hexose-1-phosphate uridyl transferase (hek´sōs-wŭn-fos´fāt u´ri-dīl trans´fer-ās) An enzyme system that promotes the interconversion of glucose 1-phosphate and galactose 1-phosphate with simultaneous interconversion of UDP glucose and UDP galactose. Also called uridyl transferase.

hexulose (hek´su-lōs) A ketohexose, such as fructose.

hexylresorcinol (hek-sĭl-rĕ-sor´sĭ-nol) A crystalline phenol used as an anthelminthic.

hiatus (hi-a´tus) An opening, aperture, or fissure.

aortic h. The opening in the diaphragm through which the aorta and thoracic duct pass.

esophageal h. The opening in the diaphragm through which the esophagus and the two vagus nerves pass.

sacral h. The normal gap at the lower end of the sacrum; provides access into the epidural space for introduction of anesthetic solutions.

hiccup (hik´up) A spasm of the diaphragm causing inhalation, followed by sudden closure of the glottis.

hidradenitis (hi-drad ĕ-ni´tis) Inflammation of a sweat gland.

h. suppurativa Chronic, relapsing, infectious disease of the apocrine sweat glands; marked by the

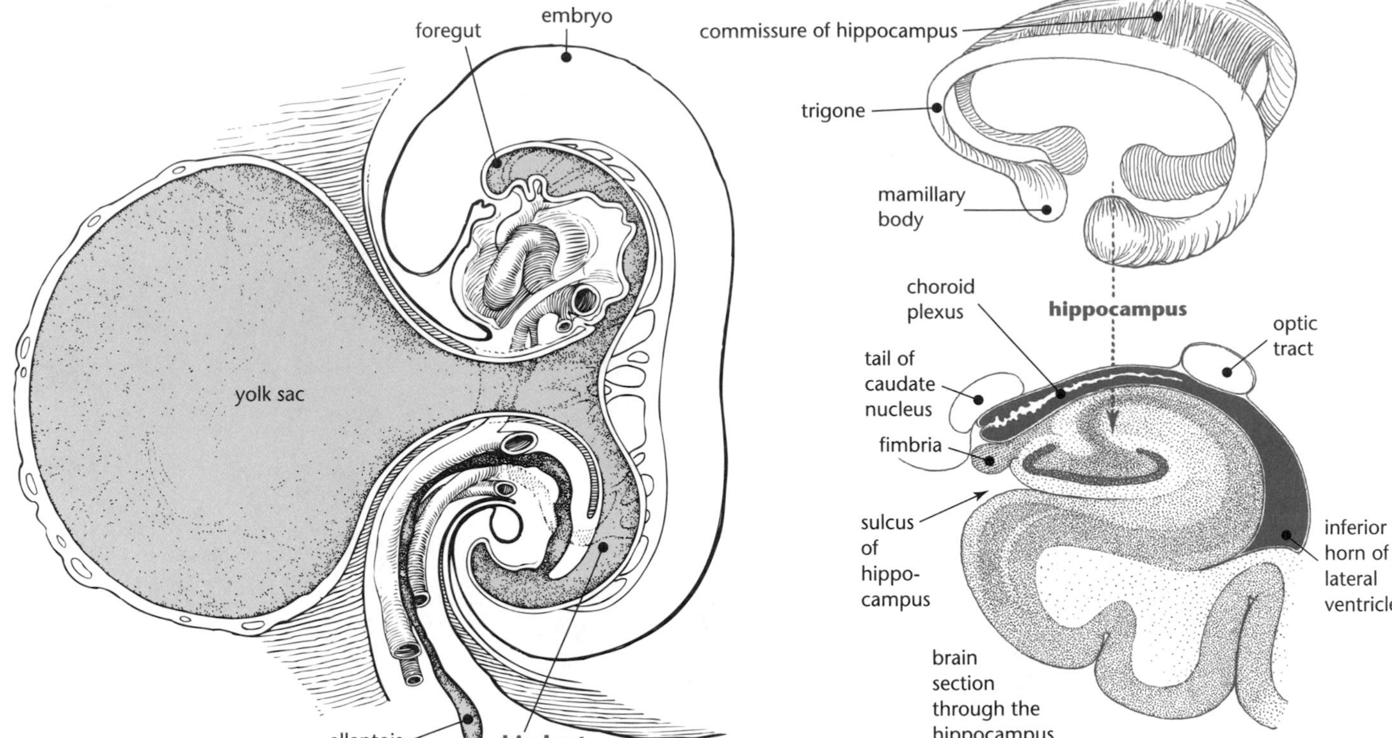

development of one or more cutaneous pea-sized nodules that undergo softening and suppuration; it occurs most commonly in the genital and perianal regions and in the armpits.

hidradenoma (hi-drad-ĕ-no´mă) A relatively infrequent benign tumor of sweat gland origin; may be solid or cystic. Also written hydradenoma.

hidroa (hi-dro´ă) See hydroa.

hidrocystoma (hi-dro-sis-to´mă) The cystic deformation of sweat glands.

hidropoiesis (hi-dro-poi-e´sis) The formation of sweat.

hidrosis (hi´dro-sis) **1.** Excessive perspiration. **2.** Any sweat gland disorder.

high (hī) Colloquial term for a state of drug induced intoxication, as from a narcotic, alcohol, or hallucinogenic agent.

hilar dance (hi´lar dans) Strong pulsations of the pulmonary arteries seen on fluoroscopic examination in patients with congenital left-to-right shunt.

hilum (hi´lum) The point at which nerves and vessels enter and leave an organ. Also called hilus.

hindbrain (hīnd´brān) See rhombencephalon.

hindfoot (hīnd´fo͞ot) **1.** The rear portion of the foot consisting of the talus and calcaneus. **2.** One of the back feet of a quadruped animal.

hindgut (hīnd´gut) The caudal part of the embryonic alimentary canal.

hip (hip) The lateral area of the body from the waist to the thigh.

hipbone (hip´bōn) A large, flattened, irregularly shaped bone that forms the anterior and lateral walls of the pelvic cavity; consisting of three parts (ilium, ischium, and pubis). Formerly called innominate bone.

Hippel-Lindau disease (hip´l-lin´dou dĭ-zēz´) See von Hippel-Lindau disease.

hippocampus (hip-o-kam´pus) One of two curved bands of a very special type of cortex about 5 cm long, on the floor of the inferior horn of the lateral ventricle on each side of the brain.

Hippocrates (hĭ-pok´ră-tēz) A Greek physician known as the "Father of Medicine"; his medical science principles were laid down about 400 years before the birth of Christ.

aphorisms of H. A collection of observations, rules, and brief statements of clinical wisdom found in Books I to III of the hippocratic writings.

hippocratic oath (hip-o-krat´ik ōth) A code of ethical conduct for the medical profession attributed to Hippocrates.

hippus (hip´us) Abnormal, spasmodic, rhythmic contraction and dilatation of the pupil.

Hirschsprung's disease (hirsh´sproongz dĭ´zēz´) Congenital disorder of early infancy characterized by extreme distention of the colon, resulting from absence of ganglion cells of the myenteric plexuses of the rectum and lower colon. Also called congenital megacolon.

hirsute (hir´soot) **1.** Hairy. **2.** Relating to hair.

hirsutism (hir-soot´iz-m) Excessive hair on cheek, chin, lip, or chest, especially in women.

hirudin (hĭ-roo´din) An anticoagulant substance secreted by the salivary glands of leeches which prevents coagulation of the blood while the leech is sucking.

histamine (his´tă-mēn) A white crystalline amine, $C_5H_9N_3$, occurring in all animal and plant tissue; formed from histidine by decarboxylation and by the action of putrefactive bacteria; its release within the body causes bronchiolar constriction, arteriolar dilatation, increased gastric secretion, and a fall in blood pressure.

histidine (his´tĭ-dēn) (His) α-Amino-β-(4-imidazole) propionic acid; a basic amino acid found in most proteins.

histiocyte (his´te-o-sīt) A large mononuclear phagocyte or macrophage; a tissue cell.

histiocytoma (his-te-o-si-to´mă) See dermatofibroma.

histiocytosis (his-te-o-si-to´sis) Abnormal proliferation of histiocytes.

acute disseminated Langerhans-cell h. An acute progressive and wasting disease of infants and young children characterized by invasion of the spleen, liver, and bone marrow by proliferating histiocytes, with involvement of the lymph nodes and enlargement of the spleen and liver; frequently present are a purpuric rash, anemia, and chronic inflammation of the middle ear. Formerly called Letterer-Siwe disease.

Langerhans-cell h. General term for a group of histiocytoses that are distinct clinicopathologic entities but with one predominant feature in common: the proliferating cell is the Langerhans cell. Formerly called histiocytosis X.

multifocal Langerhans-cell h. Disease of childhood, usually in children under 5 years old; marked by diffuse eruptions, frequent bouts of upper respiratory infections, otitis media, exophthalmos, diabetes insipidus, and destruction of bone (especially of the skull). Formerly called Hand-Schuller-Christian disease; Schuller disease.

sinus h. Disease of the lymph nodes in which the lymphatic sinusoids become distended due to hypertrophy of cells within the sinusoid lining and infiltration with histiocytes; frequently seen in cancers involving the lymph nodes.

unifocal Langerhans-cell h. A relatively benign disorder affecting children and young adults, especially males; marked by a single lesion involving one or several bones; may cause no symtoms or produce pain and tenderness and may heal spontaneously. Formerly called eosinophilic granuloma.

h. X See Langerhans-cell histiocytosis.

histochemistry (his-to-kem´is-tre) The chemistry of cell components and tissues.

histocompatibility (his-to-kom-pat-ĭ-bil´ĭ-te) The state of being histocompatible.

histocompatible (his-to-kom-pat´ĭ-bl) Relating to a donor and recipient who have a sufficient number of identical or similar histocompatibility antigens (i.e., human leukocyte antigens [HLAs]) so that the transplanted tissue is accepted.

histofluorescence (his-to-flo͞o-res´ens) Fluorescence of the tissues produced by exposure to ultraviolet rays after injection of a fluorescent substance.

histogenesis (his-to-jen´ĕ-sis) **1.** The origin and development of body tissues from undifferentiated cells of the embryonic germ layers. **2.** In myology, the development of muscle fibers from primitive cells.

histogram (his´to-gram) A columnar or bar chart used in descriptive statistics showing the relationship of two or more factors.

histologic (his-to-loj´ik) Pertaining to histology.

histologist (his-tol´ŏ-jist) A specialist in histology.

histology (his-tol´o-je) The branch of anatomy dealing with the microscopic structure of tissues. Also called microscopic anatomy; microanatomy.

histolysis (his-tol´ĭ-sis) The disintegration or breakdown of tissue.

histone (his´tōn) Any of several simple water soluble proteins containing a large proportion of basic amino acids (e.g., the globin of hemoglobin).

histophysiology (his-to-fiz-e-ol´ŏ-je) The physiology of body tissues.

Histoplasma (his-to-plaz´mă) A genus of fungi; some species cause disease in humans.

H. capsulatum Yeastlike fungus occurring in soil; when present in tissue it appears to be encapsulated; the cause of histoplasmosis.

histoplasmin (his-to-plaz´min) A concentrate of the growth products of the fungus *Histoplasma capsulatum*; used as a dermal reactivity indicator to

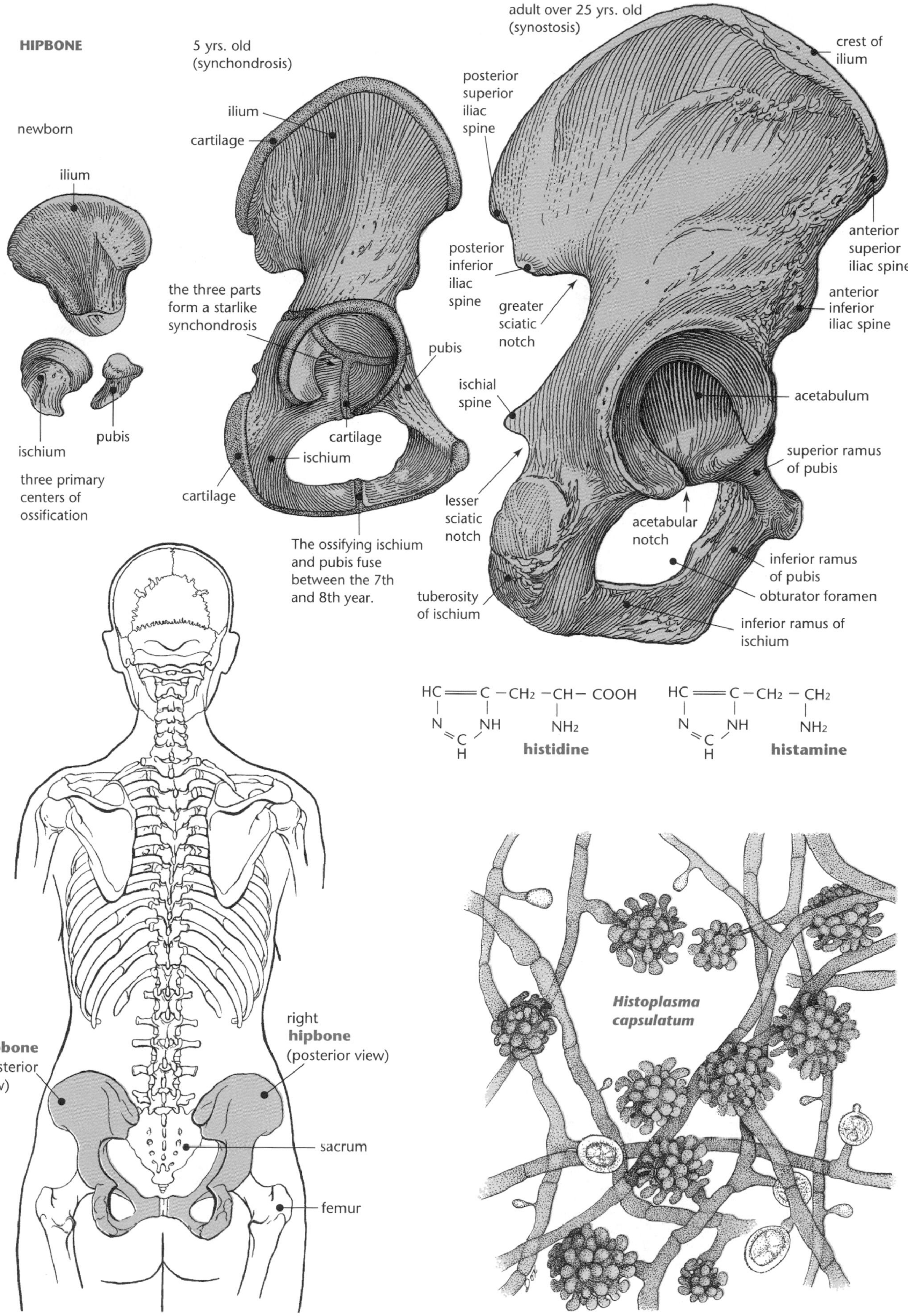
HIPBONE
newborn
ilium
ischium
pubis
three primary centers of ossification
5 yrs. old (synchondrosis)
ilium
cartilage
the three parts form a starlike synchondrosis
pubis
cartilage
ischium
cartilage
The ossifying ischium and pubis fuse between the 7th and 8th year.
adult over 25 yrs. old (synostosis)
crest of ilium
posterior superior iliac spine
posterior inferior iliac spine
greater sciatic notch
anterior superior iliac spine
anterior inferior iliac spine
ischial spine
acetabulum
superior ramus of pubis
lesser sciatic notch
acetabular notch
inferior ramus of pubis
obturator foramen
tuberosity of ischium
inferior ramus of ischium
left hipbone (posterior view)
right hipbone (posterior view)
sacrum
femur
HC ═ C − CH2 − CH − COOH
N NH NH2
C H
histidine
HC ═ C − CH2 − CH2
N NH NH2
C H
histamine
Histoplasma capsulatum

H

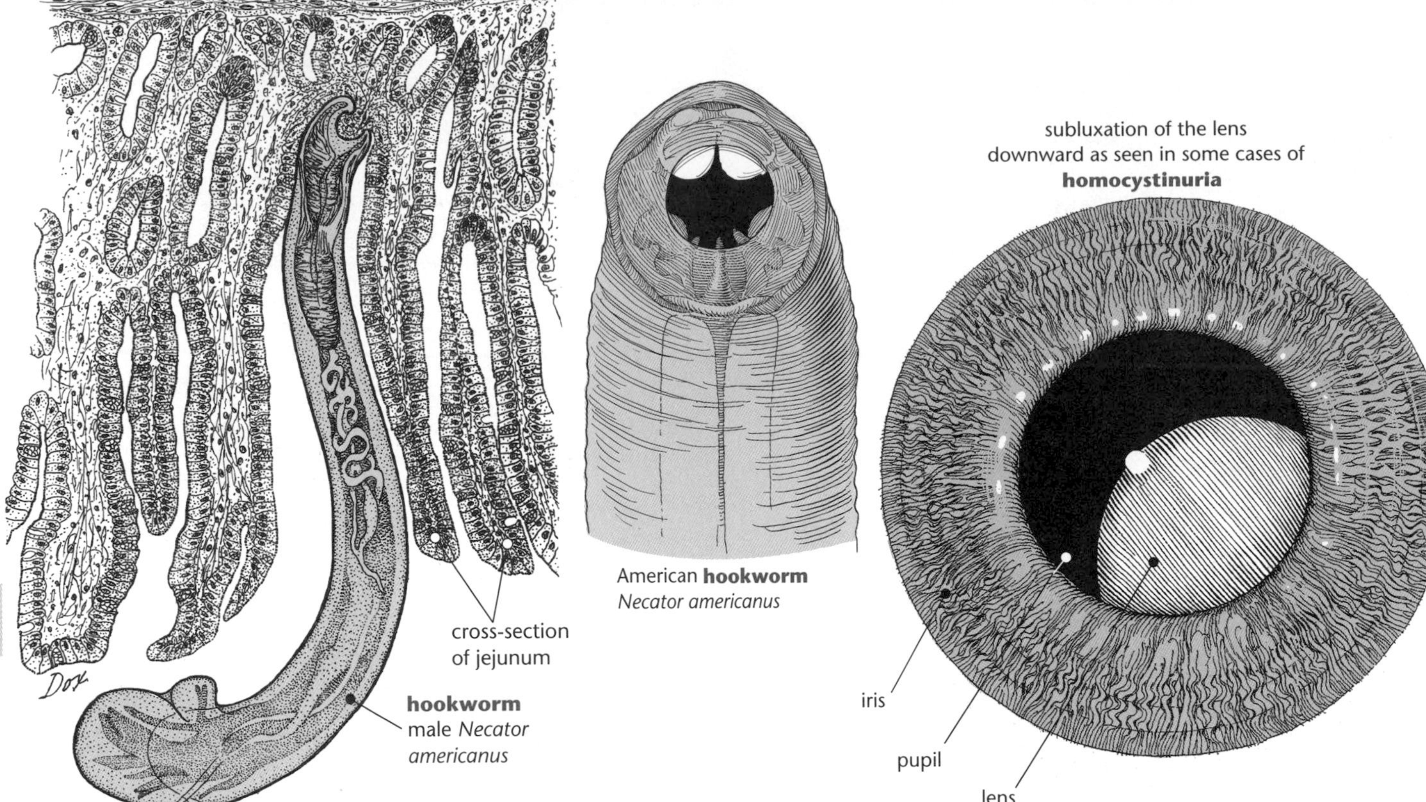

detect histoplasmosis.

histoplasmosis (his-to-plaz-mo´sis) A fungal disease caused by *Histoplasma capsulatum*; usually asymptomatic but may produce a benign, mild pulmonary illness; it is a frequent cause of pulmonary nodules; the infection may spread throughout the body, and this disseminated form, though uncommon, is quite serious.

histotope (his-to-tōp) The part of a major histocompatibility complex molecule (the antigen) that interacts with the antigen receptor of a T cell (the antibody).

HIV disease (HIV dĭ-zēz´) Disease resulting from infection with a strain of the human immunodeficiency virus (HIV 1 or HIV 2), divided on the basis of degree of immunosuppression into: *early stage* ($CD4^+$ T cell count greater than 500/microliter), *intermediate stage* ($CD4^+$ T cell count between 200 and 500/microliter), and *advanced stage* ($CD4^+$ T cell count less than 200/microliter). See also AIDS; HIV infection, under infection.

hives (hīvz) Eruption of transitory pruritic wheals, often due to hypersensitivity to foods or drugs or to emotional factors.

HMO See health maintenance organization.

hoarseness (hōrs´nes) A harsh, rough, grating quality of the voice.

Hodgkin's disease (hoj´kinz dĭ-zēz´) A disease of lymphatic tissue characterized by painless enlargement of the lymph nodes with or without systemic symptoms such as fever, sweats, weight loss, and lassitude; if untreated the disease may spread to involve the spleen and other organs; treatment and prognosis depend on the clinical staging.

Hoffmann's sign (hawf´manz sīn) Snapping the nail of the middle finger leads to flexion of thumb and fingers; a sign of a pyramidal tract lesion.

holandric (hol-an´drik) Occurring only in males; denoting a character determined by a gene on the Y chromosome.

holarthritis (hol-ar-thri´tis) Inflammation of all or most of the joints.

holoblastic (hōl-o-blas´tik) Denoting the complete division of the entire ovum into individual blastomeres.

holocrine (ho´lo-krin) Wholly secretory; relating to a gland whose secretion is composed of the disintegrated secreting cell in addition to its accumulated secretion (e.g., sebaceous glands).

holodiastolic (hōl-o-di-ă-stol´ik) Relating to or occupying all of diastole, from the second heart sound to the succeeding first heart sound.

holoenzyme (hōl-o-en´zīm) An enzyme possessing a chemical group that is non-amino acid in nature.

hologram (hōl´o-gram) A three-dimensional pattern exposed by holography on a photosensitive surface and then photographically developed.

holography (hōl-og´ră-fe) The use of lasers to record on a photographic plate the diffraction pattern of an object from which a three-dimensional image can be constructed.

acoustic h. A technique for detecting breast cancer by transmitting sound waves through breast tissue.

holosystolic (hōl-o-sis-tol´ik) See pansystolic.

Homans' sign (ho´manz sīn) Pain in the calf or the back of the knee when the foot is dorsiflexed, suggesting the presence of a deep venous thrombosis in the calf.

homeomorphous (ho-me-o-mor´fus) Of similar shape.

homeopathist (ho-me-op´ă-thist) One who practices homeopathy.

homeopathy (ho-me-op´ă-the) A system of therapeutics based on the use of small doses of a drug that in large doses is capable of producing symptoms in healthy individuals which are similar to those of the disease being treated.

homeoplasia (ho-me-o-pla´zhă) The formation of new tissue similar to that already existing in, and normal to, the part.

homeostasis (ho-me-o-sta´sis) A state of physiologic equilibrium in the living body (temperature, blood pressure, chemical content, etc.) under variations in the environment.

homeotherapy (ho-me-o-ther´ă-pe) Treatment or prevention of a disease with a substance similar to, but not identical with, the causative agent of the disease (e.g., vaccination). See also homeopathy.

homeothermal (ho-me-o-ther´mal) See homeothermic.

homeothermic (ho-me-o-ther´mik) Having a relatively constant body temperature despite variations in ambient temperature. Also called homeothermal; homothermal; homothermic.

homicidal (hom´ĭ-sīd´l, hō´mĭ-sīd-l) Having a tendency to kill another human being.

hominid (hom´ĭ-nid) **1.** A member of the family Hominidae. **2.** Relating to the family Hominidae.

Hominidae (ho-min´ĭ-de) A family of mammals (order Primates) that includes modern and prehistoric man.

Hominoidea (hom-ĭ-noi´de-ă) **1.** In some classifications, a major division of the order Primates, which segregates man from the great apes. **2.** A superfamily (suborder Anthropoidea) that includes the great apes and the fossil hominids.

Homo (ho´mo) A genus of the order Primates that includes the extinct and existing species of man.

H. sapiens The present-day human species.

homoblastic (ho-mo-blas´tik) Developing from only one type of tissue.

homocentric (ho-mo-sen´trik) Having the same center, as rays originating from one source.

homocysteine (ho-mo-sis´tēn) A sulfur-containing amino acid, $HSCH_2CH_2CHNH_2COOH$.

homocystine (ho-mo-sis´tēn) A sulfur-containing amino acid $(SCH_2CH_2CHNH_2COOH)_2$ formed by oxidation of homocysteine.

homocystinuria (ho-mo-sis-tin-u´re-ă) Genetically determined disorder of metabolism resulting from deficient activity of the enzyme cystathionine synthase; marked by elevated concentrations of methionine and homocystine in the blood, homocystine in the urine (not detectable in normal urine), mental retardation, dislocation of the ocular lenses, skeletal abnormalities (dolichostenomelia, genu valgum, osteoporosis), increased stickiness of platelets in the blood, thromboembolic episodes, and abnormality of the palate with crowding of the teeth.

homoeroticism (ho-mo-ĕ-rot´ĭ-siz-m) Homosexuality.

homogametic (ho-mo-gă-met´ik) Producing only one kind of germ cell; especially possessing an X chromosome in cell gametes. Also called monogametic.

homogenate (ho-moj´ĕ-nāt) A substance that has been homogenized; in biochemistry, tissue that has been reduced to a creamy consistency and that has disintegrated cell structure.

homogeneous (ho-mo-je´ne-us) Composed of similar elements throughout; of uniform quality.

homogenization (ho-moj-ĕ-nĭ-za´shun) The process of making diverse elements homogenous.

homogenize (ho-moj´ĕ-nīz) To blend diverse elements into a mixture that is uniform in structure or consistency throughout.

homogenous (ho-moj´ĕ-nus) **1.** In biology, correspondence of parts because of common descent. **2.** Homogeneous.

homogentisate oxygenase (ho-mo-jen-tis´āt ok´sĭ-jen-ās) An iron-containing enzyme that promotes the cleavage of the benzene ring in homogentistic acid; congenital absence of this enzyme causes alkaptonuria. Also called homogentisic acid oxidase.

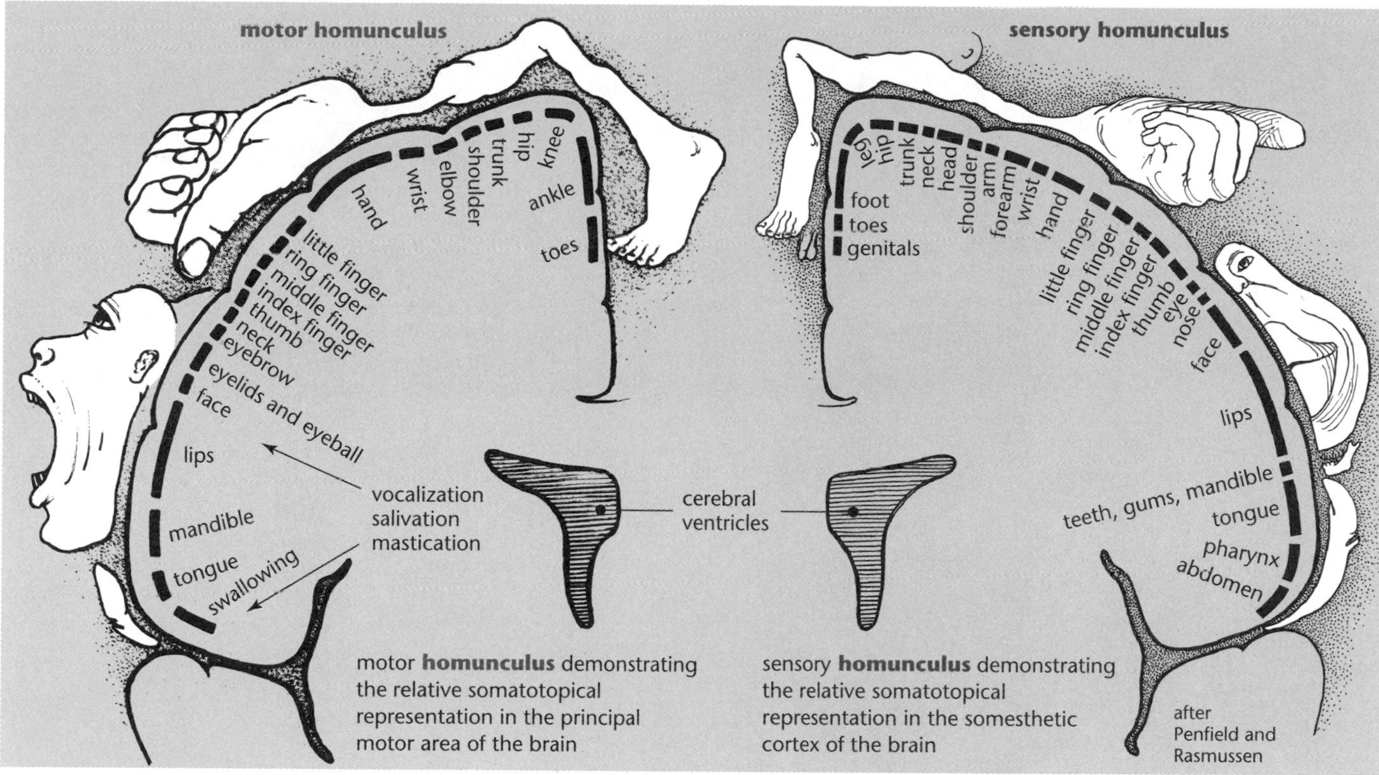

motor **homunculus** demonstrating the relative somatotopical representation in the principal motor area of the brain

sensory **homunculus** demonstrating the relative somatotopical representation in the somesthetic cortex of the brain

homogentisic acid (ho-mo-jen-tis´ik as´id) An intermediate in the metabolism of the amino acid tyrosine, excreted in the urine of persons afflicted with alkaptonuria. Also called alkapton.

h. a. oxidase See homogentisate oxygenase.

homolateral (ho-mo-lat´er-al) See ipsilateral.

homologous (ho-mol´o-gus) Corresponding in structure, position, development, and evolutionary origin, as the wing of a bird, the flipper of a seal, and the human arm.

homologue, homolog (ho´mo-log) Any structure or organ homologous to another.

homology (ho-mol´ŏ-je) Correspondence in structure, evolutionary origin, or position.

homolysin (ho-mol´ĭ-sin) Isohemolysin.

homolysis (ho-mol´ĭ-sis) See isohemolysis.

homomorphic (ho-mo-mor´fik) Denoting structures of similar size and form.

homonomous (ho-mon´ŏ-mus) Denoting parts that are similar in function and structure, such as fingers and toes.

homonymous (ho-mon´ĭ-mus) **1.** Relating to the same right or left side of the two visual fields (e.g., the nasal half of one visual field and the temporal half of the other). **2.** Having the same name.

homoplasty (ho´mo-plas-te) Repair of a defect with a graft from another member of the same species.

homopolymer (ho-mo-pol´ĭ-mer) A polymer composed of identical units of a single monomer.

homopolypeptide (ho-mo-pol-e-pep´tīd) A peptide chain containing only one type of amino acid residue, such as polyglycine, polyalanine, and polyglutamic acid.

homosexual (ho-mo-sek´shoo-al) **1.** Relating to homosexuality. **2.** Characterized by homosexuality.

homosexuality (ho-mo-sek-shoo-al´ĭ-te) Sexual interest in or relationship with members of the same sex.

homothermal, homothermic (ho-mo-ther´mal, ho-mo-ther´mik) See homeothermic.

homotype (hom´o-tīp) A part or organ having the same structure or function as another.

homozoic (ho-mo-zo´ik) Pertaining to the same animal or the same species of animal.

homozygosis (ho-mo-zi-go´sis) The formation of a zygote by the union of genetically identical gametes.

homozygosity (ho-mo-zi-gos´ĭ-te) The state of having identical alleles at one or more loci of homologous chromosomes.

homozygote (ho-mo-zi´gōt) An individual exhibiting homozygosity.

homunculus (ho-munk´u-lus) **1.** The proportional representation of various parts of the body in the motor or sensory areas of the cerebral cortex. **2.** A minute body imagined by 16th and 17th century biologists to be present in the sperm, from which the human body was supposed to be developed.

motor h. One in which the parts of the figure are roughly proportional to the extent of the excitable motor cortex associated with evoking movements of the pads; the figure is generally illustrated upside down on the brain, with the lower extremity on the medial surface of the paracentral lobule and with the head near the lateral cerebral fissure.

sensory h. One in which the parts of the figure are proportional to the amount of cortical area associated with sensory innervation density of the body areas, rather than to the size of the area (e.g., the tongue and thumb have a relatively large representation).

honk (hongk) Term used in medical parlance to describe sounds resembling the call of a goose.

systolic h. A loud, vibratory, often musical heart murmur of relatively clear pitch, usually occurring in late systole; believed to originate in the mitral (left atrioventricular) valve. Also called systolic whoop.

hook (ho͝ok) A metal instrument with a curved or sharply bent tip, used for traction or fixation of a part.

blunt h. Hook used to make traction upon the groin of a dead infant during a difficult breech presentation.

palate h. Hook used to pull forward the soft palate to facilitate posterior rhinoscopy.

tracheotomy h. A right-angled book for holding the trachea steady during tracheotomy.

hooklets (ho͝ok´let) Small horny residues from *Echinococcus* larval infestation, found in the walls of *Echinococcus* cysts.

hookworm (ho͝ok´werm) Any parasitic roundworm of the genera *Ancylostoma* and *Necator*.

American h. *Necator americanus*.

Old World h. *Ancylostoma duodenale*.

hora decubitus (or´ă de-ku´bĭ-tus) (h.d.) Latin for at bedtime.

hora somni (or´ă som´ne) (h.s.) Latin for at hour of sleep.

hordeolum (hor-de´o-lum) A common staphylococcal inflammation of the sebaceous gland of an eyelash, marked by a painful, swollen, erythematous lesion of the external surface of the eyelid. Also called stye.

hormonal (hor-mo´nal) Relating to hormones.

hormone (hor´mōn) A chemical secretion produced by specialized cells in endocrine glands and other tissues (e.g., gastrointestinal tract) and carried in the bloodstream to a specific target organ or tissue elsewhere in the body to either stimulate or retard its function.

adrenocortical h.'s Hormones (steroids) secreted by the human adrenal cortex; the principal ones are cortisol, aldosterone, and corticosterone.

adrenocorticotropic h. (ACTH) A hormone elaborated by the anterior lobe of the pituitary gland (adenohypophysis), which stimulates the adrenal cortex to functional activity. Also called adrenocorticotrophin.

adrenomedullary h.'s Any of the hormones formed by the adrenal medulla (e.g., epinephrine, norepinephrine).

androgenic h. Any of the masculinizing hormones including testosterone, the most potent one.

antidiuretic h. (ADH) See vasopressin.

chorionic growth h. See human placental lactogen, under lactogen.

corticotropin-releasing h. (CRH) Hormone of hypothalamic origin capable of accelerating pituitary secretion of corticotropin.

follicle-stimulating h. (FSH) A glycoprotein hormone of the anterior lobe of the pituitary gland (adenohypophysis), which stimulates normal cyclic growth of the ovarian follicle in females and stimulates the seminiferous tubules to produce spermatozoa in males.

follicle-stimulating hormone-releasing h. (FSHRH) A hypothalamic hormone capable of accelerating pituitary secretion of follicle-stimulating hormone.

gastrointestinal h. Any secretion of the gastrointestinal mucosa affecting the timing of various digestive secretions (e.g., secretin).

gonadotropin-releasing h. (GnRH, GRH) A decapeptide secreted by the hypothalamus that stimulates the pituitary gland to produce luteinizing hormone and follicle-stimulating hormone.

growth h. (GH) Hormone secreted by the anterior lobe of the pituitary gland (adenohypophysis), which promotes fat mobilization, inhibits glucose utilization, and affects the rate of skeletal and visceral growth; diabetogenic when present in excess. Also called somatotrophic hormone; somatotropin.

growth hormone-releasing h. (GH-RH) A hormone from the hypothalamus that stimulates release of growth hormone by the anterior lobe of the pituitary. Formerly called growth hormone-

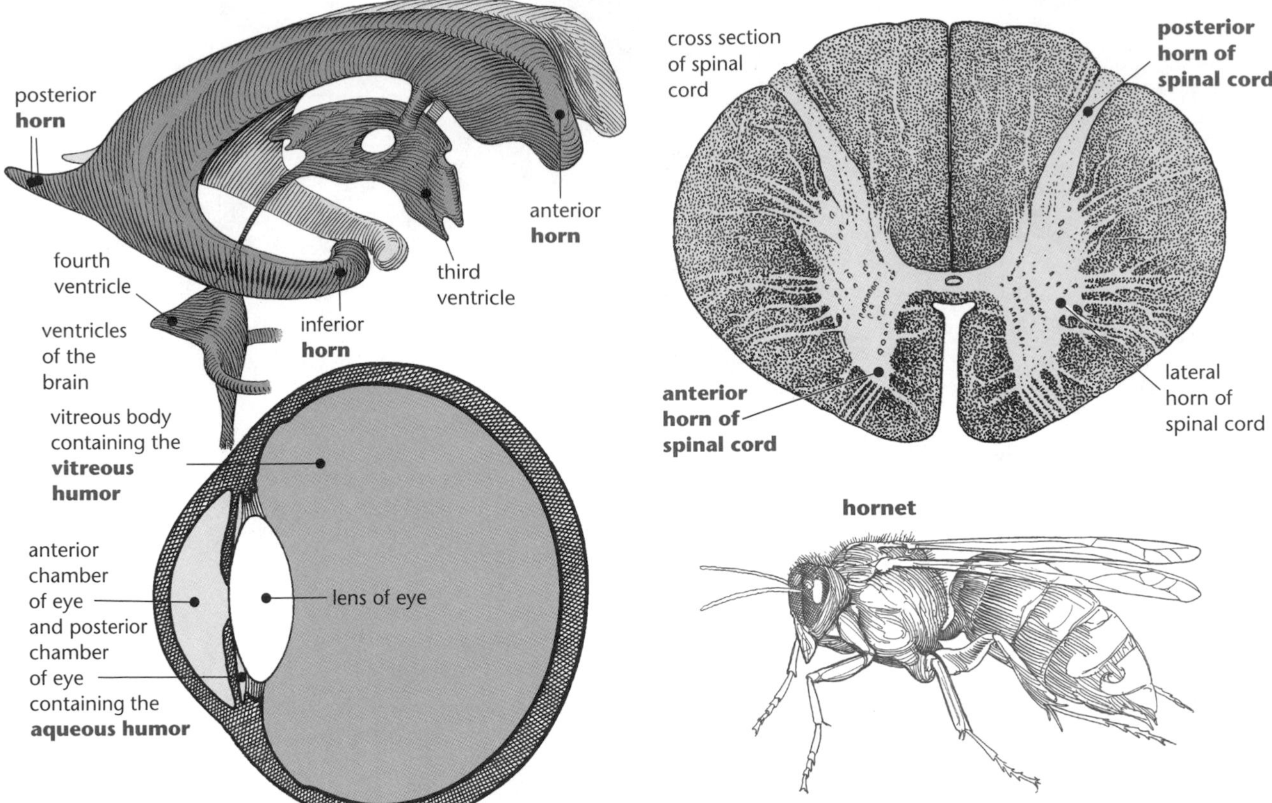

releasing factor.

interstitial cell stimulating h. (ICSH) An anterior pituitary gland secretion which stimulates testicular interstitial cells to produce androgen; ICSH in the male is identical with luteinizing hormone (LH) in the female, which is essential for ovulation and formation of the corpus luteum in the ovary.

luteinizing h. (LH) A glycoprotein hormone of the anterior pituitary gland that promotes maturation of an ovarian follicle, its secretion of progesterone, its rupture to release the egg, and the conversion of the ruptured follicle into the corpus luteum. Also called lutein-stimulating hormone (LSH).

luteinizing hormone-releasing h. (LH-RH, LRH) Hypothalamic hormone capable of accelerating pituitary secretion of luteinizing hormone.

lutein-stimulating h. (LSH) See luteinizing hormone.

melanocyte-stimulating h. (MSH) A secretion of the middle lobe of the pituitary gland that increases deposition of melanin by the melanocytes.

natriuretic h. A non-peptide substance of less than 500 daltons, isolated from plasma after volume expansion; thought to be released from the brain, it inhibits sodium-potassium ATPase throughout the body and is both natriuretic and vasoconstrictor; possible cause of essential hypertension. Also called endoxin because it binds to digoxin antibodies.

ovarian h.'s Hormones secreted by the human ovary including estradiol, estrone, estriol, and progesterone.

parathyroid h. (PTH) A protein biosynthesized and secreted into the bloodstream by the four parathyroid glands which are located in the neck behind the thyroid gland; it acts on the cells of bone, kidney, and intestinal tract to maintain a constant concentration of calcium in the blood.

pituitary growth h. (PGH) The growth hormone of the anterior lobe of the pituitary gland.

placental h. Any of the hormones secreted by the placenta (human chorionic gonadotropin, estrogen, progesterone, and human placental lactogen).

progestational h. Progesterone.

prolactin-inhibiting h. Hormone of hypothalamic origin capable of inhibiting the synthesis and release of prolactin by the anterior pituitary gland.

prolactin-releasing h. (PRH) A hypothalamic hormone that stimulates pituitary secretion of prolactin.

releasing h. (RH) Releasing factor; see under factor.

sex h.'s Estrogens (female sex hormones) and androgens (male sex hormones) formed by ovarian, testicular, and adrenocortical tissues.

somatotrophic h. See growth hormone.

testicular h.'s Hormones elaborated by the human testis, especially testosterone.

thyroid h. A term that commonly refers to thyroxin, but may also include triiodothyronine.

thyroid-stimulating h. (TSH) See thyrotropin.

thyrotrophic h. See thyrotropin.

thyrotropic h. See thyrotropin.

thyrotropin-releasing h. (TRH) A tripeptide hormone from the hypothalamus that stimulates pituitary secretion of thyrotropin.

hormonogenic (hor-mo-no-jen′ik) Denoting any agent that stimulates the production of a hormone.

hormonotherapy (hor-mo-no-ther′ă-pe) Medical treatment with hormones.

horn (horn) Any horn-shaped structure or excrescence.

anterior h. of spinal cord The anterior column of the spinal cord as seen in cross sections.

cutaneous h. A horny growth of the skin. Also called warty horn.

posterior h. of spinal cord The posterior column of the spinal cord as seen in cross sections.

pulp h. A prolongation of vital pulp tissue of a tooth directly under a cusp.

warty h. See cutaneous horn.

hornet (hōr′nit) Any of several stinging wasps, chiefly of the genera *Vespa* and *Vespula*, having a slender, spindle-shaped body with an elongated waist; they usually construct papier-mâché hives; the antigens responsible for hypersensitivity are present in both the venom sac and body of the insect.

hospice (hos′pis) An institution that is organized to provide coordinated multidisciplinary services to dying patients and their families; staff is composed of professionals in physical, psychological, social, and spiritual care.

hospital (hos′pĭ-tal) An institution whose primary aim is caring for or treating patients.

base h. Hospital located in a large military base for the care of patients received from smaller units near the battle front.

closed h. Hospital in which only members of the attending and consulting staff may admit and treat patients.

day h. Hospital that provides treatment during the day enabling patients to return home at night; it may be a special facility within a large hospital.

evacuation h. A mobile military hospital where patients are taken and cared for until they can be evacuated to a general hospital.

general h. **1.** Any large civilian hospital for the care of medical, surgical, and maternity cases. **2.** A permanent, large military hospital that receives patients from smaller evacuation hospitals.

maternity h. A hospital for the care of women immediately before, during, and shortly after childbirth and for the care of newborn babies.

mobile Army surgical h. (MASH) See surgical hospital.

private h. Hospital controlled by a legal entity rather than an agency of a government.

proprietary h. Hospital owned and operated for profit by an individual or corporation.

special h. Hospital for the treatment of patients with specific diseases.

surgical h. A mobile military hospital for the immediate care of serious casualties.

host (hōst) **1.** An organism that harbors and provides nourishment for another organism (parasite). **2.** The recipient of an organ or tissue transplant from a donor.

alternate h. Intermediate host.

definitive h. The organism in which a parasite lives during its adult and sexual phase.

intermediate h. The organism in which a parasite lives during its larval or asexual phase.

primary h. The organism in which the mature parasite lives when it has two or more stages of existence in different organisms.

reservoir h. An animal that serves as a host to species of parasites that are also parasitic in humans and from which humans may be infested, either directly through ingestion or indirectly through a carrier, such as a mosquito.

secondary h. Intermediate host.

housefly (hous′flī) A common, widely distributed member of the insect order Dipter, *Musca domestica*; it breeds in filth and decaying organic waste, and is a transmitter of numerous disease-causing organisms.

Houssay syndrome (o-sī′ sin′drōm) Abatement of diabetes mellitus resulting from surgical removal of, or a destructive lesion in, the pituitary gland.

hum (hum) Descriptive term for a low-pitched sound.

venous h. A continuous murmur due to altered flow patterns in veins; heard on auscultation over the large veins at the base of the neck when the patient is in a sitting position and looking to the opposite side; commonly heard in association with a goiter. Also called humming-top murmur.

Humalog Fast-acting hormone used to treat diabetes mellitus; begins lowering blood sugar within 15 minutes after injection, peaks 1 to 2 hours later, and

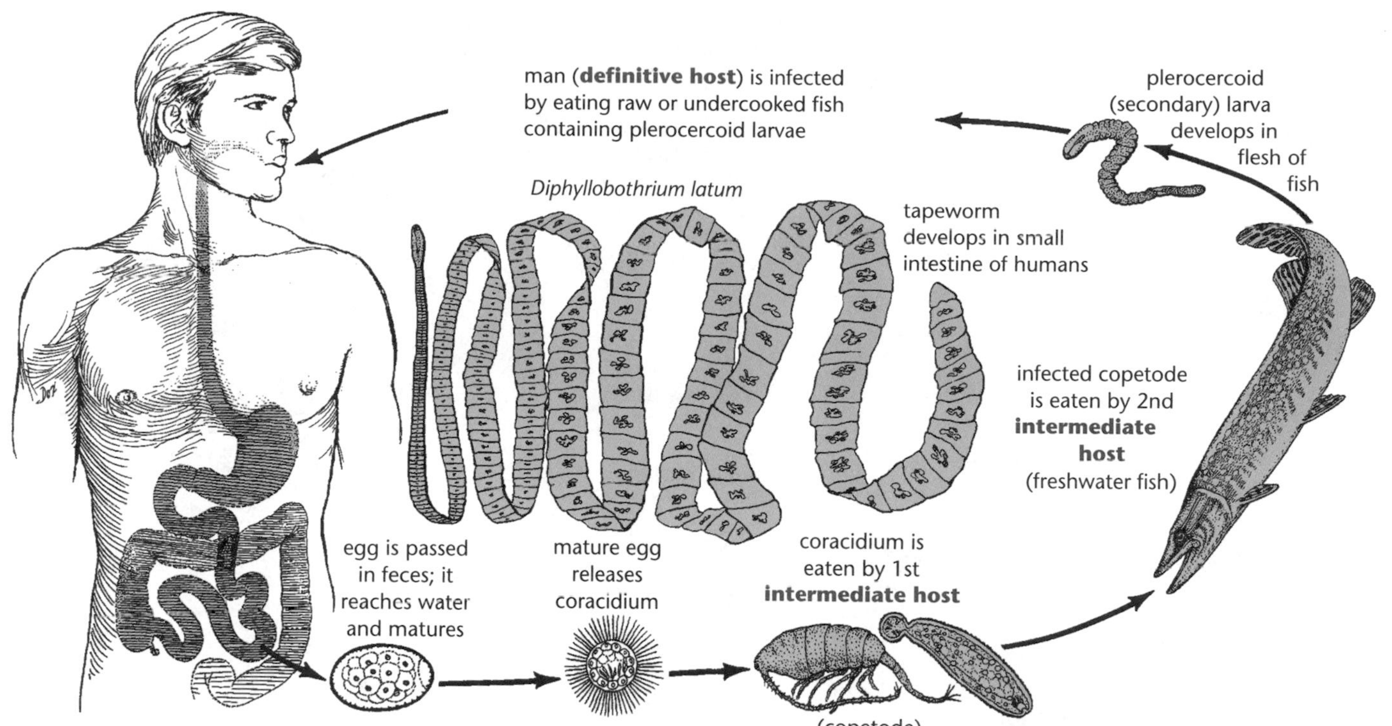

man (**definitive host**) is infected by eating raw or undercooked fish containing plerocercoid larvae
plerocercoid (secondary) larva develops in flesh of fish
Diphyllobothrium latum
tapeworm develops in small intestine of humans
infected copetode is eaten by 2nd **intermediate host** (freshwater fish)
egg is passed in feces; it reaches water and matures
mature egg releases coracidium
coracidium is eaten by 1st **intermediate host**
(copetode)

lasts up to 5 hours. Also called insulin lispro.

humectant (hu-mek´tant) A substance that helps to retain moisture.

humeral (hu´mer-al) Relating to or located in the proximity of the humerus.

humerus (hu´mer-us) The long bone of the upper arm that extends from the shoulder to the elbow. See table of bones.

humidity (hu-mid´ĭ-te) Dampness.

absolute h. The amount of water vapor present in the air when saturated at a given temperature, expressed in grains per cubic feet.

relative h. (RH) The percentage of water vapor present in the atmosphere, as compared to the amount necessary to cause saturation at a specific temperature.

humor (hu´mor) Any fluid or semifluid occurring normally in the body.

aqueous h. The clear, watery fluid filling the anterior and posterior chambers of the eye.

vitreous h. The fluid component of the vitreous body.

hump (hump) A rounded protuberance or mass.

buffalo h. A soft tissue protuberance of the upper back and shoulder associated with excess corticosteroids (e.g., cortisol).

dowager's h. Popular term for a protuberance on the upper vertebrae, caused by osteoporosis.

Humulin (hu´mu-lin) Trade name for human insulin produced by recombinant DNA technology.

hunchback, humpback (hunch´bak, hump´bak) See kyphosis.

hunger (hung´ger) **1.** A strong craving for nourishment. **2.** A strong desire for anything.

air h. The panicky, shallow, and uncoordinated breathing of patients with chronic obstructive pulmonary disease (COPD); a gasping for air.

Hunter's canal (hun´terz kă-nal´) See adductor canal, under canal.

Hunter's syndrome (hun´terz sin´drōm) A hereditary, X-linked recessive condition characterized by stiff joints, enlargement of the liver and spleen, cardiac involvement, mild retardation, and progressive deafness. Also called type II mucopolysaccharidosis.

Huntington's chorea (hunt´ing-tonz kor´e-ă) See hereditary chorea, under chorea.

Huntington's disease (hunt´ing-tonz dĭ-zēz´) An inherited disorder of the nervous system transmitted by an autosomal dominant gene and marked by degeneration of the basal ganglia and cerebral cortex; manifestations include choreiform movements, intellectual deterioration, and personality changes; onset is usually insidious and occurs in middle life; the disease is often fatal within 5 to 15 years after onset.

Hurler's syndrome (hŭr´lerz sin´drōm) An inherited metabolic disorder marked by skeletal deformities, mental retardation, and early death; characterized by an accumulation of an abnormal intracellular material, a deficiency of the enzyme alpha-L-iduronidase, and excretion of chondroitin sulfate B and heparitin sulfate in the urine. Also called type I mucopolysaccharidosis; lipochondrodystrophy.

hyalin (hi´ă-lin) **1.** The homogeneous matrix of hyaline cartilage. **2.** A clear homogeneous substance, occurring in degenerative diseases.

hyaline (hi´ă-lēn) Glassy or translucent in appearance.

hyaline membrane disease of newborn (hi´ă-lēn mem´brān dĭ-zēz´ ŭv noo´born) (HMD) See respiratory distress syndrome of newborn.

hyalitis (hi-ă-li´tis) Inflammation of the vitreous body.

hyaloid (hi´ă-loid) **1.** See hyaline. **2.** Relating to the vitreous body.

hyalomere (hi´ă-lo-mēr) The pale, homogeneous, nonrefractile portion of a blood platelet; found in it are elements of chromatomeres, microtubules, mitochondria, microfilaments, and Golgi vesicles.

hyalosis (hi-ă-lo´sis) Eye condition marked by degenerative changes of the vitreous body.

hyaluronic acid (hi-ă-lo͞o-ron´ik) A mucopolysaccharide present in the form of a gelatinous material in the tissue spaces, thus binding cells together and holding water in the tissues; it has the property of increasing the slipperiness of fluids and of the lubricating and shock absorbing system of joints.

hyaluronidase (hi-ă-lo͞o-ron´ĭ-dās) An enzyme, found in sperm, snake and bee venom, and pathogenic bacteria; it causes the breakdown of hyaluronic acid in the tissue spaces, thus enabling the invading agent to enter cells and tissues.

hybaroxia (hi-bar-ok´se-ă) Oxygen therapy with pressures greater than one atmosphere applied in a room or chamber.

hybrid (hi´brid) The offspring (plant or animal) of parents who are genetically dissimilar.

hybridization (hi-brid-ĭ-za´shun) In somatic cell genetics, the fusing of somatic cells from two different species; may result in hybrid cells (with one fused nucleus) or heterokaryons (with two or more genetically different nuclei); important in mapping of chromosomes.

***in situ* h.** Molecular hybridization of a cloned DNA sequence, which has been labeled by radioactivity or fluorescence, to a chromosome spread on a microscope slide; a direct way of mapping a gene.

hybridoma (hi-brid-o´mă) A cell culture composed of fused cells of different kinds, cloned for the purpose of producing antibody of a single specificity.

hydatid (hi´dă-tid) **1.** A cystic structure containing the embryo of *Taenia echinococcus*; a hydatid cyst. **2.** Any structure resembling a cyst.

h. of Morgagni **1.** See testicular appendage, under appendage. **2.** See vesicular appendage of uterine tube, under appendage.

hydatid disease (hi´dă-tid dĭ-zēz´) See echinococcosis.

hydatidiform (hi-dă-tid´ĭ-form) Resembling a hydatid.

hydralazine hydrochloride (hi-dral´ă-zēn hi-dro-klor´īd) An adrenergic blocking agent that lowers blood pressure by acting directly on arteriolar smooth muscle; it may also increase renal blood flow; Apresoline®.

hydramnios, hydramnion (hi-dram´ne-os, hi-dram´ne-on) The presence of an excessive quantity of amniotic fluid.

hydrargyrism, hydrargyria (hi-drar´jĭ-riz-m, hi-drar-jir´e-ă) See mercury poisoning, under poisoning.

hydrargyrum (hi-drar´jĭ-rum) Latin for mercury.

hydrarthrosis (hi-drar-thro´sis) Collection of fluid in a joint.

hydrase (hi´drās) An enzyme that promotes the addition of water, or its removal from a molecule.

hydrate (hi´drāt) Any compound containing water which is retained in its molecular state.

hydrated hi´drā-tid) Combined with water.

hydration (hi-drā´shun) The combination of a substance with water.

hydrencephalocele (hi-dren-sef´ă-lo-sēl) Brain tissue and cerebrospinal fluid protruding through a defect in the skull. Also called hydrocephalocele; hydroencephalocele.

hydrencephalomeningocele (hi-dren-sef-ă-lo-mĕ-ning´o-sēl) Hernial protrusion of the meninges, brain substance, and cerebrospinal fluid through a defect in the skull.

hydrencephalus (hi-dren-sef´ă-lus) See internal hydrocephalus, under hydrocephalus.

hydride (hi´drīd) A compound of hydrogen with a more positive element or group, thus assuming a formal negative charge.

hydroa (hid-ro´ă) Any vesicular skin eruption.

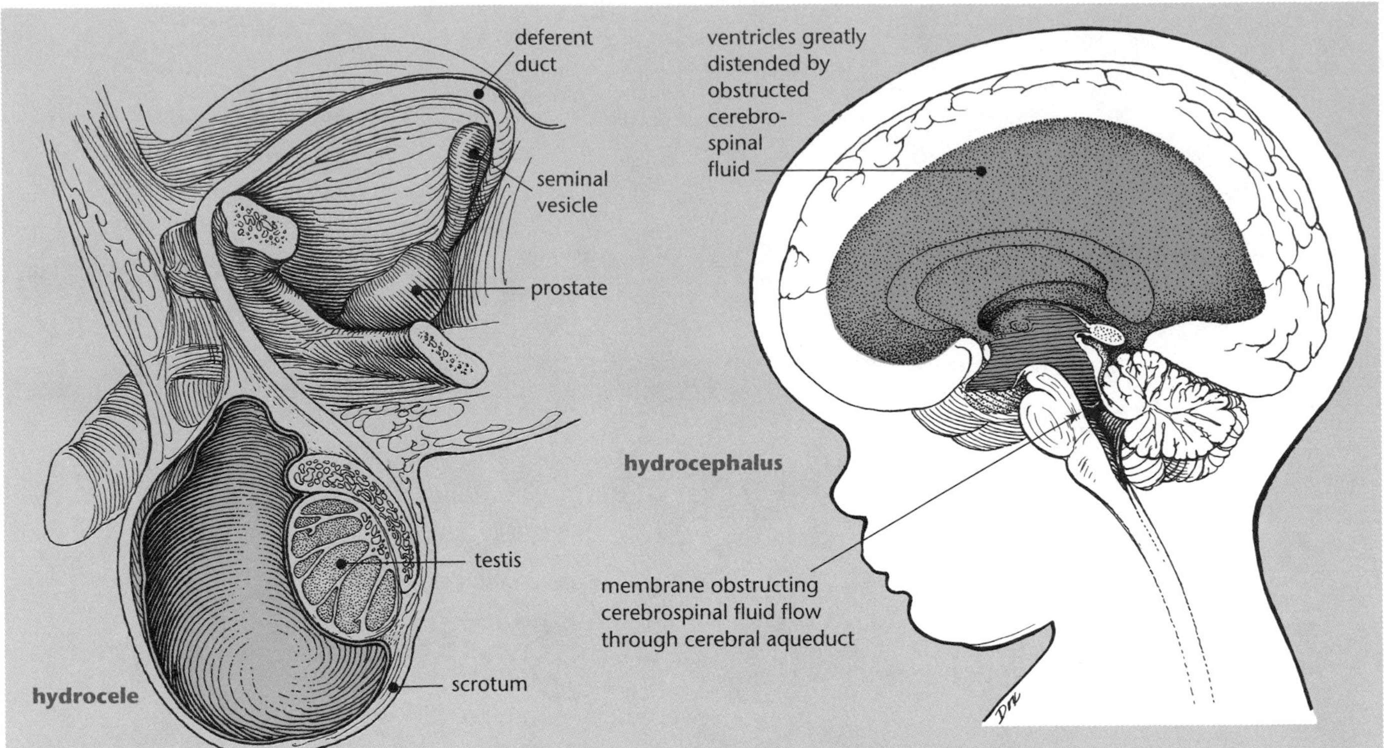

h. aestivale See hydroa vacciniforme.

h. febrilis See herpes simplex, under herpes.

h. gestationis See herpes gestationis, under herpes.

h. herpetiforme See dermatitis herpetiformis, under dermatitis.

h. puerorum See hydroa vacciniforme.

h. vacciniforme A recurrent form occurring during the summer months. Also called hydroa aestivale; hydroa puerorum.

hydroappendix (hi-dro-ă-pen´diks) Distention of the vermiform appendix with a serous fluid.

hydroblepharon (hi-dro-blef´ă-ron) Edema of the eyelid.

hydrocarbon (hi-dro-kar´bon) A compound containing hydrogen and carbon only.

hydrocele (hi´dro-sēl) Abnormal collection of fluid in any sacculated cavity in the body, especially under the serous covering of the testis or along the spermatic cord.

hernia h. Hydrocele in which the hernial sac is filled with a fluid.

hydrocelectomy (hi-dro-se-lek´tŏ-me) Surgical removal of a hydrocele.

hydrocephalic (hi-dro-sĕ-fal´ik) Relating to hydrocephalus.

hydrocephalocele (hi-dro-sef´ă-lo-sēl) See hydrencephalocele.

hydrocephalus (hi-dro-sef´ă-lus) Excessive accumulation of cerebrospinal fluid in the ventricles of the brain, causing compression of the brain and, in infants and children under the age of 2, enlargement of the head.

communicating h. Hydrocephalus occurring when the cerebrospinal fluid flows freely through the openings between ventricles but is improperly drained at the subarachnoid space or at the arachnoid granulations. Also called external hydrocephalus.

noncommunicating h. See obstructive hydrocephalus.

obstructive h. Hydrocephalus occurring as a result of a block within the ventricular system (i.e., at any of the openings between ventricles). Also called noncommunicating hydrocephalus.

hydrochloric acid (hi-dro-klor´ik as´id) A colorless compound of hydrogen chloride (HCl); the acid secreted by the stomach to facilitate digestion.

hydrochloride (hi-dro-klor´īd) Compound formed by the reaction of hydrochloric acid with an organic base.

hydrochlorothiazide (hi-dro-klor-o-thi´ă-zīd) A thiazide compound used as an oral diuretic.

hydrocolloid (hi-dro-kol´oid) A gelatinous colloid in unstable equilibrium with its contained water, used in dentistry as an elastic impression material.

irreversible h. A hydrocolloid such as alginate, whose physical condition is changed by an irreversible chemical reaction when mixed with water; used in making diagnostic casts of teeth and partial denture impressions.

reversible h. A hydrocolloid of agar base whose physical state is altered to a liquid by the application of heat and then changed to that of an elastic gel by cooling.

hydrocolpocele, hydrocolpos (hi-dro-kol´po-sēl, hi-dro-kol´pos) An accumulation of fluid in the vagina.

hydrocortisone (hi-dro-kor´tĭ-sōn) A steroid hormone isolated from the adrenal cortex or produced synthetically; of the naturally occurring adrenal cortical hormones, hydrocortisone is most capable of correcting by itself the effects of adrenalectomy; provides resistance to stresses and maintains a number of enzyme systems. Also called cortisol.

hydrocyanic acid (hi-dro-si-an´ik as´id) See hydrogen cyanide, under hydrogen.

hydrodynamics (hi-dro-di-nam´iks) The branch of physics concerned with fluids in motion and the forces affecting the motion.

hydroencephalocele (hi-dro-en-sef´ă-lo-sēl) See hydrencephalocele.

hydrogel (hi´dro-jel) A gel having water as its dispersion medium. COMPARE: hydrosol.

hydrogen (hi´dro-jen) A colorless, flammable, gaseous element; the lightest of all known chemical elements; symbol H, atomic number 1, atomic weight 1.0079.

h. acceptor **1.** Hydrogen carrier. **2.** A metabolite that transports hydrogen during metabolism.

activated h. Hydrogen removed from a compound (donor) by a dehydrogenase.

h. carrier A molecule that carries hydrogen from one substance (oxidant) to another (reductant) or to molecular oxygen to form water (H_2O).

h. cyanide A colorless, volatile, poisonous compound with an almond odor (HCN); used as an insecticide and disinfectant. Also called hydrocyanic acid; prussic acid.

h. donor Substance that gives up hydrogen atoms to another substance.

heavy h. See hydrogen-2.

h. ion The positively charged nucleus of the hydrogen atom, H° or H^+, formed by removal of the electron; it exists in aqueous solution as a hydronium ion, OH_3^+.

h. number A measure of the amount of unsaturated fatty acids in fat, equal to the quantity of hydrogen that 1 g of fat will absorb.

h. sulfide H_2S; a colorless, flammable, poisonous gas with a rotten egg odor; used as a reagent and in chemical manufacturing. Also called sulfuretted hydrogen.

sulfuretted h. See hydrogen sulfide.

h. transport The transfer of hydrogen from one substance to another; the former is thus oxidized and the latter is reduced.

hydrogen-1 (^1H) The hydrogen isotope that makes up about 99 percent of the hydrogen atoms occurring in nature; a mass 1 isotope. Also called protium.

hydrogen-2 (^2H) An isotope of hydrogen having an atomic weight of 2.0141, consisting of one proton and one neutron in the nucleus; a mass 2 isotope. Also called deuterium; heavy hydrogen.

hydrogen-3 (^3H) The heaviest of the three isotopes of hydrogen with an atomic mass of 3; weakly radioactive; half-life 12.4 years; a mass 3 isotope, made artificially by bombardment of other species. Also called tritium.

hydrogenation (hi-dro-jen-ā´shun) The combination of an unsaturated compound with hydrogen.

hydrokinetics (hi-dro-kĭ-net´iks) The study of fluids in motion under a force.

hydrolabyrinth (hi-dro-lab´ĭ-rinth) Abnormal increase in the amount of endolymph in the labyrinth of the inner ear; thought to be the cause of aural vertigo.

hydrolase (hi´dro-lās) An enzyme that promotes the hydrolysis of a compound.

hydrolysate (hi-drol´ĭ-zāt) Any product produced by hydrolysis.

protein h. A mixture of amino acids produced by splitting the protein molecule with acid, alkali, or enzyme; used in diets of infants allergic to milk or in special diets for individuals unable to eat ordinary food proteins.

hydrolysis (hi-drol´ĭ-sis) The decomposition or splitting of a compound into simpler substances by the addition of the elements of water; a hydrogen is added to one portion and a hydroxyl group to the other.

hydrolytic (hi-dro-lit´ik) Relating to hydrolysis.

hydrolyze (hi´dro-līz) To subject to hydrolysis.

hydromassage (hi-dro-mă-sahzh´) Massage effected with streams of water.

hydrometer (hi-drom´ĕ-ter) An instrument used to measure the specific gravity of a liquid such as urine. Also called gravimeter.

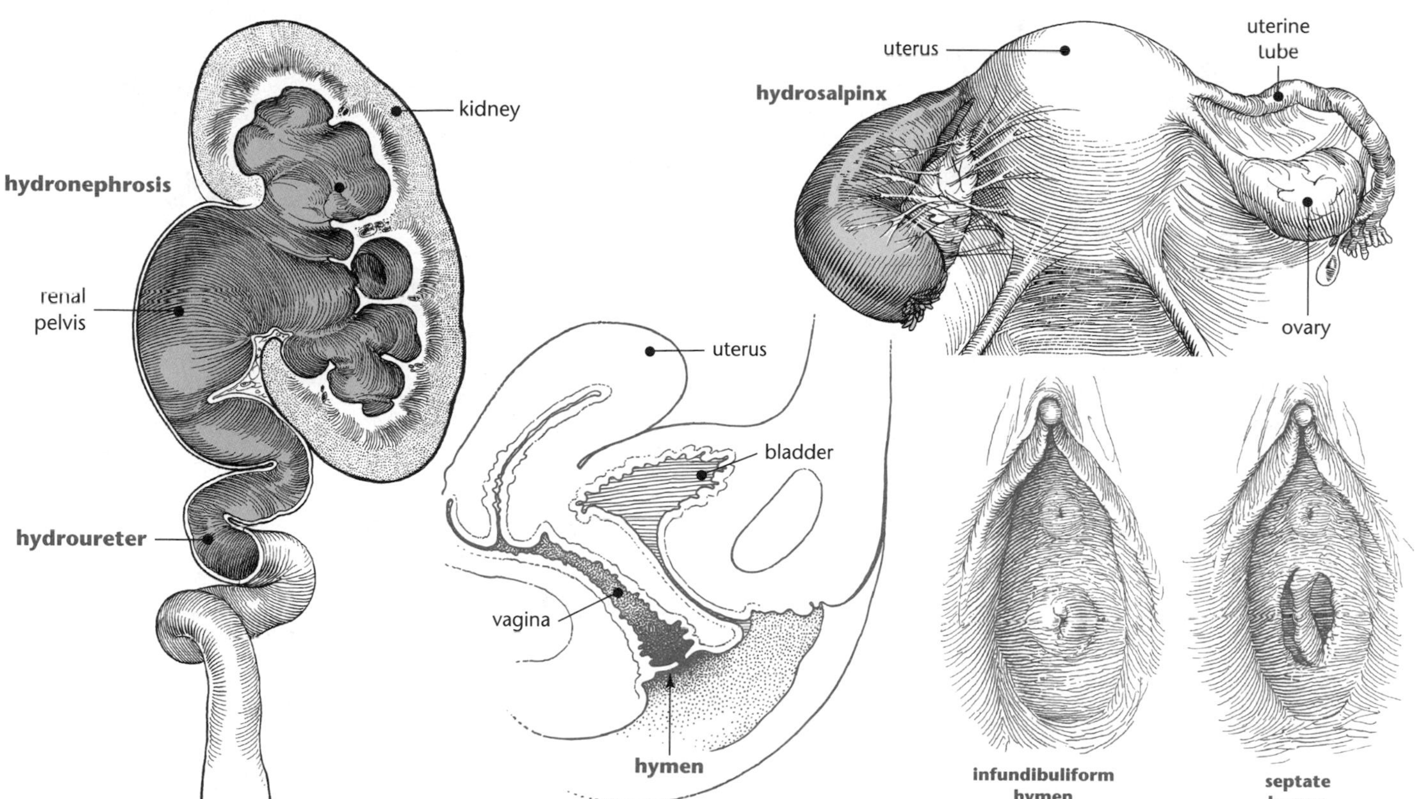

hydrometra (hi-dro-me´trǎ) Abnormal accumulation of a fluid in the uterus.

hydrometrocolpos (hi-dro-me-tro-kol´pos) Abnormal accumulation of fluid in the uterus and vagina.

hydrometry (hi-drom´ě-tre) Determination of the specific gravity of a fluid.

hydromphalus (hi-drom´fǎ-lus) A cystlike tumor of the umbilicus.

hydromyelia (hi-dro-mi-e´le-ǎ) Distention of the central canal of the spinal cord with accumulated cerebrospinal fluid.

hydromyelocele (hi-dro-mi-ě-lo-sēl) A fluid-filled saclike protrusion of the spinal cord through a spina bifida.

hydronephrosis (hi-dro-ně-fro´sis) Distention of the pelvis and calyces of one or both kidneys with urine as a result of obstruction to the urine outflow.

hydronium (hi-dro´ne-um) See hydronium ion, under ion.

hydropenia (hi-dro-pe´ne-ǎ) Condition marked by insufficient content of water in the body.

hydropericardium (hi-dro-per-ĭ-kar´de-um) Abnormal accumulation of serous fluid in the sac around the heart (pericardium).

hydroperitoneum (hi-dro-per-ĭ-to-ne´um) See ascites.

hydrophilia (hi-dro-fil´e-ǎ) Affinity for water.

hydrophilic, hydrophile (hi-dro-fil´ik, hi´dro-fīl) Readily absorbing water; opposite of hydrophobic.

hydrophobia (hi-dro-fo´be-ǎ) See rabies.

hydrophobic (hi-dro-fo´bik) **1.** Relating to rabies (hydrophobia). **2.** Tending to repel water; opposite of hydrophilic.

hydrophthalmos (hi-drof-thal´mos) See buphthalmos.

hydropneumopericardium (hi-dro-noo-mo-per-ĭ-kar´de-um) The collection of serous effusion and gas within the pericardial cavity.

hydropneumothorax (hi-dro-noo-mo-thor´aks) The presence of both gas and serous fluids in the pleural cavity. Also called pneumohydrothorax.

hydrops (hi´drops) Excessive accumulation of clear fluid in body tissues or cavities.

endolymphatic h. See Ménière's disease.

fetal h., h. fetalis Hydrops of the fetus, as seen in severe hemolytic disease.

h. of gallbladder Hydrops of the gallbladder due to long-term obstruction of the cystic duct.

hydropyonephrosis (hi-dro-pi-o-ně-fro´sis) The collection of urine and pus in the pelvis and calices of the kidney, usually caused by obstruction of the ureter.

hydrorchis (hi-dro-or´kis) Collection of fluid within the serous covering of the testis.

hydrorrhea (hi-dro-re´ǎ) Profuse watery secretion.

h. gravidarum Uncommon condition in which a pregnant woman passes a clear fluid from the vagina; usually a scant amount throughout the pregnancy, occasionally as much as 500 ml as a one-time occurrence; cause is not known.

hydrosalpinx (hi-dro-sal´pinks) Accumulation of serous fluid in the uterine (fallopian) tube.

hydrosol (hi´dro-sol) A colloid in aqueous solution; a sol in which the dispersing medium is water. COMPARE: hydrogel.

hydrospirometer (hi-dro-spi-rom´ě-ter) A spirometer in which the force of the expired air (air pressure) is indicated by the rise and fall of a column of water.

hydrostatic (hi-dro-stat´ik) Relating to the pressures exerted by liquids at rest; opposed to hydrokinetic.

hydrotherapy (hi-dro-ther´ǎ-pe) The therapeutic application of water in the treatment of certain diseases.

hydrothermal (hi-dro-ther´mal) Relating to hot water.

hydrothorax (hi-dro-thor´aks) Noninflammatory accumulation of serous fluid in the pleural cavity.

hydrotropism (hi-drot´ro-piz-m) Growth or movement of an organism toward a moist surface (positive hydrotropism) or away from a moist surface (negative hydrotropism).

hydroureter (hi-dro-u-re´ter) Distention of a ureter with retained urine due to obstruction to urine outflow.

hydrous (hi´drus) Containing water.

hydroxide (hi-drok´sīd) Any chemical compound of hydroxyl (OH) with another element or radical.

hydroxyapatite (hi-drok-se-ap´ǎ-tīt) A mineral compound used in chromatography of nucleic acids.

25-hydroxycholecalciferol (hi-drok-se-ko-le-kal-sif´ě-rol) See calcidiol.

hydroxycortisone (hi-drok-se kor´tĭ-sōn) Cortisol.

hydroxyl (hi-drok´sil) The univalent radical or group OH.

hydroxylysine (hi-drok-se-li´sēn) A basic amino acid found, thus far, only in collagen and gelatin.

β-hydroxy-β-methylglutaryl-CoA (ba´tǎ-hi-drok´se-ba´tǎ-meth-ĭl-gloo´tǎ-ril-ko-ā) (HMG-CoA) An intermediate in the production of ketone bodies and steroids.

hydroxyphenyluria (hi-drok-se-fen-ĭl-u-re´ǎ) Excretion of tyrosine and phenylalanine in the urine, usually resulting from ascorbic acid deficiency.

hydroxyproline (hi-drok-se-pro´lēn) 4-Hydroxy-2-pyrrolidinecarboxylic acid; $C_5H_9NO_3$; a nutritionally nonessential amino acid found among the hydrolysis products of collagen; not found in proteins other than those of connective tissue.

hydroxyprolinemia (hi-drok-se-pro-lĭ-ne´me-ǎ) An inborn error of metabolism characterized by increased blood levels and urinary excretion of free hydroxyproline; associated with severe mental retardation.

5-hydroxytryptamine (hi-drok-se-trip´tǎ-mēn) (5-HT) See serotonin.

hygiene (hi´jēn) The science concerned with the methods of achieving or maintaining good health.

oral h. The proper care of the mouth and teeth for the prevention of disease.

hygienic (hi-jen´ik, hi-jē-en´ik) **1.** Of or relating to hygiene. **2.** Sanitary clean.

hygienist (hi-jen´ist, hi-jē-en´ist) One who is skilled in the science of health and the prevention of disease.

dental h. A person trained in the techniques of removing plaque from teeth and other preventive treatments.

hygieology (hi-je-ol´ŏ-je) **1.** The study of hygiene. **2.** The sum of all measures for the dissemination and popularization of public health knowledge.

hygroma (hi-gro´mǎ) A bursa or cyst containing fluid.

cystic h. See cavernous lymphangioma, under lymphangioma.

subdural h. A hygroma beneath the dura mater (subdural space).

hygrometer (hi-grom´ě-ter) Any of several devices for measuring the atmospheric moisture.

hygroscopic (hi-gro-skop´ik) Readily absorbing moisture.

hymen (hi´men) The membranous fold which partly or completely closes the vaginal orifice in the virgin.

cribriform h. Hymen with a number of small perforations.

denticular h. Hymen in which the opening has serrated edges.

imperforate h. Hymen which completely closes the vaginal orifice.

infundibuliform h. A protruding hymen with a central opening.

septate h. Hymen in which the opening is divided by a narrow band of tissue.

hymenal (hi´men-al) Relating to the hymen.

hymenectomy (hi-men-ek´tŏ-me) Excision of the hymen.

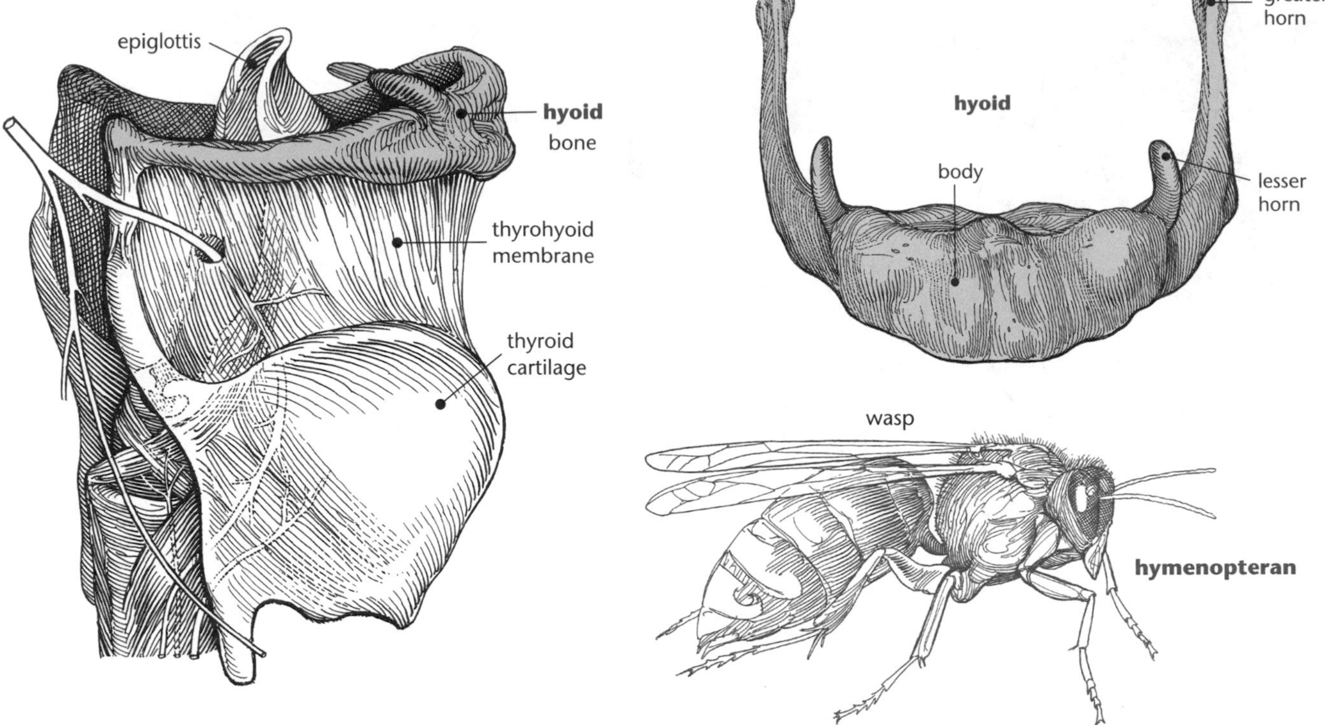

Hymenolepis (hi-mĕ-nol´ĕ-pis) A genus of tapeworms of the class Cestoda.

H. nana A small tapeworm (7 to 10 mm long) parasitic in rats, mice, and children. Also called dwarf tapeworm; dwarf mouse tapeworm.

Hymenoptera (hi-men-op´ter-ă) An order of membrane-winged insects that includes many common stinging members such as the honeybee, yellow jacket, wasp, hornet, and fire ant; the stings are capable of causing severe hypersensitivity reactions and, in some cases, death.

hymenopteran (hi-men-op´ter-an) Any of the membrane-winged insects of the order Hymenoptera, including bees, wasps, and ants.

hymenorrhapy (hi-men-or´ă-fe) **1.** Closing of the vagina by suturing the hymen. **2.** Suture of any membrane.

hymenotomy (hi-men-ot´ŏ-me) Surgical cut through the hymen, especially an imperforate hymen.

hyoepiglottic (hi-o-ep-ĭ-glot´ik) Relating to the hyoid bone and the epiglottis.

hyoglossal (hi-o-glos´al) **1.** Relating to the hyoid bone and the tongue, especially to the hyoglossal muscle from the hyoid bone to the side of the tongue. **2.** The 12th cranial nerve. See table of nerves.

hyoid (hi´oid) U-shaped, specifically, the horseshoe-shaped bone in the throat between the thyroid cartilage and the root of the tongue.

hyoscyamine (hi-o-si´ă-mēn) A poisonous alkaloid, $C_{17}H_{23}NO_3$, occurring in plants such as belladonna, duboisia, hyoscyamus, and stramonium; isometric with atropine; used as an antispasmodic, analgesic, and sedative. Also called daturine.

hypacusis (hi-pă-koo´sis) Impairment of hearing; reduction in ability to perceive sound, usually attributable to conductive or neurosensory deficiency in the peripheral organs of hearing. Also called hypoacusis; hypacusia.

hypalgesia (hi-pal-je´ze-ă) Decreased sensitivity to pain.

hypamnios, hypamnion (hi-pam´ne-os, hi-pam´ne-on) The presence of an abnormally small amount of fluid in the amniotic sac.

hypencephalon (hi-pen-sef´ă-lon) The midbrain, pons, and medulla.

hyperabduction syndrome (hi-per-ab-duk´shun) Pain and numbness of the arm and hand occurring after prolonged abduction of the arm, as during sleep, which compresses the axillary vessels and brachial plexus.

hyperacidity (hi-per-ă-sid´ĭ-te) An excessive degree of acidity.

hyperactivity (hi-per-ak-tiv´ĭ-te) Excessively increased activity.

hyperacusis, hyperacusia (hi-per-ă-koo´sis, hi-per-ă-koo´zhă) Exaggerated hearing acuteness. Also called auditory hyperesthesia.

hyperadrenalism (hi-per-ă-dre´nă-liz-m) Abnormally increased function of the adrenal cortex, with excessive output of steroid hormones. Also called hyperadrenocorticism; hypercorticism.

hyperadrenocorticism (hi-per-ă-dre-no-kor´tĭ-siz-m) See hyperadrenalism.

hyperaldosteronism (hi-per-al-dos´tĕ-ro-niz-m) See aldosteronism.

hyperalgesia (hi-per-al-je´zhă) Excessive sensitiveness to pain.

hyperalimentation (hi-per-al-ĭ-men-ta´shun) Overfeeding for therapeutic purposes.

parenteral h. The continuous administration of fluids containing nutrients (particularly a solution of amino acids and sugar) into the superior vena cava through a catheter.

hyperbaric (hi-per-bar´ik) Relating to or occurring at pressures greater than atmospheric pressure (e.g., a hyperbaric chamber).

hyperbarism (hi-per-bar´iz-m) Condition resulting from the pressure of ambient gases in excess of that within the body.

hyperbetalipoproteinemia (hi-per-ba-tă-lip-o-pro-tēn-e´me-ă) See type II familial hyperlipoproteinemia, under hyperlipoproteinemia.

hyperbilirubinemia (hi-per-bil-ĭ-roo-bĭ-ne´me-ă) The presence of an abnormally large amount of bilirubin in the blood.

hypercalcemia (hi-per-kal-se´me-ă) Abnormally high concentration of calcium in the blood.

idiopathic h. of infants Persistent hypercalcemia affecting infants, associated with osteosclerosis, renal insufficiency, and sometimes hypertension.

hypercalcinuria (hi-per-kal-sĭ-nu´re-ă) See hypercalciuria.

hypercalciuria (hi-per-kal-sĭ-u´re-ă) Elevated amounts of calcium in the urine, usually a result of hypercalcemia, as in hyperparathyroidism, bone neoplasm, and vitamin D intoxication. Also called hypercalcinuria.

idiopathic h. Condition of elevated amounts of calcium in the urine not explained by hypercalcemia.

hypercapnia, hypercarbia (hi-per-kap´ne-ă, hi-per-kar´be-ă) The presence of an abnormally high concentration of carbon dioxide in the blood.

hypercementosis (hi-per-se-men-to´sis) Overdevelopment of cementum over the root surface of teeth.

hyperchloremia (hi-per-klor-e´me-ă) Abnormal increase of chloride in the blood.

hyperchlorhydria (hi-per-klor-hi´dre-ă) Excessive secretion of gastric juice; may be due to a temporary disturbance of stomach function; chronic hyperchlorhydria may be associated with peptic ulcer.

hypercholesterolemia, hypercholesteremia (hi-per-ko-les-ter-ol-e´me-ă, hi-per-ko-les-ter-e´ me-ă) The presence of an excessive amount of cholesterol in the blood.

hypercholia (hi-per-ko´le-ă) A condition in which an excessive amount of bile is secreted by the liver.

hyperchromasia (hi-per-kro-ma´zhă) See hyperchromatism.

hyperchromatic (hi-per-kro-mat´ik) Overpigmented; having excessive coloration; said especially of a cell that stains more intensely than normal.

hyperchromatism (hi-per-kro´mă-tiz-m) **1.** Excessive pigmentation. **2.** Degeneration of a cell nucleus which becomes filled with an excessive amount of pigment particles.

hyperchromia (hi-per-kro´me-ă) **1.** Abnormal increase in the hemoglobin content of red blood cells, usually seen in macrocytic cells where the concentration of hemoglobin is normal but the quantity is increased because the cells are larger than normal. **2.** See hyperchromatism.

hyperchromic (hi-per-kro´mik) **1.** Overpigmented. **2.** Relating to an increase in light absorption.

hyperchylia (hi-per-ki´le-ă) An excessive secretion of gastric juice.

hyperchylomicronemia (hi-per-ki-lo-mi-kro-ne´me-ă) Type I familial hyperlipoproteinemia; see under hyperlipoproteinemia.

hypercoagulability (hi-per-ko-ag-u-lă-bil´ĭ-te) Abnormal tendency to form clots.

hypercoagulable (hi-per-ko-ag´u-lă-bl) Characterized by increased clot formation.

hypercorticoidism, hypercorticism (hi-per-kor´tĭ-koi-diz-m, hi-per-kor´tĭ-siz-m) Condition caused by an excess of one or more steroids of the adrenal cortex, or by the administration of large quantities of steroids having glucocorticoid qualities.

hypercryalgesia, hypercryesthesia (hi-per-kri-al-je´zhă, hi-per-kri-es-the´zhă) Excessive sensitivity to cold.

hypercupremia (hi-per-ku-pre´me-ă) Abnormally high copper content in the blood.

hypercythemia (hi-per-si-the´me-ă) The presence of an abnormally large number of erythrocytes in the circulating blood.

CLASSIFICATION OF **HYPERLIPOPROTEINEMIA**

Type and prevalence	I RARE	II COMMON	III FAIRLY COMMON	IV COMMON	V UNCOMMON
Appearance of plasma	creamy layer over clear infranatant on standing	clear or only slightly turbid	clear, cloudy or milky	clear to grossly turbid	creamy layer over turbid infranatant on standing
Cholesterol level	↑	↑	↑	↑	↑
Triglyceride level	↑	↑	↑	↑	↑
Signs and symptoms	abdominal pain hepatosplenomegaly lipemia retinalis eruptive xanthomas	tendon xanthomas tuberous xanthomas corneal arcus accelerated atherosclerosis	tendon, tuboeruptive and planar xanthomas accelerated atherosclerosis	accelerated coronary atherosclerosis abnormal glucose tolerance	abdominal pain hepatosplenomegaly lipemia retinalis eruptive xanthomas abnormal glucose tolerance

hypercytosis (hi-per-si-to´sis) Any condition in which there is an abnormal increase in the number of blood cells, especially of leukocytes.

hyperdipsia (hi-per-dip´se-ă) Intense thirst.

hyperdistention (hi-per-dis-ten´shun) Extreme distention.

hyperdynamia (hi-per-di-na´me-ă) Extreme muscular activity or restlessness; exaggeration of function.

hyperdynamic (hi-per-di-nam´ik) Marked by hyperdynamia.

hyperechoic (hi-per-ĕ-ko´ik) In ultrasonography, producing many or stronger echoes.

hyperemesis (hi-per-em´ĕ-sis) Excessive vomiting.

h. gravidarum Pernicious vomiting of pregnancy.

hyperemia (hi-per-e´me-ă) Excess of blood in an area of the body; congestion.

active h. Hyperemia caused by increased inflow of arterial blood resulting in dilatation of arterioles and capillaries, as in inflammation.

collateral h. Increased blood flow through collateral vessels due to an arrest of the flow through the main artery.

passive h. Hyperemia resulting from an obstruction to the outflow of blood from the affected area.

hyperesthesia (hi-per-es-the´zhă) Abnormally increased sensitivity to sensory stimuli.

hyperextension (hi-per-ek-sten´shun) Extension of a part of the body beyond the normal limit. Also called overextension.

hyperflexion (hi-per-flek´shun) Flexion of a limb or part beyond the normal limit. Also called superflexion.

hypergammaglobulinemia (hi-per-gam-ă-glob-u-lĭ-ne´me-ă) Excess of gamma globulin in the blood.

hypergenitalism (hi-per-jen´ĭ-tal-izm) Overdeveloped genitalia for age of the individual.

hyperglobulinemia (hi-per-glob-u-lĭ-ne´me-ă) Excess of globulin in the blood.

hyperglycemia (hi-per-gli-se´me-ă) Abnormally high concentration of sugar (glucose) in the blood.

hyperglycorrhachia (hi-per-gli-ko-ra´ke-ă) An excessive amount of sugar (glucose) in the cerebrospinal fluid (CSF).

hypergonadism (hi-per-go´nad-iz-m) Abnormally increased physiologic activity of the gonads (testes or ovaries) with enhanced secretion of gonadal hormones, marked by growth, and precocious sexual development.

hyperhidrosis (hi-per-hi-dro´sis) Excessive perspiration.

hyperhydration (hi-per-hi-dra´shun) Excess of fluids in the body; may result from the intravenous administration of unduly large amounts of glucose solution. Also called overhydration.

hyperinsulinism (hi-per-in´su-lin-iz-m) **1.** Excessive secretion of insulin by the islets of Langerhans, causing the level of sugar in the blood to fall considerably. **2.** Insulin shock from excess dosage of insulin.

hyperkalemia (hi-per-kă-le´me-ă) An elevated potassium concentration in the blood; it may cause changes in cardiac function leading to cardiac arrest. Also called hyperpotassemia.

hyperkeratosis (hi-per-ker-ă-to´sis) Overgrowth of the horny layer of the skin.

hyperkinesis, hyperkinesia (hi-per-ki-ne´sis, hi-per-ki-ne´zhă) Abnormally increased muscular activity, as seen in some psychiatric disorders, especially in children.

hyperkinetic (hi-per-ki-net´ik) Relating to hyperkinesia.

hyperkinetic syndrome (hi-per-ki-net´ik sin´drōm) Condition marked by excessive energy, emotional instability, and short attention span; may be seen in children with attention deficit disorder, brain injury, or certain types of epilepsy. Also called hyperactivity syndrome.

hyperlactation (hi-per-lak-ta´shun) Excessive or prolonged secretion of milk.

hyperlipidemia, hyperlipemia (hi-per-lip-ĭ-de´me-ă, hi-per-lĭ-pe´me-ă) The presence of an abnormally large amount of fats in the blood. Also called lipemia; lipidemia.

hyperlipoproteinemia (hi-per-lip-o-pro-te-ne´me-ă) Disorder of fat metabolism marked by high concentrations of lipoproteins in the blood.

type I familial h. Rare disorder marked by accumulation of chylomicrons in the blood and increased cholesterol and triglyceride levels; causes fatty nodules in skin, abdominal pain, and inflammation of pancreas; an autosomal recessive inheritance.

type II familial h. A group of disorders of autosomal inheritance marked by increased plasma concentration of low-density lipoprotein (LDL), cholesterol, and phospholipids, with normal to slightly elevated levels of triglyceride; associated with fatty nodules in the Achilles, patellar, and digital extensor tendons, and susceptibility to atherosclerosis; usually detected in infants and young children.

type III familial h. A rare form considered an autosomal recessive inheritance, marked by increased plasma levels of very-low-density lipoprotein (VLDL) and cholesterol, flat, yellowish-orange fatty nodules (usually on the palmar and digital creases), glucose intolerance, and premature atherosclerosis; usually detected in young adults.

type IV familial h. Common disorder, usually detected in middle age, probably an autosomal recessive inheritance; marked by increased levels of plasma triglyceride of hepatic origin and very-low-density lipoprotein (VLDL) with normal cholesterol levels, and by a predisposition to atherosclerosis.

type V familial h. A rare form with characteristics of both type I and type IV, which include increased plasma levels of chylomicrons, very-low-density lipoprotein (VLDL), and triglycerides while on ordinary diets, with eruptive fatty nodules in the skin and recurrent acute pancreatitis; occurs chiefly during adolescence and middle age, probably as an autosomal recessive inheritance.

hyperlucent (hi-per-lo͞o´sent) Characterized by increased transmission of x rays or other forms of radiation (e.g., a darker than normal area on an x-ray film).

hyperlysinemia (hi-per-li-se-ne´me-ă) A hereditary metabolic disorder in which there is an abnormal increase of lysine in the circulating blood; associated with physical and mental retardation, anemia, hypotonia, convulsions, and impaired sexual development; autosomal recessive inheritance.

hyperlysinuria (hi-per-li-se-nu´re-ă) An abnormally high concentration of lysine in the urine.

hypermagnesemia (hi-per-mag-ne-se´me-ă) Abnormally large amount of magnesium in the blood.

hypermastia (hi-per-mas´te-ă) Overdevelopment of the mammary glands.

hypermenorrhea (hi-per-men-o-re´ă) See menorrhagia.

hypermetabolism (hi-per-mĕ-tab´o-liz-m) An unusually high metabolic rate; heat production by the body above normal, as in thyrotoxicosis.

hypermetria (hi-per-me´tre-ă) A manifestation of ataxia characterized by voluntary muscular movement overreaching the intended goal.

hypermetropia (hi-per-me-tro´pe-ă) (H) See hyperopia.

hypermorph (hi´per morf) A tall, usually slender person whose standing height is great in proportion to the sitting height, owing to very long legs.

hypermyotonia (hi-per-mi-o-to´ne-ă) Marked development of muscular tonicity.

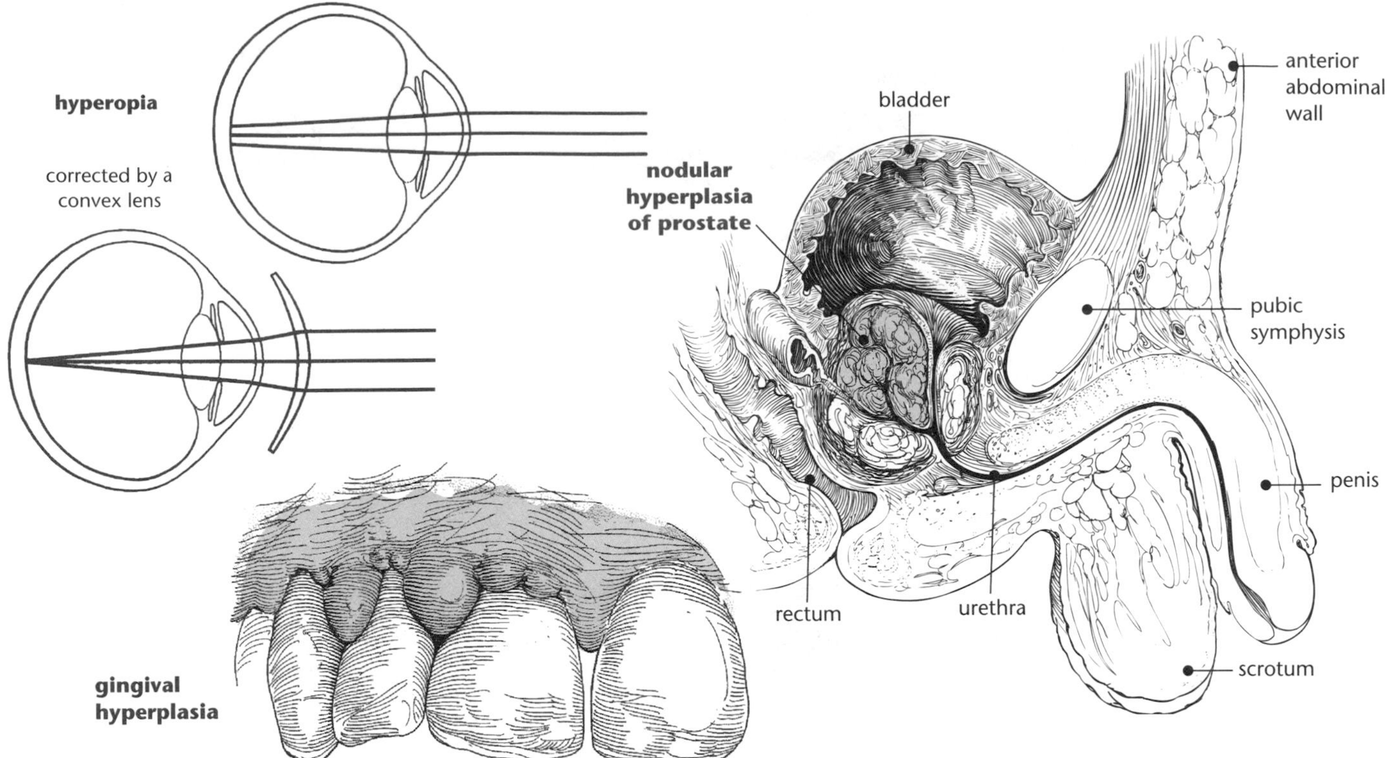

hypermyotrophy (hi-per-mi-ot´ro-fe) Marked development of muscular tissue. Also called muscular hypertrophy.

hypernatremia (hi-per-nă-tre´me-ă) Abnormally high sodium concentration in the blood.

hypernephroma (hi-per-ne-fro´mă) See renal adenocarcinoma, under adenocarcinoma.

hyperoncotic (hi-per-ong´kot-ik) Denoting an oncotic pressure higher than normal.

hyperonychia (hi-per-o-nik´e-ă) Hypertrophy of the nails.

hyperope (hi´per-ōp) One afflicted with hyperopia.

hyperopia (hi-per-o´pe-ă) A condition of the eye in which parallel light rays (rays of light from distant objects) entering the eyeball focus behind the retina, because the eyeball is short or the refractive power of the lens is weak. Also called hypermetropia; farsightedness; far sight.

latent h. (Hl) The portion of the total hyperopia that is not revealed because it is compensated for by the tonicity of the ciliary muscle.

manifest h. (Hm) The portion of the total hyperopia that may be measured by the relaxation of accommodation.

total h. (Ht) The sum of the latent and the manifest hyperopia.

hyperosmia (hi-per-oz´me-ă) An exaggerated sense of smell.

hyperosmotic (hi-per-oz-mot´ik) Having a greater concentration of osmotically active solutes than another fluid.

hyperostosis (hi-per-os-to´sis) **1.** Hypertrophy or abnormal growth of bone tissue. **2.** See exostosis.

ankylosing h. See diffuse idiopathic skeletal hyperostosis.

diffuse idiopathic skeletal h. (DISH) A degenerative joint disease, variant of osteoarthritis, characterized by ossification of ligaments along the anterior aspect of the vertebral column. Also called ankylosing hyperostosis.

h. frontalis interna Abnormal deposition of bone on the internal surface of the frontal bone.

hyperovarianism (hi-per-o-var´e-ăn-iz-m) Abnormally increased functional activity of the ovaries, usually leading to sexual precocity in young girls.

hyperoxaluria (hi-per-ok-să-lu´re-ă) An unusually large amount of oxalic acid or oxalates in the urine.

primary h. Genetic disorder affecting the metabolism of glyoxylic acid, which forms oxalate rather than glycine; becomes evident before age 10 and is a common causes of kidney stones (nephrolithiasis) and scattered kidney calcifications (nephrocalcinosis) in children.

hyperoxia (hi-per-ok´se-ă) Excessive amount of oxygen in the tissues.

hyperparathyroidism (hi-per-par-ă-thi´roid-iz-m) Excessive secretion of parathyroid hormone.

primary h. Hyperparathyroidism resulting from an adenoma in one parathyroid gland or diffuse hyperplasia of all four glands; classic laboratory findings are high serum calcium and low serum phosphate.

secondary h. Hyperparathyroidism occurring as a compensatory process carried out by slightly enlarged but otherwise normal parathyroid glands to correct a lowered serum level of calcium (as in chronic kidney disease, vitamin D deficiency, and intestinal malabsorption).

hyperpathia (hi-per-path´e-ă) Exaggerated response to pain.

hyperpepsia (hi-per-pep´se-ă) **1.** Excessive rapid digestion. **2.** Impaired digestion with hyperchlorhydria.

hyperpepsinia (hi-per-pep-sin´e-ă) Excessive secretion of pepsin in the stomach.

hyperperistalsis (hi-per-per-ĭ-stal´sis) Increase in the rate of peristalsis; peristaltic unrest; excessive rapidity of the passage of food through the stomach and intestine.

hyperphagia (hi-per-fa´jă) Overeating.

hyperphoria (hi-per-for´e-ă) Tendency of one eye to deviate upward.

hyperphosphatemia (hi-per-fos-fă-te´me-ă) Abnormally large amount of phosphates in the blood.

hyperpigmentation (hi-per-pig-men-ta´shun) Excessive coloration or pigmentation in a tissue or part.

hyperpituitarism (hi-per-pĭ-too´ĭ-tă-riz-m) Excessive production of growth hormone by the pituitary gland due to a tumor, causing gigantism in children and acromegaly in adults.

hyperplasia (hi-per-pla´zhă) The increased size of an organ or part due to the excessive but regulated increase in the number of its cells. COMPARE: neoplasm; hypertrophy.

adenomatous h. See endometrial hyperplasia.

benign prostatic h. (BPH) See nodular hyperplasia of prostate.

congenital adrenal h. (CAH) Adrenal hyperplasia with excessive secretion of androgens resulting from enzymatic defects in the biosynthesis of corticosteroids; there are four major types: a virilizing form; a sodium-losing form; one causing high blood pressure; and a 3-beta-hydroxysteroid dehydrogenase defect that may produce feminization of male genitals.

cystic h. of breast See fibrocystic change of breast, under change.

endocervical h. Development of small groups of benign, proliferating submucosal glands in the uterine cervix, usually occurring in women taking progesterone-containing oral contraceptives.

endometrial h. Hyperplasia of the uterine lining (endometrium) usually due to excessive estrogenic stimulation, especially when not opposed by progesterone secretion, causing irregular, often profuse uterine bleeding. Considered benign when there is no evidence of atypical changes in the glandular epithelium (the lining cells of the uterine glands) and, depending on the degree of glandular crowding and disordered growth pattern, may be called *simple h.* or *complex h.* Considered premalignant and designated *atypical h.* when the glandular epithelium of the hyperplastic glands exhibits cellular atypia (classified as *mild, moderate,* or *severe atypical h.).* Also called adenomatous hyperplasia; glandular hyperplasia.

fibromuscular h. Fibrosis and hyperplasia of the arterial muscular layer, usually involving the renal arteries.

gingival h. Cellular proliferation of the gingiva resulting in swelling.

glandular h. See endometrial hyperplasia.

nodular h. of prostate Enlargement of the prostate with formation of large nodules that may press against the urethra and obstruct the flow of urine; a common disorder of men over 50 years of age. Also called benign prostatic hyperplasia; benign prostatic hypertrophy (a misnomer).

hyperplastic (hi-per-plas´tik) Relating to or characterized by hyperplasia.

hyperpnea (hi-perp-ne´ă) Abnormally rapid and deep breathing.

hyperpolarization (hi-per-po-lar-ĭ-za´shun) An increase in the positive charges normally present at the surface of a nerve cell membrane.

hyperpotassemia (hi-per-po-tă-se´me-ă) See hyperkalemia.

hyperprebetalipoproteinemia (hi-per-pre-ba-tă-lip-o-pro-te-ne´me-ă) See type IV familial hyperlipoproteinemia, under hyperlipoproteinemia.

hyperprolactinemia (hi-per-pro-lak-tin-e´me-ă) Increased amounts of prolactin in the blood; normal only during lactation; may be caused by certain medications or some pituitary tumors.

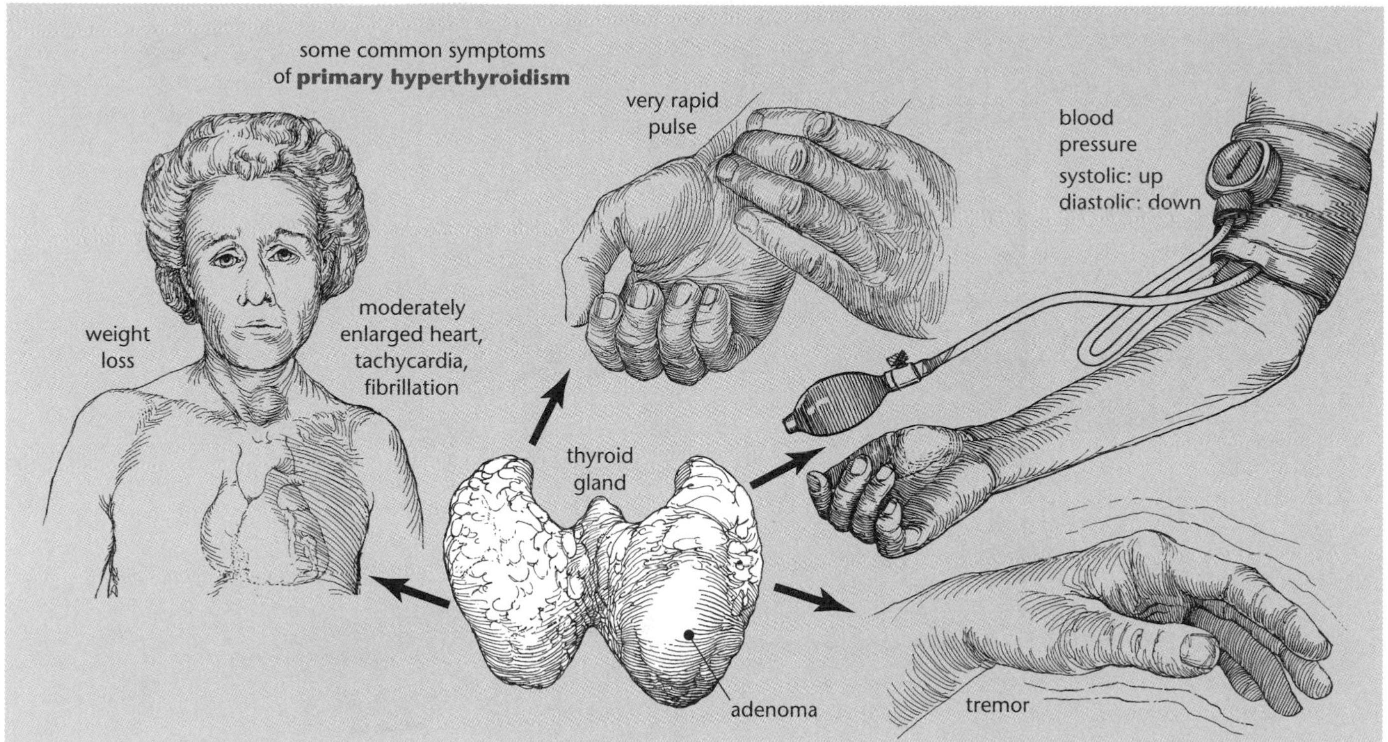

hyperprolinemia (hi-per-pro-lĭ-ne´me-ă) An inherited metabolic disorder marked by increased proline in the plasma and excretion of proline, hydroxyproline, and glycine.

hyperproteinemia (hi-per-pro-te-ne´me-ă) The presence of excessive protein in the blood.

hyperptyalism (hi-per-ti´al-iz-m) See hypersialosis.

hyperpyretic (hi-per-pi-ret´ik) Relating to high fever. Also called hyperpyrexial.

hyperpyrexia (hi-per-pi-rek´se-ă) Extremely high fever, usually 105.0°F or more.

hyperpyrexial (hi-per-pi-rek´se-al) See hyperpyretic.

hyperreflexia (hi-per-re-flek´se-ă) Exaggerated deep tendon reflexes.

hyperresonance (hi-per-rez´o-nans) An extreme or exaggerated degree of resonance on percussion as heard in pulmonary emphysema.

hypersecretion (hi-per-se-kre´shun) Excessive secretion.

hypersensitive (hi-per-sen´sĭ-tiv) Overreactive to a stimulus.

hypersensitivity (hi-per-sen-sĭ-tiv´ĭ-te) **1.** The altered reactivity to a substance, which can result in pathologic reactions upon subsequent exposure to that particular substance. Also called allergy. **2.** Excessive response to a stimulus.

delayed-type h. (DHT) T cell mediated immune reactivity to an antigen applied topically or injected subcutaneously; cellular infiltration and swelling are maximal at about 48 hours.

hypersensitization (hi-per-sen-sĭ-ti-za´shŭn) The process of creating an abnormally sensitive state.

hypersialosis (hi-per-si-ă-lo´sis) Excessive secretion of saliva. Also called hyperptyalism.

hypersomatotropism (hi-per-so-mat-o-trop´iz-m) Abnormally increased secretion of pituitary growth hormone.

hypersomia (hi-per-so´me-ă) Gigantism.

hypersomnia (hi-per-som´ne-ă) Abnormal condition in which the individual sleeps for excessive periods of time.

hypersonic (hi-per-son´ik) Relating to speeds equal to or exceeding five times the speed of sound (speeds less than hypersonic but greater than the speed of sound are called supersonic).

hypersplenism (hi-per-splen´iz-m) A disorder in which the formed elements of the blood are destroyed by the excessively increased activity of the spleen; it may result in anemia, neutropenia, thrombocytopenia, or a combination of these states.

hypersteatosis (hi-per-ste-ă-to´sis) Excessive sebaceous secretion.

hypertelorism (hi-per-te´lor-iz-m) Abnormally increased distance between paired organs or parts.

ocular h. Developmental malformation marked by enlarged sphenoid bone, causing extreme distance between the eyes; seen in craniofacial dysostosis.

hypertensin (hi-per-ten´sin) See angiotensin.

hypertensinogen (hi-per-ten-sin´o-jen) See angiotensinogen.

hypertension (hi-per-ten´shun) High arterial blood pressure; in adults, usually defined as pressures exceeding 140/90 mmHg.

accelerated h. A significant recent blood pressure increase occurring over previous hypertensive levels; blood vessel damage can be observed in the fundus of the eye.

essential h. Hypertension without a known cause. Also called idiopathic hypertension; primary hypertension.

high-normal h. Blood pressure in the range of 130–139 / 85–89 mmHg. Formerly called borderline hypertension.

idiopathic h. See essential hypertension.

malignant h. Severe hypertension that causes degenerative changes in the walls of the blood vessels throughout the body; hemorrhages occur in the retina, the kidney, and other areas; cerebral function is altered.

portal h. Increased pressure in the portal venous system; it may result from: intrahepatic causes, such as cirrhosis of the liver; suprahepatic causes, such as heart failure; infrahepatic causes, such as portal vein thrombosis.

primary h. See essential hypertension.

pulmonary h. Hypertension in the pulmonary circulation resulting from primary lung disease (e.g., fibrosis of the lung) or from heart disease (e.g., mitral stenosis).

renal h. Hypertension secondary to kidney disease.

renovascular h. Hypertension caused by obstruction of blood flow to the kidney.

hypertensive (hi-per-ten´siv) Marked by or afflicted with high blood pressure.

hyperthecosis (hi-per-the-ko´sis) Hyperplasia of the theca cells of the vesicular ovarian (graafian) follicles.

hyperthelia (hi-per-the´le-ă) See polythelia.

hyperthermia (hi-per-ther´me-ă) Extremely high body temperature.

hyperthrombinemia (hi-per-throm-bĭ-ne´me-ă) The presence of excessive thrombin in the blood.

hyperthymia (hi-per-thi´me-ă) State of increased emotivity or overactivity.

hyperthyroidism (hi-per-thi´roi-diz-m) Condition caused by excessive production or ingestion of thyroid hormone; the most common symptoms include weight loss, increased appetite, rapid heart rate, tremor, and fatigue; when exophthalmos is present, the disease is known as exophthalmic goiter.

primary h. A form originating within the thyroid gland.

secondary h. A form caused by abnormal stimulation of the thyroid gland due to a disorder of the pituitary gland.

hypertonia (hi-per-to´ne-ă) Excessive tension of the muscles or arteries.

hypertonic (hi-per-ton´ik) **1.** Characterized by abnormally increased tension. **2.** Having the greater osmotic pressure of two solutions; frequently, the comparison is to the osmotic concentration of plasma.

hypertonicity (hi-per-to-nis´ĭ-te) The state of being hypertonic.

hypertrichosis, hypertrichiasis (hi-per-tri-ko´sis, hi-per-tri-ki´ă-sis) Growth of hair in excess of normal for that particular area of the body (e.g., the face in women).

hypertriglyceridemia (hi-per-tri-glis-ĕ-ri-de´me-ă) Excessive concentration of triglyceride in the blood.

familial h. Any one of two heritable forms of the disease: (a) exogenous or fat-induced, occurring after meals of normal or high lipid content; (b) endogenous or carbohydrate-induced, occurring after meals rich in carbohydrates.

hypertrophy (hi-per´tro-fe) The enlargement of an organ or part due to the increase in size of the cells composing it; the overgrowth meets a demand for increased functional activity. COMPARE: neoplasm; hyperplasia.

adaptive h. Thickening of the walls of a hollow organ, such as the urinary bladder, when the outflow is obstructed.

asymmetrical septal h. (ASH) See idiopathic hypertrophic subaortic stenosis, under stenosis.

compensatory h. of the heart Thickening of the walls of the heart, occurring when a chamber must pump against an increased resistance (e.g., valvular disease or in hypertension), thus increasing the power of the heart to compensate for the increased resistance.

concentric h. Thickening of the walls of a hollow organ with little or no change in the size of its cavity;

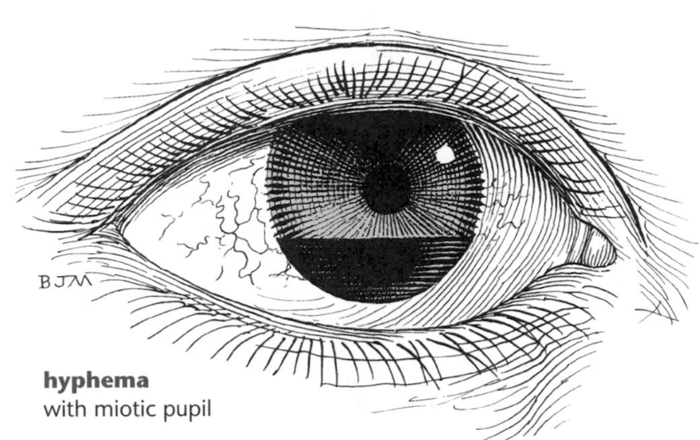

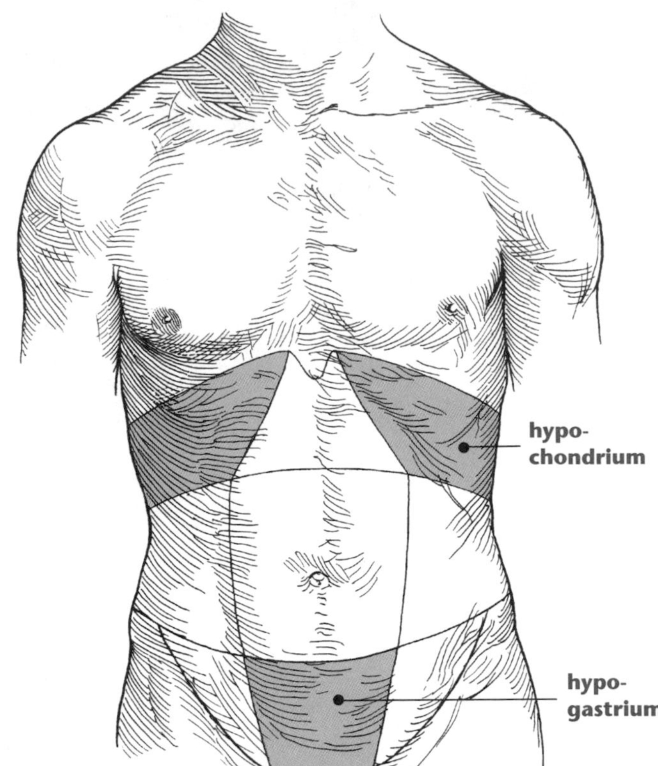

seen in left ventricular hypertrophy associated with essential hypertension or aortic stenosis.

eccentric h. Enlargement of the walls of a hollow organ as well as its cavity; seen in left ventricular hypertrophy of volume overload, as in aortic or mitral regurgitation.

left ventricular h. Hypertrophy of the muscle of the left ventricle of the heart.

physiologic h. Temporary hypertrophy of an organ to meet the demand of a natural increase in functional activity, as in the female breast during pregnancy and lactation.

right ventricular h. Hypertrophy of the muscle of the right ventricle of the heart.

ventricular h. Hypertrophy of the muscular wall of either the right (RVH) or the left (LVH) ventricle of the heart.

vicarious h. Hypertrophy of an organ due to dysfunction of another organ of allied activity.

hypertropia (hi-per-troʹpe-ă) Upward deviation of one eye not controllable by fixational efforts; unlike hyperphoria, the condition is continuous.

hyperuricemia (hi-per-u-rĭ-seʹme-ă) Excess of uric acid in the blood.

hyperuricosuria, hyperuricuria (hi-per-u-rĭ-ko-suʹre-ă, hi-per-u-rĭ-seʹme-ă) Excretion of excessive amounts of uric acid in the urine.

hyperventilation (hi-per-ven-tĭ-laʹshŭn) A condition marked by fast deep breathing, which tends to remove increased amounts of carbon dioxide from the body and lower the partial pressure of the gas, causing buzzing in the ears, tingling of the lips and fingers, and sometimes fainting. Also called over-ventilation.

central neural h. A pattern of irregular hyper-ventilation, usually seen in comatose individuals with a midbrain lesion.

hyperventilation syndrome (hi-per-ven-tĭ-la ʹshŭn sinʹdrōm) A syndrome that is almost always a manifestation of acute anxiety, characterized by difficult, deep, and rapid respiration accompanied by tightness of the chest and a feeling of suffocation; lightheadedness is commonly present and tingling of the hands may appear as a result of marked diminution of carbon dioxide in the blood (hypocapnia), produced by the excessive respiration; it may last half an hour or longer and may recur a few times a day; the attacks may be controlled somewhat by breath-holding or breathing in a paper bag.

hyperviscosity syndrome (hi-per-vis-kosʹĭ-te) Visual impairment, neurologic problems, spontaneous bleeding, sluggish blood flow, and organ congestion consequent to increased blood viscosity.

hypervitaminosis (hi-per-vi-tă-mĭ-noʹsis) Condition caused by ingestion of excessive amounts of a vitamin preparation.

hypervolemia (hi-per-vo-leʹme-ă) Abnormal increase in the volume of blood, as seen during pregnancy and in some cases of hydatidiform mole.

hypesthesia (hīp-es-theʹzhă) See hypoesthesia.

hypha (hiʹfă), *pl.* **hyphae** One of the hairlike structures forming the substance of a fungus.

hyphema, hyphemia (hi-feʹmă, hi-feʹme-ă) Collection of blood in the anterior chamber of the eye.

hyphidrosis (hīp-hi-droʹsis) Diminished or deficient perspiration; abnormally scanty perspiration.

hypnagogic (hipʹnă-goj-ik) **1.** Denoting the transitional state produced by sleep, such as mental images occurring just before sleep. **2.** Inducing sleep. Also called hypnotic.

hypnagogue (hipʹnă-gog) An agent that induces sleep.

hypnoanalysis (hip-no-ă-nalʹĭ-sis) Psychoanalysis conducted while the patient is under hypnosis.

hypnogenesis (hip-no-jenʹĕ-sis) The process of inducing sleep or a hypnotic state.

hypnology (hip-nolʹŏ-je) The study of sleep or hypnosis.

hypnophobia (hip-no-foʹbe-ă) Abnormal fear of falling asleep.

hypnopompic (hip-no-pomʹpik) Relating to the partially conscious state between the stages of sleep and complete awakening.

hypnosis (hip-noʹsis) An artificially induced state in which the individual becomes receptive to the hypnotist's suggestions; it may vary in degree from mild suggestibility to a deep sleeplike state with total surgical anesthesia.

hypnotherapy (hip-no-therʹă-pe) Treatment using hypnosis.

hypnotic (hip-notʹik) **1.** A drug that depresses the central nervous system (CNS), inducing a state that resembles natural sleep. COMPARE: sedative. **2.** Relating to hypnosis.

hypnotism (hipʹno-tiz-m) **1.** The practice of inducing hypnosis. **2.** Hypnosis.

hypnotist (hipʹno-tist) One who induces hypnosis.

hypnotize (hipʹno-tīz) To put into a hypnotic state.

hypo (hiʹpo) **1.** A popular designation for hypodermic injection. **2.** See sodium thiosulfate, under sodium.

hypoacidity (hi-po-ă-sidʹĭ-te) Deficiency of normal acidity. Also called subacidity.

hypoacusis (hi-po-ă-kuʹsis) See hypacusis.

hypoadrenalism (hi-po-ă-dreʹnal-iz-m) Reduced or deficient adrenocortical function.

hypoadrenocorticism (hi-po-ă-dre-no-korʹtĭ-siz-m) Abnormally low secretion of hormones of the adrenal cortex.

hypoadrenocortism (hi-po-ă-dre-no-korʹtĭz-m) Hypoadrenocorticism.

hypoalbuminemia (hi-po-al-bu-min-eʹme-ă) Abnormally low concentration of albumin in the blood.

hypoalimentation (hi-po-al-ĭ-men-taʹshun) Insufficient nourishment.

hypobaric (hi-po-barʹik) Relating to or occurring at pressures less than atmospheric pressure.

hypobaropathy (hi-po-bar-opʹă-the) Condition caused by greatly reduced air pressure and decreased oxygen intake. See also altitude sickness, under sickness.

hypocalcemia (hi-po-kal-seʹme-ă) A marked reduction of calcium in the blood.

hypocalcification (hi-po-kal-sĭ-fĭ-kaʹshun) Diminished calcification, especially of tooth enamel, producing opaque white spots.

hereditary enamel h. A hereditary defect of tooth enamel development affecting the primary and secondary teeth; it causes a breaking off of the enamel after tooth eruption, exposing the dentin, which gives the teeth a yellow appearance.

hypocapnia (hi-po-kapʹne-ă) Marked diminution in the amount of carbon dioxide in the blood. Also called acapnia.

hypochloremia (hi-po-klor-eʹme-ă) A marked reduction of chloride in the blood.

hypochlorhydria (hi-po-klor-hiʹdre-ă) Abnormally low amount of hydrochloric acid in the gastric juice.

hypochlorite (hi-po-klorʹīt) A salt of hypochlorous acid.

hypochlorous acid (hi-po-klorʹus asʹid) An unstable acid, HOCl; used as a bleach and disinfectant.

hypocholesterolemia (hi-po-ko-les-tĕ-reʹme-ă) An abnormally small amount of cholesterol in the blood.

hypochondria (hi-po-konʹdre-ă) See hypochondriasis.

hypochondriac (hi-po-konʹdre-ak) An individual afflicted with hypochondriasis.

hypochondriasis (hi-po-kon-driʹă-sis) The persistent neurotic preoccupation with one's health

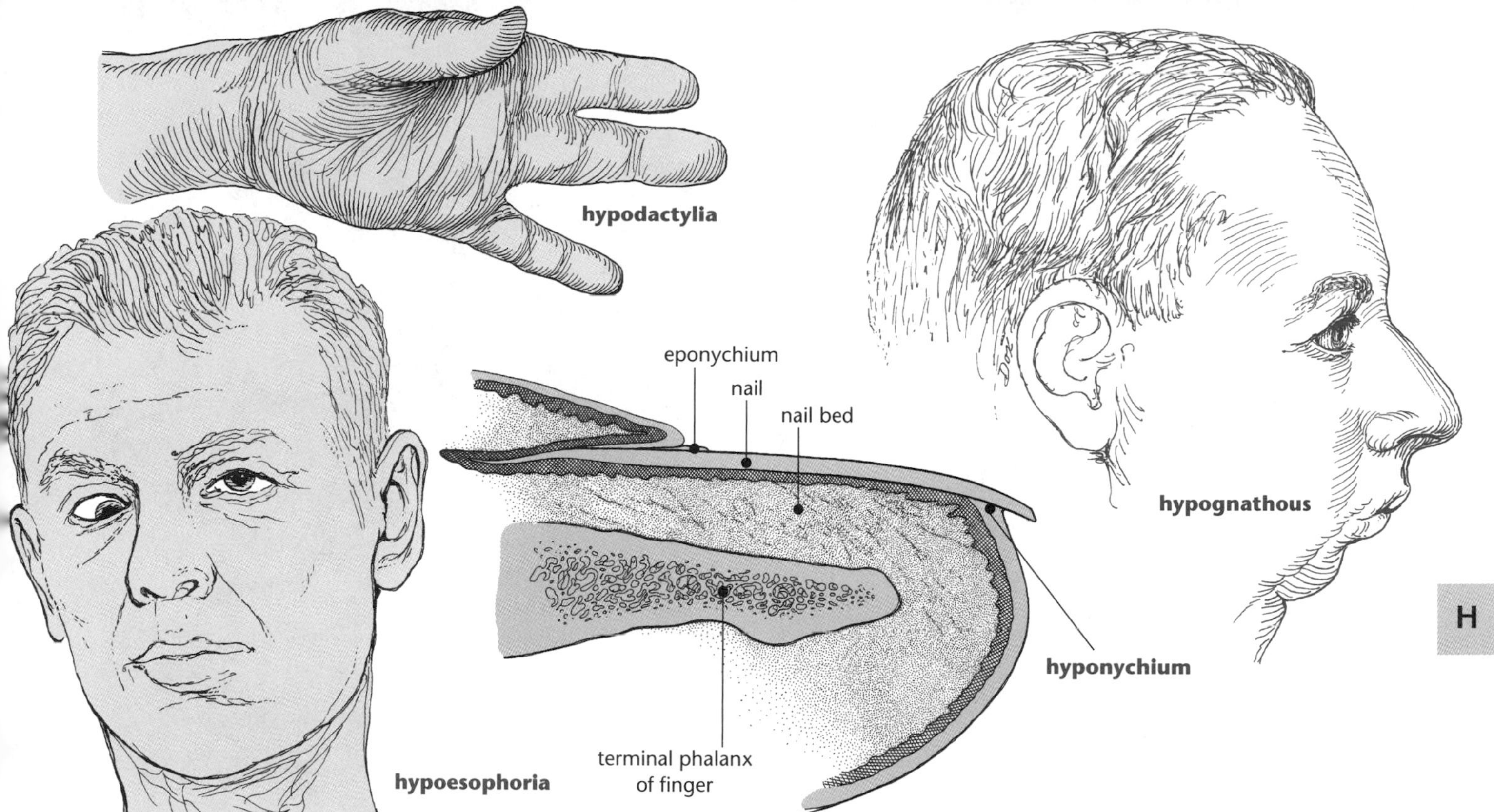

and fear of presumed diseases that persist despite reassurances; an exaggerated concern over physical health in absence of organic disease. Also called hypochondria.

hypochondrium (hi-po-kon´dre-um) Any of two lateral regions of the upper zone of the abdomen.

hypochromatic (hi-po-kro-mat´ik) Containing a small amount of pigment, or less than the normal amount for the individual tissue; abnormally deficient pigmentation.

hypochromemia (hi-po-kro-me´me-ă) Anemia characterized by an abnormally low color index of the blood.

hypochromia (hi-po-kro´me-ă) Abnormal decrease in the hemoglobin content of red blood cells.

hypochromic (hi-po-kro´mik) **1.** Having less than the normal amount of pigment. **2.** Relating to a decrease in light absorption.

hypochylia (hi-po-ki´le-ă) Abnormally low amount of chyle.

hypocomplementemia (hi-po-kom-plĕ-men-te´me-ă) A condition of the blood characterized by a lack, or decreased activity, of complement or any of the complement components of blood; may be hereditary or acquired. The condition has been postulated to be a factor in increased susceptibility to certain infections.

hypocorticism (hi-po-kor´tĭ-siz-m) See adrenocortical insufficiency, under insufficiency.

hypocorticoidism (hi-po-kor-tĭ-koi´diz-m) See adrenocortical insufficiency, under insufficiency.

hypocupremia (hi-po-ku-pre´me-ă) Abnormally low concentration of copper in the blood.

hypodactylia, hypodactyly (hi-po-dak-til´e-ă, hi-po-dak´tĭ-le) The presence of less than the normal number of digits on the hand or foot.

hypodermic (hi-po-der´mik) See subcutaneous.

hypodermis, hypoderm (hi-po-der´mis, hi´po-derm) See subcutaneous fascia, under fascia.

hypodermoclysis (hi-po-der-mok´lĭ-sis) The infusion of fluid into the subcutaneous space.

hypodontia (hi-po-don´shă) Congenital absence of one or more teeth. Also called oligodontia.

hypodynamia (hi-po-di-na´me-ă) Markedly diminished power.

hypodynamic (hi-po-di-nam´ik) Denoting diminished force, as of muscular contraction.

hypoechoic (hi-po-ĕ-ko´ik) In ultrasonography, producing fewer or weaker echoes.

hypoesophoria (hi-po-es-o-for´e-ă) Combined downward (hypophoria) and inward (esophoria) deviation of the eyeball.

hypoesthesia (hi-po-es-the´zhă) Abnormally decreased sensitiveness of the skin. Also called hypesthesia.

hypofibrinogenemia (hi-po-fi-brin-o-jĕ-ne´me-ă) Deficiency of fibrinogen in the blood, usually below 100 mg%; may occur in amniotic fluid embolism, fetal death, abruptio placentae, and occasionally intra-amniotic instillation of hypertonic saline.

hypofunction (hi-po-funk´shun) Diminished or inadequate functioning of an organ or part.

hypogalactia (hi-po-gă-lak´she-ă) Insufficient milk production.

hypogammaglobulinemia (hi-po-gam-ă-glob-u-lĭ-ne´me-ă) Lack of gamma globulin in the blood; a deficiency state manifested by recurrent infections; primary forms result from diminished rates of synthesis; secondary forms result from increased catabolism.

hypogastrium (hi-po-gas´tre-um) The middle region of the lower zone of the abdomen.

hypogenitalism (hi-po-jen´ĭ-tal-iz-m) Underdevelopment of the genitalia.

hypogeusia (hi-po-goo´zhă) Diminished sensitivity to taste.

hypoglossal (hi-po-glos´al) Located beneath the tongue.

hypoglottis (hi-po-glot´is) The undersurface of the tongue.

hypoglycemia (hi-po-gli-se´me-ă) A condition marked by lower than normal level of sugar (glucose) in the blood; characterized clinically by sweating, trembling, palpitation, hunger, weakness, and lightheadedness; the symptoms may vary in duration and often disappear rapidly after eating a snack or a sweet, or drinking a glass of milk; may result from excessive production of insulin by the pancreas or excessive administration of insulin to a diabetic person.

hypoglycemic (hi-po-gli-se´mik) **1.** Relating to hypoglycemia. **2.** An agent that tends to reduce the sugar (glucose) level in the blood.

hypognathous (hi-pog´nă-thus) Having an underdeveloped lower jaw.

hypogonadism (hi-po-go´nad-iz-m) Insufficient hormone secretion or defective response to hormonal activity by the target tissues. In immature individuals, it leads to decreased physical development of sexual characteristics.

h. with anosmia A genetic disorder, usually in males, associated with loss of the sense of smell due to failure of development of olfactory lobes; X-linked inheritance. Also called Kallmann's syndrome.

hypergonadotropic h. Hypogonadism occurring in spite of the presence of elevated levels of gonadotropins; may be due to defective steroid receptors in target tissues.

hypogonadotropic h. Hypogonadism resulting from insufficient pituitary secretion of gonadotropins.

testicular h. Condition caused by a decrease of the internal secretion of the testis, marked by the loss of secondary sexual characteristics.

hypohidrosis (hi-po-hi-dro´sis) Abnormally reduced perspiration.

hypokalemia (hi-po-ka-le´me-ă) Abnormally low level of potassium in the blood; may result in nephropathy, muscle weakness, gastric atony, paralysis of the muscles of respiration, and arrhythmias. Also called hypopotassemia.

hypokinemia (hi-po-ki-ne´me-ă) Abnormally reduced cardiac output; reduced circulation rate.

hypokinesia (hi-po-ki-ne´zhă) Diminished movement.

hypomagnesemia (hi-po-mag-nĕ-se´me-ă) Abnormally low concentration of magnesium in the blood.

hypomania (hi-po-ma´ne-ă) A moderate form of manic activity, usually marked by slightly abnormal elation and overactivity.

hypomastia (hi-po-mas´te-ă) Abnormal smallness of the breasts.

hypomenorrhea (hi-po-men-o-re´ă) Scanty menstrual flow, possibly with shortening of the duration of the menstrual period.

hypometabolism (hi-po-mĕ-tab´o-liz-m) Reduced metabolism.

hypometria (hi-po-me´tre-ă) Loss of power of muscular coordination manifested by failure to reach an intended goal; decreased range of voluntary movements.

hypomorph (hi´po-morf) **1.** A person who has short legs. **2.** In genetics, a mutant gene that acts in the same direction as the normal allele, but at a lower level of effectiveness.

hyponatremia (hi-po-nă-tre´me-ă) Low concentration of sodium in the blood.

hyponychial (hi-po-nik´e-al) Relating to the hyponychium.

hyponychium (hi-po-nik´e-um) The thickened horny zone of the epidermis beneath the free border of the nail.

hypo-ovarianism (hi-po o-va´re-an-iz-m) Diminished secretion of ovarian hormones.

hypoparathyroidism (hi-po-par-ă-thi´roid-iz-m)

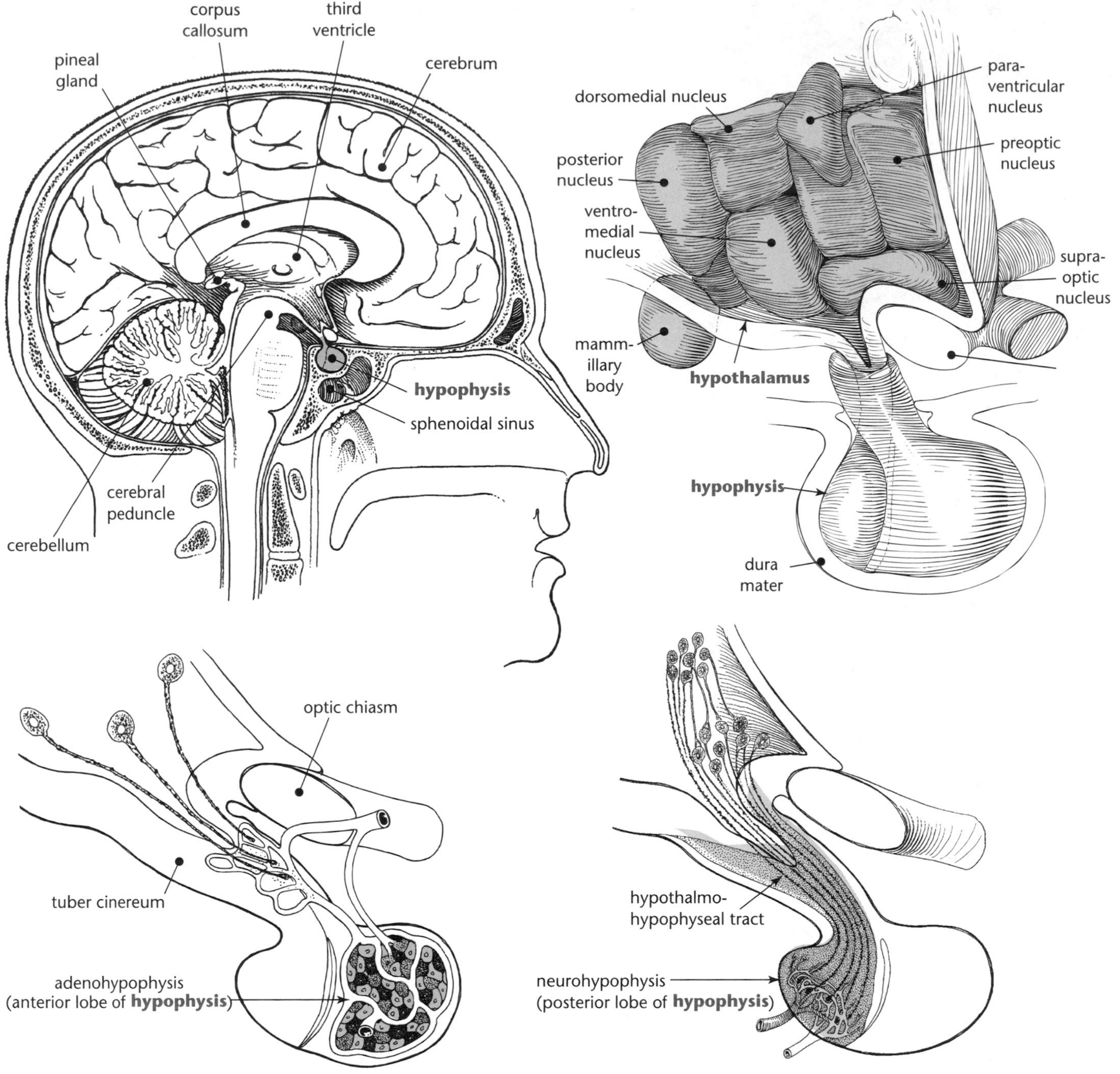

Condition caused by lack of parathyroid secretion, resulting in reduced plasma calcium level and increased plasma phosphate level.

hypophalangism (hi-po-fă-lan´jiz-m) Congenital absence of a phalanx on a finger or toe.

hypophoria (hi-po-for´e-ă) Latent condition in which one eye tends to deviate downward.

hypophosphatasia (hi-po-fos-fă-ta´zhă) Lack of alkaline phosphatase in the blood; a rare inherited disorder characterized by rickets and osteomalacia.

hypophosphatemia (hi-po-fos-fă-te´me-ă) Deficiency of phosphate in the blood.

hypophyseal (hi-pof-ĭ-ze-al, hi-po-fiz´e-al) Relating to the hypophysis (pituitary gland). Also spelled hypophysial.

hypophysectomize (hi-po-fiz-ek´to-mīz) To remove or destroy the hypophysis (pituitary gland).

hypophysectomy (hi-pof-ĭ-sek´tŏ-me) Surgical removal of the hypophysis (pituitary gland).

hypophysial, (hi-pof-ĭ-ze´al, hi-po-fiz´e-al) See hypophyseal.

hypophysis (hi-pof´ĭ-sis) A gland of internal secretion situated in the hypophysial fossa of the sphenoid bone, attached to the base of the brain by a short stalk; it consists of two main parts, anterior lobe (adenohypophysis) and posterior lobe (neurohypophysis); its secretions are of vital importance to growth, maturation, and reproduction. Also called pituitary gland.

hypopituitarism (hi-po-pĭ-too´ĭ-tă-riz-m) A condition due to abnormally diminished production of anterior pituitary hormones; caused by destruction of the pituitary gland; it leads to atrophy of the thyroid and adrenal glands and the gonads.

hypoplasia (hi-po-pla´zhă) Defective or incomplete development of an organ or a part.

hypoplastic (hi-po-plas´tik) Relating to or characterized by hypoplasia.

hypopnea (hi-pop´ne-ă) Abnormally shallow breathing.

hypopotassemia (hi-po-pot-ă-se´me-ă) See hypokalemia.

hypoproteinemia (hi-po-pro-te-ne´me-ă) Abnormally small amounts of protein in the blood.

hypoproteinosis (hi-po-pro-tēn-o´sis) Dietary deficiency of protein.

hypoprothrombinemia (hi-po-pro-throm-bĭ-ne´me-ă) Deficiency of prothrombin (blood clotting factor II) in the blood.

hypopyon (hi-po´pe-on) The presence of pus in the anterior chamber of the eye, secondary to inflammation of the cornea, iris, or ciliary body.

hyporeflexia (hi-po-re-flek´se-ă) A condition of weakened reflexes.

hyporeninemia (hi-po-re-nin-e´me-ă) Low levels of the enzyme renin in the blood.

hyporiboflavinosis (hi-po-ri-bo-fla-vin-o´sis) Disease caused by insufficient intake of riboflavin. Also called ariboflavinosis.

hyposalivation (hi-po-sal-ĭ-va´shun) Diminished flow of saliva.

hyposensitivity (hi-po-sen-sĭ-tiv´ĭ-te) The condition of less than normal sensitivity; one in which the response to a stimulus is unusually delayed or lessened in degree.

hyposensitization (hi-po-sen-sĭ-ti-za´shun) See desensitization (1).

hyposmia (hi-poz´me-ă) Reduced sense of smell. Also called hyposphresia.

hypospadias (hi-po-spa´de-as) A congenital defect in the male in which the urethra opens on the undersurface of the penis; it occurs in approximately 1 in 500 births; there is also a similar defect in the female in which the urethra opens into the vagina.

hypostasis (hi-pos´tă-sis) **1.** A sediment or deposit.

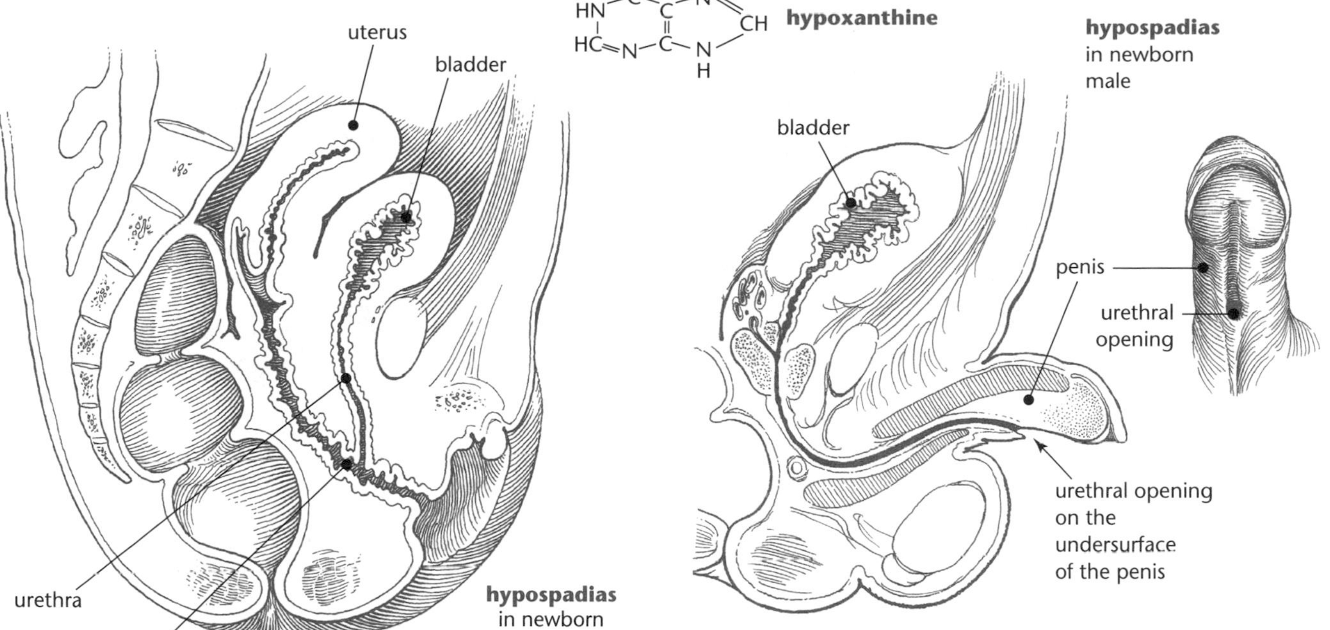

2. Blood congestion in a part.

hyposthenia (hi-pos-the´ne-ă) A weakened state; decrease or lack of strength.

hyposthenuria (hi-pos-thĕ-nu´re-ă) Impairment of ability to concentrate the urine.

hypostosis (hip-os-to´sis) Inadequate development of bone.

hyposulfite (hi-po-sul´fīt) See sodium thiosulfate, under sodium.

hypotaxia (hi-po-tak´se-ă) Condition marked by imperfect coordination.

hypotelorism (hi-po-tel´ŏ-riz-m) Abnormally small distance between two organs or parts such as the eyes.

hypotension (hi-po-ten´shun) Abnormally low blood pressure.

orthostatic h. Hypotension occurring upon arising suddenly from a recumbent position or when standing still. Also called postural hypotension.

postural h. Orthostatic hypotension.

hypotensive (hi-po-ten´siv) Marked by or causing low blood pressure.

hypothalamus (hi-po-thal´ă-mus) A deep-lying part of the brain situated just below the thalamus; it forms the floor and part of the lateral walls of the third ventricle; it includes the mammillary bodies, tuber cinereum, infundibulum, and the optic chiasm; the hypothalamic nuclei are concerned with visceral control (e.g., regulation of water balance and body temperature).

hypothenar (hi-poth´ĕ-nar) The fleshy portion of the palm of the hand, at its medial side.

hypothermal (hi-po-ther´mal) Relating to a body temperature below normal.

hypothermia (hi-po-ther´me-ă) Abnormally low body temperature, usually below 97°F (36°C).

hypothesis (hi-poth´ĕ-sis) A tentative theory subject to verification.

Lyon h. The concept that in each somatic cell of normal females only one of the two X-chromosomes is active during interphase; as inactivation of the other X-chromosome takes place randomly, females heterozygous for an X-linked mutant gene may show patches of tissue with the phenotype of the mutant gene while the majority of tissue remains normal.

Michaelis-Menten h. The assumption that an intermediate complex is formed between an enzyme and its substrate; it is further assumed that the complex decomposes to yield free enzyme and the reaction products, and that the latter rate determines the over-all rate of substrate-product conversion.

null h. The assumption that the results of a study, experiment, or test are no different than what could have occurred as a result of chance alone.

sequence h. The concept that the amino acid sequence of a protein is determined by a particular sequence of nucleotides in a definite portion of the DNA of the organism producing the protein.

sliding filament h. The assumption that a contracting muscle shortens because two sets of filaments slide past each other.

Starling's h. The rate of fluid exchange between extracapillary tissue and capillary depends on the hydrostatic and osmotic pressures on both sides of the capillary wall, considering the wall as a semi-permeable membrane.

zwitter h. The supposition that an ampholytic molecule (i.e., that behaves as an acid and as a base) yields, in an electrically neutral condition, equal numbers of basic and acid ions, thus becoming an ion (zwitter ion) with an equal number of positive and negative charges.

hypothrombinemia (hi-po-throm-bĭ-ne´me-ă) Abnormally small amount of thrombin in the blood, resulting in a tendency to bleed.

hypothyroid (hi-po-thi´roid) **1.** Manifested by reduced thyroid function. **2.** A person afflicted with hypothyroidism.

hypothyroidism (hi-po-thi´roid-iz-m) Condition caused by deficient production of thyroid hormone, characterized by a lessened rate of metabolism; clinical features may include cold intolerance, dry skin, hair loss, puffy face, constipation, slow speech, slow heart rate, and retarded mentality; when present at birth it causes cretinism; the severe form is known as myxedema.

hypotonia (hi-po-to´ne-ă) Lack of muscle tone.

ocular h. Abnormally low tension in the eyeball.

hypotonic (hi-po-ton´ik) **1.** Having an abnormally reduced tension. **2.** Having the lesser osmotic pressure of two solutions, usually compared to the osmotic concentration of plasma.

hypotoxicity (hi-po-tok-sis´ĭ-te) Reduced toxicity.

hypotrichosis (hi-po-trĭ-ko´sis) Scanty hair on the head and body. Also called oligotrichosis.

hypotropia (hi-po-tro´pe-ă) Downward deviation of one eye not controllable by fixational efforts; unlike hypophoria, the condition is constant.

hypoventilation (hi-po-ven-tĭ-la´shun) Reduced quantity of air entering the lungs.

hypovitaminosis (hi-po-vi-tă min-o´sis) Condition marked by deficiency of one or more essential vitamins.

hypovolemia (hi-po-vo-le´me-ă) Markedly diminished blood volume.

hypovolia (hi-po-vo´le-ă) Reduced water content of a particular compartment.

hypoxanthine (hi-po-zan´thēn) A purine present in muscles and other tissues; normally metabolized to uric acid by oxidation, after first being oxidized to xanthine. Also called 6-hydroxypurine.

hypoxemia (hi-pok-se´me-ă) Abnormally low content of oxygen in arterial blood.

hypoxia (hi-pok´se-ă) Abnormal reduction of oxy-gen in body tissues. Also called oxygen deficiency.

cell h. Decreased oxygen content at the cellular level.

hypsarrhythmia (hip-să-rith´me-ă) Abnormal chaotic encephalogram sometimes observed in infants with spasms.

hysteralgia (his-ter-al´jă) Pain or discomfort in the uterus. Also called hysterodynia.

hysteratresia (his-ter-ă-tre´zhă) Pathologic closure of the uterine cavity.

hysterectomy (his-ter-ek´tŏ-me) Removal of the uterus.

abdominal h. Removal of the uterus through an incision in the abdominal wall.

cesarean h. Delivery of a baby through an abdominal and uterine incision, followed by removal of the uterus through the abdominal incision.

extended h. Hysterectomy classified into five progressively expanding procedures: *Class I,* removal of all cervical tissue; *class II,* includes removal of medial half of cardinal and uterosacral ligaments, and upper third of vagina; *class III,* includes removal of the entire cardinal and utero-sacral ligaments, and upper third of vagina; *class IV,* includes removal of all connective tissue adjacent to the ureters, the superior vesical artery, and three-fourths of the vagina; *class V,* includes removal of the bladder and distal portions of the ureters.

laparoscopically assisted vaginal h. (LAVH) Operation devised to reduce the morbidity of major gynecologic surgery by converting an abdominal procedure into a vaginal one. Begins with evaluation of the pelvic viscera through a laparoscope to treat conditions that would have precluded the vaginal approach; then the hysterectomy is completed vaginally.

Meigs h. See modified radical hysterectomy.

modified radical h. Procedure for early cervical cancer with minimal stromal involvement (i.e., less than 3 mm deep); usually includes removal of the uterus, vaginal cuff, medial half of the uterosacral ligaments, and pelvic lymph nodes below the level of

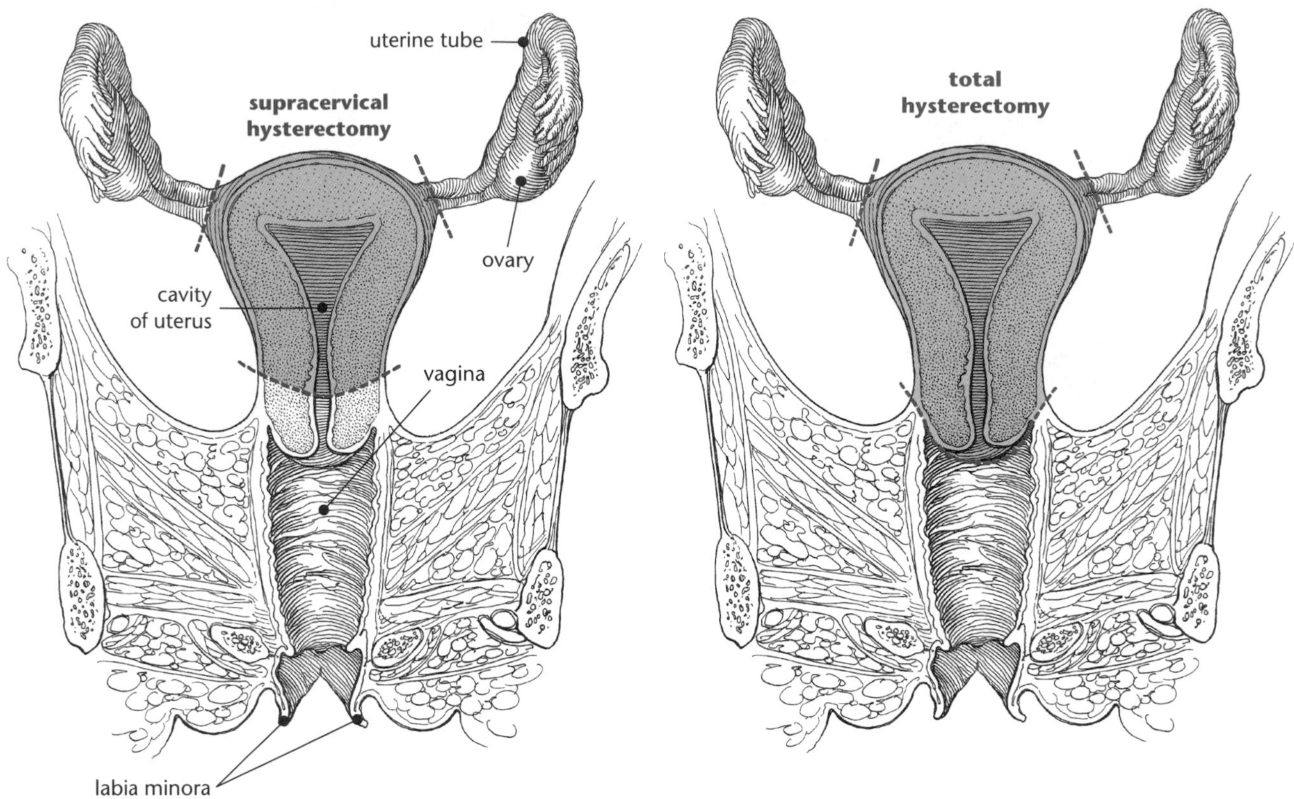

the ovaries; the ovaries and fallopian tubes may or may not be removed. The extent of tissue removed is tailored to the specific condition of the patient. Also called Meigs hysterectomy; Okabayashi hysterectomy; Wertheim hysterectomy.

Okabayashi h. See modified radical hysterectomy.

radical h. Removal of the uterus, upper third of vagina, entire uterosacral and uterovesical ligaments, connective tissue surrounding the uterus, fallopian tubes, ovaries, and all pelvic lymph nodes.

subtotal h. See supracervical hysterectomy.

supracervical h. Operation in which only the main body of the uterus is removed, to the level of the internal os, leaving the cervix in place. Also called subtotal hysterectomy.

total h. Removal of the entire uterus.

vaginal h. Removal of the uterus through the vagina.

Wertheim h. See modified radical hysterectomy.

hysteresis (his-tĕ-re´sis) **1.** The failure of coincidence of two associated phenomena, such as the difference between the solidification temperature and the melting temperature of a reversible hydrocolloid. **2.** The lag of a magnetic effect behind its cause.

hysteria (his-ter´e-ă) See conversion disorder, under disorder.

conversion h. See conversion disorder, under disorder.

hysterical (his-ter´ĭ-kal) Characterized by or pertaining to hysteria.

hysterics (his-ter´iks) Colloquial term for an uncontrollable emotional outburst.

hysterocolposcope (his-ter-o-kol´po-skōp) Instrument for inspecting the uterine cavity and vagina.

hysterodynia (his-ter-o-din´e-ă) See hysteralgia.

hysterogram (his´ter-o-gram) An x-ray picture of the uterus made after filling its cavity with radiopaque material.

hysterography (his-ter-og´ră-fe) The making of a hysterogram.

hysterolith (his´ter-o-lith) A calculus of the uterus.

hysterometer (his-tĕ-rom´ĕ-ter) A graduated sound for measuring the depth of the uterine cavity.

hysteromyoma (his-ter-o-mi-o´mă) A benign tumor of the uterine wall.

hysteromyomectomy (his-ter-o-mi-o-mek´tŏ-me) Surgical removal of a myoma from the uterus.

hysteromyotomy (his-ter-o-mi-ot´ŏ-me) Incision into the muscular wall of the uterus.

hystero-oophorectomy (his-ter-o o-of-ŏ-rek´tŏ-me) Surgical removal of the uterus and ovaries.

hysteropathy (his-tĕ-rop´ă-the) Any disease of the uterus.

hysterorrhaphy (his-ter-or´ă-fe) Surgical repair of a ruptured or lacerated uterus.

hysterorrhexis (his-ter-o-rek´sis) Rupture of the uterus. Also called metrorrhexis.

hysterosalpingectomy (his-ter-o-sal-pin-jek´tŏ-me) The surgical removal of the uterus and at least one uterine (fallopian) tube.

hysterosalpingogram (his-ter-o-sal-pin´gŏ-gram) A roentgenogram, detailing the internal structures of the uterus and uterine (fallopian) tubes.

hysterosalpingography (his-ter-o-sal-ping-gog´ră-fe) (HSG) Roentgenography of the uterus and uterine tubes following the injection of a radiopaque material.

hysterosalpingo-oophorectomy (his-ter-o-sal-ping´go o-of-ŏ-rek´tŏ-me) Surgical removal of the uterus, uterine tubes, and ovaries. Also called hysterosalpingo-oothecectomy.

hysterosalpingostomy (his-ter-o-sal-pin-gos´tŏ-me) Operation to restore the patency of an obstructed uterine (fallopian) tube.

hysteroscope (his´ter-o-skōp) A uterine endoscope used for direct visual examination of the cavity of the uterus and cervix.

hysterostomatomy (his-ter-os-to-mat´ŏ-me) See Dührssen's incisions, under incision.

hysterotomy (his-ter-ot´ŏ-me) Surgical incision of the uterus. Also called laparohysterotomy; matrotomy; uterotomy.

hysterotrachelectomy (his-ter-o-tra-kel-ek´tŏ-me) Surgical removal of the uterine cervix.

I

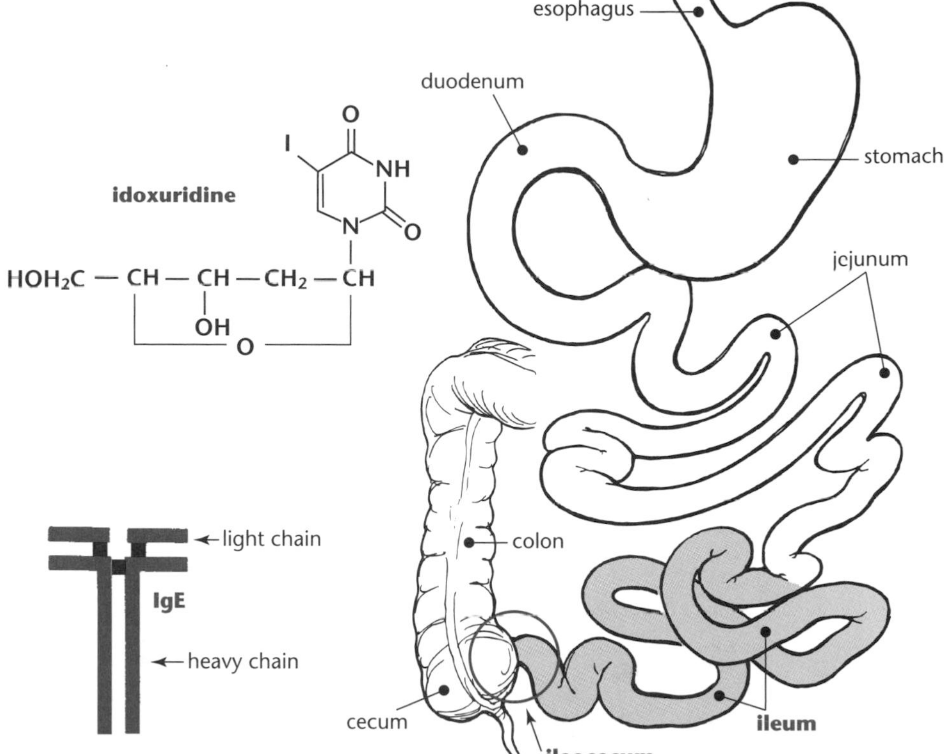

iatrogenic (i-at-ro-jen´ik) Caused by a physician; said of an illness unwittingly induced in a patient by the physician's attitude, treatment, or comments.
iatrogeny (i-ă-troj´ĕ-ne) Abnormal condition caused by a physician.
iatrotechnique (i-at-ro-tek-nēk´) Medical and surgical techniques.
ibuprofen (i-bu-pro´fen) A propionic acid derivative having anti-inflammatory properties; an inhibitor of prostaglandin synthetase.
Iceland disease (īs´land dĭ-zēz´) See epidemic neuromyasthenia, under neuromyasthenia.
ichor (ī´kōr) A watery discharge from a wound or ulcer.
ichthyism (ik-the-iz-m) Poisoning resulting from eating spoiled fish.
ichthyoid (ik´the-oid) Fishlike.
ichthyosiform (ik-the-o´sĭ-form) Resembling ichthyosis.
ichthyosis (ik-the-o´sis) Disease marked by dry, rough, scaly skin, caused by a hereditary defect of the horny layer of the skin; may affect the eyelids, conjunctiva, and cornea. Also called alligator skin; fish skin; sauriasis.
acquired i. Dry thickening and scaling of the skin that may herald the occurrence of a cancerous disease or may be associated with severe nutritional deficiencies.
lamellar i. Condition of autosomal recessive inheritance with onset at birth, marked by large, coarse scales over the body with severe involvement of the palms and soles.
i. vulgaris Condition of autosomal dominant inheritance with onset in childhood, marked by fine scales over the trunk and especially the limbs, sparing the flexural areas, and by deep creases on the palms and soles.
X-linked i. Condition of x-linked recessive inheritance affecting males with onset at birth, marked by thick scales that darken with age, sparing the soles and palms; the mother is carrier of the defective gene; both mother and offspring have small cataracts; most patients lack the enzyme steroid sulfatase.
ichthyotoxin (ik-the-o-tok´sin) A toxic substance present in or derived from fish.
icosanoid (i-ko-să´noid) See eicosanoid.
ictal (ik´tal) Relating to a convulsion.
icteric (ik-ter´ik) Relating to jaundice.
icterogenic (ik-ter-o-jen´ik) Causing jaundice.
icterus (ik´ter-us) See jaundice.
physiologic i. See physiologic jaundice, under jaundice.
scleral i. A yellow pigmentation of the sclera caused by an elevated level of bilirubin in the blood, usually over 2.5 mg/dl.
ictus (ik´tus), *pl.* **ic´tuses** A stroke, beat, or sudden convulsion.
i. epilepticus An epileptic convulsion.
id (ĭd) **1.** In psychoanalytic theory, the part of the personality structure associated with the unconscious instinctive impulses and primitive needs of the individual. **2.** See id reaction, under reaction.
idea (i-de´ă) A conception existing in the mind as the product of mental activity.
compulsive i. An inappropriate idea that recurs and persists despite reason.
fixed i. A loosely used term to describe a compulsive drive, an obsession, or a delusion. Also called idée fixe.
ideal (i-de´al) A conception regarded as a standard of perfection.
ego i. The part of the personality comprising the goals of the self; it usually refers to the emulation of significant individuals with whom the person has identified.
ideation (i-de-a´shun) The formation of ideas or conceptions; indicative of an individual's ability to think.
paranoid i. Unfounded suspicious thinking or an unfounded belief that one is being persecuted or singled out for unfair treatment.
idée fixe (e-da´fēks) French for fixed idea.
identification (i-den-tĭ-fi-ka´shun) A psychologic defense mechanism in which a person unconsciously tries to pattern himself after another; distinguished from imitation, which is a conscious process.
identity (i-den´tĭ-te) The role of a person in society and his perception of it.
ego i. A unified sense of one's own, personal identity.
gender i. The anatomic-sexual identity of an individual.
ideology (i-de-ol´o-je, id-e-ol´o-je) The intellectual-moral ideas of reflecting the needs and aspirations of an individual or group.
ideomotion (i-de-o-mo´shun) Muscular movements influenced by a dominant idea.
idioagglutinin (id-e-o-ă-gloo´tĭ-nin) An agglutinin occurring normally in the blood of a person or an animal.
idiogenesis (id-e-o-jen´ĕ-sis) The origin of an idiopathic disease (one without apparent cause).
idiogram (id´e-o-gram) A diagrammatic representation of the chromosomal constitution (karyotype) of an organism.
idioheteroagglutinin (id-e-o-het-ĕr-o-ă-gloo´tĭ-nin) An agglutinin occurring normally in the blood of one animal (idioagglutinin), but capable of combining with the antigen of another species.
idioisoagglutinin (id-e-o-i-so-ă-gloo´tĭ-nin) An agglutinin occurring in the blood of an animal (idioagglutinin) of a certain species, capable of agglutinating the cells from animals of the same species.
idiolysin (id-e-ol´ĭ-sin) An antibody occurring naturally in the blood of a person or an animal.
idionodal (id-e-o-no´dal) Arising in the atrioventricular (A-V) node of the heart.
idiopathic (id-e-o-path´ik) Denoting a disease of unknown cause.
idiophrenic (id-e-o-fren´ik) Relating to or originating in the mind or brain exclusively (i.e., neither reflex nor secondary).
idiosyncrasy (id-e-o-sin´kră-se) **1.** A characteristic (physical or behavioral) particular to an individual. **2.** A genetically determined abnormal response to a drug.
idiosyncratic (id-e-o-sin-krat´ik) Relating to an idiosyncrasy.
idiotope (id´ĭ-o-tōp) One of several antigenic determinants in the variable region of an antibody molecule. It can be recognized as antigen by the combining site (receptor) of another antibody in the same species.
idiot-savant (e-dyo´sah-vahn´) A mentally retarded individual capable of performing certain remarkable mental tasks (e.g., solving difficult mathematical problems almost instantly, playing a classical composition on the piano after hearing it only once).
idiotype (id´ĭ-o-tīp) The collection of idiotopes in the variable region of an antibody molecule; invests the variable region with its individual antigenic characteristics.
idioventricular (id-e-o-ven-trik´u-lar) Relating to the cardiac ventricles alone, as a cardiac rhythm originating from a ventricular focus.
idoxuridine (i-doks-ūr´ĭ-dēn) (IDV) An antiviral agent used locally for the treatment of herpes simplex infection of the eye.
IgA Abbreviation for immunoglobulin A (gamma A globulin); see under immunoglobulin.
IgE Abbreviation for immunoglobulin E (gamma E globulin); see under immunoglobulin.
IgG Abbreviation for immunoglobulin G (gamma G globulin); see under immunoglobulin.
IgM Abbreviation for immunoglobulin M (gamma M globulin); see under immunoglobulin.
ileal (il´e-al) Relating to the ileum.
ileitis (il-e-i´tis) Inflammation of the ileum.
backwash i. Inflammation and ulceration of the ileum occurring as an extension of ulcerative colitis.
regional i. See regional enteritis, under enteritis.
terminal i. See regional enteritis, under enteritis.
ileocecal (il-e-o-se´kal) Relating to the ileum and cecum.
ileocecostomy (il-e-o-se-kos´tŏ-me) Surgical connection of the ileum and the cecum.
ileocecum (il-e-o-se´kum) The ileum and cecum taken as a whole.
ileocolic (il-e-o-kol´ik) Relating to the ileum and the colon.
ileocolitis (il-e-o-ko-li´tis) Inflammation of the ileum and colon.
ileocolostomy (il-e-o-ko-los´tŏ-me) Surgical connection of the ileum and colon.
ileoileostomy (il-e-o-il-e-os´tŏ-me) Surgical connection of two noncontinuous portions of the ileum.
ileojejunitis (il-e-o-jĕ-joo-ni´tis) Inflammation of the ileum and jejunum.
ileostomy (il-e-os´tŏ-me) Surgical construction of an external opening into the ileum through the abdominal wall.
ileotomy (il-e-ot´ŏ-me) Surgical incision of the ileum.
ileotransversostomy (il-e-o-trans-vers-os´tŏ-me) Surgical joining of the ileum and transverse colon.
ileum (il´e-um) The portion of the small intestine

I

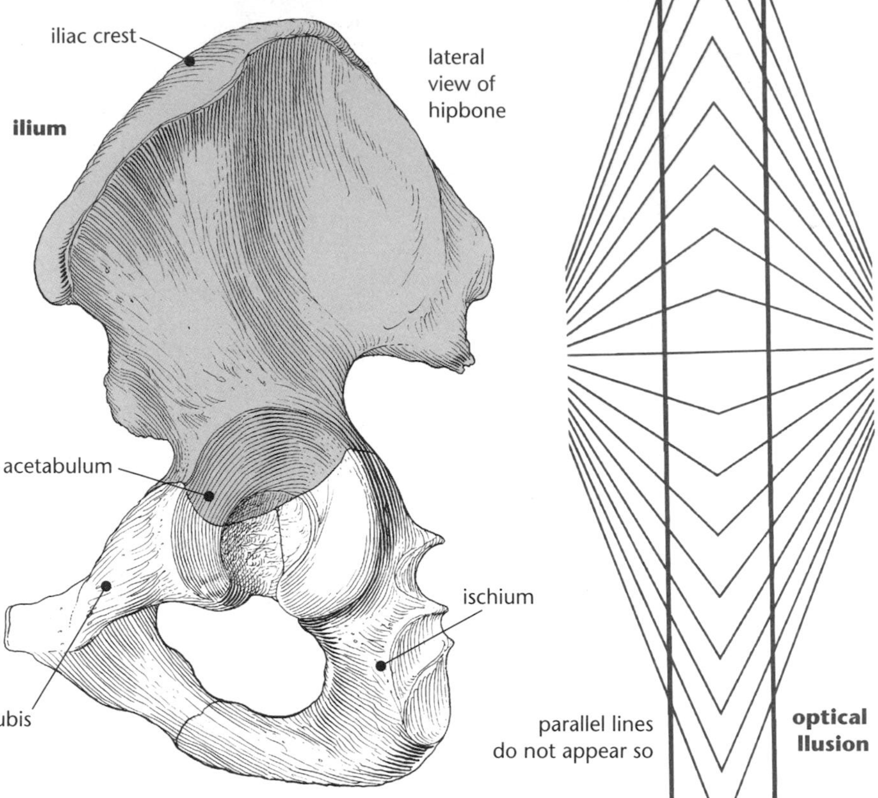

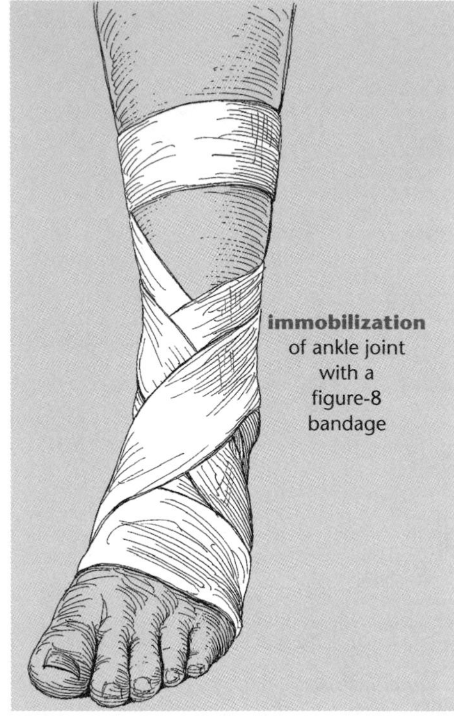

between the jejunum and the cecum; the preferred site for vitamin B_{12} absorption.

ileus (il´e-us) Obstruction of the intestines accompanied by severe colicky pain, vomiting, and sometimes fever.

adynamic i. Ileus resulting from decreased or absent propulsive activity of the intestinal walls, usually causing abdominal distention and vomiting but little or no pain; causes include peritonitis, abdominal surgery, bowel trauma, and damage to mesenteric arteries. Also called paralytic ileus.

gallstone i. A mechanical intestinal obstruction caused by impaction of one or more gallstones within the bowel lumen.

meconium i. Ileus in the newborn due to obliteration of the bowel lumen by excessively thick meconium; frequently the first evidence of cystic fibrosis.

obstructive i. Ileus caused by any mechanical reduction or obliteration of the bowel lumen (e.g., by constrictive postoperative adhesions, pressure against the bowel by a tumor, torsion of a bowel segment, or by impaction of any material within the intestine); it is usually associated with persistent vomiting and abdominal cramps.

paralytic i. See adynamic ileus.

iliac (il´e-ak) Relating to the ilium.

iliofemoral (il-e-o-fem´or-al) Relating to the ilium and the femur.

ilioinguinal (il-e-o-in´gwĭ-nal) Relating to the iliac region and the groin.

iliolumbar (il-e-o-lum´bar) Relating to the iliac and the lumbar regions.

iliopectineal (il-e-o-pek-tin´e-al) Relating to the ilium and pubic bones.

ilium (il´e-um) The superior, broad portion of the hipbone comprising one of the lateral halves of the pelvis.

illness (il´nes) Disease.

functional i. See functional disorder, under disorder.

mental i. See mental disorder, under disorder.

terminal i. A sickness that ends in death.

illumination (ĭ-loo-mĭ-na´shun) **1.** The process by which light is made to fall on a surface. **2.** In microscopy, the light thrown upon the object to be examined.

critical i. In microscopy, the focusing of the light source directly on the specimen, creating a narrow, intense light beam.

dark-field i. Illumination of a microscopic specimen by a hollow cone of light; the vertically directed light rays are blocked by a black circular shield and the peripheral rays are directed toward the specimen; the object appears bright on a dark background.

direct i. Illumination in which the object is illuminated by a beam of light falling almost perpendicularly upon it. Also called vertical illumination.

vertical i. See direct illumination.

illuminator (ĭ-loo-mĭ-na´tor) In a microscope, the source of light that illuminates the specimen to be viewed.

illusion (ĭ-loo´zhun) A false perception of reality.

optical i. An erroneous interpretation of a visual sensation.

image (im´ij) **1.** A reproduction of the appearance of an object formed by the rays of light emanating or reflected from it. **2.** A representation or picture of someone or something not present, formed in the mind from memory.

after-i. See afterimage.

double i. Two images of a single object, as formed perceptually in diplopia.

hypnopompic i. Imagery occurring after the sleeping state and before complete awakening, as when a dream figure persists in waking life.

mental i. Image (2).

mirror i. An image with right and left parts reversed, as the relationship of an object to its image in a mirror.

real i. An image, formed by converging light rays, which can be seen by inserting a screen, such as a ground glass, into the optical system, or which can be recorded on a photographic plate; the opposite of virtual image.

retinal i. The image formed on the surface of the retina by the refracting system of the eye.

virtual i. An image in which light, originating from a point on the object, and having traversed an optical system, appears to be diverging; it cannot be demonstrated on a screen or photographic plate as in the case of a real image.

image intensifier (im´ij in-ten-sĭ-fī´er) In radiology, an electronic device for intensification of the fluoroscopic image.

imaging (im´ă-jing) Creation of images of body parts.

functional magnetic resonance i. High speed magnetic resonance imaging techniques that measure changes in blood volume and flow, thereby producing functional MRI maps of brain activity.

magnetic resonance i. (MRI) The making of cross-sectional images of body parts by means of nuclear magnetic resonance. The patient is placed in a magnetic field within a cylindrical magnet, which causes the nuclei of the body's hydrogen atoms to line up parallel to each other, like rows of tiny magnets. Radiofrequency pulses are then applied to knock the nuclei out of alignment. As they fall back into alignment, the nuclei produce detectable signals, which are translated into images by computer.

SPECT i. See single photon emission computed tomography, under tomography.

imbibition (im-bĭ-bish´un) The absorption of a fluid, as in the taking up of water by a gel.

imbrication (im-brĭ-ka´shun) **1.** An overlapping of the free edges of tissue in the closure of a wound or the repair of a defect. **2.** A regular overlapping of a surface, such as the slight, horizontal, scalelike ridges on the cervical third of the labial surface of some anterior teeth.

imidazole (im-id-az´ōl) A functional component of histidine.

imide (im´id) Any compound containing the radical group =NH attached to one bivalent acid radical or two univalent acid radicals.

imino acids (im´ĭ-no as´idz) Compounds containing both an acid group and an imino group.

imipramine hydrochloride (im-ip´ră-mēn hi-dro-klor´id) A white crystalline tricyclic substance, soluble in water; used to treat depression; Tofranil®.

immersion (ĭ-mer´zhun) The submerging of an object in a liquid.

oil i. In microscopy, the use of a layer of oil between the objective and the specimen.

water i. In microscopy, the use of a layer of water between the objective and the specimen.

immiscible (ĭ-mis´ĭ-bl) Incapable of being mixed (e.g., oil and water).

immobilization (ĭ-mo-bil-ĭ-za´shun) The act of impeding movement.

immobilize (ĭ-mo´bil-īz) To render incapable of being moved; to fix.

immune (ĭ-mūn´) The state of being secure against harmful effects from pathogenic agents or influences; having immunity.

immune complex disease (ĭ-mūn´ kom´pleks dĭ-zēz´) (ICD) A hypersensitivity reaction marked by deposition of antigen-antibody-complement complexes within tissues, especially vascular endothelium.

immune deficiency syndrome (ĭ-mūn´ de-fish´en-se sin´drōm) A group of signs and symptoms indicating impairment of one or more of the major

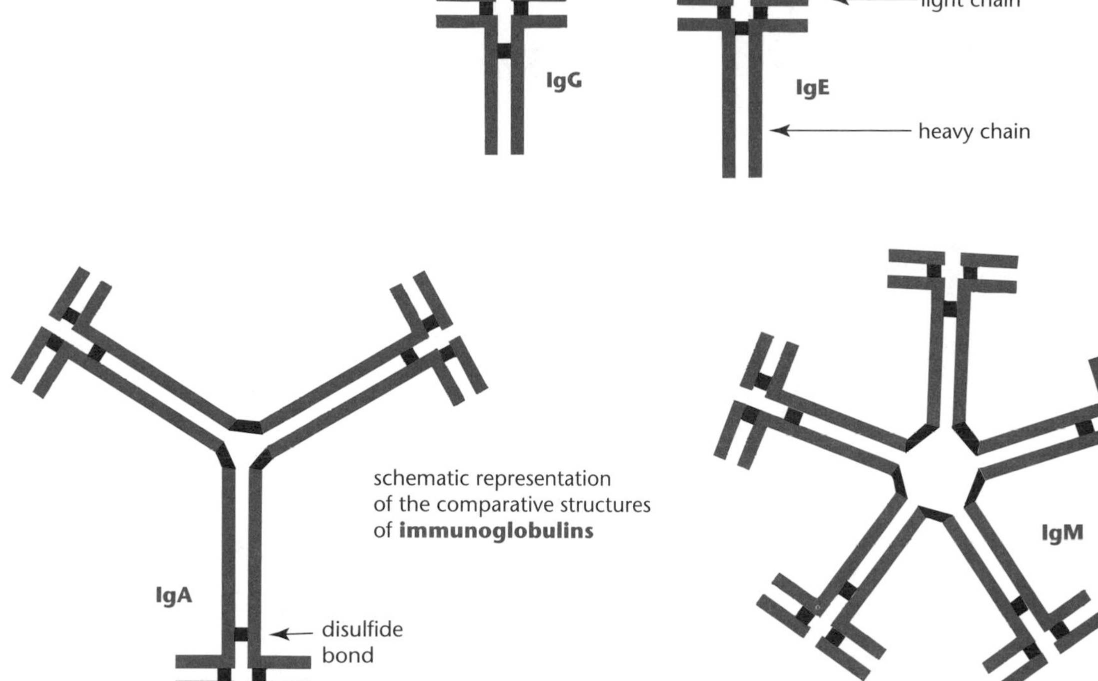

functions of the immune system; i.e., protection against infection (defense), preservation of uniformity of a given cell type (homeostasis), or the removal of malignant cells (surveillance).

immunity (ĭ-mu'nĭ-te) **1.** The physiologic state that enables the body to recognize materials that are not of itself and to neutralize, eliminate, or metabolize them with or without injury to its own tissues. **2.** An inherited or acquired (naturally or artificially) or induced conditioning to a specific pathogen.

acquired i. Immunity acquired after birth; may be active or passive.

active i. Immunity acquired as the result of having had a given infectious disease, or by deliberate inoculation with a modified form of the causative agent (vaccination).

adoptive i. Immunity produced by the administration of immune lymphoid cells.

cell-mediated i. (CMI) Specific immune response conducted by antigen-sensitized T lymphocytes. Also called cellular immunity.

humoral i. Immunity in which the involvement of blood-circulating antibodies (immunoglobulins) is predominant.

innate i. Resistance to certain infections that has not been acquired through vaccination or previous infection; included is the species-determined immunity (e.g., resistance of humans to the virus of canine distemper). Also called natural immunity.

natural i. See innate immunity.

passive i. Immunity due to receipt of maternal antibody or injection of antibody.

specific i. Acquired active immunity against a particular disease obtained through vaccination or natural infection.

immunization (im-u-nĭ-za'shun) The act or process by which a person becomes resistant or immune to a harmful agent.

active i. The promotion of antibodies when the injected antigen comes in contact with the plasma cells, reticuloendothelial cells, and large lymphocytes.

passive i. Transient immunization obtained by injection of serum or gamma globulin from an animal or human already rendered immune.

immunize (im'u-nīz) The process of making an individual resistant or immune to a harmful agent.

immunoagglutination (im-u-no-ă-gloo-tĭ-na'shun) Agglutination brought about by antibody.

immunoassay (im-u-no-as'a) Technique (e.g., ELISA) for detection of specific protein in body tissue or blood by means of antigen-antibody reactions.

immunoblotting (im-u-no-blot'ing) See Western blot analysis, under analysis.

immunochemistry (im-u-no-kem'is-tre) The chemistry of immunologic processes.

immunocompetence (im-u-no-kom'pĕ-tens) Ability to produce antibodies or cell-mediated immunity when exposed to an antigen (i.e., any substance recognized by the body as being nonself).

immunocompromised (im-u-no-kom'pro-mīzd) Reduced immune response due to immunosuppressive drugs, chemotherapy, irradiation, disease, or malnutrition.

immunoconglutinin (im-u-no-kon-gloo'tĭ-nin) Autoantibody (usually an IgM) that reacts with C3 and C4 components of complement; found in increased levels in autoimmune disease, certain infections, and after immunization with many antigens. Distinguished from conglutinin.

immunocyte (im'u-no-sīt) Any lymphoid cell that can form antibodies, or elaborate cells that form antibodies, when reacting with antigens (e.g., an inducer cell). Also called I cell; immunocompetent cell; antigen-sensitive cell.

immunocytochemistry (im-u-no-si-to-kem'is-tre) Any technique (e.g., the use of fluorescent antibodies) for analyzing cells and tissues to identify particulate antigens.

immunodeficiency (im-u-no-dĕ-fish'en-se) Any impairment of immune response. Also called immune deficiency.

common variable i. (CVI) General term for a group of disorders (hereditary or acquired) with onset at any age; characterized by low levels of all or some of the immunoglobulin classes, but with the number of B lymphocytes in peripheral blood usually within normal range; the deficiency leads to recurrent bacterial infections and an increased incidence of autoimmune disease.

severe combined i. (SCID) A group of congenital diseases of autosomal recessive or X-linked inheritance, characterized by dysfunction of both antibody formation and cellular immunity; affected infants seldom survive beyond the first year of life.

immunodiffusion (im-u-no-di-fu'zhun) A technique for the study of immune reactions that involves diffusion of antibody or antigen through a semisolid substance (e.g., a gel).

immunoelectrophoresis (im-u-no-e-lek-tro-fo-re'sis) (IE) A form of electrophoresis which in addition employs immune precipitation (antigen-antibody reaction). Also called immunophoresis.

immunofluorescence (im-u-no-floo-o-res'ens) The use of fluorescein-labeled antibodies to identify antigenic material specific for the labeled antibody.

immunogen (im'u-no-jen) See antigen.

immunogenetics (im-u-no-jĕ-net'iks) The study of all the factors controlling immunologic reactions and the transmission of antigenic specificities from generation to generation.

immunogenic (im-u-no-jen'ik) See antigenic.

immunogenicity (im-u-no-je-nis'i-te) See antigenicity.

immunoglobulin (im-u-no-glob'u-lin) (Ig) A protein molecule functioning as a specific antibody; it has two main functions: one region of the molecule binds to antigen (e.g., bacterial cells), another mediates the binding of the molecule to host tissues (including immune system cells and phagocytic cells).

i. A (IgA) The second most abundant class of immunoglobulins; present in secretions and produced especially by lymphoid tissues in the lining of the respiratory, gastrointestinal, and urogenital tracts.

i. D (IgD) A class of immunoglobulins present on the surface of lymphocytes, especially of newborns.

i. E (IgE) A reaginic antibody that has ability to attach to the skin and initiate immediate hypersensitivity reactions.

i. G (IgG) The most abundant class of immunoglobulins; present in human serum; they provide immunity to bacteria, viruses, parasites, and fungi that have a blood-borne dissemination.

i. M (IgM) A class of immunoglobulins composed of the largest immunoglobulins; they are transported across the placenta, play an important role in protecting newborns against infection and agglutinate particular antigens (e.g., bacteria, red blood cells).

monoclonal i.'s Immunoglobulins derived from a single clone of plasma cells proliferating abnormally and appearing as a narrow spike on electrophoresis of plasma.

secretory i. Immunoglobulin (usually IgA) that is linked to and transported across the cell membrane by a polypeptide produced by secretory epithelial cells; found in mucous secretions.

immunohematology (im-u-no-hēm-ă-tol'o-je) The branch of hematology concerned with antigen-antibody reactions and their effect on the blood.

immunolocalization (im-u-mo-lo-kal-ĭ-za'shun) The use of immunologic techniques to determine the location of molecules or structures within cells.

immunologist (im-u-nol'o-jist) A specialist in immunology.

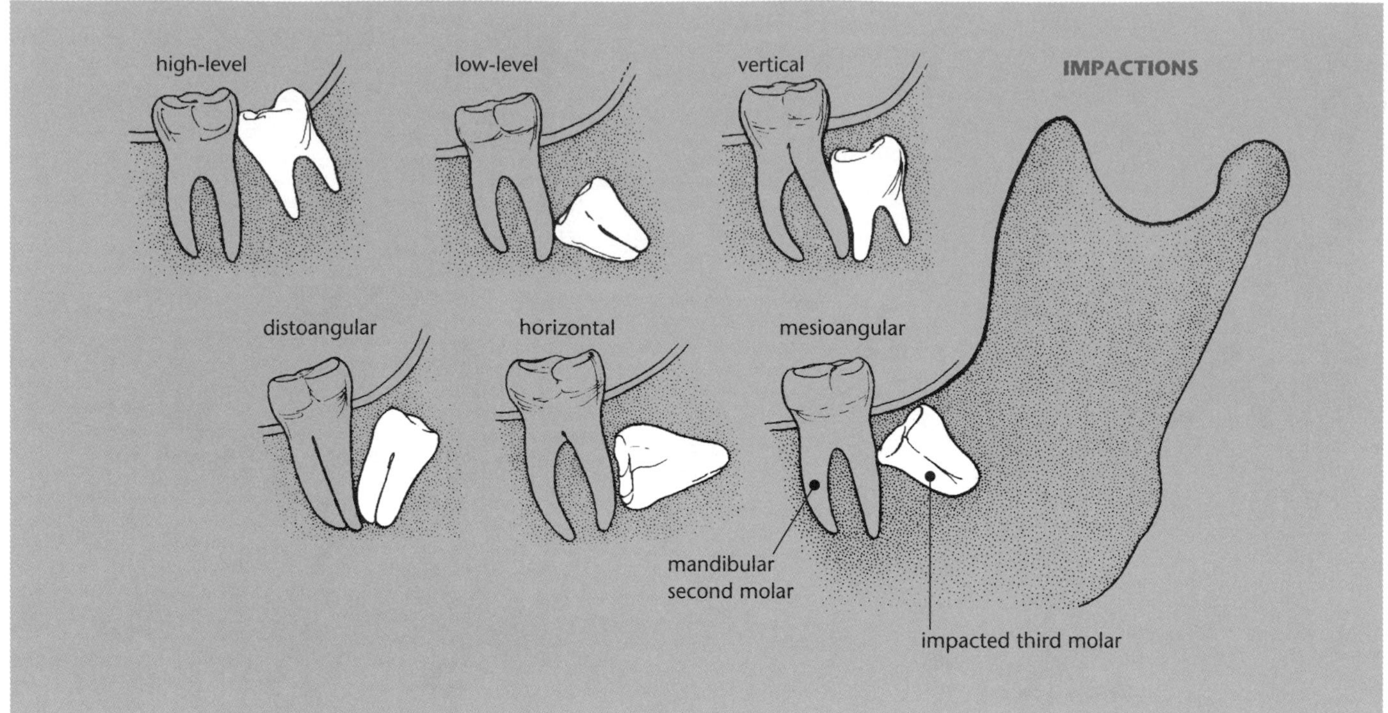

immunology (im-u-nol′o-je) The study of specific processes by which the host maintains constancy of his internal environment when confronted by substances which are recognized as foreign, whether generated from within the host or introduced from the outside.

immunomodulation (im-u-no-mod-u-la′shun) Any of various methods for therapeutic manipulation of the body's immune response to an antigen.

immunopathic (im-u-no-path′ik) Relating to damage inflicted upon cells, tissues, or organs by immune responses.

immunopathology (im-u-no-pă-thol′o-je) The study of disorders caused by antigen-antibody reactions.

immunoprophylaxis (im-u-no-pro-fĭ-lak′sis) Prevention of disease through the use of vaccines.

immunoreaction (im-u-no-re-ak′shun) See immune response, under response.

immunoselection (im-u-no-sĕ-lek′shun) Selective death or survival of fetuses of different genotypes depending on immunologic incompatibility with the mother.

immunosuppression (im-u-no-sŭ-presh′un) Diminution of the body's immune response; may occur due to infection or be produced by any of several techniques (e.g., drugs, radiation, lymphocyte depletion) as a way to prevent rejection of a transplant.

immunosuppressive (im-u-no-sŭ-pres′iv) Capable of inducing immunosuppression.

immunosurveillance (im-u-no-sur-va′lans) The concept that the immune system recognizes and destroys malignant cells as they arise.

immunotherapy (im-u-no-ther′ă-pe) **1.** Passive immunization with serum or gamma globulin; a temporary protection to one host by introducing antibodies actively produced in another. **2.** Transplantation of immunocompetent tissues (e.g., bone marrow, fetal thymus) into an immunodeficient patient. **3.** Treatment with immunosuppressive drugs or biological products. **4.** See desensitization.

impact (im′pakt) The sudden striking of one body against another.

impact (im-pakt′) To press firmly together.

impaction (im-pak′shun) Tightly wedged together or firmly lodged so as to be immovable.

ceruminal i. Accumulation of earwax in the external auditory canal.

dental i. Condition in which a tooth is so placed in the alveolus as to be incapable of complete eruption.

fecal i. A mass of compressed, hardened feces retained in some part of the bowel, usually the sigmoid colon or rectum.

impairment (im-pār′ment) Damage resulting from injury or disease.

hearing i. Reduction of hearing ability due to either malfunctioning of nerve elements or interference with conduction of sound to the end organ.

mental i. Intellectual defect as manifested by psychologic tests and diminished effectiveness (social and vocational).

impalpable (im-pal′pă-bl) Imperceptible to the touch; unable to be grasped or felt.

impatent (im-pa′tent) Closed.

impedance (im-pe′dans) (Z) A measure of the total opposition to the flow of electric current in an alternating-current circuit.

imperforate (im-per′fŏ-rāt) Abnormally closed.

impermeable (im-per′me-ă-bl) Not allowing the entrance of fluids or particular types of ionic or nonionic substances.

impetigo (im-pĕ-ti′go) Contagious skin disease marked by the formation of pustules and caused by staphylococci or streptococci; it occurs mainly in children; the lesions appear as small reddish spots which readily become vesicles and burst, forming a characteristic crust; touching the blisters usually spreads the infection.

impetus (im′pĕ-tus) In psychoanalysis, the motor constituent of an instinct.

implant (im′plant) **1.** To graft. **2.** The material grafted.

breast i. A silicone bag filled with silicone gel, saline, air, or a combination thereof, placed either behind the breast or behind the pectoral muscle to increase breast size (augmentation mammoplasty) or to reconstruct the breast after mastectomy.

cochlear i. A device inserted under the skin adjacent to the ear of persons with total sensory deafness; electrodes of the device leading to the cochlear nerve create the sensation of sound.

dental i. Any nonliving material placed in a dental socket to substitute for a damaged or missing tooth.

endosseous dental i. An implant made of biocompatible materials for insertion into the socket of a missing tooth, where it becomes directly attached to the jawbone; it functions as the tooth root, providing support for a subsequently inserted post bearing the artificial tooth or teeth.

intraocular i. Plastic lens inserted in the eye to replace a diseased natural lens removed in a cataract operation.

penile i. See penile prosthesis, under prosthesis.

powder burn i.'s Descriptive term applied to the characteristic peritoneal lesions of endometriosis.

subdermal contraceptive i. A reversible female contraceptive implanted under the skin; effective for an extended period of time (usually five years); Norplant®.

implantation (im-plan-ta′shun) **1.** Tissue grafting. **2.** The embedding of the fertilized ovum, normally to the inner wall of the uterus.

implant denture substructure (im′plant den′chur sub′struk-chur) A metal framework inserted deeply and in contact with the bone to serve as support for an implant denture superstructure.

implant denture superstructure (im′plant den′chur soo-per-struk′chur) A denture placed on, and stabilized by, the implant denture substructure.

impotence (im′pŏ-tens) **1.** Lack of power. **2.** Term traditionally used to describe the inability to attain and maintain erection of the penis sufficiently to permit satisfactory sexual intercourse. Currently, the term "erectile dysfunction" has been suggested as more precise to describe the condition. See erectile dysfunction, under dysfunction.

impregnate (im-preg′nāt) **1.** To render pregnant. **2.** To saturate.

impression (im-presh′un) An imprint made on a surface by pressure.

complete denture i. An impression of the arch for the purpose of making a complete denture.

dental i. A negative likeness of the teeth or other structures of the oral cavity, made of a setting plastic material which is later filled with plaster of Paris, thus obtaining an exact copy of the structures.

final i. In dentistry, the impression used for making the master cast. Also called secondary impression.

secondary i. See final impression.

impulse (im′puls) **1.** A sudden urge to act. **2.** The transference of energy from one neuron to another; a brief action potential in nerve fibers.

cardiac i. The movement of the chest wall produced by cardiac contraction; the point of maximal impulse (PMI) is normally in the fifth intercostal space, on the midclavicular line or somewhat medial.

inactivate (in-ak′tĭ-vāt) To render anything inactive or inert; may be done by using heat or other methods.

inadequacy (in-ad′ĕ-kwă-se) **1.** A state of being deficient. **2.** A failing.

sexual i. Insufficient sexual response (constant or

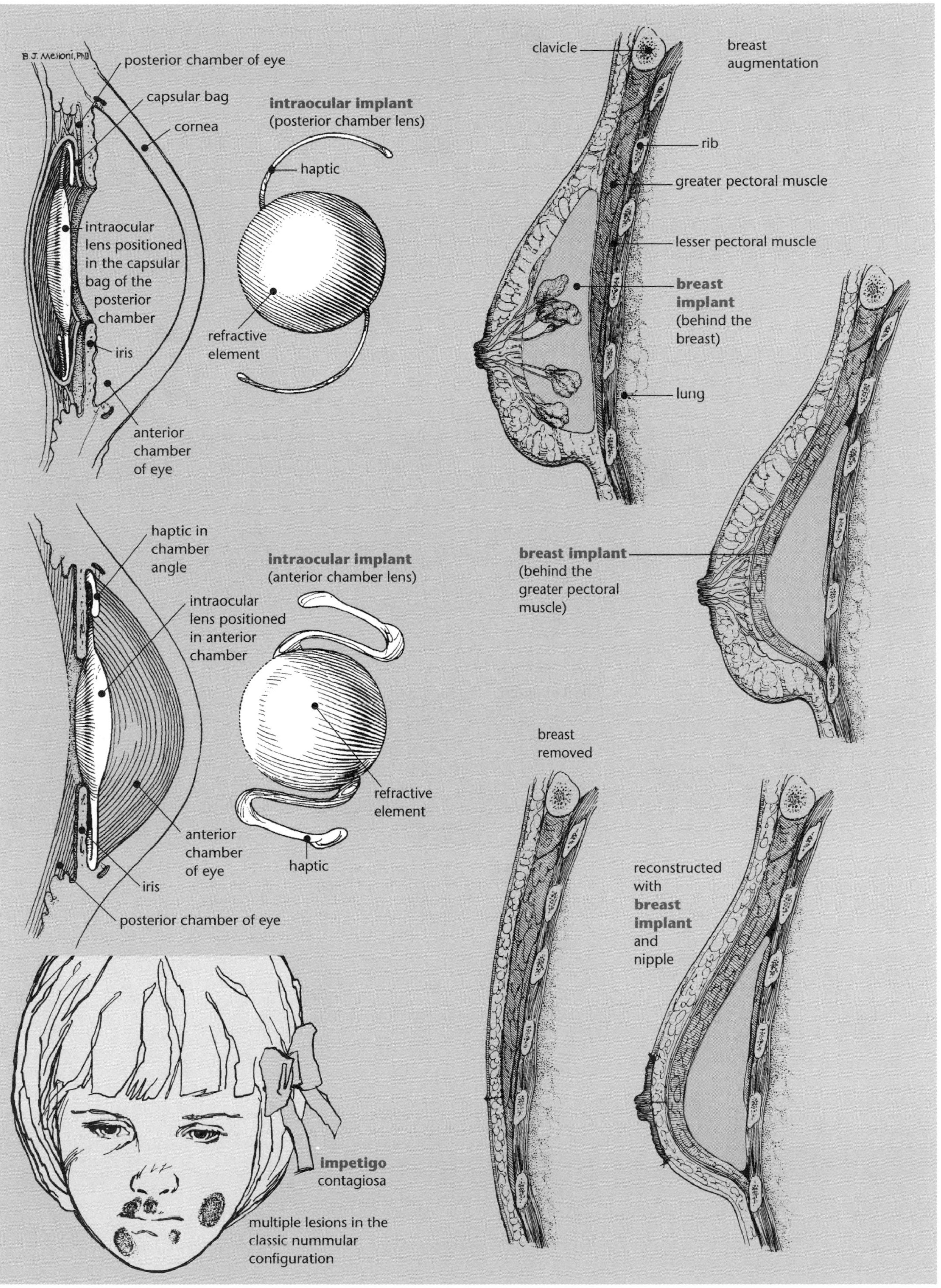
B.J. Melloni, PhD
posterior chamber of eye
capsular bag
cornea
intraocular implant
(posterior chamber lens)
haptic
intraocular
lens positioned
in the capsular
bag of the
posterior
chamber
refractive
element
iris
anterior
chamber
of eye
haptic in
chamber
angle
intraocular implant
(anterior chamber lens)
intraocular
lens positioned
in anterior
chamber
refractive
element
anterior
chamber
of eye
haptic
iris
posterior chamber of eye
impetigo
contagiosa
multiple lesions in the
classic nummular
configuration
clavicle
breast
augmentation
rib
greater pectoral muscle
lesser pectoral muscle
breast
implant
(behind the
breast)
lung
breast implant
(behind the
greater pectoral
muscle)
breast
removed
reconstructed
with
breast
implant
and
nipple

I

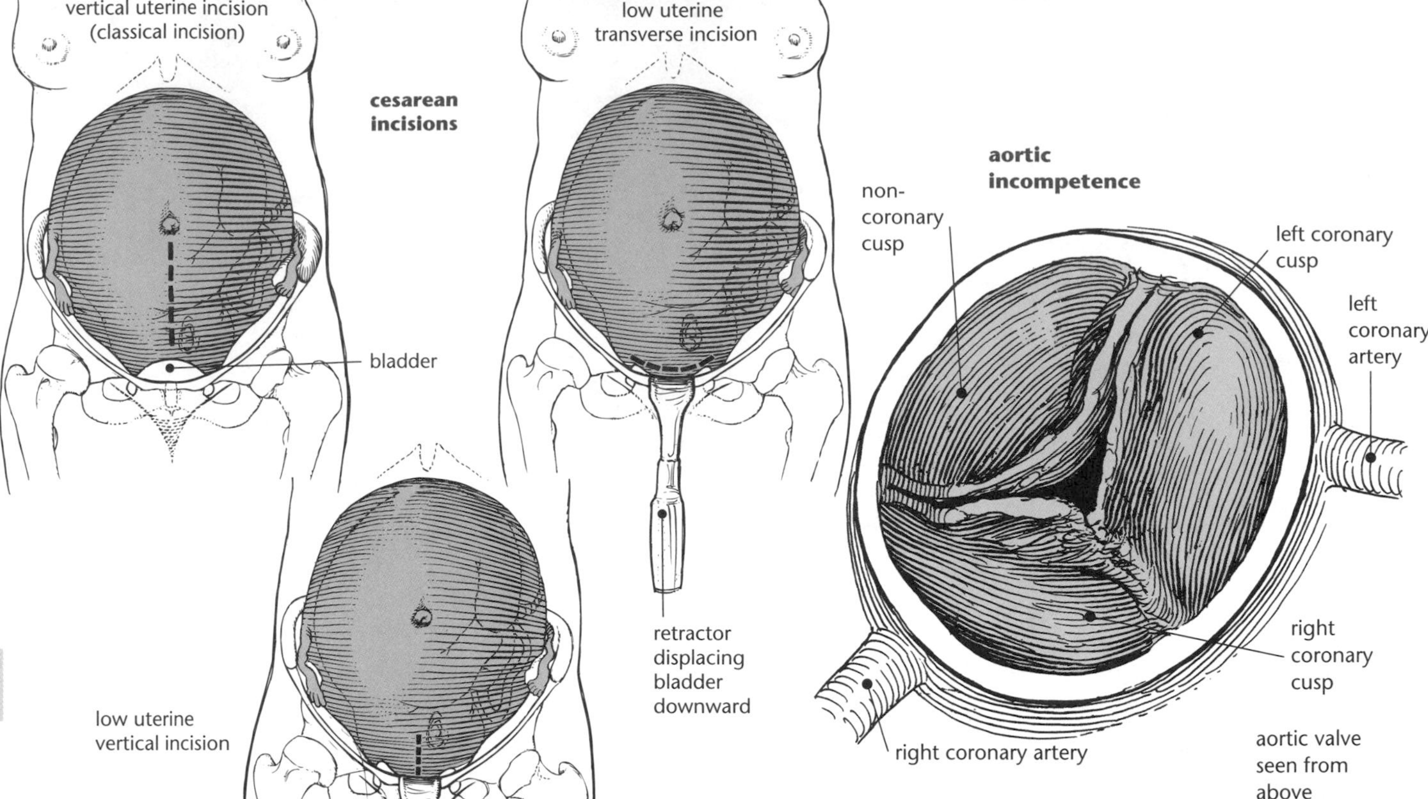

transitory).

inanimate (in-an´ĭ-mĭt) Without life.

inanition (in-ă-nish´un) Debility resulting from lack of food or defect in assimilation.

inapparent (in-ă-par´ent) Not apparent; said of certain infections.

inarticulate (in-ar-tik´u-lĭt) **1.** Not articulate; speechless. **2.** Not joined; not having functional joints.

inattention (in-ă-ten´shun) Lack of attention.

selective i. In psychiatry, failure to pay attention to a part of the perceived situation.

inborn (in´born) Ambiguous term generally meaning acquired genetically; inherited. Distinguished from congenital (present at birth).

i. error of metabolism See under error.

inbreeding (in´brēd-ing) The mating of closely related individuals, occurring naturally or as a deliberate process for the purpose of preserving desirable characters.

incaparina (in-kap-ă-re´nă) Generic name for a mixture of cereal grains and oilseed meals of a given general range of protein quality, fortified with vitamins and minerals.

incarcerated (in-kar´ser-āt-ed) Confined; held fast, as an irreducible hernia.

incest (in´sest) Sexual intercourse or sexual activity between persons closely related by blood (e.g., parents and offspring, brothers and sisters).

incestuous (in-ses´chu-us) Relating to incest.

incidence (in´sĭ-dens) The frequency at which an event occurs, such as the number of cases of a disease.

incident (in´sĭ-dent) **1.** A distinct occurrence or event. **2.** Falling upon, as incident rays.

incipient (in-sip´e-ent) Beginning to appear; in an initial stage.

incisal (in-si´zal) Cutting; pertaining to the cutting edges of the anterior teeth.

incise (in-sīz´) To cut with a knife.

incision (in-sizh´un) A surgical cut into soft tissue.

Battle's i. Vertical incision along the outer border of the abdominal rectus muscle, with division of the rectus sheath and retraction of the rectus muscle inward. Also called lateral rectus incision.

buttonhole i. A small incision made for drainage purposes.

cesarean i. Any incision through the anterior abdominal wall and the uterus; made to approach the fetus or fetuses for delivery.

Dührssen's i.'s Two or three longitudinal incisions made in the cervix when it is fully effaced and more than 17.6 cm dilated to facilitate vaginal delivery of the fetal head; performed in current practice only in extreme emergencies (e.g., impaction of an aftercoming head of a premature viable infant in breech presentation). Also called hysterostomatomy.

Halsted's i. See Halsted's operation, under operation (a).

McBurney's i. An oblique abdominal incision parallel to the fibers of the external oblique muscle, approximately 1.5 cm from the anterior superior iliac spine; used in appendectomy.

lateral rectus i. See Battle's incision.

median i. A surgical incision in the midline of the anterior abdominal wall; designated *lower median i.*, when made below the navel to expose the pelvic organs; or *upper median i.*, when made above the navel to expose the stomach and transverse colon. Also called midline incision.

midline i. See median incision.

paramedian i. A vertical incision about 1.5 cm from the midline of the anterior abdominal wall that permits the retraction of the abdominal rectus muscle laterally.

Pfannenstiel's i. A curved, transverse abdominal incision through the skin, just above the pubic symphysis; generally followed by a vertical midline incision of the fascia and peritoneum.

relief i. A skin incision made away from a wound to relax the tension of the skin so that it can be stretched to cover the wound.

incisor (in-sī´zor) Any of the eight front cutting teeth, four in each jaw.

central i. The tooth closest to and on either side of the midsagittal plane of the head, on either jaw.

lateral i. The second tooth, mandibular or maxillary, on either side of the midsagittal plane of the head.

incisura (in-si-su´ră), *pl.* **incisu´rae** A notch or indentation on any structure. Also called incisure.

incisure (in-si´zhur) See incisura.

inclination (in-klĭ-na´shun) **1.** A trend or disposition toward a particular condition. **2.** The state of being inclined; a leaning or sloping. **3.** In dentistry, the angle of the long axis of a tooth from the perpendicular.

inclusion (in-kloo´zhun) The act of enclosing or the state of being enclosed.

cell i. Transient substance in a cell that does not participate in the cell's function; e.g., pigmented granules, crystals, lipids.

fetal i. Unequal conjoined twins in which the less developed one is enclosed within the body of the other.

lipid i. See lipid droplet, under droplet.

incoherent (in-ko-hēr´ent) Disoriented; confused.

incompatible (in-kom-pat´ĭ-bl) Incapable of being mixed or used simultaneously without undergoing chemical changes or producing undesirable effects, as two types of blood or certain drugs.

incompetence, incompetency (in-kom´pe-tens, in-kom´pe-ten-se) **1.** The state of lacking functional ability; applied to an organ or body part. **2.** The state of lacking the legal qualifications to participate in a legal proceding (e.g., to legally give consent, make a contract, stand trial, make a will, testify as a witness).

aortic i. Failure of the aortic valve to close tightly, allowing regurgitation of blood into the left ventricle during diastole.

mental i. Legal term denoting defects of intellectual functioning such that comprehension of, or ability to discharge, required duties is inadequate.

mitral i. Defective closure of a mitral (left atrioventricular) valve, allowing regurgitation of blood into the left atrium during systole.

muscular i. Defective action of the papillary muscles of the heart, resulting in imperfect closure of a normal valve.

pulmonary i. Imperfect closure of a pulmonary valve, allowing regurgitation of blood into the right ventricle during diastole.

pyloric i. A relaxed state of the pylorus, allowing food to pass from the stomach into the intestine before gastric digestion is completed.

tricuspid i. Imperfect closure of a tricuspid (right atrioventricular) valve, allowing regurgitation of blood into the right atrium during systole.

valvular i. Failure of one or more heart valves to close completely.

inconstant (in-kon´stant) **1.** Variable; irregular. **2.** In anatomy, denoting a structure that may or may not be present, may have a tendency to change, or is given to change of location.

incontinence (in-kon´tĭ-nens) **1.** Inability to control the passage of urine or feces. **2.** Lack of self-control.

anorectal i. Involuntary passage of flatus or feces, which may occur as a complication of operative vaginal delivery; caused by faulty repair or healing of third- and fourth-degree perineal lacerations (which involve the anal sphincter muscles and lowest portion of the rectum).

bypass i. Diversion and leakage of urine through an abnormal channel (e.g., fistula, ectopic urethral opening, ectopic ureter); may also be the result of an overflow of urine retained within a urethral

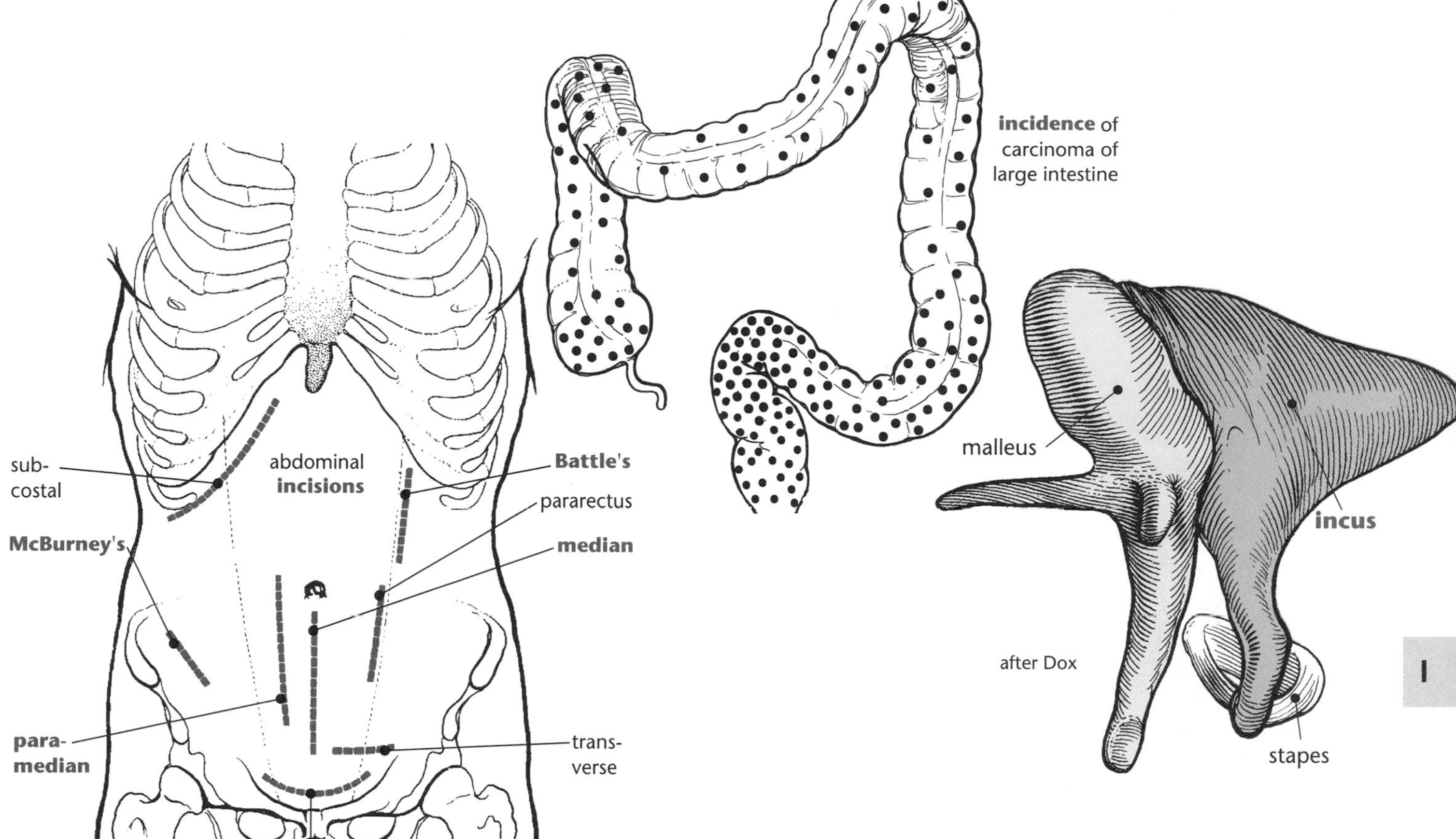

INCUBATION PERIODS OF VARIOUS DISEASES		
disease	**incubation periods**	**rash**
diphtheria	2–5 days	–
scarlet fever	1–5 days	1–5 days
measles	10–15 days	10–15 days
rubella	14–21 days	14–21 days
chickenpox	14–21 days	14–21 days
mumps	7–26 days	–
gonorrhea	1–8 days	–
hepatitis A	15–45 days	–
hepatitis B	4–26 weeks	–
	(typically 6–8 weeks)	–
hepatitis C	8–12 weeks	–
hepatitis D	30–120 days	–
	(typically 60 days)	–
hepatitis E	14–60 days	–
	(typically 40 days)	–
syphilis	1–6 weeks	6 weeks

CLASSIFICATION OF OVERWEIGHT AND OBESITY BY BODY MASS INDEX	
Underweight	< 18.5
Normal	18.5–24.9
Overweight	25.0–29.9
Obesity	
I	30.0–34.9
II	35.0–39.9
III	> 40

diverticulum or from pelvic surgery or irradiation.

overflow i. Leakage of urine occurring when the bladder is over-distended and its sphincters are overcome.

stress i. See stress urinary incontinence.

stress urinary i. (SUI) Involuntary passage of urine occurring usually on straining, coughing, or sneezing. Also called stress incontinence.

urge i. Inability to postpone voiding because the urge to urinate is abrupt and uncontrollable.

incoordination (in-ko-or-dĭ-na´shun) Inability to produce harmonious voluntary muscular movements.

incorporation (in-kor-por-a´shun) The act of making something part of oneself, either by eating and digesting food or by taking in and adopting knowledge or the attitudes of another person (especially in psychoanalysis).

incrustation (in-krus-ta´shun) **1.** The formation of a scab. **2.** A scab.

incubation (in-ku-ba´shun) **1.** The maintenance of optimal conditions of the environment, such as the proper temperature and gas content, for bacterial growth or the development of a premature newborn. **2.** The phase of an infectious disease from the time of introduction to the appearance of the first symptoms.

incubator (in´ku-ba-tor) One of a variety of apparatuses designed to maintain a constant temperature; used to preserve the life of a premature baby, to grow bacterial cultures, etc.

incurable (in-ku´ră-bl) Not curable.

incus (ing´kus) The middle of the three auditory ossicles in the middle ear chamber, situated between the malleus and the stapes.

indentation (in-den-ta´shun) **1.** A notch, dent, or impression. **2.** The act of indenting or notching.

Independent Practice Association (in-dĭ-pen´dent prak´tis ă-so-se-ā´shun) (IPA) An association composed of physicians who have joined to contract with HMOs, PPOs, or other payers while continuing to provide fee-for-service care.

index (in´deks), *pl.* **in´dexes, in´dices** **1.** The forefinger or second digit. **2.** A value expressing the ratio of one measurement to another. **3.** A mold used to record or maintain the relative position of teeth to one another and/or to a cast. **4.** A guide used to reposition teeth, casts, or parts.

Arneth i. A value obtained by adding the percentages of polymorphonuclear neutrophils with one or two lobes in their nuclei plus one-half the percentage of those with three lobes; the normal value is 60%.

body mass i. (BMI) A measure of body mass calculated by dividing weight (in kilograms) by the square of height (in meters). BMI = wt / ht^2.

cardiac i. The quantity of blood ejected by the heart in a given time (expressed in minutes), divided by the body surface (expressed in square meters).

cardiothoracic i. The ratio of the maximal transverse diameter of the heart shadow on an x-ray image to the maximal transverse diameter of the chest, normally less than one-half.

cephalic i. The ratio of the maximal width to the maximal length of the head. Also called length-breadth index.

chemotherapeutic i. The ratio of the minimal effective dose of a drug to the maximal tolerated dose.

chest i. See thoracic index.

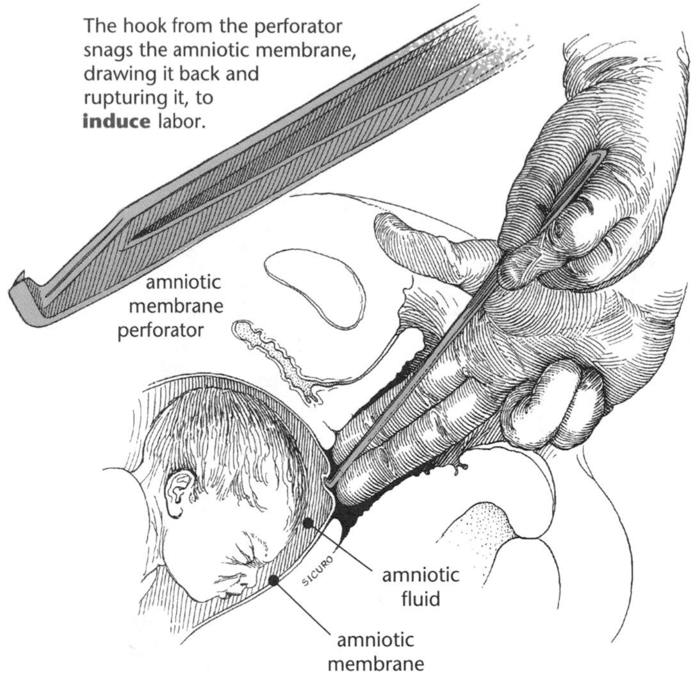

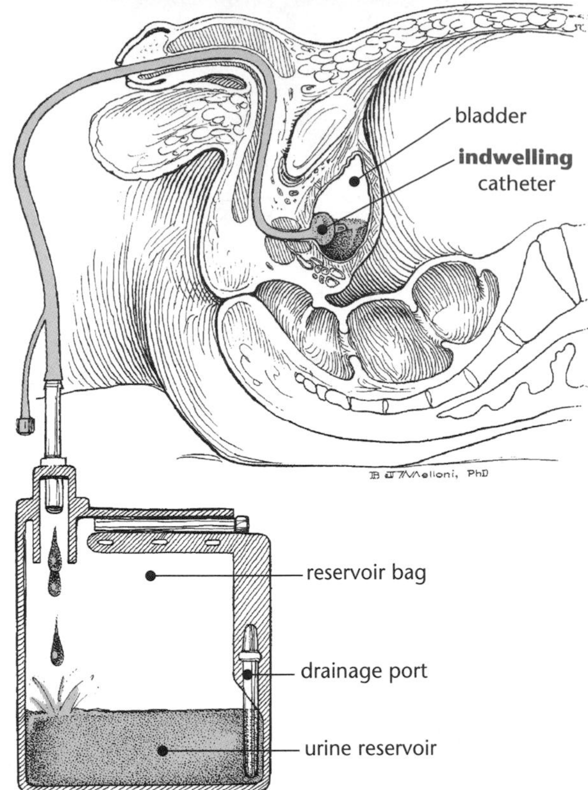

color i. (Ci) The ratio of the amount of hemoglobin to the number of red blood cells. Also called blood quotient; globular value.

fetopelvic i. A value based on the differences in certain maternal pelvic dimensions obtained by x-ray pelvimetry, and certain fetal vertex dimensions obtained by ultrasonography; used to evaluate fetomaternal relationships that may be predictive of a difficult labor (dystocia).

hemizona assay i. (HZI) In testing the functional capacity of sperm: the ratio of the number of zona-bound sperm for the test sample to the number of zona-bound sperm for the fertile donor sample.

icterus i. An index indicating the relative amount of bilirubin in the blood.

length-breadth i. See cephalic index.

maturation i. An index used to detect estrogenic activity by indicating the percentage of mature cells exfoliated from the vagina; the action of an estrogen matures vaginal epithelium; therefore, the higher percentage of mature cells exfoliated suggests increased estrogenic activity.

nasal i. The ratio of the greatest width of the nose to its length.

orbital i. The ratio of the height of the orbit to its width.

periodontal disease i. (PDI) An index for determining disease of tissues surrounding and supporting the teeth (periodontal disease), based on the condition of representative teeth regarding gum inflammation, pockets, plaques, lack of contact, and mobility.

refractive i. (n) The ratio of the speed of light in a medium of reference (vacuum, air, etc.) to the speed of light in a given medium.

Schilling's i. See Schilling's blood count, under count.

therapeutic i. The ratio of the dose that is fatal to 50 percent of test animals (LD_{50}) to the dose that produces the desired effect in 50 percent of test animals (ED_{50}); used in quantitative comparison of drugs.

thoracic i. The ratio of the anteroposterior to the transverse diameter of the chest. Also called chest index.

vital i. The ratio of births to deaths in a given population during a given time.

indican (in´dĭ-kan) **1.** A water-soluble glucoside that hydrolyzes to glucose and indoxyl, present in plants yielding the blue dye indigo. **2.** Potassium indoxyl sulfate, a product of decomposition of the amino acid tryptophan; formed in the intestines and excreted in the urine.

indicant (in´dĭ-kant) Serving to indicate, as a symptom that indicates a mode of treatment.

indicanuria (in-dĭ-kă-nu´re-ă) The presence of increased indican in the urine; a sign of protein putrefaction mainly in the intestines.

indication (in-dĭ-ka´shun) Anything that suggests the proper treatment of a disease.

indicator (in´dĭ-ka-tor) In chemistry, any of various substances (e.g., litmus) that, by means of changing color, indicate the presence, absence, or concentration of a substance, or the degree of completion of a chemical reaction between two or more substances.

indigenous (in-dij´ĕ-nus) Occurring naturally in an area. Also called native.

indigestible (in-di-jes´tĭ-bl) **1.** Not capable of being digested. **2.** Difficult to digest.

indigestion (in-dĭ-jes´chun) **1.** Discomfort caused by a temporary inability to digest food properly. **2.** Failure of digestion.

nervous i. Indigestion caused by emotional disturbances.

indigo (in´dĭ-go) A blue dye obtained from plants of the genus *Indigofera* or produced synthetically.

i. carmine A blue dye, sodium indigotindisulfonate.

indium (in´de-um) A soft, silvery-white metallic element; symbol In, atomic number 49, atomic weight 114.82.

indium-111 (^{111}In) A gamma-emitting radionuclide used primarily as a tag for labeling white blood cells in locating occult abcesses.

individuation (in-dĭ-vid-u-a´shun) The process of forming or becoming a separate person differentiated from the family or community.

indocyanine green (in-do-sī´ă-nin grēn) A dye used in a variety of blood flow, volume and function studies; most commonly used to measure cardiac output.

indole (in´dōl) A normal product of protein decomposition in the large intestine. Also called ketol.

indolent (in´do-lent) **1.** Sluggish. **2.** Causing little or no pain.

indolic acids (in´do-lik as´idz) Products of metabolism of the amino acid tryptophan.

indomethacin (in-do-meth´ă-sin) A nonsteroidal anti-inflammatory compound; an inhibitor of prostaglandin synthetase; used in the treatment of rheumatoid arthritis, osteoarthritis, acute gout, and other musculoskeletal disorders; Indocin®.

induce (in-dōōs´) **1.** To bring on or about by stimulation; to cause; to effect. **2.** In psychology, to arouse by indirect influence.

inducer (in-dōōs´er) A small molecule, usually a substrate of a specific enzyme pathway, capable of combining with the repressor to form an inactive complex that cannot combine with the operator, and as a result permits mRNA synthesis.

inductance (in-duk´tans) (L) A circuit element, typically a conducting coil in which a magnetic field is associated with the circuit when the circuit is carrying current; the unit of induction is the henry (H).

induction (in-duk´shun) Causing to occur.

enzyme i. Stimulation of the synthesis of an enzyme from amino acids programmed by a structural gene in the presence of a small inducer molecule.

i. of labor Stimulation of uterine contractions before the spontaneous onset of labor for the purpose of accomplishing delivery.

inductor (in-duk´tor) An agent that brings about induction.

inductorium (in-duk-tor´e-um) Instrument designed to generate currents of electricity for stimulation of a nerve or a muscle.

indurated (in´dōō-rāt-ed) Hardened; denoting normally soft tissues that have become abnormally firm.

induration (in-dōō-rā´shun) **1.** The hardening of a tissue. **2.** An abnormally hard spot or area.

brown i. of lung Term applied to a brown pigmentation and hardening of lung tissue due to long-standing congestion of the lungs resulting from heart disease.

cyanotic i. Induration caused by chronic venous congestion of an organ.

indwelling (in-dwel´ing) Remaining in place; denoting a catheter or drainage tube that is fixed and held in position for a period of time.

inebriant (in-e´bre-ant) Any intoxicating agent; an intoxicant.

inebriation (in-e-bre-a´shun) The condition of being intoxicated.

inert (in-ert´) **1.** Slow to move or act; sluggish. **2.** Resisting action. **3.** Devoid of chemical activity, as the inert gases. **4.** Denoting a compound or drug that has no therapeutic action.

inertia (in-er´shă) **1.** Resistance offered by a mass to a change in its position of rest or motion. **2.** Denoting inability to move unless stimulated by an external force.

colonic i. Sluggish muscular activity of the colon.

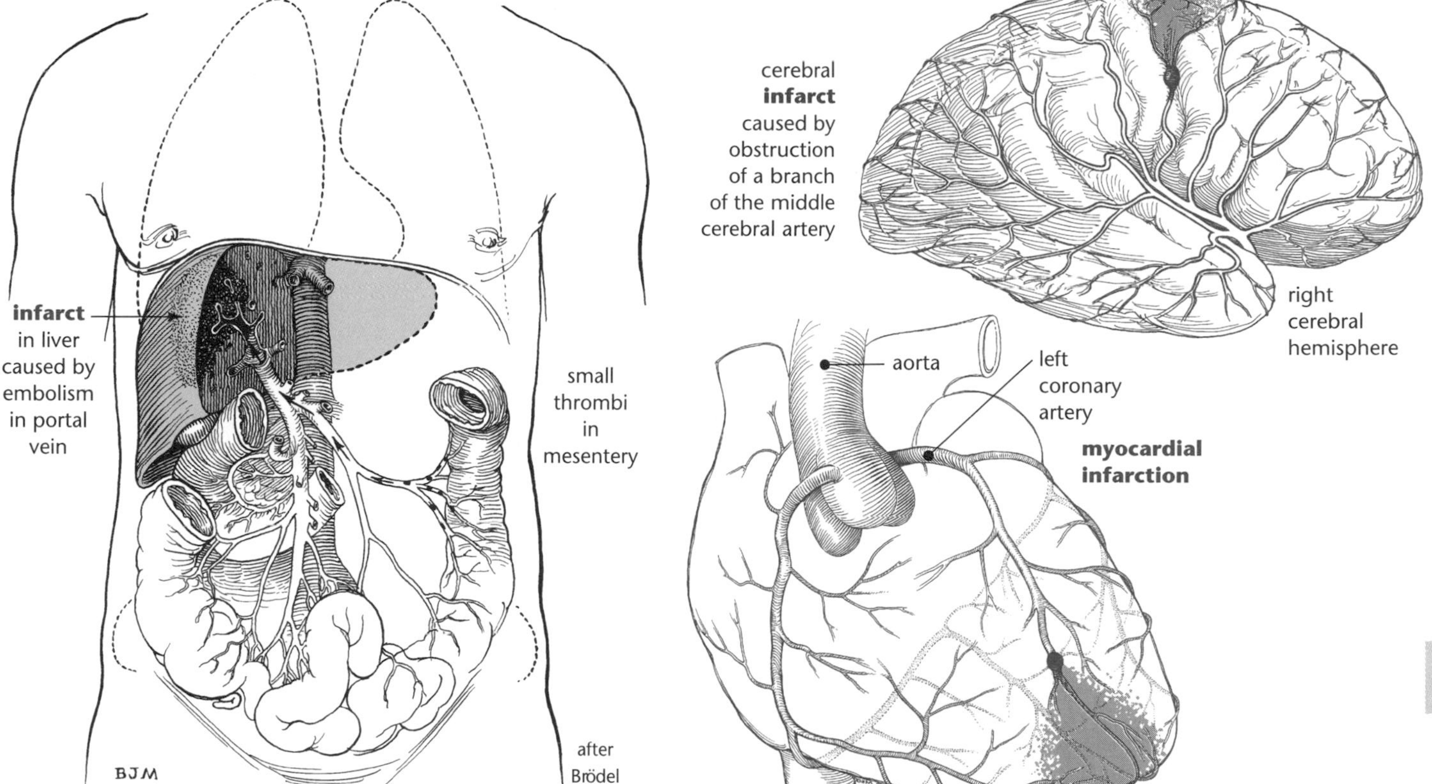

uterine i. Absence of effective uterine contractions during labor.

in extremis (in ek-strē´mis) Latin for at the point of death.

infancy (in´fan-se) Babyhood; the first two years of life.

infant (in´fant) A child under the age of two years.

appropriate-for-gestational-age i., AGA i. An infant whose weight is between the 10th and 90th percentiles when compared with other infants of the same gestational age.

dysmature i. See postmature infant.

excessive-size i. An infant who at the time of birth weighs over 4500 g (9.9 lbs).

extremely low-birth-weight i. See very low birth weight infant.

floppy i. See infantile spinal muscular atrophy, under atrophy.

immature i. An infant born at20 to28 weeks of gestation, weighing 500 to 1000 g (1.1 to2.2 lbs).

large-for-gestational-age i., LGA i. An infant whose weight is greater than the 90th percentile of that particular gestational age or 2 standard deviations above the mean weight for gestational age.

live-born i. An infant who, after being expelled or extracted from the mother, breathes or shows other evidence of life (such as beating of the heart, pulsation of the umbilical cord, and definite movements of involuntary muscles) whether the umbilical cord has been cut or the placenta has detached.

low-birth-weight i., LBW i. An infant weighing 2500 g (5.5 lbs) or less at birth.

postmature i. A postterm infant whose placenta has diminished capacity for sufficient exchange resulting in cutaneous and nutritional changes. Also called dysmature infant.

postterm i. An infant born after 42 or more completed weeks of gestation. Also called postdates infant.

premature i. An infant born between 28 and 38 weeks of gestation, weighing 1000 to 2500 g (2.2 to5.5 lbs). Popularly called preemie.

preterm i. General term for an infant born at any time through the 37th week of gestation (259 days).

small-for-gestational-age i., SGA i. An infant whose weight is less than the 10th percentile for all infants at that particular gestational age or more than 2 standard deviations below the mean for gestational age. Also called undergrown infant.

stillborn i. An infant who shows no signs of life at birth.

term i., i. at term An infant born no earlier than 38 weeks but not later than 42 weeks of gestation. Also called mature infant.

very low-birth-weight i., VLBW i. An infant weighing less than 1000 g (2.2 lbs) at birth. Also called extremely low-birth-weight infant.

infanticide (in-fan´tĭ-sīd) The killing of an infant by a willful act of commission or omission.

infantile (in´fan-tīl) Relating to an infant.

infantile polycystic disease of kidneys (in´fan-tīl pol-e-sis´tik dĭ-zēz´ ŭv kid´nez) See polycystic kidney disease.

infantilism (in´fan-tĭ-liz-m) Extremely slow development of mind or body, or both.

infarct (in´farkt) An area of necrosis in a tissue caused by obstruction in the artery supplying the area.

anemic i. See pale infarct.

bland i. An infarct that is not infected.

hemorrhagic i. A red and swollen infarct due to infiltration of blood into the dead tissue. Also called red infarct.

lacunar i. A small area (2 to 12 mm) of dead tissue deep in the brain (thalamus, putamen, base of pons, or white matter of cerebral hemisphere), resulting from occlusion or narrowing of the penetrating branches of the anterior cerebral, posterior cerebral, or basilar arteries.

pale i. Infarct caused by obstruction of the circulation in a terminal artery; seen in solid organs that lack collateral circulation (e.g., kidney, spleen). Also called anemic or white infarct.

red i. See hemorrhagic infarct.

septic i. Infarct into which a bacterial infection has spread; occurs usually when microorganisms are present in the occluding blood clot, frequently transforming the infarct into an abscess.

white i. See pale infarct.

infarction (in-fark´shun) **1.** The formation of an infarct. **2.** Infarct.

myocardial i. (MI) Deterioration and/or death of a portion of the heart muscle as a result of deprivation of its blood supply, usually due to occlusion of the artery supplying blood to the area; the occlusion may or may not be due to a thrombus (blood clot).

placental i. Degenerative lesions in the placenta varying in size, location, and degree of degeneration; caused by impairment of the uteroplacental circulation, usually by blood clots obstructing the blood flow through the spiral arteries.

pulmonary i. An airless area of lung tissue filled with blood cells as a result of the interruption of the blood supply to the tissues by a clot.

subendocardial myocardial i. Infarction limited to the layer of muscle adjacent to the inner lining of the heart ventricles.

transmural myocardial i. Infarction involving the whole thickness of the heart muscle, extending through all layers of the myocardium.

infect (in-fekt´) **1.** To invade and become established in the body; applied to microorganisms. **2.** To contaminate with harmful agents.

infection (in-fek´shun) Invasion of the body by living microorganisms; it may or may not result in an illness.

clinical i. An infection that has become sufficiently active to give rise to signs and symptoms of a disease (infectious disease).

focal i. An infection in which the microorganisms remain in a limited area.

guinea worm i. See dracunculiasis.

HIV i. Infection with a strain of the human immunodeficiency virus (HIV 1 or HIV 2); marked by active virus replication, progressive immunologic impairment throughout its course, and AIDS (the final stage). See also AIDS; HIV disease.

hospital-acquired i. See nosocomial infection.

inapparent i. An infection that is not sufficiently active to give rise to recognizable signs and symptoms of disease. Also called subclinical infection.

latent i. A persistent inapparent infection in which the presence of the organism cannot be detected by currently available methods; it flares up from time to time under certain conditions; e.g., a herpes simplex infection (cold sore).

MAC i. See *Mycobacterium avium* complex bacteremia, under bacteremia.

nosocomial i. An infection acquired as a result of hospitalization or treatment received at a hospital and that was not present or incubating at the time of exposure to the hospital environment. Also called hospital-acquired infection.

perinatal i. Any infection occurring during the time of life between the completion of 20 weeks of gestation and the first 28 days after birth (i.e., during the perinatal period).

pyogenic i. A pus-producing infection caused by certain bacteria (e.g., *Staphylococcus aureus* and *Streptococcus pyogenes*).

retrograde i. An infection of a tubular structure that spreads in a direction opposite the natural flow of secretions.

secondary i. An infection occurring in an individual already suffering from a previous infection by another microorganism.

SOME CONDITIONS THAT CAUSE **INFERTILITY**

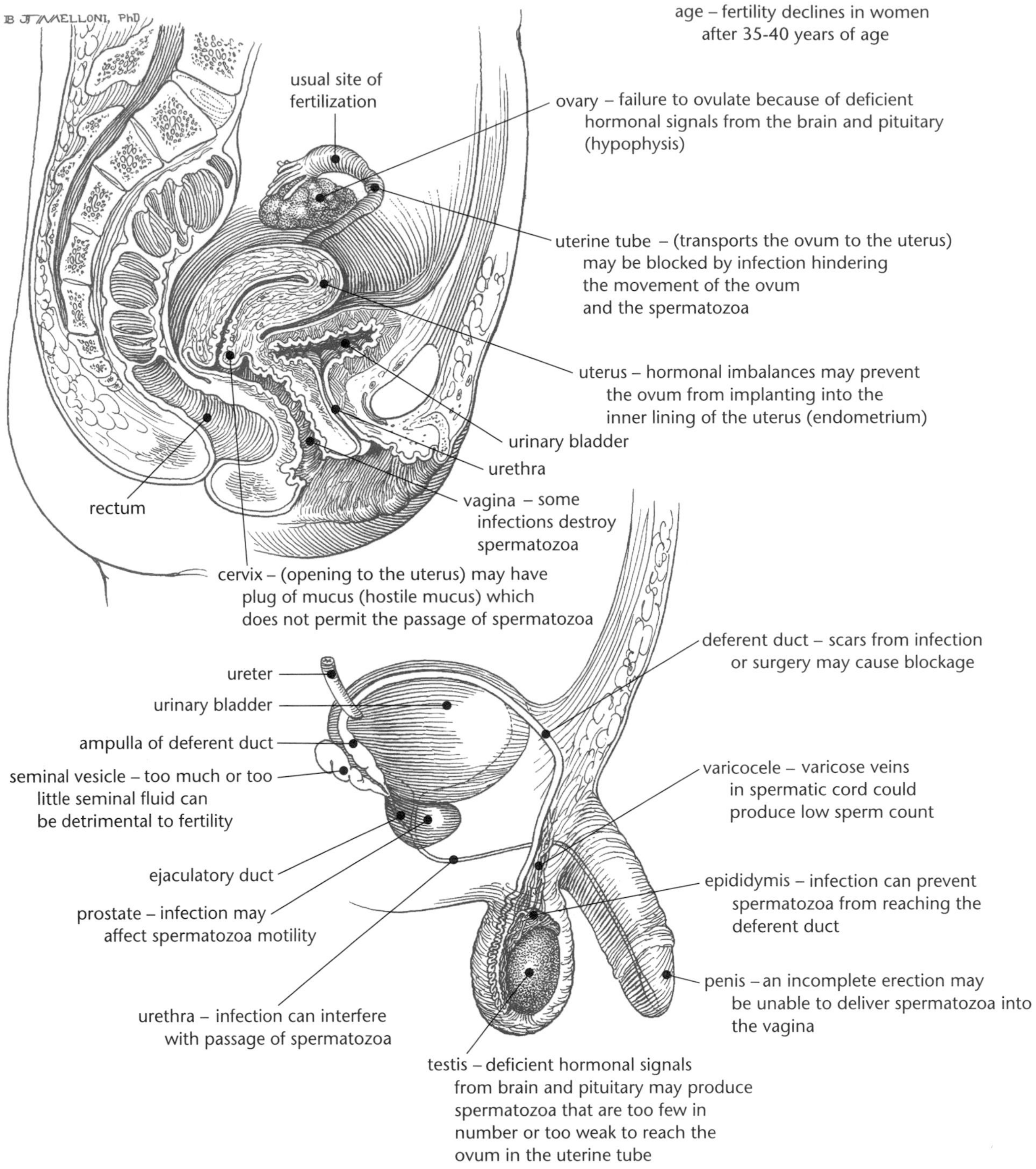

age – fertility declines in women after 35-40 years of age

usual site of fertilization

ovary – failure to ovulate because of deficient hormonal signals from the brain and pituitary (hypophysis)

uterine tube – (transports the ovum to the uterus) may be blocked by infection hindering the movement of the ovum and the spermatozoa

uterus – hormonal imbalances may prevent the ovum from implanting into the inner lining of the uterus (endometrium)

urinary bladder

urethra

rectum

vagina – some infections destroy spermatozoa

cervix – (opening to the uterus) may have plug of mucus (hostile mucus) which does not permit the passage of spermatozoa

ureter

urinary bladder

ampulla of deferent duct

seminal vesicle – too much or too little seminal fluid can be detrimental to fertility

deferent duct – scars from infection or surgery may cause blockage

varicocele – varicose veins in spermatic cord could produce low sperm count

ejaculatory duct

prostate – infection may affect spermatozoa motility

epididymis – infection can prevent spermatozoa from reaching the deferent duct

penis – an incomplete erection may be unable to deliver spermatozoa into the vagina

urethra – infection can interfere with passage of spermatozoa

testis – deficient hormonal signals from brain and pituitary may produce spermatozoa that are too few in number or too weak to reach the ovum in the uterine tube

subclinical i. See inapparent infection.

terminal i. An acute infection occurring toward the end of another disease (usually chronic) and generally causing death.

Vincent's i. See acute necrotizing ulcerative gingivitis, under gingivitis.

infectious (in-fek´shus) Capable of being transmitted with or without direct contact.

infecundity (in-fe-kun´dĭ-te) Inability of a woman to bear children.

inference, statistical (in´fer-ens, stă-tis´tĭ-kal) In biostatistics, the procedure in which a conclusion is made on the basis of a drawn sample; usually a statistic is computed and, from that, a conclusion is formed about the corresponding parameters.

inferior (in-fēr´e-or) Located in a lower position in relation to another structure.

infertility (in-fer-til´ĭ-te) **1.** Inability to produce offspring. In males, inability to fertilize the ovum; in females, inability to conceive after one year of regular intercourse without use of contraceptives. Infertility may or may not be reversible. COMPARE: sterility. **2.** Inability of a woman to carry a pregnancy to term. Also called impaired fertility.

primary i. Infertility occurring without previous pregnancies.

secondary i. Infertility in which a prior pregnancy (not necessarily a live birth) has occurred.

infest (in-fest) To attack or live on a host as a parasite.

infestation (in-fes-ta´shun) Presence of parasites on the body (e.g., ticks, mites, lice), or in the organs (e.g., worms).

infiltrate (in-fil´trāt) **1.** To pass into the interstices of a tissue or substance, as a cancer. **2.** The material that has infiltrated into the tissue (e.g., a pulmonary infiltrate noted on chest x ray).

infiltration (in-fil-trā´shun) **1.** Seepage or diffusion into tissue of substances that are not ordinarily present in that tissue or invasion by cells that are not normal to the location. **2.** Injection of a solution into a tissue (e.g., an anesthetic).

fatty i. Abnormal accumulation of fat globules in the cells.

infirm (in-firm´) Weak condition of the body due to disease or old age.

infirmary (in-fir´mă-re) A dispensary for the care of the sick or injured, especially in a school or camp.

infirmity (in-fir´mĭ-te) **1.** A disabling state of the mind or body. **2.** A disease or condition causing bodily debilitation.

inflammation (in-flă-ma´shun) A tissue reaction to irritation, infection, or injury, marked by localized heat, swelling, redness, pain, and sometimes loss of function.

inflammatory (in-flam´ă-tor-e) Relating to, marked by, resulting from, or causing inflammation.

inflation (in-fla´shun) The act of distending or the state of being distended by a gas or liquid.

inflection, inflexion (in-flek´shun) The act of turning inward, or a state of being turned inward.

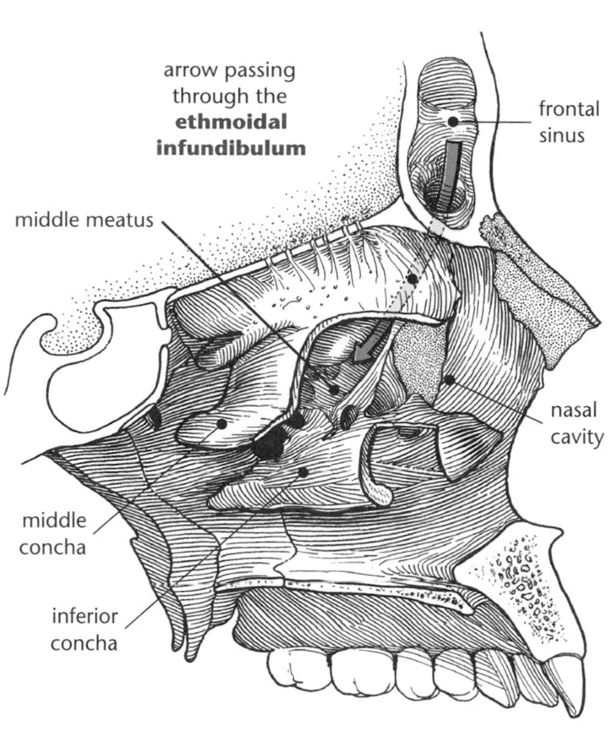

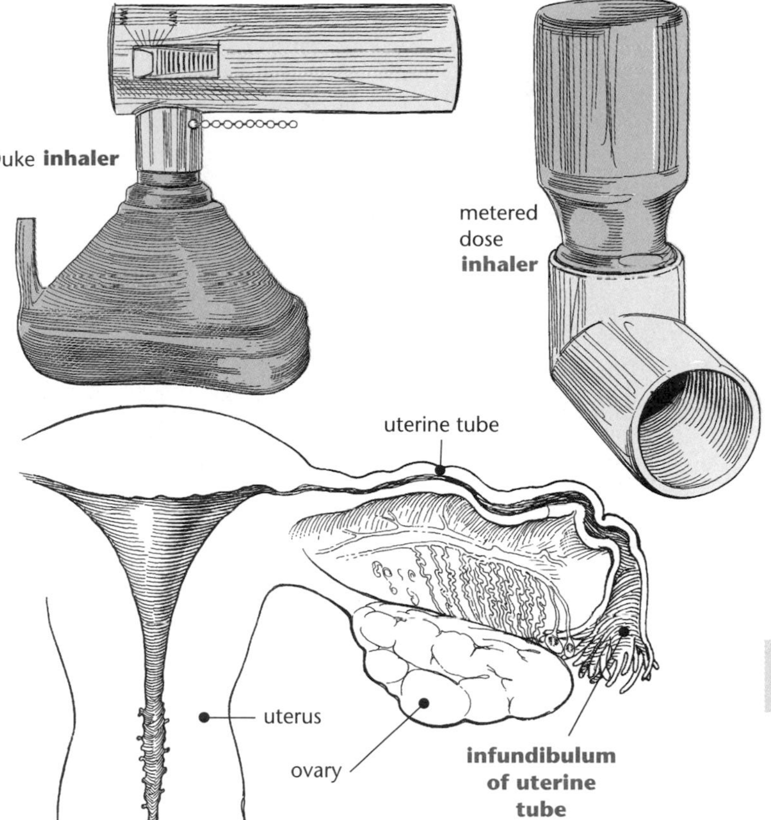

infliximab (in-flik´sĭ-mab) Monoclonal antibody that inhibits tissue coagulation and necrosis; used to treat fistulas caused by Crohn's disease.

influenza (in-floo-en´ză) Acute infection of the respiratory tract caused by inhalation of influenza viruses (family Orthomyxoviridae); marked by fever, headache, pain in the back and limbs, and inflammation of the respiratory tract; it occurs in epidemics and sometimes pandemics (world epidemics). Popularly called flu; formerly, grippe.

Influenzavirus (in-floo-en´ză-vi-rus) Genus of viruses (family Orthomyxoviridae) that includes serotypes A and B (probably C), and several subgroups of strains, classified on the basis of their surface antigens; the cause of respiratory infections.

infold (in-fōld´) To fold inward.

infraclavicular (in-fră-klă-vik´u-lar) Situated below a clavicle (collarbone).

infraclusion (in-fră-kloo´zhun) Condition in which a tooth fails to erupt. Also called infraocclusion.

infradian (in-fra-de´an) Relating to biorhythms occurring in cycles less frequent than 24 hours.

infrahyoid (in-fră-hi´oid) Located below the hyoid bone.

inframandibular (in-fră-man-dib´u-lar) Below the lower jaw.

infranatant (in-fră-nā´tant) The clear fluid seen after the flotation of particulate matter in a suspension.

infraocclusion (in-fră-o-kloo´zhun) See infraclusion.

infraorbital (in-fră-or´bĭ-tal) Beneath or on the floor of the orbit.

infrapatellar (in-fră-pă-tel´ar) Below the patella (kneecap), such as a bursa.

infrared (in-fră-red´) The electromagnetic radiation beyond the red end of the spectrum with wavelengths that are too long (greater than 7700 Å) to be seen by the human eye.

infrascapular (in-fră-skap´u-lar) Below the scapula (shoulder blade).

infraspinous (in-fră-spi´nus) Below a spinous process.

infrasplenic (in-fră-splen´ik) Below or beneath the spleen.

infrasternal (in-fră-ster´nal) Below the sternum (breastbone).

infratrochlear (in-fră-trok´le-ar) Located below the pulley (trochlea) of the superior oblique muscle of the eye.

infraumbilical (in-fră-um-bil´ĭ-kal) Below the navel.

infundibuliform (in-fun-dib´u-lĭ-form) Shaped like a funnel.

infundibulum (in-fun-dib´u-lum) Latin for funnel; most commonly refers to the funnel-shaped stalk of the pituitary gland (hypophysis).

ethmoidal i. The long, curved, funnel-shaped passage connecting the anterior ethmoid cells and the frontal sinus with the nasal cavity.

i. of uterine tube The lateral, funnel-shaped extremity of the uterine (fallopian) tube.

infusible (in-fu´zĭ-bl) **1.** Resistant to changes by heat. **2.** Capable of being infused.

infusion (in-fu´zhun) **1.** The introduction of a fluid into a vessel. **2.** The soaking or steeping of a substance in water in order to extract its soluble parts. **3.** The resulting liquid.

ingestion (in-jes´chun) **1.** The swallowing of food, drink, or medicines. **2.** Process by which a cell or a unicellular organism takes in foreign material.

inguinal (ing´gwĭ-nal) Pertaining to the groin.

inhalant (in-ha´lant) A remedy taken by inhalation.

inhalation (in-hă-la´shun) The act of breathing in; breathing in of a gas or a medication or a noxious substance.

inhale (in-hāl´) To draw into the body by breathing; to inspire.

inhaler (in-hāl er) A device that permits medicinal material in vapor form to be inhaled.

inherent (in-hĕr´ent) Belonging naturally to a person.

inheritance (in-her´ĭ-tans) **1.** In genetics, the process of transmitting genetic characters from parent to offspring. **2.** The characters so transmitted.

dominant i. See dominant gene, under gene.

hologynic i. Transmission of a trait from mother to all her daughters but not to her sons (i.e., occurring only in females).

mendelian i. See Mendel's laws, under law.

mitochondrial i. Inheritance encoded in a gene of a mitochondrial chromosome.

mosaic i. Inheritance characterized by the dominance of paternal influence in one group of cells and the dominance of the maternal in another.

recessive i. See recessive gene, under gene.

X-linked i. Inheritance determined by a gene carried on the X chromosome.

Y-linked i. Inheritance determined by a gene carried on the Y chromosome.

inhibin (in-hib´in) A polypeptide hormone synthesized and secreted by male and female gonads that specifically inhibits the release of pituitary follicle-stimulating hormone (FSH).

inhibition (in-hĭ-bish´un) The restriction or arrest of a function or specific activity.

competitive i. Blocking of enzyme activity by a compound that binds to the free enzyme, thus preventing the enzyme from binding to the substance upon which it is supposed to act.

inhibitor (in-hib´ĭ-tor) An agent or nerve that represses physiologic activity.

allosteric i. A substance that decreases enzymatic activity through noncompetitive binding to the enzyme molecule at a site (allosteric site) other than the active site of the enzyme.

ACE i. See angiotensin-converting enzyme inhibitor.

angiotensin-converting enzyme i. (ACEI) Any of a class of drugs that inhibit the action of the enzyme kininase II, which converts angiotensin I to angiotensin II; used in the treatment of high blood pressure and congestive heart failure. Use of ACEIs during pregnancy increases the risk for fetal death. Also called ACE inhibitor.

cyclooxygenase i., COX i. An agent that prevents production of prostaglandin (PG) from arachidonic acid.

cyclooxygenase-1 i.'s, COX-1 i.'s Inhibitors preventing production of a variety of prostaglandins (PGs) that cause pain and inflammation, as well as those PGs that protect the stomach.

cyclooxygenase-2 i.'s, COX-2 i.'s Inhibitors that prevent production of pain-causing prostaglandins (PGs) but not those that protect the stomach.

glucosidase i.'s A group of drugs that reduce intestinal absorption of carbohydrates. Popularly called starch blockers.

HMG-CoA reductase i.'s A group of drugs that hinder the formation of cholesterol in the body; used to treat hyperlipidemia. Referred to as "statins" because of their chemical names (e.g., lovastatin, pravastatin).

inion (in´e-on) The most prominent point of the external occipital protuberance of the skull; used as a fixed craniometric point.

initiator (ĭ-nish´e-a-tor) A substance necessary for the process of building certain giant molecules, helping to bring about such reactions; unlike a catalyst, it is altered in the process and may appear in the final product.

inject (in-jekt´) To drive a fluid into a part.

injectable (in-jek´tă-bl) Any substance that may be injected.

injection (in-jek´shun) **1.** The act of forcing or driving a fluid into a part, such as the subcutaneous tissue or a bodily cavity. **2.** The fluid injected. **3.**

placing of sperm close to the opening of the uterine tube
in vivo fertilization
numerous mature ova are available for potential fertilization
transcervical route of **intrauterine insemination** (to bypass the cervix when infertility is due to a cervical condition)
superovulation induced by administration of human chorionic gonadotrophin (hCG)
hyperextension
hyperflexion
forcible and sudden bending backward (hyperextension) followed immediately by forcible and sudden bending forward (hyperflexion) resulting in **whiplash injury**

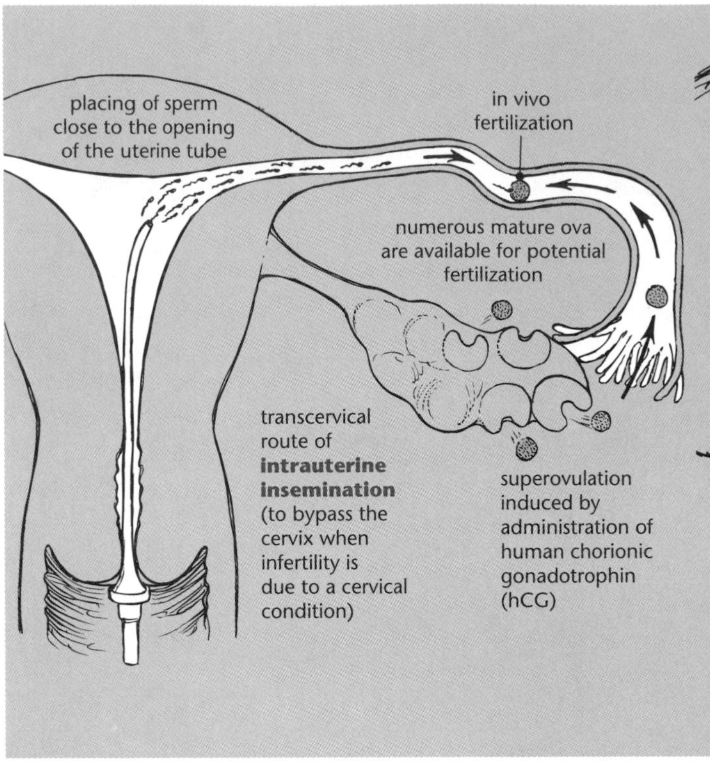

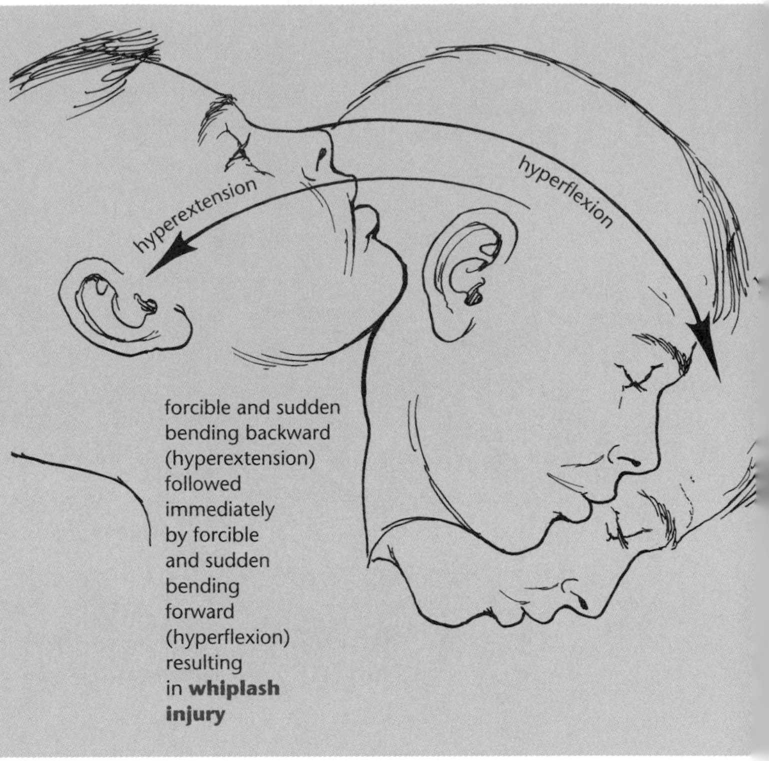

Popular term for a state of visible congestion (e.g., of the eye blood vessels).

hypodermic i. See subcutaneous injection.

intracytoplasmic sperm i. (ICSI) An *in vitro* fertilization procedure in which a single sperm is introduced directly into the cytoplasm of the ovum. See also insemination.

intramuscular (IM) i. Injection into a muscle.

intrathecal i. Injection into the subarachnoid space (e.g., of an anesthetic solution to induce spinal anesthesia).

intravenous (IV) i. Injection into a vein.

subcutaneous i. Injection into the loose tissue just beneath the skin. Also called hypodermic injection; popularly called hypo.

retrograde i. Introduction of a solution into an organ against the normal direction of flow (e.g., injection of a radiopaque solution into the kidney via the ureter).

injector (in-jek´tor) A device for administering injections.

jet i. A machine that, through high pressure, forces a liquid through a small orifice at high velocity; the liquid is thus able to penetrate the unbroken skin without causing pain.

injure (in´jur) To wound or hurt.

injury (in´ju-re) A specific bodily damage or wound. Also called trauma.

blast i. Rupture of lungs or abdominal organs caused by a blast of air, as from explosion of a bomb.

countercoup i. of brain Injury to the brain at a site opposite to the point of impact.

cumulative i. See cumulative trauma, under trauma.

hyperextension-hyperflexion i. See whiplash injury.

reperfusion i. Impairment of heart functioning, usually accompanied by irregular heartbeat, following surgical reopening of a blocked artery.

repetitive motion i. (RMI) Damage to muscles, nerves, or bones from performing activities for prolonged periods.

whiplash i. A nonspecific term applied to an injury of the spine, usually at the junction of the fourth and fifth cervical vertebrae, caused by an abrupt jerking motion of the head. Also called hyperextension-hyperflexion injury.

inlay (in´la) A solid restorative material (gold, fired porcelain, plastic) that is fitted and cemented to a tapered cavity preparation in a tooth.

inlet (in´let) A passage that leads to a cavity.

pelvic i. See pelvic plane of inlet, under plane.

innate (in´nāt) Present at birth.

innervation (in-er-va´shun) The nerve supply of a given area or structure.

innidiation (ĭ-nid-e-a-shun) The multiplication of cells in a location where they have been carried by lymph or the bloodstream.

innocent (in´o-sĕnt) Benign; said of a tumor.

innocuous (ĭ-nok´u-us) Harmless.

innominate (ĭ-nom´ĭ-nāt) Unnamed. Formerly applied to certain anatomic structures.

innominate artery (ĭ-nom´ĭ-nit ar´ter-e) See brachiocephalic trunk, under trunk.

innominate bone (ĭ-nom´ĭ-nit bōn) See hipbone.

innominate vein (ĭ-nom´ĭ-nit vān) See table of veins.

inoculable (ĭ-nok´u-lă-bl) **1.** Transmissible by inoculation. **2.** Susceptible to a disease which is transmissible by inoculation.

inoculate (ĭ-nok´u-lāt) To introduce a virus into the body; to introduce vaccines, immune sera, or other antigenic material into the body in order to prevent, cure, or experiment.

inoculation (ĭ-nok-u-la´shun) The introduction of disease-causing microorganisms into the body.

therapeutic i. The introduction of an antiserum for curative purposes.

inoculum (ĭ-nok´u-lum) Material containing microorganisms introduced by inoculation.

inoperable (in-op´er-ă-bl) Not suitable for any surgical procedure.

inorganic (in-or-gan´ik) Neither composed of nor derived from organic matter (animal or vegetable); designating compounds that do not contain carbon.

inosine 5´-diphosphate (in´o-sēn di´fos-fāt) (IDP) A nucleotide that participates in high-energy phosphate transfer.

inositol (ĭ-no´sĭ-tol) A substance classified as a member of the vitamin B complex; found in plant and animal tissue.

inotropic (in-o-trop´ik) Influencing or affecting muscular contraction.

negatively i. Weakening the action of muscles.

positively i. Strengthening the action of muscles.

inotropism (in-ot´ro-piz-m) The quality of influencing muscular contraction.

inpatient (in´pā´shent) A patient staying overnight in a hospital.

insalivation (in-sal-ĭ-va´shun) The mixing of food with saliva in chewing.

insane (in-sān´) In legal contexts, relating to insanity, or to one who is of unsound mind. The term is no longer used in psychiatry.

insanity (in-san´ĭ-te) In medicine, the term has not been used in the United States since the 1920s. In law, it denotes a mental state in which one is legally nonresponsible or incompetent for some or all purposes; the law defines different kinds or degrees of insanity (e.g., for making a will, making a business contract, committing criminal acts, or reasonable likelihood of imminent danger to oneself or others); insanity for one act may not necessarily mean insanity for other kinds of acts.

communicated i., double i. See folie à deux, under folie.

inscription (in-skrip´shun) The part of a prescription that stipulates the names and amounts of ingredients to be used by the pharmacist. See also superscription; subscription; signature.

insectarium (in-sek-tar´e-um) A place in which living insects are kept and bred for scientific purposes.

insecticide (in-sek´tĭ-sīd) Any agent that kills insects.

insemination (in-sem-ĭ-na´shun) **1.** Introduction of seminal fluid into the vagina. **2.** Fertilization of an ovum.

artificial i. Deposit of sperm in the vagina, cervix, or within the uterine cavity by means other than sexual intercourse.

artificial insemination by donor (AID) See heterologous insemination.

artificial insemination by husband (AIH) See homologous insemination.

direct intraperitoneal i. (DIPI) Injection of washed, processed sperm into the peritoneal cavity, in the area of the rectouterine pouch, via puncture of the posterior vaginal cul-de-sac; performed at the expected time of ovulation.

donor i. See therapeutic insemination.

heterologous i. Artificial insemination with sperm from a donor other than the woman's husband.

homologous i. Artificial insemination with sperm from the woman's husband.

intrauterine i. (IUI) The direct placement of sperm in the intrauterine cavity using a washed and concentrated specimen (i.e., sperm that has been diluted and centrifuged to remove the prostaglandin-containing seminal fluid); usually performed to bypass the uterine cervix when infertility is due to a cervical condition, either with its structure or its secretions. Also called washed intrauterine insemination.

subzonal i. (SUZI) An *in vitro* fertilization technique in which five to ten spermatozoa are

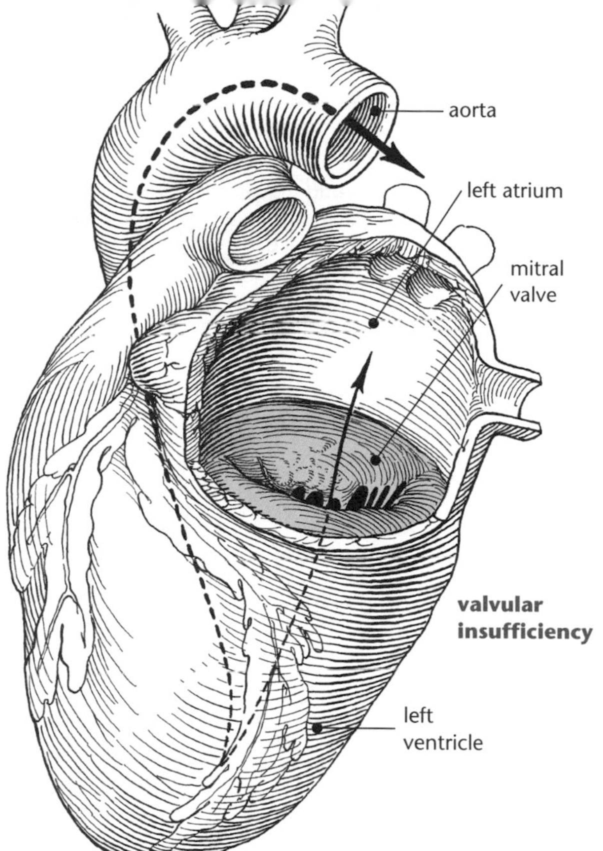

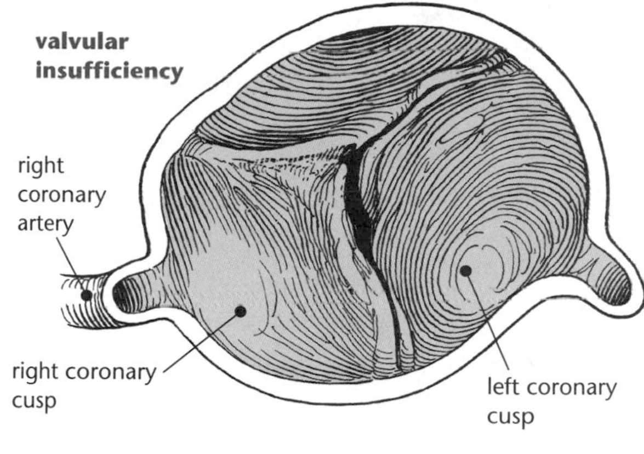

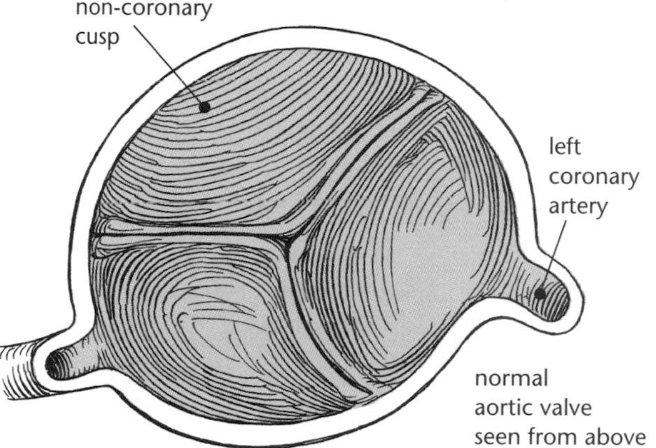

injected, with a microneedle, under the zona pellucida of the ovum (i.e., into the perivitelline space); employed in cases of sperm factor infertility. Also called subzonal insertion; direct ovum fertilization.

therapeutic i. Procedure in which fresh sperm, either husband's (TIH) or donor's (TID), is placed in a woman's vagina, cervix, or uterus; performed in the periovulatory part of the menstrual cycle. Also called donor insemination.

washed intrauterine i. See intrauterine insemination (IUI).

insensible (in-sen´sĭ-bl) **1.** Imperceptible by the senses. **2.** Unconscious.

insert (in´sert) Anything implanted or put into another thing (e.g., additional base pairs into a segment of DNA, or amino acids into a protein).

insertion (in-ser´shun) **1.** The site of attachment of a muscle to a bone which is more movable than the one from which it originated. **2.** The act of introducing or implanting. **3.** A chromosomal abnormality in which a DNA segment from one chromosome breaks loose and becomes attached into a break of a nonhomologous chromosome.

velamentous cord i. Umbilical cord insertion at the periphery of the placenta, with the umbilical vessels spread across the fetal membranes devoid of Wharton's jelly, thus at risk for rupture and hemorrhage.

insidious (in-sid´e-us) Spreading or developing harmfully in a subtle or imperceptible way; applied to certain diseases.

insight (in´sīt) **1.** The ability to understand the real nature of a situation. **2.** Self-understanding.

in situ (in si´tu) Latin for in place; in its original or normal position. The term is applied especially to an early stage in cancerous tumor development in which abnormal cells are still restricted to the site of origin (i.e., they have not invaded tissues beyond their original confines). Sometimes used synonymously with precancerous.

insoluble (in-sol´u-bl) Not capable of entering into solution.

insomnia (in-som´ne-ă) Inability to sleep under normal conditions; three varieties are recognized: (a) inability to fall asleep upon retiring; (b) intermittent waking after falling asleep; (c) early awakening.

insomniac (in-som´ne-ak) A person suffering from insomnia.

inspiration (in-spĭ-ra´shun) Inhalation; breathing in.

inspiratory (in-spi´ră-tor-e) Relating to inhalation.

inspire (in-spīr´) To inhale; to breathe in.

inspissation (in-spis-a´shun) The process of thickening as by evaporation of fluid.

inspissator (in-spis´a-tor) A device used to air-dry fluids.

instep (in´step) The arched middle part of the dorsum of the human foot.

instillation (in-stĭ-la´shun) The gradual, drop by drop, pouring of a liquid.

instinct (in´stinkt) An inherent drive or tendency to act in a certain way without the aid of reason.

instrumentation (in-stroo-men-ta´shun) The use of instruments in any therapeutic procedure.

insudate (in-soo´dāt) Substance passed into, and accumulated in, arterial walls.

insufficiency (in-sŭ-fish´en-se) Inability to perform a normal function; said of an organ or structure.

acute adrenocortical i. Inadequate secretion of adrenocortical hormone causing nausea, vomiting, hypotension, and collapse; may result from lesions in the adrenal cortex but most commonly occurs as a complication of corticosteroid therapy; may also occur in massive adrenal hemorrhage, as in the Waterhouse-Friderichsen syndrome. Also called addisonian crisis; adrenal crisis.

adrenocortical i. Reduced function of the adrenal cortex. Also called hypocorticoidism; hypocorticism.

aortic i. See valvular insufficiency.

cardiac i. See heart failure, under failure.

coronary i. Insufficient blood flow to the cardiac muscle, leading to prolonged pain or discomfort (angina).

mitral i. See valvular insufficiency.

posttraumatic pulmonary i. See adult respiratory distress syndrome.

primary chronic adrenocortical i. See Addison's disease.

pulmonary i. See valvular insufficiency.

renal i. Defective kidney function, especially a decrease in glomerular filtration manifested by a consequent increase in blood levels of urea and creatinine.

tricuspid i. See valvular insufficiency.

valvular i. Failure of a heart valve to close tightly, thus allowing regurgitation of blood; named according to the valve involved (i.e., aortic, mitral, pulmonary, or tricuspid).

venous i. Inadequate drainage of blood from a part, resulting in edema.

insufficiency disease (in-sŭ-fish´en-se dĭ-zēz´) See deficiency disease, under disease.

insufflate (in-sŭf´lāt) **1.** To blow into, as in artificial respiration. **2.** To inject a gas (e.g., carbon dioxide) into a body cavity.

insufflation (in-sŭ-fla´shun) The act of insufflating.

insufflator (in´sŭ-fla-tor) An instrument used in insufflation.

insula (in´su-lă) The central lobe of the cerebrum, lying deeply in the lateral cerebral fissure (fissure of Sylvius). Also called Reil's island; central lobe.

insular (in´su-lar) Relating to an insula, especially the central lobe of the cerebrum (Reil's island).

insulate (in´su-lāt) To prevent the passage of heat, sound, or electricity from one body or region to another by interposing material with nonconductive properties.

insulation (in-su-la´shun) **1.** The act of insulating. **2.** The material used to insulate. **3.** The state of being insulated.

insulator (in´su-la-tor) Any nonconductive material used to effect insulation.

insulin (in´su-lin) A hormone produced by the beta cells of the islets of Langerhans in the pancreas and secreted in response to increased blood sugar (glucose) levels, vagus nerve stimulation, and other factors; it is concerned with regulating carbohydrate, lipid, and protein metabolism. Deficiency of insulin results in diabetes mellitus.

human i. Insulin in which the amino acid sequence is identical to that of the human hormone; produced semisynthetically or by recombinant DNA techniques.

intermediate-acting i. Any insulin preparation that has a 2-4 hour onset of action after injection, lasting 18-24 hours, with 8–10 hours of peak action (e.g., NPH insulin; lente insulin).

isophane i. See NPH insulin.

lente i. A preparation of intermediate action, consisting of a mixture of 30 percent semilente and 70 percent ultralente insulin.

long-acting i. Any insulin preparation that has a 4–5 hour onset of action after injection, lasting 25–36 hours, with 8–14 hours of peak action (e.g., ultralente insulin; protamine zinc insulin).

NPH i. An intermediate-acting suspension of insulin, protamine, and zinc. N denotes a neutral solution; P, the protamine zinc insulin content; H, its developer (Hans C. Hagerdorn, MD). Also called

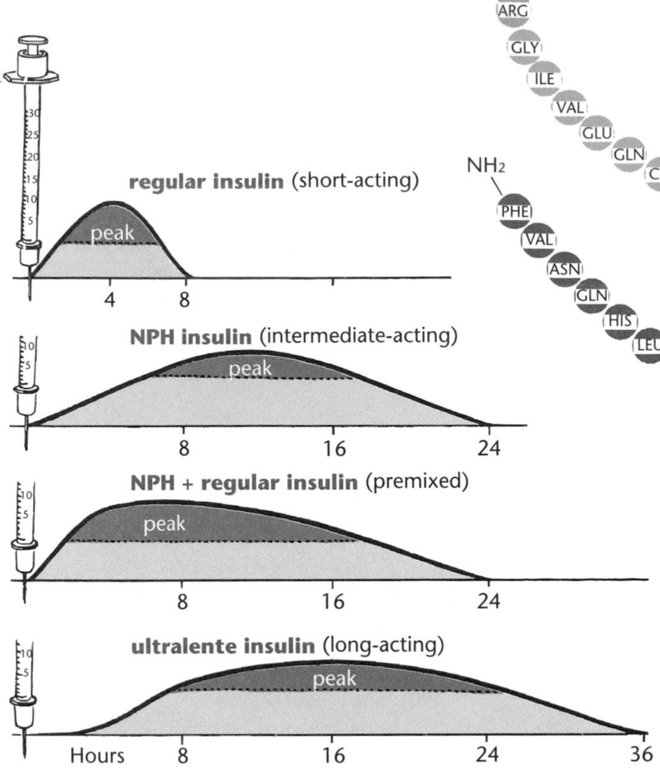

regular insulin (short-acting)
peak
4 8

NPH insulin (intermediate-acting)
peak
8 16 24

NPH + regular insulin (premixed)
peak
8 16 24

ultralente insulin (long-acting)
peak
Hours 8 16 24 36

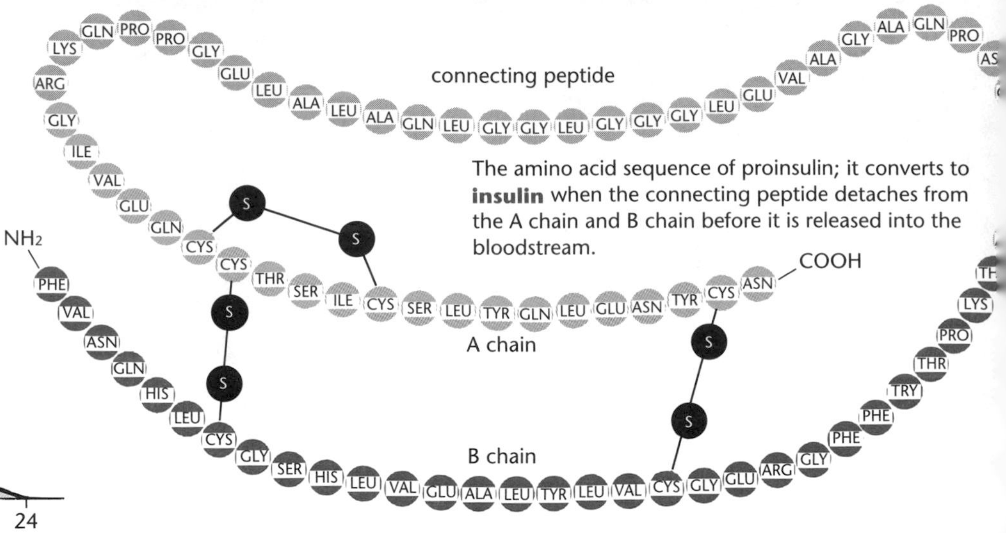

connecting peptide

The amino acid sequence of proinsulin; it converts to **insulin** when the connecting peptide detaches from the A chain and B chain before it is released into the bloodstream.

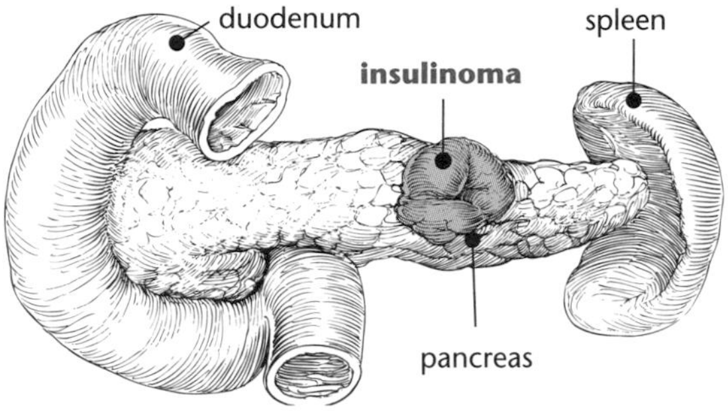

NH2 COOH A chain B chain

duodenum spleen **insulinoma** pancreas

isophane insulin.

premixed i. A preparation containing both a short-acting (regular) and an intermediate-acting (NPH) insulin. The preparation has a 15 to 30 minute onset of action after injection lasting 18 to 24 hours, with 10 to 12 hours of peak action.

protamine zinc i. (PZI) A long-acting preparation consisting of a suspension of insulin, protamine, and zinc chloride. A seldom used preparation in the U.S.A.

regular i. A short-acting aqueous solution of crystalline zinc insulin; its action begins within 15 minutes after subcutaneous injection, peaking at 1–3 hours, and lasting 5–7 hours; can be injected intravenously or used in continuous subcutaneous pumps.

semilente i. A short-acting preparation consisting of an amorphous form of insulin and zinc in acetate buffer.

short-acting i., rapid-acting i. Any insulin preparation that begins to act 15–30 minutes after injection, lasting 5–7 hours, with 1–3 hours of peak action (e.g., regular insulin; semilente insulin).

ultralente i. A long-acting preparation containing a suspension of large insulin crystals.

insulinoma, insuloma (in-su-lin-o´mă, in-su-lo´mă) An insulin-producing tumor of the islet cells of the pancreas.

insulinopenia (in-su-lin-o-pe´ne-ă) Decreased or inadequate level of insulin in the blood.

insulitis (in-su-li´tis) Destruction of beta cells of the pancreas by the patient's own immune system (autoimmunity), as occurs in type I diabetes; thought to be due to a genetic mechanism or triggered by an environmental agent (e.g., virus).

insult (in´sult) An injury or irritation.

integration (in-tĕ-gra´shun) **1.** The condition of being combined. **2.** The process of bringing all parts together to form a whole, as the building up of living substance by assimilation of nutritive material.

integrin (in´te-grin) Any of a family of glycoproteins that are bound to the cell membrane, promote cell adhesion, and participate in many important processes (e.g., embryological development, wound healing, and immune, nonimmune defense activities).

beta 1-i.'s, β 1-i.'s A family of cell surface receptors that mediate cell-matrix interactions (i.e., between the outside of cells and their interior) and play a critical role in tissue development and in post-injury tissue remodeling.

integument (in-teg´u-ment) A covering or coat, as the skin or the membrane covering an organ. Also called tegument.

intelligence (in-tel´ĭ-jens) **1.** The faculty of thought, reason, and understanding. **2.** The ability to acquire and apply knowledge.

abstract i. The ability to acquire and understand abstract ideas and symbols.

artificial i. (AI) Computer programming that includes certain features usually associated with human intelligence.

i. quotient (IQ) See under quotient.

mechanical i. The ability to acquire knowledge and understanding of technical mechanisms.

social i. Ability to understand and manage social relationships.

intemperance (in-tem´per-ans) Lack of self-restraint, as in the indulgence of alcoholic beverages.

intensity (in-ten´sĭ-te) Degree of activity, tension, strength, etc., usually implying a large measure.

intensive (in-ten´siv) Characterized by intensity; applied to an exhaustive and concentrated form of treatment.

intensivist (in-ten´si-vist) A physician who specializes in intensive care.

intention (in-ten´shun) **1.** A process. **2.** Objective.

healing by first i. See under healing.

healing by second i. See under healing.

healing by third i. See under healing.

interacinous (in-ter-as´ĭ-nus) Between the acini of a gland.

interaction (in-ter-ak´shun) Reciprocal action.

cognate i. In immunology, direct interaction between a processed antigen on the surface of a B lymphocyte and T lymphocyte receptor and eventual antibody production.

interalveolar (in-ter-al-ve´o-lar) Between alveoli.

interarticular (in-ter-ar-tik´u-lar) Between two joints or joint surfaces.

interatrial (in-ter-a´tre-al) Between the atria of the heart.

intercadence (in-ter-ka´dens) The occurrence of an extra pulse beat, between two regular beats.

intercalary (in-ter´kă-lar-e) Occurring between parts.

intercalate (in-ter´kă-lāt) To interpose or insert between others; to interpolate.

interclavicular (in-ter-clă-vik´u-lar) Between the clavicles (collarbones).

intercondylar, intercondyloid (in-ter-kon´dĭ-lar, in-ter-kon´dĭ-loid) Located between two condyles.

intercostal (in-ter-kos´tal) Between successive ribs.

intercourse (in´ter-kors) Interchange between individuals.

sexual i. See coitus.

intercristal (in-ter-kris´tal) Located between two crests.

intercurrent (in-ter-kur´ent) Occurring during the course of an already existing disease.

interdental (in-tĕr-den´tal) Between the teeth.

interdentium (in-ter-den´she-um) The space between two adjacent teeth.

interdigital (in-ter-dij´ĭ-tal) Between the fingers or toes.

interdigitation (in-ter-dij-ĭ-ta´shun) **1.** Interlocking of structures by means of finger-like processes. **2.** The processes so interlocked.

interepithelial (in-ter-ep-ĭ-the´le-al) Situated or passing between epithelial cells.

interface (in´ter-fās) A surface forming a common boundary between two bodies.

interfacial (in-ter-fa´shal) Relating to an interface.

interference (in-ter-fēr´ens) **1.** The coming together of waves in various media in such a way that the crests of one series correspond to the hollows of the other; when they cross, they reinforce each other at certain points and neutralize each other at other points. **2.** The collision of two waves of excitation in the myocardium, seen in fusion beats. **3.** In A-V (atrioventricular) dissociation, the disturbance of the rhythm of the heart ventricles by a conducted impulse from the atria. **4.** Superinfection, as occurs when cells are exposed to two viruses.

interferon (in-ter-fēr´on) (INF) A protein substance produced by body cells in response to invasion by viruses and other intracellular parasites; it interferes with the synthesis of new virus and is effective against certain protozoal parasitic infections, such as malaria; may also inhibit oncogenic virus growth.

interictal (in-ter-ik´tal) Denoting the interval between convulsions.

interleukin (in-ter-loo´kin) (IL) Name given to a group of hormonelike protein molecules (cytokines) once their amino acid structure is known.

interleukin-1 (IL) Cytokine derived from monocytes, macrophages, natural killer (NK) cells, endothelial cells, fibroblasts, astrocytes, and keratinocytes; increases proliferation of helper T lymphocytes, growth and differentiation of B lymphocytes, and growth of fibroblasts; can release proteolytic

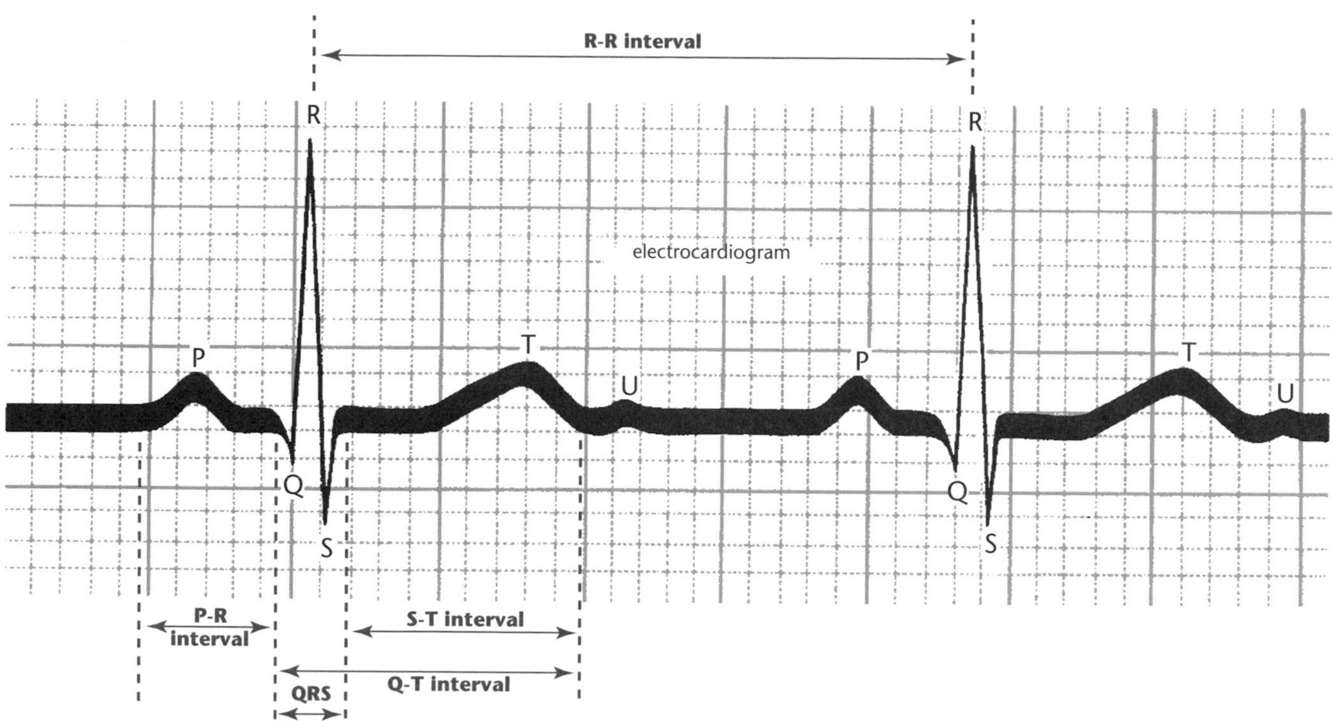

enzymes, cause fever, and initiate tissue catabolism.

interleukin-2 (IL) Cytokine derived from activated T lymphocytes and natural killer (NK) cells; causes growth of T lymphocytes and proliferation of B cells; increases natural killer (NK) cell activity and monocyte cytotoxicity.

interleukin-3 (IL-3) Cytokine derived from activated T lymphocyte clones; causes growth of multipotential stem cells. Also called multi-colony-stimulating factor.

interleukin-4 (IL-4) Cytokine derived from activated T lymphocytes; increases proliferation of B lymphocytes.

interleukin-5 (IL-5) Cytokine derived from activated T lymphocytes; increases secretion of IgA and IgM (immunoglobulins) by activation of B lymphocytes.

interleukin-6 (IL-6) Cytokine derived from activated T lymphocytes, monocytes, fibroblasts, and carcinoma and sarcoma cells; increases production of immunoglobulins by B lymphocytes.

interleukin-7 (IL-7) Cytokine derived from stromal cells isolated from the thymus; causes proliferation of $CD4^+$ or $CD8^+$ T lymphocytes, stimulates proliferation of $CD4^-$ $CD8^-$ thymocytes.

interleukin-8 (IL-8) Cytokine derived from endothelial cells, keratinocytes, fibroblasts, monocytes, and T lymphocytes; causes migration of neutrophils (e.g., toward an inflammation site).

interleukin-9 (IL-9) Cytokine derived from activated $CD4^+$ T lymphocytes; causes growth of helper T lymphocytes and stimulates growth of a human megakaryoblastic leukemia cell line.

interleukin-10 (IL-10) Cytokine derived from activated helper T lymphocytes and B lymphocytes; causes growth of murine T lymphocytes and differentiation of murine cytotoxic T lymphocytes; inhibits synthesis of cytokines.

interleukin-11 (IL-11) Cytokine derived from stromal cells in bone marrow (i.e., endothelial cells, macrophages, preadipocytes); causes growth of murine B lymhocytes and murine progenitors; inhibits fat formation on stromal cells of bone marrow.

interleukin-12 (IL-12) Cytokine derived from B lymphocytes; causes proliferation of T lymphocytes and natural killer (NK) cells.

interleukin-13 (IL-13) Cytokine derived from activated helper T lymphocytes; inhibits mononuclear cell inflammation.

interleukin-14 (IL-14) Cytokine derived from activated T lymphocytes; blocks immunoglobulin production.

interleukin-15 (IL-15) Cytokine derived from activated T lymphocytes and other cell types (e.g., peripheral blood mononuclear cells, epithelial cells, fibroblasts); causes proliferation of T lymphocytes and activation of natural killer (NK) cells.

interlobar (in-ter-lo´bar) Between two lobes.

interlobular (in-ter-lob´u-lar) Between two lobules.

intermediate (in-ter-me´de-it) **1.** Occurring between two extremes. **2.** A substance formed in the course of chemical reactions which then proceeds to participate rapidly in further reactions, so that at any given moment it is present in minute concentrations only.

metabolic i.'s Substances that appear in the course of the reactions involved in metabolism.

intermediate coronary syndrome (in-ter-me´de-it kor´ŏ-nar-e sin´drōm) Episodes of precordial pain that are too severe or protracted to be called angina, yet are not accompanied by the symptoms of a myocardial infarction. Also called acute coronary insufficiency.

intermenstrual (in-ter-men´stroo-al) Denoting the interval between two consecutive menstrual periods.

intermittency, intermittence (in-ter-mit´en-se, in-ter-mit´ens) The quality of being recurrent (often at regular intervals); not continuous.

intermuscular (in-ter-mus´ku-lar) Located between muscles.

intern (in´tern) A medical school graduate receiving supervised practical training by assisting in the medical and surgical care of patients at a hospital. Also called postgraduate year-1 resident; PGY-1 resident; resident intern (RI).

internal (in-ter´nal) Located within or on the inside; away from the surface.

internalization (in-ter-nal-ĭ-za´shun) In psychiatry, an unconscious process of taking into one's sense of self aspects of significant persons.

International System of Units (in-ter-nash´on-al sis´tem ŭv u´nitz) (SI) See under system

interneuron (in-ter-noo´ron) See internuncial neuron, under neuron.

internist (in-ter´nist) A specialist in internal medicine.

internodal (in-ter-no´dal) Between two nodes; applied to the segment of a nerve fiber between two successive nodes.

internuncial (in-ter-nun´she-al) Denoting a connecting agent or part, as a nerve cell connecting two other nerve cells.

interoceptor (in-ter-o-sep´tor) Any one of the sensory nerve endings located in, and receiving stimuli from, visceral tissues and blood vessels.

interosseous (in-ter-os´e-us) Connecting or lying between bones.

interphalangeal (in-ter-fă-lan´je-al) Between two contiguous bones of fingers or toes.

interphase (in-ter-fāz) The interval between two successive mitotic divisions; the phase when the cell is not dividing but is actively synthesizing DNA. Formerly called resting stage.

interplanting (in-ter-plant´ing) In experimental embryology, the transferring of an embryonic part from one embryo to an indifferent environment in another embryo.

interpretation (in-ter-prĕ-ta´shun) In psychoanalysis, the process by which the therapist explains to the patient the meaning of a particular aspect of the patient's problems.

interproximal (in-ter-prok´sĭ-mal) Between adjacent surfaces, as the space between adjacent teeth in the same dental arch.

interradicular (in-ter-ră-dik´u-lar) Between the roots of a tooth.

interscapular (in-ter-skap´u-lar) Between the scapulas (shoulder blades).

interseptal (in-ter-sep´tal) Between two tissue partitions (septa).

intersex (in´ter-seks) See hermaphrodite.

intersexuality (in-ter-seks-u-al´ĭ-te) See hermaphroditism.

interspace (in´ter-spās) Space between two similar structures.

interspinal (in-ter-spi´nal) Between the spinous processes of the vertebrae. Also called interspinous.

interstice (in-te´stis) A minute space in the substance of an organ or tissue.

interstitial (in-ter-stish´al) Relating to the spaces within a tissue.

interstitium (in-ter-stish´e-um) A small gap or space in the substance of an organ.

intertriginous (in-ter-trij´ĭ-nus) Characterized by or related to intertrigo.

intertrigo (in-ter-tri´go) Inflammatory skin eruption occurring between two adjacent surfaces, as between the scrotum or the vulva and the thigh.

intertrochanteric (in-ter-tro-kan-ter´ik) Located between the two trochanters of the femur.

interval (in´ter-val) **1.** The lapse of time between two events or between the recurrence of similar

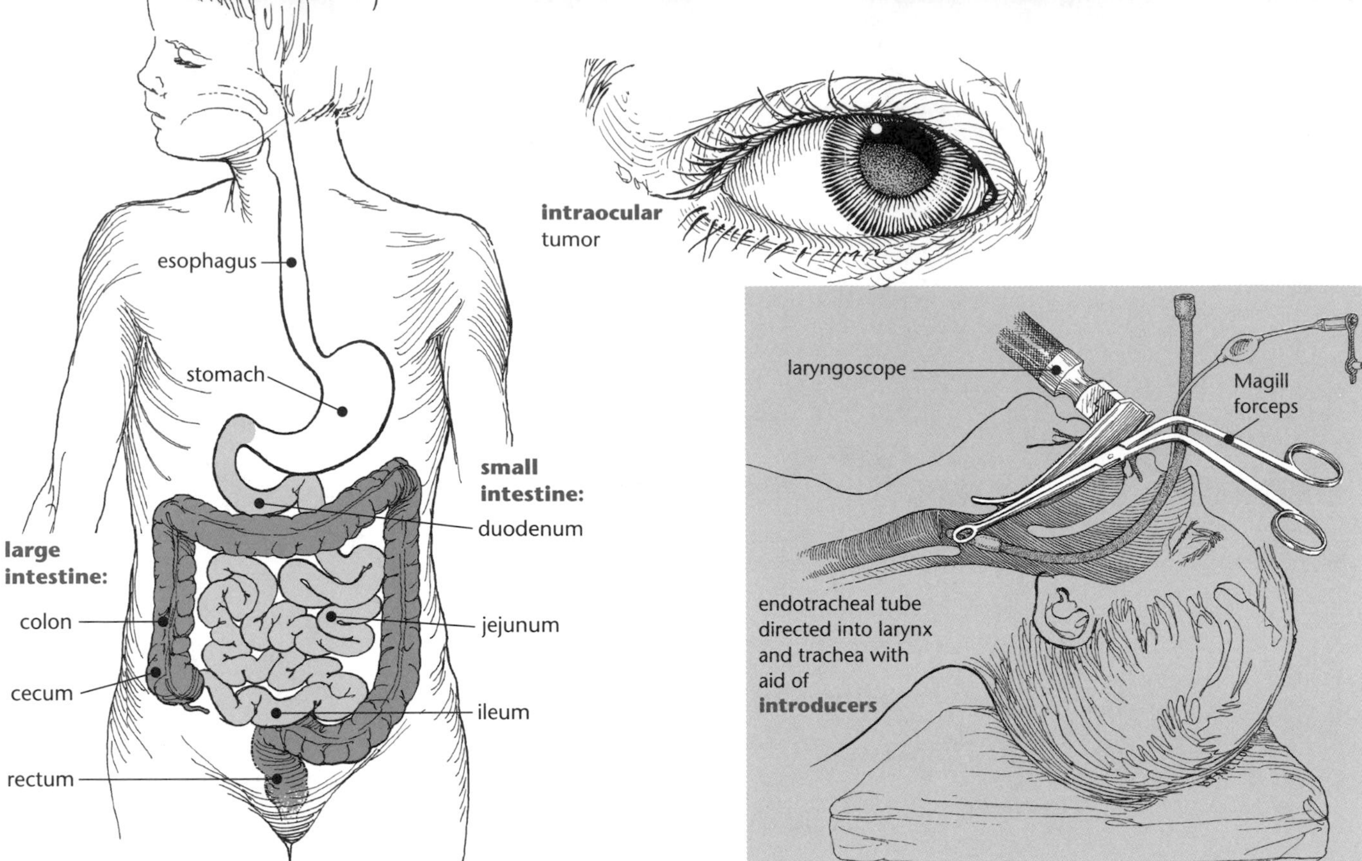

I

episodes of a disease. **2.** A distance between two objects. **3.** A gap in a continuous process.

coupling i. The interval between a premature heart beat and the normal beat preceding it.

lucid i. (a) A period of normal brain function immediately following a head injury in which a ruptured artery bleeds slowly into the space between skull and dura mater; no neurological signs or clouding of consciousness occurs until accumulated blood compresses the brain. (b) A period of mental clarity occurring in the course of a mental disorder.

P-P i. The distance between the same points on two consecutive P waves of the electrocardiogram.

P-R i. The atrioventricular conduction time, measured from the beginning of the P wave to the beginning of the QRS complex of the electrocardiogram; it includes the time required for atrial depolarization and repolarization plus the normal delay of excitation in the atrioventricular node.

Q-R i. The interval from the beginning of the QRS complex to the peak of the R wave in the electrocardiogram.

QRS i. The duration of the QRS complex, representing the measurement of total ventricular depolarization.

Q-T i. The interval between the onset of the Q wave and the end of the T wave of the electrocardiogram; it measures the duration of electrical systole.

R-R i. The interval between two consecutive QRS complexes of the electrocardiogram.

S-T i. Interval from the S wave to the end of the T wave of the electrocardiogram.

intervertebral (in-tĕr-ver´te-bral) Between two vertebrae.

intervillous (in-ter-vil´us) Located among villi.

intestinal (in-tes´tĭ-nal) Relating to the intestine or bowel.

intestine (in-tes´tin) The portion of the alimentary canal between the stomach and the anus.

large i. The portion of intestine between the ileum and the anus, composed of three parts: cecum, colon, and rectum and forming an arch over the convolutions of the small intestine.

small i. The convoluted portion of the intestine between the stomach and the cecum; divisible into three portions: duodenum, jejunum, and ileum.

intima (in´tĭ-mă) The inner layer of a blood vessel.

intoe (in´to) The turning in of the feet on walking; may be a minor self-correcting condition of toddlers, or may be a physical sign of other disorders. Popularly called pigeon toe.

intolerance (in-tol´er-ans) Unfavorable reaction to a substance.

hereditary fructose i. Metabolic defect due to an autosomal recessive inheritance; marked by a deficiency of fructose 1-phosphate aldolase, causing vomiting and hypoglycemia upon ingestion of fructose; repeated ingestion of fructose by infants with this disorder may result in severe disease.

lactose i. Intolerance to lactose due to presence of less than the normal amount of the enzyme lactase; manifested by abdominal cramps and diarrhea upon ingestion of milk and milk products.

pregnancy-induced glucose i. See gestational diabetes mellitus, under diabetes.

intorsion, intortion (in-tor´shun) The real or apparent inward turning of one or both eyes.

intortor (in´tor-ter) A muscle, such as an extraocular muscle, that turns a part inward.

intoxicant (in-tok´sĭ-kant) An intoxicating agent, especially alcohol.

intoxication (in-tok-sĭ-ka´shun) **1.** Stimulation or stupefaction produced by a chemical substance (e.g., alcohol). **2.** Poisoning.

water i. Excessive water content of the body resulting in salt depletion and a variety of associated symptoms.

intra-abdominal (in-tră-ab-dom´ĭ-nal) Situated within the abdomen.

intra-articular (in-tră-ar-tik´u-lar) Located within a joint's cavity.

intrabronchial (in-tră-brong´ke-ăl) See endobronchial.

intracapsular (in-tră-kap´su-lar) Within a capsule, especially the capsule of a joint.

intracardiac (in-tră-kar´de-ak) Located within the heart.

intracartilaginous (in-tră-kăr—tĭ-laj´ĭ-nus) See endochondral.

intracatheter (in-tră-kath´ĕ-ter) A slender plastic tube inserted into a vein for injection, infusion, or venous pressure monitoring.

intracellular (in-tră-sel´u-lar) Within a cell or cells.

intracerebral (in-tră-ser´e-bral) Within the cerebrum.

intracostal (in-tră-kos´tal) Situated on the inner surface of a rib or ribs.

intracranial (in-tră-kra´ne-al) Within the skull.

intractable (in-trak´tă-bl) Resistant to therapy.

intracutaneous (in-tră-ku-ta´ne-us) Within the layers of the skin.

intradermal (in-tră-der´mal) Within the dermis (deep layer of skin).

intradural (in-tră-doo´ral) Within the dura mater, the outermost membrane surrounding the brain and spinal cord.

intraepithelial (in-tră-ep-ĭ-the´le-al) Situated within, or passing through, epithelial cells.

intrahepatic (in-tră-hĕ-pat´ik) Within the liver.

intraictal (in-tră-ik´tal) Occurring during a convulsion or seizure.

intraluminal (in-tră-lu´mĭ-nal) Within the lumen of a tubule or tubular structure.

intramedullary (in-tră-med´u-lar-e) Within the bone marrow, the spinal cord, or the medulla oblongata.

intramembranous (in-tră-mem´bră-nus) Between layers of a membrane.

intramolecular (in-tră-mo-lek´u-lar) Occurring or located within a molecule.

intramural (in-tră-mu´ral) Within the wall of an organ or cavity.

intramuscular (in-tră-mus´ku-lar) (IM) Within the substance of a muscle.

intranasal (in-tră-na´zal) Within the nasal cavity.

intraneural (in-tră-nōōr´al) Within a nerve.

intraocular (in-tră-ok´u-lar) Within the eyeball.

intraoral (in-tră-or´al) Within the mouth.

intraorbital (in-tră-or´bĭ-tal) Within the orbit (eye socket).

intraosseous (in-tră-os´e-us) Within bone tissue.

intraperitoneal (in-tră-per-ĭ-to-ne´al) (IP) Within the peritoneal cavity.

intrapsychic (in-tră-sĭ´kik) Taking place within the mind.

intrapulmonary (in-tră-pul´mo-nar-e) Within the lungs.

intrarenal (in-tră-re´nal) Located within a kidney.

intrathecal (in-tră-the´kal) Within a sheath.

intrathoracic (in-tră-tho-ras´ik) Within the chest cavity.

intrauterine (in-tră-u´ter-in) Within the uterus.

intravascular (in-tră-vas´ku-lar) Within the blood or lymphatic vessels.

intravenous (in-tră-ve´nus) (IV) Within a vein.

intraventricular (in-tră-ven-trik´u-lar) Within a ventricle of the heart or brain.

intrinsic (in-trin´sik) Belonging or situated entirely within a part.

introducer (in-trŏ-doo´ser) Instrument used to intro-

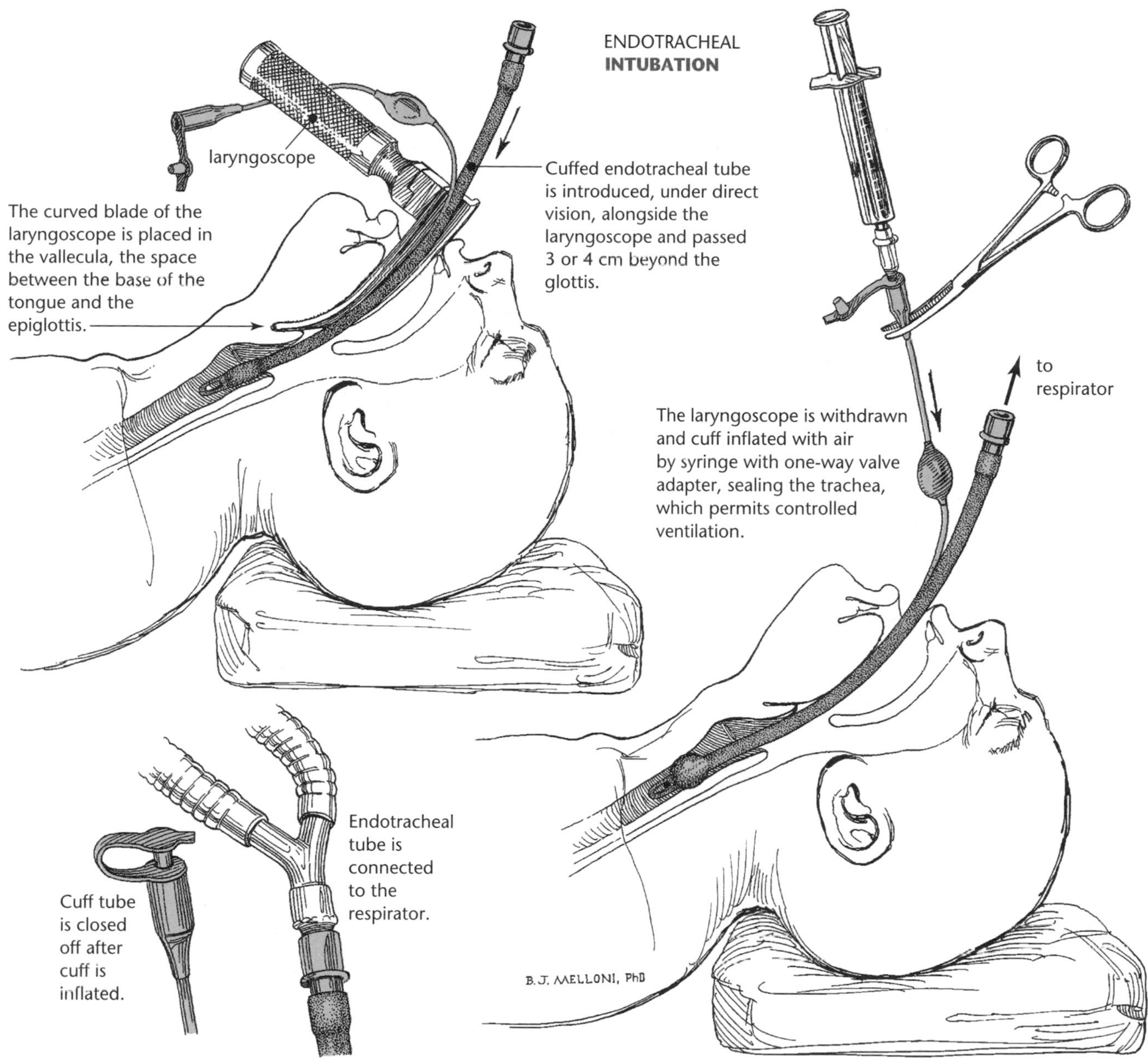
ENDOTRACHEAL
INTUBATION
laryngoscope
The curved blade of the laryngoscope is placed in the vallecula, the space between the base of the tongue and the epiglottis.
Cuffed endotracheal tube is introduced, under direct vision, alongside the laryngoscope and passed 3 or 4 cm beyond the glottis.
to respirator
The laryngoscope is withdrawn and cuff inflated with air by syringe with one-way valve adapter, sealing the trachea, which permits controlled ventilation.
Endotracheal tube is connected to the respirator.
Cuff tube is closed off after cuff is inflated.
B.J. MELLONI, PhD

duce a tube into the trachea. Also called intubator.

introitus (in-tro´ĭ-tus) Entrance into a cavity or hollow organ.

introjection (in-tro-jek´shun) The unconscious symbolic assimilation of a loved or hated object, making it a part of the self.

intromission (in-tro-mish´un) Insertion; introduction.

intron (in´tron) A region of DNA that is located between two exons, is transcribed into DNA as usual but later is spliced out; therefore, it is not expressed as protein in protein synthesis. Also called intervening sequence.

introspection (in-tro-spek´shun) Examination of one's own mental processes.

introversion (in-tro-ver´zhun) **1.** Preoccupation with one's own interests and experiences and concomitant reduction of outside interests. **2.** The process of turning an organ or part inward.

introvert (in´tro-vert) **1.** One whose thoughts are predominantly about himself. **2.** (in-tro-vert´) To turn inward.

intubate (in´too-bāt) To introduce a tube into the trachea or the larynx.

intubation (in-too-bā´shun) **1.** Introduction of a tube into any canal. **2.** Insertion of a tube into the trachea to allow air to enter the lungs.

intubator (in´too-ba-tor) See introducer.

intumesce (in-too-mes´) To swell.

intumescence (in-too-mes´ĕns) A swelling.

intumescent (in-too-mes´ĕnt) Enlarging; swelling.

intussuscept (in-tu-sŭ-sept´) To turn inward.

intussusception (n-tu-sŭ-sep´shun) Condition in which one part of the intestine becomes pushed into the lumen of an adjoining segment; it occurs chiefly at the iliocecal junction, causing acute abdominal symptoms; seen most commonly among children.

intussusceptum (in-tu-sŭ-sep´tum) The inner or ensheathed segment of intestine in an intussusception.

intussuscipiens (in-tu-sŭ-sip´e-ens) The outer portion of intestine surrounding the inner segment in an intussusception.

inulin (in´u-lin) A fructose polysaccharide found in the roots and underground stems of several plants; used in kidney function tests as a measure of glomerular filtration rate since it is filtered at the glomerulus, and is neither secreted nor reabsorbed by the tubules.

inunction (in-ungk´shun) **1.** The rubbing or smearing of a drug, in ointment form, into the skin. **2.** Ointment.

in utero (in u´ter-o) Latin for within the uterus.

in vacuo (in vak´u-o) Latin for in a vacuum.

invaginate (in-vaj´ĭ-nāt) To turn within or enclose; to ensheathe; to infold one part within another part of the same structure.

invagination (in-vaj-ĭ-na´shun) Ensheathing or infolding of a part within itself.

invalid (in´vă-lid) A person disabled by a chronic illness or infirmity.

invasion (in-va´zhun) **1.** The spread of a malignant tumor to adjacent tissues. **2.** The beginning of a disease.

stromal i. Spread of malignant cells from the superficial layer into the deeper, connective tissue of an organ (e.g., the spread of carcinoma *in situ* of the cervix, from the epithelium to and beyond the basement membrane into the cervical stroma).

invasive (in-va´siv) Having a tendency to spread or to invade healthy tissue.

inventory (in´ven-tor-e) In psychology, a list of questions.

personality i. A psychological test for evaluation of personal characteristics; usually a checklist about, and answered by, the patient.

inversion (in-ver´zhun) **1.** A turning inside out. **2.** Any reversal of the normal relation with other organs. **3.** In genetics, a chromosome aberration resulting from fragmentation of a chromosome by two breaks, followed by a turning end for end of the fragment and refusion.

i. of nipple Failure of the nipple to protrude from the breast.

i. of the uterus A turning of the uterus inside out, exposing the lining membrane (endometrium).

invert (in´vert) To turn upside down or inside out.

invertase (in-ver´tās) An enzyme that converts sucrose into glucose and fructose; found in the small intestine. Also called sucrase.

invertebrata (in-ver-tĕ-bra´tă) A division of the animal kingdom composed of animals without spinal columns.

invertebrate (in-ver´tĕ-brāt) An animal that does not have a spinal column.

invertor (in-ver´tor) A muscle that turns a part inward.

invest (in-vest´) To envelop; to cover completely.

investing (in-vest´ing) **1.** In dentistry, the process of covering an object, such as a wax pattern of a tooth restoration or a denture, with a refractory investment material before casting or curing. **2.** In psychoanalysis, affecting an object with psychic energy or cathexis.

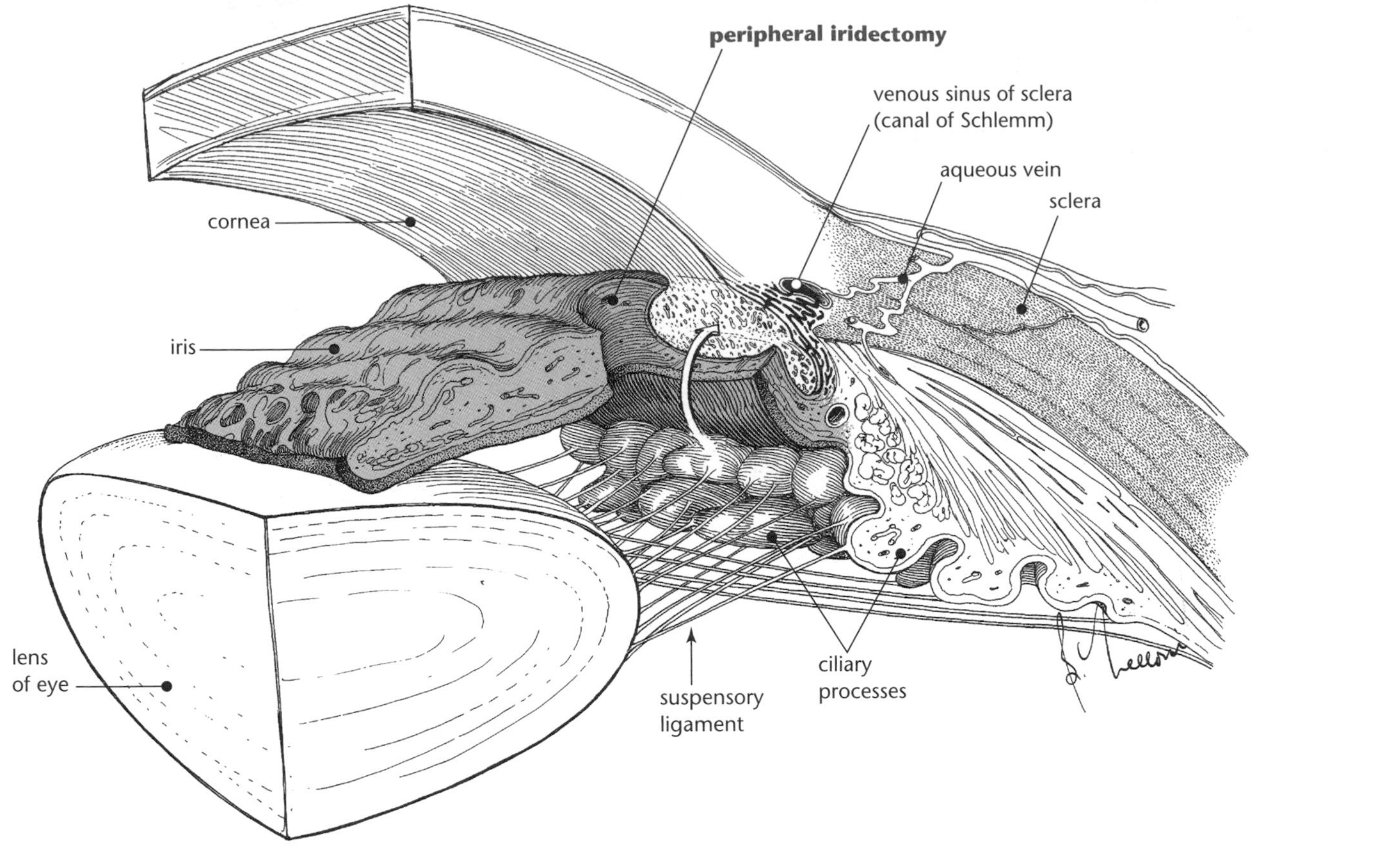

vacuum i. Forming a mold around a pattern in a vacuum to avoid trapping air in the investment material.

investment (in-vest´ment) Any material used to invest an object.

in vitro (in ve´tro) In an environment outside of the body, usually in a test tube or other similar artificial environment.

in vivo (in ve´vo) Within the living body.

involucrum (in-vo-loo´krum) An enveloping sheath of new bone, such as that developed around a necrosed bone as a response to infection.

involuntary (in-vol´un-tar-e) **1.** Performed independently of one's own free will. **2.** Not performed willingly.

involution (in-vo-loo´shun) A retrograde process resulting in lessening in the size of a tissue, as the return to normal size of the uterus after childbirth, or the shrinking of organs and tissues in old age.

involutional (in-vo-loo´shun-al) Relating to involution.

iodate (i´o-dāt) **1.** A salt of iodic acid. **2.** To iodize.

ioderma (i-o-der´mă) Any cutaneous reaction caused by iodine and compounds thereof; lesions may vary from mild acneform to granulomatous.

iodic acid (i-o´dik as´id) A white or colorless crystalline powder, HIO_3; used as an antiseptic and deodorant.

iodide (i´o-dīd) A compound of iodine with another element, especially with potassium or sodium.

iodimetry (i-o-dim´ĕ-tre) See iodometry.

iodine (i´o-dīn) A lustrous, grayish black, corrosive, nonmetallic element; symbol I, atomic number 53, atomic weight 126.91; used as an antiseptic and in the diagnosis and treatment of thyroid disease; it has no natural isotopes; its most widely used artificial isotopes are ^{131}I and ^{125}I.

protein-bound i. (PBI) Thyroid hormone in its circulating form, consisting of one or more of the iodothyronines bound to one or more of the serum proteins.

iodine-125 (^{125}I) Radioisotope used as a label in radioimmunoassay; has a half-life of 60 days.

iodine-131 (^{131}I) A beta-emitting radioactive isotope with a half-life of 8 days; used to deliver therapeutic doses of radiation to the thyroid gland and to certain types of tumors; it has limited use in imaging the thyroid and adrenal glands.

iodism (i´o-diz-m) Poisoning from the prolonged use of iodine or an iodide.

iodize (i´o-dīz) To treat or combine with iodine.

iodoform (i-o´do-form) A lemon-yellow iodine compound used as an antiseptic.

iodohippurate sodium (i-o-do-hip´u-rāt so´de-um) A radiopaque compound used in radiography of the urinary tract.

iodometry (i-o-dom´ĕ-tre) The volumetric determination of the amount of iodine in a compound. Also called iodimetry.

iodophilia (i-o-do-fil´e-ă) Affinity for iodine; said of certain cells.

iodopsin (i-o-dop´sin) A color-sensitive violet pigment composed of a vitamin A derivative and a protein; present in the cones of the retina and important in color vision. Also called visual violet.

ion (i´on) An atom or group of atoms or molecules having acquired an electric charge by gaining (cations) or losing (anions) electrons.

dipolar i. An ion that carries both a positive and a negative charge; amino acids are the most notable dipolar ions, containing the positively charged NH_3 group and the negatively charged COO group. Also called zwitterion.

hydronium i. The hydrated hydrogen ion, H_3O^+, as it exists in water.

ion exchange (i´on eks-chānj´) Chemical reaction between an insoluble solid and a solution surrounding the solid through which ions of like charge are interchanged; used in the separation of radioactive isotopes and in water softening.

ion exchanger (i´on eks-chānj´er) **1.** A solid substance used in ion exchange. **2.** Apparatus used to effect ion exchange.

ionic (i-on´ik) Containing, or relating to, an ion or ions.

ionization (i-on-ĭ-za´shun) **1.** Production of ions (electrically charged atoms or molecules) from neutral atoms or molecules; radiation creates ions by dislocating negatively charged electrons from the atoms they impinge upon. **2.** See iontophoresis.

ionize (i´on-īz) To separate into ions, totally or partially.

ionophore (i-on´ŏ-for) A molecule (e.g., of an antibiotic drug) that increases the permeability of cell membranes (e.g., of bacterial cells).

ion pair (i´on pār) Two particles of opposite charge formed during the interaction of radiation and matter.

iontophoresis (i-on-to-fŏ-re´sis) Introduction of the ions of a medication through intact skin by means of an electric current. Also called ionization; ionic medication; iontotherapy.

iontotherapy (i-on-to-ther´ă-pe) See iontophoresis.

ipecac, ipecacuanha (ip´ĕ-kak, ip-e-kak-u-an´ă) The dried root of *Cephaelis ipecacuanha* or *Cephaelis acuminata*, a shrub of South America; used as an emetic, as an expectorant, and in the treatment of amebic dysentery.

i. syrup A suspension of ipecac alkaloids that induces vomiting; available without prescription.

ipsilateral (ip-sĭ-lat´er-al) Occurring or located on the same side (e.g., symptoms occurring on the same side of a brain lesion).

iridectomy (ir-ĭ-dek´tŏ-me) Surgical removal of a portion of the iris.

laser i. Treatment for narrow angle glaucoma, using a laser attached to a slitlamp for making a small hole on the iris at its root to reestablish free flow of aqueous humor.

peripheral i. Surgical removal of a minute portion of the periphery of the iris, as in the treatment of narrow angle glaucoma.

iridemia (ir-ĭ-de´me-ă) Bleeding from the iris.

iridencleisis (ir-ĭ-den-kli´sis) One of the filtering operations for glaucoma in which a portion of the iris is cut and trapped (incarcerated) in an incision on the border of the cornea; thus a channel is created for draining fluid (aqueous humor) from the anterior and posterior chambers of the eye.

irides (i´rĭ-dēz) Plural of iris.

iridescent (ir-ĭ-des´ent) Displaying a changeable, colorful, metallic luster.

iridesis (i-rid´ĕ-sis) Surgical procedure in which a portion of the iris is brought out through an incision in the cornea and fixed with a suture.

iridic (i-rid´ik) Relating to the iris.

iridium (ĭ-rid´e-um) A whitish-yellow metallic element, symbol Ir, atomic number 77, atomic weight 192.2; of all chemical elements, it has the greatest resistance to corrosion.

iridization (ir-ĭ-di-za´shŭn) The multicolor halo around a bright light observed by persons afflicted with glaucoma.

iridocapsulitis (ir-ĭ-do-kap-su-li´tis) Inflammation of the iris and the capsule of the lens of the eye.

iridocele (i-rid´o-sēl) Protrusion of a portion of the iris through a defect or wound in the cornea.

iridochoroiditis (ir-ĭ-do-ko-roi-di´tis) Inflammation of both the iris and the vascular coat (choroid)

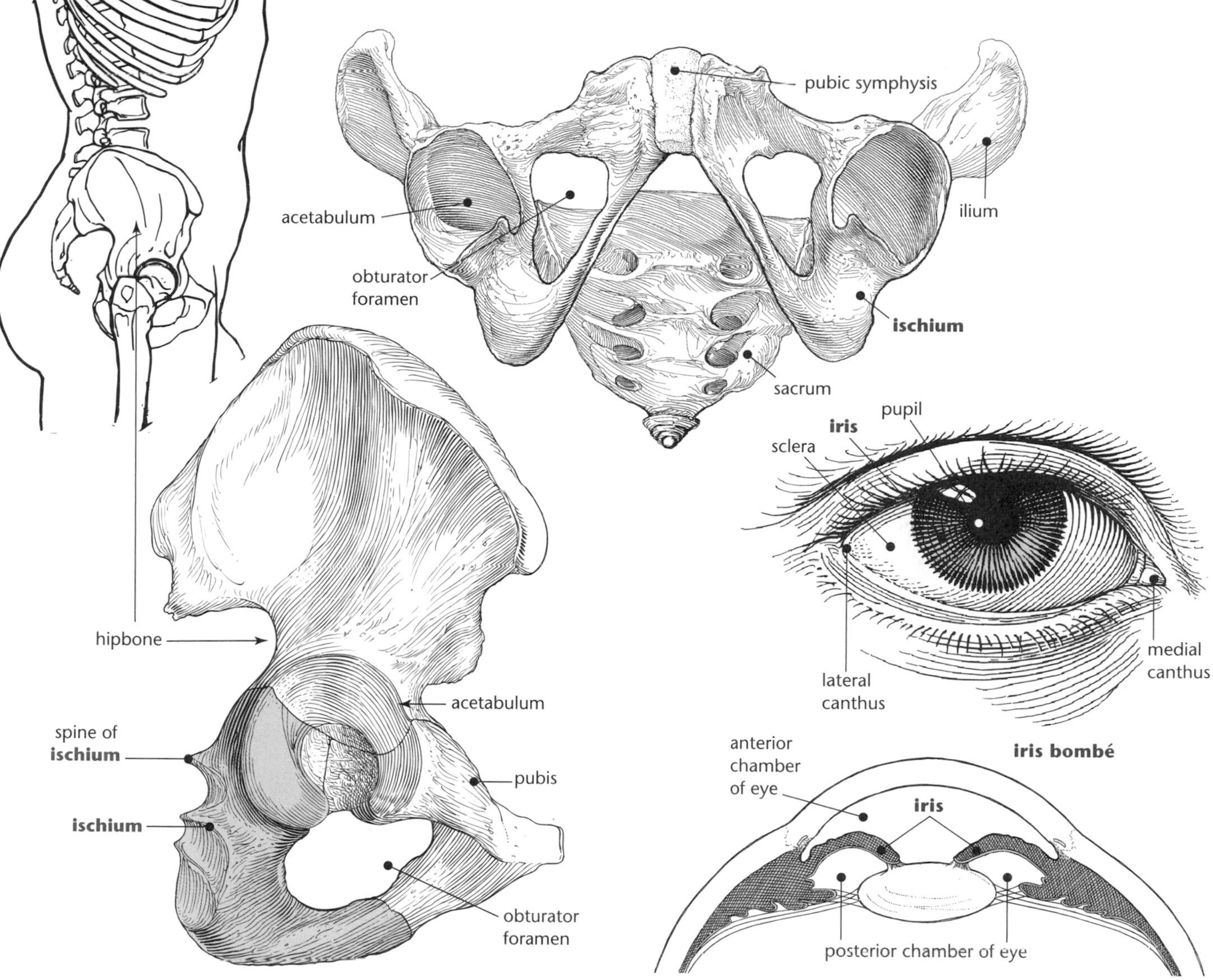

I

of the eyeball.

iridocoloboma (ir-ĭ-do-kol-o-bo´mă) Congenital absence of a portion of the iris.

iridoconstrictor (ir-ĭ-do-kon-strik´tor) **1.** Anything that causes contraction of the pupil, such as a nerve or a chemical. **2.** The circular muscle fibers of the iris.

iridocyclectomy (ir-ĭ-do-si-klek´to-me) Surgical removal of the iris and ciliary body.

iridocyclitis (ir-ĭ-do-si-kli´tis) Inflammation of the iris and the ciliary body. Also called anterior uveitis.

iridocyclochoroiditis (ir-ĭ-do-si-klo-ko-roi-di´tis) Inflammation of the iris, ciliary body, and choroid.

iridodialysis (ir-ĭ-do-di-al´ĭ-sis) Separation or rupture of a portion of the iris from its attachment to the ciliary body.

iridodilator (ir-ĭ-do-di-la´tor) Stimulating dilation of the pupil; denoting the sympathetic ciliary nerve fibers that innervate the pupillary dilator muscle or any chemical that causes constriction of that muscle.

iridodonesis (ir-ĭ-do-do-ne´sis) Abnormal trembling of the iris upon movement of the eye, as may occur in partial dislocation (subluxation) of the lens.

iridokeratitis (ir-ĭ-do-ker-ă-ti´tis) Inflammation of the iris and cornea.

iridokinesis, iridokinesia (ir-ĭ-do-ki-ne´sis, ir-ĭ-do-ki-ne´zhă) The movement of the iris resulting in dilatation and contraction of the pupil.

iridomalacia (ir-ĭ-do-mă-la´shă) Degenerative softening of the iris as a result of disease.

iridoplegia (ir-ĭ-do-ple´jă) Paralysis of the iris.

iridosclerotomy (ir-ĭ-do-skle-rot´ŏ-me) Incision into the sclera and the margin of the iris.

iridotomy (ir-ĭ-dot´ŏ-me) Incision into the iris.

laser i. See laser iridectomy, under iridectomy.

iris (i´ris), *pl.* **i´rides** The doughnut-shaped part of the eye, situated between the cornea and the crystalline lens, and separating the anterior and posterior chambers; the contraction of the iris alters the size of the pupil; the amount of pigment in it determines the color of the eye.

i. bombé A bulging forward of the iris caused by pressure from the aqueous humor in the posterior chamber, which cannot pass to the anterior chamber because of adhesion of the pupillary border of the iris to the anterior surface of the lens.

iritic (i-rit´ik) Relating to iritis.

iritis (i-ri´tis) Inflammation of the iris.

iron (i´ĕrn) A metallic element, symbol Fe, atomic number 26, atomic weight 55.85; present in the body as a component of hemoglobin, myoglobin, cytochrome, and the proteins catalase and peroxidase; its role in the body is predominantly concerned with cellular respiration.

iron-59 (^{59}Fe) A radioactive beta-emitter iron isotope with a half-life of 45.1 days; used as a tracer for erythrocyte studies and ferrokinetics.

iron storage disease (i´ĕrn stōr´ij dĭ-zēz´) Accumulation of excess iron in the tissues of many organs, especially the liver and pancreas, leading to fibrosis and functional insufficiency. Also called hemochromatosis.

irradiate (i-ra´de-āt) To treat with or expose to radiation.

irradiation (i-ra-de-a´shun) **1.** Exposure to the action of rays. **2.** The condition of having been subjected to radiation. **3.** Therapy by exposure to radiation.

external i. Radiation treatment in which the radiation source (e.g., x-ray machine) is placed at a distance from the body.

internal i. See interstitial irradiation.

interstitial i. Local irradiation in which the radiation source is placed within the tissue under treatment, usually in the form of pellets or needles.

local i. Therapeutic irradiation from a source in direct proximity to the tissues under treatment.

irrational (ĭ-rash´un-al) Contrary to reason or to the principles of logic.

irreducible (ĭr-ĭ-dōō´sĭ-bl) Incapable of being reduced in size or made simpler.

irresponsibility (ĭr-ĭ-spon´sĭ-bil´ĭ-te) The state of not being responsible.

criminal i. The state of not being responsible for one's own criminal acts, due to a mental defect or disorder.

irrigate (ir´ĭ-gāt) To wash out a wound or body cavity with water or a medicated liquid.

irrigation (ir-ĭ-gā´shun) The washing out of a wound or a body cavity with a stream of fluid.

irritability (ir-ĭ-tă-bil´ĭ-te) **1.** Responsiveness to stimuli. **2.** Exaggerated responsiveness to a stimulus.

irritable (ir´ĭ-tă-bl) Capable of reacting, or tending to overreact, to a stimulus.

irritable bowel syndrome See irritable colon, under colon.

irritant (ir´ĭ-tant) **1.** Causing irritation. **2.** A stimulus.

irritation (ir-ĭ-ta´shun) **1.** Incipient inflammation of a body part. **2.** The act of eliciting a reaction (normal or exaggerated) in the tissues.

ischemia (is-ke´me-ă) Lack of blood in an area of the body due to mechanical obstruction or functional constriction of a blood vessel.

myocardial i. Ischemia of the heart muscle, usually due to coronary heart disease.

ischemic (is-kem´ik) Relating to local deficiency of blood.

ischia (is´ke-ă) Plural of ischium.

ischial (is´ke-al) Relating to the ischium.

ischialgia (is-ke-al´jă) Pain in the hip.

ischiodynia (is-ke-o-din´e-ă) See ischialgia.

ischium (is´ke-um), *pl.* **is´chia** The lowest of three bones comprising each half of the hipbone; the bone on which the body rests when sitting.

ischuria (is-ku´re-ă) Suppression or retention of the urine.

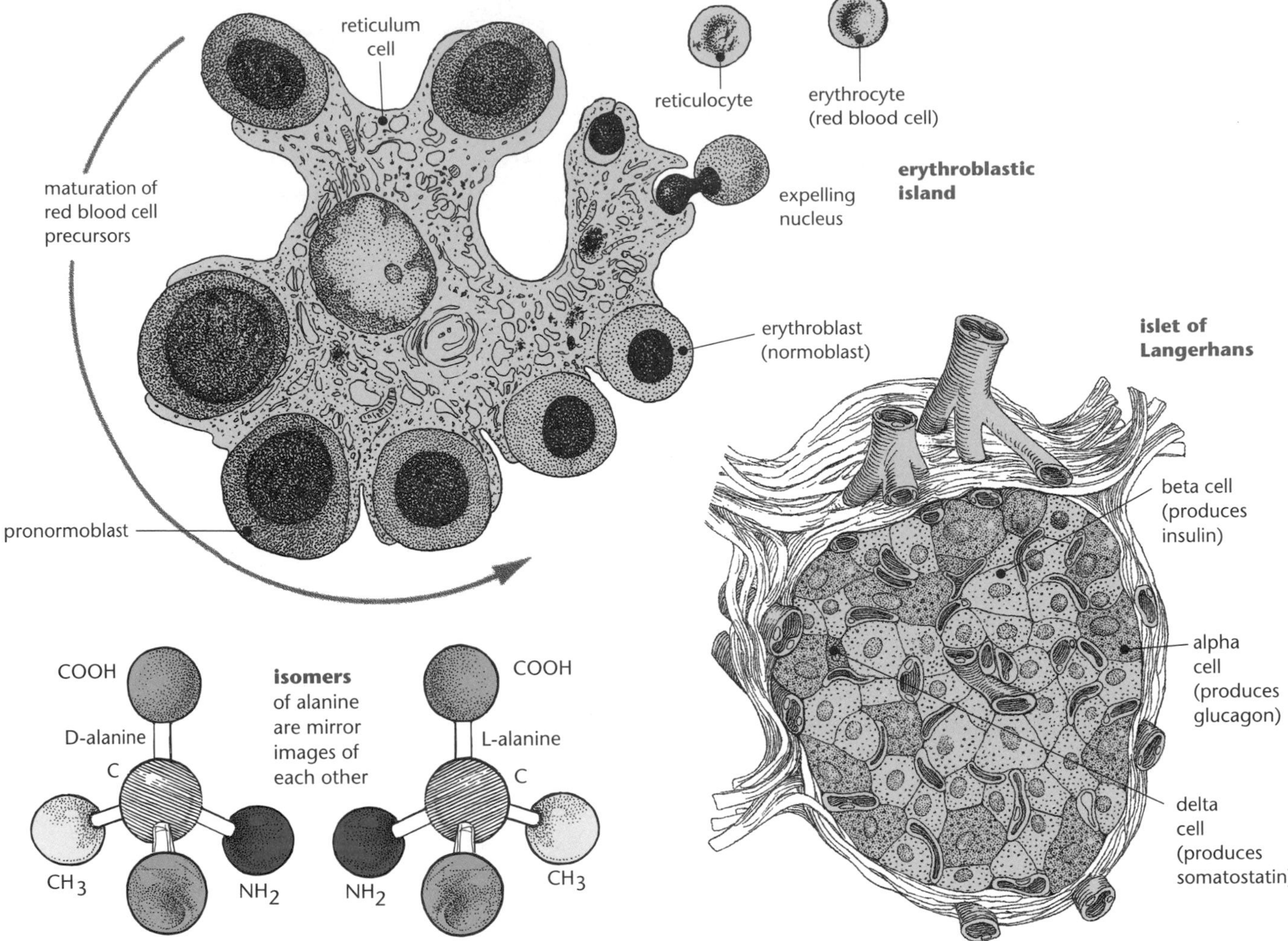

island (i´land) An isolated structure or cluster of cells.

erythroblastic i. One or two central reticulum cells of the bone marrow surrounded by normoblasts at various stages of development; the reticulum cells phagocytize the ejected nuclei of the developing normoblasts just prior to their release into the marrow capillaries as erythrocytes; they also ingest worn out or damaged red blood cells, conserving their iron as ferritin.

i. of Langerhans See islet of Langerhans, under islet.

pancreatic i. See islet of Langerhans, under islet.

Reil's i. See insula.

islet (i´let) Small island.

i. of Langerhans A cluster of cells in the pancreas that produce insulin. Also called island of Langer-hans; pancreatic island.

isoagglutinin (i-so-ă-gloo´tĭ-nin) An antibody directed against antigenic sites on the red blood cells of individuals of the same species and causing agglutination of the cells.

isoantibody (i-so-an´tĭ-bod-e) See alloantibody.

isoantigen (i-so-an´tĭ-jen) See alloantigen.

isobar (i´so-bar) **1.** Any one of two or more atomic species that have the same atomic weight but not necessarily the same atomic number. **2.** A line on a chart connecting two points of equal barometric pressure at a given time.

isobaric (i-so-băr´ik) Denoting atoms having the same weight.

isocellular (i-so-sel´u-lăr) Composed of similar cells.

isochromatic (i-so-kro-mat´ik) Of uniform or equal color.

isochromosome (i-so-kro´mo-sōm) A chromosome with two identical arms, resulting from transverse rather than longitudinal division of the centromere during meiosis.

isocoria (i-so-kor´e-ă) Equal size of the two pupils.

isocortex (i-so-kor´teks) The non-olfactory, phylogenetically younger part of the cerebral cortex; so called because its cellular and fibrous layers are distributed in a uniform pattern. Also called neocortex; neopallium.

isodynamic (i-so-di-nam´ik) Of equal strength.

isoelectric (i-so-e-lek´trik) Having an equal number of positive and negative charges; electrically neutral; said of certain molecules.

isoenzyme (i-so-en´zīm) See isozyme.

isoflurophate (i-so-flo͞or´o-fāt) A potent cholinergic agent used topically in the treatment of glaucoma and strabismus. Also called diisopropyl flurophosphate.

isogamete (i-so-gam´ēt) A gamete that has the same size as the one with which it unites.

isogamy (i-sog´ă-me) Conjugation or fusion of morphologically identical gametes.

isogenic, isogeneic (i-so-jen´ik, i-so-jĕ-ne´ik) Genetically alike. Also called isologous; isoplastic.

isograft (i´so-graft) A tissue transplant involving two genetically identical or near-identical individuals, such as identical twins or highly inbred animals. Also called isogeneic graft; isologous graft; isoplastic graft; syngeneic graft; isotransplant; syngraft.

isohemagglutinin (i-so-hem-ă-gloo´tĭ-nin) See isoagglutinin.

isohemolysin (i-so-he-mol´ĭ-sin) A specific antibody from one individual that reacts with antigen in red blood cells of another individual of the same species, resulting in cell destruction. Also called homolysin.

isohemolysis (i-so-he-mol´ĭ-sis) Dissolution of red blood cells caused by reaction between specific antigens present in the cells and antibodies (isohemolysins) from another individual of the same species. Also called hemolysis.

isohydric (i-so-hi´drik) Having the same pH.

isoimmunization (i-so-im-u-nĭ-za´shun) The development of a significant concentration of specific antibody stimulated by the presence of antigens from another individual of the same species, as when fetal cells or other proteins gain access to the maternal circulation, with resulting maternal immunization to the paternal antigens present in the fetal material.

isolation (i-so-lā´shun) **1.** Separation from a group, such as the placing of a patient in quarantine and segregation of his body fluids and clotting to prevent transmission of infection. **2.** In microbiology, identification and separation of a pure strain of microorganisms from a mixed source such as a clinical specimen. **3.** Dissociation of experiences or memories from the emotions pertaining to them, so as to render them a matter of indifference; an unconscious psychological defense mechanism against anxiety.

isoleucine (i-so-loo´sēn) An essential amino acid formed by the hydrolysis of fibrin and other proteins.

isologous (i-sol´o-gus) See isogenic.

isomer (i´so-mer) One of two or more compounds that have the same percentage composition and molecular weight but different physical or chemical properties due to a different arrangement of the atoms in the molecule.

isomerase (i-som´er-ās) An enzyme that catalyzes the conversion of a substance to an isomeric form (e.g., glucosephosphate isomerase).

isomeric (i-so-mer´ik) Relating to or displaying isomerism.

isomerism (i-som´ĕ-riz-m) The existence of a compound in two or more forms having the same percentage composition and molecular weight but differing in chemical and physical properties, and also in the arrangement of the atoms within the molecule.

chain i. A form of structural isomerism in which the linkages in the basic chain of carbon atoms vary.

geometric i. An isomerism in which free rotation about a carbon bond is restricted.

optical i. Stereoisomerism involving the arrangement of substituents about asymmetric carbon

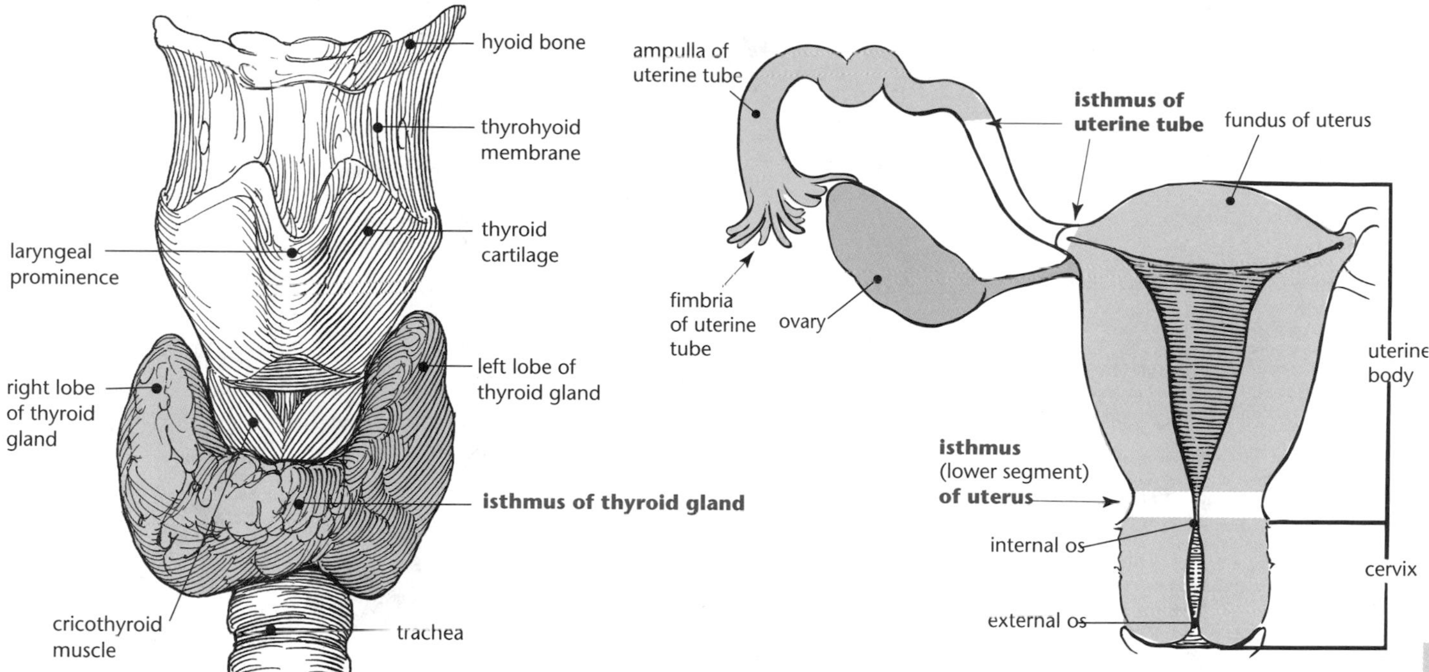

atoms which can rotate the plane of polarized light passing through the substance.

structural i. Isomerism involving the same atoms in different structural formulas.

isomerization (i-som-er-ĭ-za´shun) The process in which an isomer is converted into another, as in the action of isomerases.

isometric (i-so-met´rik) **1.** Denoting the contraction of a muscle in which its tension is increased without shortening its length; opposed to isotonic. **2.** Of equal dimensions.

isometropia (i-so-mĕ-tro´pe-ă) Equality in the refractive state of the two eyes.

isomorphism (i-so-mor´fiz-m) Similarity of shape or structure.

isoniazid (i-so-ni´ă-zid) Isonicotinic acid hydrazide (INH); used in the treatment of tuberculosis.

isoplastic (i-so-plas´tik) See isologous.

isopropyl alcohol (i-so-pro´pl al´ko-hol) A secondary toxic alcohol, $(CH_3)_2CHOH$; used in the preparation of cosmetics and medicines for external use.

isoproterenol sulfate (i-so-pro-tĕ-re´nol sul´fāt) A compound used as an inhalation in the treatment of asthma and emphysema.

isopter (i-sop´ter) A contour line in a visual field representing the area in which the visual acuity is the same as that measured with a specific test target.

isosexual (i-so-sek´shoo-al) **1.** Relating to characteristics of both sexes in one person. **2.** Denoting the traits of an individual which are characteristic of the sex to which the individual belongs.

isosmotic (i-sos-mot´ik) Having the same osmotic pressure as another fluid.

Isospora (i-sos´po-ră) A genus of coccidia (family Eimeriidae); some species are parasitic in humans, causing disease.

I. belli Protozoan parasite infecting the small intestine of humans; occurs most commonly in the tropics.

isosporiasis (i-sos-po-ri´ă-sis) Infection by *Isospora belli* usually causing mild, self-limiting diarrhea except in cases of AIDS, where it causes chronic watery diarrhea and weight loss.

isosthenuria (i-sos-thĕ-nu´re-ă) Lack of variation in the specific gravity of urine, regardless of amount of fluid intake; inability to concentrate or dilute the urine above or below, respectively, the osmolality of plasma, generally corresponding to a specific gravity of 1.010. A sign of advanced kidney failure.

isotherapy (i-so-ther´ă-pe) Prevention of disease by using the agent that causes the disease (i.e., vaccines).

isothermal (i-so-ther´mal) Relating to or of the same temperature.

isotonic (i-so-ton´ik) Of equal tension or osmotic pressure, usually referring to the osmotic concentration of blood plasma.

isotonicity (i-so-to-nis´ĭ-te) **1.** Equality of tension, as between two muscles. **2.** Equality of osmotic pressure, as between two solutions.

isotope (i´so-tōp) One of two or more chemical elements in which all atoms have the same atomic number but varying atomic weights, due to unequal numbers of neutrons in their nuclei; many are radioactive; designated by the chemical symbol and a superscript number representing the atomic weight, as ^{12}C (isotope of carbon with atomic weight of 12).

radioactive i. An isotope with an unstable nucleus that emits ionizing radiation in stabilizing itself.

stable i. An isotope of a chemical element that shows no inclination to undergo radioactive breakdown; a nonradioactive nuclide.

isotoxin (i-so-tok´sin) A poison in the blood or tissues of an animal that only has toxic effects on other animals of the same species, not on that animal itself.

isotransplant (i-so-trans´plant) See isograft.

isotropic, isotropous (i-so-trop´ik, i-sot´rŏ-pus) Equal in all directions.

isotypes (i´so-tīps) Antigenic determinants of immunoglobulin heavy chains that define classes and subclasses of immunoglobulins.

isovalericacidemia (i-so-vă-ler-ik-as-ĭ-de´me-ă) Disorder of leucine metabolism characterized by elevated serum isovaleric acid upon protein ingestion or during infectious episodes; associated with recurrent episodes of coma, acidosis, and malodorous sweat; autosomal recessive inheritance.

isovolumic, isovolumetric (i-so-vŏ-loo´mik, i-so-vol-u-met´rik) Equal or unchanged volume; occurring without an associated alteration in volume, as when, in early ventricular systole, the muscle fibers initially increase their tension without shortening so that ventricular volume remains unchanged.

isozyme (i´so-zīm) One of a group of enzymes that catalyze the same chemical reaction but have different physical properties. Also called isoenzyme.

isthmus (is´mus) **1.** A narrow section of tissue connecting two larger parts. **2.** A narrow passage connecting two larger cavities or tubular structures.

i. of aorta A slight constriction of the aorta between the left subclavian artery and the ligamentum arteriosum.

i. of auditory tube The narrowest part of the auditory (eustachian) tube, at the junction of the bony and cartilaginous portions.

i. of cingulate gyrus The narrow posterior portion of the cingulate gyrus that joins the hippocampal gyrus. Also called isthmus of the limbic lobe.

i. of external auditory meatus The narrowest portion of the external auditory canal near the junction of the bony and cartilaginous parts.

i. of limbic lobe See isthmus of cingulate gyrus.

i. of nasopharynx The opening between the free edges of the soft palate and the posterior pharyngeal wall.

i. of oropharynx The constricted aperture by which the mouth is connected with the pharynx; located at the interval between the two palatoglossal arches.

i. of prostate The anterior portion of the base of the prostate gland.

i. of rhombencephalon A marked constriction of the embryonic brain from which the anterior medullary velum is formed; it connects the rhombencephalon with the mesencephalon.

i. of thyroid The narrow, central portion connecting the two lateral lobes of the thyroid gland.

i. of urethra The slightly constricted junction of the urethra between the cavernous and membranous portions.

i. of uterine tube The narrow, medial portion of the uterine tube at its junction with the uterus.

i. of uterus The elongated constricted part of the uterus between the cervix and the uterine body; it is about 1 cm in length.

Vieussens' i. The ring or margin of the fossa ovalis.

itch (ich) **1.** A skin sensation and/or irritation causing a desire to scratch. **2.** Common name for scabies.

barber's i. See tinea barbae.

jock i. See tinea cruris, under tinea.

swimmer's i. An itchy rash caused by penetration of the skin by the larvae of the worm *Schistosoma mansoni* during immersion in contaminated freshwater.

iter (i´ter) A passageway leading from one anatomic part to another.

IUD See intrauterine device, under device.

Ixodes (iks-o´dēz) A genus of parasitic ticks (family Ixodidae); transmitters of viral and bacterial diseases to humans and animals.

I. dammini The deer tick; chief vector of *Borrelia burgdorferi,* the spirochete causing Lyme disease.

I. holocyclus A species prevalent in Australia and South Africa; vector of tick paralysis in sheep, cattle, dogs, and occasionally humans.

I. pacificus The black-legged tick of California; it infests cattle and deer; may bite humans, causing severe reactions.

I. persulcatus The vector of Russian spring-summer encephalitis.

I. ricinus The castor bean tick; it infects cattle, sheep, and wild animals and transmits tularemia, infectious encephalomyelitis, and Russian spring-summer encephalitis.

ixodiasis (ik-so-di´ă-sis) Skin lesions and fever caused by ticks, particularly those of the family Ixodidae (hard-bodied ticks).

ixodic (ik-sod´ik) Relating to ticks.

Ixodidae (ik-sod´ĭ-de) A family of hard-bodied ticks (order Acarina); transmitters of several diseases. Also called hard ticks.

J

jacket (jak′et) An outer casing, bandage, or garment, especially one extending from the shoulders to the hips.
Minerva j. A plaster of Paris cast extending from the chin to the hips for immobilization of the lower cervical or upper thoracic spine.
porcelain j. In dentistry, a porcelain jacket crown.
strait j. See straitjacket.
jackscrew (jak′skroo) A device used to approximate or separate teeth or jaw segments.
Jackson's syndrome (jak′sonz sin′drōm) Paralysis of one side of the tongue, palate, and larynx. Also called syndrome of vago-accessory-hypoglossal paralysis.
jactitation (jak-tĭ-ta′shun) The tossing to and fro of a distressed patient in bed; extreme restlessness.
Jansky-Bielschowsky disease (yahn′ske-bēl-shov′ske dĭ-zēz′) See cerebral sphingolipidosis, under sphingolipidosis.
Janus green B (jā′nŭs grēn bē) An azo dye used as a supravital stain for the demonstration of mitochondria.
jargon (jar′gon) **1.** Language peculiar to a trade, profession, class, etc. **2.** Incoherent, meaningless utterance. See also paraphasia.
jaundice (jawn′dis) Yellow pigmentation of the skin and/or sclera caused by high levels of bilirubin in the blood. Also called icterus.
breast milk j. Jaundice occurring in some full-term newborn infants who are breast fed, resulting from elevated unconjugated bilirubin.
chronic idiopathic j. See Dubin-Johnson syndrome.
familial nonhemolytic j. Jaundice in the absence of liver damage, biliary obstruction, or hemolysis; the unconjugated bilirubin is elevated; believed to be due to an inborn error of metabolism. Also called Gilbert's disease.
hemolytic j. Jaundice resulting from excessive breakdown of red blood cells.
hepatocellular j. A form due to disease of the liver cells.
infectious spirochetal j. See Weil's disease.
obstructive j. Jaundice caused by obstruction of the bile ducts.
physiologic j. Mild jaundice of the newborn, primarily due to immaturity of the liver; disappears within one week after birth. Also called physiologic icterus.
jaundiced (jawn′dist) **1.** Marked by jaundice. **2.** Yellowish.
jaw (jaw) One of the two bones supporting the teeth; the upper one is the maxilla and the lower one is the mandible.
lock-j. See trismus.
lumpy j. See actinomycosis.
jawbone (jaw′bōn) See mandible.
jaw-winking syndrome (jaw-wingk′ing sin′drōm) Involuntary unilateral lowering of the upper eyelid, occurring while chewing; the person appears to be winking. Also called Gunn's syndrome.
jejunal (jĕ-joo′nal) Of or relating to the jejunum.
jejunectomy (jĕ-joo-nek′tŏ-me) Surgical removal of the jejunum, or a portion of it.
jejunitis (jĕ-joo-ni′tis) Inflammation of the jejunum.
jejunocolostomy (jĕ-joo-no-ko-los′tŏ-me) Operation in which a communication between the jejunum and the colon is established.
jejunoileitis (jĕ-joo-no-il-e-i′tis) Inflammation of the jejunum and ileum.
jejunoileostomy (jĕ-joo-no-il-e-os′tŏ-me) Surgical connection between the jejunum and a noncontinuous segment of the ileum.
jejunojejunostomy (jĕ-joo-no-jĕ-joo-nos′tŏ-me) Surgical joining of two noncontinuous segments of the jejunum.
jejunoplasty (jĕ-joo′no-plas-te) Corrective surgery on the jejunum.
jejunostomy (jĕ-joo-nos′tŏ-me) The formation of a permanent opening through the abdominal wall into the jejunal part of the small intestine.
jejunotomy (jĕ-joo-not′ŏ-me) Cutting into the jejunum.
jejunum (je-joo′nŭm) The portion of the small intestine between the duodenum and the ileum; in the adult, it is about 2.5 m in length, with a diameter of approximately 4 cm.

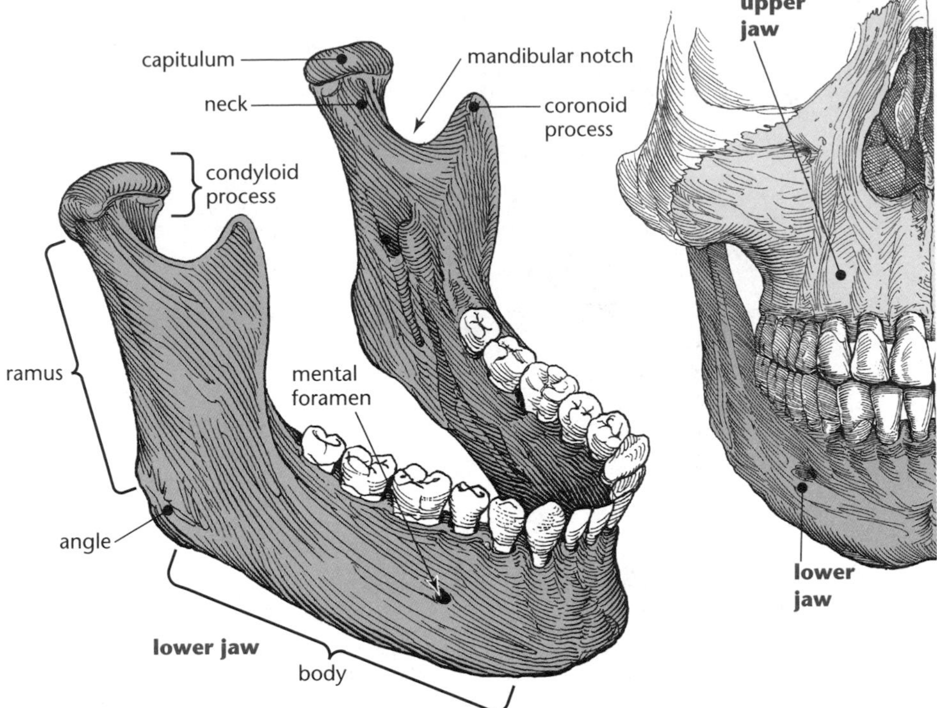

Jellinek's sign (yel′ĭ-neks sīn) Brownish pigmentation of the eyelids, seen in people afflicted with Graves' disease.
jelly (jel′e) A semisolid substance having resilient consistency.
petroleum j. See petrolatum.
Wharton's j. The soft, homogenous connective tissue comprising the matrix of the umbilical cord and supporting the umbilical vessels.
jellyfish (jel′e-fish) A member of the class Hydrozoa, which includes the small acorn-shaped species and the umbrella-shaped type with tentacles equipped with stinging organs; some are poisonous; the poison injected into a victim's skin can produce reactions ranging from rashes to anaphylactic shock.
Jensen's disease (yen′senz dĭ-zēz′) See chorioretinitis.
jerk (jerk) **1.** A sudden abrupt movement or reflex.
ankle j. See Achilles reflex, under reflex.
crossed j. See crossed reflex, under reflex.
elbow j. See triceps reflex, under reflex.
knee j. See patellar reflex, under reflex.
jigger (jig′ĕr) See chigoe.
jimsonweed (jim′son-wēd) See *Datura stramonium.*
jitteriness (jit′ĕ-re-nes) Condition similar to seizure activity observed in some newborn infants; marked by fine, tremorlike movements of the extremities which, unlike the coarse jerky movements of seizures, will cease if the child's hands are grasped and are not accompanied by abnormal eye movements.
jitters (jit′ĕrz) Extreme nervousness.
joint (joint) The point of connection between two or more bones; an articulation.
acromioclavicular j. Articulation between the lateral end of the collarbone (clavicle) and the acromion of the shoulder blade (scapula).
amphiarthrodial j. Joint in which the articulating surfaces are united by a disk of fibrocartilage, allowing only slight movement (e.g., the articulation between two vertebrae). Also called amphiarthrosis; cartilaginous joint.
ankle j. See talocrural joint.
anterior talocalcanean j. See talocalcaneonavicular joint.
arthrodial j. See plane joint.
atlantoaxial j. Either of two articulations between the first and second cervical vertebrae (atlas and axis).
atlantoepistrophic j. Either of two joints at the neck: *Lateral atlantoepistrophic j.*, the junction between the inferior articular processes of the first cervical vertebra (atlas) and the superior articular processes of the second cervical vertebra (axis). *Median atlantoepistrophic j.*, the junction between the dens of the second cervical vertebra (axis) and the anterior arch and transverse ligament of the first cervical vertebra (atlas).
ball and socket j. A type of diarthrodial joint in which the globular end of one bone fits into the cuplike cavity of the other, permitting extensive movement in any direction, as seen in the hip and shoulder. Also called enarthrosis; spheroidal joint.
bicondylar j. Synovial joint in which two rounded condyles of one bone fit into two shallow cavities of another bone, as in the knee or temporomandibular joints, allowing all movement except rotation. Also called condylar joint; condyloid joint.
calcaneocuboid j. A saddle-shaped joint in the posterior portion of the foot between the front surface of the heel bone (calcaneus) and the back surface of the cuboid bone.
capitular j. Articulation between the head of a rib and the bodies of two adjacent thoracic vertebrae.
carpometacarpal j. The plane joints between the carpal bones of the wrist and the second, third, fourth, and fifth metacarpal bones of the hand.
carpometacarpal j. of thumb Joint between the trapezium of the wrist and the first metacarpal bone of the hand.
cartilaginous j. See amphiarthrodial joint.
Charcot's j. Swollen, unstable but painless joint, frequently with destruction of intra-articular ligaments and consequent abnormally increased range of motion; caused by loss of sensory innervation; the lack of sensation deprives the joint of protective reactions to undue stresses; considered a complication of a neurologic disorder (e.g., tabes dorsalis, diabetic neuropathy). Also called neuropathic joint.
Chopart's j. See transverse tarsal joint.
coccygeal j. See sacrococcygeal joint.
condylar j. See bicondylar joint.
condyloid j. See bicondylar joint.
costochondral j. Cartilaginous articulation between the anterior end of a rib and the lateral end of a costal cartilage.
cricothyroid j. Synovial joint between the side of the cricoid cartilage and the inferior horn of the thyroid cartilage, permitting gliding and rotational

RESULTS OF LABORATORY TESTS IN COMMON JAUNDICE DISORDERS

DISORDER	SERUM TRANSAMINASES		ALKALINE PHOSPHATASE	ALBUMIN-GLOBULIN RATIO	PROTHROMBIN TIME	OTHER
	SGOT*	SGPT*				
Viral hepatitis	Moderate or great increase	Moderate or great increase	Slight or moderate increase	Usually normal	Decreased	Cephalin-cholesterol flocculation positive, dark urine, pale stool
Cirrhosis	Slight increase	Normal, occasional slight increase	Slight or moderate increase	Albumin decreased, globulin increased	Decreased	Cephalin-cholesterol flocculation positive, dark urine, pigmented stool
Carcinoma of pancreas and ampulla of Vater	Normal or slight increase	Normal or slight increase	Moderate or great increase	Normal	Normal or decreased	Prothrombin increased after vitamin K, pale stool
Choledocholithiasis	Normal, slight or moderate increase	Normal or slight increase	Slight to great increase	Normal	Normal or decreased	Fever, leukocytosis, intermittent pale stool
Drug cholestasis	Slight or moderate increase	Normal or slight increase	Moderate or great increase	Normal	Normal or slightly decreased	Cholesterol increased, eosinophilia, pale stool
Drug necrosis	Moderate or great increase	Moderate or great increase	Slight increase	Normal or slight albumin decrease	Decreased	Cephalin-cholesterol flocculation positive, dark urine, pale stool
Biliary cirrhosis	Slight or moderate increase	Slight or moderate increase	Moderate or great increase	Normal	Normal or decreased	Cholesterol and phospholipids increased, steatorrhea
Hemolytic **jaundice**	Normal	Normal	Normal	Normal	Normal	Anemia, reticulocystosis, acholuria, stool pigment increase

*Slight increase: 40–200; moderate: 200–1000; great: over 1000 units

American Family Physician

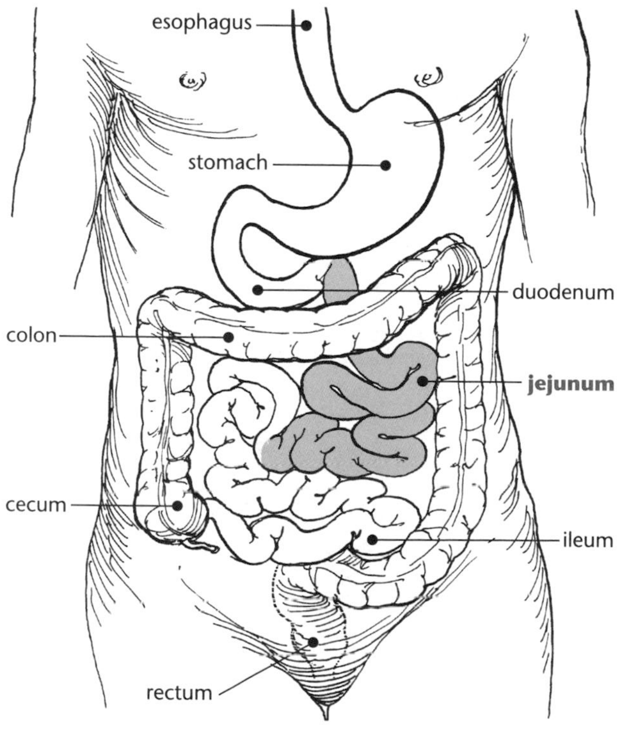

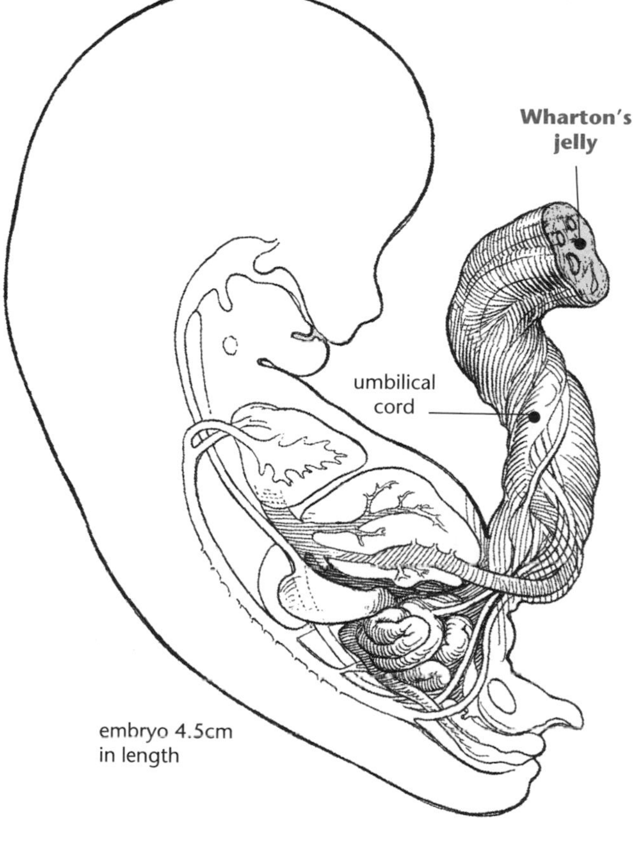

J

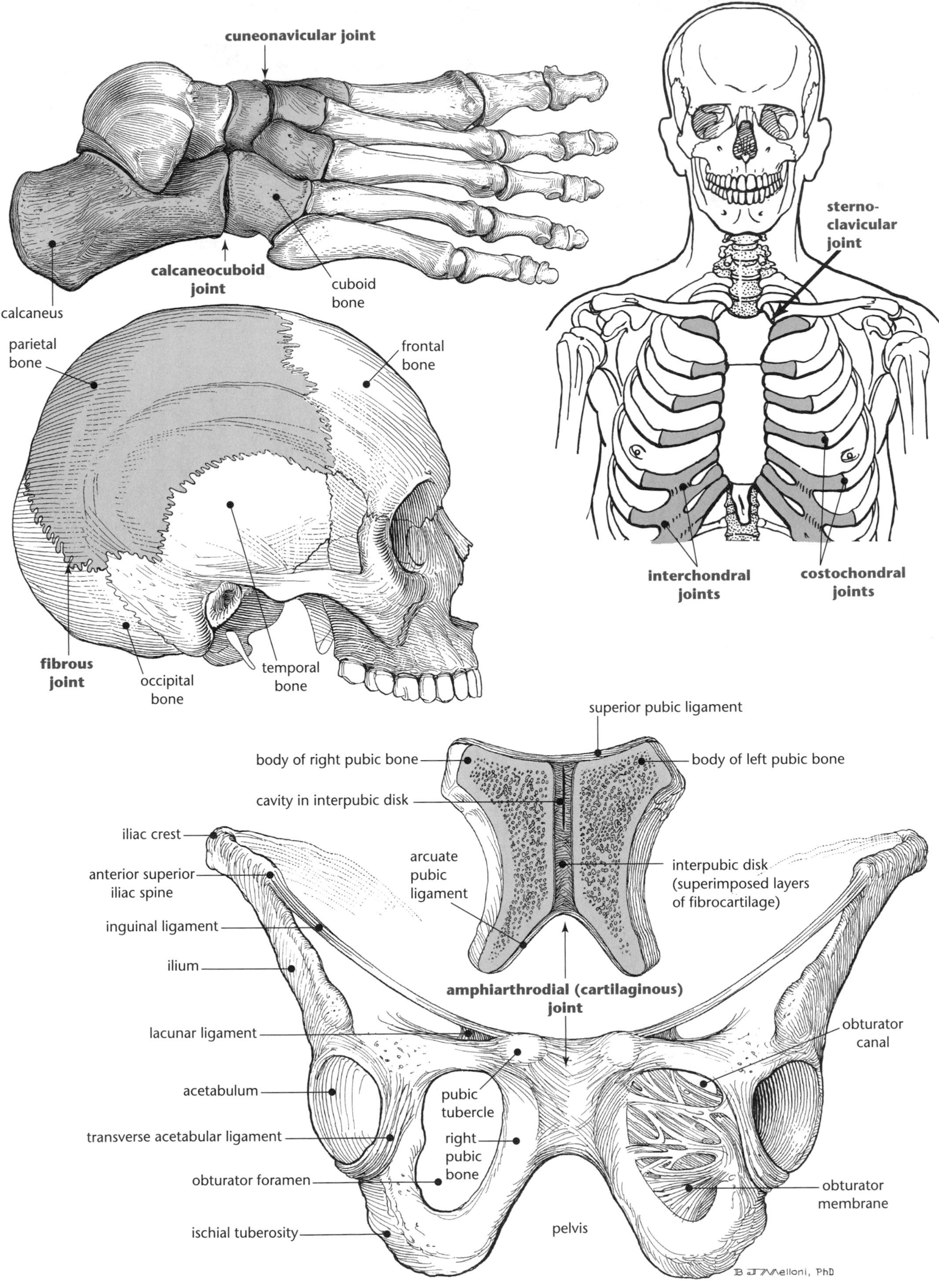
cuneonavicular joint
calcaneocuboid joint
calcaneus
cuboid bone
sterno-clavicular joint
parietal bone
frontal bone
fibrous joint
occipital bone
temporal bone
interchondral joints
costochondral joints
superior pubic ligament
body of right pubic bone
body of left pubic bone
cavity in interpubic disk
iliac crest
anterior superior iliac spine
arcuate pubic ligament
interpubic disk (superimposed layers of fibrocartilage)
inguinal ligament
ilium
amphiarthrodial (cartilaginous) joint
lacunar ligament
obturator canal
acetabulum
pubic tubercle
transverse acetabular ligament
right pubic bone
obturator foramen
obturator membrane
ischial tuberosity
pelvis
B J Melloni, PhD

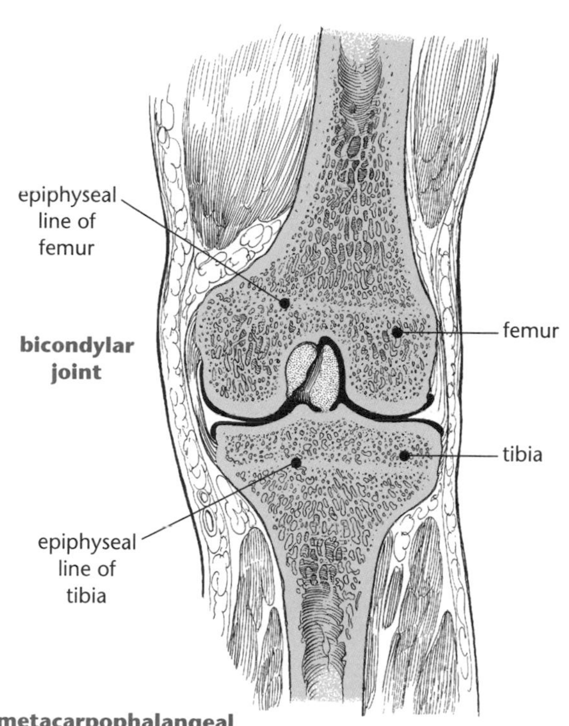
epiphyseal line of femur
bicondylar joint
femur
tibia
epiphyseal line of tibia

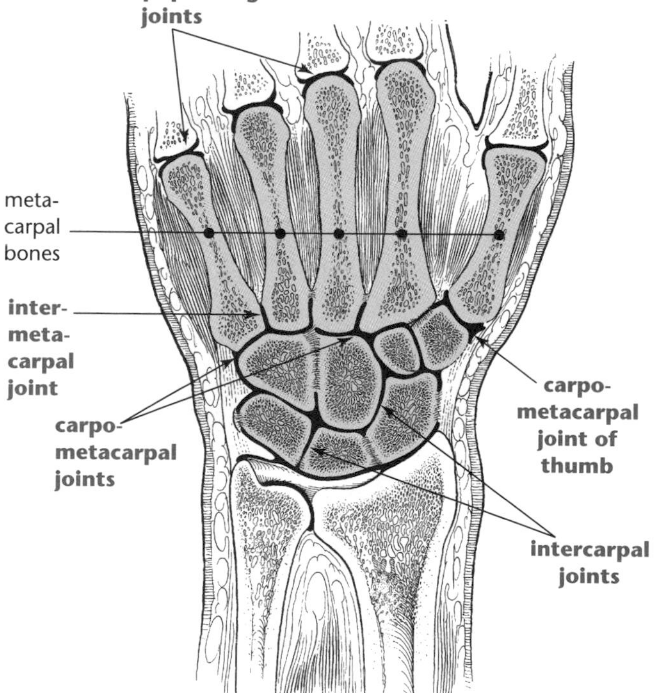
metacarpophalangeal joints
meta-carpal bones
inter-meta-carpal joint
carpo-metacarpal joints
carpo-metacarpal joint of thumb
intercarpal joints

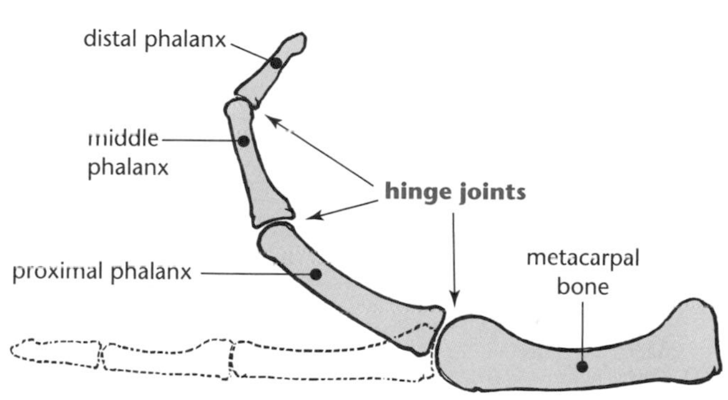
distal phalanx
middle phalanx
hinge joints
proximal phalanx
metacarpal bone

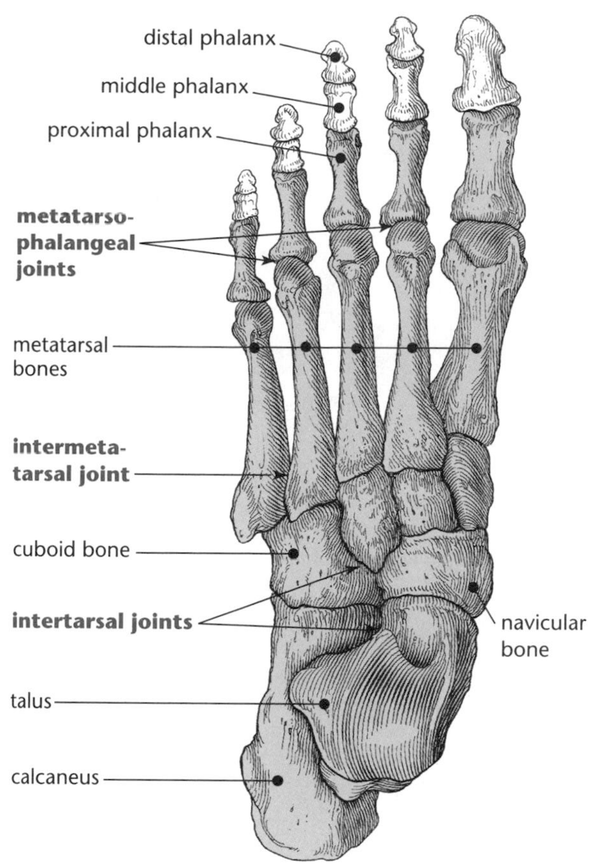
distal phalanx
middle phalanx
proximal phalanx
metatarso-phalangeal joints
metatarsal bones
intermeta-tarsal joint
cuboid bone
intertarsal joints
navicular bone
talus
calcaneus

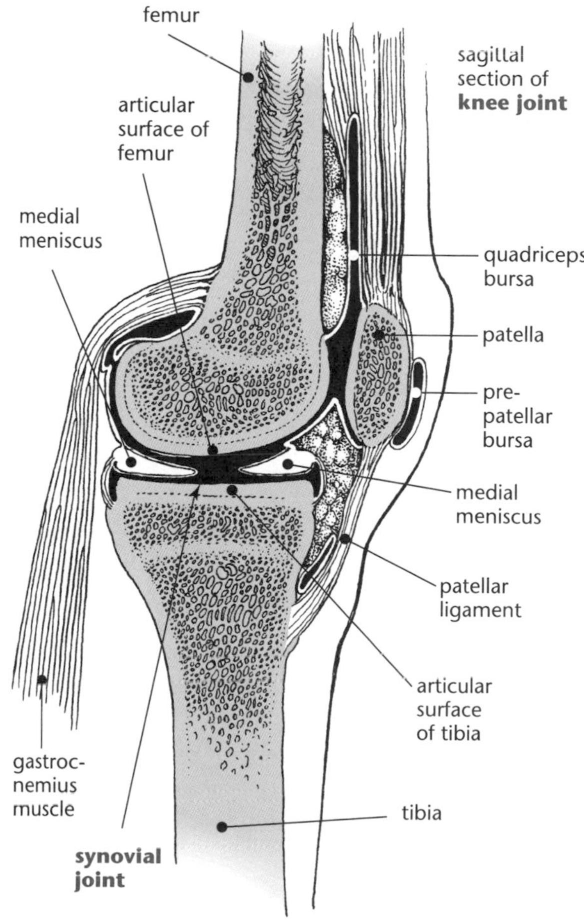
femur
sagittal section of knee joint
articular surface of femur
medial meniscus
quadriceps bursa
patella
pre-patellar bursa
medial meniscus
patellar ligament
articular surface of tibia
gastroc-nemius muscle
tibia
synovial joint

J

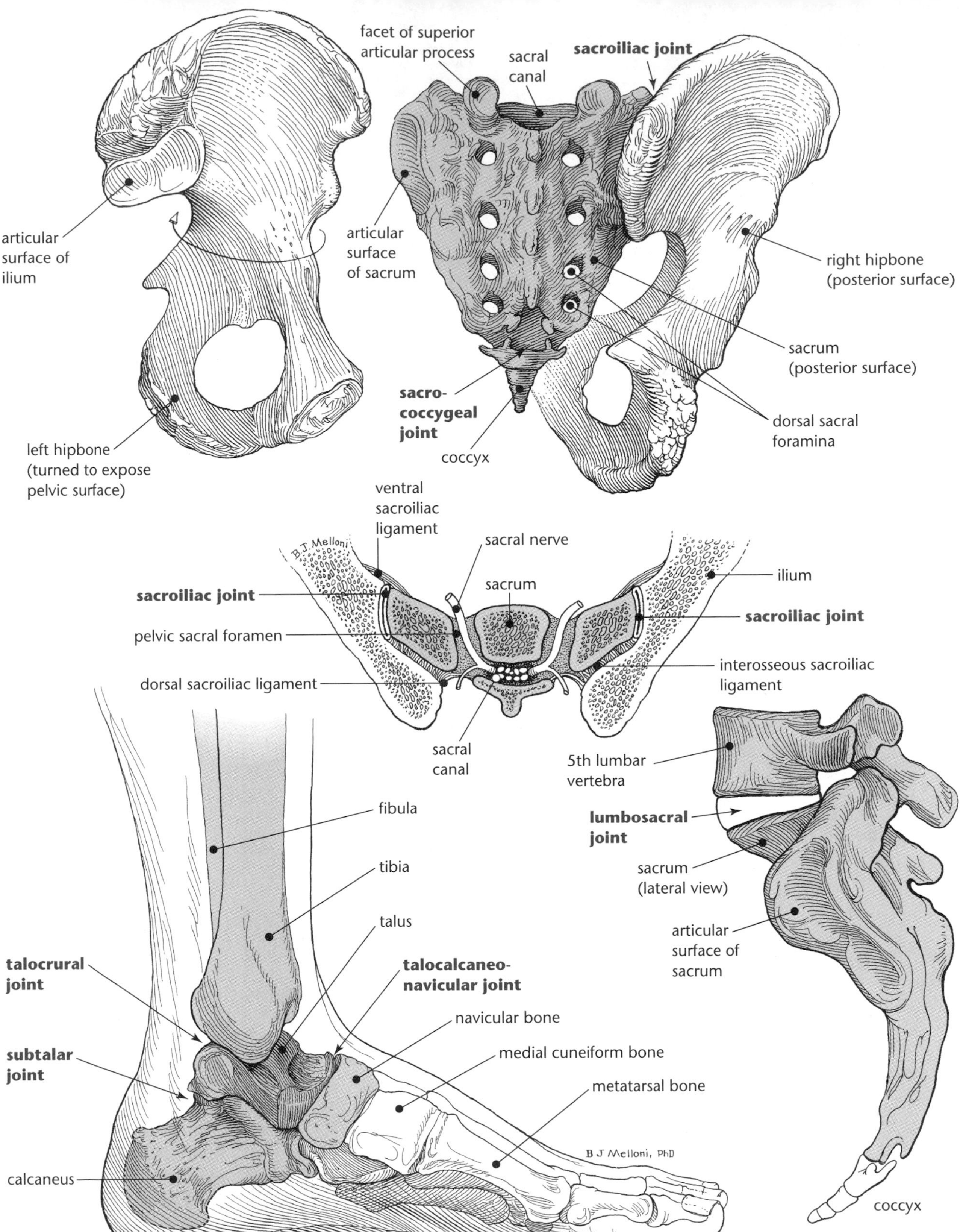

movements.

cuneometatarsal j.'s See tarsometatarsal joints.

cuneonavicular j. Articulation in the posterior portion of the foot between the front surface of the navicular bone and the back surfaces of the three cuneiform bones.

diarthrodial j. See synovial joint.

ellipsoidal j. A joint with an oval-shaped part that fits into an elliptic cavity permitting all types of movement except pivotal.

false j. See pseudarthrosis.

femoropatellar j. The part of the knee joint formed by the articulation between the back surface of the kneecap (patella) and corresponding anterior surface of the femur.

fibrous j. A type of joint such as syndesmosis, suture, and gomphosis in which fibrous tissue unites two bones (e.g., the joints between the skull bones). Also called immovable joint; synarthrodial joint; synarthrosis.

frozen j. See ankylosis.

ginglymoid j. See hinge joint.

gliding j. A type of diarthrodial joint in which the apposed surfaces are more or less flat, permitting a gliding motion (e.g., between the articular processes of vertebrae). Also called arthrodia; plane joint.

hinge j. A type of diarthrodial joint that permits only a forward and backward movement, as the hinge of a door (e.g., the interphalangeal joints). Also called ginglymoid joint; ginglymus.

hip j. The ball-and-socket joint between the head of the femur and the acetabulum of the hipbone.

humeroradial j. The joint at the elbow between the humerus and the head of the radius.

humeroulnar j. The joint at the elbow between the trochlea of the humerus and the trochlear notch of the ulna.

immovable j. See fibrous joint.

intercarpal j.'s Joints between the carpal bones

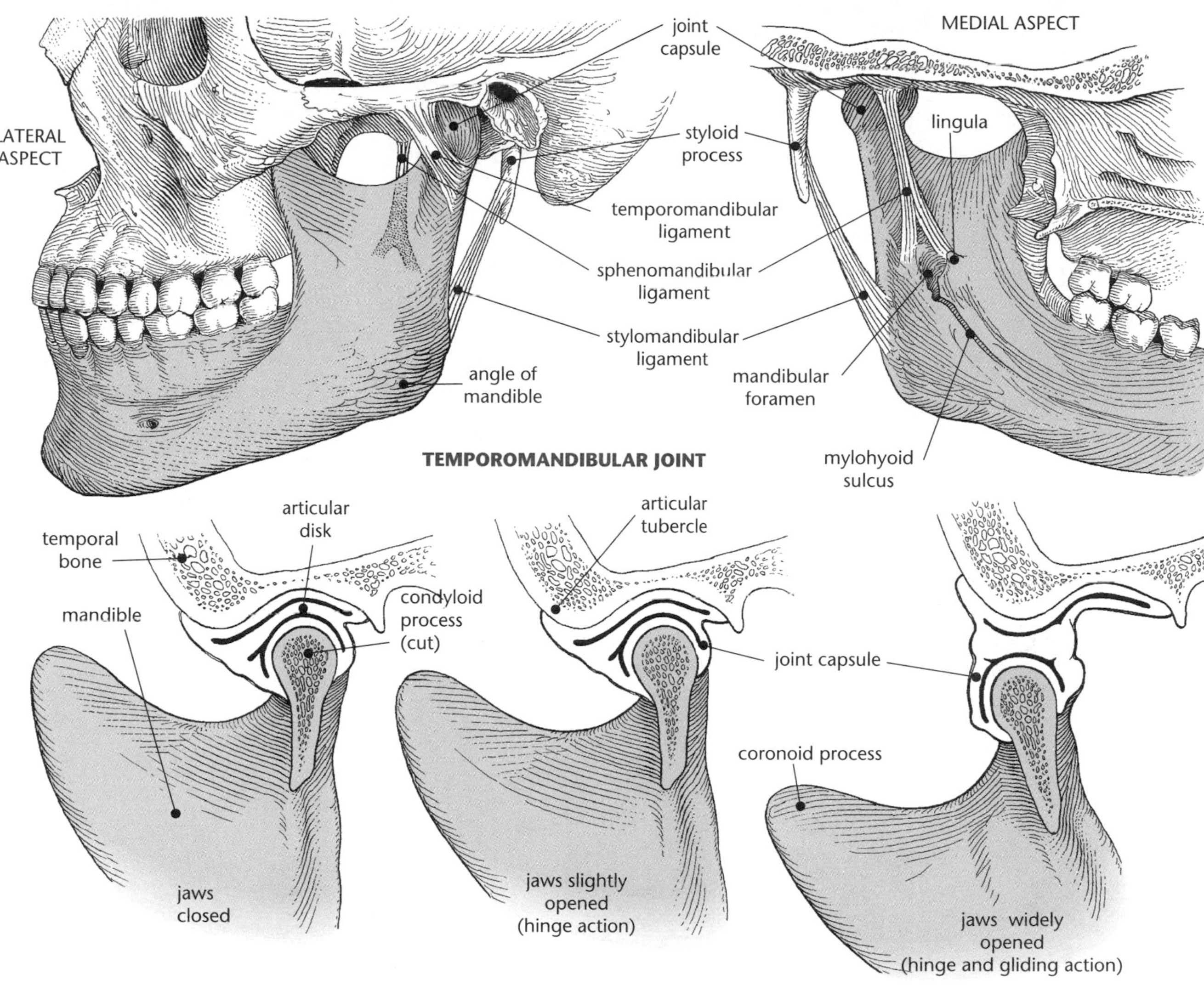

of the wrist.

interchondral j.'s Joints between the contiguous surfaces of the fifth through tenth costal cartilages.

intermetacarpal j.'s The plane joints between adjoining bases of the second through fifth metacarpal bones of the hand.

intermetatarsal j.'s The plane joints between adjoining bases of the five metatarsal bones of the foot.

interphalangeal j.'s Hinge joints between the phalanges of each finger and toe.

intertarsal j.'s Joints between the tarsal bones in the posterior portion of the foot. Also called tarsal joints.

knee j. A compound condylar joint formed by the two condyles and patellar surface of the femur, the posterior surface of the kneecap (patella), and the superior articular surface of the tibia.

Lisfranc's j.'s See tarsometatarsal joints.

lumbosacral j. The joint between the fifth lumbar vertebra and the sacrum.

metatarsophalangeal j.'s Ellipsoid joints at the front of the foot between the heads of the five metatarsal bones and the concave bases of the corresponding proximal phalanges.

midtarsal j. See transverse tarsal joint.

movable j. See synovial joint.

neuropathic j. See Charcot's joint.

pivot j. See rotary joint.

plane j. A synovial joint in which the opposing articular surfaces are either flat planes or slightly curved; it allows gliding movements, as in the intermetacarpal joints. Also called arthrodial joint; gliding joint.

radiocarpal j. The ellipsoid joint at the wrist between the radius and its articular disk, and the scaphoid, lunate, and triangular bones. Also called wrist joint.

radioulnar j.'s The two articulations between the radius and the ulna: *Distal radioulnar j.*, the joint between the rounded head of the ulna and the ulnar notch of the radius at the distal end of the forearm, near the wrist; also called inferior radioulnar joint. *Proximal radioulnar j.*, the joint between the head of the radius and the radial notch of the ulna within the annular ligament of the radius at the proximal end of the forearm, near the elbow. Also called superior radioulnar joint.

rotary j. A type of diarthrodial joint in which a pivot-like process fits and rotates within a ring that is formed partly of bone and partly of ligaments, as the proximal radioulnar articulation. Also called pivot joint; trochoid joint.

sacrococcygeal j. The joint between the sacrum and the tailbone (coccyx). Also called coccygeal joint.

sacroiliac j. Joint between the vertebral column and the pelvis, specifically between the two auricular surfaces on the upper part of the sacrum and each ilium on the posterior part of the pelvis.

saddle j. A type of synovial joint in which the articular surface of one bone is concave in one direction and convex in a direction at right angles to the first, with the articular surface of the other bone reciprocally convex and concave (e.g., the carpometacarpal joint of the thumb).

spheroidal j. See ball and socket joint.

sternoclavicular j. Joint formed by the medial end of the collarbone (clavicle), the manubrium of the breastbone (sternum), and the cartilage of the first rib.

subtalar j. The joint between the inferior surface of the ankle bone (talus) and the superior surface of the heel bone (calcaneus). Also called talocalcanean joint.

synarthrodial j. See fibrous joint.

synovial j. A joint that usually permits free movement, composed of a layer of hyaline cartilage or fibrocartilage and a synovial cavity between the bones (a fluid-containing cavity lined by a synovial membrane); includes most of the joints of the body. Also called diarthrosis; diarthrodial joint; movable joint.

talocalcanean j. See subtalar joint.

talocalcaneonavicular j. Joint formed by the rounded head of the ankle bone (talus), the concave surface of the navicular bone, the upper surface of the heel bone (calcaneus), and the plantar calcaneonavicular ligament. Also called anterior talocalcanean joint.

talocrural j. Hinge joint formed by the tibia and fibula and the ankle bone (talus). Also called ankle joint.

tarsal j.'s See intertarsal joints.

tarsometatarsal j.'s The three joints between the tarsal and metatarsal bones of the foot, involving a medial joint between the first metatarsal bone and the medial cuneiform bone; an intermediate joint between the second and third metatarsal bones and the intermediate and lateral cuneiform bones; and a lateral joint between the fourth and fifth metatarsal bones and the cuboid bone. Also called cuneometatarsal joints; Lisfranc's joints.

temporomandibular j. (TMJ) Synovial joint between the condyle of the mandible inferiorly and the mandibular fossa and articular tubercle of the temporal bone superiorly; separated by a thin articular disk into two cavities, each of which is lined by a synovial membrane.

tibiofibular j., superior Plane joint between the lateral condyle of the tibia and the head of the fibula, near the knee.

transverse tarsal j. Joint between the heel bone (calcaneus) and cuboid bones, and the ankle bone (talus) and navicular bones of the foot. Also called Chopart's joint; midtarsal joint.

trochoid j. See rotary joint.

ureteropelvic j. (UPJ) The site at which the funnel-shaped renal pelvis ends and the ureter begins; may be marked by a slight constriction.

wrist j. See radiocarpal joint.

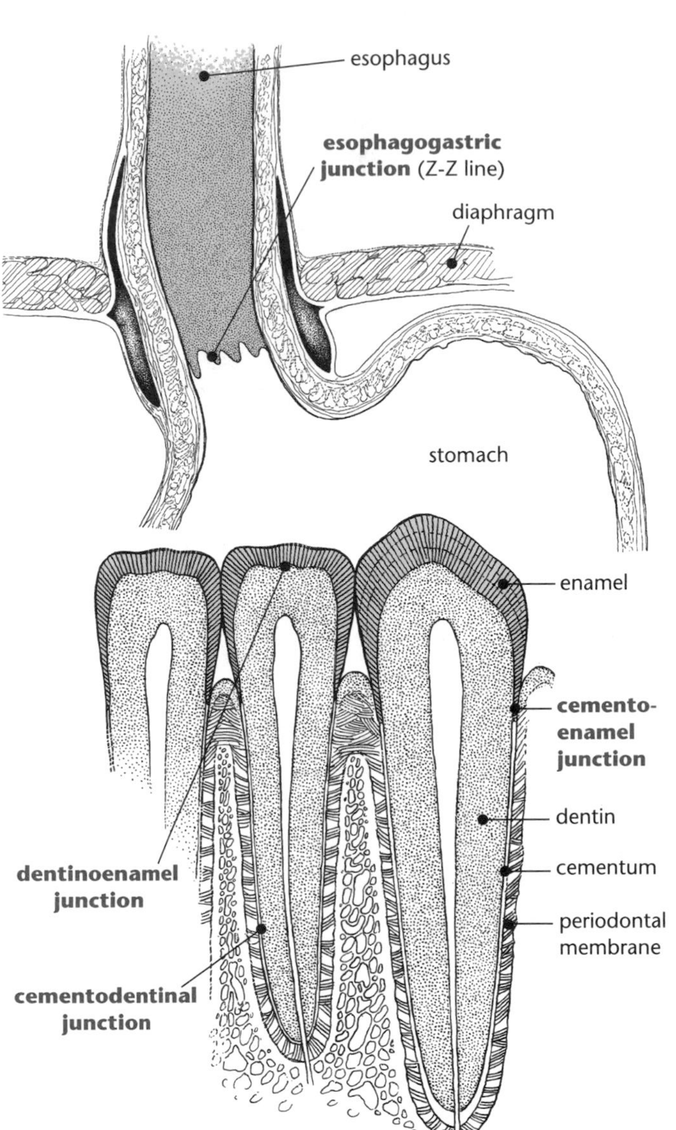

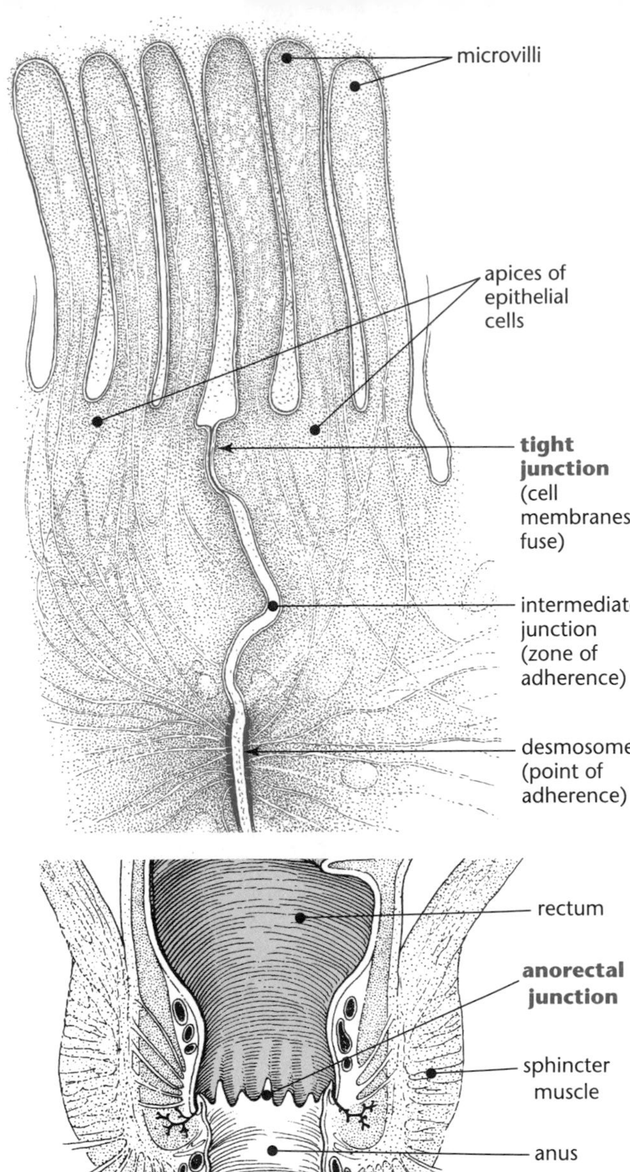

joule (jo͞ol) (J) **1.** A unit of energy equivalent to that expended when a current of 1 ampere is passed through a resistance of 1 ohm for 1 second. **2.** A unit of energy equivalent to the work done in moving a body 1 meter against a force of 1 newton.

jugal (jo͞o´gal) **1.** Connecting. **2.** Relating to the cheek.

jugular (jug´u-lar) **1.** Relating to the neck. **2.** Denoting certain structures in the neck.

jugulum (jug´u-lum) The neck or throat.

jugum (jo͞o´gum), *pl.* **ju´ga** A ridge connecting two structures.

juga alveolaria Eminences on the front of the alveolar processes of the maxilla and mandible, produced by the roots of incisors and cuspids within.

j. sphenoidale The elevated smooth front part of the body of the sphenoid bone that connects the lesser wings of the bone; it forms part of the anterior cranial fossa.

juice (jo͞os) A digestive secretion (e.g., gastric juice, pancreatic juice).

junction (junk´shun) **1.** A joint or articulation. **2.** The line of union of two parts or surfaces.

anorectal j. The region where the rectum ends and the anal canal begins, in front of, and slightly below the tip of the coccyx.

cardioesophageal j. See esophagogastric junction.

cementodentinal j. The surface at which the cementum and dentin of a root of a tooth meet.

cementoenamel j. The line around a tooth where the enamel of its crown and the cementum of its root meet. Also called cervical line.

communicating j. See gap junction.

conjunctivocorneal j. The area of the eye, at the limbus, where the fibrous membrane of the conjunctiva ends and only the epithelium continues centrally to cover the cornea.

costochondral j. The point of articulation between the sternal end of a rib and the lateral end of its cartilage.

dentinoenamel j. The surface at which the dentin and the enamel of the crown of a tooth meet.

electrical j. See gap junction.

esophagogastric j. The junction of the esophagus and the stomach. Also called cardioesophageal junction.

gap j. Intercellular space containing channels which connect adjacent cells; seen between certain nerve cells; and in cardiac and smooth muscles.

J j. The point at the end of the QRS complex of the electrocardiogram (principal deflection) and the beginning of the ST segment (segment immediately following the QRS complex). Also called J point.

mucocutaneous j. The area of transition from a mucous membrane to the epidermis.

myoneural j. See neuromuscular junction.

myotendinal j. The region between the end of the muscle fibers and their tendinous attachment.

neuromuscular j. The area of contact between the motor nerve and the muscle; the end of the nerve broadens into an end-plate that fits into a depression in the skeletal muscle fiber. Also called myoneural junction.

occluding j. See tight junction.

sclerocorneal j. See limbus of cornea, under limbus.

tight j. An annular junction around the apices of epithelial cells, present at sites requiring a barrier to diffusion through the intercellular space; at the junction, the membranes are in firm contact, obliterating the space between them and thereby creating a barrier to the movement of molecules. Also called occluding junction; zona occludens; zonula occludens.

ureteropelvic j. (UPJ) The site at which the funnel-shaped renal pelvis ends and the ureter begins; may be marked by a slight constriction.

junctura (jŭnk-too´ră), *pl.* **junctu´rae** Latin for a joining. Also called articulation.

jurisprudence (jo͝or-is-pro͞o´dens) The science or philosophy of a particular system of law.

dental j. See forensic dentistry.

medical j. See forensic medicine.

jury-mast (jo͝or´ē mast) An upright bar used in conjunction with a plaster of Paris jacket to serve as a head support in cases of diseases of the spine (e.g., in Pott's disease).

juxtaepiphyseal (juks-tă-ep-ĭ-fĭz´e-al) Near or next to an end (epiphysis) of a long bone.

juxtaglomerular (juks-tă-glo-mer´u-lar) Near or adjacent to a glomerulus of the kidney.

j. apparatus See under apparatus.

juxtacrine (juks´tă-krin) Hormone action that depends on direct contact between the cell producing the hormone and the target cell.

juxtamedullary (juks-tă-med´u-lar-e) Referring to that portion of the inner cortex of the kidney adjacent to the medulla (e.g., juxtamedullary glomeruli).

juxtapose (juks´tă-pōz) To position side by side.

juxtaposition (juks-tă-pŏ-zish´un) The state of being side by side; the act of placing side by side.

juxtapyloric (juks-tă-pi-lor´ik) Located near the pylorus.

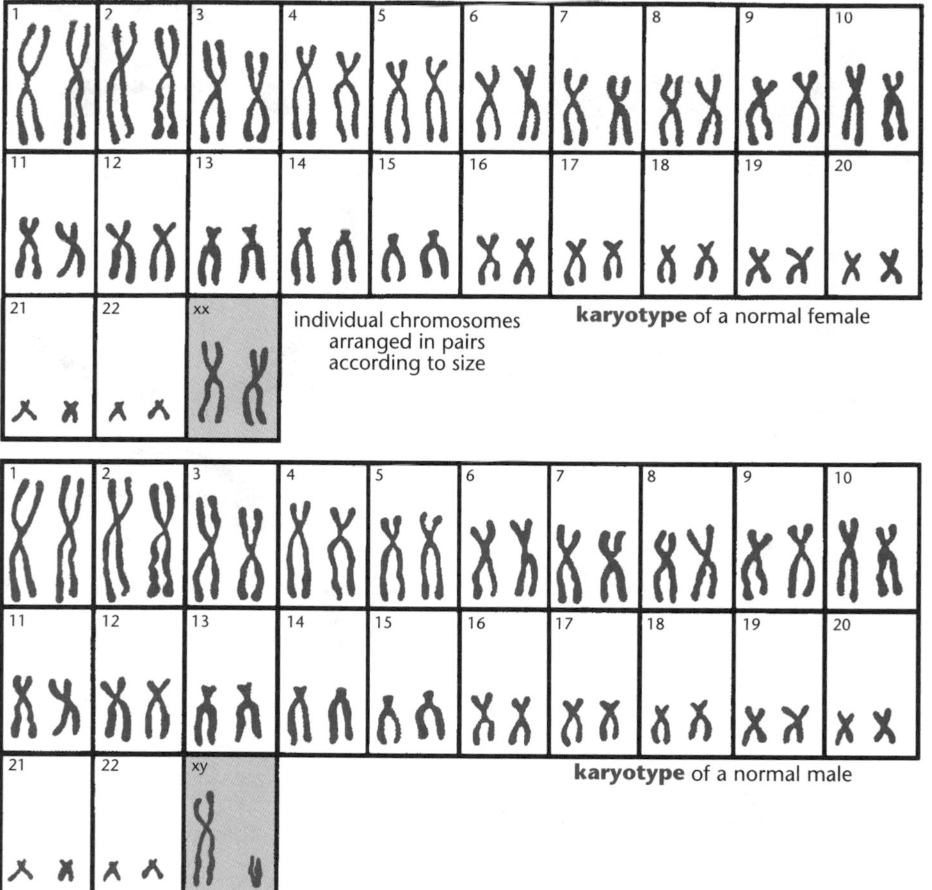

karyotype of a normal female

karyotype of a normal male

K

K

Κ (kap´ă) Kappa.

kala azar (kă´lă ă-zar´) See visceral leishmaniasis, under leishmaniasis.

kaliopenia (ka-le-o-pe´ne-ă) Potassium deficiency in the body.

kalium (ka´le-um) Latin for potassium.

kaliuresis (ka-le-u-re´sis) Increased excretion of potassium in the urine. Also called kaluresis.

kaliuretic (ka-le-u-ret´ik) **1.** Relating to kaliuresis. **2.** An agent that induces kaliuresis.

kallikrein (kal-ĭ-kre´in) A peptidase which acts on alpha$_2$ globulins in plasma or in glands to produce kinins.

Kallmann's syndrome (kahl´mahnz sin´drōm) See hypogonadism with anosmia, under hypogonadism.

kaluresis (kal-u-re´sis) See kaliuresis.

K and k blood groups See Kell blood group.

kaolin (ka´o-lin) A fine, whitish clay used as a demulcent and adsorbent. Also called aluminum silicate.

kappa (kap´ă) **1.** The tenth letter of the Greek alphabet, κ. **2.** The tenth in a series. **3.** In chemistry, a position on the tenth atom from the carboxyl or other functional group. **4.** In statistics, the degree of nonrandom agreement between measurements of the same variable.

Kartagener's syndrome (kahr-tag´ĕ-nerz sin´drōm) Displacement of the viscera to the opposite side of the body (situs inversus) associated with dilatation of the bronchial tubes (bronchiectasis) and chronic sinusitis.

karyochrome (kar´e-o-krōm) A nerve cell having a nucleus that stains deeply.

karyocyte (kar´e-o-sīt) A nucleated cell; usually referring to a young nucleated red blood cell (normoblast).

karyogamy (kar-e-og´ă-me) Fusion of the nuclei of two cells during cell conjugation.

karyogenesis(kar-e-o-jen´ĕ-sis) The formation of a cell nucleus.

karyogram (kar´e-o-gram) See karyotype.

karyokinesis (kar-e-o-ki-ne´sis) See mitosis.

karyolobic (kar-e-o-lo´bik) Having a lobulated nucleus.

karyolymph (kar´e-o-limf) The clear homogeneous liquid part of a cell nucleus.

karyolysis (kar-e-ol´ĭ-sis) The destruction or dissolution of the nucleus of a cell.

karyomere (kar´e-o-mēr) A cellular structure usually formed during an abnormal cell division; consists of a vesicle containing a small portion of the cell nucleus.

karyomitome (kar-e-o-mi´tōm) See chromatin.

karyomorphism (kar-e-o-mor´fiz-m) **1.** Development of a cell nucleus. **2.** Referring to the nuclear shapes of cells.

karyon (kar´e-on) The cell nucleus.

karyoplasm (kar´e-o-plaz-m) The protoplasm of the cell nucleus. Also called nucleoplasm.

karyopyknosis (kar-e-o-pik-no´sis) Shrinkage of cell nuclei and condensation of the chromatin.

karyorrhexis (kar-e-o-rek´sis) Fragmentation of the cell nucleus.

karyosome (kar´e-o-sōm) One of the spherical masses of chromatin resembling a knot in the chromatin network of a resting nucleus during mitosis. Also called net knot; chromatin nucleolus; false nucleolus.

karyotype (kar´e-o-tīp) **1.** The chromosome constitution of an individual. **2.** A systematized presentation of individual chromosomes of a single cell, photomicrographed during the metaphase stage of mitosis and arranged in pairs according to size. **3.** To make such an arrangement.

karyotyping (kar-e-o-tīp´ing) Analysis of chromosomes.

Kawasaki disease (kă-wă-să´ke dĭ-zēz´) Mucocutaneous lymph node syndrome.

Kell blood group (kel blud grōōp) A blood group of clinical importance because of its immunogenicity; consists of a series of codominant antigens determined by alleles at a site that is thought to be on the short arm of chromosome 2; first detected through antiserum produced by a Mrs. Kell.

keloid (ke´loid) A nodular, nonencapsulated, highly hyperplastic mass of scar tissue.

keloidosis (ke-loi-do´sis) The presence of multiple keloids.

keloplasty (ke´lo-plas-te) Surgical removal of a scar or keloid.

Kennedy's syndrome (ken´ĕ-dēz sin´drōm) The association of unilateral loss of the sense of smell and atrophy of the optic disk of the same side with swelling of the optic disk of the opposite side; caused by a tumor (meningioma) at the base of the frontal lobe. Also called Foster Kennedy's syndrome.

keratalgia (ker-ă-tal´jă) Pain in the cornea.

keratectomy (ker-ă-tek´to-me) Surgical removal of the superficial layers of the cornea affected by scarring or degeneration, without replacing the excised tissue with a graft.

photorefractive k. (PRK) Procedure for correcting nearsightedness and astigmatism by reshaping the curvature of the cornea with the excimer laser (which uses an invisible, high energy light); a portion of the epithelium (the thin superficial layer of the cornea) is removed and the exposed corneal surface is flattened; the epithelium usually regenerates within one week.

keratic (ker-at´ik) **1.** Horny. **2.** Relating to the cornea.

keratin (ker´ă-tin) The protein present largely in, and forming the main components of, epidermal structures such as hair, nails, horns, feathers, etc.

alpha-k. Keratin in its folded form (as in normal hair).

beta-k. Keratin in its extended form (as in stretched hair).

keratinization (ker-ă-tin-i-za´shun) The formation of keratin or a horny layer.

keratinize (ker´ă-tin-īz) To become horny.

keratinosome (kĕ-rat´ĭ-no-sōm) One of several ovoid cytoplasmic granules in the spinous cells of the epidermis about 300 nm in diameter, bound by a double-layered membrane, and filled with lamellae; considered by some to be a specialized epidermal lysosome. Also called lamellated granule; membrane-coating granule.

keratinous (kĕ-rat´ĭ-nŭs) Relating to or consisting of keratin.

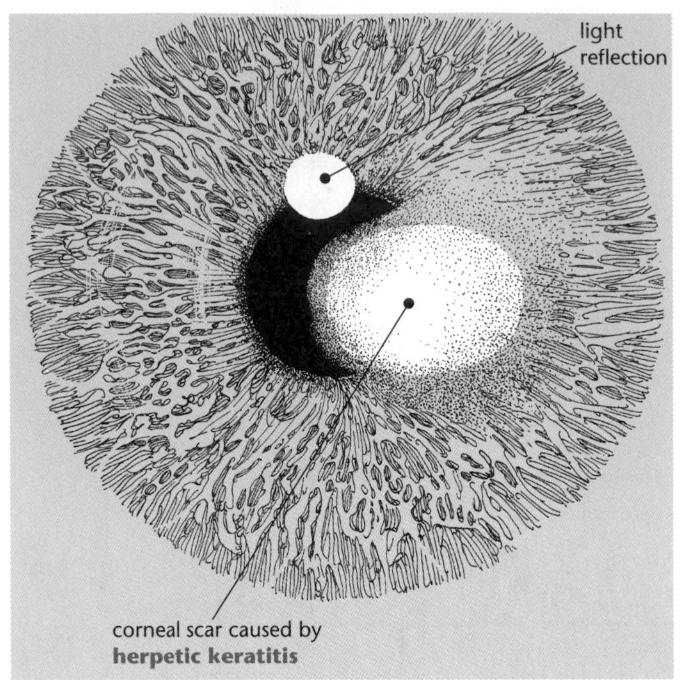

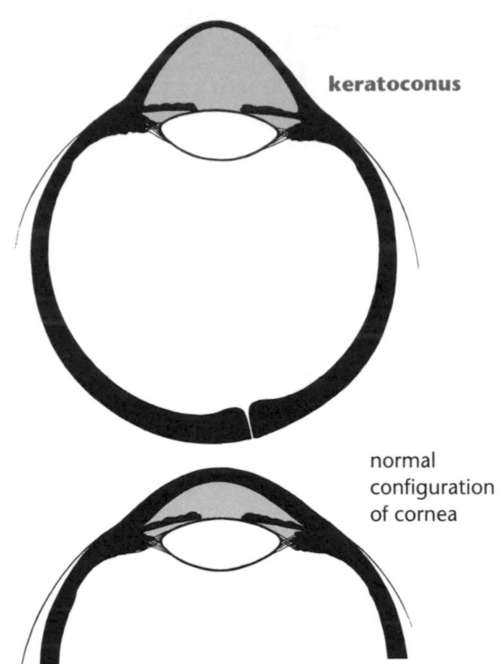

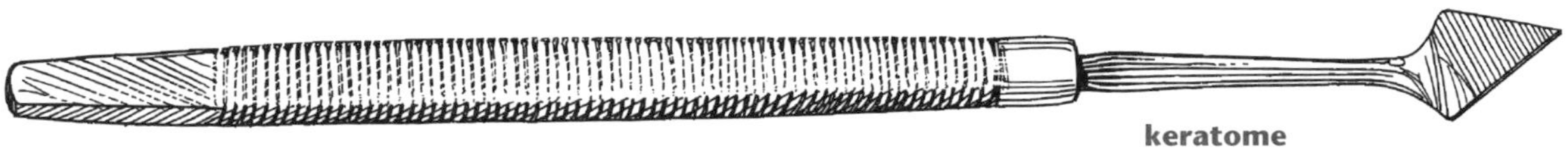

keratometry

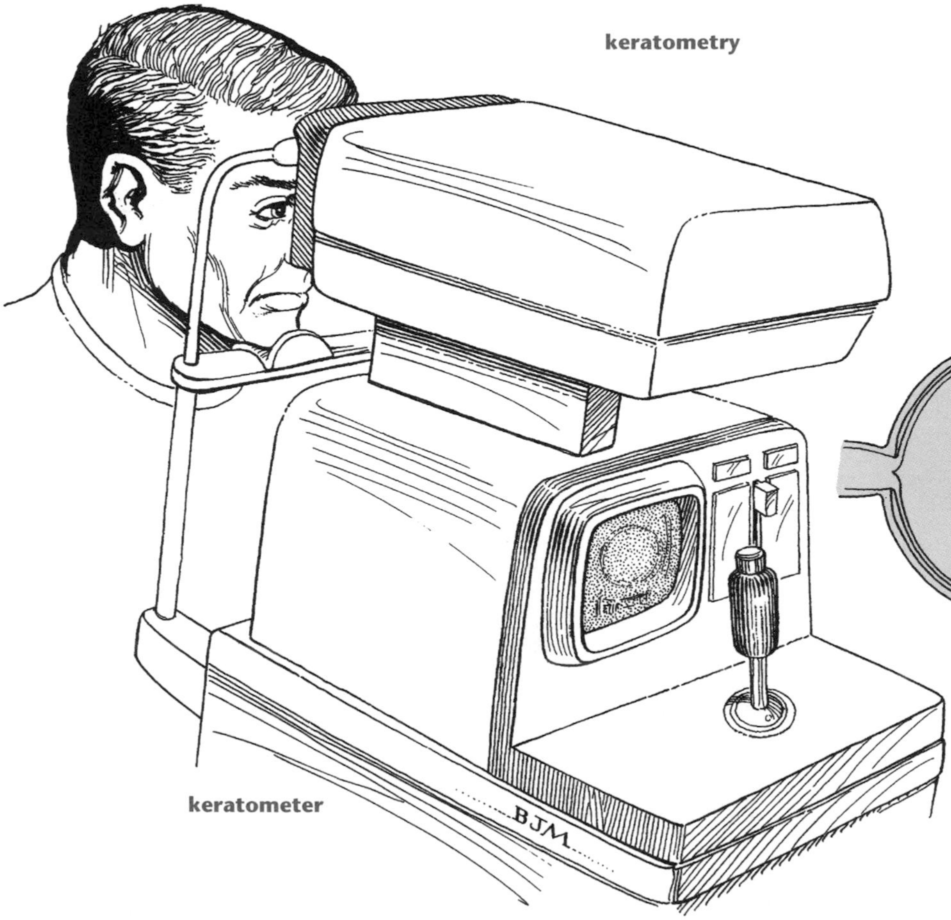

The curvature of the corneal refractive surface is accurately measured by **keratometry.**

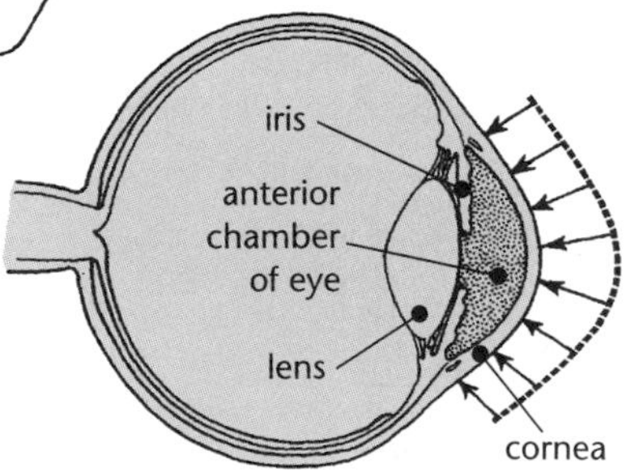

iris

anterior chamber of eye

lens

cornea

keratometer

BJM

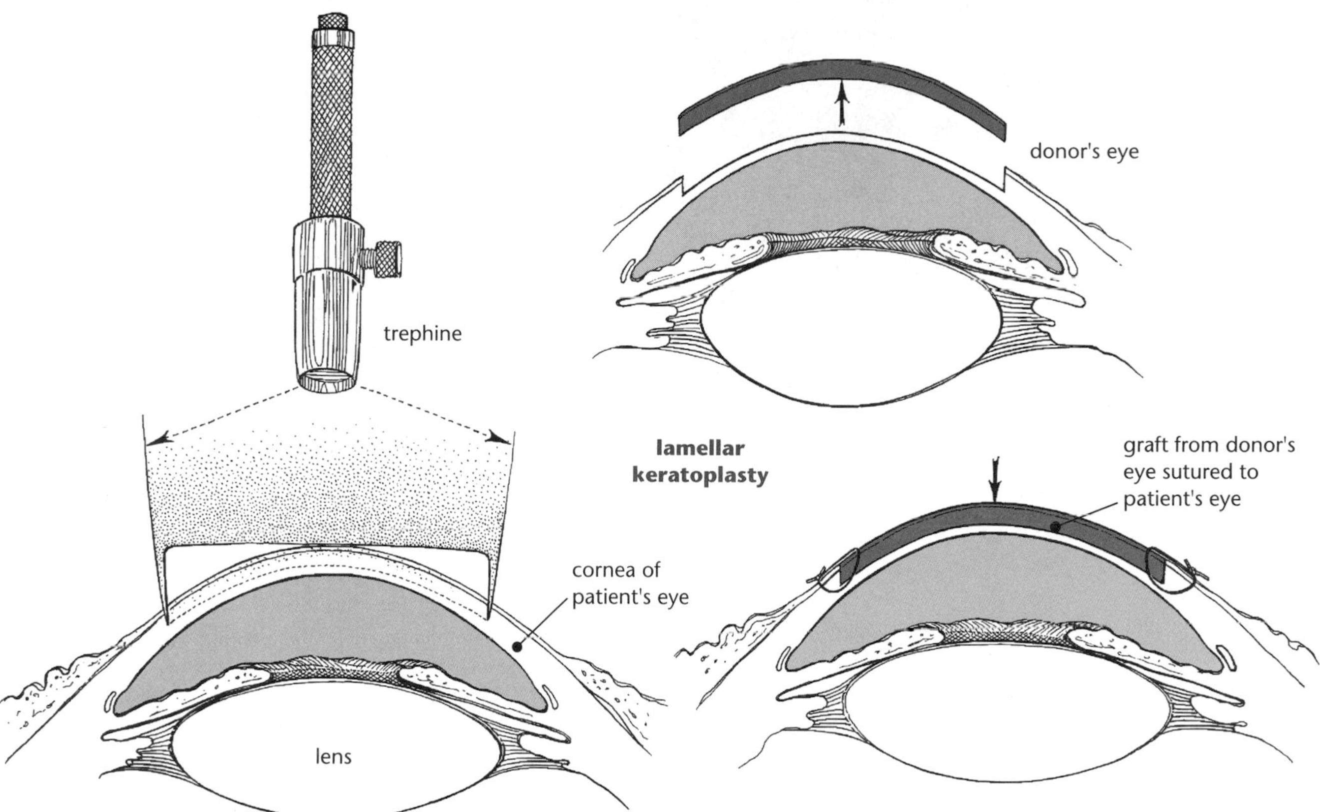

K

keratitis (ker-ă-ti´tis) Inflammation of the cornea. Also called corneitis.

fascicular k. Superficial corneal ulcer that moves from the periphery to the center of the cornea, carrying with it a narrow band of blood vessels from the conjunctiva; it remains superficial and terminates in a linear opacity; secondary to phlyctenular keratitis.

herpetic k., herpes simplex k. Herpes simplex infection of the cornea.

interstitial k. Deep inflammation and vascularization of the cornea involving primarily the middle layer; found chiefly in children and young adults as a late manifestation of congenital syphilis.

laser-assisted *in situ* k. (LASIK) Procedure in which reshaping of the cornea is performed with the excimer laser (which uses an invisible, high energy light); a hinged flap of corneal tissue is cut and a thin layer of tissue is removed from the exposed corneal surface, then the flap is placed back in its original position.

phlyctenular k. Small gray nodules that break down forming a shallow ulcer; seen most commonly in the corneal periphery.

k. sicca (KCS) See keratoconjunctivitis sicca, under keratoconjunctivitis.

keratoacanthoma (ker-ă-to-ak-an-tho´mă) A rapidly growing benign skin nodule, usually with a central depression, histologically resembling squamous cell carcinoma and occurring chiefly on the face.

keratocele (ker´ă-to-sēl) Hernia of the posterior limiting (Descemet's) membrane of the cornea.

keratochromatosis (ker-ă-to-kro-mă-to´siš) Discoloration of the cornea.

keratoconjunctivitis (ker-ă-to-kon-junk-tĭ-vi´tis) Inflammation of the cornea and conjunctiva.

epidemic k. A contagious form caused by a type 8 adenovirus, occurring mainly in persons exposed to dust and trauma in industry. Also called shipyard eye.

phlyctenular k. A delayed hypersensitivity to proteins from microorganisms, including those from tubercle bacillus, *Candida albicans, Chlamydia lymphogranulomatis,* and especially *Staphylococcus aureus,* characterized by formation of minute, ulcerating nodules (phlyctenules) primarily on the conjunctiva and cornea, especially around its periphery. Those occurring on the cornea may cause scarring.

k. sicca (KCS) Condition of the corneal and conjunctival epithelium, marked by absence of tears, increased sensitivity to light, and formation of thick mucous strands. Also called dry eye syndrome; keratitis sicca.

keratoconometer (ker-ă-to-ko-nom´ĕ-ter) An instrument for determining the degree of keratoconus.

keratoconus (ker-ă-to-ko´nus) A degenerative, noninflammatory, central, conical protrusion of the cornea; usually bilateral; inherited as an autosomal recessive trait. Also called conical cornea.

keratocyte (ker´ă-to-sīt) **1.** A ruptured or mutilated red blood cell (erythrocyte). **2.** One of the flattened cells between the lamellae of the cornea. Also called corneal corpuscle.

keratodermia (ker-ă-to-der´me-ă) Thickening of the horny layer of the skin.

k. blennorrhagica See keratosis blennorrhagica, under keratosis.

k. palmoplantar Thickening of the skin occurring in symmetrical patches on the palms and soles. Also called keratodermia symmetrica.

k. symmetrica See palmoplantar keratodermia.

keratoectasia (ker-ă-to-ek-ta´zhă) Protrusion or bulging of the cornea due to a thinning or weakening of the corneal tissue.

keratogenesis (ker-ă-to-jen´ĕ-sis) The formation of horny tissue.

keratogenous (ker-ă-toj´ĕ-nŭs) Causing the production of horny tissue such as nails, feathers, etc.

keratohelcosis (ker-ă-to-hel-ko´sis) Ulceration of the cornea.

keratohemia (ker-ă-to-he´me-ă) The presence of blood deposits in the cornea.

keratoid (ker´ă-toid) **1.** Horny. **2.** Resembling the cornea.

keratoiridoscope (ker-ă-to-i-rid´o-skōp) Instrument used to examine the cornea and the iris.

keratoiritis (ker-ă-to-i-ri´tis) Inflammation of the cornea and iris.

keratoleptynsis (ker-ă-to-lep-tin´sis) Plastic surgery of the eye; removal of the anterior surface of the cornea and replacement by bulbar conjunctiva.

keratolysis (ker-ă-tol´ĭ-sis) The peeling and shedding of the epidermis.

keratolytic (ker-ă-to-lit´ik) Causing scaling of the epidermis. Also called desquamative.

keratomalacia (ker-ă-to-mă-la´zhă) Dryness, softening, and dissolution of the cornea caused by severe deficiency of vitamin A.

keratome (ker´ă-tōm) A surgical knife for incising the cornea. Also called keratotome.

keratometer (ker-ă-tom´ĕ-ter) An instrument for measuring the curvature of the cornea.

keratometry (ker-ă-tom´ĕ-tre) The measuring of the anterior curvature of the cornea with a keratometer.

keratomileusis (ker-ă-to-mĭ-loo´sis) Surgical reshaping of a deep layer of the cornea for correction of nearsightedness and astigmatism.

keratomycosis (ker-ă-to-mi-ko´sis) Fungus infection of the cornea.

keratonosus (ker-ă-ton´o-sus) Any disease of the cornea.

keratonyxis (ker-ă-to-nik´sis) Surgical puncture of the cornea, as for needling the lens for soft cataract.

keratopathy (ker-ă-top´ă-the) A noninflammatory disease of the cornea, distinguished from keratitis.

bullous k. Excessive accumulation of fluid in the cornea; occurs occasionally after intraocular operations (e.g., in cataract procedures).

calcific band k. Horizontal opacity of the cornea caused by deposition of calcium salts in its anterior layer; associated with certain inflammatory, metabolic, and degenerative disorders, especially juvenile rheumatoid arthritis.

climatic k. Corneal degeneration beginning as minute, subepithelial, yellow droplets in the corneal periphery which, as the disorder progresses, extend toward the center, causing blurred vision; seen mainly in persons who spend a great deal of time outdoors; believed to be caused by prolonged exposure to ultraviolet light.

keratoplasty (ker´ă-to-plas-te) Operation in which all, or part, of a defective cornea is removed and replaced with a healthy cornea. Also called corneal transplantation; corneal graft.

lamellar k. Procedure in which only the superficial layer of the cornea is removed for the treatment of superficial corneal opacities or recurrent superficial lesions.

penetrating k. Procedure in which the entire corneal thickness is removed.

refractive k. Surgical reshaping of the cornea to correct refractive errors (e.g., myopia), which prevent images from focusing on the retina. Also called keratorefractive surgery.

keratoprosthesis (ker-ă-to-pros-the´sis) Plastic corneal implant.

keratorrhexis (ker-ă-to-rek´sis) Rupture of the cornea due to a perforating ulcer or to injury.

keratoscleritis (ker-ă-to-skle-ri´tis) Inflammation of the cornea and the sclera.

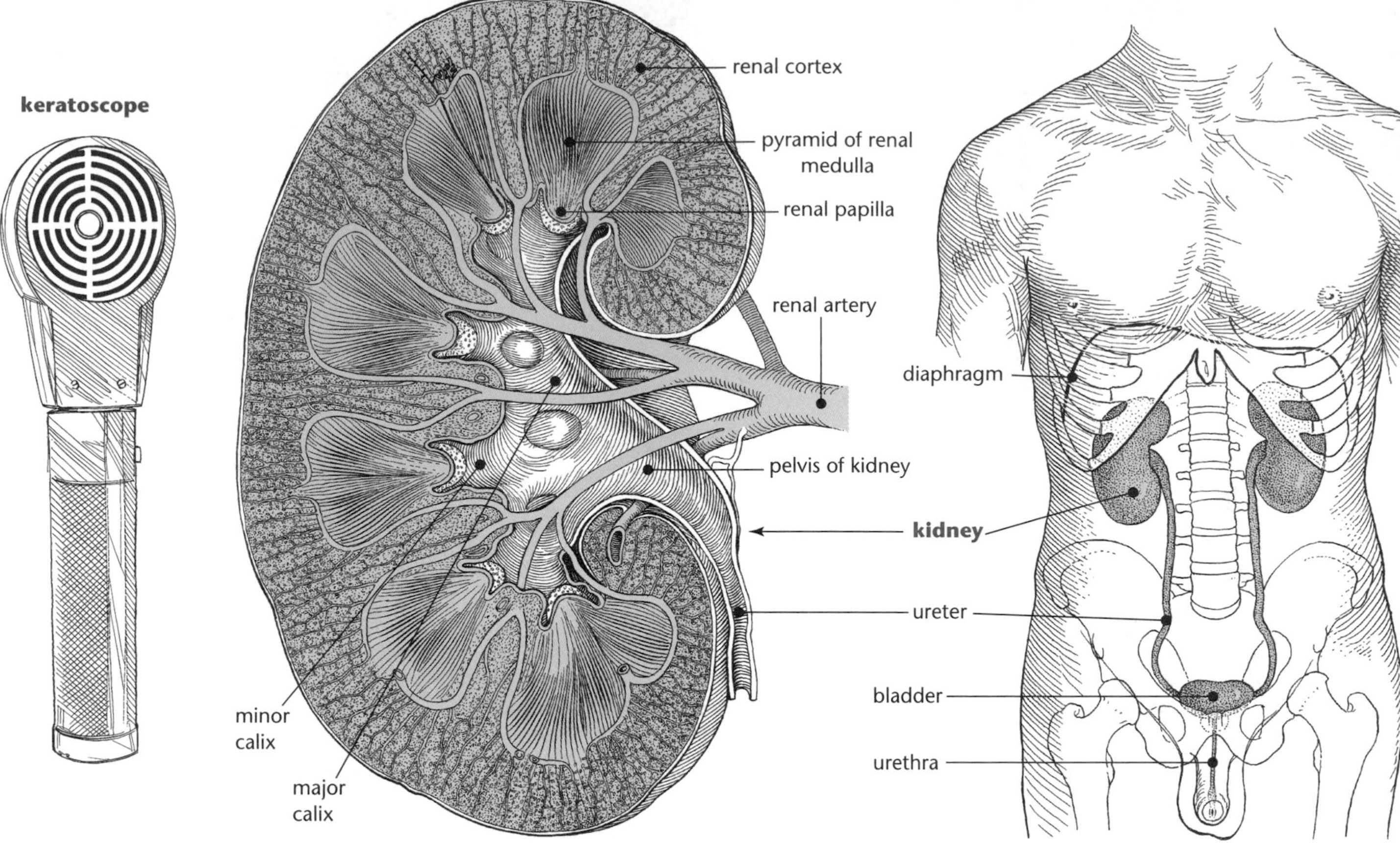

keratoscope (ker′ă-to-skōp) Instrument containing a disc of concentric rings used to examine the curvature of the cornea.

keratoscopy (ker-ă-tos′ko-pe) Inspection of the anterior surface of the cornea with a keratoscope.

keratose (ker′ă-tos) **1.** Relating to or marked by keratosis. **2.** Horny; applied to certain types of skin lesions.

keratosis (ker-ă-to′sis) A circumscribed overgrowth of the horny layer of the epidermis.

actinic k. See senile keratosis.

arsenical k. Keratosis resulting from chronic arsenic poisoning.

k. blennorrhagica Pustules and crusts associated with Reiter's disease. Also called keratodermia blennorrhagica.

k. pilaris A recurring form of keratosis limited to the hair follicles; most often seen on the upper outer arms and thighs of children and young women.

seborrheic k. Flat, warty, benign lesions seen in persons after the third decade of life.

senile k. Premalignant warty lesions occurring on the sun-exposed parts of the aged. Also called actinic keratosis.

keratotome (ker′ă-to-tōm) See keratome.

keratotomy (ker-ă-tot′o-me) Surgical incision through the cornea.

radial k. Flattening of the cornea by means of a series of incisions from its outer edge to its center in a spokelike pattern; used to correct myopia.

keraunophobia (ke-raw-no-fo′be-ă) Abnormal fear of thunder and lightning.

kerectomy (ke-rek′tŏ-me) See keratectomy.

kerion (ke′re-on) Suppurative inflammation of the scalp, a complication of ringworm; it may simulate a carbuncle, with follicular pustules, exudate, and crusting.

Kerley lines (ker′le līnz) See B lines of Kerley, under line.

kernicterus (ker-nik′ter-us) The neurologic complication of unconjugated hyperbilirubinemia in the infant, causing staining of nuclear masses in the brain and spinal cord by bile pigment, with associated degenerative changes; the clinical signs include spasticity, opisthotonos, twitching, and convulsions.

Kernig's sign (ker′nigz sīn) Inability to extend the leg completely when lying on the back with thigh flexed at right angles with the trunk; seen in meningitis.

keroid (ker′oid) See keratoid.

keto acid (ke′to as′id) An acid having the general formula RCO-COOH.

ketoacidosis (ke-to-ă-sĭ-do′sis) The presence of an excessive amount of ketone bodies (acetoacetic acid, beta-hydroxybutyrate, and acetone) in the tissues and body fluids; occurs in such conditions as diabetes and starvation.

ketoaciduria (ke-to-as-ĭ-du′re-ă) Excessive ketonic acids in the urine.

branched-chain k. See maple syrup urine disease.

ketoconazole (ke-to-kon′ă-zol) A broad-spectrum antifungal agent, administered orally or topically for the treatment of fungal infections.

ketogenesis (ke-to-jen′ĕ-sis) The production of ketone bodies (acetone substances).

ketol (ke′tol) See indole.

ketone (ke′tōn) Any of a group of compounds having a carbonyl group (CO) linking to hydrocarbon groups.

ketonemia (ke-to-ne′me-ă) The presence of ketone bodies in the blood.

ketones (ke′tōns) See ketone bodies, under body.

ketonization (ke-to-ni-za′shŭn) Conversion into a ketone.

ketonuria (ke-to-nu′re-ă) The presence of ketone bodies (acetoacidic acid, beta-hydroxybutirate, and acetone) in the urine.

ketose (ke′tōs) A carbohydrate containing a ketone group in its molecule.

ketosis (ke-to′sis) Abnormally large amounts of ketone (acetone) bodies in the tissues and fluids.

17-ketosteroid (ke-to-ster′oid) A steroid hormone with a ketone radical on the seventeen carbon, derived from the adrenal glands or the gonads; present in the urine of adults and in excess in certain tumors of the adrenal cortex; normal values in the urine are 6 to18 mg/24 hours in the male and 4 to13 mg/24 hours in the female.

ketosuccinic acid (ke-to-suk-sin′ik) See oxaloacetic acid.

kick (kĭk) A forceful thrust.

atrial k. A forceful atrial contraction that tends to improve the performance of the ventricle when the ventricular wall has become stiffened; usually occurs in aortic stenosis or in ischemic heart disease.

Kidd blood group (kid blud grōōp) The red blood cell antigens, specified by the Jk gene, that react with the antibodies designated anti-Jk^a and anti-Jk^b; named after a Mrs. Kidd, in whose blood the antibodies were discovered.

kidney (kid′ne) One of two bean-shaped organs located in the posterior part of the abdomen, behind the peritoneum, on either side of the spine; it serves to filter the blood, regulate acid-base concentration and water balance in the tissues, and discharge metabolic wastes as urine.

artificial k. See hemodialyzer.

Ask-Upmark k. An anomalous kidney that failed to develop fully, with deep transverse grooving on its superficial layer and a decreased number of renal lobes and pyramids (six or less); may be the result of reflux nephropathy early in life.

contracted k. A small scarred kidney due to abnormally large amounts of fibrous tissue.

crush k. Degeneration of renal tubule epithelium following crushing injuries of muscle.

ectopic k. A permanently abnormally placed kidney; distinguished from a floating kidney.

floating k. The excessively mobile kidney in nephroptosia; distinguished from ectopic kidney. Also called movable kidney; wandering kidney.

Goldblatt k. Kidney with impaired arterial blood supply, causing arterial hypertension.

horseshoe k. Kidney resulting from the fusion of the lower extremities of the two kidneys across the body midline.

medullary sponge k. Congenital defect marked by cyst formation of the pyramids of the kidney, occasionally associated with dilatation of the collecting tubules and formation of stones; often asymptomatic and not generally a cause of renal failure. See also cystic disease of renal medulla.

movable k. See floating kidney.

polycystic k. A kidney whose substance has been largely replaced by tightly packed cysts of varying sizes resembling a bunch of grapes. See also polycystic kidney disease.

wandering k. See floating kidney.

Kikuchi's disease (kĭ-kōō′chĭz dĭ-zēz′) Disease of unknown cause, chiefly affecting young women; marked by unilateral, usually painless, enlargement of lymph nodes in the neck. Also called histiocytic necrotizing lymphadenitis.

kilobase (kil′o-bās) (kb) One thousand base pairs in a DNA sequence.

kilocalorie (kil′o-kal-o-re) (Kcal) See large calorie, under calorie.

kilocycle (kil′o-si-kl) A thousand cycles per second.

kilogauss (kil′o-gows) (Kg) In magnetic resonance imaging (MRI), the unit of magnetic field strength equal to 103 gauss.

kilogram (kil′o-gram) (kg) One thousand grams,

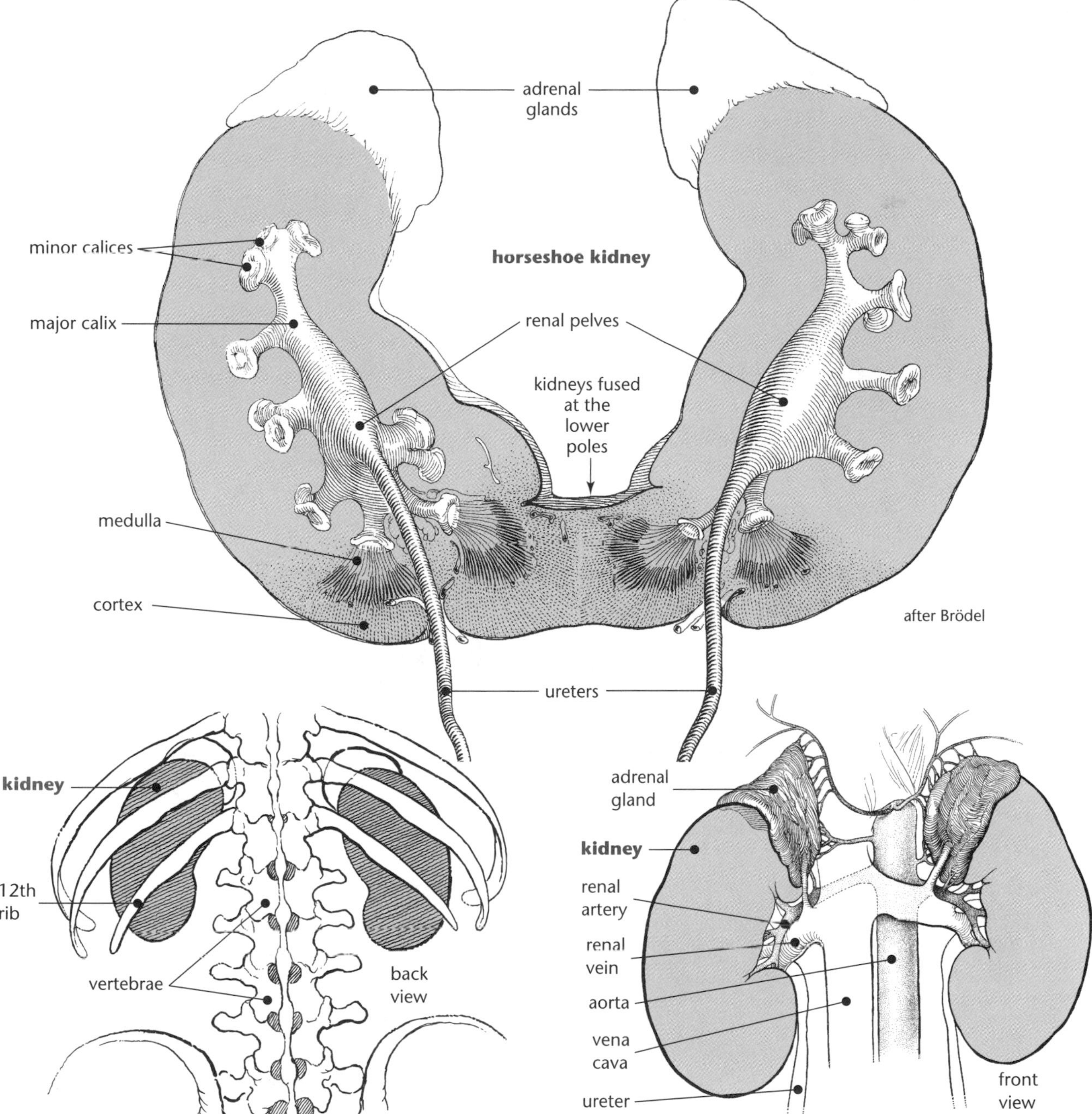

K

or 2.2046 pounds.

kilovolt (kil´o-vōlt) (kv) A thousand volts.

Kimmelstiel-Wilson disease (kim´ĕl-stēl-wil´sŏn dĭ-zēz´) See Kimmelstiel-Wilson syndrome.

Kimmelstiel-Wilson syndrome (kim´ĕl-stēl-wil´son sin´drōm) Disorder occurring in patients with diabetes mellitus of several years' duration, marked by hypertension, edema, and proteinuria associated with intercapillary glomerulosclerosis. Also called Kimmelstiel-Wilson disease.

kinanesthesia (kin-an-es-the´zhă) Loss of ability to perceive sensation of movement.

kinase (ki´nās) An enzyme that activates pro-enzymes or zymogens (inactive enzymes).

kindling (kind´ling) A phenomenon of the central nervous system characterized by the enduring reduction in threshhold needed to activate a repeated stimulus. Posttraumatic stress disorder is a clinical example of this phenomenon.

kindred (kin´drid) An extended group of genetically related persons. Distinguished from pedigree. Also called family group; clan; tribe.

degree of k. The level of kindred between two members of a family group; *first degree* (sibs, parent and child); *second degree* (aunts, uncles, nephews); etc.

kinematics (kin-ĕ-mat´iks) The science of motion, particularly of the body parts, exclusive of the influences of mass or force.

kinesalgia (kin-ĕ-sal´jă) Pain brought on by muscular movement.

kinescope (kin´ĕ-skōp) Instrument for testing the refraction of the eye; consisting of a disk with a slit, moved across the front of the eye, through which the patient observes a fixed object.

kinesia (ki-ne´zhă) Motion sickness.

kinesiatrics (ki-ne-se-at´riks) See kinesitherapy.

kinesics (ki-ne´siks) The study of nonverbal body motion as a form of communication, as in shrugs, waves, crossing of arms.

kinesin (ki-ne´sin) A mechanochemical, cytoplasmic protein that converts the chemical energy of adenosine triphosphate (ATP) into mechanical force for movement of cellular components along microtubules; it may function in organelle transport, endoplasmic reticulum extension, and mitosis.

kinesiology (ki-ne-se-ol´ŏ-je) The study of muscular movement as it applies to treatment.

kinesis (ki-ne´sis) Motion.

kinesitherapy (ki-ne-sĭ-ther´ă-pe) Treatment employing movement, exercise, or massage as the mode of therapy. Also called kinethiatrics.

kinesthesia (kin-es-the´zhă) The perception of one's own muscular movement and position of the body.

kinetic (kĭ-net´ik) Relating to or produced by motion.

kinetics (kĭ-net´iks) The study of all aspects of motion and forces affecting motion.

chemical k. The study of the rate and velocity of chemical reactions.

first-order k. The kinetics characteristic of a reaction whose rate of movement is proportional to the concentration of a single substance.

zero-order k. The kinetics characteristic of a reaction that proceeds at a constant rate regardless of the concentrations of reactants.

kinetocardiogram (kĭ-ne-to-kăr´de-o-gram) Graphic representation of chest wall vibrations caused by heart activity.

kinetochore (ki-ne´to-kōr) See centromere.

kinetoplasm (ki-ne´to-plaz-m) **1.** The chromophil substance of nerve cells. **2.** The most contractile portion of a cell.

kinetoplast (ki-ne´to-plast) A rod-shaped structure, located at the base of the flagellum of parasitic flagellates; it divides independently prior to the division of the nucleus.

kinin (ki´nin) Any of various small peptides with proinflammatory properties (e.g., increasing blood flow or permeability of blood vessels); they are usually breakdown products of larger precursor molecules (kininogens), which do not have proinflammatory properties in their intact state.

kink (kink´) **1.** A bend. **2.** A muscle spasm, usually painful.

kissing disease (kis´ing dĭ-zēz´) See infectious mononucleosis, under mononucleosis.

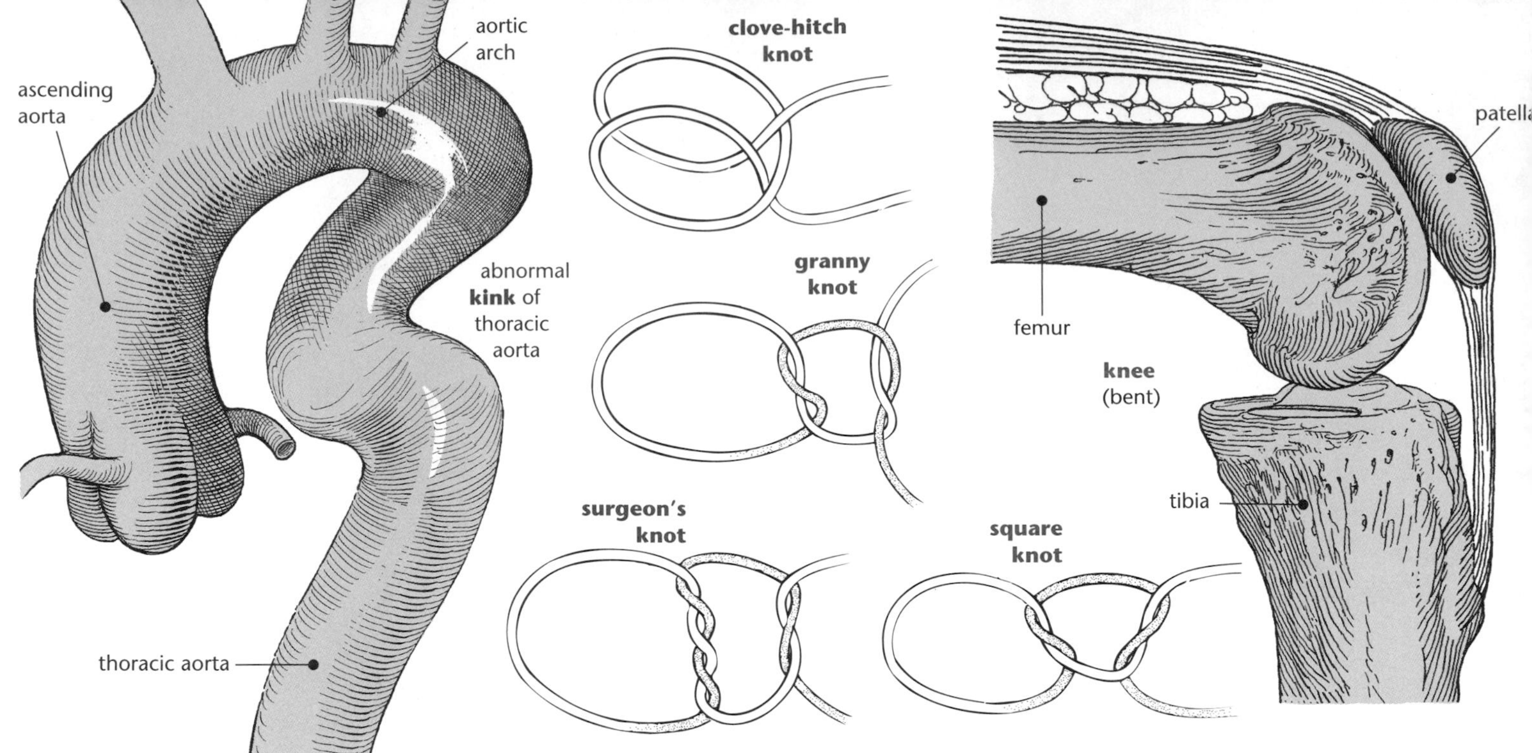

K

Klebsiella (kleb-se-el′ă) A genus of coliform bacteria (family Enterobacteriaceae), composed of motile and nonmotile gram-negative microorga-nisms.
K. pneumoniae The causative agent of Friedländer's pneumonia; normally found in the nose, mouth, and intestinal tract of healthy persons; it causes less than 10 percent of all acute bacterial pneumonias and is frequently present as a secondary invader in the lungs of individuals with chronic pulmonary diseases. Also called Friedländer's bacillus.
K. rhinoscleromatis A species causing rhinoscleroma.
kleptomania (klep-to-ma′ne-ă) A morbid compulsion to steal.
Klinefelter's syndrome (klīn′fel-terz sin′drōm) Genetic disease of males, usually characterized by abnormally long legs, extremely small testes, enlarged breasts, eunuchoid body, lack of sperm production, and a general deficiency of secondary male features (e.g., deep voice, beard); syndrome exhibits a classic pattern of 47 XXY karyotype (an extra X chromosome). Also called XXY syndrome; seminiferous tubule dysgenesis.
Klippel-Feil syndrome (klĭ-pel′fīl sin′drōm) Congenital defect marked primarily by fusion of one or more cervical vertebrae (at the neck), resulting in a characteristic short, thick neck with limited movements. Also called cervical fusion syndrome.
knee (ne) The articulation between the femur and the tibia.
housemaid's k. Inflammation of the bursa in front of the patella (kneecap), usually due to repeated trauma. Also called prepatellar bursitis.
jumper's k. Inflammation of the patellar or quadriceps tendons, causing discomfort, tenderness, or pain, especially at the tendon-kneecap attachment; may occur in athletes after jumping, kicking, climbing, or running.
knock k. See genu valgum.
locked k. Limited motion of the knee due to the presence of loose tissue, such as cartilage, in the joint.
runner's k. Pain or discomfort around the kneecap (patella); seen most commonly (not exclusively) in recreational joggers and long distance runners; may occur also when sitting with the knee flexed for long periods, or when walking up or down stairs.
kneecap (ne′kap) See patella.
knife (nīf) A cutting instrument.
Bard-Parker k. A surgical knife with a disposable blade.
Blair k. A knife with a long sharp blade used to cut skin grafts.
Buck k. A periodontal knife with a spearlike point, used for incising the gums between the teeth.
cautery k. A knife connected to an electric battery that sears tissue while cutting, to control bleeding.
chemical k. See reactive endonuclease, under endonuclease.
gamma ray k. A beam of high energy gamma rays; used in radiation therapy.
Merrifield k. A gingivectomy knife with a long, narrow, triangular blade.
needle k. A fine pointed knife used in surgical procedures of the eye. Also called discission needle.
knitting (nit′ing) The union or growing together of the fragments of a broken bone.
knob (nob) A protuberance; a nodule.
knock (nok) A sharp short sound.
pericardial k. Heart sound occurring early during diastole, after the second heart sound but earlier than the normal physiologic third sound; common in patients with constrictive pericarditis. Also called early diastolic sound; third heart sound of constrictive pericarditis.
knot (not) **1.** An intertwining of the ends of one or two cords, tapes, sutures, etc., so that they cannot be separated. **2.** A node or circumscribed swelling. **3.** To join the ends.
clove-hitch k. A knot made with two continuous loops around a part.
flat k. See square knot.
granny k. An insecure double knot in which the two stretches of cord do not pass together under the loop but are separated by it.
net k. See karyosome.
primitive k. See primitive node, under node.
reef k. See square knot.
square k. A double knot in which the free ends are parallel to the standing ends of the first knot. Also called flat knot; reef knot.
surgeon's k. Knot in which the thread is passed twice through the loop of the first knot with a simple knot tied over the first.
knuckle (nuk′īl) The dorsal part or region around a joint of the finger, especially of the metacarpophalangeal joints of the flexed fingers.
koilocytosis (koi-lo-si-to′sis) A condition of superficial or intermediate squamous cells having a large perinuclear cavity ("halo") which is thought to be indicative of human papillomavirus infection.
koilonychia (koi-lo-nik′e-ă) A rarely seen symptom of iron deficiency anemia in which the nails are concave or spoon-shaped.
koilosternia (koi-lo-ster′ne-ă) See pectus excavatum, under pectus.
kola nut (ko′lă nut) The large caffeine-containing seed of the *Cola acuminata* tree; its extract is used in beverages.
Korsakoff's syndrome (kor′să-kofs sin′drōm) Severe impairment of recent memory and inability to learn new information, seen in disorders predominantly affecting the hippocampal-mammillary system in the brain, especially thiamine deficiency; confabulation is usually a prominent feature; often associated with Wernicke's disease and called by some the Wernicke-Korsakoff's syndrome. Also called Korsakoff's psychosis.
Krabbe's disease (kră′bez dĭ-zēz′) A disease of late infancy marked by progressive cerebral demyelination and large globoid phagocytic cells in the white matter of the brain and spinal cord; the development of the infant usually ceases; an autosomal recessive inheritance. Also called globoid cell leukodystrophy.
kraurosis vulvae (kraw-ro′sis vul′vă) See lichen sclerous, under lichen.
Krebs' cycle (krebz sī′kl) See tricarboxylic acid cycle, under cycle.
krypton (krip′ton) One of the inert gaseous elements found in the atmosphere; symbol Kr, atomic number 36, atomic weight 83.80.
krypton-85 (^{85}Kr) A radioactive form of krypton used as a tracer (e.g., in studies of regional blood flow).
Kufs' disease (koofs dĭ-zēz′) See cerebral sphingolipidosis, under sphingolipidosis.
kuru (koo′roo) A progressive dementing illness seen in certain natives of New Guinea; related to cannibalism; caused by a prion. Initial symptoms of headache progress to ataxia, dysarthria, tremors, and dementia.
Kussmaul's sign (koos′moulz sīn) Great increase in jugular venous distention and pressure during inspiration; seen in patients with cardiac tamponade.
kwashiorkor (kwash-e-or′kor) A nutritional deficiency syndrome of children due to inadequate intake of proteins relative to the caloric intake; marked by edema, apathy, anorexia, diarrhea, and skin lesions with characteristically low serum protein, especially albumin.
kymograph (ki′mo-graf) An instrument for graphically recording pressure variations.
kymoscope (ki′mo-skōp) Apparatus for measuring pulse waves or the variations in blood pressure.
kynurenic acid (kin-u-ren′ik as′id) A crystalline compound; product of trypotophan metabolism.
kyphos (ki′fos) Greek for hump.
kyphoscoliosis (ki-fo-sko-le-o′sis) Abnormal backward and lateral curvature of the spine; it not only deforms but progressively disables, impairing first lung function and then heart function.
kyphosis (ki-fo′sis) Abnormal backward increase in the curvature of the thoracic spine; may be caused by a variety of spinal disorders.
kyrtorrhachic (kir-to-rak′ik) Relating to curvature of the lumbar spine with the concavity backward.

L

λ (lam´dă) The eleventh letter of the Greek alphabet, lambda.

L+ The lethal plus dose; symbol for a toxin-antitoxin mixture of diphtheria containing a fatal dose in excess, which will kill an experimental animal in four days.

la belle indifference (lă bel an-dif-er-ahns´) French term meaning a constant unjustified state of complacency and indifference, often seen in patients with conversion hysteria.

labia (la´be-ă) Plural of labium.

labial (la´be-al) Relating to lips.

labile (la´bīl) **1.** Unstable or easily changed, as drugs or preparations that are readily altered when exposed to heat. **2.** In psychiatry, emotionally unstable.

lability (lă-bil´ĭ-te) Instability or the condition of being changeable.

labiochorea (la-be-o-ko-re´ă) Spasm and stiffening of the lips during speech.

labiogingival (la-be-o-jin´jĭ-val) Relating to the area of junction of the lips and the gums.

labiograph (la´be-o-graf) Device used to record the movements of the lips in speaking.

labiomental (la-be-o-men´tal) Relating to the lower lip and the chin.

labionasal (la-be-o-na´zal) Relating to the lips and nose.

labioplacement (la-be-o-plās´ment) The abnormal position of a tooth toward the lips.

labioplasty (la´be-o-plas-te) Plastic surgery of the lips. Also called cheiloplasty.

labioversion (la-be-o-ver´zhun) Deviation of teeth toward the lips.

labium (la´be-um), *pl.* **la´bia** A lip or liplike structure.

l. anterius The anterior portion of the uterine cervix; it is shorter and thicker than the posterior portion. Also called anterior lip. See also labia uteri.

l. majus, *pl.* **labia majora** The two mounds of tissue forming the lateral boundaries of the vulva. Embryologically, they correspond to the scrotum of the male. Commonly called major lips.

l. minus, *pl.* **labia minora** The two narrow folds between the labia majora, on either side of the urethral and vaginal openings. Anteriorly, each labium minus splits into two layers; the upper layers meet over the free end of the clitoris (forming the prepuce of the clitoris), the lower ones meet under the clitoris (forming the frenulum of the clitoris). Also called lesser lips of pudendum; nymphae; commonly called minor lips.

l. posterius The posterior portion of the uterine cervix; it is longer and thinner than the anterior portion. Also called posterior lip. See also labia uteri.

labia uteri The anterior and posterior margins of the uterine cervix surrounding its vaginal opening (external os); most prominently seen in women who have borne children, in whom the originally round opening becomes a transverse slit. See labium anterius; labium posterius.

labor (la´bor) The coordinated sequence of involuntary contractions of the uterus that increase in regularity, intensity, and duration, resulting in effacement and dilatation of the cervix and voluntary bearing-down efforts leading to expulsion of the fetus and placenta via the vagina. Also called true labor.

disordered l. General term for inefficient progress of labor occuring secondary to various factors (e.g., uterine hypofunction, effects of analgesia or anesthesia, fetopelvic disproportion).

dry l. Labor occurring after premature breaking of the amniotic sac and escape of most of the fluid that surrounds the fetus. Also called xerotocia.

false l. Irregular brief uterine contractions, typically with abdominal and/or back pain, occurring in late pregnancy; they are inconsistent in interval, duration, and strength and cause no cervical change. See also Braxton Hicks contractions, under contraction.

first stage of l. Interval between onset of labor to full dilatation of the cervix (10 cm).

induced l. Labor brought on by artificial means.

precipitate l. Labor of abnormally short duration, usually lasting three hours or less; frequently a result of abnormally low resistance of the maternal soft structures or abnormally strong contractions of the uterus and abdominal muscles.

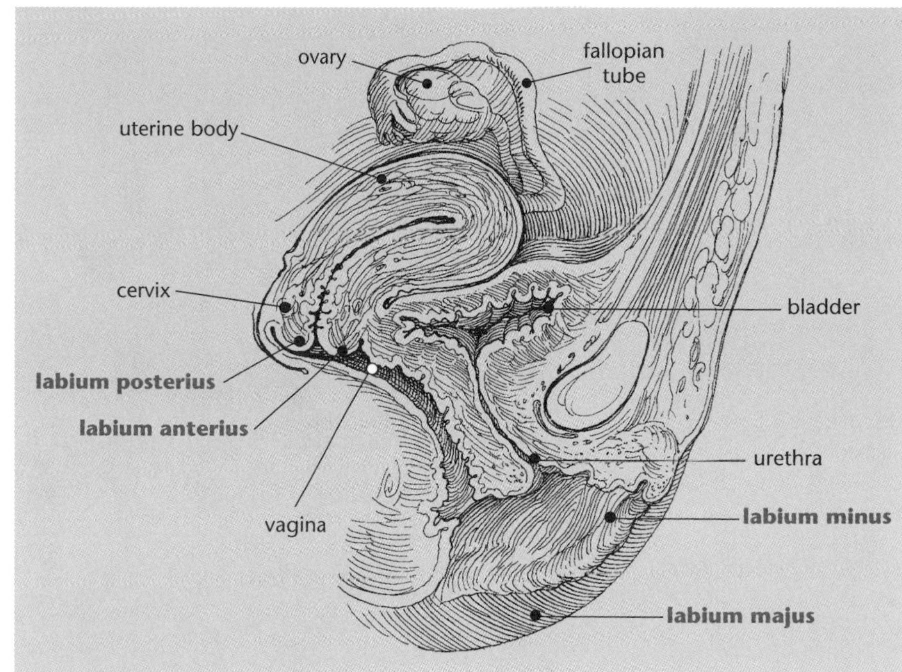

premature l. See preterm labor.

preterm l. Labor occurring after 20 but before 36 weeks of gestation. Also called premature labor.

prolonged l. Labor lasting longer than 18 hours.

second stage of l. Stage of childbirth beginning with complete dilatation of the cervix and ending with delivery of the baby.

third stage of l., placental stage of l. Interval between delivery of the infant through delivery of the placenta.

laboratory (lab´ră-tor-e) **1.** A room or building equipped with scientific equipment for conducting experiments, tests, etc. **2.** A place used for the manufacture of drugs and chemicals.

labrum (la´brum), *pl.* **la´bra** A lip, edge, or liplike structure.

labyrinth (lab´ĭ-rinth) **1.** A group of intercommunicating canals. **2.** Inner ear.

bony l. A series of cavities in the petrous portion of the temporal bone that houses the membranous labyrinth. Also called osseous labyrinth.

ethmoidal l. The labyrinth in the lateral part of the ethmoid bone consisting of thin-walled cavities or cells. Also called ectethmoid.

membranous l. A system of communicating membranous canals, lying within the bony labyrinth of the inner ear.

osseous l. See bony labyrinth.

labyrinthine (lab-ĭ-rin´thēn) Relating to a labyrinth, especially of the inner ear.

labyrinthitis (lab-ĭ-rin-thi´tis) Inflammation of the labyrinth of the inner ear. Also called otitis interna.

labyrinthotomy (lab-ĭ-rin-thot´ŏ-me) Incision into the labyrinth of the inner ear.

lac (lak), *pl.* **lac´ta** Any whitish, milky fluid.

laceration (las-er-a´shun) A wound made by tearing of the tissue.

lacinia (la-sin´e-ă) Fringe; fimbria.

lacrimal (lak´rĭ-mal) Relating to tears.

lacrimation (lak-rĭ-ma´shun) The secretion, especially excessive, of tears.

lacrimatory (lak´rĭ-mă-tor-e) Causing discharge of tears.

lacrimotomy (lak-rĭ-mot´ŏ-me) The operation of incising the lacrimal sac or duct.

lactacidemia (lak-tas-ĭ-de´me-ă) See lacticacidemia.

lactalbumin (lak-tal-bu´min) An albumin of milk.

lactase (lak´tās) An intestinal enzyme that catalyzes the conversion of lactose to glucose and galactose; a sugar-splitting enzyme; a deficiency of lactase may lead to gastrointestinal symptoms such as bloating, flatulence, and diarrhea following ingestion of milk or milk products.

lactate (lak´tāt) **1.** To secrete milk. **2.** Any salt or ester of lactic acid.

l. dehydrogenase (LDH) See lactic acid dehydrogenase.

lactation (lak-ta´shun) The production of milk.

lacteal (lak´te-al) **1.** A lymph vessel that conveys chyle from the small intestine. **2.** Relating to milk.

lactescent (lak-tes´ens) **1.** Milky. **2.** Producing a milky fluid, as certain plants and insects.

lactic (lak´tik) Relating to milk.

lactic acid (lak´tik ăs´id) A colorless syrupy substance formed by the fermentation of milk sugar (lactose); an end product of anaerobic glycolysis in the body.

lactic acid dehydrogenase (lak´tik ăs´id de-hi-droj´en-ās) (LDH) An enzyme that may be measured in serum for diagnosis of some diseases (e.g., acute myocardial infarction, liver disease). Also called lactate dehydrogenase.

lacticacidemia (lak-tik-as-ĭ-de´me-ă) The presence of lactic acid in the circulating blood. Also called lactacidemia.

lactiferous (lak-tif´er-us) Secreting or conveying milk.

lactifugal (lak-tĭ-fūj´al) See galactophygous.

lactifuge (lak´tĭ-fūj) An agent that arrests the secretion of milk.

lactigenous (lak-tij´ĕ-nus) Producing milk.

lactin (lak´tin) Lactose.

lactinated (lak´tĭ-nāt-ed) Containing lactose.

Lactobacillus (lak-to-bă-sil´us) (L) A genus of rod-shaped, non-motile microorganisms (family Lactobacillacea) that produce lactic acid in the fermentation of carbohydrates, especially in milk.

L. acidophilus A species found in the feces of milk-fed infants and individuals on a diet with a high content of milk, lactose, or dextrin.

lactobezoar (lak-to-be´zor) A coagulum in the stomach formed by the prolonged ingestion of powdered milk which is mixed with an insufficient amount of water.

lactocele (lak´to-sēl) See milk retention cyst, under cyst.

lactoflavin (lak-to-fla´vin) The original name of riboflavin.

lactogen (lak´to-jen) Any agent that stimulates the production of milk.

human placental l. (HPL; hPL) A polypeptide hormone appearing in the serum of pregnant women at about the sixth week of gestation and rising steadily thereafter; it disappears from the blood immediately after delivery; it is produced by the syncytiotrophoblast (in placenta) and is intimately involved in carbohydrate metabolism of both mother and fetus. Also called human chorionic somatomammotropin; chorionic growth hormone.

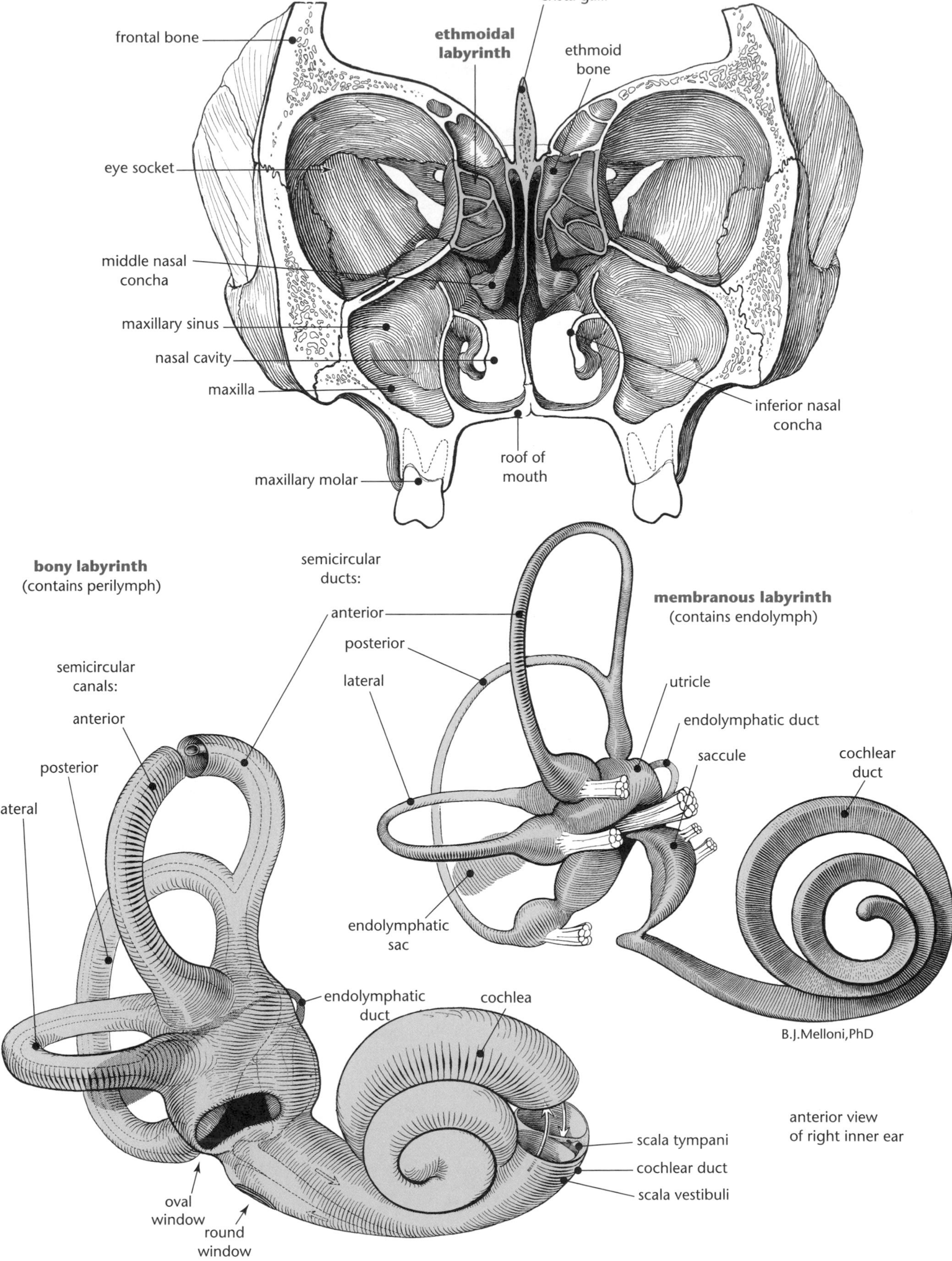

crista galli
frontal bone
ethmoidal labyrinth
ethmoid bone
eye socket
middle nasal concha
maxillary sinus
nasal cavity
maxilla
inferior nasal concha
roof of mouth
maxillary molar
L
bony labyrinth
(contains perilymph)
semicircular ducts:
anterior
posterior
lateral
membranous labyrinth
(contains endolymph)
semicircular canals:
anterior
posterior
lateral
utricle
endolymphatic duct
saccule
cochlear duct
endolymphatic sac
endolymphatic duct
cochlea
B.J.Melloni,PhD
anterior view of right inner ear
scala tympani
cochlear duct
scala vestibuli
oval window
round window

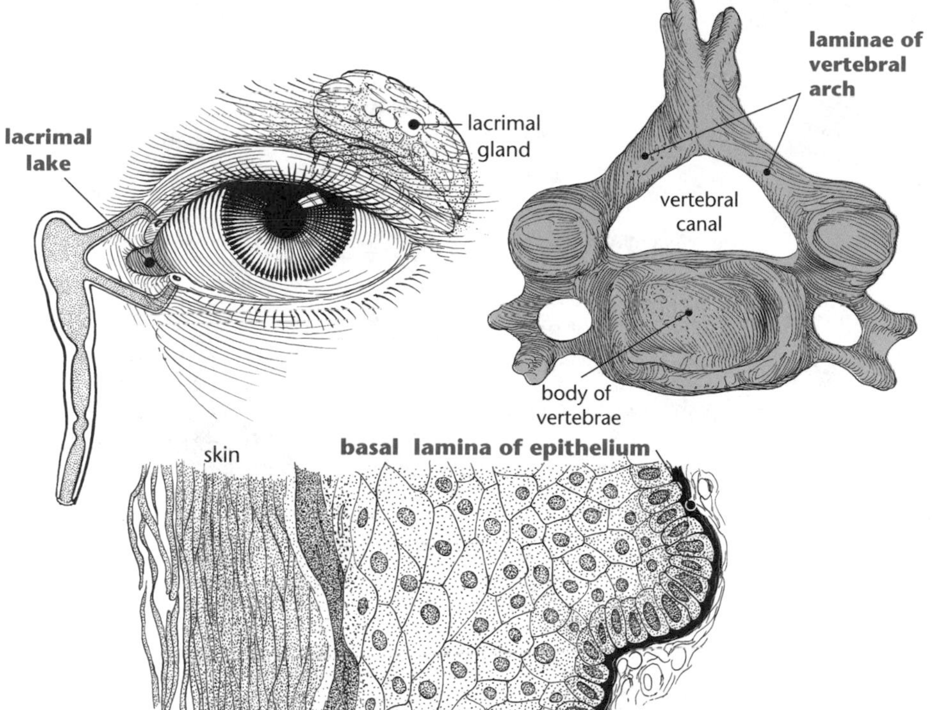

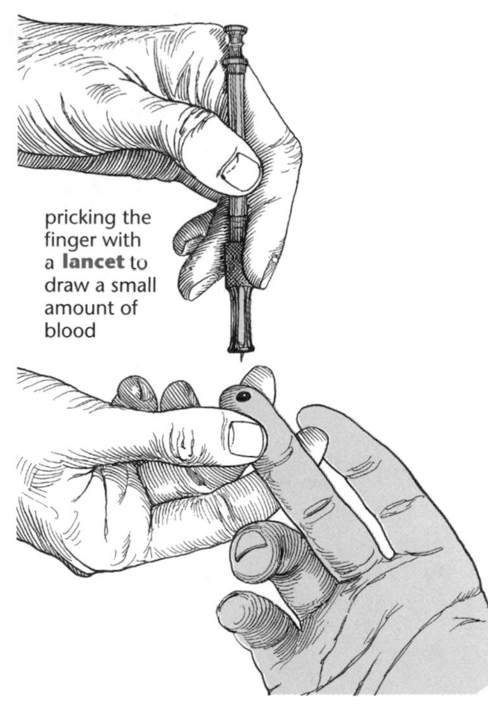

lactogenic (lak-to-jen´ik) Inducing milk production.
lactoglobulin (lak-to-glob´u-lin) A simple protein found in milk.
lactone (lak´tōn) A salt of a hydroxyl acid, formed by the removal of water from the acid.
lactoprotein (lak-to-pro´tēn) Protein normally present in milk.
lactorrhea (lak-to-re´ă) See galactorrhea.
lactose (lak´tōs) A sugar formed by the mammary glands and constituting about 5% of cow's milk; it yields glucose and galactose on hydrolysis. Also called milk sugar.
lactosuria (lak-to-su´re-ă) The presence of lactose in the urine; occurring sometimes in premature newborn infants.
lactovegetarian (lak-to-vej-ĕ-tār´e-an) One who lives on a diet of vegetables, milk, and milk products.
lactulose (lak´tū-lōs) Compound used to treat constipation.
lacuna (lă-ku´nă), *pl.* **lacu´nae** **1.** A small anatomic cavity or depression. **2.** A defect or gap.
Howship's l. See resorption lacuna.
resorption l. A depression in bone caused by resorption of bone tissue by osteocytes. Also called Howship's lacuna.
Laënnec's cirrhosis (la-en-neks´ sĭ-ro´sis) See alcoholic cirrhosis, under cirrhosis.
lag (lag) **1.** A slowness. **2.** The time interval between a change and its effect (e.g., of a stimulus or action).
lid l. See Graefe's sign.
lagophthalmos, lagophthalmia (lag-of-thal´mos, lag-of-thal´me-ă) Condition in which the eyelids cannot be closed completely.
lake (lāk) **1.** A small accumulation of fluid. **2.** To cause blood plasma to become red as a result of the release of hemoglobin from the erythrocytes.
lacrimal l. The area of the conjunctiva, between the medial margins of the eyelids at the inner angle, in which the tears collect after bathing the anterior surface of the eyeball; the caruncle lies on its floor.
lalling (lal´ing) Infantile speech; babbling.
lalopathy (lă-lop´ă-the) Any speech defect (seldom used term).
laloplegia (lal-o-ple´jă) Paralysis of muscles involved in the production of speech.
lambda (lam´dă) (λ) A craniometric point at the junction of the sagittal and lambdoid sutures.
lambdoid (lam´doid) Resembling the shape of the Greek letter lambda (λ); denoting the deeply serrated suture in the skull between the occipital bone and the two parietal bones.
lambert (lam´bert) (L) Unit of brightness, equal to the uniform brightness of a perfectly diffusing surface emitting or reflecting light at the rate of 1 lumen per square centimeter.
lamella (lă-mel´ă), *pl.* **lamel´lae** **1.** A thin layer or plate, as of bone. **2.** A medicated gelatin disk, used under the eyelid in place of solutions.
lamellar (lă-mel´ar) **1.** Scaly. **2.** Relating to lamellae.
lamina (lam´ĭ-nă), *pl.* **lam´inae** A thin layer of flat plate, as of muscle or bone.
basal l. of choroid The transparent, inner layer of the choroid in contact with the pigmented layer of the retina. Also called Bruch's membrane; lamina vitrea.
basal l. of epithelium A relatively thin layer, about 300 to 1,200 Å in thickness, composed of slender filamentous material enmeshed in a mucopolysaccharide matrix; it occurs at the base of epithelial cells where it blends with the reticular lamina to form the basement membrane.
basement l. See basement membrane, under membrane.
choriocapillary l. The layer of the choroid between the basal lamina and the vascular lamina. Also called choriocapillary layer.
l. cribrosa sclerae The sievelike portion of the sclera through the holes of which pass the fibers of the optic nerve. Also called perforated layer of sclera.
external cranial l. The outer plate of the flat bones of the skull.
l. fusca sclerae A layer consisting of a delicate mesh of elastic fibers connecting the sclera and choroid.
internal cranial l. The inner plate of the flat bones of the skull.
lateral l. of pterygoid plate See lateral pterygoid plate, under plate.
medial l. of pterygoid plate See medial pterygoid plate, under plate.
reticular l. A relatively thin layer of reticular and collagenous fibers embedded in a mucopolysaccharide matrix; together with the basal lamina of epithelium, it makes up the basement membrane which holds the basal cells of the epithelium firmly to the underlying connective tissue; it also encloses fat cells, muscle cells, and Schwann cells of peripheral nerves.
spiral l. A double plate of bone spiraling around the modiolus of the inner ear, dividing the spiral canal of the cochlea into the scala tympani and the scala vestibuli.
suprachoroidal l. A layer of loose connective tissue forming the external layer of the choroid.
vascular l. of choroid The layer of the choroid between the suprachoroid and choriocapillary, containing the largest choroidal blood vessels.
laminae of vertebral arch Two broad plates directed dorsally and medially from the pedicles of a vertebra; their posterior midline fusion forms the vertebral arch.
l. vitrea See basal lamina of choroid.
laminar (lam´ĭ-nar) **1.** Arranged in layers. **2.** Relating to a bony plate.
Laminaria digitata (lam-ĭ-na´re-ă dij-ĭ-tă´tă) A species of seaweed from which tents are made by drying and sterilizing the stems; the dry stem is capable of expanding to about five times its original diameter; used for atraumatic dilatation of the uterine cervix (e.g., as a preoperative procedure in abortion and prior to induction of labor at or near term). See also laminaria tent, under tent.
lamination (lam-ĭ-na´shun) An arrangement in layers.
laminectomy (lam-ĭ-nek´tŏ-me) Surgical removal of the posterior arch of a vertebra.
laminin (lam´ĭ-nin) A polypeptide glycoprotein with adhesive properties; a component of basement membrane that plays a role in the attachment of epithelial cells to underlying connective tissue.
laminotomy (lam-ĭ-not´ŏ-me) The surgical division of the lamina of a vertebra.
lamp (lamp) Any device for producing light, heat, or therapeutic radiation.
annealing l. An alcohol lamp with a soot-free flame used for heating and purifying gold leaf intended as a filling for tooth cavities.
argon l. A lamp radiating chiefly in the near ultraviolet area around 360 nm; used chiefly in conjunction with fluorescein in fitting of contact lenses.
Eldridge-Green l. A color perception test lamp containing a single light with color filters mounted in rotating disks.
Kromayer's l. A U-shaped quartz lamp of mercury vapor that generates ultraviolet rays.
mignon l. A small electric lamp used in the cystoscope.
slit-l. See slitlamp.
ultraviolet l. Lamp that emits rays in the ultraviolet band of the spectrum.
uviol l. An electric lamp with a globe of uviol glass producing light with a high content of ultraviolet rays; used in phototherapy.
lanatoside A, B, C (lă-nat´o-sīd ā, bē, sē) Digilanid A, B, and C, the three natural glycosides of *Digitalis lanata*.
lance (lans) To cut into a part, as into a boil.
lancet (lan´set) A small, pointed, double-edged surgical knife.
lancinating (lan´sĭ-nāt-ing) Denoting a piercing or cutting pain.
Landry's paralysis (lah-drēz´ pă-ral´ĭ-sis) See acute ascending paralysis, under paralysis.
language (lang´gwĭj) The use of vocal sounds in articulate, meaningful patterns, as a form of communication.
body l. Expression of thoughts and feelings by

L

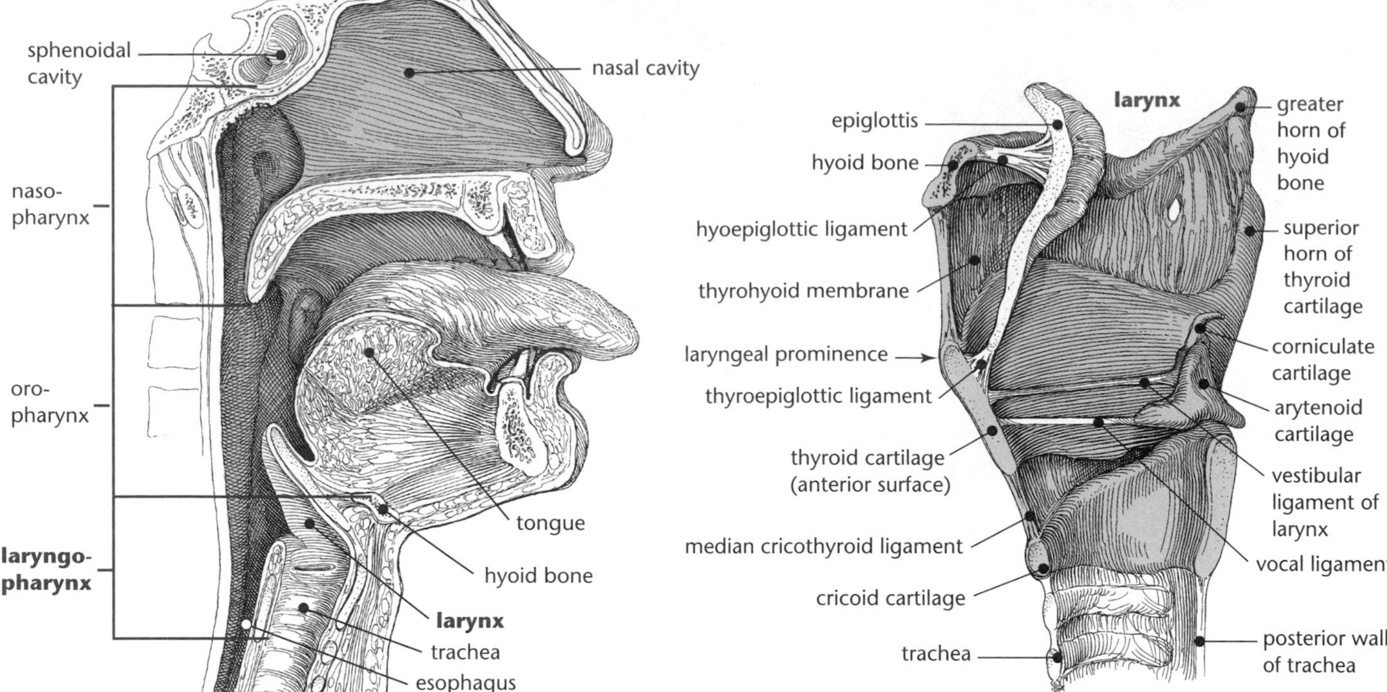

means of bodily movements.

lanolin (lan´o-lin) Fat obtained from sheep's wool; used in the preparation of ointments.

anhydrous l. See wool fat.

lanthanum (lan´thă-num) Metallic rare earth element; symbol La, atomic number 57, atomic weight 138.92.

lanuginous (lă-noo´jĭ-nus) Covered with fine, soft, downlike hair (lanugo).

lanugo (la-noo´go) The fine soft hair covering the body of the newborn. Also called embryonic hair; primary hair.

laparohysterectomy (lap-ă-ro-his-ter-ek´tŏ-me) Removal of the uterus through an incision of the abdominal wall.

laparohysterotomy (lap-ă-ro-his-ter-ot´ŏ-me) Incision of the uterus through an incision of the abdominal wall.

laparoscope (lap´ă-ro-skōp) Instrument for visualizing the peritoneal cavity. Also called peritoneoscope.

laparoscopy (lap-ă-ros´kŏ-pe) Visualization of the contents of the abdominal cavity by means of an endoscope. Also called celioscopy; peritoneal endoscopy; peritoneoscopy.

operative l. See laparoscopic surgery, under surgery.

laparotomy (lap-ă-rot´ŏ-me) Surgical incision into the flank or through any part of the abdominal wall. Also called celiotomy; abdominal section.

larva (lar´vă), *pl.* **lar´vae** The wormlike early stage in the development of certain animals, bearing little or no resemblance to the adult form.

larva migrans (lar´vă mī´granz) Larval worms existing for a period of time in the tissues of a host other than the one to which they are adapted.

cutaneous l. m. A subcutaneous creeping eruption of the skin caused by wandering larvae of *Ancylostoma braziliense* and other domestic animal hookworms; acquired through contact with soil containing contaminated dog or cat feces. Also called creeping eruption.

visceral l. m. Disease caused by the presence of larvae of *Toxocara canis* (intestinal parasite of dogs) that penetrate the intestinal wall and wander through organs, especially the liver; acquired through consumption of raw vegetables contaminated with eggs of the parasite.

larvicide (lar´vĭ-sīd) An agent destructive to larvae.

laryngeal (lă-rin´je-al) Relating to the larynx.

laryngectomee (lar-in-jek´tŏ-me) A person who has had the larynx removed.

laryngectomy (lar-in-jek´tŏ-me) Removal of the larynx.

laryngismus (lar-in-jiz´mus) Spasmodic contraction of the larynx.

l. stridulus A disease of children marked by sudden attacks of spasm of the larynx, lasting a few seconds, with a crowing noise on inspiration and cyanosis. Also called pseudocroup.

laryngitis (lar-in-ji´tis) Inflammation of the larynx.

acute l. Laryngitis caused by infection or by mechanical irritation; infectious forms are frequently associated with sore throat and cough; characterized by hoarseness that may progress to complete loss of voice.

atrophic l. A chronic form leading to atrophy of the glands of the mucous membrane, diminished secretions, and formation of crusts.

laryngocele (lă-ring´go-sēl) A congenital anomaly of the larynx; a sac formed by the outpocketing of the laryngeal mucosa reaching upward and outward between the true and false vocal cords.

laryngocentesis (lă-ring-go-sen-te´sis) A small surgical incision or puncture of the larynx.

laryngofissure (lă-ring-go-fish´ur) Surgical incision of the larynx, usually through the midline, for the removal of a tumor. Also called median laryngotomy.

laryngograph (lă-ring´go-graf) Instrument used to make tracings of the movements of the larynx.

laryngology (lar-ing-gol´ŏ-je) The study of the larynx and treatment of its diseases.

laryngoparalysis (lă-ring-go-pă-ral´ĭ-sis) Paralysis of the larynx.

laryngopharyngeal (lă-ring-go-fă-rin´je-al) Relating to both the larynx and pharynx.

laryngopharyngectomy (lă-ring-go-far-ĭn-jek´tŏ-me) Removal of the larynx and pharynx.

laryngopharynx (lă-ring-go-far´ĭnks) The lower portion of the pharynx from the hyoid bone to the esophagus, with which it is continuous. Also called pars laryngea pharyngis. See also pharynx.

laryngoplasty (lă-ring´go-plas-te) Reparative surgery of the larynx.

laryngoscope (lă-ring´gŏ-skōp) Any tubular instrument used in examining the interior of the larynx.

laryngoscopy (lar-ing-gos´kŏ-pe) Examination of the larynx with a laryngoscope.

indirect l. Examination of the larynx by an instrument giving a reflected view.

laryngospasm (lă-ring´go-spaz-m) A reflex contraction of the laryngeal muscles.

laryngostenosis (lă-ring-go-stě-no´sis) Stricture or narrowing of the larynx.

laryngostomy (lar-in-gos´tŏ-me) Creation of a permanent opening into the larynx.

laryngotome (lă-ring´go-tōm) Instrument used to make an incision into the larynx.

median l. See laryngofissure.

laryngotomy (lar-ing-got´ŏ-me) Surgical incision into the larynx.

laryngotracheobronchitis (lă-ring-go-tra-ke-o-brong-ki´tis) Acute inflammation of the upper respiratory passages, occurring as a primary infection or attending a systemic disease (e.g., diphtheria, whooping cough).

larynx (lar´inks) The organ of voice production, located at the upper end of the trachea; it is composed of a cartilaginous and muscular frame, lined with mucous membrane, and contains the vocal cords. Popularly called voice box.

Lasègue's sign (lah-segz´ sīn) Pain along the course of the sciatic nerve when the patient, lying on his back, flexes the thigh on his abdomen and then extends the leg at the knee; it indicates disease of the sciatic nerve.

laser (la´zer) Device that converts light of mixed frequencies into an intense narrow beam of nondivergent monochromatic light (electromagnetic radiation); used in surgical, diagnostic, and physiological procedures; the term is an acronym for light amplification by stimulated emission of radiation.

lassitude (las´i-tōōd) Weakness or weariness.

latah (lă´tă) Nervous disorder marked by imitative behavior and extreme response to suggestion.

latent (la´tent) Present but not manifest; concealed.

lateral (lat´er-al) Located on the side; farther from the middle.

laterality (lat-er-al´ĭ-te) A tendency to use either the right or the left parts of the body; right or left dominance of the cerebral cortex.

laterodeviation (lat-er-o-de-ve-a´shun) Displacement to one side.

lateroduction (lat-er-o-duk´shun) Movement to one side, as of a limb.

lateroflexion (lat-er-o-flek´shun) Bending to one side.

lateropulsion (lat-er-o-pul´shun) Involuntary movement toward one side, occurring in certain nervous disorders.

laterotorsion (lat-er-o-tor´shun) Rotation of the eye around its anteroposterior axis.

lateroversion (lat-ĕr-o-ver´shun) The displacement of an organ to one side.

lathyrism (lath´ĭ-riz-m) Disease due to poisoning with some species of peas of the genus *Lathyrus*; neurologic symptoms predominate.

Latin square (lat´n skwār) In statistics, a square design consisting of rows and columns; used to prevent or remove errors in an experiment (e.g., in experimental treatments).

latissimus (lă-tis´ĭ-mus) Broadest; widest.

Latrodectus (lat-ro-dek´tus) A genus of highly poisonous spiders.

L. mactans See black widow.

lattice (lat´is) A regular configuration of ions or

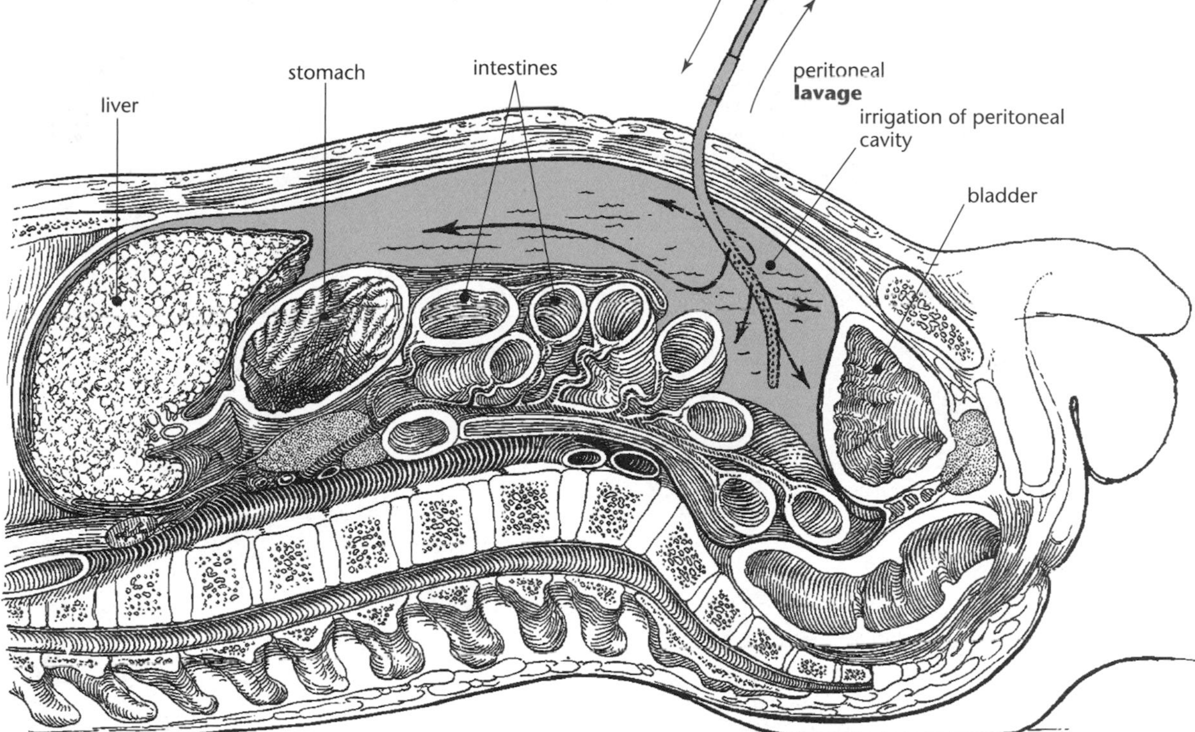

molecules in a definite geometric arrangement.

latus (la´tus), *pl.* **la´tera** The side of the body between the ribs and the pelvis; the flank.

laudanum (law´dă-num) A tincture of opium.

Laurence-Moon-Biedl syndrome (law´rens-mo͞on-be´dil sin´drōm) A recessive hereditary disorder marked by some or all of the following: mental retardation, obesity, polydactyly, hypogonadism, and visual disturbances (retinitis pigmentosa). Also called Laurence-Biedl syndrome; Laurence-Moon-Biedl-Bardet syndrome.

lauric acid (law´rik as´id) A fatty acid present in milk and especially in coconut oil. Also called dodecanoic acid.

Lauth's violet (lawths vi´o-lit) See thionin.

lavage (lă-vahzh´) The washing out of a cavity or a hollow organ.

law (law) **1.** A principle, rule, or formula expressing a fact based on observed recurrence, order, relationship, or interactions of natural processes or actions. **2.** A generalization based on the repetition of events.

all-or-none l. See Bowditch's law.

Arrhenius' l. Only those solutions which have high osmotic pressures are electrically conductive.

Avogadro's l. Equal volumes of gases contain equal numbers of molecules (pressure and temperature being the same).

Beer's l. The intensity of a light ray is inversely proportional to the depth of liquid through which it is transmitted (the absorption is dependent upon the number of molecules in the ray's path).

Bowditch's l. The heart muscle will contract to the fullest extent, even if the stimulus is weak, or it will not contract at all. Also called all-or-none law; all-or-none.

Boyle's l. At a fixed temperature, the volume of confined gas varies inversely with the pressure upon it.

Charles' l. All gases expand and contract equally on heating and cooling. Also called Gay-Lussac law.

Courvoisier's l. If the gallbladder is enlarged, obstruction is usually due to causes other than gallstones, such as carcinoma of the head of the pancreas. When obstruction of the bile duct is caused by gallstones, the gallbladder is likely to be contracted due to scarring and inflammation. Also called Courvoisier's sign.

Dalton's l. Each gas in a mixture of gases exerts a pressure proportionate to the percentage of its volume in the mixture as if that were the only gas dissolved. Also called law of partial pressure.

Dalton-Henry l. In dissolving a mixture of gases, a fluid will absorb as much of each gas in the mixture as if that were the only gas dissolved.

Einthoven's l. In electrocardiography, the potential difference in lead II is equal to the sum of the potential differences of leads I and III. Also called Einthoven's equation.

Faraday's l.'s (a) In electrolysis, the amount of an ion liberated by an electric current is proportional to the strength of the current. (b) When the same current is passed through several electrolytes, the amounts of different substances decomposed are proportioned to their chemical equivalents.

Fick's l. of diffusion The direction of movement of a substance in solution is always from the highest to the lowest concentration, and the increase of its concentration is directly proportional to the change in the concentration gradient.

Galton's l. While offspring generally tend to resemble their parents, the offspring of parents of extreme types tend to regress toward the mean of the population. Also called law of regression.

Gay-Lussac l. See Charles' law.

l. of the heart See Starling's law.

Henry's l. The amount of gas that can be dissolved in a liquid solution is proportional to the partial pressure of the gas; when the pressure is doubled, twice as much gas passes into solution.

l. of independent assortment Mendel's second law.

inverse square l. A law which is especially applied to all point sources of radiation; the intensity of radiation is inversely proportional to the square of the distance.

Laplace's l. The relationship between transmural pressure difference (ΔP), wall tension (T), and diameter (D) related to surface tension in a concave surface: $\Delta P = (4\ T/D)$.

l. of mass action The speed of a chemical reaction is proportional to the active masses (molar concentration) of the reacting material.

Mendel's l.'s The principles of heredity summarized in two laws and expressed in modern times as: (a) First law or law of segregation: paired hereditary units (genes) in the offspring (one from each parent) do not mix or alter one another, therefore they are able to separate during the formation of sex cells (gametes) in meiosis and are transmitted independently from generation to generation. (b) Second law or law of independent assortment: the corresponding hereditary units in a pair of gametes unite in the offspring to form new combinations and recombinations according to the laws of chance, provided that the two pairs of genes do not lie on the same chromosome. Also called mendelian laws.

Mendeleeff's l. See periodic law.

mendelian l.'s See Mendel's laws.

Newton's l. All bodies attract each other with a force directly proportional to their masses and inversely proportional to the square of the distance between them. Also called law of universal gravitation.

Ohm's l. The electric current in a circuit is equal to the electromotive force divided by the resistance: amperes = volts/ohms.

l. of partial pressure See Dalton's law.

Pascal's l. Fluids at rest transmit pressure equally in every direction.

periodic l. The elements when arranged in the order of their atomic weights display a periodic variation of their properties; every element of the series is related in its properties to the eighth element before and after it. Also called Mendeleef's law.

Poiseuille's l. Speed of fluid flowing in a tube is proportional to the cross-sectional area of the tube.

l. of refraction For two given media, the sine of the angle of incidence is constantly related to the sine of the angle of refraction.

l. of regression See Galton's law.

l. of segregation Mendel's first law.

Sherrington's l. Every dorsal spinal nerve root supplies a special area of the skin (dermatome), although the area may be overlapped by fibers from adjacent spinal segments.

Starling's l. The energy liberated by the contracting heart muscle depends on the length of the muscle fibers at the end of diastole; within limits, the stroke volume of the heart is determined by the change in myocardial fiber length associated with ventricular filling in diastole. Also called law of the heart.

l. of universal gravitation See Newton's law.

van't Hoff's l.'s (a) In stereochemistry, all optically active substances form an unsymmetrical arrangement in space, owing to their having multivalent atoms united to four different atoms or radicals. (b) The osmotic pressure of a substance in a dilute solution is the same that the same substance would exert if present in the state of an ideal gas occupying the same volume as the solution. (c) The velocity of chemical reactions increases between twofold and threefold for each 10°C rise in temperature.

wallerian l. A nerve fiber loses its normal structure and function when continuity with its cell of origin is interrupted.

lawrencium (law-ren´se-um) Synthetic transuranic element; symbol Lw, atomic number 103, atomic weight 257.

laxative (lak´să-tiv) An agent that stimulates evacuation of a soft formed stool by increasing peristalsis or simply through hydration of the stool; distinguished from a cathartic, which produces a stronger effect.

layer (la´er) A sheetlike coating, or stratum, covering a surface. Also called stratum; lamina.

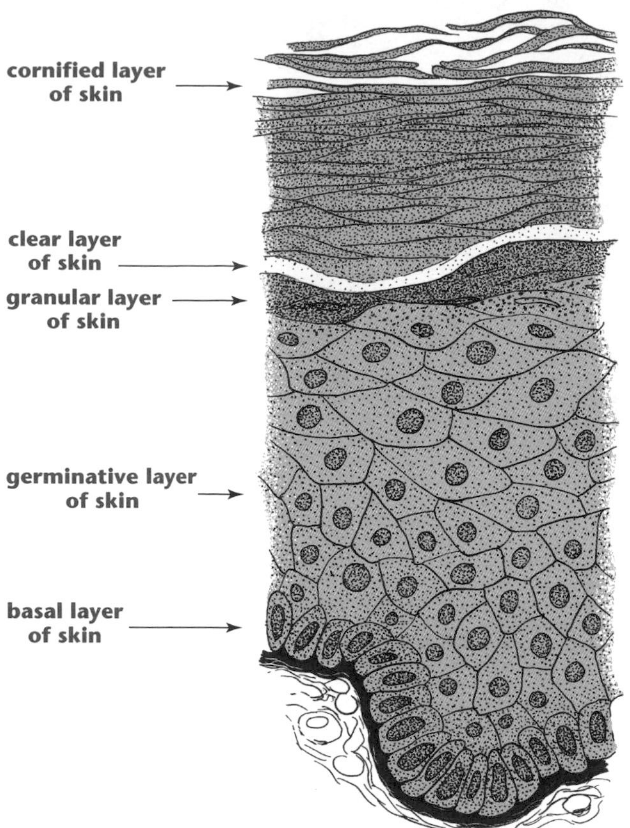

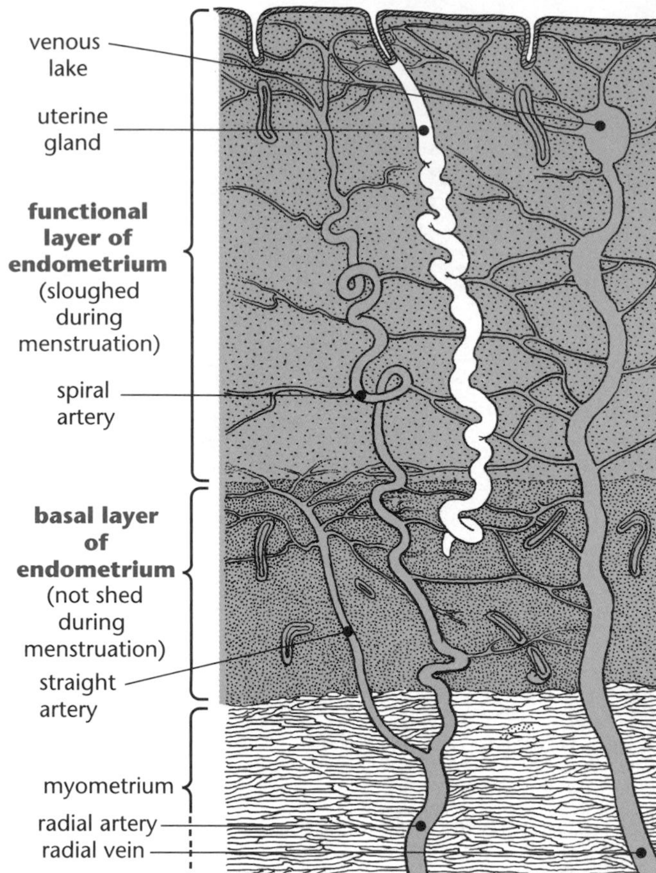

anterior elastic l. of cornea See Bowman's membrane, under membrane.
bacillary l. See layer of rods and cones.
basal l. of endometrium The deepest layer of the uterine mucosa (endometrium); it accommodates the blind ends of the tubelike uterine glands; it is not shed during menstruation or at parturition.
basal l. of epidermis See basal layer of skin.
basal l. of skin The single layer of the epidermis adjacent to the basement membrane, from which all other cells of the skin are derived by mitotic division of its cells. Also called basal layer of epidermis; malpighian layer.
l.'s of cerebellar cortex Three distinct layers of the cerebellar cortex that, from the surface inward, are: molecular layer, Purkinje cell layer, and granular layer; the granular layer is adjacent to the cerebellar white matter.
l.'s of cerebral cortex Six not too obvious layers of the cerebral cortex that tend to blend into each other; from the surface inward, they are: molecular layer, outer granular layer, pyramidal cell layer, inner granular layer, ganglionic layer, and the multiform layer.
choriocapillary l. See choriocapillary lamina, under lamina.
clear l. of skin A narrow homogeneous layer of the skin between the cornified and granular layers; consists of a few rows of clear, flat, dead cells containing a refractile substance (eleidin) that eventually is transformed to keratin; nuclei and cell boundaries are not visible; generally only seen in the thick skin of palms and soles.
compact l. of endometrium The layer of endometrium nearest the inner surface of the uterus; it is adjacent to the spongy layer, with which it forms the functional endometrial layer; contains the neck of the uterine glands and is shed during menstruation and parturition.
conjunctival l. of bulb The mucous membrane investing the anterior surface of the sclera, terminating at the margin of the cornea.
conjunctival l. of eyelids The mucous membrane that lines the posterior surface of the eyelids; it is continuous with the bulbar conjunctiva.
cornified l. of skin The outer layer of the epidermis consisting of several layers of flat keratinized nonnucleated cells.
functional l. of endometrium The compact and spongy layers of the endometrium considered as a functional unit; becomes markedly engorged during the secretory phase of the endometrial cycle and is shed during menstruation.
ganglion cell l. of retina The eighth layer of the retina composed of multipolar nerve cells, between the innermost layer of optic nerve fibers and the inner plexiform layer.
germ l. Any of three primary layers formed in the early development of the embryo, the ectoderm, mesoderm or endoderm, that give rise to specific tissues of the body.
germinative l. of skin The growing part of the skin containing several rows of cells undergoing active mitosis; composed of a deep row of columnar cells (basal layer) and a superficial layer of variable thickness composed of polyhedral cells (prickle-cell layer).
granular l. of skin The layer just under the clear layer of skin, composed of flattened cells with pyknotic nuclei; surrounded by conspicuous granules of keratohyalin and associated with keratinization.
inner nuclear l. of retina The sixth layer of the retina, between the outer plexiform layer and the layer of ganglion cells; composed of cell bodies of the retinal bipolar, horizontal, and amacrine neurons, and retinal gliocytes.
inner plexiform l. of retina The seventh layer of the retina, between the inner nuclear layer and the ganglion cell layer; composed of interconnecting neurites of bipolar, amacrine, and ganglionic neurons.
malpighian l. See basal layer of skin.
nerve fiber l. of retina The ninth layer of the retina, composed of the axons of ganglion cells converging toward the optic disk from all parts of the retina.
oblique l. of muscles of stomach The incomplete, innermost oblique muscular layer of the stomach that is strongly developed in the fundus region and becomes progressively thinner as it approaches the pylorus; totally absent at the lesser curvature of the stomach and quite sparse at the greater curvature.
odontoblastic l. The layer of odontoblast cells lining the pulpal surface of the dentin of teeth; it extends protoplasmic processes into the dentin.
outer nuclear l. of retina The fourth layer of the retina, between the membrane and the outer plexiform layer; composed of the portions of rod and cone cells that are internal to the external limiting membrane. Also called external nuclear lamina of retina.
outer plexiform l. of retina The fifth layer of the retina, composed of an intricate zone of multiple synaptic areas of rod and cone cells and of dendrites and axons of the bipolar and horizontal neurons.
perforated l. of sclera See lamina cribrosa sclerae, under lamina.
pigment l. of retina A single layer of flat cells that constitutes the outermost (first) layer of the retina; it serves as a mechanism for preventing reflections by absorbing light, and as mechanical support for the retinal photoreceptor cells (rods and cones).
posterior elastic l. of cornea See Descemet's membrane, under membrane.
prickle-cell l. of skin The thick layer of the skin (epidermis) between the basal layer and the granular layer, composed of several rows of flattened rhombic cells with their long axis parallel with the skin; thought to represent the transitional stage in the formation of soft keratin; the cells contain conspicuous granules of keratohyalin; the prickle-cell layer provides most of the mechanical coherence of the skin. Also see germinative layer of skin.
Purkinje l. The middle of three layers of the cerebellar cortex consisting of large neuron cell bodies.
l. of rods and cones of the retina A layer of the retina between the pigment epithelium and the external limiting membrane, containing the visual receptors (rod and cone cells). Also called bacillary layer.
spongy l. of endometrium Layer of the endometrium between the compact and basal layers; contains the uterine glands which, during the late proliferative stage of the endometrial cycle, become greatly engorged and tortuous.
subendothelial l. The thin layer of connective tissue between the endothelium and elastic lamina of the intima of large and medium-sized blood vessels, and under the endocardium.

layering (la´er-ing) An arrangement in layers.

leaching (lēch´ing) The process of washing out soluble matter from a substance by a percolating

retinal arteriole, branch of central retinal artery (blood supply to inner two-thirds of retina)
nerve fibers converging to form optic nerve
retinal venule
nerve fiber layer of retina
ganglion cell layer of retina
inner plexiform layer of retina
inner nuclear layer of retina
outer plexiform layer of retina
outer nuclear layer of retina (contains nuclei of rods and cones)
layer of rods and cones
pigment layer of retina (rich in melanin)
basal lamina of choroid (Bruch's membrane)
sclera
choroid
choriocapillaries (blood supply nourishes avascular outer third of the retina)

LAYERS OF THE RETINA

germ layers

lacunae
syncytiotrophoblast
cytotrophoblast
extraembryonic mesoderm
amniotic cavity
ectoderm
endoderm
celom
endometrial epithelium
primitive yolk sac

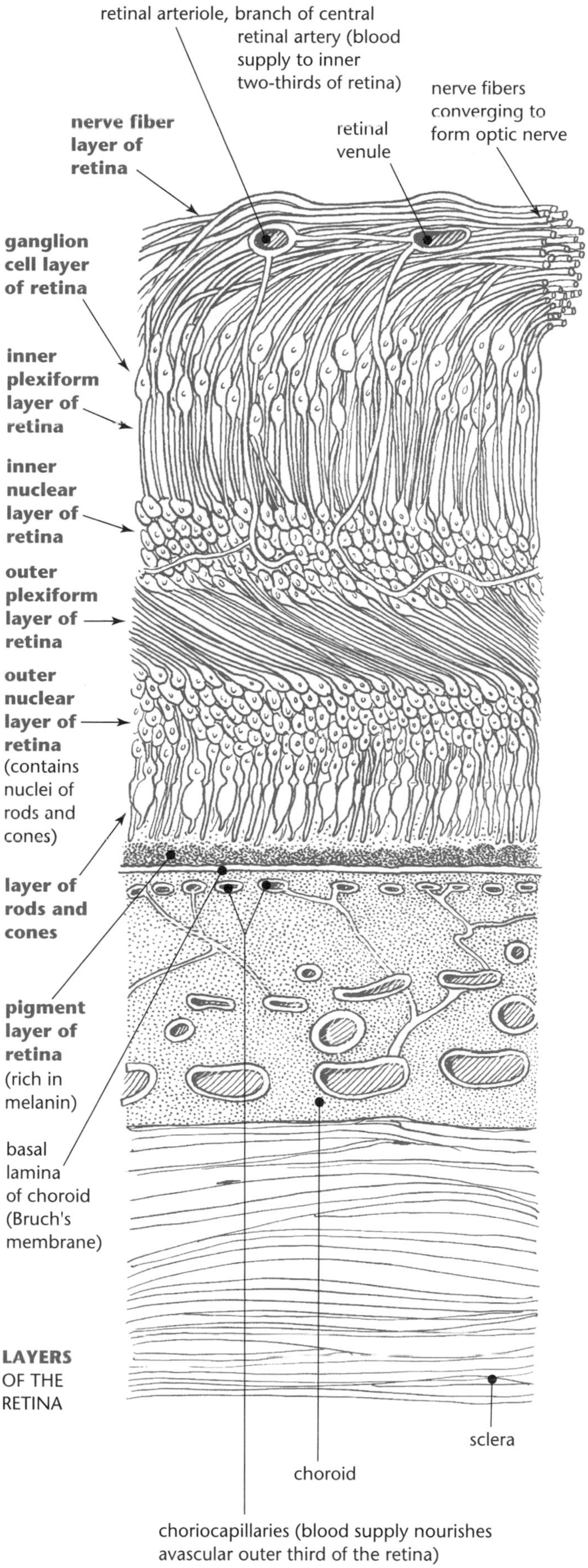

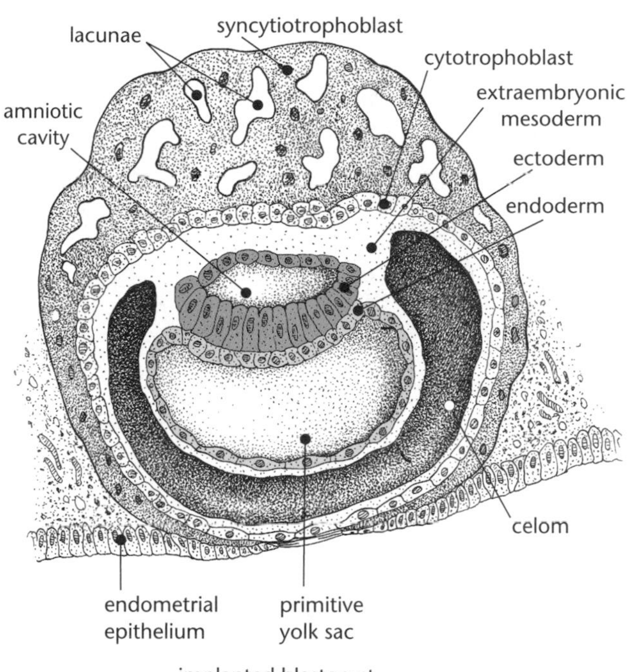

implanted blastocyst during second week of development

longitudinal layer of muscles of esophagus
circular layer of muscles of stomach
cardiac incisura
circular layer of muscles of esophagus
oblique layer of muscles of stomach
longitudinal layer of muscles of stomach
lesser curvature
greater curvature
duodenum
jejunum
BJ7VA

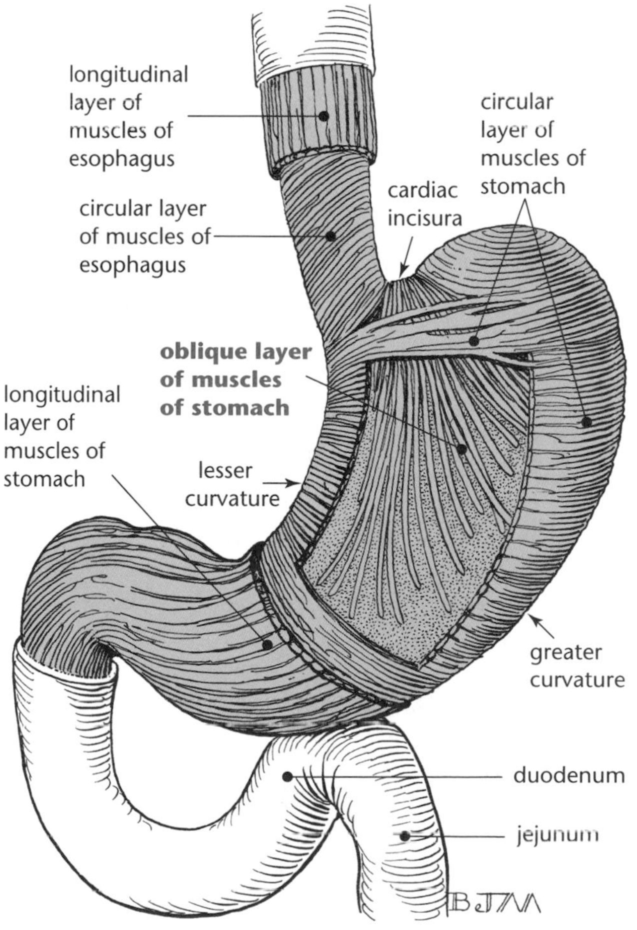

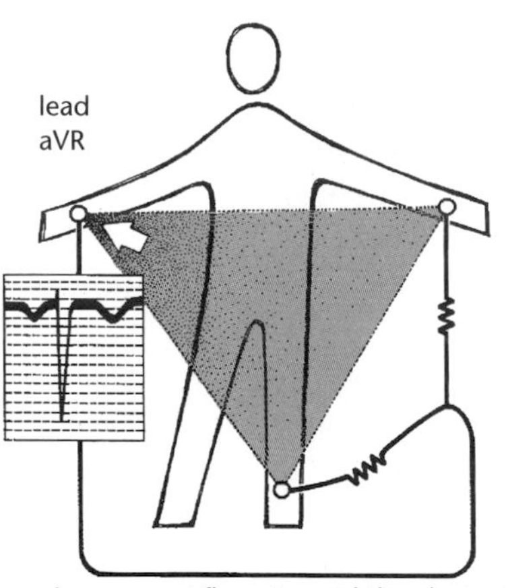

augmented limb leads

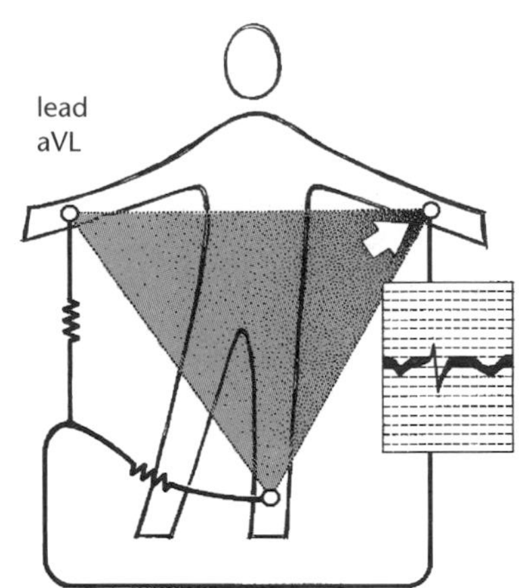

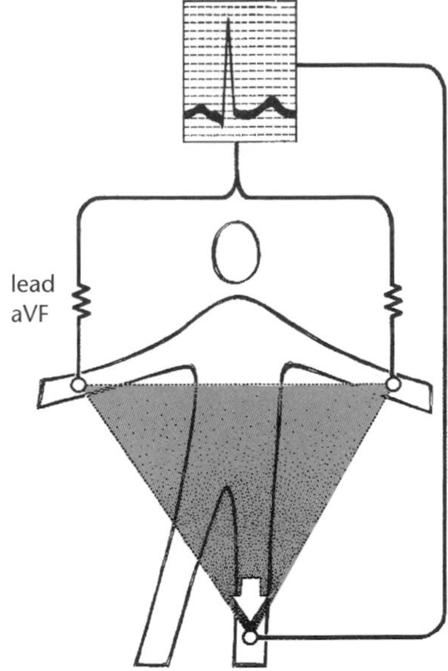

• when current flows toward the electrodes, upward deflection occurs in the ECG
• when current flows away from the electrodes, downward reflection occurs in the ECG

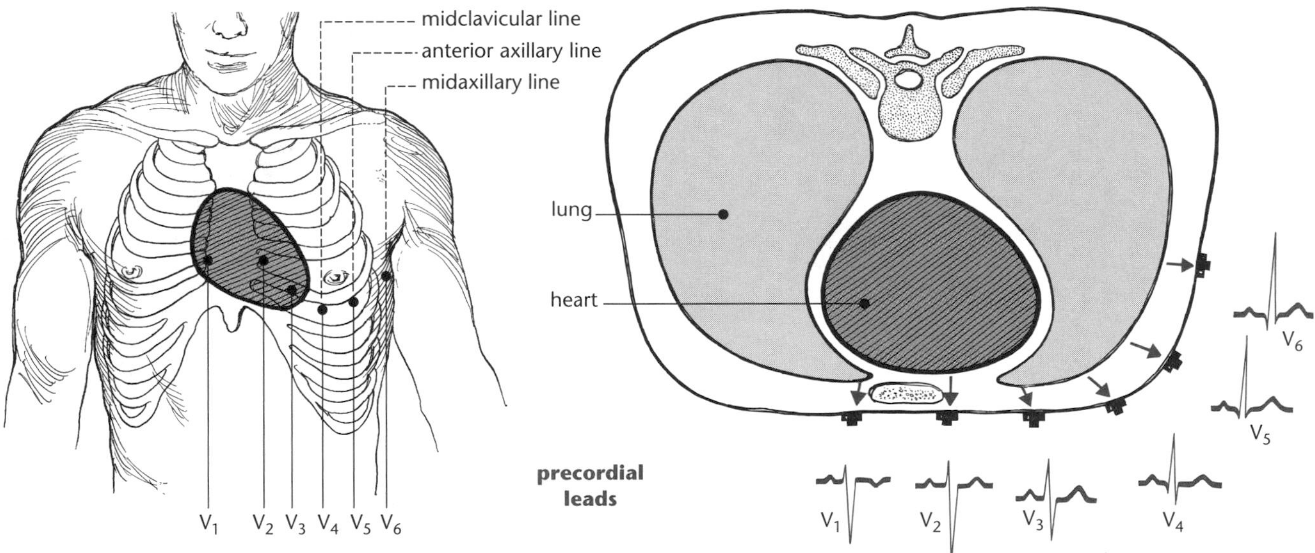

precordial leads

liquid. Also called lixiviation.

lead (led) A malleable, bluish gray, dense metallic element, extracted chiefly from lead sulfide; symbol Pb (plumbum), atomic number 82, atomic weight 207.19.

l. carbonate A poisonous white powder, $PbCO_3$, used largely in the manufacture of paint.

l. chromate A poisonous lemon-yellow powder, $PbCrO_3$, used as a paint pigment.

l. sulfide (PbS) The natural form in which lead is usually found. Also called galena.

lead (lēd) A specific array of electric connections (electrodes) used for recording the electric potential created by a functioning organ, such as the heart (electrocardiography) or brain (electroencephalography).

augmented limb l. One of three unipolar leads for registering the variations in electric potentials at one point (right arm, aVR; left arm, aVL; or left leg, aVF) with respect to a point which does not vary significantly in electric activity during contraction of the heart; the lead is augmented (increased) by virtue of an electric connection which increases the amplitude; lead aVR records the electric potentials of the right arm with reference to a junction made by connecting the wires from the left arm and the left leg; lead aVL records the potentials at the left arm in reference to a junction made by connecting the wires from the right arm and the left foot; lead aVF records the potentials at the left foot in reference to a junction made by connecting the wire from the left and right arms.

bipolar l. A lead in which the electrodes detect electric variations at two points and record the difference.

chest l. See precordial lead.

direct l. A lead recorded with the exploring electrode placed directly on the surface of the exposed heart.

esophageal l. An exploring electrode introduced into the lumen of the esophagus in order to improve visualization of atrial deflections on the electrocardiogram (ECG); useful in the recognition of arrhythmias.

intracardiac l. A lead recorded with the exploring electrode placed in one of the heart's chambers, usually by means of cardiac catheterization.

limb l. One of the three bipolar standard leads or one of the three unipolar augmented limb leads (aVR, aVL, aVF).

precordial l. One in which the exploring electrode is on the chest overlying the heart or its vicinity; unipolar chest lead recorded in positions V_1 through V_6 (the V designation denotes that the movable electrode registers the electric potential under the electrode with respect to a V or central terminal connection, which is made by connecting wires from the right arm, left arm, and left leg; the electric potential of the central terminal connection does not vary significantly throughout the cardiac cycle; as a result, the recordings made with the V connection show the electric variations that are taking place under the movable precordial electrode; position V_1 is at the fourth intercostal space at the right sternal border; V_2 is at the fourth intercostal space at the left sternal border; V_4 is at the left midclavicular line in the fifth intercostal space; V_3 is equidistant between V_2 and V_4; V_5 is the fifth intercostal space in the anterior axillary line; V_6 is at the fifth intercostal space in the left midaxillary line.

standard l. One of the original bipolar limb leads designated I, II, and III; it detects the electric variations at two points and displays the difference; lead I records the potential difference between the right and left arms; lead II records the difference between right arm and left leg; lead III records the difference between left arm and left leg.

unipolar l.'s Leads in which the exploring electrode records the variations in electric potential at one point with reference to a point that does not vary significantly in electric activity during cardiac contraction.

V l. A chest lead with the central terminal as the indifferent electrode.

leaflet (lēf′lit) A structure resembling a small leaf, such as the cusps of a heart valve.

lecithin (les′ĭ-thin) (L) One of a group of phospholipids having a yellowish or brown waxy appearance; found in nerve tissue, egg yolks, and cells (both animal and vegetable).

lecithinase (les-ĭ-thin′ās) See phospholipase.

lectin (lek′tin) A protein found predominantly in seeds, particularly those of the legumes; it binds to specific carbohydrate-containing receptor sites on the red blood cell surface and can cause the cells to agglutinate. Also called phytoagglutinin.

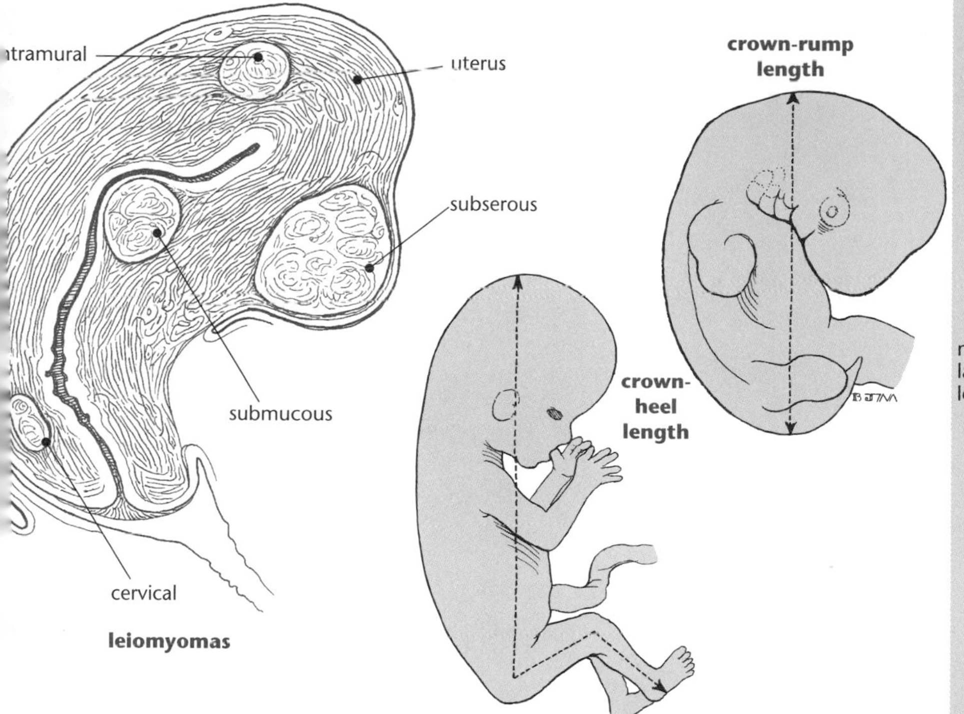

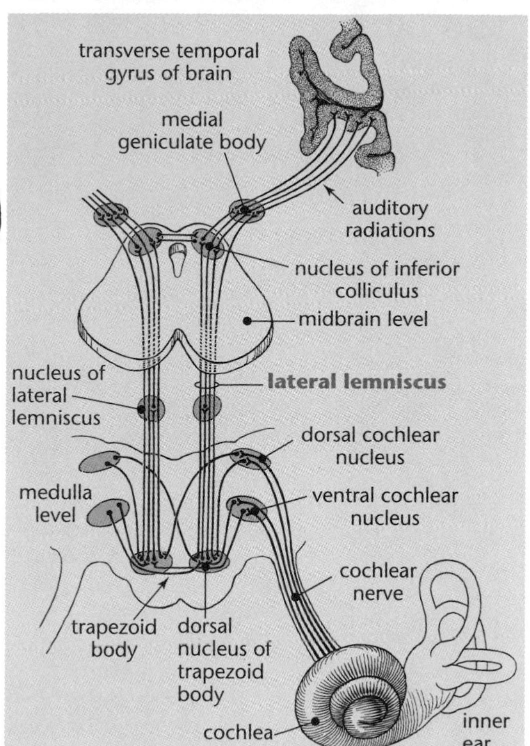

leech (lēch) Any of various annelid worms (class Hirudinea) of which one blood sucking species, *Hirudo medicinalis* (German leech), was used for bleeding patients.

leg (leg) The lower limb, especially between the knee and the ankle.

milk l. See puerperal thrombophlebitis, under thrombophlebitis.

Legg-Calvé-Perthes disease (leg-kal-va´per´tez dĭ-zēz´) See epiphysial aseptic necrosis, under necrosis.

Legionella pneumophila (le-jŭ-nel´ă noo-mo´fil-ă) A gram-negative, rod-shaped bacterium; the cause of legionnaire's disease.

legionnaire's disease (le-jun-ārz dĭ-zēz´) Infectious disease caused by *Legionella pneumophila* (a gram-negative bacillus); symptoms include high fever, headache, abdominal pain, and pneumonia; the liver, kidneys and nervous system may also be affected.

legumin (lĕ-gu´min) Protein found in peas and beans.

leiomyofibroma (li-o-mi-o-fi-bro´mă) See leiomyoma.

leiomyoma (li-o-mi-o´mă) A benign tumor derived from smooth muscle and containing varying amounts of collagen; may occur anywhere in the body but is most frequently seen in the uterus, with a tendency to grow rapidly during pregnancy. Also called fibromyoma; leiomyofibroma; fibroid.

leiomyomatosis (li-o-mi-o-mă-to´sis) The state of having multiple benign tumors of smooth muscle (leiomyomas).

leiomyomectomy (li-o-mi-o-mek´tŏ-me) Removal of a leiomyoma.

leiomyosarcoma (li-o-mi-o-sar-ko´mă) A malignant neoplasm in which smooth (nonstriated) muscle cells proliferate into a fleshy mass.

Leishmania (lēsh-ma´ne-ă) A genus of flagellated parasitic protozoa (family Trypanosomidae) transmitted to humans by the bite of infected sandflies.

L. braziliensis Species causing mucocutaneous leishmaniasis.

L. donovani Intracellular parasite causing visceral leishmaniasis (kala azar).

L. tropica Species causing cutaneous leishmaniasis.

leishmaniasis, leishmaniosis (lēsh-ma-nī´ă-sis, lēsh-ma-ni-o´sis) Infection with a species of *Leishmania*.

American l. See mucocutaneous leishmaniasis.

cutaneous l. Chronic skin lesions with a tendency to ulcerate produced by *Leishmania tropica*; prevalent in tropical and subtropical areas. Also called oriental sore; Old World leishmaniasis.

mucocutaneous l. Skin lesions often associated with ulcerative lesions of the mucous membranes of the nose, mouth, and pharynx; caused by *Leishmania braziliensis*. Also called American leishmaniasis; New World leishmaniasis.

New World l. See mucocutaneous leishmaniasis.

Old World l. See cutaneous leishmaniasis.

visceral l. A disease characterized by chronic fever, splenomegaly, anemia, leukopenia, and hyperglobulinemia; caused by *Leishmania donovani*; transmitted by the bite of a sandfly. Also called kala azar; tropical splenomegaly.

leishmanid (lēsh´man-īd) Any lesion that may be infected with a species of the genus *Leishmania*.

lema (le´mă) The normal sebaceous secretion of the meibomian glands in the eyelids, collected at the inner angle of the eye.

lemniscus (lem-nis´kus), *pl.* **lemnis´ci** A band or bundle of nerve fibers in the central nervous system.

lateral l. The major auditory pathway to the brainstem; it consists of a band of longitudinal ascending fibers that pass through the pons (in the lateral tegmentum) to the level of the midbrain, where most of the fibers terminate in the inferior colliculus with a few projecting directly to the medial geniculate body.

medial l. A bundle of ascending fibers that originates in the nuclei of the lower brainstem and terminates in the ventral posterolateral nucleus of the thalamus.

trigeminal l. A band of fibers in the brainstem passing from the sensory nuclei of the trigeminal nerve to the posterior part of the ventral nucleus of the thalamus.

length (lengkth) Distance between two points.

bond l. The average distance between the nuclei of two atoms linked by a bond.

crown-heel l., C-H l. The length of an embryo from the top of the head to the heel.

crown-rump l., C-R l. The length of an embryo from the top of the head to the bottom of the buttocks.

lenitive (len´ĭ-tiv) **1.** A soothing agent. **2.** Soothing.

lens (lenz) **1.** A transparent object (made of glass, plastic, quartz, etc.) having two polished surfaces of which at least one is curved, usually with a spherical curvature, shaped so that light rays on passing through it are made to diverge or converge. **2.** The lens of the eye; the biconvex transparent structure of the eye located between the iris and the vitreous body.

achromatic l. A compound lens that eliminates or reduces chromatic aberration; made of two kinds of glass with different dispersive powers.

acoustic l. A lens used in ultrasonography to focus or diverge a sound beam.

acrylic l. A lens made of acrylic material; used to replace a cataractous lens.

aplanatic l. A lens that corrects spherical aberration.

apochromatic l. A lens that corrects both spherical and chromatic aberrations.

bifocal l. Lens having one portion (usually the upper and larger portion) suited for distant vision and the other suited for near vision.

compound l. Optical system having two or more lenses.

concave l. A lens that disperses light rays. Also called minus, diverging, myopic, negative, or reducing lens.

concavoconvex l. Lens having one concave and one convex surface. Also called positive meniscus lens.

contact l. A molded plastic lens that rests directly on the eye in contact with the cornea; used to correct refractive errors.

convex l. A lens that converges or focuses light rays. Also called plus, converging, hyperopic, or magnifying lens.

convexoconcave l. Lens having one convex and one concave surface. Also called negative meniscus lens.

crystalline l. See lens (2).

cylindrical l. (cyl) A lens in which one or both surfaces have the curve of a cylinder, either concave or convex; used to correct astigmatism.

eye l. The lens in an eyepiece that is nearest the eye; it renders light rays from the objective lens parallel prior to entrance into the eye. Also called ocular lens.

field l. The lens nearest the objective lens in an eyepiece; it increases the field of view in a microscopic or telescopic system.

gas-permeable l. A hard contact lens that allows atmospheric oxygen to pass directly through to reach the cornea, which renders the lens comfortable to wear for long periods of time.

hard contact l. A contact lens made of a substance that absorbs little or no water, thus the lens remains rigid when worn. Also called hydrophobic contact lens; rigid contact lens.

immersion l. The lens in a microscope nearest the object, designed so that it can be lowered into contact with a fluid which is placed on the cover glass.

meniscus l. A crescent-shaped lens; one that is concave on one surface and convex on the other.

minus l. See concave lens.

non-gas permeable l. A hard contact lens that, as it moves up and down with each blink of the eyelid, allows oxygen-carrying tears to bathe the cornea.

objective l. The lens in a microscope or telescope nearest the object; it converges light rays from the field of view.

planoconcave l. A lens that is flat on one surface

L

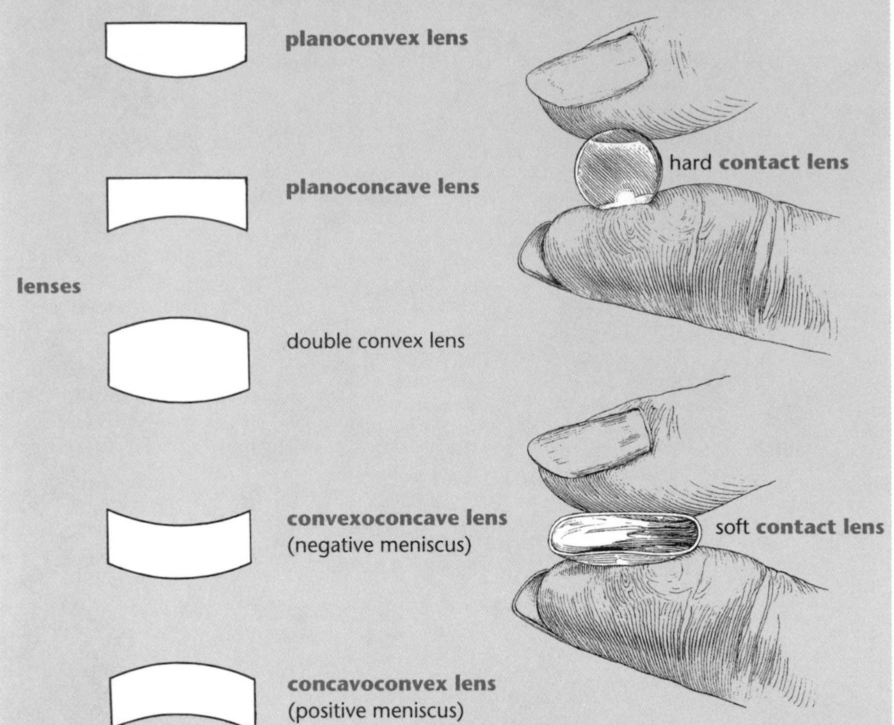

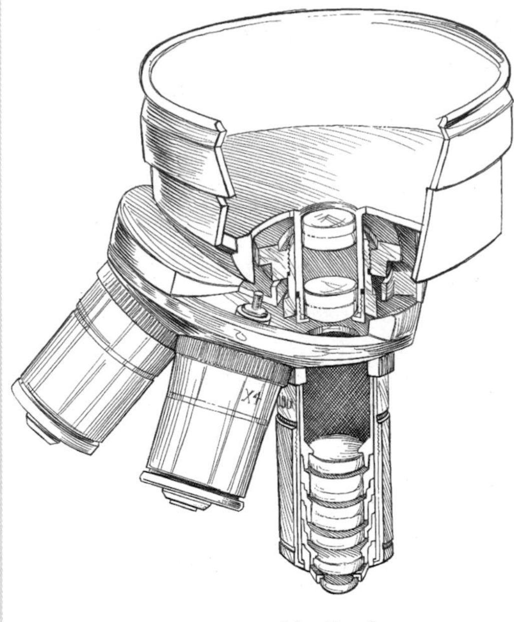

objective lens

and concave on the other.

planoconvex l. A lens that is flat on one surface and convex on the other.

plus l. See convex lens.

soft contact l. A flexible contact lens made of a water-absorbing substance. Also called hydrophilic contact lens.

spherical l. A lens in which all refractive surfaces are spherical.

sphericocylindrical l. A lens in which one surface is spherical and the other is cylindrical.

trifocal l. A lens having three portions with different focal powers serving for distant, intermediate, and near vision.

lensometer (lenz-om´ĕ-ter) An optical instrument used to determine the refractive power, optical center, cylinder axis, and prismatic effect of ophthalmic lenses.

lens system (lenz sis´tem) Two or more lenses arranged to work in conjunction with one another in order to accomplish a required function (e.g., microscope, projection lens system).

lenticonus (len-ti-ko´nus) A conical protrusion on either the anterior or posterior surface of the lens of the eye, usually affecting only one eye.

lenticular (len-tik´u-lar) **1.** Relating to a lens. **2.** Shaped like a lentil.

lenticulostriate (len-tik-u-lo-stri´āt) Relating to the lentiform nucleus and the corpus striatum of the brain.

lentiform (len´tĭ-form) **1.** Lenticular. **2.** Shaped like a lens.

lentigo (len-ti´go), *pl.* **lentigines** A flat, tan or brown spot on the skin which is to be differentiated from a freckle; an early junctional nevus.

malignant l. See melanoma *in situ*, under melanoma.

senile l. A brown discoloration on the exposed area of the skin occurring in elderly people. It is not a premalignant lesion. Popularly called liver spot.

leontiasis (le-on-ti´ă-sis) The lionlike appearance of the face in some cases of advanced leprosy (i.e., ridges and furrows on the forehead and cheeks).

LEOPARD syndrome A hereditary (autosomal dominant) disorder. The name is an acronym of the characteristic abnormalities: lentigines, electrocardiographic (disturbances), ocular (hypertelorism), pulmonary (stenosis), abnormalities (of genitals), retardation (of growth), and (neural) deafness.

leper (lep´er) An individual afflicted with leprosy.

lepidosis (lep-ĭ-do´sis) Any scaly eruption of the skin.

lepothrix (lep´ō-thriks) See trichomycosis axillaris, under trichomycosis.

leprid (lep´rid) The early skin lesion of leprosy.

leprology (lep-rol´ŏ-je) The study of leprosy.

leproma (lep-ro´mă) The characteristic lesion of the focus of infection with *Microbacterium leprae*.

lepromatous (lep-ro´mă-tus) Relating to a leproma.

lepromin (lep´ro-min) Extract made from tissue containing the leprosy bacillus (*Mycobacterium leprae*), used in skin tests to determine resistance to leprosy.

leprosarium (lep-ro-sar´e-um) A special hospital for the care and treatment of those afflicted with leprosy.

leprosary (lep´ro-sar-e) A leper colony.

leprostatic (lep-ro-stat´ik) An agent that inhibits the growth of the leprosy bacillus (*Mycobacterium leprae*).

leprosy (lep´rŏ-se) A chronic infectious disease caused by the bacillus *Mycobacterium leprae* with a patient-to-patient transmission; produces granulomatous lesions of the skin and mucous membranes, with involvement of the peripheral nervous system. Its severity can range from benign forms (tuberculoid leprosy) to highly contagious malignant forms (lepromatous leprosy) marked by mutilation. Also called Hansen's disease.

leprous (lep´rus) Relating to leprosy.

leptocyte (lep´to-sīt) A thin red blood cell having a pigmented border surrounding a clear area with a pigmented center.

leptocytosis (lep-to-si-to´sis) The presence of leptocytes in the blood, occurring in certain disorders, including thalassemia.

leptodermic (lep-to-der´mik) Thin-skinned.

leptomeningeal (lep-to-mĕ-nin´je-al) Relating to the leptomeninges.

leptomeninges (lep-to-mĕ-nin´jēz) The pia mater and arachnoid considered as one functional unit; the pia-arachnoid.

leptomeninx (lep-to-men´inks) Singular of leptomeninges.

leptomonad (lep-to-mo´nad) **1.** A member of the genus *Leptomonas*. **2.** See promastigote.

Leptospira (lep-to-spi´ră) A genus of spiral, hook-ended spirochetes, bacteria of the order Spirochaetales.

leptospire (lep´to-spīr) Any organism belonging to the genus *Leptospira*.

leptospirosis (lep-to-spi-ro´sis) Infection with bacteria of the genus *Leptospira*; the clinical picture may vary from a mild fever to a fulminating toxic illness with jaundice and renal failure; specific syndromes include aseptic meningitis and pretibial fever, the latter associated with a pretibial eruption and splenomegaly.

l. icterohemorrhagia See Weil's disease.

leptotene (lep´to-tēn) In meiosis, the first stage of prophase in which the chromosomes appear as individual, slender threads, well separated from each other.

Leptotrichia (lep-to-trik´e-ă) A genus of anaerobic, nonmotile bacteria indigenous to the oral cavity of humans.

Leptotrombidium (lep-to-trom-bid´e-um) Genus of mites (family Trombiculidae); transmit tsutsugamushi disease.

Leriche's syndrome (lĕ-rēsh´as sin´drōm) See aortoiliac occlusive disease.

lesbian (lez´be-an) **1.** A homosexual female. **2.** Relating to lesbianism.

lesbianism (lez´be-ă-niz-m) Female homosexuality.

Lesch-Nyhan syndrome (lesh-ni´an sin´drōm) Disorder of purine metabolism and excessive uric acid; clinical features include severe mental retardation and compulsive, self-mutilating behavior; death usually occurs during childhood due to kidney failure; an X-linked recessive inheritance.

lesion (le´zhun) Any morbid change in the structure or function of tissues due to injury or disease.

coin l. A round shadow the size of a small coin seen in radiographs of the lungs; may indicate tuberculosis, cancer, or other diseases.

Councilman's l. See Councilman's bodies, under body.

Ghon's primary l. The primary lesion of pulmonary tuberculosis, appearing in the roentgenogram as a small sharply defined shadow. Also called Ghon's focus.

Janeway l. A small hemorrhagic lesion on the palm or sole, occurring in some cases of bacterial endocarditis.

lethal (le´thal) (L) Deadly.

lethargy (leth´ar-je) A state of drowsiness and sluggishness.

Letterer-Siwe disease (let´er-ĕr-si´we dĭ-zēz´) See acute disseminated Langerhans-cell histiocytosis, under histiocytosis.

leucine (loo´sēn) (Leu) An essential amino acid formed by the hydrolysis of protein; found in many tissues, especially the pancreas and spleen.

leucovorin (loo-ko-vo´rin) See folinic acid.

leukapheresis (loo-kă-fĕ-re´sis) Procedure in which white blood cells are removed from withdrawn blood, which is then retransfused into the patient.

leukemia (loo-ke´me-ă) Disease characterized by proliferation of large numbers of immature and abnormal white blood cells in bone marrow, where they impair production of normal white blood cells, red blood cells, and platelets; in most cases these malignant cells are also present in peripheral blood and may also infiltrate other tissues and organs. Classified as acute or chronic depending (in part) on the rapidity of its course and (primarily) on the degree of immaturity of predominant cells; may also be classified on the basis of the dominant cell involved (e.g., granulocytic, lymphocytic, monocytic).

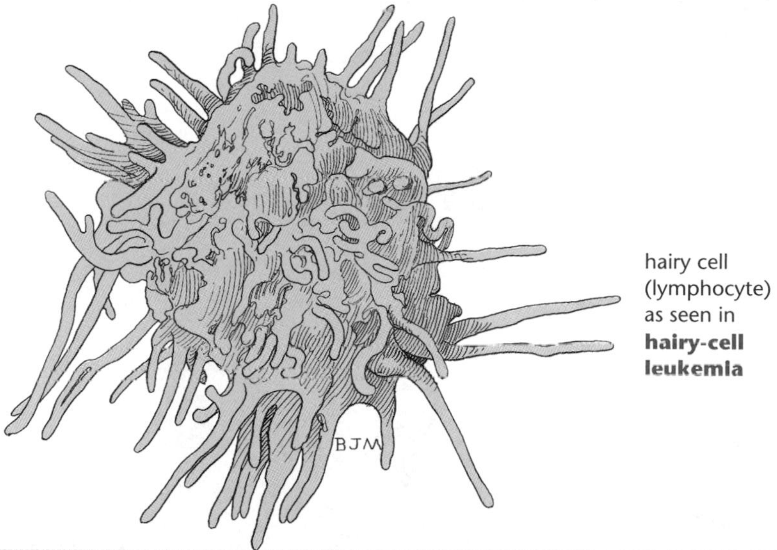

hairy cell (lymphocyte) as seen in **hairy-cell leukemia**

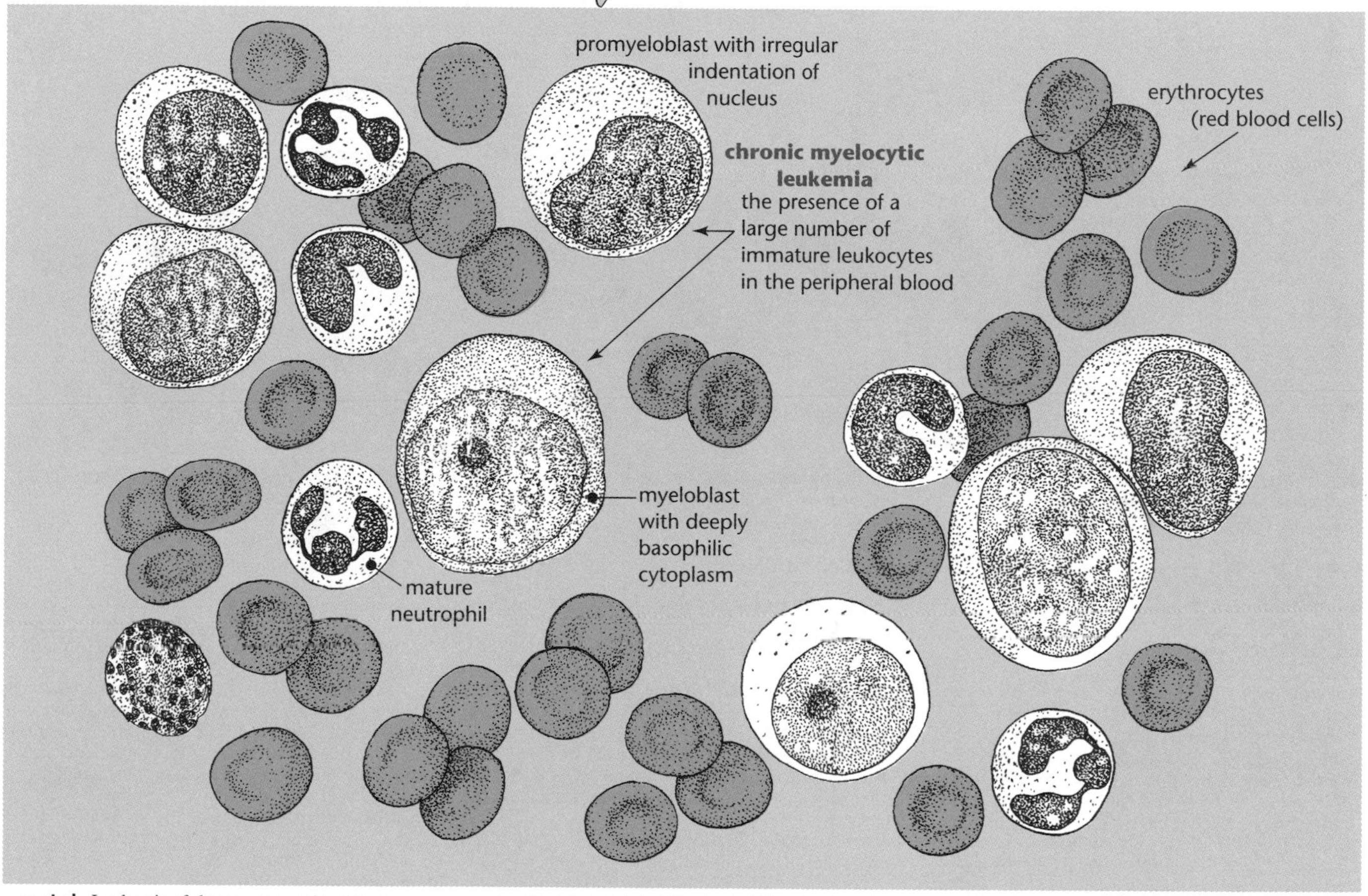

promyeloblast with irregular indentation of nucleus

erythrocytes (red blood cells)

chronic myelocytic leukemia
the presence of a large number of immature leukocytes in the peripheral blood

myeloblast with deeply basophilic cytoplasm

mature neutrophil

acute l. Leukemia of abrupt onset and rapid course leading to death if untreated; characterized by proliferation of primitive undifferentiated cells ("blasts") that mature little, if at all; bone marrow is the primary site of the disease; clinical features include: rapidly developing anemia (often severe), fatigue, fever, susceptibility to infections, abnormal bleeding (of gums, nose, and subcutaneous tissues), enlargement of lymph nodes (usually) and organs (sometimes), and bone pain and tenderness; may involve the central nervous system, causing associated symptoms (e.g., headache, stiff neck, vomiting, lethargy, swelling of optic disks).

acute granulocytic l. (AGL) See acute myeloblastic leukemia.

acute lymphoblastic l. (ALL) Leukemia occurring predominantly in children, with peak incidence at three to four years of age; constitutes 80% of childhood acute leukemias. Most of the blood cells involved are B lymphocytes (80%), others are T lymphocytes. Also called acute lymphocytic leukemia.

acute lymphocytic l. See acute lymphoblastic leukemia.

acute myeloblastic l. (AML) Leukemia originating from any white blood cell of the granulocyte series. Also called acute granulocytic leukemia (AGL); acute myelocytic leukemia; acute myeloid leukemia.

acute myelocytic l. See acute myeloblastic leukemia.

acute myeloid l. See acute myeloblastic leukemia.

chronic l. Leukemia characterized by an insidious onset and a slow clinical course; patients often survive many years, sometimes without treatment; characterized by proliferation of immature cells that are more mature than those of acute leukemia; white blood cell counts in peripheral blood are usually very high; clinical features include a slowly developing anemia (sometimes over years), generalized lymph node enlargement (in some types) and massive enlargement of spleen and liver (in others). The condition is frequently discovered accidently.

chronic granulocytic l. (CGL) See chronic myelocytic leukemia.

chronic lymphocytic l. (CLL) Leukemia occurring primarily in persons over the age of 50 years, most commonly in men; cells involved are B lymphocytes; clinical features include: fatigability and appetite and weight loss, with generalized lymph node and liver enlargement. Median survival rate after onset is usually 4 to 5 years.

chronic myelocytic l. (CML) Leukemia primarily affecting adults 25–60 years old, with peak incidence in the fourth and fifth decades of life; dominant cells involved are myelocytes, metamyelocytes, and granulocytes; symptoms include fatigability, weakness, and appetite and weight loss, with a typical dragging sensation in the abdomen caused by massive enlargement of the spleen. Some patients develop an accelerated phase (blast crisis) for which all forms of treatment are ineffective. Also called chronic granulocytic leukemia; chronic myeloid leukemia.

hairy-cell l. A rare form of chronic B lymphocyte leukemia in which the abnormal cells have fine, hairlike projections; affects primarily males over 50 years of age; most prominent symptom is massive enlargement of the spleen. Median survival is 4 years.

leukemic (loo-ke´mik) Relating to leukemia.

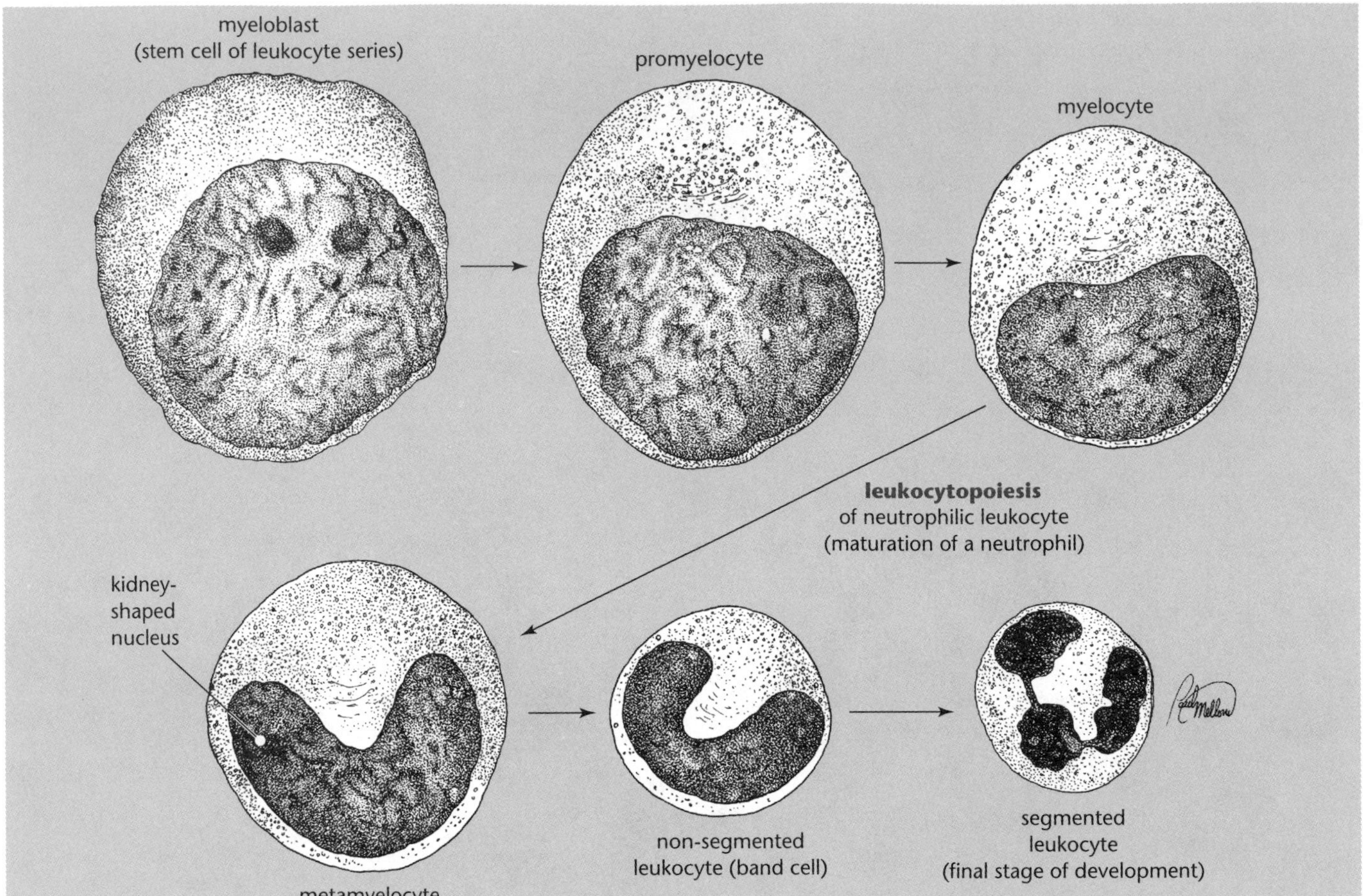

L

leukemogenesis (loo-ke-mo-jen´ĕ-sis) The cause and development of a leukemic disease.

leukemoid (loo-ke´moid) Resembling the blood changes of leukemia.

leukoagglutinin (loo-ko-ă-gloo-tĭ-nin) Antibody that agglutinates white blood cells.

leukoblast (loo´ko-blast) An immature white blood cell.

leukocytactic (loo-ko-si-tak´tik) See leukocytotactic.

leukocytaxia (loo-ko-si-tak´se-ă) See leukocytotaxia.

leukocyte (loo´ko-sīt) Any colorless cell of the blood generally called white blood cell; may be: *granular*, containing readily stainable cytoplasmic granules and lobulated nuclei (neutrophilic, eosinophilic, and basophilic leukocytes) or *nongranular*, containing minute cytoplasmic granules, not detectable with ordinary methods (lymphocytes and monocytes).

basophilic l. Leukocyte containing large granules that stain readily with basic dyes (e.g., methylene blue); constitutes about 0.5% of total white blood cell count. Also called basophil; mast leukocyte.

eosinophilic l. Phagocytic leukocyte with a bilobed nucleus and numerous large cytoplasmic granules that stain intensely with acid dyes (e.g., eosin) and are rich in protein highly toxic to parasites; constitutes 2 to5% of total white blood cell count. Also called eosinophil; acidophil; oxyphil.

mast l. See basophilic leukocyte.

neutrophilic l. Mature granular leukocyte containing granules that stain with a mixture of acid and basic dyes, has a nucleus of three to five distinct lobes joined by either thin strands or wide bands of chromatin, and constitutes about 50 to 75% of total white blood cell count; its primary function is to ingest and digest particulate matter, especially virulent bacteria. Also called neutrophil; neutrophilic granulocyte; polymorphonuclear leukocyte; PMN.

polymorphonuclear (PMN) l. See neutrophilic leukocyte.

leukocytoblast (loo-ko-sī´to-blast) General term denoting any immature white blood cell.

leukocytogenesis (loo-ko-sī-to-jen´ĕ-sis) The formation of white blood cells.

leukocytolysin (loo-ko-sī-tol´ĭ-sin) Any agent causing dissolution of white blood cells.

leukocytolysis (loo-ko-sī-tol´ĭ-sis) The dissolution of white blood cells. Also called leukolysis.

leukocytometer (loo-ko-sī-tom´ĕ-ter) A standardized glass slide used to count leukocytes.

leukocytopenia (loo-ko-sī-to-pe´ne-ă) See leukopenia.

leukocytopoiesis (loo-ko-sī-to-poi-e´sis) The formation of white blood cells.

leukocytosis (loo-ko-sī-to´sis) Abnormal increase in the number of white corpuscles in the blood.

leukocytotactic (loo-ko-sī-to-tak´tik) Relating to leukocytotaxia. Also called leukocytactic; leukotactic.

leukocytotaxia (loo-ko-sī-to-tak´se-ă) The tendency of white blood cells to move either toward (positive leukocytotaxia) or away from (negative leukocytotaxia) certain microorganisms and substances formed in inflamed tissue. Also called leukocytaxia; leukotaxis.

leukocytoxin (loo-ko-sī-tok´sin) Any agent that causes destruction of leukocytes.

leukoderma (loo-ko-der´mă) Absence of pigment in the skin. Also called achromoderma.

acquired l. See vitiligo.

congenital l. See albinism.

leukodystrophy (loo-ko-dis´trŏ-fe) Disease occurring early in life and affecting primarily the white matter of the brain, especially the cerebral hemispheres; thought to be a congenital defect in the formation or maintenance of myelin.

globoid cell l. See Krabbe's disease.

metachromatic l. Progressive disorder of sphingolipid metabolism in which sulfatide accumulates in the tissues; it affects the central and peripheral nervous systems, causing blindness, deafness, muteness, and quadriplegia; death usually follows a few years from onset; most commonly seen in infants and young children. Also called sulfatide lipidosis.

leukoencephalitis (loo-ko-en-sef-ah-li´tis) Inflammation of the white matter of the brain.

leukoencephalopathy (loo-ko-en-sef-ă-lop´ă-the) Disease of the white matter of the brain.

progressive multifocal l. (PML) Disease of insidious onset and fatal outcome affecting immunocompromised patients; marked by widespread but focal disintegration of myelin in the brain; features include organic brain dysfunction, hemiplegia, partial loss of vision, and language difficulties; caused by the JC virus.

subtotal l. Diffuse loss of white matter, axons, and myelin deep in the cerebral hemispheres, with hardening (sclerosis) of the manute penetrating arteries of the brain; often involves arteriosclerosis and/or infarcts in other regions of the brain; may be associated with progressive dementia.

leukoerythroblastosis (loo-ko-ĕ-rith-ro-blas-to´sis) Any anemic condition resulting from destruction of blood cell-forming (hemopoietic) tissues by space-occupying lesions of bone marrow, especially metastatic cancer. Also called myelophthisic anemia; myelopathic anemia.

leukokoria (loo-ko-kor´e-ă) Any eye condition that causes a white reflection from behind the clear crystalline lens, giving the appearance of a white pupil.

leukolysis (loo-kol´ĭ-sis) See leukocytolysis.

leukoma (loo-ko´mă) An opaque white spot on the cornea.

leukomyelitis (loo-ko-mi-ĕ-li´tis) Inflammation of the white tracts of the spinal cord.

leukomyelopathy (loo-ko-mi-ĕ-lop´ă-the) Any disease that involves the white tracts of the spinal cord.

leukonychia (loo-ko-nik´e-ă) Unduly white nails; especially white spots or patches under the nails.

l. striata Leukonychia in which the nail plate is marked by horizontal streaks of whiteness.

l. totalis Leukonychia in which the entire nail is white.

leukopathia, leukopathy (loo-ko-path´e-ă, loo-kop´ă-the) See leukoderma.

leukopedesis (loo-ko-pĕ-de´sis) Movement of white blood cells through the capillary walls into the

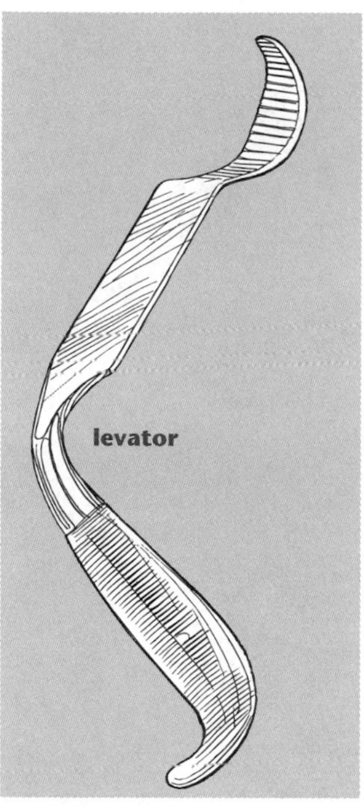

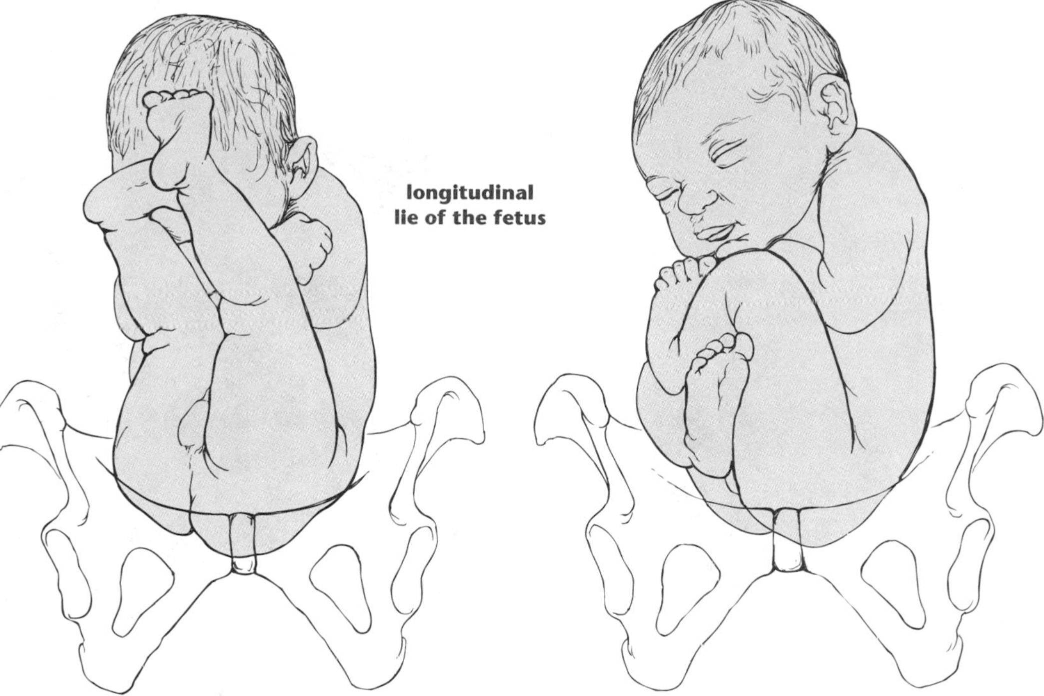

tissues.

leukopenia (loo-ko-pe´ne-ă) Abnormal reduction in the number of white corpuscles in the blood. Also called leukocytopenia.

monocytic l. See monocytopenia.

leukoplakia (loo-ko-pla´ke-ă) A white, irregular lesion in mucous membranes, most commonly of the lips, oral cavity, and genitals; may be simply an increased thickness of the keratin layer of tissues due to chronic irritation, or it may be precancerous. Popularly called smoker's patch when it occurs on the lips.

atrophic l. See lichen sclerosus, under lichen.

leukopoiesis (loo-ko-poi-e´sis) The production of white blood cells.

leukoprotease (loo-ko-pro´te-ās) An enzyme, the product of polynuclear leukocytes, formed in an area of inflammation and causing liquefaction of dead tissue.

leukorrhea (loo-ko-re´ă) An abnormal, white, or yellowish discharge from the vagina, containing mucus and pus cells.

leukosis (loo-ko´sis) Abnormal proliferation of tissues that form white blood cells.

leukotactic (loo-ko-tak´tik) See leukocytotactic.

leukotaxine (loo-ko-tak´sēn) A crystalline nitrogenous substance prepared from inflammatory exudates and injured degenerating tissue.

leukotaxis (loo-ko-tak´sis) See leukocytotaxia.

leukotomy (loo-kot´ŏ-me) Surgical incision into the white matter of the frontal lobe of the brain.

prefrontal l. See prefrontal lobotomy, under lobotomy.

transorbital l. See transorbital lobotomy, under lobotomy.

leukotriene (loo-ko-tri´ēn) Any 20-carbon unsaturated fatty acid derived from arachidonic acid that contains three alternating double bonds; leukotrienes trigger smooth muscle contraction, as in asthma, and have important roles in the inflammatory response.

levallorphan tartrate (lev-ă-lor´fan tar´trāt) White, bitter, crystalline, antianalgesic substance; used in the treatment of narcotics overdose.

levamisole (le-vam´ĭ-sōl) Drug used, along with other drugs, to stimulate the immune system in cancer patients.

levan (lev´an) See fructosan.

levarterenol bitartrate (lev-ar-tĕ-re´nol bi-tar´trāt) A white, crystalline, sympathomimetic substance that is soluble in water. Also called L-norepinephrine bitartrate.

levator (le-va´tor) **1.** Denoting a muscle that raises a body part. **2.** Surgical instrument used to lift a structure or a depressed part such as that of a fractured skull.

level (lev´l) A standard.

Clark's l. See Clark's classification, under classification.

hearing l. The measure of hearing ability as read on the hearing loss scale of the audiometer.

l. of significance The probability that an observed difference is due to some factor or factors other than chance.

toxic blood l. Level of concentration of a drug in the blood at which toxic symptoms are seen.

levodopa, L-Dopa (le-vo-do´pă, ĕl-do´pă) A crystalline powder, 3-hydroxy-L-tyrosine, used to treat Parkinson's disease.

levorotatory (le-vo-ro´tă-tor-e) Denoting the property of certain substances, such as levulose, that turn the plane of polarized light counterclockwise.

levulan (lev´u-lan) See fructosan.

levulin (lev´u-lin) See fructosan.

levulose (lev´u-lōs) See fructose.

levulosuria (lev-u-lo-soo´rĭ-ă) See fructosuria.

Lewis blood group (loo´is blud groop) (La) Antigens of red blood cells, saliva, and other body fluids, specified by the Le gene, that react with the antibodies designated anti-Le^a and anti-Le^b; named after a Mrs. Lewis in whose blood the antibodies were discovered.

lewisite (loo´i-sīt) An oily liquid, $C_2H_2AsCl_3$, used to make a highly poisonous war gas.

libido (lĭ-be´do, lĭ-bi´do) **1.** The emotional energy associated with primitive biologic impulses. **2.** In psychoanalysis, the term is applied to the motive force of the sexual instinct.

library (li´brer-e) **1.** An organized collection of materials kept for information, study, reference, etc. **2.** A building or space where such a collection is kept. **3.** A systematically arranged collection of substances.

chromosome-specific l. A gene library that contains only clones from a specific human chromosome; constructed by the cloning of DNA from chromosomes separated on the basis of size from all other chromosomes; used for screening or isolating a particular gene of interest from a chromosome.

gene l. A set of independently cloned DNA fragments containing the gene of interest and, theoretically, one copy of all the genes of the original source from which the DNA was obtained.

lichen (li´ken) Any eruption of small firm papules on the skin or mucous membranes. Also spelled liken.

l. planus (LP) An eruption of flat papules with depressed purplish centers; the extremities are most commonly involved; may occur also in the oral mucosa as whitish lesions.

l. sclerosus (LS) Chronic condition marked by formation of papules or macules on the mucous membrane of the vulva that eventually coalesce to form whitish plaques of thin, glistening parchment-like patches; usually occurs in postmenopausal women; cause is unknown. Also called kraurosis vulvae; atrophic leukoplakia.

lichenification (li-ken-ĭ-fi-ka´shun) Hardening and thickening of the skin resulting from long-continued irritation.

licorice (lik´o-ris) See glycyrrhiza.

lidocaine hydrochloride (li´do-kān hi-dro-klor´īd) A widely used local anesthetic; also used in the treatment of cardiac arrhythmias; Xylocaine Hydrochloride®.

lie of the fetus (lī ŭv thĕ fe´tus) The relationship that the long axis of the fetus bears to that of the mother.

longitudinal l. Relationship in which the long axis of the fetus is roughly parallel to the long axis of the mother, noted in about 99 percent of all labors at term.

transverse l. Relationship in which the long axis of the fetus is at right angles to that of the mother.

lien (li´en) Latin for spleen.

lienorenal (li-e-no-re´nal) See splenorenal.

life (līf) The state or quality manifested by active metabolism; also called vitality.

life support (līf sup-port´) The act of keeping a person alive.

advanced l.s. (ALS) Emergency medical care, including the use of drugs, electrical stimulation of the heart and respiratory support, to maintain ventilation and blood circulation.

basic l.s. (BLS) Emergency treatment that includes basic first aid, cardiopulmonary resuscitation, and treatment of shock.

ligament (lig´ă-ment) **1.** Any band of thickened white fibrous tissue that connects bones and forms the capsule of joints. **2.** Any membranous fold, sheet, or cordlike structure that holds an organ in position.

acromioclavicular l. Ligament extending from the acromion process of the scapula to the lateral end of the clavicle; it covers the upper part of the capsule of the acromioclavicular joint at the shoulder.

alar l. One of two short, rounded cords connecting the second vertebra (axis) to the occipital bone of the skull. Also called odontoid ligament.

alveolodental l. See periodontal ligament.

annular l. of base of stapes A ring of elastic fibers encircling the base of the stapes (innermost ear ossicle), attaching it to the circumference of the oval window; it permits movement of the ossicle during the transmission of sound vibrations from the eardrum (tympanic membrane) to the inner ear; it also serves as a hinge in response to the contraction of the stapedius muscle.

annular l. of radius An osseofibrous band encircling the head of the radius at the elbow, holding

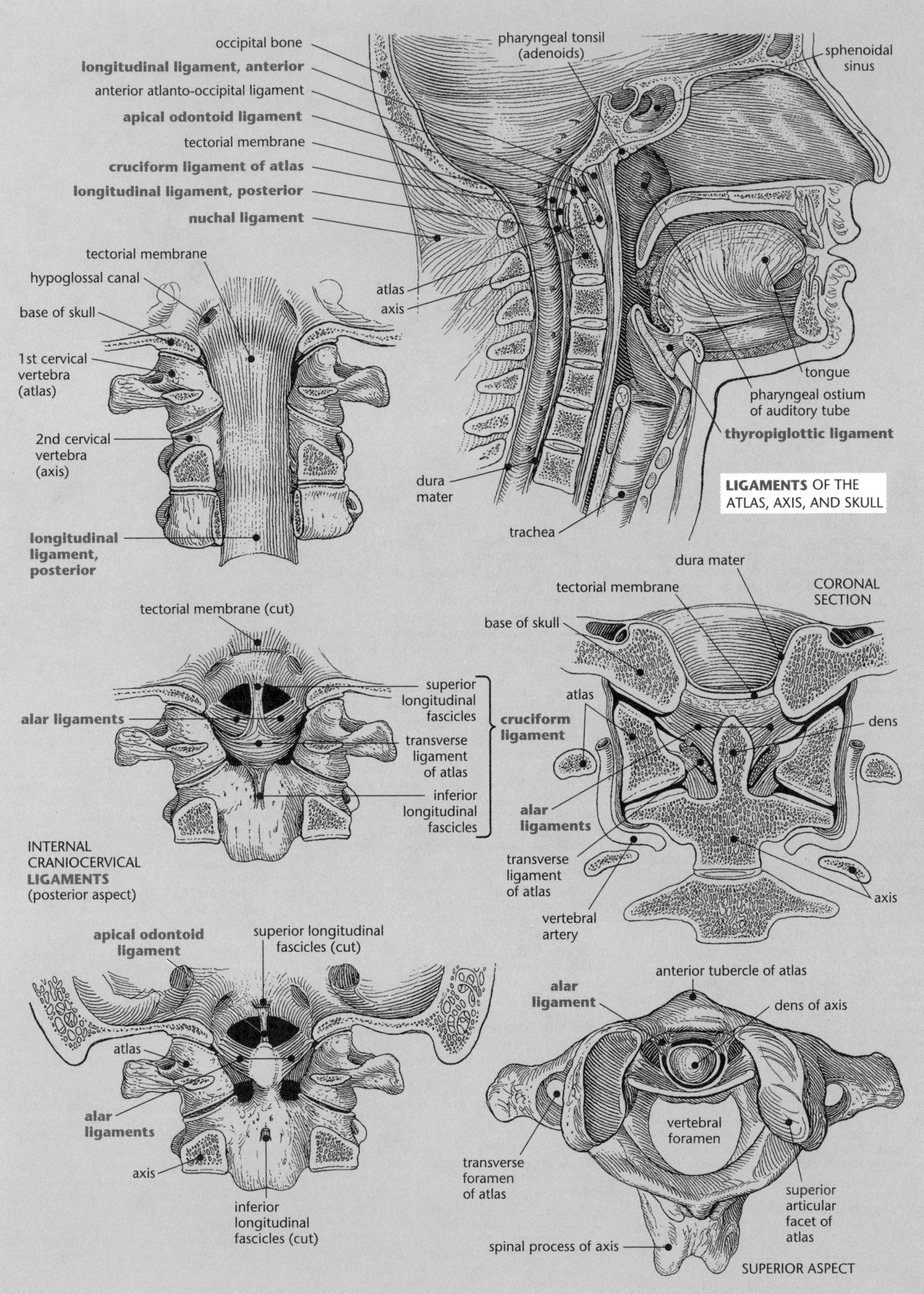
occipital bone
longitudinal ligament, anterior
anterior atlanto-occipital ligament
apical odontoid ligament
tectorial membrane
cruciform ligament of atlas
longitudinal ligament, posterior
nuchal ligament
pharyngeal tonsil (adenoids)
sphenoidal sinus
atlas
axis
tongue
pharyngeal ostium of auditory tube
thyropiglottic ligament
dura mater
trachea
LIGAMENTS OF THE ATLAS, AXIS, AND SKULL
tectorial membrane
hypoglossal canal
base of skull
1st cervical vertebra (atlas)
2nd cervical vertebra (axis)
longitudinal ligament, posterior
tectorial membrane (cut)
alar ligaments
superior longitudinal fascicles
transverse ligament of atlas
inferior longitudinal fascicles
cruciform ligament
INTERNAL CRANIOCERVICAL LIGAMENTS (posterior aspect)
dura mater
tectorial membrane
CORONAL SECTION
base of skull
atlas
dens
alar ligaments
transverse ligament of atlas
vertebral artery
axis
apical odontoid ligament
superior longitudinal fascicles (cut)
atlas
alar ligaments
axis
inferior longitudinal fascicles (cut)
anterior tubercle of atlas
alar ligament
dens of axis
vertebral foramen
transverse foramen of atlas
superior articular facet of atlas
spinal process of axis
SUPERIOR ASPECT

L

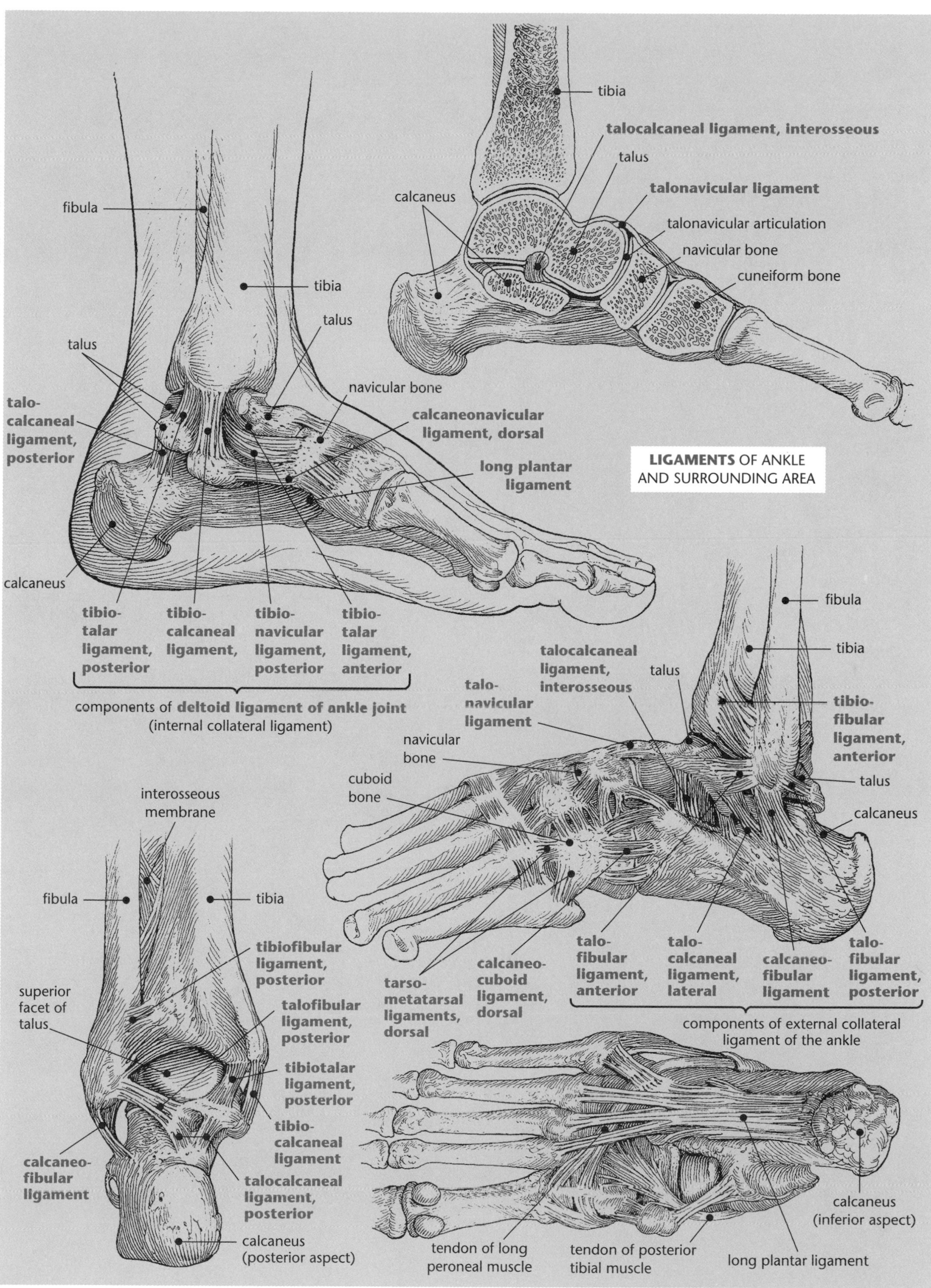
fibula
tibia
talus
talus
talo-calcaneal ligament, posterior
navicular bone
calcaneonavicular ligament, dorsal
long plantar ligament
calcaneus
tibio-talar ligament, posterior
tibio-calcaneal ligament,
tibio-navicular ligament, posterior
tibio-talar ligament, anterior
components of deltoid ligament of ankle joint (internal collateral ligament)
tibia
talocalcaneal ligament, interosseous
talus
talonavicular ligament
calcaneus
talonavicular articulation
navicular bone
cuneiform bone
LIGAMENTS OF ANKLE AND SURROUNDING AREA
fibula
tibia
talocalcaneal ligament, interosseous
talus
talo-navicular ligament
tibio-fibular ligament, anterior
navicular bone
talus
cuboid bone
calcaneus
talo-fibular ligament, anterior
talo-calcaneal ligament, lateral
calcaneo-fibular ligament
talo-fibular ligament, posterior
components of external collateral ligament of the ankle
tarso-metatarsal ligaments, dorsal
calcaneo-cuboid ligament, dorsal
interosseous membrane
fibula
tibia
tibiofibular ligament, posterior
superior facet of talus
talofibular ligament, posterior
tibiotalar ligament, posterior
tibio-calcaneal ligament
calcaneo-fibular ligament
talocalcaneal ligament, posterior
calcaneus (posterior aspect)
calcaneus (inferior aspect)
tendon of long peroneal muscle
tendon of posterior tibial muscle
long plantar ligament

L

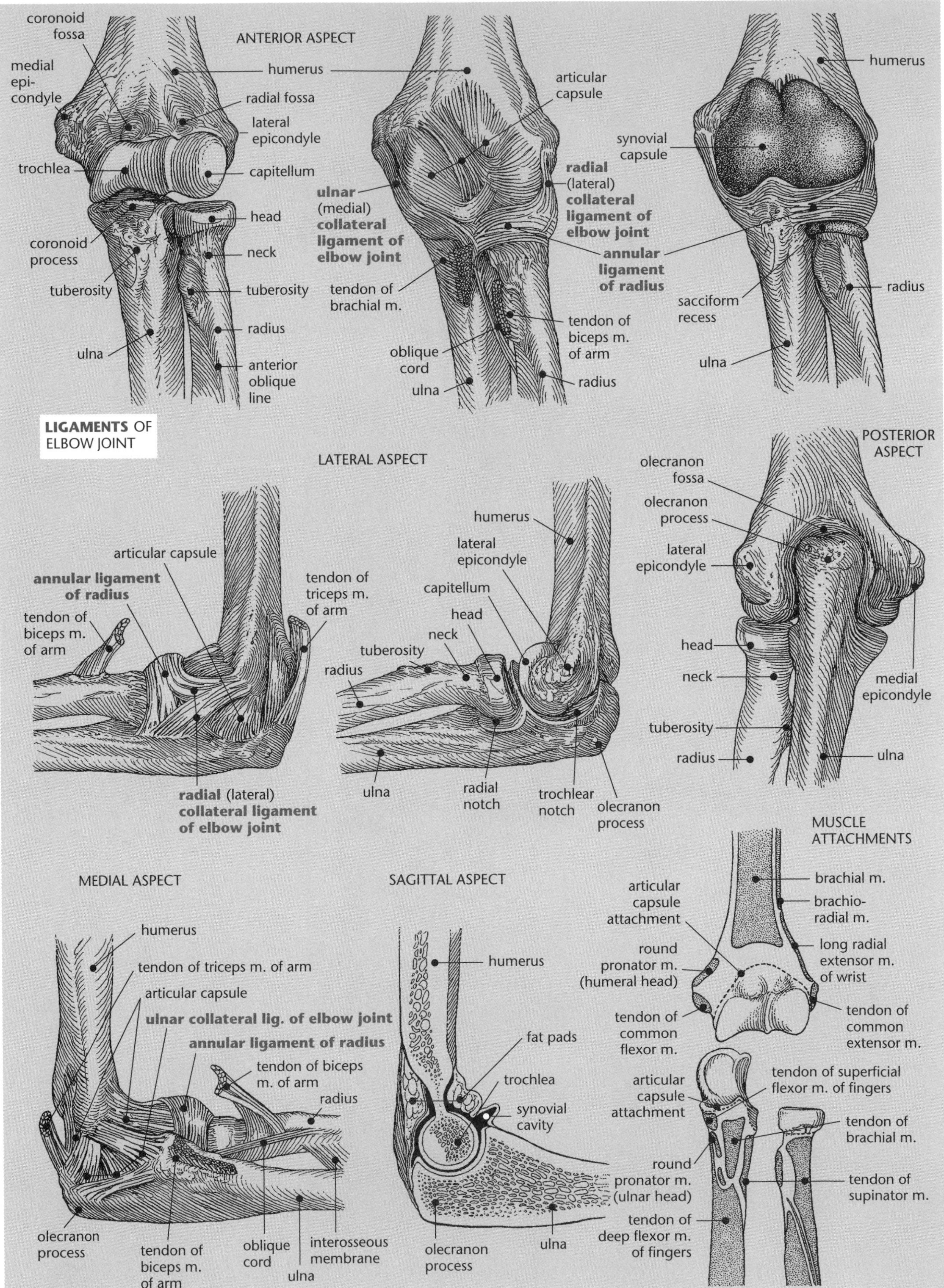
LIGAMENTS OF ELBOW JOINT
ANTERIOR ASPECT
coronoid fossa
medial epi-condyle
trochlea
coronoid process
tuberosity
ulna
humerus
radial fossa
lateral epicondyle
capitellum
head
neck
tuberosity
radius
anterior oblique line
articular capsule
ulnar (medial) collateral ligament of elbow joint
radial (lateral) collateral ligament of elbow joint
annular ligament of radius
tendon of brachial m.
oblique cord
ulna
tendon of biceps m. of arm
radius
humerus
synovial capsule
sacciform recess
ulna
radius
LATERAL ASPECT
articular capsule
annular ligament of radius
tendon of biceps m. of arm
tendon of triceps m. of arm
radial (lateral) collateral ligament of elbow joint
humerus
lateral epicondyle
capitellum
head
neck
tuberosity
radius
ulna
radial notch
trochlear notch
olecranon process
POSTERIOR ASPECT
olecranon fossa
olecranon process
lateral epicondyle
head
neck
tuberosity
radius
medial epicondyle
ulna
MEDIAL ASPECT
humerus
tendon of triceps m. of arm
articular capsule
ulnar collateral lig. of elbow joint
annular ligament of radius
tendon of biceps m. of arm
radius
olecranon process
tendon of biceps m. of arm
oblique cord
ulna
interosseous membrane
SAGITTAL ASPECT
humerus
fat pads
trochlea
synovial cavity
olecranon process
ulna
MUSCLE ATTACHMENTS
articular capsule attachment
round pronator m. (humeral head)
tendon of common flexor m.
brachial m.
brachio-radial m.
long radial extensor m. of wrist
tendon of common extensor m.
articular capsule attachment
round pronator m. (ulnar head)
tendon of deep flexor m. of fingers
tendon of superficial flexor m. of fingers
tendon of brachial m.
tendon of supinator m.
L

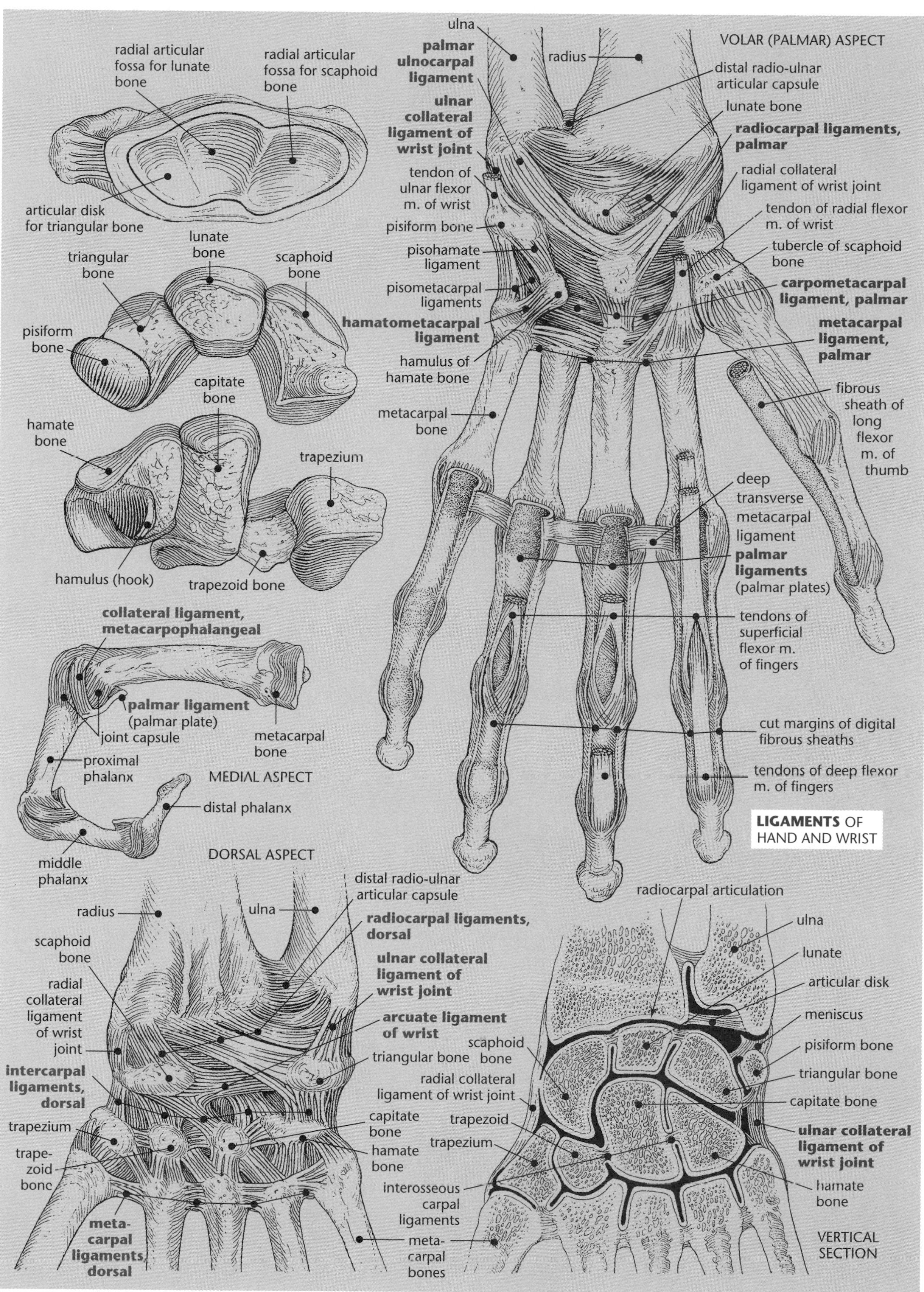
radial articular fossa for lunate bone
radial articular fossa for scaphoid bone
articular disk for triangular bone
lunate bone
triangular bone
scaphoid bone
pisiform bone
capitate bone
hamate bone
trapezium
hamulus (hook)
trapezoid bone
collateral ligament, metacarpophalangeal
palmar ligament (palmar plate)
joint capsule
metacarpal bone
proximal phalanx
MEDIAL ASPECT
distal phalanx
middle phalanx
ulna
radius
VOLAR (PALMAR) ASPECT
palmar ulnocarpal ligament
distal radio-ulnar articular capsule
lunate bone
ulnar collateral ligament of wrist joint
radiocarpal ligaments, palmar
tendon of ulnar flexor m. of wrist
radial collateral ligament of wrist joint
pisiform bone
tendon of radial flexor m. of wrist
pisohamate ligament
tubercle of scaphoid bone
pisometacarpal ligaments
carpometacarpal ligament, palmar
hamatometacarpal ligament
metacarpal ligament, palmar
hamulus of hamate bone
fibrous sheath of long flexor m. of thumb
metacarpal bone
deep transverse metacarpal ligament
palmar ligaments (palmar plates)
tendons of superficial flexor m. of fingers
cut margins of digital fibrous sheaths
tendons of deep flexor m. of fingers
LIGAMENTS OF HAND AND WRIST
DORSAL ASPECT
distal radio-ulnar articular capsule
radius
ulna
radiocarpal ligaments, dorsal
scaphoid bone
ulnar collateral ligament of wrist joint
radial collateral ligament of wrist joint
arcuate ligament of wrist
intercarpal ligaments, dorsal
triangular bone
trapezium
capitate bone
hamate bone
trapezoid bone
metacarpal ligaments, dorsal
meta-carpal bones
radiocarpal articulation
ulna
lunate
articular disk
meniscus
scaphoid bone
pisiform bone
triangular bone
radial collateral ligament of wrist joint
capitate bone
trapezoid
ulnar collateral ligament of wrist joint
trapezium
interosseous carpal ligaments
hamate bone
VERTICAL SECTION

L

L

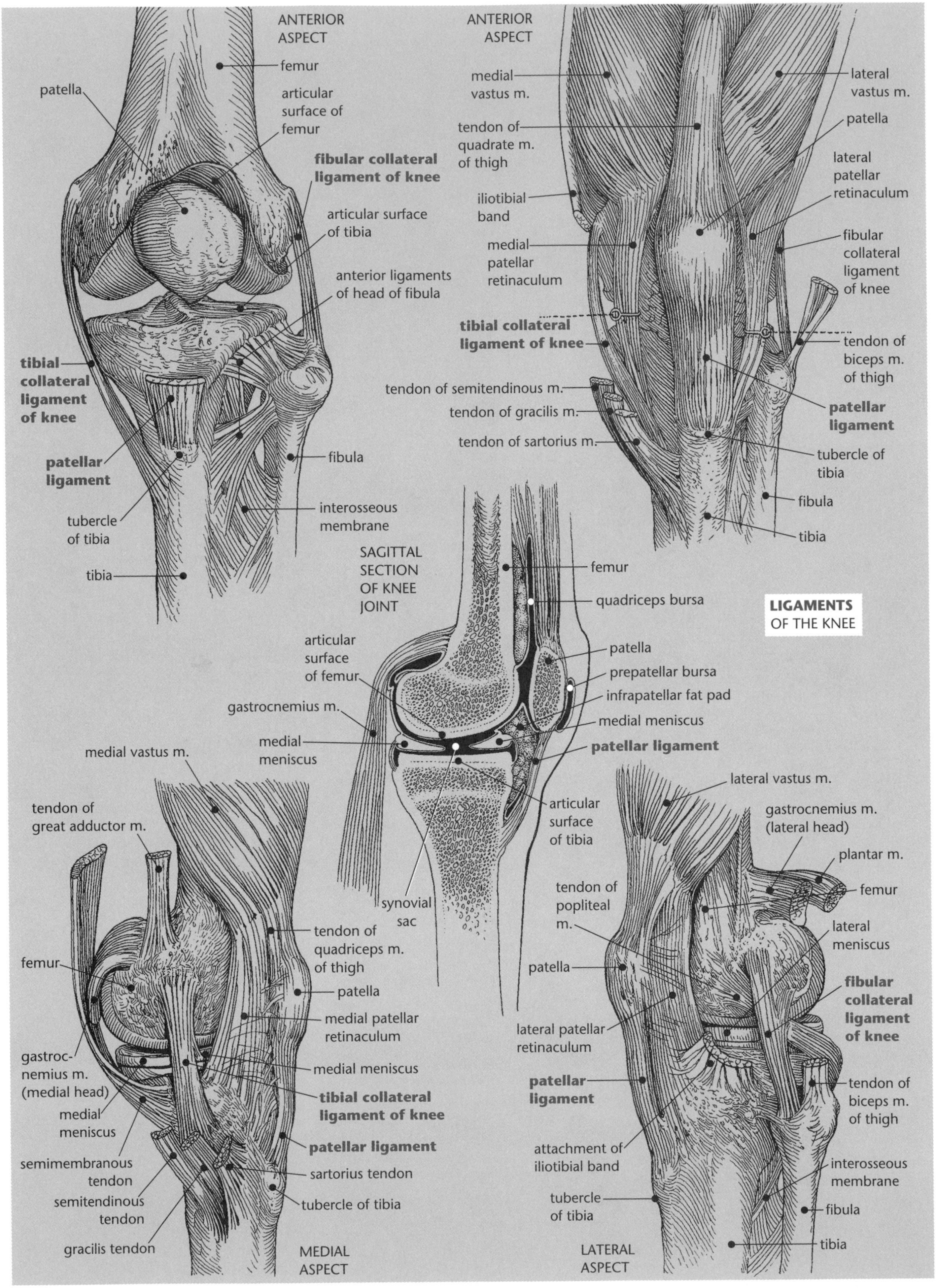

LIGAMENTS OF THE KNEE

ANTERIOR ASPECT

femur
patella
articular surface of femur
fibular collateral ligament of knee
articular surface of tibia
anterior ligaments of head of fibula
tibial collateral ligament of knee
patellar ligament
fibula
interosseous membrane
tubercle of tibia
tibia

ANTERIOR ASPECT

medial vastus m.
lateral vastus m.
patella
tendon of quadrate m. of thigh
lateral patellar retinaculum
iliotibial band
medial patellar retinaculum
fibular collateral ligament of knee
tibial collateral ligament of knee
tendon of biceps m. of thigh
tendon of semitendinous m.
tendon of gracilis m.
patellar ligament
tendon of sartorius m.
tubercle of tibia
fibula
tibia

SAGITTAL SECTION OF KNEE JOINT

femur
quadriceps bursa
patella
articular surface of femur
prepatellar bursa
infrapatellar fat pad
gastrocnemius m.
medial meniscus
medial meniscus
patellar ligament
articular surface of tibia
synovial sac

MEDIAL ASPECT

medial vastus m.
tendon of great adductor m.
tendon of quadriceps m. of thigh
femur
patella
medial patellar retinaculum
gastrocnemius m. (medial head)
medial meniscus
medial meniscus
tibial collateral ligament of knee
patellar ligament
semimembranous tendon
sartorius tendon
semitendinous tendon
tubercle of tibia
gracilis tendon

LATERAL ASPECT

lateral vastus m.
gastrocnemius m. (lateral head)
plantar m.
tendon of popliteal m.
femur
lateral meniscus
patella
fibular collateral ligament of knee
lateral patellar retinaculum
patellar ligament
tendon of biceps m. of thigh
attachment of iliotibial band
interosseous membrane
tubercle of tibia
fibula
tibia

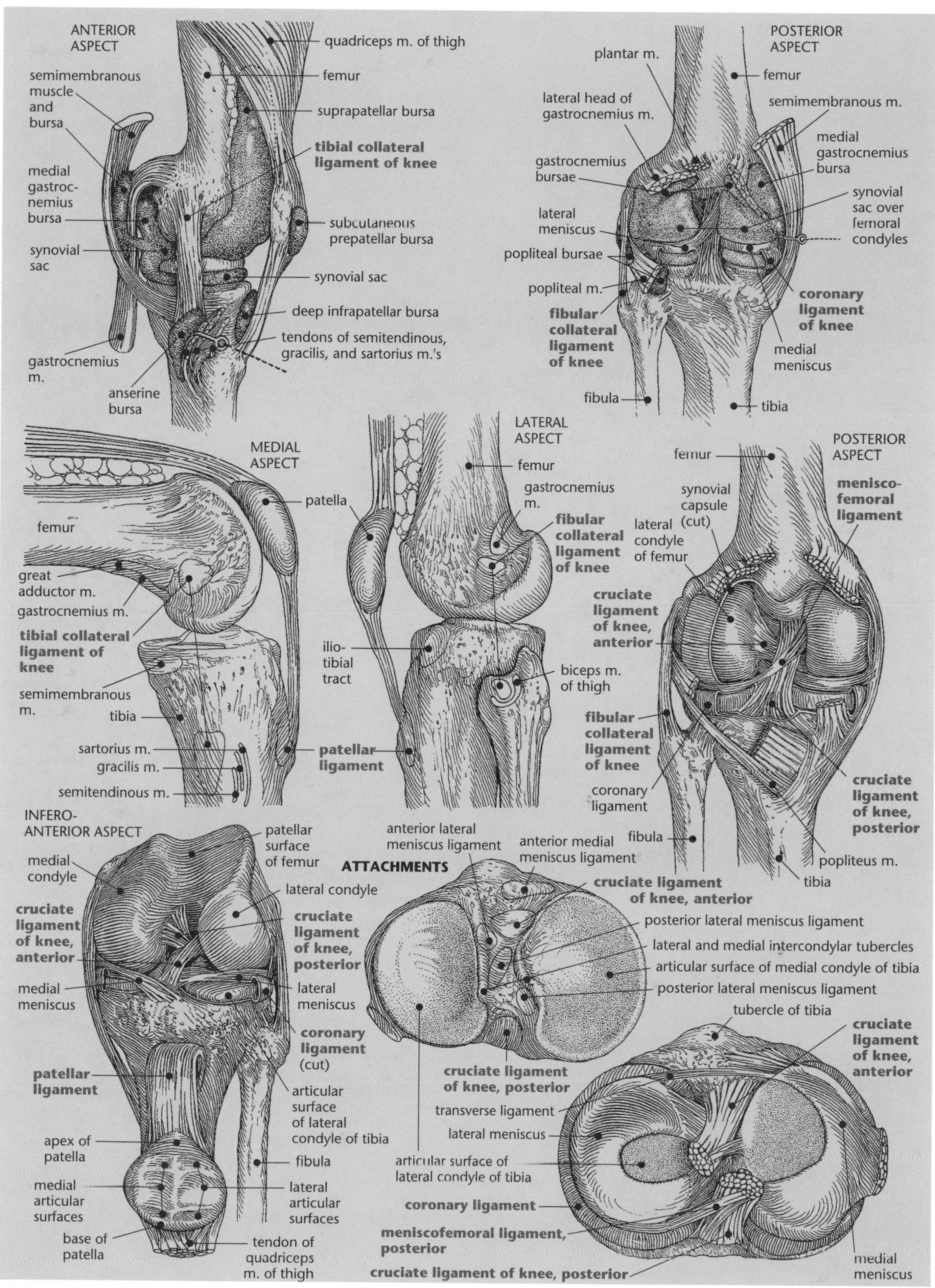

ANTERIOR ASPECT
quadriceps m. of thigh
femur
semimembranous muscle and bursa
suprapatellar bursa
tibial collateral ligament of knee
medial gastrocnemius bursa
subcutaneous prepatellar bursa
synovial sac
synovial sac
deep infrapatellar bursa
tendons of semitendinous, gracilis, and sartorius m.'s
gastrocnemius m.
anserine bursa
POSTERIOR ASPECT
plantar m.
femur
lateral head of gastrocnemius m.
semimembranous m.
medial gastrocnemius bursa
gastrocnemius bursae
synovial sac over femoral condyles
lateral meniscus
popliteal bursae
popliteal m.
coronary ligament of knee
fibular collateral ligament of knee
medial meniscus
fibula
tibia
MEDIAL ASPECT
patella
femur
great adductor m.
gastrocnemius m.
tibial collateral ligament of knee
semimembranous m.
tibia
sartorius m.
gracilis m.
semitendinous m.
patellar ligament
LATERAL ASPECT
femur
gastrocnemius m.
fibular collateral ligament of knee
ilio-tibial tract
biceps m. of thigh
POSTERIOR ASPECT
femur
synovial capsule (cut)
menisco-femoral ligament
lateral condyle of femur
cruciate ligament of knee, anterior
fibular collateral ligament of knee
coronary ligament
fibula
cruciate ligament of knee, posterior
popliteus m.
tibia
INFERO-ANTERIOR ASPECT
patellar surface of femur
medial condyle
lateral condyle
cruciate ligament of knee, anterior
cruciate ligament of knee, posterior
medial meniscus
lateral meniscus
coronary ligament (cut)
patellar ligament
articular surface of lateral condyle of tibia
apex of patella
fibula
medial articular surfaces
lateral articular surfaces
base of patella
tendon of quadriceps m. of thigh
ATTACHMENTS
anterior lateral meniscus ligament
anterior medial meniscus ligament
cruciate ligament of knee, anterior
posterior lateral meniscus ligament
lateral and medial intercondylar tubercles
articular surface of medial condyle of tibia
posterior lateral meniscus ligament
tubercle of tibia
cruciate ligament of knee, anterior
cruciate ligament of knee, posterior
transverse ligament
lateral meniscus
articular surface of lateral condyle of tibia
coronary ligament
meniscofemoral ligament, posterior
cruciate ligament of knee, posterior
medial meniscus
L

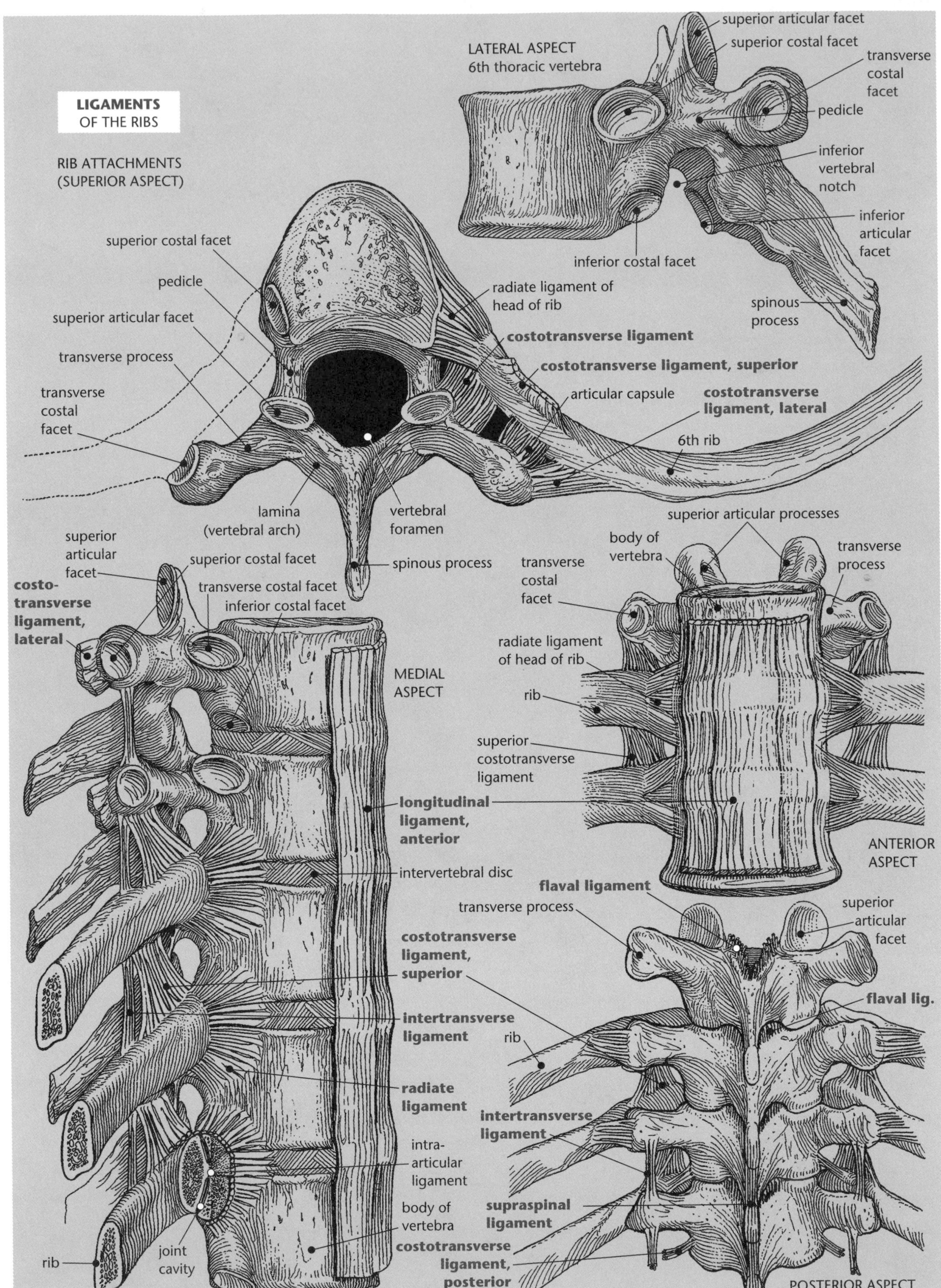
LIGAMENTS
OF THE RIBS
RIB ATTACHMENTS
(SUPERIOR ASPECT)
superior costal facet
pedicle
superior articular facet
transverse process
transverse
costal
facet
lamina
(vertebral arch)
vertebral
foramen
spinous process
radiate ligament of
head of rib
costotransverse ligament
costotransverse ligament, superior
articular capsule
costotransverse
ligament, lateral
6th rib
LATERAL ASPECT
6th thoracic vertebra
superior articular facet
superior costal facet
transverse
costal
facet
pedicle
inferior
vertebral
notch
inferior
articular
facet
inferior costal facet
spinous
process
superior
articular
facet
costo-
transverse
ligament,
lateral
superior costal facet
transverse costal facet
inferior costal facet
MEDIAL
ASPECT
longitudinal
ligament,
anterior
intervertebral disc
costotransverse
ligament,
superior
intertransverse
ligament
radiate
ligament
intra-
articular
ligament
body of
vertebra
rib
joint
cavity
superior articular processes
body of
vertebra
transverse
process
transverse
costal
facet
radiate ligament
of head of rib
rib
superior
costotransverse
ligament
ANTERIOR
ASPECT
flaval ligament
transverse process
superior
articular
facet
flaval lig.
rib
intertransverse
ligament
supraspinal
ligament
costotransverse
ligament,
posterior
POSTERIOR ASPECT

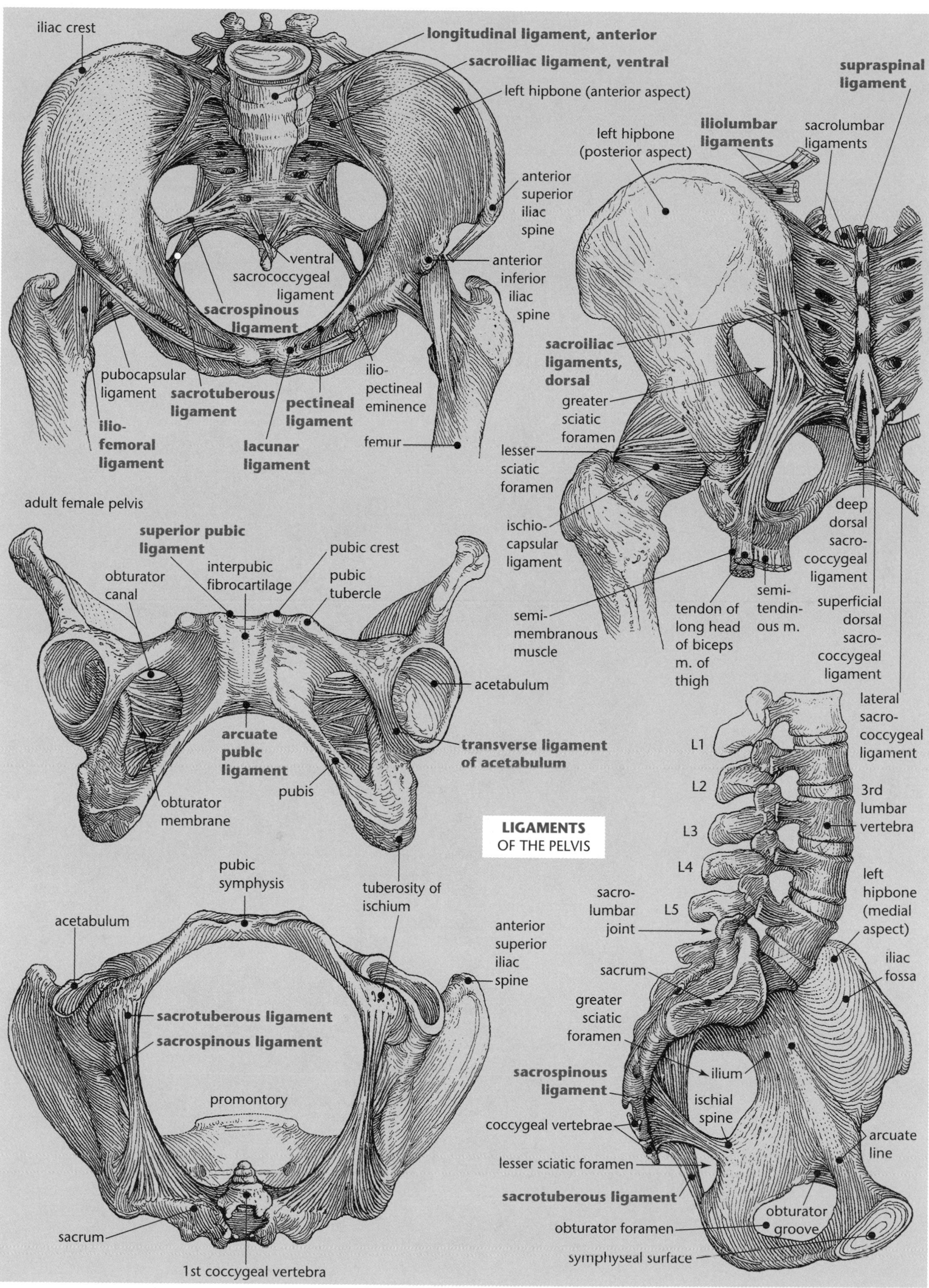
iliac crest
longitudinal ligament, anterior
sacroiliac ligament, ventral
left hipbone (anterior aspect)
anterior superior iliac spine
ventral sacrococcygeal ligament
anterior inferior iliac spine
sacrospinous ligament
pubocapsular ligament
sacrotuberous ligament
pectineal ligament
ilio-pectineal eminence
ilio-femoral ligament
lacunar ligament
femur
adult female pelvis
supraspinal ligament
left hipbone (posterior aspect)
iliolumbar ligaments
sacrolumbar ligaments
sacroiliac ligaments, dorsal
greater sciatic foramen
lesser sciatic foramen
ischio-capsular ligament
semi-membranous muscle
tendon of long head of biceps m. of thigh
semi-tendin-ous m.
deep dorsal sacro-coccygeal ligament
superficial dorsal sacro-coccygeal ligament
lateral sacro-coccygeal ligament
superior pubic ligament
interpubic fibrocartilage
pubic crest
obturator canal
pubic tubercle
acetabulum
arcuate pubic ligament
transverse ligament of acetabulum
pubis
obturator membrane
LIGAMENTS OF THE PELVIS
L1
L2
L3
L4
L5
3rd lumbar vertebra
left hipbone (medial aspect)
pubic symphysis
tuberosity of ischium
acetabulum
anterior superior iliac spine
sacro-lumbar joint
iliac fossa
sacrotuberous ligament
sacrospinous ligament
sacrum
greater sciatic foramen
ilium
sacrospinous ligament
ischial spine
promontory
coccygeal vertebrae
arcuate line
lesser sciatic foramen
sacrotuberous ligament
obturator groove
obturator foramen
sacrum
symphyseal surface
1st coccygeal vertebra

L

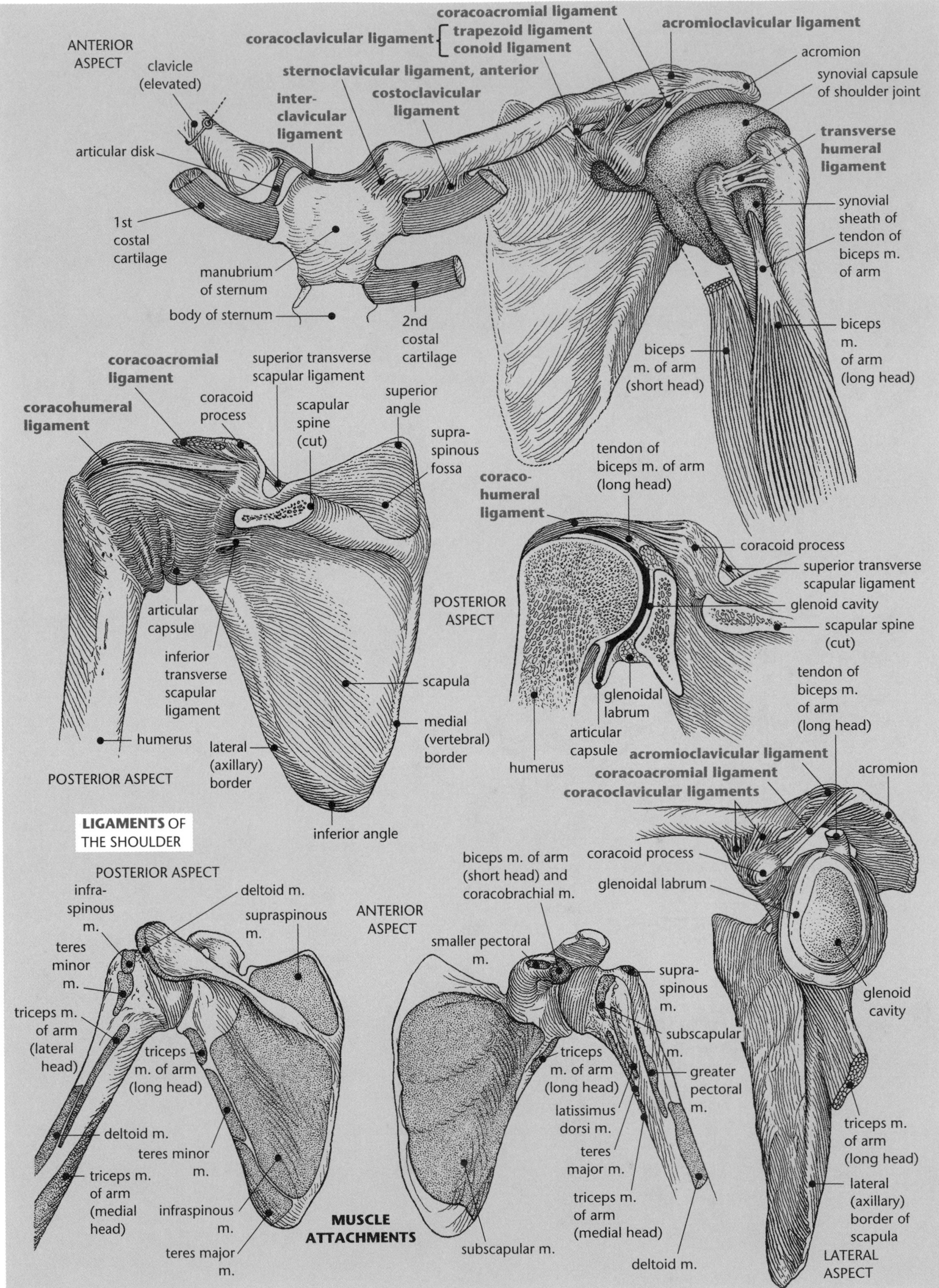
ANTERIOR ASPECT
clavicle (elevated)
articular disk
1st costal cartilage
inter-clavicular ligament
sternoclavicular ligament, anterior
coracoclavicular ligament
trapezoid ligament
conoid ligament
coracoacromial ligament
acromioclavicular ligament
costoclavicular ligament
manubrium of sternum
body of sternum
2nd costal cartilage
acromion
synovial capsule of shoulder joint
transverse humeral ligament
synovial sheath of tendon of biceps m. of arm
biceps m. of arm (short head)
biceps m. of arm (long head)
coracoacromial ligament
coracohumeral ligament
coracoid process
superior transverse scapular ligament
scapular spine (cut)
superior angle
supra-spinous fossa
articular capsule
inferior transverse scapular ligament
scapula
humerus
lateral (axillary) border
medial (vertebral) border
inferior angle
POSTERIOR ASPECT
tendon of biceps m. of arm (long head)
coraco-humeral ligament
coracoid process
superior transverse scapular ligament
glenoid cavity
scapular spine (cut)
POSTERIOR ASPECT
glenoidal labrum
articular capsule
humerus
tendon of biceps m. of arm (long head)
acromioclavicular ligament
coracoacromial ligament
coracoclavicular ligaments
acromion
coracoid process
glenoidal labrum
glenoid cavity
triceps m. of arm (long head)
lateral (axillary) border of scapula
LATERAL ASPECT
LIGAMENTS OF THE SHOULDER
POSTERIOR ASPECT
infra-spinous m.
teres minor m.
deltoid m.
supraspinous m.
triceps m. of arm (lateral head)
triceps m. of arm (long head)
deltoid m.
teres minor m.
triceps m. of arm (medial head)
infraspinous m.
teres major m.
MUSCLE ATTACHMENTS
ANTERIOR ASPECT
smaller pectoral m.
biceps m. of arm (short head) and coracobrachial m.
supra-spinous m.
subscapular m.
triceps m. of arm (long head)
greater pectoral m.
latissimus dorsi m.
teres major m.
triceps m. of arm (medial head)
subscapular m.
deltoid m.

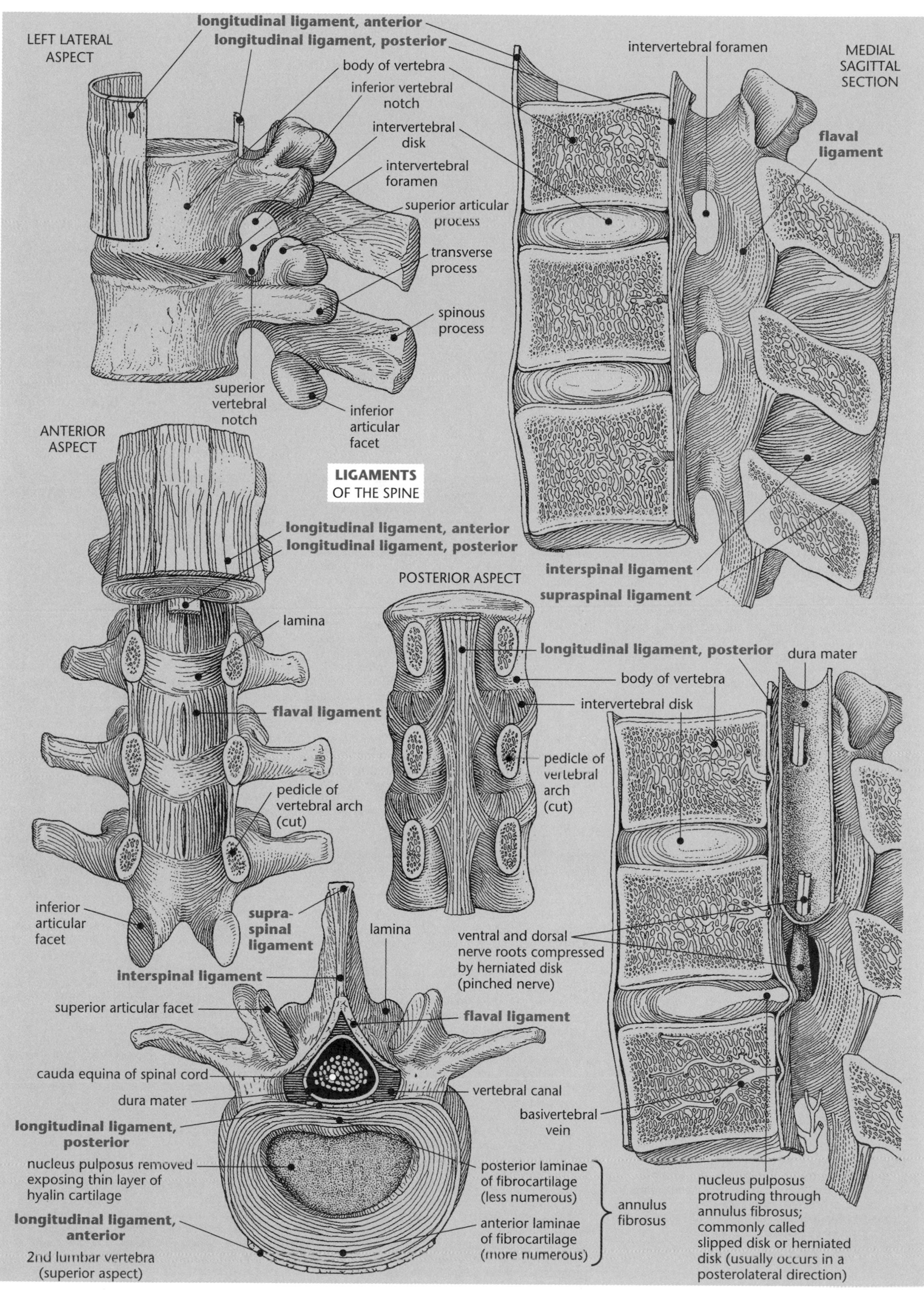
LEFT LATERAL ASPECT
longitudinal ligament, anterior
longitudinal ligament, posterior
body of vertebra
inferior vertebral notch
intervertebral disk
intervertebral foramen
superior articular process
transverse process
spinous process
superior vertebral notch
inferior articular facet
intervertebral foramen
MEDIAL SAGITTAL SECTION
flaval ligament
interspinal ligament
supraspinal ligament
ANTERIOR ASPECT
LIGAMENTS OF THE SPINE
longitudinal ligament, anterior
longitudinal ligament, posterior
lamina
flaval ligament
pedicle of vertebral arch (cut)
inferior articular facet
POSTERIOR ASPECT
longitudinal ligament, posterior
body of vertebra
intervertebral disk
pedicle of vertebral arch (cut)
dura mater
supra-spinal ligament
lamina
interspinal ligament
superior articular facet
flaval ligament
cauda equina of spinal cord
dura mater
vertebral canal
longitudinal ligament, posterior
nucleus pulposus removed exposing thin layer of hyalin cartilage
longitudinal ligament, anterior
2nd lumbar vertebra (superior aspect)
posterior laminae of fibrocartilage (less numerous)
anterior laminae of fibrocartilage (more numerous)
annulus fibrosus
ventral and dorsal nerve roots compressed by herniated disk (pinched nerve)
basivertebral vein
nucleus pulposus protruding through annulus fibrosus; commonly called slipped disk or herniated disk (usually occurs in a posterolateral direction)

L

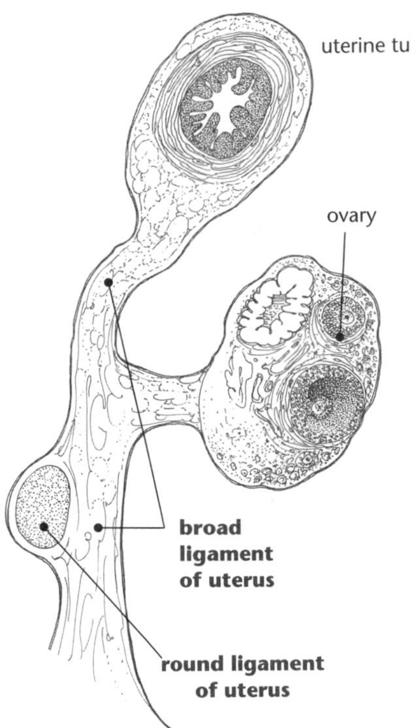

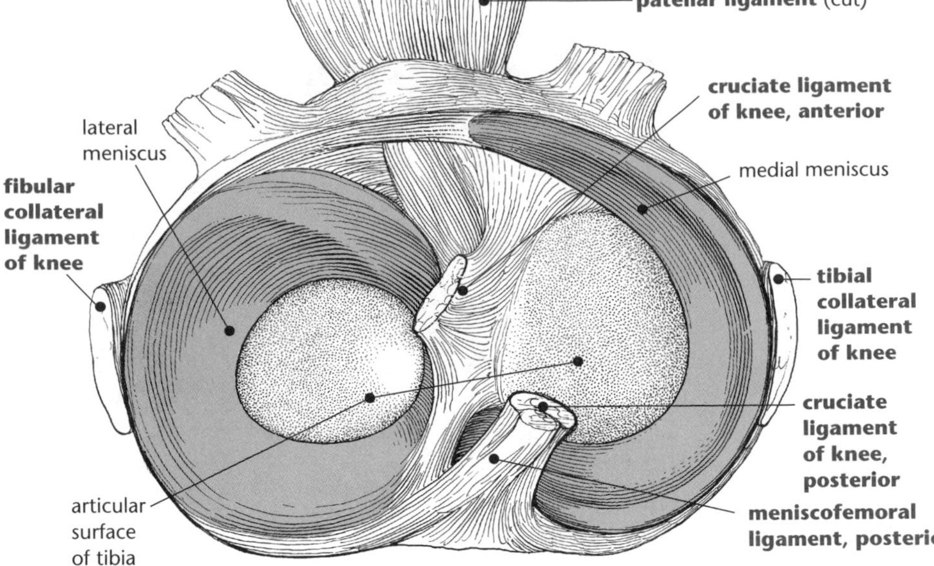

it in contact with the radial notch of the ulna.

anococcygeal l. A mass of fibrous and muscular tissue between the anal canal and the tip of the coccyx to which some of the fibers of the levator ani muscle are attached.

anterior talotibial l. See tibiotalar ligaments.

anterior l. of uterus. See uterovesical fold, under fold.

apical odontoid l. A ligament extending from the tip of the odontoid process (dens) of the second cervical vertebra (axis) to the anterior margin of the foramen magnum of the skull.

arcuate l.'s Two arched ligaments (lateral and medial) that attach the diaphragm to the first lumbar vertebra and the twelfth rib on either side, serving as the origin of the diaphragm.

arcuate l. of knee See arcuate popliteal ligament.

arcuate popliteal l. Y-shaped capsular fibers, with the stem attached to the head of the fibula, the posterior limb arched medially over the tendon of the popliteus muscle, and the anterior limb extending to the lateral epicondyle of the femur. Also called arcuate ligament of knee.

arcuate pubic l. A thick arch of ligamentous fibers connecting the lower border of the pubic symphysis, where it intermingles with the interpubic disk of the symphysis; it forms the upper border of the pubic arch.

arcuate l. of wrist A band stretching transversely from the triquetral bone to the scaphoid bone on the dorsal aspect of the wrist.

atlantoaxial l. The ligament extending from the anteroinferior margin of the first cervical vertebra (atlas) down to the anterosuperior margin of the second cervical vertebra (axis).

bifurcated l. A strong band attached to the front of the upper surface of the calcaneus (heel bone) and dividing anteriorly to form the calcaneonavicular and calcaneocuboid ligaments, attached respectively to the navicular and cuboid bones of the foot.

broad l. of uterus One of two fibrous sheets extending from the lateral surface of the uterus, on either side, to the lateral walls of the pelvis; together with the uterus, it forms a partition across the lesser pelvis, dividing it into an anterior part (containing the bladder) and a posterior one (containing the rectum and part of the sigmoid colon).

calcaneocuboid l. The medial part of the bifurcated ligament that connects the anterior part of the upper surface of the calcaneus (heel bone) to the dorsal part of the cuboid bone of the foot.

calcaneofibular l. A long cordlike band extending from the tip of the lateral malleolus of the fibula downward to the lateral side of the calcaneus (heel bone).

calcaneonavicular l. The lateral part of the bifurcated ligament that connects the calcaneus (heel bone) to the navicular bone of the foot.

calcaneotibial l. See tibiocalcaneal ligament.

capsular l. The fibrous membrane of a joint capsule.

cardinal l. See transverse cervical ligament.

carpometacarpal l. A series of ligaments in the hand reinforcing the joints between the distal row of carpal bones and the second to fifth metacarpal bones: *Dorsal carpometacarpal l.,* strong bands extending from the carpal to the metacarpal bones on their dorsal surface. *Interosseous carpometacarpal l.,* short, thick fibers connecting the capitate and hamate bones (distal row of carpus) to the adjacent surfaces of the third and fourth metacarpal bones. *Palmar carpometacarpal l.,* bands extending from the carpal to the metacarpal bones on their palmar surfaces.

collateral l.'s Collateral ligaments of the hand and foot: *Interphalangeal collateral l.,* strong bands running obliquely along the sides of the phalangeal joints of both hand and foot. *Metacarpophalangeal collateral l.,* strong bands running obliquely along the sides of the joints between the metacarpal bones and adjoining phalanges of the hand. *Metatarsophalangeal collateral l.,* strong bands running obliquely along the sides of the joints between the metatarsal bones and adjoining phalanges of the foot.

conoid l. Part of the coracoclavicular ligament extending from the root of the coracoid process of the scapula (adjacent to the scapular notch) upward to the undersurface of the lateral end of the clavicle.

Cooper's l. (a) See suspensory ligament of breast. (b) See pectineal ligament.

coracoacromial l. A triangular band on the scapula extending from the tip of the acromion to the lateral edge of the coracoid process; it forms a protective arch over the shoulder joint.

coracoclavicular l. A band that connects the coracoid process of the scapula with the overlying undersurface of the lateral end of the clavicle; composed of two parts: the conoid and trapezoid ligaments.

coracohumeral l. A band of fibers extending from the root of the coracoid process to the front of the greater tuberosity of the humerus; it blends with the capsule of the shoulder joint.

coronary l. of knee The part of the fibrous capsule of the knee joint that extends downward to the peripheral margins of the condyle of the tibia and firmly encapsulates the periphery of each meniscus.

costoclavicular l. A short, flattened band extending downward from the bottom of the medial end of the clavicle to the upper surface of the first costal cartilage and adjoining rib.

costotransverse l.'s Ligaments that reinforce the joints between the ribs and the vertebrae: *Lateral costotransverse l.,* the ligament extending from the nonarticular part of the tubercle of each rib (costal tubercle) to the tip of the thoracic transverse process of the corresponding vertebra. *Superior costotransverse l.* the ligament extending from the neck of each rib to the transverse process of the vertebra above.

cricothyroid l. The median part of the cricothyroid membrane; a well defined band of elastic tissue that extends in the midline from the lower border of the thyroid cartilage down to the upper border of the cricoid cartilage. Also called cricovocal membrane.

cruciate l.'s of knee Two ligaments of considerable strength in the middle of the knee joint; they cross each other like the letter X and stabilize the tibia and femur in their anteroposterior glide upon one another: *Anterior cruciate l. of knee,* a band attached below to the front of the intercondylar area of the tibia and above to the back of the medial surface of the lateral condyle of the femur; it partly blends with the anterior end of the lateral meniscus; it is tight on extension and limits excessive anterior mobility of the tibia against the femur. *Posterior cruciate l. of knee,* a band (stronger, shorter and less oblique than the anterior ligament) attached below to the back of the intercondylar area of the tibia and above to the lateral surface of the medial condyle of the femur; it partly blends with the posterior end of the lateral meniscus; it limits posterior mobility and is tight on flexion.

cruciform l. of atlas A cross-shaped ligament consisting of two parts; a thick transverse band that arches within the ring of the first cervical vertebra and divides the vertebral foramen into two unequal parts, and a vertical band extending upward from the transverse band to the anterior margin of the foramen magnum and downward from the transverse band to the back of the body of the second cervical vertebra.

crural l. Inguinal ligament.

deep transverse metacarpal l.'s Three short, wide, flattened bands in the hand that connect transversely the palmar ligaments of the 2nd, 3rd, 4th, and 5th metacarpophalangeal joints to one another.

deep transverse metatarsal l.'s Four short, wide, flattened bands in the foot that connect the plantar ligaments of the 1st, 2nd, 3rd, 4th, and 5th metatarsophalangeal joints to one another.

deltoid l. of ankle joint The medial reinforcing ligament of the ankle joint, composed of the tibiocalcaneal, anterior tibiotalar, posterior tibiotalar, and tibionavicular ligaments; they pass downward from the medial malleolus of the tibia to the navicular bone, calcaneus and talus, respectively. Also called internal collateral ligament of ankle; medial collateral

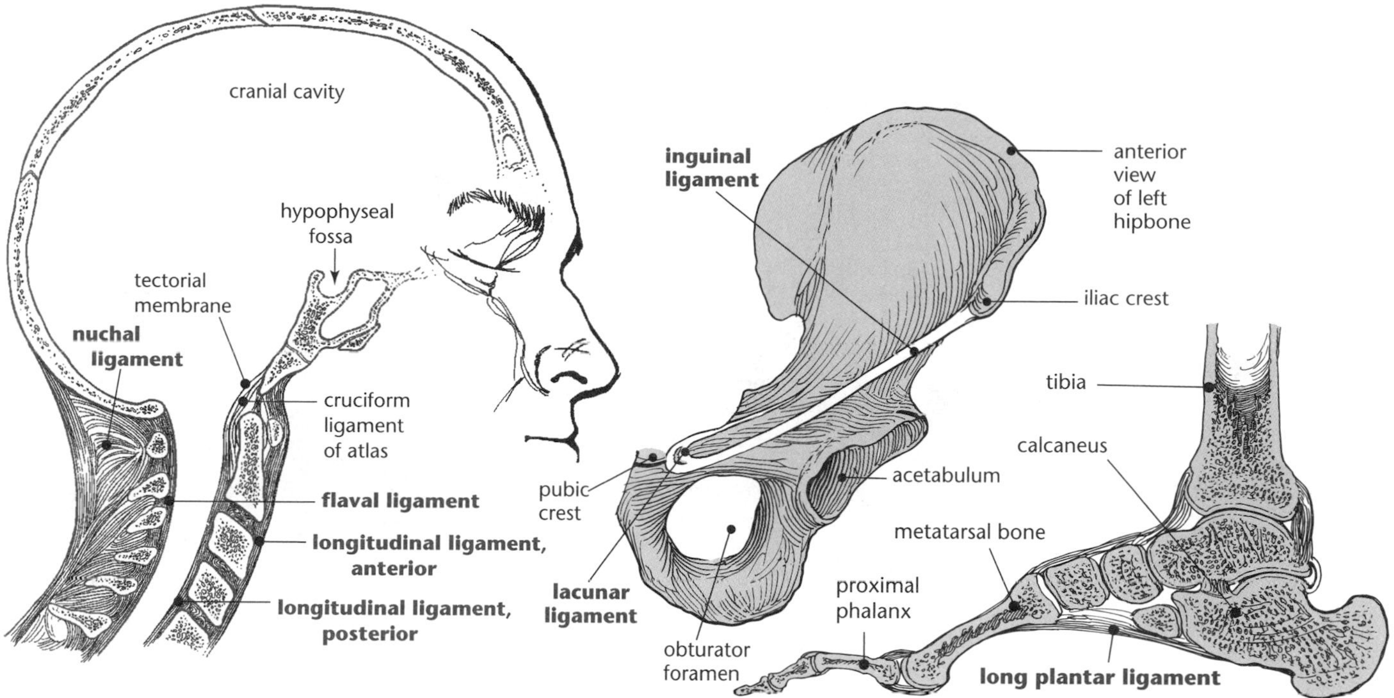

ligament of ankle.

external collateral l. of ankle See lateral collateral ligament of ankle.

falciform l. of liver A median sickle-shaped ligament composed of two layers of peritoneum connecting the liver to the diaphragm and anterior abdominal wall as low as the level of the umbilicus; it contains the round ligament of the liver between its layers.

fibular collateral l. of knee A strong, round, fibrous cord on the lateral side of the knee joint, extending from the lateral epicondyle of the femur to the lateral side of the head of the fibula. Also called lateral collateral ligament of knee.

flaval l.'s A series of yellow elastic bands that bind together the laminae of adjacent vertebrae from the first cervical vertebra to the first sacral vertebra; they serve to maintain the upright position.

fundiform l. of penis A thickened fibroelastic tissue that is intimately adherent to the lower part of the linea alba and the top of the pubic symphysis and extends to the dorsum of the penis.

glenohumeral l.'s Three thick fibrous bands (superior, middle, and inferior) overhanging the anterior portion of the shoulder joint capsule, extending from the anterior border of the glenoid cavity to the lesser tuberosity and neck of the humerus.

hamatometacarpal l. A ligament that passes from the palmar aspect of the hook of the hamate bone of the wrist to the base of the 5th metacarpal bone.

l. of head of femur A flattened intracapsular band at the hip joint originating from the head of the femur and attaching by two bands to the acetabulum, one on each side of the acetabular notch; it blends with the transverse ligament of acetabulum. Also called round ligament of femur.

hyoepiglottic l. A short triangular elastic band uniting the anterior surface of the upper epiglottic cartilage to the upper part of the hyoid bone.

iliofemoral l. A strong triangular ligament overlying the hip joint and blending with its capsule; it extends from the bottom of the anterior inferior iliac spine, broadening out as it descends to the trochanteric line of the femur.

iliolumbar l.'s Strong bands extending from the transverse processes of the 4th and 5th lumbar vertebrae to the inner lip of the posterior iliac crest and the lateral side of the upper sacrum; they blend below with the ventral sacroiliac ligament.

inguinal l. The thickened upturned lower margin of the aponeurosis of the external oblique muscle, extending from the anterior superior spine of the ilium to the tubercle of the pubic bone. Also called Poupart's ligament.

intercarpal l.'s A series of dorsal, interosseous and palmar ligaments that unite the wrist (carpal) bones with one another.

interclavicular l. A strong band of curved fibers connecting the medial (sternal) ends of the two clavicles across the suprasternal notch.

interfoveolar l. The thickened portion of the transverse fascia that lies medial to the deep inguinal ring, connecting the transverse muscle of the abdomen to the inguinal ligament and pectineal fascia; it is inconstant. Also called Hesselbach's ligament.

internal collateral l. of ankle See deltoid ligament of ankle joint.

interspinal l.'s A series of short ligaments connecting the spinous processes of adjoining vertebrae; they abut the flaval ligament in front and the supraspinal ligament behind.

intertransverse l.'s A series of weak ligaments connecting the tips of adjacent transverse processes of vertebrae, mainly in the lumbar region.

lacunar l. A triangular band extending horizontally from the medial end of the inguinal ligament to the iliopectineal line of the hipbone.

lateral collateral l. of ankle The lateral reinforcing ligament of the ankle joint, consisting of the posterior talofibular ligament, calcaneofibular ligament, and the anterior talofibular ligament. Also called external collateral ligament of ankle.

lateral collateral l. of elbow See radial collateral ligament of elbow joint.

lateral collateral l. of knee See fibular collateral ligament of knee.

longitudinal l.'s Long, broad, flat bands of fibers reinforcing the articulations of the vertebral bodies: *Anterior longitudinal l.,* a band of fibers extending along the anterior surface of the vertebral bodies from the base of the skull to the upper part of the sacrum; it is firmly fixed to the intervertebral disks and is thickest in the thoracic area. *Posterior longitudinal l.,* a band of fibers on the posterior surface of the vertebral canal, extending from the second cervical vertebra to the upper part of the sacrum; it is attached to the intervertebral disks.

long plantar l. A thick band (the longest of the tarsal ligaments) extending from the plantar surface of the calcaneus and dividing into deep fibers, which attach to the plantar surface of the cuboid bone, and superficial fibers which attach to the proximal ends of the 2nd, 3rd, 4th metatarsal bones; it limits the flattening of the lateral longitudinal arch of the foot.

medial collateral l. of elbow See ulnar collateral ligament of the elbow joint.

medial collateral l. of knee See tibial collateral ligament of knee.

medial collateral l. of wrist See ulnar collateral ligament of wrist joint.

medial umbilical l.'s Two fibrous cords passing along the bladder to the navel; formed by the remains of the obliterated umbilical arteries.

median umbilical l. A fibrous cord extending on the midline from the apex of the bladder to the navel; formed by the remains of the obliterated urachus. Also called middle umbilical ligament; urachal ligament.

meniscofemoral l.'s Meniscus ligaments of the knee joint: *Anterior meniscofemoral l.,* an inconstant oblique band passing from the posterior end of the lateral meniscus in the knee joint to the medial condyle of the femur; it passes anterior to the posterior cruciate ligament. *Posterior meniscofemoral l.,* a strong band passing upward and medially from the posterior end of the lateral meniscus in the knee to the medial condyle of the femur; it passes behind the posterior cruciate ligament.

metacarpal l.'s Ligaments that strengthen the proximal metacarpal articulations of the hand: *Dorsal metacarpal l.'s,* short transverse bands uniting the dorsal surface of the bases of the 2nd, 3rd, 4th, and 5th metacarpal bones with one another. *Interosseous metacarpal l.'s.,* short bands connecting the contiguous surfaces of the metacarpal bones of the hand. *Palmar metacarpal l.'s,* short transverse bands uniting the palmar surface of the bases of the 2nd to 5th metacarpal bones with one another.

middle umbilical l. See median umbilical ligament.

nuchal l. A broad, somewhat triangular membranous septum in the back of the neck extending from the tips of the cervical spinous processes to the external occipital crest of the skull: it forms a septum for attachment of muscles on either side of the neck.

oblique posterior l. of knee A ligament from the tendon of the semimembranous muscle (near its insertion), extending obliquely to the posterior part of the knee joint capsule.

odontoid l. See alar ligament.

ovarian l. A cordlike bundle of fibers between the layers of the broad ligament of uterus, joining the uterine end of the ovary to the lateral margin of the uterus, on either side, immediately behind the attachment of the uterine (fallopian) tube.

palmar l.'s Fibrocartilaginous plates on the palmar surfaces of the metacarpophalangeal joints, firmly united to the bases of the proximal phalanges and loosely connected to the metacarpal bones.

palmar ulnocarpal l. A rounded fibrous band passing downward and laterally from the base of the styloid process of the ulna and the front of the articular disk of the distal radioulnar joint to the palmar surface of the hamate and triquetral bones (proximal row of wrist bones).

palpebral l.'s Ligaments of the eyelids: *Lateral*

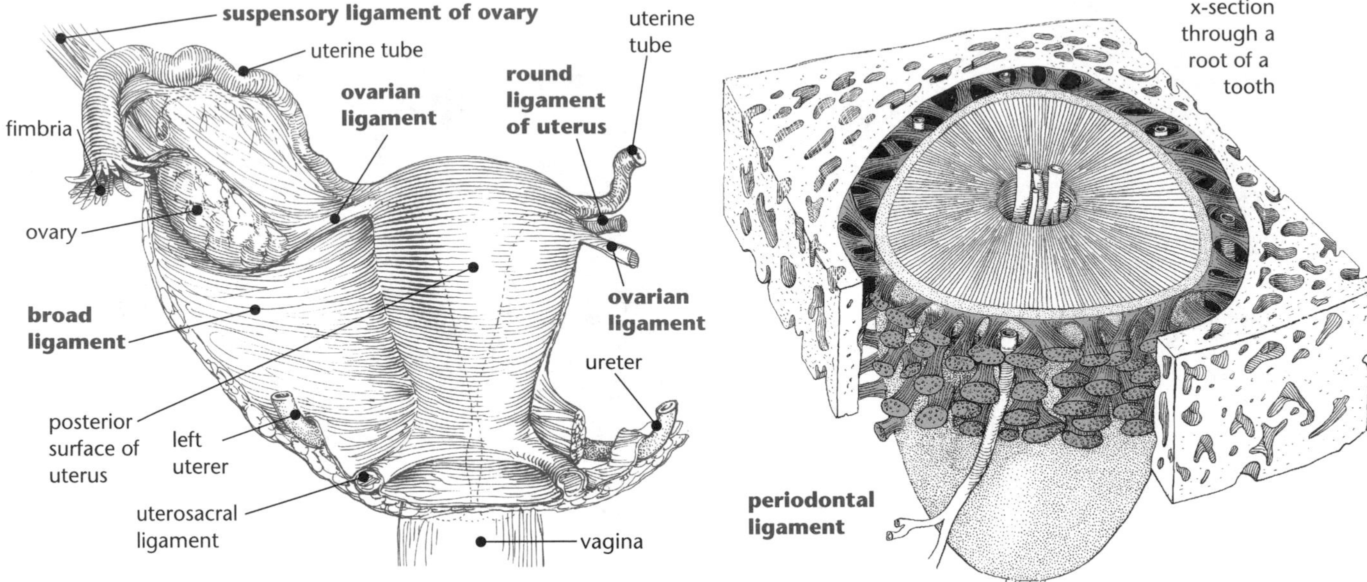

palpebral l., a thin band connecting the lateral ends of the tarsal plates of the eyelids to the zygomatic bone, just within the orbital margin. *Medial palpebral l.,* a tendinous band connecting the medial ends of the tarsal plates of the eyelids to the frontal process of the maxilla, in front of the nasolacrimal groove.

patellar l. The continuation of the strong, flattened common tendon of the quadriceps muscle of thigh from the patella (kneecap) downward to the tuberosity of the tibia; in the adult it is about 8 cm in length.

pectineal l. A strong fibrous band extending from the upper border of the pectineal surface of the hipbone to the medial end of the lacunar ligament at the groin, with which it is continuous. Also called Cooper's ligament.

periodontal l. Connective tissue fibers that attach the root of a tooth to the bone of its socket. Also called alveolodental ligament; periodontal membrane.

phrenicocolic l. A fold of peritoneum attaching the left flexure of the colon to the diaphragm, on which rests the base of the spleen.

posterior talotibial l. See tibiotalar ligaments.

posterior l. of uterus See rectovaginal fold, under fold.

Poupart's l. See inguinal ligament.

pubic l.'s (a) See arcuate pubic ligament. (b) See superior pubic ligament.

radial collateral l. of elbow joint A fan-shaped ligament extending from the bottom part of the lateral epicondyle of the humerus to the annular ligament of the radius and the upper end of the supinator crest of the ulna. Also called lateral collateral ligament of elbow.

radiate l. A fan-shaped band extending from the side of the bodies of two adjoining vertebrae to the head of the rib with which it articulates. Also called radiate ligament of head of rib.

radiate l. of head of rib See radiate ligament.

radiocarpal l.'s Ligaments of the wrist joint: *Dorsal radiocarpal l.,* a thin sheath of ligamentous tissue overlying the wrist joint, extending from the distal end of the radius to the dorsal surface of the proximal row of wrist bones (triquetral, lunate, and scaphoid bones); it blends with the underlying articular disk of the inferior radioulnar articulation. *Palmar radiocarpal l.,* a broad membranous band extending from the anterior aspects of the lower end of the radius and its styloid process to the anterior surface of the proximal row of wrist bones (triquetral, lunate, and scaphoid bones), and occasionally to the capitate bone.

reflected inguinal l. A small, frequently absent, triangular sheet extending from the medial part of the inguinal ring to the linea alba.

round l. of femur See ligament of head of femur.

round l. of liver A fibrous cord (the remains of the fetal umbilical vein) extending from the anterior abdominal wall at the level of the umbilicus to the inferior surface of the liver.

round l. of uterus A fibromuscular ligamentous cord that extends from the lateral margin of the uterus, on either side, traverses the inguinal canal and attaches to the connective tissue of the labium majus.

sacrococcygeal l.'s The five ligaments uniting the lower portion of the sacrum and the coccyx: *anterior sacrococcygeal l., deep posterior sacrococcygeal l., superficial posterior sacrococcygeal l.,* and two *lateral sacrococcygeal l.'s.*

sacroiliac l.'s Ligaments that bind the sacrum with the ilium of the hipbone: *Dorsal (posterior) sacroiliac l.,* a set of thick fibrous bands overlying the interosseous sacroiliac ligament, consisting of a lower, superficial group (long posterior sacroiliac ligament) that extends from the posterior superior iliac spine of the hipbone to the transverse tubercles of the third and fourth segments of the sacrum (the bands blend with the sacrotuberous ligament); and an upper, deep group (short posterior sacroiliac ligament) that extends from the posterior inferior iliac spine and adjacent part of the ilium to the back of the sacrum. *Interosseous sacroiliac l.,* short, thick bundles of fibers interconnecting the sacral and iliac tuberosities, posterior to their articular surfaces. *Ventral (anterior) sacroiliac l.,* a thin, wide, fibrous layer reinforcing the anterior part of the articular capsule of the sacroiliac joint and stretching from the ala and pelvic surface of the sacrum to the adjoining parts of the ilium.

sacrospinous l. A strong triangular ligament attached by its apex to the spine of the ischium of the hipbone and by its base to the lateral part of the lower sacrum and coccyx.

sacrotuberous l. A long, strong triangular ligament extending from the tuberosity of the ischium of the hipbone to the lateral part of the sacrum and coccyx and to the superior and inferior posterior iliac spine.

sphenomandibular l. A flat, thin fibrous band that extends from the spine of the sphenoid bone, becoming broader as it descends to the lingula of the mandibular foramen.

sternoclavicular l.'s Ligaments that reinforce the sternoclavicular joint: *Anterior sternoclavicular l.,* a short, broad band overlying the front of the sternoclavicular joint, extending from the medial end of the clavicle to the front of the upper sternum and adjoining costal cartilage. *Posterior sternoclavicular l.,* a short, broad band overlying the back of the sternoclavicular joint, extending from the medial end of the clavicle to the back of the upper sternum and adjoining costal cartilage.

stylomandibular l. A condensed band of deep cervical fascia extending from the tip of the styloid process, downward to the posterior margin of the angle of the lower jaw.

superior pubic l. A transverse band that binds the two pubic bones superiorly, and extends as far as the pubic tubercles; it is firmly attached to the interpubic disk at the midline.

supraspinal l. A strong fibrous band that connects the tips of the spinous processes from the 7th cervical vertebra to the sacrum; it blends with the interspinous ligament. From the 7th cervical vertebra to the base of the skull, it expands to form the nuchal ligament.

suspensory l. of breast One of numerous fibrous bands distributed between the lobes of the mammary glands, extending from the overlying skin to the underlying pectoral fascia. Also called Cooper's ligament.

suspensory l. of lens See ciliary zonula, under zonula.

suspensory l. of ovary A band of peritoneum arising from the ovary and extending upward over the iliac vessels to become continuous with the lateral wall of the pelvis; it contains the ovarian vessels and nerves.

talocalcaneal l.'s Fibrous bands reinforcing the two articulations between the talus (ankle bone) and the calcaneus (heel bone): *Anterior talocalcaneal l.,* a band extending from the upper anterior part of the neck of the talus to the upper surface of the calcaneus. *Interosseous talocalcaneal l.,* a strong, broad, flattened band extending obliquely from the deep groove of the talus to the deep groove of the calcaneus. *Lateral talocalcaneal l.,* a short, flattened band extending from the lateral process of the talus and passing downward and backward to the lateral surface of the calcaneus. *Medial talocalcaneal l.,* a band extending from the medial tubercle of the talus to the medial surface of the calcaneus; it blends with the deltoid ligament. *Posterior talocalcaneal l.,* a short, wide band extending from the posterior process of the talus, downward to the adjacent calcaneus.

talofibular l.'s Ligaments of the ankle joint: *Anterior talofibular l.,* a ligament stretching from the anterior margin of the lateral malleolus of the fibula to the lateral aspect of the neck of the talus. *Posterior talofibular l.,* a ligament stretching from the posterior margin of the lateral malleolus of the fibula to the posterior process of the talus.

talonavicular l. A broad, thin band, extending from the neck of the talus (ankle bone) to the dorsal surface of the adjoining navicular bone of the foot.

tarsometatarsal l.'s Ligaments reinforcing the

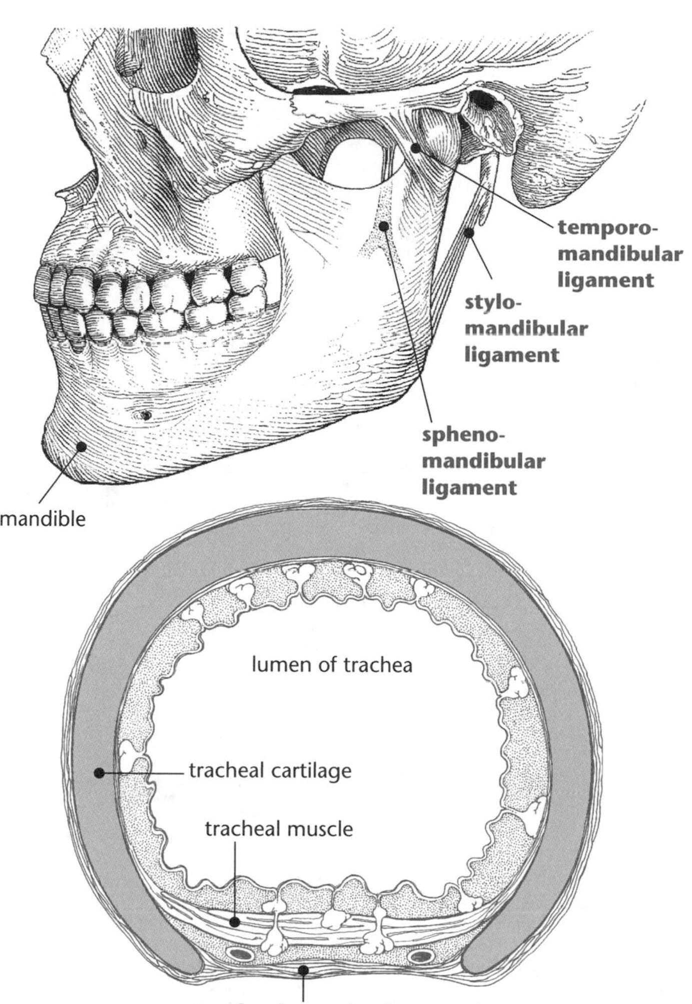

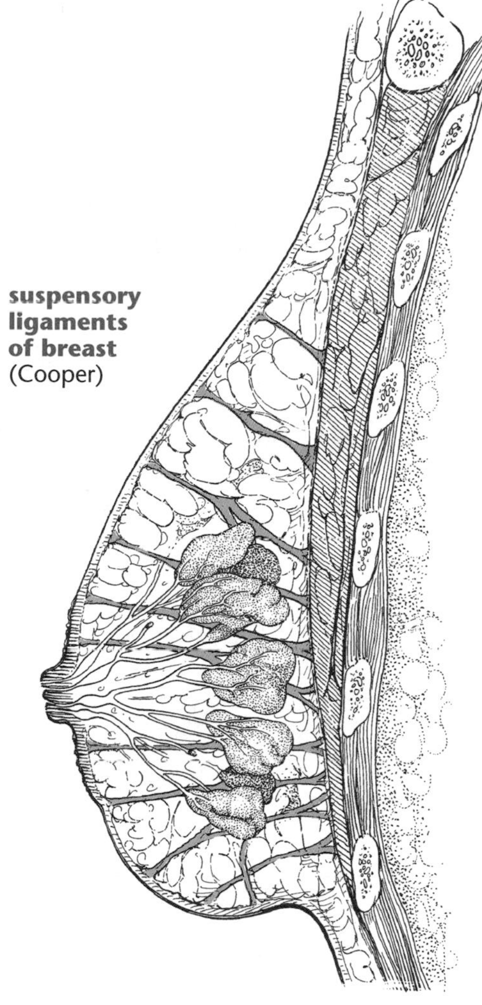

joints between the tarsus and the metatarsal bones of the foot: *Dorsal tarsometatarsal l.'s,* strong, flat bands connecting the dorsal surface of the proximal metatarsal bones to the distal tarsus (cuboid and three cuneiform bones). *Interosseous tarsometatarsal l.'s,* bands from the first and third cuneiform bones to the second and fourth metatarsal bones, respectively. *Plantar tarsometatarsal l.'s,* oblique bands connecting the plantar surface of the proximal metatarsal bones to the distal tarsus (cuboid and three cuneiform bones).

temporomandibular l. An oblique band extending downward and backward from the lower surface of the zygomatic process to the posterolateral surface margin of the neck of the lower jaw.

thyroepiglottic l. An elastic ligament that attaches the stalk (petiole) of the lower end of the epiglottic cartilage to the back of the thyroid cartilage, just below the notch.

tibial collateral l. of knee A broad, flat membranous band, posteromedial to the knee joint, extending from the medial epicondyle of the femur to the medial condyle and medial surface of the tibia; consists of two parts: a short, deep, thick posterior band, and a longer anterior band, extending from the femoral epicondyle and fanning out into a broad expansion on the anteromedial surface of the tibia. Also called medial collateral ligament of knee.

tibiocalcaneal l. The widest part of the deltoid ligament of the ankle joint extending from the medial malleolus of the tibia to the median projection (sustentaculum tali) of the calcaneus. Also called calcaneotibial ligament.

tibiofibular l.'s Ligaments connecting the tibia and fibula at the proximal and distal ends: *Anterior (superior) tibiofibular l.,* flat bands that extend from the front of the head of the fibula to the front of the lateral condyle of the tibia. *Anterior (inferior) tibiofibular l.,* a flattened oblique band extending downward and laterally from the distal end of the front of the tibia to the adjoining fibula. *Posterior (superior) tibiofibular l.,* thick band that extends from the back of the head of the fibula to the back of the lateral condyle of the tibia. *Posterior (inferior) tibiofibular l.,* a strong oblique band extending downward and laterally from the distal end of the back of the tibia to the adjoining fibula; its lowest part extends transversely from the fibula to the talus (ankle bone).

tibionavicular l. The part of the deltoid ligament of the ankle joint extending from the medial malleolus of the tibia to the tubercle on the dorsal side of the navicular bone.

tibiotalar l.'s Parts of the deltoid ligament of the ankle joint: *Anterior tibiotalar l.,* the deep part extending from the medial malleolus of the tibia to the medial surface of the talus. Also called anterior talotibial ligament. *Posterior tibiotalar l.,* the part that extends from the medial malleolus of the tibia, posteriorly to the medial side of the ankle bone (talus) and its tubercle. Also called posterior talotibial ligament.

tracheal annular l. The fibroelastic membrane that connects the ends of the incomplete tracheal rings posteriorly.

transverse l. of acetabulum A strong flattened ligament that is attached to the margin of the acetabulum and crosses the acetabular notch, forming a foramen at the hip joint for the passage of nerves and vessels.

transverse carpal l. A broad ligament bridging over the carpal tunnel of the wrist extending from the pisiform and hamate bones to the scaphoid and trapezium bones of the wrist.

transverse cervical l. A fibrous band attached to each side of the uterine cervix and to the lateral fornices of the vagina; it is continuous with the tissue surrounding the pelvic blood vessels. Formerly called cardinal ligament.

transverse humeral l. The lowest part of the capsule of the shoulder joint, extending from the lesser to the greater tubercle of the humerus; it serves as a retinaculum for the tendon of the long head of the biceps muscle of the arm (biceps brachii) as it emerges from the capsule to enter the intertubercular sulcus of the humerus.

trapezoid l. Part of the coracoclavicular ligament extending from the upper surface of the coracoid process upward to the undersurface of the lateral end of the clavicle.

l. of Treitz Suspensory muscle of duodenum. See table of muscles.

ulnar collateral l. of elbow joint A strong triangular ligament on the medial side of the elbow joint, composed of anterior and posterior bands united by a thin oblique band; the anterior band extends from the front of the medial epicondyle of the humerus to the medial margin of the coronoid process of the ulna; the posterior band extends from the lower part of the medial epicondyle to the medial surface of the olecranon; the oblique band stretches from the olecranon to the coronoid process. Also called medial collateral ligament of elbow.

ulnar collateral l. of wrist joint A fibrous band that extends from the styloid process of the ulna and divides into two parts to attach to two bones of the wrist, the triquetral and the pisiform bones. Also called medial collateral ligament of wrist.

urachal l. See median umbilical ligament.

uterosacral l. Fibromuscular band that extends backward on either side from the uterine cervix, along the lateral wall of the pelvis to the front of the sacrum. It passes by the sides of the rectum and can be palpated on rectal examination.

venous l. of liver A thin fibrous cord, the remains of the obliterated ductus venosus of the fetus, lying in a fossa on the posterior part of the diaphragmatic surface of the liver.

vestibular l. of larynx A thin fibrous band in the ventricular fold of the larynx, extending from the thyroid cartilage, anteriorly, to the arytenoid cartilage, posteriorly.

vocal l. The elastic tissue band that extends on

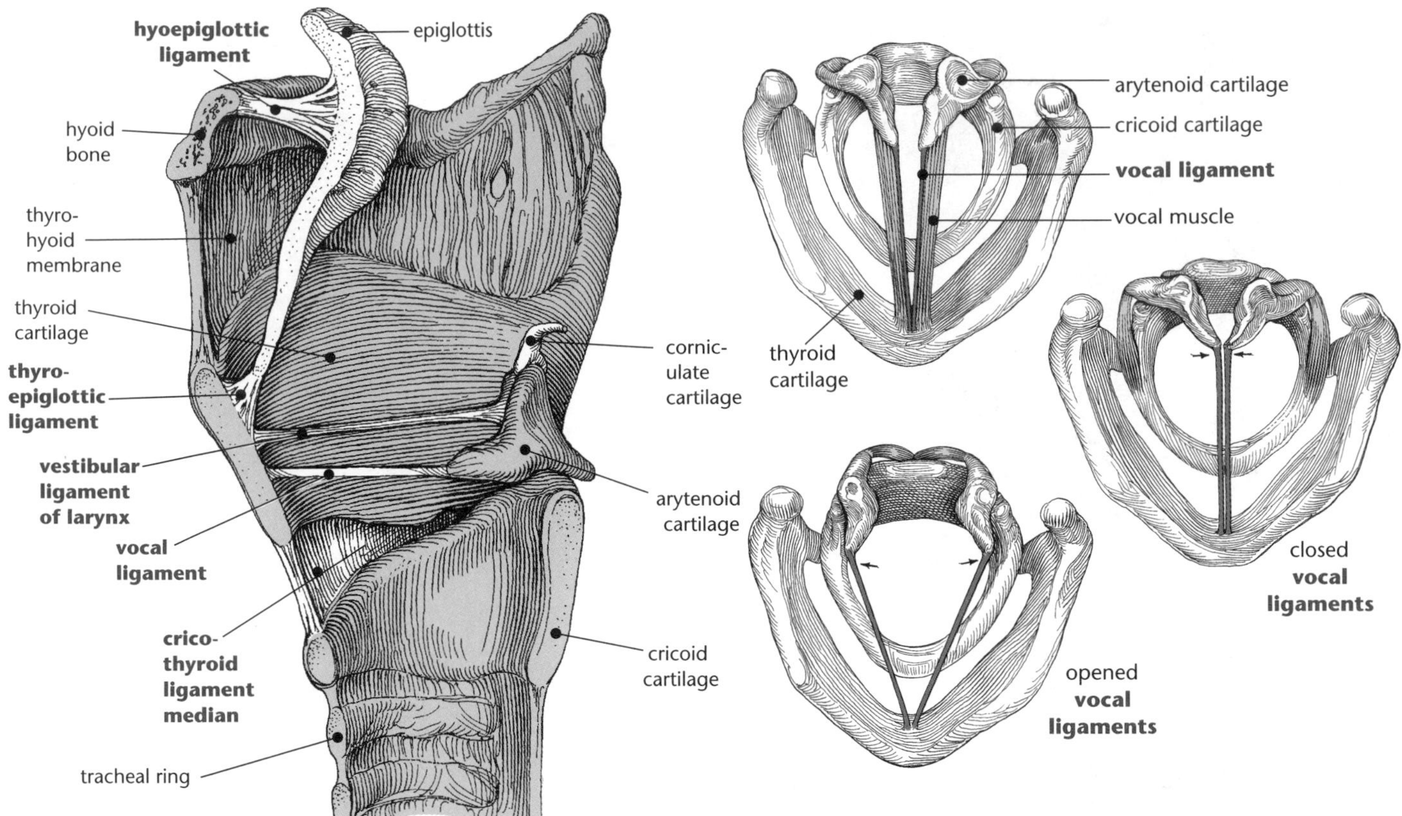

L

either side from the thyroid cartilage in front, to the vocal process of the arytenoid cartilage behind; it is situated within the vocal fold, just below the vestibular ligament of larynx; it represents the upper border of the conus elasticus of the larynx.

l. of Zinn See common annular tendon, under tendon.

ligamentous (lig-ă-men´tus) Of the nature of a ligament.

ligamentum (lig-ă-men´tum) Latin for ligament.

l. arteriosum A short fibrous cord, the remains of the fetal ductus arteriosus, extending from the pulmonary artery to the arch of the aorta.

l. venosum A fibrous cord, the remains of the fetal ductus venosus, lying in a groove on the diaphragmatic surface of the liver.

ligand (li´gand) **1.** Any molecule (especially a small one) that binds specifically to another molecule (e.g., an antigen to an antibody, hormone to a receptor, or substrate to an enzyme). **2.** An organic molecule attached to a central metal ion by multiple coordination bonds, as oxygen is bound to the central iron atom of hemoglobin.

ligase (li´gās) Enzyme that catalyzes the joining of two molecules coupled with the breakdown of ATP or some other nucleoside triphosphate.

ligate (li´gāt) To constrict a blood vessel, a duct, or the pedicle of a tumor by means of a tightly tied thread (ligature).

ligation (li-ga´shun) The tying of a blood vessel.

ligator (li-ga´tor) An instrument used for ligating blood vessels that are generally deep or nearly inaccessible.

ligature (lig´ă-chur) A thread used for tying vessels.

light (līt) An electromagnetic radiation capable of inducing visual sensation through the eye; radiant energy, approximately between 380 and 760 nm.

axial l. Rays of light parallel to each other and to the axis of an optical system.

coherent l. Electromagnetic radiation in which waves have a continuous relationship among phases.

cold l. **1.** Light producing little or no heat, as that by certain luminous insects. **2.** Any visible light essentially devoid of infrared radiation.

diffused l. Light whose rays have no predominant directional component.

infrared l. See infrared rays, under ray.

polarized l. Light of which the vibrations are all in one plane, transverse to the ray, instead of in all planes.

reflected l. Light whose rays have been bent by a mirror-like surface and which continues to travel in the altered direction.

refracted l. Light whose pathway is altered from its original direction as a result of passing from one transparent medium to another of different density.

transmitted l. Light which passes or has passed through a transparent medium.

ultraviolet l. Ultraviolet rays; see under ray.

Wood's l. Ultraviolet radiation in the region near the visible spectrum, produced by the Wood's lamp; used in diagnosis and treatment of skin diseases, detection of corneal abrasions, and evaluation of the fit of contact lenses.

lightening (līt´en-ing) The sinking of the fetal head into the pelvic inlet causing the uterus to descend to a lower level and fall forward, thus relieving pressure on the diaphragm and making breathing easier.

Lignac-Fanconi syndrome (le-nyahk´fahng-ko ´ne sin´drōm) A childhood form of cystinosis; a rare genetic disorder marked by widespread deposits of cystine throughout the body and dysfunction of the renal tubules, associated with vitamin D-resistant rickets, acidosis, dwarfism, glycosuria, and albuminuria.

limb (lim) An extremity; an arm or leg.

lower l. The lower extremity that includes the hip, buttock, thigh, leg, and foot.

phantom l. A phenomenon often experienced by amputees in which sensations, sometimes painful, seem to originate in the amputated limb.

upper l. The upper extremity that includes the shoulder, arm, forearm, and hand.

limbic (lim´bik) **1.** Relating to a limbus or border. **2.** Relating to the limbic system of the brain, comprising the cortex and related nuclei; thought to control emotional and behavioral patterns.

limbus (lim´bus), *pl.* **lim´bi** A border.

l. of cornea The highly vascular band at the junction of the cornea and sclera.

lime (līm) Calcium oxide, CaO; a white caustic powder used in waste treatment, insecticides, and several industries.

limen (li´men), *pl.* **li´mina** A threshold; a border; the beginning point; the entrance to a structure.

l. insulae Threshold of the insula (island of Reil) of the brain; a narrow tongue of insular cortex extending ventromedially toward the anterior perforated substance; it receives fibers from the lateral olfactory stria.

l. nasi The threshold of the nose; the curved ridge that forms the superior and posterior boundary between the nasal cavity proper and the vestibule, where the skin is replaced by mucous membrane.

liminal (lim´ĭ-nal) Having the lowest amount of strength necessary to elicit a response; said of a stimulus.

liminometer (lim-ĭ-nom´ĕ-ter) Instrument to measure a stimulus that has the lowest amount of strength necessary to produce a reflex response.

limp (limp) **1.** To walk unevenly, with a yielding step. **2.** An uneven gait, favoring one leg. **3.** Flaccid.

lincomycin (lin-ko-mi´sin) Substance produced by *Streptomyces lincolnensis*; it has antibacterial action against gram-positive organisms.

lindane (lin´dān) A compound that repels ticks and kills lice.

Lindau's disease (lin´dowz dĭ-zēz´) See von Hippel-Lindau disease.

line (līn) **1.** A thin, continuous strip, mark, or ridge. **2.** A skin crease; a wrinkle. **3.** An imaginary mark connecting landmarks on the body or passing through them. **4.** A boundary or limit. **5.** A succession of ancestors or descendants.

absorption l.'s Numerous dark lines in a spectrum due to absorption of specific wavelengths of light by the substance through which it passes.

l. of accommodation The linear extent to which an object can be moved closer to or away from the eye in a given state of refraction without causing noticeable blurriness.

axillary l. One of three imaginary vertical lines associated with the axilla; the anterior axillary line passes through the anterior fold of the axilla; the posterior passes through the posterior fold; the midaxillary passes through the center of the axilla.

B l.'s of Kerley Horizontal lines in the chest x ray (above the costophrenic angle) of individuals with pulmonary hypertension secondary to mitral stenosis.

blue l. See lead line.

cell l. In tissue culture, cells derived from a primary culture, growing *in vitro* in the first and subsequent subcultures.

cervical l. See cementoenamel junction, under junction.

cleavage l.'s Definite linear clefts in the skin indicative of the direction of the underlying sub-

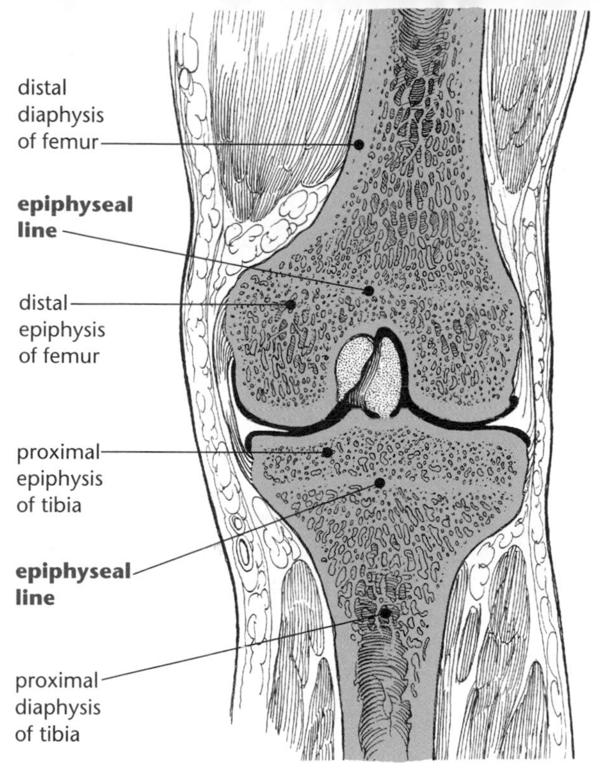

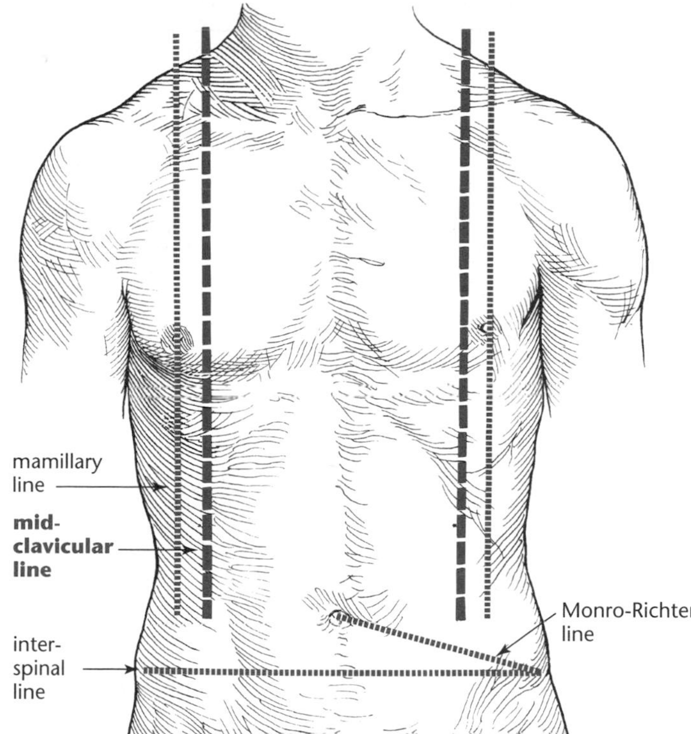

cutaneous fibrous connective tissue bundles. Also called Langer's lines.

dentate l. See pectinate line.

epiphysial l. The line of junction of the epiphysis and diaphysis of an adult long bone.

Fleischner l.'s Linear shadows on a chest x-ray, indicating foci of atelectasis.

fulcrum l. An imaginary line of dental appliance rotation. Also called rotational axis.

germ l. The genetic material carried by ova and spermatozoa; contains the genes that parents pass to their offspring.

gingival l. The position of the margin of the gingiva as it extends onto a tooth. Also called gum line.

gluteal l. One of three rough curved lines on the outer surface of the iliac part of the hipbone, designated anterior, posterior, and inferior.

gum l. See gingival line.

Hampton l. In radiography, a line of decreased density surrounding a benign stomach ulcer.

iliopectineal l. An oblique ridge on the surface of the ilium and continued on the pelvis, forming the lower boundary of the iliac fossa; it separates the true from the false pelvis.

Langer's l. See cleavage lines.

lead l. A dark bluish area of abnormal pigmentation of the gingival tissues, usually 1 mm from the gingival crest, associated with lead poisoning. Also called blue line.

M l. A line formed by the nodular thickenings of the myofilament (myosin) bisecting the H zone of striated muscle myofibrils.

median l. A vertical center line dividing the body surface into right and left parts.

Mees' l.'s White lines on fingernails occurring in arsenic poisoning. Also called Mees' stripes.

mercurial l. A linear discoloration of the gingival tissues associated with mercury poisoning and seen along the gingival margin; it can be bluish, purplish, or muddy red in coloration.

midaxillary l. An imaginary vertical line passing through the middle of the axilla.

midclavicular l. A vertical line passing through the midpoint of the clavicle on either side; it corresponds closely to a perpendicular line passing through the nipple.

milk l. The line or ridge of thickened epithelium in the embryo, extending from the axillary to the inguinal region, along which the mammary glands are developed.

Muehrcke's l.'s Parallel, transverse white lines in fingernails and toenails; associated with chronic hypoalbuminemia.

nipple l. A vertical line passing through the nipple on either side.

nuchal l.'s Three lines or ridges (inferior, superior, and highest) on the exterior surface of the occipital bone of the skull.

l. of occlusion The alignment of the occluding surface of the teeth in the horizontal plane.

pectinate l. The line between the rectal mucosa and the skin lining the anus. Also called dentate line.

pectineal l. The line on the superior ramus of the pubic bone from the pubic tubercle to the iliopubic eminence. Also called pecten pubis.

pure l. A strain of laboratory animals inbred for many generations, homozygous for certain specific genes.

scapular l. An imaginary vertical line passing through the lower angle of the scapula on either side.

Schwalbe's annular l. See anterior limiting ring of eye, under ring.

simian l. See simian crease, under crease.

survey l. (a) A line inscribed on a cast of a tooth by a surveyor scriber; it marks the greatest height of contour in relation to the chosen path of insertion of the restoration. (b) The line denoting the height of contour of a tooth after the cast has been positioned according to the chosen path of insertion. Also called clasp guideline.

temporal l.'s The two curved lines (inferior and superior) on the outer surface of the parietal bones of the skull.

visual l. See visual axis, under axis.

Wagner's l. A narrow line representing the area of preliminary calcification, at the junction of the epiphysis and diaphysis of a long bone.

Z l. One of the transverse septa dividing the myofibrils of skeletal muscle into longitudinally arranged sarcomeres; the region between two Z lines consists of overlapping thick and thin myofilaments. Also called Z band.

zigzag l. See Z-Z line.

Z-Z l. The transition line from esophageal to gastric mucosa; it appears as an irregular dentate or zigzag line. Also called zigzag line.

linea (lin´e-a), *pl.* **lin´eae** A line.

l. alba The narrow portion of the anterior aponeurosis running down the midline of the abdominal wall from the xiphoid process to the pubic symphysis. Also called white line.

l. aspera A longitudinal ridge with two prominent lips, on the posterior surface of the femur. Also called rough line.

l. nigra The dark streak on the abdomen of pregnant women, between the umbilicus and the pubic symphysis.

l. semilunaris The lateral edge of the abdominal rectus muscle; it crosses the costal margin at the tip of the ninth costal cartilage.

line breeding (līn brēding) A method of breeding designed to perpetuate the desirable traits of an animal by crossbreeding its descendants.

lingua (ling´gwă) Latin for tongue.

lingual (ling´gwal) Pertaining to the tongue.

lingually (ling´gwă-le) Toward the tongue.

lingula (ling´gu-lă) Any tongue-shaped process.

l. of cerebellum The most anterior tongue-shaped lobule of the superior vermis of the cerebellum.

l. of lung A projection from the upper lobe of the left lung just beneath the cardiac notch.

l. of mandible A projection of bone overlapping the mandibular foramen on the inner surface of the ramus of the mandible; it serves for the attachment of the sphenomandibular ligament.

lingulectomy (ling-gu-lek´to-me) Surgical removal of the lingular portion of the upper lobe of the left lung.

linguoclusion (ling-gwo-kloo´shun) Displacement of a tooth or group of teeth toward the tongue. Also called lingual occlusion.

linguo-occlusal (ling-gwo-ŏ-kloo´zal) Relating to the lingual and occlusal surfaces of a posterior tooth; usually denoting the line angle formed by the junction of the two surfaces.

linguopapillitis (ling-gwo-pap-ĭ-li´tis) Small painful ulcers around the papillae on the tongue margins.

linguoversion (ling-gwo-ver´zhun) Malposition of a tooth toward the tongue.

liniment (lin´ĭ-ment) An oily medicinal liquid applied to the skin by friction as a counterirritant.

linin (li´nin) The fine, threadlike, nonstaining (achromatic) substance of the cell nucleus that interconnects the chromatin granules.

lining (li´ning) In dentistry, a coating applied to the walls of a tooth cavity to protect the pulp from irritation by the restorative filling; most commonly used cements include zinc-oxide eugenol (ZOE), zinc phosphate, and calcium hydroxide.

linitis (lĭ-ni´tis) Inflammation of the cellular tissue of the stomach.

l. plastica Extensive thickening of the stomach wall due to infiltrating scirrhous carcinoma. Also called leather bottle stomach.

linkage (lingk´ij) **1.** The force that holds together the atoms in a chemical compound, or the symbol used to represent it. **2.** The relationship existing between two or more genes in the same chromosome that causes them to remain together from generation to generation.

sex l. Old term for X linkage.

X l. Linkage associated with a gene located on the X chromosome.

Y l. Linkage associated with a gene located on the Y chromosome.

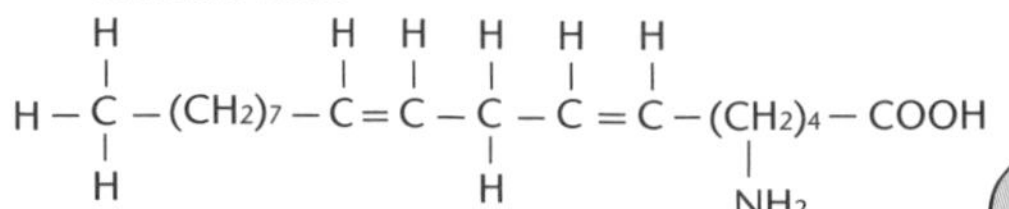

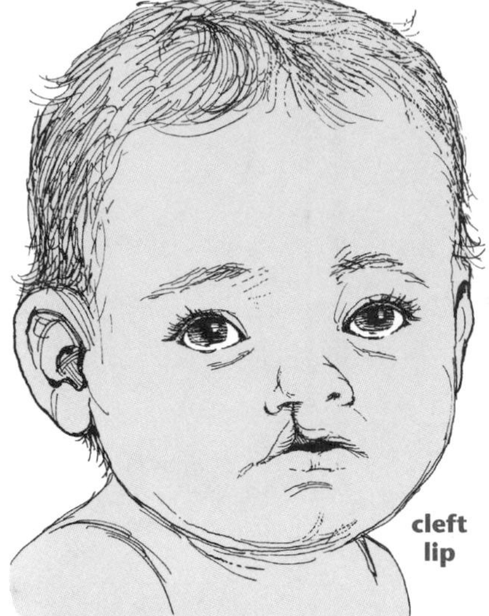

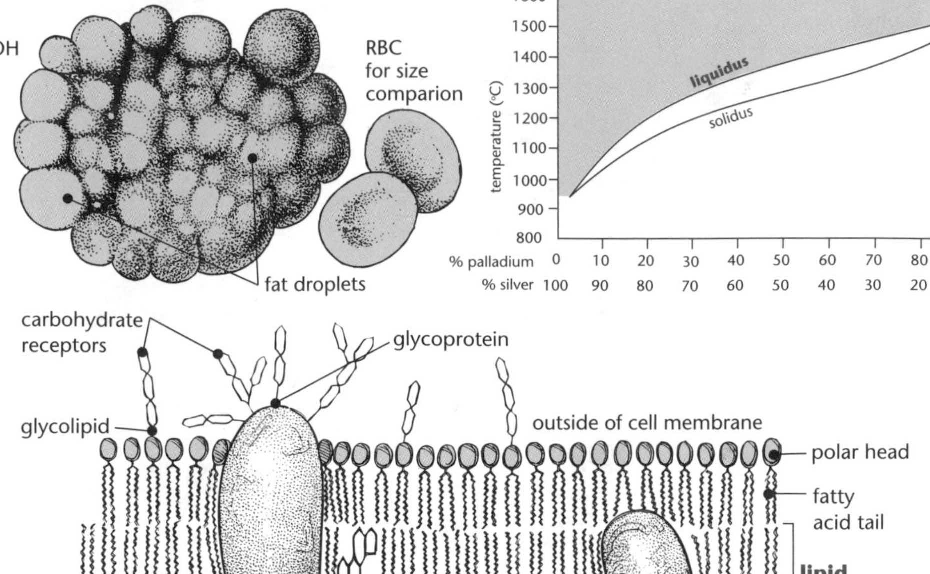

linoleic acid (lin-o-le′ik as′id) A light straw-colored polyunsaturated fatty acid, $C_{18}H_{32}O_2$, that is essential in the human diet; it strengthens capillary walls, lowers serum cholesterol, and prolongs blood clotting time.

linolenic acid (lin-o-len′ik as′id) A colorless polyunsaturated fatty acid, $C_{18}H_{30}O_2$, that is essential in the human diet.

liothyronine (li-o-thi′ro-nēn) See triiodothyronine.

lip (lip) **1.** One of the two fleshy folds forming the anterior boundary of the mouth. **2.** Any liplike structure.

anterior l. See labium anterius, under labium.

cleft l. Developmental defect of the upper lip ranging from a scarlike groove, or a notch on the lip, to a complete cleft extending into the nasal cavity; may be unilateral or bilateral and is frequently accompanied by a cleft palate. Also called cheiloschisis.

double l. An oral anomaly consisting of a fold of excess or redundant tissue on the mucosal side of the lip; the upper lip is involved more than the lower one.

lesser l.'s of pudendum See labia minora, under labium.

major l.'s See labia majora, under labium.

minor l.'s See labia minora, under labium.

posterior l. See labium posterius, under labium.

lipase (lip′ās) A fat-splitting enzyme present in pancreatic juice, blood, and many tissues.

lipoprotein l. Enzyme that promotes the breakdown of the triglycerides of chylomicrons to form free fatty acid and glycerol.

lipectomy (lĭ-pek′to-me) Surgical removal of adipose tissue, as for certain cases of obesity.

suction l. See liposuction.

lipedema (lip-ĕ-de′mă) Chronic swelling of the legs, seen most frequently in middle-aged women.

lipemia (lĭ-pe′me-ă) See hyperlipidemia.

lipid (lip′id) **1.** Generally any fat, oil, or wax, or any derivative of these materials; soluble in organic compounds like alcohol and insoluble in water. **2.** Specifically, the fats and fat-like materials which, together with carbohydrates and proteins, constitute the main structural substance in the living cell.

lipidemia (lip-ĭ-de′me-ă) See hyperlipidemia.

lipidosis (lip-ĭ-do′sis), *pl.* **lipido′ses** General term applied to disorders marked by abnormal concentration of lipids in the tissues.

ganglioside l. See gangliosidosis.

sulfatide l. See metachromatic leukodystrophy, under leukodystrophy.

lipoatrophy, lipoatrophia (li-po-at′ro-fe, li-po-at′ro-fe-ă) Atrophy of body fat, as in the loss of subcutaneous fat after repeated injections of insulin into the same area.

insulin l. Circumscribed loss of subcutaneous body fat after repeated daily injections of insulin into the same area.

lipocele (lip′o-sēl) A hernial sac containing adipose tissue. Also called adipocele.

lipochondrodystrophy (lip-o-kon-dro-dis′tro-fe) See Hurler's syndrome.

lipochrome (lip′o-krōm) Any of various naturally occurring fatty pigments such as carotene and lipofuscin.

lipocyte (lip′o-sīt) See fat cell, under cell.

lipodystrophy (lip-o-dis′tro-fe) Defective or faulty metabolism of fat.

intestinal l. See Whipple's disease.

lipofibroma (lip-o-fi-bro′mă) A benign tumor composed of fibrous connective tissue and fatty tissue.

lipofuscin (lip-o-fu′sin) A golden brown lipid-containing pigment that represents the indigestible residue of cellular lysosomal activity, associated with normal wear and tear. Sometimes called old age pigment.

lipogenesis (lip-o-jen′ĕ-sis) The formation of fat.

lipogenic (lip-o-jen′ik) Fat-producing. Also called adipogenic.

lipoid (lip′oid) Resembling fat.

lipoidosis (lip-oi-do′sis) The presence of lipid material in various organs.

lipolipoidosis (lip-o-lip-oi-do′sis) Fatty infiltration of the cells.

lipolysis (lĭ-pol′ĭ-sis) The splitting up or chemical decomposition of fat.

lipoma (lĭ-po′mă) A benign tumor composed of mature fat cells. Also called adipose tumor.

l. fibrosum See fibrolipoma.

lipomatoid (lĭ-po′mă-toid) Resembling a tumor of fatty tissue.

lipomatosis (lip-o-mă-to′sis) Deposition of fat, either local or general. Also called liposis.

lipomatous (lĭ-po′mă-tus) **1.** Of the nature of a lipoma. **2.** Marked by the presence of a lipoma.

lipophage (lip′o-fāj) A fat-absorbing cell.

lipophagic (lip-o-fa′jik) Ingesting or absorbing fat.

lipophil (lip′o-fil) Having affinity for lipids.

lipoprotein (lip-o-pro′tēn) (LP) A conjugated protein containing fat as the nonprotein substance.

high-density l. (HDL) A plasma protein of relatively small molecular weight containing proportionally more protein and less cholesterol and triglycerides. Also called alpha-lipoprotein (relating to its electrophoretic mobility).

low-density l. (LDL) A plasma protein of relatively large molecular weight containing proportionally less protein and more cholesterol and triglycerides. Also called beta-lipoprotein (relating to its electrophoretic mobility).

Lp(a) l. A low-density lipoprotein chemically modified by insertion of apolipoprotein a (a glycoprotein).

very-low-density l. (VLDL) A large plasma protein containing a relatively high percentage of triglycerides. Also called pre-beta-lipoprotein (relating to its electrophoretic mobility).

l. X An abnormal lipoprotein associated with obstructive jaundice.

lipoprotein lipase (lip-o-pro′tēn lip′as) Enzyme promoting the breakdown of fat to fatty acid and glycerol.

liposarcoma (lip-o-sar-ko′mă) A rare malignant tumor usually found in the retroperitoneal and mediastinal fat deposits of elderly people.

liposis (lĭ-po′sis) See lipomatosis.

liposome (lip′o-sōm) A bilayered vesicle formed by a phospholipid when exposed to aqueous medium in tissues.

liposuction (li-po-suk′shun) Removal of subcutaneous fat with a vacuum device.

lipotropic (lip-o-trop′ik) Relating to lipotropy.

lipotropy (lĭ-pot′ro-pe) **1.** Prevention of excessive accumulation of fat in the liver. **2.** Affinity of basic dyes for fatty tissue.

lipoxygenase (lĭ-pok′se-jĕ-nās) Enzyme that promotes oxidation of polyunsaturated fatty acids.

lipping (lip′ing) The formation of a liplike border at the articular end of a bone in degenerative bone disease.

lipuria (lĭ-pu′re-ă) The presence of fat in the urine.

liquefacient (lik-wĕ-fa′shent) An agent that causes a solid to dissolve or become liquid.

liquefaction (lik-wĕ-fak′shun) **1.** The act of liquefying. **2.** The state of being converted into a liquid form.

liquescent (lik-wes′ent) Tending to liquefy.

liquid (lik′wid) A substance, neither solid nor gaseous, that exhibits a characteristic readiness to flow, like water.

liquidus (lik′wid-us) The temperature line on a constitution diagram above which the indicated metal element or alloy turns to liquid.

liquor (lik′er), *pl.* **liq′uores** **1.** A liquid substance. **2.** A solution of a nonvolatile substance in water.

l. folliculi See follicular fluid, under fluid.

Listeria (lis-te′re-ă) A genus of bacteria (family Corynebacteriaceae) containing small, gram-positive, aerobic rods; found in feces, sewage, and vegetation.

L. monocytogenes A species causing meningitis, septicemia, abscesses, and local purulent lesions.

listeriosis (lis-ter-e-o′sis) Infection with bacteria of the genus *Listeria*; commonly occurring in animals,

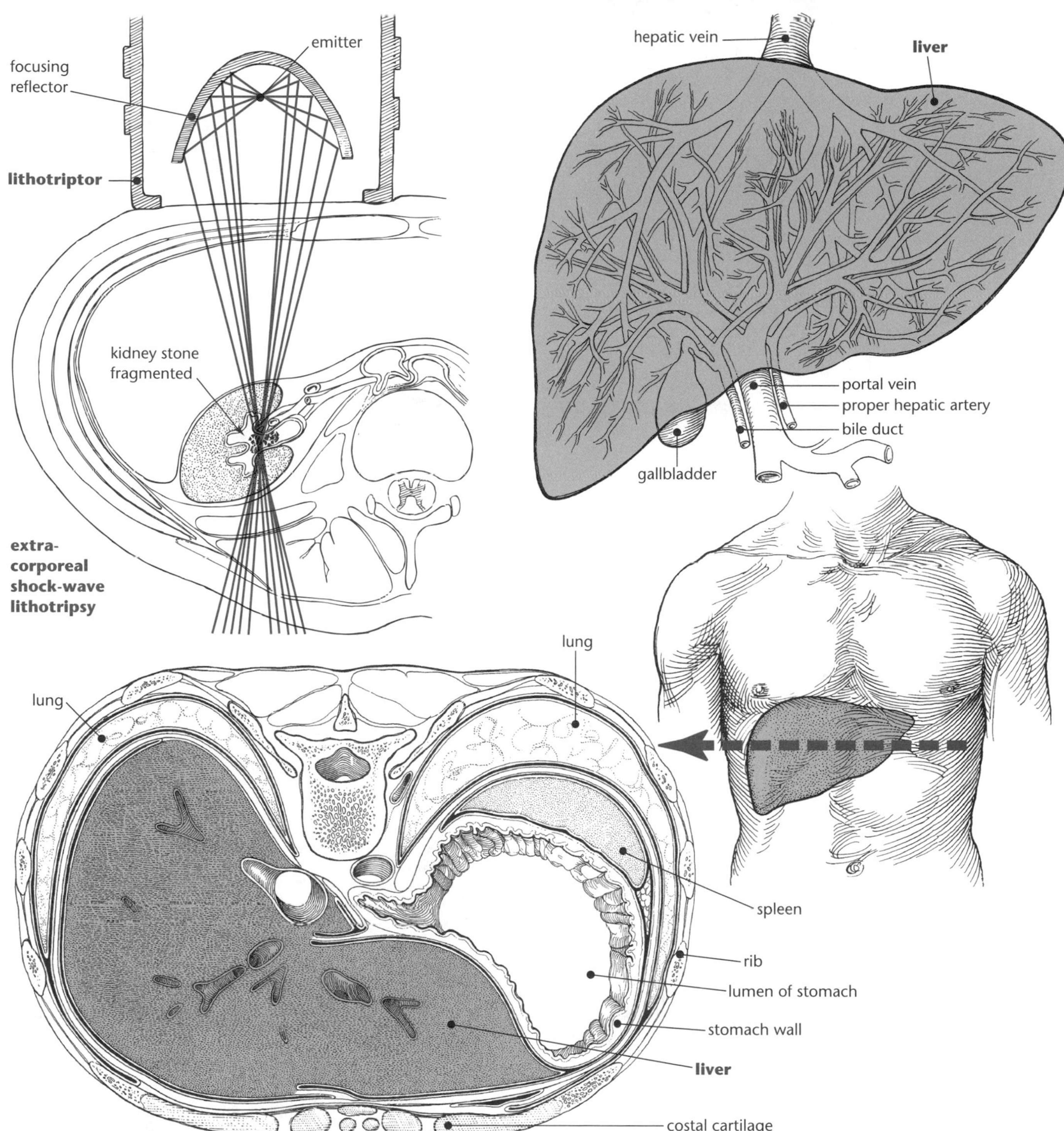

but occasionally transmitted to man, where it may produce a clinical picture resembling infectious mononucleosis or an acute meningitis.

neonatal l. Listeriosis occurring in the newborn, usually acquired through maternal infection during passage through the birth canal or by aspiration of infected amniotic fluid; occasionally acquired from the hospital nursery; the condition may become evident the first or second day after birth (early onset), or approximately 7 days afterward (late onset); complications include respiratory distress, skin lesions, abscesses in several organs, and meningitis.

liter (le´ter) (l) A metric unit of capacity equal to a cubic decimeter, or 1000 cubic centimeters; approximately 1.056 liquid quarts.

lites (līts) Colloquial term for low-weight infants.

lithagogue (lith´ă-gog) An agent that causes the dislodging or expulsion of a calculus, especially of a urinary calculus.

lithectasy (lĭ-thek´to-me) The extraction of a bladder stone through the previously dilated urethra.

lithiasis (lĭ-thi´ă-sis) The formation of stones, especially biliary or urinary stones.

lithic acid (lith´ik as´id) See uric acid.

lithium (lith´e-um) A silvery, soft, highly reactive metallic element; symbol Li, atomic number 3, atomic weight 6.939; lithium salts are used to treat mental disorders, particularly in bipolar disorders.

lithocystotomy (lith-o-sis-tot´o-me) Removal of stones from the bladder.

lithodialysis (lith-o-di-al´ĭ-sis) The crushing or dissolving of a stone in the bladder.

lithogenic (lith-o-jen´ik) Promoting the formation of stones in the body.

lithogenous (lĭ-thoj´ĕ-nus) Causing the formation of stones in the body.

litholapaxy (lĭ-thol´ă-pak-se) See lithotripsy.

litholysis (lĭ-thol´ĭ-sis) Dissolution of stones.

lithometra (lith-o-me´tră) Calcification of the tissue of the uterus.

lithonephria (lith-o-nef´re-ă) Stone in the kidney.

lithopedion (lith-o-pe´de-on) The calcified remnants of an ectopic pregnancy.

lithotomy (lĭ-thot´o-me) Operation for the removal of a stone, especially from the bladder.

lithotresis (lith-o-tre´sis) The boring of holes in a calculus to facilitate its crushing and removal.

lithotripsy (lith´o-trip-se) Fragmentation of stones within the urinary tract, followed by washing out of the fragments. Also called litholapaxy.

electrohydraulic shock wave l. (ESWL) Lithotripsy in which a high-voltage spark is created by two electrodes at the tip of a probe, directed toward a fluid-filled organ.

extracorporeal shock wave l. (ESWL) Lithotripsy conducted by positioning the patient in contact with a water cushion and in the path of shock waves focused on the stones with the aid of fluoroscopy or ultrasound.

lithotriptic (lith-o-trip´tik) **1.** Relating to lithotripsy. **2.** An agent that dissolves a calculus.

lithotriptor (lith´o-trip-tor) Device for breaking up urinary stones by extracorporeal shock-wave litho-

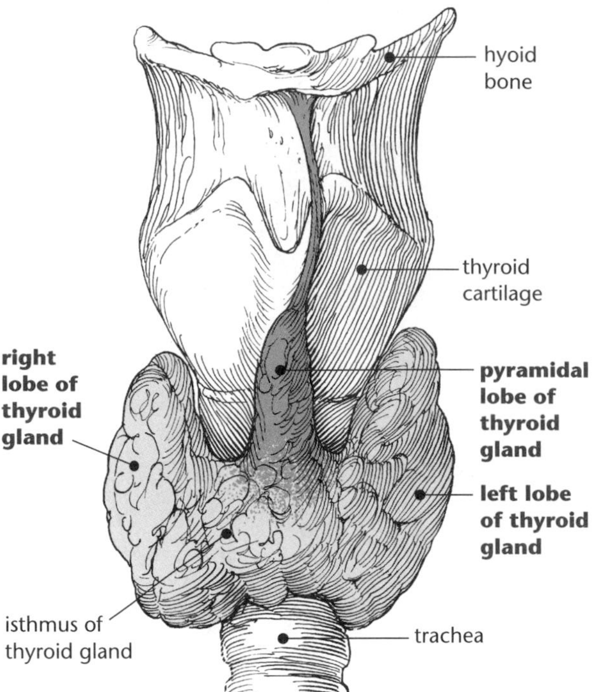

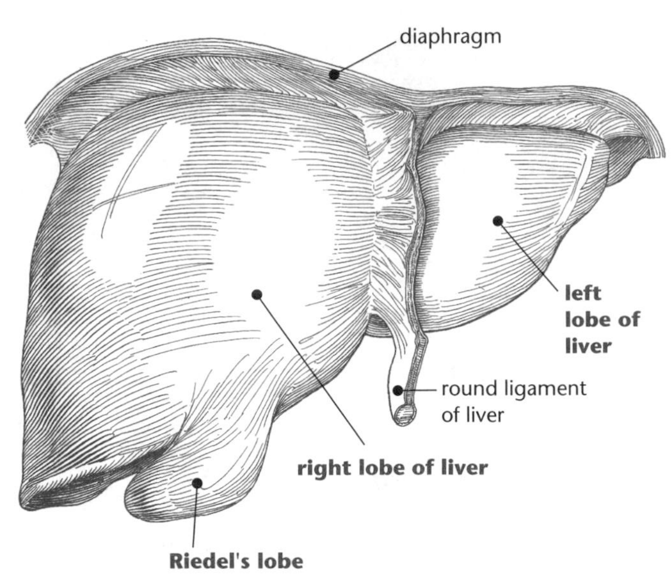

tripsy.

lithotrite (lith′o-trīt) Instrument for crushing stones in the bladder.

lithous (lith′us) Relating to a calculus or stone.

lithuresis (lith-u-re′sis) The passage of minute stones or sand in the urine.

lithuria (lith-u′re-ă) A condition marked by excess uric acid or urates in the urine.

litmus (lit′mus) A blue pigment, obtained from *Roccella tinctoria* and other lichens, that turns red with increasing acidity and blue with increasing alkalinity.

litmus paper (lit′mus pa′per) White paper impregnated with litmus powder and used as a test for acidity and alkalinity; the acid-base pH range is from 4.5 to 8.3.

litter (lit′er) A stretcher for transporting the disabled.

littritis (lit-tri′tis) Inflammation of the urethral (Littre's) glands in the penile portion of the male urethra.

livedo reticularis (lĭ-ve′do rĕ-tik-u-lar′is) Circulatory disorder of unknown origin causing constant bluish discoloration on large areas of the extremities.

liver (liv′er) A large, dark red gland that produces and secretes bile, playing an important role in the metabolism of carbohydrates, fats, protein, minerals, and vitamins; located beneath the entire right dome of the diaphragm and approximately one-third of the left dome, it is the largest glandular organ in the body, weighing from 1200 to 1600 g in the adult (about 1/40 the weight of the body); on the basis of the internal distribution of the blood vessels and bile ducts, the liver may be divided into nearly equal right and left lobes.

cirrhotic l. See cirrhosis.

fatty l. An enlarged, doughy liver due to fatty degeneration and infiltration (fatty metamorphosis); it may develop as a complication of any disease in which malnutrition, especially protein deficiency, is present; commonly seen in the early stages of alcoholic cirrhosis or in diabetes.

fibrotic l. A liver marked by an increase in connective tissue without disturbance of the lobular architecture.

nutmeg l. A liver presenting a mottled or polymorphic appearance when sectioned.

polycystic l. See polycystic liver disease.

livid (liv′id) Black and blue; denoting a bluish gray coloration (e.g., from congestion or bruising).

lixiviation (liks-iv-e-a′shun) See leaching.

lixivium (liks-iv′e-um) See lye.

load (lōd) **1.** The quantity borne or sustained by an organism or a part. **2.** A deviation from normal of any body contents (water, salt, etc.); positive load is more than normal and negative load is less than normal. **3.** To introduce a defined quantity for some test purpose or to achieve a desired blood level.

Loa loa (lo′ă lo′ă) The eyeworm; a threadlike roundworm that infests subcutaneous tissues, causing tumefactions; the worms migrate readily and are usually noticed when passing through the conjunctiva across the eyeball or over the bridge of the nose; indigenous to the western part of equatorial Africa.

lobar (lo′bar) Relating to a lobe.

lobate (lo′bāt) Composed of or divided into lobes; lobed.

lobe (lōb) **1.** A fairly well defined portion of an organ or gland bounded by structural borders such as fissures, sulci, or septa. **2.** A rounded anatomic projecting part, such as the fatty lobule of the human ear. **3.** One of the main divisions of the crown of a tooth, formed from a distinct point of calcification.

anterior l. of hypophysis See adenohypophysis.

azygos l. of lung An occasional small triangular lobe on the mediastinal surface at the apex of the right lung, which is delimited by the arch of the azygos vein embedded in the lung substance.

caudate l. of liver A small lobe of the liver situated posteriorly between the inferior vena cava and the fissure for the ligamentum venosum.

central l. See insula.

l.'s of cerebellum *Anterior l.*, the anterior part of the upper portion of the cerebellum lying in front of the primary fissure; consists of the lingula, central lobule, culmen, alae of the central lobules, and quadrangular lobules. *Middle l.*, the major part of the body of the cerebellum lying behind the primary fissure, between the anterior and flocculonodular lobe; consists of the declive, folium vermis, tuber vermis, pyramid, uvula, lobuli simplices, biventral lobules, semilunar lobules, and cerebellar tonsils. *Flocculonodular l.*, the lobe of the cerebellum that includes both flocculi, their peduncles, and the nodule.

ear l. The lower fleshy part of the auricle.

frontal l. of cerebrum The portion of each cerebral hemisphere bounded behind by the central and below by the lateral sulci.

l. of liver, hepatic l. Any of the liver lobes, designated right, left, caudate, and quadrate.

limbic l. A general term that usually denotes the cingulate and parahippocampal gyri along with the olfactory bulb and stalk and the parolfactory and olfactory gyri.

l.'s of mammary gland The 15 to 20 milk producing lobes of the female breast, each drained by a lactiferous duct that opens at the nipple (papilla).

occipital l. of cerebrum The most posterior portion of each cerebral hemisphere, bounded anteriorly by the parieto-occipital sulcus and the line joining it to the preoccipital notch.

olfactory l. A general term that usually denotes the olfactory bulb, tract, and trigone plus the anterior perforated substance.

parietal l. of cerebrum The upper central portion of each cerebral hemisphere between the frontal and occipital lobes, and above the temporal lobe; it is separated from the frontal lobe by the central sulcus.

posterior l. of hypophysis See neurohypophysis.

pyramidal l. of thyroid gland An inconstant, narrow, somewhat cone-shaped lobe of the thyroid gland that arises from the upper border of the isthmus and extends upward; occasionally it arises from the adjacent part of either lobe (most commonly the left), or may be completely detached; sometimes it is attached to the hyoid bone by a fibrous band.

Riedel's l. A tongue-shaped mass of tissue occasionally extending downward from the right lobe of the liver.

quadrate l. of liver A small lobe on the inferior surface of the liver between the gallbladder and the ligamentum teres.

temporal l. of cerebrum A long lobe on the outer side and under surface of each cerebral hemisphere; it is bounded above by the lateral sulcus.

l.'s of thyroid gland Two lobes of the thyroid gland on either side of the larynx, connected near their bases by a narrow band of tissue (isthmus) lying across the upper anterior trachea.

lobectomy (lo-bek′to-me) Surgical removal of a lobe.

lobelia (lo-be′le-ă) The dried leaves and tops of *Lobelia inflata*; contains several alkaloids including lobeline, norlobelanine, and isolobelanine.

lobeline (lob′e-lin) A mixture of alkaloids derived from plants of the genus *Lobelia*; it has actions similar to those of nicotine, but less potent.

lobotomy (lo-bot′o-me) Surgical incision into a lobe.

prefrontal l. A psychosurgical procedure consisting of division of the fibers in the brain connecting the prefrontal and frontal lobes with the thalamus. Also called prefrontal leukotomy.

transorbital l. Lobotomy through the roof of the orbit. Also called transorbital leukotomy.

lobulated (lob′u-lāt-ed) Consisting of or divided into lobules.

lobule (lob′ūl) A small lobe.

lobulet, lobulette (lob-u-let′) A very small lobule or a section or subdivision of a lobule.

lobulus (lob′u-lus), *pl.* **lob′uli** Latin for lobule.

lobus (lo′bus), *pl.* **lo′bi** Latin for lobe.

local (lo′kal) Confined to a limited area of the body.

localization (lo-kă-li-za′shun) **1.** Restriction of a process to a limited area. **2.** Determination of the site of a morbid process.

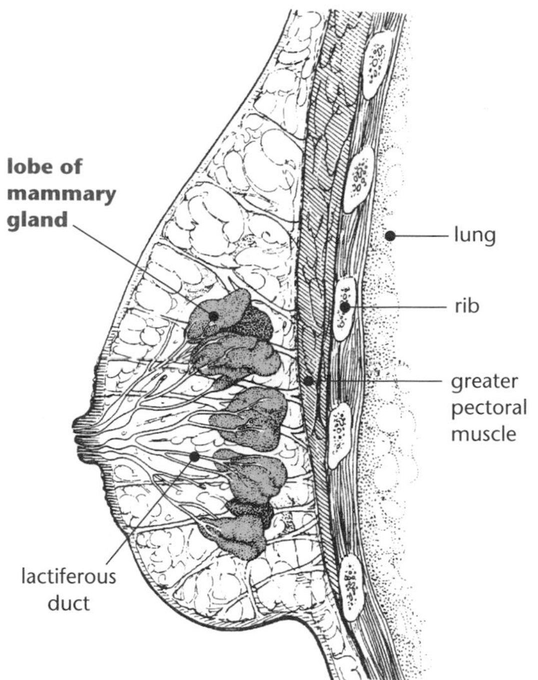

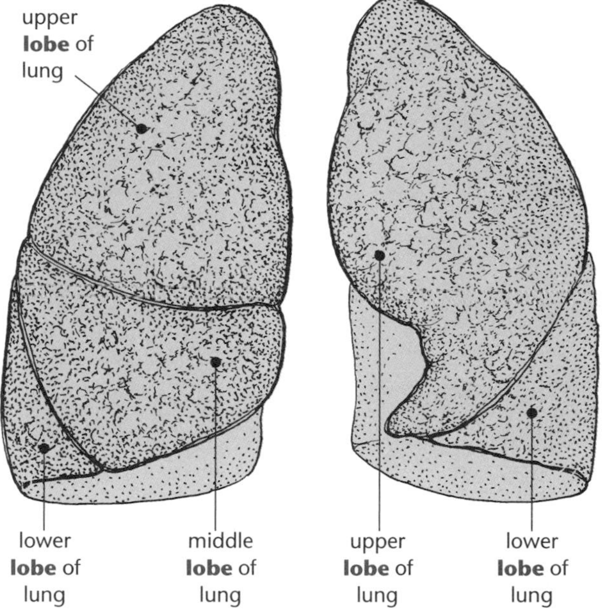

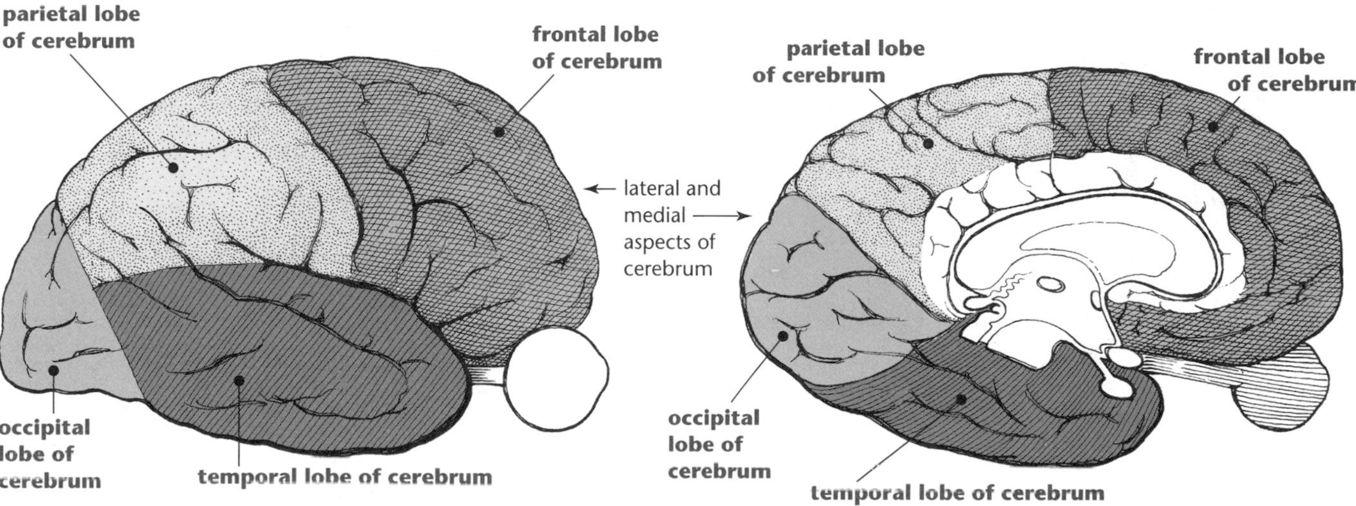

localized (lo´kal-īzd) Limited to a definite part; generally applied to changes that are restricted or confined to a particular area or part of the body.
localizer (lo´kal-īz-er) A visual training instrument used in the treatment of amblyopia or anopsia.
lochia (lo´ke-ă) The bloody discharge from the uterus following childbirth.
lochiometra (lo-ke-o-me´tră) Distention of the uterus with retained blood and mucus (lochia) following childbirth, due to blocking of the cervical canal; associated with inflammation of the uterine lining. Commonly called lochia block.
lochiometritis (lo-ke-o-me-trī´tis) Inflammation of the uterus following childbirth.
lochiorrhea (lo-ke-o-re´ă) Excessive flow of discharges after childbirth.
loci (lo´si) Plural of locus.
locked-in syndrome (lokd-in-sin-drōm) Difficult swallowing and inability to speak, move the limbs and facial muscles, and move the eyes sideways; the patient retains consciousness, breathing ability, and vertical movement of the eyes; caused by blocked circulation to, or hemorrhage into, the anterior portion of the pons (at the base of the brain).
lockjaw (lok´jaw) See trismus.
locomotor (lo-ko-mo´tor) Relating to motion.
locular (lok´u-lar) Of or relating to a loculus.
loculate, loculated (lok´u-lāt, lok-u-lā´ted) Divided into or containing numerous loculi.
loculation (lok-u-lā´shun) **1.** A structure or tissue having numerous small cavities. **2.** The formation of small cavities (loculi).
loculus (lok´u-lus), *pl.* **loc´uli** A small cavity.
locum tenens (lo´kum tĕnenz) One who temporarily assumes the place of another (e.g., a practitioner assuming someone else's practice during an illness or vacation).
locus (lo´kus), *pl.* **lo´ci** A place or spot, such as the specific site occupied by a gene in a chromosome.
l. ceruleus A bluish gray area in the floor of the fourth ventricle.
Löffler's disease (lef´lerz dĭ-zēz´) See Löffler's endocarditis, under endocarditis.
Löffler's syndrome (lef´lerz sin´drōm) See simple pulmonary eosinophilia, under eosinophilia.
logopathy (log-op´ă-the) Any disorder of speech.
logoplegia (log-o-ple´jă) Paralysis of the speech organs.
logorrhea (log-o-re´ă) Excessive, uncontrollable talking.
log roll (log´rol) Colloquialism for a procedure using a drawsheet to turn a patient in bed (as if the patient were a rigid log) to prevent injury to the spine; it usually involves three persons, two on one side of the bed, the other on the opposite side.
loiasis (lo-ī´ă-sis) Disease caused by *Loa loa* worms.
loin (loin) The part of back and sides of the body between the ribs and the pelvis.
loop (lo͞op) **1.** A bend in a cord or cordlike structure. **2.** A platinum wire attached to a handle at one end and bent into a circle at the other; used to transfer bacterial cultures.
Henle's l. See nephronic loop.
nephronic l. The thin U-shaped tubule between the ascending and descending limbs of the intermediate renal tubule. Also called Henle's loop.
lophotrichous (lo-fot´rĭ-kus) Referring to a bacterial cell with two or more flagella or cilia at one or both poles.
lordoscoliosis (lor-do-sko-le-o´sis) An abnormal backward and lateral curvature of the spine.
lordosis (lor-do´sis) Abnormally increased forward curvature of the lumbar spine. Also called sway-back.
lordotic (lor-dot´ik) Relating to lordosis.
lotion (lo´shun) **1.** Any of various medicated liquids for external application, especially those containing one or more insoluble substances in suspension. **2.** Any of various liquid cosmetic preparations, usually applied to the face and hands.
calamine l. A preparation of mineral oil with zinc oxide, ferric oxide, glycerin, bentonite magma, and calcium hydroxide solution.
Lou Gehrig's disease (loo ger´igz dĭ-zēz´) See amyotrophic lateral sclerosis, under sclerosis.
loupe (lo͞op) A small magnifying lens, usually set in an eyepiece.
louse (lous), *pl.* **lice** **1.** Any of various small, wingless, flat-bodied, parasitic insects of the orders Anoplura and Mallophaga. **2.** Common name for *Pediculus humanus capitis*.
body l. *Pediculus*.
crab l. See *Phthirus pubis*, under *Phthirus*.
head l. *Pediculus*.
pubic l. See *Phthirus pubis*, under *Phthirus*.
Lowe's syndrome (lōz sĭn´drōm) See oculocerebrorenal syndrome.
Loxosceles reclusa (loks-os´sĕ-lēs re-kloo´să) North American brown recluse spider; volume for volume its venom is more potent than a rattlesnake's; its bite is potentially about as lethal as that of the black widow spider.
loxoscelism (lok-sos´sĕ-liz-m) Condition resulting

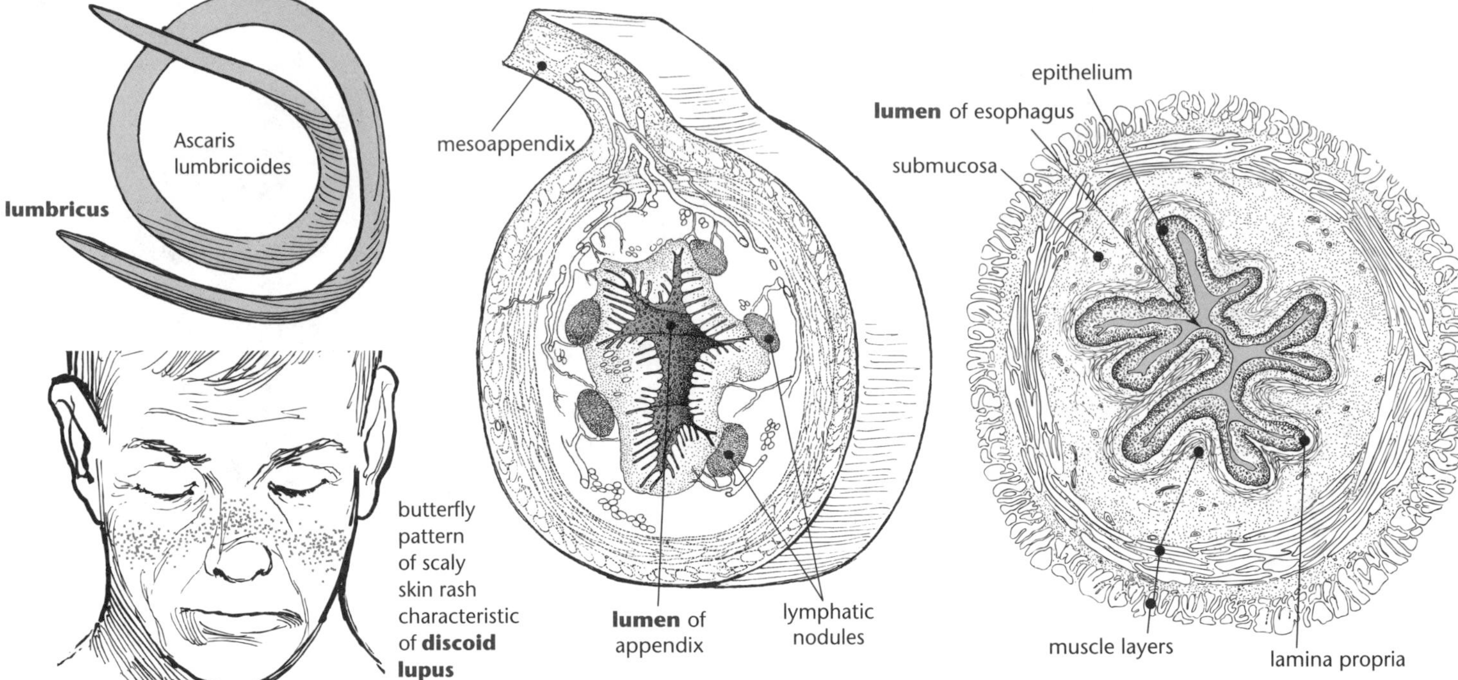

from the bite of the North American brown recluse spider, *Loxosceles reclusa*, and other members of the *Loxosceles* genus; characterized by gangrenous slough at the bite site, sometimes with nausea, vomiting, malaise, fever, and muscular weakness.

loxotomy (lok-sot´o-me) Surgical amputation by means of an oblique incision through the soft tissue; distinguished from a circular amputation.

lozenge (loz´enj) A medicated disk-shaped tablet for local treatment of the mouth or throat. Also called troche.

lub-dub (lub dub´) Commonly used term to describe the normal sounds made by the closing heart valves.

lucifugal (loo-sif´u-gal) Avoiding light.

lues (loo´ēz) Syphilis.

luetic (loo-et´ik) Syphilitic.

lumbago (lum-ba´go) Backache in the lumbar region.

lumbar (lum´bar) (1) Relating to the loins (i.e., the part of the back between the lowest rib and the pelvic bone on either side of the spine).

lumbarization (lum-ber-i-za´shun) Fusion between the transverse processes of the lowest lumbar and the adjacent sacral vertebrae.

lumbosacral (lum-bo-sa´kral) Relating to the lumbar portion of the spine and the sacrum.

lumbrical (lum´brĭ-kal) Resembling an earthworm; applied to certain muscles. See table of muscles.

lumbricoid (lum´brĭ-koid) Resembling an earthworm.

lumbricus (lum-bri´kus) A worm parasitic in the intestine, *Ascaris lumbricoides*.

lumen (loo´men) **1.** The interior space of a tubular structure, such as a blood vessel or the esophagus. **2.** A unit of emitted light; one lumen equals 0.001946 watt.

lumina (loo´min-ă) Plural of lumen.

luminal (loo´mĭ-nal) Relating to the lumen of a blood vessel, intestine, or other tubular structure.

luminescence (loo-mĭ-nes´ens) The property of giving off light by processes that derive energy from essentially non-thermal sources.

luminiferous (loo-mĭ-nif´er-us) Producing, conveying, or transmitting light.

luminophore (loo´mĭ-no-fōr) **1.** Any substance that emits light at room temperature. **2.** An organic radical that produces or increases the property of luminescence of certain organic compounds.

luminous (loo´mĭ-nus) Emitting or reflecting light.

lumirhodopsin (loo-mĭ-ro-dop´sin) An intermediate product in the bleaching process of rhodopsin (a retinal pigment) by the action of light prior to the formation of metarhodopsin and retinene.

lumpectomy (lum-pek´tŏ-me) Surgical removal of a hard mass and a margin of tissue, especially from the breast.

lunacy (loo´nă-se) Obsolete word for a major mental disorder.

lung (lung) The paired organ of respiration occupying the chest cavity (together with the heart) and enveloped by the pleura; generally the right lung is slightly larger than the left and is divided into three lobes, while the left has but two; the primary purpose of the lung is the uptake of oxygen and the elimination of carbon dioxide; it is accomplished by the following processes: (a) ventilation (inspired air reaches the alveoli and is distributed evenly to the millions of alveoli in the lungs); (b) diffusion (oxygen and carbon dioxide pass across the alveolar capillary membranes); (c) pulmonary capillary blood flow (flow is distributed evenly to all the ventilated alveoli).

black l. A form of pneumoconiosis common in coal mines, characterized by heavy deposit of coal dust in the lung; chronic bronchitis and emphysema may be associated with the condition. Also called coal miner's lung.

brown l. See byssinosis.

coal miner's l. See black lung.

farmer's l. An acute reaction or condition due to inhalation of moldy hay dust, usually from handling grains, particularly in threshing; thought to be of allergic origin; the symptoms are distressing dyspnea, cyanosis, and a dry cough. Also called thresher's lung.

honeycomb l. A lung marked by a spongy or honeycomb appearance from numerous small cysts resulting from diffuse fibrosis and cystic dilatation of bronchioles. Cause is unknown.

hyperlucent l. The appearance of a lung in an x-ray film; marked by areas of less than normal density; may be due to decreased blood flow or air trapped in a bronchus.

iron l. A popular name for the Drinker respirator; see under respirator.

miner's l. Black lung.

pump l. See adult respiratory distress syndrome.

rheumatoid l. Infiltrates in the lung associated with rheumatoid arthritis.

shock l. See adult respiratory distress syndrome.

silo-filler's l. Acute bronchitis occurring while working in freshly filled silos; thought to be caused by inhalation of high levels of nitrogen dioxide.

thresher's l. See farmer's lung.

welder's l. Relatively benign form of pneumoconiosis due to deposition of fine metallic particles in the lung; occupational hazard among welders.

wet l. Accumulation of fluid in the lung as in pulmonary edema.

lunula (loo´nu-lă) The pale semicircle at the root of each nail. Popularly called half moon.

lupoid (loo´poid) Resembling lupus.

lupus (loo´pus) A general term denoting any of several diseases manifested by characteristic skin lesions; used with a qualifying adjective.

discoid l. erythematosus (DLE) Disease confined to the skin, marked by a scaly rash, usually in a butterfly pattern over the nose and cheeks, sometimes extending to the scalp and causing baldness.

drug-induced l. Systemic lupus erythematosus, including the presence of antinuclear antibodies but only rarely involving the kidneys, precipitated by drugs used to lower high blood pressure (e.g., hydralazine), or to control cardiac arrhythmias (e.g., procainamide). Withdrawal of the drug reverses the condition.

l. pernio Sarcoid lesions of the hands and face, especially the ears and nose, resembling frostbite.

systemic l. erythematosus (SLE) A progressive, often severe, condition involving multiple systems (including skin, blood vessels, joints, heart, nervous system, and kidneys); thought to be of autoimmune origin. It is characterized by the presence of antinuclear antibodies (ANA) and other autoantibodies, including rheumatoid factor; antibodies producing false positive VDRL (syphilis) tests; antibodies against plasma coagulating protein; and antibodies against antigens on red and white blood cells and platelets, leading to immune destruction of these cells. Clinical features of the disease are diverse, depending on the location of the immune injury.

l. vulgaris Infection of the skin with the bacillus of tuberculosis, causing red-brown nodular lesions most frequently on the face.

lusitropy Relaxation of cardiac muscle.

luteal (loo´te-al) Relating to the corpus luteum of the ovary.

lutein (loo´tēn) The yellow pigment of egg yolks, corpus luteum, and fat cells.

luteinization (loo-tēn-ĭ-za´shun) The formation of luteal tissue; process in which the mature ovarian follicle, after discharging the egg, becomes hypertrophied and yellow, thus forming the corpus luteum.

luteinized unruptured follicle syndrome (loo´tēn-īzed un-rup´churd fol´lĭ-kl sĭn´drōm) Failure of a mature ovarian follicle to release an ovum; may impair fertility if the condition becomes chronic.

luteinizing (loo-tēn-i´zing) See luteogenic.

Lutembacher's syndrome (loo´tem-bak-erz sĭn´drōm) Congenital abnormality of the heart marked by an atrial septal defect, mitral stenosis, and enlargement of the right atrium.

luteogenic (loo-te-o-jen´ik) Inducing the development of corpora lutea. Also called luteinizing.

luteoma (loo-te-o´mă) An uncommon ovarian enlargement, usually occurring during pregnancy and regressing after childbirth.

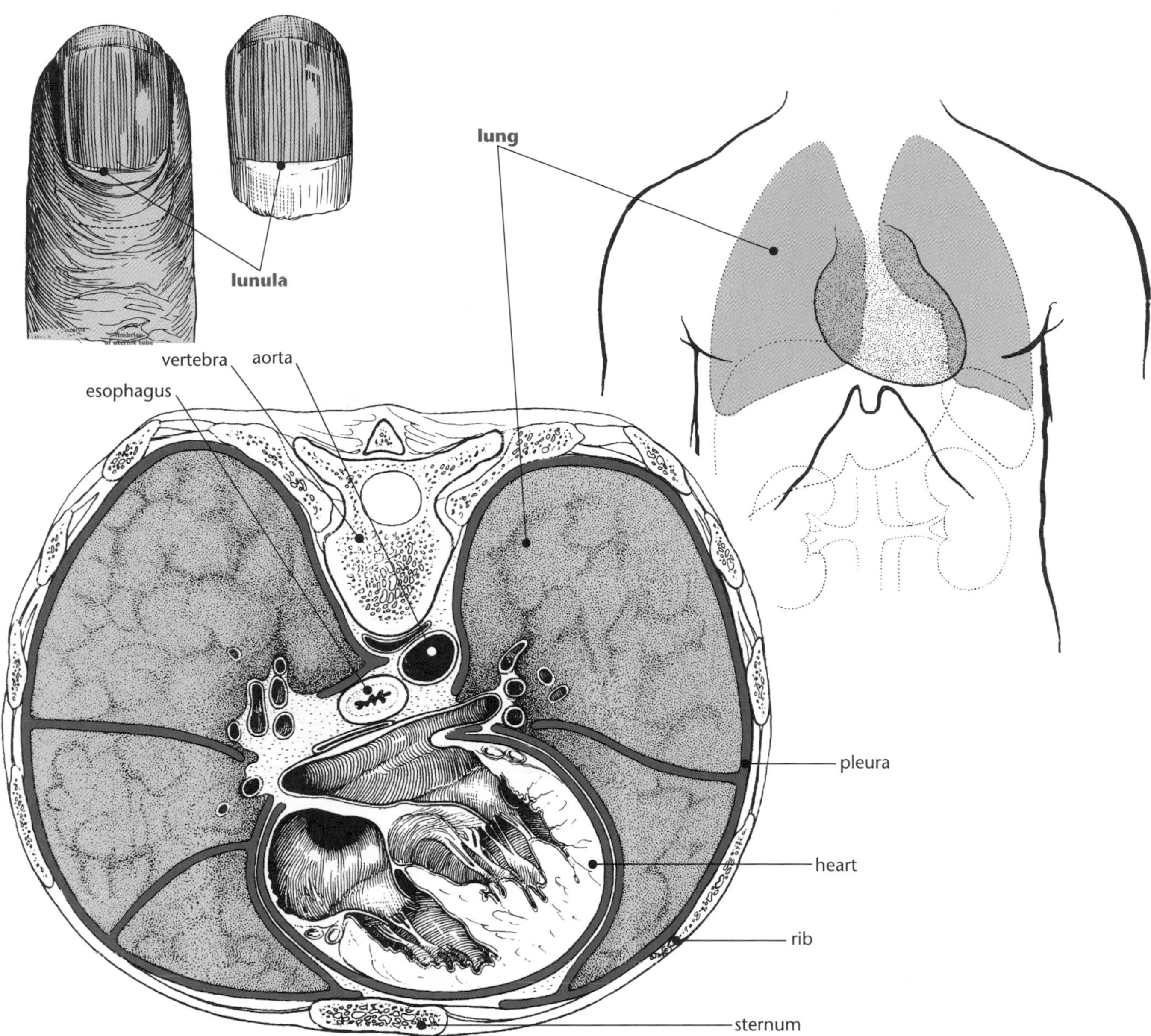

luteotropic (loo-te-o-trop´ik) Having a stimulating action on the development and function of the corpus luteum.

lutetium (loo-te´she-um) A silvery-white rare earth element, symbol Lu, atomic number 71, atomic weight 174.97; the final member of the lanthanide rare earth series; used in nuclear technology.

Lutheran blood group (loo´ther-an blud gro͞op) Antigens of red blood cells, specified by the Lu gene, that react with antibodies designated anti-Lu[a] and anti-Lu[b]; first detected in the serum of an individual who had received many transfusions and who developed antibodies against the erythrocytes of a donor named Lutheran.

lux (luks) A unit of illumination, equal to 1 lumen per square meter.

luxation (luk-sa´shun) Dislocation.

lycopene (li´ko-pēn) A tomato-derived antioxidant that may have anticancer properties.

lye (li) The liquid resulting from leaching wood ashes. Household lye is a mixture of sodium hydroxide and sodium carbonate. Also called lixivium.

lying-in (li-ing-in´) Popular term for the period from childbirth through the first few weeks afterwards.

Lyme disease (līm dĭ-zēz´) Disorder caused by a spirochete (*Borrelia burgdorferi)* transmitted by a tick (*Ixodes dammini)*; usually begins with an expanding red spot on the skin (stage 1, localized infection); days to weeks later the spirochete may spread via the bloodstream to other organs (stage 2, disseminated infection) possibly causing secondary skin lesions, meningitis, neuritis, or musculoskeletal pain; months to years later chronic arthritis or chronic neuritis may develop (stage 3, persistent infection). Also called Lyme borreliosis.

lymph (limf) A transparent or slightly opalescent fluid containing a clear liquid portion, a varying number of white blood cells, chiefly lymphocytes, and a few red blood cells; it is absorbed from the tissue spaces by the lymphatic capillaries (a system of closed tubes), conveyed, and eventually returned to the bloodstream by the lymphatic vessels, after it flows through a filtering system (lymph nodes).

inflammatory l. The slightly yellow fluid collecting on the surface of an acutely inflamed surface wound or membrane.

lymphaden (lim´fă-den) Lymph node; see under node.

lymphadenectasia (lim-fad-ĕ-nek´tă-zhă) Enlargement of lymph nodes with excessive lymph.

lymphadenectomy (lim-fad-ĕ-nek´tŏ-me) Surgical removal of lymph nodes.

lymphadenitis (lim-fad´ĕ-ni-tis) Inflammation of the lymph nodes.

histiocytic necrotizing l. See Kikuchi's disease.

lymphadenography (lim-fad-ĕ-nog´ră-fe) Roentgenographic examination of a lymph node after injection of a radiopaque medium.

lymphadenopathy (lim-fad-ĕ-nop´ă-the) Any disorder of the lymph nodes.

lymphadenosis (lim-fad-ĕ-no´sis) Generalized enlargement of the lymph nodes and lymphatic tissues.

benign l. See infectious mononucleosis, under mononucleosis.

lymphagogue (lim´fă-gog) An agent that increases the formation and flow of lymph.

lymphangiectasis, lymphangiectasia (lim-fan-je-ek-ta´sis, lim-fan-je-ek-ta´zha) Abnormal dilatation of lymphatic vessels. Also called lymphectasia.

lymphangiectomy (lim-fan-je-ek´to-me) Surgical excision of a lymph vessel.

lymphangioendothelioma (lim-fan-je-o-en-do-the-le-o´mă) A tumor composed of small masses of endothelial cells and aggregations of tubular structures thought to be lymph vessels.

lymphangiography (lim-fan-je-og´ră-fe) Roentgenographic visualization of lymphatic vessels after injection of a contrast medium. Also called lymphography.

lymphangiology (lim-fan-je-ol´o-je) The study of lymph vessels.

lymphangioma (lim-fan-je-o´mă) A benign tumorlike mass of dilated lymphatic vessels.

capillary l. See simple lymphangioma.

cavernous l. A poorly demarcated mass observed at birth or shortly thereafter, usually at the neck or in the armpit and often reaching up to 15 cm in diameter. It is a common feature of Turner's syndrome. Also called cystic hygroma.

simple l. Lymphangioma occurring typically in the head and neck as a rubbery cutaneous nodule 1 to 2 cm in diameter; may also occur within connective tissue of any organ. Also called capillary lymphangioma.

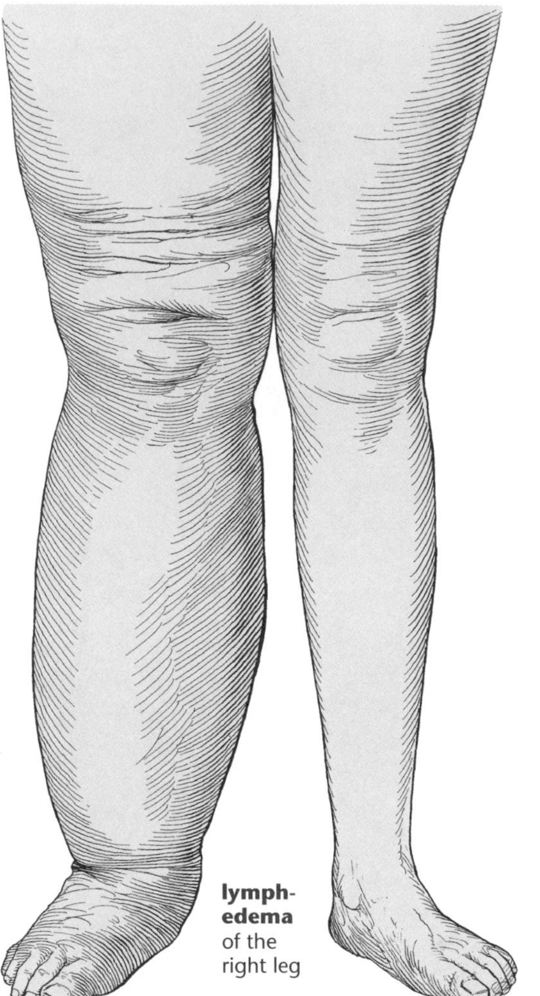
lymph-edema of the right leg

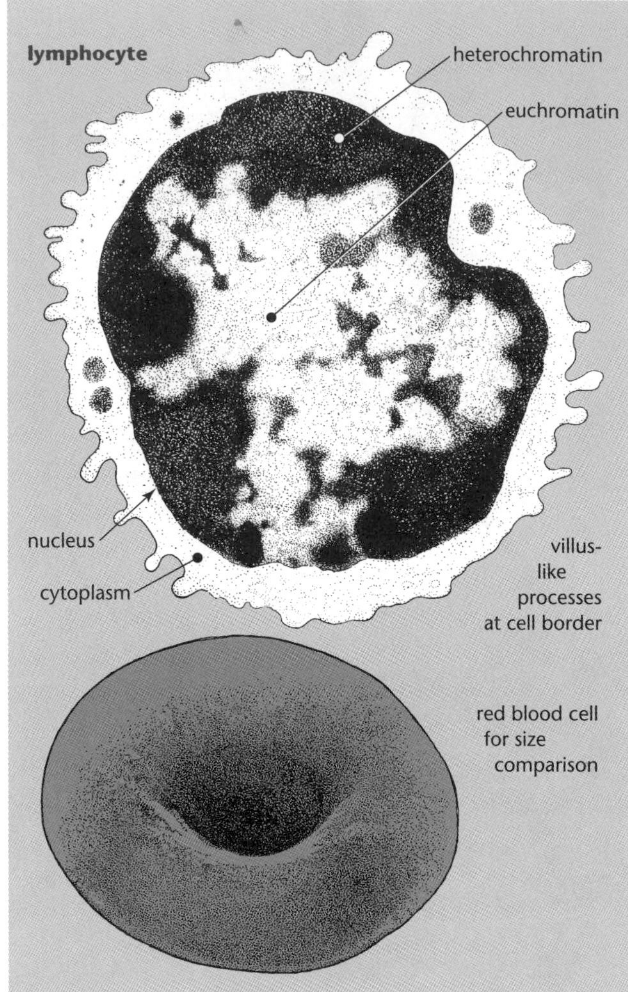

lymphangiosarcoma (lim-fan-je-o-sar-ko´mă) A rarely occurring cancerous tumor arising from the inner lining of lymphatic vessels.

lymphangitis (lim-fan-ji´tis) Inflammation of the lymphatic vessels; a common manifestation of a bacterial infection, usually caused by the hemolytic streptococcus.

lymphatic (lim-fat´ik) Relating to lymph, lymph nodes, or lymph vessels.

lymphectasia (lim-fek-ta´zhă) See lymphangiectasis.

lymphedema (lim-fĕ-de´mă) Chronic unilateral or bilateral swelling of the extremities caused by obstruction of the lymphatic vessels or disease of the lymph nodes.

lymphoblast (lim´fo-blast) An immature cell that is the precursor of the lymphocyte. Also called lymphocytoblast.

lymphoblastic (lim-fo-blas´tik) Relating to lymphoblasts or the production of lymphocytes.

lymphoblastoma (lim-fo-blas-to´mă) A tumor arising in a lymph node or group of nodes, composed mainly of lymphoblasts; a form of malignant lymphoma.

lymphoblastosis (lim-fo-blas-to´sis) Excess of lymphoblasts in the blood.

lymphocele (lim´fo-sēl) A cystic mass that contains lymph. Also called lymphocyst.

lymphocyst (lim´fo-sĭst) See lymphocele.

lymphocyte (lim´fo-sīt) A white blood cell formed in lymphoid tissue and constituting normally from 25 to 33 percent of all white blood cells in adult peripheral blood. Also called lymph cell.

B l.'s Lymphocytes derived from bone marrow; they interact chiefly with the humoral immune system which involves substances such as antibodies, antigens, and serum complement enzymes in the blood; analogous to the lymphocytes of birds governed by the bursa of Fabricius. Also called B cells.

B1 l.'s A minor population of B lymphocytes that secrete polyspecific low-affinity IgM antibodies. Also called B1 cells.

B2 l.'s The main population of B lymphocytes arising from stem cells in the bone marrow and secreting highly specific antibody within the secondary lymphoid tissues. Also called B2 cells.

cytotoxic T l. (CTL) Lymphocyte that kills its target cell by releasing a protein (perforin) to perforate the target-cell membrane after recognizing an antigen on the target-cell membrane. Also called cytotoxic T cell.

helper T l. A T lymphocyte that secretes the hormone-like proteins (cytokines) required for the functional activities of other cells in the immune system; usually expresses CD4 on its cell surface. Also called helper T cell.

NUL l. See null cell, under cell.

T l.'s Lymphocytes derived from the thymus; they play a large role in the cellular immune system by responding to antigens and triggering reactions in other cells, such as macrophages. Also called T cells.

type1 helper T l. A T lymphocyte that secretes the cytokines interleukin-2 and interferon-γ, inhibits type 2 helper T lymphocytes, and is chiefly involved in cell-mediated immunity (i.e., activation of macrophages and cytotoxic T cells). Also called type 1 helper T cell.

type 2 helper T l. A helper T lymphocyte that secretes the cytokines interleukin-4, 5, 6, and 10, inhibits type 1 helper T cells, and is chiefly involved in humoral immunity (i.e., production of antibody by B cells). Also called type 2 helper T cell.

virgin l. See inducible cell, under cell.

lymphocytic (lim-fo-sit´ik) Relating to lymphocytes.

lymphocytoblast (lim-fo-si´to-blast) See lymphoblast.

lymphocytoma (lim-fo-sī-to´mă) A tumor of low grade malignancy, arising in a lymph node or group of nodes; made up chiefly of adult lymphocytes.

lymphocytopenia (lim-fo-si-to-pe´ne-ă) See lymphopenia.

lymphocytopoiesis (lim-fo-si-to-poi-e´sis) The formation of lymphocytes.

lymphocytosis (lim-fo-si-to´sis) Excessive number of lymphocytes in the blood.

lymphoepithelioma (lim-fo-ep-ĭ-the-le-o´mă) A malignant tumor derived from the epithelium of the area around the tonsils and nasopharynx, and containing abundant lymphoid tissue.

lymphogenesis (lim-fo-jen´ĕ-sis) The production of lymph.

lymphogenous (lim-foj´ĕ-nus) **1.** Originating from lymph. **2.** Producing lymph.

lymphogranuloma venereum (lim-fo-gran-u-lo´mă ve-ne´re-um) (LGV) A chlamydial infection marked by the appearance of a transient ulcer on the genitalia and enlargement of the lymph nodes of the groin in the male and the pararectal nodes in the female. Also called tropical bubo; lymphogranuloma inguinale; venereal lymphogranuloma. Formerly called lymphopathia venereum.

lymphography (lim-fog´ră-fe) See lymphangiography.

lymphoid (lim´foid) Pertaining to or resembling lymph or lymphatic tissue.

lymphoidectomy (lim-foi-dek´to-me) Surgical excision of lymphoid tissue, such as adenoids.

lymphokine (lim´fo-kīn) A hormone-like peptide produced by sensitized lymphocytes when they come in contact with the antigen to which they were sensitized; acts as an intercellular messenger to regulate immune and inflammatory responses.

lymphokinesis (lim-fo-ki-ne´sis) **1.** Circulation of lymph through the lymphatic vessels and nodes. **2.** The movement of endolymph in the membranous labyrinth of the inner ear.

lymphology (lim-fol´o-je) The science of the lymphatic system comprising lymph, lymphocytes,

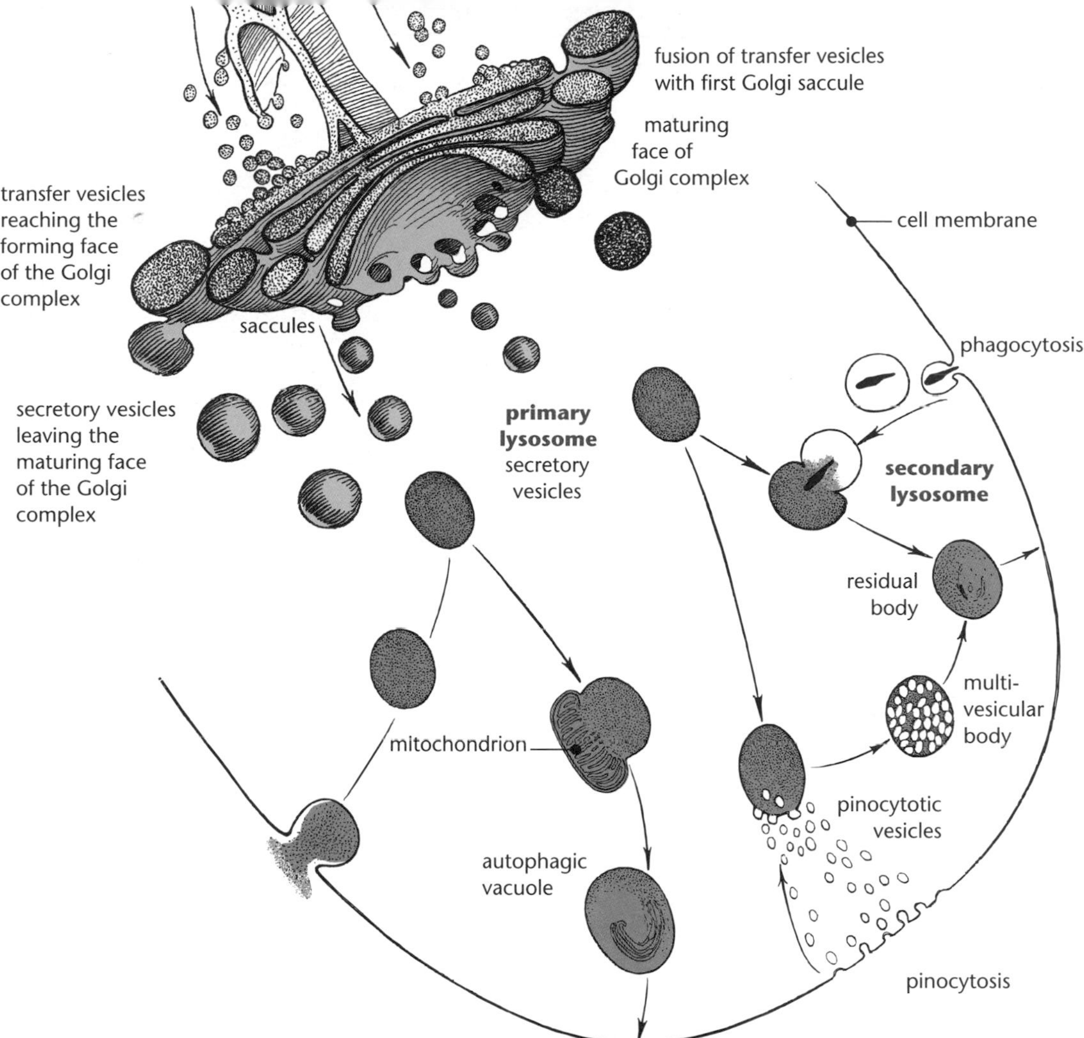

lymph nodes, and lymph vessels.

lymphoma (lim-fo´mă) Any of a group of malignant diseases originating in the lymphoreticular system, usually in the lymph nodes. Formerly called malignant lymphadenosis.

Burkitt's l. A malignant tumor primarily of the jaw and abdominal area, usually affecting children and young adults of the middle African regions and, sporadically, other parts of the world. Also called African lymphoma.

histiocytic l. Malignant lymphoma in which the abnormal cells are a mixture of large histiocytes and smaller cells resembling lymphocytes.

Hodgkin's l. See Hodgkin's disease.

nodular l. A type of non-Hodgkin's lymphoma marked by a growth pattern in which the tumor cells aggregate and form nodules.

non-Hodgkin's l. (NHL) A group of malignant lymphomas that typically begin as painless enlargement of a lymph node; some spread to other lymph nodes and eventually involve the spleen, liver, and bone marrow; others, after becoming widespread, disseminate to the circulating blood, creating a leukemia-like condition in the peripheral blood. Classified by the Working Formulation for Clinical Use as low-, intermediate-, and high-grade.

lymphomatosis (lim-fo-mă-to´sis) Any condition characterized by the presence of multiple lymphoid tissue tumors (lymphomas).

lymphopathia venereum (lim-fo-path´e-ă vě-ne´re-um) Old term for lymphogranuloma venereum.

lymphopathy (lim-fop´ă-the) Any disease of the lymphatic system.

lymphopenia (lim-fo-pe´ne-ă) Reduction in the number of lymphocytes in the blood. Also called lymphocytopenia.

lymphopoiesis (lim-fo-poi-e´sis) The formation of lymphocytes.

lymphoreticular (lim-fo-rĕ-tik´u-lar) Relating to a tissue containing a variety of cell types involved in the elaboration of a cell product when confronted with a substance which is recognized as foreign; the tissue is located within the thymus gland, lymph nodes, spleen, and the lining of the lymphatic and vascular channels, as well as in bodily tracts exposed to the outside.

lymphosarcoma (lim-fo-sar-ko´mă) Malignant tumor of lymph nodes, composed of lymphoblasts and lymphocytes.

lymphoscintigraphy (lim-fo-sin-tig´ră-fe) Scanning of the lymph vessels and nodes after injection of radioactively labeled colloid.

lymphostasis (lim-fos´tă-sis) Obstruction of the normal flow of lymph.

lyophil (li´o-fil) Any substance that easily goes into solution.

lyophilic (li-o-fil´ik) Dissolving readily due to having a pronounced affinity for the dissolving medium (solvent); applied to colloids.

lyophilization (li-of-ĭ-li-za´shun) The process of freeze-drying; the act of separating a solid substance from solution by freezing the solution and evaporating the ice under vacuum; used for preservation of a variety of tissues and bacteria.

lyophilize (li-of´ĭ-līz) To separate a solid from solution by rapid freezing and dehydration under vacuum; to freeze-dry.

lyophobic (li-o-fo´bik) Lack of affinity for a solvent; applied to colloids.

lyotropic (li-o-trop´ik) Readily soluble.

lyse (līz) To effect lysis (disintegration of cells).

lysergic acid (li-sur´jik as´id) A crystalline compound derived from ergot.

lysergic acid diethylamide (LSD) A hallucinogenic drug derived from lysergic acid.

lysin (li´sin) An antibody that destroys cells by dissolving them, as hemolysin and bacteriolysin which destroy blood cells and bacteria, respectively.

lysine (li´sēn) (Lys) One of the essential amino acids; produced by the hydrolysis of casein and other proteins.

lysis (li´sis) **1.** Destruction of cells by a specific lysin **2.** The gradual recovery from an acute disease.

lysogen (li´so-jen) An antigen (e.g., bacterial cell) that stimulates the formation of a lysin (e.g., antibody) that is specific to that antigen.

lysogenesis (li-so-jen´ĕ-sis) The production of antibodies that cause dissolution of cells and tissues.

lysogeny (li-soj´e-ne) A form of viral parasitism in which viral DNA becomes incorporated in a cell (bacterial) genome, without destroying the cell, thereby permitting the transmission of the virus to the subsequent generation.

lysokinase (li-so-ki´nās) An activator agent of the fibrinolytic system, such as streptokinase or staphylokinase, that produces plasma by indirect or multiple-stage action on plasminogen.

lysolecithin (li-so-les´ĭ-thin) A lecithin (phosphatidyl choline) from which the unsaturated fatty acid residue has been removed by partial hydrolysis; it has strong hemolytic properties and is a good detergent and emulsifier of dietary lipid.

lysophosphatidic acid (li-so-fos-fă-tid´ik) (LPA) A lipid, intermediate in the production of phosphatidic acid, that appears to be a promoter of cancer cell growth; present in accumulated abdominal fluid (ascites) of patients with ovarian cancer. It is a possible marker for ovarian cancer. Also called ovarian cancer activating factor.

lysosomal (li-so-sōmal) Relating to lysosomes.

lysosome (li´so-sōm) One of the large cytoplasmic particles in a cell containing a powerful digestive juice (hydrolyzing enzyme or lysozyme) capable of breaking down most of the constituents of living matter; it is present in all animal cells, being particularly large and abundant in white blood cells.

primary l. A lysosome that has not engaged in any digestive activity.

secondary l. A vacuolated lysosome that is the site of current or previous digestive activity.

lysozyme (li´so-zīm) An antibacterial enzyme naturally present in tear fluid, sweat, saliva, and nasal secretions. Also called mucopeptide gluco-hydrolase.

lytic (lit´ik) Relating to or causing disintegration of cells.

M

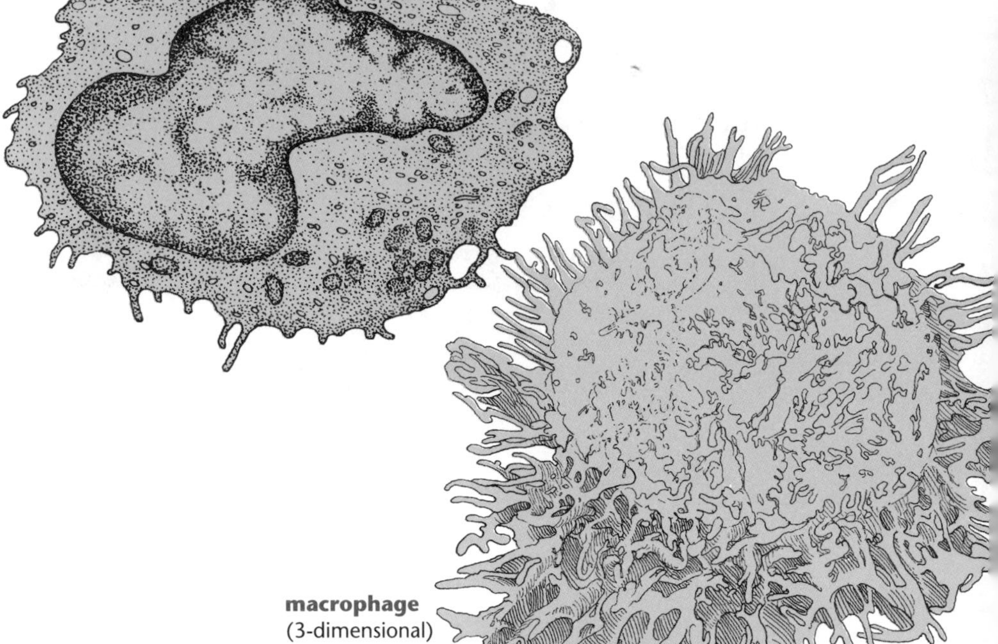

µ (myōō) The 12th letter of the Greek alphabet.

MAC disease (mak dī-zēz′) See *Mycobacterium avium* complex bacteremia, under bacteremia.

Macaca mulatta (mă-kak′ă mōō-lat′ă) The rhesus monkey; a species (genus *Macaca*, family Cercopithecidae) of Southeast Asia that is frequently used as a laboratory animal.

Mace, **MACE** (mās) Trademark for a type of tear gas used in an aerosol form as a defensive weapon; causes intense eye pain and respiratory distress.

macerate (mas′er-āt) To soften a solid or a tissue by soaking in a fluid.

maceration (mas-er-a′shun) **1.** The softening of a tissue or other solid or the separation of its constituents by soaking it in a liquid. **2.** In obstetrics, the softening and disintegration of a fetus remaining in the uterus after its death.

machine (mă-shēn′) A device that accomplishes a specific objective.

anesthesia m. In inhalation anesthesia, apparatus for delivering quantified volumes of anesthetic gases and oxygen to the patient's breathing circuit for inducement of general anesthesia; includes vaporizers, flowmeters, and sources of compressed gases.

heart-lung m. Any of various machines that make it possible to support the circulation with oxygenated blood while keeping the heart essentially free of blood and permitting surgery within the heart, coronary arteries, and ascending arch of the aorta under direct vision; venous blood ordinarily returning to the right atrium is diverted to an oxygenator (artificial lung) where it takes up oxygen and gives off carbon dioxide; the oxygenated blood is pumped into the individual's arterial system.

Holtz m. A device for developing high-voltage static electricity by multiplication of an induced charge.

kidney m. See hemodialyzer.

panoramic rotating m. An x-ray machine capable of radiographing all the teeth and surrounding structures by using a reciprocating motion of the tube and extraoral film.

Van de Graaf m. An electrostatic machine that produces high potential; used for generating high-voltage x rays.

Wimshurst's m. A machine capable of converting mechanical energy into electrical energy by electrostatic action.

Macracanthorhynchus hirudinaceus (mak-ră-kan-tho-ring′kus hir-u-dĭ-na′se-us) A species of thorn-headed worms (class Acanthocephala) between 5 and 65 cm in length; a parasite of hogs and, occasionally, of humans.

macrencephaly, macrencephalia (mak-ren-sef′ă-le, mak-ren′sĕ-fa′le-ă) The state of having an oversized brain.

macroamylase (mak-ro-am′ĭ-lās) A form of serum amylase in which the enzyme occurs as a complex joined to a globulin.

macrobrachia (mak-ro-bra′ke-ă) Condition of having abnormally long arms.

macrocephalous (mak-ro-sef′ă-lus) Having an abnormally large head. Also called megalocephalous.

macrocephaly (mak-ro-sef′ă-le) An abnormally large head circumference of an infant, i.e., two or more standard deviations (SDs) above the mean for its age and sex; it may or may not be associated with hydrocephalus; other causes include slow subdural effusions (usually from trauma) and large cystic defects.

macrochemistry (mak-ro-kem′is-tre) Chemistry in which the reactions are visible to the naked eye.

macrochilia (mak-ro-ki′le-ă) **1.** Unusually large lips. **2.** A condition of permanently enlarged oral lips, usually due to the presence of distended lymph spaces.

macrochiria (mak-ro-ki′re-ă) Abnormally large hands. Also called megalochiria.

macroconidium (mak-ro-ko-nid′e-um) A large exospore or conidium.

macrocornea (mak-ro-kor′ne-ă) See megalocornea.

macrocrania (mak-ro-kra′ne-ă) Abnormal general enlargement of the cranium of an infant (i.e., circumference greater than 98th percentile).

macrocryoglobulinemia (mak-ro-kri-o-glob-u-lin-e′me-ă) The presence of cold precipitating macroglobulins (cold hemagglutinins) in the peripheral blood.

macrocyte (mak′ro-sīt) A large red blood cell at least 2 µm larger than normal; can be seen in the blood of individuals with pernicious anemia, folic acid deficiency, and other anemias. Also called macroerythrocyte.

macrocythemia (mak-ro-si-the′me-ă) See macrocytosis.

macrocytosis (ak-ro-si-to′sis) A condition in which the red blood cells are larger than normal. Also called macrocythemia.

macrodactyly (mak-ro-dak′tĭ-le) A condition in which fingers or toes are abnormally large. Also called dactylomegaly; megadactyly; megalodactylism.

macrodont (mak′ro-dont) **1.** An abnormally large tooth. **2.** Denoting a skull with a dental index over 44.

macrodontia (mak-ro-don′shă) The condition of having abnormally large teeth.

macroencephaly (mak-ro-en-sef′ă-le) See macrencephaly.

macroerythrocyte (mak-ro-ĕ-rith′ro-sīt) See macrocyte.

macrogamete (mak-ro-gam′ēt) The female of certain unicellular organisms.

macrogametocyte (mak-ro-gă-me′to-sīt) A mother cell producing the females or macrogametes of certain protozoa.

macrogenitosomia (mak-ro-jen-ĭ-to-so′me-ă) Disorder of the adrenal cortex most commonly affecting male children; characterized by excessive and early development of sexual organs, associated with rapid maturation of the musculoskeletal system, which results in abnormally short stature.

macrogingivae (mak-ro-jin-ji′ve) Abnormal enlargement of the gums.

macroglia (mak-rog′le-ă) The astrocyte and oligodendrocyte, the two neuroglial elements of ectodermal origin.

macroglobulin (mak-ro-glob′u-lin) Unusually large plasma globulin (protein); molecular weight is often about 1 million.

macroglobulinemia (mak-ro-glob-u-lĭ-ne′me-ă) The presence of macroglobulins in the circulating blood.

Waldenström's m. A malignancy predominantly seen in people over 60 years of age; marked by diffuse infiltration of bone marrow by certain cells (lymphocytes, plasma cells, and lymphocytoid plasma cells) that secrete an abnormal protein (M component, a monoclonal immunoglobulin); cells may also infiltrate lymph nodes, spleen, and liver; symptoms include weakness, weight loss, visual impairment, dizziness, and deafness. Also called Waldenström's syndrome.

macroglossia (mak-ro-glos′e-ă) Enlargement of the tongue. Also called megaloglossia.

macrognathia (mak-ro-na′the-ă) Abnormal largeness of the jaw.

macrogyria (mak-ro-ji′re-ă) A congenital malformation in which the convolutions of the cerebral cortex are larger than normal due to a reduction in the number of sulci.

macrolides (mak′ro-līdz) A group of antibiotics having molecules made up of large-ring lactones (e.g., erythromycin).

macromastia, macromazia (mak-ro-mas′te-ă, mak-ro-ma′ze-ă) Abnormally large breasts.

macromelia (mak-ro-me′le-ă) Abnormally large size of one or more of the extremities. Also called megalomelia.

macromethod (mak′ro-meth-od) A chemical test using ordinary (not minute) quantities.

macromolecule (mak-ro-mol′ĕ-kūl) Any molecule composed of several monomers, notably proteins, nucleic acids, polysaccharides, glycoproteins, and glycolipids.

macronucleus (mak-ro-nu′kle-us) **1.** A nucleus that occupies a large area of the cell. **2.** The larger, nonreproductive nucleus in ciliated protozoa.

macro-orchidism (mak-ro-or′kĭ-diz-m) Abnormally large testes.

macroparasite (mak-ro-par′ă-sīt) A parasite that is visible to the unaided eye (e.g., a louse).

macropathology (mak-ro-pă-thol′o-je) Gross anatomic changes caused by disease.

macrophage (mak′ro-fāj) A large mononuclear cell which ingests degenerated cells and blood tissue; found in large numbers throughout the body, with the greatest accumulation in the spleen, where they remove damaged or aging red blood cells from the circulation; in the brain and spinal cord they are known as microglia; in the blood they are called monocytes.

activated m. A mature macrophage that has been made cytotoxic to certain cells (e.g., tumor cells) by exposure to a particular hormone-like intercellular

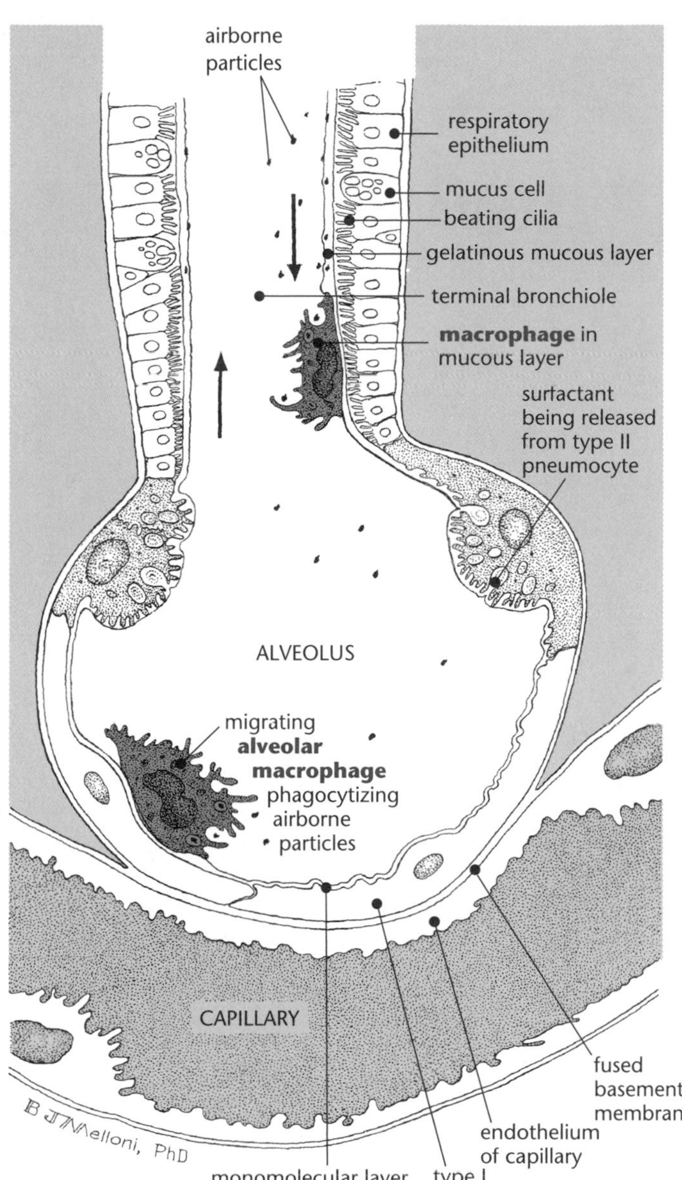

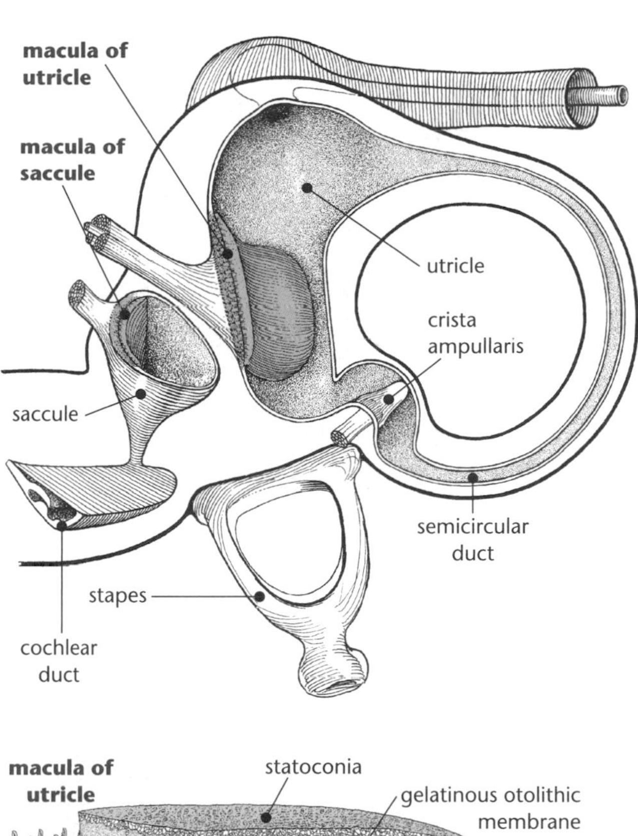

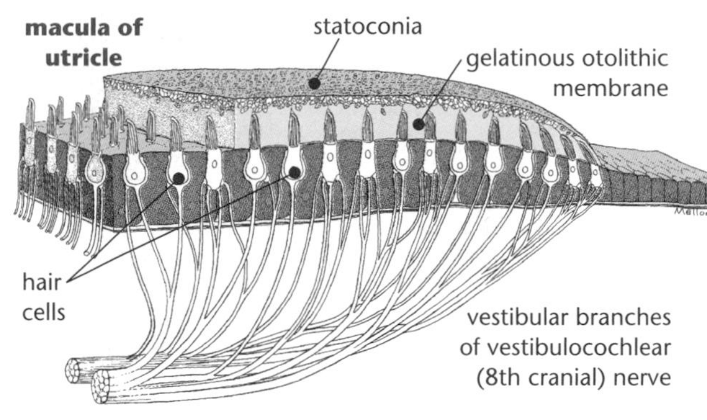

mediator (cytokine).

alveolar m. A cell that moves about on the alveolar surface of the lung engulfing airborne particles that reach the alveolus; derived from the hematogenous monocyte. Also called dust cell; alveolar phagocyte.

macrophthalmia (mak-rof-thal′me-ă) See megalophthalmos.

macropolycyte (mak-ro-pol′e-sīt) An extremely large polymorphonuclear neutrophilic leukocyte having a nucleus with numerous segments.

macropsia (mă-krop′se-ă) The condition of seeing objects as larger than their actual sizes. Also called megalopsia.

macrorhinia (mak-ro-rin′e-ă) The condition of having an abnormally large nose.

macroscopic (mak-ro-skop′ik) Visible with the naked eye, without need of magnifying equipment.

macrosomia (mak-ro-so′me-ă) Abnormally large size of the body, such as that of a newborn infant of a diabetic mother.

macrospore (mak′ro-spōr) See megaspore.

macrostomia (mak-ro-sto′me-ă) Developmental malformation occurring when the embryonic maxillary and mandibular swellings fail to fuse, resulting in extension of the mouth toward the ear; the defect may be bilateral or unilateral.

macrostructure (mak-ro-struk′chur) A structure visible with the unaided eye.

macrotia (mak-ro′she-ă) Abnormal largeness of the ears.

macula (mak′u-lă), *pl.* **maculae** A small area differing in appearance from the surrounding tissue.

m. adherens See desmosome.

m. communis The thickened portion of the medial wall of the auditory vesicle in the embryo; eventually it divides to form the macula sacculi and the macula utriculi.

corneal m. A moderately dense whitish opacity of the cornea.

m. densa That portion of the distal convoluted tubule of the kidney contacting the wall of the afferent arteriole just before the latter enters the glomerulus; the cells are narrow and slightly taller than those around them; part of the juxtaglomerular apparatus.

m. of follicle A relatively avascular area on the surface of an ovary where a vesicular ovarian follicle ruptures, forcing the enclosed egg, cumulus, some detached follicular (granulosa) cells, and follicular fluid out into the peritoneal cavity; usually the rupture point is rapidly sealed off.

m. of gonorrhea The red, inflamed opening of the duct of the greater vestibular gland, seen in gonorrheal vulvitis.

m. lutea See macula retinae.

m. retinae A small oval yellowish depression on the retina, lateral to and slightly below the optic disk; it contains the fovea centralis. Also called macula lutea; yellow spot.

m. of saccule The oval neuroepithelial sensory area in the medial wall of the saccule that houses the terminal arborizations of vestibular nerve fibers.

m. of utricle The neuroepithelial sensory area in the lateral wall of the utricle that houses the terminal arborizations of vestibular nerve fibers.

macular, maculate (mak′u-lar, mak′u-lāt) Relating to macules.

maculation (mak-u-la′shun) The formation of macules or spots on the skin.

macule (mak′ūl) A nonelevated, discolored lesion on the skin; a spot on the skin.

maculocerebral (mak-u-lo-ser′e-bral) Relating to the brain and the macula lutea of the retina.

maculoerythematous (mak-u-lo-er-ĭ-them′ă-tus) Both red and spotted; said of certain lesions.

maculopapular (mak-u-lo-pap′u-lar) Related to maculopapules.

maculopapule (mak-u-lo-pap′ūl) A raised lesion (papule) on a discoloration or spot (macule) on the skin.

maculopathy (mak-u-lop′ă-the) Any disease of the macula retinae. Also called macular retinopathy.

mad (mad) Colloquial term for one who is suffering from a mental disorder.

madarosis (mad-ă-ro′sis) Loss of the eyelashes or of the eyebrows.

mad-cow disease (mad-kou dĭ-zēz′) See bovine spongiform encephalopathy (BSE), under encephalopathy.

Madurella (mad-u-rel′ă) A genus of fungi (family Dematiaceae); some species cause maduromycosis.

maduromycosis (mă-du-ro-mi-ko′sis) Also called mycetoma.

Maffucci's syndrome (mă-fu′chēz sin′drōm) The combination of multiple cutaneous hemangiomas and dyschondroplasia; the vascular malformations are manifested by extensive birthmarks and dilatation of the veins (phlebectasias) in the form of soft, tender, purple tumors in subcutaneous tissue, lips, and palate; deformities of the hands and feet are usually evident.

maggot (mag′ot) A legless, soft-bodied grub that is the larva of various insects of the order Diptera, such

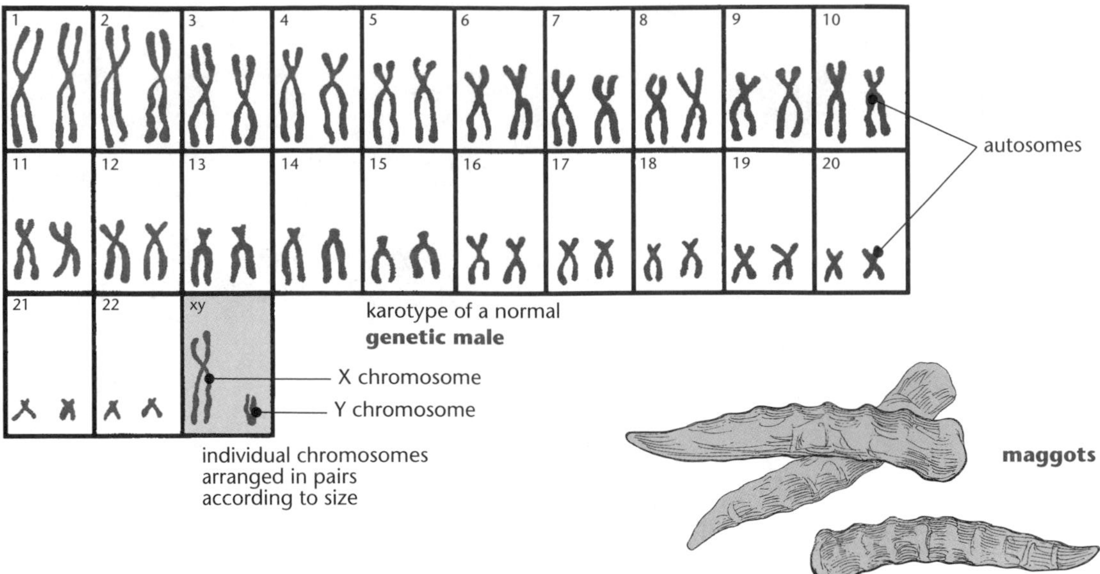

as the housefly; it develops usually in dead organic matter.

magma (mag´mă) A soft inert mass composed of finely divided solids in an aqueous medium; a paste or salve.

magnesia (mag-ne´zhă) Magnesium oxide.

citrate of m. See magnesium citrate, under magnesium.

m. magma See milk of magnesia.

milk of m. (MOM) An aqueous suspension of magnesium hydroxide; used as a laxative and antacid. Also called magnesia magma.

magnesium (mag-ne´ze-um) A light, moderately hard, metallic element with a silvery luster; symbol Mg, atomic number 12, atomic weight 24.31, valence 2; it is an essential nutritional substance.

m. carbonate A very light, white powdery compound, $MgCO_3$, used in gastric and intestinal acidity and as a laxative; it is insoluble in water.

m. citrate A colorless crystalline powder, $Mg_3(C_6H_5O_7)_2 \cdot 14H_2O$, used in solution as a laxative. Also called citrate of magnesia.

m. hydroxide A white powdery compound, $Mg(OH)_2$, practically insoluble in water, used as an antacid and laxative.

m. oxide A white powdery compound, MgO, insoluble in water; used as an antacid and laxative. Also called magnesia.

m. sulfate A colorless, crystalline compound, $MgSO_4$, soluble in water; effective cathartic, particularly useful in certain poisonings; the form $MgSO_4 \cdot 7H_2O$ is Epsom salt.

magnetism (mag´nĕ-tiz-m) **1.** The property of mutual attraction or repulsion produced by a magnet or by an electric current. **2.** The force exhibited by a magnetic field.

magneton (mag´nĕ-ton) A unit of measure of the magnetic movement of an atomic or subatomic particle.

magnification (mag-nĭ-fi-ka´shun) An enlargement of an object by an optical element or instrument.

maieusiophobia (ma-u-sio-fo´biă) Abnormal fear of childbirth.

maim (mām) To disable, mutilate, or cripple.

main (măn) French for hand.

m. d'accoucheur See accoucheur's hand, under hand.

m. en crochet Permanent flexure of the fourth and fifth fingers, resembling the position of a person's hand while crocheting.

m. an griffe See clawhand.

m. an lorgnette See opera glass hand, under hand.

mainlining (mān´līn-ing) Term used by drug addicts denoting intravenous injection of heroin or other drugs.

mainstreaming (mān´strēm-ing) **1.** Placement of a child with physical or mental disabilities in a regular classroom while providing supplemental services and educational programs. **2.** Any effort to deinstitutionalize a person with an affliction (e.g., mental disorder).

Majocchi's disease (mă-yok´ēz dĭ-zēz´) See annular telangiectatic purpura, under purpura.

mal (mahl) French for disease.

grand m. See generalized epilepsy, under epilepsy.

petit m. See childhood absence epilepsy, under epilepsy.

mala (ma´lă) Latin for cheekbone, the cheek.

malabsorption (mal-ab-sorp´shun) Inadequate or imperfect absorption.

m. syndrome Condition marked by weight loss, weakness, pallor, protuberant abdomen, bleeding tendency and other symptoms and signs, caused by any disease that impairs the absorption of nutrients.

malachite green (mal´ă-kīt grēn) Green crystalline substance, soluble in water, used as a pH indicator; it changes at pH 1.0 from yellow (acid) to blue-green (alkaline); used also for staining bacteria and as an antiseptic. Also called Victoria green.

malacia (mă-la´shă) Abnormal softening of tissues.

malacoplakia (mal-ă-ko-pla´ke-ă) See malakoplakia.

maladie (mal-ă-de´) French for malady.

m. de Roger See Roger's disease.

malady (mal´ă-de) Illness; disease.

malaise (mal-āz´) A vague general discomfort or feeling of illness.

malakoplakia (mal-ă-ko-pla´ke-ă) The formation of soft, fungus-like growths on the mucous membrane of a hollow organ, especially the urinary bladder. Also written malacoplakia.

malalignment (mal-ă-līn´ment) The displacement of a tooth, or teeth, from normal position.

malar (ma´lar) Relating to the cheek or cheek bone.

malaria (mă-la´re-ă) Infectious disease caused by any of four species of a protozoan parasite of the genus *Plasmodium*; transmitted by the bite of an infected female mosquito of the genus *Anopheles*; usual symptoms include extreme exhaustion, paroxysms of high fever, sweating, shaking chills, anemia, and enlargement of the spleen; the typical fever may occur on alternate days, every third day, or daily, depending on the time required for a new generation of parasites to complete its life cycle. See also *Plasmodium*.

benign tertian m. See vivax malaria.

estivoautumnal m. See falciparum malaria.

falciparum m. A form caused by the most invasive of all malarial parasites, *Plasmodium falciparum*, causing infected blood cells to clump and block capillaries; the paroxysms of fever usually occur every other day but frequently at indefinite intervals; in severe cases cerebral, renal, gastrointestinal, or pulmonary complications may develop. Also called malignant tertian malaria; estivoautumnal malaria.

malariae m. A form caused by *Plasmodium malariae*; the paroxysms of fever usually occur every third day. Also called quartan malaria.

malignant tertian m. See falciparum malaria.

quartan m. See malariae malaria.

quotidian m. A form in which the paroxysms occur daily; usually caused by two groups of *Plasmodium vivax* parasites reproducing alternately every 48 hours; may also be caused by a combination of *Plasmodium falciparum* and *Plasmodium vivax* or by two generations of *Plasmodium falciparum*.

relapsing m. A type in which exoerythrocytic forms of the parasite persist after the initial incubation period; if not destroyed, these forms act as a reservoir for repeated clinical episodes due to invasion of the red blood cells.

tertian m. See vivax malaria.

vivax m. A form caused by *Plasmodium vivax* or *Plasmodium ovale*; the paroxysms occur every other day. Also called tertian or benign tertian malaria.

malarial (mă-la´re-al) Relating to malaria.

Malassezia (mal-ă-sa´zĭ-ă) A genus of fungi.

M. furfur The species of fungus that causes tinea versicolor.

malate (ma´lāt) A salt of malic acid.

malathion (mal-ă-thi´on) Substance used as an insecticide and, in veterinary medicine, against external parasites.

male (māl) **1.** One who produces spermatozoa. **2.** Masculine.

genetic m. An individual with a normal male karyotype, one X and one Y chromosome.

malformation (mal-for-ma´shun) A defect or deformity.

Arnold-Chiari m. Extrusion of brain tissue through the foramen magnum down into the upper cervical canal, usually associated with spina bifida; ranges from mild, with herniation of the posteroinferior portion of the cerebellum and little or no downward displacement of the 4th ventricle, to severe, with extrusion of the 4th ventricle, medulla oblongata, and cerebellar vermis into the cervical canal. Also called Arnold-Chiari syndrome.

congenital m. One evident at birth, either genetic or of environmental origin. Commonly called birth defect.

malfunction (mal-funk´shun) Abnormal or inadequate function.

malic acid (mal´ik as´id) An intermediate in carbohydrate metabolism; present in unripe apples, cherries, tomatoes, etc.

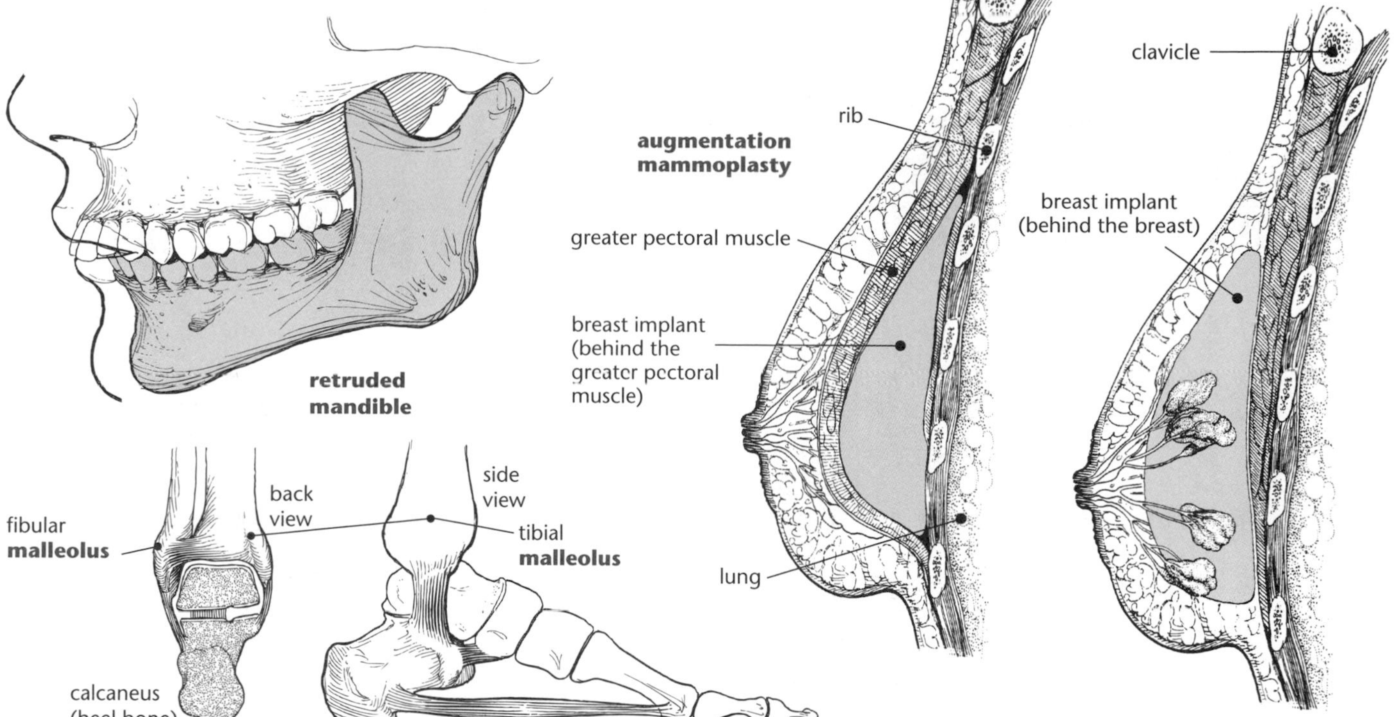

malignancy (mă-lig′nan-se) The condition of being malignant.

malignant (mă-lig′nant) **1.** Denoting any disease resistant to treatment and of a fatal nature. **2.** Denoting a tumor of uncontrollable growth and dissemination.

malingering (ma-ling′ger-ing) A faking of illness or voluntary production of symptoms for a rationally determined gain (e.g., monetary compensation, avoidance of responsibility).

malleable (mal′e-ă-bl) Capable of being made into thin sheets; said of certain metals.

malleation (mal-e-a′shun) A spasmodic movement of the hands, as of hammering.

malleolar (mal-e′o-lar) Relating to one or both prominences on either side of the ankle.

malleolus (mă-le′o-lus), *pl.* **malle′oli** One of two projections (one on the tibia and one on the fibula) on either side of the ankle joint.

malleus (mal′e-us) The club-shaped and most lateral of the three auditory ossicles in the middle ear chamber, which is firmly attached to the tympanic membrane (eardrum) and articulates with the incus.

Mallory-Weiss syndrome (mal′o-rē-wīs′ sin′ drōm) Lacerations of the lower esophagus with vomiting of blood, usually following protracted, severe, incoordinate vomiting and retching; frequently seen in alcoholics.

malnutrition (mal-noo-trish′un) Faulty nutrition due to inadequate diet (e.g., consuming inadequate amounts or the wrong proportions of nutrients), or to a metabolic abnormality.

malocclusion (mal-o-kloo′zhun) Abnormal contact of opposing teeth (mandibular and maxillary), so as to interfere with the efficient movement of the jaws during mastication.

close bite m. Condition in which the edges of the anterior mandibular teeth extend lingually toward the gums of the opposing teeth when the jaws are closed.

open bite m. A condition marked by the failure of opposing teeth to establish contact when the jaws are closed.

malonyl (mal′o-nil) The bivalent radical of malonic acid.

malposition (mal-pŏ-zish′un) An abnormal or anomalous position.

malpractice (mal-prak′tis) Negligence by a professional (e.g., physician, attorney, accountant).

medical m. Negligence by a medical professional; medical care provided to a patient that falls below the accepted standards of medical practice, thereby exposing the patient to an unreasonable risk of harm. A legal claim for medical malpractice requires that the patient prove the health care professional owed the patient a duty to provide medical care within the accepted standards of medical practice, that the duty was breached, and that the breach caused injury to the patient. The injury claimed by the patient must be recognized by law as compensable.

malpresentation (mal-prez-en-ta′shun) In obstetrics, any position of the fetus at the time of birth in which the presenting part is not the usual: head first, sharply flexed with chin and chest in contact.

malrotation (mal-ro-ta′shun) Failure of a body part to undergo normal rotation (e.g., failure of intestines to rotate during embryonic development).

maltase (mawl′tās) A digestive enzyme that promotes the conversion of maltose into glucose.

maltose (mawl′tōs) $C_{32}H_{22}O_{11}$; a sugar formed by the action of a digestive enzyme on starch; it consists of two glucose moieties. Also called malt sugar.

malum (ma′lum) Latin for disease.

malunion (mal-ūn′yon) Union of a fractured bone in a faulty alignment or position.

mamelon, mammelon (mam′ĕ-lon) One of the three rounded prominences on the cutting edge of an erupting incisor tooth.

mamilla (mă-mil′ă) **1.** Nipple. **2.** Any nipple-like protuberance.

mamillaplasty (mă-mil-ă-plas′te) Reparative surgery of the nipple. Also called theleplasty.

mamillary (mam′ĭ-ler-e) Relating to or resembling a nipple.

mamillate, mammillated (mam′ĭ-lāt, mam′ĭ-lāt-ed) Having nipple-like projections.

mamillitis (mam-ĭ-li′tis) Inflammation of a nipple.

mamma (măm′ă), *pl.* **mam′mae** See breast.

mammal (mam′al) A member of the class Mammalia.

Mammalia (mă-ma′le-ă) A class of vertebrates that includes all animals that nourish their young with milk.

mammaplasty (mam′ă-plas-te) See mammoplasty.

mammary (mam′er-e) Relating to the breast.

mammectomy (mă-mek′to-me) See mastectomy.

mammitis (mam-i′tis) See mastitis.

mammogram (mam′ŏ-gram) A radiograph of the breast.

mammography (mă-mog′ră-fe) A soft tissue x-ray technique for visualization of the female breast; the making of a mammogram; used to detect nonpalpable lesions and to identify palpable lesions.

mammoplasty (mam′o-plas-te) Plastic surgery of the breasts. Also called mammaplasty; mastoplasty.

augmentative m. Increase of breast size by insertion of an implant.

reconstructive m. Introduction of an implant to replace a breast that has been removed partly or completely.

reduction m. Operation to reduce the size of the breasts.

mammotrophic (mam-o-trof′ik) Promoting the development, growth, and function of the mammary gland.

mandelate (man-del′āt) A salt of mandelic acid.

mandelic acid (man-del′ik as′id) A crystalline substance, soluble in water; used as a urinary antibacterial agent. Also called phenylglycolic acid.

mandible (man′dĭ-bl) The horseshoe-shaped bone of the lower jaw which articulates with the skull at the temporo-mandibular joint; it houses the lower teeth. Also called jawbone.

mandibular (man-dib′u-lar) Relating to the lower jaw or mandible.

mandibulectomy (man-dib-u-lek′to-me) Surgical removal of the lower jaw.

mandibulopharyngeal (man-dib-u-lo-fă-rin′je-al) Relating to the mandible and pharynx.

Mandragora (man-drag′o-ră) Genus of plants that include the *M. officinarum,* a poisonous European herb that has sedative, hypnotic, and anesthetic properties. Also called mandrake.

mandrake (man′drāk) Any plant of the genus *Mandragora.*

mandrel (man′drel) A shaft on which a working tool is mounted, and by means of which it is rotated.

disk m. A mandrel designed to hold a polishing disk.

snap-on m. A mandrel with a split end that supports a rubber polishing cup.

maneuver (mă-noo′ver) A procedure or movement requiring skill and dexterity.

Adson's m. See Adson's test, under test.

Bracht's m. In obstetrics, maneuver used in breech extraction whereby the breech is allowed to deliver spontaneously up to the umbilicus, then the baby's body is held (without pressure) against the mother's pubic symphysis and moderate suprapubic pressure is applied by an assistant.

Brandt-Andrews m. A method of delivering the placenta during the last (third) stage of labor; pressure is applied with the fingers of one hand just above the symphysis to elevate the uterus into the abdomen and at the same time express the placenta into the vagina; gentle cord traction with the other hand is used to guide the placenta into the birth canal.

Credé's m.'s (a) A method of expressing the placenta that is generally no longer recommended. (b) Application of 1 drop of a 2% solution of silver nitrate onto each eye of the newborn infant to prevent gonococcal conjunctivitis. (c) Manual pressure on the bladder, especially a paralyzed bladder, to express urine.

Heimlich m. Maneuver used to dislodge a piece of food stuck in a person's throat and obstructing the

M

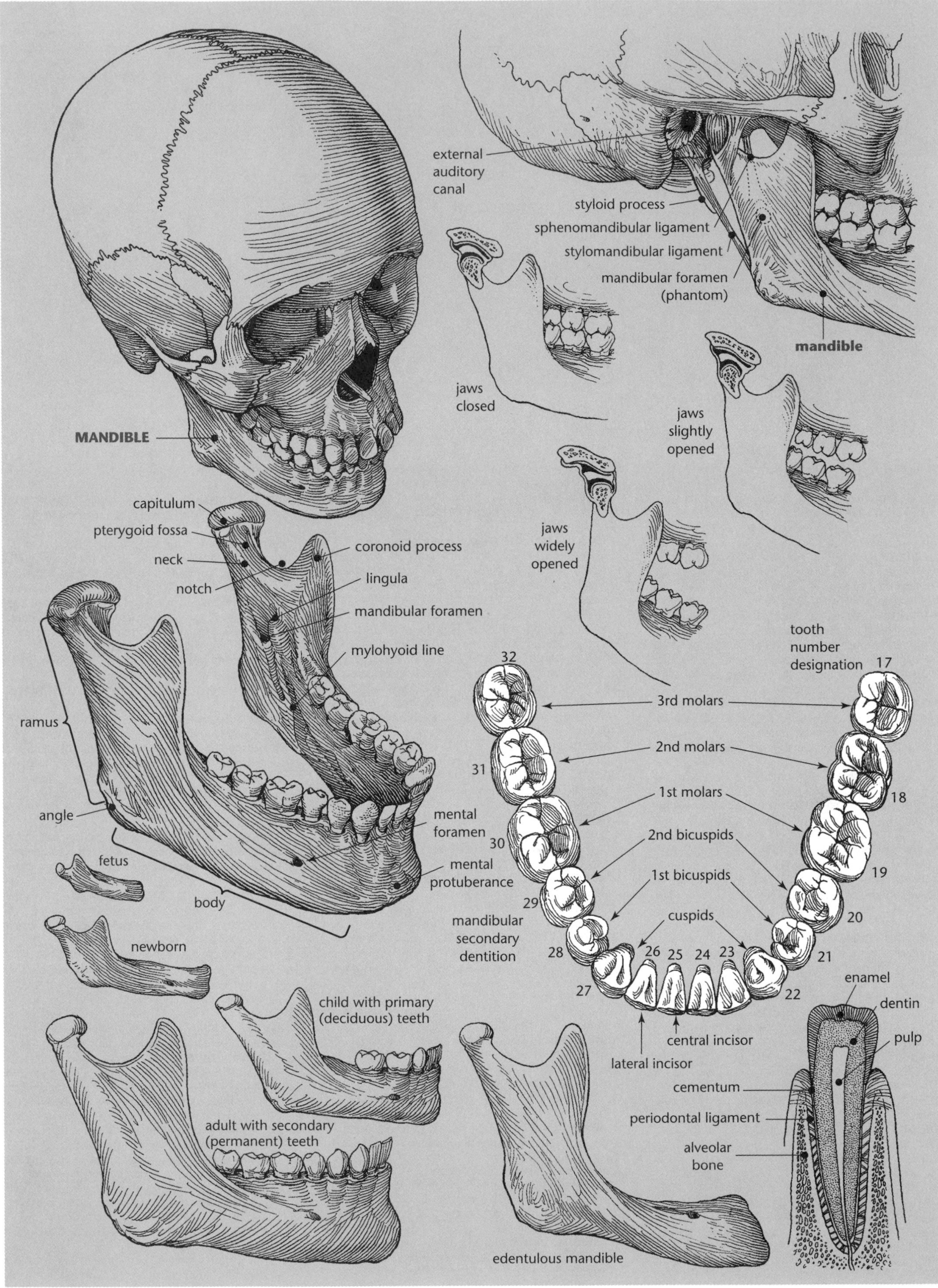
external auditory canal
styloid process
sphenomandibular ligament
stylomandibular ligament
mandibular foramen (phantom)
mandible
jaws closed
jaws slightly opened
jaws widely opened
MANDIBLE
capitulum
pterygoid fossa
neck
notch
coronoid process
lingula
mandibular foramen
mylohyoid line
ramus
angle
mental foramen
mental protuberance
body
fetus
newborn
child with primary (deciduous) teeth
adult with secondary (permanent) teeth
edentulous mandible
tooth number designation
32
17
3rd molars
2nd molars
31
18
1st molars
30
2nd bicuspids
1st bicuspids
19
29
20
cuspids
mandibular secondary dentition
28
26
25
24
23
21
27
22
central incisor
lateral incisor
enamel
dentin
pulp
cementum
periodontal ligament
alveolar bone

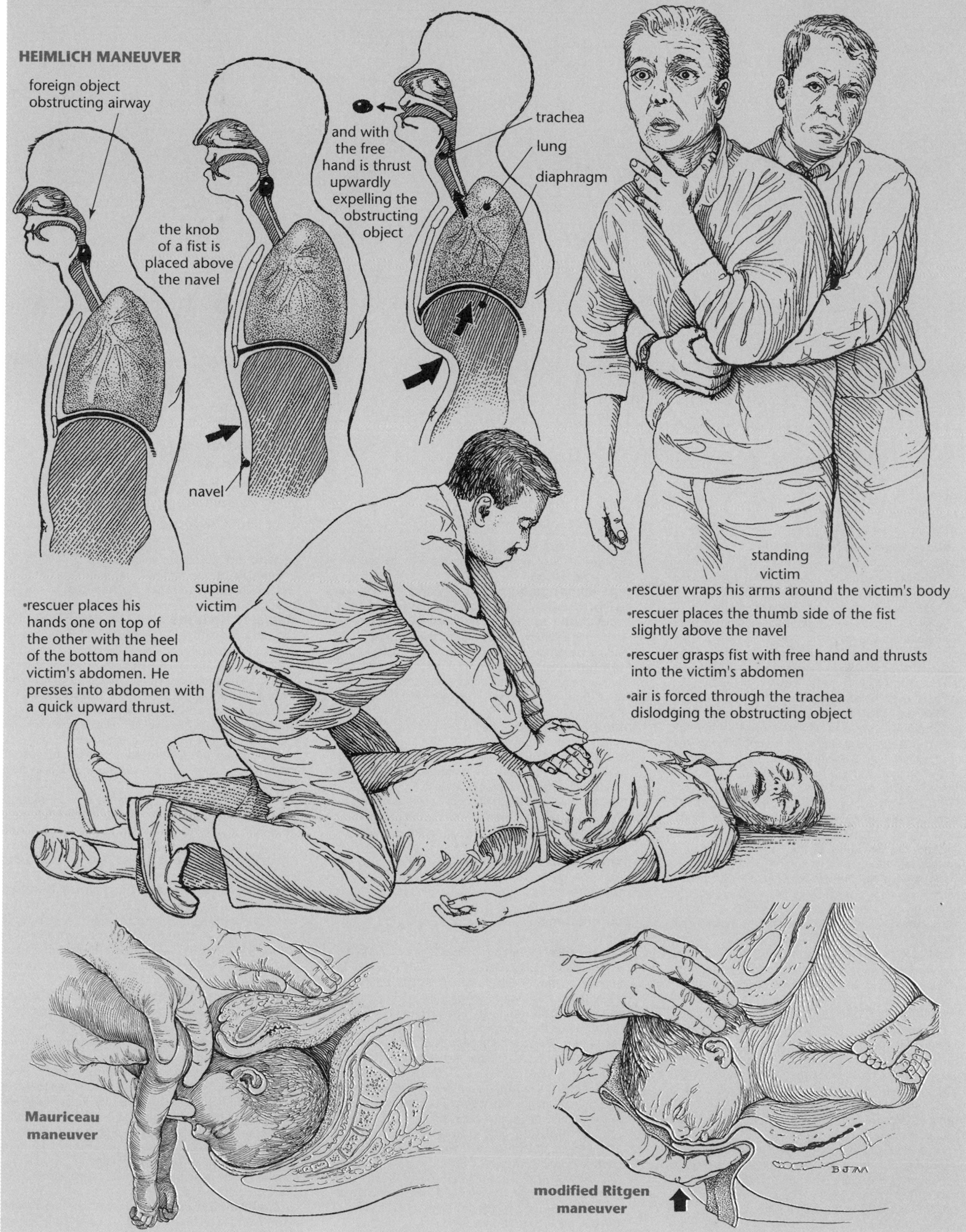
HEIMLICH MANEUVER
foreign object obstructing airway
the knob of a fist is placed above the navel
navel
and with the free hand is thrust upwardly expelling the obstructing object
trachea
lung
diaphragm
standing victim
•rescuer wraps his arms around the victim's body
•rescuer places the thumb side of the fist slightly above the navel
•rescuer grasps fist with free hand and thrusts into the victim's abdomen
•air is forced through the trachea dislodging the obstructing object
supine victim
•rescuer places his hands one on top of the other with the heel of the bottom hand on victim's abdomen. He presses into abdomen with a quick upward thrust.
Mauriceau maneuver
modified Ritgen maneuver
BJM

M

airway; standing in back of the victim, the rescuer places both arms around him; he makes a fist with one hand, grasps it with the other hand, and (with the thumb toward the victim) presses his fist sharply upward against the victim's abdomen, between the navel and the rib cage; this causes the diaphragm to elevate and the lungs to compress; the resulting increased air pressure forced through the trachea (windpipe) forces out the food particle.

Leopold's m.'s Four methods of abdominal palpation to determine the position of the fetus in the uterus.

Mauriceau m. Method of extracting the aftercoming head in partial breech presentation when the chin is directed posteriorly and the rest of the body has been delivered; the body of the fetus straddles the forearm of the operator, the middle and index fingers of one of the operator's hands are pressed over the maxilla to maintain flexion of the head, two fingers of the operator's other hand are placed forklike over the neck and shoulders to exert gentle downward traction until the suboccipital region appears under the maternal pubic symphysis; then the body is elevated toward the mother's abdomen until the mouth, nose, and brow are delivered over the perineum. Also called Mauriceau-Smellie-Veit maneuver.

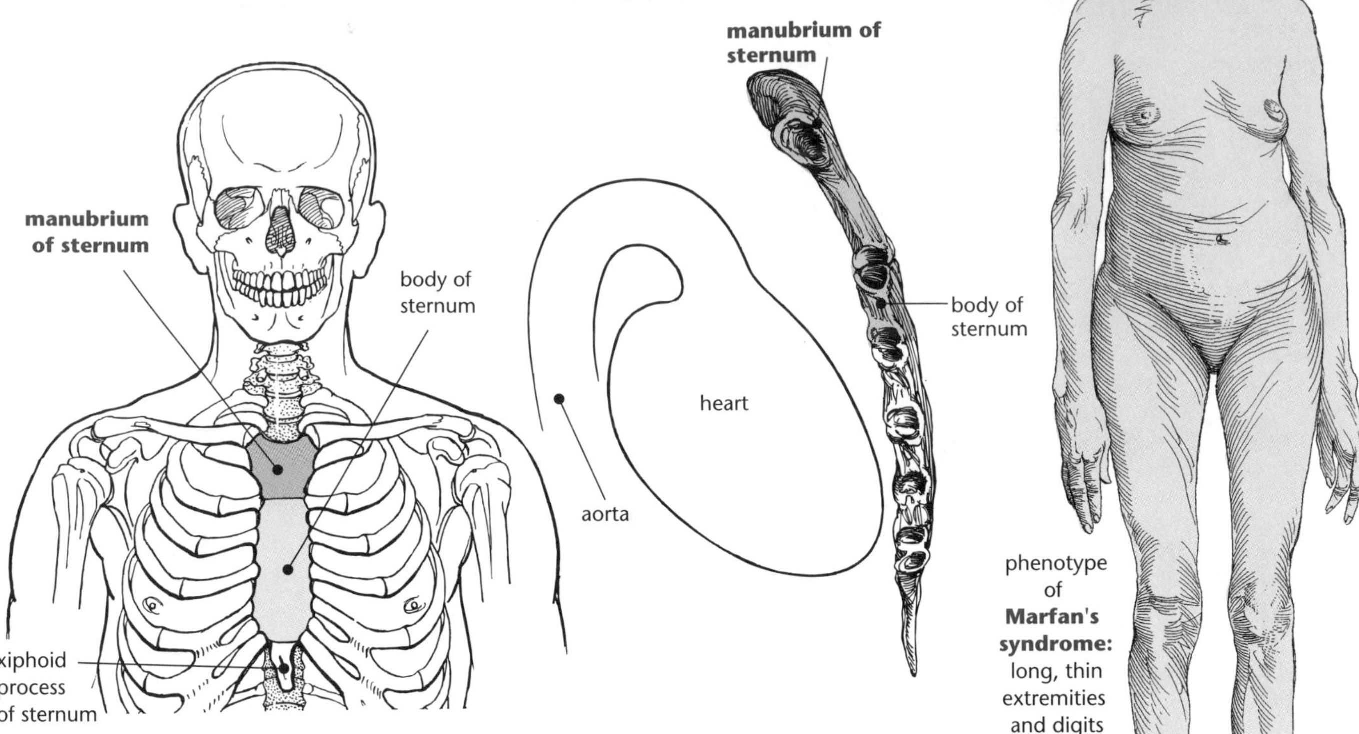

M

Mauriceau-Smellie-Veit m. See Mauriceau's maneuver.
modified Prague m. Method of delivering the fetal head in breech presentation when the back of the head remains posteriorly directed and the rest of the body has been delivered; one hand of the operator supports the shoulders from below while the other hand gently draws the body upward toward the maternal abdomen, thus flexing the head within the birth canal, which permits delivery of the back of the head over the perineum.
modified Ritgen's m. Delivery of a baby's head by applying forward pressure on the chin through the perineum with one hand while applying pressure on the head with the other hand; the maneuver is performed between contractions and allows for slow delivery of the head.
Pinard's m. Method of fetal extraction in a frank breech presentation; two fingers are passed along the fetal thigh to the knee to push it away from the midline and flex the leg; the foot is then readily grasped and brought down and out.
Scanzoni's m. Forceps rotation of the fetal head, when it presents with its back directed posteriorly, followed by removal and reapplication of the instrument for delivery to avoid injury to the maternal soft parts.
Sellick m. A technique used to facilitate endotracheal intubation in which pressure is applied to the cricoid cartilage to occlude the esophagus.
Valsalva m. **1.** Forced expiration against the closed glottis to increase pressure within the lungs. **2.** Forced expiration with mouth closed and pinched nose to clear the auditory tube.

manganese (man´gă-nēs) A grayish or silvery metallic element; symbol Mn, atomic number 25, atomic weight 54.94; some of its salts are used in medicine.

manganous (man´gă-nus) Denoting a compound containing bivalent manganese.

mange (mānj) A skin disease of animals caused by burrowing itch mites, usually *Sarcoptes chorioptes*; in humans, the disease is called scabies.

mania (man´ne-ă) Mental state characterized by episodes of excessive excitement, hyperactivity, and profuse and rapidly changing ideas; occurs in certain mental disorders.

maniac (ma´ne-ak) Common vague and misleading term for a mentally disturbed (usually violent) individual.

manic (ma´nik) Relating to mania.

manic-depressive (ma´nik-de-pres´iv) See bipolar disorder, under disorder.

manifestation (man-ĭ-fes-tā´shun) The display of characteristic signs or symptoms of a disease.
neurotic m. Defense mechanisms (e.g., phobias, displacement, conversion, dissociation) that handicap a person's daily living activities; used in an attempt to relieve anxiety.
psychophysiologic m. Symptoms that are primarily physical with a partial emotional origin.
psychotic m. The loss of contact with reality impairing a person's ability to function in society and indicating personality disintegration.

manikin (man´ĭ-kin) An anatomic model of the human body used for practicing certain manipulations (e.g., those of obstetrics). Also called simulation model.

maniphalanx (man-ĭ-fa´lanks) One of the bones (phalanx) of a finger.

manipulation (mă-nip-u-la´shun) Treatment by the skillful use of the hands, as in reducing a dislocation or changing the position of the fetus.

manna (man´ă) The dried sugary exudate of the ash tree, *Fraxinus ornus*; formerly used as a mild laxative.

mannerism (man´er-iz-m) A distinctive characteristic or behavioral trait.

mannitol (man´ĭ-tol) An alcohol, $C_6H_{14}O_6$, derived from fructose; used as an osmotic agent.

manometer (mă-nom´ĕ-ter) An instrument for measuring the pressure of gases and liquids.

manometric (man-o-met´rik) Relating to a manometer.

Mansonella (man-son-el´ă) Genus of parasitic worms, commonly called filaria; adults live mainly in body cavities or subcutaneous tissues of the host, while larvae exist in the peripheral blood.

mansonellosis (man-so-nel-o´sis) Infection with organisms of the genus *Mansonella.*

Mansonia (man-so´ne-ă) Genus of mosquitoes in tropical Asia and Africa that transmit microfilaria to man.

manubrium (mă-nu´bre-um) A structure that resembles a handle; when used alone the term refers to the manubrium of the sternum.
m. of malleus The process of the malleus attached to the inner surface of the tympanic membrane (eardrum).
m. of sternum The upper portion of the sternum articulating with the clavicles and the first and upper parts of the second costal cartilages on each side.

manus (ma´nus) Latin for hand.
m. extensa Backward deviation of the hand.
m. flexa Forward deviation of the hand.
m. valga Deviation of the hand toward the ulnar side.
m. vara Deviation of the hand toward the radial side.

map (map) A graphic representation of the relative positions of any parts or units.
chromosome m. The specific linear arrangement of genes along the chromosomes. Also called gene map.
gene m. See chromosome map.
linkage m. A chromosome map indicating the relative positions of genes, as determined by linkage studies.

maple syrup urine disease (mā´pl sir´up u´rin dĭ-zēz´) An autosomal recessive inherited disorder marked by deficient oxidative decarboxylation of α-keto acids; the urine has a characteristic maple syrup odor; hypotonia, hypoglycemia, and neurologic manifestations appear within the first week of life. Also called branched-chain keloaciduria.

mapping (map´ing) In genetics, locating the position and order of gene loci on a chromosome by analyzing the frequency of recombination between the loci.

marantic (mă-ran´tik) **1.** See marasmic. **2.** See under endocarditis.

marasmic (mă-raz´mik) Relating to marasmus.

marasmus (mă-raz´mus) Gradual, progressive wasting of the body, occurring mainly in young children; caused by protein and calorie depletion.

marble bone disease (mar´bl bōn dĭ-zēz´) See osteopetrosis.

Marburg disease, Marburg virus disease (mar´berg dĭ-zēz´, mar´berg vi´rus dĭ-zēz´) An often fatal disease marked by rash and multi-organ hemorrhages, caused by a rhabdovirus (family Filoviridae). First observed among laboratory workers in Marburg, Germany, exposed to African green monkeys.

Marchiafava-Micheli syndrome (anemia) (mar-ke-ă-fă´vă-me-ka´le sin´drōm) See paroxysmal nocturnal hemoglobinuria, under hemoglobinuria.

Marfan's syndrome (mar-făn´ sin´drōm) Disorder inherited as an autosomal dominant trait and marked by defective formation of elastic fibers that affects the skeleton, large arteries, suspensory ligaments of the lens of the eye, tendons, and joint capsules; the affected individuals have abnormally long slender extremities, spidery fingers, high palate, displacement of the lens, lax joints, and aneurysm of the aorta.

margin (mar´jin) A border or edge.
ciliary m. of iris The border of the iris attached to the ciliary body.
costal m. The curved lower portion of the thoracic wall, formed by the cartilages of the seventh through tenth ribs.
falciform m. The lower lateral border of the saphenous opening in the deep fascia (fascia lata) in front of the thigh; it lies anterior to the femoral vessels.
free gingival m. The edge of the gum tissue that is not directly attached to the tooth. Also called free gum margin.
free gum m. See free gingival margin.
gingival m. The part of the gum, not attached to

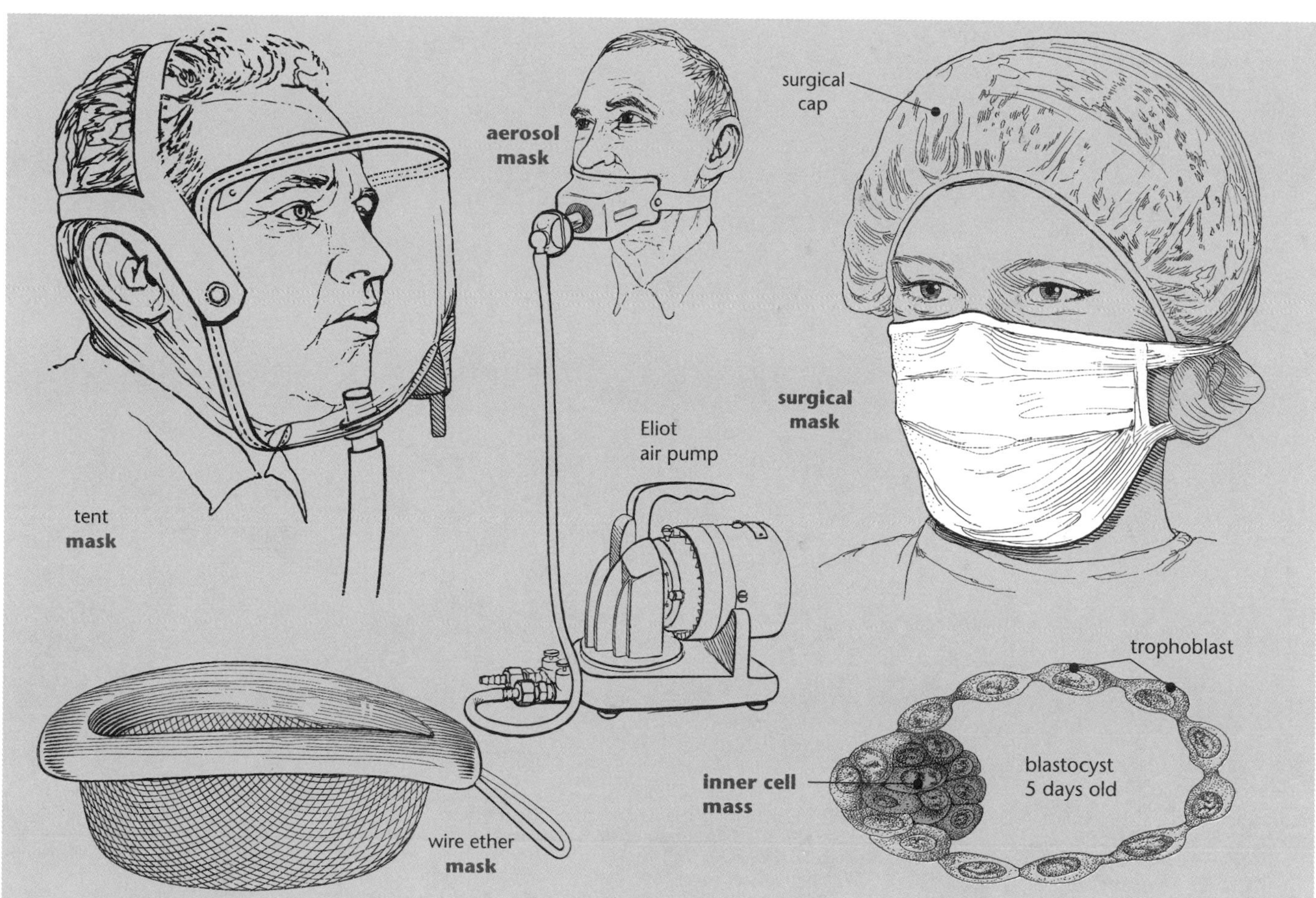

M

the tooth, facing either the lips, cheeks, or tongue.

infraorbital m. The lower border of the orbit.

orbital m. Margin of the ocular orbit bounded by the frontal bone superiorly, the zygomatic bone laterally, the maxilla inferiorly, and the process of the maxilla and frontal bone medially.

pupillary m. of iris The border of the iris forming the edge of the pupil.

right m. of heart The border between the diaphragmatic and sternocostal aspects of the heart.

supraorbital m. The superior edge of the orbit.

margination (mar-jĭ-na´shun) Adhesion of leukocytes to the interior of capillary walls during early stages of inflammation.

marginoplasty (mar-jin´o-plas-te) Plastic surgery of the eyelid border.

marijuana, marihuana (mar-ĭ-wă´nă) **1.** A tall hemp plant. **2.** The dried, chopped leaves, flowers, and stems of the common hemp plant *Cannabis sativa* (family Moraceae); smoked or mixed into food to induce euphoria; the origin of the word is obscure, but may be a composite of the Spanish names Maria and Juana (Mary and Jane).

Marie-Strümpell disease (mă-re´strim´pel dĭ-zēz´) See ankylosing spondylitis, under spondylitis.

mark (mark) A visible impression on a surface; a blemish; a spot.

port-wine m. See nevus flammeus, under nevus.

stretch m. See stria atrophica, under stria.

marker (mark´er) **1.** A characteristic or factor by which a cell or molecule can be identified or a disease can be recognized. **2.** A general term for any trait that helps to throw light on the genetic nature of a disorder, such as a defect of structure or a deviant enzyme.

cutaneous m. Any of various skin changes that serve as a sign of an internal (frequently malignant) disease.

genetic m. In general, any character that serves as a signpost of the presence or location of a gene in an individual or a given population. Specifically, a locus (site) on a chromosome that has easily classifiable alleles and can be used in genetic studies.

tumor m. A substance secreted by a tumor and released into the blood and other body fluids; detection of its presence aids diagnosis of the tumor; examples include alphafetoprotein (AFP) for hepatoma and chorionic embryonic antigen (CEA) for colon cancer.

marmot (mar´mot) A rodent that sometimes carries the plague bacillus and ticks that transmit Rocky Mountain spotted fever. Also called groundhog; woodchuck.

Maroteaux-Lamy syndrome (mă-ro-to´lă-me´ sin´drōm) A form of mucopolysaccharidosis characterized by dwarfism, chest deformities, knock knees, stiff joints, corneal clouding, short hands and fingers and excessive dermatan sulfate excretion in the urine; inherited as an autosomal recessive trait. Also called type VI mucopolysaccharidosis.

marrow (mar´o) The soft material filling a central cavity, especially of bones.

bone m. The soft tissue in the cavities of bones; produces most cells circulating in the blood (erythrocytes, leukocytes, and megakaryocytes). Also called marrow; medulla of bone.

red m. Bone marrow containing blood cells in different stages of development; found chiefly within the cancellous (spongy) tissue of bones, including small bones, and within the ends of long bones; it is the site where red blood cells and granular white blood cells are produced.

yellow m. Bone marrow found chiefly within the large cavities of long bones; consists mainly of fat cells and a few immature blood cells.

marsupialization (mar-soo-pe-al-ĭ-za´shun) Surgical procedure for eradication of a cyst, such as a pilonidal cyst, in which the sac is incised and emptied: its edges are then stitched to the edges of the external incision.

masculine (mas´ku-lin) Relating to the male sex

masculinization (mas-ku-lin-ĭ-za´shun) **1.** The normal development of secondary male characteristics. **2.** See virilization.

maser (ma´zer) A device that converts incident electromagnetic radiation of various frequencies into a beam of highly amplified monochromatic radiation at a frequency within the microwave region; the term is an acronym for microwave amplification by stimulated emission of radiation.

optical m. See laser.

mask (mask) **1.** A covering for the face, or a portion of it, for the administration of anesthetics or oxygen, or as an antiseptic measure. **2.** An expressionless appearance or a pigmentation of the face characteristic of certain conditions. **3.** A facial bandage.

aerosol m. A face mask used in inhalation therapy.

m. of pregnancy See melasma gravidarum, under melasma.

surgical m. A covering for the mouth and nose, made of gauze or plastic material; used by hospital personnel in operating rooms or when caring for patients with communicable diseases or impaired defenses against infection.

masking (mask´ing) **1.** Introduction of a noise in one ear to prevent that ear from hearing a test given to the other ear. **2.** The opaque material placed over the metal or any other part of a dental prosthesis.

masochism (mas´o-kiz-m) **1.** A form of sexual perversion in which satisfaction depends largely on being subjected to physical or psychological pain. **2.** The infliction of physical or psychological pain upon oneself to relieve guilt.

masochist (mas´o-kist) **1.** The passive partner in the practice of masochism. **2.** One who for psychological purposes exposes himself unnecessarily to suffering.

mass (mas) **1.** A body of coherent material. **2.** In pharmacology, a soft pasty mixture of drugs suitable for rolling into pills.

inner cell m. An aggregation of cells that stick together and collect at the embryonic pole of the blastocyst and that give rise to the tissues of the embryo. Also called embryoblast.

lateral m. of atlas The solid parts of the atlas (first vertebra) on either side, articulating above with the occipital condyles of the skull and below with the axis (second vertebra).

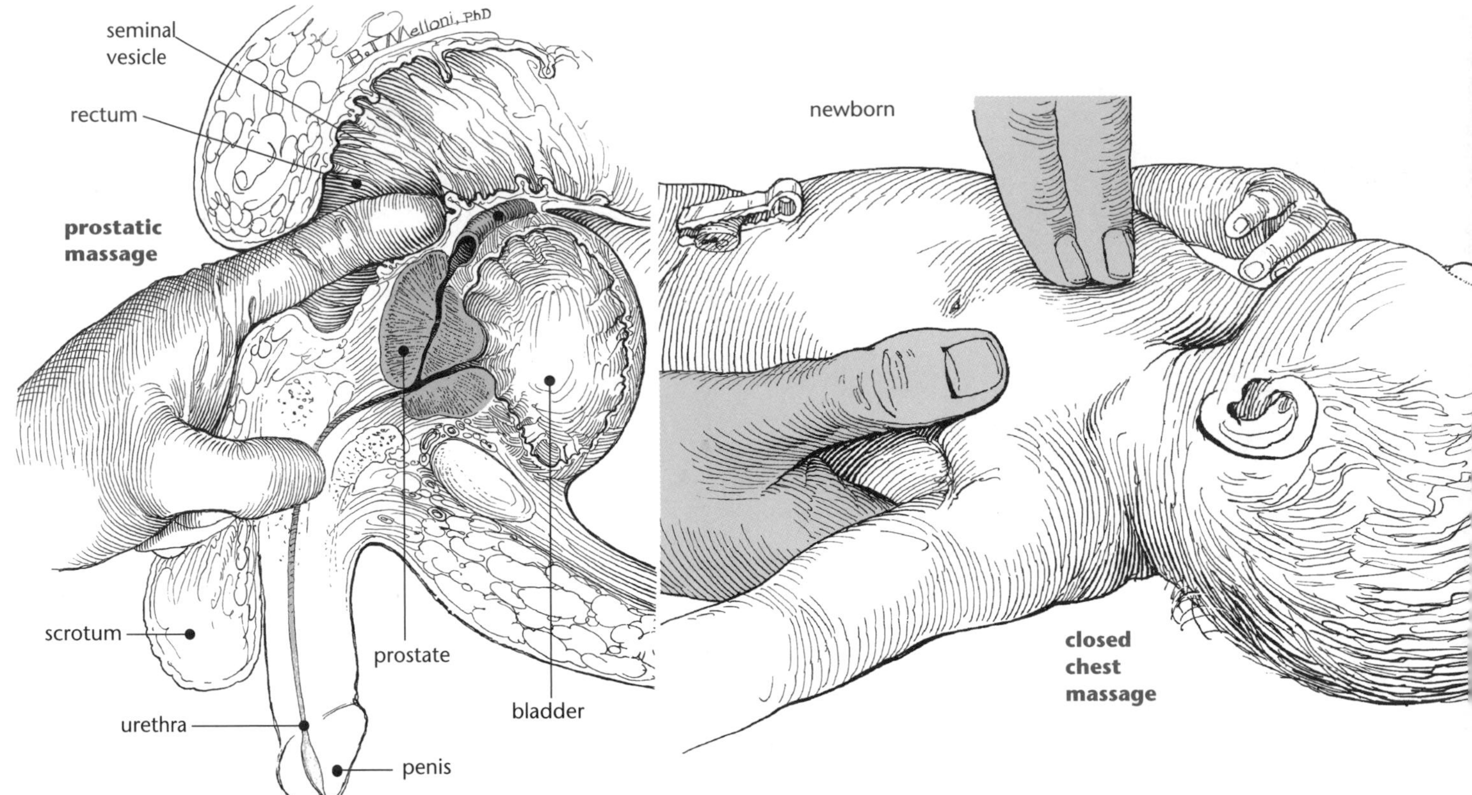

massage (mă-sahzh´) The therapeutic rubbing, kneading, or tapping of areas of the body (e.g., to relieve painful muscle spasms, reduce swelling due to water retention in tissues, and increase blood circulation).

cardiac m. The application of manual rhythmic compression of the heart to restore circulation; may be external (open chest m.) or internal (closed chest m.).

closed chest m. Cardiac massage conducted by applying rhythmic pressure on the sternum approximately 60 times per minute. Also called external cardiac massage.

external cardiac m. See closed chest massage.

gingival m. Stimulation of the gums by rubbing or pressing.

open chest m. Cardiac massage conducted by applying rhythmic pressure to the ventricles of the heart with the hand inside the chest cavity.

prostatic m. Pressing the prostate with the pad of the index finger to express secretions into the urethra for diagnostic and therapeutic purposes.

masseter (mas-se´ter) See table of muscles.

massotherapy (mas-o-ther´ă-pe) The therapeutic use of massage.

mastadenitis (mas-tad-ĕ-ni´tis) See mastitis.

Mastadenovirus (mas-tad-ĕ-no-vi´rus) Genus of the family Adenoviridae containing 34 species (types) which infect man, causing respiratory diseases, conjunctivitis, and epidemic keratoconjunctivitis. Also called mammalian adenoviruses.

mastalgia (mas-tal´jă) See mastodynia.

mastatrophy, mastatrophia (mas-tat´rŏ-fe, mas-tă-tro´fe-ă) Atrophy of the breasts.

mastectomy (mas-tek´tŏ-me) Surgical removal of a breast. Also called mammectomy.

extended radical m. Radical mastectomy and, in addition, removal of the internal mammary chain of lymph nodes.

Halsted m. See radical mastectomy.

modified radical m. Removal of breast, axillary lymph nodes, and connective tissue covering the pectoral muscles, without removing the muscles.

partial m. See segmental mastectomy.

radical m. Removal of breast, chest muscles, axillary lymph nodes, and associated skin and subcutaneous tissues. Also called Halsted mastectomy.

segmental m. Removal of a growth in the breast, along with only enough healthy tissue to ensure that the margins of the removed specimen are free of tumor. Also called breast conservation treatment; partial mastectomy.

simple m. See total mastectomy.

total m. Removal of breast only. Also called simple mastectomy.

masthelcosis (mas-thel-ko´sis) Ulcers on the breast.

masticate (mas´tĭ-kāt) To chew.

mastication (mas-tĭ-ka´shun) The process of chewing food for swallowing.

Mastigophora (mas-tĭ-gof´o-ră) A subphylum of Protozoa composed of organisms with one or more flagella and a single nucleus; some species are parasitic in man. *Trypanosoma* and *Leishmania* are included in this subphylum.

mastitis (mas-ti´tis) Inflammation of the breast. Also called mammitis: mastadenitis.

chronic cystic m. See fibrocystic change of breast, under change.

infectious m. Acute condition, primarily occurring in lactating women, in which one breast becomes tender, reddened, swollen, and hot; caused by infection with a microorganism (usually *Staphylococcus aureus*) entering through cracks in the nipple made during the breast-feeding process. Also called lactational mastitis; postpartum mastitis; puerperal mastitis.

interstitial m. Inflammation of the connective tissue of the breast.

lactational m. See infectious mastitis.

phlegmonous m. Diffuse inflammation of the breast, sometimes accompanied by abscess formation.

plasma cell m. Benign condition characterized chiefly by dilatation and occlusion of mammary ducts with indurated masses of secretion and plasma cells.

postpartum m., puerperal m. See infectious mastitis.

mastocytogenesis (mas-to-si-to-jen´e-sis) The formation of mast cells.

mastocytoma (mas-to-si-to´mă) A nodule resembling a tumor, composed chiefly of mast cells.

mastocytosis (mas-to-si-to´sis) Abnormal proliferation of mast cells in a variety of tissues. See also urticaria pigmentosa, under urticaria.

diffuse m. Mastocytosis usually involving the bone marrow, liver, spleen, and gastrointestinal lining and causing a variety of manifestations, ranging from fever and weight loss to gastrointestinal bleeding and hypotension. Also called systemic mastocytosis.

diffuse cutaneous m. See urticaria pigmentosa, under urticaria.

systemic m. See diffuse mastocytosis.

mastodynia (mas-to-din´e-ă) Pain in the breast. Also called mastalgia.

mastoid (mas´toid) The downward projection of the temporal bone, located behind the ear.

mastoidectomy (mas-toi-dek´to-me) Removal of the mastoid cells; formerly indicated in the presence of persistent or recurrent mastoiditis and otitis; rarely indicated since the advent of antibiotics.

mastoiditis (mas-toi-di´tis) Inflammation of the mastoid process.

mastoidotomy, mastoideocentesis (mas-toi-dot´o-me, mas-toi-de-o-sen-te´sis) Surgical creation of an opening into the mastoid cells.

mastopathy (mas-top´ă-the) Any disease of the breast.

mastopexy (mas´to-pek-se) Surgical procedure for correction of sagging breasts.

mastoplasty (mas´to-plas-te) See mammoplasty.

mastoptosis (mas-to-to´sis) Sagging or pendulous breasts.

mastotomy (mas-tot´ŏ-me) Surgical incision into a breast.

masturbation (mas-tur-ba´shun) Self-manipulation of the genital organs to produce sexual excitement.

materia (mă-te´re-ă) Latin for matter or substance.

m. alba Whitish, loosely adhered deposits on the teeth or dental appliances, composed of mucus, epithelial cells, food debris, and bacteria.

m. medica (a) The science concerned with drugs used in medicine, their origin, preparation, and usage. (b) Any substance used medically.

maternal (mă-ter´nal) Relating to or derived from the mother.

maternity (mă-ter´nĭ-te) **1.** The state of being pregnant or a mother. **2.** Pertaining to childbirth.

mating (māt´ing) The pairing of male and female for reproduction.

assortative m. Mating that is not random but involves individuals of specific characteristics, which may be similar (positive) or opposite (negative).

random m. Mating without regard to the genetic constitution of the mate. Also called panmixis.

matrilineal (ma-trĭ-lin´e-al) Relating to inheritance of traits through the maternal line rather than the

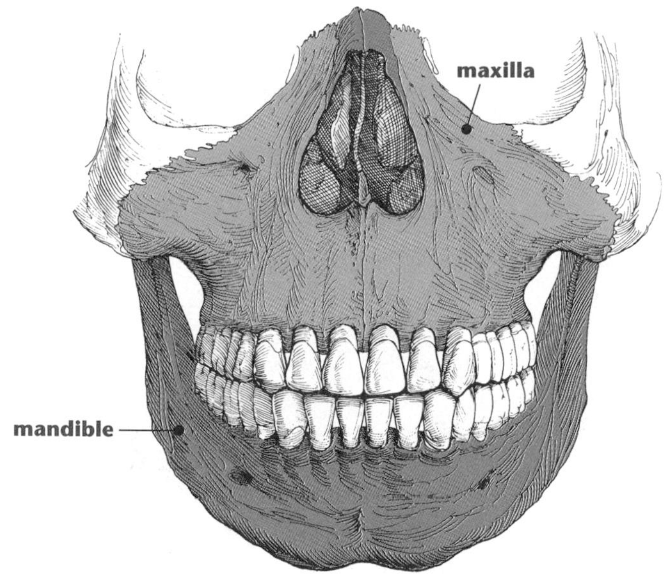

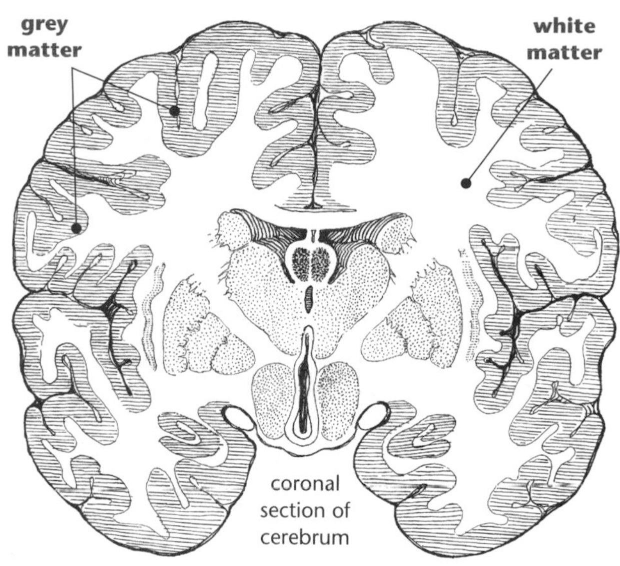

paternal.

matrix (ma´triks), *pl.* **ma´trices** **1.** The basic material from which any structure develops. **2.** The homogeneous intercellular substance of any tissue. **3.** A mold in which a cast is made.

nail m. The thick portion of the nail bed, beneath the nail root, from which the nail develops.

matter (mat´er) **1.** Substance. **2.** Waste from a living organism.

gray m. The gray portion of the brain and spinal cord composed of cell bodies. Also called gray substance.

white m. The white portion of the brain and spinal cord consisting of nerve fibers. Also called white substance.

matting (mat´ing) A cohesive, enlarged state, as of lymph nodes in certain infections (e.g., tuberculosis).

maturate (mach´u-rāt) To mature.

maturation (mach-u-ra´shun) **1.** The process of becoming mature. **2.** A stage of cell division in which the number of chromosomes in the sex cells is reduced to one-half the number that is characteristic of the species. **3.** Pus formation.

sexual m. See puberty.

mature (mă-chur´) **1.** Complete in natural development; ripe (e.g., the reproductive cell which has undergone the process of meiosis). **2.** Relating to or marked by full development, either mental or physical. **3.** To achieve full development.

maturity (mă-chur´rĭ-te) The state of being mature.

maxilla (mak-sil´ă) One of a pair of irregularly shaped bones forming the upper jaw; it houses the upper teeth. See table of bones.

maxillary (mak´sĭ-ler-e) Relating to the upper jaw (maxilla).

maxillofacial (mak-sil-o-fa´shal) Pertaining to the upper jaw and the face.

maximum (mak´sĭ-mum) **1.** The greatest quantity, value, or degree. **2.** The height of a fever or any acute state. Also called fastigium.

glucose transport m. (glucose Tm) The maximum rate at which the kidneys can reabsorb glucose (approximately 300 mg per minute).

transport m., tubular m. (Tm) The maximum ability of the renal tubules either to reabsorb or to secrete a given substance.

maze (māz) An intricate labyrinth of walled pathways frequently used to study the learning process in experimental animals.

McArdle's disease (mă-kahr´d'lz dĭ-zēz´) See type V glycogenosis, under glycogenosis.

meal (mēl) Food.

Boyden m. Meal used to test the evacuation time of the gallbladder; consists of flour, egg yolks, and milk mixed with sugar or port wine.

test m. Bland food (e.g., toast or crackers and tea) given before analysis of stomach secretions.

mean (mēn) The numerical average.

arithmetic m. In statistics, the sum of numerical data divided by the number of items.

regression to the m. If a measurement is repeated, on average the second reading will be closer to the mean than the first.

standard error of the m. (SEM) In statistics, an index of the probability that the mean of a given sample represents the mean of the population from which the sample was taken.

measle (me´zel) The larva of the tapeworm.

measles (me´zelz) An acute contagious viral disease marked by fever, inflammation of the mucous membrane of the respiratory tract, and an eruption of red spots on the skin; the incubation period is usually 10 to 12 days. Also called rubeola.

German m. See rubella.

slapped-cheek m. See erythema infectiosum, under erythema.

three-day m. See rubella.

measly (me´zle) Containing tapeworm larvae.

measure (mezh´er) **1.** The dimensions, quantity, or capacity of something that can be determined by measuring (e.g., length, area, volume, etc.). **2.** The act of determining such dimensions, quantity or capacity. **3.** A device used for measuring (e.g., a graduated container or a marked tape).

measurement (mezh´er-ment) The dimensions, quantity, or capacity of something determined by measuring.

measures of central tendency (mezh´ers ŭv sen´tral ten´den-sē) In biostatistics, the tendency of statistical data to group about an average value.

meatal (me-a´tal) Relating to a meatus or body opening.

meatometer (me-ă-tom´ĕ-ter) An instrument for measuring the size of a meatus, as that of the urethra.

meatoplasty (me-ă-to-plas´te) Reconstructive surgery of the external auditory canal or the urethral meatus.

meatoscope (me-at´o-skōp) Instrument for visualization of the urethral meatus.

meatoscopy (me-ă-tos´ko-pe) Examination of the urethral meatus with a meatoscope.

meatotome (me-at´o-tōm) Knife used in meatotomy.

meatotomy (me-ă-tot´o-me) Incision for the enlargement of the urethral opening.

meatus (me-a´tus), *pl.* **mea´tus, mea´tuses** A body channel or its opening.

external auditory m. See external auditory canal, under canal.

inferior meatus of nose See inferior nasal meatus.

inferior nasal m. The space under the inferior nasal concha that extends downward to the floor of the nasal cavity (almost the entire length of the lateral wall of the nose) into which the nasolacrimal duct opens. Also called inferior meatus of nose.

internal auditory m. See internal auditory canal, under canal.

middle meatus of nose See middle nasal meatus.

middle nasal m. The passage between the middle and inferior conchae, with which the frontal and maxillary sinuses and the anterior ethmoidal cells communicate in the nasal cavity. Also called middle meatus of nose.

nasopharyngeal m. See nasopharyngeal passage, under passage.

superior m. of nose. See superior nasal meatus.

superior nasal m. The narrow passageway below the superior concha where the posterior ethmoidal cells communicate with the nasal cavity. Also called superior meatus of nose.

urethral m. See external orifice of urethra, under orifice.

mechanical (me-kan´ĭ-kal) **1.** Produced with the aid of a machine or apparatus. **2.** Automatic.

mechanics (me-kan´iks) The branch of physics dealing with energy and forces acting on bodies (solid, liquid, or gaseous) either in motion or at rest; divided into statics, dynamics, and fluid mechanics.

body m. The study of the action of muscles on the body in motion and at rest.

mechanism (mek´a-niz-m) **1.** An aggregation of parts that interact in order to perform a specific or common function. **2.** The means by which an effect is obtained.

m. of action Process through which a substance (e.g., drug, hormone) produces its effects.

association m. Mental process through which the memory of past experiences may be related to or compared with present ones.

cough m. A mechanism for the removal of foreign material from the respiratory tract, consisting of a short inspiration, closure of the glottis, forcible expiratory effort, and then release of the glottis with a rush of air at flow rates of usually 3000 to 4000 ml/sec.

countercurrent m. A mechanism essential to the production of an osmotically concentrated urine; it involves two basic processes, countercurrent multiplication in the nephronic (Henle's) loop and countercurrent exchange in the medullary blood vessels, the vasa recta.

defense m. (a) Any of various techniques, usually unconscious, that serve as a protection against awareness of conflicts or anxiety. (b) The immune system.

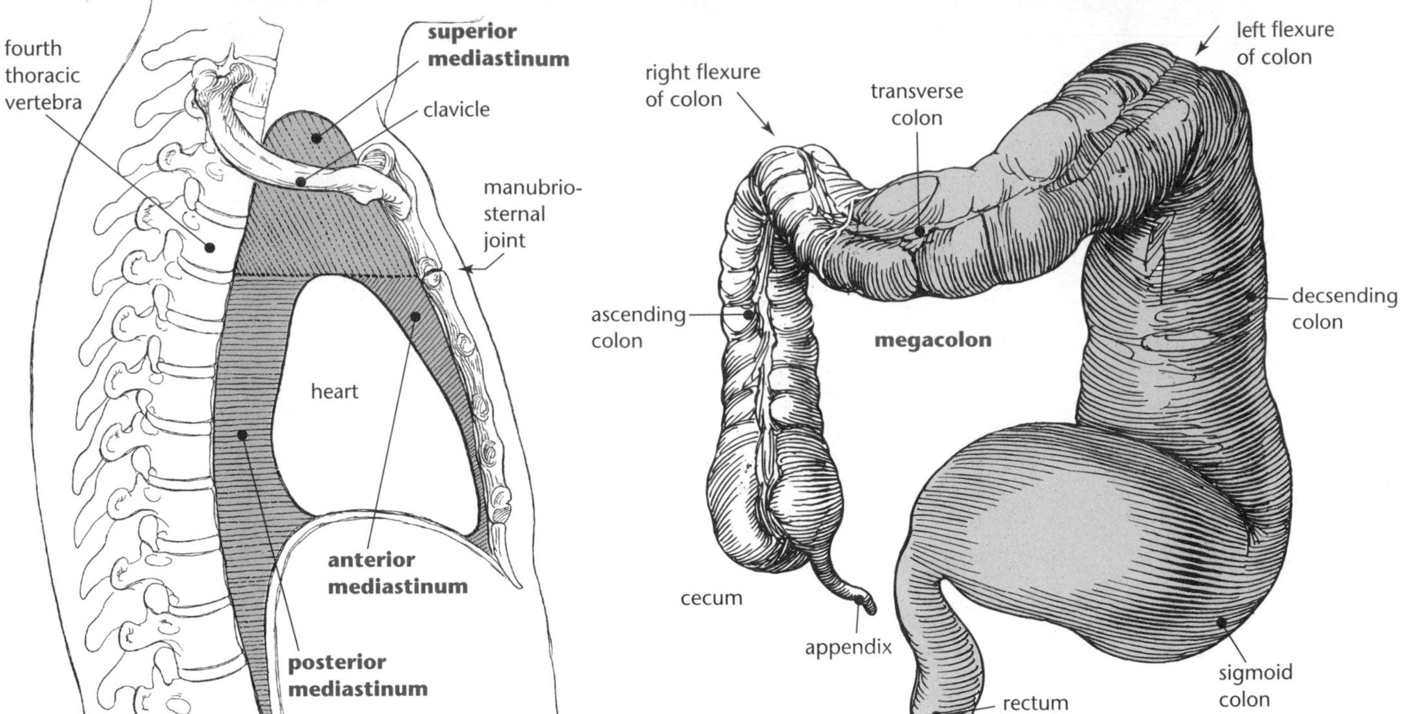

pressoreceptive m. Mechanism whereby the pressoreceptive areas (especially the carotid sinuses and aortic arch) react to a stimulus such as a rise in arterial blood pressure.

proprioceptive m. Process by which the body regulates its muscular movements and maintains its equilibrium.

mechanocardiography (mek-ă-no-kar-de-og´ră-fe) The use of tracings that represent the mechanical effects of the heart beat.

mechanoreceptor (mek-ă-no-re-sep´tor) A receptor that responds to the stimulation of mechanical pressure. Also called mechanicoreceptor.

mechlorethamine hydrochloride (mek-lor-eth´ă-mēn hi-dro-klo´rīd) HN_2; an alkylating agent used in the treatment of Hodgkin's disease; Mustargen Hydrochloride®.

meclizine hydrochloride (mek´lĭ-zēn hi-dro-klo´rīd) Preparation used in the prevention and treatment of motion sickness; Bonine®.

meconiorrhea (mĕ-ko-ne-o-re´ă) The passage of an abnormally large amount of meconium by the newborn infant.

meconium (mĕ-ko´ne-um) The dark green intestinal contents formed before birth and present in a newborn child.

m. ileus (mĕ-ko´ne-um il´e-us) See meconium ileus, under ileus.

meconium aspiration syndrome (MAS) An intense inflammatory reaction and air obstruction resulting in severe respiratory distress of the newborn; caused by fetal aspiration of meconium-stained amniotic fluid during intrauterine life or during the birth process.

meconium plug syndrome Total blockage of the lower intestinal tract of the newborn with a mass of hard meconium, causing abdominal distention.

media (me´de-ă) Plural of medium.

mediad (me´de-ad) Directed toward the midline.

medial (me´de-al) Relating to the middle; near the median plane of the body or an organ.

median (me´de-an) **1.** Situated in the middle, as certain nerves and blood vessels. Also called central. **2.** In statistics, denoting the middle value in a distribution, i.e., the point in a series at which half of the plotted values are on one side and half on the other.

mediastinal (me-de-as-ti´nal) Relating to the mediastinum.

mediastinitis (me-de-as-tĭ-ni´tis) Inflammation of the tissues in the central compartment of the chest (mediastinum).

mediastinography (me-de-as-tĭ-nog´ră-fe) X-ray examination of the mediastinum.

mediastinopericarditis (me-de-as-tĭ-no-per-ĭ-kar-di´tis) Inflammation of the sac enveloping the heart (pericardium) and the tissues and organs between the sternum and vertebral column (mediastinum).

mediastinoscope (me-de-ă-sti´no-skōp) An instrument for visual inspection of the mediastinum through an incision above the suprasternal notch.

mediastinoscopy (me-de-as-tĭ-nos´ko-pe) Exploration of the mediastinum, under anesthesia, through a transverse suprasternal incision (usually 2 cm above the suprasternal notch); it allows access to the lymph nodes overlying the trachea for surgical biopsy.

mediastinotomy (me-de-as-tĭ-not´o-me) Incision into the mediastinum.

mediastinum (me-de-as-tĭ´num), *pl.* **mediastĭ´na** **1.** The central space in the chest bounded anteriorly by the sternum, posteriorly by the vertebral column, and laterally by the pleural sacs. **2.** A septum between two parts of an organ.

anterior m. The division of the lower mediastinum located in front of the pericardium and behind the body of the sternum; it contains, among other structures, part of the thymus gland, a few lymph nodes, and loose areolar tissue.

inferior m. See lower mediastinum.

lower m. The part of the mediastinum below the plane that extends from the manubriosternal joint in front to the lower border of the fourth vertebra behind; it is subdivided into anterior, middle, and posterior mediastina. Also called inferior mediastinum.

middle m. The broadest division of the lower mediastinum; it contains, among other structures, the pericardium and heart and the adjacent parts of the great vessels.

posterior m. The division of the lower mediastinum located in back of the pericardium and in front of the vertebral column; it contains, among other structures, the esophagus, many lymph nodes, thoracic aorta, thoracic duct, and vagus nerves.

superior m. The division of the mediastinum above the plane that extends from the manubriosternal joint in front to the lower border of the fourth vertebra behind; it contains, among other structures, the aortic arch with its branches, the brachiocephalic veins and the upper half of the superior vena cava, the vagus, phrenic, cardiac, and left recurrent laryngeal nerves, the trachea, esophagus, thoracic duct, thymus gland, and some lymph nodes. Also called upper mediastinum.

upper m. The superior mediastinum.

medicable (med´ĭ-kă-bl) Potentially curable by drug therapy.

medical (med´ĭ-kal) **1.** Relating to medicine. **2.** Medicinal.

medicament (med´ĭ-kă-ment) A remedy; a healing agent.

medicamentosus (med-ĭ-kă-men-to´sus) Relating to a drug.

medicate (med´ĭ-kāt) **1.** To treat disease with a medicinal substance. **2.** To impregnate with a medicinal substance.

medicated (med´ĭ-kāt-ed) **1.** Permeated with a medicinal substance. **2.** Treated medically.

medication (med-ĭ-ka´shun) **1.** A medicine or drug. **2.** The act or process of administering remedies.

medicinal (me-dis´ĭ-nal) Having curative properties.

medicine (med´ĭ-sin) **1.** A drug. **2.** The science of diagnosing and treating general diseases or those involving the internal parts of the body, distinguished from surgery.

alternative m. A broad range of approaches to the promotion of health and treatment of disease (e.g., acupuncture, biofeedback, chiropractic, diets, homeopathy, massage, osteopathy, faith healing); may be based on anatomic observations, medications, and some form of clinical practice.

chiropractic m. See chiropractic.

clinical m. The study and practice of medicine at the bedside as opposed to theoretical and laboratory investigation.

community m. The medical specialty dealing with the study and solution of in-depth community health problems.

critical care m. Medical subspecialty concerned with the care of medical and surgical patients whose conditions are life-threatening and require comprehensive care and constant monitoring. Also called intensive care medicine.

family m. The medical specialty dealing with first patient contact, long-term care, and a broad responsibility to all members of a family regardless of age.

folk m. Treatment of disease in the home with remedies and techniques passed on from generation to generation.

forensic m. The branch of medicine concerned with the application and practice of medical knowledge to the solution of problems associated with the administration of justice. Also called legal medicine; medical jurisprudence.

geriatric m. Medical specialty concerned with the diagnosis, treatment, and prevention of disease in the elderly. Also called geriatrics.

holistic m. Medical care provided from the perspective that organisms function as complete integrated units instead of aggregates of separate parts.

hyperbaric m. Therapeutic use of high barometric pressure.

intensive care m. See critical care medicine.

internal m. The branch of medicine concerned with the nonsurgical aspects of diseases.

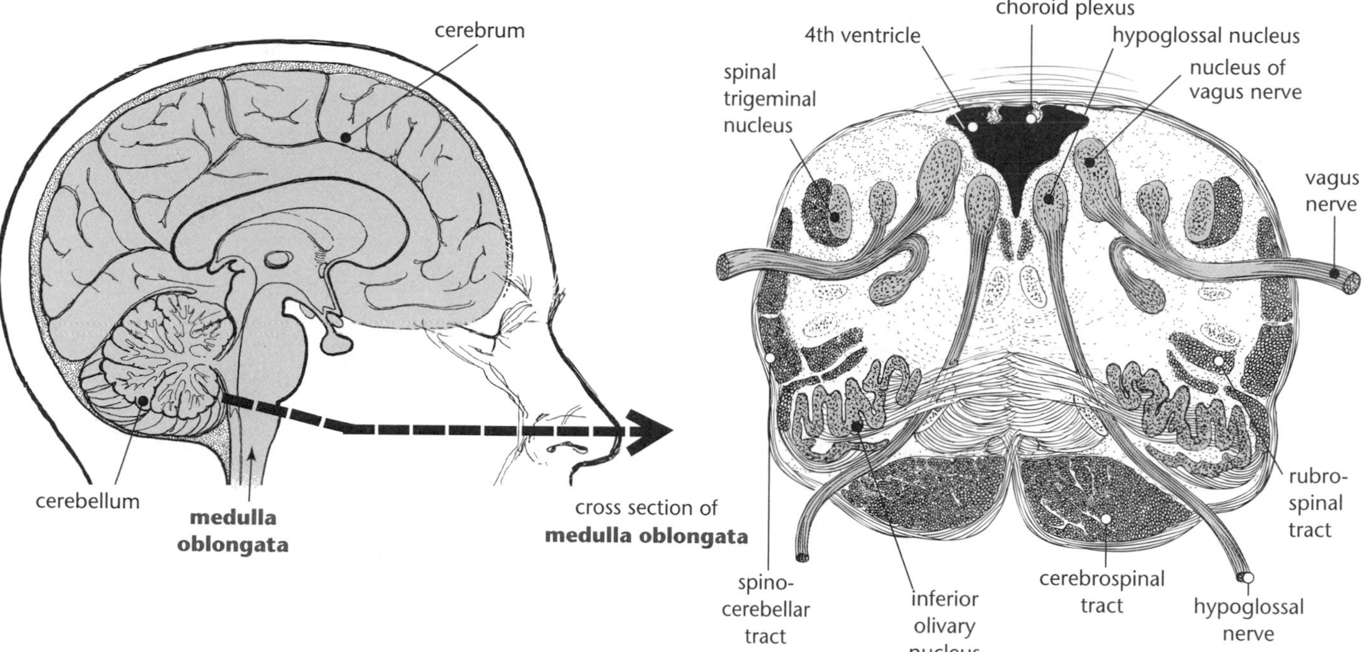

legal m. See forensic medicine.
nuclear m. The application of nuclear energy in the diagnosis and treatment of disease; (e.g., the use of radioisotopes as tracers).
perinatal m. See perinatology.
physical m. and rehabilitation The branch of medicine concerned with treatment and restoration of function of the neuromusculoskeletal systems with the aid of physical elements (i.e., heat, cold, water, electricity).
preventive m. The study and practice of measures aimed at preventing disease.
primary care m. The care a patient receives during his initial contact with a health practitioner or health-service system; it implies an ongoing responsibility for the patient regardless of the presence or absence of disease and includes that aspect of preventive medicine that can be practiced at the family level.
proprietary m. A medicinal preparation that is the property of the maker and, by patent or trade mark, is protected against imitation.
socialized m. The control of medical practice by a branch of the government.
space m. The branch of medicine concerned with disorders occurring in humans and animals exposed to the conditions of space travel.
transfusion m. A subspecialty of either clinical pathology or internal medicine that is concerned with the therapeutic administration of blood or blood products; it involves relevant areas of hematology, immunology, and infectious diseases. Legal issues of transfusion medicine center around the purity of the transfused product (i.e., whether it is free of infectious material, especially hepatitis and human immunodeficiency virus), or whether a person has the right to refuse a medically appropriate and potentially life-saving transfusion. Also called blood banking.
veterinary m. The diagnosis and treatment of the diseases of animals.

medicolegal (med-ĭ-ko-le´gal) Relating to the health professions and the law; applied especially to damages brought before a court of law, which may include injuries due to medical negligence or malpractice, medical evidence of injury in a civil action, mental competence of people who have drawn legal documents, commitment of the mentally ill to mental institutions, and the use of tests for determining paternity; may also relate to a person's right to die, sterilization, artificial insemination, *in vitro* fertilization, surrogacy, and the right to confidentiality.

medionecrosis (me-de-o-nĕ-kro´sis) Necrosis of the middle layer of an arterial wall.
m. of the aorta See cystic medial necrosis, under necrosis.

meditation (med-ĭ-ta´shun) Concentration on one thing (e.g., an object, word, or idea) with the intention of inducing an altered state of mind.
transcendental m. (TM) An exercise of contemplation that induces a temporary sense of well being and complete relaxation associated with changes in physiologic function, including reduction in oxygen consumption, decrease in cardiac output, and altered brain wave activity.

medium (me´de-um), *pl.* **me´dia** **1.** A means. **2.** Any substance through which something is transmitted. **3.** Any substance used for the cultivation of bacteria. Also called culture medium.
clearing m. A substance used in histology to make specimens transparent.
contrast m. Any substance (e.g., barium) opaque to x rays, used to facilitate visual examination of internal organs. Also called radiopaque medium; contrast agent.
culture m. See medium (3).
iodine-containing contrast media Water-soluble triiodinated derivatives of benzoic acid; in high concentration, they provide x-ray attenuation.
nonionic contrast m. A nonionic hydrophilic moiety used to provide radiographic contrast; it is used in lower osmolality and it may lower the incidence of adverse effects from contrast media.
radiopaque m. See contrast medium.
rich m. Culture medium containing various kinds of nutrients.
selective m. Culture medium containing components that limit growth to organisms of a specific type.
separating m. A substance used in dentistry to coat impressions to facilitate removal of the cast.
Thayer-Martin m. See Thayer-Martin agar, under agar.

MEDLARS (Medical Literature Analysis and Retrieval System) The National Library of Medicine's computerized system of online databases containing citations of the world's biomedical literature; available through a network of centers at universities, medical schools, hospitals, government agencies, and commercial organizations; terminals at these institutions are connected via commercial telephone to the library's computers. To retrieve references, a user types in successive queries until the needed references are identified.

MEDLINE (MEDLARS-online) A segment of MEDLARS; contains references to biomedical journal articles published in the current and two preceding years in the U.S. and foreign countries, and indexed by the National Library of Medicine; coverage of previous periods (from 1966) is provided by backfiles which are searchable online; MEDLINE is updated monthly.

medroxyprogesterone acetate (med-rok-se-pro-jes´ter-ōn as´ĕ-tāt) Preparation used in combination with ethynyl estradiol as an oral contraceptive.

medulla (mĕ-dul´ă) Any centrally located soft tissue.
adrenal m. The inner, reddish-brown portion of the adrenal gland that produces epinephrine and norepinephrine.
m. oblongata The oblong, caudal portion of the brainstem extending from the lower margin of the pons to, and continuous with, the spinal cord.
m. of bone See bone marrow, under marrow.
m. of kidney The inner, darker portion of the kidney containing the vasa rectae, nephronic (Henle's) loops, and collecting tubules and ducts.
m. of ovary The inner part of the ovary composed of loose connective tissue containing lymphatics, nerves, and a mass of large contorted blood vessels.

medullary (med´u-lār-e) Relating to the medulla or marrow.

medullated (med´u-lat-ed) Containing, or covered with, a soft marrow-like substance.

medullation (med-u-la´shun) The formation of marrow or a medullary sheath.

medullization (med-u-li-za´shun) The replacement of bone tissue by marrow, as in rarefying osteosis.

medulloblast (mĕ-dul´o-blast) An undifferentiated cell of the embryonic neural tube.

medulloblastoma (mĕ-dul-o-blas-to´mă) A rapidly growing tumor, usually of the vermis of the cerebellum, composed of undifferentiated preneuroglial cells.

megabladder (meg-ă-blad´er) See megalocystis.

megacolon (meg-ă-ko´lon) Abnormally large colon.
congenital m. Megacolon observed in young infants, resulting from absence of ganglion cells of the myenteric plexuses of the rectum and lower colon; the aganglionic area of the intestine is unable to relax during normal peristaltic activity, producing constriction and constipation. Also called Hirschsprung's disease.
idiopathic m. A form having its onset in childhood, characterized chiefly by constipation and distention of colon (sometimes the entire colon) with feces, without constriction or absence of ganglion cells.
toxic m. Marked dilatation of the colon in acute fulminating ulcerative colitis.

megadactyly (meg-ă-dak´tĭ-lē) See macrodactyly.

megadyne (meg´ă-dīn) Unit of force equal to one million dynes.

megaelectron volt (meg-ă-e-lek´tron vōlt) (mev) One million electron volts.

megaesophagus (meg-ă-ĕ-sof´ă-gus) Abnormal enlargement of the lower esophagus.

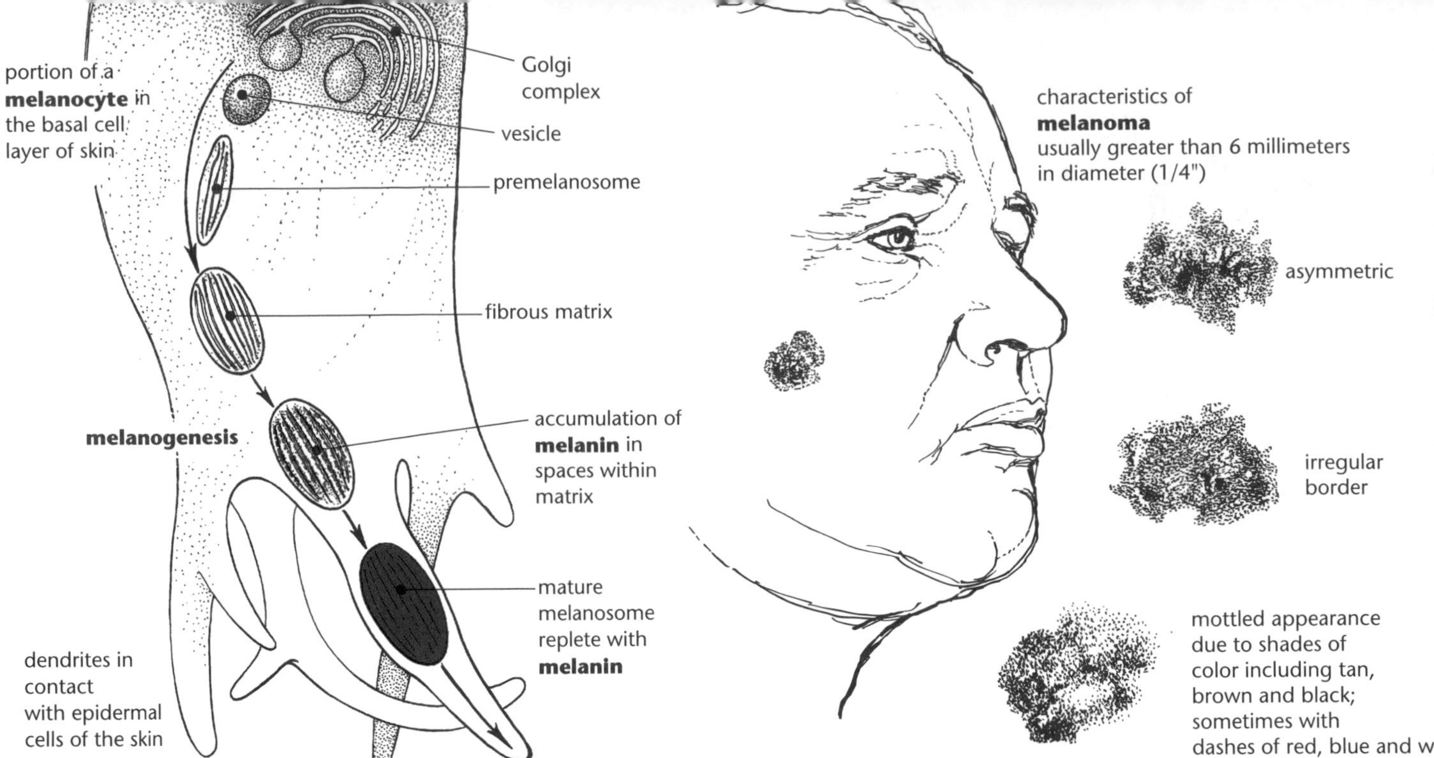

megakaryoblast (meg-ă-kar´e-o-blast) A primitive cell of the megakaryocyte series about 25 to 30 μm in diameter with a large oval or kidney-shaped nucleus and scanty cytoplasm; it develops into a promegakaryocyte before finally differentiating into a megakaryocyte.

megakaryocyte (meg-ă-kar´e-o-sīt) A giant cell with a usually multilobed nucleus, the precursor of platelets; the largest cell in the bone marrow (up to 100 μm in diameter).

megaloblast (meg´ă-lo-blast) An embryonic red blood cell of large size, found in the bone marrow in pernicious anemia and folic acid deficiency states.

megalocardia (meg-ă-lo-kar´de-ă) See cardiomegaly.

megalocheiria (meg-ă-lo-kī´re-ă) See macrochiria.

megalocornea (meg-ă-lo-kor´ne-ă) Developmental eye anomaly in which an otherwise normal cornea is abnormally large at birth and continues to grow in diameter; the pressure within the eye remains normal, which distinguishes this condition from buphthalmos. Also called macrocornea.

megalocystis (meg-ă-lo-sis´tis) An abnormally enlarged or distended bladder. Also called megabladder.

megalodactylism (meg-ă-lo-dak´tĭ-liz-m) See macrodactyly.

megalogastria (meg-ă-lo-gas´tre-ă) Abnormally large size of the stomach.

megaloglossia (meg-ă-lo-glos´e-ă) See macroglossia.

megalomania (meg-ă-lo-ma´ne-ă) A psychopathologic condition marked by unfounded conviction of one's own great importance and power.

megalomelia (meg-ă-lo-me´le-ă) See macromelia.

megalopenis (meg-ă-lo-pe´nis) Abnormally large penis.

megalophthalmos (meg-ă-lof-thal´mos) Abnormal enlargement of the eyeballs. Also called macrophthalmia.

megalosplenia (meg-ă-lo-sple´ne-ă) See splenomegaly.

megaloureter (meg-ă-lo-u-re´ter) Excessive distention of a ureter without obstruction. Also called megaureter.

megarectum (meg-ă-rek´tum) Abnormally distended rectum.

megasigmoid (meg-ă-sig´moid) An extremely distended sigmoid colon.

megaspore (meg´ă-spōr) The larger of the spores of certain protozoans or heterosporous plants. Also called macrospore.

megaureter (meg-ă-u-re´ter) See megaloureter.

megavitamin (meg-ă-vi´tă-min) Any quantity of a vitamin far in excess of minimal daily requirement.

megavolt (meg-ă-vōlt) (MV) A unit of electromotive force, equal to 1 million volts.

megavoltage (meg-ă-vol´tij) Electromotive force in the range of 2 to 10 million electron volts (mev); used in radiation therapy.

meglumine (meg´lu-mēn) *N*-methylglucamine, a substance used in the preparation of radiopaque compounds.

megohm (meg´ōm) Unit of electric resistance, equal to 1 million ohms.

meibomianitis, meibomitis (mi-bo-me-ă-ni´tis, mi-bo-mi´tis) Inflammation of the meibomian (tarsal) glands on the inside of the eyelid.

Meig's syndrome (mehzh´ez sin´drōm) The presence of a benign ovarian fibroma associated with the formation of ascites and pleural effusion.

meiosis (mi-o´sis) The special process of cell division during maturation of the sex cells in which two nuclear cell divisions occur in rapid succession, thus forming four gametes, each containing half the number of chromosomes found in the general body cells; when the ovum unites with the sperm in fertilization, the resulting cell then has the normal diploid number of chromosomes (46).

meiotic (mi-ot´ik) Relating to meiosis.

mel (mel) Honey, especially the refined form used in pharmaceutical preparations.

melalgia (mel-al´jă) Pain in the lower extremity.

melancholia (mel-an-kó le-ă) Major depression characterized by loss of pleasure in almost all usual activities; symptoms include excessive or inappropriate guilt, psychomotor retardation or agitation, anorexia, and disordered sleep.

melanic (mel´ă-nik) Having a dark color.

melaniferous (mel-ă-nif´er-us) Containing any dark pigment.

melanin (mel´ă-nin) Black or dark brown pigment found in the skin, hair, and retina.

melanism (mel´ă-niz-m) See melanosis.

melanoameloblastoma (mel-ă-no-ă-mel-o-blas-tó mă) See melanotic neuroectodermal tumor, under tumor.

melanoblast (mel´ă-no-blast) A cell that when developed to maturity (melanocyte) is capable of producing melanin.

melanocyte (mel´ă-no-sīt) Mature pigment cell of the skin that produces melanin.

melanoderma (mel-ă-no-der´mă) Any abnormal dark pigmentation of the skin predominantly resulting from accumulation of the pigment melanin; usually associated with other conditions.

melanodermatitis (mel-ă-no-der-mă-ti´tis) Excessive deposit of melanin in an area of dermatitis.

melanogen (mĕ-lan´o-jen) Colorless substance that, under certain conditions, may be transformed to melanin.

melanogenemia (mel-ă-no-jen-e´me-ă) The presence of melanin precursors in the blood.

melanogenesis (mel-ă-no-jen´ĕ-sis) The production of melanin by living cells.

melanoma (mel-ă-no´mă) Malignant tumor that grows and metastasizes rapidly, is derived from pigment-producing cells (melanocytes), occurs usually in the skin and less commonly in other areas (the eye, oral cavity, genitalia), and ranges from light brown and white to red and bluish black. Melanomas vary in appearance but have four distinguishing characteristics in common called the ABCD of melanoma: *Asymmetry*, one half of the tumor is unlike the other half; *Border*, irregular, scalloped and poorly circumscribed; *Color*, varies from one area of the tumor to another; *Diameter*, larger than 6 mm (diameter of a pencil eraser). Also called malignant melanoma.

acral lentiginous m. (ALM) A subtype of melanoma occurring as a darkly pigmented, flat to nodular lesion on palms, soles, and beneath nails (subungual). Formerly called melanotic whitlow.

early m. Either melanoma *in situ* or a thin invasive melanoma less than 1 mm in depth.

m. *in situ* Flat or elevated lesions with histologic features identical to those of melanoma but confined to the full thickness of the superficial layer of the skin (epidermis) and its surrounding outermost layer (epithelium). Has been called malignant lentigo; lentigo maligna; atypical melanotic proliferation; pagetoid melanotic proliferation.

lentigo maligna m. (LMM) A subtype of early melanoma occurring as a flat, nonpalpable pigmentation less than 1 cm in diameter (macule), on sun-exposed skin (head, neck); often seen in elderly persons.

malignant m. Term used interchangeably with melanoma.

nodular m. (NM) A subtype of early melanoma consisting of an elevated or polypoid lesion on any anatomic site; may be uniform in pigmentation and frequently shows ulceration when advanced.

superficial spreading m. (SSM) The most common subtype of early melanoma, occurring on any anatomic site, and with typical asymmetry, border irregularity, color variegation, and diameter greater than 6 mm (the ABCDs of melanoma).

melanomatosis (mel-ă-no-mă-tó sis) The presence of numerous melanomas.

melanonychia (mel-ă-no-nik´e-ă) Black discoloration of the nails.

melanopathy (mel-ă-nop´ă-the) Any disease characterized by black pigmentation of the skin.

melanophage (mel´ă-no-fāj) A phagocytic cell that engulfs particles of melanin.

melanophore (mel´ă-no-fōr) **1.** In human histology and pathology, a pigment cell carrying melanin. **2.**

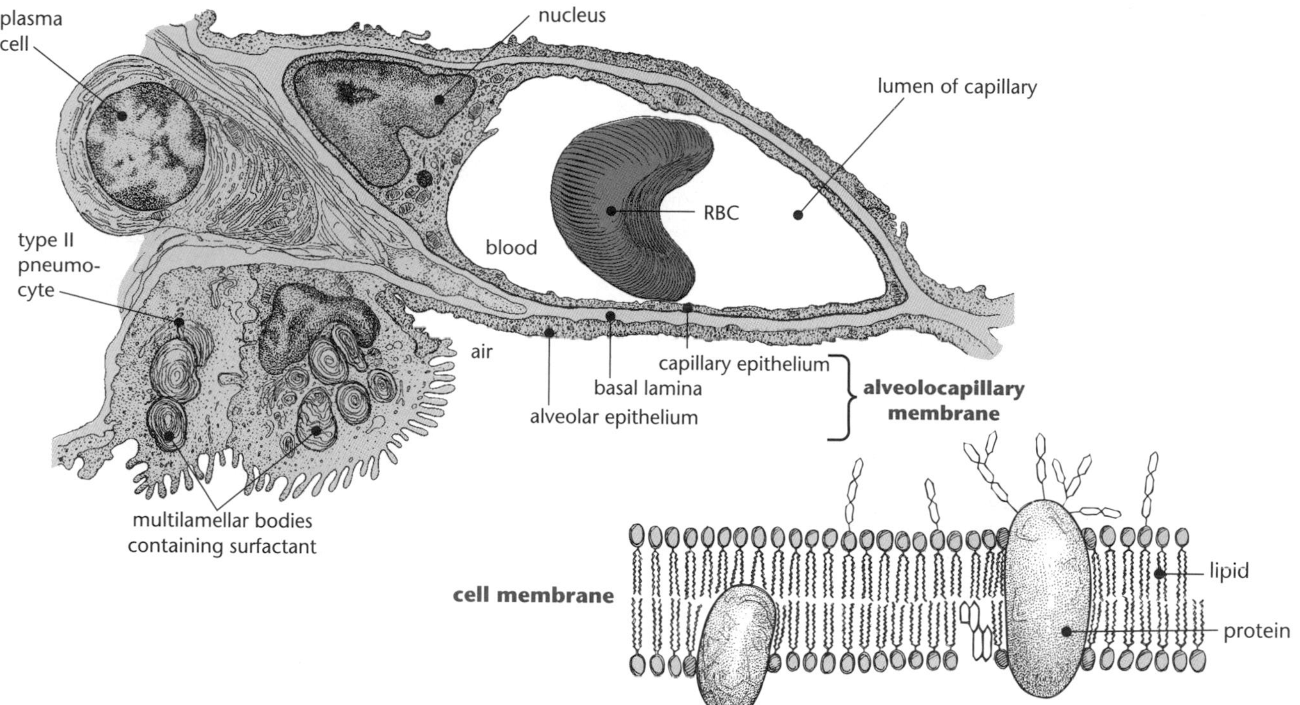

In general biology, a cell that produces melanin.

melanoplakia (mel-ă-no-pla´ke-ă) Pigmented patches on the tongue and oral mucosa.

melanoprotein (mel-ă-no-pro´tēn) A protein complex with melanin.

melanorrhagia, melanorrhea (mel-ă-no-ra´jă, mel-ă-no-re´ă) See melena.

melanosis (mel-ă-no´sis) Abnormal deposits of dark pigment in various organs or tissues. Also called melanism.

melanosome (mel´ă-no-sōm) A single melanin-containing organelle that has finished synthesizing melanin.

melanotic (mel-ă-not´ik) Pertaining to melanosis or to a darkened or blackened condition.

melanuria (mel-ă-nu´re-ă) Presence of melanin or other dark pigment in the urine; usually caused by malignant melanoma.

melasma (mĕ-laz´mă) Areas of brown patches on the skin, most commonly of the face and neck; caused by hormonal action (e.g., while using oral contraceptives). Also called chloasma.

m. gravidarum Increased pigmentation on the forehead and across the cheeks and nose occurring sometimes during pregnancy. Also called chloasma of pregnancy; mask of pregnancy.

melatonin (mel-ă-to´nin) A hormone chiefly produced by the pineal gland.

melena (mĕ-le´nă) The passage of dark, tarry stools due to blood, usually originating in the upper intestinal tract. Also called melanorrhagia; melenorrhea.

m. spuria Melena in nursing babies in which the blood originates from fissures in the nipples of the mother.

melenemesis (mel-ĕ-nem´ĕ-sis) Vomiting of dark colored material.

melioidosis (me-le-oi-do´sis) Infectious, glanders-like disease of wild rodents of Southeast Asia; caused by the bacillus *Pseudomonas pseudomallei* (*Actinobacillus pseudomallei*); in humans it may appear acutely or insidiously and is often associated with fever, cough, purulent sputum, and abscess formation.

melitensis (mel-ĭ-ten´sis) See brucellosis.

melitis (mĕ-li´tis) Inflammation of the cheek.

melitose (mel´ĭ-tōs) See raffinose.

mellitum (mĕ-li´tum), *pl.* **melli´ta** Any pharmaceutical preparation having honey as the excipient.

mellitus (mĕ-li´tus) Latin for honeyed.

meloplasty, melonoplasty (mel´o-plas-te) Plastic surgery of the cheek.

melphalan (mel´fă-lan) A compound, derivative of nitrogen mustard sometimes used in the management of multiple myeloma.

membrana (mem-bră´nă), *pl.* **membra´nae** Latin for membrane.

membrane (mem´brān) A thin sheet of tissue that covers a surface, envelopes a part, lines a cavity, divides a space, or connects two structures.

abdominal m. Peritoneum.

alveolocapillary m. The blood-air barrier in the lung consisting of the alveolar epithelium, basal lamina, and the capillary endothelium.

anterior limiting m. One of the five layers forming the cornea (between the epithelium and the substantia propria), consisting of fine, closely interwoven fibrils. Also called anterior elastic lamina of cornea; Bowman's membrane.

atlantooccipital m. Any of two membranes (anterior and posterior) extending from the border of the foramen magnum to the atlas (first vertebra).

basement m. A thin transparent noncellular layer under the epithelium of mucous membranes and secreting glands.

basilar m. of the cochlear duct Membrane extending from the osseous spiral lamina to the basilar crest of the cochlea; it forms the floor of the cochlear duct and supports the spiral organ of Corti.

Bowman's m. See anterior limiting membrane.

Bruch's m. See basal lamina of choroid, under lamina.

cell m. A delicate structure about 90 Å in thickness that encloses the cell, separating the contents of the cell from the surrounding environment; it is composed of lipids and proteins and regulates the passage of substances into and out of the cell. Also called plasmalemma; plasma membrane.

cricothyroid m. A broad, thin membrane originating from the upper border of the cricoid cartilage, and extending to the vocal process of the arytenoid cartilage and to the thyroid cartilage.

decidual m. See decidua.

Descemet's m. See postrior limiting membrane.

diphtheritic m. See false membrane.

external limiting m. The third of ten layers of the retina; it has the form of chicken wire, allowing the ample passage of the rod and cone cells.

false m. A tough fibrous exudate on a mucous membrane, as seen in the pharynx of patients with diphtheria. Also called diphtheritic membrane; pseudomembrane; neomembrane.

fetal m.'s Extraembryonic membranes concerned with the respiration, excretion, nutrition, and protection of the embryo; they include the amnion, chorion, allantois, yolk sac, decidua, and placenta.

glomerular filtration m. The capillary wall of the renal corpuscle; it allows ultrafiltration of the blood by delivering the plasma as primary urine to the urinary space within the nephronic (Bowman's) capsule; it does not allow the formed elements of the blood to pass through.

hyaline-like m. The eosinophilic, homogeneous, transparent membrane lining the alveoli and air passages of newborn infants (particularly premature) afflicted with respiratory distress syndrome of newborn.

internal limiting m. The innermost of the ten layers of the retina forming both the inner limit of the retina and the outer boundary of the vitreous body.

mucous m. Membrane lining tubular structures, including the alimentary, respiratory, and genitourinary tracts; consists of epithelium, basement membrane, lamina propria, and lamina muscularis.

Nasmyth's m. An extremely thin membrane covering the enamel of recently erupted teeth; it is soon abraded by mastication.

nuclear m. (n.m.) An ordered membrane interface regulating the exchange of material between the nucleus and cytoplasm of the cell.

obturator m. Membrane that almost completely closes the obturator foramen of the hipbone; it leaves a small canal for the passage of structures from the pelvis to the thigh.

perineal m. The inferior layer of fascia of the urogenital diaphragm filling in the gap of the pubic arch of the pelvis.

periodontal m. See periodontal ligament, under ligament.

plasma m. See cell membrane.

posterior limiting m. One of the five layers of the cornea covering the posterior surface of the substantia propria: it is elastic, transparent, homogeneous, and extremely thin. Also called posterior elastic lamina of cornea; Descemet's membrane.

postjunctional m. See postsynaptic membrane.

postsynaptic m. The portion of the cell membrane at the site of the synapse, sensitive to neurotransmitter substances. Also called postjunctional membrane.

prejunctional m. See presynaptic membrane.

presynaptic m. The cell membrane of an axon at the site of the synapse, through which neurotransmitter substances pass into the synaptic cleft. Also called prejunctional membrane.

Reissner's m. Vestibular membrane of cochlear duct.

secondary tympanic m. The membrane that closes the round window between the blind end of the scala tympani of the inner ear and the middle ear chamber.

semipermeable m. A membrane that permits the passage of water or other solvent but prevents the passage of a dissolved substance (solute) or colloidal matter.

serous m. Membrane composed of mesothelium and fibroelastic connective tissue lining the pleural, peritoneal, and pericardial cavities and exposed

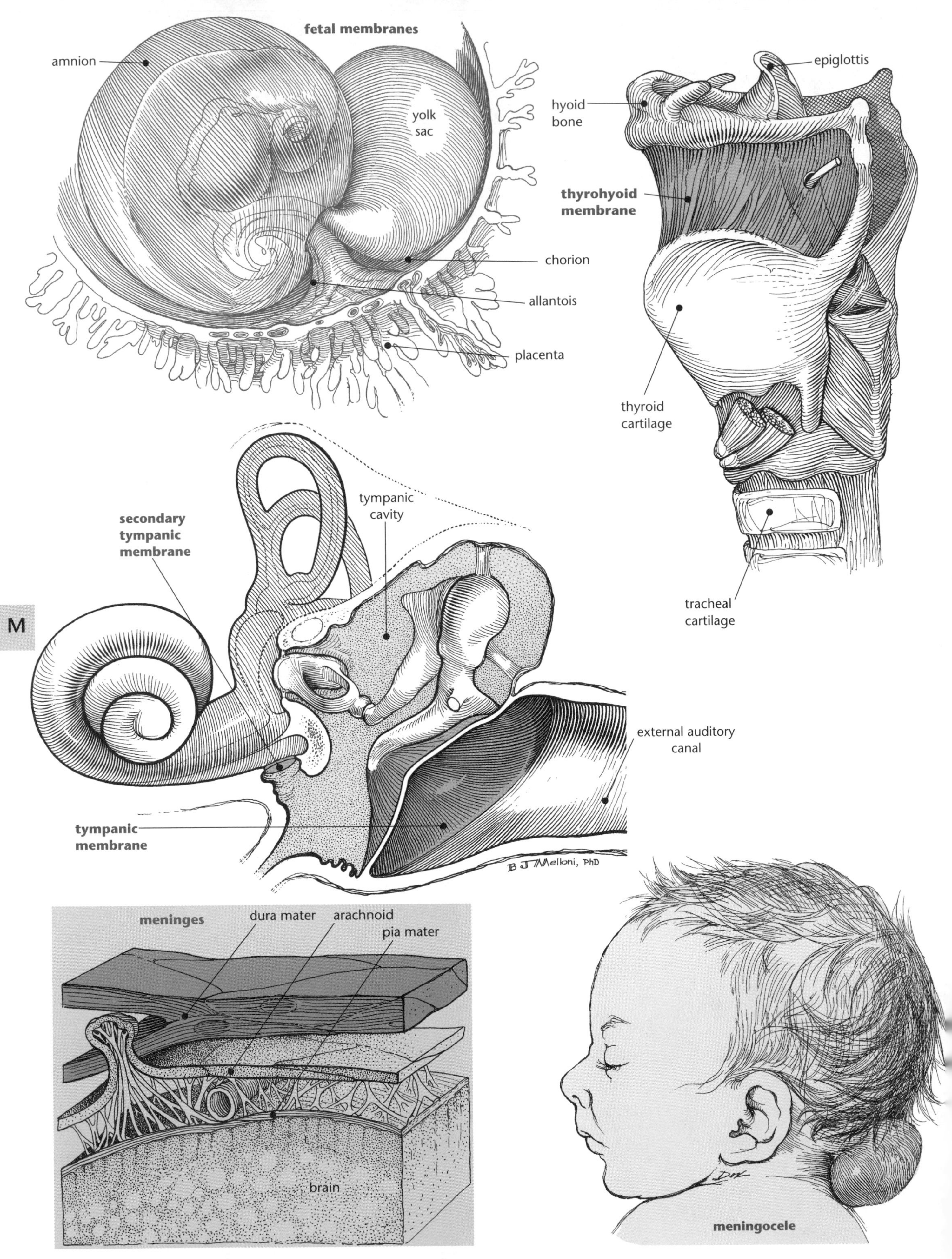
fetal membranes
amnion
yolk sac
chorion
allantois
placenta
epiglottis
hyoid bone
thyrohyoid membrane
thyroid cartilage
tracheal cartilage
secondary tympanic membrane
tympanic cavity
external auditory canal
tympanic membrane
B J Melloni, PhD
meninges
dura mater
arachnoid
pia mater
brain
meningocele
M

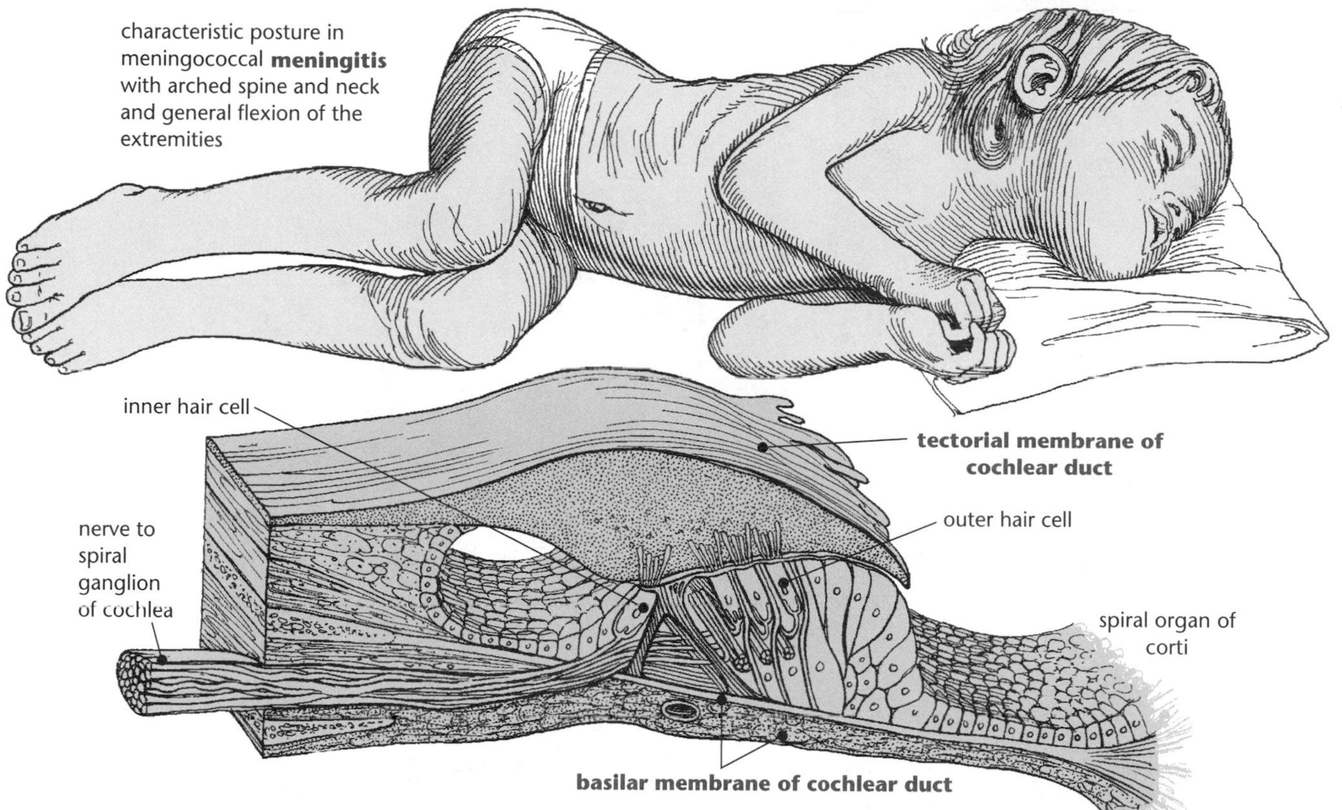

surfaces of protruding organs; a film of thin fluid covers its surface. Also called serosa.

suprapleural m. A dense, tent-shaped fascial layer attached from the inner part of the first rib and costal cartilage to the transverse process of the seventh cervical vertebra; it helps to close the thoracic inlet.

synaptic m. The cell membrane of a neuronal ending (presynaptic membrane) in relation to the postsynaptic membrane of the adjacent neuron, usually separated by a 200 Å synaptic cleft.

synovial m. The connective tissue membrane that lines the cavity of a synovial joint and produces the lubricating fluid.

tectorial m. of cochlear duct A delicate gelatinous membrane positioned on the spiral organ of Corti of the inner ear.

thyrohyoid m. A broad fibroelastic sheet that fills in the interval between the hyoid bone and thyroid cartilage.

tympanic m. (TM) The membrane separating the external auditory canal from the middle ear chamber; it is kept tense for better reception of vibrations by the tensor muscle of the tympanum (tensor tympani); during ordinary conversation the tympanic membrane is displaced only the diameter of a molecule of hydrogen. Also called eardrum.

undulating m. An organelle of locomotion of certain flagellate parasites consisting of a finlike extension of the limiting membrane with a wavelike flagellar sheath.

vestibular m. of cochlear duct The delicate membrane in the inner ear separating the cochlear duct from the scala vestibuli. Also called Reissner's membrane.

virginal m. See hymen.

Zinn's m. The outermost layer of the iris.

membranelle (mem-bră-nel′) A minute membrane composed of fused cilia, seen in certain ciliate organisms.

membranocartilaginous (mem-bră-no-kar-tĭ-laj ′ĭ-nus) Partly membranous and partly cartilaginous.

membranous (mem′bră-nus) Relating to a membrane.

memory (mem′o re) The neural mechanism involved in the storage and representation of an experience; the "read-in phase" of learning; the mental faculty of retaining in the subconscious an impression or idea of which the mind has once been conscious.

immunologic m. The ability of the immune system to recall an encounter with a specific antigen and to mount a secondary immune response on reencountering the antigen.

menacme (mĕ-nak′me) The period of menstrual activity in a woman's life.

menadione (men-ă-dī′ōn) A synthetic preparation having vitamin K properties; used in the treatment of hemorrhagic disorders caused by low prothrombin content of blood.

menarche (mĕ-nar′ke) The first menstrual period.

menarchal (mĕ-năr′kal) Relating to menarche.

mendelevium (men-dĕ-le′ve-um) Radioactive element; symbol Md, atomic number 101, atomic weight 256.

Menétrièr's disease (mān-a-tre-ārz′ dĭ-zēz′) A disease of unknown cause, characterized by huge gastric rugae and pseudopolyps, which may be associated with ulcer-like symptoms, bleeding, or idiopathic hypoproteinemia.

Ménière's disease (men-e-ārz′ dĭ-zēz′) Paroxysmal labyrinthine vertigo, characterized by recurrent episodes of severe vertigo associated with deafness and tinnitis, due to an unexplained increase in pressures of the endolymph. Also called endolymphatic hydrops; auditory vertigo.

meningeal (mĕ-nin′je-al) Relating to the membranes that cover the brain and spinal cord.

meningeorrhaphy (mĕ-nin-je-or′ă-fe) Surgical repair of a membrane, especially of those covering the brain and spinal cord (meninges).

meninges (mĕ-nin′jēz) Specifically, the membranes covering the brain and spinal cord (pia mater, arachnoid, and dura mater). Also called membranes.

meningioma (mĕ-nin-je-o′mă) An intracranial tumor arising from the arachnoid, usually occurring in adults over 30 years of age.

meningism, meningismus (mĕ-nin′jiz-m, men-in-jis′mus) Irritation of the brain or spinal cord producing symptoms similar to those of meningitis, but without inflammation of the meninges.

meningitis (men-in-ji′tis) Inflammation of the meninges (membranes covering the brain and spinal cord). The infection may occur via retrograde thrombophlebitis, bloodstream and spinal fluid pathways or directly from a local infection.

acute bacterial m. Meningitis generally characterized by headache, irritability, fever, lethargy, neck stiffness, presence of large numbers of polymorphonuclear leukocytes in a cloudy (normally clear) cerebrospinal fluid; caused by a variety of bacteria, especially *Escherichia coli* (affecting chiefly newborn infants), *Haemophilus influenzae, Neisseria meningitidis* (the cause of epidemics), and *Streptococcus pneumoniae* (affecting most frequently infants and old people and those with head injuries). If untreated, the disease may be fatal. Also called acute pyogenic meningitis.

acute chemical m. Meningitis caused by irritating substances introduced or released into the cerebrospinal fluid (e.g., certain spinal anesthetics or contents of intradural cysts).

acute lymphocytic m. See aseptic meningitis.

acute nonpyogenic m. See aseptic meningitis.

acute pyogenic m. See acute bacterial meningitis.

aseptic m. Meningitis characterized by intense headache, nausea, vomiting, neck stiffness, an increase of lymphocytes in the cerebrospinal fluid, normal glucose levels, and absence of bacteria; usually caused by viruses, most frequently by coxsackieviruses, echoviruses, and the genital herpes (Herpes simplex II) virus. Also called acute lymphocytic meningitis; acute nonpyogenic meningitis.

chronic m. Meningitis characterized by a progression of headache, malaise, mental confusion, and vomiting; caused by bacteria, especially those of tuberculosis (*Mycobacterium tuberculosis*) and by fungi (e.g., species of *Candida* and *Coccidioides*); most common site of infection is the base of the brain, causing obstruction of cerebrospinal fluid circulation and (in children) hydrocephalus.

meningocele (mĕ-ning′go-sēl) A congenital saclike, skin-covered protrusion of the meninges (membranes of the brain and spinal cord) through a defect in the skull or vertebral column; the most frequent sites are the midoccipital area of the head and the lumbosacral area of the spine.

meningococcemia (mĕ-ning-go-kok-se′me-ă) Presence of meningococci in the blood; may be associated with petechial lesions, cardiovascular collapse, and/or meningitis; the causative agent is the gram-negative coccus *Neisseria meningitidis*.

acute fulminating m. See Waterhouse-Friderichsen syndrome.

meningococcus (mĕ-ning-go-kok′us) *Neisseria meningitidis*; a microorganism that causes an infectious form of meningitis.

meningocortical (mĕ-ning-go-kor′tĭ-kal) Relating to the membranes and the cortex of the brain.

meningocyte (mĕ-ning′go-sīt) A mesenchymal epithelial cell of the subarachnoid space.

meningoencephalitis (mĕ-ning-go-en-sef-ă-li′tis) Inflammation of the brain and its membranes. Also called encephalomeningitis.

primary amebic m. Invasive infection with the

M

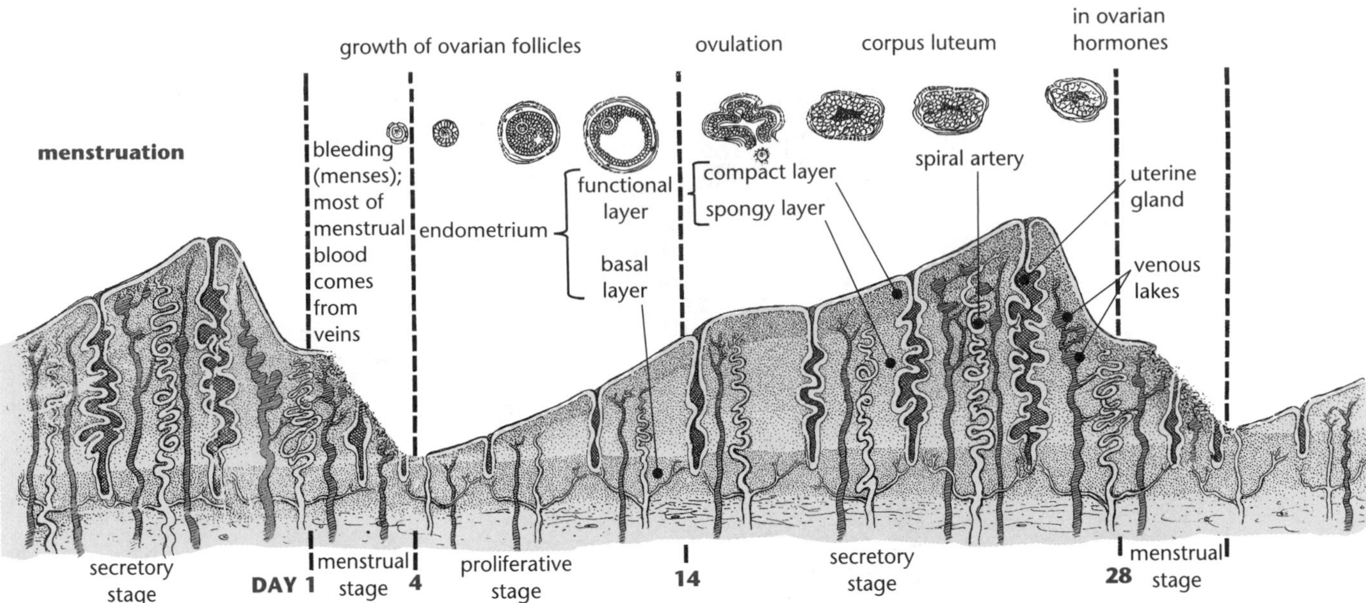

ameba *Naegleria fowleri*; symptoms include cough, nausea, fever, and neck rigidity; the amebae enter the brain through the nasal cavity, frequently from swimming in infested waters. Death occurs within a few days after onset.

meningoencephalocele (mě-ning-go-en-sef´ă-lo-sēl) Congenital defect consisting of an outpouching of the brain and its coverings (meninges) through a large gap in the skull, usually in the midoccipital area.

meningoencephalomyelitis (mě-ning-go-en-sef-ă-lo-mi-ě-li´tis) Inflammation of the brain and spinal cord and their membranes.

meningoencephalopathy (mě-ning-go-en-sef-ă-lop´ă-the) Any disease of the brain and its membranes.

meningohydroencephalocele (mě-ning-go-hi-dro-en-sef´ă-lo-sēl) Congenital defect consisting of a saclike protrusion of the brain and its membranes (meninges) containing part of a ventricle filled with cerebrospinal fluid; the outpouching occurs through a large gap in the skull, usually in the midoccipital area.

meningomalacia (mě-ning-go-mă-la´shă) Softening of the meninges.

meningomyelitis (mě-ning-go-mi-ě-li´tis) Inflammation of the spinal cord and its membranes, most commonly the arachnoid and pia mater.

meningomyelocele (mě-ning-o-mi´ě-lo-sēl) An outpouching of the meninges (membranes covering the brain and spinal cord), containing spinal cord and/or nerve roots, through an abnormal gap in the vertebral column (spina bifida); the protrusion is devoid of a skin cover. Also called myelomeningocele.

meningoradiculitis (mě-ning-go-ră-dik-u-li´tis) Inflammation of the meninges and nerve roots.

meningovascular (mě-ning-go-vas´ku-lar) Concerning the meninges and adjacent blood vessels.

meninx (me´ninks), *pl.* **me´ninges** A membrane, especially one of the membranes covering the brain and spinal cord. See also meninges.

meniscectomy (men-ĭ-sek´to-me) Surgical removal of an interarticular cartilage, especially from the knee joint.

meniscitis (men-ĭ-si´tis) Inflammation of any interarticular cartilage.

meniscocyte (mě-nis´ko-sīt) See sickle cell, under cell.

meniscus (mě-nis´kus), *pl.* **menis´ci** A crescent-shaped structure, such as the fibrocartilage serving as a cushion between two bones articulating in a joint.

lateral m. of knee joint A nearly circular, crescent-shaped fibrocartilage attached to the lateral articular surface of the superior end of the tibia.

medial m. of knee joint A crescent-shaped fibrocartilage attached to the medial articular surface of the superior end of the tibia.

temporomandibular m. See temporomandibular articular disk, under disk.

menometrorrhagia (men-o-met-ro-ra´jă) Uterine bleeding occurring at irregular intervals and in varying amounts and duration of flow.

menopausal (men-o-paw´zal) Relating to the menopause.

menopause (men´o-pawz) The permanent cessation of menstruation. The term is commonly used interchangeably with climacteric. Popularly called change of life. See also climacteric.

artificial m. See iatrogenic menopause.

iatrogenic m. Permanent cessation of menstruation resulting from surgical procedures (removal of the ovaries or the uterus, or both) or from radiation therapy or chemotherapy. Also called artificial menopause; surgical menopause.

natural m. See physiologic menopause.

physiologic m. Permanent cessation of menstruation resulting from the normal cessation of ovarian function, usually between the ages of 45 and 55 years. Also called natural menopause.

premature m. Cessation of ovarian function at an abnormally early age.

surgical m. See iatrogenic menopause.

menorrhagia (men-o-ra´jă) Excessive or prolonged menstrual flow. Also called hypermenorrhea.

menoschesis (mě-nos´kě-sis) Suppression of the menses.

menses (men´sēz) See menstruation.

menstrual (men´stroo-al) Relating to the menses.

menstruate (men´stroo-āt) To undergo menstruation.

menstruation (men-stroo-a´shun) Bleeding that occurs with the cyclic breakdown and shedding of the uterine mucosa in the absence of pregnancy; it is normally preceded by discharge of an ovum from the ovary and usually occurs approximately every 28 days (from the start of one menstrual period to the start of the next) and lasts three to five days. Also called menses. See also menstrual cycle, under cycle.

anovular m., anovulatory m. Menstruation without ovulation; occurs normally from the first through the following 12 to 18 menstruations and just before the menopause.

painful m. See dysmenorrhea.

vicarious m. Bleeding from sites other than the uterus (e.g., the nose), occurring at the time when normal menstruation takes place.

mensual (men´su-al) Monthly.

mensuration (men-su-ra´shun) Measurement by immediate comparison.

mental (men´tal) **1.** Relating to the mind. **2.** Relating to the chin.

mentation (men-ta´shun) Mental activity.

menthol (men´thol) Peppermint camphor, an organic compound derived from peppermint oil or prepared synthetically; used as a nasal decongestant, minor local anesthetic, and to relieve itching.

menton (men´ton) The lowermost point of the median plane of the lower jaw.

mentoplasty (men´to-plas-te) Plastic surgery of the chin.

mentum (men´tum) Latin for chin.

meperidine hydrochloride (mě-per´ĭ-dēn hi-dro-klor´id) A widely used narcotic and analgesic; may produce addiction; Demerol®.

meprobamate (mě-pro´bă-māt) A minor tranquilizer used to allay anxiety; Equanil®; Miltown®.

mepyrapone (mě-pi´ră-pōn) See metyrapone.

meralgia (me-ral´jă) Pain in the thigh.

m. paresthetica Burning, tingling, pricking, or numbness of the lateral side of the thigh due to compression of the lateral femoral cutaneous nerve in the fascia lata.

meralluride (mer-al´u-rīd) An organic mercurial diuretic.

merbromin (me-bro´min) A green crystalline compound, used in aqueous solution as a germicide and antiseptic; Mercurochrome®.

mercaptan (mer-kap´tan) **1.** Any substance containing the radical –SH bound to carbon; analogous to alcohols and phenols but containing sulfur instead of oxygen. Also called thioalcohol. **2.** The basic ingredient of the polysulfide polymer in rubber-based materials; used in dentistry as an elastic impression compound.

mercaptopurine (mer-kap-to-pū´rēn) A yellow crystalline compound that is an analog of purine; Purinethol®.

mercurial (mer-ku´re-al) **1.** Relating to mercury. **2.** Denoting any pharmaceutical preparation of mercury.

mercurialism (mer-ku´re-al-iz-m) Poisoning by mercury or its compounds.

mercuric (mer-ku´rik) Denoting a compound containing bivalent mercury.

mercurous (mer´ku-rus) Relating to or containing monovalent mercury.

mercury (mer´ku-re) A heavy, silvery, poisonous metallic element, liquid at room temperature; symbol Hg, atomic number 80, atomic weight 200.59, specific gravity 13.546; used in thermometers, barometers, manometers, vapor lamps, and batteries, and in the preparation of some pharmaceuticals. Also called quicksilver.

mercury-197 (^{197}Hg) A radioactive mercury isotope used in brain tumor localization and in the study of renal function.

meridian (mě-rid´e-an) A line surrounding a spherical body, passing through both poles, or half

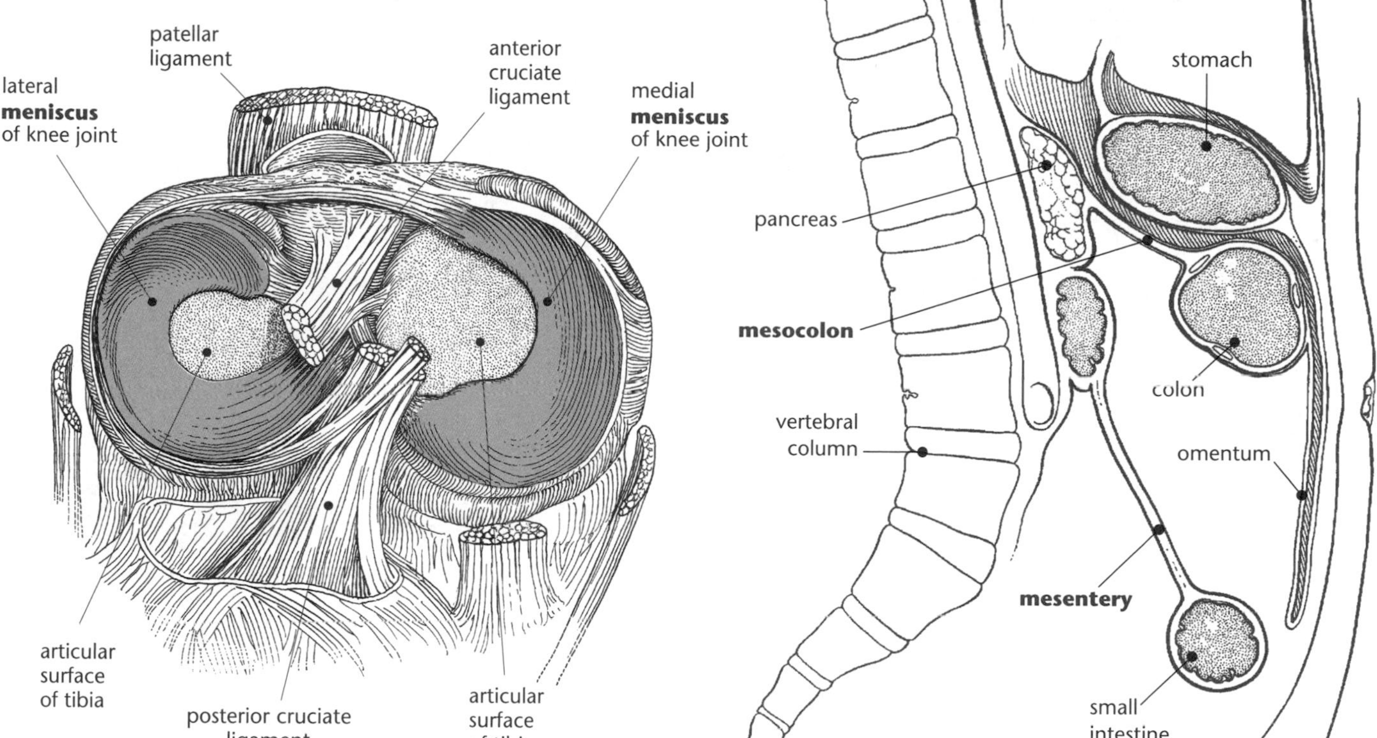

of such a circle, containing both poles.

m. of cornea Any line bisecting the cornea through the apex.

m. of eye Any line surrounding the surface of the eyeball and passing through both poles.

merocrine (mer´o-krīn) Denoting secreting cells that remain intact during discharge of the secretory products, as those in the salivary glands.

meromelia (mer-o-me´le-ă) Congenital absence of any part of a limb.

merotomy (mĕ-rot´o-me) Cutting into parts.

merozoite (mer-o-zo´īt) A small ameboid cell produced by schizogeny (asexual division) of a protozoan (e.g., the infective malarial parasite) capable of initiating either a new asexual or a sexual cycle of development. Also called schizozoite.

mesad (me´sad) Toward the middle.

mesal (me´sal) Median.

mesangial (mes-an´je-al) Relating to the mesangium.

mesangium (mes-an´je-um) The supporting stalk of the glomerulus, a specialized form of connective tissue present in the renal glomerulus (in the center of each lobule); it stabilizes the capillary loops both physically and chemically and consists of a few cells and a small amount of matrix produced by the cells.

mesaortitis (mes-a-or-ti´tis) Inflammation of the muscular coat of the aorta.

mesarteritis (mes-ar-ter-i´tis) Inflammation of the muscular coat of an artery.

mesaxon (mes-ak´son) A supporting cell membrane that folds in and completely surrounds the axon; it generally elongates and encircles the axon like a jelly roll, forming the myelin lamellae.

mescaline (mes´kă-lin) A hallucinatory, addictive alkaloid derived from the peyote cactus; also prepared synthetically.

mescalism (mes´kă-liz-m) Addiction to mescaline.

mesencephalon (mes-en-sef´ă-lon) The embryonic midbrain; the second cephalic dilatation of the neural tube that develops into the corpora quadrigemina, cerebral peduncles, and cerebral aqueduct (aqueduct of Sylvius).

mesenchyme (mes´eng-kīm) Embryonic connective tissue; a loose network formed by a group of widely separated cells in contact with one another by long processes; the space between the cells is filled with a ground substance. The mesenchymal cell is multipotential (i.e., it can develop into many kinds of connective tissue).

mesenteric (mes-en-ter´ik) Relating to the mesentery.

mesenteritis (mes-en-tĕ-ri´tis) Inflammation of the mesentery.

mesentery (mez´en-ter-e) A double layer of peritoneum attaching various organs to the body wall and conveying to them their blood vessels and nerves; commonly used in reference to the peritoneal fold attaching the small intestine to the posterior body wall.

meshwork (mesh´werk) See network.

mesial (me´ze-al) Toward the middle, as toward the middle line or apex of the dental arch.

mesiobuccal (me-ze-o-buk´al) Pertaining to the mesial and buccal surfaces of a tooth; usually denoting the line angle formed by the junction of the two surfaces.

mesiobucco-occlusal (me-ze-o-buk-o-ŏ-kloo´zal) Relating to the mesial, buccal, and occlusal surfaces of a posterior tooth; usually denoting the point angle formed by the junction of the three surfaces.

mesiocervical (me-ze-o-ser´vĭ-kal) Relating to the mesial surface of the neck of a tooth. Also called mesiogingival.

mesioclusion (me-ze-o-kloo´zhun) Malocclusion in which the lower dental arch is anterior to the upper.

mesiodens (me´ze-o-denz) An accessory tooth located between two upper incisors.

mesiodistal (me-ze-o-dis´tal) Denoting the plane of a tooth from its mesial surface across to its distal surface.

mesiogingival (me-ze-o-jin´jĭ-val) See mesiocervical.

mesiolabioincisal (me-ze-o-la-be-o-in-si´zal) Relating to the mesial, labial, and incisal surfaces of an anterior tooth; usually denoting the point angle formed by the junction of the three surfaces.

mesiolingual (me-ze-o-ling´gwal) Relating to the mesial and lingual surfaces of a tooth; usually denoting the line angle formed by the junction of the two surfaces.

mesiolinguoincisal (me-ze-o-ling-gwo-in-si´zal) Relating to the mesial, lingual, and incisal surfaces of an anterior tooth; usually denoting the point angle formed by the junction of the three surfaces.

mesiolinguo-occlusal (me-ze-o-ling-gwo-ŏ-kloo´zal) Relating to the mesial, lingual, and occlusal surfaces of a posterior tooth; usually denoting the point angle formed by the junction of the three surfaces.

mesio-occlusal (me-ze-o-ŏ-kloo´zal) Relating to the mesial and occlusal surfaces of a posterior tooth; usually denoting the line angle formed by the junction of the two surfaces.

mesioversion (me-ze-o-ver´zhun) **1.** Position of a tooth closer to the midline than normal. **2.** Position of a jaw (upper or lower) anterior to its normal position.

mesmerism (mes´mer-iz-m) Early name for hypnosis.

mesoappendix (mes-o-ă-pen´diks) The mesentery of the appendix; the small, double-layered fold of peritoneum connecting the appendix to the mesentery of the ileum.

mesoblast (mez´o-blast) The mesoderm in its early stage of development; the middle of the three germinal layers of the embryo.

mesoblastic (mez-o-blas´tik) Relating to the mesoblast.

mesobronchitis (mez-o-brong-ki´tis) Inflammation of the middle or muscular layer of the bronchi.

M

mesocardium (mez-o-kar´de-um), *pl.* **mesocar´dia** The double layer of mesoderm attaching the embryonic heart to the wall of the pericardial cavity.

mesocecum (mes-o-se´kum) The mesentery of the cecum; it is frequently absent.

mesocephalic (mez-o-sĕ-fal´ik) Denoting a skull with a cephalic index between 75 and 80. Also called normocephalic.

mesocolic (mez-o-kol´ik) Relating to the mesocolon.

mesocolon (mez-o-ko´lon) The double layer of peritoneum attaching the colon to the posterior abdominal wall.

mesoderm (mez´o-derm) The middle layer of embryonic cells, between the ectoderm and the endoderm; it gives rise to the dermis, connective tissues, vascular and urogenital systems, and most skeletal and smooth muscles.

mesoepithelium (mez-o-ep-ĭ-the´le-um) See mesothelium.

mesogaster (mez-o-gas´ter) See mesogastrium.

mesogastrium (mez-o-gas´tre-um) The broad primitive mesentery which encloses the enteric canal (future stomach) in the embryo, and from which the greater omentum is developed. Also called mesogaster.

mesognathic (mez-og-na´thik) Having a slightly projecting upper jaw with a gnathic index between 98 and 103.

mesognathion (mez-o-na´thĭ-on) The part of the maxilla bearing the lateral incisor tooth.

mesometrium (mez-o-me´tre-um) The broad ligament of the uterus below the attachment of the ovary; it extends to the lateral wall of the pelvis.

mesomorph (mez´o-morf) A body build in which tissues derived from the mesoderm prevail (i.e., prominent musculature, heavy bone structure, and proportioned trunk and limbs).

meson (mes´on) Subatomic particle with a mass between that of the electron and the proton.

mesonephroma (mes-o-ne-fro´mă) Rare ovarian tumor believed to be formed from displaced mesonephric tissue.

mesonephros (mes-o-nef´ros) An intermediate excretory organ of the embryo; it is replaced by the metanephros and eventually by the permanent kidney,

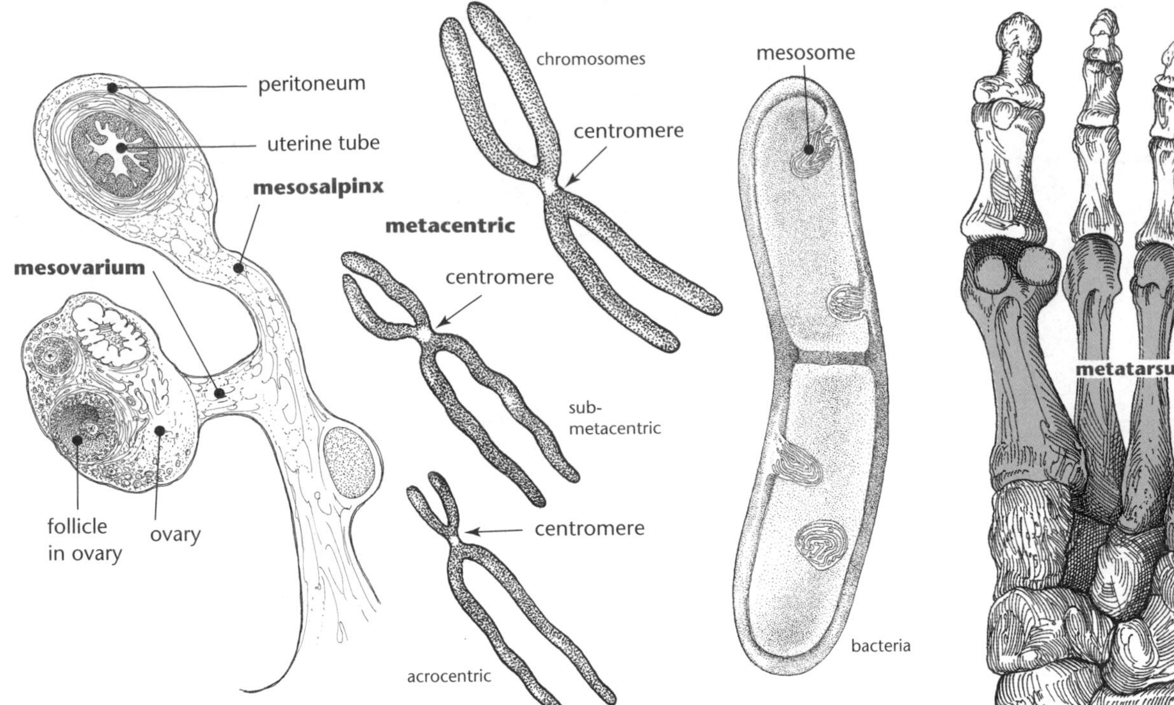

while its duct system is retained in the male as the epididymis and deferent duct. Also called wolffian body.

mesorchium (mes-or´ke-um) **1.** The fold of peritoneum in the fetus that attaches the developing testis to the developing urinary system (mesonephros) **2.** A fold of peritoneum in the adult between the testis and epididymis.

mesorectum (mes-o-rek´tum) The short peritoneal fold investing the upper part of the rectum and connecting it to the sacrum.

mesorrhine (mes´o-rin) Having a nose of moderate width with a nasal index from 47 to 51 on the skull.

mesosalpinx (mez-o-sal´pinks) The upper free portion of the broad ligament, above the attachment of the ovary and investing the uterine tube.

mesosigmoid (mes-o-sig´moid) Denoting the portion of peritoneum attaching the sigmoid colon to the posterior abdominal wall.

mesosome (mes´o-sōm) A structure present in some bacterial cells, 2,500 to 5,000 Å in diameter, derived from the invagination of the plasma membrane; thought to play a role in the formation of a membrane septum and a crosswall.

mesosternum (mes-o-ster´num) The body or main portion of the sternum (breastbone).

mesotendineum, mesotendon (mes-o-ten-din´e-um, mes-o-ten´don) The connective tissue covered by synovial membrane extending from a tendon to the wall of its synovial tendon sheath; it conveys blood vessels and nerve fibers.

mesothelioma (mes-o-the-le-o´mă) Tumor composed of spindle cells or fibrous tissue, formed most frequently in the lining of the lung.

benign m. A well-defined, solitary, fibrous growth on the pleura, often attached to the lung by a pedicle; it does not invade other tissues.

malignant m. A cancerous growth arising from the pleura and spreading diffusely over the surface of the lung, forming a firm grayish sheath over it, and frequently invading both lungs and the chest wall; symptoms include cough, chest pain, and breathing difficulty; also occurs less frequently in the peritoneum and other organs.

mesothelium (mes-o-the´le-um) A single layer of large flattened cells, derived from the mesoderm, which forms the epithelium lining the internal surface of closed body cavities, such as the pericardium, pleura, and peritoneum. Also called mesoepithelium.

mesovarium (mez-o-va´re-um) The short fold of peritoneum attaching the ovary to the posterior wall of the broad ligament.

messenger (mes´en-jer) A conveyor of information.

first m. A hormone that interacts with a mediator (second messenger) at or near the cell membrane.

second m. Cyclic adenosine monophosphate or cyclic guanosine monophospate; functioning as mediator of enzyme action; found on cell membranes.

messenger RNA See under ribonucleic acid.

mestranol (mes´tră-nol) Estrogen used in the preparation of various oral contraceptives.

meta-analysis (met-ă-ă-nal´ĭ-sis) A method of statistically examining the findings of two or more studies, often used when there are conflicting data between independent trials and when effects from single studies are too small to be statistically significant.

metabiosis (met-ă-bi-o´sis) The dependence of an organism upon the pre-existence (and influence on the environment) of another for its development and flourishing.

metabolism (mĕ-tab´o-lizm) A general term applied to the chemical processes taking place in living tissues, necessary for the maintenance of the living organism. See also catabolism; anabolism.

basal m. The minimum amount of energy required to maintain vital functions in an individual at complete physical and mental rest. Also called basal metabolic rate (BMR).

inborn error of m. See under error.

protein m. The breakdown and manufacture of proteins in the tissues.

metabolite (mĕ-tab´o-līt) Any product of metabolism.

essential m. The substrate of an essential metabolic reaction.

metacarpophalangeal (met-ă-kar-po-fă-lan´je-al) Relating to the articulations between the metacarpal bones and the phalanges.

metacarpus (met-ă-kar´pus) The five bones of the hand between the carpus and the phalanges.

metacentric (met´ă-sen´trik) Pertaining to a chromosome with the centromere in the middle.

metachromasia (met-ă-kro-ma´zha) **1.** The property by which certain cells stain in a color different from the dye with which they are stained. **2.** The property through which a single dye stains different tissue elements in different colors.

metachromatic (met-ă-kro-mat´ik) Term applied to cells and dyes exhibiting metachromasia.

metachrosis (met-ă-kro´sis) The ability to change color, possessed by certain animals.

metacresol (met-ă-kre´sol) (m-Cresol) $CH_3C_6H_4$; a local antiseptic.

metacryptozoite (met-ă-krip-to-zo´īt) A member of a second or subsequent generation of the exoerythrocytic, tissue-dwelling malarial parasite; it develops from the sporozoite, without intervening blood-parasitic generations.

metacyesis (met-ă-si-e´sis) See ectopic pregnancy, under pregnancy.

metafemale (me-tă-fe´māl) A female with three X chromosomes and two sets of autosomes, characterized by short stature and a certain degree of obesity; many are mildly retarded. Also called superfemale; trisomy X.

Metagonimus (met-ă-gon´ĭ-mus) Genus of small flukes that may infect humans upon eating raw or undercooked contaminated fish.

M. yokogawai One of the smallest flukes (1.0 to 1.5 mm long) infecting human intestines; prevalent in the Far East and the Balkan states.

metainfective (met-ah-in-fek´tiv) Occurring after an infection.

metakinesis (met-ă-ki-ne´sis) The separation of the two chromatids of a chromosome during the anaphase of mitosis.

metal (met´l) (M) Any of a group of elements that have a characteristic luster, are usually malleable and ductile, are conductors of electricity and heat, and tend to lose electrons in chemical reactions.

alkali-earth m. See alkaline earth, under earth.

noble m. Metal that cannot be oxidized by heat alone, nor readily dissolved by acid.

rare-earth m. Any metallic element of atomic number 57 through 71.

metaldehyde (met-al´de-hīd) A polymer of acetaldehyde formerly used as an antiseptic.

metalloenzyme (mĕ-tal-o-en´zīm) An enzyme having a metal ion as an integral part of its active structure.

metallophilia (mĕ-tal-o-fil´e-ă) Having an affinity for metal salts; said of certain cells.

metalloporphyrin (mĕ-tal-o-por´fĭ-rin) Compound containing a porphyrin and a metal; e.g., hematin (iron), chlorophyll (magnesium).

metalloprotein (mĕ-tal-o-pro´tēn) A protein containing a more or less tightly bound metal ion or ions (e.g., hemoglobin).

metallotherapy (mĕ-tal-o-ther´ă-pe) Treatment of disease by the use of metals or metal compounds.

metamale (met´ă-māl) A male with one X chromosome and two Y chromosomes, usually tall and somewhat lean, and often having a tendency toward aggressive behavior. Also called supermale; XYY syndrome.

metamere (met´ă-mēr) One of a series of homologous body segments.

metamerism (me-tam´er-iz-m) The state of having a series of structures arranged in a repetitive pattern.

metamorphosis (met-ă-mor´fō-sis) A change in form and/or function, as in the phases in the development of certain insects from larva to adult.

metamyelocyte (met-ă-mi´ĕ-lo-sīt) An immature, early stage of a granular white blood cell (granulocyte) derived from a myelocyte; its cytoplasm contains fine specific granules, and azurophilic

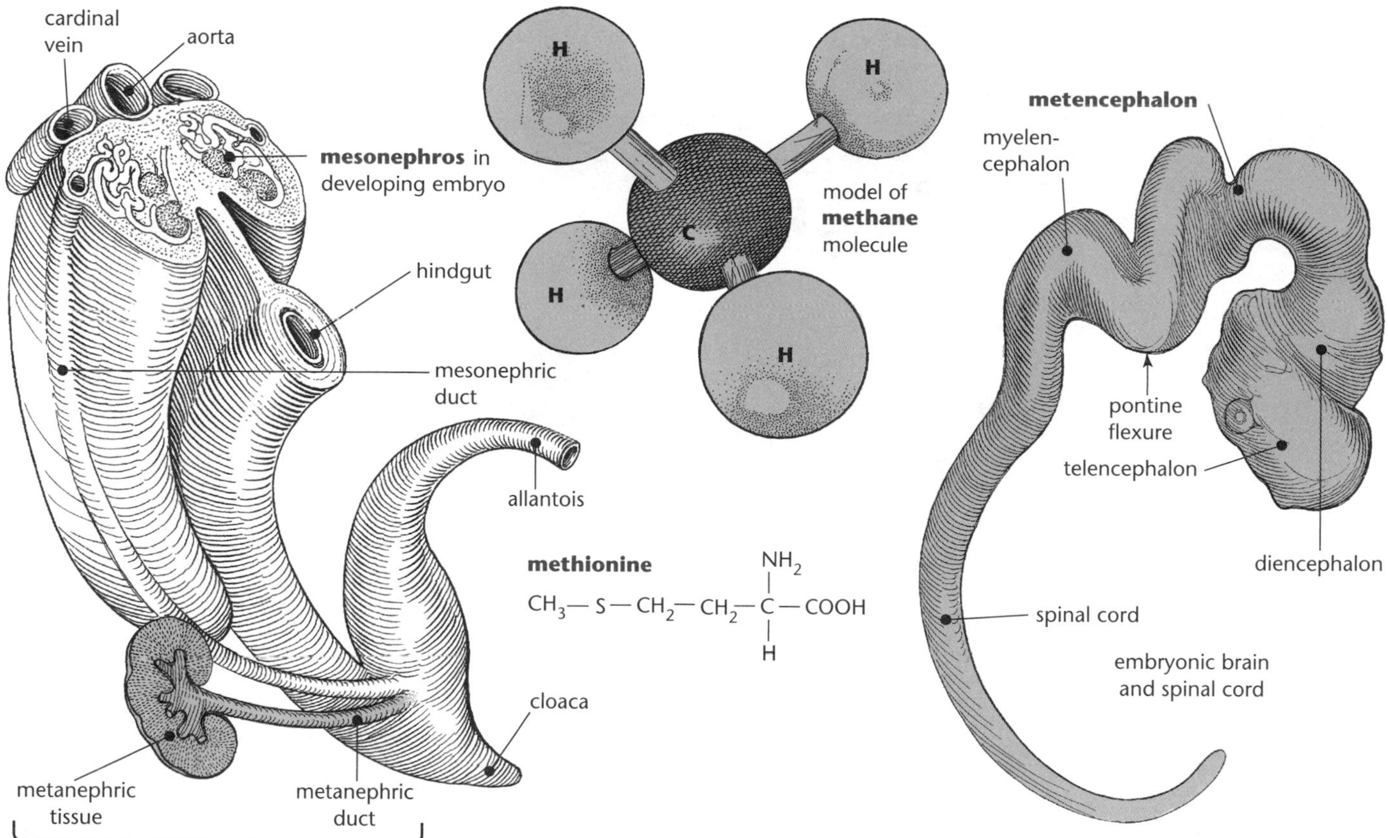

granules; its nucleus is indented or kidney-shaped.

metanephrine (met-ă-nef′rin) One of the products of catabolism of epinephrine excreted in the urine.

metanephros (met-ă-nef′ros) The tubular excretory system of the embryo representing the permanent embryonic kidney; its formation follows the regression of the mesonephros.

metaneutrophil (met-ă-nu′tro-fil) Not staining normally with neutral histologic dyes.

metaphase (met′ă-fāz) The second stage of cell division by mitosis, during which the chromatids are aligned along the equatorial plane of the cell and attached by spindle fibers to the centromere.

metaphysis (mĕ-taf′ĭ-sis) The line of junction of the epiphysis with the shaft (diaphysis) of a long bone.

metaplasia (met-ă-pla′zhă) The development of adult tissue from cells that normally produce a different type of tissue.

metapsychology (met-ă-si-kol′o-je) A systematic, but usually speculative, attempt to describe what lies beyond the empirical facts of psychology.

metaraminol bitartrate (met-ă-ram′ĭ-nol bi-tahr′trāt) A sympathomimetic compound used to elevate the blood pressure in acute hypotensive conditions.

metarubricyte (met-ă-roo′brĭ-sīt) See orthochromatic normoblast, under normoblast.

metastable (met′ă-sta-bl) Denoting an intermediate, unstable, or transient state, as of a supersaturated solution or the excited state of an atomic nucleus.

metastasis (mĕ-tas′tă-sis), *pl.* **metas′tases** **1.** The process by which cancerous cells form secondary tumors that are discontinuous with the primary tumor, in parts of the body distant from the original site; it is the most important feature distinguishing malignant from benign tumors. **2.** The secondary cancerous tumor thus formed.

metastasize (mĕ-tas′tă-sīz) To spread by metastasis.

metatarsal (met-ă-tar′sal) Relating to the metatarsus.

metatarsophalangeal (met-ă-tar-so-fă-lan′je-al) Relating to the metatarsus and the bones of the toes.

metatarsus (met-ă-tar′sus) The five bones in the anterior part of the foot between the tarsus, at the back of the foot, and the bones of the toes (phalanges).

m. adductus Foot deformity in which only the front part of the foot (at the tarsometatarsal joints) is drawn toward the midline; a common cause of the toe-in gait. Also called metatarsus varus.

m. varus See metatarsus adductus.

metathalamus (met-ă-thal′ă-mus) The part of the thalamencephalon comprising the medial and lateral geniculate bodies.

Metazoa (met-ă-zo′ă) The subkingdom of animals composed of multicellular individuals in which cells are differentiated into tissues; includes all animals except the protozoa.

metencephalon (met-en-sef′ă-lon) The portion of the embryonic brain from which develop the pons, cerebellum, and pontine part of the fourth ventricle; together with the myelencephalon it makes up the hindbrain or rhombencephalon.

meteorism (me′te-ŏ-riz-m) See tympanites.

meter (me′ter) (M) **1.** Measure of length, equal to 39.37 inches. **2.** A measuring instrument.

dose-rate m. In radiology, an instrument that displays the rate of a radiation dose.

rate m. Device that indicates the magnitude of events averaged over differing time intervals.

total solids m. A calibrated refractometer used for determining the total solids in a drop of fluid, such as urine or serum.

metformin (met-for′min) A pharmaceutical agent taken orally to reduce sugar (glucose) level in the blood. It has replaced phenformin in the USA because it is less likely to produce lactic acidosis.

methadone (meth′ă-don) A synthetic narcotic compound, used as an analgesic and in the treatment of heroin addiction.

methamphetamine hydrochloride (meth-am-fet′ă-mēn hi-dro-klo′rīd) A potent sympathomimetic agent that stimulates the central nervous system and depresses the motility of the digestive tract, thus allaying hunger; taken orally or intravenously by drug abusers; produces strong psychic dependence. Also known by the slang terms meth; speed.

methane (meth′ān) Odorless, colorless gas, CH_4; produced by the decomposition of organic matter; it is the smallest and lightest hydrocarbon, and with its next-larger relative, ethane, makes up as much as 90 percent of natural gas. Also called marsh gas.

methanol (meth′ă-nol) CH_3OH; a colorless, flammable liquid, soluble in water or ether; used as an industrial solvent and in the manufacture of formaldehyde; can cause severe acidosis and blindness when ingested. Also called methyl alcohol; wood alcohol; pyroxylic spirit.

methaqualone (mĕ-thă′kwhă-lōn) A short-acting sedative; Quaalude®.

methemalbumin (met-hem-al-bu′min) Compound formed by the combination of heme with plasma albumin; found in the blood of individuals with malarial hemoglobinuria or paroxysmal nocturnal hemoglobinuria.

methemoglobin (met-he′mo-glo-bin) (MetHb) A dark brown compound sometimes formed in the red blood corpuscles by the action of certain drugs on hemoglobin; equivalent to but chemically different from oxygenated hemoglobin; its oxygen is in firm union with iron and is not available to the tissues.

methemoglobinemia (met-he-mo-glo-bi-ne′me-ă) An excessive amount of methemoglobin in the blood.

methenamine (meth-en′ă-mēn) $C_6H_{12}N_4$; a urinary antiseptic that acts by releasing formaldehyde in an acid medium; effective against *Escherichia coli*, a common cause of urinary tract infections.

m. hippurate A compound of methenamine and hippuric acid.

m. mandelate A compound of methenamine and mandelic acid.

methicillin sodium (meth-ĭ-sil-in so′de-ŭm) A semisynthetic penicillin derivative used as an antibiotic in staphylococcal infections resistant to penicillin.

methionine (mĕ-thi′o-nin) (Met) An essential amino acid, $C_5H_{11}NO_2S$, present in proteins such as egg albumin.

method (meth′ŏd) A mode of performing an act, especially a systematic way of performing an examination, operation, or test. See also technique; procedure.

activated sludge m. A method of treating sewage waste by adding 15% bacterially active liquid sludge; it causes the colloidal material of the sewage to coagulate and undergo sedimentation.

M

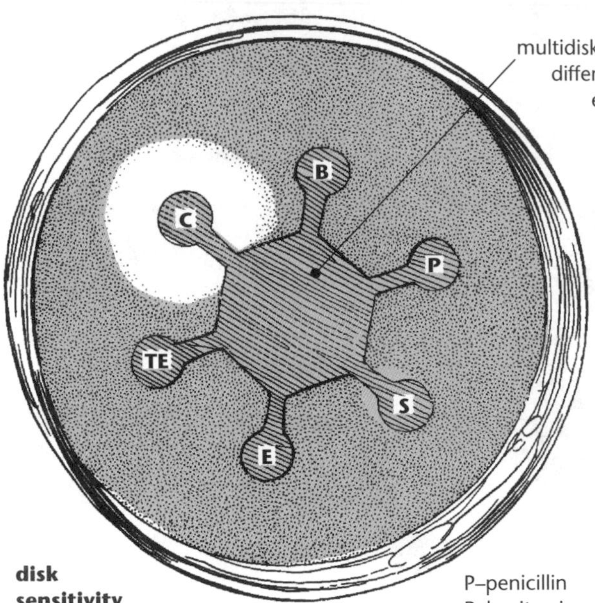

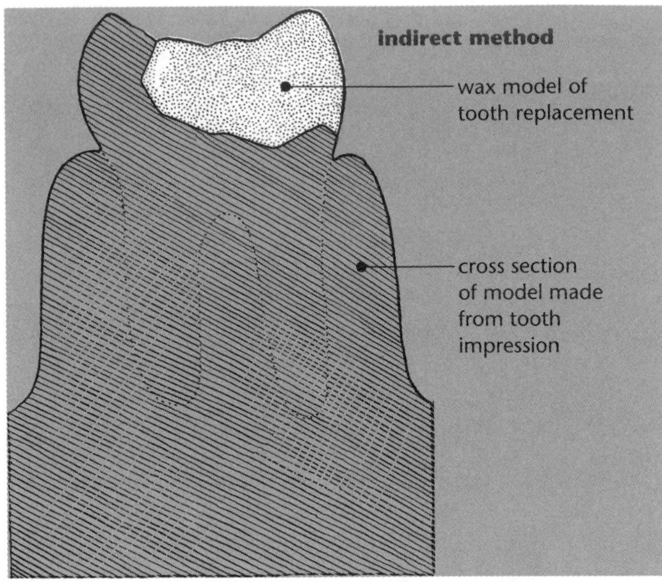

barrier m. Method of contraception that relies on the use of any device to prevent entrance of sperm into the cervical canal and uterine cavity (e.g., male and female condoms, diaphragm, cervical cap, spermicidal agents).

Credé's m.'s (a) The application of 1 drop of a 2% solution of silver nitrate onto each eye of the newborn infant to prevent gonococcal conjuncti-vitis. (b) Use of manual pressure on the bladder, particularly a paralyzed bladder, to express urine.

direct m. In dentistry, a technique of fabricating a wax pattern of lost tooth structure directly in the prepared cavity in the tooth; an inlay technique.

disk sensitivity m. A procedure for determining the relative effectiveness of various antibiotics; small disks of paper are impregnated with known antibiotics and then placed in a Petri dish, on the surface of the medium that was inoculated with the organism being tested; after a period of incubation the lack of growth in areas around the various disks indicates the relative effectiveness of the antibiotics.

Fick m. Calculation of cardiac output by dividing oxygen consumption in a period of time by the arteriovenous oxygen difference across the lungs.

flash m. A method of pasteurizing milk by quickly heating it to a temperature of 178°F, holding it there for a brief time, and then reducing it rapidly to 40°F.

immunofluorescence m.'s Any method in which a fluorescent labeled antibody is used to detect the presence or determine the location of the corresponding antigen.

indirect m. In dentistry, the fabrication of an inlay entirely on a cast made from an impression of the prepared tooth cavity.

Kjeldahl m. A method of determining the amount of nitrogen in an organic compound by heating it with strong sulfuric acid in the presence of appropriate catalysts; the nitrogen is thereby converted to ammonia which is distilled off, titrated, and measured, and from this the amount of nitrogen is estimated.

Lamaze m. A method of psychophysiologic preparation for the birth process; it involves educating the pregnant woman about her body functions and the physiology of labor, emphasizing exercise, breathing techniques, and relaxation; usually requires the assistance of a partner or "coach."

Lee-White m. A method of determining the coagulation time of venous blood by placing it in tubes of standard bore at body temperature.

micro-Kjeldahl m. A modified Kjeldahl procedure designed for the analysis of nitrogenous compounds in relatively small quantities, such as 1 or 2 mg.

Nissl's m. A histologic technique using basic dyes to demonstrate the presence of Nissl bodies or aggregated RNA in the cytoplasm of nerve cells. Also called Nissl's stain.

Ouchterlony m. Double diffusion, a method of double immunodiffusion using a Petri dish of agar in which antigen and antibody are placed in separate wells cut into the gel; during incubation, both antigen and antibody diffuse from the wells and interact to form precipitins in the agar; as diffusion progresses, concentration gradients are established; distinct bands or lines of precipitate form where diffused specific antigen and antibody meet in optimal proportions; the precipitin reaction is a useful analytic technique for the identification of unknown antibodies or antigens.

reference m. An analytic procedure that is used as a standard against which other procedures are validated because of its relatively high degree of accuracy.

rhythm m., periodic abstinence m. Birth control by abstaining from sexual intercourse for a few days before, during, and after the expected day of ovulation. Also called natural family planning.

Schick's m. A method of producing immunity to diphtheria by the injection of a mixture of toxin and antitoxin of that disease.

silver cone m. The method in which a prefitted silver cone is placed into the apex of the root canal of a tooth and then sealed.

Sippy's m. A method formerly used for treating peptic ulcer by neutralizing the free acid of the gastric juice with foods (milk and cream especially) administered frequently in small amounts.

split cast m. A method of indexing dental casts on an articulator to facilitate their removal and replacement on the instrument.

Westergren m. A method for estimating the sedimentation rate of red blood cells in blood; after mixing 4.5 ml of venous blood with 0.5 ml of 3.8% aqueous solution of sodium citrate, a standard pipet (2-mm bore, 300 mm in length, and graduated at 1-mm intervals from 0 to 200) is filled to the zero mark and kept in an upright position; in 1 hour the fall of the red blood cells is recorded; the average rate for males is 0 to 15 mm and for females, 0 to 20 mm.

Wintrobe m. A method of determining the sedimentation rate of red cells in blood mixed with an anticoagulant, by the use of the narrow-bore Wintrobe tube; the amount of sedimentation is noted after 1 hour, then the sample is centrifuged and the measured volume of packed red cells is used to modify the first reading using a standard table; corrected normal value for males is 0 to 10 mm and for females 0 to 20 mm in 1 hour.

withdrawal m. See coitus interruptus, under coitus.

methotrexate (meth-o-trek´sāt) A folic acid antagonist used in the treatment of choriocarcinoma.

methoxyflurane (meth-ok-se-floo´rān) 2,2-Dichloro-1,1-difluoroethyl methyl ether; a clear, colorless liquid with a fruity odor; nonflammable and nonexplosive in air or oxygen; used as a slow anesthetic; Penthrane®.

methscopolamine bromide (meth-sko-pol´ă-mēn bro´mīd) A gastrointestinal antispasmodic agent of prolonged action (about eight hours); used chiefly in the treatment of gastrointestinal diseases; Pamine Bromide®.

methyl (meth´il) The radical $-CH_3$.

m. chloride See chloromethane.

m. methacrylate An acrylic resin; a plastic material.

m. salicylate A colorless liquid, insoluble in water; used in ointments to relieve muscle pain. Also called oil of Wintergreen.

methylate (meth´ĭ-lāt) **1.** To combine with methyl alcohol or the methyl radical. **2.** A compound of methyl alcohol and a metal.

methylated (meth´ĭ-lāt-ed) Combined with or containing methyl alcohol.

methylbenzene (meth-il-ben´zēn) See toluene.

methylcellulose (meth-il-sel´u-lōs) A bulk-forming cellulose derivative with laxative properties; available in powder, granules, or capsule forms and used for constipation and occasionally as an appetite depressant in the management of obesity; the synthetic form is used to prolong the duration of contact in ophthalmic drops.

methylcholanthrene (meth-il-ko-lan´thrēn) A cancer-producing hydrocarbon.

methyldopa (meth-il-do´pă) A drug used in the treatment of hypertension; Aldomet®.

methylene (meth´ĭ-lēn) The organic radical CH_2.

methylene blue (meth´ĭ-lēn blu) Methylthionine chloride, an aniline dye which when dissolved in water forms a deep blue liquid; formerly used as a urinary antiseptic; now used in the treatment of methemoglobinemia, as an antidote for cyanide poisoning, and as a staining agent, especially for demonstrating basophilic and metachromatic substances. Also called toluidine blue.

3,4-methylene dioxyamphetamine (meth-ĭ-lēn di-oks-ĭ-am-fet´ă-min) (MDA) A hallucinogen commonly referred to as the love drug.

methylglucamine diatrizoate (meth-il-gloo´kă-mīn di-ă-tri-zo´āt) An organic compound used as a contrast medium in the making of x-ray transparencies.

methylmalonic acid (meth-il-mă-lon´ik as´id) (MMA) An intermediate in fatty acid metabolism; elevated levels are found in vitamin B_{12} deficiency.

methylmalonic aciduria (meth-il-mă-lon´ik as-ĭ-du´re-ă) Excretion of excessive amounts of

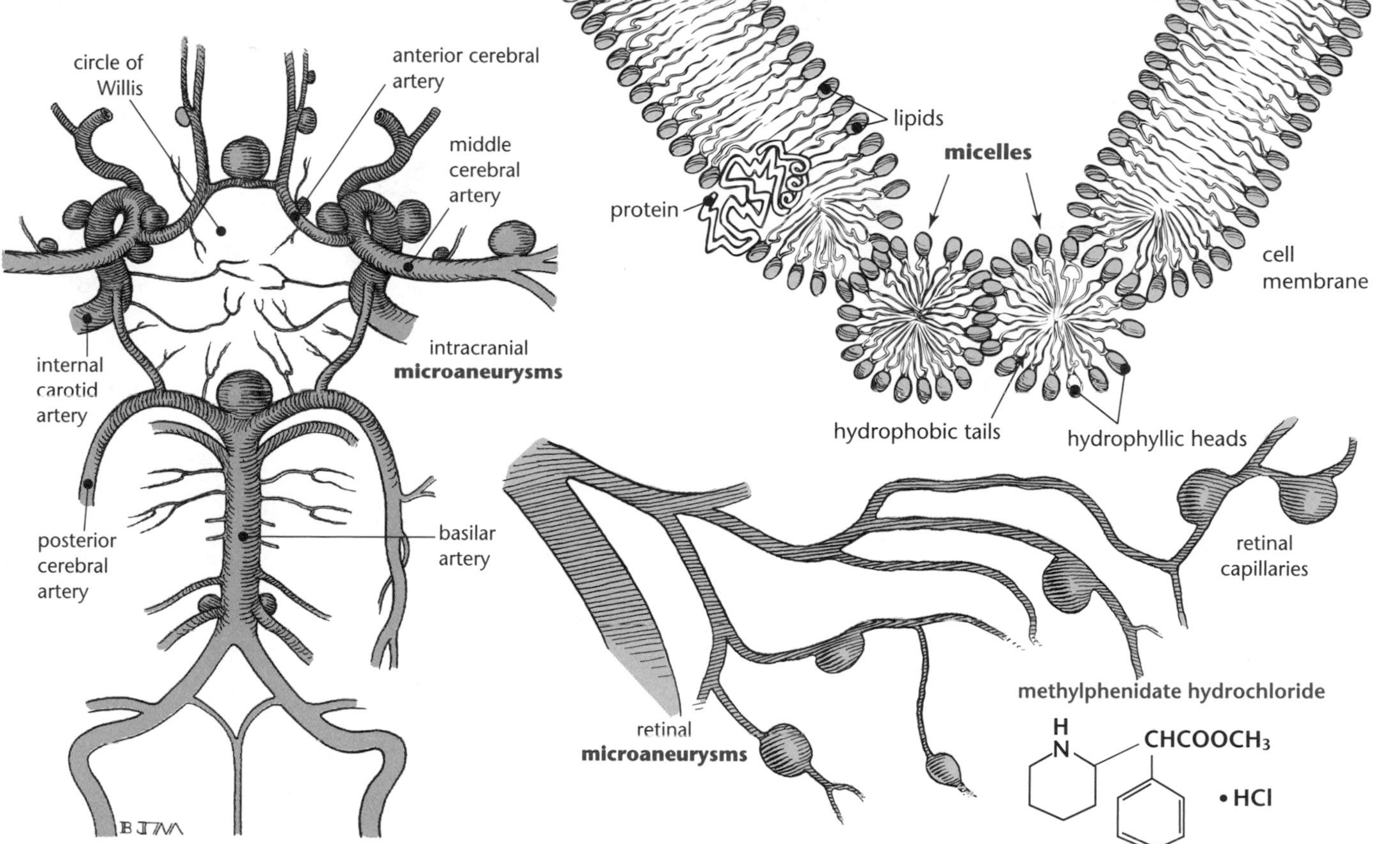

methylmalonic acid in urine.

methyl orange (meth´il or´anj) Sodium salt of helianthin; yellow-orange powder used as an indicator with a pH range from 3.2 to 4.4 (yellow at 3.2, pink at 4.4).

methylparaben (meth-il-par´ă-ben) An antifungal preservative; Niapagin®.

methylphenidate hydrochloride (meth-il-fen´ĭ-dāt hi-dro-klor´īd) A mild central nervous system stimulant similar to amphetamine; used in the management of hyperkinetic syndrome in children and attention deficit disorder; Ritalin®.

methylprednisolone (meth-il-pred´nĭ-so-lōn) A corticosteroid drug used in the treatment of asthma and in replacement therapy for pituitary and adrenal hormone deficiencies. Adverse effects include weight gain and high blood pressure (hypertension).

methyl red (meth´il red) A red compound, $C_{15}H_{15}O_2N_3$, soluble in alcohol; used as an indicator with a pH range of 4.4 to 6 (red at 4.4, yellow at 6).

methyltestosterone (meth-il-tes-tos´ter-ōn) A methyl derivative of testosterone.

methyltransferase (meth-il-trans´fer-ās) An enzyme that transfers a methyl group from one compound to another. Also called transmethylase.

methyl violet (meth´il vi´o-let) See crystal violet.

methysergide maleate (meth-ĭ-ser´jīd mal´e-āt) Compound used in the preventive treatment of migraine and cluster headaches; prolonged use may be associated with retroperitoneal fibrosis; Sansert®.

metmyoglobin (met-mi-o-glo´bin) (MetMb) A reddish brown pigment resulting from the oxidation of myoglobin.

metoclopramine (met-o-klo´prah-men) Drug used to relieve nausea and vomiting associated with anticancer drugs and radiation therapy. Adverse effects may include dryness of mouth, irritability, and agitation.

metolazone (me-tol´ah-zon) Diuretic drug used in the treatment of high blood pressure (hypertension) and to reduce fluid retention (edema) in such conditions as kidney disorders, heart failure, and premenstrual syndrome. Possible side effects include weakness and lethargy.

metopic (me-top´ik) Relating to the forehead.

metopion (me-to´pe-on) Craniometric point on the sagittal plane between the two frontal eminences.

metopism (met´o-piz-m) Persistence of the frontal suture in the adult skull.

metopoplasty (met´o-po-plas-te) Plastic or reconstructive surgery of the skin of the forehead and/or underlying bone.

metoprolol (mĕ-to´pro-lōl) A $beta_1$-adrenergic blocking agent.

metopyrone (mĕ-to-pi´rōn) See metyrapone.

metoxenous (mĕ-tok´sĕ-nus) See heterecious.

metra (me´tra) Greek for uterus.

metratonia (me-tră-to´ne-ă) Lack of tone of the uterine wall after childbirth.

metrectomy (mĕ-trek´to-me) See hysterectomy.

metria (me´tre-ă) Any inflammatory condition of the uterus following childbirth.

metric (met´rik) Relating to or based on the meter as a standard of measurement.

metritis (mĕ-tri´tis) Inflammation of the uterus.

metrodynamometer (me-tro-di-nă-mom´ĕ-ter) Instrument used to measure the strength of uterine contractions.

metromalacia (me-tro-mă-la´she-ă) Abnormal softening of the uterus.

metropathia hemorrhagica (me-tro-path´e-ă hem-o-raj´ik-ă) Profuse and prolonged bleeding from the uterus associated with cyst formation of the endometrium.

metropathic (me-tro-path´ik) Related to disease of the uterus.

metropathy (mĕ-trop´ă-the) Any disease of the uterus.

metrophlebitis (mĕ-tro-flĕ-bi´tis) Inflammation of the uterine veins, usually occurring only during pregnancy and immediately after childbirth.

metroptosis (mĕ-tro-to´sis) See prolapse of uterus, under prolapse.

metrorrhagia (mĕ-tro-ra´jhă) Irregular bleeding from the uterus occurring any time between menstrual periods; at midcycle, it may be due to ovulation; other causes include acute inflammation of the cervix, a benign tumor, and endometrial or cervical cancer.

metrorrhea (me-tro-re´ă) Discharge of pus or mucus from the uterus.

metrorrhexis (me-tro-rek´sis) See hysterorrhexis.

metrosalpingitis (me-tro-sal-pin-ji´tis) Inflammation of the uterus and one or both uterine (fallopian) tubes.

metroscope (me´tro-skōp) See hysteroscope.

metrostaxis (me-tro-stak´-sis) A slight continuous bleeding from the uterus.

metrostenosis (me-tro-stĕ-no´sis) Constriction of the uterine cavity.

metrotomy (me-trot´ŏ-me) See hysterotomy.

metyrapone (mĕ-ter´ă-pōn) $C_{14}H_{14}N_2O$; 2-methyl-1,2-di-3-pyridyl-1-propanone; an inhibitor of adrenocortical steroid C-11 β hydroxylation; administered orally or intravenously as a diagnostic test to determine the capability of the pituitary (hypophysis) to increase its production of corticotropin. Also called mepyrapone; metopyrone.

micelle (mi-sel´) **1.** A formation of approximately 50 to 100 amphipathic molecules arranged spherically, usually with the hydrophobic moiety on the inside and the hydrophilic groups on the outside. **2.** A hypothetical submicroscopic particle thought to be the unit of living matter, capable of growth and division.

microabscess (mi-kro-ab´ses) A minute collection of leukocytes in solid tissues; a very small abscess.

microadenoma (mi-kro-ad-ĕ-no´ma) A noncancerous glandular tumor, smaller than 10 mm in diameter, such as those occurring in the anterior pituitary gland.

microaerophil, microaerophile (mi-kro-ar´o-fil, mi-kro-ar´o-fīl) A microorganism that requires very little free oxygen.

microaerosol (mi-kro-ar´ŏ-sōl) A suspension in air of particles between 1 and 10 µm in diameter.

microalbuminuria (mi-kro-al-bu-mĭ-nu´re-ă) Urinary excretion of albumin just above the normal range, that is, 30 to 300 milligrams (mg) per day or 20 to 200 micrograms (µg) per minute.

microanalysis (mi-kro-ă-nal´ĭ-sis) Special analytic technique involving quantities weighing 1 mg or less.

microanatomy (mi-kro-ă-nat´o-me) See histology.

microaneurysm (mi-kro-an´u-riz-m) A minute aneurysm of a small vessel as seen in diabetic retinopathy.

microangiography (mi-kro-an-je-og´ră-fe) The making of x-ray pictures of the smallest blood vessels.

microangiopathy (mi-kro-an-je-op´ă-the) Any disorder of the small blood vessels.

diabetic m. Diffuse thickening of the basement membrane of blood vessels, especially of capillaries of the skin and medulla of the kidney.

thrombotic m. A combination of arteriolar thrombosis and capillary wall thickening resulting in a narrow lumen.

microbalance (mi´kro-bal-ans) A scale designed to weigh minute amounts of materials.

microbe (mi´krōb) A microorganism; a one-celled animal or plant that causes disease.

microbial, microbic (mi-kro´be-al, mi-kro´bik) Relating to a microorganism.

microbicide (mi-kro´bĭ-sīd) Anything that destroys

M

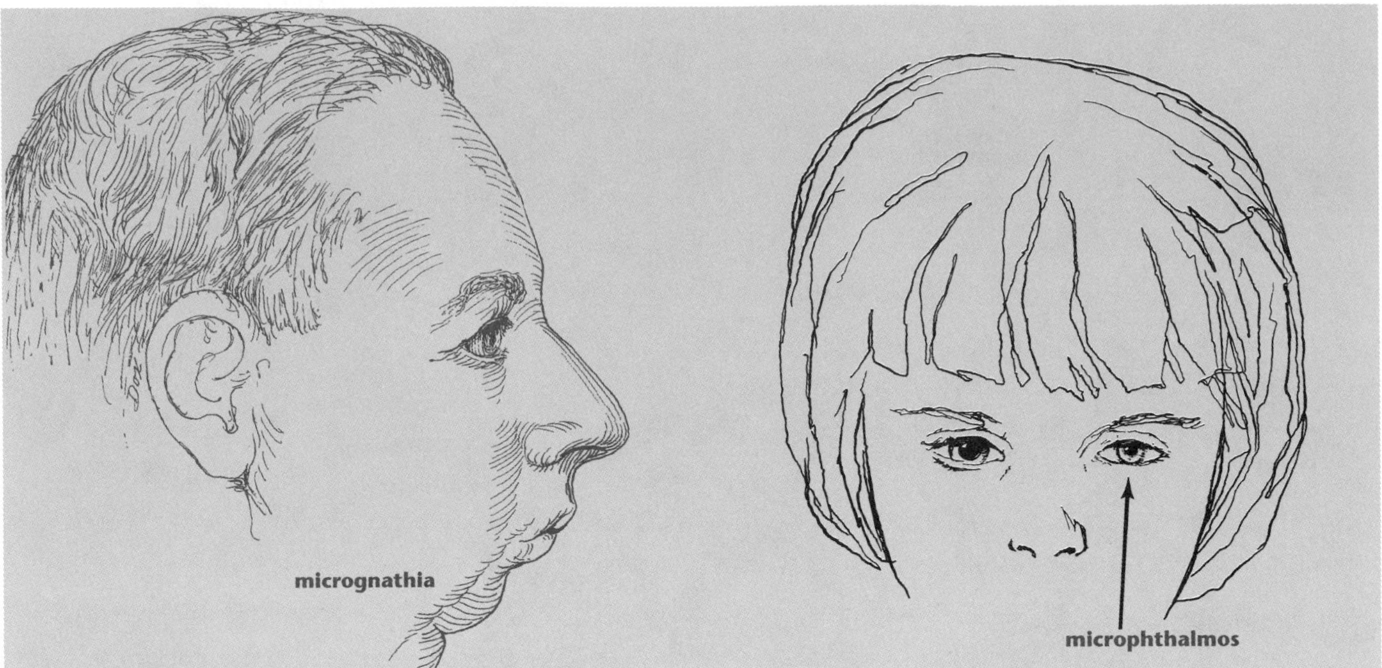

microorganisms.

microbiologic (mi-kro-bi-o-loj´ik) Relating to microbiology.

microbiologist (mi-kro-bi-ol´o-jist) A specialist in microbiology.

microbiology (mi-kro-bi-ol´o-je) The branch of science concerned with the study of microorganisms and their effect on other living organisms.

microblast (mi´kro-blast) A small nucleated red blood cell.

M

microbody (mi-kro-bod´e) See peroxisome.

microbrachia (mi-kro-bra´ke-ă) Abnormal smallness of the arms.

microcarcinoma (mi-kro-kar-sĭ-no´mă) An early stage in the spread of cancer in which stromal infiltration is limited but there are multiple and confluent malignant projections, with a high risk of lymphatic involvement; the tumor is no larger than 10 mm long and 5 mm wide.

microcardia (mi-kro-kar´de-ă) Abnormal smallness of the heart.

microcephaly (mi-kro-sef´ă-le) Abnormal smallness of the head. Also called nanocephaly.

microchemistry (mi-kro-kem´is-tre) The use of minute amounts (in the range of one milligram) of substances in chemical reactions.

microcirculation (mi-kro-sir-ku-la´shun) Blood circulation in the capillaries, arterioles, and venules.

Micrococcaceae (mi-kro-kok-ka´se-e) A family of gram-positive spherical or elliptical bacteria that divide in two or three planes, forming pairs, tetrads, or masses of cells; includes some pathogenic species; the type genus is *Micrococcus*.

micrococcus (mi-kro-kok´us), *pl* **micrococ´ci** Any member of the genus *Micrococcus*.

microcoria (mi-kro-ko´re-ă) Congenital smallness of the pupil.

microcornea (mi-kro-kor´ne-ă) Abnormal smallness of the cornea.

microcoulomb (mi-kro-koo´lom) (µC) A microunit of electric quantity; one-millionth (10^{-6}) of a coulomb.

microcrania (mi-kro-kra´ne-ă) Abnormally small cranium.

microcurie (mi-kro-ku´re) (µCi) A measure of radioactivity, one-millionth (10^{-6}) of a curie.

microcyst (mi´kro-sist) A tiny cyst, usually undetected by the unaided eye.

microcyte (mi´kro-sīt) A small red blood cell at least 2 µm smaller than normal; can be seen in the blood of individuals with iron deficiency anemia.

microcythemia, microcytosis (mi-kro-si-the´me-ă, mi-kro-si-to´sis) Condition in which the red blood cells are abnormally small.

microdactyly (mi-kro-dak´tĭ-le) Abnormal smallness of the fingers or toes.

microdissection (mi-kro-di-sek´shun) Dissection with the aid of a microscope or enlarging lens.

microdontia, microdentism (mi-kro-don´shă, mi-kro-den´tiz-m) Abnormal smallness of the teeth.

microelectrode (mi-kro-e-lek´trōd) A fine caliber electrode used in physiologic experiments.

microfarad (mi-kro-far´ad) (µF) A microunit of electrical capacity; one-millionth (10^{-6}) of a farad.

microfilament (mi-kro-fil´ă-ment) Any of several rodlike structures (4–6 nm in diameter) within cells composed of the proteins actin and myosin; involved in movement of cellular elements within and of the cell itself.

microfilaremia (mi-kro-fil-ah-re´me-ah) Presence of microfilariae in the blood.

microfilaria (mi-kro-fi-la´re-ă) The prelarval or embryonic forms of filarial worms.

microgastria (mi-kro-gas´tre-ă) Congenital smallness of the stomach.

microgenia (mi-kro-jen´e-ă) Abnormal smallness of the chin.

microgenitalism (mi-kro-jen´ĭ-tal-izm) Abnormal smallness of the external genital organs.

microglia (mi-krog´le-ă) The smallest neuroglial cells; the macrophages of the brain and spinal cord; they help remove the cellular debris of the central nervous system.

microglobulin (mi-kro-glob´u-lin) Any globulin, or fraction of a globulin, of low molecular weight.

beta 2-m. (β_2m) A protein (molecular weight 11,600) that functions as a structural portion of the histocompatibility antigens; present on the outer membrane of many cells, including lymphocytes, and in elevated levels in Wilson's disease and AIDS patients.

microglossia (mi-kro-glos´e-ă) Abnormal smallness of the tongue.

micrognathia (mi-kro-na´the-ă) Abnormal smallness of the jaw, especially the lower jaw, usually resulting in a recessive, birdlike profile.

primary m. See Pierre Robin syndrome.

microgonioscope (mi-kro-go´ne-o-skōp) Instrument used to measure minute angles, such as the filtration angle of the anterior chamber of the eye.

microgram (mi´kro-gram) (mcg, µg) A unit of weight equivalent to one-millionth (10^{-6}) of a gram.

microgyria (mi-kro-jir´e-ă) Abnormal narrowness of the convolutions of the brain.

microhm (mi´kro-ōm) A microunit of electrical resistance equivalent to one-millionth (10^{-6}) of an ohm.

microincineration (mi-kro-in-sin-er-a´shun) The combustion of a tissue section in order to examine the remaining mineral ashes under a dark-field microscope. Also called spodography.

microincision (mi-kro-in-sizh´un) See micropuncture (2).

microinvasion (mi-kro-in-va´zhun) The earliest, limited stage in the spread of a cancerous tumor to adjacent tissues to a depth no greater than 3 mm, with no confluent extensions and no lymphatic or blood vessel invasion.

microkymatotherapy (mi-kro-ki-ma-to-ther´ă-pe) Treatment of disease with high frequency radiation. Also called microwave therapy.

microliter (mi´kro-le-ter) (µl) One-millionth (10^{-6}) of a liter.

microlith (mi´kro-lith) A minute stony concretion (calculus).

microlithiasis (mi-kro-lĭ-thi´ă-sis) The presence of many minute concretions.

micromanipulation (mi-kro-mă-nip-u-la´shun) Dissection, injection, teasing apart, etc. of microscopic structures (e.g., tissue cells) with the aid of a microscope and micromanipulators.

micromanipulator (mi-kro-mă-nip´u-la-tor) An attachment to a microscope for maneuvering minute instruments while performing micromanipulations.

micromelia (mi-kro-me´le-ă) The state of having abnormally small limbs.

micrometer (mi´kro-me-ter) (µm) One-millionth (10^{-6}) of a meter. Formerly called micron.

micrometer (mi-krom´ĕ-ter) Instrument for measuring microscopic objects.

micromethod (mi-kro-meth´od) Chemical analysis or techniques involving minimal amounts of material or the use of a microscope.

micrometry (mi-krom´e-tre) Measurement with a micrometer.

micromicrogram (mi´kro-mi´kro-gram) (µµg) See picogram.

micromicron (mi-kro-mi´kron) (µµ) See picometer.

micromolar (mi-kro-mo´lar) Having a concentration of one millionth of a mole.

micromole (mi´kro-mōl) (µmol) One-millionth (10^{-6}) of a mole.

micromyelia (mi-kro-mi-e´le-ă) Congenital smallness or shortness of the spinal cord.

micron (mi´kron) (µ) See micrometer.

micronucleus (mi-kro-nu´kle-us) **1.** The smallest of the nuclei in a multinuclear cell. **2.** The smaller (reproductive) of the two nuclei in ciliates dividing mitotically, the larger being the vegetative nucleus.

micronutrients (mi-kro-nu´tre-ents) Essential compounds required by the body only in minute amounts (e.g., vitamins).

microorganic (mi-kro-or-gan´ik) Relating to a microorganism.

microorganism (mi-kro-or´gan-iz-m) A microscopic animal or plant.

micropathology (mi-kro-pă-thol´o-je) **1.** The microscopic study of disease-caused changes in the

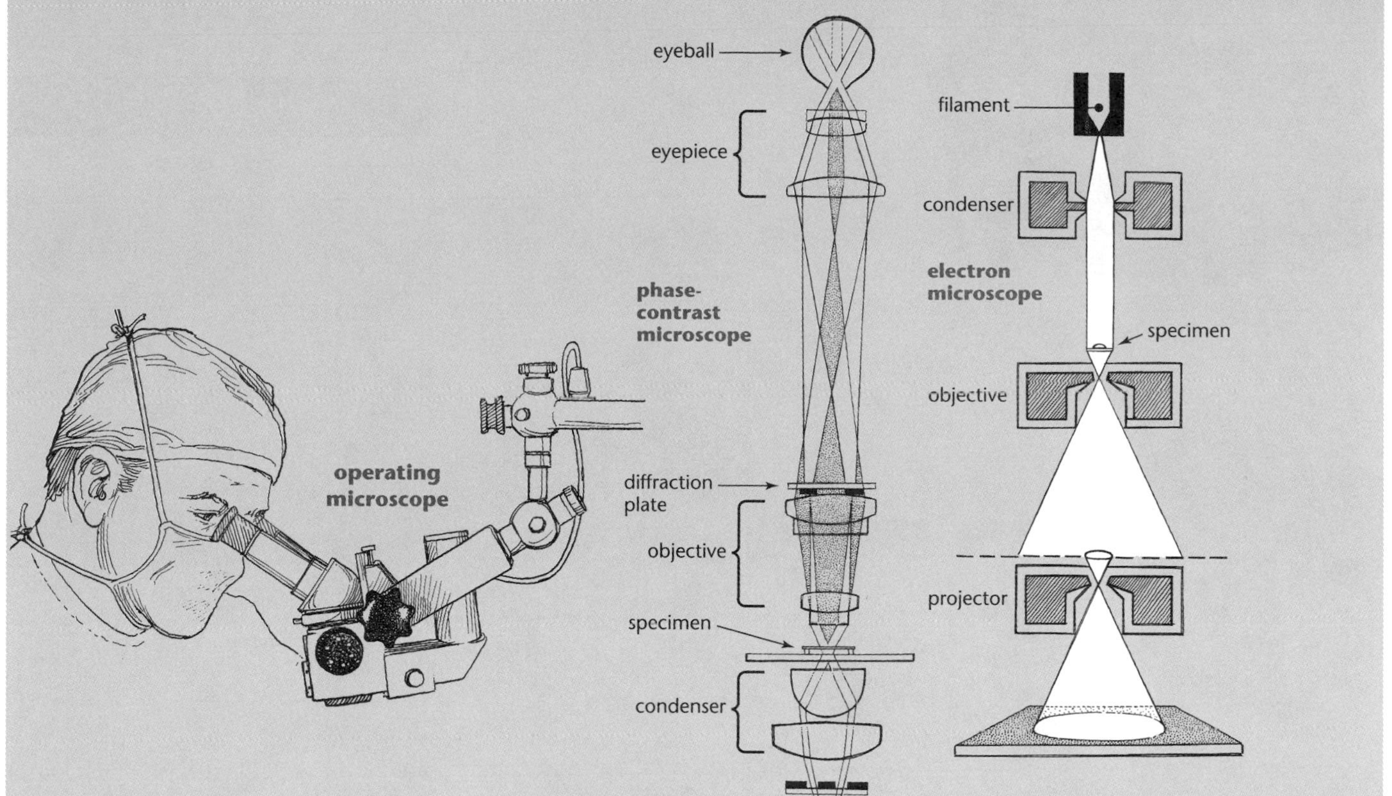

tissues. **2.** The study of disease caused by microorganisms.

micropenis (mi-kro-pe´nis) An abnormally small penis; in the newborn, one less than 2 cm in length from the pubic bone to the tip.

microphage (mi´kro-fāj) A small neutrophil that leaves the bloodstream to phagocytose bacteria and small particles; contrasted with the larger macrophage that characteristically engulfs large particles.

microphobia (mi-kro-fo´be-ă) Abnormal fear of microorganisms.

microphthalmos, microphthalmia (mi-krof-thal´mus, mi-krof-thal´me-ă) Abnormal smallness of the eyeballs.

micropipet, micropipette (mi-kro-pi-pet´) Any variously shaped, calibrated glass tubes designed to transfer minute volumes of liquid or cells.

microplasia (mi-kro-pla´zhă) Arrested growth.

microplethysmography (mi-kro-pleth-is-mog´ră-fe) Recording of changes in the size of a body part resulting from the flow of blood into and out of it.

microprobe (mi´kro-prob) An ultrafine probe used in microsurgery.

micropsia (mi-krop´se-ă) The condition of seeing objects as smaller than their actual sizes.

micropuncture (mi´kro-punk-chur) **1.** A technique for studying the function of the kidney by placement of a micropipette within a tubule and/or blood vessel of the kidney in order to sample the composition of fluid, measure the pressure, or determine the electric potential at different sites. **2.** Destruction of the organelles of a cell by a ruby laser beam. Also called microincision.

microscope (mi´kro-skōp) An instrument with a combination of lenses used to observe small objects or substances under magnification.

atomic force m. (AFM) A microscope that allows examination of cellular structures under physiologic (aqueous) conditions (unlike the electron microscope, which uses a vacuum).

binocular m. Microscope with two eyepiece tubes, permitting observation with both eyes simultaneously.

bright field m. Microscope that makes an object visible by passing light through it (transillumination).

compound m. Microscope with an objective and an eyepiece at opposite ends of an adjustable cylinder.

confocal m. Microscope that allows visualization of a specimen (usually fluorescent molecules) on a single plane for a sharper focus. Three-dimentional reconstruction can be obtained by the use of optical sectioning and a computer to record the serial sections.

dark field m. Microscope that permits illumination of the specimen from the side; details of the specimen appear light against a dark background.

electron m. (EM) Microscope that uses electrons rather than visible light, thereby allowing a much greater magnification than a light microscope. The image may be seen on a fluorescent screen or it may be photographed. Also called transmission electron microscope.

interference m. Microscope in which the emerging light is split into two beams that pass through the object and are recombined in the image plane, where transparent and refractile details of the specimen become visible as intensity differences; useful in the examination of living or unstained cells.

laser m. Microscope that uses a laser beam to vaporize a portion of the specimen; the resulting vapor is then analyzed by means of a microspectrometer.

operating m., surgical m. Microscope used in the operating room for magnifying the surgical field.

phase-contrast m., phase m. Microscope that makes use of two paths of light (light entering the microscope objective directly through the specimen and light entering the objective after being diffracted by the specimen), so that the refraction differences within the specimen become visible as variations of intensity; useful for examining transparent specimens (e.g., living cells).

polarizing m. Microscope especially equipped to illuminate the specimen with polarized light and a means to examine the alterations of the polarized light by the specimen; useful in the identification of crystals.

scanning electron m. (SEM) Microscope in which a beam of electrons scans over the specimen, giving the surface image a three-dimensional quality.

stereoscopic m. Microscope with double eyepieces and objectives, designed to give a three-dimensional view of the specimen; magnifying power is usually limited to about 150 diameters.

transmission electron m. (TEM) See electron microscope.

ultraviolet m. Microscope in which the image is formed by ultraviolet radiation and visualized by ultraviolet-transmitting lenses.

x-ray m. A microscope that produces magnified images by recording the differences in the structure's absorption or emission of x-rays.

microscopic (mi-kro-skop´ik) **1.** Visible only with the aid of a microscope. **2.** Relating to the microscope.

microscopic colitis syndrome A syndrome of unknown cause marked by chronic watery diarrhea, a normal or near normal appearance of the colon lining, infiltration of the lamina propia of the bowel with inflammatory cells (lymphocytes and plasmacytes), and intraepithelial lymphocytosis.

microscopy (mi-kros´ko-pe) The study of minute objects or organisms by means of a microscope.

fluorescence m. Microscopy of natural fluorescent materials or of specimens treated with a fluorescent solution, which emit visible light when exposed to blue or ultraviolet rays.

microsecond (mi´kro-sek-und) One-millionth (10^{-6}) of a second.

microsome (mi´kro-sōm) Any of a group of lipoprotein-rich vesicles formed from ruptured endoplasmic reticulum after disruption and centrifugation of cells.

microspherocyte (mi-kro-sfe´ro-sīt) A smaller than normal red blood cell having a spherical shape, present in hemolytic diseases.

microspherocytosis (mi-kro-sfe-ro-si-to´sis) Presence of a large number of small spherical red blood cells (spherocytes) in the blood; associated with hemolysis.

microsporidia (mi-kro-spo-rid´e-ă) General term for a group of protozoa of the phylum Microsporidia, which infect vertebrates and invertebrates, especially insects; the genera *Encephalitozoon, Enterocytozoon, Nosema, Pleistophora,* and *Septata* cause human disease in those with compromised immune systems.

Microsporum (mi-kros´po-rum) A genus of fungi causing skin infections.

M. audouini Fungus causing ringworm, especially ringworm of the scalp.

microsurgery (mi´kro-ser-jer-e) Surgery aided by stereoscopic magnification that permits precise observation, differentiation, and delicate manipulation of tissues.

microsuture (mi-kro-su´chur) Suture material 40 μm or less in diameter; used in microsurgery.

microsyringe (mi-kro-sir´inj) Syringe designed to measure accurately minute amounts of fluid for injection.

microtia (mi-kro´she-ă) Abnormal smallness of the auricle of the ear, sometimes associated with an incompletely developed or absent ear canal.

microtome (mi´kro-tōm) An instrument for slicing thin sections of tissue for microscopic examination.

microtomy (mi-krot´o-me) The slicing of tissue into thin sections with a microtome.

microtonometer (mi-kro-to-nom´ĕ-ter)

M

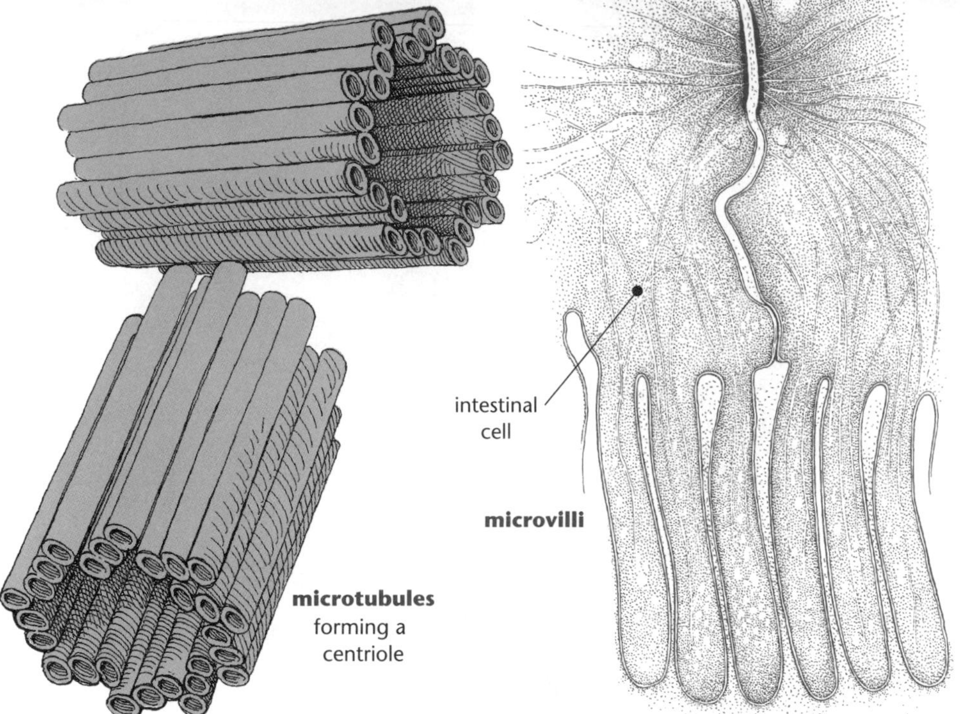

Composition of MILK (per 100g)	Human	Cow's
protein	2g	3.5g
carbohydrate	7g	5g
fat	4g	3.5g
calcium	25mg	120mg
phosphorus	16mg	95mg
iron	0.1mg	0.1mg
thiamine	17µg	40µg
riboflavin	30µg	150µg
nicotinic acid	170µg	80µg
ascorbic acid	3.5µg	2.0µg
vitamin A	170IU	150IU
vitamin D	1.0IU	1.5IU
calories	70	66

Instrument designed to determine the tensions of oxygen and carbon dioxide in arterial blood.

microtubules (mi-kro-tu´būl) Long, slender, delicate cylindrical organelles, about 250 Å in diameter, made up of a protein, the amino acid of which resembles the muscle protein actin; they are scattered throughout the cytoplasm of almost every cell type; during cell division they increase greatly in number to form the mitotic spindle; they also form the framework of the basal body and the centriole, and the cores of cilia, flagella, and sperm tails; they play an important role in intracellular movements and in maintaining cell shape.

microvilli (mi-kro-vil´i) Submicroscopic finger-like projections on the surface of the cell membrane which greatly increase the surface area.

microvolt (mi´kro-volt) (µV) One-millionth (10^{-6}) of a volt.

microwave (mi´kro-wāv) Any electromagnetic radiation having a very short wavelength between 1 mm and 30 cm; wavelengths shorter than 1 mm are in the infrared region, while those above 30 cm are radiowaves. Also called microelectric wave.

micrurgical (mi-krur´jik-al) Relating to procedures performed on minute structures with the aid of a microscope.

micturate (mik´tu-rāt) To urinate.

micturition (mik-tu-rish´un) The act of urinating. Also called urination.

midazolam hydrochloride (mi-daz´o-lam hi-dro-klo´rid) Short-acting depressant of the central nervous system, used as a preoperative sedative. It rapidly crosses the placenta into the fetus.

midbrain (mid´brān) The upper portion of the brainstem, connecting the pons and cerebellum with the hypothalamus; it contains the cerebral aqueduct.

midclavicular (mid-klah-vik´u-lar) Relating to the middle of the clavicle (collarbone).

middle lobe syndrome (mid´l lōb sin´drōm) A form of chronic atelectasis marked by collapse of the middle lobe of the lung resulting from compression of the bronchus by surrounding lymph nodes, often due to tumor involvement; symptoms include chronic cough, wheezing, recurrent respiratory infections, and chest pains. Also called Brock's syndrome.

midfoot (mid´foot) The middle portion of the foot consisting of the navicular, cuboid, and cuneiform bones.

midgut (mid´gut) **1.** The middle portion of the embryonic digestive tract between the foregut and the hindgut from which the ileum and the jejunum develop. **2.** The small intestine.

midmenstrual (mid-men´stroo-al) Midway between two menstrual periods.

midpelvis (mid-pel´vis) The area of the pelvis extending from the posterior inferior aspects of the symphysis in a line through the ischial spines to the sacrum, intersecting it at about the second and third vertebrae.

midsection (mid-sek´shun) A section or division through the center of an organ or a part.

midwife (mid´wīf) A woman who attends women in childbirth.

certified nurse m. A formally trained and credentialed person in obstetrics, usually a registered nurse, who provides care to a woman during pregnancy and childbirth and cares for both mother and infant immediately following childbirth, usually with physician backup in case of emergencies or complications.

lay m. A person without formal training in obstetrics who attends a woman in childbirth and the puerperium.

midwifery (mid-wif´ĕ-re, mid-wi´fer-e) The care provided by a midwife in a hospital, birthing center, or home.

mifepristone (mif-pris´tōn) A progestational and glucocorticoid antagonist; may be used to induce menses before the missed period, as an abortifacient in early pregnancy, or to treat hypercortisolism in patients with nonpituitary Cushing's syndrome. Trade name: RU486.

migraine (mi´grān) A recurrent, intense headache, usually confined to one side of the head and associated with nausea, vomiting, and visual disturbances. Also called blind headache; sick headache; vascular headache.

classic m. Unilateral headache preceded by a characteristic scotoma, a visual disturbance appearing as a flashing blind spot with luminous edges, lasting 20 to 25 minutes and disappearing when headache begins.

common m. Migraine in which the headache is not limited to one side and neurologic disturbances (i.e., hypersensitivity to light and sound, nausea, and vomiting) do not precede the headache but occur during its course; relief is usually produced by sleep.

migration (mi-gra´shun) Passing from one part of the body to another.

Mikulicz's syndrome (mik´u-lich-ez sin´drōm) Painless enlargement of the salivary and lacrimal glands, usually bilateral, accompanied by dryness of mouth and decreased lacrimation; may be caused by immune-mediated destruction of the glands or by complication of tuberculosis, leukemia, lymphoma, or sarcoidosis.

miliaria (mil-e-a´re-ă) A skin eruption due to retention of sweat in the sweat follicles.

m. rubra See prickly heat, under heat.

miliary (mil´e-a-re) Having a millet seed size (about 2 mm), such as the nodules of miliary tuberculosis.

milieu (me-lyuh´) French for environment or surroundings.

m. intérieur The internal environment; the fluids bathing the tissue cells of multicellular animals.

milium (mil´e-um) A minute whitish or yellowish papule on the skin caused by retention of fatty material. Popularly called whitehead.

milk (milk) **1.** A white or yellowish liquid secreted by the mammary glands of female mammals for the nourishment of the young; contains proteins, sugar, and lipids. **2.** A milklike liquid.

m. of magnesia See under magnesia.

uterine m. Secretion produced by uterine glands.

witch's m. The milklike fluid sometimes secreted by the breasts of newborn babies of either sex.

milk-alkali syndrome (milk-al´kă-li sin´drōm) Hypercalcemia without hypercalcuria or hypophosphaturia, induced by the prolonged ingestion of large amounts of milk and soluble alkali, usually as therapy for peptic ulcer; it is reversible in its early stages, but if undetected leads to renal failure. Also called Burnett's syndrome.

milking (milk´ing) Removal of the contents of a tubular structure by gently running a finger along the length of the structure.

Milkman's syndrome (milk´manz sin´drōm) Osteoporosis causing multiple fractures; seen most frequently in postmenopausal women.

Millard-Gubler syndrome (mil´ard-goob´ler sin´drōm) Paralysis of facial muscles on one side and of the extremities on the opposite side, produced by a unilateral lesion of the brainstem.

milliampere (mil-e-am´pēr) (ma, mA) One-thousandth (10^{-3}) of an ampere.

millicurie (mil-ĭ-ku´re) (mCi) One thousandth (10^{-3}) of a curie.

milliequivalent (mil-ĭ-e-kwiv´ă-lent) (mEq) An expression of concentration of substance per liter of solution, calculated by dividing the concentration in milligrams per 100 milliliters by the molecular weight.

milligram (mil´ĭ-gram) (mg) One-thousandth (10^{-3}) of a gram.

milliliter (mil´ĭ-le-ter) (ml) One-thousandth (10^{-3}) of a liter; one cubic centimeter.

millimeter (mil´ĭ-me-ter) (mm) One-thousandth (10^{-3}) of a meter.

millimicrogram (mil-ĭ-mi´kro-gram) See nanogram (ng).

millimicron (mil´ĭ-mi-kron) (mµ) See nanometer (nm).

millimole (mil´ĭ-mōl) (mmol) One-thousandth (10^{-3}) of a mole.

milling-in (mil´ing-in) The placing of abrasives between the occlusal surfaces of dentures while rubbing them together in the mouth or on the

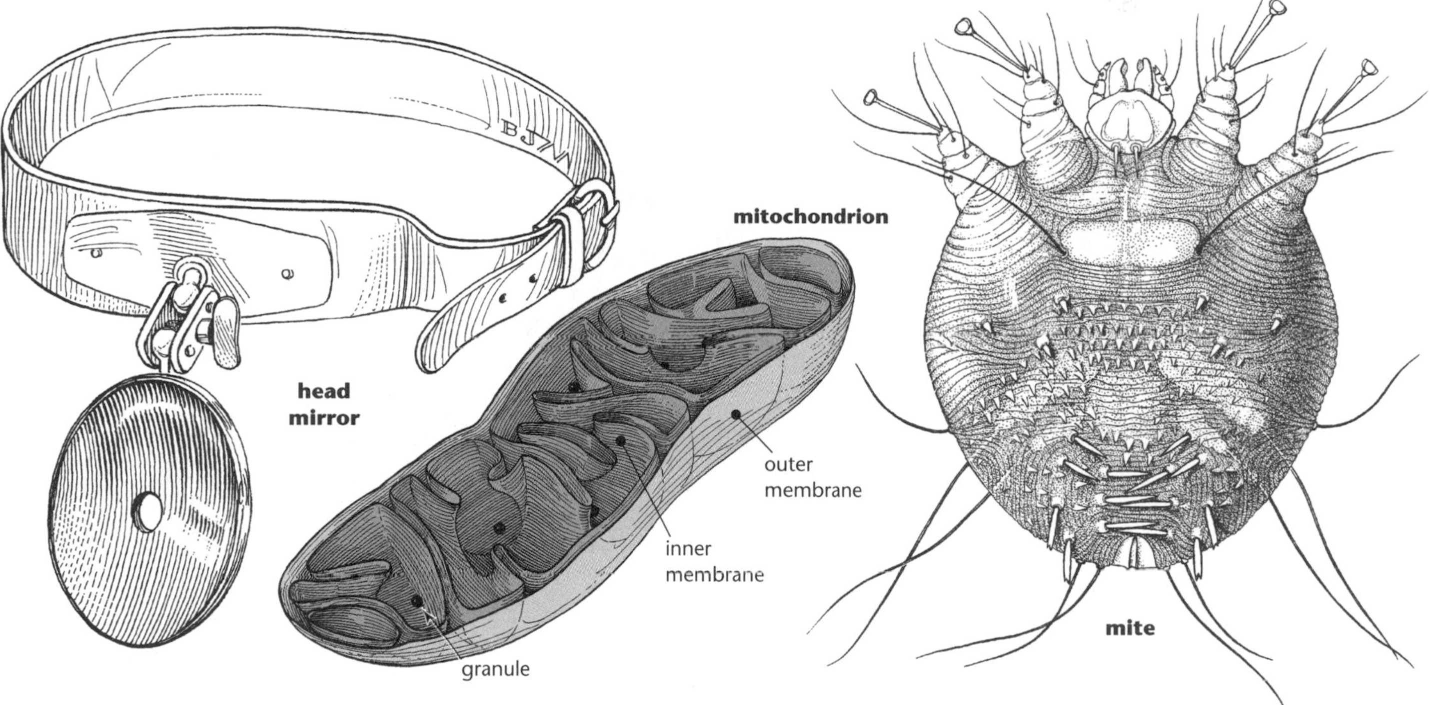

articulator; used to perfect the occlusion.

milliosmole (mil-ĭ-os ´mōl) (mOsm) One-thousandth (10^{-3}) of an osmole; the osmotic pressure exerted by the concentration of a substance in solution; expressed as milligrams per kilogram divided by atomic weight for an ionized substance, or divided by molecular weight for nonionized solutes; normal plasma osmolality is 280 to 300 mOsm/kg.

millirad (mil´ĭ-rad) (mrad) One-thousandth (10^{-3}) of a rad.

millirem (mil´ĭ-rem) (mrem) One-thousandth (10^{-3}) of a rem.

milliroentgen (mil´ĭ-rent-gen) (mr) One-thousandth (10^{-3}) of a roentgen.

millisecond (mil-ĭ-sek´ond) (msec) One-thousandth (10^{-3}) of a second.

millivolt (mil´ĭ-vōlt) (mV) One-thousandth (10^{-3}) of a volt.

Milroy's disease (mil´rois dĭ-zēz´) Familial and congenital swelling of subcutaneous tissues (usually confined to the extremities) with large accumulation of lymph.

mimesis (mi-me´sis) State in which one disease presents the symptoms of another. Also called imitation.

mind (mīnd) The totality of conscious and unconscious processes serving to adjust the individual to the demands of the environment. Also called the psyche.

mineral (min´er-al) Any naturally occurring homogeneous inorganic substance, having a characteristic crystalline structure and chemical composition.

mineralocorticoid (min-er-al-o-kor´tĭ-koid) One of the steroids in the adrenal cortex that controls salt metabolism.

minilaparotomy (min-e-lap-ah-rot´o-me) Technique for gaining access into the abdominopelvic cavity through a minute incision in the abdominal wall (e.g., to ligate the uterine tubes for female sterilization).

minim (min´im) A unit of fluid measure; in the United States, 1/60 of a fluid dram; about a drop.

minimal change disease (min´ĭ-mal chānj dĭ-zēz´) (MCD) A form of nephrotic syndrome in which minimal or no glomerular abnormalities are noted by light microscopy and the major abnormality on electron microscopy is fusion of epithelial foot processes. Also called lipoid nephrosis; nil (nothing in light microscopy) disease.

miosis (mi-o´sis) Reduction in the size of the pupil of the eye.

miotic (mi-ot´ik) Denoting any agent that causes contraction of the pupil.

miracidium (mi-ră-sid´e-um), *pl.* **miracid´ia** A free-swimming ciliated larva of a trematode that penetrates a small intermediate host where it develops into a sporocyst.

mire (mēr) One of the luminous objects in the ophthalmometer, used in measuring the anterior curvature of the cornea.

mirror (mir´or) A polished surface that forms optical images by reflection.

head m. A circular concave mirror attached to a headband, used to illuminate a bodily cavity.

misandry (mis´an-dre) Hatred of men.

misanthropy (mis-an-throp´pe-ă) Aversion to people.

miscarriage (mis-kar´ij) See spontaneous abortion, under abortion.

miscarry (mis-kar´e) To deliver a nonviable fetus.

misce (mis´e) (M) Latin for mix.

misce et signa (mis´e-ĕt sig´nă) Latin for mix and label.

miscible (mis´ĭ-bl) Capable of being mixed.

misdiagnosis (mis-di-ag-no´sis) A wrong diagnosis.

misogyny (mĭ-soj´ĭ-ne) Hatred of women.

misophobia (mis-o-fo´be-ă) An abnormal fear of contamination.

missense (mis´sens) See missense mutation, under mutation.

mite (mīt) Any of various minute arachnids that are often parasitic on humans and animals; they may infest food and carry disease.

harvest m. See chigger.

hay itch m. See *Pyemotes tritici.*

itch m. See *Sarcoptes scabiei.*

northern fowl m. See *Ornithonyssus sylviarum.*

mithridatism (mith´rĭ-da-tiz-m) Immunity to a poison achieved by taking gradually increased doses of it.

miticide (mi´tĭ-sīd) An agent that kills mites.

mitochondria (mi-to-kon´dre-ă) Plural of mitochondrion.

mitochondrion (mi-to-kon´dre-on), *pl.* **mitochon´dria** One of numerous compartmentalized, self-reproducing organelles present in the cytoplasm of most cells; has its own DNA and is responsible for generating usable energy by the formation of adenosine triphosphate (ATP). The average cell contains several hundred mitochondria, each about 15,000 Å in length.

mitogen (mi´to-jen) A substance that stimulates cell mitosis and lymphocyte transformation.

pokeweed m. (PWM) A mitogen for B lymphocytes, derived from the plant *Phytolacca americana.*

mitogenesis (mi-to-jen´ĕ-sis) The induction of mitosis in a cell.

mitogenic (mi-to-jen´ik) Causing or inducing cell mitosis.

mitosis (mi-to´sis) Multiplication or division of a cell that results in the formation of two daughter cells normally receiving the same chromosome and deoxyribonucleic acid (DNA) content as that of the original cell. Also called karyokinesis.

mitotic (mi-tot´ik) Relating to mitosis or cell division.

mitral (mi´tral) Relating to the left atrioventricular valve of the heart.

mitralization (mi-tral-i-za´shun) In radiography, straightening of the left border of the heart shadow with protrusion of the atrial appendage and/or the pulmonary salient.

mittelschmerz (mit´el-shmarts) Intermenstrual pain, specifically at the time of ovulation.

mixture (miks´chur) **1.** An aggregation of two or more substances that are not chemically combined. **2.** A pharmaceutical preparation consisting of an insoluble substance suspended in a liquid by means of a viscid material (e.g., sugar or glycerol).

binary m. One containing two substances.

Brompton m. See Brompton cocktail.

explosive m. One capable of instantaneous combustion.

Ringer's m. See Ringer's solution, under solution.

M-mode (ĕm-mōd) A diagnostic ultrasound presentation of echo changes in which a B-mode tracing is moved to indicate the pattern of echo motion (M) as a function of time (T). Also called TM-mode.

mnemonic (ne-mon´ik) Relating to or assisting the memory.

mnemonics (ne-mon´iks) A system for improving the memory.

MNSs blood group (blud´ grōōp) A system of erythrocyte antigens determined by the allelic genes M, N, and S, s; first demonstrated by injecting human blood into rabbits, which developed antibodies against it; originally defined to include antigens to antibodies anti-M and anti-N and later extended to include those reacting to antibodies anti-S and anti-s; the group is primarily used to solve identification problems such as disputed paternity and for genetic linkage population studies.

mobilization (mo-bĭ-li-za´shun) **1.** Making a part movable. **2.** Starting a sequence of physiologic activity.

stapes m. Surgical procedure through which the footplate of the stapes is liberated from adhesions or overlapping bony tissue caused by otosclerosis or middle ear infection.

mobilize (mo´bĭ-līz) To cause stored substances in the body to participate in physiologic activity; to liberate material from storage sites.

Möbius' sign (me´be-us sīn) Convergence weakness of the eyes occurring in Graves' disease.

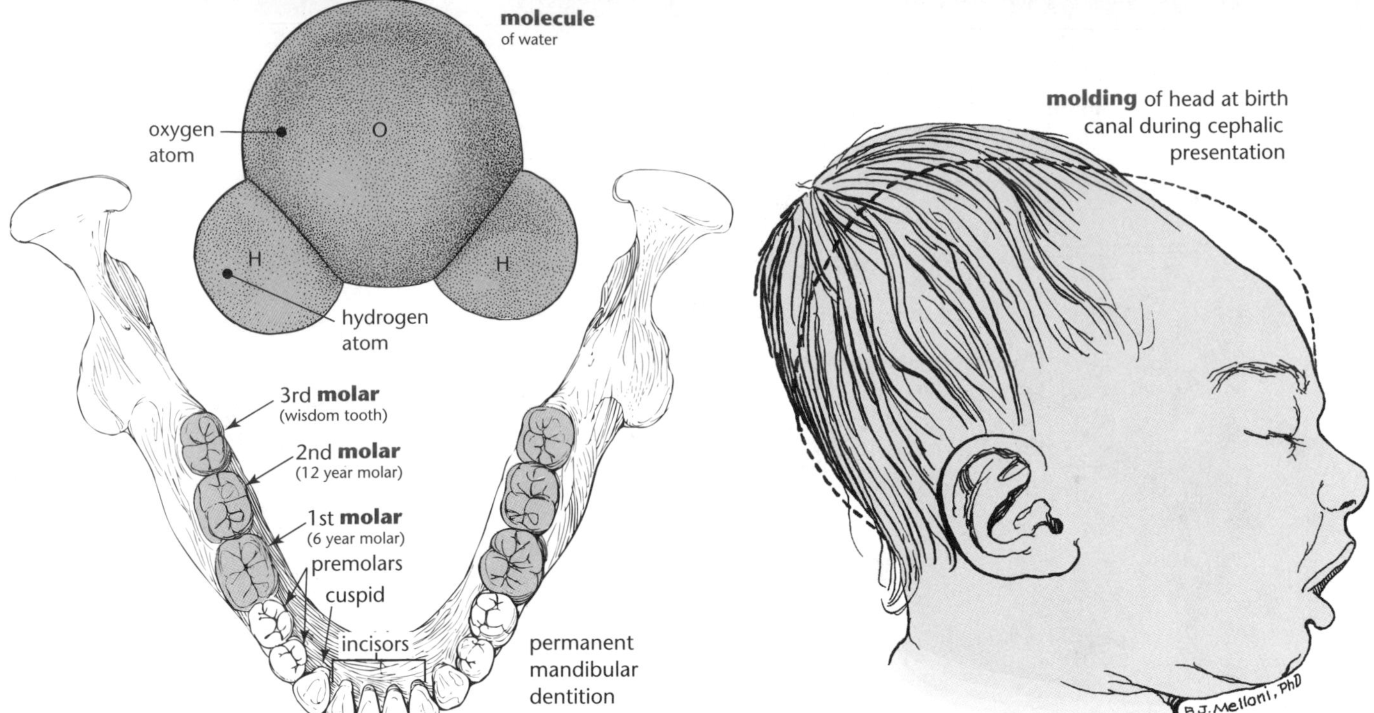

M

Möbius' syndrome (me´be-us sin´drōm) A congenital disorder characterized by bilateral paralysis of both external rectus muscles and face muscles and sometimes associated with other musculoskeletal anomalies or neurologic disorders. Also called congenital facial diplegia; congenital oculofacial paralysis.

modality (mo-dal´ĭ-te) **1.** Any of several forms of therapy (e.g., diathermy). **2.** Any of the main forms of sensation (e.g., hearing).

mode (mōd) In statistics, the value occurring most often.

model (mod´el) A three-dimensional shape representing a likeness of some existing structure, used for study, experimentation, or diagnosis. Also called replica.

ball and stick m. A three-dimensional schematic representation of a molecular structure.

disease m. The artificial creation of an abnormality in an experimental animal in order to allow further study of the entity.

simulation m. See manikin.

study m. In dentistry, a replica of the teeth and adjoining oral structures, used as a diagnostic aid. Also called diagnostic cast.

modification (mod-ĭ-fĭ-ka´shun) A change in an organism that is acquired, not inherited.

behavior m. The systematic use of techniques (e.g., desensitization and biofeedback) to modify or eliminate selected undesirable behaviors, attitudes, or phobias. Also called behavior modification therapy.

modifier (mod-ĭ-fi´ĕr) Agent that alters form or character without transforming (e.g., a gene that alters the phenotypic effect of another gene).

modiolus (mo-di´o-lus) The central pillar or column of bone around which the spiral canals of the cochlea turn.

modulation (mod-u-la´shun) The changes that take place in response to changes in the environment, such as the temporary change of osteoblasts into osteocytes and back to osteoblasts in response to altered conditions in the environment.

mogigraphia (moj-ĭ-graf´ĭ-ă) See writer's cramp, under cramp.

moiety (moi´ĕ-te) **1.** One of two more or less equal parts. **2.** A part or portion of indefinite size.

molal (mo´lal) Containing 1 mole of solute per 1000 grams of solvent. COMPARE: molar (2).

molality (mo-lal´ĭ-te) The concentration of a solution expressed as the number of moles of solute per 1000 kilograms of solvent.

molar (mo´lar) (M) **1.** A posterior tooth for grinding and pulverizing food. **2.** Containing 1 gram-molecular weight (1 mole) of solute per 1000 milliliters of solution. COMPARE: molal. **3.** Relating to a body of matter; not molecular.

deciduous m. One of eight posterior teeth in the deciduous (primary) dentition.

first permanent m. Largest permanent tooth in the mouth; first permanent tooth to erupt, usually at the age of 6 years. Also called six-year molar.

impacted m. A molar unable to erupt properly.

permanent m. One of 12 posterior teeth in the permanent (secondary) dentition.

second permanent m. A permanent molar immediately distal to the first molar; usually erupts at the age of 12 years. Also called twelve-year molar.

third permanent m. Last permanent posterior tooth in the mouth; erupts usually between the ages of 17 and 21 years. Also called wisdom tooth.

molarity (mol-ar´ĭ-te) The concentration of a solution expressed as the number of moles of solute per liter of solution.

mold (mōld) **1.** Any of a group of fungi usually growing on decaying organic matter. **2.** A receptacle for shaping any cast material (e.g., wax, plastic). **3.** To shape.

molding (mōld´ing) **1.** The process of shaping. **2.** The temporary change in shape of the fetal head as it passes through the birth canal. Also called configuration.

compression m. In dentistry, the pressing of a plastic material to the negative form of a mold.

mole (mōl) (mol) The quantity of a chemical substance with as many elementary entities as there are carbon atoms in 12 grams of carbon 12 (^{12}C).

mole (mōl) **1.** Popular term for a nevocellular nevus; see under nevus. **2.** Intrauterine mass.

atypical m. An acquired pigmented lesion of the skin that has clinical and histologic characteristics different from a typical common mole (nevocellular nevus); may have macular and/or papular components; has well-defined irregular borders; is typically larger than most acquired common moles (over 6 mm) with pigment variegation, ranging from tan to dark brown; and occurs on both sun-exposed and nonexposed areas of the body, especially on the trunk. Also called dysplastic nevus.

hydatid m. See hydatidiform mole.

hydatidiform m. An abnormal pregnancy in which a mass of clear vesicles resembling a bunch of grapes grows within the uterus from proliferation of placental tissues; initial symptoms are usually those of early pregnancy; characteristic symptoms include bleeding (usually during the first trimester), passage of vesicles, and a uterus too large for the estimated time of gestation; designated *complete hydatidiform m.* when there is no fetus present, and *incomplete hydatidiform m.* when a fetus is present in addition to the mole. Also called hydatid mole; molar pregnancy.

invasive m. A hydatidiform mole that invades the uterine wall; it may completely penetrate the wall and be associated with uterine rupture. Also called chorioadenoma destruens; chorioadenocarcinoma.

molecular (mo-lek´u-lar) Relating to, or consisting of, molecules.

molecular weight (mo-lek´u-lar wāt) (mol wt, MW) The sum of the atomic weights of all the atoms making up a molecule; e.g., hydrogen (H) has an atomic weight of one and chlorine (Cl) has an atomic weight of 35.5; thus, a molecule of hydrochloric acid (HCl) has a molecular weight of 36.5.

molecule (mol´ĕ-kūl) The smallest unit of a substance (composed of two or more atoms) which can exist in a free state and still retain the chemical properties of the substance.

costimulatory m. A molecule that provides signals for lymphocyte activation in addition to those provided through the antigen receptor.

cyclic m. A molecule that appears in organic compounds, and whose atoms are arranged in a ring or polygon.

molimen (mo-li´men), *pl.* **moli´mina** (mo-lim´ĭ-nă) The effort required by a normal physiologic function, especially the menstrual flow.

molluscum (mo-lus´kum) A skin disease marked by the presence of soft rounded tumors.

m. contagiosum An infectious disease of the skin, marked by small wartlike lesions containing a substance resembling curds; caused by a poxvirus.

molt (mōlt) To cast off.

molybdate (mo-lib´dāt) A salt of molybdic acid.

molybdenum (mo-lib´dĕ-num) Metallic element; symbol Mo, atomic number 42, atomic weight 95.95; it has several isotopes.

molybdic (mo-lib´dik) Denoting a salt of trivalent or hexavalent molybdenum.

molybdic acid (mo-lib´dik as´id) Any of two acids, H_2MoO_4 (colorless needles), or $H_2Mo_4{\cdot}4H_2O$, a yellow crystalline substance, soluble in ammonia and used as a reagent.

momism (mom´is-m) The state of being excessively dependent on or subordinate to one's mother or her substitute.

monad (mon´ad) **1.** A univalent element, radical, or atom. **2.** A unicellular organism. **3.** The single chromosome formed after the second division in meiosis.

monarthritis (mon-ar-thri´tis) Arthritis of one joint.

monarticular (mon-ar-tik´u-lar) Denoting a single joint.

monaural (mon-aw´ral) Relating to one ear.

Monday disease (mun´dā dĭ-zēz´) The return of symptoms after a weekend away from work, as in the case of an allergic reaction to a substance encountered while at work.

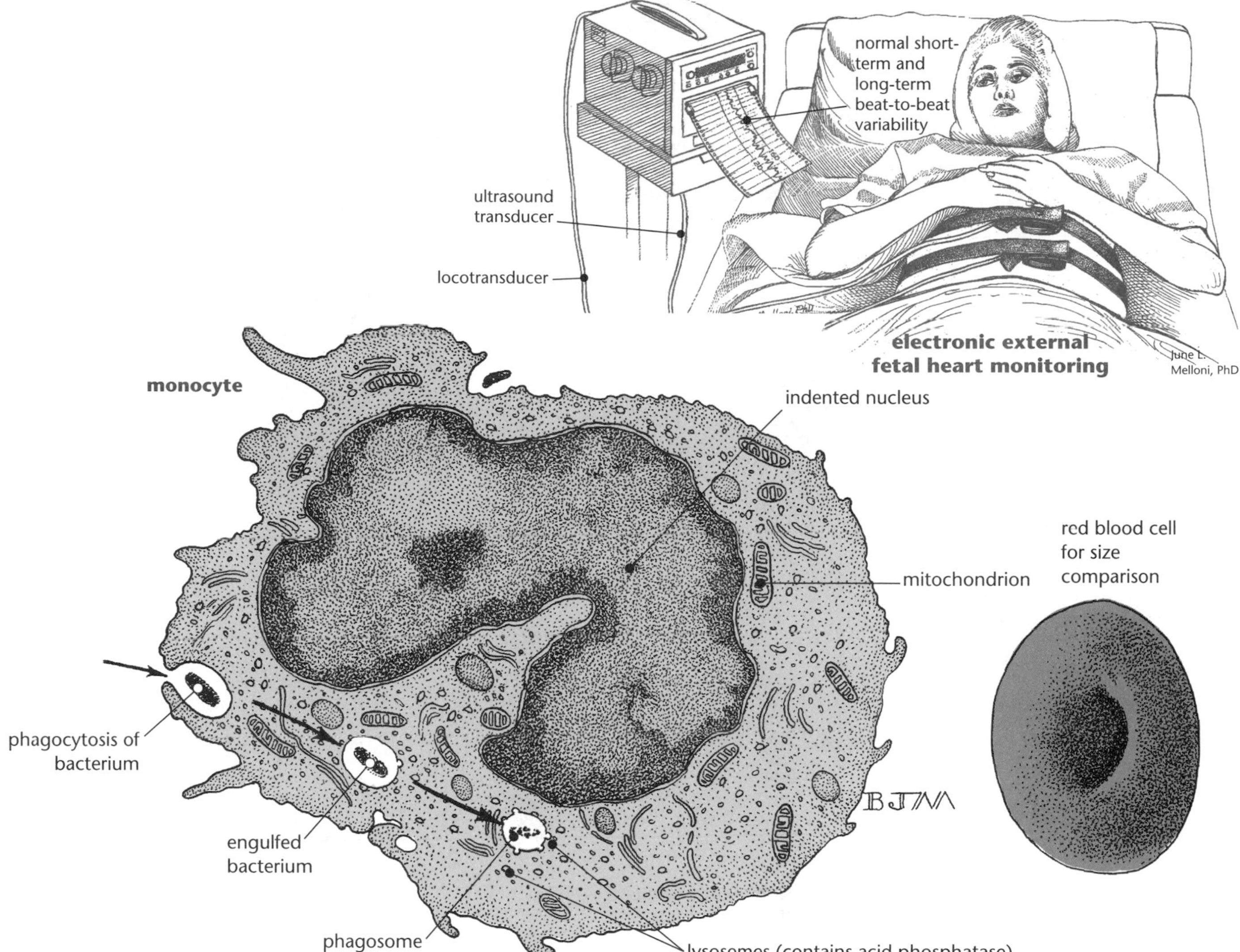

Mondor's disease (mon´dorz dĭ-zēz´) Inflammation of the subcutaneous veins of the chest and breast, usually extending from the epigastric region to the axilla and occurring in both males and females.
mongolism (mong´gŏ-liz-m) Obsolete term. See Down syndrome.
monilethrix (mo-nil´e-thriks) Beaded hair, an anomalous condition in which the hair shafts exhibit nodosities or points of thickening alternating with normal or constricted girth, giving the appearance of a string of fusiform beads.
Monilia (mo-nil´e-ă) A genus of molds or fungi commonly called fruit molds; formerly included in this genus was a similar group of organisms now called *Candida.*
monilial (mo-nil´e-al) Relating to the fruit molds; frequently used incorrectly with reference to *Candida.*
moniliasis (mon-ĭ-lī´ă-sis) See candidiasis.
moniliform (mo-nil´ĭ-form) Shaped like a string of pearls.
monitor (mon´ĭ-tor) **1.** To maintain a close, constant watch on a patient's condition. **2.** In laboratory medicine, a part of an instrument for detecting physical or chemical changes in electromagnetic radiation. **3.** Any device used in monitoring.
cardiac m. An electronic device used for observation of each heartbeat of a person.
monitoring (mon´ĭ-tor-ing) Constant observation.
auscultatory fetal m. Assessment of the fetal heart tones with a head stethoscope (fetoscope) during labor.
constant cardiac m. Prolonged observation of the electrocardiogram with the aid of an oscilloscope to detect irregularities in the heart rhythm.
electronic fetal heart rate m. Monitoring of the fetal heart rate with any of various electronic devices; may be *external* (indirect), performed through the maternal abdominal wall, usually by pulsed ultrasonography (Doppler ultrasound); or it may be *internal* (direct), performed during labor with a spiral electrode attached directly on the scalp of the fetus.
mono (mon´o) Colloquialism for mononucleosis.
monoamine (mon-o-am´ēn) Compound containing only one amine group.
m. oxidase (MAO) An enzyme that catalyzes the oxidation of a wide variety of physiologic amines to the corresponding aldehydes and NH_3.
m. oxidate inhibitors (MAOI) Derivatives of hydrazine and hydrazide that inhibit the action of monoamine oxidases.
monoamniotic (mon-o-am-ne-ot´ik) Sharing one amniotic sac in the uterus; applied to twins.
monoblast (mon´o-blast) An immature cell of the monocytic series, from 18 to 22 µm in diameter, which has several nucleoli; formed primarily in the spleen and lymphoid tissues.
monochromat (mon-o-kro´mat) A totally color blind individual who sees colors as different shades of gray.
monochromatic (mon-o-kro-mat´ik) **1.** Having one color. **2.** Indicating a spectral color of a single wavelength.
monoclonal (mon-o-klōn´al) Derived from a single clone of cells.
monocrotic (mon-o-krot´ik) Forming a smooth single crest on the downward line of a curve; said of a pulse.
monocular (mon-ok´u-lar) Relating to, having, or used by one eye.
monocyte (mon´o-sīt) A large mononuclear white blood cell, generally 15 to 25 µm in diameter, with a round, kidney-shaped, or lobulated nucleus and a cytoplasm that stains a gray-blue color with Wright's stain; it is the largest cell found in normal blood; when it leaves the bloodstream, it becomes a macrophage (phagocyte).
monocytopenia (mon-o-sī-to-pe´ne-ă) Reduction of monocytes in the blood. Also called monocytic leukopenia; monopenia.
monocytosis (mon-o-si-to´sis) Increased number of monocytes in the blood, at least 15 or more monocytes per 100 white blood cells; common reaction to inflammation.
monodactylism (mon-o-dak´tĭl-iz-m) The presence of only one finger on the hand or one toe on the foot.
monogametic (mon-o-gam-et´ik) See homogametic.
monogenic (mon-o-jen´ik) Relating to an inherited characteristic or process that is determined by a single gene.
monogenous (mon-o-jen´us) Produced asexually.
monograph (mon´o-graf) A detailed written account of one particular subject, one class of subjects, or a small area of a special field of learning.
monohybrid (mon-o-hi´brid) A cross between parents that differ in one character.
monoiodotyrosine (mon-o-i-o-do-ti´ro-sēn) (MIT) An amino acid formed by the iodination of tyrosine; an initial step in the formation of thyronine, a component of thyroxin.
monokine (mon´o-kīn) A hormone-like factor produced by activation of monocytes; acts as an intercellular messenger to regulate immunologic and inflammatory responses.
monolayer (mon-o-la´er) A film consisting of a single layer of molecules, formed on a water surface by certain substances (e.g., proteins, fatty acids) in which some atoms are soluble, others insoluble, in

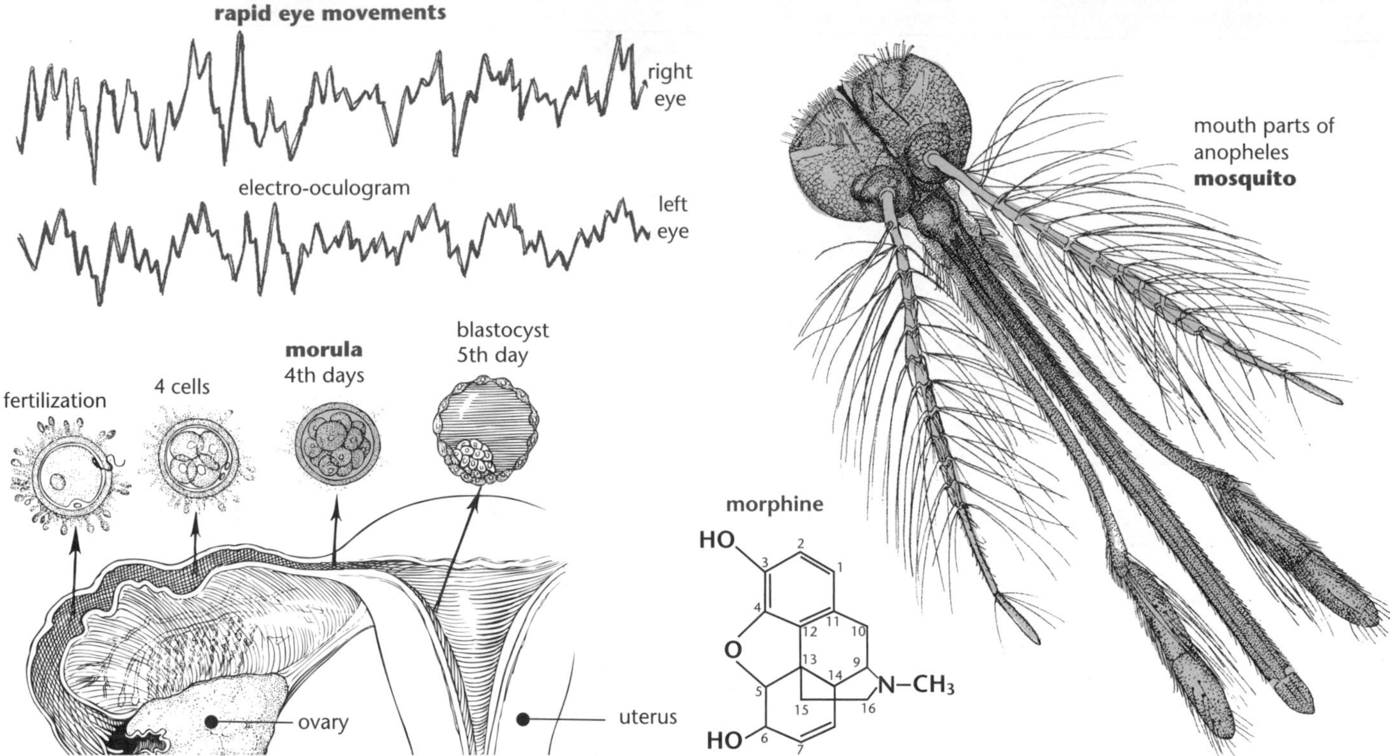

water.

monolocular (mon-o-lok′u-lar) Having only one cavity. Also called unicameral.

monomania (mon-o-ma′ne-ă) Pathologic preoccupation with one idea.

monomer (mon′o-mer) A simple molecule of low molecular weight that, when repeated in a chain, forms a polymer (e.g., ethylene is the monomer of polyethylene).

M

monomorphic (mon-o-mor′fik) Having but one shape.

mononeuritis (mon-o-nu-ri′tis) Inflammation or degeneration of a single nerve trunk or some of its branches.

m. multiplex Neuritis involving single nerves at several distant sites.

mononuclear (mon-o-nu′kle-ar) Uninuclear.

mononucleosis (mon-o-noo-kle-o′sis) Abnormal increase of mononuclear white blood cells (monocytes) in the blood.

cytomegalovirus (CMV) **m.** Infectious disease resembling infectious mononucleosis but without throat and cervical node involvement; caused by CMV with incubation period of 20–60 days; marked by prolonged high fevers, headache, malaise, profound fatigue, muscle pains, and enlargement of the spleen; may follow transplant of organs from donors with prior CMV infections.

infectious m. An infectious febrile disease caused by the EB virus (Epstein-Barr virus); marked by fever, sore throat, enlargement of the spleen and lymph nodes, and the presence in the blood of an abnormally large number of atypical lymphocytes that resemble monocytes; the virus can be carried in the mouth and throat of afflicted individuals for several months after the disappearance of clinical illness. Sometimes called glandular fever. Popularly called mono; kissing disease.

mononucleotide (mon-o-noo′kle-o-tīd) See nucleotide.

monophasia (mon-o-fa′zhă) Disorder in which the individual's vocabulary is limited to a single word or sentence.

monophenol monooxygenase (mon-o-fe′nol mon-o-ok′si-je-nas) A copper-containing enzyme that promotes the oxidation of phenols such as tyrosine; it is involved in the eventual conversion of tyrosine to melanin; its absence in the body tissues is linked to albinism. Also called tyrosinase.

monoplegia (mon-o-ple′jă) Paralysis of only one limb or part.

monorchid (mon-or′kid) An individual with only one visible testicle.

monorchism, monorchidism (mon′or-kiz-m, mon-or′kid-iz-m) The condition of having or appearing to have only one testicle, the other being absent or undescended.

monosaccharide (mon-o-sak′ă-rīd) A carbohydrate which is not further broken down by hydrolysis; a simple sugar.

monosodium glutamate (mon-o-so′de-um glu′tă-māt) (MSG) A white crystalline compound used in cooking to enhance flavor. Also called sodium glutamate.

monosome (mon′o-sōm) A chromosome without its homologous chromosome.

monosomy (mon′o-so-me) Condition in which one chromosome of a pair of homologous chromosomes is missing.

monosubstituted (mon-o-sub′stĭ-tūt-ed) Having only one atom in each molecule replaced.

monotrichous (mon-ot′rĭ-kus) Denoting a unicellular organism having a single flagellum.

monovalent (mon-o-val′lent) See univalent.

monoxide (mon-ok′sīd) An oxide containing only one oxygen atom.

monozygotic (mon-o-zi-got′ik) Denoting identical twins (i.e., twins derived from a single fertilized egg).

mons (monz), *pl.* **mon′tes** In anatomy, a slight prominence or elevation.

m. pubis The fleshy prominence formed by a pad of fatty tissue over the pubic symphysis in the female.

m. ureteris A slight prominence on the wall of the bladder at the entrance of the ureter.

mood (mōōd) A prevailing emotional state of mind.

Moraxella (mo-rak-sel′ă) A genus of bacteria containing gram-negative, short, rod-shaped cells; aerobic and parasitic; sometimes found on human mucous membranes.

M. catarrhalis A species causing upper respiratory infections, especially in immunocompromised people. Also called *Branhamella catarrhalis; Neisseria catarrhalis.*

morbid (mor′bid) Relating to disease; pathologic.

morbidity (mor-bid′ĭ-te) **1.** The condition of being diseased. **2.** The ratio of disease to the population of a given area.

morbilli (mor-bil′i) Measles.

morbilliform (mor-bil′ĭ-form) Resembling measles.

Morbillivirus (mor-bil-ĭ-vi′rus) Genus of the family Paramyxoviridae that includes the measles and canine distemper viruses; all members produce both intranuclear and cytoplasmic inclusion bodies.

morbillous (mor-bil′us) Relating to measles.

morbus (mor′bus) Latin for disease.

mordant (mor′dant) A substance used in bacteriology to fix a dye or stain.

morgan (mor′gan) (M) The unit of map distance on a chromosome.

Morganella (mor-gă-nel′ă) Genus of gram-negative, anaerobic, motile bacteria; normally found in soil, water, and sewage and as part of the normal fecal flora.

M. morganii The single species of *Morganella;* causes infections of the blood, respiratory and urinary tracts, and wounds in debilitated patients.

morgue (morg) A place where the dead are kept pending autopsy and burial.

moribund (mor′ĭ-bund) Dying.

morphea (mor-fe′ă) A skin disease marked by indurated white or yellow lesions surrounded by a violet ring; occurring chiefly on the chest, face, or neck.

morphine (mor′fēn) An alkaloid compound extracted from opium, used in medicine as an analgesic; prolonged use causes addiction.

morphogenesis (mor-fo-jen′ĕ-sis) The embryonic differentiation of cells leading to the establishment of the characteristic structure and form of the organism or its parts.

morphologic (mor-fo-loj′ik) Relating to the structure or form of organisms.

morphology (mor-fol′o-je) The study of the configuration or structure of living organisms.

Morquio's syndrome (mor-ke′ōz sin′drōm) A form of mucopolysaccharidosis characterized chiefly by dwarfism, deformed wrist and hands, knock knees, pectus carinatum, osteoporosis, flat vertebrae, and corneal clouding; keratosulfate is excreted in the urine; transmitted as an autosomal recessive trait. Also called type IV mucopolysaccharidosis.

mors (morz) Latin for death.

mortal (mor′tal) **1.** Subject to death. **2.** Deadly.

mortality (mor-tal′ĭ-te) The quality of being mortal.

reproductive m. The sum of deaths related to pregnancy and deaths caused by techniques used to prevent pregnancy (i.e., intrauterine devices and oral contraceptives).

mortar (mor′tar) A small receptacle in which substances are crushed or pulverized with a pestle.

morula (mor′u-lă) A cluster of cleaving blastomeres resulting from the early division of the zygote; a stage in the development of the embryo prior to the blastula.

morulation (mor-u-la′shun) The formation of a morula.

mosaic (mo-za′ik) An individual or tissue affected with mosaicism.

mosaicism (mo-sa′ĭ-sizm) The presence of two or more populations of cells within one person, some with a normal set of chromosomes, others with extra or missing chromosomes; caused by errors of cell division in the fertilized egg (zygote). Predominance of abnormal cells gives rise to chromosomal abnormality syndromes (e.g., Down's syndrome, Turner's syndrome).

SOME DIFFERENTIAL FEATURES OF INFECTIOUS MONONUCLEOSIS

	infectious mononucleosis	infectious hepatitis (hepatitis A)	tonsillitis
usual age	15 to 25 years	15 to 25 years	5 to 20 years
incubation period	30 to 50 days	15 to 45 days	usually 3 to 5 days
fever	irregular; usually about 2 weeks	moderate; disappears when jaundice develops	moderate to high; usually under 5 days
sore throat	marked; whitish-gray exudate	none	constant; yellow or white exudate
adenopathy (enlargement of lymph nodes)	most commonly: anterior and posterior cervical chains; often generalized	minimal; usually cervical	submandibular; anterior cervical
splenomegaly (enlargement of spleen)	approximately 50%	less than 10%	none
hepatomegaly (enlargement of liver)	approximately 10%	over 80%	none

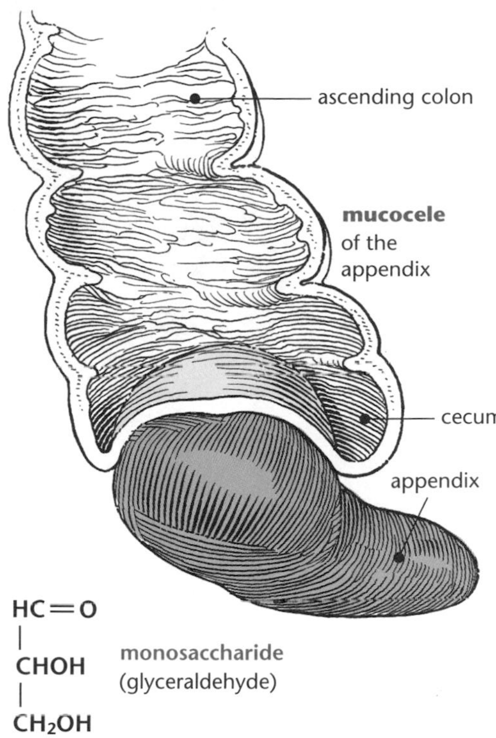

Moschowitz's disease (mos´ko-witz dī-zēz´) See thrombotic thrombocytopenic purpura, under purpura.

mosquito (mos-ke´to) Any of various blood-sucking, winged insects (family Culicidae), some species of which are responsible for the transmission of various diseases such as malaria and yellow fever.

motile (mo´tĭl) Having the capacity to move spontaneously.

motilin (mo-til´in) A polypeptide hormone of 22 amino acids produced in the mucosa of the lower stomach, duodenum, and upper jejunum; it stimulates motility of the stomach and intestines.

motivation (mo-tĭ-va´shun) An incentive to act or the reason for an attitude.

motor (mo´tor) Producing movement; denoting nerves that convey impulses from the nerve centers to the muscles.

plastic m. An artificial point of attachment on an amputation stump through which motion is provided to an artificial limb.

mottling (mot´ling) Macular lesions of varying shades or hues on the skin.

moulage (mo͞o-läzh´) A mold of a body structure, especially for identification, prosthetics, and teaching purposes.

mounting (mownt´ing) Dental laboratory procedure in which a maxillary and/or mandibular cast is attached to an articulator.

mouse (mows), *pl.* **mice** Any of numerous small rodents of the genus *Mus*.

cancer-free white m. (CFW) A mouse used in cancer research.

knockout m. A mouse in which a specific gene has been intentionally deleted thorugh homologous recombination.

New Zealand black m. (NZB) An inbred strain exhibiting (in the adult form) immune hemolytic anemia and renal disease.

transgenic m. A mouse that is the product of bioengineering (i.e., one produced to mimic human diseases by *in vitro* transfer of genes of interest into the mouse embryo); it serves as a model for studying human diseases.

mousepox (mows´poks) See ectromelia.

mouth (mowth) The body opening through which an individual takes in food; the upper portion of the digestive tract, including the lips, tongue, teeth, and related parts; the oral cavity.

dry m. See xerostomia.

trench m. See acute necrotizing ulcerative gingivitis, under gingivitis.

mouthwash (mowth´wosh) A solution for rinsing the mouth and teeth; it generally contains sodium borate, thymol, potassium bicarbonate, eucalyptol, methyl salicylate, alcohol, glycerin, and water. Also called collutorium.

movement (mo͞ov´ment) **1.** Change of place or position. **2.** Popular name for defecation.

associated contralateral m. An involuntary movement occurring on the affected side of a hemiplegic patient, induced by a voluntary movement on the normal side.

bowel m. (BM) See defecation.

brownian m. Erratic motion of microscopic particles suspended in a liquid or gas, resulting from collision with molecules in the suspending medium.

cardinal ocular m.'s The six principal eye movements: to the right and left, upward to the right and left, and downward to the right and left; used in diagnosis of certain neurologic disorders.

ciliary m. Rhythmic motion of the cilia of epithelial cells or protozoa.

circus m. The movement of an excitation wave continuing uninterrupted around a ring of muscle or through the wall of the heart. Also called circus rhythm.

conjugate m. of the eyes Movement of the two eyes in one direction.

non-rapid eye m. (NREM) The slow oscillating movement of the eyes during sleep.

passive m. Movement of the body or any of its parts effected by an external force.

rapid eye m.'s (REMs) The short, quick movements of the eyes during sleep. This phase lasts from five to 60 minutes and is associated with dreaming. See under sleep.

saccadic m. A rapid, abrupt movement of the eyes, as occurs in changing fixation from one point to another.

streaming m. The characteristic movement of the protoplasm of certain white cells or unicellular organisms.

mover (moo´ver) One that sets something in motion.

prime m. See agonistic muscle, under muscle.

moxa (mok´să) A small mass of combustible material placed near the skin or on an acupuncture needle and ignited to produce a counterirritation.

moxibustion (mok-sĭ-bus´chun) Counterirritation by means of a moxa; used in traditional Chinese and Japanese medicine.

mu (mu) **1.** The twelfth letter of the Greek alphabet, μ. **2.** A micron.

mucid (mu´sid) Slimy.

muciferous (mu-sif´er-us) See muciparous.

muciform (mu´sĭ-form) Resembling mucus.

mucigenous (mu-sij´ĕ-nus) See muciparous.

mucilage (mu´sĭ-lij) In pharmacology, a thick viscous liquid; a water solution of the mucilaginous principles of certain vegetable substances.

mucin (mu´sin) A substance secreted by mucous membranes, containing an organic compound (mucopolysaccharide); the main constituent of mucus.

mucinase (mu´sĭ-nās) Any enzyme (e.g., lysozyme) that promotes the breakdown of mucin.

mucinoid (mu´sĭ-noid) Resembling mucin.

mucinosis (mu-sĭ-no´sis) A condition in which mucin is present in abnormal amounts.

mucinous (mu´sĭ-nus) Relating to or containing mucin.

muciparous (mu-sip´ă-rus) Secreting mucus. Also called muciferous; mucigenous.

mucocele (mu´ko-sēl) **1.** A retention cyst of a mucous gland. **2.** Distention of a hollow organ or part (e.g., gallbladder, appendix) with mucin-containing secretions.

mucocutaneous (mu-ko-ku-ta´ne-us) Relating to mucous membrane and skin, especially the line of meeting of those tissues as in the nasal, oral, and anal orifices.

mucocutaneous lymph node syndrome (mu-ko-ku-ta´ne-us limf nōd sin´drōm) Condition affecting mainly infants and young children; marked by fever, conjunctivitis, reddening of oral cavity and lips, pharyngitis, and enlargement of lymph nodes of the neck; accompanied by reddening and peeling of the hands and feet; cause is unknown. Also called Kawasaki disease.

mucoenteritis (mu-ko-en-ter-ī´tis) Inflammation of the intestinal mucous membrane.

mucoid (mu´koid) **1.** Resembling mucus. **2.** A mucus-like conjugated protein or polysaccharide of animal origin.

mucolipidosis (mu-ko-lip-ĭ-do´sis) Any of a group of hereditary metabolic disorders in which mucopolysaccharides and lipids accumulate in the tissues, but urinary patterns of these substances are normal; an autosomal recessive inheritance.

mucolytic (mu-ko-lit´ik) Capable of dissolving mucus.

mucomembranous (mu-ko-mem´bră-nus) Relating to a mucous membrane.

mucoperiosteum (mu-ko-per-e-os´te-um) Periosteum with a closely adhered mucous membrane.

mucopolysaccharide (mu-ko-pol-e-sak´ă-rīd) Polysaccharide components (e.g., hyaluronic acid and chondroitin sulfate) attached to a polypeptide component through weak chemical bonding; a ubiquitous macromolecular complex that forms the amorphous component of intercellular material in the body.

mucopolysaccharidosis (mu-ko-pol-e-sak-ă-rī-do´sis) (MPS) A group of genetic diseases characterized by defective metabolism of mucopolysaccha-

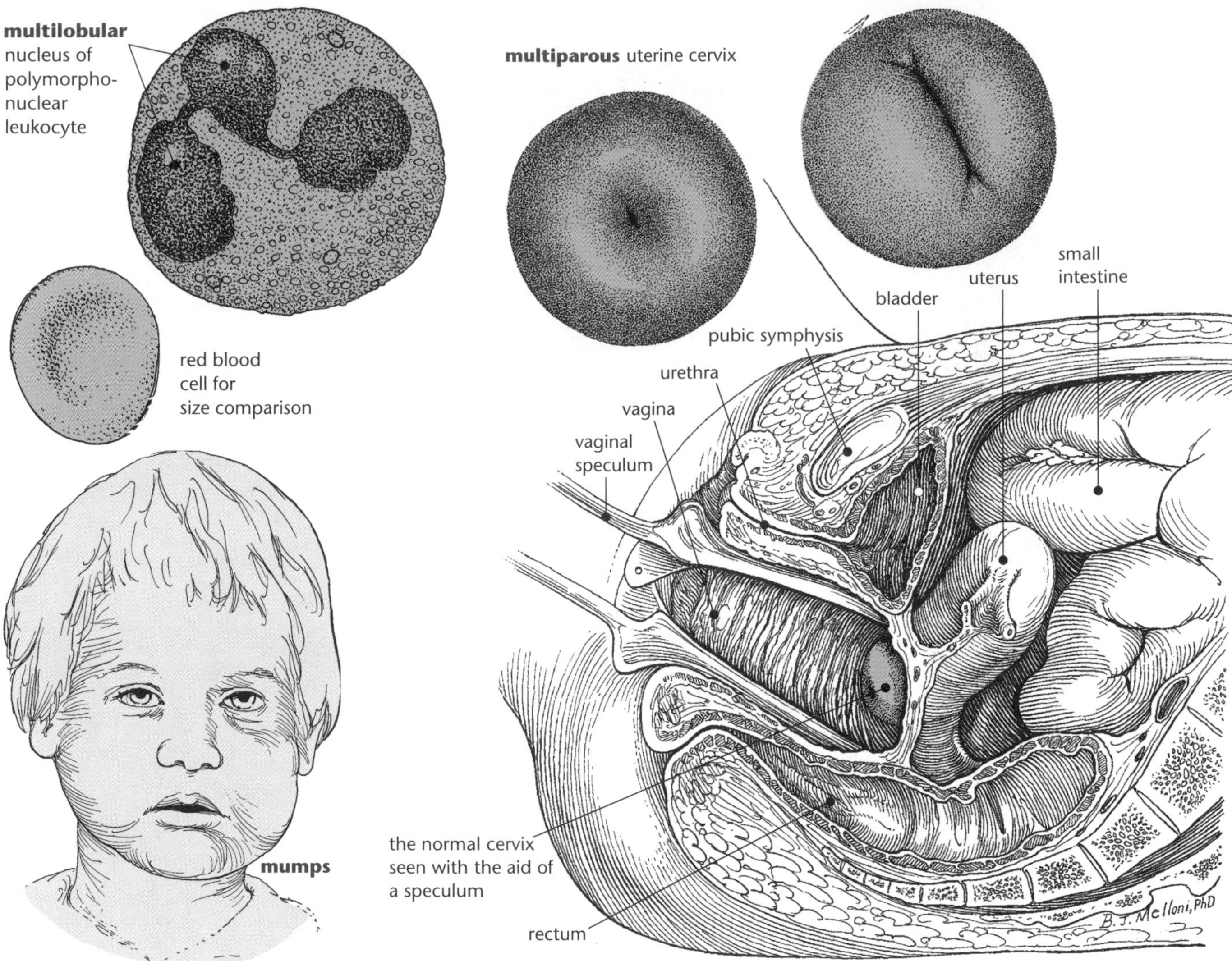

rides, causing accumulation of these substances in the cells.

m. I See Hurler's syndrome.

m. II See Hunter's syndrome.

m. III See Sanfilippo's syndrome.

m. IV See Morquio's syndrome.

m. V Former name for Scheie's syndrome.

m. VI See Maroteaux-Lamy syndrome.

m. VII A type caused by beta-glucuronidase deficiency; it resembles a mild form of Hurler's syndrome, transmitted as an autosomal recessive trait.

mucoprotein (mu-ko-pro´tēn) A group of organic compounds containing proteins and mucopolysaccharides.

mucopurulent (mu-ko-pu´roo-lent) Containing mucus and pus.

mucopus (mu´ko-pus) Discharge composed of mucus and pus.

Mucor (mu´kor) Genus of fungi (class Zygomycetes); some species cause human diseases.

Mucoraceae (mu-ko-ra´se-e) A family of molds (order Mucorales) having a branching, nonsegmented mycelium; some species destroy food products (bread, fruits, and vegetables).

mucormycosis (mu-kor-mi-ko´sis) See phycomycosis.

mucosa (mu-ko´să) See mucous membrane, under membrane.

mucosanguineous (mu-ko-sang-gwin´e-us) Containing mucus and blood; said of a discharge.

mucoserous (mu-ko-se´rus) Relating to or containing mucus and serum or plasma.

mucosin (mu-ko´sin) A mucin peculiar to the more tenacious, adhesive variety of mucus, as that of the nasal cavity.

mucous (mu´kus) Relating to mucus.

mucoviscidosis (mu-ko-vis-ĭ-do´sis) See cystic fibrosis, under fibrosis.

mucus (mu´kus) The slippery suspension of mucin, desquamated cells, inorganic salts, and water secreted by glands in mucous membranes; it moistens and protects the membrane.

cervical m. Mucus secreted by glands within the lining of the cervical canal; it undergoes periodic changes under hormonal influence and, during pregnancy, becomes abundant and thick and forms a plug that completely fills and seals the canal.

muliebria (mu-le-eb´re-ă) The female genital organs.

muliebris (mu-le-eb´ris) Relating to a female.

multangular (mul-tang´gu-lar) Having many angles; said of certain bones.

multiarticular (mul-tĭ-ar-tik´u-lar) Relating to many joints.

multicellular (mul-tĭ-sel´u-lar) Composed of many cells.

multifactorial (mul-tĭ-fak-to´re-al) Determined by several genetic and nongenetic factors. COMPARE: polygenic.

multifid (mul´tĭ-fid) Divided into many segments by clefts.

multifocal (mul-tĭ-fo´kal) Arising from several sites.

multiform (mul´tĭ-form) Occurring in many forms or shapes; polymorphic.

multigravida (mul-tĭ-grav´ĭ-dă) A woman who has been pregnant more than once.

multi-infarct (mul-tĭ-in´farkt) Several areas of cell death resulting from lack of blood supply.

multilobular (mul-tĭ-lob´u-lar) Having many lobules.

multilocular (mul-tĭ-lok´u-lar) Having several cells or compartments.

multimammae (mul-tĭ-mam´e) See polymastia.

multinuclear (mul-tĭ-nu´kle-ar) Having more than one nucleus. Also called polynuclear.

multipara (mul-tip´ă-ră) A woman who has completed two or more pregnancies in which each fetus reached the stage of viability, regardless of whether the infants were live or stillborn.

multiparity (mul-tĭ-par´ĭ-te) The condition of being a multipara.

multiparous (mul-tip´ă-rus) Relating to a multipara.

multiple (mul´tĭ-pl) **1.** Having more than one part or component. **2.** Occurring in several sites at the same time.

multiple organ dysfunction syndrome (mul´tĭ-pl or´gan dis-funk´shun sin´drōm) (MODS) Altered organ function present in an acutely ill patient.

multipolar (mul-tĭ-po´lar) Having more than two poles, as certain nerve cells.

multivalence (mul-tĭ-va´lens) The property of having the capacity to combine with two or more hydrogen atoms. Also called polyvalence.

multivalent (mul-tĭ-va´lent) Having the capacity to combine with more than one hydrogen atom, usually more than two. Also called polyvalent.

mummifaction (mum-ĭ-fĭ-ka´shun) **1.** See dry gangrene, under gangrene. **2.** Drying and compression of a dead fetus retained in the uterus, so that it resembles parchment.

mumps (mumps) An acute contagious disease caused by an RNA myxovirus, affecting primarily the parotid glands and less often the sublingual and submaxillary glands; characterized by glandular swelling and fever; may also involve the pancreas, testes, or central nervous system; incubation period is about three weeks. Also called epidemic parotitis.

Münchausen syndrome (men-chow´zenz sin´drōm) Continual fabrication of clinically convincing

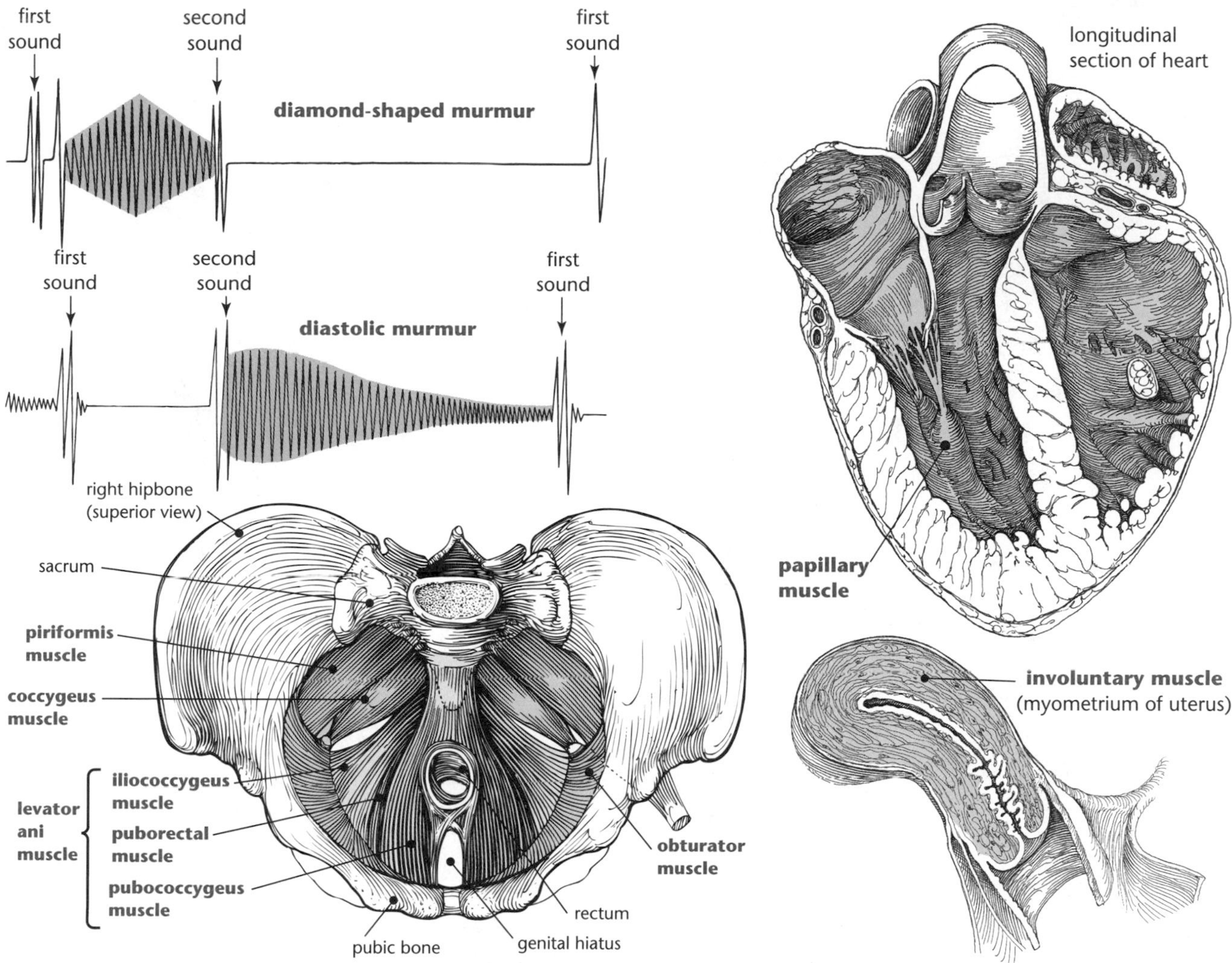

M

simulation of disease; may include self-induced fits, faints, anesthesias, hallucinations, or delusions; the individual's history usually shows a long record of hospitalization.

Münchausen-by-proxy syndrome Condition of a parent or caretaker of a child (usually the mother) who frequently and persistently reports illnesses in the child which are fabricated, or even induced by the adult, to obtain medical attention.

mural (mu´ral) Relating to the wall of a cavity or hollow organ.

muramic acid (mu-ram´ik as´id) A component of the murein molecule of bacterial cell walls.

muramidase (mu-ram´ĭ-dās) Mucopeptide glucohydrolase, an enzyme that promotes the hydrolysis of muramic acid-containing mucopeptides in bacterial cell walls (e.g., lysozyme).

murein (mu´re-in) The bag-shaped macromolecule that encases a bacterial cell.

muriatic (mu-re-at´ik) Hydrochloric.

murine (mu´rin) Relating to animals of the family Muridae, especially rats and mice.

murmur (mur´mur) A relatively prolonged series of auditory vibrations resulting from turbulent blood flow.

aortic m. Murmur arising from the aortic orifice.

Austin Flint's m. See Flint's murmur.

cardiac m. Murmur arising from the heart.

continuous m. Murmur that begins in systole and continues without interruption into all or part of the diastole.

crescendo m. Murmur that increases in intensity and stops suddenly.

Cruveilhier-Baumgarten m. Murmur heard on the abdominal wall over collateral veins connecting portal and caval venous systems.

diamond-shaped m. Murmur that increases in loudness and then decreases in such a manner as to produce a diamond-shaped curve on the phonocardiogram.

diastolic m. Murmur beginning with or after the second heart sound and ending before the first heart sound (i.e., during diastole).

Duroziez's m. A double murmur heard over the femoral artery in cases of aortic insufficiency.

dynamic m. Murmur due to a condition other than diseased heart valves.

early diastolic m. Murmur beginning with the second heart sound (at the time of aortic valve closure); the typical murmur of aortic incompetence.

ejection m. A diamond-shaped murmur occurring when blood is ejected across the aortic or pulmonary valves, from the left or right ventricles into the ascending aorta or pulmonary trunk.

extracardiac m. Murmur heard over the heart area but originating from another structure.

Flint's m. A mid-diastolic or presystolic rumble, similar to the murmur of mitral stenosis, which appears to originate at the anterior leaflet of the mitral valve when the normal and abnormal streams of blood enter the left ventricle in cases of aortic incompetence. Also called Austin Flint's murmur.

functional m. Murmur due to causes other than cardiac disorders. Also called inorganic murmur; innocent murmur.

Graham Steell's m. An early diastolic, high-pitched murmur; caused by pulmonary incompetence due to pulmonary hypertension.

hemic m. A cardiac or vascular murmur occurring in anemic individuals without heart disease.

holosystolic m. See pansystolic murmur.

humming-top m. See venous hum, under hum.

innocent m. See functional murmur.

inorganic m. See functional murmur.

late diastolic m. See presystolic murmur.

machinery m. The continuous murmur typical of patent ductus arteriosus.

mid-diastolic m. Murmur beginning soon, but at a clear interval, after the second heart sound; originating at the atrioventricular valves, usually due either to constriction of the valve orifices or to abnormal patterns of atrioventricular blood flow.

mitral valve m. A murmur produced at the mitral valve; caused by either constriction of the valve orifice or backward flow of blood through the valve.

musical m. Murmur having a musical quality.

organic m. Murmur caused by organic disease (i.e., a valvular deformity or a septal defect) in contrast to a functional murmur.

pansystolic m. Murmur lasting throughout systole, from the first to the second heart sound. Also called holosystolic murmur.

presystolic m. A short, usually crescendo murmur heard during atrial systole, due most often to obstruction of one of the atrioventricular orifices. Also called late diastolic murmur.

pulmonary m., pulmonic m. Murmur heard at the orifice of the pulmonary trunk.

regurgitant m. Murmur originating at the valvular orifices of the heart, due to leakage or backward flow of blood.

Roger's m. A loud pansystolic murmur with maximal intensity at the left sternal border caused by a small ventricular septal defect. Also called bruit de Roger.

sea gull m. A musical murmur similar to the cry of a gull.

seesaw m. See to-and-fro murmur.

systolic m. Murmur beginning with or after the first heart sound and ending at or before the second sound (i.e., during systole).

to-and-fro m. Murmur heard in both systole and diastole. Also called seesaw murmur.

tricuspid m. Murmur originating at the orifice of the tricuspid valve.

muscae volitantes (mus´ke vol-ĭ-tan´tez) See floaters.

muscarine (mus´kă-rēn) A poisonous alkaloid present in certain mushrooms, causing inhibition of the heart action and gastrointestinal stimulation.

muscarinic (mus-kă-rin´ik) **1.** Producing postganglionic parasympathetic stimulation, an effect resembling that of muscarine. **2.** An agent that produces such an effect.

muscle (mus´el) Tissue that serves to produce motion, composed primarily of contractile cells. See

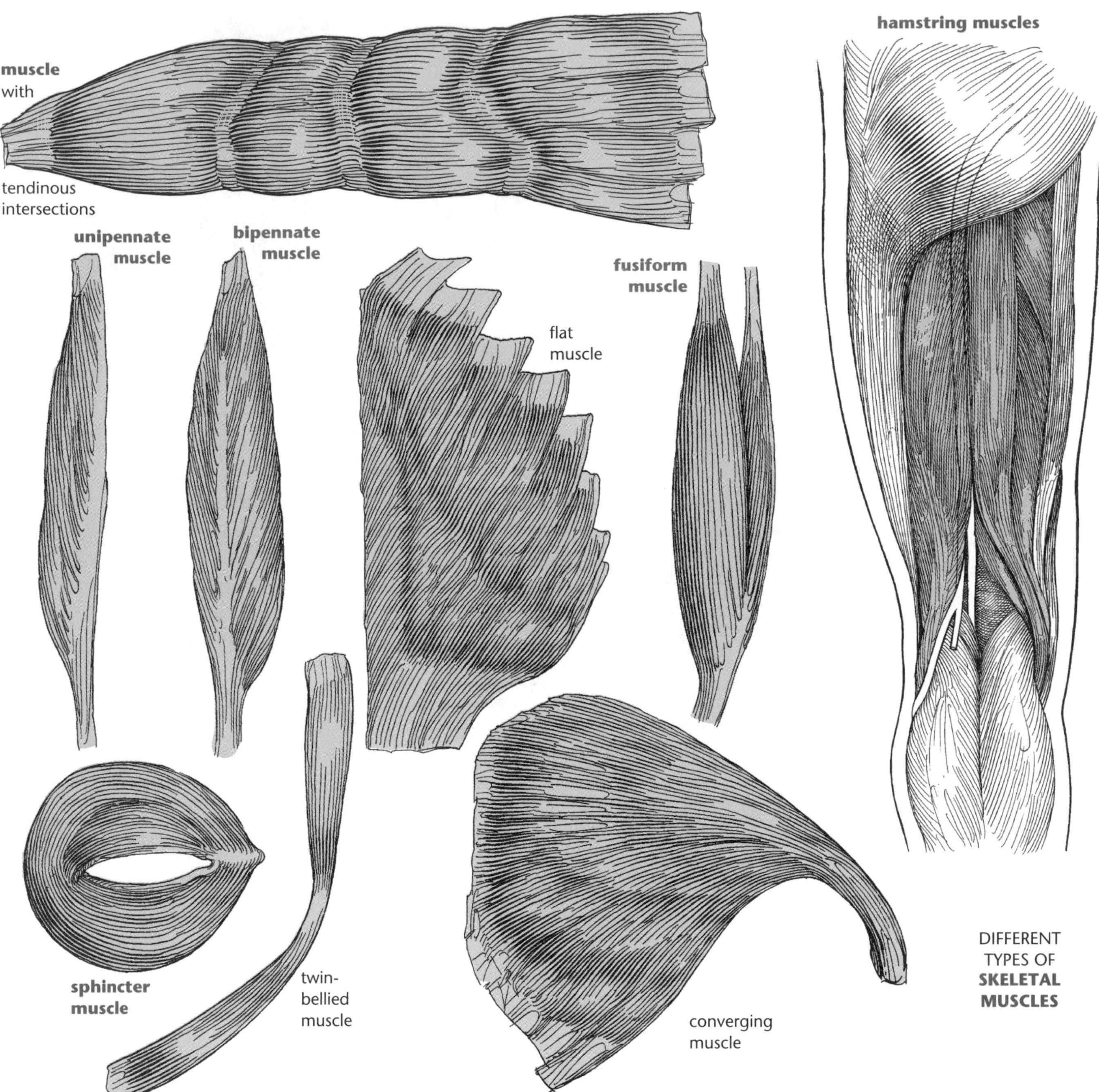

M

table of muscles for individual muscles.

agonistic m. A muscle that is continuously active in both the initiation and maintenance of a particular movement of an anatomic part (e.g., the brachial muscle in flexion of the forearm at the elbow joint); the action of the agonistic muscle can be opposed by that of another (the antagonistic) muscle. Also called prime mover.

antagonistic m. A muscle with opposing force that counteracts the action of another (the agonistic) muscle, or that initiates and maintains a movement opposite to that of the agonist.

antigravity m.'s Those maintaining the posture characteristic of a given species.

bipennate m. Muscle with a central tendon (e.g., rectus muscle of thigh).

cardiac m. Muscle of the heart (myocardium), composed of striated fibers.

fixation m.'s See fixator muscles.

fixator m.'s Agonistic and antagonistic muscles collaborating in stabilizing the position of a joint or part; they contract together to hold the joint in position when powerful external forces are encountered. Also called fixation muscles.

fusiform m. Muscle with a fleshy belly tapering at either end. Also called spindle-shaped muscle.

hamstring m.'s Three muscles at the back of the thigh; the biceps muscle of the thigh (biceps femoris), the semitendinous muscle, and the semimembranous muscle; they flex the leg and rotate it medially and laterally at the knee joint, and extend the thigh at the hip joint. Also called posterior femoral muscles.

involuntary m. See smooth muscle.

papillary m.'s The fleshy columns in the ventricles of the heart to which the chordae tendinae are attached; participate in the movement of the atrioventricular valves.

skeletal m. A striated voluntary muscle that is attached to bones. Also called voluntary muscle.

smooth m. Muscle that is not under voluntary control; it responds to the autonomic nervous system. Also called involuntary muscle.

sphincter m. A circular band of muscle (e.g., sphincter muscle of anus).

spindle-shaped m. See fusiform muscle.

strap m. Any flat muscle, especially those of the neck associated with the hyoid bone and thyroid cartilage.

striated m. Skeletal and cardiac muscle in which cross striations occur in the fibers; with the exception of the cardiac muscle, striated muscles are voluntary, as opposed to the smooth muscles, which are under autonomic control.

synergistic m.'s Muscles having a mutually helpful action.

unipennate m. Muscle with a tendon attached along one side (e.g., extensor muscle of little finger).

voluntary m. Muscle whose action is under voluntary control.

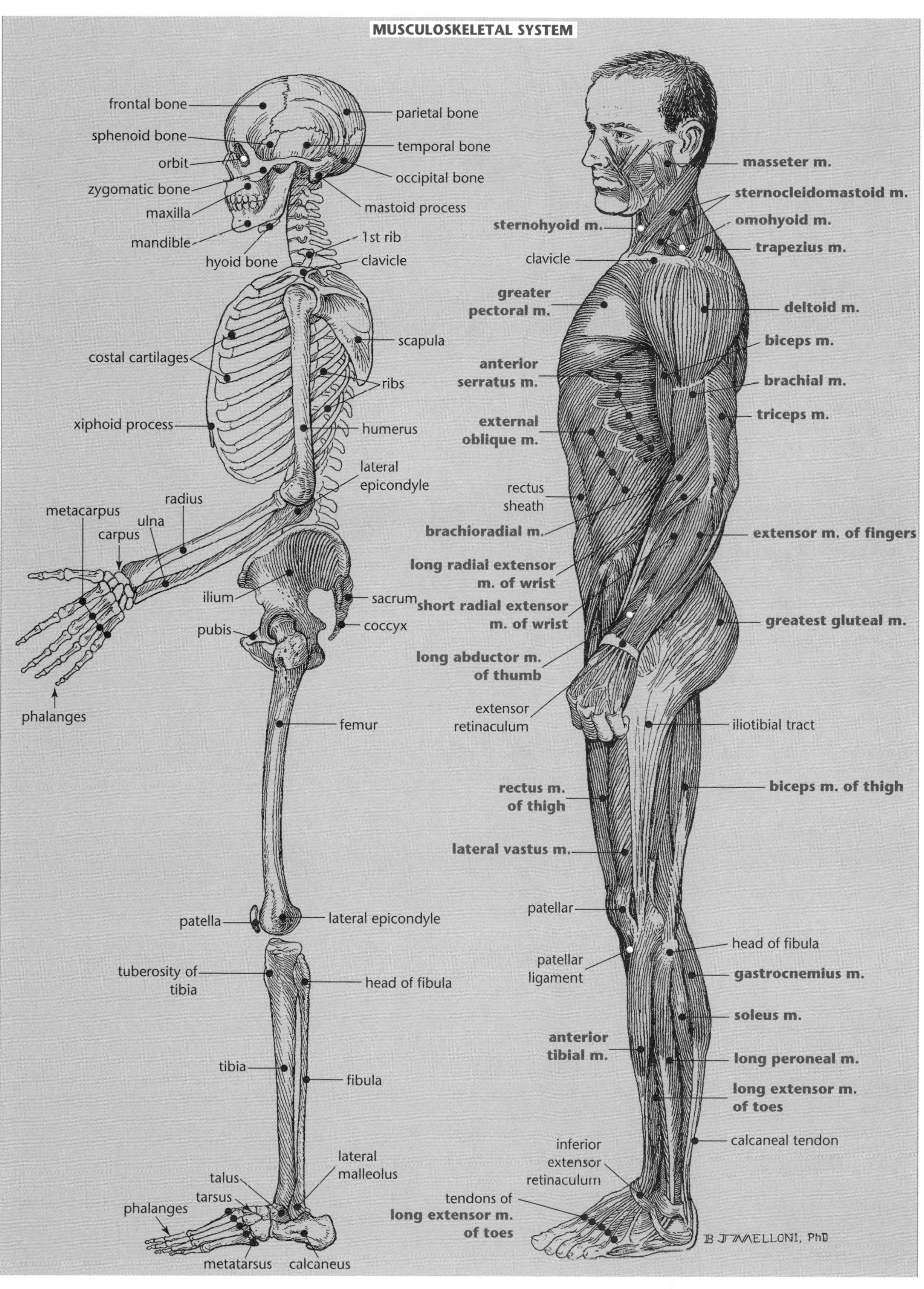
MUSCULOSKELETAL SYSTEM
frontal bone
parietal bone
sphenoid bone
temporal bone
orbit
occipital bone
zygomatic bone
mastoid process
maxilla
mandible
1st rib
hyoid bone
clavicle
scapula
costal cartilages
ribs
xiphoid process
humerus
lateral epicondyle
radius
metacarpus
ulna
carpus
ilium
sacrum
pubis
coccyx
phalanges
femur
patella
lateral epicondyle
tuberosity of tibia
head of fibula
tibia
fibula
lateral malleolus
talus
tarsus
phalanges
metatarsus
calcaneus
masseter m.
sternocleidomastoid m.
sternohyoid m.
omohyoid m.
trapezius m.
clavicle
greater pectoral m.
deltoid m.
biceps m.
anterior serratus m.
brachial m.
triceps m.
external oblique m.
rectus sheath
brachioradial m.
extensor m. of fingers
long radial extensor m. of wrist
short radial extensor m. of wrist
greatest gluteal m.
long abductor m. of thumb
extensor retinaculum
iliotibial tract
rectus m. of thigh
biceps m. of thigh
lateral vastus m.
patellar
head of fibula
patellar ligament
gastrocnemius m.
soleus m.
anterior tibial m.
long peroneal m.
long extensor m. of toes
calcaneal tendon
inferior extensor retinaculum
tendons of long extensor m. of toes
B J MELLONI, PhD
M

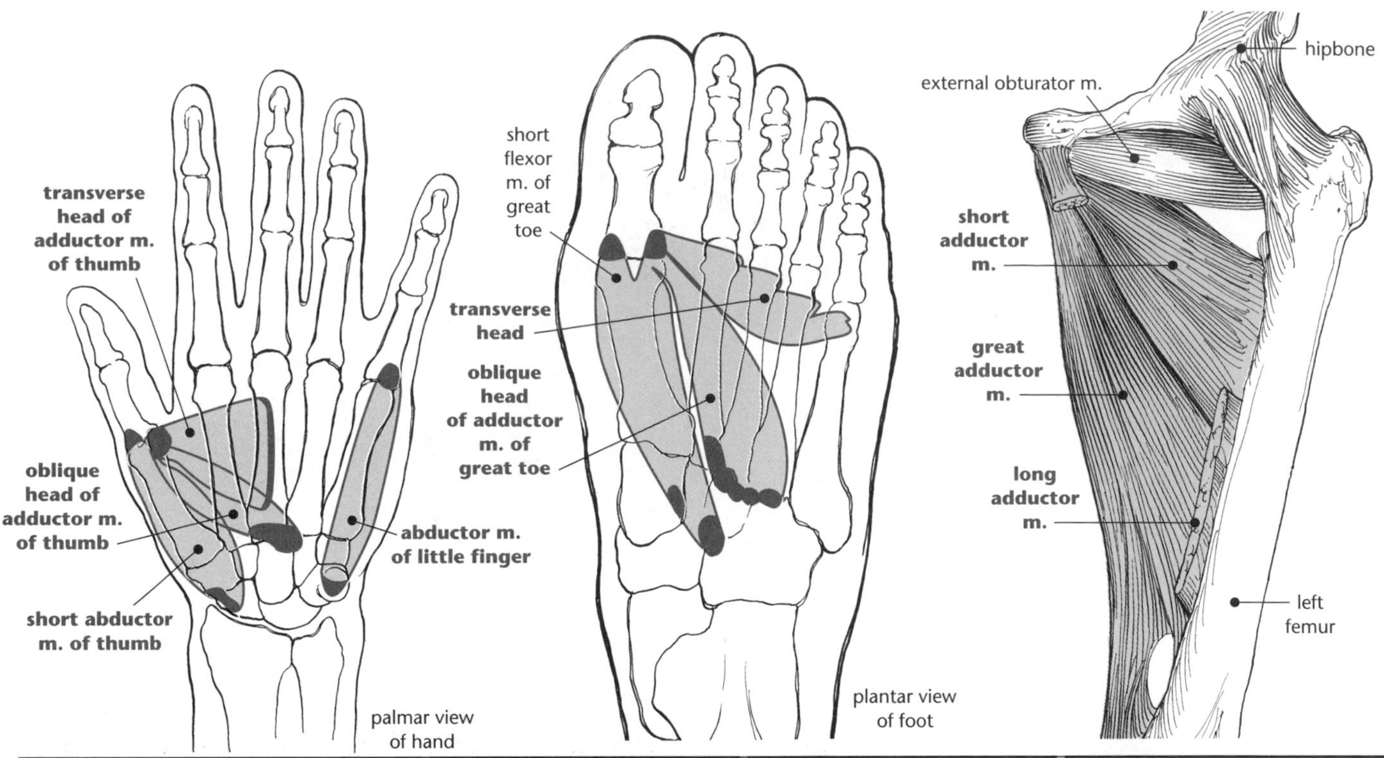

MUSCLE	ORIGIN	INSERTION	ACTION
abductor m. of great toe m. abductor hallucis	calcaneus, plantar aponeurosis	proximal phalanx of great toe (joined by short flexor m. of great toe)	abducts and aids in flexion of great toe
abductor m. of little finger *m. abductor digiti minimi manus*	pisiform bone, tendon of ulnar flexor m. of wrist	proximal phalanx of fifth digit	abducts little finger
abductor m. of little toe *m. abductor digiti minimi pedis*	lateral tubercle of calcaneus, plantar aponeurosis	proximal phalanx of little toe	abducts and flexes little toe
abductor m. of thumb, long *m. abductor pollicis longus*	posterior surface of ulna, middle third of radius	first metacarpal bone	abducts and extends thumb
abductor m. of thumb, short *m. abductor pollicis brevis*	flexor retinaculum of hand, scaphoid and trapezium	proximal phalanx of thumb	abducts and aids in flexion of thumb
adductor m., great *m. adductor magnus*	*adductor part:* inferior ramus of pubis, ramus of ischium; *extensor part:* ischial tuberosity	*adductor part:* linea aspera of femur; *extensor part:* adductor tubercle of femur	adducts, flexes, and rotates thigh medially
adductor m., long *m. adductor longus*	pubis, below pubic crest	linea aspera of femur	adducts, flexes, and rotates thigh medially
adductor m., short *m. adductor brevis*	pubis, below origin of the long adductor m.	upper part of linea aspera of femur	adducts, flexes, and rotates thigh laterally
adductor m., smallest m. adductor minimus	the proximal portion of the great adductor m. when it forms a distinct muscle		
adductor m. of great toe *m. adductor hallucis*	*oblique head:* bases of middle three metatarsal bones; *transverse head:* metatarsophalangeal ligaments of lateral three toes	proximal phalanx of great toe (joined by flexor m. of great toe)	*oblique head:* adducts and flexes great toe; *transverse head:* supports transverse arch, adducts great toe
adductor m. of thumb *m. adductor pollicis*	*oblique head:* capitate, second, and third metacarpal bones; *transverse head:* third metacarpal bone	proximal phalanx of thumb; medial sesamoid bone	adducts and aids in apposition of thumb
anconeus m. *m. anconeus*	back of lateral epicondyle of humerus	olecranon process, posterior surface of ulna	extends forearm, abducts ulna in pronation of wrist
antitragus m. *m. antitragicus*	outer surface of antitragus of ear	caudate process of helix and antihelix	thought to be vestigial
arrector m.'s of hair *mm. arrectores pilorum*	dermis	hair follicles	elevate hairs of skin; aid in discharging sebum
articular m. of elbow *m. articularis cubiti*	lower part of triceps m. of arm	posterior aspect of elbow joint capsule	elevates capsule in extension of elbow joint
articular m. of knee *m. articularis genus*	lower part of anterior surface of femur	upper part of synovial membrane of knee joint	elevates capsule of knee joint during extension of leg

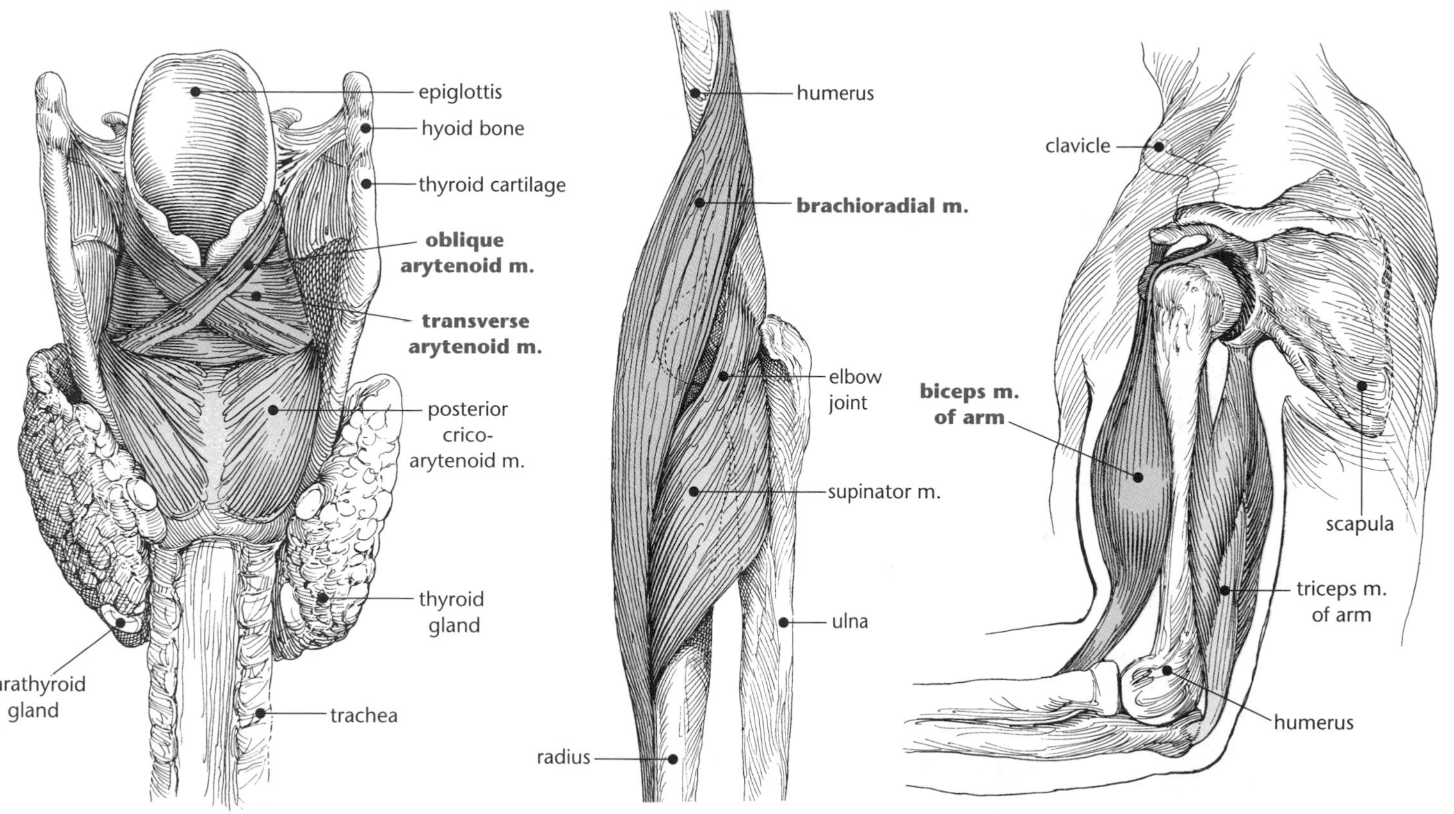

MUSCLE	ORIGIN	INSERTION	ACTION
aryepiglottic m. *m. aryepiglotticus*	apex of arytenoid cartilage	lateral margin of epiglottis	narrows inlet of larynx by lowering epiglottis
arytenoid m., oblique *m. arytenoideus obliquus*	muscular process of arytenoid cartilage	apex of opposite arytenoid cartilage, prolonged as aryepiglottic m.	helps to close inlet of larynx by approximating arytenoid cartilages
arytenoid m., transverse (only unpaired m. of the larynx) *m. arytenoideus transversus*	posterior surface of arytenoid cartilage	posterior surface of opposite arytenoid cartilage	approximates arytenoid cartilages; constricts entrance to larynx during swallowing
auricular m., anterior *m. auricularis anterior*	superficial temporal fascia	cartilage of ear	feeble forward movement of auricle
auricular m., posterior *m. auricularis posterior*	mastoid process	cartilage of ear	feeble backward movement of auricle
auricular m., superior *m. auricularis superior*	temporal fascia, epicranial aponeurosis	cartilage of ear	feeble elevation of auricle
auricular m., transverse *m. auricularis transversus*	upper surface of auricle	circumference of auricle	retracts helix
biceps m. of arm *m. biceps brachii*	*long head:* supraglenoid tubercle of scapula; *short head:* apex of coracoid process	tuberosity of radius; posterior border of ulna, through bicipital aponeurosis	flexes forearm and arm, supinates hand
biceps m. of thigh *m. biceps femoris*	*long head:* ischial tuberosity; *short head:* linea aspera and second supracondylar ridge of femur	head of fibula, lateral condyle of tibia	flexes knee, rotates leg laterally; long head extends thigh
brachial m. *m. brachialis*	anterior surface of distal two-thirds of humerus	coronoid process of ulna	flexes forearm
brachioradial m. *m. brachioradialis*	lateral supracondylar ridge and intermuscular septum of humerus	lower end of radius	flexes forearm
bronchoesophageal m. *m. bronchoesophageus*	m. fibers arising from wall of left bronchus	musculature of esophagus	reinforces esophagus
buccinator m. *m. buccinator*	pterygomandibular raphe, alveolar processes of jaws	orbicular m. *(orbicularis oris)* at angle of mouth	retracts angle of mouth by compressing cheek; accessory m. of mastication
bulbocavernous m. *m. bulbospongiosus*	*female:* central tendon of perineum; *male:* median raphe over bulb of penis, central tendon of perineum	*female:* dorsum of clitoris, urogenital diaphragm; *male:* corpus spongiosum, root of penis	*female:* compresses vaginal orifice; *male:* compresses urethra, assists in ejaculation

M

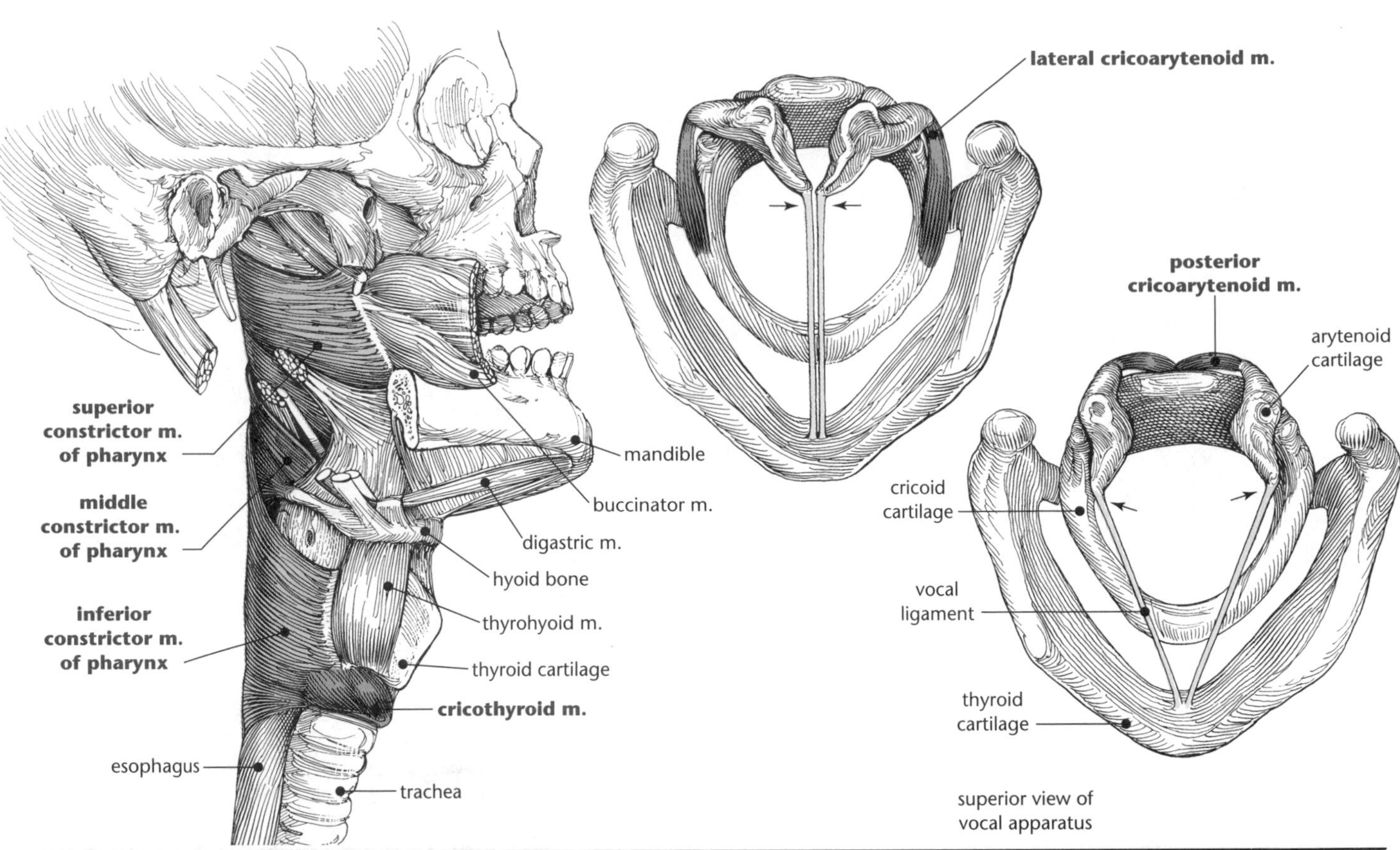

M

MUSCLE	ORIGIN	INSERTION	ACTION
canine m. *caninus m.*		see levator m. of angle of mouth	
ceratocricoid m. *m. ceratocricoideus*	lower margin of cricoid cartilage	inferior horn (cornu) of thyroid cartilage	helps posterior cricoarytenoid m. separate vocal cords
chin m. *m. mentalis*	incisive fossa of mandible	skin of chin	raises and protrudes lower lip
chondroglossus m. *m. chondroglossus*	lesser horn (cornu) and body of hyoid bone	side of tongue	depresses tongue
ciliary m. *m. ciliaris*	*meridional part:* scleral spur; *circular part:* sphincter of ciliary body	ciliary process	makes lens more convex in accommodation for near vision
coccygeal m. ischiococcygeus m. *m. coccygeus*	ischial spine and sacrospinous ligament	coccyx, lower part of lateral border of sacrum	aids in raising and supporting pelvic floor
constrictor m. of pharynx, inferior *m. constrictor pharyngis inferior*	cricoid cartilage, oblique line of thyroid cartilage, inferior horn of thyroid cartilage	median raphe of posterior wall of pharynx	narrows lower part of pharynx in swallowing
constrictor m. of pharynx, middle *m. constrictor pharyngis medius*	stylohyoid ligament and horns of hyoid bone	median raphe of posterior wall of pharynx	narrows pharynx in swallowing
constrictor m. of pharynx, superior *m. constrictor pharyngis superior*	medial pterygoid plate, pterygoid hamulus, pterygomandibular raphe, mandible, side of tongue	median raphe of posterior wall of pharynx; pharyngeal tubercle of skull	narrows pharynx in swallowing
coracobrachial m. *m. coracobrachialis*	coracoid process of scapula (shoulder blade)	midway along inner side of humerus	flexes, adducts arm
corrugator m. m. corrugator	brow ridge of frontal bone	skin of eyebrow	draws eyebrows together, wrinkles forehead
cremaster m. *m. cremaster*	inferior border of internal oblique abdominal m.	spermatic cord	elevates testis in male, encircles round ligament in female
cricoarytenoid m., lateral *m. cricoarytenoideus lateralis*	upper margin of arch of cricoid cartilage	muscular process of arytenoid cartilage	approximates vocal cords so they meet in midline for phonation
cricoarytenoid m., posterior *m. cricoarytenoideus posterior*	posterior surface of lamina of cricoid cartilage	muscular process of arytenoid cartilage	separates vocal cords, opening the glottis
cricothyroid m. *m. cricothyroideus*	anterior surface of arch of cricoid cartilage	lamina and inferior horn of thyroid cartilage	lengthens, stretches, and tenses vocal cords

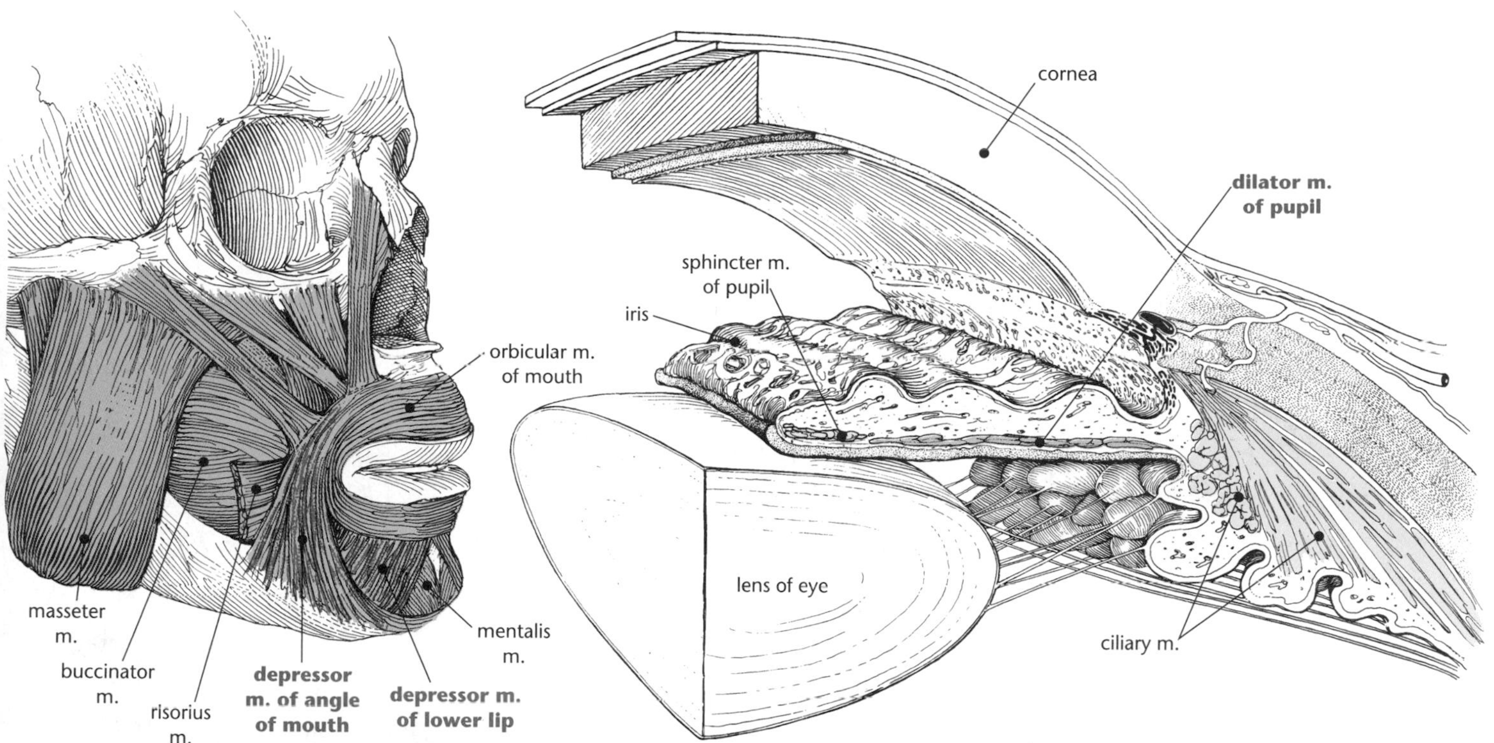

MUSCLE	ORIGIN	INSERTION	ACTION
deltoid m. *m. deltoideus*	lateral third of clavicle, acromion, and spine of scapula	deltoid tuberosity of shaft of humerus	abductor of arm; aids in flexion, extension, and lateral rotation of arm
depressor m., superciliary *m. depressor supercilii*	orbicular fibers of eye; medial palpebral ligament	skin of eyebrow	pulls eyebrow downward
depressor m. of angle of mouth triangular m. *m. depressor anguli oris*	oblique line of mandible	angle of mouth	pulls corner of mouth downward
depressor m. of lower lip quadrate m. of lower lip m. depressor labii inferioris	mandible adjacent to mental foramen	skin of lower lip	draws lower lip downward and slightly laterally
depressor m. of nasal septum *m. depressor septi nasi*	incisive fossa of maxilla (over roots of incisor teeth)	ala and septum of nose	widens the nostrils in deep inspiration
detrussor m. of urinary bladder *m. detrussor vesicae*	in wall of urinary bladder, consisting of three layers of nonstriated m. fibers		empties urinary bladder
detrusor urinae m.	see detrusor m. of urinary bladder		
diaphragm diaphragmatic m. *diaphragma*	xiphoid process, six lower costal cartilages, four lower ribs, lumbar vertebrae, arcuate ligaments	central tendon of diaphragm	increases capacity of thorax in inspiration (main m. of inhalation)
diaphragm m., pelvic	composed of the coccygeal and levator ani m.'s sheathed in a superior and inferior layer of fasciaviscera		forms floor to support pelvic
digastric m. *m. digastricus*	digastric notch at mastoid process; mandible near symphysis	tendon bound to hyoid bone by fascia	raises hyoid bone and base of tongue, lowers mandible
dilator m. of nose *m. dilator naris*	nasal notch of maxilla	ala cartilage at margin of nostril	widens nostril
dilator m. of pupil *m. dilator pupillae*	ciliary margin	near margin of pupil	dilates pupil
epicranial m. *m. epicranius*	the muscular and tendinous layer of the scalp composed of the occipitofrontal and temporoparietal m.'s connected by the epicranial aponeurosis (galea aponeurotica)		elevates eyebrows, draw scalp forward and backward, tightens scalp
erector m. of penis	see ischiocavernous m.		
erector m. of spine *m. erector spinae*	deep m. arising from the broad and thick tendon attached to the middle crest of sacrum, spinous processes of lumbar and 11th and 12th thoracic vertebrae; and back part of the iliac crest; it splits in the upper lumbar region into three columns of m's.; iliocostal (lateral division), longissimus (intermediate division), and spinal (medial division)		
extensor m. of fingers *m. extensor digitorum*	lateral epicondyle of humerus	phalanges of digits 2 to 5; via dorsal digital expansion	extends fingers, hand, and forearm
extensor m. of great toe, long *m. extensor hallucis longus*	middle of fibula, interosseous membrane	distal phalanx of great toe	extends great toe, dorsiflexes foot

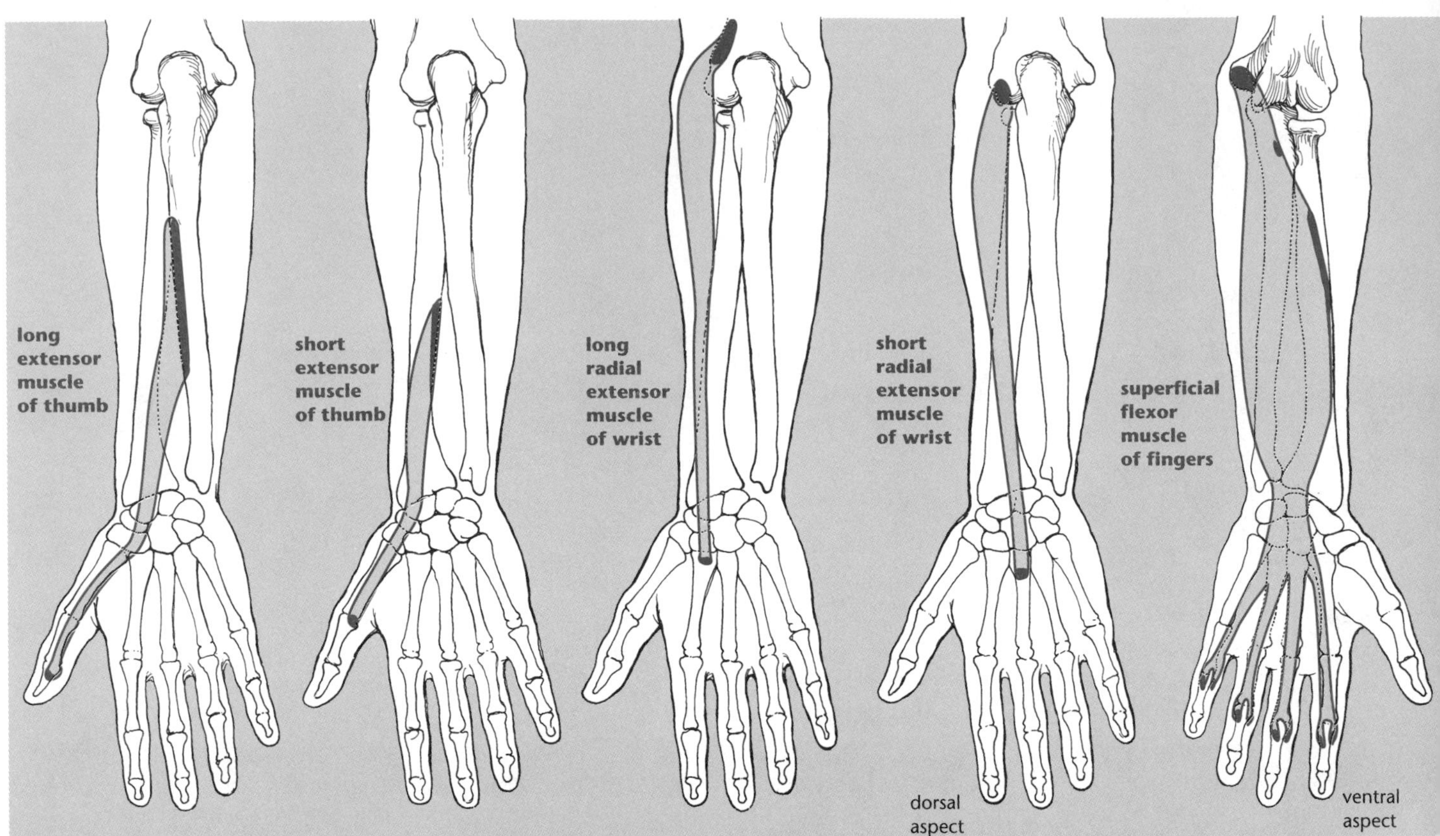

M

MUSCLE	ORIGIN	INSERTION	ACTION
extensor m. of great toe, short *m. extensor hallucis brevis*	dorsal surface of calcaneus	base of proximal phalanx or great toe	dorsiflexes great toe
extensor m. of index finger *m. extensor indicis*	posterior surface of ulna, interosseous membrane	extensor expansion of index finger	extends index finger and hand
extensor m. of little finger *m. extensor digiti minimi manus*	lateral epicondyle of humerus	extensor expansion of little finger	extends little finger
extensor m. of thumb, long *m. extensor pollicis longus*	middle third of ulna, adjacent interosseous membrane	distal phalanx of thumb	extonds distal phalanx of thumb, abducts hand
extensor m. of thumb, short *m. extensor pollicis brevis*	middle third of radius, interosseous membrane	proximal phalanx of the thumb	extends thumb and abducts hand
extensor m. of toes, long *m. extensor digitorum longus pedis*	lateral condyle of tibia, upper three-fourths of fibula, interosseous membrane	extensor expansion of four lateral toes (by four slips)	extends toes and dorsiflexes foot
extensor m. of toes, short *m. extensor digitorum brevis pedis*	dorsal surface of calcaneus	extensor tendons of second, third, and fourth toes	extends toes
extensor m. of wrist, radial, long *m. extensor carpi radialis longus*	lateral supracondylar ridge of humerus	second metacarpal bone	extends wrist, abducts hand
extensor m. of wrist, radial, short *m. extensor carpi radialis brevis*	lateral epicondyle of humerus, radial collateral ligament of elbow joint	third metacarpal bone	extends wrist, abducts hand
extensor m. of wrist, ulnar *m. extensor carpi ulnaris*	*humeral head:* lateral epicondyle of humerus; *ulnar head*: posterior border of ulna	fifth metacarpal bone	extends wrist, abducts hand
fibular m.		see peroneal m.	
flexor m. of fingers, deep *m. flexor digitorum profundus manus*	proximal three-fourths of ulna and adjacent interosseous membrane	distal phalanges of fingers	flexes terminal phalanges of lateral four digits; aids in flexing wrist
flexor m. of fingers, superficial *m. flexor digitorum superficialis manus*	*humeroulnar head:* medial epicondyle of humerus, coronoid process of ulna; *radial head:* anterior border of radius	middle phalanges of fingers	flexes phalanges and wrist
flexor m. of great toe, long *m. flexor hallucis longus*	lower two-thirds of posterior surface of fibula, intermuscular septum, interosseous membrane	distal phalanx of great toe	flexes great toe and plantarflexes foot

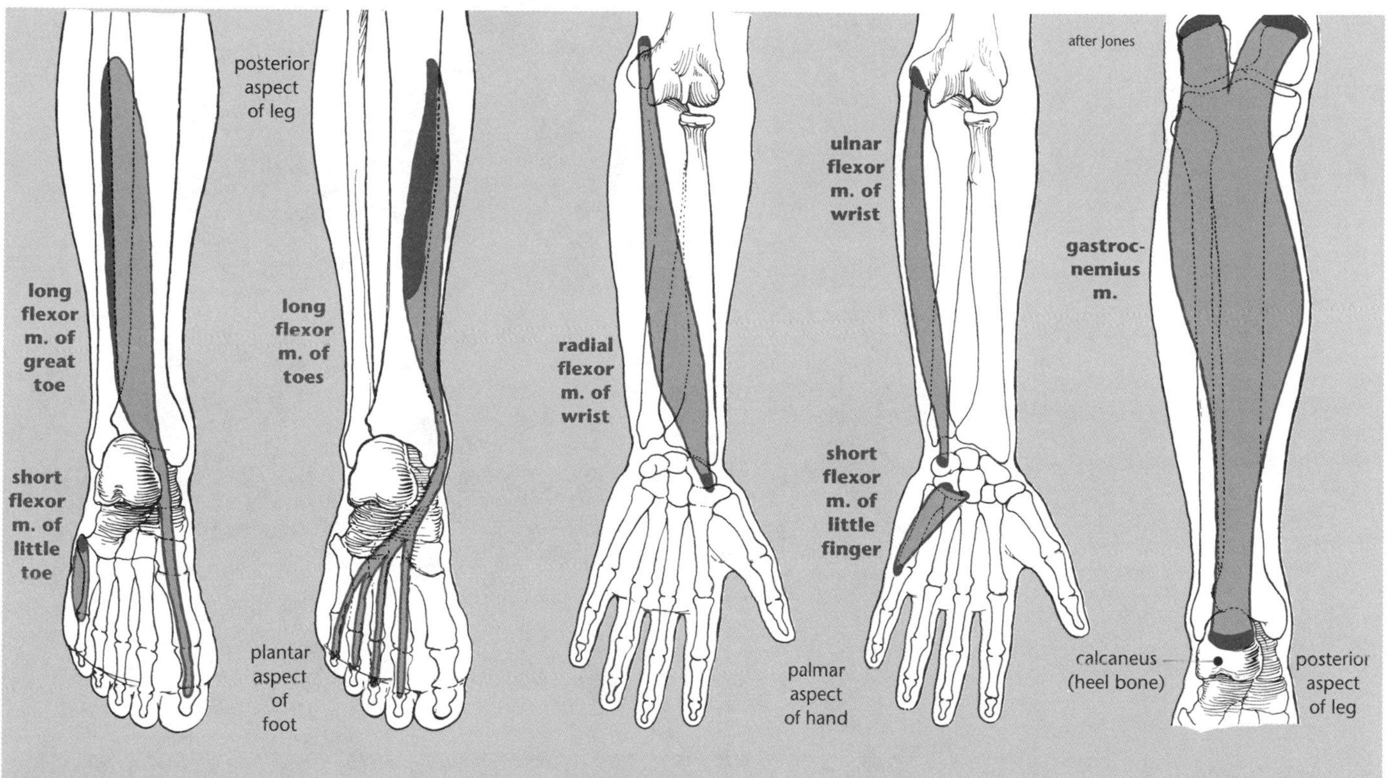

MUSCLE	ORIGIN	INSERTION	ACTION
flexor m. of great toe, short *m. flexor hallucis brevis*	cuboid and third cuneiform bones	both sides of proximal phalanx of great toe	flexes great toe
flexor m. of little finger, short *m. flexor digiti minimi brevis manus*	hook of hamate, flexor retinaculum	proximal phalanx of little finger	flexes proximal phalanx of little finger
flexor m. of little toe, short *m. flexor digiti minimi brevis pedis*	base of fifth metatarsal and plantar fascia	lateral surface of proximal phalanx of little toe	flexes little toe
flexor m. of thumb, long *m. flexor pollicis longus*	radius, adjacent interosseous membrane, coronoid process of ulna	distal phalanx of thumb	flexes thumb
flexor m. of thumb, short *m. flexor pollicis brevis*	trapezium, trapezoid, and capitate bones of wrist	proximal phalanx of thumb	flexes thumb
flexor m. of toes, long *m. flexor digitorum longus pedis*	middle half of tibia	distal phalanges of lateral four toes (by four tendons)	flexes second to fifth toes and plantarflexes foot
flexor m. of toes, short *m. flexor digitorum brevis pedis*	tuberosity of calcaneus and plantar fascia	middle phalanges of four lateral toes	flexes four lateral toes
flexor m. of wrist, radial *m. flexor carpi radialis*	medial epicondyle of humerus; antibrachial fascia	bases of second and third metacarpal bones	flexes wrist; aids in pronation and abduction of hand
flexor m. of wrist, ulnar *m. flexor carpi ulnaris*	*humeral head:* medial epicondyle of humerus; *ulnar head:* olecranon and posterior border of ulna	pisiform, hamate, and fifth metacarpal bones; flexor retinaculum	flexes wrist; adducts hand
frontal m.		see occipitofrontal m.	
gastrocnemius m. *m. gastrocnemius*	*medial head:* popliteal surface of femur, upper part of medial condyle of femur; *lateral head:* lateral condyle of femur	calcaneus via calcaneal tendon (tendo calcaneus) (in common with soleus m.)	flexes leg and plantarflexes foot
gemellus m., inferior *m. gemellus inferior*	lower margin of lesser sciatic notch	greater trochanter via internal obturator tendon	rotates thigh laterally
gemellus m., superior *m. gemellus superior*	spine if ischium	greater trochanter via internal obturator tendon	rotates thigh laterally; abducts flexed thigh
genioglossus m. *m. genioglossus*	mental spine of the mandible	ventral surface of tongue and body of hyoid bone	protrudes, retracts, and depresses tongue, elevates hyoid bone
geniohyoid m. *m. geniohyoideus*	mental spine (genial tubercle) of the mandible	body of hyoid bone	elevates hyoid bone and draws it forward

M

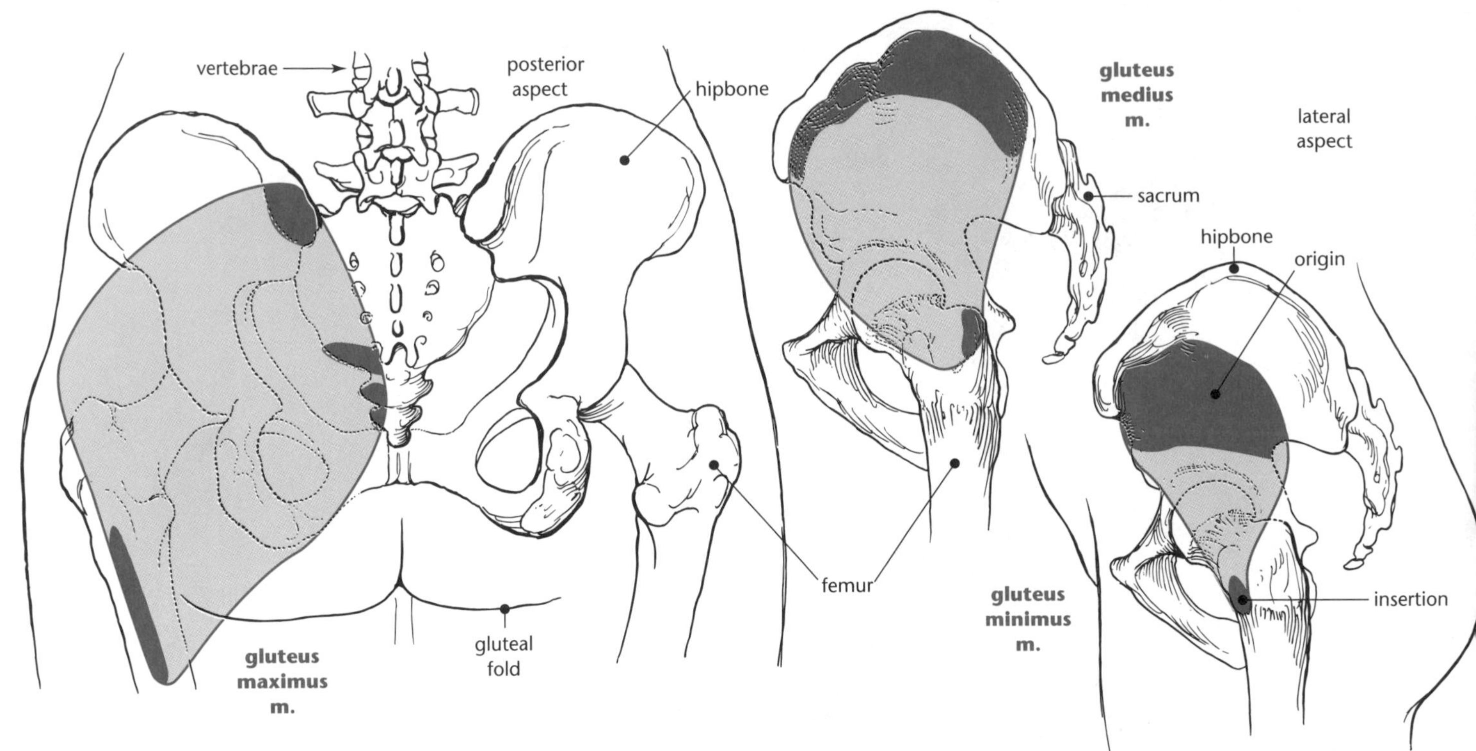

MUSCLE	ORIGIN	INSERTION	ACTION
glossopalatine m.	see palatoglossus m.		
gluteus maximus m. greatest gluteal m. *m. gluteus maximus*	upper portion of ilium, sacrum and coccyx, sacro-tuberous ligament, gluteus aponeurosis	gluteal tuberosity of femur, iliotibial tract (band of fascia lata)	chief extensor, powerful lateral rotator of thigh
gluteus medius m. middle gluteal m *m. gluteus medius*	midportion of outer surface of ilium	greater trochanter and oblique ridge of femur	abducts, rotates thigh medially; tilts pelvis to raise opposite foot from floor
gluteus minimus m. least gluteal m. *m. gluteus minimus*	lower portion of outer surface of ilium	greater trochanter of femur, capsule of hip loint	abducts, rotates thigh medially
gracilis m. *m. gracilis*	lower half of pubis	medial side of uper part of tibia	adducts thigh, flexes and rotates leg medially
helix m. larger *m. helicis minor*	spine of helix	anterior border of helix	thought to be vestigal
helix m., smaller *m. helicis minor*	anterior rim of helix	crux of helix	thought to be vestigial
hyoglossus m. hyoglossal m. *m. hyoglossus*	body and greater horn (cornu) of hyoid bone	side of tongue	retracts, depresses tongue
iliac m. *m. iliacus*	iliac fossa, lateral aspect of sacrum	greater psoas tendon, lesser trochanter of femur	flexes thigh
iliococcygeal m. *m. iliococcygeal*	ischial spine and arching tendon over internal obturator m.	coccyx and perineal body between tip of coccyx and anal canal	supports pelvic viscera
iliocostal m. *m. iliocostalis*	the lateral division of erector m. of spine composed of three parts: ilicostal m. of loins, ilicostal m. of neck, ilicostal m. of thorax		extends vertebral column and assists in lateral movements of trunk
iliocostal m. of loins *m. iliocostalis lumborum*	iliac crest and thoracolumbar fascia	transverse processes of lumbar vertebrae, angles of lower seven ribs	extends lumbar vertebral column and flexes it laterally
iliocostal m. of neck *m. iliocostalis cervicis*	angles of third, fourth, fifth, and sixth ribs	transverse processes of fourth, fifth, and sixth cervical vertebrae	extends cervical vertebral column and flexes it laterally
iliocostal m. of thorax *m. iliocostalis thoracis*	lower six ribs, medial to angles of the ribs	angles of upper six ribs, transverse process of seventh cervical vertebra	extends thoracic vertebral column and flexes it laterally
iliopsoas m. *m. iliopsoas*	a compound m. consisting of the iliac and greater psoas m.'s, which join to form the iliopsoas tendon and insert to the lesser trochanter of femur		
incisive m.'s of lower lip *mm. incisivi labii inferioris*	portion of orbicular m. of mouth (orbicularis oris)	angle of mouth	make vestibule of mouth shallow; aid in articulation

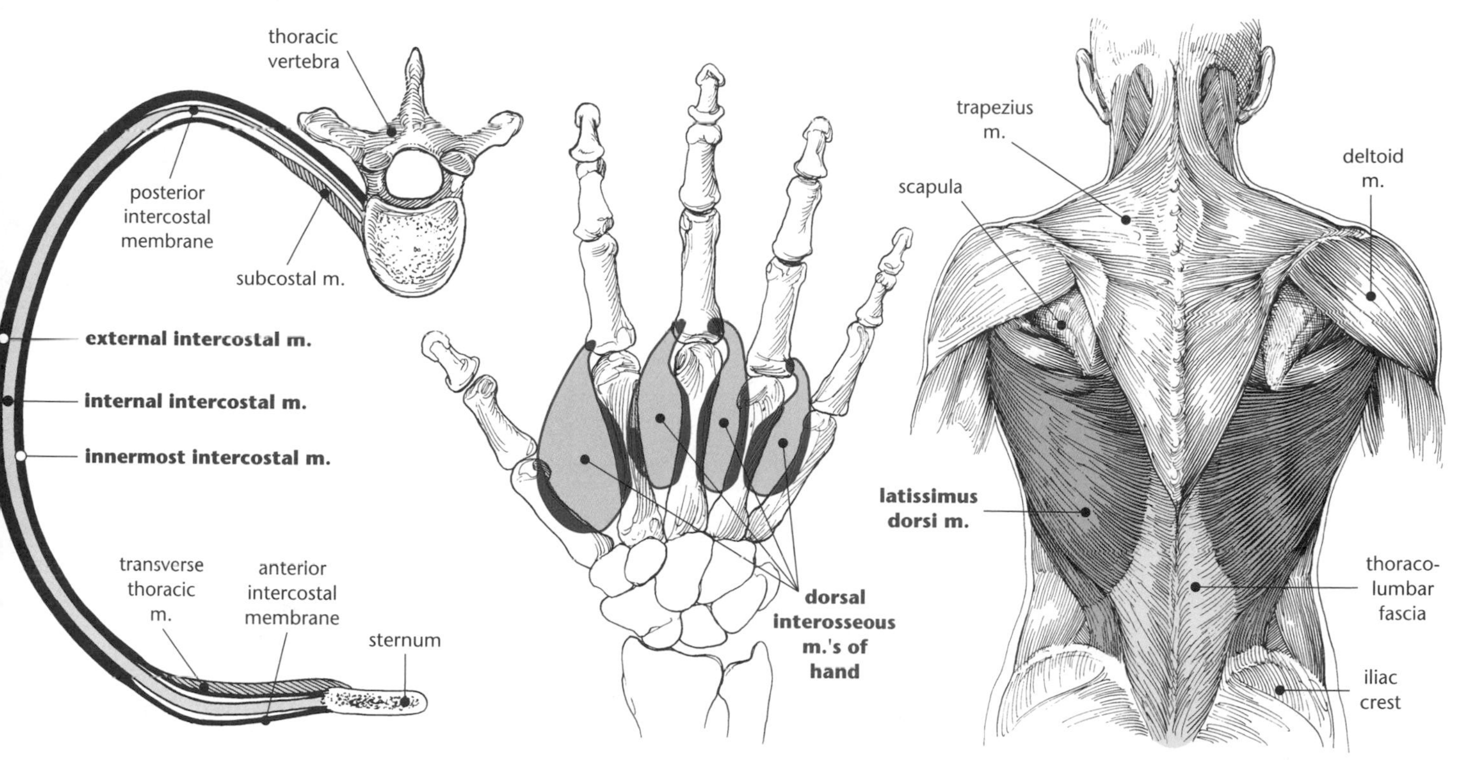

MUSCLE	ORIGIN	INSERTION	ACTION
incisive m.'s of upper lip *mm. incisivi labii superioris*	portion of orbicular m. of mouth (*orbicularis oris*)	angle of mouth	make vestibule of mouth shallow; aid in articulation
infrahyoid m.'s *mm. infrahyoidei*	the ribbon-like m.'s below the hyoid bone including the omohyoid, sternohyoid, sternothyroid, and thyrohyoid m.'s		
infraspinous m. *m. infraspinatus*	infraspinous fossa of scapula	midportion of greater tubercle of humerus	rotates arm laterally
intercostal m.'s, external *mm. intercostales externi*	inferior border of rib	superior border of rib below origin	draw ribs together
intercostal m.'s, innermost *mm. intercostales intimi*	superior border of rib	inferior border of rib above origin	draw ribs together
intercostal m.'s, internal *mm. intercostales interni*	inferior border of rib, costal cartilage	superior border of rib below origin, costal cartilage	draw ribs together
interosseous m.'s, palmar (three in number) *mm. interossei palmares*	medial side of second, lateral side of fourth and fifth metacarpals	base of proximal phalanx in line with its origin	adduct second, fourth, and fifth fingers; aid in flexing proximal phalanges
interosseous m.'s, plantar (three in number) *mm. interossei plantares*	medial side of third, fourth, and fifth metatarsal bones	medial side of proximal phalanges of third, fourth, and fifth toes	adduct three lateral toes toward second toe; flex toes
interosseous m.'s of foot, dorsal (four in number) *mm. interossei dorsales pedis*	adjacent sides of metatarsal bones	proximal phalanges of both sides of second toe, lateral side of third and fourth toes	abduct lateral toes, move second toe from side to side; flex proximal phalanges
interosseous m.'s of hand, dorsal (four in number) *mm. interossei dorsales manus*	adjacent sides of metacarpal bones	extensor tendons of second, third, and fourth fingers	abduct second, third, and fourth fingers, spread fingers; flex phalanges
interspinal m.'s *mm. interspinales*	short m.'s between the spinous processes of contiguous vertebrae on either side of the interspinous ligament		extend vertebral column
intertransverse m.'s *mm. intertransversarii*	small paired m.'s between the transverse processes of contiguous vertebrae		aid in maintaining erect posture by extension; lateral flexion, and rotation of the body
ischiocavernous m. erector m. of penis *m. ischiocavernosus*	ramus of ischium adjacent to crus of penis or clitoris	crus near pubic symphysis	maintains erection of penis or clitoris
ischiococcygeal m.	see coccygeal m.		
latissimus dorsi m. *m. latissimus dorsi*	spinous processes of vertebrae, T7 to S3; throacolumbar fascia, iliac crest; lower four ribs; inferior angle of scapula	floor or intertubercular groove of humerus	adducts, extends, and medially rotates arm

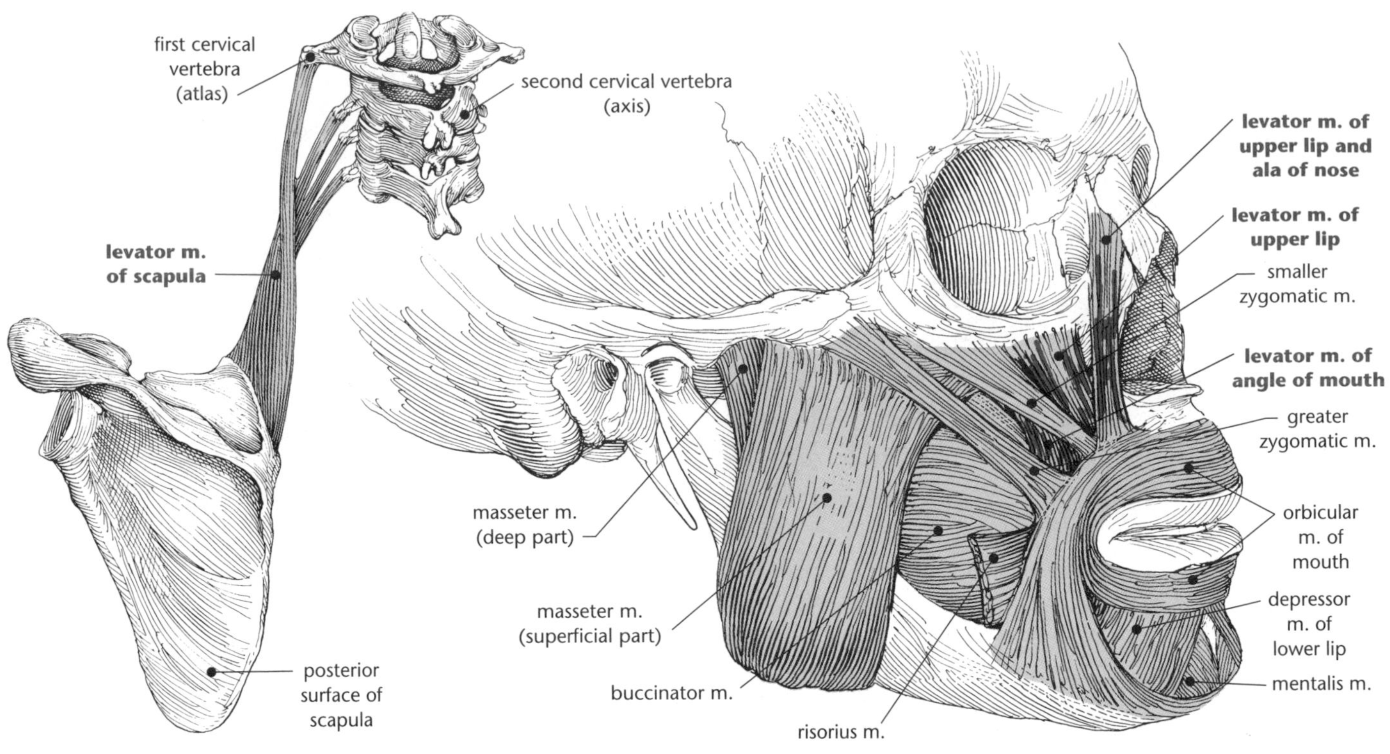

MUSCLE	ORIGIN	INSERTION	ACTION
levator ani m. *m. levator ani*	the main m. of the pelvic floor within the lesser pelvis; composed of pubococcygeal, iliococcygeal, and puborectal m.'s as well as the levator m. of prostate in the male		supports pelvic viscera and separates it from the perineum; constricts lower end of rectum and vagina
levator m. of angle of mouth caninus m. canine m. *m. levator anguli oris*	maxilla next to cuspid fossa just below infraorbital foramen	corner of mouth	raises angle of mouth
levator m. of soft palate *m. levator veli palatini*	apex of petrous part of temporal bone and undersurface of cartilaginous part of auditory tube	aponeurosis of soft palate	raises soft palate in swallowing; aids in opening orifice of auditory tube
levator m. of prostate *m. levator prostatae*	pubic symphysis	fascia of prostate gland	elevates and compresses prostate gland
levator m.'s of ribs *mm. levatores costarum*	transverse processes of seventh cervical and first 11 thoracic vertebrae	angle of rib below	aid in raising ribs; extend vertebral column
levator m. of scapula *m. levator scapulae*	transverse processes of first four cervical vertebrae	vertebral (medial) border of scapula	raises scapula; aids in rotating the neck
levator m. of thyroid gland (inconstant muscle) *m. levator glandulae thyroideae*	isthmus or pyramidal lobe of thyroid gland	body of hyoid bone	stabilizes thyroid gland
levator m. of upper eyelid *m. levator palpebrae superior*	roof of orbital cavity above optic canal	skin and tarsal plate of upper eyelid, and superior fornix of conjunctiva	raises upper eyelid
levator m. of upper lip quadrate m. of upper lip *m. levator labii superioris*	maxilla and zygomatic bone above level of infraorbital foramen	muscular substance of upper lip and margin of nostril	raises upper lip, dilates nostril
levator m. of upper lip and ala of nose *m. levator labii superioris alaeque nasi*	frontal process of maxilla	skin of upper lip, ala of nose	raises upper lip, dilates nostril (m. of facial expression)
long m. of head *m. longus capitis*	transverse processes of third to sixth cervical vertebrae	basal part of occipital bone	flexes head
long m. of neck *m. longus colli*	*superior oblique part:* anterior tubercle of transverse processes of third, fourth, and fifth cervical vertebrae;	*superior oblique part:* anterolateral surface of tubercle on anterior arch of first vertebra (atlas);	bends neck forward and slightly rotates cervical portion of vertebral column

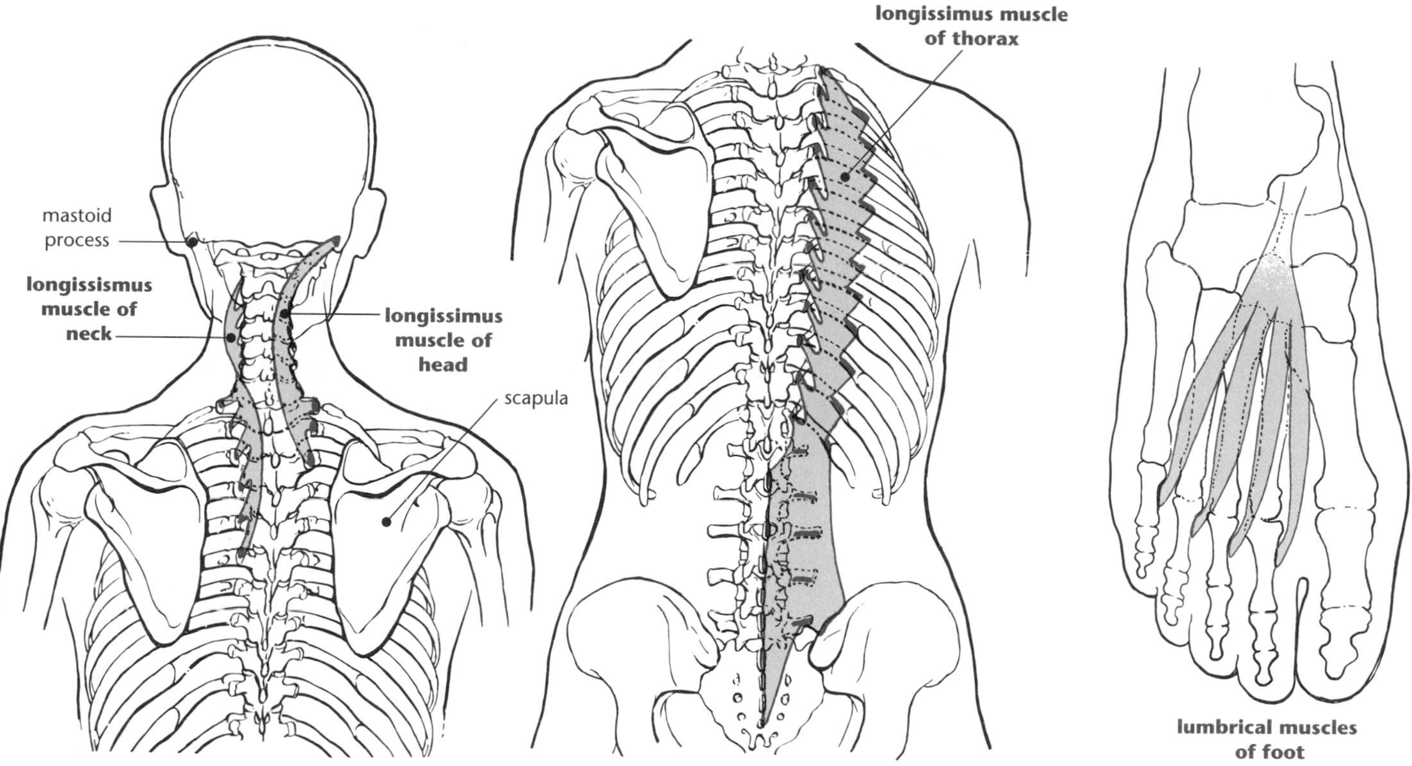

M

MUSCLE	ORIGIN	INSERTION	ACTION
long m. of neck (cont'd)	*inferior oblique part:* front of bodies of first two or three thoracic vertebrae; *vertical part:* front of bodies of first three thoracic and last three cervical vertebrae	*inferior oblique part:* anterior tubercle of transverse processes of fifth and sixth cervical vertebrae; *vertical part:* front of bodies of second, third, and fourth cervical vertebrae	
longissimus m. of head trachelomastoid m. *m. longissimus capitis*	transverse processes of cervical and thoracic vertebrae C3 to T4	mastoid process of temporal bone	draws head backward, rotates head
longissimus m. of neck *m. longissimus cervicis*	transverse processes of upper six thoracic vertebrae	transverse processes of second through sixth cervical vertebrae	bends vertebral column backward and laterally
longissimus m. of thorax longissimus dorsi m. *m. longissimus thoracis*	thoracolumbar fascia, transverse processes of lower six thoracic and first two lumbar vertebrae	transverse processes of lumbar and thoracic vertebrae, inferior borders of lower 9 or 10 ribs	bends vertebral column backward and laterally
longitudinal m. of tongue, inferior *m. longitudinalis inferior linguae*	undersurface of tongue at base	tip of tongue	acts to alter shape of tongue
longitudinal m. of tongue, superior *m. longitudinalis superior linguae*	submucosa and median septum of tongue	margins of tongue	acts to alter shape of tongue
lumbrical m.'s of foot *mm. lumbricales pedis*	tendons of long flexor m.'s of toes	medial side of proximal phalanges and extensor tendon of four lateral toes	flex proximal, extend middle and distal phalanges
lumbical m.'s of hand (four in number) *mm. lumbricales manus*	tendons of deep flexor m.'s of fingers	extensor tendons of four lateral fingers	flex proximal, extend middle and distal phalanges
masseter m. *m. masseter*	*superficial part:* zygomatic process and arch; *deep part:* zygomatic arch	*superficial part:* ramus and angle of lower jaw; *deep part:* upper half of ramus, coronoid process of lower jaw	closes mouth, clenches teeth (m. mastication)
mentalis m. *m. levator menti*	incisor fossa of mandible	skin of chin	raises and protrudes lower lip
multifidus m. *m. multifidus*	sacrum and transverse processes of lumbar, thoracic, and lower cervical vertebrae	spinous processes of lumbar, thoracic, and lower cervical vertebrae	extends, rotates vertebral column; maintains posture

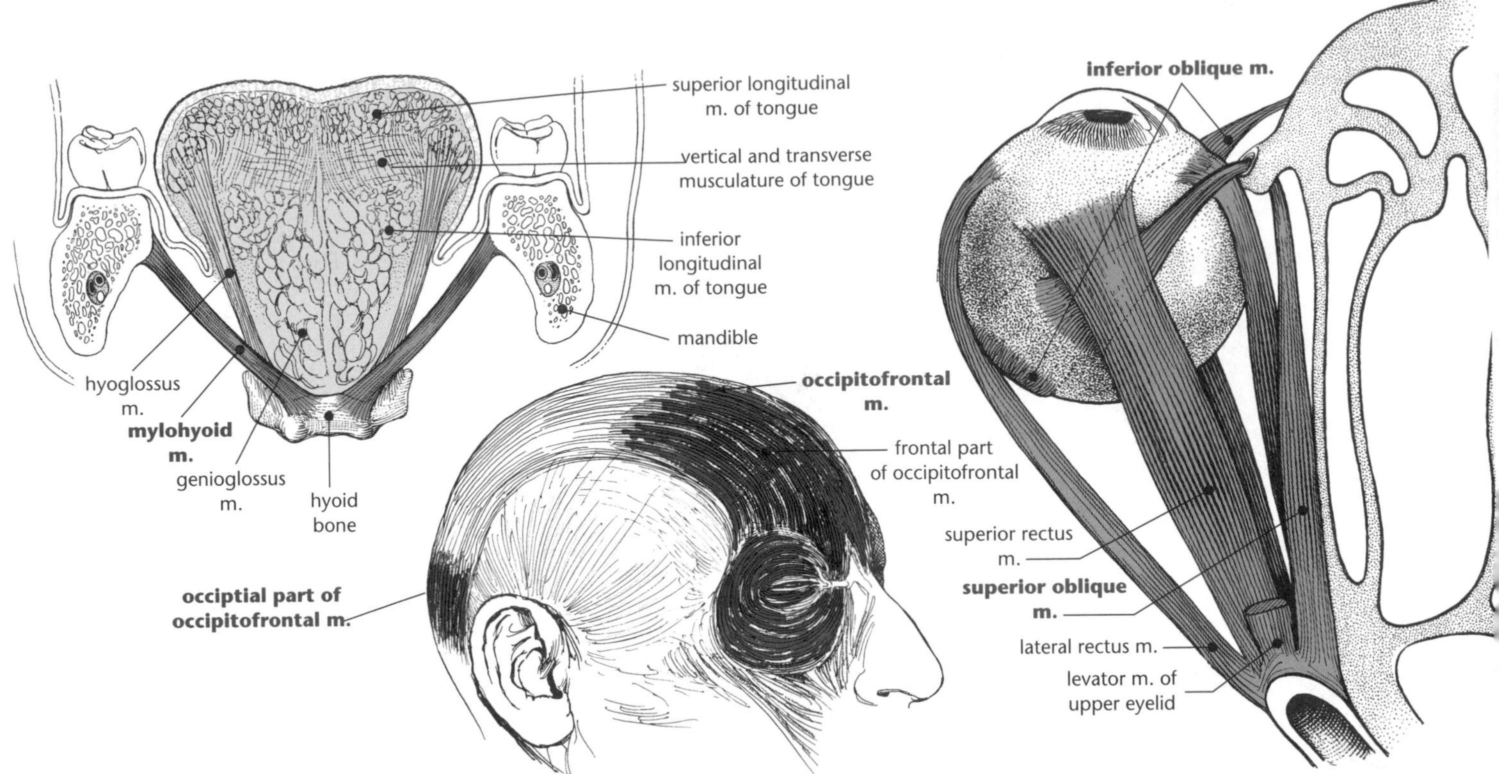

MUSCLE	ORIGIN	INSERTION	ACTION
m. of Treitz		see suspensory m. of duodenum	
mylohyoid m. *m. mylohyoideus*	mylohyoid line of mandible	median raphe and hyoid bone	elevates floor of mouth and tongue; elevates hyoid bone and larynx; depresses mandible
nasal m. *m. nasalis*	maxilla adjacent to cuspid and incisor teeth	side of nose above nostril	draws margin of nostril toward septum
oblique m. of abdomen, external *m. obliquus externus abdominis*	inferior borders of lower eight ribs	anterior half of crest of ilium, linea alba through rectus sheath, inguinal ligament	flexes and rotates vertebral column, tenses abdominal wall; aids in defecation and micturation
oblique m. of abdomen, internal *mm. obliquus internus abdominis*	iliac crest, thoracolumbar fascia, inguinal ligament	lower three or four costal cartilages, linea alba by conjoint tendon to pubis	flexes and rotates vertebral column, tenses abdominal wall
oblique m. of auricle *m. obliquus auriculae*	eminence of concha (media surface)	convexity of the helix (medial surface)	thought to be vestigial
oblique m. of eyeball, inferior *m. obliquus interior bulbi*	floor of orbital cavity at anterior margin	between insertion of superior and lateral recti	rotates eyeball upward and outward
oblique m. of eyeball, superior *m. obliquus superior bulbi*	lesser wing of sphenoid above the optic canal	after passing through a fibrous pulley, reverses direction to insert on sclera deep to superior rectus m.	rotates eyeball downward and outward
oblique m. of head, inferior *m. obliquus capitis inferior*	spine of second vertebra (axis)	transverse process of first vertebra (atlas)	rotates head laterally
oblique m. of head, superior *m. obliquus capitis superior*	transverse process of first vertebra (atlas)	outer third of inferior curved line of occipital bone	rotates head laterally; bends head backward
obturator m., external *m. obturatorius externus*	external margin of obturator foramen of pelvis, obturator membrane	trochanteric fossa of femur	flexes and rotates thigh laterally
obturator m., internal *m. obturatorius internus*	pelvic surface of hipbone and internal margin of obturator foramen, obturator membrane	greater trochanter of femur	abducts and rotates thigh laterally
occipital m.		see occipitofrontal m.	
occipitofrontal m. *m. occipitofrontalis*	*frontal part:* epicranial aponeurosis; *occipital part:* highest nuchal line of occipital bone; mastoid process	*frontal part:* skin of eyebrow, root of nose; *occipital part:* epicranial aponeurosis	*frontal part:* elevates eyebrows, wrinkles forehead; *occipital part:* draws scalp backward

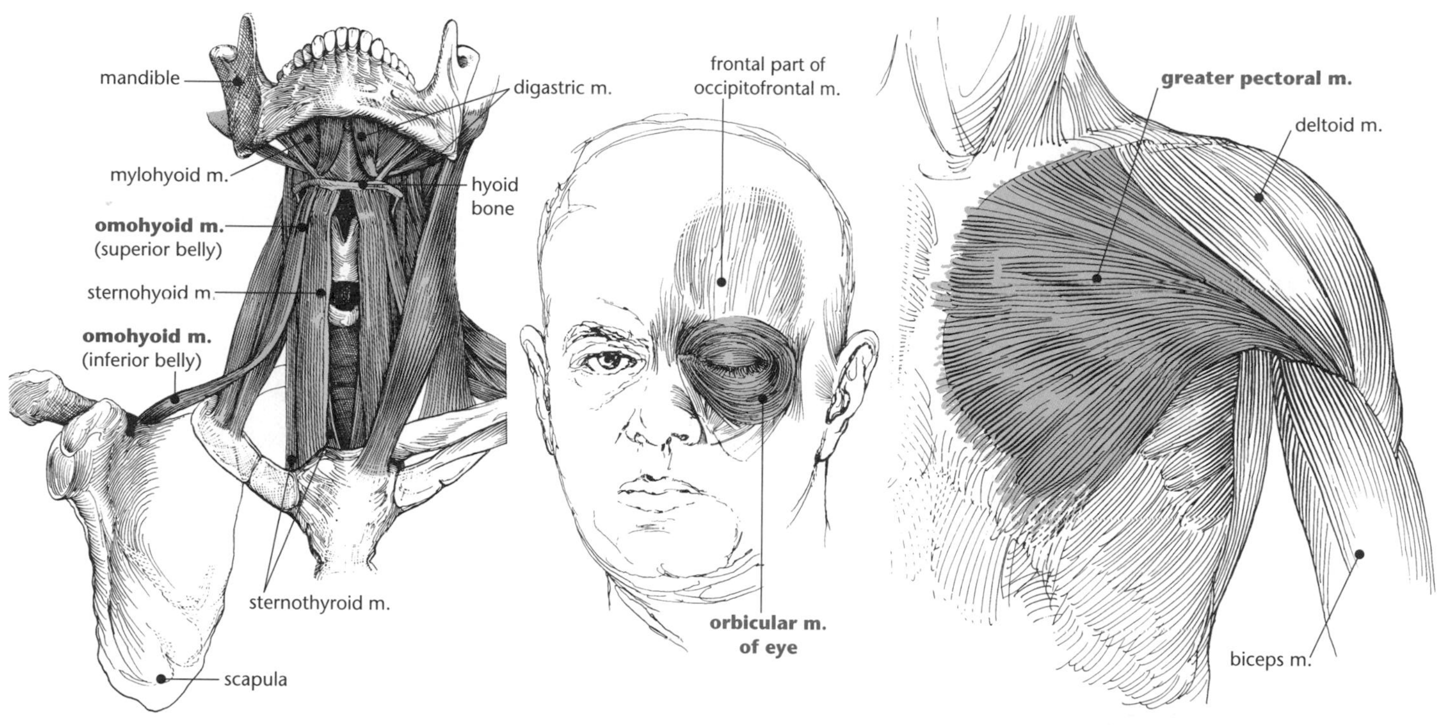

MUSCLE	ORIGIN	INSERTION	ACTION
omohyoid m. *m. omohyoideus*	medial tip of suprascapular notch on upper scapula	lower border of body of hyoid bone	depresses and retracts hyoid bone
opposing m. of little finger *m. opponens digiti minimi manus*	hook of hamate bone, flexor retinaculum	fifth metacarpal	draws fifth metacarpal bone toward palm, opposes thumb
opposing m. of thumb *m. opponens pollicis*	tubercle of trapezium, flexor retinaculum	lateral border of first metacarpal bone	draws first metacarpal bone toward palm
orbicular m. of eye *m. orbicularis oculi*	*orbital part:* frontal process of maxilla, adjacent portion of frontal bone; *palpebral part:* medial palpebral ligament; *lacrimal part:* posterior lacrimal ridge of lacrimal bone	near origin after encircling orbit lateral palpebral raphe; superior and inferior tarsi	closes eyelids, tightens skin of forehead, compresses lacrimal sac
orbicular m. of mouth *m. orbicularis oris*	m. adjacent to mouth	m.'s interlace to encircle mouth	closes and purses lips
orbital m. *m. orbitalis*	bridges inferior orbital groove and sphenomaxillary fissure		thought to be rudimentary; may feebly protrude the eyeball
palatoglossus m. glossopalatine m. *m. palatoglossus*	undersurface of soft palate	dorsum and side of tongue	elevates back of tongue and narrows fauces
palatopharyngeal m. *m. palatopharyngeus*	soft palate; back of hard palate	posterior wall of thyroid cartilage and wall of pharynx	elevates pharynx and shortens it during swallowing; narrows fauces
palmar m., long *m. palmaris longus*	medial epicondyle of humerus	flexor retinaculum, palmar aponeurosis	flexes hand
palmar m., short *m. palmaris brevis*	flexor retinaculum; medial side of plmar aponeurosis	skin of palm over hypothenar eminence	aids in deepening hollow of palm, wrinkles skin of palm
pectinate m.'s *mm. pectinati*	a number of muscular columns projecting from the inner walls of the atria of the heart		contract the atria of the heart during systole
pectineal m. *m. pectineus*	pectineal line of pubis	pectineal line of femur between lesser trochanter and linea aspera	adducts and aids in flexion of thigh
pectoral m., greater *m. pectoralis major*	medial half of clavicle, sternum, and costal cartilages; aponeurosis of external oblique muscle of abdomen; sixth rib	lateral lip of intertubercular groove of humerus	flexes, adducts, and rotates arm medially

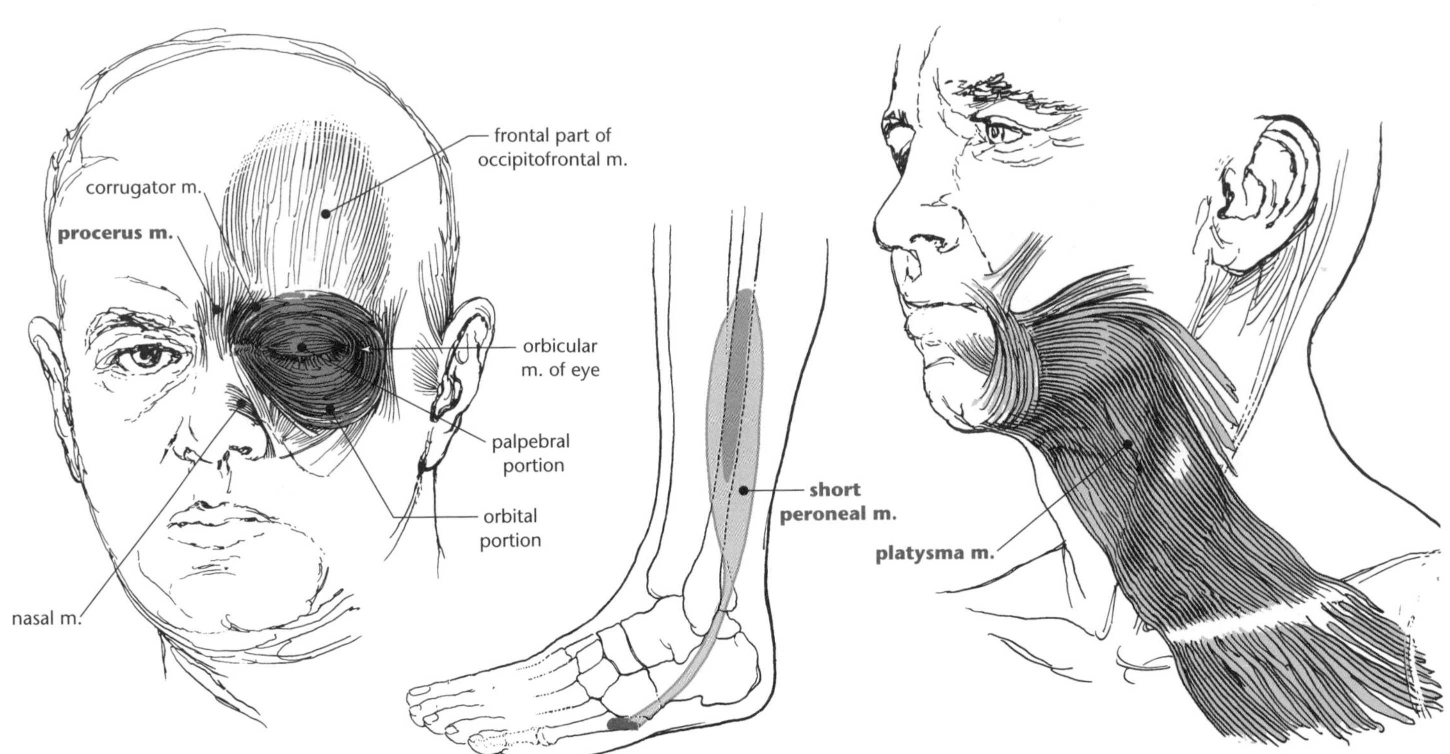

MUSCLE	ORIGIN	INSERTION	ACTION
pectoral, m., smaller *m. pectoralis minor*	anterior aspect of third through fifth ribs, near costal cartilages	coracoid process of scapula	draws scapula downward, elevates ribs
pectoralis major m.	see pectoral m. greater		
pectoralis minor m.	see pectoral m. smaller		
peroneal m., long fibular m. long *m. peroneuos longus*	upper two-thirds of fibula; crural septum	first metatarsal bone, medial cuneiform bone	aids in plantar flexion and everts foot; helps maintain transverse arch of foot
peroneal m., short fibular m., short *m. peroneus brevis*	lower two-thirds of fibula; crural septum	tuberosity of fifth metatarsal bone	aids in plantar flexion; everts foot; aids in preventing over-inversion of foot
peroneal m., third *m. peroneus tertius*	distal third of fibula; crural fascia	fascia of fifth metatarsal bone on dorsum of foot	dorsiflexes and everts foot
piriform m. *m. prirformis*	internal aspect of sacrum, sacrotuberous ligament	upper portion of greater trochanter of femur	rotates thigh laterally
plantar m. *m. plantaris*	supracondylar line just above lateral condyle of femur; oblique popliteal ligament	posterior part of calcaneus (along with calcaneal tendon)	plantar flexion of foot
platysma m. *m. platysma*	superficial fascia of upper chest	skin over mandible and neck	depresses lower jaw and lower lip, wrinkles skin of neck and upper part of chest; draws down angle of mouth
pleuroesophageal m. m. pleuroesophageus			reinforces musculature of esophagus
popliteal m. *m. popliteus*	popliteal groove of lateral condyle of femur; arcuate popliteal ligament	upper part of posterior surface of tibia	flexes and rotates leg medially
procerus m. *m. procerus*	fascia covering bridge of nose	skin between eyebrows	wrinkles skin over bridge of nose (assists frontal muscle)
pronator m., quadrate *m. pronator quadratus*	distal fourth of shaft of ulna	distal fourth of shaft of radius	pronates forearm
pronator m., round *m. pronator teres*	humeral part: medial epicondyle of humerus; ulnar part: coronoid process of ulna	lateral aspect of radius bone at point of maximum convexity	pronates and flexes forearm
psoas m., greater *m. psoas major*	transverse processes and bodies of lumbar vertebrae; body of 12th thoracic vertebra	lesser trochanter of femur	flexes and medially rotates thigh
psoas m., smaller *m. psoas minor*	bodies of last thoracic and first lumbar vertebrae	pectineal line of hipbone	flexes vertebral column

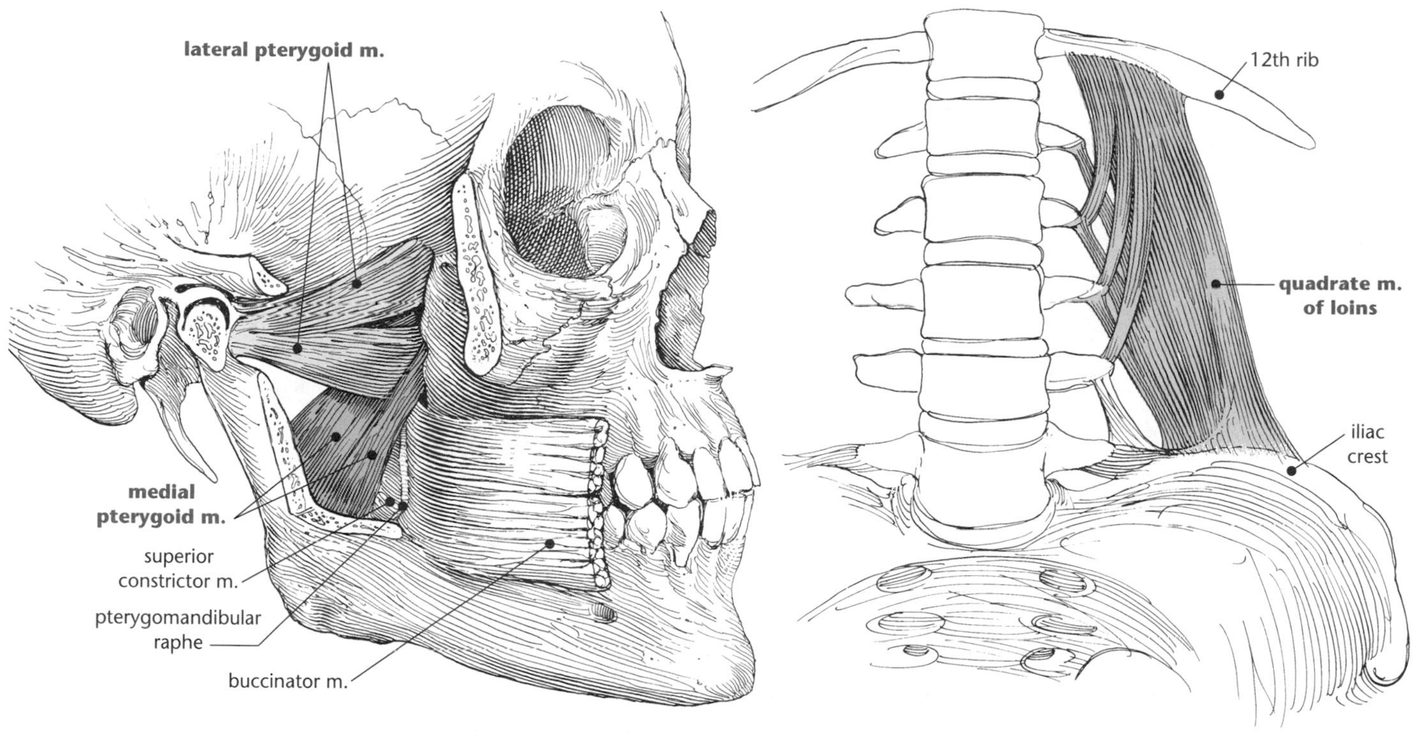

MUSCLE	ORIGIN	INSERTION	ACTION
pterygoid m., lateral *external pterygoid m.* *m. pterygoideus lateralis*	lateral pterygoid plate and greater wing of sphenoid	condyle of mandible, capsule of temporomandibular joint	opens and protrudes mandible
pterygoid m., medial internal pterygoid m. *m. pterygoideus medialis*	maxillary tuberosity and lateral pterygoid plate, tubercle of palatine bone	medial surface of ramus and angle of mandible	closes and protrudes mandible and moves it side to side
pubococcygeal m. *m. pubococcygeus*	back of pubis and obturator fascia	coccyx and perineal body	supports pelvic floor
puborectal m. *m. puborectalis*	back of pubis and pubic symphysis	interdigitates to form a sling which passes behind the rectum	holds anal canal at right angle to rectum
pubovaginal m. *m. pubovaginalis*		part of levator ani m. in the female	
pubovesical m. *m. pubovesicalis*	posterior surface of body of pubis	*female:* around fundus of bladder to front of vagina; *male:* around fundus of bladder to prostate gland	strengthens musculature of urinary bladder; secures base of bladder
pyramidal m. *m. pyramidalis*	pubis and pubic symphysis	linea alba	tenses abdominal wall
quadrate m. of loins *m. quadratus lumborum*	iliac crest, transverse processes of lumbar vertebrae, iliolumbar ligament	12th rib, transverse processes of upper lumbar vertebrae	draws rib cage inferiorly, bends vertebral column laterally
quadrate m. of lower lip *m. quadratus labli inferioris*		see depressor m. of lower lip	
quadrate m. of sole accessory flexor m. *m. quadratus plantae*	calcaneus and plantar fascia	tendons of long flexor muscle of toes (*m. flexor digitorum longus*)	aids in flexing all toes except the big toe
quadrate m. of thigh *m. quadratus femoris*	proximal part of external border of tuberosity of ischium	proximal part of linea quadrata (line extending vertically and distally from intertrochanteric crest of femur)	rotates thigh laterally
quadrate m. of upper lip *m. quadratus labii superioris*		see levator m. of upper lip	
quadratus lumborum m.		see quadrate m. of loins	
quadriceps m. of thigh *m. quadriceps femoris*	the large four-headed fleshy mass that covers the front and sides of the femur, consisting of the rectus m. of thigh (*m. rectus femoris*), lateral vastus (*m. vastus lateralis*), medial vastus m. (*m. vastus medialis*), and intermediate vastus m. (*m. vastus intermedius*)		great extensor m. of leg

M

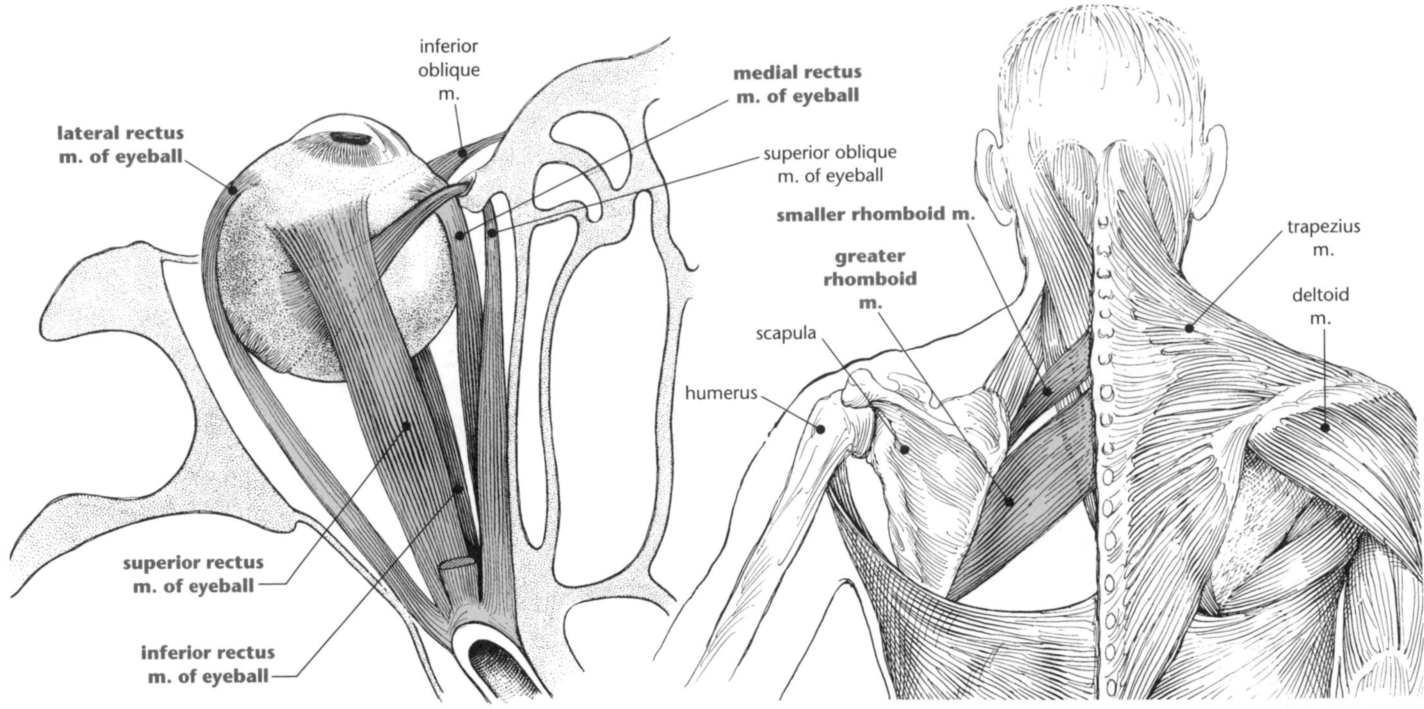

MUSCLE	ORIGIN	INSERTION	ACTION
rectococcygeal m. *m. rectococcygeus*	smooth m. fibers in the pelvic fascia between the coccyx and rectum		secures rectum
rectourethral m. *m. rectourethralis*	smooth m. fibers in the pelvic fascia between the rectum and membranous urethra of male		secures urethra
rectouterine m. *m. rectouterinus*	bundle of smooth m. fibers in pelvic fascia between rectum and cervix of uterus		secures uterus
rectus m. of abdomen *m. rectus abdominis*	pubic crest, pubic symphysis	xiphoid process, fifth to seventh costal cartilages	tenses abdominal wall, draws thorax downard, flexes vertebral column
rectus m. of eyeball, inferior *m. rectus inferior bulbi*	common tendon ring around the optic canal	lateral part of sclera just posterior to corneoscleral junction	rotates eyeball downward and somewhat medially
rectus m. of eyeball, lateral *m. rectus lateralis bulbi*	common tendon ring around the optic canal	lateral part of sclera just posterior to corneoscleral junction	rotates eyeball laterally
rectus m. of eyeball, medial *m. rectus medialis bulbi*	common tendon ring around the optic canal	medial part of sclera just posterior to corneoscleral junction	rotates eyeball medially
rectus m. of eyeball, superior *m. rectus superior bulbi*	common tendon ring around the optic canal	top part of sclera just posterior to corneoscleral junction	rotates eyeball upward and somewhat medially
rectus m. of head, anterior *m. rectus capitis anterior*	lateral portion of first vertebra (atlas)	basilar portion of occipital bone, in front of foramen magnum	flexes and supports head
rectus m. of head, lateral *m. rectus capitis lateralis*	transverse process of first vertebra (atlas)	jugular process of occipital bone	aids in lateral movements of head, supports head
rectus m. of head, posterior, greater *m. rectus capitis posterior major*	spinous process of second vertebra (axis)	occipital bone	extends head
rectus m. of head, posterior, smaller *m. rectus capitis posterior minor*	posterior tubercle of first vertebra (atlas)	occipital bone	extends head
rectus m. of thigh *m. rectus of femoris*	anterior inferior iliac spine, rim of acetabulum	base of patella (kneecap)	extends leg and flexes thigh
rhomboid m., greater *m. rhomboideus major*	spinous processes of second through fifth thoracic vertebrae	lower two-thirds of vertebral margin of scapula	adducts and laterally rotates scapula
rhomboid m., smaller *m. rhomboideus minor*	spinous processes of seventh cervical and first thoracic vertebrae and lower part of nuchal ligament	vertebral margin of scapula above spine	adducts and laterally rotates scapula
risorius m. *m. risorius*	fascia over masseter m.; platysma m.	skin at angle of mouth	retracts angle of mouth

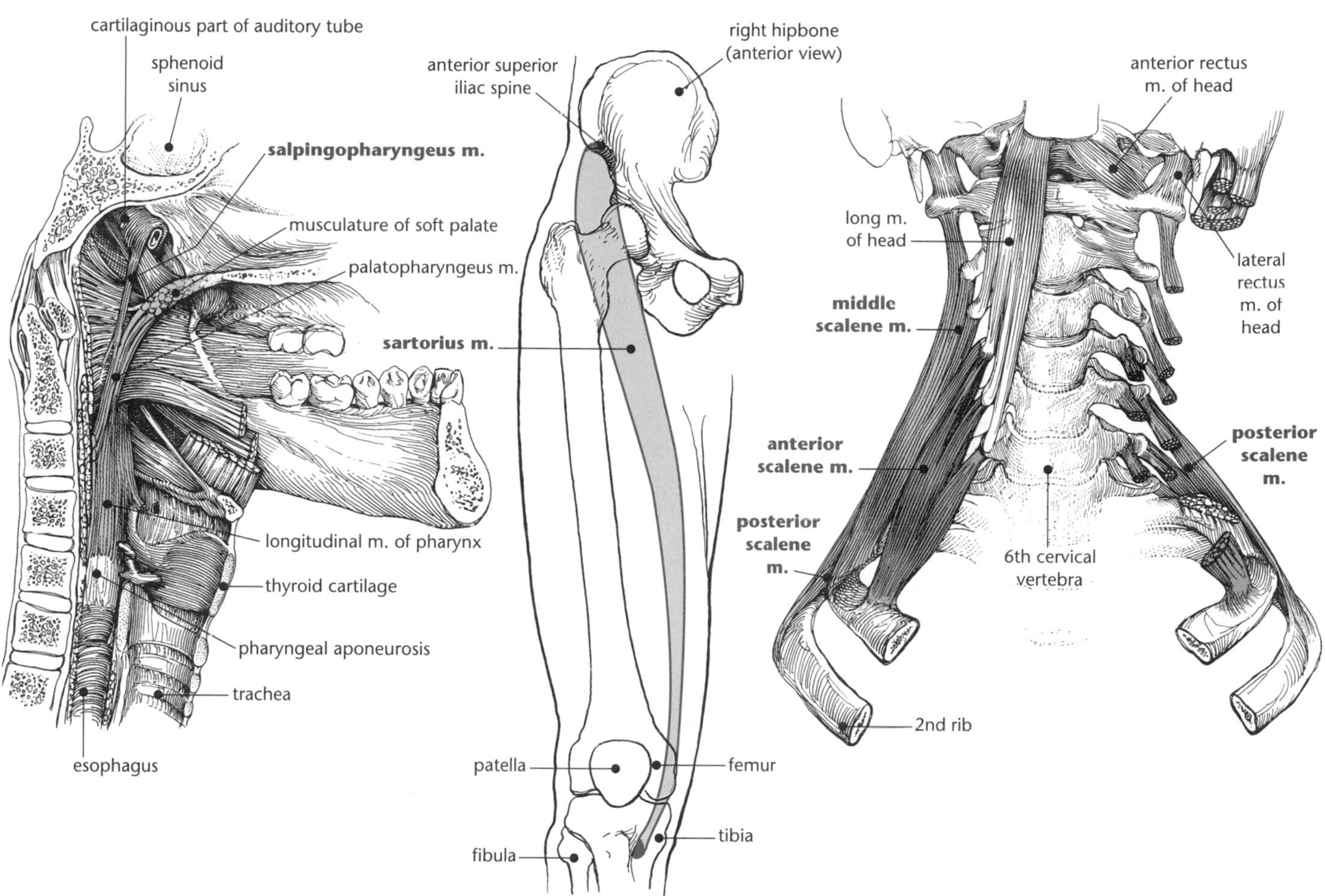

M

MUSCLE	ORIGIN	INSERTION	ACTION
rotator m.'s *mm. rotatores*	transverse processes of all vertebrae below second cervical	lamina above vertebra of origin	extend and rotate the vertebral column toward opposite side
sacrococcygeal m., dorsal *m. sacrococcygeus dorsalis*	a muscular slip from the dorsal aspect of the sacrum to the coccyx		feebly protects sacrococcygeal joint
sacrococcygeal m., ventral *m. sacrococcygeus ventralis*	a muscular slip from the ventral aspect of the sacrum		feebly protects sacrococcygeal joint
sacrospinal m.	see erector m. of spine		
salpingopharyngeal m. *m. salpingopharyngeus*	cartilage of auditory tube near nasopharyngeal orifice	wall of pharynx	elevates nasopharynx
sartorius m. *m. sartorius*	anterior superior iliac spine	upper medial surface of tibia	flexes thigh and leg; rotates thigh laterally
scalene m., anterior *m. scalenus anterior*	transverse processes of third to sixth cervical verebrae	scalene tubercle of first rib	raises first rib, stabilizes or inclines neck to the side
scalene m., middle *m. scalenus medius*	transverse processes of first six cervical vertebrae	upper surface of first rib	raises first rib, stabilizes or inclines neck to the side
scalene m., posterior *m. scalenus posterior*	transverse processes of fifth to seventh cervical vertebrae	outer surface of upper border of second rib	raises second rib, stabilizes or inclines neck to the side
scalene m., smallest *m. scalenus minimus*	occasional extra m. fibers or slip of posterior scalene m.		tenses dome of pleura
semimembranous m. *m. semimembranosus*	tuberosity of ischium	medial condyle of tibia; oblique popliteal ligament	extends thigh, flexes and rotates leg medially
semispinal m. of head *m. semispinalis capitis*	transverse processes of six upper thoracic and four lower cervical vertebrae	occipital bone between superior and inferior nuchal lines	rotates head and draws it backward
semispinal m. of neck *m. semispinalis cervicis*	transverse processes of upper six thoracic vertebrae	spinous processes of second through sixth cervical vertebrae	extends and rotates vertebral column
semispinal m. of thorax *m. semispinalis thoracis*	transverse processes of lower six thoracic vertebrae	spinous processes of upper six thoracic and lower two cervical vertebrae	extends and rotates vertebral column

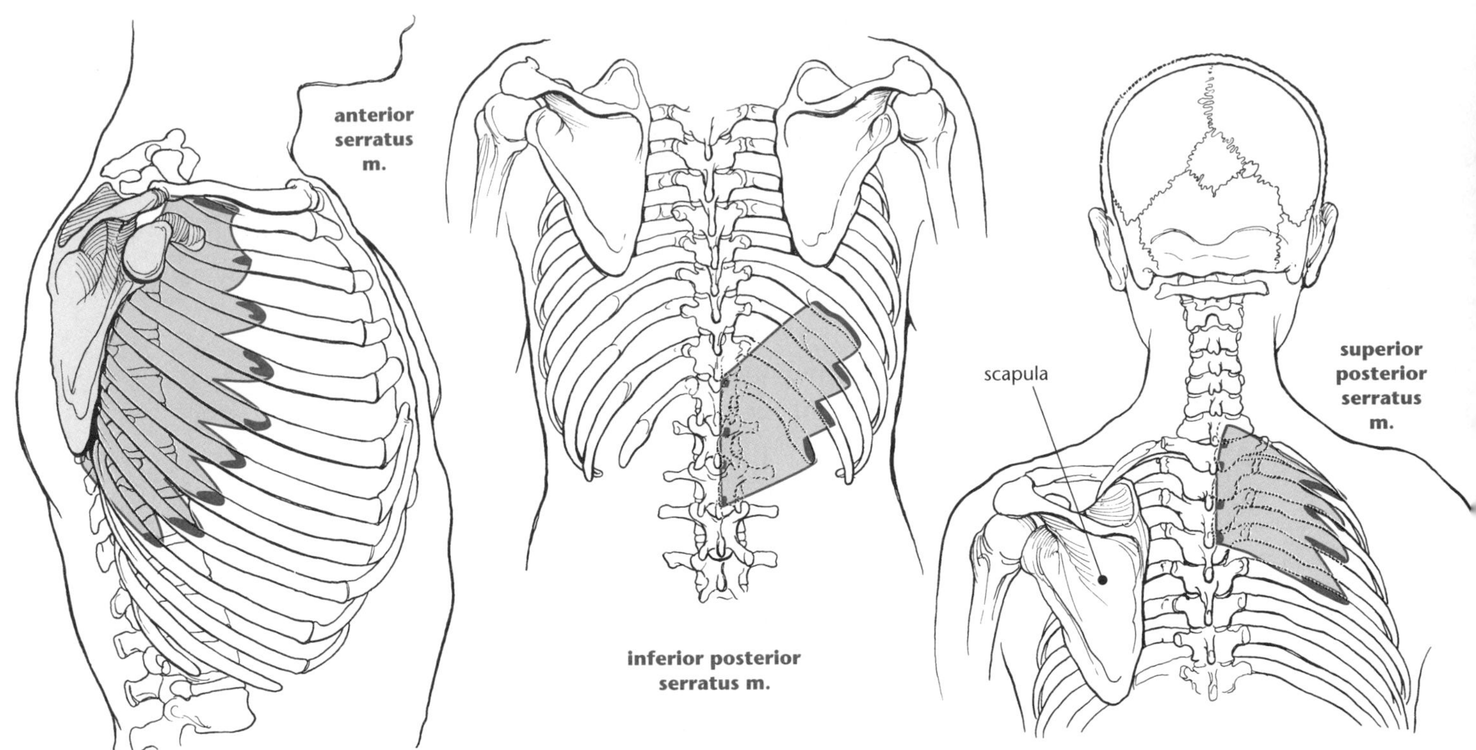

M

MUSCLE	ORIGIN	INSERTION	ACTION
semitendinous m. *m. semitendinosus*	tuberosity of ischium (in common with biceps m. of thigh)	upper part of tibia near tibial tuberosity	flexes and rotates leg medially, extends thigh
serratus m., anterior *m. serratus anterior*	lateral surface of eight or nine uppermost ribs	anterior surface of vertebral border of scapula	draws scapula forward and laterally, rotates scapula in raising arm
serratus m., posterior, inferior *m. serratus posterior interior*	spinous processes of last two thoracic and first two or three lumbar vertebrae, supraspinal ligament	inferior borders of the last four ribs, slightly beyond their angles	draws the ribs outward and downward (counteracting the inward pull of the diaphragm)
serratus m posterior, superior *m. serratus posterior superior*	caudal part of nuchal ligament, spinous processes of the seventh cervical and first two or three thoracic vertebrae, supraspinal ligament	upper borders of the second, third, fourth, and fifth ribs, slightly beyond their angles	raises the ribs
soleus m. *m. soleus*	upper third of fibula, soleal line of tibia, tendinous arch	calcaneus by calcaneal tendon (*tendo calcaneus*)	plantarflexes foot
sphincter m. of anus, external *m. sphincter ani externus*	tip of coccyx, anococcygeal ligament	central tendon of perineum, skin	closes anal canal and anus
sphincter m. of anus, internal *m. sphincter ani internus*	1-cm-thick muscular ring surrounding approximately 2.5 cm of the upper part of the anal canal, about 6.0 mm from the orifice of the anus		aids in occlusion of anal aperture and expulsion of feces
sphincter m. of bile duct *m. sphincter choledochi*	a circular m. around lower part of the bile duct within the wall of the duodenum (part of the sphincter m. of hepatopancreatic ampulla)		constricts lower part of common bile duct
sphincter m. of hepatopancreatic ampulla sphincter of Oddi *m. sphincter ampullae hepatopancreaticae*	circular m. around terminal part of main pancreatic duct and common bile duct, including the duodenal ampulla (papilla of Vater)		constricts both lower part of common bile duct and main pancreatic duct
sphincter m. of pupil *m. sphincter pupillae*	circular fibers of iris arranged in a narrow band about 1 mm in width		constricts pupil
sphincter m. of pylorus *m. sphincter pylori*	thick muscular ring at the end of the stomach, near opening of the duodenum		acts as valve to close lumen
sphincter m. of urethra external urethral sphincter m. *m. sphincter urethrae*	ramus of pubis	fibers interdigitate around urethra	compresses urethra
sphincter m. of urinary bladder *m. sphincter vesicae urinariae*	thick muscular ring towards the lower part of bladder around internal urethral orifice		acts as valve to close internal urethral orifice

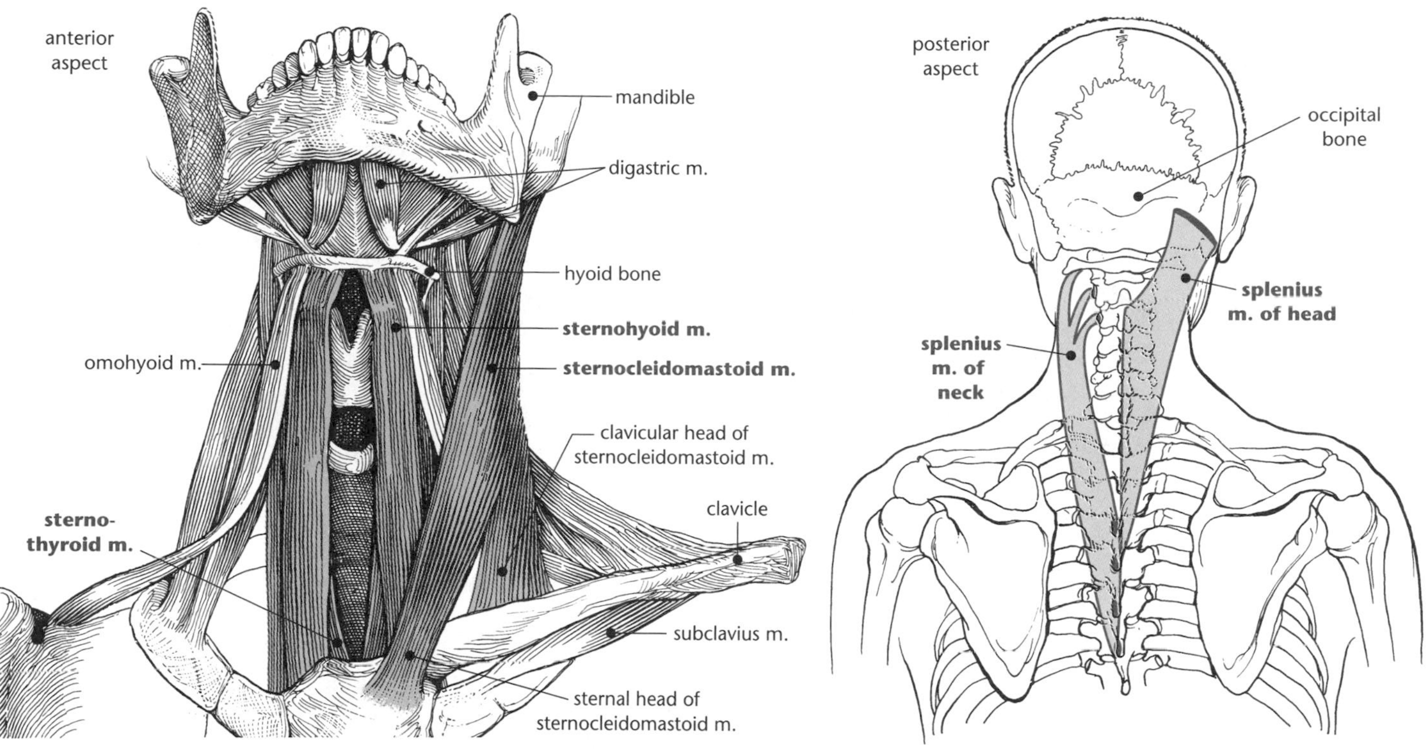

MUSCLE	ORIGIN	INSERTION	ACTION
sphincter m. of vagina *m. sphincter vaginae*	pubic symphysis	interdigitates around and interlaces into vaginal barrel	constricts vaginal orifice
sphincter of Oddi	see sphincter m. of hepatopancreatic ampulla		
spinal m. of head biventer cervicis m. *m.spinalis capitis*	spinous processes of vertebrae C6 to T2	occipital bone between superior and inferior nuchal lines	extends head
spinal m. of neck *m. spinalis cervicis*	spinous processes of vertebrae C7 to T2	spinous processes of second, third, and fourth cervical vertebrae	extends vertebral column
spinal m. of thorax *m. spinalis thoracis*	spinous processes of upper two lumbar and lower two thoracic vertebrae, nuchal ligament	spinous processes of second through seventh thoracic vertebrae	extends vertebral column
splenius m. of head *m. splenius capitis*	spinous processes of upper thoracic vertebrae	mastoid process and superior nuchal line	inclines and rotates head
splenius m. of neck splenius colli m. *m. splenius cervicis*	nuchal ligament, spinous processes of third to sixth thoracic vertebrae	posterior tubercles of the transverse processes of upper two or three cervical vertebrae	extends head and neck, turns head toward the same side
stapedius m. *m. stapedius*	bony canal in pyramidal eminence on posterior wall of middle ear chamber	posterior surface of neck of stapes	dampens excessive vibrations of stapes by tilting the baseplate
sternal m. *m. sternalis*	small superficial muscular band at sternal end of greater pectoral m. (*m. pectoralis major*) parallel with the margin of sternum		protects sternum
sternocleidomastoid m. *m. sternocleidomastoideus*	*sternal head:* anterior surface of manubrium; *clavicular head:* medial third of clavicle	mastoid process, superior nuchal line of occipital bone	rotates and extends head, flexes vertebral column
sternocostal m.	see transverse m. of thorax		
sternohyoid m. *m. sternohyoideus*	medial end of clavicle, posterior surface of manubrium, first costal cartilage	lower border of body of hyoid bone	depresses hyoid bone and larynx from elevated position during swallowing
sternothyroid m. *m. sternothyroideus*	dorsal surface of upper part of sternum and medial edge of first costal cartilage	oblique line on lamina of thyroid cartilage	draws thyroid cartilage downward from elevated position during swallowing
styloglossus m. *m. styloglossus*	lower end of styloid process, upper end of stylomandibular ligament	*longitudinal part:* side of tongue near dorsal surface; *oblique part:* over hyoglossus muscle	raises and retracts tongue

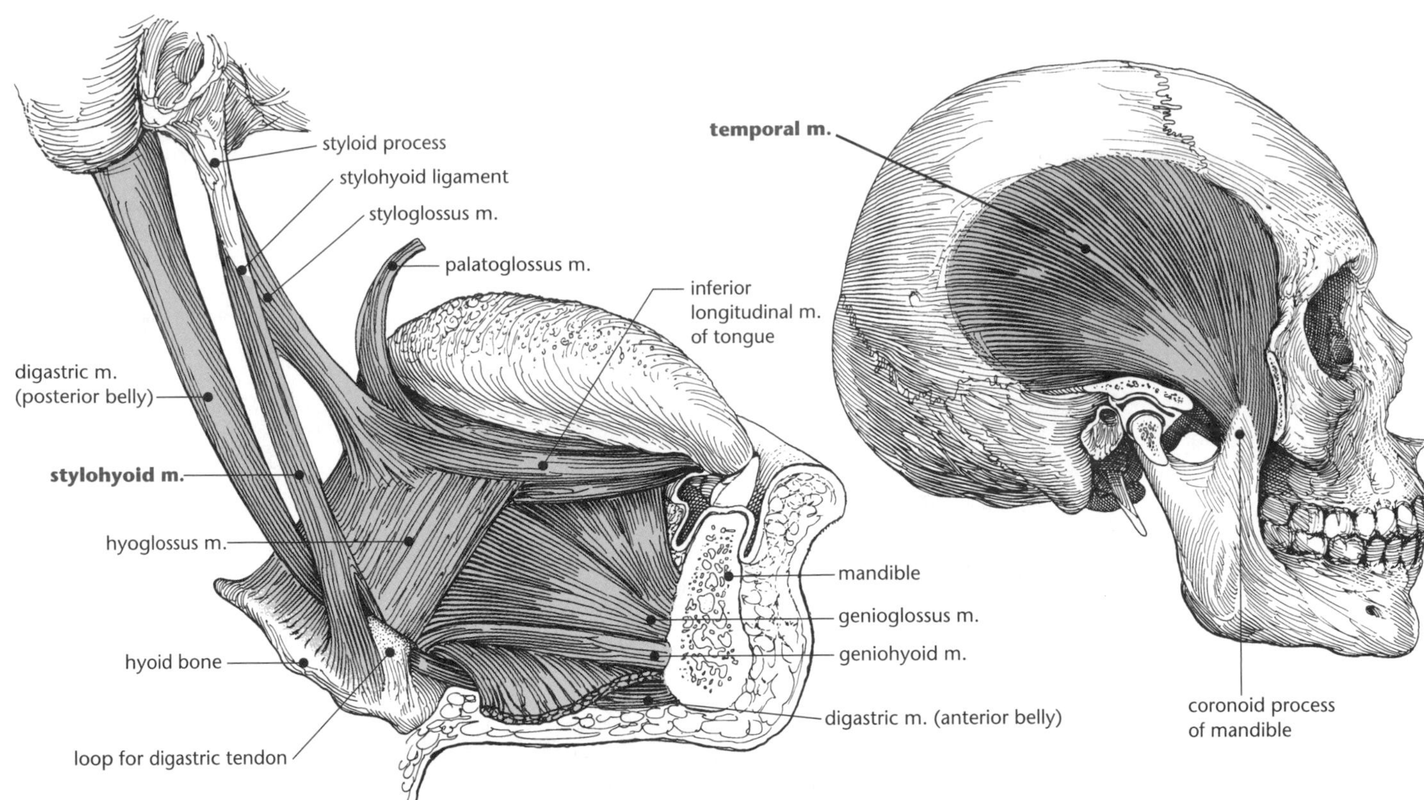

MUSCLE	ORIGIN	INSERTION	ACTION
stylohoid m. *m. stylohyoideus*	posterior and lateral surfaces of the styloid process near the base	hyoid bone at junction of greater horn and body	draws hyoid bone upward and backward
stylopharyngeal m. *m. stylopharyngeus*	root of styloid process of temporal bone	borders of thyroid cartilage, wall of pharynx	elevates and opens pharynx
subclavius m. *m. subclavius*	junction of first rib and costal cartilages	lower surface of clavicle	depresses lateral end of clavicle
subcostal m.'s *mm. subcostales*	inner surface of ribs near their angles	lower inner surface of second or third rib below rib of origin	draw adjacent ribs together; depresses lower ribs
subscapular m. *m. subscapularis*	subscapular fossa	lesser tubercle of humerus	rotates arm medially
supinator m. *m. supinator*	lateral epicondyle of humerus, supinator crest of ulna	upper third of radius	supinates the forearm by rotating radius
suprahyoid m.'s *mm. suprahyoidei*	the group of m.'s attached to the upper part of the hyoid bone from the skull; includes the digastric, stylohyoid, mylohyoid, and geniohyoid m.'s		elevates hyoid bone
supraspinous m. *m. supraspinatus*	supraspinous fossa	superior aspect of greater tubercle of humerus	abducts arm
suspensory m. of duodenum ligament of Treitz suspensory ligament of duodenum m. of Treitz *m. suspensorius duodeni*	connective tissue around celiac artery and right crus of diaphragm	superior border of duodenojejunal junction, part of ascending duodenum	acts as suspensory ligament of the duodenum
tarsal m., inferior *m. tarsalis inferior*	aponeurosis of inferior rectus m. of eyeball	lower border of tarsal plate of lower eyelid	widens palpebral fissure by depressing lower eyelid
tarsal m., superior lamina profundus m. *m. tarsalis superior*	aponeurosis of levator m. of upper eyelid	upper border of tarsus plate of upper eyelid	widens palpebral fissure by raising upper eyelid
temporal m. *m. temporalis*	temporal fossa on side of cranium	coronoid process of mandible	closes mouth, clenches teeth, retracts lower jaw
temporoparietal m. *m. temporoparietalis*	temporal fascia above ear	frontal part of epicranial aponeurosis	tightens scalp
tensor m. of fascia lata *m. tensor fasciae latae*	iliac crest; anterior superior iliac spine, fascia lata	iliotibial tract of fascia lata	extends knee with lateral rotation of leg
tensor m. of soft palate *m. tensor veli palatini*	spine of sphenoid, scaphoid fossa of pterygoid process, cartilage and membrane of the auditory tube	midline of aponeurosis of soft palate, wall of auditory tube	elevates palate and opens auditory tube

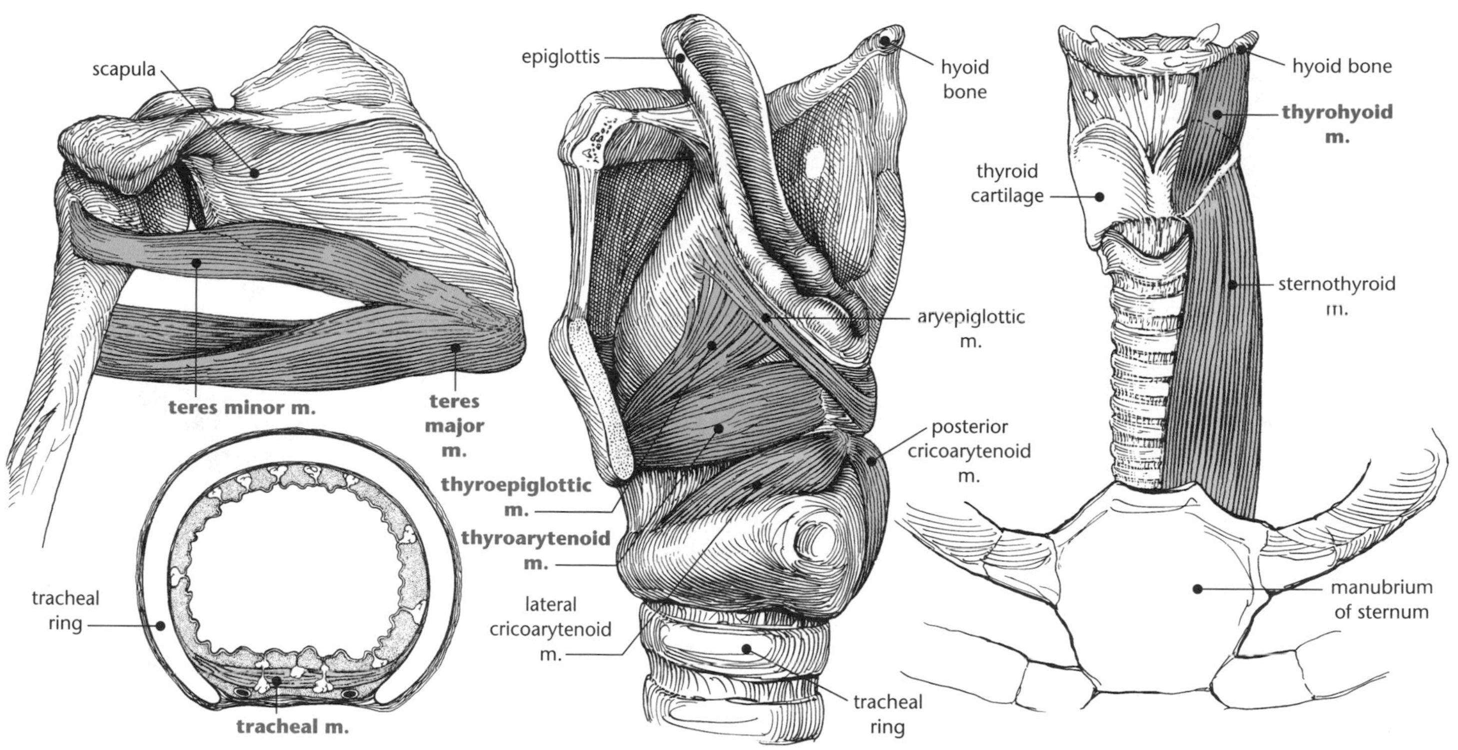

MUSCLE	ORIGIN	INSERTION	ACTION
tensor m. of tympanum tensor m. of tympanic membrane (eardrum) *m. tensor tympani*	cartilaginous portion of auditory (eustachian) tube and adjoining part of great wing of sphenoid bone	manubrium of malleus near its root	draws tympanic membrane medially, thus increasing its tension
teres major m. *m. teres major*	inferior axillary border of scapula	crest of lesser tubercle of humerus	adducts and rotates arm medially
teres minor m. *m. teres minor*	axillary border of scapula	inferior aspect of greater tubercle of humerus	rotates arm laterally, and weakly adducts it
thyroarytenoid m. *m. thyroarytneoideus*	inside of thyroid cartilage	lateral surface of arytenoid cartilage	aids in closure of laryngeal inlet, relaxes vocal ligament
thyroepiglottic m. *m. thyroepiglotticus*	inside of thyroid cartilage	margin of epiglottis	depresses the epiglottis, widens inlet of larynx
thyrohyoid m. *m. thyrohyoideus*	oblique line of thyroid cartilage	greater horn (cornu) of hyoid bone	elevates larynx, depresses hyoid bone
tibial m., anterior *m. tibialis anterior*	upper two-thirds of tibia, interosseous membrane	first metatarsal bone, medial cuneiform bone	dorsiflexes and inverts foot
tibial m., posterior *m. tibialis posterior*	tibia, fibula, and interosseous membrane	navicular, with slips to three cuneiform bones; cuboid, second, third, and fourth metatarsals	principal inverter of foot, aids in plantarflexion of foot
tracheal m. *m. trachealis*	anastomosing transverse muscular bands connecting the ends of the tracheal rings		reduces size of tracheal lumen
trachelomastoid m.	see longissimus m. of head		
tragus m. *m. tragicus*	a short band of vertical muscular fibers on the outer surface of the tragus of the ear		slightly alters shape of ear
transverse m. of abdomen *m. transversus abdominis*	7th through 12th costal cartilages, thoracolumbar fascia, iliac crest, inguinal ligament	xiphoid process, linea alba, conjoint tendon to pubis	supports abdominal viscera tenses abdominal wall
transverse m. of auricle *m. transversus auriculae*	see auricular m., transverse		
transverse m. of chin *m. transversus menti*	superficial muscular fibers of depressor m. of angle of mouth (triangular m.) which turn back and cross to the opposite side below the chin		aids in drawing angle of mouth downward
transverse m. of nape *m. transversus nuchae*	an occasional m. passing between the tendons of the trapezius and sternocleidomastoid m.'s		moves scalp feebly
transverse m. of perineum, deep *m. transversus perinei profundus*	inferior ramus of ischium	central tendon of perineum, external anal sphincter	suports pelvic viscera

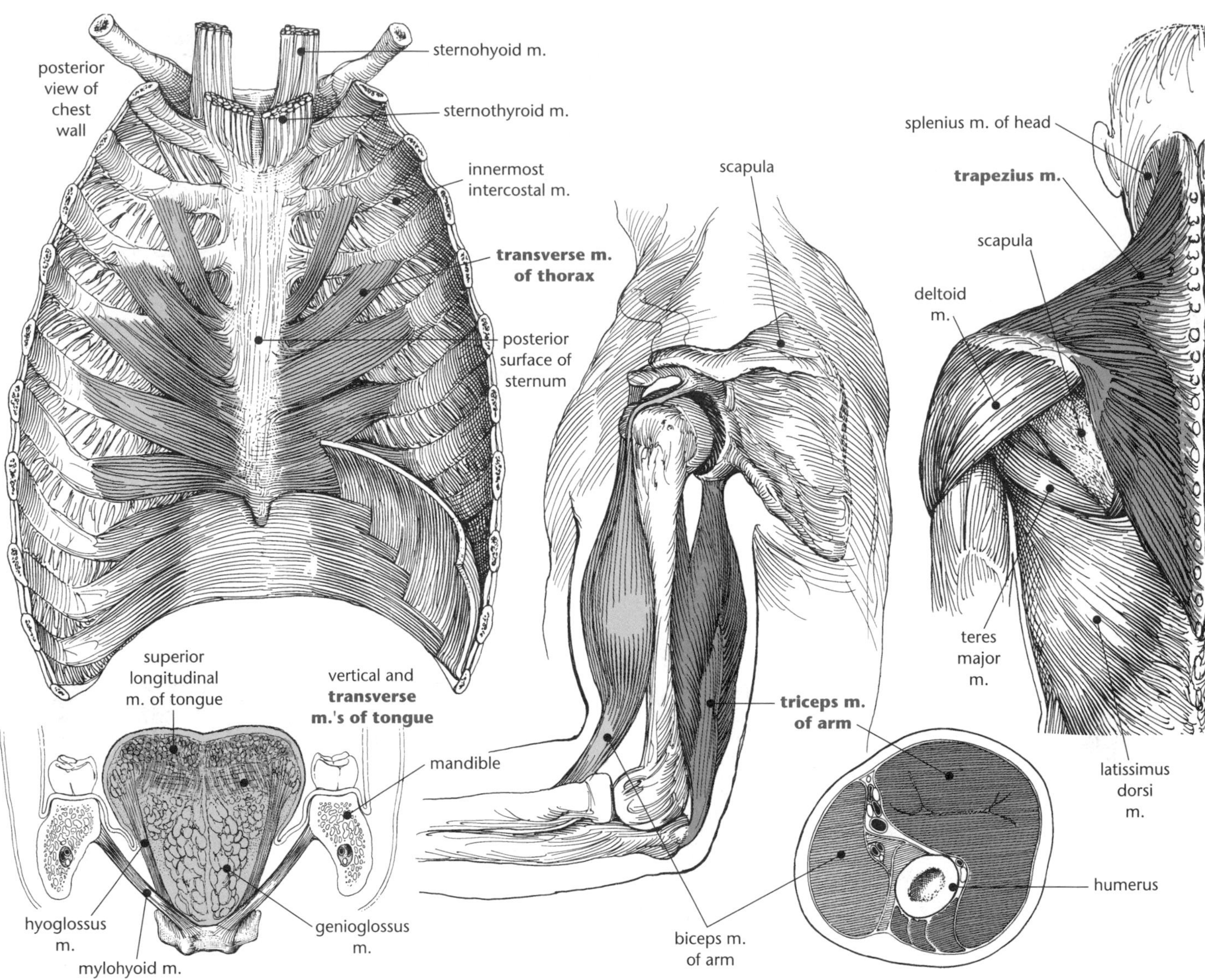

MUSCLE	ORIGIN	INSERTION	ACTION
transverse m. of perineum, superficial *m. transversus perinei superficialis*	ramus of ischium near tuberosity	central tendon of perineum	supports pelvic viscera
transverse m. of thorax sternocostal m. *m. transversus thoracis*	xiphoid process, posterior surface of lower part of sternum, adjacent costal cartilages	second to sixth costal cartilages (inner surface)	narrows chest, draws costal cartilages downward
transverse m. of tongue *m. transversus linguae*	median fibrous septum of tongue	submucous fibrous tissue at sides of tongue	narrows and elongates tongue
trapezius m. *m. trapezius*	superior nuchal line of occipital bone, nuchal ligament, spinous processes of seventh cervical and all thoracic vertebrae, external occipital protruberance	*superior part:* posterior border of lateral third of clavicle; *middle part:* medial margin of acromion, superior lip of posterior border of scapular spine; *inferior part:* tubercle at apex of medial end of scapular spine	elevates shoulder, rotates scapula to raise shoulder in full abduction and flexion of arm, draws scapula backward
triangular m.	see depressor m. of angle of mouth		
triceps m. of arm *m. triceps brachii*	*long head:* infraglenoid tubercle of scapula; *lateral head:* proximal portion of humerus; *medial head:* distal half of humerus	posterior part of superior surface of olecranon process of ulna; adjacent deep fascia; articular capsule of elbow joint	main extensor of forearm

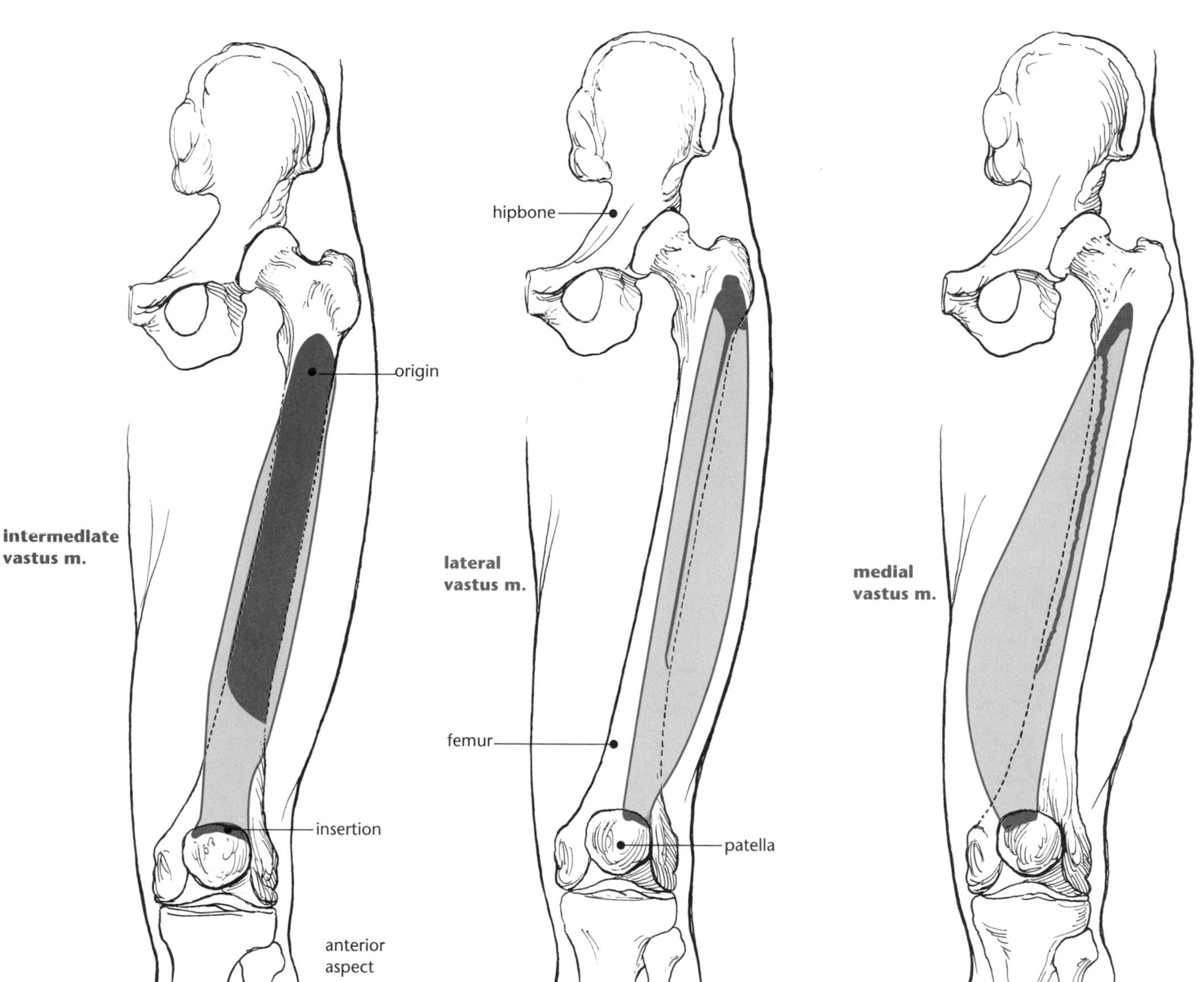

M

MUSCLE	ORIGIN	INSERTION	ACTION
triceps m. of calf *m. triceps surae*	combined gastrocnemius and soleus m.'s; its tendon of insertion is the calcaneal tendon		plantar flexes foot
uvula m. *m. uvulae*	palatine aponeurosis and posterior nasal spine of palatine bone	mucous membrane and connective tissue of uvula	elevates uvula
vastus m., intermediate *m. vastus intermedius*	anterior and lateral surface of the upper two-thirds of femur	common tendon of quadriceps m. of thigh, patella	extends leg
vastus m., lateral *m. vastus lateralis*	lateral aspect of upper part of femur	common tendon of quadriceps m. of thigh, patella	extends leg
vastus m., medial *m. vastus medialis*	medial aspect of femur	common tendon of quadriceps m. of thigh, patella	extends leg
vertical m. of tongue *m. verticalis linguae*	dorsal fascia of tongue	undersurface of tongue	aids in mastication, swallowing, and speech by altering shape of tongue
vocal m. *m. vocalis*	inner surface of thyroid cartilage near midline	vocal process of arytenoid cartilage	adjusts tension of vocal cords
zygomatic m., greater *m. zygomaticus major*	zygomatic arch	angle of mouth	draws upper lip upward and laterally
zygomatic m., smaller *m. zygomaticus minor*	malar surface of zygomatic bone	upper lip	aids in forming nasolabial furrow (m. of facial expression)

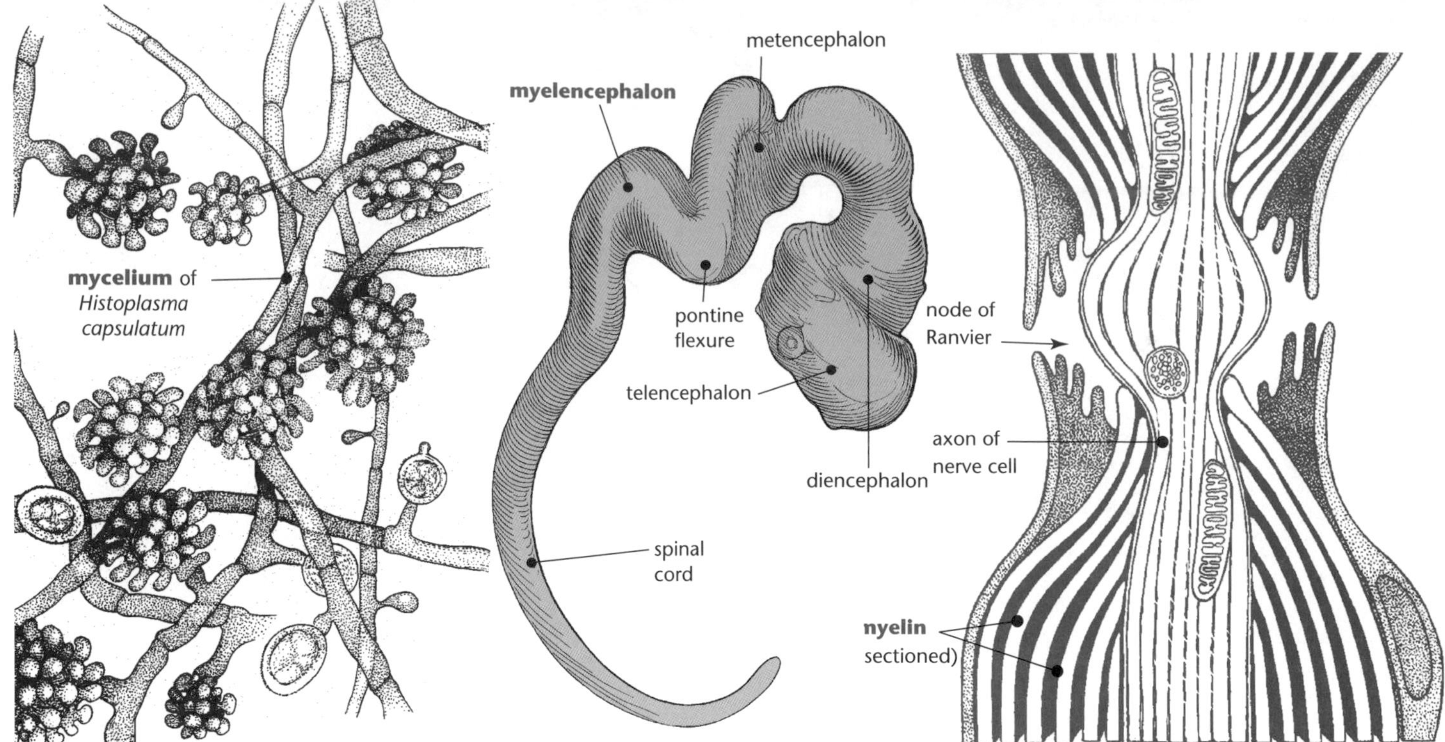

musculor (mus´ku-lar) **1.** Relating to muscles. **2.** Having well-developed muscles.

musculature (mus´ku-lă-chur) The system of muscles in the body or a body part.

musculoaponeurotic (mus-ku-lo-ap-o-nu-rot´ik) Relating to muscle and aponeurosis.

musculocutaneous (mus-ku-lo-ku-ta´ne-us) Relating to muscle and skin, as certain nerves that supply both structures.

musculomembranous (mus-ku-lo-mem´bră-nus) Relating to or composed of muscular and membranous tissues.

musculoskeletal (mus-ku-lo-skel´ĕ-tal) Relating to the muscles and skeleton.

musculospiral (mus-ku-lo-spi´ral) Denoting the distribution of certain nerves (e.g., the radial nerve, which crosses obliquely across the back of the humerus, then spirals around the bone to enter the anterior compartment of the arm).

musculotropic (mus-ku-lo-trop´ik) Acting upon muscle tissue.

Musset's sign (mu-sāz sīn) Rhythmic nodding of the head, occurring in incompetence of the aortic valve.

mutagen (mu´tă-jen) Any agent that causes a permanent, heritable change mutation in the genetic material of a cell (e.g., radioactive substances, certain chemicals).

mutagenesis (mu-tă-jen´ĕ-sis) The formation of a mutation.

mutagenic (mu-tă-jen´ik) Causing mutation.

mutant (mu´tant) An organism or cell differing from the parental strain due to having a gene that has undergone a permanent structural change.

mutase (mu´tās) One of various enzymes that promote the apparent migration of a phosphate group from one hydroxyl group to another of the same molecule.

mutation (mu-ta´shun) **1.** A permanent, heritable, structural change in a gene. **2.** The modified gene.

frameshift m. In genetics, a mutation resulting from deletion or addition that is not an exact multiple of 3 base pairs in a coding gene sequence, thus changing the reading frame of the gene. The altered grouping of 3 bases causes formation of either an elongated or a truncated protein.

missense m. Substitution of one codon for another during protein synthesis, causing the insertion of a different amino acid in the growing polypeptide chain, which results in an altered protein. Frequently called missense.

nonsense m. A single DNA base substitution resulting in a chain-termination codon in the middle of the polypeptide chain.

point m. Mutation involving minute sections of a chromosome (the purine or pyrimidine bases of a single gene), as seen in sickle cell anemia.

reading-frameshift m. See frameshift mutation.

mute (mūt) A person who is unable to speak, or one who refuses to speak for conscious or unconscious reasons.

mutilation (mu-tĭ-la´shun) **1.** Damaging or removing an essential part of the body. **2.** The state of being mutilated.

mutism (mu´tiz-m) Inability to speak.

mutualism (mu´tu-al-iz-m) A state in which two dissimilar organisms live together with mutual benefit; a form of symbiosis.

myalgia (mi-al´jă) Muscle pain.

myasthenia (mi-as-the´ne-ă) Weakness of muscle.

m. gravis (MG) Neuromuscular disorder of autoimmune origin marked by variable degrees of muscular weakness, which may progress to paralysis; it frequently begins in the muscles of the eyes, often associated with abnormalities of the thymus. There is evidence that specific antibodies interfere with the action of the neurotransmitter acetylcholine (Ach) in passing nerve impulses to muscles at the neuromuscular junctions.

myasthenic (mi-as-then´ik) Relating to myasthenia.

myatonia, myatony (mi-ă-to´ne-ă, mi-at´ŏ-ne) Absence of muscle tone.

myatrophy (mi-at´ro-fe) See myoatrophy.

mycelial (mi-se´le-al) Relating to mycelium; having the filamentous appearance of a mold colony.

mycelium (mi-se´le-um) The network of threadlike filaments (hyphae) constituting the body or vegetative portion of a fungus.

mycete (mi´sēt) A fungus.

mycetism, mycetismus (mi´sē-tiz-m, mi-sĕ-tiz´mus) Mushroom poisoning.

mycetogenic, mycetogenous (mi-sĕ-to-jen´ik, mi-sĕ-toj´ĕ-nus) Caused by fungi.

mycetoma (mi-sĕ-to´mă) A chronic disease affecting chiefly the feet, marked by the formation of yellow, white, red, or black granules, draining sinuses, suppuration, and swelling; caused by fungi, especially *Madurella mycetomi.* Also called maduromycosis. Formerly called Madura foot after a city in India where it was first observed.

mycetozoa (mi-se-to-zo´ă) The slime animals; microscopic animal forms, similar to fungi and often regarded as such.

mycid (mi´sid) A secondary lesion occurring in certain mycotic infections.

mycobacteria (mi-ko-bak-te´re-ă) Microorganisms of the genus *Mycobacterium.*

group I m. A group of organisms that produce a bright yellow pigment when grown in the presence of light; some cause a tuberculosis-like disease. Also called photochromogens.

group II m. Mycobacteria that produce a yellow to orange pigment and grow in dead animal or plant tissues. Also called scotochromogens.

group III m. Mycobacteria that either are colorless or produce a light yellow pigment when grown in the presence of light. Also called nonchromogens.

Mycobacterium (mi-ko-bak-te´re-um) A genus (family Mycobacteriaceae) of aerobic gram-positive, acid-fast, nonmotile, rod-shaped bacteria.

***M. avium* complex** (MAC) A bacterial complex that includes several strains of *Mycobacterium avium* and the immunologically related *Mycobacterium intracellulare*; most frequently found in respiratory secretions from persons with a tuberculous-like lung disease; it is the cause of a disseminated blood infection (MAC bacteremia) in AIDS patients. Distinguished from *Mycobacterium avium*, which causes disease primarily in birds. See also *Mycobacterium avium* complex bacteremia, under bacteremia.

M. avium-intracellulare (MAI) Species causing a nontuberculous lung disease in humans, similar to tuberculosis; occurs primarily in persons with underlying lung disease and as an opportunistic infection in AIDS patients.

M. leprae The causative agent of Hansen's disease (leprosy). Also called Hansen's bacillus; leprosy bacillus.

M. marinum Species causing warty skin nodules (granulomas) that may ulcerate; transmitted through contaminated aquariums, swimming pools, or natural bodies of water.

M. tuberculosis The causative agent of tuberculosis in man and animals. Also called Koch's bacillus; tubercle bacillus (human).

mycodermatitis (mi-ko-der-mă-ti´tis) Any fungal infection of the skin.

mycogastritis (mi-ko-gas-tri´tis) Inflammation of the stomach caused by a fungus.

mycologist (mi-kol´o-jist) A specialist in fungi and fungal diseases.

mycology (mi-kol´o-je) The branch of science concerned with the study of fungi.

mycophenolate mofetil (mi-ko-fe´no-lāt mo´fe-til) (MMF) An antibiotic that inhibits maturation of lymphocytes (a type of white blood cell). Used in transplant patients to treat rejection of transplanted tissue.

Mycoplasma (mi-ko-plaz´mă) A genus of bacteria lacking a rigid cell wall, having instead a triple-layered membrane (thus occurring in many shapes); the smallest freeliving organisms presently known, being intermediate in size between viruses and

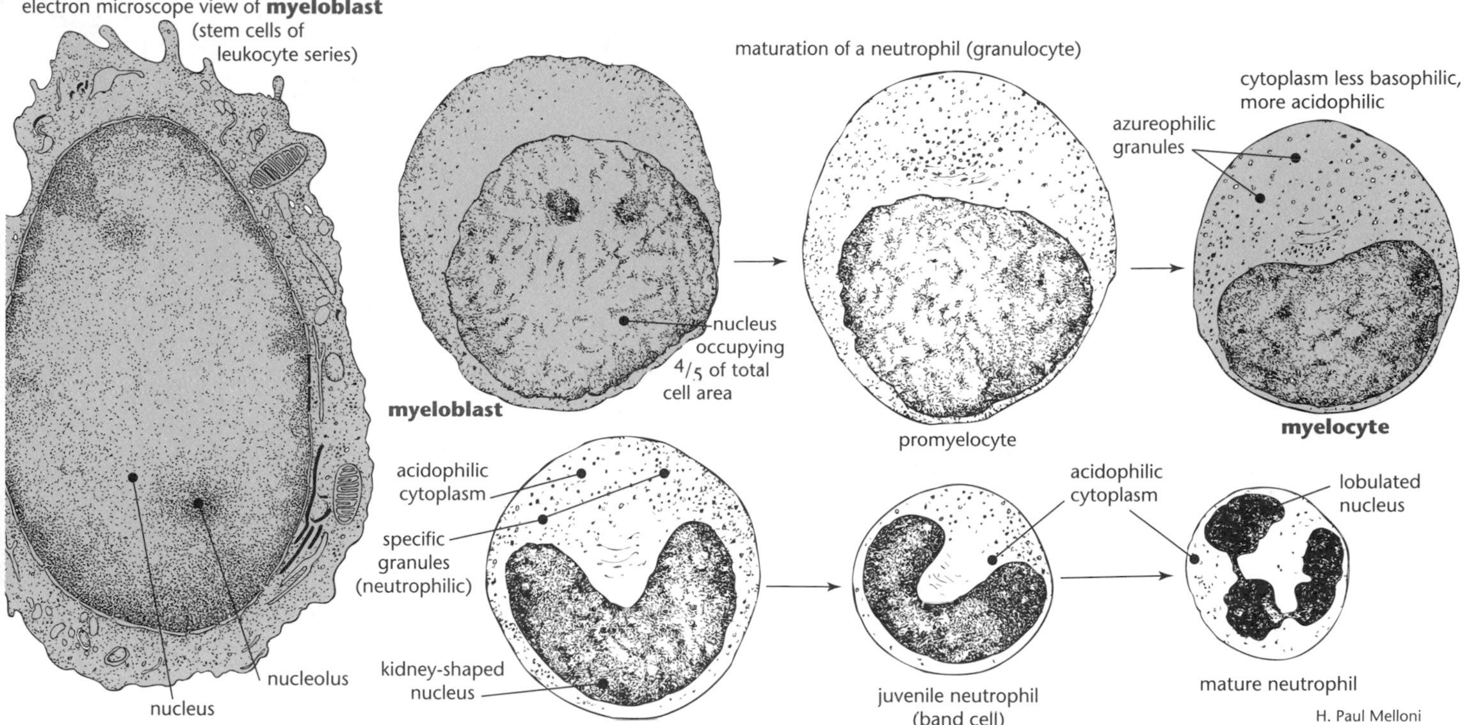

bacteria; some species are pathogenic.

M. pneumoniae A species that is one of the main causes of primary atypical pneumonia in humans. Also called Eaton agent.

mycoplasma (mi-ko-plaz′mă) Any organism of the genus *Mycoplasma*.

T-m.'s Microorganisms known to inhabit the urinary tracts of a large percentage of individuals; they have the capacity to attach to mammalian cells and to aggregate mucoproteins; so called because they form tiny colonies in agar (about 20 μm in diameter).

mycosis (mi-ko′sis) Disease caused by a fungus.

deep m. See systemic mycosis.

systemic m. A serious disease, often fatal, caused by various fungi that can invade the subcutaneous tissues and spread throughout the organism. Also called deep mycosis.

mycotic (mi-kot′ik) Relating to mycosis or any disease caused by fungi or vegetable microorganisms.

mydriasis (mĭ-dri′ă-sis) Dilatation of the pupil.

mydriatic (mid-re-at′ik) Any agent that dilates the pupil.

myectomy (mi-ek′to-me) Surgical removal of a portion of a muscle.

myelencephalon (mi-el-en-sef′ă-lon) The portion of the embryonic brain from which develop the medulla oblongata and the bulbar part of the fourth ventricle; together with the metencephalon, it makes up the hindbrain (rhombencephalon).

myelic (mi′ĕl-ik) **1.** Relating to the spinal cord. **2.** Relating to bone marrow.

myelin (mi′ĕ-lin) Fatty substance that is a major component of the sheath surrounding and insulating the axon of some nerve cells.

myelinated (mĭ′ĕ-lĭ-nāt-ed) Having a myelin sheath.

myelination (mi-ĕ-lĭ-na′shun) The formation of a medullary sheath around a nerve fiber.

myelinolysis (mi-ĕ-lin-ol′ĭ-sis) Demyelination; destruction of the myelin sheath of nerve fibers.

central pontine m. Demyelination distributed about the midbase of the pons.

myelinopathy (mi-ĕ-lĭ-nop′ă-the) Any disorder of the myelin of peripheral nerves.

myelitis (mi-ĕ-li′tis) **1.** Inflammation of the spinal cord. **2.** Inflammation of the bone marrow.

acute necrotizing m. Myelitis causing sensory abnormalities and upper motor neuron weakness leading to paralysis, associated with a necrotizing lesion.

compression m. A progressive form of myelitis due to pressure on the spinal cord, as from a hemorrhage or tumor.

concussion m. Inflammation following concussion of the spinal cord. Also called traumatic myelitis.

disseminated m. Inflammation of several distinct areas of the spinal cord. Also called multiple focal myelitis.

radiation m. Myelitis caused by excessive exposure to x rays.

transverse m. Inflammation extending across the whole thickness of the spinal cord.

traumatic m. See concussion myelitis.

myeloarchitectonics (mi-ĕ-lo-ar-kĭ-tek-ton′iks) The study of the arrangement of nerve fibers in the cerebral cortex.

myeloblast (mi-ĕ-lo-blast) A white blood cell in its earliest stage of development, occurring normally in bone marrow; the first recognizable cell of the granulocytic (myeloid) series; it has a large, oval nucleus that occupies about four-fifths of the cell, usually containing two to five nucleoli; it can differentiate into a neutrophilic, eosinophilic, or basophilic granulocyte. Also called granuloblast.

myeloblastemia (mi-ĕ-lo-blas-te′me-ă) The presence of myeloblasts in the circulating blood.

myeloblastoma (mi-ĕ-lo-blas-to′mă) A nodular accumulation of myeloblasts.

myeloblastosis (mi-ĕ-lo-blas-to′sis) The presence of a large number of myeloblasts in the blood or tissues, as in acute leukemia.

myelocele (mi′ĕ-lo-sēl) Developmental defect in which the vertebral arches are absent, leaving an open groove lined with imperfect spinal cord tissue through which cerebrospinal fluid drains.

myelocyst (mi′ĕ-lo-sist) A cyst originating from a rudimentary medullary canal in the central nervous system.

myelocystic (mi-ĕ-lo-sis′tik) Relating to or of the nature of a myelocyst.

myelocystocele (mi-ĕ-lo-sis′to-sēl) Hernial protrusion of spinal cord substance through a defect in the vertebral column.

myelocyte (mi′ĕ-lo-sīt) **1.** A young cell of the granulocytic (myeloid) series, developed from the promyelocyte and occurring normally in red bone marrow; characterized by a cytoplasm containing specific neutrophilic granules, an oval nucleus with the nuclear chromatin appearing as thick strands, and no discernible nucleoli. **2.** A nerve cell in the gray matter of the brain or spinal cord.

myelocytosis (mi-ĕ-lo-si-to′sis) The increase of myelocytes in circulating blood, above the normal range.

myeloencephalic (mi-ĕ-lo-en-sĕ-fal′ik) Relating to the spinal cord and brain.

myeloencephalitis (mi-ĕ-lo-en-sef-ă-lī′tis) Acute inflammation of the brain and spinal cord. Also called encephalomyelitis.

myelofibrosis (mi-ĕ-lo-fi-bro′sis) A myeloproliferative disorder marked by fibrosis of the bone marrow; may occur as a primary disease or associated with other conditions (e.g., polycythemia vera, or chronic myelocytic leukemia). Also called myelosclerosis; osteomyelofibrotic syndrome.

myelogenesis (mi-ĕ-lo-jen′ĕ-sis) Development of the bone marrow.

myelogenic, myelogenous (mi-ĕ-lo-jen′ik, mi-ĕ-loj′ĕ-nus) Developed in the bone marrow.

myelogram (mi′ĕ-lo-gram) A radiographic record of the spinal cord.

cervical m. Myelogram of the spinal cord in the neck area.

myelography (mi-ĕ-log′ră-fe) Radiography of the spinal cord after introduction of a radiopaque substance into the spinal arachnoid space.

myeloid (mi′ĕ-loid) **1.** Relating to bone marrow. **2.** Relating to the spinal cord.

myeloma (mi-ĕ-lo′mă) Tumor composed of cell types normally found in bone marrow.

multiple m. Disease characterized by the appearance of scattered malignant tumors in various bones of the body; associated with the production of abnormal globulins and the presence of Bence Jones protein in the urine; the condition occurs mostly in persons in the sixth to eighth decade of life and affects males more often than females. Also called multiple plasmacytoma; myelomatosis; plasma cell myeloma.

plasma cell m. See multiple myeloma.

myelomalacia (mi-ĕ-lo-mă-la′shă) Softening of the spinal cord.

myelomatosis (mi-ĕ-lo-mă-to′sis) See multiple myeloma, under myeloma.

myelomeningitis (mi-ĕ-lo-men-in-ji′tis) Inflammation of the spinal cord and its membranes.

myelomeningocele (mi-ĕ-lo-mĕ-ning′go-sēl) See meningomyelocele.

myelon (mi′ĕ-lon) The spinal cord.

myeloneuritis (mi-ĕ-lo-nu-ri′tis) Inflammation of the spinal cord and one or more peripheral nerves.

myelonic (mi-ĕ-lon′ik) Of, or relating to, the spinal cord.

myelopathy (mi-ĕ-lop′ă-the) Any disease of the spinal cord.

myelophthisis (mi-ĕ-lof′thĭ-sis) **1.** Atrophy or wasting of the spinal cord. **2.** Insufficiency of the cell-forming activity of the bone marrow.

myeloplast (mi′ĕ-lo-plast) A leukocyte of the bone marrow.

myelopoiesis (mi-ĕ-lo-poi-e′sis) The formation of bone marrow or the blood cells derived from it.

myeloproliferative (mi-ĕ-lo-pro-lif′er-ă-tiv) Relating to proliferation of blood-forming elements in bone marrow.

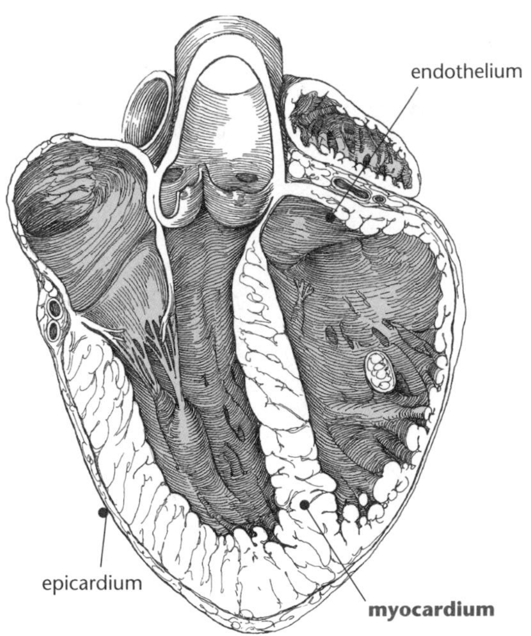

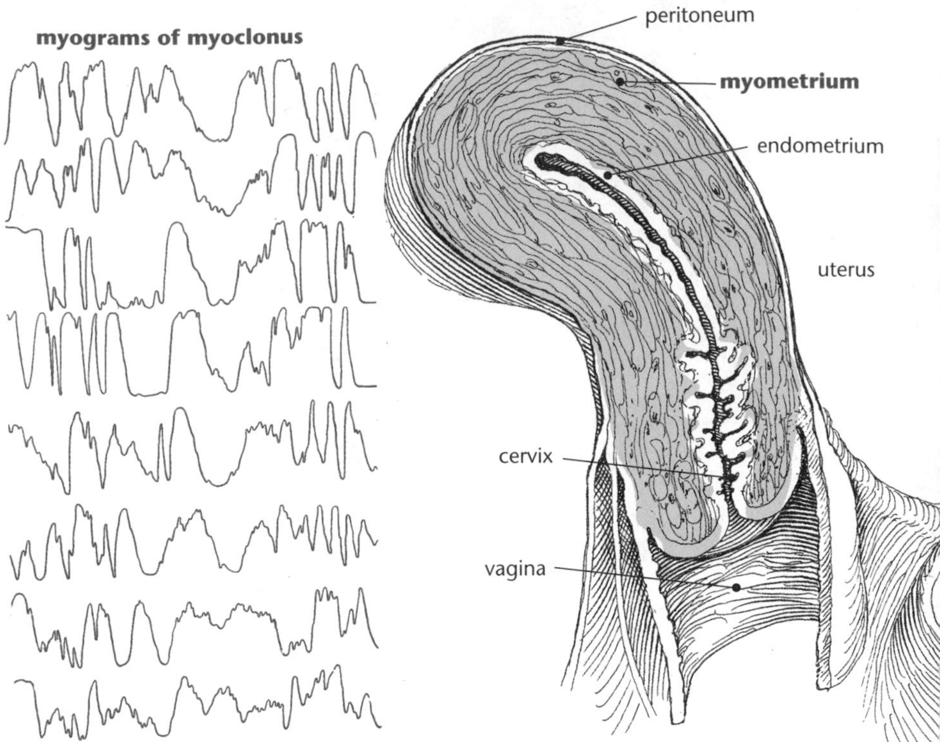

myeloproliferative diseases (mi-ĕ-lo-pro-lif′er-ă-tiv dĭ-zēz′ĕz) A group of disorders characterized by abnormal proliferation of one or more types of bone marrow cells; includes myelofibrosis, polycythemia vera, idiopathic thrombocytosis, and chronic myelogenous leukemia.

myeloradiculitis (mi-ĕ-lo-ră-dik-u-li′tis) Inflammation of the spinal cord and the roots of the spinal nerves.

myeloradiculodysplasia (mi-ĕ-lo-ră-dik-u-lo-dis-pla′zhă) Congenital abnormal development of the spinal cord and spinal nerve roots.

myeloradiculopathy (mi-ĕ-lo-ră-dik-u-lop′ă-the) Disease involving the spinal cord and spinal nerve roots.

myelorrhagia (mi-ĕ-lo-ra′jă) See hematomyelia.

myelosarcoma (mi-ĕ-lo-sar-ko′mă) Malignant tumor derived from bone marrow cells.

myeloschisis (mi-ĕ-los′kĭ-sis) Cleft spinal cord resulting from failure of the normal closing of the neural tube.

myelosclerosis (mi-ĕ-lo-skle-ro′sis) See myelofibrosis.

myelosis (mi-ĕ-lo′sis) Condition marked by abnormal proliferation of blood-forming cells in bone marrow and other organs.

chronic nonleukemic m. Condition characterized primarily by undue proliferation of elements giving rise to white blood cells, the total count remaining normal; a variant of myelofibrosis.

erythremic m. See erythroleukemia.

myelotomy (mi-ĕ-lot′o-me) The cutting of nerve fibers in the spinal cord.

myelotoxic (mi-ĕ-lo-tok′sik) **1.** Destructive to bone marrow. **2.** Relating to diseased bone marrow.

myenteric (mi-en-ter′ik) Relating to the muscular layer (myenteron) of the intestinal wall.

myenteron (mi-en′ter-on) The muscular layer of the intestinal wall.

myesthesia (mi-es-the′zhă) Sensation felt within a muscle.

myiasis (mi′yă-sis) Any infection resulting from infestation of human tissue by fly maggots or flies, usually by deposition of ova by flies in open wounds.

mylohyoid (mi-lo-hi′oid) Relating to the posterior portion of the lower jaw and to the hyoid bone.

myoarchitectonic (mi-o-ar-ke-tek-ton′ik) Relating to the structure of muscles.

myoatrophy (mi-o-at′ro-fe) Wasting away of muscles due to lack of use. Also called myatrophy.

myoblast (mi′o-blast) The embryonic cell which becomes a muscle cell.

myoblastoma (mi-o-blas-to′mă) Tumor composed of immature muscle cells.

granular cell m. See granular cell tumor, under tumor.

myocardial (mi-o-kar′de-al) Pertaining to the heart muscle (myocardium).

myocardiograph (mi-o-kar′de-o-graf) An instrument for graphically recording the action of the heart muscle.

myocardiopathy (mi-o-kar-de-op′a-the) See cardiomyopathy.

myocardiorraphy (mi-o-kar-de-or′ă-fe) Surgical suture of the muscular wall of the heart.

myocarditis (mi-o-kar-di′tis) Inflammation of the heart muscle.

acute isolated m. Acute myocarditis of unknown cause. Also called Fiedler's myocarditis.

Fiedler's m. See acute isolated myocarditis.

myocardium (mi-o-kar′de-um) The middle and thickest layer of the heart wall composed of specialized striated muscle cells and intervening connective tissue; each cell possesses a central nucleus, a plasma membrane (sarcolemma), and numerous contractile myofibrils that are separated by varying amounts of sarcoplasm.

infarcted m. Dead heart muscle resulting, usually, from an occluded artery.

myocele (mi′o-sēl) Herniation of a muscle.

myocellulitis (mi-o-sel-u-li′tis) Inflammation of muscle (myositis) and cellular tissue (cellulitis).

myoclonia (mi-o-klo′ne-ă) Any disorder characterized by twitching or spasmodic contraction of muscles.

myoclonic (mi-o-klon′ik) Marked by myoclonus.

myoclonus (mi-ok′lo-nus, mi-o-klo′nus) A sudden rapid twitch resulting from the sudden contraction of one or more muscle groups.

myocyte (mi′o-sīt) A muscle cell.

myodynamometer (mi-o-di-nă-mom′ĕ-ter) An instrument used to measure muscular strength.

myodystony (mi-o-dis′tŏ-ne) A succession of minute contractions during slow relaxation of a muscle following electrical stimulation.

myoedema (mi-o-ĕ-de′mă) **1.** Swelling of a muscle. **2.** The localized contraction (forming a lump) of a degenerating muscle when struck. Also called mounding.

myoelectric (mi-o-e-lek′trik) Relating to the electric attributes of muscles.

myoendocarditis (mi-o-en-do-kar-di′tis) Inflammation of the wall and lining of the cardiac cavities.

myoepithelium (mi-o-ep-ĭ-the′le-um) Tissue composed of contractile epithelial cells that resemble smooth muscle cells.

myofascial syndrome (mi-o-fash′e-al sin′drōm) A painful condition of muscle that can be elicited by pressure on one or more discrete hypersensitive areas termed trigger points; these trigger points produce pain in the area of the patient's symptoms, which may occur anywhere in the body; a typical example is the temporomandibular joint (TMJ).

myofibril (mi-o-fi′bril) One of the fine longitudinal fibrils present in muscle fiber; each myofibril is divided into a series of repeating units, the sarcomeres, which are the fundamental structural and functional units of contraction.

myofibroma (mi-o-fi-bro′mă) A benign tumor containing fibrous and muscular tissues.

myofibrosis (mi-o-fi-bro′sis) Chronic inflammation of a muscle with excessive formation of connective tissue, resulting in atrophy of the muscular tissue.

myofilaments (mi-o-fil′ă-ments) The microscopic structures that make up the fibrils of striated muscle.

myogen (mi′o-jen) A mixture of proteins, extractable from skeletal muscle with cold water, consisting largely of glycolytic enzymes.

myogenic (mi-o-jen′ik) Of muscular origin.

myoglia (mi-og′le-ă) A fine network of fibrils formed by muscle cells. Also called muscle cement.

myoglobin (mi-o-glo′bin) (MB) An oxygen-transporting protein found in muscle fibers, similar to hemoglobin.

myoglobinuria (mi-o-glo-bin-u′re-ă) The presence of myoglobin in the urine, usually after crush injuries or occasionally after very vigorous exercise. Also called myoglobulinuria.

paroxysmal idiopathic m. See rhabdomyolysis.

myoglobulin (mi-o-glob′u-lin) (Mb) A globulin present in muscle tissue.

myoglobulinuria (mi-o-glob-u-lin-u′re-ă) See myoglobinuria.

myogram (mi′o-gram) A tracing produced by myography.

myograph (mi′o-graf) An instrument for graphically recording muscular contractions.

myography (mi-og′ră-fe) A technique used to record muscular activity.

myoid (mi′oid) Resembling muscle.

myoischemia (mi-o-is-ke′me-ă) Lack of blood supply to localized areas of muscle tissue.

myokymia (mi-o-kim′e-ă) A twitching or tremor of individual fasciculi (bundles of fibers) of a muscle.

myolipoma (mi-o-li-po′mă) A benign tumor composed chiefly of adipose and muscle tissues.

myology (mi-ol′o-je) The study of muscles.

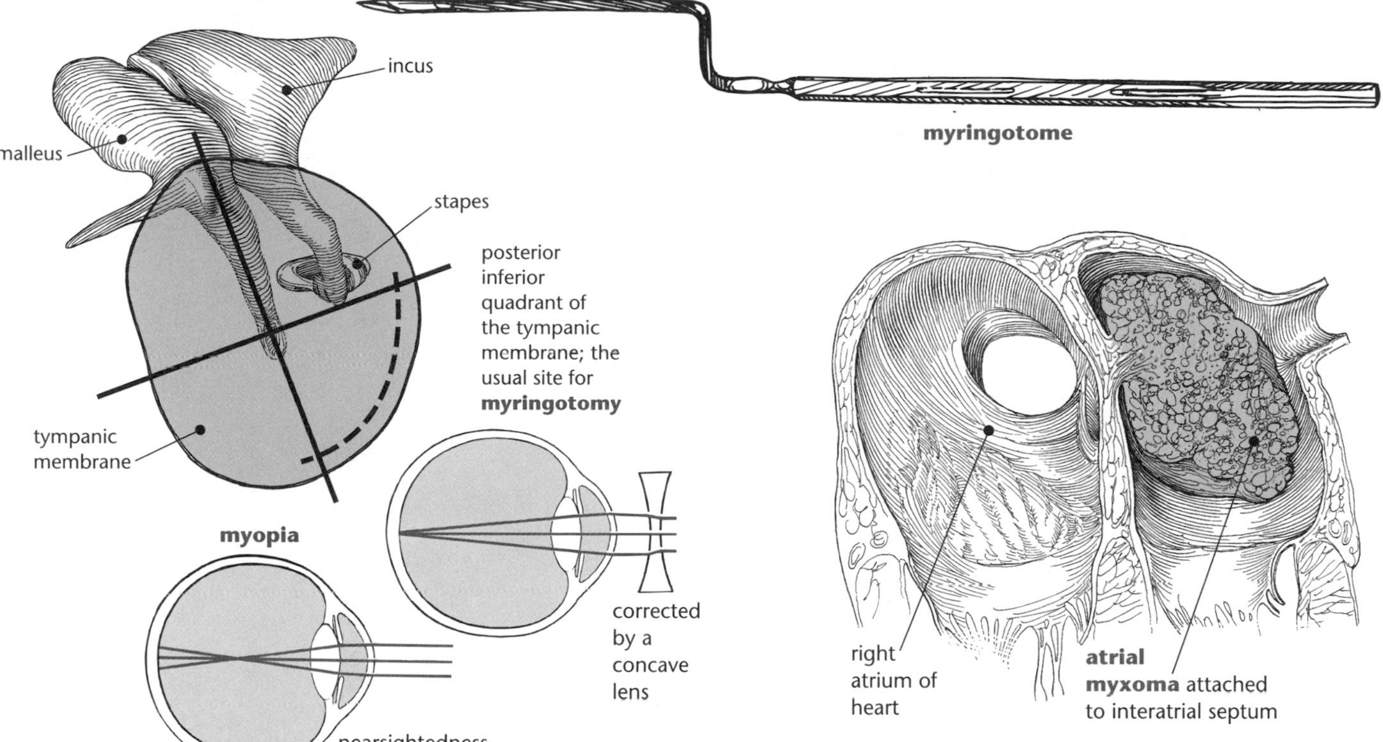

myolysis (mi-ol´ĭ-sis) Disintegration of muscle tissue.

myoma (mi-o´mă) A benign tumor consisting of muscle tissue.

myomalacia (mi-o-mă-la´shă) Abnormal softening and degeneration of muscular tissue.

myomatous (mi-o´mă-tus) Resembling a myoma.

myomectomy (mi-o-mek´to-me) Surgical removal of a myoma, especially of the uterus.

myometer (mi-om´ĕ-ter) An apparatus for determining the strength of a muscular contraction.

myometritis (mi-o-mĕ-tri´tis) Inflammation of the muscular layer of the uterine wall.

myometrium (mi-o-me´tre-um) The thick, smooth muscle forming the middle layer of the uterine wall.

myon (mi´on) A functional unit consisting of a muscle fiber with its basal membrane, together with the associated blood capillaries and nerves.

myonecrosis (mi-o-ne-kro´sis) Death of muscle tissue.

myoneural (mi-o-nu´ral) Relating to muscle and nerve, as the nerve endings that terminate in muscular tissue.

myopathy (mi-op´ă-the) Any disease of muscular tissue.

myopericarditis (mi-o-per-ĭ-kar-di´tis) Inflammation of the muscle tissue of the heart and the enveloping membrane (pericardium).

myopia (mi-o´pe-ă) (M, My) Condition in which light rays entering the eyeball from a distance focus in front of the retina, causing only near objects to be seen in focus. Also called near sight; nearsightedness; shortsightedness.

myopic (mi-op´ik) Relating to or afflicted with myopia.

myoplasm (mi´o-plaz-m) The contractile part of a muscle cell.

myoplasty (mi´o-plas-te) Surgical repair of a muscle.

myorrhaphy (mi-or´ă-fe) Suture of a muscle wound.

myorrhexis (mi-o-rek´sis) The tearing or rupturing of a muscle.

myosarcoma (mi-o-sar-ko´mă) A general term for a malignant neoplasm or sarcoma derived from muscular tissue.

myosclerosis (mi-o-skle-ro´sis) Chronic inflammation of a muscle with overgrowth of the interstitial connective tissue, resulting in hardening of the muscle.

myosin (mi´o-sin) The thick filaments of polymerized protein molecules in the myofibril which, along with the protein actin, are responsible for muscular contraction; they comprise the dark A bands seen microscopically; called "A" bands because they are anisotropic to polarized light.

myosis (mi-o´sis) Miosis.

myositis (mi-o-si´tis) Inflammation of a muscle, usually a voluntary muscle.

m. ossificans Condition in which muscular tissue is replaced by bone; it may be localized following an injury or, rarely, it may be generalized, progressive (beginning in childhood), and due to unknown causes.

myospasm (mi´o-spaz-m) Spasmodic contraction of a muscle or group of muscles.

myostatin (mi-o-sta´tin) Member of a family of tumor growth factors that limit muscle size.

myotactic (mi-o-tak´tik) Relating to the muscular proprioceptive sense; denoting any reflex elicited by tapping the belly or tendon of a muscle.

myotasis (mi-ot´ă-sis) The stretching of muscle.

myotatic (mi-o-tat´ik) Relating to the stretching of a muscle.

myotome (mi´o-tōm) **1.** Knife used in surgery to divide muscle. **2.** In embryology, the portion of the mesodermic somite from which skeletal muscle develops.

myotomy (mi-ot´o-me) **1.** Dissection of muscles. **2.** Surgical division of a muscle.

myotonia (mi-o-to´ne-ă) Temporary rigidity of a muscle or group of muscles.

m. atrophica See myotonic dystrophy, under dystrophy.

m. congenita Hereditary condition marked by temporary tonic spasm of certain muscles whenever a voluntary movement is attempted. Also called myotonia hereditaria; Thomsen's disease.

m. hereditaria See myotonia congenita.

myotonic (mi-o-ton´ik) Characterized by myotoma.

myringectomy (mir-in-jek´to-me) Surgical removal of the tympanic membrane (eardrum).

myringitis (mir-in-ji´tis) Inflammation of the tympanic membrane.

myringoplasty (mĭ-ring´go-plas-te) A surgical procedure performed to close a perforation of the eardrum acquired through injury or infection. Also called type I tympanoplasty.

myringorupture (mĭ-ring-go-rup´chur) The tearing or rupturing of the tympanic membrane (eardrum).

myringotome (mĭ-ring´go-tōm) A knife used for puncturing the tympanic membrane.

myringotomy (mir-in-got´o-me) Surgical incision of the tympanic membrane (eardrum) to allow drainage of the middle ear chamber. Also called ototomy; tympanotomy.

mysophobia (mi-so-fo´be-ă) Morbid fear of contamination, manifested by constant hand washing.

mythomania (mith-o-ma´ne-ă) An abnormal compulsion to tell lies.

myxadenoma (miks-ad-ĕ-no´mă) Benign tumor derived from glandular epithelial tissue.

myxedema (mik-sĕ-de´mă) A severe form of hypothyroidism occurring in juveniles and adults; caused by insufficient circulating thyroid hormone, marked by dry skin, brittle hair, swelling of the face, puffy eyelids, dull expression, and muscle weakness.

pretibial m. A bulging over the lateral aspect of the lower leg above the lateral malleolus, due to localized mucoid deposits in subcutaneous tissues; usually associated with Graves' disease.

myxedematous (mik-sĕ-dem´ă-tus) Relating to myxedema.

myxochondrofibrosarcoma (mik-so-kon-fro-fi-bro-sar-ko´mă) A malignant tumor derived from fibrous connective tissue.

myxochondroma (mik-so-kon-dro´mă) A benign tumor composed chiefly of cartilaginous tissue.

myxocyte (mik´so-sīt) One of the stellate or polyhedral cells found in mucous tissue.

myxofibroma (mik-so-fi-bro´mă) A benign tumor of connective tissue containing portions that resemble primitive mesenchymal tissue.

myxoid (mik´soid) Resembling or containing mucus.

myxolipoma (mik-so-li-po´mă) A benign tumor of adipose tissue containing portions that resemble primitive mesenchymal tissue.

myxoma (mik-so´mă) A benign tumor composed of connective tissue embedded in a soft, mucoid matrix.

atrial m. Myxoma arising from the lining of the atria and resembling a polyp; it may cause murmurs that change with shifts in body position or simulate mitral or tricuspid stenosis.

myxoneuroma (mik-so-nu-ro´mă) Tumor resulting from proliferation of Schwann cells in which degenerative changes produce areas that resemble primitive mesenchymal tissue.

myxopoiesis (mik-so-poi-e´sis) The formation of mucus.

myxosarcoma (mik-so-sar-ko´mă) A malignant tumor derived from connective tissue.

myxospore (mik´so-spōr) A spore embedded in a gelatinous mass.

myxovirus (mik-so-vi´rus) General term for a group of viruses that include the influenza, mumps, and Newcastle disease viruses.

M

N

nacreous (na´kre-us) Having a mother-of-pearl luster; iridescent.

nadolol (na-do´lol) A long-acting β_1- and β_2-adrenergic blocking agent.

nafcillin (naf-sil´in) A semisynthetic penicillin that is not readily destroyed by gastric acids.

nail (nāl) **1.** The keratinous structure at the end of a finger (fingernail) or toe (toenail), composed of several layers of flat, clear cells. Also called unguis. **2.** A metal rod for fixation of a fractured bone.

hippocratic n. A deformed overhanging fingernail associated with the clubbing of terminal phalanges in certain pulmonary and cardiac conditions.

ingrown n. A toenail with its edges growing abnormally into the soft tissues. Also called onychocryptosis.

nailing (nāl´ing) The fastening of a fractured bone with a nail.

nail-patella syndrome (nāl-pă-tel´ă sin´drōm) Autosomal dominant inheritance marked by bilateral underdevelopment of the kneecap, deformity and dislocation of the head of the radius, and dystrophy of fingernails.

nalorphine (nal´or-fēn, nal-or´fēn) $C_{19}H_{21}NO_3$; narcotic antagonist used as an antidote to narcotic overdosage; capable of causing withdrawal symptoms in narcotic addicts; Nalline®.

naloxone (nal-oks´ōn) Narcotic antagonist used in treating respiratory depression suspected of being produced by a narcotic; Narcan®.

name (nām) A word that designates and distinguishes one entity from another.

brand n. See trade name.

chemical n. A scientific name that indicates a precise chemical structure; e.g., 2-(diphenylmethoxy)-*N*,*N*-dimethylethylamine hydrochloride (Benadryl®). Also called systematic name.

N

generic n. Strictly defined, a name that designates a family relationship among drugs, e.g., antihistamine, barbiturate; often used as a synonym for nonproprietary name, e.g., diphenhydramine (Benadryl®).

nonproprietary n. A name assigned to a drug (by the United States Adopted Name Council) when it is found to have therapeutic value; it indicates the chemical composition of the drug and is not protected by trademark registration; e.g., diphenhydramine (Benadryl®). Also called official name.

official n. See nonproprietary name.

proprietary n. See trade name.

semisystematic n., semitrivial n. A name used in the sciences, especially chemistry, composed of two parts, one of which relates to a scientific (systematic) name, the other to a common (trivial) name; e.g., cortisone, derived from cortex and the suffix *-one* (indicating an aldehyde group).

systematic n. See chemical name.

trade n. A name selected by the pharmaceutical company that manufactures and sells the drug; it is registered and protected by a trademark and is usually followed by an encircled superscript R (e.g., Benadryl®). Also called brand name; proprietary name.

trivial n. A common name that tells nothing about the structure of the organism or chemical it designates (e.g., water, caffeine).

nanocephaly (na-no-sef´ă-le) See microcephaly.

nanocormia (na-no-kor´me-ă) Abnormal smallness of the body in relation to the head and extremities.

nanogram (na´no-gram) (ng) A unit of weight equal to one-billionth of a gram; 10^{-9} gram.

nanomelia (na-no-me´le-ă) Abnormal smallness of the extremities.

nanomelus (na-nom´ĕ-lus) Individual characterized by nanomelia.

nanometer (na-no-me´ter, na-nom´ĕ-ter) (nm) A unit of linear measure equal to one- thousandth of a micron; 10^{-9} meter. Also called millimicron.

nanosecond (na-no-sek´ond) (nsec) A unit of time equal to one-billionth of a second; 10^{-9} second.

nanosomia, nanosoma (nan-o-so´me-ă, nan-o-som´ă) See dwarfism.

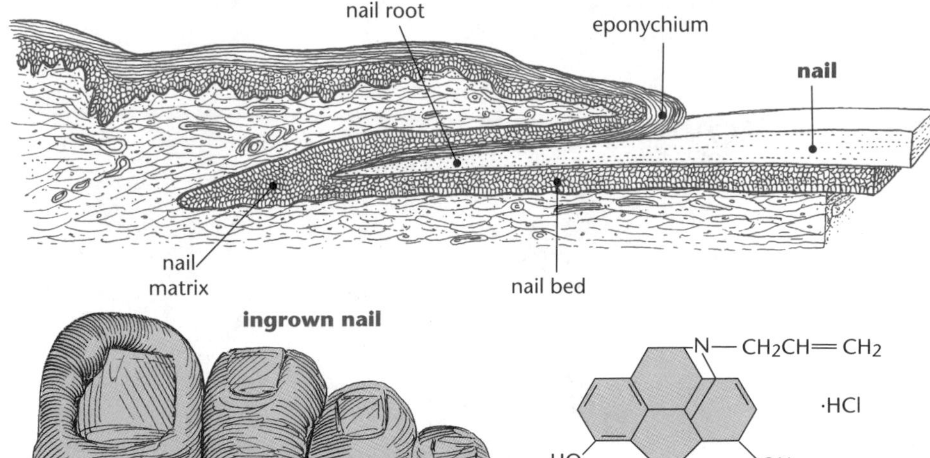

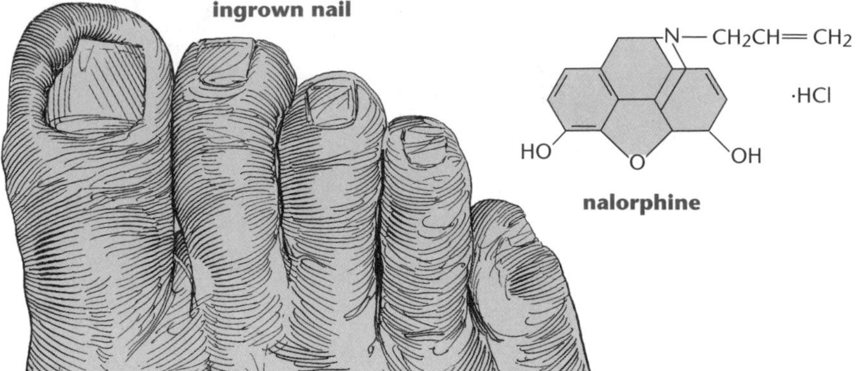

nanus (nă´nus) See dwarf.

nape (nāp) The back of the neck. Also called nucha.

naphthalene (naf´thă-lēn) Tar camphor, a crystalline hydrocarbon derived from coal tar, insoluble in water, and soluble in alcohol; used as an insecticide (mothballs) and antiseptic, and in the manufacture of indigo and lampblack.

naphthol (naf´thol) A crystalline, antiseptic derivative of naphthalene.

α-naphthol (al´fa-naf´thol) Colorless crystals, soluble in water; used in microscopy. Also written alpha-naphthol.

narcissism (nar´sĭ-siz-m) Self-love, as opposed to object-love or love of another person; the term is derived from Narcissus, a figure in Greek mythology who fell in love with his own reflected image.

narcoanalysis (nar-ko-an-al´ĭ-sis) Psychotherapeutic treatment conducted with the aid of a partial anesthetic. Also called narcosynthesis.

narcolepsy (nar´ko-lep-se) Condition characterized by paroxysmal episodes of sleep lasting from minutes to hours; frequently accompanied by transient muscular weakness, sleep paralysis, and hallucinations during the period between sleep and wakefulness. Also called paroxysmal sleep; sleep epilepsy.

narcomania (nar-ko-ma´ne-ă) An uncontrollable craving for narcotics.

narcosis (nar-ko´sis) A deep stuporous state produced by certain chemical and physical agents.

narcosynthesis (nar-ko-sin´thĕ-sis) See narcoanalysis.

narcotherapy (nar-ko-ther´ă-pe) Psychotherapy conducted after a state of complete relaxation is induced by injecting a barbiturate drug intravenously (either sodium amytal or sodium pentothal). Under this therapy some individuals have a capacity to communicate thoughts previously repressed.

narcotic (nar-kot´ik) **1.** Producing narcosis. **2.** Generally, any physical or chemical agent that produces narcosis. **3.** A drug intended for the relief of pain that also tends to produce insensibility, stupor, and sleep; with prolonged use it may become addictive.

narcotism (nar´ko-tiz-m) Addiction to a narcotic drug.

narcotize (nar´ko-tīz) To subject to the influence of a narcotic.

naris (na´ris), *pl.* **na´res** See nostril.

posterior n. See choana.

nasal (na´zal) Relating to the nose.

nascent (nas´ent, na´sent) Beginning to exist; denoting an atom or element at the moment it is liberated from a compound.

nasion (na´ze-on) A craniometric point: the midline of the nasofrontal suture. Also called nasal point.

nasoantral (na-zo-an´tral) Relating to the nose and the maxillary sinus (antrum).

nasoendoscope (na-zo-en´do-skōp) Instrument for examining of the nasal cavity and postnasal space; it has a self-contained illumination and magnifying lens that is passed through the nostril.

nasofrontal (na-zo-frun´tal) Relating to the nose and frontal bones.

nasolabial (na-zo-la´be-al) Relating to the nose and lip.

nasolacrimal (na-zo-lak´rĭ-mal) **1.** Relating to the nasal and lacrimal bones. **2.** Relating to the nose and the structures producing and conveying tears.

naso-oral (na-zo-o´ral) Relating to the nose and mouth.

nasopalatine (na-zo-pal´ă-tīn) Relating to the nose and palate.

nasopharyngeal (na-zo-fă-rin´je-al) Relating to the nasopharynx.

nasopharyngitis (na-zo-far-in-jī´tis) Inflammation of the nasopharynx.

nasopharyngoscope (na-zo-fă-rin´go-skōp) An instrument for visual examination of the nasal passages and the nasopharynx.

nasopharynx (na-zo-far´inks) The uppermost part of the pharynx immediately behind the nasal cavity, above the level of the soft palate. Also called rhinopharynx.

nasoscope (na´zo-skōp) See rhinoscope.

nasoseptal (na-zo-sep´tal) Pertaining to the septum of the cavity of the nose.

nasoseptitis (na-zo-sep-tī´tis) Inflammation of the lining of the nasal septum.

nasosinusitis (na-zo-si-nu-sī´tis) Inflammation of the lining of the nasal cavity and adjacent sinuses.

nasus (na´sus) Latin for nose.

nasute (na´soot) **1.** Having a long or large nose. **2.** Possessing a keen sense of smell.

natal (na´tal) Relating to birth.

natality (na-tal´ĭ-te) The birth rate.

nates (na´tēz) The buttocks.

natiform (na´tĭ-form) Shaped like the buttocks.

natimortality (na-tĭ-mor-tal´ĭ-te) See fetal death rate, under rate.

National Formulary (nash´ĭn-ăl for´mu-ler-ē) (NF) An official publication of the American Pharmaceutical Association that provides authoritative information on drugs.

National Institutes of Health (nash´ĭn-ăl in´stĭ-toots ŭv hĕlth) (NIH) An agency of the United States Public Health Service; consists of eighteen health institutes that support integrated programs of research, clinical trials, and demonstrations relating to cause, diagnosis, and treatment of disease.

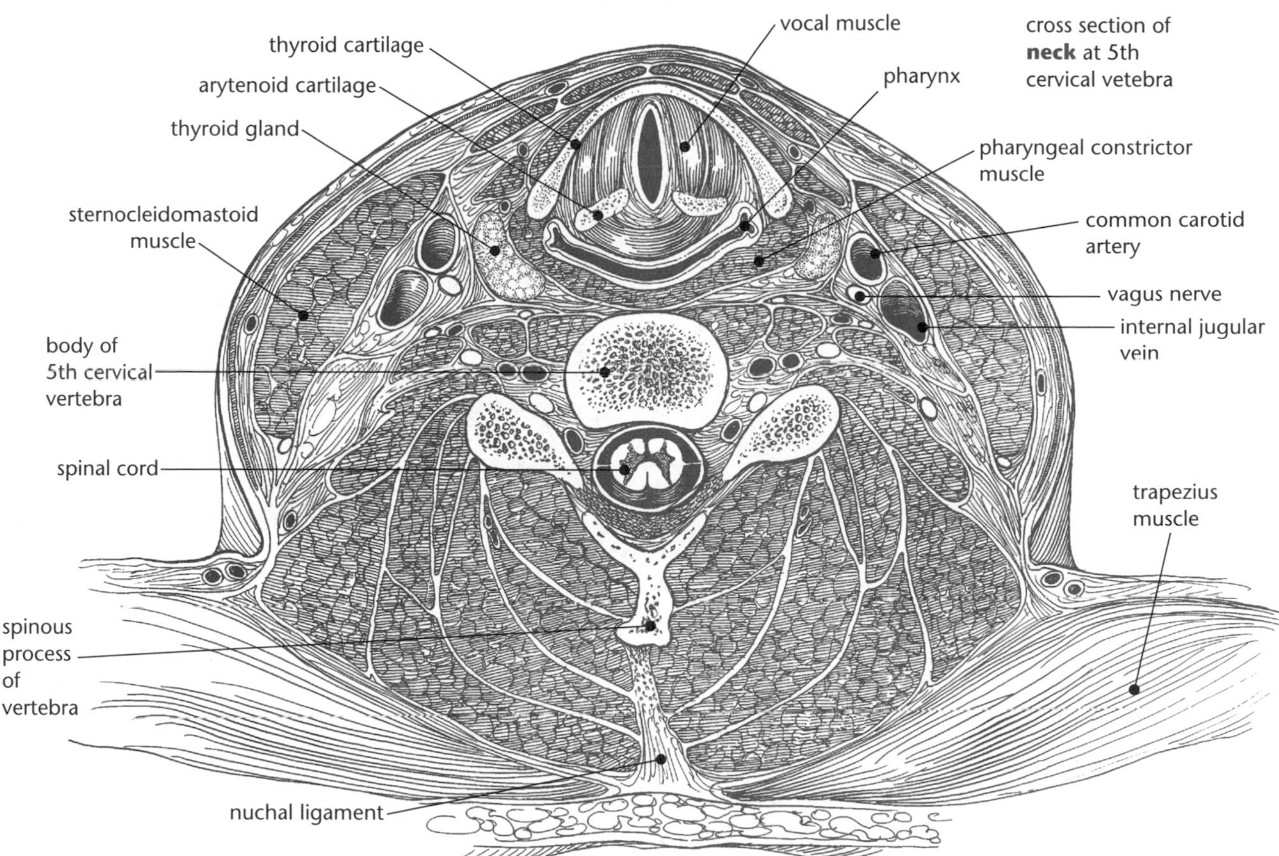

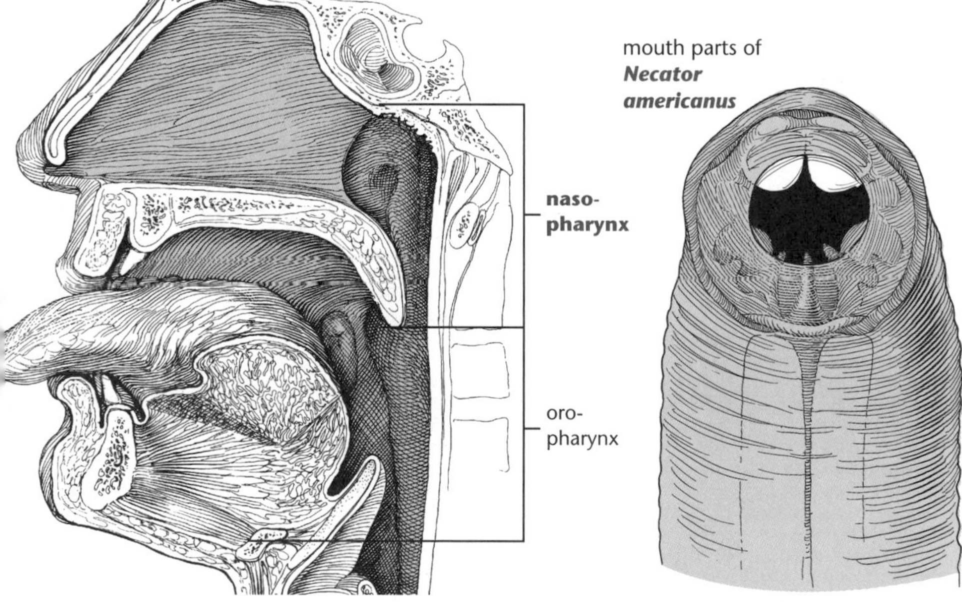

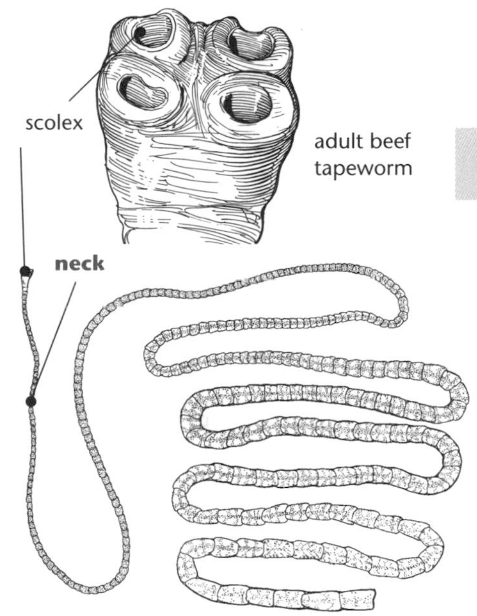

N

natrium (na´tre-um) Latin for sodium (Na).

natriuresis (na-tre-u-re´sis) Increased sodium excretion in the urine.

natriuretic (na-tre-u-ret´ik) **1.** Relating to the excretion of sodium in the urine. **2.** An agent promoting excretion of sodium.

naturopath (na´tūr-o-path) One who practices naturopathy.

naturopathy (na-tūr-op´ă-the) An alternative treatment of disease by using the forces of nature (e.g., light, heat, water, cold) supplemented with massage and diet.

nausea (naw´ze-ă) A feeling of the need to vomit.

n. gravidarum Nausea occurring in some pregnant women.

nauseant (naw´ze-ant) **1.** Nauseating; inducing a feeling of the need to vomit. **2.** Any agent that induces nausea.

nauseate (naw´ze-āt) To cause a desire to vomit.

nauseous (naw´shus) Relating to or causing nausea.

navel (na´vel) See umbilicus.

navicular (nă-vik´u-lar) Boat-shaped. See table of bones.

nearsightedness (nēr´sīt-ed-nes) See myopia.

nebula (neb´u-lă) A slight opacity of the cornea.

nebulization (neb-u-li-za´shun) The process of nebulizing.

nebulize (neb´u-līz) **1.** To create a fine spray from a liquid. **2.** To medicate through a fine spray.

nebulizer (neb´u-līz-er) An apparatus for dispersing a liquid in the form of a fine spray.

Necator (ne-ka´tor) A genus of hookworms of the class Nematoda.

N. americanus A nematode parasite that produces the human hookworm disease (necatoriasis). Also called American hookworm; New World hookworm.

necatoriasis (ne-ka-to-rī´ă-sis) Human hookworm disease caused by the nematode parasite *Necator americanus*.

neck (nek) **1.** The part of the body between the head and the trunk. **2.** Any relatively constricted portion of a structure or organ. **3.** The germinative portion of an adult tapeworm; the region of cestode segmentation behind the scolex. **4.** The portion of a tooth between the crown and root.

anatomic n. of humerus A narrow groove separating the head of the humerus from its tubercles; it affords attachment to the capsular ligament of the shoulder-joint.

n. of femur A more or less conical portion of bone separating the head and shaft of the femur.

stiff n. See torticollis.

surgical n. of humerus The constriction below the tubercles of the humerus; a frequent site of fractures.

n. of talus A constriction separating the head

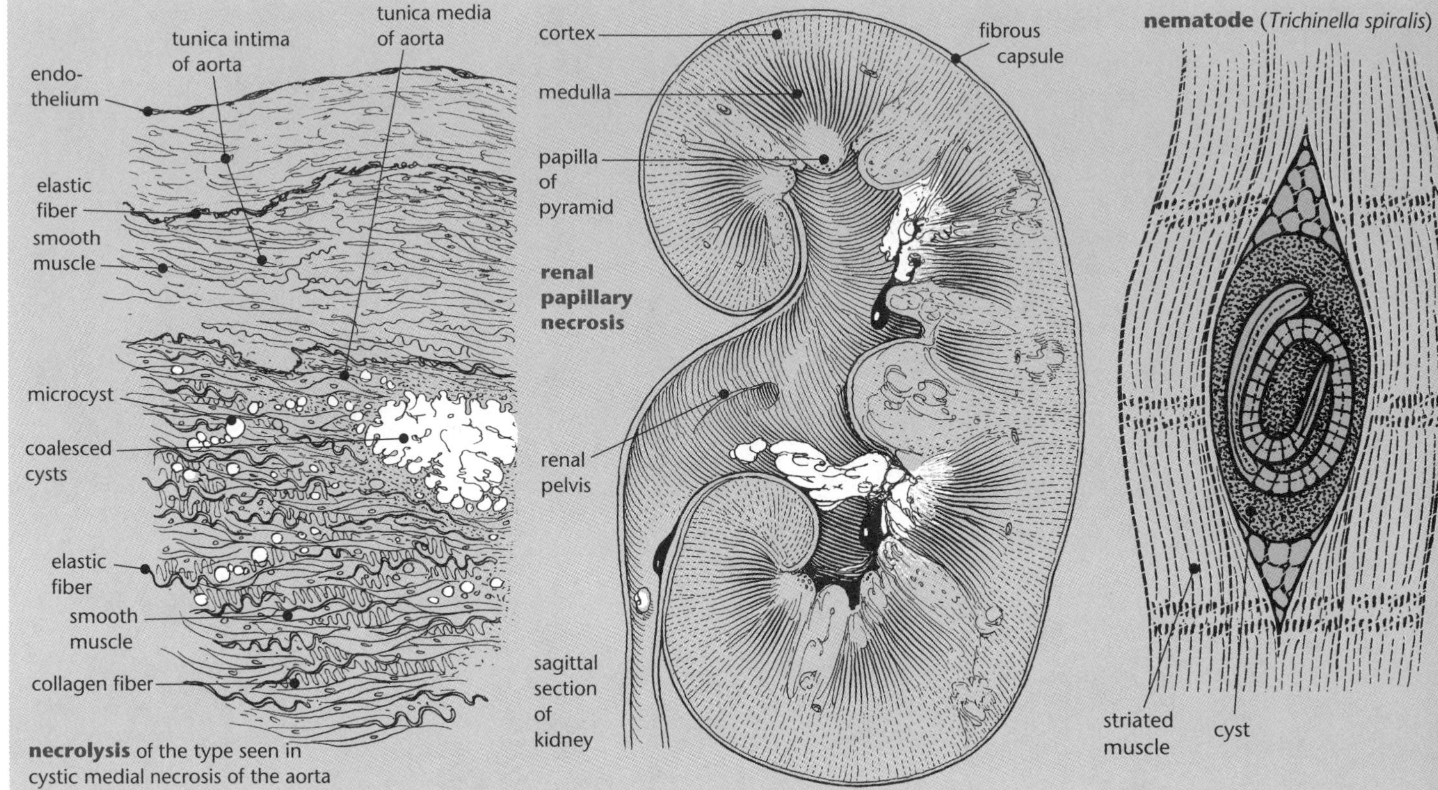

necrolysis of the type seen in cystic medial necrosis of the aorta

from the body of the ankle bone (talus).

webbed n. A neck with lateral folds extending from the head to the clavicles, giving it a broad, short appearance.

n. of womb See uterine cervix, under cervix.

necrobiosis (nek-ro-bi-o′sis) The natural death of tissue with the concurrent replacement thereof.

n. diabeticorum A condition characterized by patchy degeneration of the skin in which fat tissue is extensively involved in the concurrent degeneration and reparative process; usually, but not exclusively, associated with diabetes mellitus.

necrocytosis (nek-ro-si-to′sis) Abnormal degeneration and death of cells.

necrogenic (nek-ro-jen′ik) Originating in dead matter.

necrology (nĕ-krol′o-je) **1.** A record of people who have died, especially during a specific period of time. **2.** The study of death statistics.

necrolysis (nĕ-krol′ĭ-sis) Loosening or separation of tissue due to death and decay of cells.

toxic epidermal n. (TEN) Acute desquamative condition marked by formation of large blisters and/or loss of diffuse sheets of skin; may occur as a reaction to systemic drugs; may also be due to unknown causes.

necromania (nek-ro-ma′ne-ă) Morbid interest in death or dead bodies.

necroparasite (nek-ro-par′a-sīt) See saprophyte.

necrophile (nek′ro-fīl) One afflicted with necrophilia.

necrophilia (nek-ro-fil′e-ă) An abnormal fascination with the dead; especially erotic attraction for contact with dead bodies.

necrophilous (nĕ-krof′ĭ-lus) Feeding on dead tissue; said of certain bacteria.

necrophobia (nek-ro-fo′be-ă) A morbid fear of death or dead bodies.

necropsy (nek′rop-se) See autopsy.

necroscopy (nĕ-kros′ko-pe) See autopsy.

necrose (nek′rōs) To cause or undergo irreversible damage, decomposition, and death; said of cells, tissues, and organs. Also called necrotize.

necrosis (nĕ-kro′sis) Death of tissue within a circumscribed area.

acute tubular n. (ATN) A form of acute renal failure usually caused by a toxic agent or associated with a hypotensive period, especially from shock, sepsis, or trauma; characterized classically by absent or scanty urine followed by gradually increasing flow of dilute urine, often reaching very large amounts.

aseptic n. Necrosis occurring without infection. See also epiphyseal aseptic necrosis.

avascular n. (AVN) Necrosis caused by deficient blood supply; may occur anywhere in the body.

caseous n. Necrosis in which the tissue becomes soft, dry, and cheeselike, as in the lesions of tuberculosis.

central n. Necrosis involving the inner portion of a part, as necrosis in the cells surrounding the central veins of the liver.

coagulation n. Necrosis induced by loss of arterial blood supply to a tissue, leading to denaturation and coagulation of cell protein. Also called ischemic necrosis.

colliquative n. See liquefactive necrosis.

cystic medial n. (CMN) Focal accumulation of mucopolysaccharide in the middle layer of the aortic wall with fragmentation of connective tissue; affects especially the ascending aorta. Also called medionecrosis of aorta; mucoid medial degeneration.

epiphyseal aseptic n. Avascular necrosis affecting long bones, most commonly occurring in the femur (near the hip joint). Also called Legg-Calvé-Perthes disease.

fat n. Destruction of fatty tissue characterized by the formation of small, white, chalky areas. Also called adiponecrosis; steatonecrosis.

ischemic n. See coagulation necrosis.

liquefactive n. Complete and rapid dissolution of cells (including cell membranes) by enzymes, forming circumscribed areas of softened tissue with a semifluid exudate; characteristic of abscesses and infarcts of the brain. Also called colliquative necrosis.

renal papillary n. Ischemic necrosis of the renal papillae, usually occurring in patients with diabetes mellitus and pyelonephritis, in individuals who have habitually ingested large quantities of analgesic medicines, in sickle cell disease, and in the presence of obstructive uropathy and infection. Also called necrotizing papillitis.

necrospermia (nek-ro-sper′me-ă) Condition in which the semen contains a high percentage of nonmotile spermatozoa.

necrotic (nĕ-krot′ik) Relating to dead tissue.

necrotize (nĕ-kro′tīz) See necrose.

necrotomy (nĕ-krot′o-me) Surgical removal of a dead portion of a bone (sequestrum). Also called necrectomy.

needle (ne′dl) **1.** A slender, pointed implement for stitching or puncturing. **2.** To separate tissues. **3.** To puncture the lens capsule to allow absorption of the lens substance, a surgical procedure for the treatment of soft cataract.

acupuncture n. A fine needle, usually 76.2 to 127.0 mm in length, used to perform acupuncture.

aneurysm n. A needle with a curved blunt end for passing a ligature around a blood vessel.

aspirating n. A long, hollow needle used to withdraw fluid from a cavity.

atraumatic n. An eyeless surgical needle.

biopsy n. A hollow needle used to obtain tissue for microscopic examination.

caudal n. A long, hollow needle used to inject an anesthetic into the epidural space via the sacral hiatus.

discission n. See needle knife, under knife.

exploring n. A grooved needle which is thrust into a tumor or cavity to determine the presence or absence of fluid.

hypodermic n. A hollow needle for injecting fluids beneath the skin.

lumbar puncture n. A needle designed for entering the spinal canal to remove cerebrospinal fluid or to introduce medication.

Menghini n. A needle designed to obtain tissue, especially from the liver, for biopsy; the tissue core is obtained and held in with the aid of suction applied to the end of the needle.

spinal n. A long, hollow needle used to inject an anesthetic into the spinal subarachnoid space.

stop n. A needle with a shoulder permitting insertion to a predetermined depth.

surgical n. Any sewing needle used in a surgical operation.

Vim-Silverman n. Needle provided with a stylet and tweezer-like cutters for obtaining a small core of tissue for biopsy.

needling (nēd′ling) A surgical technique in which the lens capsule is punctured to permit absorption of a soft cataract.

negative (neg′ă-tiv) **1.** Denoting absence of a condition, or microorganism, or failure of a response to occur, especially one being tested. **2.** Denoting a quantity less than zero.

negativism (neg′ă-tiv-iz-m) Persistent opposition to suggestions or advice; a symptom of certain psychiatric disorders which also occurs normally in

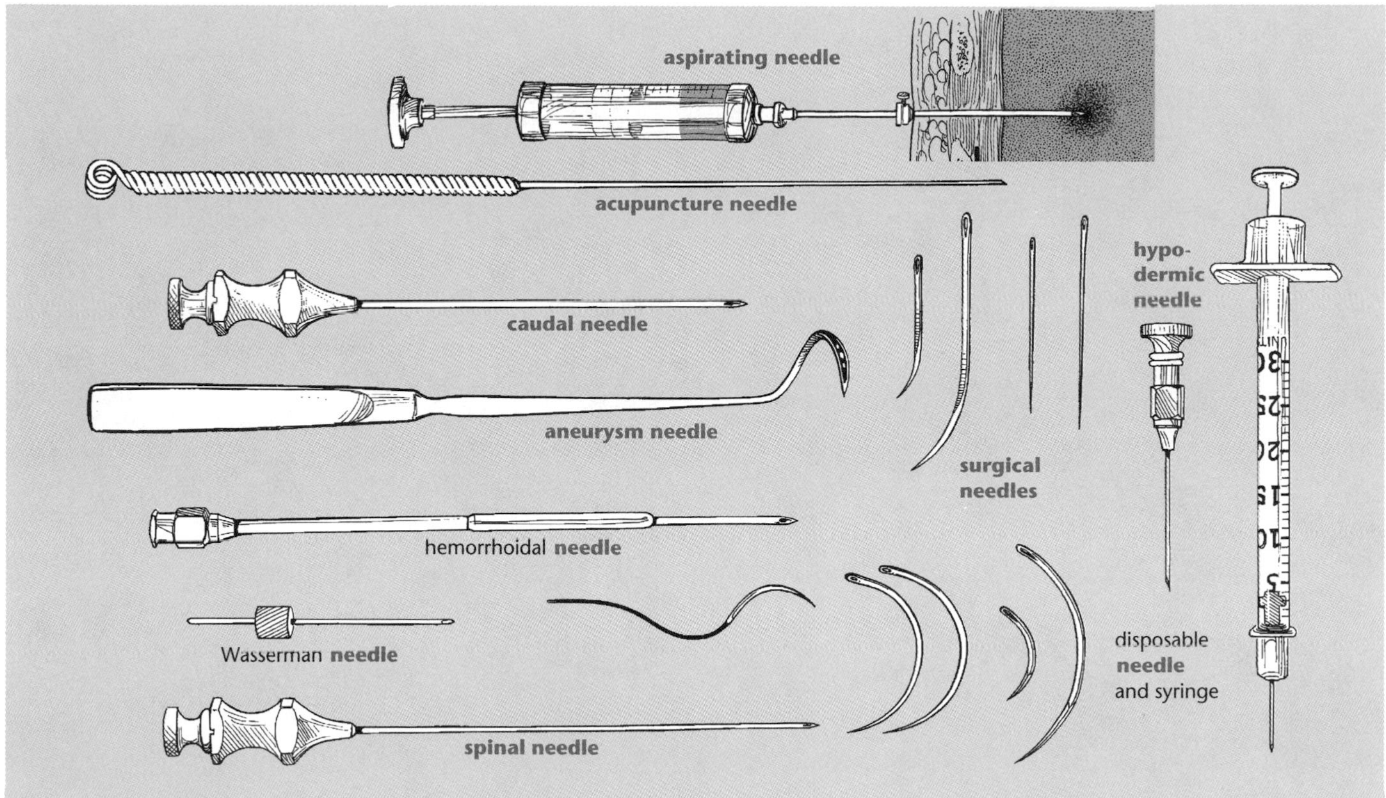

late infancy.

negatron (neg´ă-tron) See electron.

negligence (neg´lĭ-jens) Failure to use care that a reasonably prudent person would exercise under similar circumstances, thereby exposing another to an unreasonable risk of harm. In order to have a legal claim against another for a negligent act, one must prove that a duty to exercise reasonable care was owed to the claimant, that the duty was breached, and that the breach of duty caused a legally compensable injury to the claimant.

comparative n. The apportioning of the negligence of all parties (including the claimant) when determining responsibility for the claimant's losses.

contributory n. An affirmative defense in a negligence claim wherein the claimant is proven to have contributed to his own loss by his own acts of negligence. In medical malpractice, failure of the patient to exercise reasonable care in following the physician's instructions concurrent with the physician's negligent conduct, and constituting a part of the proximate cause of the injury or loss for which compensation is being sought.

Neisseria (ni-se´re-ă) A genus of bacteria (family Neisseriaceae) composed of small, gram-negative organisms occurring in pairs, each having a coffee-bean shape, flattened at the site of contact with its mate; parasitic (some pathogenic) in man.

N. catarrhalis See *Moraxella catarrhalis,* under *Moraxella.*

N. gonorrhoeae Species that causes gonorrhea and ophthalmia neonatorum.

N. meningitidis Intracellular species that causes meningococcal meningitis.

nemathelminth (nem-ă-thel´minth) A member of the phylum Nemathelminthes.

Nemathelminthes (nem-ă-thel-min´thēz) A phylum of roundworms, including the class Nematoda, characterized by cylindrical bodies with pointed ends.

nematocide (nĕ-mat´ĭ-sīd) An agent that kills roundworms.

nematocyst (nem´ă-to-sist) One of many minute stinging organelles in various marine coelenterates, such as sea nettle, Portuguese man-of-war, and hydra; when stimulated, it ejects a potent venom.

Nematoda (nem-ă-to´dă) A phylum of roundworms; some species are parasitic in humans (e.g., the intestinal roundworms and the threadworms of blood, lymphatic tissues, and viscera).

nematode (nem´ă-tōd) Any worm of the phylum Nematoda. Also called roundworm.

nematodiasis (nem-ă-to-di´ă-sis) Infestation with nematode (roundworm) parasites.

nematoid (nem´ă-toid) Relating to, or resembling roundworms.

nematology (nem-ă-tol´o-je) The science that deals with nematode worms.

neoarthrosis (ne-o-ar-thro´sis) See pseudarthrosis.

neoblastic (ne-o-blas´tik) Relating to or originating in new tissue.

neocerebellum (ne-o-ser-ĕ-bel´um) The lateral lobes of the cerebellum; so called because it is the last part of the cerebellum to develop.

neocinetic (ne-o-si-net´ik) See neokinetic.

neocortex (ne-o-kor´teks) See isocortex.

neocystostomy (ne-o-sis-tos´tŏ-me) Surgical procedure whereby a ureter or a segment of the ileum is inserted into the bladder.

neodymium (ne-o-dim´e-um) A silvery, rare-earth metallic element; symbol Nd, atomic number 60, atomic weight 144.27.

neogenesis (ne-o-jen´ĕ-sis) See regeneration.

neokinetic (ne-o-ki-net´ik) Denoting the area of the cerebral cortex that regulates motor activities.

neolalism (ne-o-lal´iz-m) Abnormal usage of neologisms.

neologism (ne-ol´o-jiz-m) Any new word or phrase or old word used in a new way; the coining of bizarre neologisms is a common symptom of certain psychoses.

neomembrane (ne-o-mem´brān) See false membrane, under membrane.

neomorph (ne´o-morf) **1.** New formation; a part or organ that is not evolved from a similar structure in an ancestor. **2.** A mutant gene producing an effect not produced by any nonmutant gene in the same locus.

neomycin (ne´o-mi-sin) An antibacterial substance produced by the metabolism of the bacterium *Streptomyces fradiae*; belongs to the group of aminoglycoside antibodies.

neon (ne´on) A rare, inert, gaseous element in the atmosphere; symbol Ne, atomic number 10, atomic weight 20.183.

neonatal (ne-o-na´tal) Pertaining to the first 4 weeks of life.

neonate (ne´o-nāt) A newborn infant, from birth through the first 28 days of life. Also called newborn.

neonatologist (ne-o-na-tol´ŏ-jist) A specialist in neonatology.

neonatology (ne-o-na-tol´ŏ-je) The branch of medicine concerned with disorders of the newborn infant from birth through the first 28 days of life. Also called neonatal medicine.

neopallium (ne-o-pal´le-um) See isocortex.

neoplasia (ne-o-pla´zhă) The abnormal process that results in the formation and growth of a tumor (neoplasm). See also dysplasia.

cervical intraepithelial n. (CIN) See cervical dysplasia, under dysplasia.

gestational trophoblastic n. (GTN) See gestational trophoblastic disease.

multiple endocrine n., type 1 (MEN 1) Association of parathyroid, pancreatic islet, and pituitary hypoplasia or neoplasia.

multiple endocrine n., type 2 (MEN 2) Association of medullary thyroid carcinoma and pheochromocytoma with multiple mucosal neuromas. Also called Sipple's syndrome.

vaginal intraepithelial n. (VAIN) Abnormal cell growth occurring as single or multiple lesions within the epithelium of the vagina; it may progress and develop into carcinoma and occur with or without cervical or vulvar involvement. Depending on the thickness of epithelium involved, it is classified as VAIN I (mild), VAIN II (moderate), or VAIN III (severe); VAIN III is sometimes called carcinoma *in situ.*

vulvar intraepithelial n. (VIN) See vulvar dysplasia, under dysplasia.

neoplasm (ne´o-plaz-m) An abnormal mass of tissue characterized by excessive growth that is uncoordinated with that of the surrounding normal tissues and persists in the same excessive manner after cessation of the stimuli that initiated the change. Also called tumor.

borderline malignant n. Term used to describe tumors of low malignancy potential.

neoplastic (ne-o-plas´tik) **1.** Relating to neoplasia. **2.** Containing a neoplasm.

neostomy (ne-os´tŏ-me) Surgical creation of a new artificial opening.

neovagina (ne-o-vaj-ĭ´nă) A surgically constructed vagina using a split thickness skin graft, or a bowel segment.

neovascularization (ne-o-vas-ku-lar-ĭ-za´shun)

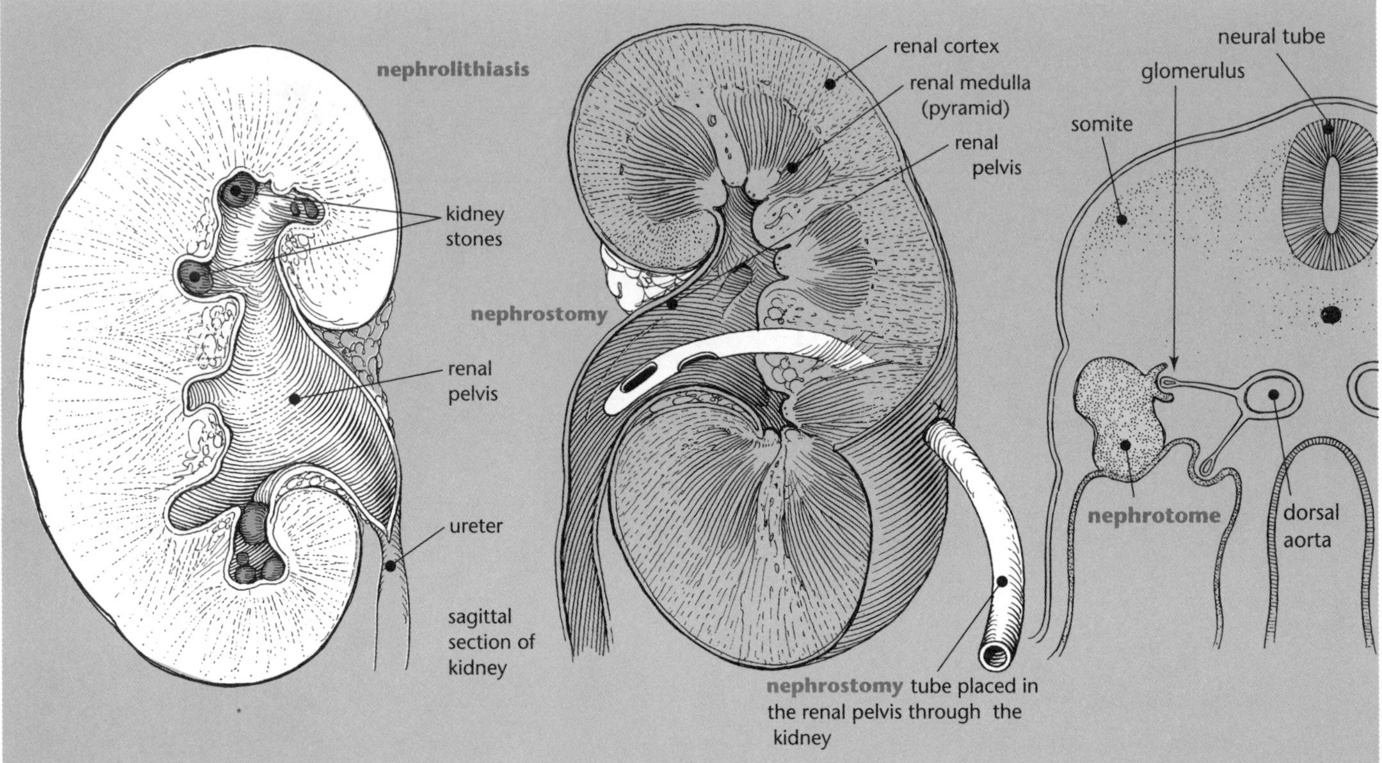

Abnormal formation of new blood vessels in any tissue.

neoxanthoendothelioma (ne-o-zan-tho-en-do-the-le-o´mă) See juvenile xanthogranuloma, under xanthogranuloma.

nephelometer (nef-ĕ-lom´ĕ-ter) Instrument used in nephelometry.

nephelometry (nef-ĕ-lom´ĕ-tre) Measurement of light scattered from the main beam of a transmitted light source; used to detect precipitation between antigen and antibody. In dilute solutions, the reaction increases the scattering of light.

nephrectasia, nephrectasy (nef-rek-ta´zha, nef-rek-ta´sē) Abnormal distention of the pelvis of the kidney.

nephrectomy (nĕ-frek´to-me) Surgical removal of a kidney.

nephric (nef´rik) See renal.

nephridium (nĕ-frid´e-um) One of the excretory tubules of invertebrates.

nephritic (nĕ-frit´ik) Relating to nephritis.

nephritis (nĕ-fri´tis) Inflammation of the kidneys; a nonspecific term, often used to indicate glomerulonephritis.

acute n. See acute proliferative glomerulonephritis; under glomerulonephritis.

acute interstitial n. Acute inflammation of the interstitial tissues of the kidney, generally with involvement of the tubules and relative sparing of the glomeruli; commonly caused by reaction to a drug.

analgesic n. Degeneration of a kidney papilla with inflammation of the tubules and supporting tissues, caused by long-term intake of large amounts of nonsteroidal analgesics and anti-inflammatory drugs. Also called analgesic abuse nephropathy.

analgesic n. Necrosis of the kidney papillae and inflammation of the tubules and supporting tissues, caused by long-term intake of large amounts of nonsteroidal analgesics and anti-inflammatory drugs; symptoms include passage of blood in the urine, hemolytic anemia, gastrointestinal disturbances, and high blood pressure. Also called analgesic abuse nephropathy.

chronic n. See chronic glomerulonephritis, under glomerulonephritis.

chronic interstitial n. Fibrotic interstitial tissue accompanied by chronic inflammatory cells; thought to be caused by many different agents, including chronic drug reaction, heavy metal toxicity, and gout.

hereditary n. Hereditary kidney disease progressing to chronic kidney failure, sometimes associated with cataracts, lens dislocation, and corneal dystrophy; becomes evident in childhood by excretion of blood in the urine. When associated with nerve deafness, it is called Alport's syndrome.

IgA n. See IgA nephropathy, under nephropathy.

potassium-losing n. Unusual potassium loss in the urine; may be seen, uncommonly, as a manifestation of renal tubular acidosis and chronic pyelonephritis.

salt-losing n. Tendency of some individuals with chronic renal disease to excrete a high percentage of filtered sodium; most likely to occur with chronic pyelonephritis, polycystic kidneys, analgesic nephropathy, or medullary cystic disease.

nephritogenic (nĕ-frit-o-jen´ik) Producing nephritis.

nephroblastoma (nef-ro-blas-to´mă) See Wilm's tumor, under tumor.

nephrocalcinosis (nef-ro-kal-si-no´sis) Condition marked by calcifications scattered throughout the kidneys. Also called renal calcinosis.

nephrocardiac (nef-ro-kar´de-ak) See cardiorenal.

nephrogenic (nef-ro-jen´ik) Originating in the kidney.

nephrogram (nef´ro-gram) X-ray picture of the kidney structures made after infusion of a radiopaque substance.

nephrography (nĕ-frog´ră-fe) The process of making a nephrogram.

nephroid (nef´roid) Resembling a kidney.

nephrolith (nef´ro-lith) See kidney stone, under stone.

nephrolithiasis (nef-ro-lĭ-thi´ă-sis) Condition marked by the presence of stones in the kidney.

nephrolithotomy (nef-ro-lĭ-thot´o-me) Cutting through the kidney for the removal of kidney stones.

nephrologist (nĕ-frol´o-jist) A specialist in nephrology.

nephrology (nĕ-frol´o-je) The study of the kidney and its diseases.

nephrolysin (nĕ-frol´ĭ-sin) An antibody that causes specific destruction of kidney cells.

nephromalacia (nef-ro-mă-la´shă) Softening of the kidneys.

nephromere (nef´ro-mēr) In embryology, a portion of the intermediate mesoderm from which the kidney develops.

nephron (nef´ron) The functional unit of the kidney, located mostly within the renal cortex; it consists of the filtering unit (glomerulus), convoluted tubules (proximal and distal), intermediate tubule, Henle's (nephronic) loop, and connecting tubule. There are approximately 1 million nephrons in each kidney, the number declining with increasing age; three processes work together in each nephron to carry out the excretory and regulatory functions of the kidney, namely: filtration at the glomerulus; selective resorption of many materials (e.g., water, glucose, amino acids, phosphate, chloride, sodium, calcium, bicarbonate) from the filtrate as it passes along the nephron; and secretion of various substances (e.g., hydrogen ions, ammonium, organic acids) into the filtrate by the cells of the tubules.

nephropathy (nĕ-frop´ă-the) Any disease of the kidney.

analgesic abuse n. See analgesic nephritis, under nephritis.

diabetic n. A complication of diabetes mellitus (either diabetes 1 or diabetes 2) resulting from long-term high glucose levels in the blood; chief features include hypertension, damage to the filtration system of the kidney, and eventual kidney failure.

IgA n. Condition marked by deposition of IgA in the central portions of the glomeruli and recurrent excretion of blood in the urine; affects chiefly children and young adults. Also called Berger's disease.

reflux n. Kidney damage caused by backing up of infected urine from ureter and bladder.

nephropexy (nef´ro-pek-se) Surgical fixation of a displaced kidney.

nephrophthisis (nĕ-frof´thĭ-sis) Suppurative inflammation of the kidney with wasting of kidney substance.

nephroptosis, nephroptosia (nef-rop-to´sis, nef-rop-to´se-ă) Downward displacement of a kidney.

nephropyelitis (nef-ro-pi-ĕ-li´tis) Inflammation of the renal pelvis.

nephropyeloplasty (nef-ro-pi´ĕ-lo-plas-te) Reparative surgery of the kidney pelvis.

nephropyosis (nef-ro-pi-o´sis) Suppuration of a kidney.

nephrorrhagia (nef-ro-ra´jhă) Hemorrhage from or into the kidney.

nephrorrhaphy (nef-ror´ă-fe) Suturing of a kidney.

nephrosclerosis (nef-ro-skle-ro´sis) Renal impairment secondary to arteriosclerosis or hypertension.

arterial n. Atrophy and scarring of the kidney due to arteriosclerotic thickening of the walls of large

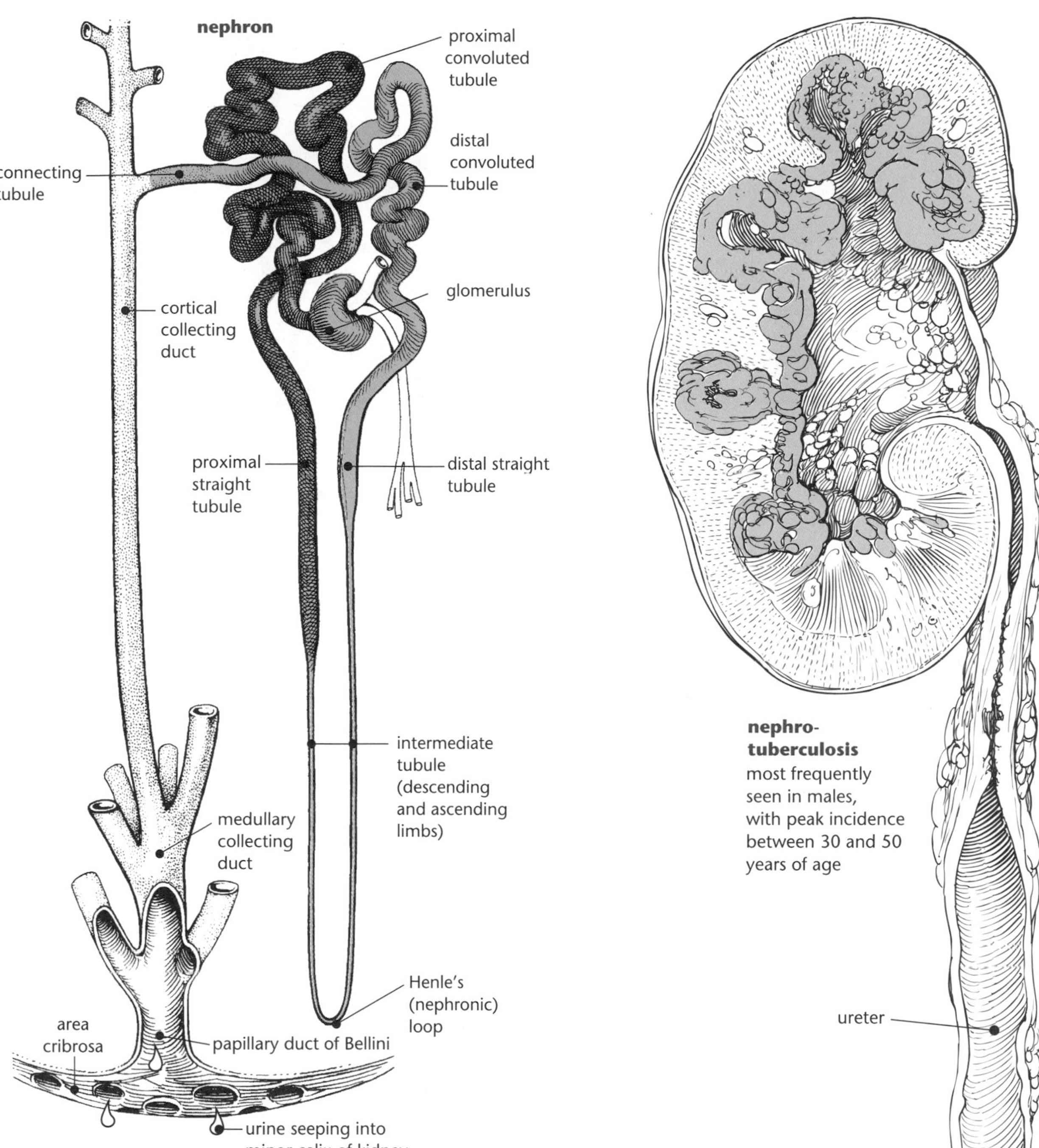

nephrotuberculosis most frequently seen in males, with peak incidence between 30 and 50 years of age

N

branches of the renal artery; may cause hypertension. Also called arterionephrosclerosis.

arteriolar n. Renal changes associated with hypertension in which the arterioles thicken and the areas they supply undergo ischemic atrophy and interstitial fibrosis. Also called arteriolonephrosclerosis; benign nephrosclerosis.

benign n. See arteriolar nephrosclerosis.

malignant n. Rapid deterioration of renal function caused by inflammation of renal arterioles; it accompanies malignant hypertension.

nephrosclerotic (nef-ro-skle-rot´ik) Relating to nephrosclerosis.

nephroscope (nef´ro-skōp) Instrument for viewing the interior of the kidney pelvis.

nephrosis (nĕ-fro´sis) **1.** General term denoting a noninflammatory disease of the kidneys. **2.** See nephrotic syndrome.

lipoid n. See minimal change disease.

lower nephron n. Acute tubular necrosis.

nephrospasis (nef-ro-spas´is) See floating kidney, under kidney.

nephrostome, nephrostoma (nef´ro-stōm, nĕ-fros´to-mă) In embryology, one of the ciliated funnels connecting the embryonic uriniferous tubules with the celomic cavity.

nephrostomy (nĕ-fros´tŏ-me) Surgical creation of an opening into the kidney pelvis, performed through the renal cortex and an inferior calix, for introduction of a drainage tube.

percutaneous n. Introduction of a drainage tube directly into the kidney pelvis through a skin incision and under the guidance of ultrasonography.

nephrotic (nĕ-frot´ik) Relating to nephrosis.

nephrotic syndrome (nĕ-frot´ik sin´drōm) (NS) Clinical symptom complex caused by various kidney diseases, characterized by generalized edema, low plasma albumin concentration, and severe proteinuria; seen in minimal change disease, membranous glomerulonephritis, and varieties of chronic proliferative glomerulonephritis. It also may be secondary to lupus erythematosus, diabetes mellitus, or amyloid; or to a number of infections or allergies. Also called nephrosis.

nephrotome (nef´ro-tōm) The plate of embryonic mesenchyme of the somites of a vertebrate embryo from which the kidney tubules develop.

nephrotomogram (nef-ro-to´mo-gram) Sectional x-ray images (tomogram) of the kidney following injection of radiopaque material.

nephrotomography (nef-ro-to-mog´ră-fe) X-ray examination of the kidney by means of tomography.

nephrotomy (nĕ-frot´o-me) Incision of the kidney.

nephrotoxic (nef-ro-tok´sik) Destructive to the cells of the kidney.

nephrotoxin (nef-ro-tok´sin) A substance (cytotoxin) that is destructive to kidney cells.

nephrotropic (nef-ro-trop´ik) See renotrophic.

nephrotuberculosis (nef-ro-tu-ber-ku-lo´sis) Tuberculosis of the kidney.

nephroureterectomy (nef-ro-u-re-ter-ek´to-me) Removal of a kidney with complete or partial removal of its ureter.

neptunium (nep-tu´ne-um) A radioactive metallic element; symbol Np, atomic number 93, atomic weight 237; prepared artificially by the neutron bombardment of uranium atoms.

nerve (nerv) A cordlike structure of one or more fascicles of nerve tissue that carries impulses

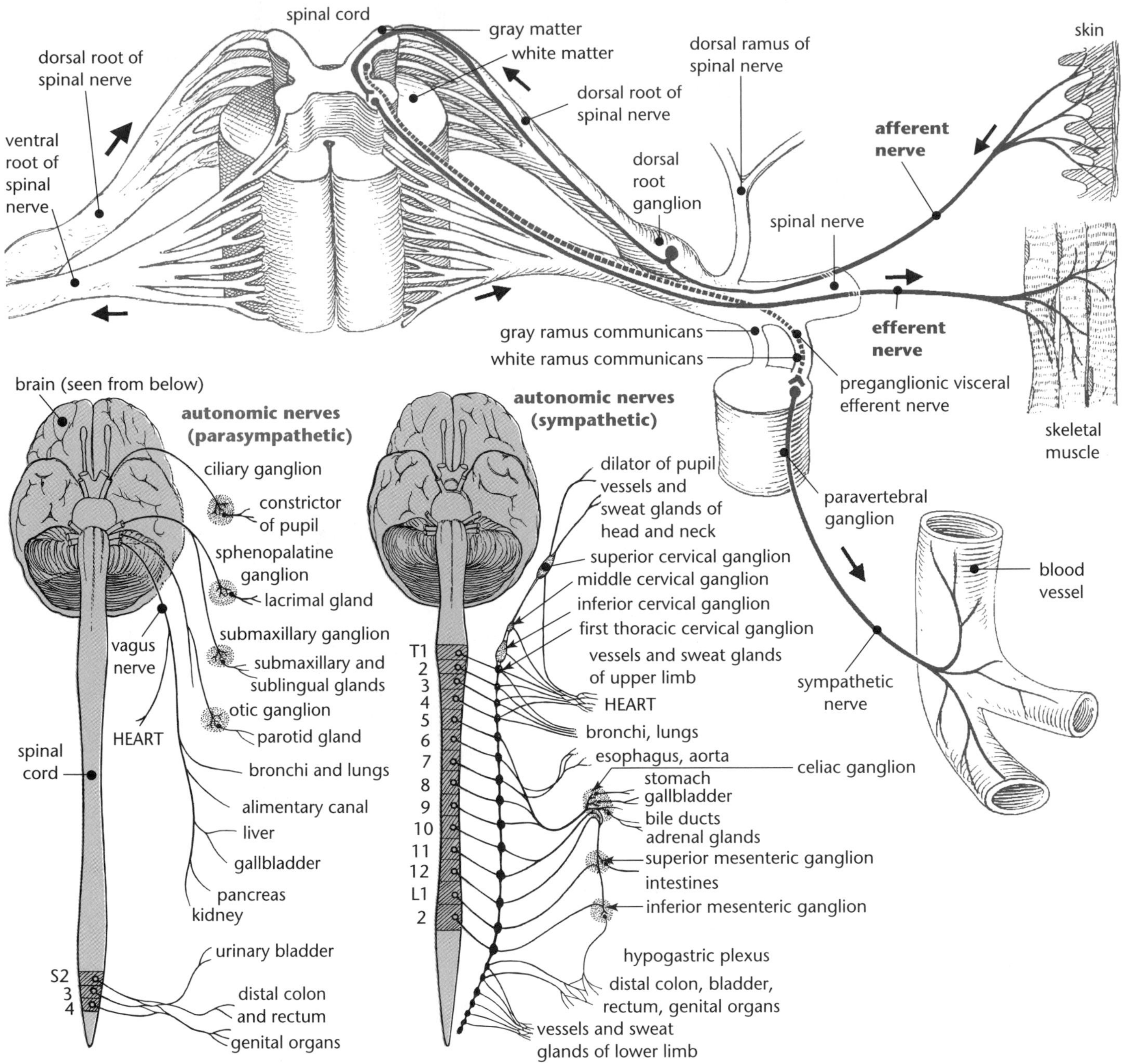

(transmissions) from the central nervous system (brain and spinal cord) to the various structures of the body and from the structures to the central nervous system. For specific nerves, see table of nerves.

accelerator n.'s Nerve fibers arising from the hypothalamus and brainstem which reach the heart via the cardiac nerves and increase the rate of its beat; they are part of the sympathetic division of the autonomic nervous system.

afferent n. A nerve that carries an impulse from the periphery to the central nervous system where it is interpreted into the consciousness of sensation; those arising from the skin, muscles, and joints are called somatic afferent nerves; those from the viscera are known as visceral afferent nerves. Also called sensory nerve.

augmentor n.'s Nerves that increase the force as well as the rate of the heart beat.

autonomic n. A bundle of nerve fibers relating to the activity of cardiac muscle, smooth muscle, and glands; they belong to the autonomic nervous system.

cranial n.'s Nerves directly connected with the brain. See table of nerves.

dead n. A misnomer for a functionless tooth pulp.

depressor n. A nerve that causes depression of a motor center, or one that reduces the function of an organ.

efferent n. A nerve that conveys impulses from the central nervous system to the periphery; those that terminate at skeletal muscles are called somatic efferent nerves; those that terminate at smooth muscles, cardiac muscles, and gland cells are called visceral efferent (autonomic) nerves. Also called motor nerve.

inhibitory n. A nerve that carries impulses which diminish functional activity of a structure.

mixed n. A nerve composed of both afferent and efferent fibers.

motor n. See efferent nerve.

peripheral n.'s The cranial and spinal nerves with their branches; in general, they carry both afferent and efferent fibers.

pressor n. An afferent nerve which when stimulated excites vasoconstriction, thereby increasing blood pressure.

sensory n. See afferent nerve.

somatic n. The afferent (sensory) and efferent (motor) nerves that innervate skeletal muscle and somatic tissue.

spinal n.'s The 31 pairs of nerves directly connected with the spinal cord. See table of nerves.

vasomotor n. An efferent nerve that can cause blood vessels to dilate (vasodilator nerve) or to constrict (vasoconstrictor nerve).

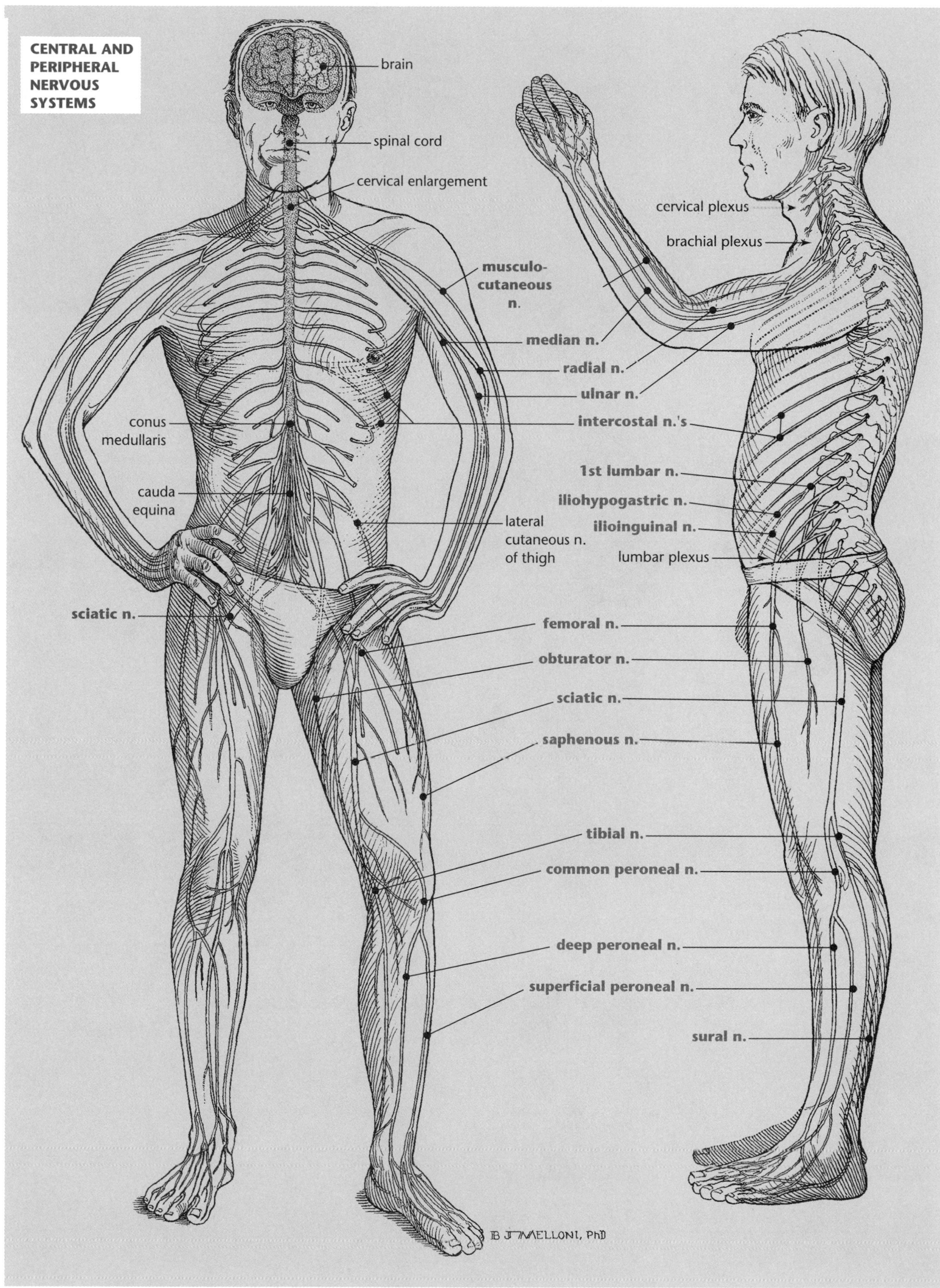

CENTRAL AND PERIPHERAL NERVOUS SYSTEMS
brain
spinal cord
cervical enlargement
musculo-cutaneous n.
median n.
radial n.
ulnar n.
intercostal n.'s
conus medullaris
cauda equina
lateral cutaneous n. of thigh
sciatic n.
femoral n.
obturator n.
sciatic n.
saphenous n.
tibial n.
common peroneal n.
deep peroneal n.
superficial peroneal n.
cervical plexus
brachial plexus
1st lumbar n.
iliohypogastric n.
ilioinguinal n.
lumbar plexus
sural n.
B J MELLONI, PhD

N

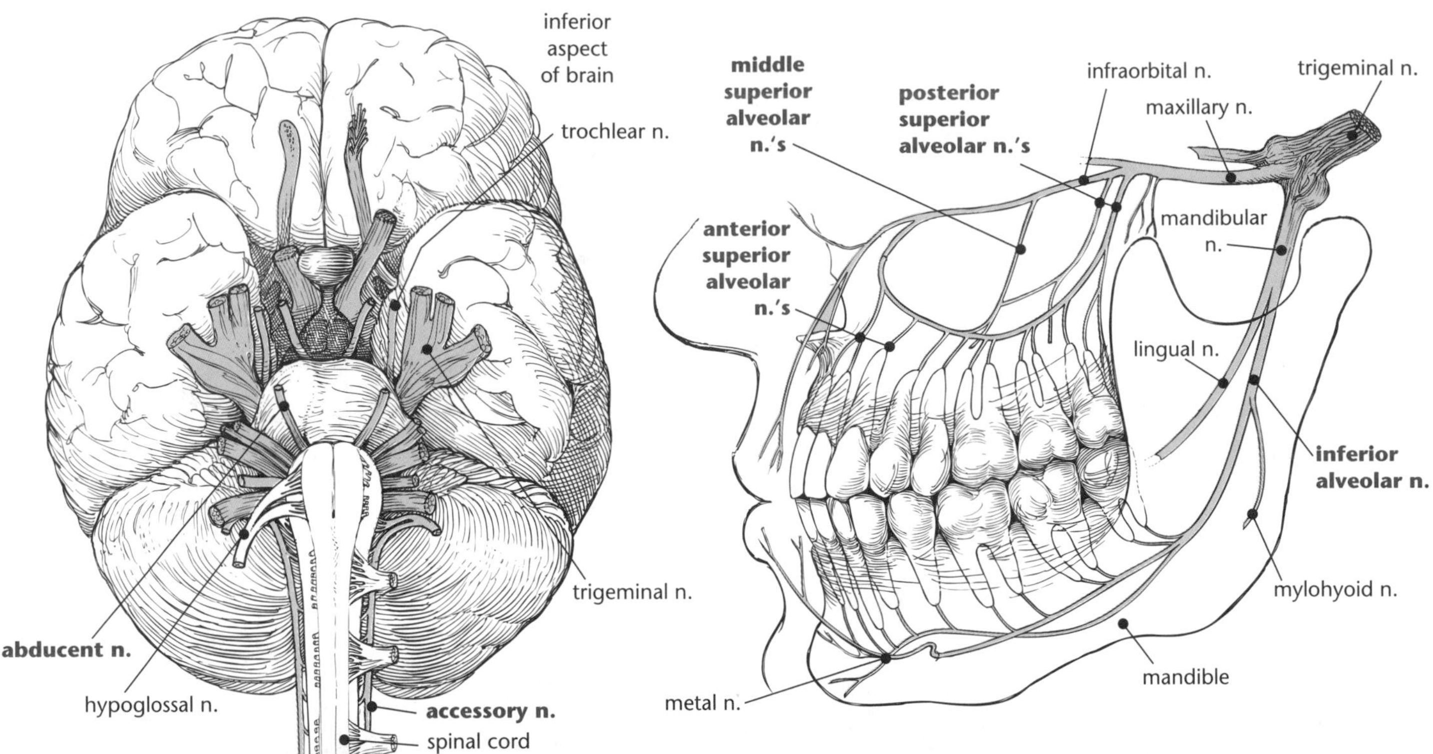

NERVE	ORIGIN	BRANCHES	DISTRIBUTION
abducent n. sixth cranial n. *n. abducens*	brainstem at inferior border of pons located in floor of fourth ventricle	filaments	lateral rectus muscle of eyeball
accessory n. spinal accessory n. eleventh cranial n. *n. accessorius*	*cranial part:* side of medulla oblongata; *spinal part:* first five cervical segments of spinal cord	internal branch external branch	striate muscles of larynx, pharynx, and soft palate sternocleidomastoid and trapezius muscles
acoustic n.		see vestibulocochlear nerve	
acoustic meatus n., external *n. meatus acustici externi*	auriculotemporal n.	filaments	external acoutic meatus
alveolar n.'s, anterior superior anterior superior dental n.'s *nn. alveolares anterior superior*	infraorbital n.	filaments, nasal, superior alveolar	anterior teeth (incisors and cuspids), mucous membrane of anterior walls and floor of nasal cavity; nasal septum
alveolar n., inferior inferior dental n. *n. alveolaris inferior*	mandibular n.	mylohyoid, inferior alveolar, incisive, mental	mylohyoid and anterior belly of digastric muscles, lower teeth, skin of chin, mucous membrane of lower lip
alveolar n., middle superior middle superior dental n. *n. alveolaris superior medius*	infraorbital n.	filaments, superior alveolar	maxillary sinus, superior dental plexus, maxilliary bicuspid teeth
alveolar n., posterior superior posterior superior dental n. *n. alveolaris superior posterior*	maxillary n.	filaments, superior alveolar	maxillary sinus, cheek, gums, molar and bicuspid teeth, superior dental plexus
ampullary n., anterior		see ampullary n., superior	
ampullary n., lateral *n. ampullaris lateralis*	utriculoampullar n.	none	ampulla of lateral semicircular duct
ampullary n., posterior inferior ampullary n. *n. ampullaris posterior*	vestibular ganglion	none	ampulla of posterior semicircular duct
ampullary n., superior anterior ampullary n. *n. ampullaris superior*	utriculoampullar n.	none	ampulla of superior semicircular duct
anococcygeal n.'s *nn. anococcygei*	coccygeal plexus	filaments	skin over coccyx
ansa cervicalis ansa hypoglossi *ansa cervicalis*	branch from first cervical uniting with branches from second and third cervical segments of spinal cord (forming a loop)	filaments	omohyoid, sternohyoid, and sternothyroid muscles

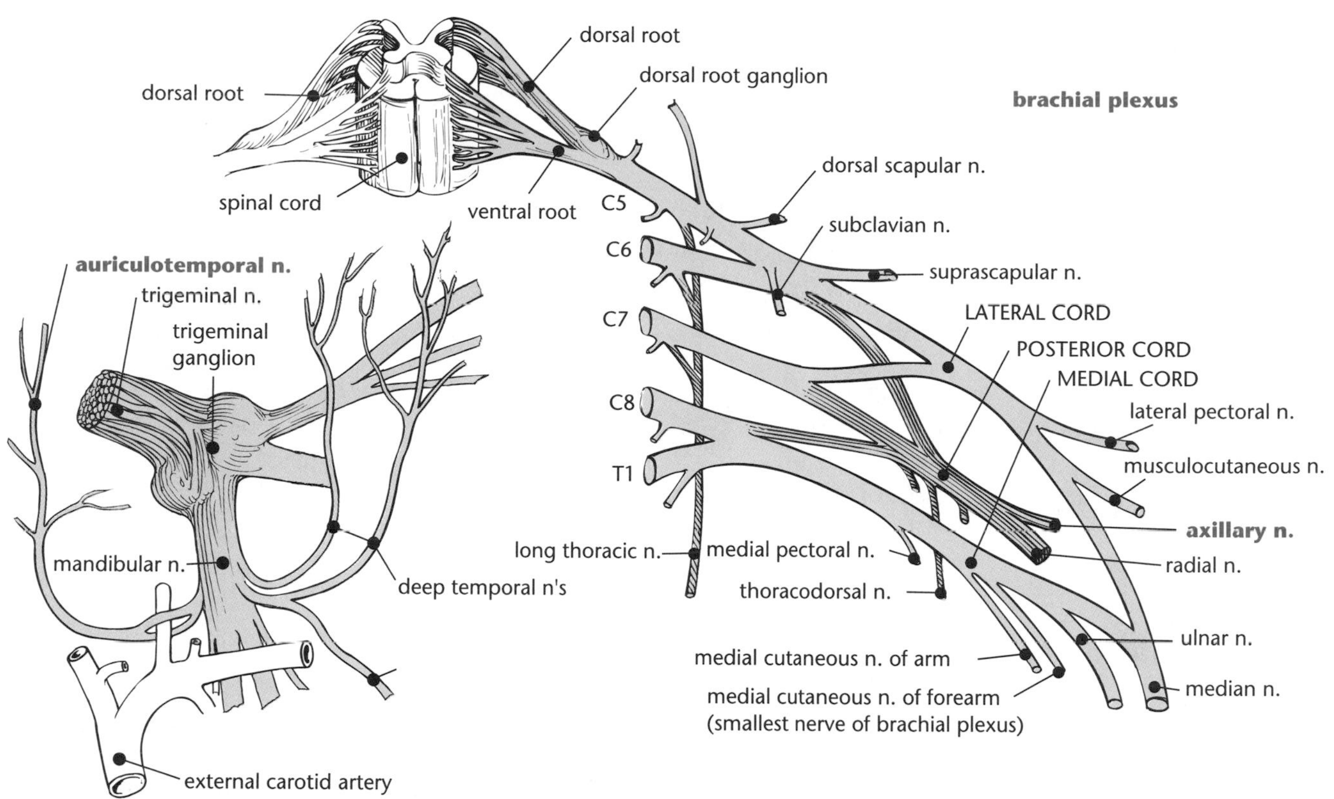

NERVE	ORIGIN	BRANCHES	DISTRIBUTION
auditory n.	see vestibulocochlear nerve		
auricular n.'s, anterior (usually two in number) *nn. auriculares anteriores*	auriculotemporal n.	filaments	skin of anteriosuperior part of external ear, principally helix and tragus
auricular n., great *n. auricularis magnus*	second and third cervical n.'s	anterior, posterior	skin over ear, mastoid process and parotid gland
auricular n., posterior *n. auricularis posterior*	facial n.	auricular, occipital	posterior auricular and occipital muscles, skin of external ear
auriculotemporal n. *n. auriculotemporalis*	mandibular division of trigeminal n.	anterior auricular, external, acoustic meatus, articular, parotid, superficial temporal, branches communicating with otic ganglion and facial n.	external meatus and skin of anterior superior part of auricle, temporomandibular joint, parotid gland, skin of temporal region
axillary n. circumflex n. *n. axillaris*	posterior cord of brachial plexus	posterior, anterior, cutaneous, articular	deltoid and teres minor muscles, and neighboring skin
brachial plexus *plexus brachialis*	ventral rami of fifth to eight cervical and first thoracic n.'s	*from cervical n.'s:* phrenic, muscular, accessory phrenic; *from roots:* dorsal scapular, long thoracic; *from trunks:* subclavius, suprascapular; *from cords:* pectoral, subscapular, thoracodorsal, axillary, medial cutaneous of forearm, medial cutaneous of arm; *terminal n.'s:* musculocutaneous, median, ulnar, radial	upper limb
buccal n. buccinator n. long buccal n. *n. buccalis*	mandibular division of trigeminal n.	filaments, branches communicating with buccal branches of facial n.	skin of cheek, mucous membranes of mouth and gums
buccinator n.	see buccal nerve		
cardiac n., inferior cervical *n. cardiacus cervicalis inferior*	inferior cervical ganglion, first thoracic ganglion, stellate ganglion, or ansa subclavia	filaments	heart

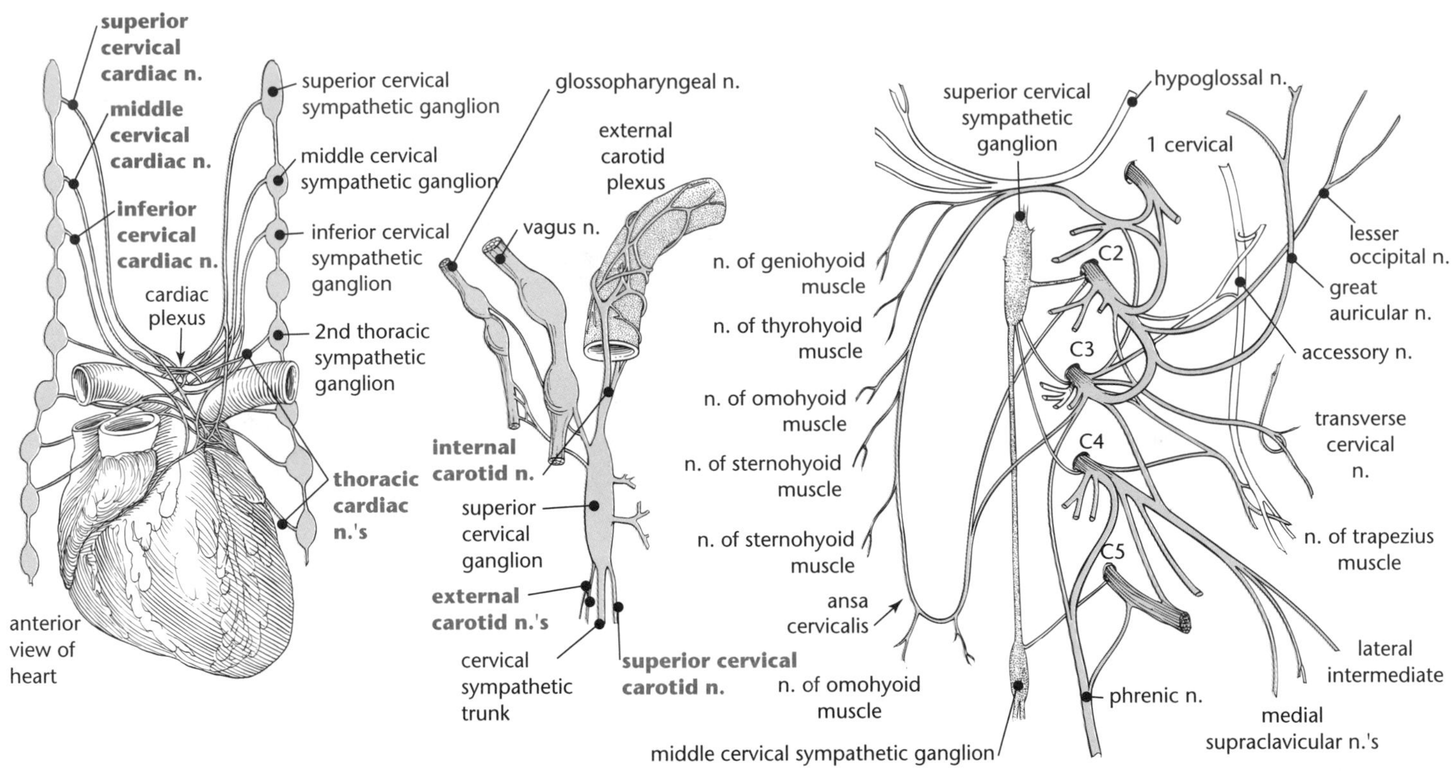

N

NERVE	ORIGIN	BRANCHES	DISTRIBUTION
cardiac n., middle cervical great cardiac n. *n. cardiacus cervicalis medius*	middle cervical ganglion	filaments	heart
cardiac n., superior cervical *n. cardiacus cervicalis superior*	lower part of superior cervical ganglion	filaments	heart
cardiac n.'s, thoracic *nn. cardiaci thoracici*	second to fifth thoracic ganglion of sympathetic trunk	filaments	heart
caroticotympanic n.'s *nn. caroticotympanici*	superior cervical sympathetic ganglion	superior, inferior	middle ear chamber, auditory tube
carotid n.'s, external *nn. carotici externi*	superior cervical ganglion	filaments	external carotid plexus, cranial blood vessels, smooth muscles and glands of head
carotid n., internal *n. caroticus internus*	cephalic end of superior cervical ganglion	medial, lateral	internal carotid plexus, cranial blood vessels, smooth muscle glands of head, cavernous plexus
carotid sinus n. carotid n. *n. caroticus*	glossopharyngeal n. just beyond its emergence from jugular foramen	filaments	carotid sinus, carotid body
cavernous n. of clitoris, greater *n. cavernosus clitoridis major*	uterovaginal plexus	filaments	corpus cavernosum of clitoris
cavernous n.'s of clitoris, lesser *nn. cavernosi clitorides minor*	uterovaginal plexus	filaments	erectile tissue of clitoris
cavernous n. of penis, greater *n. cavernosus penis major*	prostatic plexus	filaments	corpus cavernosum of penis
cavernous n.'s of penis, lesser *nn. cavernosi penis minor*	prostatic plexus	filaments	corpus spongiosum of penis and penile urethra
cervical n.'s (eight pairs of spinal nerves) *nn. cervicales*	cervical segments of spinal cord	filaments	cervical plexus and brachial plexus
cervical plexus *plexus cervicalis*	ventral rami of first to fourth cervical nerves	*cutaneous branches:* lesser occipital, great auricular, anterior cutaneous, supraclavicular; *muscular branches*: anterior and lateral rectae of head, long muscles of head and neck, geniohyoid, thyrohyoid, and omohyoid (superior belly), sternohyoid, and omohyoid	muscles and skin of neck, upper back and parts of head and chest; diaphragm

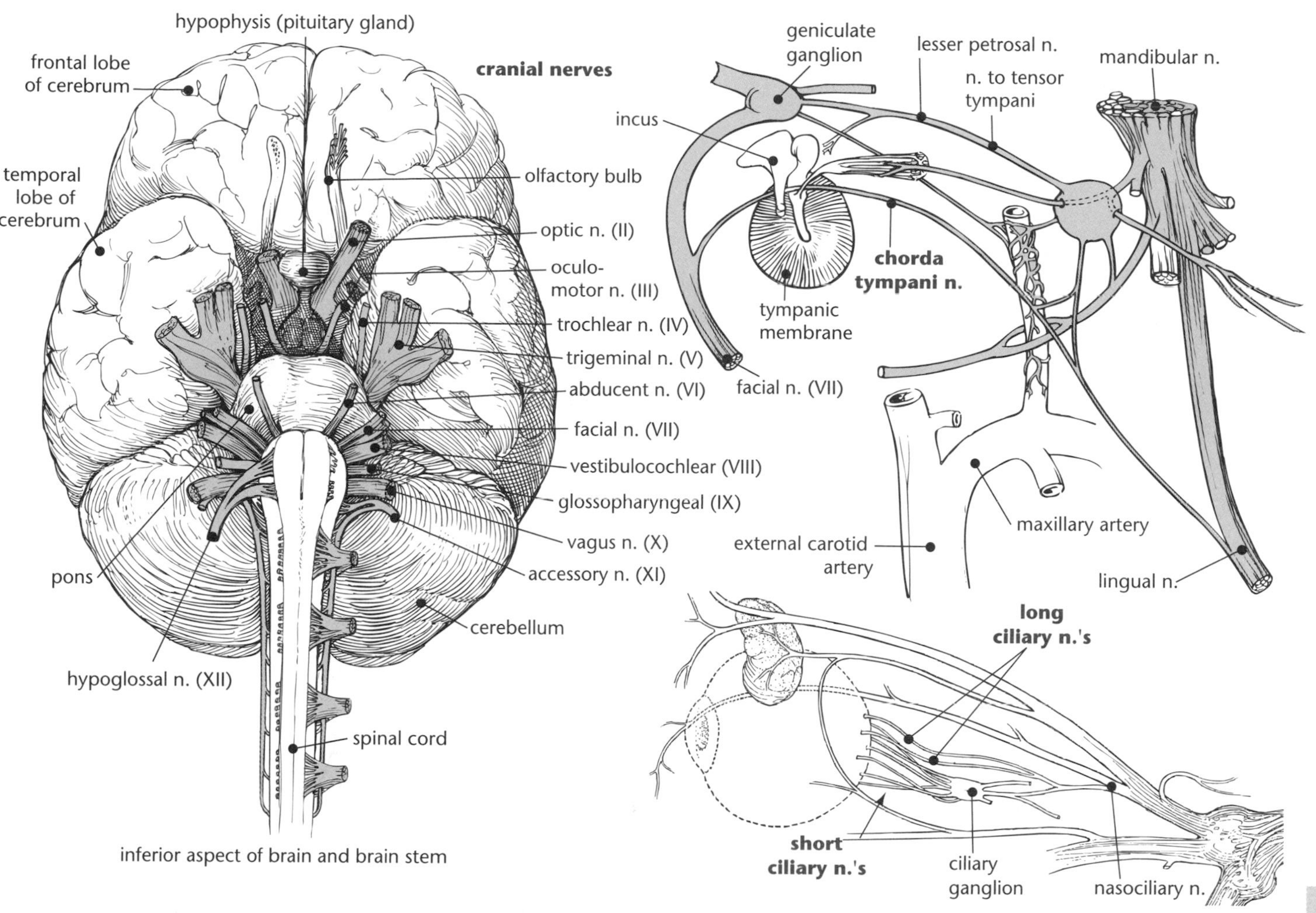

inferior aspect of brain and brain stem

N

NERVE	ORIGIN	BRANCHES	DISTRIBUTION
cervical plexus (cont'd)		(inferior belly), phrenic, sternocleidomastoid, trapezius, levator muscle of scapula, middle scalene	
chorda tympani n. *n. chorda tympani*	facial n. (intermediate) just above stylomastoid foramen	filaments	anterior two-thirds of tongue, submandibular and sublingual glands
ciliary n.'s, long (two or three in number) *nn. ciliares longi*	nasociliary n. as it crosses optic n.	filaments	iris, cornea, ciliary body
ciliary n.'s, short (6–10 in number) *nn. ciliares breves*	ciliary ganglion from oculomotor n.	filaments	ciliary body, iris, cornea, and choroid layer of eyeball
circumflex n.		see axillary nerve	
clunial n.'s, inferior *n. clunium inferiores*	posterior cutaneous n. of thigh	filaments	skin of lower and lateral gluteal region
clunial n.'s, middle *nn. clunium medii*	first, second, and third sacral n.'s	filaments	skin of medial gluteal region
clunial n.'s, superior *nn. clunium superiores*	first, second, and third lumbar n.'s	filaments	skin of upper gluteal region
coccygeal n. *n. coccygeus*	coccygeal segments of spinal cord	filaments	coccygeal plexus
coccygeal plexus *plexus coccygeus*	fourth and fifth sacral n.'s and coccygeal n.'s	anococcygeal, filaments	skin of region of the coccyx
cochlear n. n. of hearing *n. cochlearis*	vestibulocochlear n.	vestibular, filaments	through spiral ganglion of cochlea to spiral organ of Corti of internal ear
common peroneal n.		see peroneal nerve, common	
cranial n.'s cerebral n.'s *nn. craniales*	12 pairs of nerves attached to the base of the brain; they include the following: (I) olfactory; (II) optic; (III) oculomotor; (IV) trochlear; (V) trigeminal; (VI) abducent; (VII) facial; (VIII) vestibulocochlear; (IX) glossopharyngeal; (X) vagus; (XI) accessory; (XII) hypoglossal		

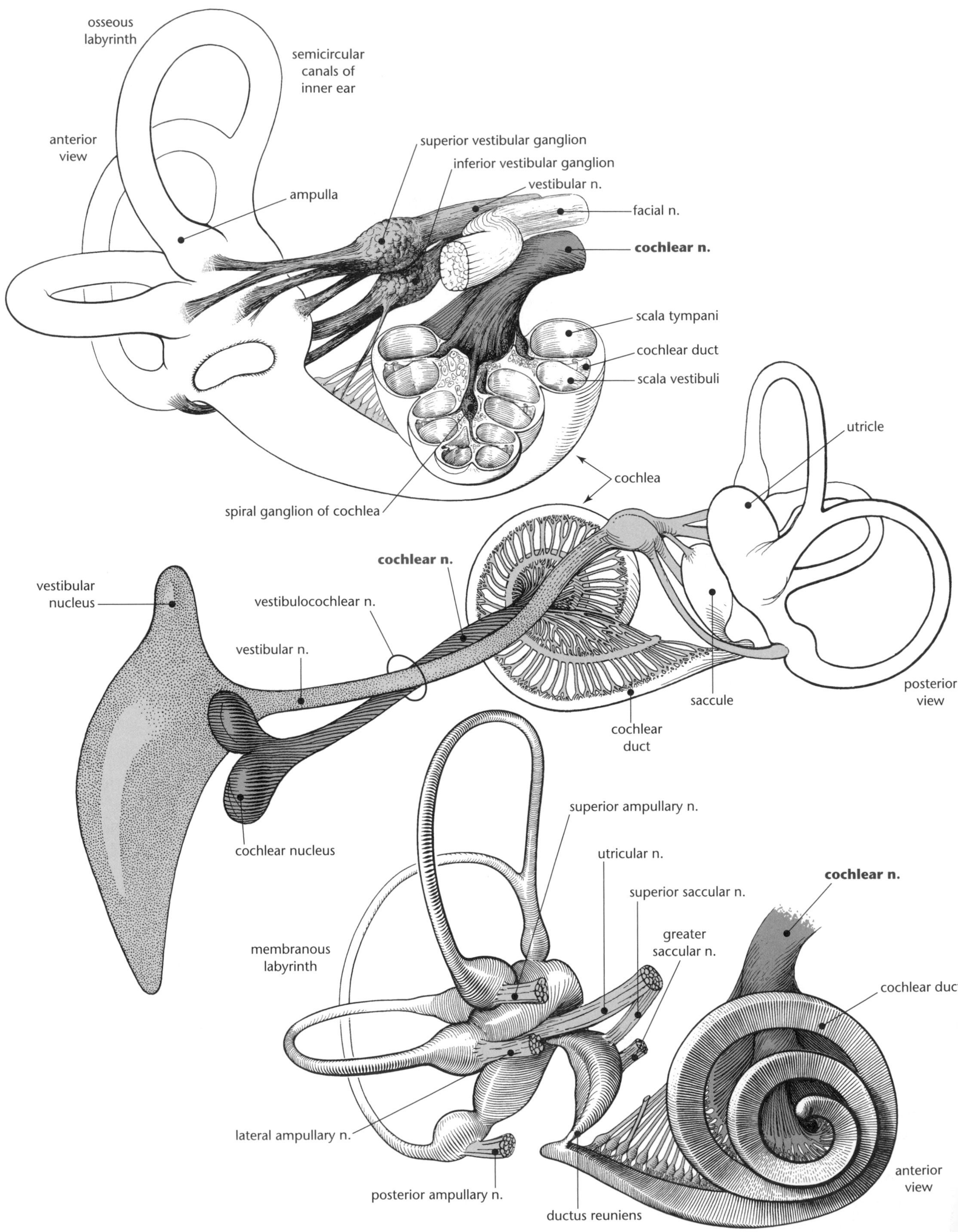
osseous
labyrinth
semicircular
canals of
inner ear
anterior
view
superior vestibular ganglion
inferior vestibular ganglion
vestibular n.
ampulla
facial n.
cochlear n.
scala tympani
cochlear duct
scala vestibuli
utricle
cochlea
spiral ganglion of cochlea
cochlear n.
vestibular
nucleus
vestibulocochlear n.
vestibular n.
saccule
posterior
view
cochlear
duct
cochlear nucleus
superior ampullary n.
utricular n.
cochlear n.
superior saccular n.
greater
saccular n.
membranous
labyrinth
cochlear duc
lateral ampullary n.
anterior
view
posterior ampullary n.
ductus reuniens

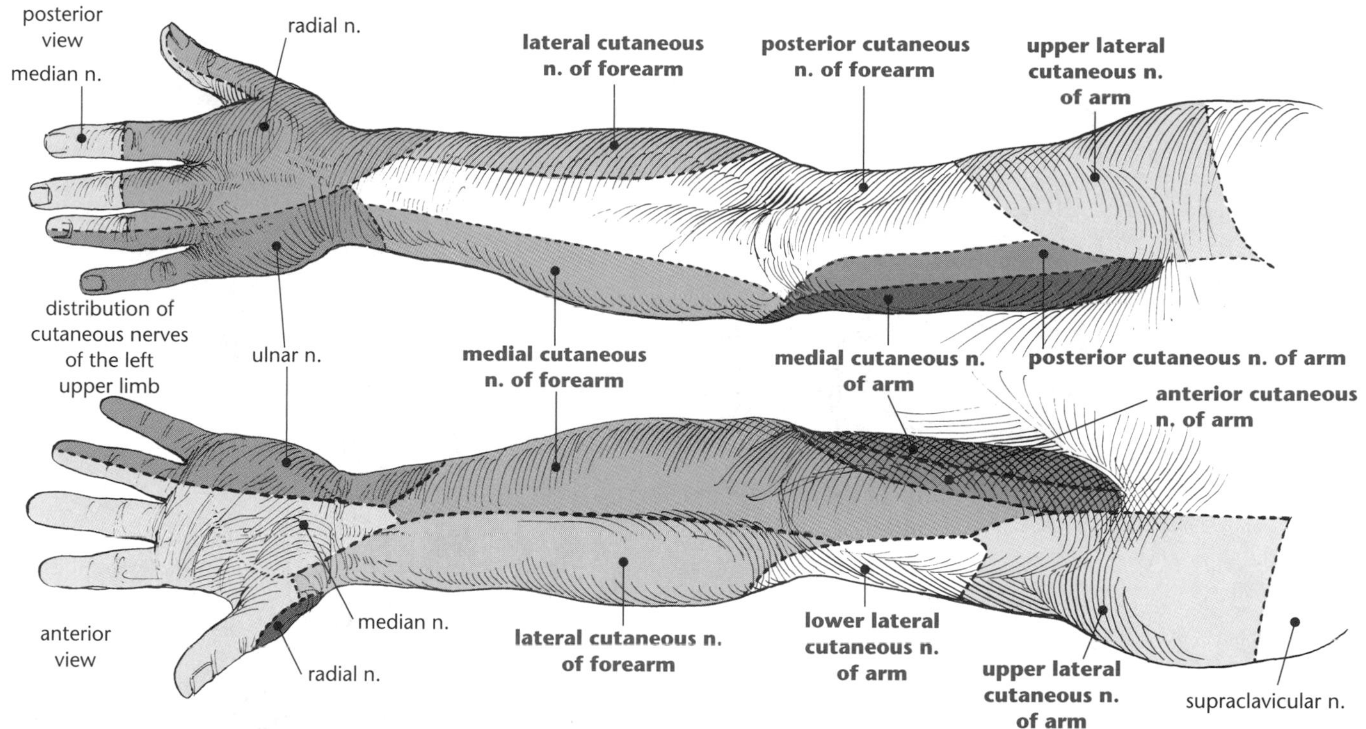

NERVE	ORIGIN	BRANCHES	DISTRIBUTION
cutaneous n. of arm, lower lateral lower lateral brachial cutaneous n. *n. cutaneus brachii lateralis inferior*	radial n.	filaments	skin on lateral aspect of lower part of arm
cutaneous n. of arm, medial medial brachial cutaneous n. *n. cutaneus brachii medialis*	medial cord of brachial plexus	filaments	skin to medial side of arm down to olecranon
cutaneous n. of arm, posterior posterior brachial cutaneous n. *n. cutaneus brachii posterior*	radial n.	filaments	skin on posterior aspect of arm nearly as far as olecranon
cutaneous n. of arm, upper lateral upper lateral brachial cutaneous n. *n. cutaneus brachii lateralis superior*	axillary n.	filaments	skin on lateral aspect of upper part of arm
cutaneous n. of calf, lateral *n. cutaneus surae lateralis*	common peroneal n.	sural, filaments	skin of lateral and posterior aspects of leg (calf)
cutaneous n. of calf, medial *n. cutaneus surae medialis*	tibial n.	sural, filaments	skin of medial and posterior aspects of leg (calf)
cutaneous n. of foot, intermediate dorsal *n. cutaneus dorsalis intermedius pedis*	superficial peroneal n.	dorsal digital (two)	skin of lateral side of ankle and dorsum of foot, and adjacent sides of third, fourth, and fifth toes
cutaneous n. of foot, lateral dorsal *n. cutaneus dorsalis lateralis pedis*	continuation of sural n.	filaments	skin of dorsolateral part of foot
cutaneous n. of foot, medial dorsal *n. cutaneus dorsalis medialis pedis*	superficial peroneal n.	medial dorsal digital, lateral dorsal digital, filaments	skin of medial side of ankle, foot and great toe, skin of adjacent sides of second and third toes
cutaneous n. of forearm, lateral lateral antebrachial cutaneous n. *n. cutaneus antebrachii lateralis*	musculocutaneous n.	anterior, posterior, filaments	skin over radial side of forearm
cutaneous n. of forearm, medial medial antebrachial cutaneous n. *n. cutaneus antebrachii medialis*	medial cord of brachial plexus	filaments, anterior, ulnar	skin over biceps muscle and of ulnar side of forearm
cutaneous n. of forearm, posterior posterior antebrachial cutaneous n. *n. cutaneus antebrachii posterior*	radial n.	proximal, distal, filaments	skin on posterior part of lower half of arm and of forearm
cutaneous n. of thigh, lateral external cutaneous n. n. *cutaneus femoris lateralis*	second and third lumbar n.'s	anterior, posterior, filaments	skin of lateral and anterior part of thigh
cutaneous n. of thigh, posterior small sciatic n. *n. cutaneus femoris posterior*	first, second, and third sacral n.'s	gluteal, perineal, femoral, sural	skin of lower gluteal region, external genitalia, perineum, and posterior aspect of thigh and leg (calf)

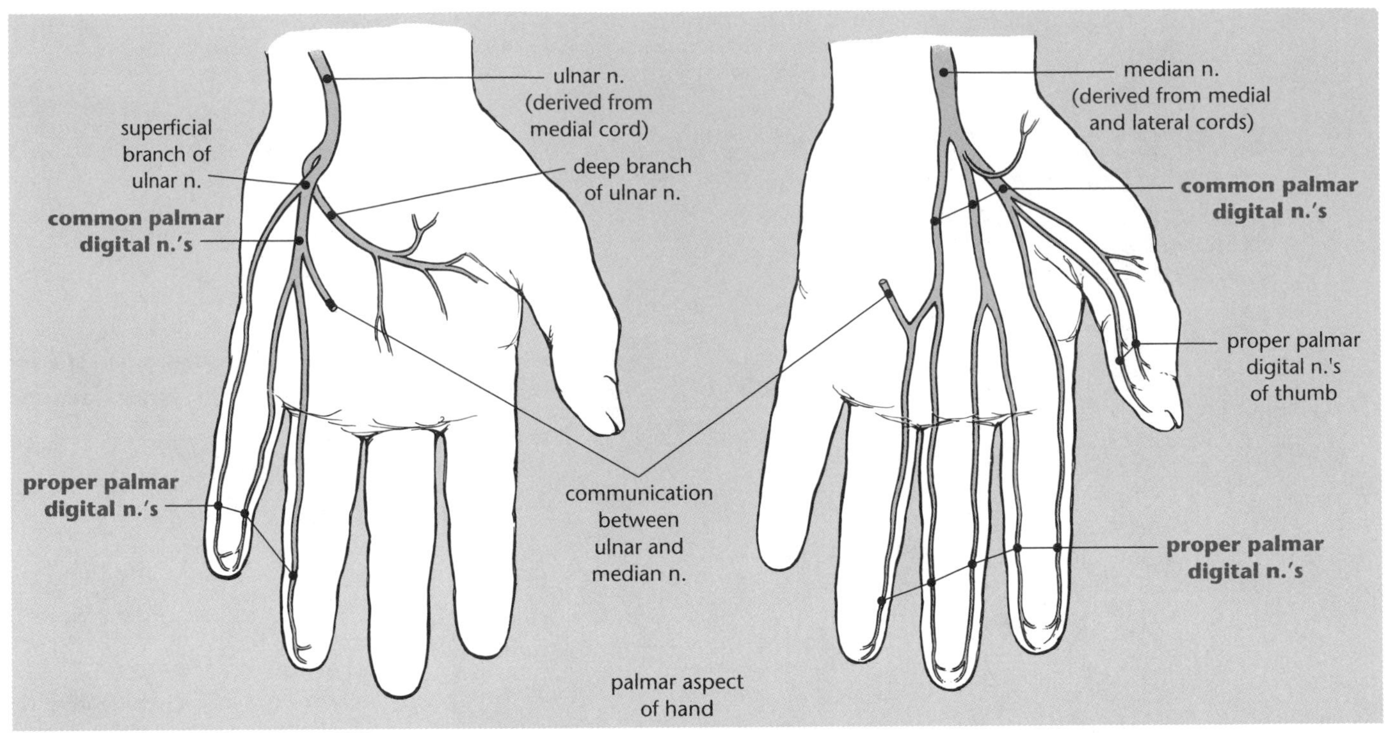

N

NERVE	ORIGIN	BRANCHES	DISTRIBUTION
dental n.'s		see alveolar nerves	
digital n.'s, common palmar *nn. digitales palmares communes*	median n. ulnar n.	proper palmar digitals	skin of palmar surface and sides of digits I–IV, first two lumbrical muscles
digital n.'s, proper palmar digital collaterals *nn. digitales palmares proprii*	common palmar digital n.'s	proper palmer digitals	skin on adjacent sides of digits; first two lumbrical muscles
digital n.'s of foot, dorsal *nn. digitales dorsales pedis*	intermediate dorsal cutaneous n. of foot	filaments	skin on adjacent sides of third, fourth, and fifth toes
digital n.'s of lateral plantar n., common plantar *nn. digitales plantares communes nervi plantaris lateralis*	superficial branch of lateral plantar n.	proper plantar digitals (medial and lateral)	adjacent sides of fourth and fifth toes; short flexor muscle of little toe
digital n.'s of lateral plantar n., proper plantar *nn. digitales plantares proprii nervi plantaris lateralis*	common plantar digital nerves of lateral plantar n.	filaments	plantar aspect of lateral toes, adjacent sides of fourth and fifth toes
digital n.'s of lateral side of great toe and medial side of second toe *nn. digitales dorsales hallucis lateralis et digiti secundi medialis*	deep peroneal n.	filaments	adjacent sides of great and second toes
digital n.'s of medial plantar n., common plantar *nn. digitales plantares communes nervi plantaris medialis*	medial plantar n.	proper plantar digitals, muscular	plantar aspect of medial toes
digital n.'s of medial plantar n., proper plantar *nn. digitales plantares proprii nervi plantaris medialis*	common plantar digital n.'s	filaments	adjacent sides of first, second, third, and forth toes
digital n.'s of radial n., dorsal *nn. digitales dorsales nervi radialis*	superficial branch of radial n.	filaments	skin of dorsum of lateral fingers
digital n.'s of ulnar n., common palmar *nn. digitales palmares communes nervi ulnaris*	superficial branch of palmar branch of ulnar n.	proper palmar digitals	skin of palmar surface and adjacent sides of fourth and fifth fingers
digital n,'s of ulnar n., dorsal *nn. digitales dorsales nervi ulnaris*	dorsal branch of ulnar n.	filaments	skin of adjoining sides of third to fifth fingers
digital n.'s of ulnar n., proper palmar *nn. digitales palmares proprii nervi ulnaris*	common palmar digital nerves of ulnar n.	filaments	adjacent sides of fourth and fifth fingers and medial side of fifth finger

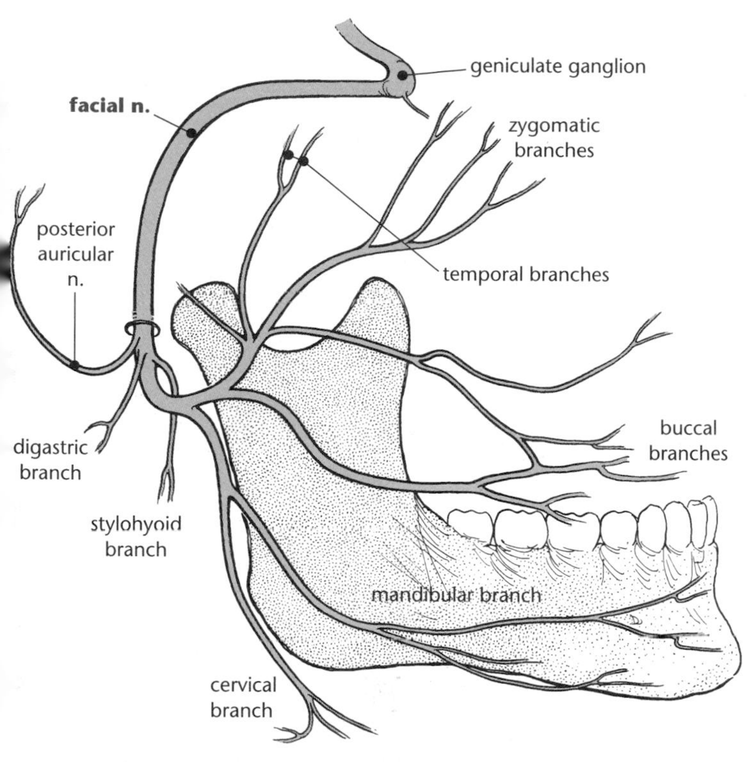

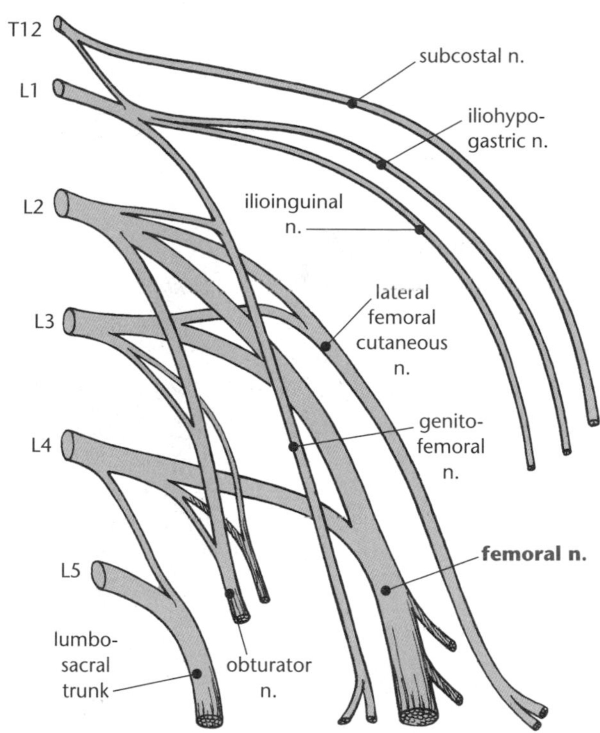

NERVE	ORIGIN	BRANCHES	DISTRIBUTION
dorsal n. of clitoris *n. dorsalis clitoridis*	pudendal n.	filaments	urethra and clitoris
dorsal n. of penis *n. dorsalis penis*	pudendal n.	filaments	urethra and penis
dorsal scapular n.		see scapular n., dorsal	
eighth cranial n.		see vestibulocochlear nerve	
eleventh cranial n.		see accessory nerve	
ethmoid n., anterior *n. ethmoidalis anterior*	continuation of nasociliary n.	internal, external, lateral, and medial nasal	mucous membrane of nasal cavity
ethmoid n. posterior *n. ethmoidalis posterior*	nasociliary n.	filaments	mucous membrane of posterior ethmoidal and sphenoidal sinuses
facial n. seventh cranial n. *n. facialis*	lower border of pons	petrosal, to tympanic plexus, stapedial, chorda tympani, muscular, auricular, temporal, zygomatic, buccal, mandibular, cervical	*motor part:* muscles of facial expression, scalp, external ear, buccinator, platysma, stapedius, stylohyoid, and posterior belly of digastric; *sensory part:* anterior two-thirds of tongue, parts of external acoustic meatus, soft palate, and adjacent pharynx; *parasympathetic part:* secretomotor fibers of submandibular, sublingual, lacrimal, nasal, and palatine glands
femoral n. anterior crural n. *n. femoralis*	second, third, and fourth lumbar n.'s	articular, muscular, saphenous, anterior cutaneous	skin of anterior and medial side of leg, hip and knee joint, quadriceps muscle of thigh, pectineal, sartorius, and iliac muscles
fifth cranial n.		see trigeminal nerve	
first cranial n.		see olfactory nerve	
fourth cranial n.		see trochlear nerve	
frontal n. *n. frontalis*	ophthalmic n.	supraorbital, supratrochlear, frontal sinus	conjunctiva, skin of upper eyelid and forehead, corrugator and frontal muscles, scalp, frontal sinus

N

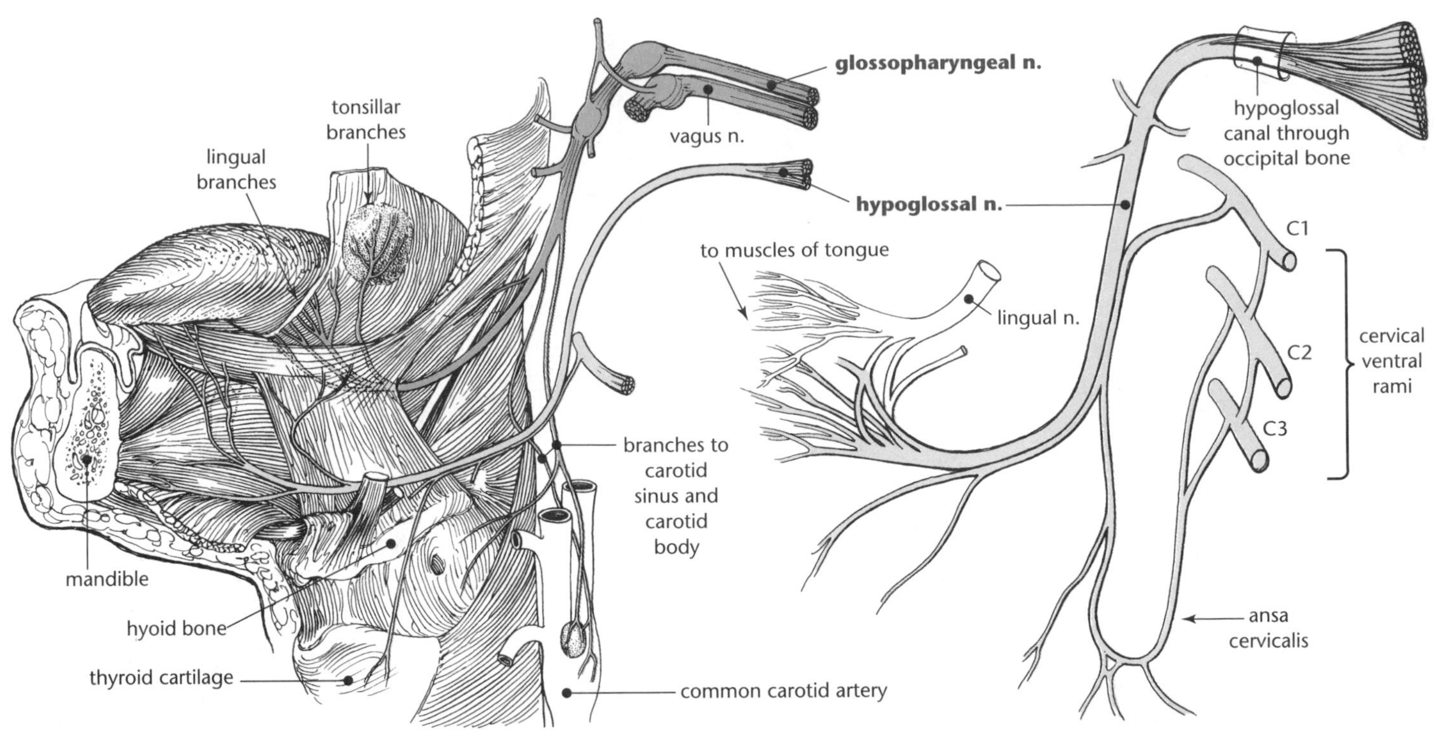

NERVE	ORIGIN	BRANCHES	DISTRIBUTION
n. of geniohyoid *n. geoiohyoideus*	first cervical n.	filaments	geniohyoid muscle
genitofemoral n. genitocrural n. *n. genitofemoralis*	first and second lumbar n.'s	genital, femoral	cremaster muscle, skin of scrotum or labium major and adjacent thigh, proximal part of anterior surface of thigh
glossopalatine n.	see intermediate nerve		
glossopharyngeal n. ninth cranial n. *n. glossopharyngeus*	upper part of medulla oblongata	tympanic, carotid sinus, pharyogeal, stylopharyngeal, tonsillar, lingual	tongue and pharynx, fauces, palatine tonsil, blood pressure receptor of carotid sinus, stylopharyngeus muscle
gluteal n., inferior *n. gluteus inferior*	fifth lumbar n. and first and second sacral n.'s	filaments	gluteus maximum muscle
gluteal n. superior *n. glureus superior*	fourth and fifth lumbar n.'s and first sacral n.	superior, inferior, filaments	gluteus minimus and medius muscles, tensor muscle of fascia lata
hemorrhoidal n.	see rectal nerve		
hypogastric n. *n. hypogastricus*	a single large n. (or several parallel bundles) which interconnects the superior hypogastric with the inferior hypogastric plexus		
hypoglossal n. twelfth cranial n. *n. hypoglossus*	series of rootlets between pyramid and olive of medulla oblongata	meningeal, descending hypoglossal, muscular, lingual	intrinsic and extrinsic muscles of tongue; dura mater
hypoglossal n., small	see lingual nerve		
iliohypogastric n. *n. iliohypogastricus*	first lumbar n.	anterior cutaneous, muscular, lateral cutaneous	abdominal muscles, skin of lower part of abdomen and gluteal region
ilioinguinal n. *n. ilioinguinalis*	first lumbar n.	anterior scrotal (male), anterior labial (female), muscular, filaments	muscles of abdominal wall, skin of proximal and medial part of thigh, root of penis (male), mons pubis and labium major (female)
infraoccipital n.	see suboccipital nerve		
infraorbital n. *n. infraorbitalis*	continuation of maxillary n. after entering orbit through inferior orbital fissure	inferior palpebral, external nasal, superior labial; posterior, middle and anterior superior alveolar	upper teeth, skin of face, mucous membrane of mouth and floor of nasal cavity
infratrochlear n. *n. infratrochlearis*	nasociliary n.	palpebral	skin of eyelids and side of nose, conjunctiva, lacrimal sac and duct

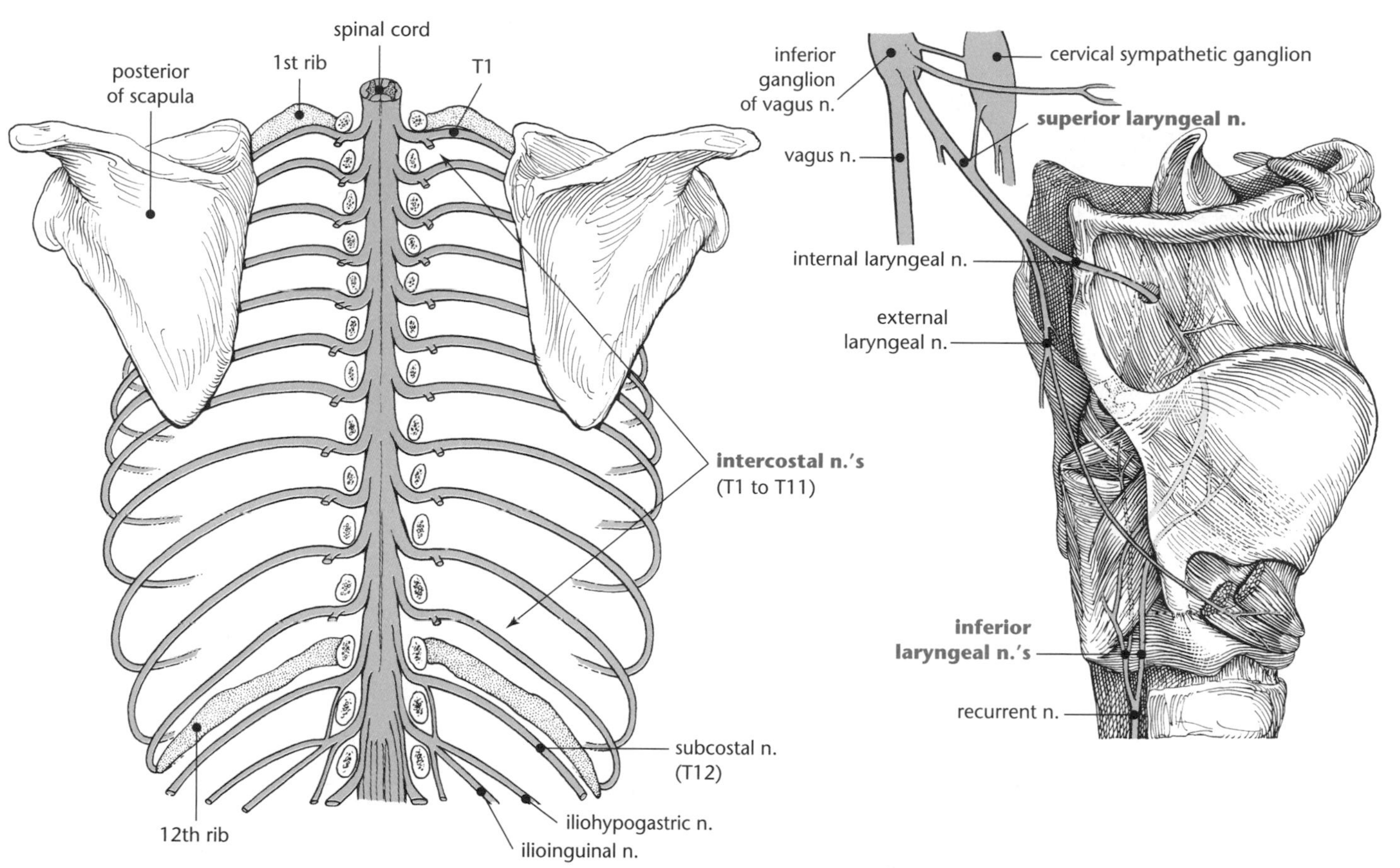

NERVE	ORIGIN	BRANCHES	DISTRIBUTION
intercostal n.'s (ventral rami of upper 11 thoracic n.'s between ribs) *nn. intercostales*	thoracic segments of spinal cord	lateral cutaneous, anterior cutaneous, collateral	first two n.'s supply fibers to upper limb and thoracic wall; next four supply thoracic wall; lower five supply thoracic and abdominal walls
intercostobrachial n. *n. intercostobrachialis*	second and frequenty third intercostal n.	filaments	skin of medial and posterior part of upper arm; axilla
intermediate n. glossopalatine n. n. of Wrisberg *n. intermedius*	brainstem at inferior border of pons	greater petrosal, chorda tympani	taste buds of anterior two-thirds of tongue, glands of soft palate and nose, sub-mandibular and sublingual glands, skin of external acoustic meatus and mastoid process
interosseous n. of forearm, anterior *n. interosseus antebrachii anterior*	median n.	muscular, filaments	most of the deep anterior muscles of forearm
interosseous n. of forearm, posterior *n. interosseus antebrachll posterior*	deep branch of radial n.	muscular, articular	wrist and intercarpal joints, deep extensor muscles of forearm, long abductor and extensor muscles of thumb
interosseous n. of leg *n. interosseus cruris*	tibial n.	filaments	ankle joints, tibia and fibula articulations
jugular n. *n. jugularis*	superior cervical ganglion	filaments	to glossopharyngeal and vagus n.'s
labial n.'s, anterior *nn. labiales anteriores*	ilioinguinal n.	filaments	skin to anterior labial area of female genitalia
labial n.'s, posterior *nn. labiales posteriores*	perineal n.	filaments	skin of posterior part of labium majus and vestibule of vagina
lacrimal n. *n. lacrimalis*	ophthalmic n.	superior palpebral, glandular, filaments	lacrimal gland and adjacent conjunctiva, skin of upper eyelid
laryngeal n., inferior *n. laryngeus inferior*	recurrent laryngeal n.	filaments	all intrinsic muscles of larynx except cricothyroid muscle

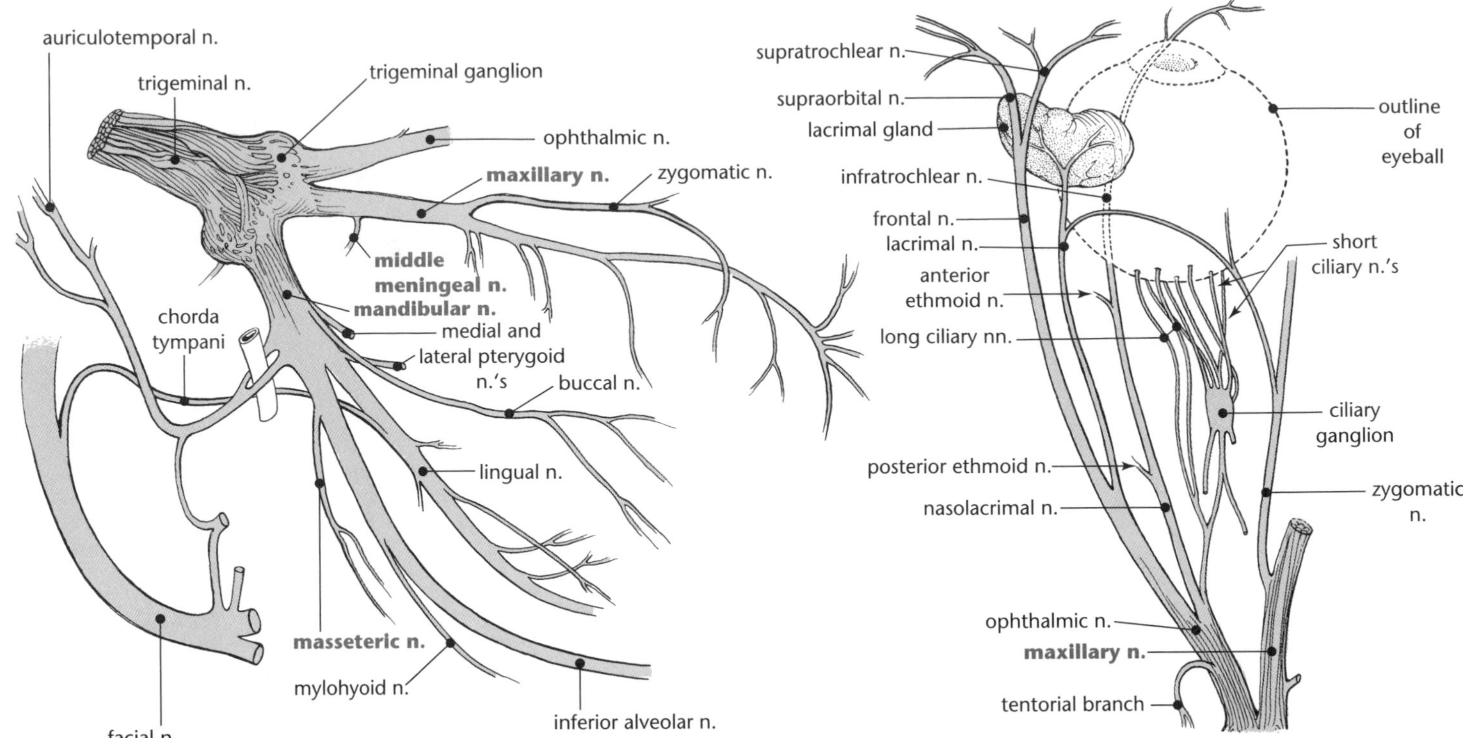

N

NERVE	ORIGIN	BRANCHES	DISTRIBUTION
laryngeal n., superior *n. laryngeus superior*	vagus n. near the inferior ganglion	external, internal	mucous membrane of larynx and epiglottis; inferior pharyngeal and cricothyroid muscles
laryngeal recurrent n.		see recurrent nerve	
lingual n. small hypoglossal n. *n. lingualis*	mandibular division of trigeminal n.	sublingual, lingual, branches communicating with hypoglossal n., chorda tympani, and submandibular ganglion	mucous membranes of anterior two-thirds of tongue, floor of mouth, gums, and sublingual glands
lumbar n.'s (five pairs of spinal n.'s) *nn. lumbales*	lumbar segments of spinal cord	ventral, dorsal	lumbar and sacral plexuses, deep muscles and skin of lower back
mandibular n. inferior maxillary n. *n. mandibularis*	trigeminal ganglion	masseteric, medial pterygoid, lateral pterygoid, deep temporal, buccal, auriculotemporal, lingual, inferior alveolar, meningeal	muscles of mastication, tensor tympani, tensor of palatal velum, anterior belly of digastric, and mylohyoid muscles, mandible, lower teeth and gums, anterior two-thirds of tongue, cheek, lower face, meninges, temporomandibular joint, skin of temporal region, external ear
masseteric n. *n. massetericus*	mandibular n.	filaments	masseter muscle, temporomandibular joint
maxillary n. superior maxillary n. *n. maxillaris*	trigeminal ganglion	middle meningeal, zygomatic, pterygopalatine, infraorbital, superior alveolar, inferior palpebral, external nasal, superior labial	skin of middle part of face, nose, lower eyelid, and upper lip; upper teeth and gums, tonsil and roof of mouth, soft palate, maxillary sinus, mucous membrane of nasopharynx
median n. *n. medianus*	by two roots from medial and lateral cords of brachial plexus	muscular, articular, anterior interosseous, common palmar digitals, proper digital	most of flexor muscles of forearm, short muscles of thumb, lateral lumbricals, skin of hand, hand joints, elbow joint, pulp under nails
meningeal n. *n. meningeus*	vagus	filaments	meninges
meningeal n., middle *n. meningeus medius*	maxillary n.	filaments	meninges, especially dura mater

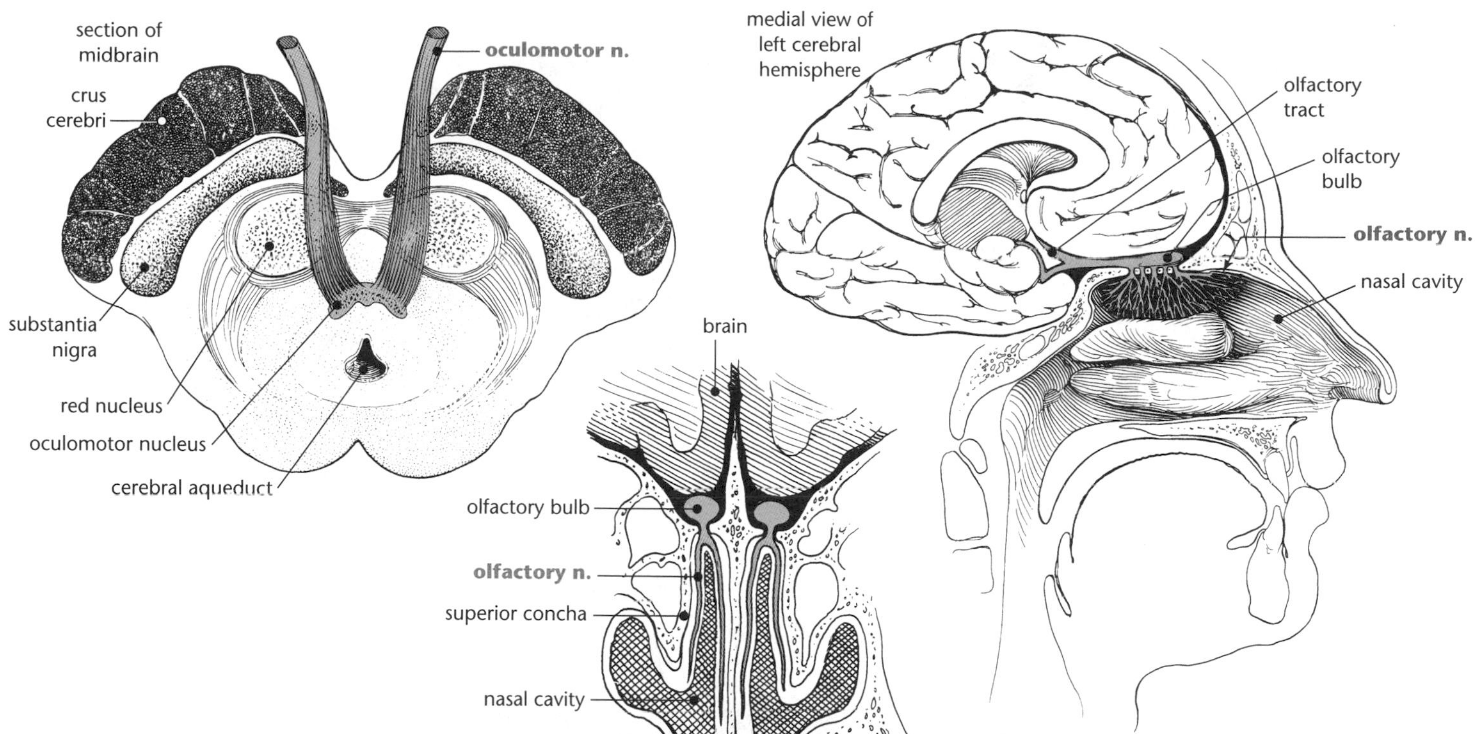

NERVE	ORIGIN	BRANCHES	DISTRIBUTION
mental n. *n. mentalis*	inferior alveolar n.	filaments	skin of chin, mucous membrane of lower lip
musculocutaneous n. *n. musculocutaneus*	lateral cord of brachial plexus	muscular, articular, filament, humeral filament, lateral cutaneous n. of forearm	coracobrachialis, brachialis and biceps muscles; skin of lateral side of forearm
musculospiral n.	see radial nerve		
mylohyoid n. *n. mylohyoideus*	inferior alveolar n. just before it enters mandibular foramen	filaments	mylohyoid and anterior belly of digastric muscles
nasal n.'s, external *nn. nasales externi*	anterior ethmoid n.	filaments	skin on side of nose
nasociliary n. nasal n. *n. nasociliaris*	ophthalmic n.	long ciliary, anterior ethmoidal, posterior ethmoidal, infratrochlear, communication with ciliary ganglion	mucous membranes of nasal cavity, anterior ethmoidal and frontal sinuses; iris, cornea, conjunctiva, lacrimal sac, skin of eyelids and side of nose
nasopalatine n. Scarpa's n. *n. nasopalatinus*	pterygopalatine ganglion and maxillary n.	filaments	mucous membrane of hard palate and nasal septum
ninth cranial n.	see glossopharyngeal nerve		
obturator n. *n. obturatorius*	second, third, and fourth lumbar n.'s	anterior, posterior, filaments	hip and knee joints, skin of medial side of thigh, gracilis muscle, great, long, and short adductor muscles
obturator n., accessory *n. obturatorius accessorius*	third and fourth lumbar n.'s	muscular, articular	pectineal muscle, hip joint
n. of obturatur, internal *n. obturatorius internus*	fifth lumbar and first and second sacral n.'s	muscular, filaments	internal obturator and superior gemelius muscles
occipital n., larger (greater) *n. occipitalis major*	median branch of dorsal division of second cervical n.	muscular, filaments, medial, lateral, auricular	scalp of top and back of head; semispinal muscle of head
occipital n., smaller (lesser) *n. occipitalis minor*	second sacral n.	auricular, filaments	skin of side of head and behind ear
occipital n., third least occipital *n.* *n. occipitalis tertius*	cutaneous part of third cervical n.	medial, lateral	skin of lower part of back of head
oculomotor n. third cranial n. *n. oculomotorius*	midbrain at medial side of cerebral peduncle	superior, inferior	levator muscle of upper eyelid, most intrinsic and extrinsic muscles of eye

N

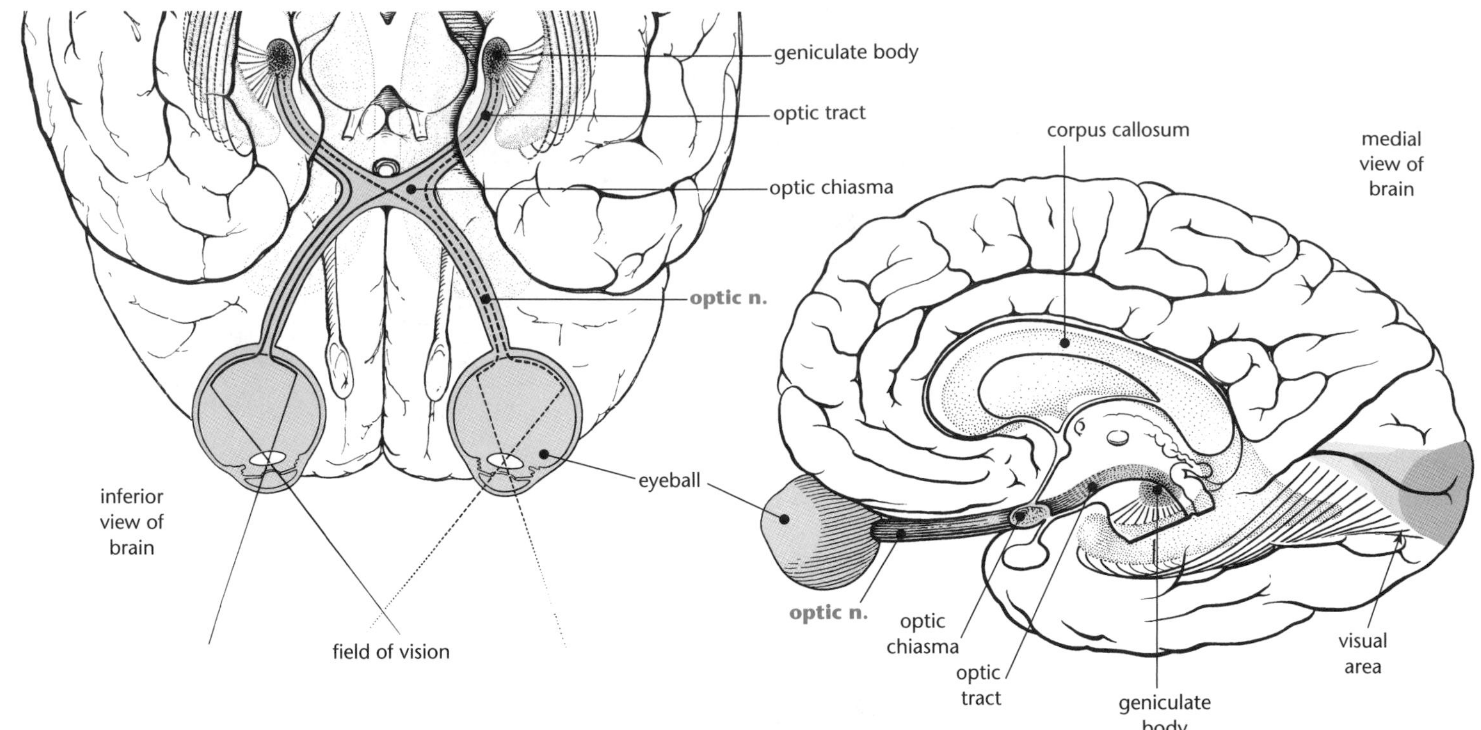

NERVE	ORIGIN	BRANCHES	DISTRIBUTION
olfactory n.'s first cranial n.'s *nn. olfactorii*	olfactory portion of nasal mucosa	filaments	olfactory bulb
ophthalmic n. *n. ophthalmicus*	trigeminal ganglion	tentorial, lacrimal, frontal, nasociliary	dura mater, eyeball, conjunctiva, lacrimal gland, mucous membrane of nose and paranasal sinuses, skin of the forehead, eyelids, and nose
optic n. second cranial n. n. of sight *n. opticus*	ganglionic layer of retina	filaments	optic chiasma
palatine n., large anterior palatine n. *n. palatinus anterior*	pterygopalatine ganglion	posterior inferior nasal, lesser palatine	gums, mucous membrane of hard and soft palates
palatine n.'s, small *nn. palatini medius et posterior*	pterygopalatine ganglion	filaments	soft palate, uvula, palatine tonsil
palpebral n., inferior *n. palpebralis inferior*	infraorbital n.	filaments	lower eyelid
palpebral n., superior *n. palpebralis superior*	lacrimal n.	filaments	upper eyelid
pectoral n., lateral *n. pectoralis lateralis*	lateral cord of brachial plexus	filaments	greater pectoral muscle
pectoral n., medial *n. pectoralis medialis*	medial cord of brachial plexus	filaments	smaller pectoral muscle and caudal part of greater pectoral muscle
perineal n. *n. perinei*	pudendal n.	muscular, posterior scrotal (male), n. to urethal bulb, labial (female)	urogenital diaphragm, skin of external genitalia, perineal muscles, mucous membrane of urethra
peroneal n., common external popliteal n. peroneal n. *n. peroneus communis*	sciatic n.	articular (three), lateral cutaneous n. of calf, deep peroneal, superficial peroneal	knee joint, skin of posterior and lateral surfaces of leg, short head of biceps muscle of thigh, leg muscles
peroneal n., deep anterior tibial n. *n. peroneus profundus*	common peroneal n.	muscular, articular, lateral terminal, medial terminal, dorsal digital	anterior tibial, long extensor of great toe, long extensor of toes, short extensor of toes, third peroneal, ankle joint, tarsal and tarsophalangeal joints of second, third, and fourth toes

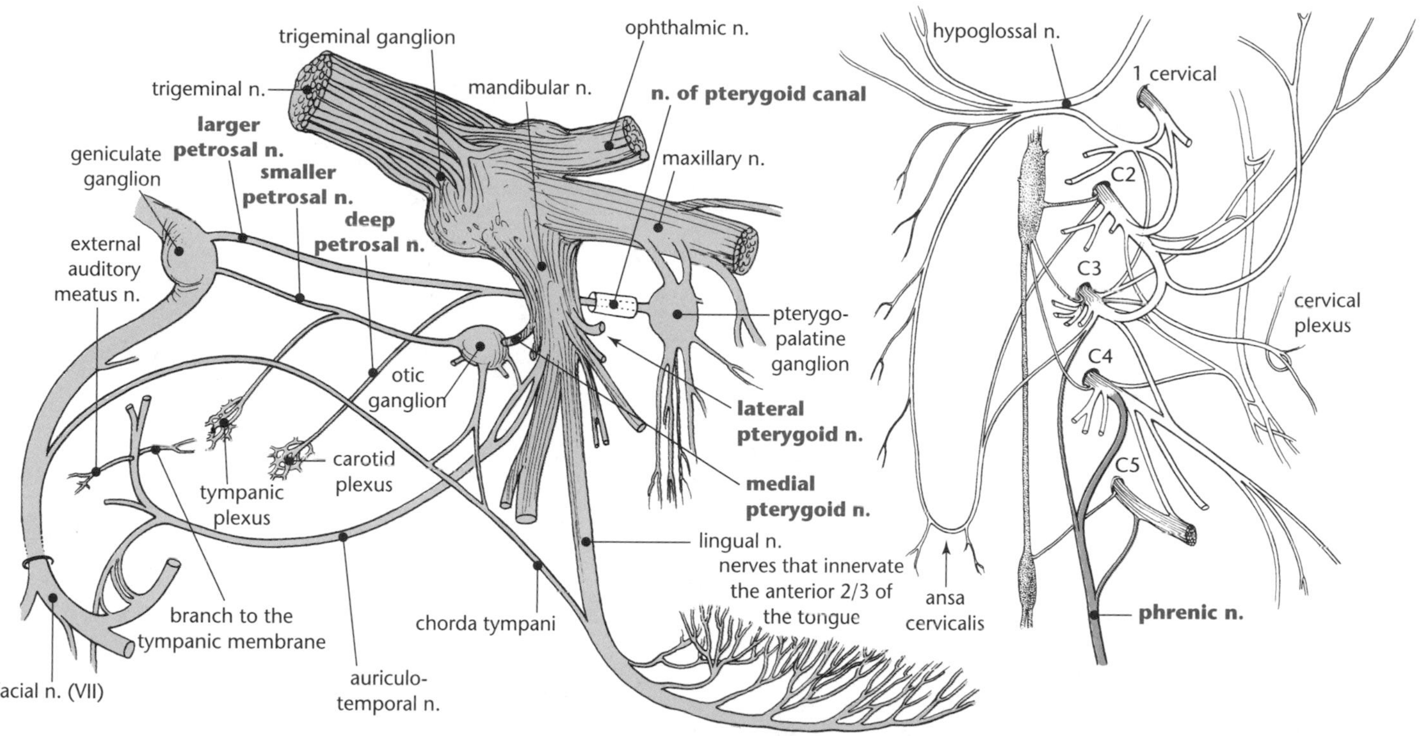

NERVE	ORIGIN	BRANCHES	DISTRIBUTION
peroneal n., superficial musculocutaneous n. *n. peroneus superficialis*	common peroneal n.	muscular, cutaneous filaments, medial dorsal cutaneous, intermediate dorsal cutaneous	long and short peroneal muscles, skin of lower part of leg, skin of medial side of foot, ankle, and side of great toe, skin of adjacent sides of second, third, fourth, and fifth toes
petrosal n., deep *n. petrosus profundus*	internal carotid plexus	joins larger petrosal n. to form n. of the pterygoid canal	glands and blood vessels of pharynx, nasal cavity, lacrimal gland, and palate
petrosal n., larger (greater) greater superficial petrosal n. *n. petrosus major*	geniculate ganglion of facial n.	joins deep petrosal n. to form n. of pterygoid canal	mucous membrane and glands of palate, nose, lacrimal gland, and naso-pharynx
petrosal n., smaller (lesser) lesser superficial petrosal n. *n. petrosus minor*	tympanic plexus	ganglionic, filaments	otic ganglion, parotid gland
phrenic n. internal respiratory n. of Bell *n. phrenicus*	third, fourth, and fifth cervical n.'s	pericardial, phrenico-abdominal	diaphragm, pericardium mediastinal pleura, sympathetic plexus
phrenic n.'s, accessory *nn. phrenici accessorii*	inconstant branch from fifth cervical n. which arises with subclavian n.	joins phrenic n.	diaphragm
n. of piriform *n. piriformis*	first and second sacral n.'s	filaments	piriform muscle
plantar n., lateral external plantar n. *n. plantaris lateralis*	tibial n.	muscular, superficial, deep	skin of fifth and lateral half of fourth toes, deep muscles of foot
plantar n., medial internal plantar n. *n. plantaris medialis*	tibial n.	common plantar digital, common digitals (three), plantar cutaneous, muscular, articular	skin of sole of foot, skin of adjacent sides of great, sec-ond, third, and fourth toes, joints of tarsus and metatar-sus, short flexor muscle of great toe, lumbrical muscles of foot
pterygoid canal, n. of Vidian n. *n. canalis pterygoidei*	formed by union of larger petrosal and deep petrosal n.'s	filaments	glands of nose, palate, and pharynx; pterygopalatine ganglion
pterygoid n., lateral *n. pterygoideus lateralis*	mandibular n.	none	deep surface of lateral pterygoid muscle
pterygoid n., medial *n. pterygoideus medialis*	mandibular n.	tensor veli palatini, tensor tympani, filaments	tensor veli palatini, tensor tympani and medial ptery-goid muscles

N

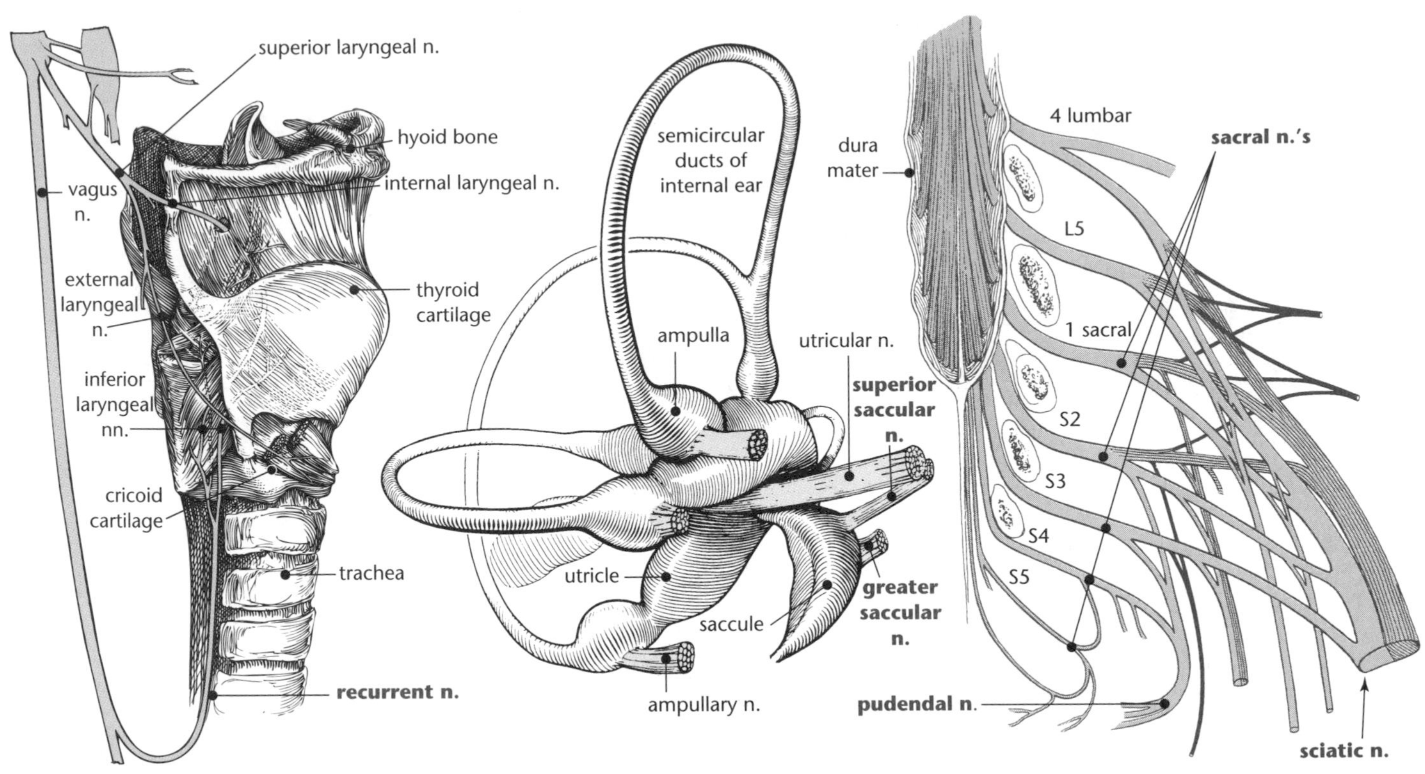

N

NERVE	ORIGIN	BRANCHES	DISTRIBUTION
pterygopalatine n.'s sphenopalatine n.'s *nn. pterygopalatini* *nn. ganglionares*	maxillary n.	orbital, greater palatine, posterior superior nasal, pharyngeal	mucous membranes of posterior ethmoidal and sphenoidal sinuses, nasal part of pharynx, and hard palate; periosteum of orbit, gums, nasal septum
pudendal n. internal pudic n. *n. pudendus*	second, third, and fourth sacral n.'s	inferior rectal, perineal, dorsal n. of penis (male) or dorsal n. clitoris (female)	urogenital diaphragm, skin around anus, skin of scrotum or labium major, external sphincter of anus, erectile tissue, muscles of perineum
n. of quadrate muscle of thigh *n. quadratus femoris*	fourth and fifth lumbar and first sacral n.'s	filaments	quadrate muscle of thigh and inferior gemellus muscle
radial n. musculospiral n. *n. radialis*	posterior cord of brachial plexus	muscular, articular, superficial, deep, cutaneous	extensor muscles of arm and forearm, and skin on back of arm, forearm, and hand
rectal n., inferior inferior hemorrhoidal *n.* *n. rectalis inferior*	pudendal n.	filaments	external sphincter of anus, skin around anus, lining of anal canal
rectal n., middle *n. rectalis medius*	hypogastric plexus	filaments	rectum
rectal n., superior *n. rectalis superior*	inferior mesenteric plexus	filaments	rectum
recurrent n. recurrent laryngeal n. inferior laryngeal n. *n. recurrens*	vagus n.	pharyngeal, inferior laryngeal, tracheal, esophageal, cardiac	all muscles of larynx except cricothyroid; cardiac plexus, trachea, esophagus
saccular n., greater *n. saccularis major*	vestibular ganglion	filaments	larger of two nerves that innervate saccule of internal ear
saccular n., superior *n. saccularis superior*	vestibular ganglion	filaments	smaller of two nerves that innervate saccule of internal ear
sacral n.'s (five pairs of spinal nerves) *nn. sacrales*	sacral segments of spinal cord	dorsal, ventral, pelvic splanchnic	deep muscles and skin of lower back, pelvic viscera, sacral plexus, coccygeal plexus
sacral plexus *plexus sacralis*	fourth and fifth lumbar and first, second, and third sacral n.'s	internal obturator, superior and inferior gluteals, posterior femoral cutaneous, quadrate muscle of thigh, piriform, sciatic, pudendal	muscle and skin of perineum and lower limb; hip joint, buttock

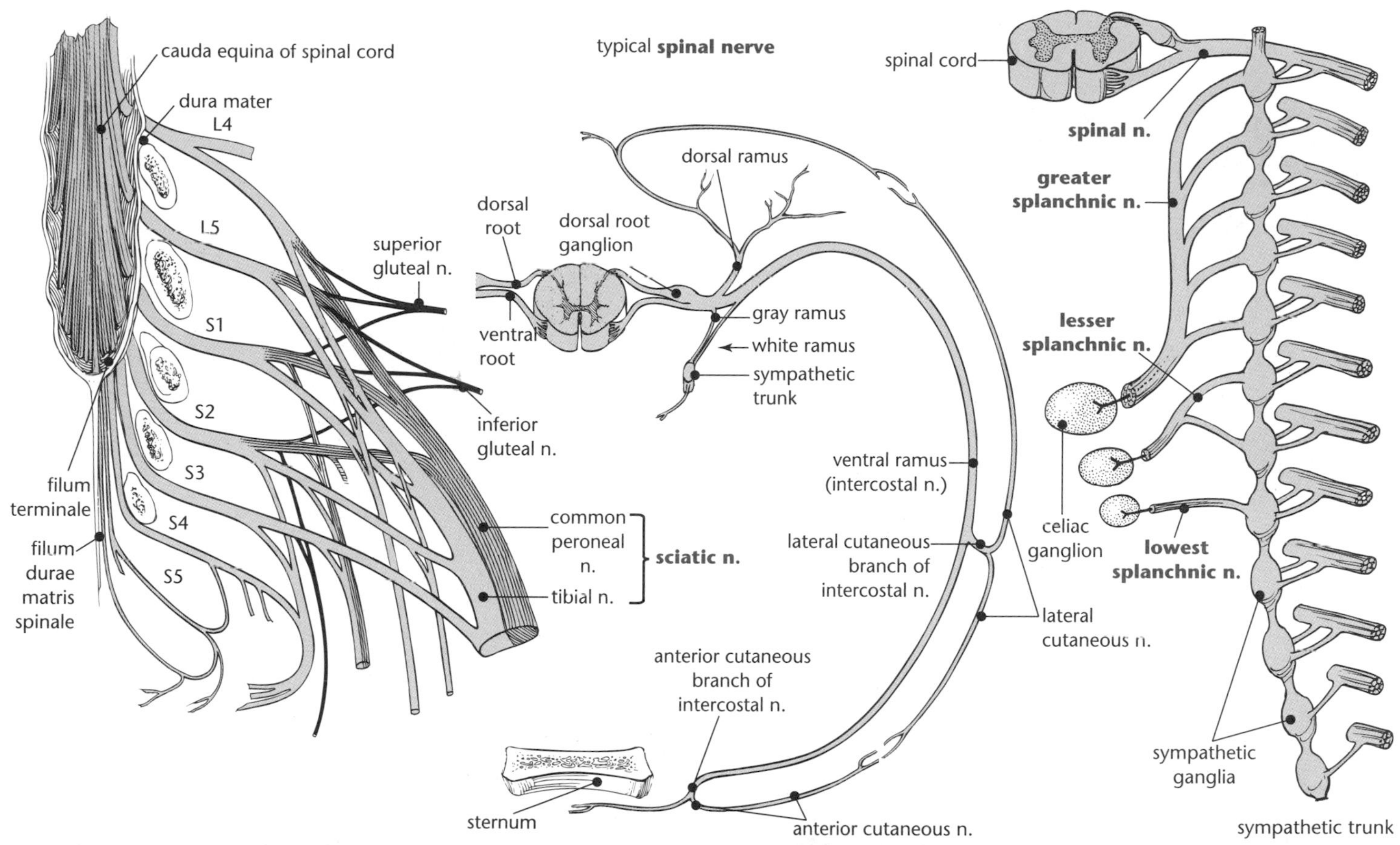

NERVE	ORIGIN	BRANCHES	DISTRIBUTION
saphenus n. *n. saphenus*	femoral n.	infrapatellar, medial crural cutaneous, filaments	skin of medial side of leg and foot, knee joint, patellar plexus
scapular n., dorsal posterior scapular n. *n. dorsalis scapulae*	fifth cervical n. near intervertebral foramen	filaments	greater and smaller rhomboid muscle, levator muscle of scapula
sciatic n. (largest n. in body) great sciatic n. *n. ischiadicus*	fourth and fifth lumbar and first, second, and third sacral n.'s	articular, muscular, tibial, common peroneal	skin of foot and most of leg, muscles of leg and foot, all joints of lower limb
sciatic n., small	see cutaneous n. of thigh, posterior		
scrotal n.'s, anterior *nn. scrotales anteriores*	ilioinguinal n.	filaments	skin of anterior scrotal area and root of penis
scrotal n.'s, posterior *nn. scrotales posteriores*	perineal n.	filaments	skin of posterior scrotal area
second cranial n.	see optic nerve		
seventh cranial n.	see facial nerve		
sixth cranial n.	see abducent nerve		
spermatic n., external *n. genitalis externi*	genitofemoral	filaments	skin of scrotum and around inguinal ring area
sphenopalatine n.	see pterygopalatine nerve		
spinal n.'s *nn. spinales*	31 pairs of n.'s arising from the spinal cord within the vertebral canal, including 8 cervical, 12 thoracic, 5 lumbar, 5 sacral, and 1 coccygeal		
splanchnic n., greater *n. splanchnicus major*	5th (or 6th) to 9th (or 10th) thoracic sympathetic ganglia	filaments	celiac ganglion, thoracic aorta, adrenal gland, aorticorenal ganglion
splanchnic n., lesser *n. splanchnicus minor*	9th and 10th thoracic sympathetic ganglia	renal, filaments	aorticorenal ganglion
splanchnic n., lowest least splanchnic n. *n. splanchnicus imus*	last thoracic sympathetic ganglion or lesser splanchnic n.	filaments	renal plexus
splanchnic n.'s, lumbar (two to four in number) *nn. splanchnici lumbales*	lumbar sympathetic trunk at level of first, second, and third lumbar vertebrae	filaments	renal intermesenteric, and hypogastric plexuses

N

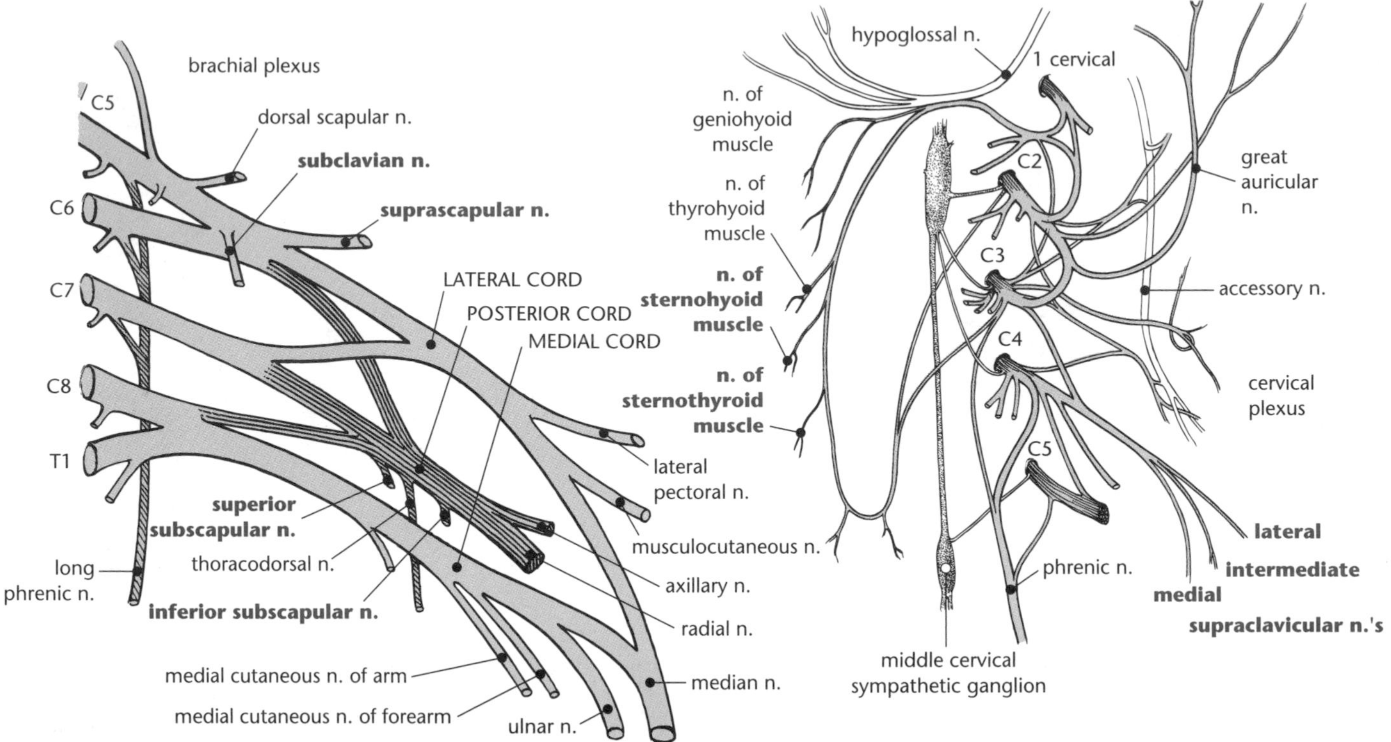

NERVE	ORIGIN	BRANCHES	DISTRIBUTION
splanchnic n.'s, sacral *nn. splanchnici sacrales*	sacral sympathetic ganglion	filaments	inferior hypogastric plexus
splanchnic n.'s, pelvic erigentes n.'s *nn. splanchnici pelvini*	second to fourth sacral n.'s	filaments	inferior hypogastric plexus, descending and sigmoid colon, pelvic viscera
n. of stapedius *n. stapedius*	facial n.	filaments	stapedius muscle
n. of sternohyoid *n. sternohyoideus*	convexity of ansa cervicalis	filaments	sternohyoid muscle
n. of sternothyroid *n. sternothyroideus*	convexity of ansa cervicalis	filaments	sternothyroid muscle
subclavian n. *n. subclavius*	superior trunk of brachial plexus	articular, filaments	subclavius muscle, sternoclavicular joint
subcostal n. *n. subcostalis*	12th thoracic n.	anterior cutaneous, lateral cutaneous	skin of lower abdominal wall and gluteal region; some abdominal muscles
sublingual n. *n. sublingualis*	lingual n.	filaments	sublingual gland and mucous membrane of floor of mouth
suboccipital n. infraoccipital n. *n. suboccipitalis*	first cervical n.	filaments	deep muscles of back of neck
subscapular n.'s (usually two in number) *nn. subscapulares*	posterior cord of brachial plexus	superior, inferior	subscapular and teres major muscles
supraclavicular n.'s, intermediate middle supraclavicular n.'s *nn. supraclaviculares intermedii*	common trunk formed by third and fourth cervical n.'s	filaments	skin over pectoral and deltoid muscles
supraclavicular n.'s, lateral posterior supraclavicular n.'s super-acromial n.'s *nn. supraclaviculares laterales*	common trunk formed by third and fourth cervical n.'s	filaments	skin of upper and dorsal parts of shoulder
supraclavicular n.'s, medial anterior supraclavicular n.'s *nn. supraclaviculares mediales*	common trunk formed by third and fourth cervical n.'s	filaments	skin of medial infraclavicular region as far as the midline, sternoclavicular joint
supraorbital n. *n. supraorbitalis*	frontal n.	medial, lateral, filaments	skin of upper eyelid and forehead, mucosa of frontal sinus, scalp
suprascapular n. *n. suprascapularis*	superior trunk of brachial plexus	supraspinous, infraspinous, articular, filaments	supraspinous and infra-spinous muscles, shoulder joint

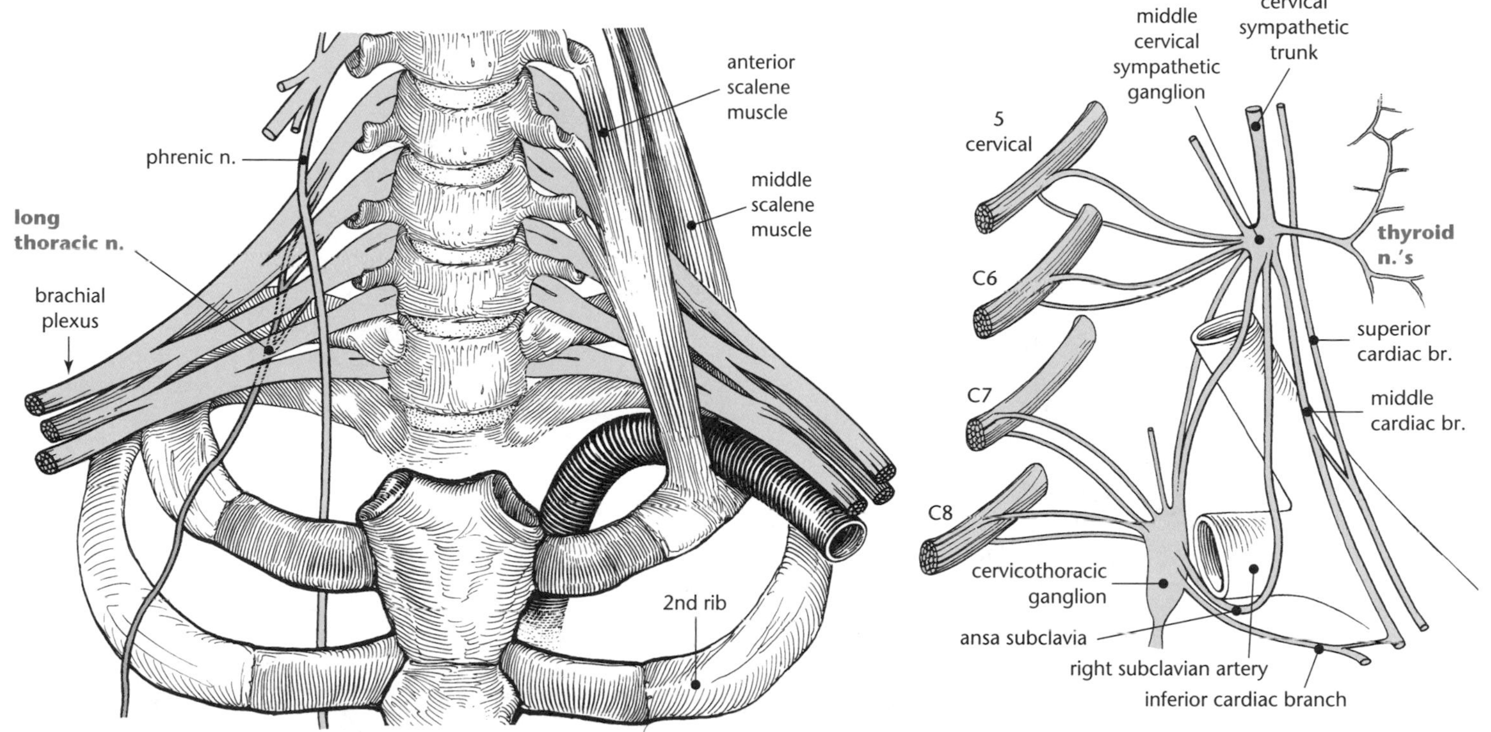

NERVE	ORIGIN	BRANCHES	DISTRIBUTION
supratrochlear n. *n. supratrochlearis*	frontal n.	filaments, ascending, descending	conjunctiva, skin of upper eyelid and forehead
sural n. short saphenous n. *n. suralis*	medial and lateral cutaneous n.'s of calf	lateral dorsal cutaneous, lateral calcaneal	skin of back of leg and lateral side of foot
temporal n.'s, deep (usually two in number) *nn. temporales profundi*	mandibular division of trigeminal n.	filaments	temporal muscle
n. to tensor tympani *n. tensoris tympani*	medial pterygoid n.	filaments	tensor muscle of tympanum
n. to tensor veli palatini *n. teosoris veli palatini*	medial pterygoid n.	filaments	tensor muscle of palatine velum
tenth cranial n.	see vagus nerve		
tentorial n. *n. tentorii*	ophthalmic n.	filaments	tentorium cerebelli
terminal n. *n. terminalis*	cerebral hemispheres near olfactory trigone	filaments	dura mater, mucous membrane of nasal septum
third cranial n.	see oculomotor nerve		
thoracic n.'s (12 pairs of spinal n.'s) *nn. thoracici*	thoracic segments of spinal cord	dorsal, ventral	thoracic and abdominal walls (parietes) and skin of the buttock
thoracic n., long n. of serratus anterior *n. thoracicus longus*	fifth, sixth, and seventh cervical n.'s	filaments	all digitations of serratus anterior muscle
thoracoabdominal intercostal n.'s *nn. thoracoabdominales intercostales*	ventral primary divisions of 7th to 11th thoracic n.'s beyond the intercostal spaces	filaments	anterior abdominal wall
thoracodorsal n. long subscapular n. n. of latissimus dorsi *n. thoracodorsalis*	posterior cord of brachial plexus	filaments	latissimus dorsi muscle
n. of thyrohyoid *n. thyrohoideus*	first cervical n. traveling with hypoglossal n.	filaments	thyrohyoid muscle
thyroid n.'s *nn. thyroideus*	middle cervical ganglion	filaments	thyroid gland, parathyroid glands
tibia n. internal popliteal n. *n. tibialis*	sciatic n.	articular, medial calcaneal, medial sural cutaneous, medial and lateral plantar	knee and ankle joints, muscles of posterior leg, plantar muscles of foot

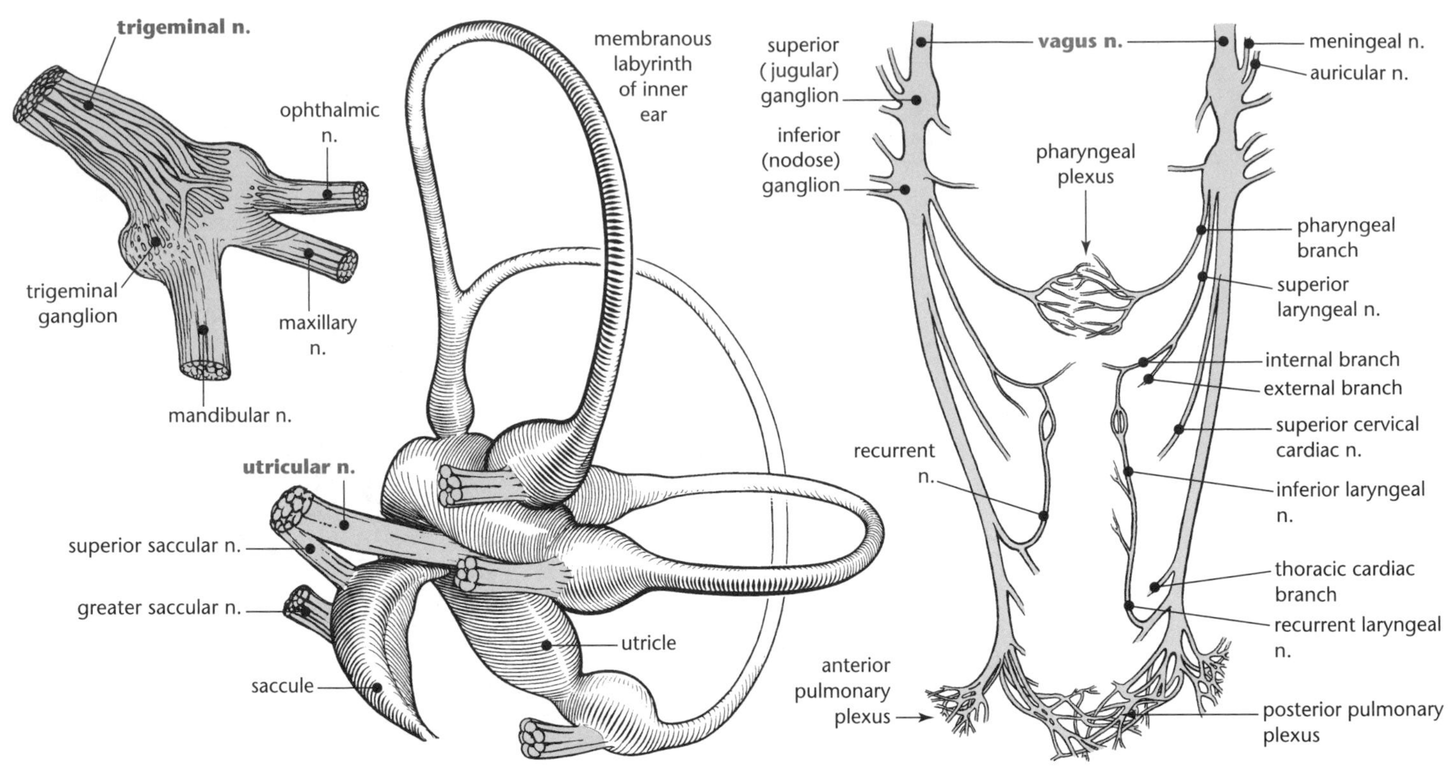

N

NERVE	ORIGIN	BRANCHES	DISTRIBUTION
tibial n., anterior	see peroneal nerve, deep		
tranverse cervical n. cervical cutaneous n. *n. transversus colli*	second and third cervical n.'s	ascending, descending	skin over anterior and lateral parts of neck
trigeminal n. (largest of the cranial n.'s) fifth n. trifacial n. *n. trigeminus*	brainstem at inferior surface of pons	two roots (motor and sensory) expand into trigeminal ganglion near apex of petrous portion of temporal bone, from which ophthalmic, maxillary, and mandibular n.'s arise	skin of face, muscles of mastication, teeth, mouth, and nasal cavity, scalp
trochlear n. (smallest of the cranial n.'s) fourth cranial n. *n. trochlearis*	midbrain immediately posterior to the inferior colliculus	filaments	superior oblique muscle of eyeball
twelfth cranial n.	see hypoglossal nerve		
tympanic n. n. of Jacobson *n. tympanicus*	glossopharyngeal n.	lesser petrosal, contributes to formation of tympanic plexus	middle ear chamber, tympanic membrane, mastoid air cells, auditory tube, parotid gland
ulnar n. cubital n. *n. ulnaris*	medial cord of brachial plexus	articular, muscular, dorsal, palmar (superficial and deep)	intrinsic muscles of hand, elbow, wrist and hand joints, skin of medial side of hand
utricular n. *n. utricularis*	utriculoampullar n.	filaments	utricle of the internal ear
utriculoampullar n. *n. utriculoampullaris*	a division of the vestibular portion of the vestibulocochlear n.; it innervates the macula of the utricle and saccule as well as the ampullae of the anterior and lateral semicircular ducts		
vaginal n.'s *nn. vaginales*	uterovaginal plexus	filaments	vagina
vagus n. tenth cranial n. pneumogastric n. *n. vagus*	side of medulla oblongata between the olive and the inferior cerebellar peduncle	meningeal, auricular, pharyngeal, superior laryngeal, superior and inferior cardiac, anterior and posterior bronchial, recurrent, esophageal, gastric, hepatic, celiac	dura mater, skin of posterior surface of external ear, voluntary muscles of larynx and pharynx, heart, nonstriated muscles and glands of esophagus, stomach, trachea, bronchi, biliary tract, and intestines, mucous membranes of pharynx, larynx, bronchi, lungs, digestive tract, and kidney

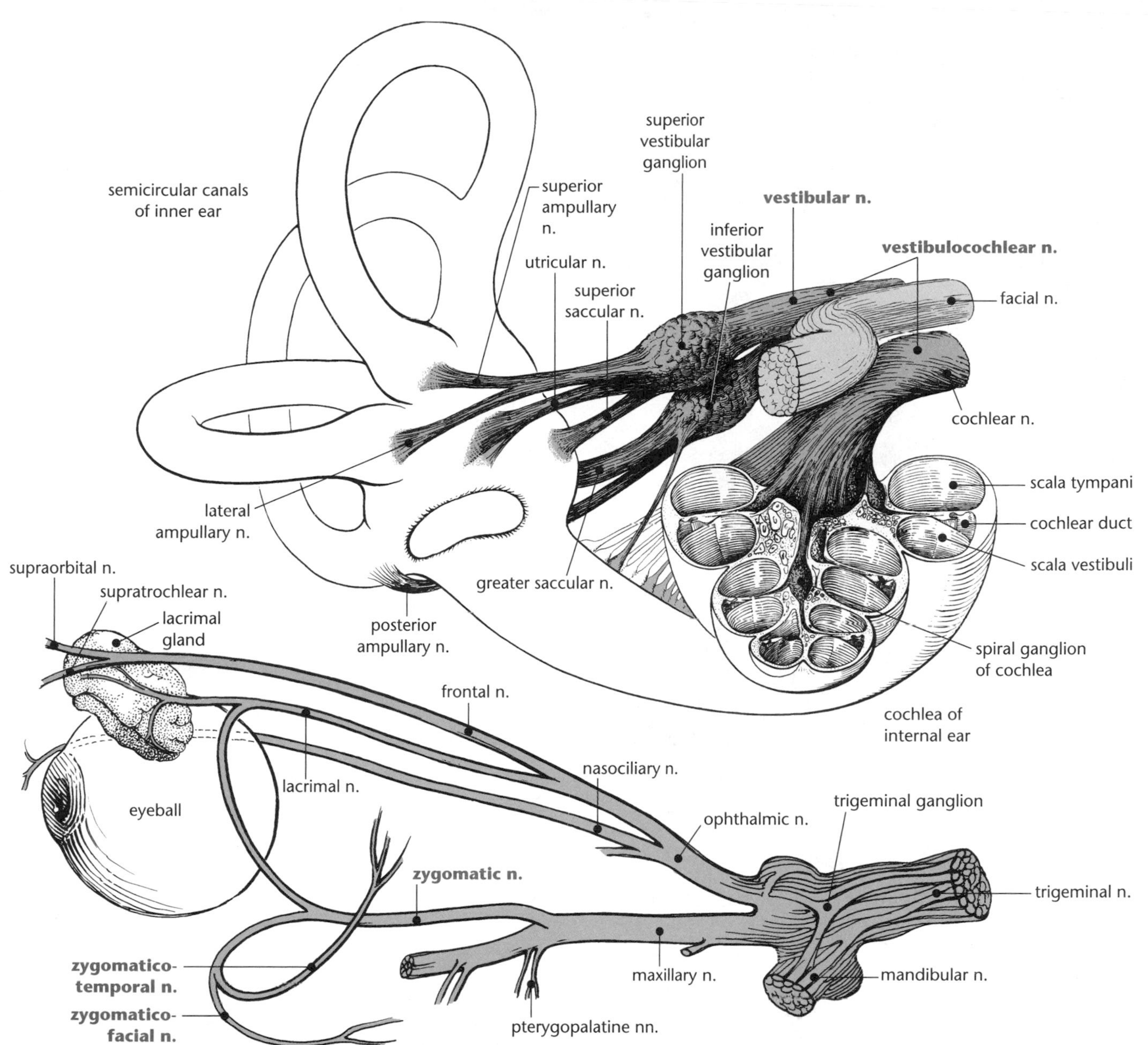

NERVE	ORIGIN	BRANCHES	DISTRIBUTION
vertebral n. *n. vertebralis*	cervicothoracic (stellate) ganglion	meningeal, filaments	meninges, joins cervical n.'s, vertibral artery
vestibular n. n. of equilibration *n. vestibularis*	vestibulocochlear n.	utricular, saccular, ampullar	through vestibular ganglion (ganglion of Scarpa) to maculae of utricle and saccule, and to ampullae of semicircular ducts)
vestibulocochlear n. eighth cranial n. auditory n. acoustic n. otic n. *n. vestibulocochlearis*	brainstem between pons and medulla oblongata formed by union of vestibular and cochlear n.'s	vestibular (medial), cochlear (lateral)	receptor organs in membranous labyrinth of inner ear
Vidian n.	see pterygoid canal, n. of		
vomernasal n. *n. vomernasalis*	present in the nasal septum of the fetus but disappears before birth		
zygomatic n. orbital n. temporomalar n. *n. zygomaticus*	maxillary n.	zygomaticotemporal, zygomaticofacial	skin of temple, skin on prominence of cheek (zygomatic arch)
zygomaticofacial n. *n. zygomaticofacialis*	zygomatic n.	filaments	skin over prominence of cheek (zygomatic arch)
zygomaticotemporal n. *n. zygomaticotemporalis*	zygomatic n.	filaments	skin on side of forehead (temple)

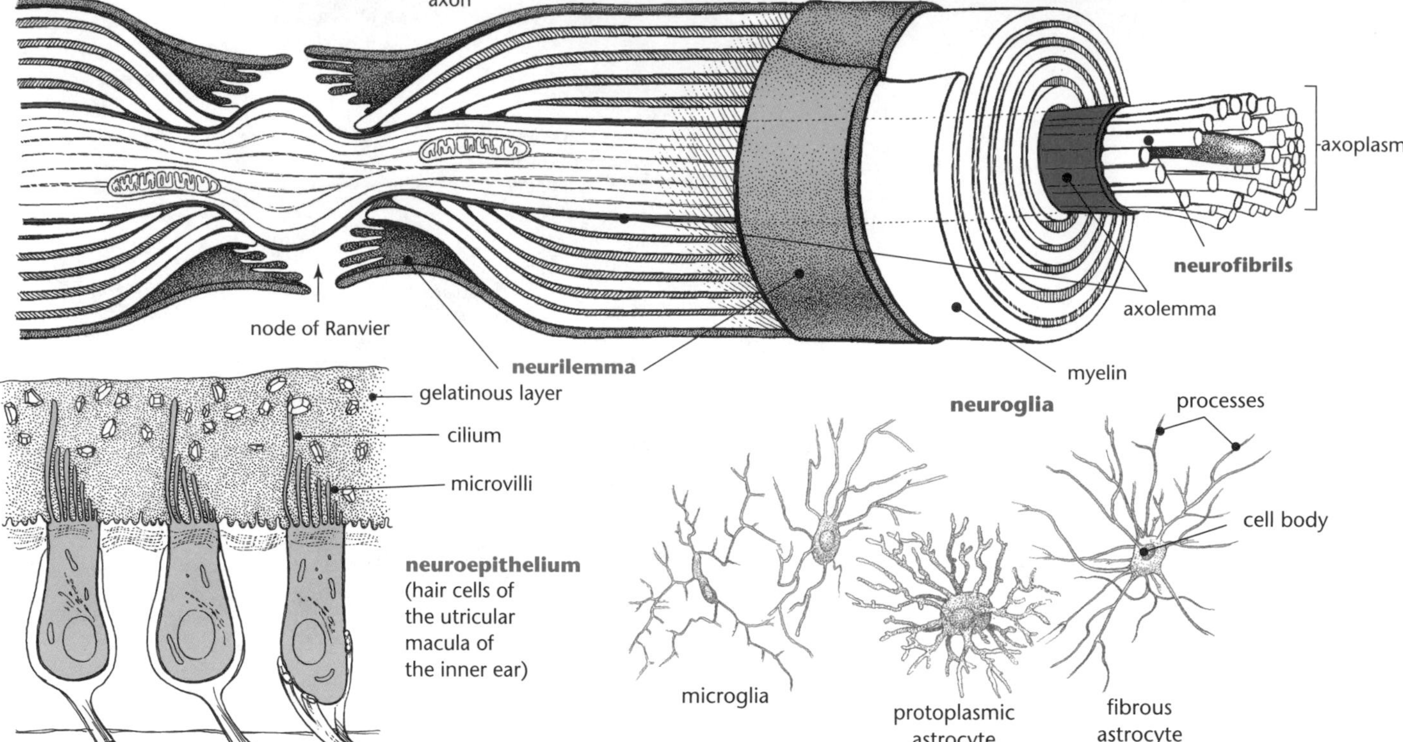

nervous (ner´vus) **1.** Relating to nerves. **2.** High-strung; excitable.
nervous breakdown (ner´vus brāk´down) Popular euphemism for mental disorder.
nervousness (ner´vus-nes) Undue irritability and excitability.
nervus (ner´vus), *pl.* **nervi** Latin for nerve.
nesslerize (nes´ler-īz) To treat a blood or urine specimen with Nessler's reagent to determine the urea nitrogen levels.
nest (nest) A collection of similar entities.
cell n.'s Small collections of a different type of cell in a tissue.
net (net) Network.
network (net´werk) A structure composed of interlocking filaments. Also called reticulum; rete; net.
chromatin n. Basophilic network in the nuclei of many cells, appearing after fixation.
Purkinje's n. Network of muscle fibers beneath the endocardium of the cardiac ventricles.
neural (nōō´ral) **1.** Relating to the nervous system. **2.** Referring to the dorsal region of an embryo.
neuralgia (nōō-ral´je-ă) Severe pain along the course of a nerve.
Morton's n. See Morton's neuroma, under neuroma.
occipital n. Piercing pain on one side of the back of the head, caused by entrapment of the greater occipital nerve as it exits from the skull.
trigeminal n. Spasmodic, piercing facial pain along the trigeminal nerve. Also called tic douloureux.
neuralgic (nōō-ral´jik) Relating to neuralgia.
neuranagenesis (nōō-ran-ă-jen´ĕ-sis) Regeneration of a nerve.
neurapraxia (nōō-ră-prak´se-ă) Injury to a nerve resulting in temporary paralysis.
neurasthenia (nōō-ras-the´ne-ă) Condition marked by fatigue, irritability, and poor concentration; originally considered to be due to exhaustion of the nervous system.
traumatic n. See posttraumatic syndrome.
neuraxis (nōō-rak´sis) **1.** The central nervous system. **2.** Axon.
neuraxon (nōō-rak´son) See axon.
neurectomy (nōō-rek´tŏ-me) Surgical removal of a nerve segment.
neurectopia, neurectopy (noor-ĕk-to-pe-ă, nōō-rek´to-pe) Abnormal location of a nerve.
neurergic (nōō-rer´jik) Relating to the action of nerves.
neurilemma (noor-ĭ-lem´ă) The thin cytoplasmic membrane of a Schwann cell enwrapping the axon of an unmyelinated nerve fiber and also the myelin layers of a myelinated nerve fiber. Also called sheath of Schwann.
neurilemmitis (noor-ĭ-lem-i´tis) Inflammation of the neurilemma.
neurilemoma (noor-ĭ-lem-o´mă) See schwannoma.
acoustic n. See vestibular schwannoma, under schwannoma.
Antoni type A n. A relatively solid tumor consisting of Schwann cells (arranged in twisting bundles) and reticulum fibers.
Antoni type B n. A relatively soft tumor consisting of Schwann cells (arranged in a haphazard way) reticulum fibers, and minute cysts.
neurinoma (noor-ĭ-no´mă) See schwannoma.
acoustic n. See vestibular schwannoma, under schwannoma.
neuritis (nōō-ri´tis) Inflammation or degeneration of a nerve.
intraocular optic n. See papillitis.
optic n. General term denoting inflammation, degeneration, or demyelinization of the optic nerve caused by any of various diseases with loss of vision as a chief symptom.
toxic n. Neuritis resulting from a chemical toxin, as in arsenic or lead poisoning.
traumatic n. Neuritis following an injury.
neuroanastomosis (noor-o-ă-nas-tă-mo´sis) Surgical union of nerves.
neuroanatomy (noor-o-ă-nat´ŏ-me) The branch of anatomy concerned with the study of the nervous system.
neurobiology (noor-o-bi-ol´ŏ-je) The integrated study of neuroanatomy and neurophysiology (i.e., of the structure and normal vital processes of the nervous system).
neurobiotaxis (noor-o-bi-o-tak´sis) The tendency of nerve cells to move in the direction of the area where most of the impulses originate.
neuroblast (noor´o-blast) An embryonic nerve cell.
neuroblastoma (noor-o-blas-to´mă) A highly malignant tumor composed of embryonic neural crest cells and seen most frequently in the medulla of the adrenal gland; it is the most common malignant tumor of childhood and infancy. Also called sympathoblastoma; sympathogonioma.
neuroborreliosis (noor-o-bŏ-rel-e-o´sis) Inflammation of the nervous system caused by bacteria of the genus *Borrelia;* seen in AIDS patients.
neurocardiac (noor-o-kar´de-ak) **1.** Relating to the nerve supply of the heart. **2.** Relating to a cardiac neurosis.
neurocele (noor´o-sēl) The ventricles of the brain and the central canal of the spinal cord.
neurochemistry (noor-o-kem´is-tre) The study of the chemical activity of nervous tissues.
neurochoroiditis (noor-o-kor-oi-di´tis) Inflammation of the optic nerve and the middle vascular coat (choroid) of the eye.
neurocladism (nōō-rok´lă-diz-m) Regeneration of a cut nerve by the outgrowth of axonal branches from the proximal stump toward the distal stump, bridging the gap.
neuroclonic (nōō-ro-klon´ik) Relating to or marked by nervous spasm.
neurocranium (noor-o-kra´ne-um) The portion of the skull containing the brain, distinguished from the facial bones.
neurocytoma (noor-o-si-to´mă) See ganglioneuroma.
neurodensin (noor-o-den´sin) A tridecapeptide released from the small intestine by entry of food; appears to relax the lower esophageal sphincter muscle and to delay stomach emptying; may enhance propulsive activity of the colon. Originally found in the brain.
neurodermatitis (noor-o-der-mă-ti´tis) Localized inflammation of the skin of nervous or psychological origin.
neurodynamic (noor-o-di-nam´ik) Relating to nervous energy.
neurodynia (noor-o-din´e-ă) Neuralgia.
neuroectoderm (noor-o-ek´to-derm) In embryology, the part of the ectoderm that gives rise to the neural tube.
neuroendocrine (noor-o-en´do-krin) Denoting a relationship between the nervous system and the endocrine glands.
neuroendocrinology (noor-o-en-do-krĭ-nol´ŏ-je) The study of the interactions of the nervous system with the endocrine glands.
neuroepithelioma (noor-o-ep-ĭ-the-le-o´mă) A type of glioma consisting primarily of cells that resemble the precursors of specialized sensory epithelium or of the brain and spinal cord.
neuroepithelium (noor-o-ep-ĭ-the´le-um) **1.** The specialized epithelium composed of cells that act as receptors of external stimuli (e.g., hair cells of the inner ear). **2.** The layer of the ectoderm from which the neural tube develops.
neurofibril (noor-o-fi´bril) A nerve fibril; one of numerous aggregates of slender filaments running parallel with one another in the axon and dendrite but crossing and intermingling in the cell body.
neurofibroma (noor-o-fi-bro´mă) A benign tumor originating in the connective tissues of nerves; it occurs most frequently in the skin, where the nodules are formed.
neurofibromatosis (noor-o-fi-bro-mă-to´sis) Inherited disorder transmitted as a dominant trait, chiefly marked by formation of multiple nerve tumors

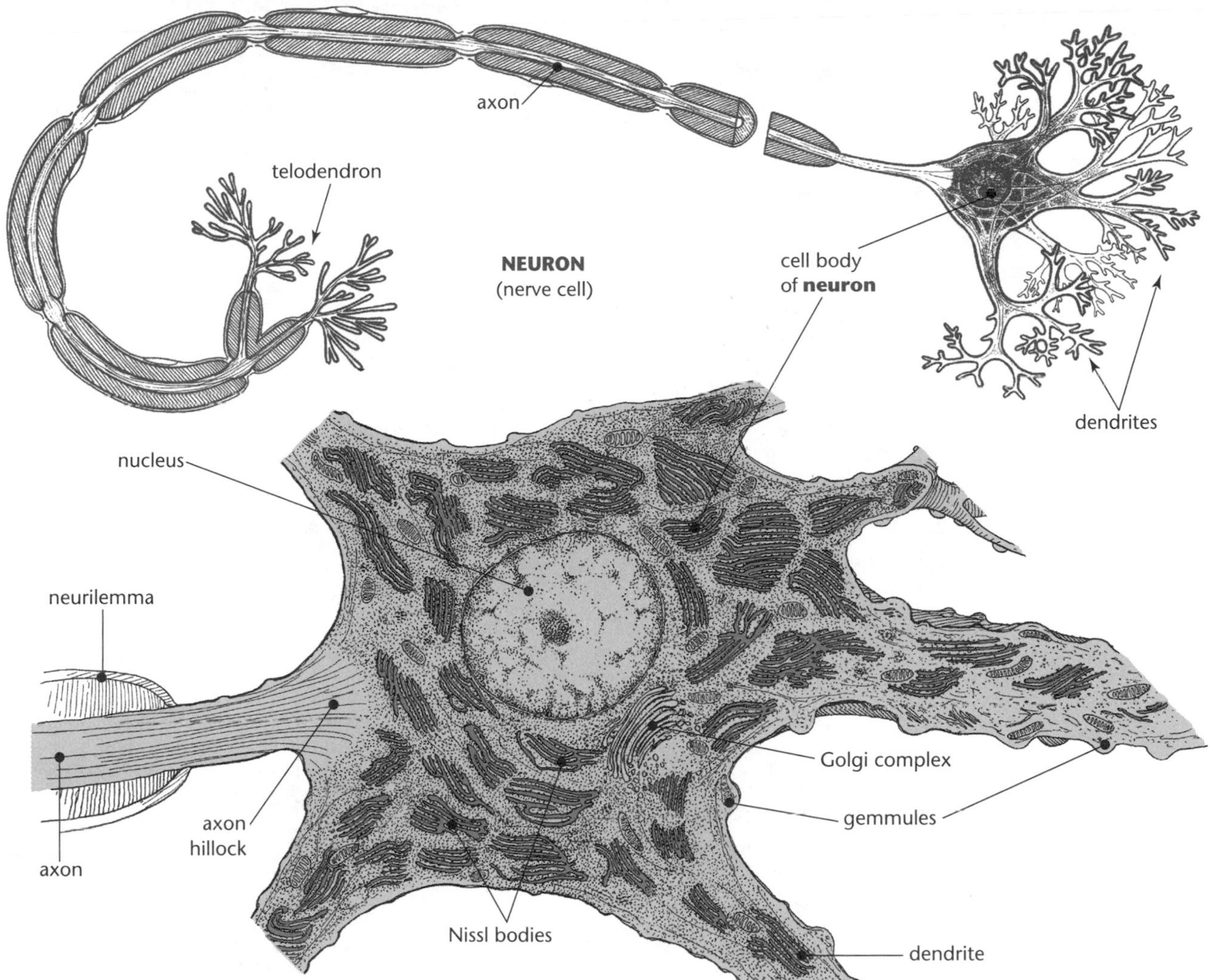

(neurofibromas); occurs in several forms that share some, not all, features.

n. I A form marked by multiple, pedunculated, soft tumors involving nerve trunks of skin and internal organs; light brown (café au lait) spots on the skin; pigmented (Lisch) nodules in the iris; may be associated with bone cysts, and erosion of bone surface and mental impairment. The defective gene is in chromosome 17. Also called Recklinghausen's disease.

n. II A central, acoustic form chiefly marked by the presence of tumors in both vestibulocochlear (eight cranial) nerves and absence of Lisch nodules in the iris. Other features may or may not be present. The defective gene is in chromosome 22.

incomplete n. Minimal manifestations of the disease (e.g., limited small tumors, café au lait spots); however, affected persons may have children with severe involvement.

neurogenesis (noor-o-jen′ĕ-sis) The formation of nerve tissue.

neurogenic, neurogenetic (noor-o-jen′ik, noor-o-jĕ-net′ik) Originating in the nervous system.

neuroglia (nŏŏ-rog′le-ă) The non-neuronal tissue of the brain and spinal cord that performs supportive and other ancillary functions; composed of various types of cells collectively called neuroglial cells or glial cells. Also called glia.

neuroglial, neurogliar (nŏŏ-rog′le-al, nŏŏ-rog′le-ar) Relating to neuroglia.

neurogliocyte (nŏŏ-rog′le-o-sīt) One of the cells composing the supporting, non-nervous portion of the nervous system.

neurogliomatosis (nŏŏ-rog-le-o-mă-to′sis) The presence of tumors of neuroglial cells in the brain or spinal cord.

neurogliosis (nŏŏ-rog-le-o′sis) **1.** Abnormal proliferation of neuroglial cells. **2.** The presence of several gliomas in the brain or spinal cord.

neurogram (noor′o-gram) The hypothesized imprint left on the brain by each mental experience, stimulation of which produces memory. Also called brain residual.

neurohistology (noor-o-his-tol′ŏ-je) Microscopic study of the nervous system.

neurohormone (noor-o-hor′mōn) A hormone whose secretion is controlled by the nervous system.

neurohumor (noor′o-hu′mor) An active chemical substance that effects the passage of nerve impulses from one cell to another at the synapse.

neurohypophyseal (noor-o-hi-po-fiz′e-al) See neurohypophysial.

neurohypophysial (noor-o-hi-po-fiz′e-al) Relating to the posterior lobe of the pituitary gland. Also written neurohypophyseal.

neurohypophysis (noor-o-hi-pof′ĭ-sis) The posterior or nervous lobe of the hypophysis; developed from the floor of the diencephalon.

neuroid (noor′oid) Resembling a nerve.

neurokeratin (noor-o-ker′ă-tin) **1.** A proteolipid network in the myelin sheath of axons. **2.** The pseudokeratin present in brain tissue.

neurolemma (noor-o-lem′ă) See neurilemma.

neuroleptic (noor-o-lep′tik) Any major tranquilizer that acts on the nervous system and has therapeutic effects on psychoses and other types of psychiatric disorders. Also called antipsychotic.

neuroleptic malignant syndrome (noor-o-lep′tik mă-lig′nant sin′drōm) Rare, life-threatening reaction to neuroleptic drugs, marked by high fever, muscle rigidity, and coma.

neurologist (nŏŏ-rol′ŏ-jist) A specialist in the nervous system and its diseases.

neurology (nŏŏ-rol′ŏ-je) The branch of medicine concerned with the nervous system and its diseases.

neurolymph (noor′o-limf) Obsolete term. See cerebrospinal fluid, under fluid.

neurolysin (nŏŏ-rol′ĭ-sin) See neurotoxin.

neurolysis (nŏŏ-rol′ĭ-sis) **1.** Destruction of nerve tissues. **2.** The removal of adhesions from a nerve.

neuroma (nŏŏ-ro′mă) General term denoting any tumor derived from nerve tissue.

acoustic n. See vestibular schwannoma, under schwannoma.

amputation n. A mass (often painful) of intertwined nerve fibers formed at the proximal end of an injured nerve. Also called traumatic neuroma.

interdigital nerve n. See Morton's neuroma.

Morton's n. Fibrosis of the sheath covering an interdigital plantar nerve, usually between the second and third toes, forming a painful tumorlike mass; caused by compression of the nerve at the metatarsophalangeal joint. Also called interdigital nerve neuroma; Morton's neuralgia.

traumatic n. See amputation neuroma.

neuromalacia (noor-o-mă-la′shă) Abnormal softening of nervous tissue.

neuromechanism (noor-o-mek′ă-niz-m) That part of the nervous system that controls the function of an organ.

neuromuscular (noor-o-mus′ku-lar) Relating to nerve and muscle, such as the nerve endings in a muscle, or the interaction of nerve and muscle.

neuromyasthenia (noor-o-mi-es-the′ne-ă) Muscular weakness, especially of emotional origin.

epidemic n. An epidemic febrile disorder generally affecting only adults, marked by stiffness of the neck and back, fever, headache, diarrhea, and localized muscular weakness. Also called Iceland disease; benign myalgic encephalomyelitis.

neuromyelitis (noor-o-mi-ă-lī′tis) Inflammation of the nerves and spinal cord.

n. optica Inflammation of the optic nerves and spinal cord; considered a type of multiple sclerosis. Also called Devic's disease.

neuromyopathy (noor-o-mi-op′ă-the) A muscular disorder due to a disease of the nerve innervating the muscle.

neuromyositis (noor-o-mi-o-si′tis) Inflammation of a nerve and the muscle it innervates.

neuron (noor′on) The basic functional and anatomic unit of the nervous system, concerned with the conduction of impulses; structurally, it is the most complex cell of the body; the human nervous system contains about 28 billion neurons. Also called nerve cell.

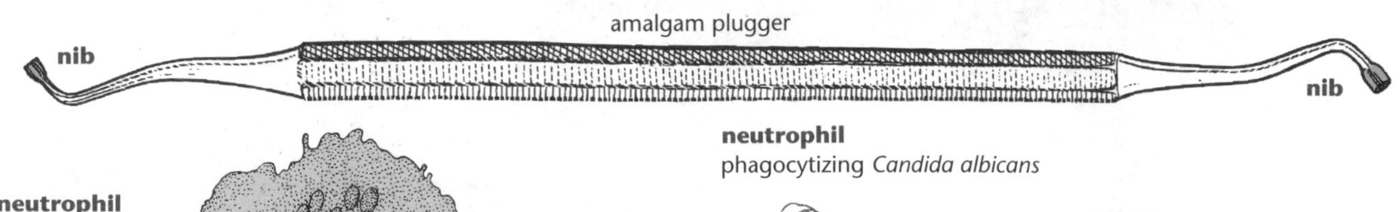

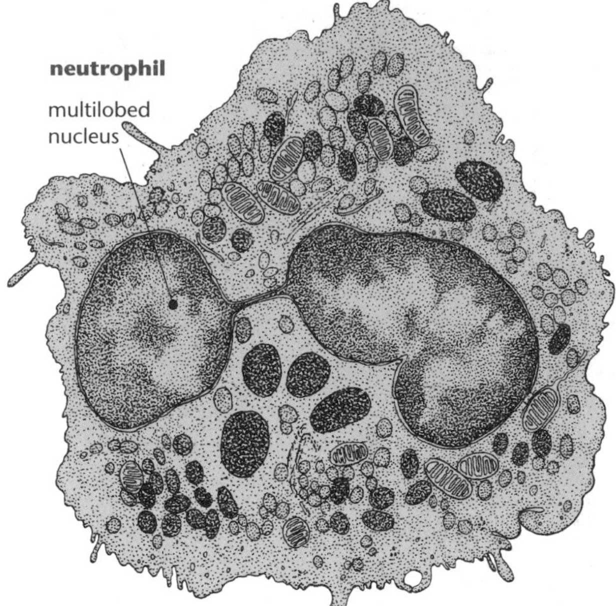

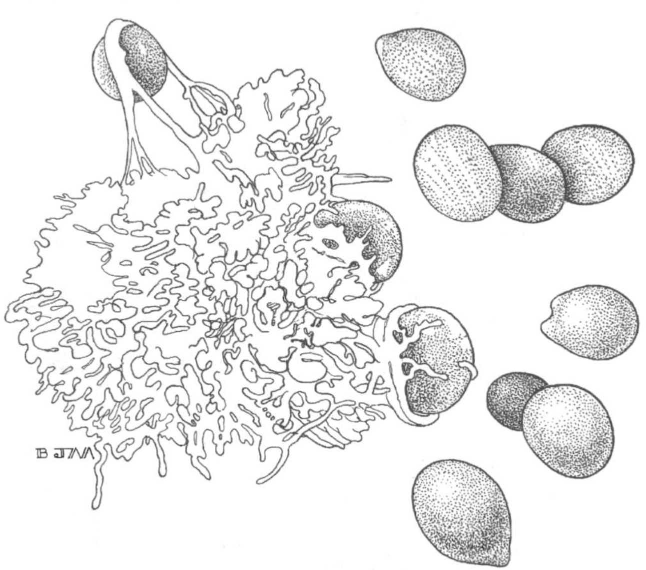

bipolar n. A neuron possessing two separate axons as in the retina, olfactory mucosa, internal ear, and taste buds.

central n. A neuron entirely within the spinal cord or brain.

Golgi type I n. A relatively large pyramidal neuron with a long axon connecting different parts of the nervous system by leaving the gray matter of the central nervous system and terminating in the periphery.

Golgi type II n. A relatively small stellate neuron with a short axon that terminates close to the cell body; in some cases the axon is absent.

intercalary n. See internuncial neuron.

internuncial n. A neuron that is interposed between two other neurons. Also called intercalary neuron; interneuron.

multipolar n. A neuron with several short processes (dendrites) and a single long axon.

unipolar n. A neuron having a single process (axon) attached to its cell body. Also called unipolar cell.

neuronal (noor´o-nal) Relating to a nerve cell.

neuronic (noor-on´ik) Relating to a nerve cell.

neuronitis (noor-o-ni´tis) Inflammation of nerve cells, especially those of the roots of spinal nerves.

neuronophage (nōō-ron´o-fāj) A white blood cell that ingests elements of injured or diseased nerve cells.

neuronophagia (noor-on-o-fa´jă) Ingestion of unwanted nerve cell debris by neuronophages.

neuronyxis (noor-o-nik´sis) See acupuncture.

neuro-ophthalmology (noor-o-of-thal-mol´ŏ-je) The branch of ophthalmology concerned with the part of the nervous system related to the eye. Also written neurophthalmology.

neuropapillitis (noor-o-pap-ĭ-li´tis) See papillitis.

neuroparalysis (noor-o-pă-ral´ĭ-sis) Paralysis due to disease of the nerve supplying the affected part.

neuropathic (noor-o-path´ik) Relating to a disease of the nervous system.

neuropathogenesis (noor-o-path-o-jen´ĕ-sis) The origin of diseases of the nervous system.

neuropathology (noor-o-pă-thol´o-je) Study of diseases of the nervous system.

neuropathy (nōō-rop´ă-the) Any disease of the nervous system.

brachial plexus n. See neuralgic amyotrophy, under amyotrophy.

compression n. Injury to a nerve caused by sustained mechanical pressure exerted upon a localized portion of the nerve.

diabetic n. A complication of diabetes mellitus; may affect the sensory nerves, especially of the lower extremities, or the autonomic nervous system, especially innervation of the bladder and bowel.

entrapment n. Any of a group of inflammatory nerve conditions (e.g., carpal tunnel syndrome) caused by traumatic pressure exerted upon the nerve by neighboring structures.

familial amyloid n. Disturbance of nerve function caused by a mutant serum protein (transthyretin) deposited as amyloid in nerve tissue; occurs in a variety of genetic diseases of autosomal dominant inheritance.

Graves' optic n. Visual dysfunction occurring in Graves' disease, due to compression of the optic nerve in the orbital apex by enlarged external muscles of the eye and by increased volume of inflammatory orbital contents.

heavy metal n. Peripheral or central nervous system disorders producing functional impairment caused by continued exposure to heavy metals (e.g., arsenic lead, mercury, thallium).

ischemic n. Injury to a peripheral nerve resulting from blockage of its blood supply.

peripheral n. A disorder of the peripheral nerves characterized by motor and sensory changes in the extremities; most commonly associated with alcoholism and/or poor nutrition.

neuropeptide (noor-o-pep´tīd) Any of various substances (e.g., endorphins, vasopressin) present in neural tissue, especially the brain.

n. Y A 36-amino acid peptide stored in sympathetic nerve fibers and released together with norepinephrine.

neuropharmacology (noor-o-făr-mă-kol´o-je) Study of drugs that affect the nervous system.

neurophthalmology (noor-of-thal-mol´o-je) See neuro-ophthalmology.

neurophthisis (nōō-rof´thĭ-sis) Wasting of nervous tissue.

neurophysin (noor-o-fi´sin) A large endocrine gland molecule produced in nerve cell bodies at the base of the brain and stored in the pituitary gland; this macromolecule with a 92-step chemical sequence transports the hormones vasopressin and oxytocin.

n. II The carrier of antidiuretic hormone in the brain, from the hypothalamus to the posterior pituitary.

neurophysiology (noor-o-fiz-e-ol´o-je) Study of the normal vital processes of the nervous system.

neuropil, neuropile (noor´o-pil, noor´o-pīl) A dense net of interwoven glia and nerve cells and their processes.

neuroplasm (noor´o-plaz-m) The cytoplasm of a nerve cell.

neuroplasticity (nu-ro-plas-tis´i-te) The ability of the brain to change in response to environmental influences (e.g., in the mechanism of posttraumatic stress disorder). See also kindling.

neuroplasty (noor´o-plas-te) Reparative surgery of the nerves.

neuroplexus (noor-o-plek´sus) A network (plexus) of nerves. See also plexus.

neuropodium (noor-o-po´de-um), *pl.* **neuropo´dia** See axon terminal, under terminal.

neuropore (noor´o-pōr) The opening at the ends of the neural tube of the developing embryo prior to complete closure around the 20 to 25 somite stage.

neuropsychiatry (noor-o-si-kī´ă-tre) The study of both organic and functional diseases of the nervous system.

neuropsychology (noor-o-si-kol´ŏ-je) The study of the relationship between the mind and the nervous system.

neuropsychopathy (noor-o-si-kop´ă-the) Functional disease of the nervous system accompanied by mental symptoms.

neuroradiology (noor-o-ra-de-ol´ŏ-je) Study of the nervous system with the aid of x-ray images.

neuroretinitis (noor-o-ret-ĭ-nī´tis) Inflammation of the head of the optic nerve and adjacent retina.

neurorrhaphy (nōō-ror´ă-fe) Suturing together the ends of a divided nerve.

neurosarcocleisis (noor-o-sar-ko-klī´sis) Operative removal of portions of the bony canal surrounding a nerve for the relief of neuralgia.

neurosclerosis (noor-o-skle-ro´sis) Hardening of nerves.

neurosecretion (noor-o-se-kre´shun) Any of several secretory products of nerve cells (e.g., of the neurohypophysis and those of the base of the hypothalamus) that enter the bloodstream and act as hormones.

neurosis (noo-ro´sis), *pl.* **neuro´ses** Emotional maladjustment that may impair thinking and judgment but causes minimal loss of contact with reality.

battle n. See war neurosis.

cardiac n. Anxiety caused by exaggerated concern with the state of one's heart in the absence of heart disease. Also called cardioneurosis.

hysterical n. See conversion disorder, under disorder.

military n. See war neurosis.

posttraumatic n. See posttraumatic stress disorder, under disorder.

war n. Any mental disorder brought about by conditions of warfare. Also called battle neurosis; military neurosis.

neuroskeleton (noor-o-skel-´ĕ-ton) The part of the skeleton surrounding the brain and spinal cord.

neurosome (noor´o-sōm) **1.** One of the minute granules in the protoplasm of a nerve cell. **2.** The

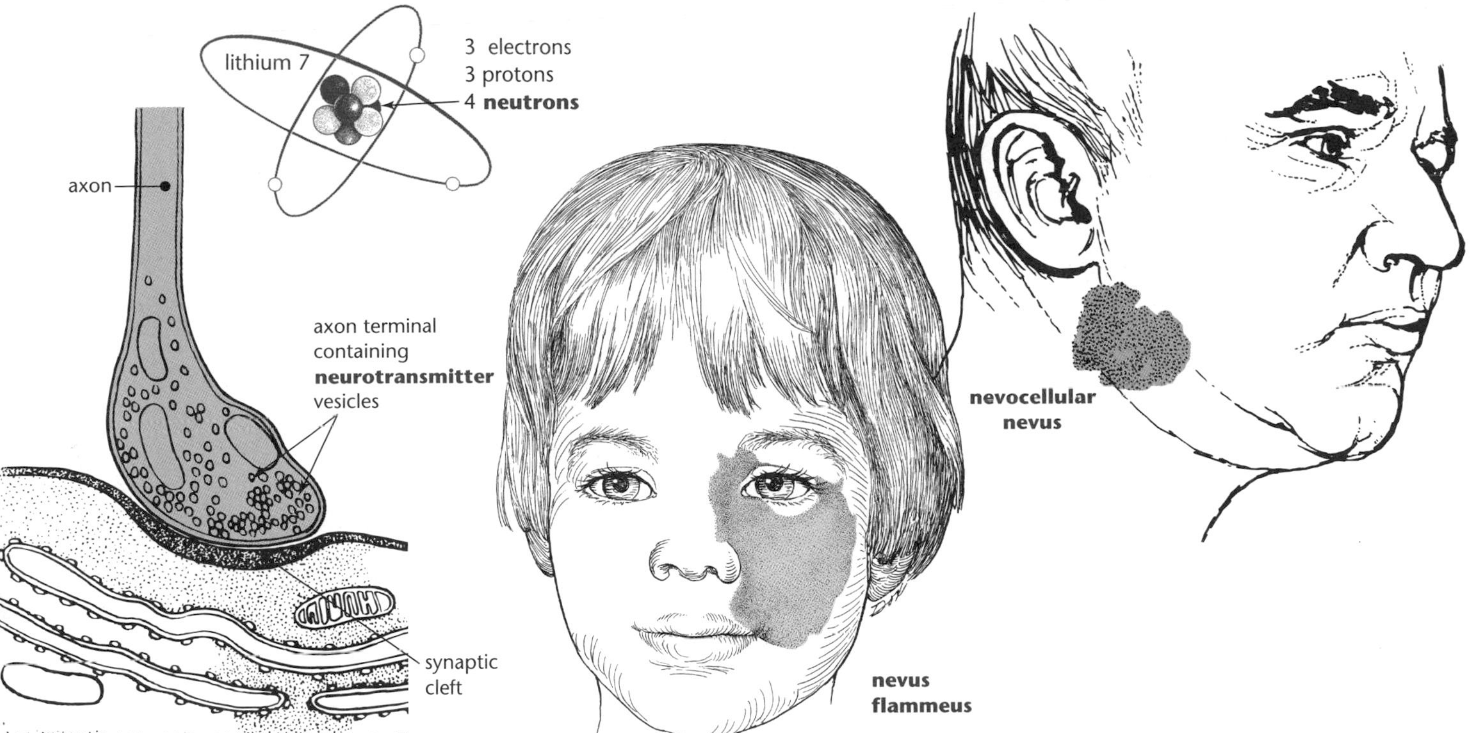

body of a nerve cell.

neurosplanchnic (noor-o-splangk´nik) Relating to the autonomic nervous system.

neurosurgeon (noor-o-sur´jun) A specialist in surgery of the nervous system.

neurosurgery (noor-o-sur´jer-e) Surgery of the nervous system.

stereotactic n. Neurosurgery involving the use of a mechanically directed probe introduced into the brain through a small hole in the skull; precise topographical coordinates are used to arrive at the desired location.

neurosyphilis (noor-o-sif´ĭ-lus) Syphilis of the nervous system; the third stage of syphilis. Forms of involvement include tabes dorsalis and general paresis.

neurotic (nŏŏ-rot´ik) Relating to or affected with a neurosis.

neurotization (nŏŏ-rot-ĭ-za´shun) Nerve regeneration.

neurotomy (nŏŏ-rot´ŏ-me) Surgical division of a nerve.

neurotonic (noor-o-ton´ik) **1.** Stimulating impaired nervous function. **2.** An agent having such an effect.

neurotoxicity (noor-o-tok-sis´ĭ-te) The property of having a harmful effect on nerve tissue.

neurotoxin (noor-o-tok´sin) Any substance that destroys or injures nerve tissue.

neurotransmitter (noor-o-trans-mit´er) Any substance that aids in transmitting impulses between two nerve cells or between a nerve and a muscle (e.g., acetylcholine).

neurotrophasthenia (noor-o-tro-fas-the´ne-ă) Condition due to under-nourishment; marked by fatigue, poor concentration, and feelings of inadequacy.

neurotropic (noor-o-trop´ik) Having an affinity for nervous tissue; said of certain histologic dyes and microorganisms.

neurula (noor´u-lar) The early vertebrate embryo during the stages when it possesses a neural plate.

neurulation (noor-u-la´shun) The formation and closure of the neural plate in the early vertebrate embryo.

neutralization (noo-tral-ĭ-za´shun) **1.** The chemical reaction between an acid and a base that yields a salt and water. **2.** The process of rendering something ineffective.

neutralize (noo´tral-īz) **1.** To render ineffective (in counteracting the effect of a drug or a toxin). **2.** To make neutral.

neutral red (noo´tral red) A dye used as an indicator with pH range of 6.8 to 8 (red at 6.8, yellow at 8).

neutrino (noo-tre´no) An uncharged subatomic particle emitted from a radioactive nucleus when a positron is emitted from, or captured by, the nucleus; it has zero mass when at rest, travels at the speed of light, and interacts with matter only in the reverse process by which it is produced.

neutron (noo´tron) (n) An uncharged subatomic particle existing along with the protons in the nucleus of an atom; slightly heavier than a proton.

fast n. A neutron with an energy level that exceeds 10^5 electron volts.

neutropenia (noo-tro-pe´ne-ă) Abnormally small number of neutrophils in the blood. Also called neutrophilic leukopenia.

neutrophil (noo´tro-fil) See neutrophilic leukocyte, under leukocyte.

neutrophilia (noo-tro-fil´e-ă) Increased number of neutrophils in the blood. Also called neutrocytosis; neutrophilic leukocytosis.

nevi (ne´vi) Plural of nevus.

nevoid (ne´void) Resembling a nevus.

nevoxanthoendothelioma (ne-vo-zan-tho-en-do-the-le-o´mă) See juvenile xanthogranuloma, under xanthogranuloma.

nevus (ne´vus), *pl.* **ne´vi** A benign lesion of the skin; may be pigmented or nonpigmented, flat or elevated, smooth or warty; may become malignant.

n. anemicus A congenital pale, well-defined area on the skin; thought to be a functional defect of blood vessels within the area, which, although otherwise normal, are hyperresponsive to vasoconstrictive stimuli.

n. araneus See spider telangiectasia, under telangiectasia.

blue n. A circumscribed, blue to black nodule in the deep layer of the skin, occurring anywhere in the body but most commonly on the dorsum of the hand and foot; chiefly composed of dopa-positive melanocytes (pigment-producing cells) containing a high concentration of melanin pigment; becomes malignant only rarely.

congenital nevocellular n. A relatively large nevus present at birth, often covered with hairs; the pigmented (melanocytic) cells are located in the deepest layers of skin and subcutaneous fat; occasionally may develop malignant potential.

dysplastic n. See atypical mole, under mole.

n. flammeus A purple-red, vascular birthmark that is level with the skin surface and usually tends to be permanent. Also called port-wine hemangioma; port-wine mark; port-wine stain.

intradermal n. A nevus occurring in the dermis (deep layer of the skin).

junctional n. Nevus occurring between the dermis and epidermis (deep and superficial layers of the skin).

melanocytic n. See nevocellular nevus.

nevocellular n. Any of various circumscribed pigmented nevi present at birth or acquired in childhood; they vary from smooth to rough and from nonpalpable to nodular. Also called pigmented nevus; melanocytic nevus; commonly called mole.

pigmented n. See nevocellular nevus.

port-wine n. See nevus flammeus.

spider n. See spider telangiectasia, under telangiectasia.

systematized n. A widely distributed congenital nevus exhibiting a pattern.

n. vasculosus See strawberry hemangioma, under hemangioma.

N

newborn (noo´born) **1.** A recently born infant. **2.** Just born.

Newcastle disease (noo´kas-ĕl dĭ-zēz´) An acute contagious disease of fowl caused by a paramyxovirus; transmissible to humans, causing respiratory and nervous symptoms.

newton (noo´ton) (N) A unit of force in the meter-kilogram-second system; the force required to accelerate a mass of one kilogram one meter per second per second.

niacin (ni´ă-sin) Official designation for nicotinic acid in its role as a vitamin. See also nicotinic acid.

niacinamide (ni-ă-sin´ă-mīd) See nicotinamide.

nib (nib) In dentistry, the working part of a condensing instrument corresponding to the blade of a cutting instrument.

niche (nich) **1.** A small recess. **2.** Eroded area, especially in the wall of a hollow organ, usually detected by contrast radiography.

nickel (nik´ĕl) A metallic element, symbol Ni, atomic number 28, atomic weight 58.71.

nicking (nik´ing) Constriction of a blood vessel of the retina.

A-V n., arteriovenous n. Depression of a retinal vein into the tissue of the retina at the point where it is crossed by an artery; usually caused by arteriolar sclerosis.

nicotinamide (nik-o-tin´ă-mīd) White crystalline compound, soluble in water; a B-complex vitamin used to treat pellagra. Also called nicotinic acid amide; niacinamide.

nicotinamide adenine dinucleotide (nik-o-tin´ă-mīd ad´ĕ-nēn di-nu´kle-o-tīd) (NAD) One of the coenzymes of the vitamin niacin (nicotinic acid); in association with any of a number of proteins, it acts as an oxidation-reduction catalyst. Also called coenzyme I; codehydrogenase I. Formerly called diphosphopyridine nucleotide (DPN).

nicotinamide adenine dinucleotide phosphate (nik-o-tin´ă-mīd ad´ĕ-nēn di-nu´kle-o-tīd´fos´fāt) (NADP) A coenzyme that participates in biological oxidation reactions; structurally and

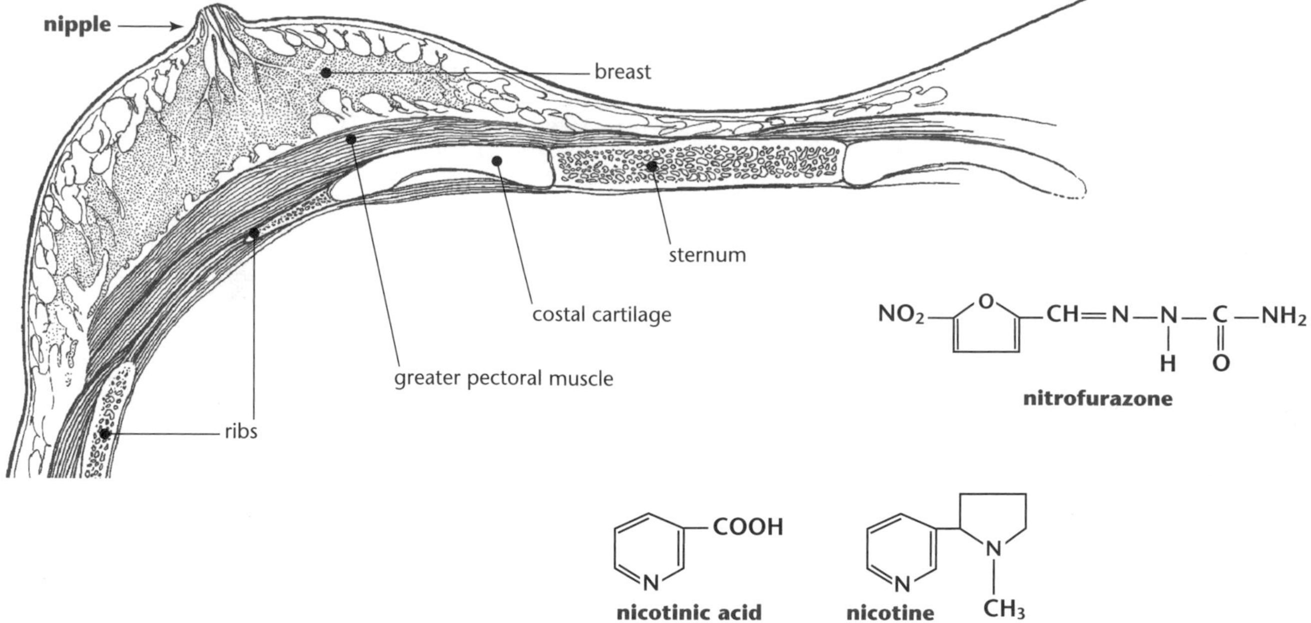

functionally similar to NAD. Also called coenzyme II; codehydrogenase II. Formerly called triphosphopyridine nucleotide (TPN).

nicotine (nik´o-tēn) An alkaloid derived from tobacco (*Nicotiana tabacum*); small doses stimulate and large doses depress autonomic ganglia.

nicotinic (nik-o-tin´ik) Resembling nicotine; denoting the action of certain agents on the nervous system.

nicotinic acid (nik-o-tin´ik as´id) An odorless, white crystalline compound, part of the vitamin B complex; used in the prevention and treatment of pellagra. Also called niacin.

nicotinic acid amide (nik-o-tin´ik as´id am´īd) See nicotinamide.

nicotinomimetic (nik-o-tin-o-mi-met´ik) Simulating the action of nicotine.

nictitation (nik-tĭ-ta´shun) Winking.

nidation (ni-da´shun) Implantation of the fluid-filled blastocyst in the lining of the uterus (endometrium); occurs approximately five days after fertilization of the ovum.

nidus (ni´dus) **1.** A nest. **2.** The point of focus of a morbid process. **3.** The point of origin or nucleus of a nerve.

n. avis A cerebellar depression between the biventral lobe and the uvula, which accommodates the cerebellar tonsil.

Niemann-Pick disease (ne´man-pik dĭ-zēz´) Disorder of lipid metabolism marked by accumulation of foam cells in the reticuloendothelial system, spleen, liver, kidneys, and pancreas; at a late stage, deposits of sphingomyelin, gangliosides, and cholesterol may be found in the brain and spinal cord; an autosomal recessive inheritance.

nifedipine (ni-fed´ĭ-pēn) A dihydropyridine calcium channel-blocking agent used in the treatment of hypertension and angina pectoris, especially variant angina.

nightmare (nīt´mār) A dream accompanied by intense anxiety, fear, oppression, and helplessness.

night terror (nīt ter´ŏr) Sleep disorder of children in which the child abruptly starts to scream and seems to be awake but does not recognize familiar faces, then gradually falls asleep and has no recollection of the event the following day.

nihilism (ni´hil-iz-m) In psychiatry, a delusion of nonexistence; it may be total (including the patient and the world as a whole) or selective (referring to a part of the patient or his environment).

therapeutic n. A disbelief in the value of any type of therapy.

Nikolsky's sign (nĭ-kol´skēz sīn) A peculiar vulnerability of the skin in pemphigus vulgaris; the superficial layer of the skin is easily rubbed off with slight friction.

nil disease (nĭl) See minimal change disease.

ninhydrin (nin-hi´drin) Triketohydrindene hydrate, a reagent widely used in the analytical determination of amino acids and related substances.

niobium (ni-o´be-um) A rare metallic element, symbol Nb, atomic number 41, atomic weight 92.906. Formerly called columbium (Cb).

nipple (nip´l) The conical protuberance at the apex of the breast in which the outlets of the milk ducts are located. Also called mammary papilla.

accessory n. A nipple that develops anywhere on the sides of the thoracoabdominal wall along the mammary lines.

nit (nit) **1.** The egg of a louse. **2.** A unit of luminance.

niter (ni´ter) See potassium nitrate.

nitrate (ni´trāt) A salt of nitric acid.

nitric (ni´trik) Relating to nitrogen.

nitric acid (ni´trik as´id) A colorless or yellowish corrosive liquid, HNO_3.

nitric oxide (ni´trik ok´sīd) (NO) A gas by-product of high-temperature combustion. Also produced in the body by a variety of cells and by the endothelium of blood vessels (endothelium-derived relaxing factor), where it acts as a cell-to-cell communicator and as a dilator of blood vessels. See also endothelium-derived relaxing factor (EDRF), under factor.

nitric oxide (NO) synthase (ni´trik ok´sīd sin´thās) Enzyme that converts L-arginine to nitric acid.

nitridation (ni-trĭ-da´shun) Formation of nitrides through the combination with nitrogen.

nitride (ni´trīd) A compound containing nitrogen and one other element, usually a more electropositive one.

nitrification (ni-trĭ-fĭ-ka´shun) **1.** The conversion of nitrogenous matter into nitrates by the action of bacteria. **2.** The treatment of a material with nitrogen or nitrogen compounds.

nitrile (ni´tril) A compound containing trivalent nitrogen attached to one carbon atom.

nitrite (ni´trīt) A salt or ester of nitrous acid.

nitritoid (ni´trĭ-toid) Resembling the reaction caused by a nitrite, such as the reaction following the intravenous administration of arsphenamine.

nitrobacteria (ni-tro-bak-te´re-ă) Bacteria that cause the conversion of nitrogenous matter into nitrites.

nitrofuran (ni-tro-fu´ran) Any of a group of compounds containing a nitro group; effective against a wide range of bacteria.

nitrofurantoin (ni-tro-fu-ran´to-in) Antibacterial compound used in the treatment of urinary tract infections.

nitrofurazone (ni-tro-fu´ră-zōn) 5-Nitro-2-furaldehyde semicarbazone; a topical antibacterial agent; Furacin®.

nitrogen (ni´tro-jen) A colorless, odorless, gaseous element forming about 47% of the atmosphere by weight; symbol N, atomic number 7, atomic weight 14.008.

blood urea n. (BUN) A constituent of normal whole blood. See urea nitrogen.

nonprotein n. (NPN) The nitrogen content of the blood exclusive of the protein bodies; normally urea contains about half of the nonprotein nitrogen in the blood.

urea n. The portion of nitrogen derived from the urea content of a biologic sample such as blood or urine.

nitrogenous (ni-troj´ĕ-nus) Containing nitrogen.

nitroglycerin (ni-tro-glis´er-in) A thick, yellow, explosive liquid, used in the production of dynamite; in medicine, the solid form is used as a vasodilator in the treatment of angina. Also called trinitroglycerin.

nitroprusside (ni-tro-prus´īd) A salt containing the radical $Fe(CN)_5NO$ (e.g., sodium nitroprusside). A potent blood pressure lowering agent.

nitrosamine (ni-trōs´ă-mēn) Any of various *N*-nitroso derivatives of secondary amines (R_2N–NO); some are thought to be carcinogenic; formed naturally from nitrites plus amines; found also in smoke.

nitrosourea (ni-tro-so-u´re-ă) An alkylating agent (destructive to cells), used in the treatment of cancerous tumors.

nitrosyl (ni´tro-sil) The univalent radical or group –NO, when attached to an electronegative element such as chlorine.

nitrous (ni´trus) Denoting a compound of nitrogen containing the smallest possible number of oxygen atoms.

nitrous oxide (ni´trus ok´sīd) A colorless gas of sweet taste, N_2O, used as a mild anesthetic. Popularly called laughing gas.

nobelium (no-be´le-um) The tenth transuranium element to be discovered; symbol No, atomic number 102, atomic weight 253.

Nocardia (no-kar´de-ă) A genus of soil bacteria (family Actinomycetes) that includes fungus-like organisms with delicate branching, often beaded, intertwining filaments that break into rod-shaped or coccoid forms; some are pathogenic.

N. asteroides Species isolated from diseases resembling pulmonary tuberculosis and brain abscesses.

N. madurae Species that is the causative agent of mycetoma.

nocardiosis (no-kar-de-o´sis) Any of several conditions caused by any species of *Nocardia*.

nociceptor (no-se-sep´tor) A peripheral nerve organ that receives and transmits painful sensations.

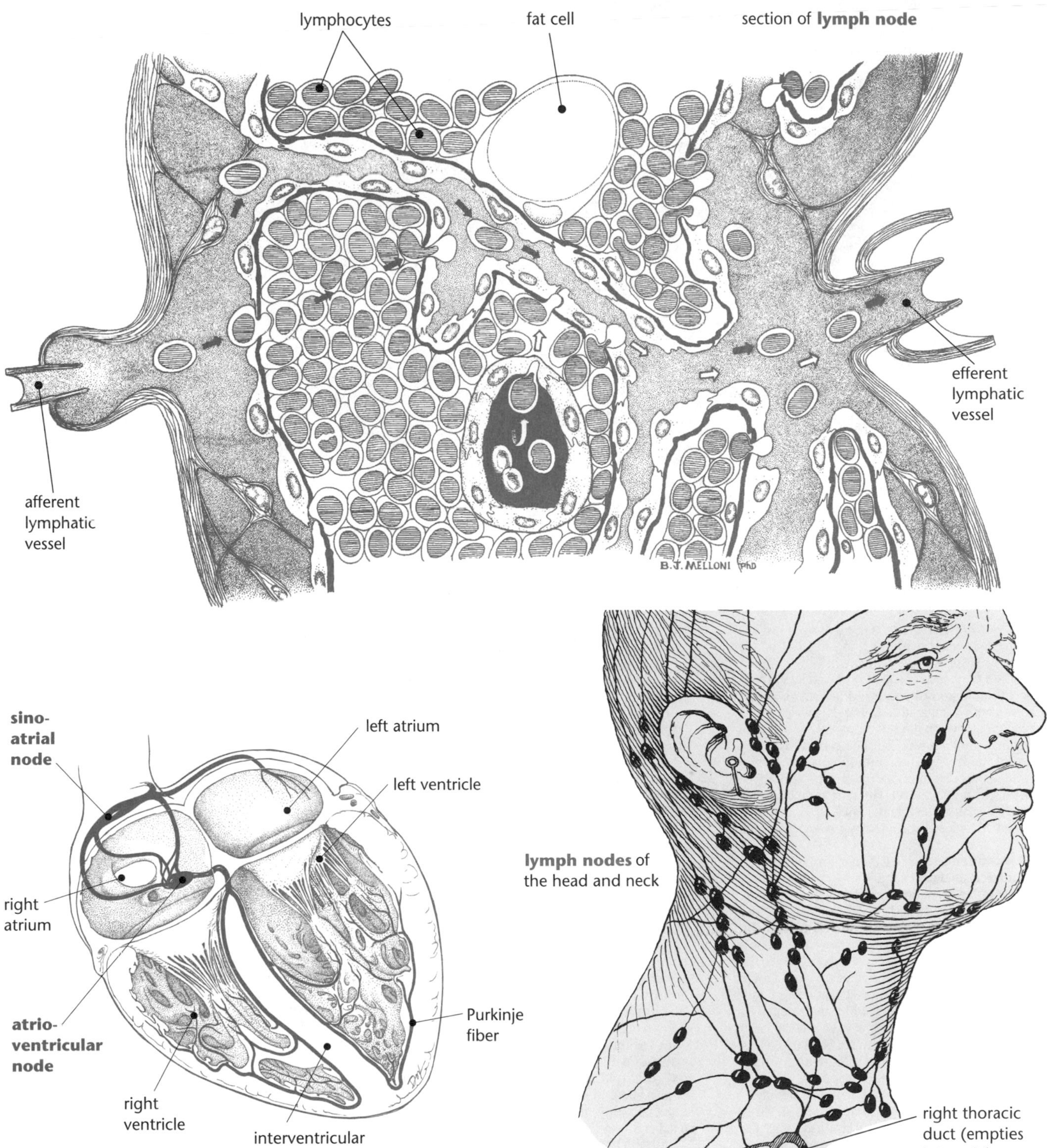

N

nociperception (no-se-per-sep´shun) Perception of painful or injurious stimuli.
noctambulism (nok-tam-bu´liz-m) See somnambulism.
noctiphobia (nok-te-fo´be-ă) An abnormal fear of night and its accompanying darkness and silence.
nocturia (nok-tu´re-ă) Voiding of urine during the night.
nocturnal (nok-ter´nal) Relating to the night-time hours; opposite of diurnal.
nodal (no´dal) Relating to a node.
node (nōd) **1.** A circumscribed mass of differentiated tissue. **2.** A swelling.
atrioventricular n. A small uncapsulated node made of thin strips of interwoven modified cardiac muscle and situated near the orifice of the coronary sinus; when normally activated by the sinoatrial node, it transmits the impulse, through the Purkinje fibers, to the ventricular muscles, causing practically simultaneous contraction. Also called A-V node.
A-V n. See atrioventricular node.
axillary lymph n.'s Twenty to thirty large nodes of the axilla extending along the axillary veins. Based on their location, designated: *anterior (pectoral)*, *apical*, *central*, *lateral*, and *posterior (subscapular)*.
Bouchard's n. A small, hard nodule located in the proximal interphalangeal joint of a finger; seen in osteoarthritis.
Cloquet's n. The highest of the deep inguinal lymph nodes, located on the lateral part of the femoral ring of the lower abdomen. Also called Rosemüller's node; highest deep inguinal lymph node.
gouty n. A concretion of sodium biurate generally occurring in the vicinity of joints in certain individuals afflicted with gout.
Heberden's n. A pea-sized swelling in the distal interphalangeal joint of a finger, seen in osteoarthritis.
Hensen's n. Primitive node.
highest deep inguinal lymph n. See Cloquet's node.
iliac lymph n.'s Nodes receiving lymph from the pelvic organs. Depending on their location, designated: *common iliac lymph n.'s*, grouped around the common iliac artery; *external iliac lymph n.'s*, along the external iliac blood vessels; *internal iliac lymph n.'s*, around the internal iliac blood vessels and roots of their branches.
lymph n.'s Oval structures located along the course of lymphatic vessels; their functions are the filtration of foreign matter from lymph and the production of lymphocytes; their enlargement may indicate a local infection, a systemic disorder, or a metastatic malignancy.
Osler's n. Small, tender, and discolored node usually appearing on the pads of fingers and toes in subacute endocarditis.
pelvic lymph n.'s The nodes receiving lymph from the pelvic organs and the wall of the pelvis; they include those of the external and internal iliac groups, which drain into the common iliac lymph

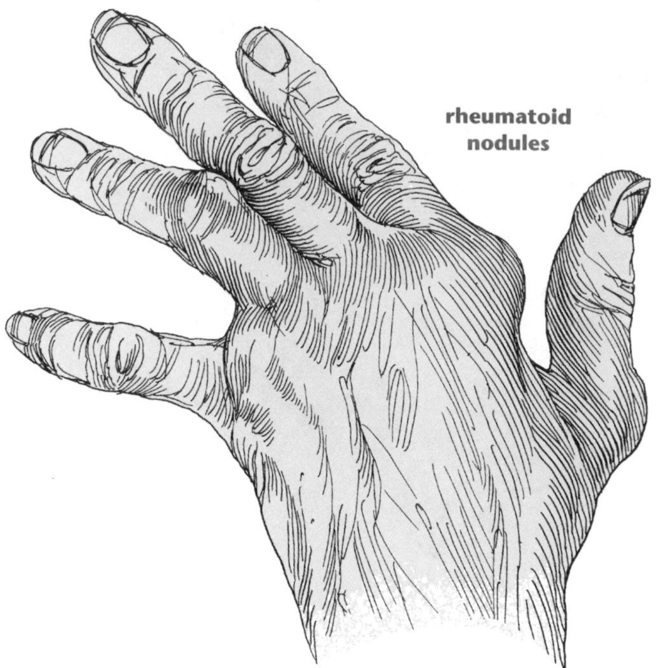

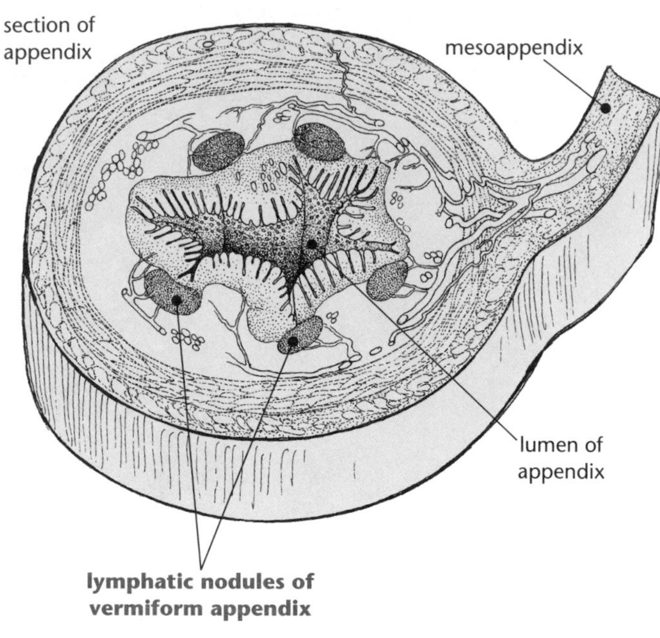

nodes.

prelaryngeal lymph n.'s Lymph nodes of the deep anterior cervical group lying in front of the larynx.

primitive n. A local thickening of ectodermal cells at the cephalic end of the primitive streak of the embryo from which a strand of cells grows toward the cranium, between the ectoderm and endoderm in the midline, until it is blocked at the prechordal plate.

Ranvier's n. An interruption or constriction occurring at regular intervals (of about 1 mm) in the myelin sheath of a nerve fiber; it is here that a collateral branch may leave the axon; the area between two nodes is occupied by a single Schwann cell.

Rosenmüller's n. See Cloquet's node.

S-A n. See sinoatrial node.

sentinel n. See sentinel lymph node; signal node.

sentinel lymph n. (SLN) The first node in a group of lymph nodes into which drains the immediate area of a primary tumor. The node's histologic constitution presumably reflects the constitution of the rest of the nodes in that group; therefore, hypothetically, if found negative for tumor invasion, the rest of the nodes will also be negative.

signal n. An enlarged, palpable, supraclavicular lymph node, usually on the left, that is often the first presumptive sign of a malignant abdominal neoplasm. Also called Virchow's node.

singer's n. See singer's nodule, under nodule.

sinoatrial n. The mass of interwoven strips of cardiac muscle fibers that normally acts as the pacemaker of the cardiac conduction system; situated in the wall of the right atrium at the upper end of the crista terminalis just at the point of entry of the superior vena cava; receives fibers from both autonomic nervous systems and is the part of the heart that originates the heartbeat. Also called S-A node.

syphilitic n. A localized swelling of bone resulting from syphilitic periostitis.

teacher's n. See singer's nodule, under nodule.

Virchow's n. See signal node.

nodose (no´dōs) Having nodes.

nodosity (no-dos´ĭ-te) **1.** A knotlike swelling. **2.** The condition of having nodes.

nodular (nod´u-lar) Relating to or having nodes.

nodulation (nod-u-la´shun) The presence or the formation of nodules.

nodule (nod´ūl) A small node or closely packed collection of cells appearing distinct from the surrounding tissue.

aggregated lymphatic n.'s Large aggregations of densely packed lymphocytes, present in the submucosa of the intestines, mainly in the ileum and distal jejunum.

Aschoff n. See Aschoff bodies, under body.

bronchial lymphatic n.'s Small lymph nodes on the larger branches of the bronchi, in the substance of the lungs.

cold n. A thyroid nodule that does not concentrate an administered dose of radioactive iodine as well as the rest of the gland.

gastric lymphatic n. Solitary mass of lymphoid tissue in the mucous membrane of the stomach.

hot n. A thyroid nodule containing a higher concentration of an administered dose of radioactive iodine than the rest of the gland; usually benign.

juxta-articular n. An inflammatory nodule situated near a joint.

Lisch n. A minute, abnormal, pigmented mass formed in the iris (iris hamartoma) of persons afflicted with neurofibromatosis I.

lymphatic n.'s of the vermiform appendix Masses of lymphoid tissue in the submucous coat of the vermiform appendix.

rheumatoid n.'s Round or ovoid masses most commonly occurring subcutaneously over pressure points and near joints, in patients with rheumatoid arthritis.

Schmorl's n. A localized protrusion of the central portion of an intervertebral disk through the cartilage plate and into the spongy bone of the vertebral body.

singer's n. A small, whitish beadlike nodule on the vocal fold, caused by chronic overuse or abuse of the vocal mechanism, as in prolonged singing, especially of high notes. Also called singer's node; teacher's node.

Sister Mary Joseph's n. A malignant nodule in the subcutaneous area of the navel, metastasized from intra-abdominal cancer.

nodulus (nod´u-lus), *pl.* **nod´uli** Latin for nodule.

Noguchia (no-goo´chē-ă) A genus of gram-negative, motile, encapsulated bacteria (family Brucellaceae) found in the conjunctiva of humans and animals affected by a follicular type of disease.

noma (no´mă) A rapidly destructive gangrenous disease of the mouth; seen in poorly nourished children and debilitated adults. Also called gangrenous stomatitis.

Nomina Anatomica (no´mĭ-nă an-ă-tom´ĭ-kă) (NA) A system of anatomic terminology prepared by the International Congress of Anatomists.

nomogram, nomograph (nom´o-gram, nom´o-graf) A graph consisting of three coplanar graduated lines of different variables arranged in such a manner that a straight line connecting two known values on two of the graduated lines intersects the unknown value on the third graduated line; used generally to estimate the surface area of a body on the basis of an individual's height and weight.

nomotopic (no-mo-top´ik) Located in the normal or usual place.

nonan (no´nan) Recurring every ninth day; said of a fever.

nonapeptide (non-ă-pep´tīd) A peptide possessing nine amino acids.

nonchromogens (non-kró´mo-jēns) See group III mycobacteria, under mycobacteria.

noncomedogenic (non-kom-ĕ-do-jen´ik) Not forming blackheads (comedones).

non compos mentis (non kom´pos men´tis) Latin for not having control of the mind (i.e., afflicted with some form of mental defect), hence legally not responsible.

nonconductor (non-kon-duk´tor) Anything that does not readily transmit electrical current, light, or heat.

nondisease (non-dĭ-zēz´) A disease suspected but not confirmed by further appropriate examinations.

nondisjunction (non-dis-junk´shun) Failure of paired chromosomes to separate at metaphase, so that both chromosomes are received by one daughter cell and none by the other, resulting in certain genetic conditions.

nonelectrolyte (non-e-lek´tro-līt) A substance that, when in solution, does not conduct an electric current.

noninfectious (non-in-fek´shus) Not spread by direct or indirect contact; not causing infection.

nonintervention (non-in-ter-ven´shun) See passive euthanasia, under euthanasia.

noninvasive (non-in-va´siv) Denoting diagnostic procedures that do not involve the use of instruments that penetrate the skin.

nonionic (non-i-on´ik) Not forming ions in solution.

nonmetal (non-met´al) Any electronegative element (e.g., iodine and fluorine) that forms oxides that produce acids and, in a solid state, is a poor conductor of heat and electricity.

non-nucleated (non-nu´kle-āt-ed) Without a nucleus.

nonocclusion (non-ŏ-kloo´zhun) Condition in which a tooth of one dental arch fails to contact its opponent of the other arch.

nonparous (non-par´us) See nulliparous.

nonpenetrance (non-pen´ĕ-trans) Failure of a genetic trait to be evident even though the genetic elements that usually produce the trait are present.

nonproprietary (non-pro-pri´ĕ-ta-re) See non-proprietary name, under name.

nonresectable (non-re-sek´tă-bl) Not capable of being cut off; said of a tumor not suitable for resection.

nonsecretor (non-se-kre´tor) A person whose body secretions do not contain antigens of the ABO blood group.

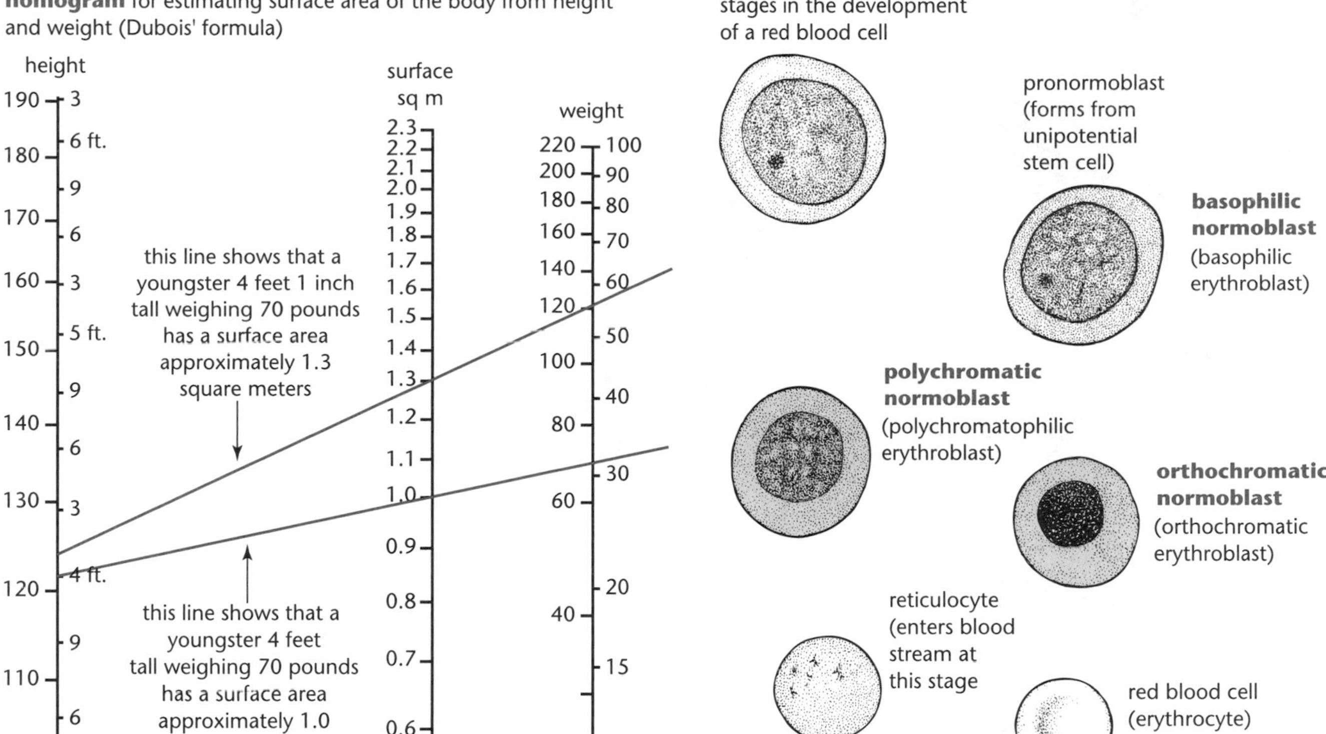

nonself (non´self) In immunology, foreign to the self; applied to molecules that are not normal constituents of the body of a given individual and are recognized as such by the individual's immune system, thereby tending to form antibodies against them.

nonsense (non´sens) See nonsense mutation, under mutation.

nonsteroidal (non-ster´oid-al) Not containing steroids. See also nonsteroidal anti-inflammatory drugs, under drug.

nonunion (non-ūn´yun) Complication of a bone fracture in which healing stops short of firm union.

nonviable (non-vī´ă-bl) Not capable of living independently.

Noonan's syndrome (noo´nanz sin´drōm) Downward slant of the eyes at the temporal angles and low-set ears associated with valvular pulmonic stenosis.

noradrenaline (nor-ă-dren´ă-lin) See norepinephrine.

norepinephrine (nor-ep-ĭ-nef´rin) (NE) A chemical substance (hormone) that produces constriction of practically all the blood vessels of the body; secreted by the postganglionic endings of the sympathetic nervous system; also produced and stored by the adrenal medulla and released upon stimulation of its sympathetic nerves. Also called levarterenol noradrenaline.

L-norepinephrine bitartrate (ĕl -nor-ep-ĭ-nef´rin bi-tar´trāt) The medicinal form of norepinephrine.

norethindrone (nor-eth´in-drōn) A progestational agent used in conjunction with estrogen as an oral contraceptive and in hormone replacement therapy; used alone to treat endometriosis and amenorrhea.

norethynodrel (nor-ĕ-thi´no-drel) A steroid structurally similar to progesterone, used in combination with mestranol as an oral contraceptive.

norm (norm) An ideal standard or pattern regarded as typical for a specific group.

norma (nor´mă) An outline of a body part, especially the skull.

normal (nor´mal) (n) **1.** Conformed to an established norm, standard, or pattern. **2.** Perpendicular; a line or plane forming a right angle with another. **3.** In bacteriology, nonimmune; denoting an animal or serum that has not been experimentally exposed to or treated with any microorganism.

normalization (nor-mal-ĭ-za´shun) **1.** The process of making normal. **2.** The process of dispersing fat homogeneously throughout milk after pasteurization.

normative (nor´mă-tiv) Relating to normal.

normetanephrine (nor-met-ă-nef´rin) A product of norepinephrine catabolism excreted in the urine.

normoblast (nor´mo-blast) A young red blood cell in its immature, nucleated stage.

acidophilic n. Orthochromatic normoblast.

basophilic n. The second stage in the development of the normoblast, following the pronormoblast. Also called basophilic erythroblast; early erythroblast; prorubricyte.

orthochromatic n. The last stage in the development of the normoblast in which 80% of the hemoglobin is synthesized. Also called metarubricyte; late erythroblast; orthochromatic erythroblast; acidophilic normoblast.

polychromatic n. The third stage in the development of the normoblast. Also called polychromatophilic erythroblast; rubricyte.

normoblastosis (nor-mo-blas-to´sis) Excessive production of normoblasts in the bone marrow.

normocephalic (nor-mo-sĕ-fal´ik) See mesocephalic.

normochromia (nor-mo-kro´me-ă) Normal color of red blood cells.

normochromic (nor-mo-kro´mik) Having normal color; said of red blood cells.

normocyte (nor´mo-sīt) A red blood cell of normal size.

normoglycemia (nor-mo-gli-se´miă) See euglycemia.

normoglycemic (nor-mo-gli-se´mik) See euglycemic.

normokalemia (nor-mo-kă-le´me-ă) A normal level of potassium in the blood.

normotensive (nor-mo-ten´siv) Denoting a normal arterial blood pressure.

normothermia (nor-mo-ther´me-ă) **1.** A normal temperature. **2.** Environmental temperature that does not affect the activity of body cells.

normotonic (nor-mo-ton´ik) Having normal muscular tone. Also called eutonic.

normotopia (nor-mo-to´pe-ă) The state of being in the normal location.

normovolemia (nor-mo-vo-le´me-ă) A normal blood volume.

nose (nōz) The external organ of the sense of smell and the beginning of the air passages; the midline prominence on the face bearing the nostrils.

pug n. A short slightly flattened nose turned up at the end; a snub nose.

saddle n. A nose with a markedly depressed bridge.

nosebleed (nōz´blēd) Bleeding from the nose. Also called epistaxis.

nosepiece (nōz´pēs) A device at the lower end of the microscope body tube for holding two or more readily interchangeable objectives.

nosocomial (nos-o-ko´me-al) Relating to or originating in a hospital.

nosogenesis, nosogeny (nos-o-jen´ĕ-sis, no-soj´ĕ-ne) See pathogenesis.

nosographer (no-sog´ră-fer) One who writes about diseases.

nosography (no-sog-ră-fe) The systematic written description of diseases.

nosology (no-sol´o-je) **1.** The science concerned with the classification of diseases. Also called nosotaxy. **2.** A classification of diseases.

nosomania (nos-o-ma´ne-ă) An unfounded, abnormal fear that one is diseased.

nosomycosis (nos-o-mi-ko´sis) A disease caused by a fungus.

nosoparasite (nos-o-par´ă-sīt) **1.** A microorganism occurring in association with, but not causing, a disease. **2.** A pathogenic microorganism living on diseased tissue.

nosophilia (nos-o-fil´e-ă) An abnormal desire to be sick.

nosophobia (nos-o-fo´be-ă) An abnormal fear of disease; a dread of having all the symptoms of all the diseases read or heard about.

nosopoietic (nos-o-poi-et´ik) See pathogenic.

nosotaxy (nos´o-tak-se) See nosology (1).

nosotoxin (nos-o-tok´sin) Any toxin associated with a disease.

nostril (nos´tril) One of the two external openings of the nose. Also called naris.

nostrum (nos´trum) A quack remedy.

notal (no´tal) Relating to the back.

notch (noch) An indentation or depression.

acetabular n. A notch in the inferior margin of the acetabulum of the hipbone; it is bridged by the transverse acetabular ligament.

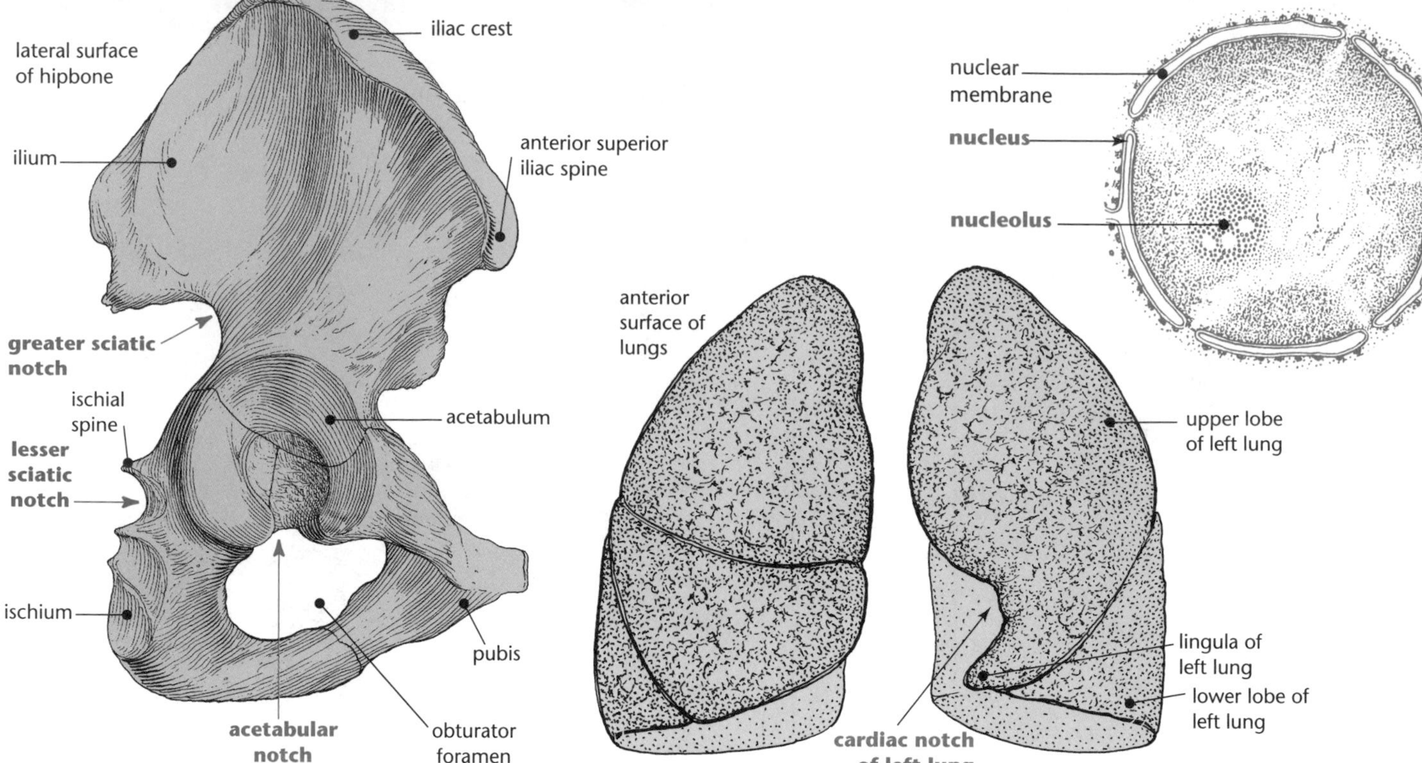

aortic n. The depression on the sphygmogram caused by the rebound at the closure of the aortic valves.

cardiac n. of left lung A notch in the anterior border of the left lung at the level of the fourth costal cartilage; it accommodates the heart.

cardiac n. of stomach A notch at the junction of the esophagus and the fundus of the stomach.

dicrotic n. The depression on the sphygmogram which precedes the dicrotic pulse wave.

Hutchinson's crescentic n. The somewhat semilunar notch on the incisal edge of upper central incisors in Hutchinson's teeth; seen also occasionally in other anterior teeth.

interclavicular n. See suprasternal notch.

jugular n. See suprasternal notch.

mandibular n. The deep semilunar notch between the condyle and coronoid process of the lower jaw (mandible).

scapular n. A semicircular notch on the superior border of the scapula (shoulder blade), at the base of the coracoid process.

sciatic n., greater The deep indentation in the posterior border of the hipbone at the junction of the ilium and ischium; it is converted into a foramen by the sacrospinal ligament.

sciatic n., lesser The notch in the posterior border of the ischium below the ischial spine; it is converted into a foramen by the sacrotuberous and sacrospinal ligaments.

supraorbital n. A notch or groove (occasionally a foramen) in the superior part of the margin of the orbit through which pass the supraorbital nerve and vessels.

suprasternal n. The notch between the sternal heads of the two sternocleidomastoid muscles. Also called interclavicular notch; jugular notch.

tentorial n. A gap in the tentorium cerebelli, through which the brain stem extends from the posterior into the middle cranial fossa.

trochlear n. A large concavity on the anterior surface of the olecranon process of the ulna which articulates with the trochlea of the humerus.

vertebral n. One of two notches above and below the pedicle of a vertebra; the notches of two adjacent vertebrae form an intervertebral foramen.

notching (noch´ing) The presence of a notch or notches.

rib n. Small grooves on the anterior aspect of ribs, occurring in children with constriction of the aorta beyond the ductus arteriosus; formed by pressure from enlarged collateral blood vessels upon the ribs.

notochord (no´to-kord) A supporting rod of cells in the embryo of all chordates; in vertebrates, it is replaced partially or wholly by the skull and vertebral column.

noxa (nok´să) Any harmful agent or influence.

noxious (nok´shus) Harmful to health.

nu (noo) Thirteenth letter of the Greek alphabet, ν; symbol for kinematic viscosity.

nubile (noo´bīl) Ready for marriage; said of a sexually mature young woman.

nucha (nu´kă) The nape.

nuchal (nu´kal) Relating to the back of the neck.

nuclear (noo´kle-ar) Of or relating to a nucleus.

nuclease (noo´kle-ās) An enzyme that promotes the breakdown of nucleic acid into nucleotides.

nucleated (noo´kle-āt-ed) Having a nucleus.

nuclei (noo´kle-i) Plural of nucleus.

nucleic acids (noo-kle´ik as´ids) Macromolecules contained in all living organisms in the form of deoxyribonucleic acid (DNA) and ribonucleic acid (RNA); they consist mainly of a sugar moiety (pentose or deoxypentose), nitrogenous bases (purines and pyrimidines), and phosphoric acid.

nucleocapsid (noo-kle-o-kap´sid) The protein coat (capsid) of a virus together with its enclosed nucleic acid.

nucleofugal (noo-kle-of´u-gal) Moving away from a cell nucleus.

nucleogram (noo-kle´o-gram) The data obtained through nucleography.

nucleography (noo-kle-og´ră-fe) A method of observing and recording the chemical composition, structure, size, etc., of a cell nucleus.

nucleohistone (noo-kle-o-his´tōn) A nucleoprotein derived from a histone; a salt between the basic protein and the nucleic acid.

nucleolonema (noo-kle-o-lo-ne´mă) A dense, coarse branching strand forming a network within the nucleolus of a cell; contains genes involved in transcription of ribosomal RNA.

nucleolus (noo-kle´ŏ-lus), *pl.* **nucle´oli** A small, spherical organelle within the nucleus of a cell; it contains RNA (ribonucleic acid) and protein and is an active center of protein and RNA synthesis, as well as an important center for the formation of ribosomes.

chromatin n. See karyosome.

false n. See karyosome.

nucleon (noo´kle-on) One of the constituent particles of an atomic nucleus (i.e., a proton or a neutron).

nucleonics (noo-kle-on´iks) The technology and application of nuclear energy.

nucleopetal (noo-kle-op´e-tal) Moving toward a cell nucleus.

nucleophile, nucleophil (noo´kle-o-fīl, noo´kle-o-fil) The electron donor in a chemical reaction.

nucleoplasm (noo´kle-o-plaz-m) The protoplasm of the cell nucleus, composed mainly of proteins, metabolites, and ions. Also called karyoplasm.

nucleoprotein (noo-kle-o-pro´tēn) A nondescript complex of compounds consisting of a simple protein and a nucleic acid; chromosomes and viruses are largely nucleoprotein in nature.

nucleoreticulum (noo-kle-o-re-tik´u-lum) Any structural network within the nucleus.

nucleorrhexis (noo-kle-o-rek´sis) The breaking up of a cell nucleus.

nucleosidase (noo-kle-o-si´dās) An enzyme that promotes the splitting of nucleosides into sugar and purine or pyrimidine base.

nucleoside (noo´kle-o-sīd) A purine or pyrimidine base attached to a sugar (pentose, ribose, or deoxyribose).

nucleotidase (noo´kle-o-tī´dās) An enzyme that catalyzes the splitting of a nucleotide into nucleosides and phosphoric acid.

nucleotide (noo´kle-o-tīd) One of the compounds into which nucleic acid splits on hydrolysis consisting of a nitrogenous base (either a purine or a pyrimidine), a sugar (either ribose or deoxyribose), and a phosphate group. Also called mononucleotide.

cyclic n. Nucleotide in which the phosphate group forms a ring.

nucleotidyltransferase (noo-kle-o-tīd-īl-trans´fer-ās) Enzymes that transfer nucleotide residues from nucleoside di- or triphosphates into dimer or polymer forms.

nucleotoxin (noo-kle-o-tok´sin) A toxin affecting cell nuclei.

nucleus (noo´kle-us), *pl.* **nu´clei** **1.** The generally oval protoplasmic body in the center of the cell that contains the chromosomes and is surrounded by a membrane; an essential organelle that controls metabolism, growth, and reproduction. **2.** A localized mass of gray matter within the brain and spinal cord, composed of nerve cells. **3.** The heavy, central, positively charged portion of the atom (composed of protons and neutrons); it constitutes the mass of the atom, about which the electrons revolve in orbit. **4.** A central part or mass.

abducens n. A cranial nerve nucleus with fibers directed anteriorly to supply the lateral rectus muscle of the eye.

ambiguous n. A motor nucleus composed of large multipolar cells that send fibers into the glossopharyngeal, vagus, and accessory nerves to supply the pharynx and larynx.

amygdaloid n. See amygdaloid body, under body.

anterior horn n. A column of cells extending the entire length of the spinal cord and organized into medial and lateral groups, each with several sub-

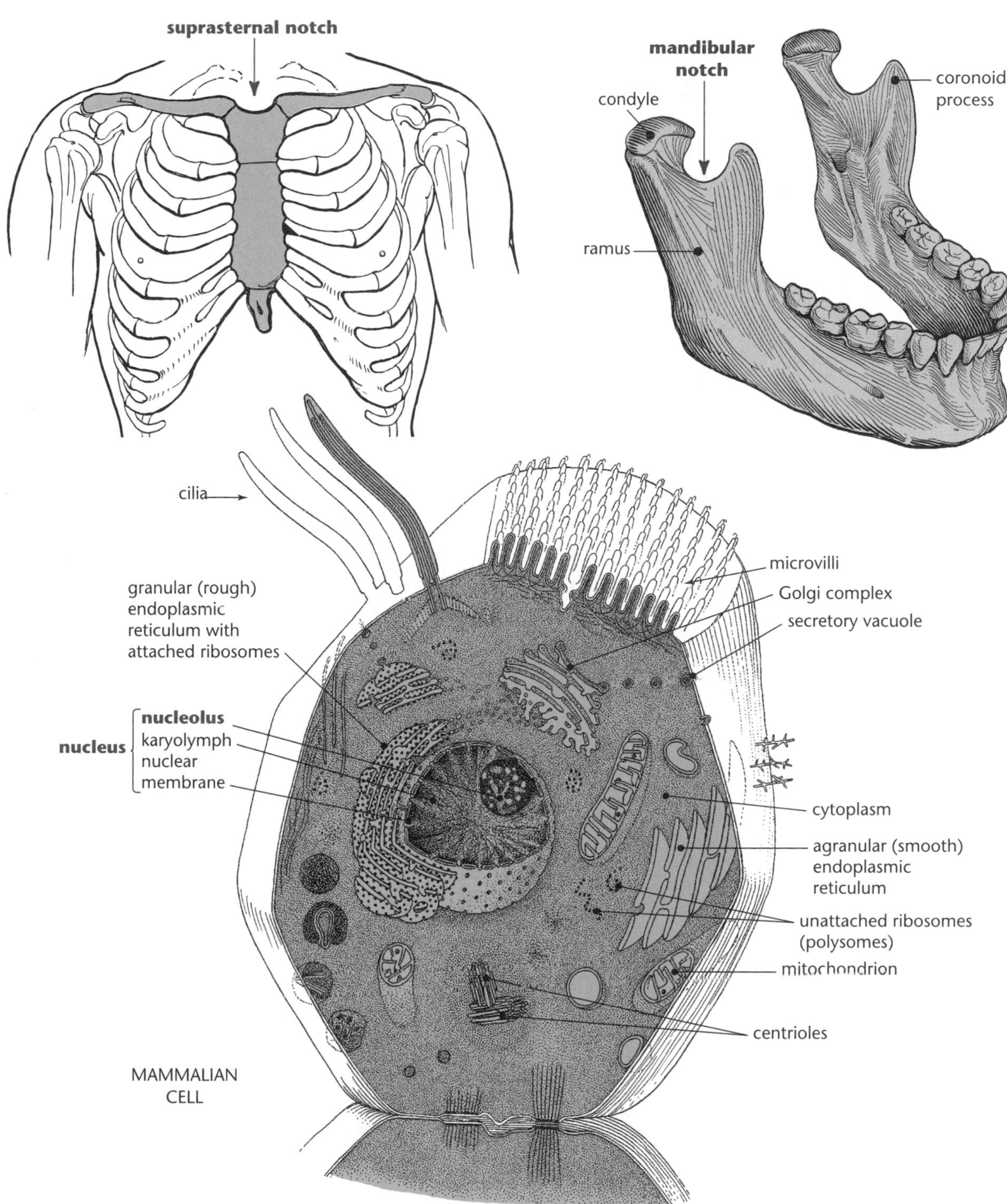

divisions.

caudate n. A long horseshoe-shaped mass of gray matter consisting of an enlarged anterior portion that occupies most of the lateral wall of the anterior horn of the lateral ventricle, a narrower body extending along the floor of the lateral ventricle, and a tapered curved tail that follows the curvature of the inferior horn of the lateral ventricle and enters the temporal lobe, terminating in the amygdaloid complex.

cochlear n. A nucleus located on the surface of the inferior cerebellar peduncle at the junction of the medulla oblongata and the pons; it receives incoming fibers from the bipolar cells in the spiral ganglion of the cochlea.

dentate n. of the cerebellum The largest of the central nuclei of the cerebellum embedded within the hemisphere of the cerebellum; its efferent fibers pass to the brainstem.

diploid n. A cell nucleus containing the diploid or normal double complement of chromosomes.

dorsal motor n. of vagus nerve A nucleus situated in the floor of the fourth ventricle which sends fibers through the medulla oblongata to the vagus and spinal accessory nerves which end in vagal sympathetic plexuses in the chest and abdomen.

dorsomedial n. of hypothalamus The dorsal portion of the two main groups of nerve cell bodies in the tuber cinereum of the hypothalamus; some of their efferent fibers pass to the posterior lobe of the hypophysis (pituitary).

Edinger-Westphal n. A circumscribed group of nerve cells whose fibers run to the oculomotor nerve and thence to the ciliary ganglion, innervating the intrinsic eye muscles.

facial n. A nucleus giving rise to fibers that innervate the voluntary facial muscles.

n. of hypoglossal nerve A cranial nerve nucleus with fibers directed to the lower border of the pyramid to supply the tongue.

inferior colliculus n. An ovoid cellular mass surrounded by a thin cortex which serves as a relay in transmitting auditory impulses to thalamic levels and is involved in acoustic reflexes.

lenticular n., lentiform n. A mass of gray matter the size and shape of a Brazil nut, deeply buried in the white matter of the cerebral hemisphere; a vertical plate of white matter divides the nucleus into a large

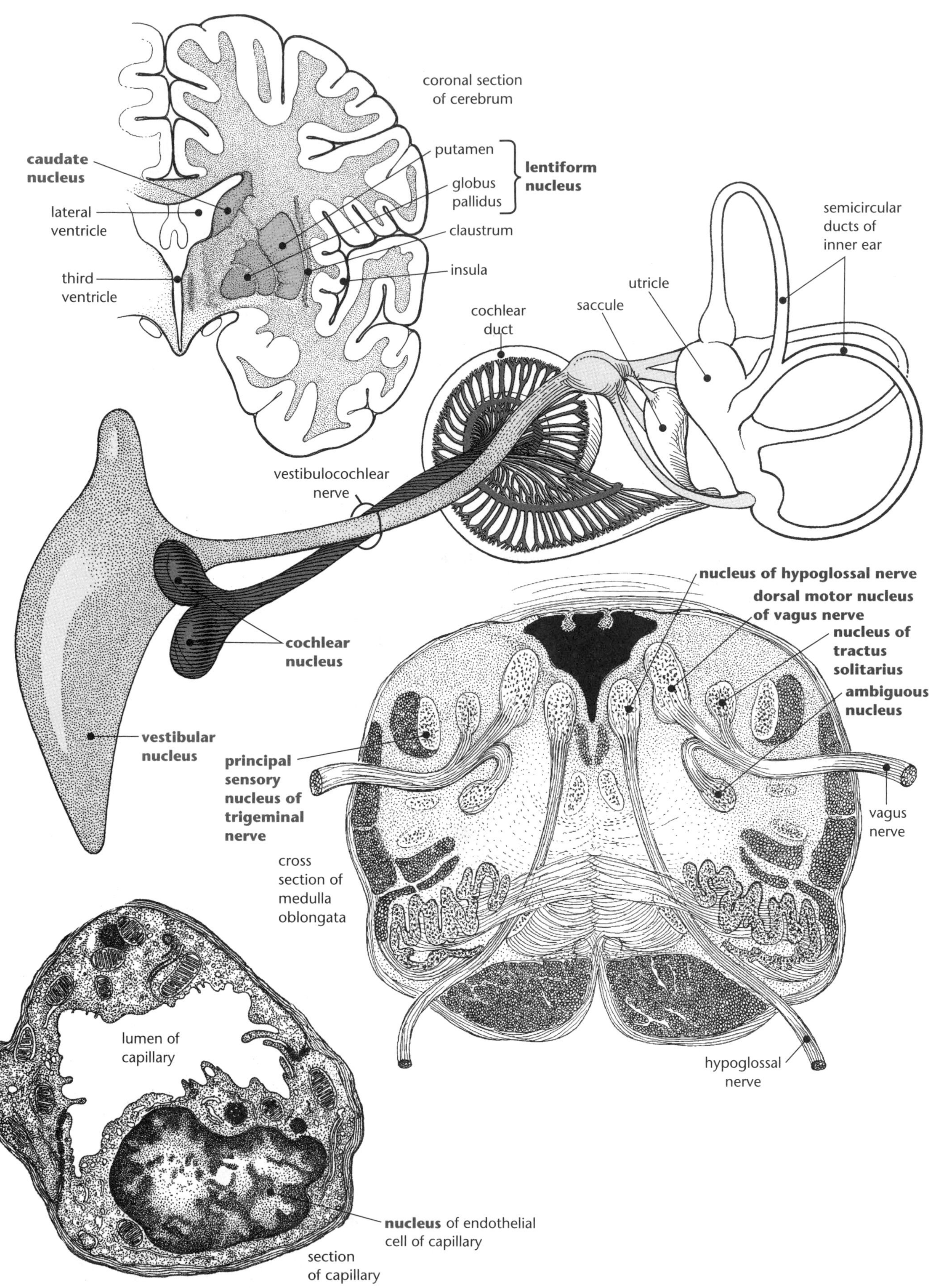
coronal section
of cerebrum
caudate
nucleus
lateral
ventricle
third
ventricle
putamen
globus
pallidus
lentiform
nucleus
claustrum
insula
semicircular
ducts of
inner ear
utricle
saccule
cochlear
duct
vestibulocochlear
nerve
cochlear
nucleus
vestibular
nucleus
nucleus of hypoglossal nerve
dorsal motor nucleus
of vagus nerve
nucleus of
tractus
solitarius
ambiguous
nucleus
principal
sensory
nucleus of
trigeminal
nerve
vagus
nerve
cross
section of
medulla
oblongata
hypoglossal
nerve
lumen of
capillary
nucleus of endothelial
cell of capillary
section
of capillary

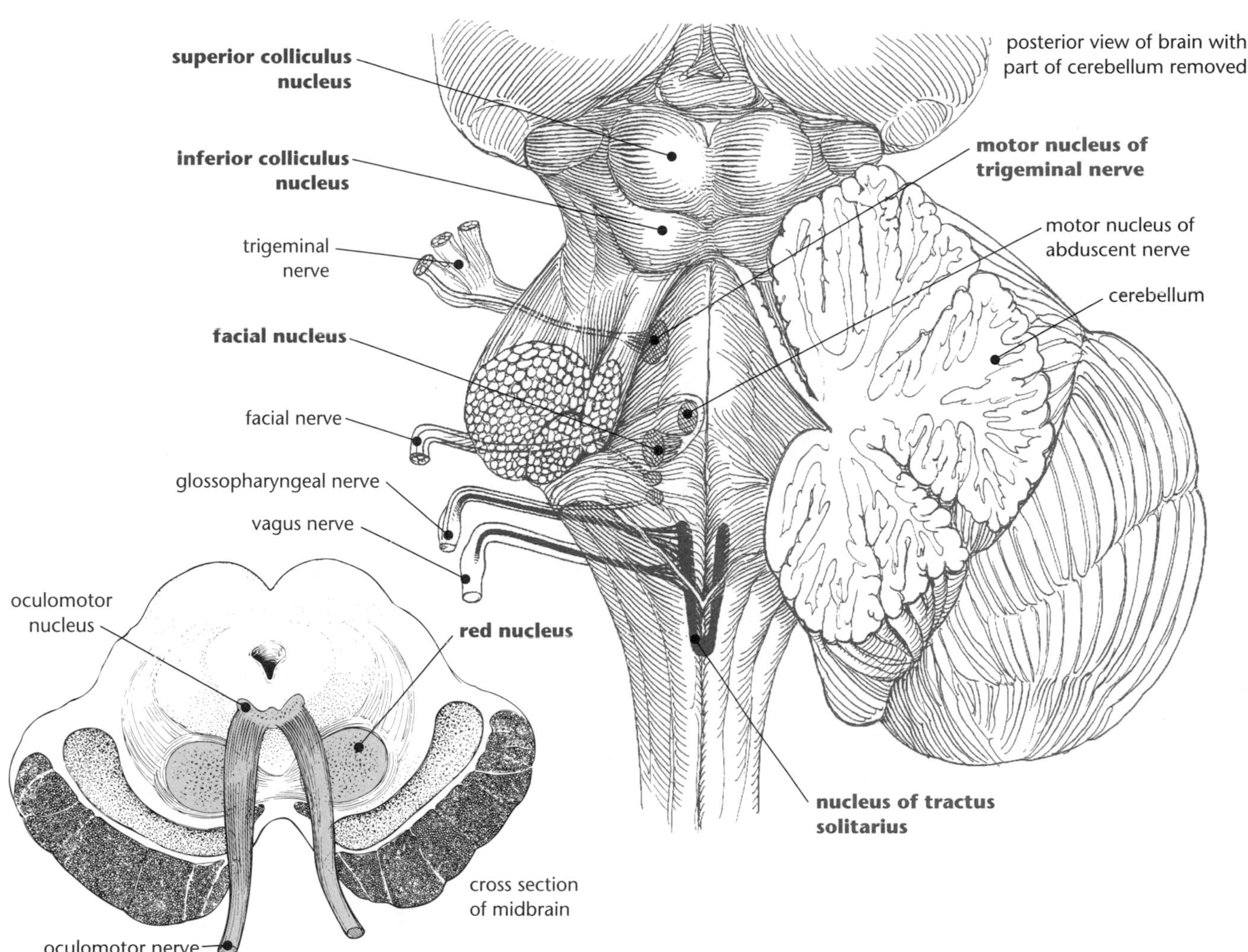

N

lateral portion, the putamen, and a smaller medial portion, the globus pallidus.

mesencephalic n. of trigeminal nerve A cranial sensory nerve nucleus that receives fibers from extrinsic eye muscles and muscles of mastication; the mesencephalic root of the trigeminal nerve arises from it.

motor n. of facial nerve See facial nucleus.

motor n. of trigeminal nerve A nucleus from which fibers run laterally with the mandibular nerve to innervate the muscles of mastication.

naked nuclei The characteristic vesicular nuclei, without cytoplasm, typically found in vaginal secretions during early pregnancy.

paraventricular n. A collection of nerve cells in the anterior part of the hypothalamus on either side of the third ventricle; it gives rise to the paraventriculohypophyseal tract that passes to the posterior lobe of the pituitary (neurohypophysis), related to the autonomic nervous system.

pontine nuclei Groups of nerve cell bodies in the pyramidal tract at the basilar part of the pons, where impulses relay from the cerebrum to the cerebellum.

principal sensory n. of trigeminal nerve A nucleus that receives fibers carrying impulses of touch, pain, and temperature from the head and face.

n. pulposus The central gelatinous part of the intervertebral disk enclosed in several layers of fibrous tissue; it generally becomes fibrocartilaginous in old age.

red n. A large oval nucleus in the midbrain, extending from the caudal margin of the superior colliculus to the subthalamic region; it receives fibers mainly from the deep cerebellar nuclei and the cerebral cortex; it is characterized by its pinkish yellow color, its central position, and its capsule-like covering formed by the fibers of the superior cerebellar peduncle.

salivary nuclei, superior and inferior Scattered nuclei in the dorsolateral reticular formation, just above the pontomedullary junction; the superior sends fibers to the submandibular and sublingual glands via the facial nerve and submandibular ganglion; the inferior sends fibers to the parotid gland via the glossopharyngeal nerve and otic ganglion.

spinal n. of trigeminal nerve A cranial sensory nerve nucleus receiving fibers that mediate pain and temperature for the head and face.

superior colliculus n. A laminated nucleus forming the top half of the tectum (roof of the midbrain); it serves as a primary relay in transmitting visual impulses.

supraoptic n. of hypothalamus One of two nuclei in the hypothalamus located on either side of the third ventricle near the optic tract; it gives rise to the supraopticohypophyseal tract which passes to the posterior lobe of the hypophysis (pituitary gland).

n. of tractus solitarius The nucleus of the solitary tract that receives visceral afferent fibers from the facial, glossopharyngeal, and vagus nerves; a slender nucleus extending the entire length of the medulla oblongata.

ventral posterolateral n. (VPL nucleus) A large mass of the thalamus that receives terminal fibers of the spinothalamic tract and medial lemniscus; it projects to the sensory cortex.

ventral posteromedial n. (VPM nucleus) A crescentic mass of the thalamus ventral to the centrum medianum that receives the secondary trigeminal tract; its axons project to the postcentral gyrus for the face.

ventromedial n. of hypothalamus The ventral portion of two main groups of nerve cell bodies in the tuber cinereum of the hypothalamus; thought to be involved in sexual behavior and the control of food intake.

vestibular n. A nucleus located in the floor of the fourth ventricle that receives fibers from the bipolar ganglion cells of the vestibular nerve.

nuclide (noo´klīd) An atom or a species of atom marked by its particular atomic number and atomic mass (A) or proton number (Z); nuclides with the same proton number are isotopes of a specific element; nuclides with the same atomic mass but different atomic numbers are isobars.

nulligravida (nul-ĭ-grav´ĭ-da) A woman who has never been pregnant.

nullipara (nŭ-lip´ă-ră) A woman who has not delivered an offspring weighing 500 g or more, or of a gestation length of 20 weeks or longer.

nulliparity (nul-ĭ-par´ĭ-te) The condition of not having borne children.

nulliparous (nŭ-lip´ă-rus) Never having borne children. Also called nonparous.

nullisomic (nul-ĭ-som´ik) Lacking both members of a single pair of chromosomes.

number (num´ber) (no) One of a series of symbols expressing a specified quantity or a definite value in a fixed order derived by counting.

accession n. A number sequentially assigned to

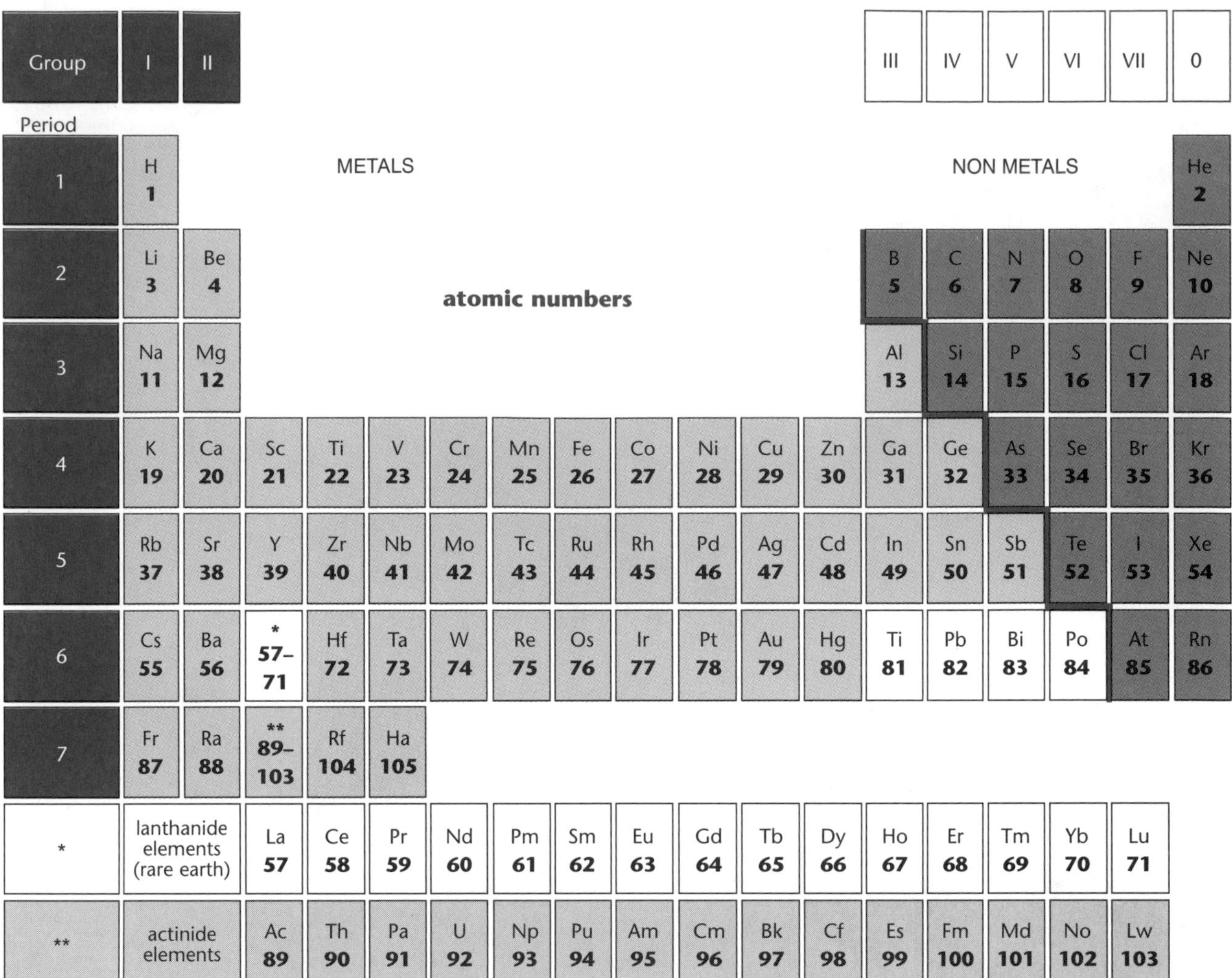

N

each order as it is entered into medical records.

atomic n. (Z) The position of an element in the periodic system; it represents the number of protons in the nucleus of an atom.

Avogadro's n. The number of molecules or particles in 1 gram mole of any compound; it equals 6.022×10^{23}.

Brinell hardness n. (BHN) A number expressing the hardness of a dental material, derived by measuring the diameter of a dent made by pressing, with the aid of the Brinell tester, a standard carbide ball into the surface of the material under a specified load.

electronic n. The number of electrons in the outermost orbit (valence shell) of an element.

Knoop hardness n. (KHN) A number representing the hardness of material (especially tooth structure and dental materials) determined by the penetration of a diamond indenting tool.

Mach n. (M) A number representing the ratio of the speed of an object to the speed of sound in the same surrounding medium.

mass n. The nearest integer to the number expressing the sum of the protons and neutrons in the atomic nucleus of an isotope, denoted as a prefix superscript (e.g., ^{16}O).

numbness (num´nes) Insensitivity in a part of the body.

nummular (num´u-lar) **1.** Shaped like a small coin; applied to a skin lesion or rash. **2.** Arranged like stacks of coins.

nummulation (num-u-la´shun) Formation of disk-shaped masses.

nurse (ners) **1.** An individual trained to care for the sick, disabled, or enfeebled. **2.** To breast-feed. **3.** To care for or tend one unable to provide for his own needs.

certified n. (CN) A registered nurse who has met the criteria for certification established by the American Nurses Association.

charge n. A nurse in charge of supervising the nursing staff of a hospital unit. Also called head nurse.

clinical n. specialist A nurse with advanced degree and training in a particular specialized area of nursing.

community health n. See public health nurse.

graduate n. A nurse who is a graduate of a school of nursing, generally applied to one who has not been licenced or registered to practice.

head n. See charge nurse.

licensed practical n. (LPN) A licensed nurse who has had one year of vocational training and is required by state law to work under the supervision of a registered nurse or a physician. Also called licensed vocational nurse (LVN).

licensed vocational n. (LVN) See licensed practical nurse.

occupational health n. A nurse who has been trained in occupational health to promote and maintain health in the workplace and to provide treatment for injury or disease when necessary; usually has more autonomy than a hospital-based nurse; functions do not include prescribing drugs or performing surgical procedures.

office n. A registered nurse employed in a physician's office either to perform or to assist in performing certain procedures.

operating room n. A member of the operating room nursing staff who provides assistance in the operating room.

practical n. A nurse who has had practical experience in nursing care; distinguished from licensed practical nurse.

private duty n., private n. A nurse who is not a member of a hospital staff but is privately employed to provide nursing care to a patient in a hospital or elsewhere.

public health n. A registered nurse employed by a public health agency to provide educational and preventive programs or treatment and diagnostic services to the community, usually working under the supervision of a public health official. Also called community health nurse.

registered n. (RN) A graduate nurse registered and licensed to practice by a state board authority.

scrub n. A nurse who dons sterile gown and gloves to assist the surgeon at the operating table.

visiting n. A nurse who provides nursing care to patients in their homes.

wet n. A woman who breast-feeds another woman's infant.

nurse-anesthetist (ners ă-nes´thĕ-tist) A registered nurse who has completed postgraduate training in the administration of anesthesia.

certified n-a. (C.R.N.A.) A registered nurse-anesthetist who has received additional education in the administration of anesthesia.

nurse-midwife (ners mid´wīf) A registered nurse formally educated to provide care to pregnant women, including delivery and related health services.

nurse practitioner (ners prak-tish´un-er) A registered nurse who has advanced skills in assessing health-illness status through history taking and physical examination and who is specially trained in designing and implementing a nursing care plan.

nursing (ners´ing) **1.** Breast-feeding. **2.** Activities that constitute the duties of a nurse.

nursing home (ners ing´hōm) A residential health care institution for providing nursing care and limited medical care (usually long-term) for persons who do not require hospitalization.

nutrient (noo´tre-ent) A nourishing component of food.

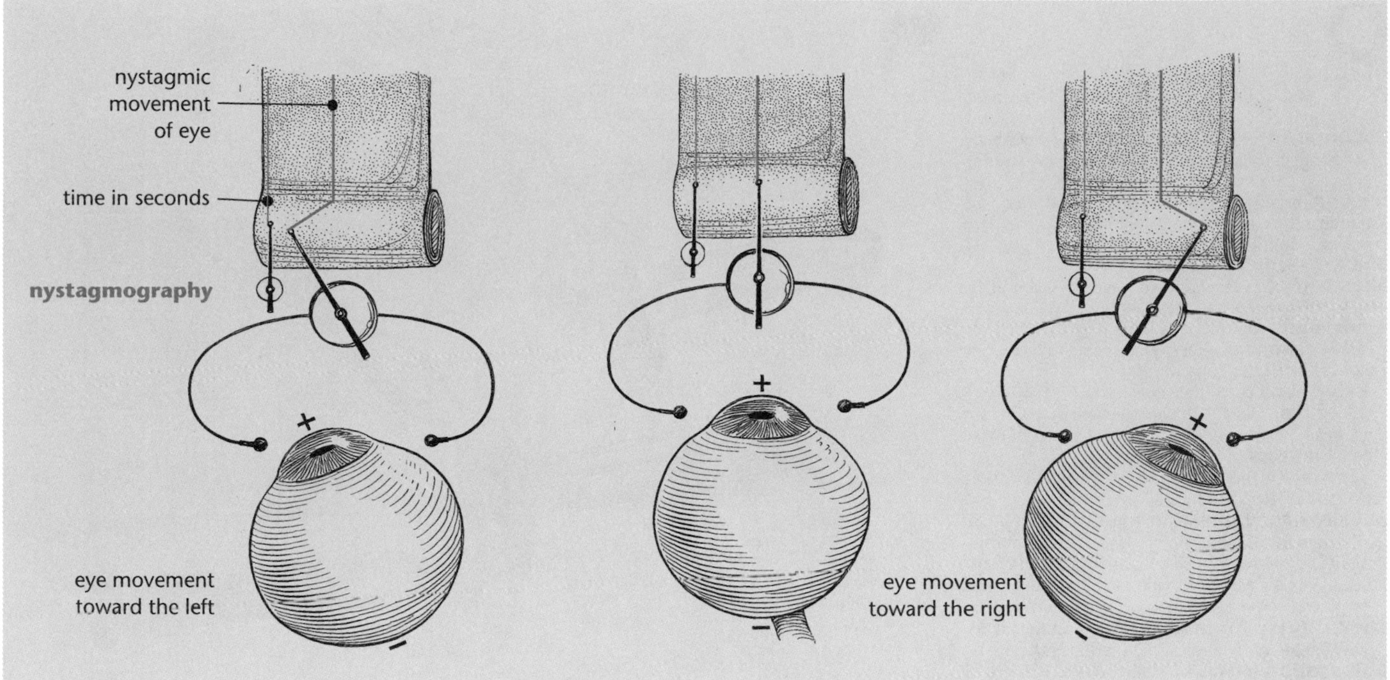

nutrition (noo-trish´un) The process in which a living organism utilizes food for growth and replacement of tissues through digestion, absorption, assimilation, and excretion.

enteral n. Introduction of nutrients via a tube inserted directly into the stomach or duodenum.

total parenteral n. (TPN) Intravenous infusion of nutrients in place of oral intake. Also called total parenteral alimentation.

nutritionist (noo-trĭ´shŏn-ist) One who applies the knowledge of nutrition to the promotion of health and control of disease.

nutriture (noo´trĭ-chur) The state of the body in regard to nourishment, especially in regard to a specific nutrient, such as protein.

nux (nuks) Latin for nut.

n. vomica A poisonous nut from *Strychnos nuxvomica*, a tree native to Southeast Asia; it is a source of two alkaloids, strychnine and brucine, and has been used as a bitter tonic, a tincture, and a central nervous system stimulant. Also called strychnos seed; poison nut; Quaker button.

nyctalopia (nik´tă-lo´pe-ă) Impaired vision in subdued light, while daylight vision is normal; generally due to vitamin A deficiency; often used incorrectly instead of hemeralopia (day blindness). Also called night blindness; day sight.

nycterohemeral (nik-ter-o-hem´er-al) See nyctohemeral.

nyctohemeral (nik-to-hem´er-al) Indicating both night and day. Also called nycterohemeral.

nyctophobia (nik-to-fo´be-ă) Exaggerated and unreasonable fear of darkness.

nymph (nimf) The wingless stage in the development of certain insects immediately after hatching.

nympha (nim´fă), *pl.* **nym´phae** See labia minora, under labium.

nympholabial (nim-fo-la´be-ă) Relating to the labia minora and the labia majora.

nymphomania (nim-fo-ma´ne-ă) Excessive sexual desire in the female.

nymphomaniac (nim-fo-ma´ne-ak) A woman affected with nymphomania.

nymphoncus (nim-fong´kus) A swelling or enlargement of one or both labia minora.

nymphotomy (nim-fot´o-me) Surgical incision into the labia minora.

nystagmic (nis-tag´mik) Relating to or affected with a jerky twitching of the eyeball.

nystagmograph (nis-tag´mo-graf) Apparatus used to record graphically the movements of the eyeball in nystagmus.

nystagmography (nis-tag-mog´ră-fe) The recording of nystagmic movements of the eyes.

nystagmus (nis-tag´mus) An involuntary movement of the eyes in either a rotatory, vertical, or horizontal direction; most commonly it is a rhythmic jerking with a fast and slow component; described by the direction of the quick component.

direction-changing positional n. (DCPN) Nystagmus that changes its direction with different body and head positions.

nystatin (nis´tă-tin, ni-stat´in) An antibiotic agent obtained from cultures of *Streptomyces noursei*; used in the treatment of monilia infections.

nyxis (nik´sis) A puncture.

O

Ω (o-meg´ă, o-me´gă) Omega, the final letter in the Greek alphabet; symbol for ohm.
obdormition (ob-dor-mish´un) Numbness of a body part due to pressure on the sensory nerve innervating it.
obelion (o-be´le-on) A point on the skull where the sagittal suture is crossed by a line joining the two parietal foramina; a craniometric point.
obese (o-bēs´) Very fat; corpulent.
obesity (o-bēs´ĭ-te) Excessive accumulation of fat in the subcutaneous tissues.
alimentary o. Simple obesity.
endogenous o. Obesity attributed to endocrine and metabolic abnormalities.
exogenous o. Simple obesity.
morbid o. Obesity that is so severe as to threaten health and limit activities; usually in excess of twice the ideal weight.
simple o. Obesity that occurs when the caloric intake is greater than the energy expenditure.
obesity-hypoventilation syndrome (o-bēs´ĭ-te-hi-po-ven-tĭ-la´shun sin´drōm) Extreme (morbid) obesity associated with respiratory insufficiency and breathlessness, carbon dioxide retention, and daytime sleepiness. Also called pickwickian syndrome.
obex (o´beks) The small, triangular lamina at the caudal angle of the roof of the fourth ventricle.
obfuscation (ob-fus-kā´shun) **1.** The process of rendering obscure or indistinct; a darkening. **2.** Confusion.
object (ob´jekt) **1.** Anything perceptible through any of the senses. **2.** A person or thing that arouses any type of emotion in an observer.
sex o. A person or thing that arouses sexual feelings in another.
test o. Device used to determine the defining power of the objective lens of a microscope.
objective (ob-jek´tiv) The lens or arrangement of lenses in a microscope or other optical system that receives light from the field of view and forms the first image; so named because it is nearest the object.
immersion o. A high-power objective designed to include oil or other liquid instead of air between its front lens and cover glass.
obligate (ob´lĭ-gāt) Capable of surviving in only one environment; said of certain parasites; opposite of facultative.
oblique (o-blēk´) Having a slanting or sloping direction; deviating from the perpendicular or the horizontal.
obliquity (ob-lik´wĭ-te) Former name for asynclitism.
obliquus (o-bli´kwus) Latin for oblique.
oblongata (ob-long-ga´tă) Having a long dimension; elongated.
obmutescence (ob-mo͞o-tes´sens) Loss of speech.
obnubilation (ob-noo-bĭ-la´shun) A confused state of mind.
observerscope (ob-zer´ver-skōp) A Y-shaped instrument that enables two observers to view simultaneously the interior of a canal or cavity.
obsession (ob-sesh´un) A persistently recurring and unwanted idea that cannot be eliminated.
obsessive-compulsive (ob-ses´iv-kom-pul´siv) Having an obsessive-compulsive disorder. See under disorder.
obstetric, obstetrical (ob-stet´rik, ob-stet´re-kal) Relating to obstetrics.
obstetrician (ob-stĕ-trish´un) A physician who specializes in obstetrics.
obstetrics (ob-stet´riks) (OB) The branch of medicine concerned principally with the management of pregnancy, labor, and the phenomena following childbirth to complete involution of the uterus.
obstipation (ob-stĭ-pa´shun) Constipation that does not respond to treatment; persistent failure to pass any stool.
obstruction (ob-struk´shun) An impedance; a blockage or clogging.
obstruent (ob´stroo-ent) **1.** Causing obstruction. **2.** An agent having such an effect.
obtund (ob-tund´) To diminish pain or touch sensations.
obtundent (ob-tun´dent) An agent that dulls perception of pain or touch.

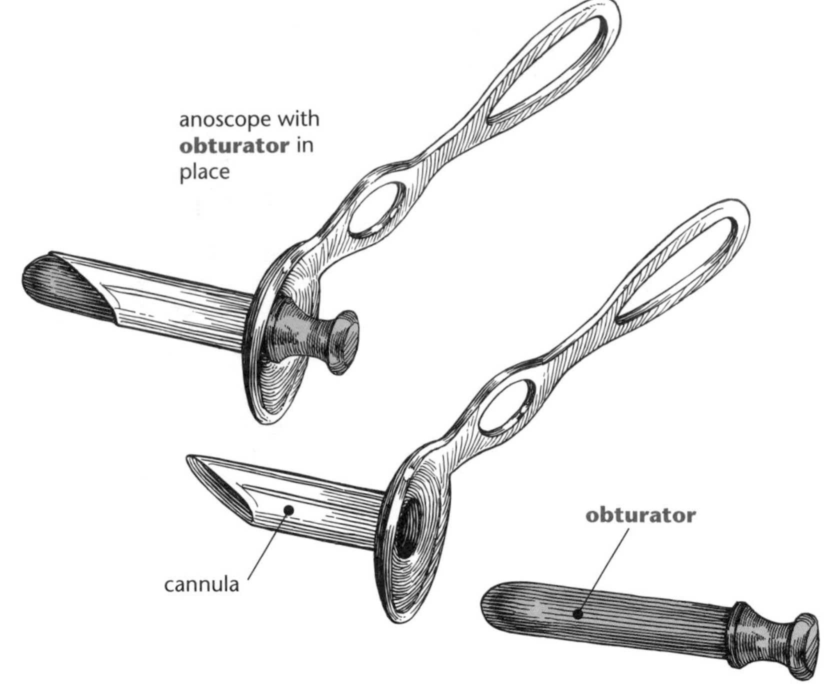

obturation (ob-tu-ra´shun) A stoppage or occlusion.
obturator (ob-tu-ra´tor) **1.** In anatomy, any structure that closes an opening. **2.** A prosthetic device for closing a defect in the hard palate. **3.** An instrument used to close the opening of a hollow tube (cannula) during its insertion into the body.
obtusion (ob-tu´zhun) Dulling of normal sensibility.
OC-125 A murine monoclonal immunoglobulin developed to detect the serum marker CA-125 in the monitoring of a wide variety of tumors.
occipital (ok-sip´ĭ-tal) Relating to the back of the head. See occipital bone in table of bones.
occipitalization (ok-sip-ĭ-tal-ĭ-za´shun) Fusion of the first cervical vertebra (atlas) and the occipital bone.
occipitoatloid (ok-sip-ĭ-to-at´loid) Pertaining to the occipital bone and the first vertebra (atlas); applied to the articulation between the two bones.
occipitobregmatic (ok-sip-ĭ-to-breg-mat´ik) Relating to the occiput and the bregma (a craniometric point).
occipitomental (ok-sip-ĭ-to-men´tal) Relating to the back of the head and the chin.
occipitoparietal (ok-sip-ĭ-to-pa-ri´ĕ-tal) Relating to the occipital and parietal bones.
occipitotemporal (ok-sip-ĭ-to-tem´po-ral) Relating to the occipital and temporal bones.
occiput (ok´sĭ-put) The lower back of the head.
occlude (ŏ-klo͞od´) **1.** To close or obstruct. **2.** In dentistry, to bring together the upper and lower teeth.
occluder (ŏ-klo͞od´er) **1.** Device placed before an eye to block vision. **2.** Device placed on a blood vessel to prevent flow; used in certain physiologic experiments in animals.
occlusal (ŏ-kloo´zal) **1.** Relating to a closure. **2.** In dentistry, relating to the contacting surfaces of teeth or occlusion rims.
occlusion (ŏ-kloo´zhun) **1.** The process of closing or the state of being closed. **2.** In dentistry, the contact of the mandibular teeth with the maxillary teeth in any functional relation. **3.** In chemistry, the absorption of a gas by a metal.
abnormal o. See malocclusion.
afunctional o. Malocclusion that prevents proper mastication.
centric o. Occlusion in which the upper and lower teeth are together in a normal, relaxed manner, and the mandible is in centric relation to the maxilla.
coronary o. Impedance of coronary circulation, usually by thrombosis.
eccentric o. Relating to teeth, any occlusion other than centric occlusion.
enteromesenteric o. Obstructed blood flow in the wall of the intestine and in the mesentery.
hepatic vein o. A rare condition characterized by blocking of the hepatic veins, usually by tumor infiltration or by thrombosis of the vessels, causing enlargement of the liver, portal hypertension, and ascites. Also called Budd-Chiari syndrome.
pathogenic o. An abnormal occlusal relationship of the teeth capable of incurring damage to supporting tissues.
protrusive o. Protrusion of the lower jaw from centric position.
occlusive (ŏ-kloo´siv) Covering; closing.
occlusometer (ok-loo-som´ĕ-ter) See gnathodynamometer.
occult (ŏ-kult´) Hidden (e.g., concealed internal bleeding).
ocellus (o-sel´us), *pl.* **ocel´li** A simple eye found in many invertebrates.
ochrodermia (o-kro-der´me-ă) Yellow discoloration of the skin.
ochronosis (o-kro-no´sis) A characteristic brown-black pigmentation of connective tissue occuring in certain metabolic disorders; a result of deposition of homogentisic acid.
ocrylate (ok´rĭ-lāt) A tissue adhesive used in surgery.
octamethyl pyrophosphoramide (ok-tă-meth´ĭl pi-ro-fos-for´ă-mīd) (OMPA) A chemical used as a plant insecticide. Commonly called schradan.
octan (ok´tan) Occuring every eighth day; said of certain fevers.
octapeptide (ok-tă-pep´tīd) A peptide compound of eight amino acid residues, such as the posterior pituitary hormones, oxytocin and vasopressin.
octavalent (ok-tă-va´lent) Having the combining power of eight hydrogen atoms.
ocular (ok´u-lar) **1.** Relating to the eye. **2.** The eyepiece of a microscope.
ocularist (ok´u-lar-ist) One who designs, constructs, and fits artificial eyes.
oculist (ok´u-list) Obsolete term for ophthalmologist.
oculocerebrorenal syndrome (ok-u-lo-ser-ē-bro-rē´nal sin´drōm) An X-linked recessive inheritance consisting of congenital cataracts and glaucoma, mental retardation, and dysfunction of the kidney tubules leading to proteinuria, glycosuria, ammoaciduria, and inability to concentrate and acidify the urine. Also called cerebro-oculorenal dystrophy; Lowe's syndrome.
oculocutaneous (ok-u-lo-ku-ta´ne-us) Relating to the eyes and the skin.
oculography (ok-u-log´ră-fe) The graphic recording of eye positions and movements.
oculogyria (ok-u-lo-ji´ră) Rotation of the eyeballs.
oculogyric (ok-u-lo-ji´rik) Relating to rotation of the eyeballs.
oculomotor (ok-u-lo-mo´tor) Relating to movements of the eyeball. See also oculomotor nerve, in

O

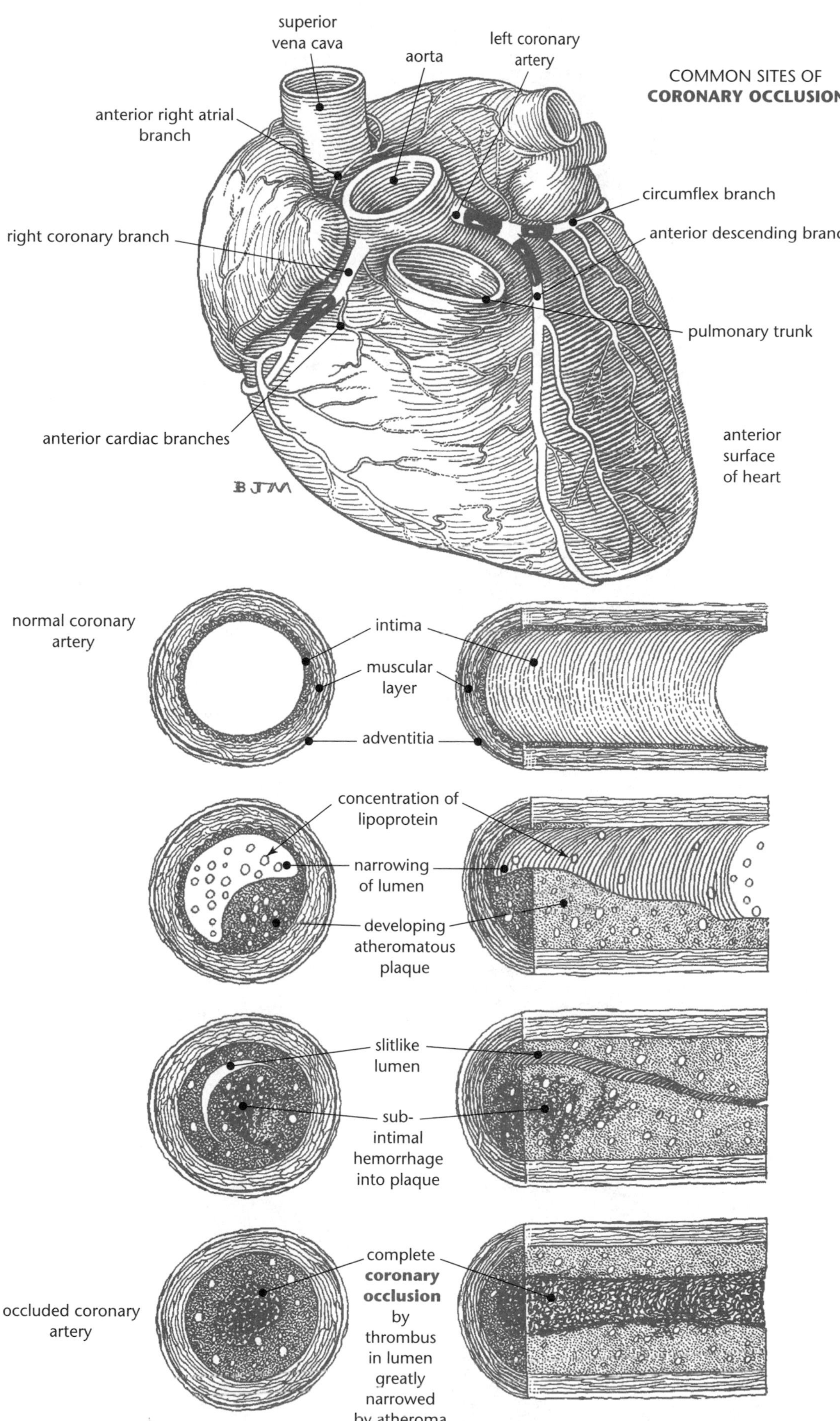
COMMON SITES OF
CORONARY OCCLUSION
superior
vena cava
aorta
left coronary
artery
anterior right atrial
branch
circumflex branch
anterior descending branch
right coronary branch
pulmonary trunk
anterior cardiac branches
anterior
surface
of heart
BJM
normal coronary
artery
intima
muscular
layer
adventitia
concentration of
lipoprotein
narrowing
of lumen
developing
atheromatous
plaque
slitlike
lumen
sub-
intimal
hemorrhage
into plaque
occluded coronary
artery
complete
coronary
occlusion
by
thrombus
in lumen
greatly
narrowed
by atheroma

O

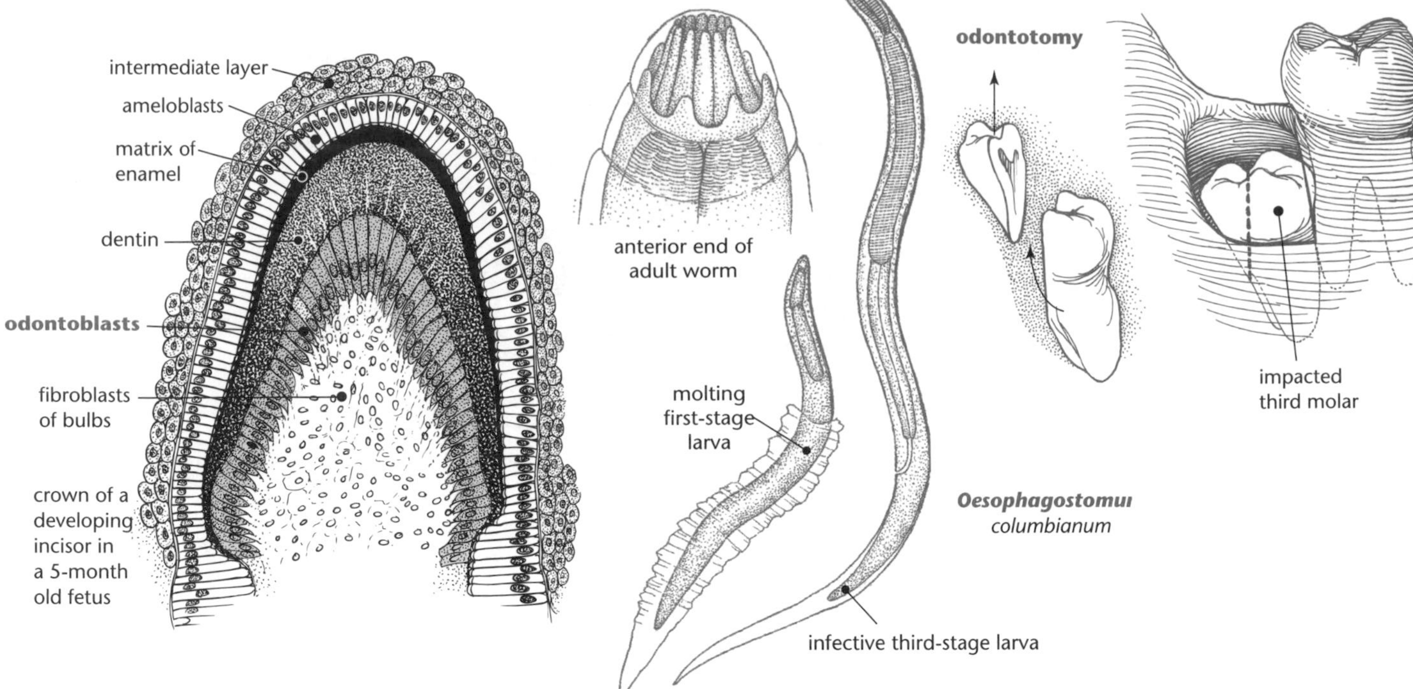

table of nerves.
oculomycosis (ok-u-lo-mi-ko′sis) See ophthalmomycosis.
oculonasal (ok-u-lo-na′zal) Relating to the eye and the nose.
oculopathy (ok-u-lop′ă-the) See ophthalmopathy.
oculus (ok′u-lus), *pl.* **oc′uli** (O) Latin for eye.
o. dexter (O.D.) Right eye.
o. sinester (O.S.) Left eye.
o. uterque (O.U.) The two eyes.
ocutome (ok′u-tom) A miniaturized surgical instrument used in closed vitrectomy to enter the back of the eye through three minute incisions; it consists of three probes; one probe provides light to view the interior of the eye, another cuts and removes tissue, and through the third one a sterile solution is poured in.
odditis (o-di′tis) Inflammation of the sphincter of the hepatopancreatic duct (sphincter of Oddi), at the junction of the duodenum and bile duct.
odontalgia (o-don-tal′jĕ) Toothache.
odontectomy (o-don-tek′tŏ-me) Extraction of a tooth by first removing the bone around its roots.
odontic (o-don′tik) Of or relating to teeth; dental.
odontoblast (o-don′to-blast) A specialized cell that takes part in the formation of dentin in teeth; odontoblasts are present in the papilla of a developing tooth, they line the pulp cavity and may form secondary dentin throughout life.
odontoblastoma (o-don-to-blas-to′mă) **1.** Tumor composed chiefly of epithelial and mesenchymal cells that may develop to produce calcified tooth substances. **2.** An odontoma in its early stage.
odontoclast (o-don′to-klast) A multinucleated cell believed to be involved in the absorption of the roots of primary teeth.
odontogenesis (o-don-to-jen′ĕ-sis) The origin and development of teeth.
o. imperfecta Developmental defect of teeth; enamel and dentin are thin and pulp cavity is large; affected teeth appear opalescent.
odontogenic (o-don-to-jen′ik) Derived from tissues involved in tooth formation; said of certain tumors.
odontogeny (o-don-toj′ĕ-ne) Development of teeth.
odontoid (o-don′toid) Shaped like a tooth (e.g., the odontoid process of the second cervical vertebra).
odontology (o-don-tol′ŏ-je) Dentistry.
forensic o. See forensic dentistry, under dentistry.
odontolysis (o-don-tol′ĭ-sis) Erosion of teeth.
odontoma (o-don-to′mă) A tumor developed from tissues involved in tooth formation.
odontopathy (o-don-top′ă-the) Any disease of the teeth.
odontoprisis (o-don-to-pri′sis) See bruxism.
odontorrhagia (o-don-to-rā′jă) Profuse bleeding from the socket after extraction of a tooth.
odontoscope (o-don′to-skōp) A small circular mirror used for inspecting the teeth.
odontotherapy (o-don-to-ther′ă-pe) Treatment of diseases of teeth.
odontotomy (o-don-tot′ŏ-me) Cutting into a tooth.
odor (o′dor) An emanation perceived by the sense of smell.
odoriferous (o-dor-if′ĕr-ŭs) Odorous; giving off an odor.
odorimeter (o-dor-im′ĕ-ter) An instrument for determining the intensity of odors.
odorimetry (o-dor-im′ĕ-tre) Measurement of relative intensity of odors.
odynacusis (o-din-ă-ku′sis) Hypersensitivity of the spiral organ of Corti (organ of hearing), so that noises cause actual discomfort. Also called painful hearing.
odynometer (o-din-om′ĕ-ter) See algesimeter.
odynophagia (od-ĭ-no-fa′jă) Pain on swallowing.
oersted (er′sted) (H) Unit of magnetic intensity, equal to the intensity of a magnetic field exerting a mechanical force of one dyne on a unit magnetic pole.
Oesophagostomum (e-sof-ă-gos′to-mum) Genus of roundworms parasitic in the intestines of ruminants, swine, and humans; larvae form nodules in the intestinal wall; adults inhabit the intestinal lumen.
oestrid (es′trĭd) A two-winged botfly, the larva of which is parasitic in man and animals.
Oestrus (es′trus) A genus of tissue-invading botflies.
official (o-fĭ′shal) In pharmacology, authorized by or listed in the U.S. Pharmacopeia or the National Formulary.
officinal (o-fis′ĭ-nal) Kept in stock; available without special preparation; said of pharmaceuticals.
ohm (ōm) (Ω) A unit of electrical resistance equal to that of any conductor allowing one ampere of current to pass from a one volt potential across its terminals.
ohmmeter (ōm′me-ter) An apparatus for direct measurement of the electric resistance (in ohms) of a conductor.
oidiomycetes (o-id-e-o-mi-se′tēz) Common name for a group of fungi that produce arthrospores (reproductive spores) through fragmentation of the mycelium.
oidium (o-id′e-um), *pl.* **oid′ia** A free, thin-walled hyphal cell frequently called arthrospore.
oil (oil) Any of several substances that are viscous, unctuous, flammable, and not miscible with water but soluble in several organic solvents; classified, according to their origin, as animal, mineral, or vegetable oils.
castor o. Oil obtained from castor-oil plant seeds (*Ricinus communis*); used as a laxative and externally as an emollient for skin disorders.
cod liver o. Oil obtained from fresh livers of cod fish; a rich source of vitamins A and D.
mineral o. Liquid petrolatum, a mixture of liquid hydrocarbons obtained from petroleum. Also called white mineral oil; liquid paraffin.
peanut o. Oil extracted from peanuts; used as a vehicle in pharmaceutical preparations. Also called arachis oil.
pine o. The volatile oil (crude turpentine) produced by the destructive distillation of pine wood; used as a deodorant and disinfectant.
rectified tar o. Oil obtained from pine tar; used in the treatment of certain skin disorders.
red o. See oleic acid.
safflower o. Oil from seeds of the safflower, *Carthamus tinctorius*, rich in polyunsaturated fats; used as a dietary supplement and in the manufacture of cosmetics.
o. of vitriol Sulfuric acid.
wheat germ o. Oil obtained from the embryo of the wheat kernel; a rich source of vitamin E.
o. of wintergreen A fragrant, volatile oil, rich in methyl salicylate, obtained from the macerated leaves of wintergreen.
ointment (oint′ment) Any of numerous soft, bland, highly viscous preparations used as a vehicle for external medication, as an emollient, or as a cosmetic; a salve.
benzoic and salicylic acid o. Ointment composed of benzoic acid and salicylic acid in a water-soluble base; used to treat athlete's foot and similar fungus infections. Also called Whitfield's ointment.
Whitfield's o. Benzoic and salicylic acid oil.
oleate (o′le-āt) **1.** A salt of oleic acid. **2.** A pharmaceutical preparation containing an alcohol or metallic base and oleic acid.
olecranon (o-lek′ră-non) Point of the elbow; the prominent curved process of the ulna forming the tip of the elbow.
olefin (o′lĕ-fin) An open-chain hydrocarbon having at least one double bond.
oleic (o-le′ik) Of or relating to oil.
oleic acid (o′le′ik as′id) A colorless unsaturated fatty acid with a lardlike aroma; a constituent of most of the common fats and oils. Also called red oil.
olein (o′le-in) The glyceryl ester of oleic acid; a colorless oily substance occuring in many natural fats and oils; the main constituent of olive oil. Also called triolein.
oleometer (o-le-om′ĕ-ter) Apparatus used to determine the specific gravity of oils.
oleoresin (o-le-o-rez′in) **1.** A natural compound of some plants (e.g., pines) containing resin and

O

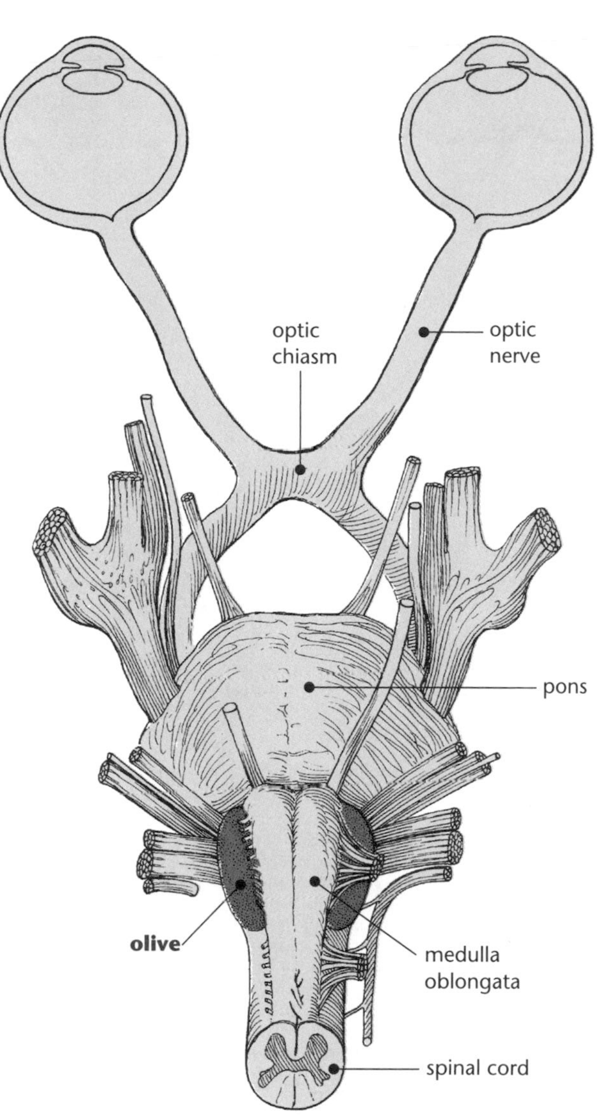

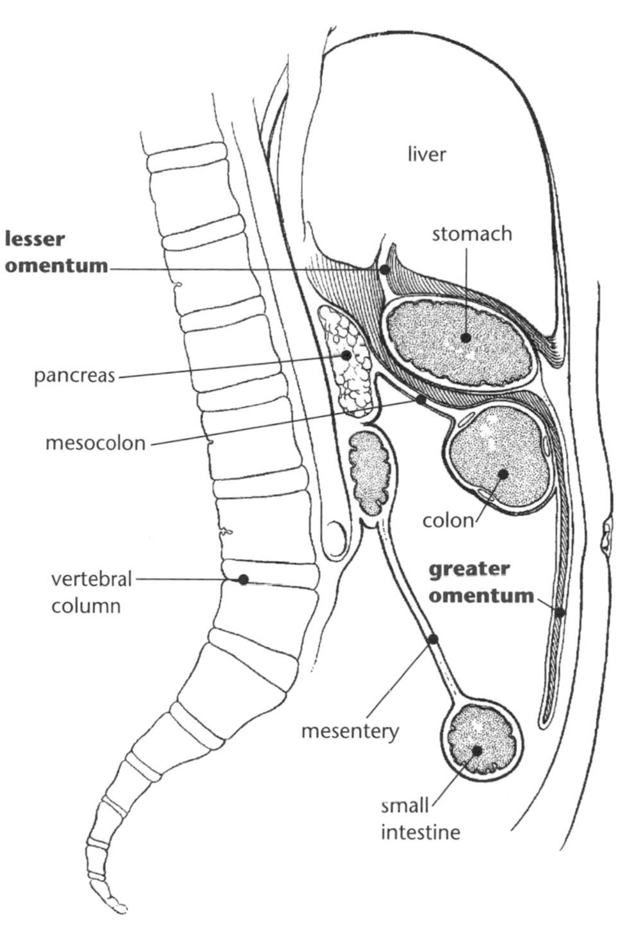

essential oils. **2.** An extract of a drug.

oleosaccharum (o-le-o-sak′ă-rum), *pl.* **oleosac′chara** A homogeneous substance made by mixing sugar with a small amount of a volatile oil; used in pharmaceutical preparations. Also called oil sugar.

oleostearate (o-le-o-ste′ar-āt) A double salt of the oleic and stearic acids.

oleotherapy (o-le-o-ther′ă-pe) Treatment of disease with oil, usually by injections. Also called eleotherapy. Also called eleothorax.

oleovitamin (o-le-o-vi′tă-min) A preparation containing an edible oil and a vitamin.

olfaction (ol-fak′shun) **1.** The sense of smell. **2.** The act of smelling.

olfactology (ol-fak-tol′ŏ-je) The science concerned with the study of the sense of smell.

olfactometer (ol-fak-tom′ĕ-ter) A device for testing the sense of smell.

olfactometry (ol-fak-tom′ĕ-tre) Determination of the degree of acuity of olfactory perception.

olfactory (ol-fak′tŏ-re) Relating to the sense of smell. Also called osmatic. See also olfactory nerve, in table of nerves.

olfacty, olfactie (ol-fak′te) An arbitrary unit of smell, used in olfactometry to determine the strength of a stimulus.

oligemia (ol-ĭ-ge′me-ă) Deficient amount of blood in the body.

olighidria (ol-ig-hid′re-ă) Scanty or diminished sweating.

oligoamnios (ol-ĭ-go-am′ne-os) See oligohydramnios.

oligocholia (ol-ĭ-go-ko′le-ă) Abnormally low secretion of bile.

oligochylia (ol-ĭ-go-ki′lē-ă) Deficiency of chyle.

oligochymia (ol-ĭ-go-ki′me-ă) A lack of chyme.

oligodactyly, oligodactylia (ol-ĭ-go-dak′tĭ-le, ol-ĭ-go-dak-tĭl′ē-ă) Congenital absence of one or more digits of a hand or foot.

oligodendria (ol-ĭ-go-den′dre-ă) See oligodendroglia.

oligodendrocyte (ol-ĭ-go-den′dro-sīt) A cell of the oligodendroglia.

oligodendroglia (ol-ĭ-go-den-drog′le-ă) Nonnervous supportive tissue (neuroglia) surrounding nerve cells and fibers of the brain and spinal cord; composed of small, angular cells (oligodendrocytes) with short, beaded processes and no fibrils; present in both white and gray matter. Also called oligodendria.

oligodendroglioma (ol-ĭ-go-den-dro-gli-o′mă) A relatively slow growing solid tumor made up of oligodendroglia, usually found in the cerebrum of adults.

oligodipsia (ol-ĭ-go-dip′se-ă) Abnormally reduced thirst.

oligodontia (ol-ĭ-go-don′she-ă) See hypodontia.

oligodynamic (ol-ĭ-go-di-nam′ik) Effective in very small quantities.

oligohydramnios (ol-ĭ-go-hi-dram′ne-os) Deficient amount of amniotic fluid in the pregnant uterus, sometimes represented by only a few milli-liters of a thick viscid fluid. Also called oligoamnios.

oligomenorrhea (ol-ĭ-go-men-o-re′ă) The occurrence of menstruation at intervals of 37 to 180 days.

oligonucleotide (ol-ĭ-go-noo′kle-o-tīd) A compound made up of a small number of nucleotides (2 to 10).

oligosaccharide (ol-ĭ-go-sak′ă-rīd) A compound made up of a small number of monosaccharide units (2 to 10).

oligospermia, oligospermatism (ol-ĭ-go-sper′me-ă, ol-ĭ-go-sper′mă-tiz-m) Deficiency in the number of spermatozoa per unit volume of semen.

oligotrichosis (ol-ĭ-go-tri-ko′sis) See hypotrichosis.

oliguria (ol-ĭ-gu′re-ă) Abnormally low excretion of urine; arbitrarily defined as less than 400 ml of urine per day for an adult of average size.

olive (ol′iv) A smooth prominent oval mass on each side of the medulla oblongata. Also called oliva.

Ollier's disease (o-le-az dĭ-zēz′) See enchondromatosis.

ololiuqui (o-lo-lyoo′kē) A substance present in the seeds of the morning-glory; has been used in ceremonies by Indians of the North American continent to produce altered states of consciousness.

omalgia (o-mal′jă) Pain in the shoulder area.

omega (o-ma′gă) Last letter of the Greek alphabet, Ω.

omental (o-men′tăl) Of or relating to the omentum.

omentectomy (o-men-tek′tŏ-me) Removal of the entire omentum, or a portion of it.

omentofixation (o-men-to-fik-sa′shun) See omentopexy.

omentopexy (o-men′to-pek-se) Suturing of the omentum to the abdominal wall. Also called omentofixation; epiplopexy.

omentorrhaphy (o-men-tor′ă-fe) Suturing of the omentum.

omentum (o-men′tum) A peritoneal fold in the abdominal cavity that connects various viscera with each other or with the abdominal wall.

greater o. A prominent double fold of peritoneum descending a variable distance from the greater curvature of the stomach to the front of the small intestine, where turning upon itself (thereby making four layers) it ascends to the top of the transverse colon; it resembles an apron and usually contains large deposits of fat.

lesser o. The fold of peritoneum extending between the liver and the lesser curvature of the stomach and the beginning of the duodenum; the portion connecting the liver to the stomach is called the hepatogastric ligament, while the portion passing from the liver to the duodenum is named the hepatoduodenal ligament; the right border of the

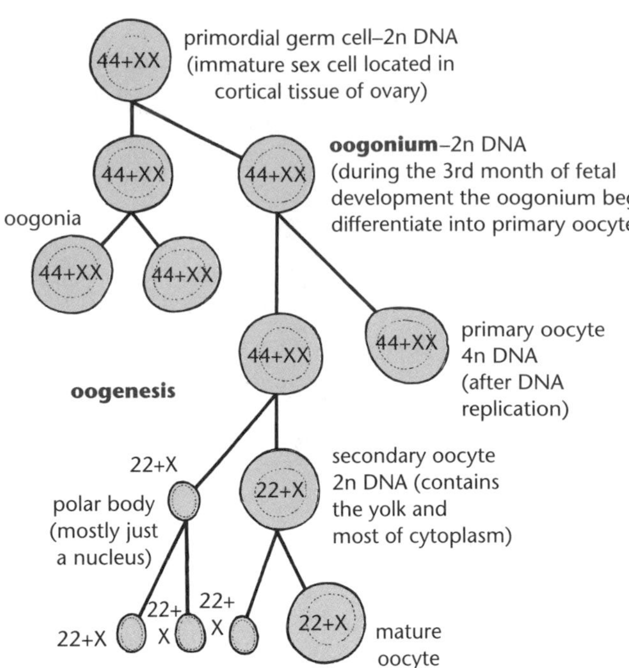

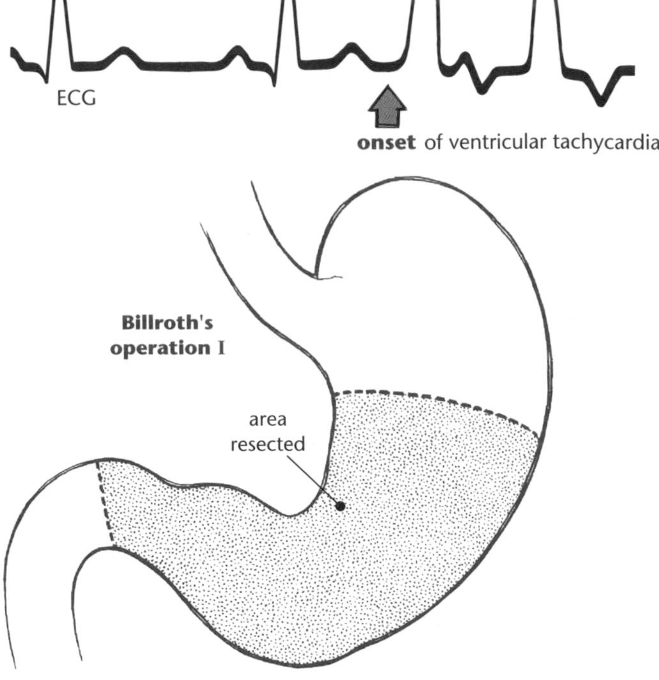

lesser omentum is free, forming the ventral margin of the epiploic foramen.

omeprazole (o-mep´ră-zōl) Drug used to reduce stomach acid secretions in the treatment of ulcers by inhibiting the proton pump that secretes hydrogen ions. A proton pump inhibitor (PPI).

omni hora (om´ne o´ră) (Omn. hor.) Latin for every hour; used in prescription writing.

omnivorous (om-niv´ŏ-rus) Living on both plant and animal food.

omoclavicular (o-mo-klă-vik´u-lar) Relating to the shoulder and the clavicle (collarbone).

omohyoid (o-mo-hi´oid) See table of muscles.

omothyroid (o-mo-thi´roid) See table of muscles.

omphalectomy (om-fă-lek´to-me) Surgical removal of the navel.

omphalic (om-fal´ik) Umbilical.

omphalitis (om-fă-li´tis) Inflammation of the navel.

omphalocele (om´fă-lo-sēl) Congenital hernia of the umbilicus; a small portion of the abdominal contents covered by a membranous sac protrudes into the base of the umbilical cord; the cord structures pass individually over the sac, coming together at its apex to form a normal-looking umbilical cord. Also called amniocele; exomphalos.

omphalomesenteric (om-fă-lo-mes-ĕn-ter´ik) Relating to the umbilicus and the mesentery.

omphalophlebitis (om-fă-lo-flĕ-bi´tis) Inflammation of the umbilical veins.

omphalorrhagia (om-fă-lo-ra´jă) Bleeding from the navel.

omphalorrhea (om-fă-lo-re´ă) A discharge from the navel.

omphalotomy (om-fă-lot´o-me) Cutting of the umbilical cord at birth.

onanism (o´nă-niz-m) See coitus interruptus, under coitus.

Onchocerca (ong-ko-ser´kă) A genus of parasitic worms of the family Onchoceridae (which includes *Wuchereria* and *Loa*); the worms inhabit connective tissues of humans and animals, usually coiled and entangled within firm nodules; two species, *Onchocerca caecutiens* and *Onchocerca volvulus*, can penetrate the skin.

onchocerciasis, onchocercosis (ong-ko-sĕr-ki´ă-sis, ong-ko-sĕr-ko´sis) Skin disease caused by infestation with a threadlike worm, *Onchocerca volvulus;* marked by irritation of the skin with corneal opacities and skin nodules; transmitted by the bite of infested flies. Also called river blindness; volvulosis.

oncocyte (on´ko-sīt) An acidophilic, granular tumor cell.

oncogene (ong´ko-jēn) A gene normally coding for proteins involved in cell growth or regulation but which, under certain conditions, becomes involved in cancer development. See also proto-oncogene.

oncogenesis (ong-ko-jen´ĕ-sis) The origin of a neoplasm.

oncogenic, oncogenous (ong-ko-jen´ik, ong-koj´ĕ-nus) **1.** Causing tumor formation. **2.** Originating from a tumor.

oncolipid (ong-ko-lip´id) A structurally altered fat from a protein molecule found in the blood of many cancer patients.

oncology (ong-kol´o-je) The scientific study of neoplasms.

oncolysis (ong-kol´ĭ-sis) **1.** Destruction of a tumor. **2.** Reduction of any abnormal mass.

oncoma (ong-ko´mă) A tumor or a swelling.

oncornavirus (ong-kor-nă-vi´rus) See oncovirus.

oncosis (ong-ko´sis) Condition characterized by the presence of tumors.

oncosphere (ong´ko-sfēr) See hexacanth.

oncotherapy (ong-ko-ther´ă-pe) Treatment of tumors.

oncotic (ong-kot´ik) Relating to edema or any swelling. See also oncotic pressure, under pressure.

oncotropic (ong-ko-trop´ik) Having an affinity for neoplastic cells.

Oncovirinae (ong-ko-vir´ĭ-ne) The RNA tumor viruses (family Retroviridae) that, on the basis of morphology and antigenicity, are grouped into types A, B, C, and D; associated with malignant diseases.

oncovirus (ong-ko-vi´rus) Any tumor virus (family Retroviridae, subfamily Oncovirinae). Also called oncornavirus.

oneirology (o-ni-rol´o-je) The study of dreams.

onlay (on´la) An extended restoration of a tooth that covers the entire occlusal surface.

onset (on´set) The start or the beginning.

ontogenesis (on-to-jen´ĕ-sis) The biologic development of the individual; distinguished from phylogenesis.

ontogeny (on-toj´ĕ-ne) See ontogenesis.

onychatrophy, onychatrophia (on-ĭ-kat´ro-fe, on-ĭ-kă-tro´fe-ă) Atrophy or underdevelopment of nails, congenital or acquired.

onychauxis (on-ĭ-kawk´sis) Marked thickening or overgrowth of nails.

onychectomy (on-ĭ-kek´to-me) Surgical removal of a nail or nail bed.

onychia (o-nik´e-ă) Inflammation of the matrix of a nail.

onychocryptosis (on-ĭ-ko-krip-to´sis) See ingrown nail, under nail.

onychodystrophy (on-ĭ-ko-dis´tro-fe) Deformity of nails.

onychogryposis (on-ĭ-ko-grĭ-po´sis) Massive curved overgrowth and thickening of a fingernail or toenail; different factors such as irritation of the nail bed by direct trauma, intermittent pressure, and infection may be possible causes.

onychoid (on´ĭ-koid) Resembling a fingernail or toenail.

onycholysis (on-ĭ-kol´ĭ-sis) Detachment, occasionally with shedding, of a nail.

onychomalacia (on-ĭ-ko-mă-la´shă) Abnormal softening of the nails.

onychomycosis (on-ĭ-ko-mi-ko´sis) See tinea unguium, under tinea.

onychopathy (on-ĭ-kop´ă-the) Any disease of the nails. Also called onychosis.

onychophagia, onychophagy (on-ĭ-ko-fa´jă, on-ĭ-kof´ă-je) Nailbiting.

onychorrhexis (on-ĭ-ko-rek´sis) Abnormal brittleness of the nails with breakage of the free edge.

onychosis (on-ĭ-ko´sis) See onychopathy.

onychotillomania (on-ĭ-ko-til-o-ma´ne-ă) A compulsive habit of picking on the cuticles or at the nails.

onychotomy (on-ĭ-kot´o-me) Surgical incision into a fingernail or toenail.

onyx (on´iks) A fingernail or a toenail.

onyxis (o-nik´sis) Ingrown nail.

oocyesis (o-o-si-e´sis) See ovarian pregnancy, under pregnancy.

oocyst (o´o-sist) The encysted zygote of sporozoans in which the infectious sporozoites are formed.

oocyte (o´o-sīt) A developing ovum in the ovary.
primary o. Oocyte derived from an oogonium.
secondary o. An oocyte resulting from the division of a primary oocyte.

oogenesis (o-o-jen´ĕ-sis) Formation of an ovum. Also called ovigenesis.

oogenetic (o-o-je-net´ik) Relating to oogenesis.

oogenic, oogenous (o-o-jen´ik, o-o-jen´us) Producing ova.

oogonium (o-o-go´ne-um), *pl.* **oogo´nia** One of the primordial cells in the embryonic ovary that proliferate and differentiate into primary oocytes (from which the ova develop).

ookinesia (o-o-kĭ-ne´ză) The movements of the ovum during maturation and fertilization.

ookinete (o-o-ki´nēt, o-o-kĭ-net´) A motile zygote; a stage in the life cycle of certain protozoan parasites (e.g., malarial parasite).

oolemma (o-o-lem´ă) The cell membrane of the ovum.

oophoralgia (o-of-or-al´jă) Pain in an ovary.

oophorectomy (o-of-o-rek´to-me) Removal of one or both ovaries. Also called ovariectomy.

oophoritis (o-of-o-ri´tis) Inflammation of one or both ovaries, usually occuring secondary to another infection such as mumps.

oophorocystectomy (o-of-o-ro-sis-tek´to-me) Removal of an ovarian cyst.

oophorocystosis (o-of-o-ro-sis-to´sis) The presence of cysts in an ovary.

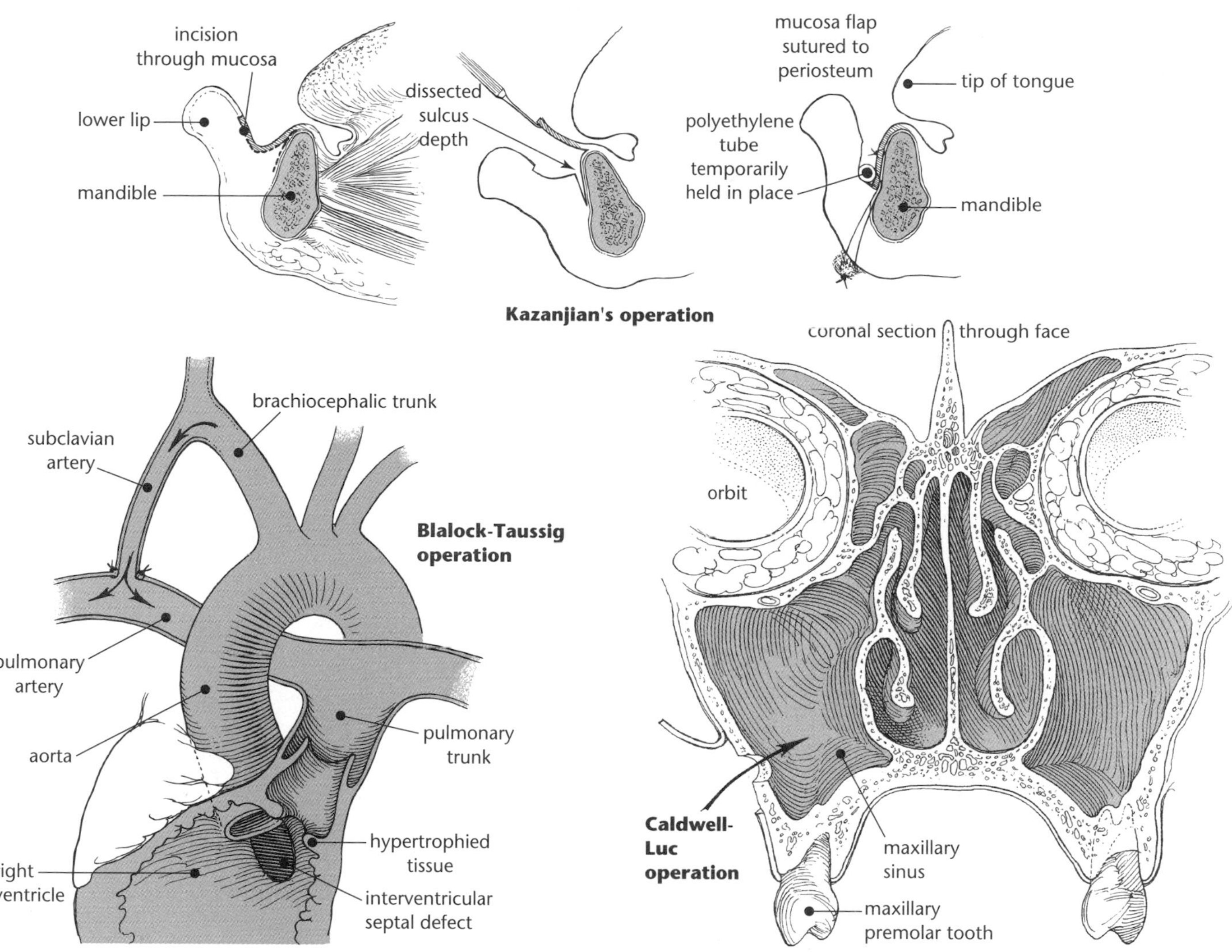

oophoron (o-of´o-ron) The ovary.

oophoropathy (o-of-o-rop´ă-the) Any disease of the ovary.

oophoroplasty (o-of´o-ro-plas-te) Reparative surgery on an ovary.

oophorotomy (o-of-o-rot´o-me) Incision into an ovary. Also called ovariotomy.

ooplasm (o´o-plaz-m) The cytoplasm of an ovum.

ootheca (o-o-the´kă) **1.** The egg case of certain insects. **2.** Ovary.

ootid (o´o-tid) One of two cells derived from the maturation division of the secondary oocyte; it corresponds to the spermatid in the male.

ooze (o͞oz) **1.** Serous discharge or exudate, as from the skin. **2.** To leak out slowly.

opacification (o-pas-ĭ-fĭ-ka´shun) The formation of opacities; the process of making opaque.

opacity (o-pas´ĭ-te) **1.** The state of being opaque. **2.** An area of a normally transparent structure (e.g., the cornea) that has lost its transparency.

opalescent (o-pal-es´ent) Exhibiting an iridescence of color resembling an opal; denoting certain bacterial cultures.

opaque (o-pāk´) Impenetrable by light rays.

opaque media (o-pāk´ me´de-ă) See contrast medium, under medium.

open (o´pen) Exposed to the air, affording unobstructed entrance; said of a wound.

operable (op´er-ă-bl) Denoting a pathologic condition that is reasonably expected to be cured by an operation.

operate (op´er-āt) To perform surgery.

operation (op-er-a´shun) Any surgical procedure for remedying a bodily injury, ailment, or dysfunction.

Abbe's o. Procedure for correcting a defect on a lip by transferring a full thickness flap from the other lip, using an arterial pedicle to insure survival of the graft.

Babcock's o. Removal of a varicosed saphenous vein by introducing a sound (usually from the groin to the ankle), fastening the cut vein to it and drawing it out.

Billroth's o.'s. Procedures for removal of part of the stomach: *Billroth I*, removal of the pylorus followed by end-to-end anastomosis of the stomach and duodenum. *Billroth II*, removal of the pylorus and most of the lesser curvature of the stomach and closure of the cut ends of the stomach and duodenum, followed by a posterior anastomosis of the stomach and jejunum.

Blalock-Hanlon o. Creation of a large interatrial opening to allow mixing of oxygenated blood; a palliative measure for abnormality of the heart in which the aorta originates from the right ventricle (instead of the left) and the pulmonary artery from the left ventricle (instead of the right).

Blalock-Taussig o. Anastomosing of the brachiocephalic trunk, or a subclavian or carotid artery to the pulmonary artery to direct blood from the systemic circulation to the lungs, in cases of congenital pulmonary stenosis with septal defect.

blind o. A procedure in which the surgeon operates by using his sense of touch and knowledge of surgical anatomy without full view of the operative field.

bloodless o. An operation performed with little or no blood loss.

Bricker's o. Diversion of urine disposal from the bladder by connecting the ureter to a pouch of isolated ileum opening onto the abdominal wall.

Caldwell-Luc o. Removal of the contents of a maxillary sinus through an opening on its facial wall above the root of the bicuspid tooth.

debulking o. Removal of a major portion of a cancerous tumor that cannot be removed completely.

exploratory o. A procedure used to establish a diagnosis by ascertaining the condition present.

fenestration o. A rarely performed operation for the treatment of conduction type deafness (e.g., otosclerosis); an opening is created between the middle ear chamber and the lateral semicircular canal as an alternate sound access, bypassing the ankylosed stapes at the oval window.

flap o. (a) Any procedure involving partial detachment of tissue. (b) In dental surgery, partial detachment of soft tissue from underlying bone to gain access to the area.

Gillies' o. Reduction of fractures of the zygoma and zygomatic arch through an incision above the hairline.

Halsted's o.'s (a) Removal of a breast for carcinoma along with the greater and smaller pectoral muscles and adjacent lymphatic structures. (b) Operation for the repair of a direct inguinal hernia.

Hofmeister o. Reestablishment of intestinal continuity after partial removal of the stomach by closure of the lesser curvature side of the stomach and the duodenal stump, followed by anastomosis of the greater curvature side of the stomach and jejunum.

Huggins' o. Removal of testes for cancer of the prostate gland.

Irving's o. A method of female sterilization; each fallopian (uterine) tube is tied with two sutures; the tubes are cut between the sutures; then, either both distal and proximal stumps are buried between the two layers of the broad ligament, or only the distal stumps are thus buried and the proximal stumps are sutured under the serous covering of the uterus. Also called Irving's procedure; Irving's technique.

Kazanjian o. A surgical procedure for extending the vestibular sulcus of edentulous ridges to increase their height and to improve denture retention.

Madlener's o. A method of female sterilization by partial resection of the fallopian (uterine) tubes; the middle third of each tube is lifted to create a loop, the loop is crushed with a clamp at its base, the

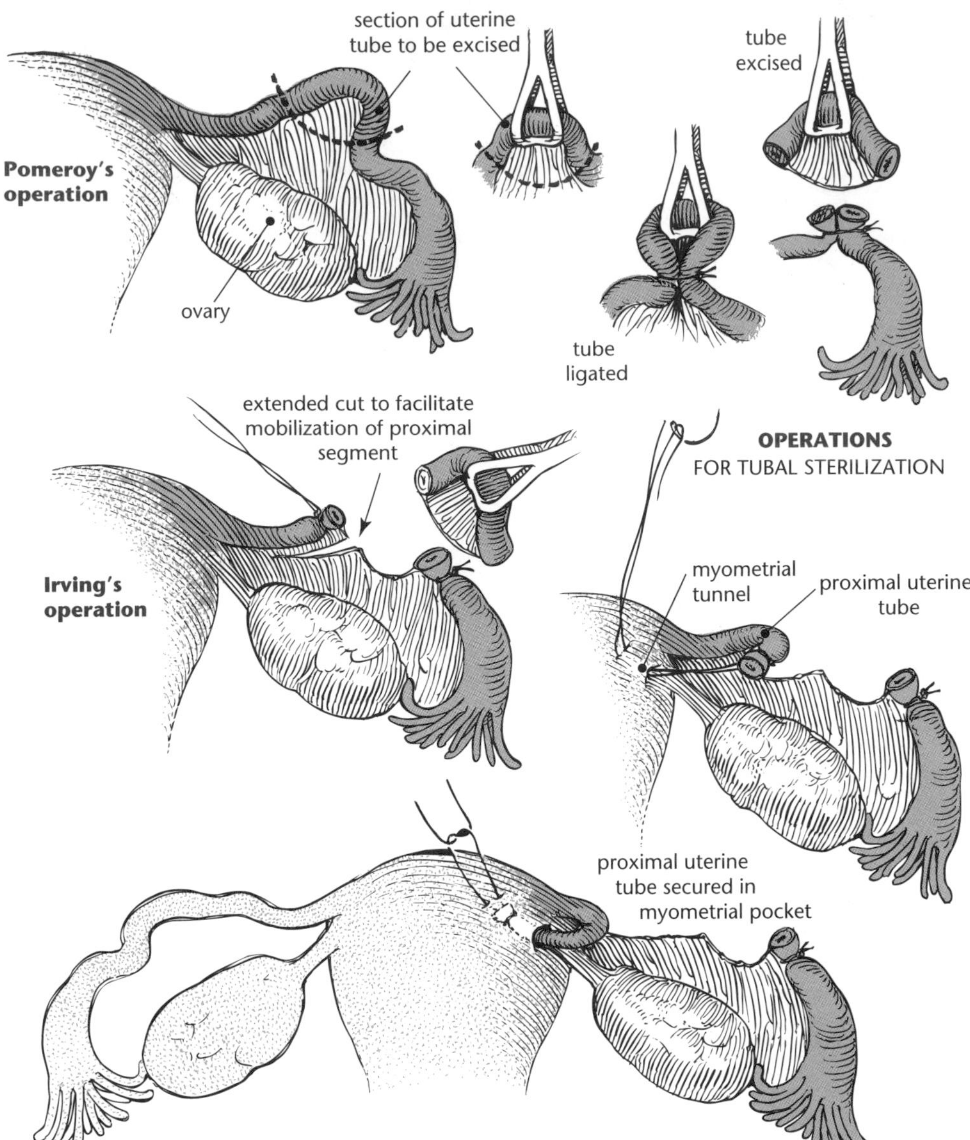

O

crushed region is ligated and covered with the round ligament to prevent adhesion formation. Also called Madlener's procedure; Madlener's technique.

Manchester o. High amputation of the uterine cervix and suturing together of the broad ligament bases in front of the shortened cervix; devised to relieve first and second degree prolapse of the uterus.

Marshall-Marchetti-Krantz o. An operation for correction of stress incontinence; the tissues on either side of the urethra are sutured together anteriorly, then to the posterior side of the pubis and to the rectus muscle.

Naftziger's o. Removal of the lateral and superior orbital walls for severe malignant exophthalmos.

open o. A procedure in which the surgeon operates with full view of the operative field.

plastic o. An operation intended to restore appearance, function, or lost parts.

Pomeroy's o. A method of female sterilization by partial resection of the fallopian (uterine) tubes; the middle third of each tube is lifted to create a loop, the loop is ligated and resected at its base, and the wound is covered with the round ligament to prevent adhesion formation. Also called Pomeroy's procedure; Pomeroy's technique.

Potts' o. Side-to-side connection between the aorta and the pulmonary artery; a palliative measure for tetralogy of Fallot.

radical o. A thorough operation aimed at complete cure of a disease or correction of a defect.

Roux-en-Y o. Procedure in which the jejunum is cut about 15 cm below its origin, the distal end is sutured to the stomach, and the end of the proximal segment is sutured to the side of the jejunum farther down.

stapes mobilization o. Freeing of stapes from overgrowth of bone to restore hearing in individuals with otosclerosis.

Whipple's o. Removal of carcinoma of the head of the pancreas.

operative (op´er-ă-tiv) **1.** Relating to an operation. **2.** Active.

operculated (o-per´ku-la-ted) Having a caplike cover (operculum).

operculum (o-per´ku-lum), *pl.* **oper´cula** **1.** Any anatomic structure resembling a lid or cover (e.g., brain tissue covering the insula). **2.** The mucus plug sealing the opening of the endocervical canal of the uterus during pregnancy. **3.** The caplike cover of the eggs of certain parasitic worms. **4.** The tissue covering an unerupted tooth. **5.** The attached portion of a retinal detachment.

o. oculi The eyelid.

operon (op´er-on) A cluster of two or more structural genes and an operator gene on a chromosome; it is the functional unit of DNA governing synthesis of enzymes of a metabolic pathway.

ophiasis (o-fi´ă-sis) Loss of hair occuring in bands partly or completely encircling the head.

ophidiasis (o-fi-di´ă-sis) Poisoning by the venom of a snake. Also called ophidism.

ophidic (o-fid´ik) Relating to snakes.

ophidiophobia (o-fid-e-o-fo´bē-ă) A morbid fear of snakes.

ophryosis (of-re-o´sis) Spasmodic twitching in the area of the eyebrow.

ophthalmalgia (of-thal-mal´jă) Pain in the eyeball.

ophthalmectomy (of-thal-mek´to-me) Surgical removal of the eyeball.

ophthalmia (of-thal´me-ă) Inflammation of the eye.

gonorrheal o. Acute purulent conjunctivitis caused by gonorrheal infection.

metastatic o. See sympathetic ophthalmia.

migratory o. See sympathetic ophthalmia.

o. neonatorum Acute purulent conjunctivitis of the newborn infant acquired during passage through the birth canal when the mother has gonorrhea. Also called neonatal conjunctivitis.

sympathetic o. Inflammation of the uveal tract of one eye followed by an identical inflammation of the other eye, leading to bilateral blindness; occurs after a perforating injury in the area of the ciliary body or retention of a foreign body in the same area. Also called sympathetic uveitis; metastatic ophthalmia; migratory ophthalmia; transferred ophthalmia.

transferred o. See sympathetic ophthalmia.

ophthalmic (of-thal´mik) Pertaining to the eyeball.

ophthalmitic (of-thal-mit´ik) Relating to inflammation of the eye.

ophthalmoblenorrhea (of-thal-mo-blen-o-re´ă) Purulent conjunctivitis.

ophthalmocentesis (of-thal-mo-sen-te´sis) Surgical puncture of the eye.

ophthalmodiaphanoscope (of-thal-mo-di-ă-fan´o-skōp) Instrument used to inspect the interior of the eye by means of transmitted light.

ophthalmodonesis (of-thal-mo-do-ne´sis) A trembling motion of the eyes.

ophthalmodynamometer (of-thal-mo-di-nă-mom´ĕ-ter) **1.** Instrument for estimating the blood pressure of the retinal vessels. **2.** Instrument for measuring the power of convergence of the eyes, applied to a near point of vision.

ophthalmodynamometry (of-thal-mo-di-nă-

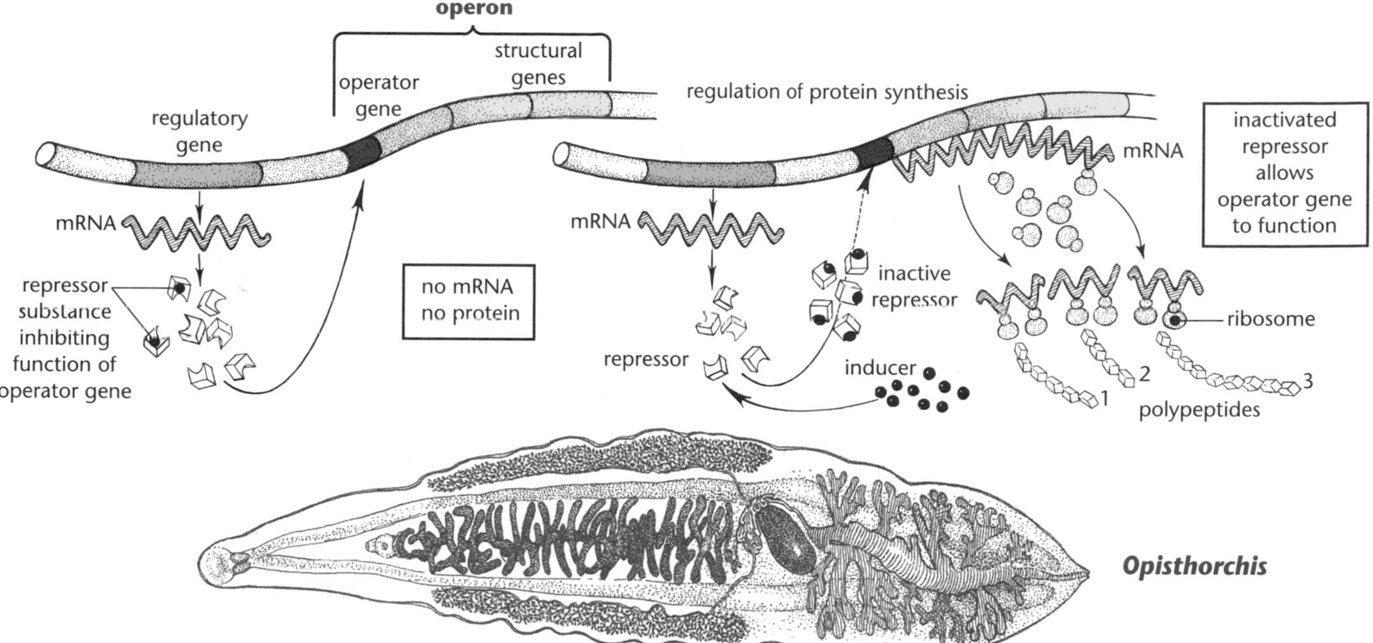

mom´ĕ-tre) Measurement of the blood pressure in the retinal circulation within the eye by means of an ophthalmodynamometer; used to determine the presence of an occluding or constricting lesion in the carotid artery system.

ophthalmodynia (of-thal-mo-din´e-ă) See ophthalmalgia.

ophthalmo-eikonometer (of-thal-mo-i-ko-nom´ĕ-ter) Instrument for measuring the ocular disorder aniseikonia.

ophthalmograph (of-thal´mo-graf) Instrument for recording eye movements during reading.

ophthalmoleukoscope (of-thal-mo-loo´ko-skōp) Instrument for testing color perception; it controls color intensities by means of filters to produce a white mixture.

ophthalmologist (of-thal-mol´o-jist) A physician who specializes in treating diseases and refractive errors of the eye.

ophthalmology (of-thal-mol´o-je) The medical and surgical specialty concerned with the eye, its diseases, and refractive errors.

ophthalmomalacia (of-thal-mo mă la´shă) Abnormally low intraocular pressure of the eyeball.

ophthalmometer (of-thal-mom´ĕ-ter) See keratometer.

ophthalmometry (of-thal-mom´ĕ-tre) See keratometry.

ophthalmomycosis (of-thal-mo-mi-ko´sis) Any fungal disease of the eye or its appendages. Also called oculomycosis.

ophthalmomyiasis (of-thal-mo-mi-i´ă-sis) Infection of the eye with the larvae of flies. Also called ocular myiasis.

ophthalmomyotomy (of-thal-mo-mi-ot´ŏ-me) Surgical division of any of the extrinsic (extraocular) eye muscles.

ophthalmoneuritis (of-thal-mo-nōō-ri´tis) Inflammation of the optic nerve.

ophthalmopathy (of-thal-mop-ă-the) Any disease of the eye. Also called oculopathy.

ophthalmophacometer (of-thal-mo-fa-kom´ĕ-ter) Instrument for measuring the curvature of the cornea and lens of the eye.

ophthalmoplasty (of-thal´mo-plas-te) Reparative surgery of the eye.

ophthalmoplegia (of-thal-mo-ple´jă) Partial or total paralysis of one or more muscles of the eyes.

chronic progressive external o. Rare condition of all three nerves supplying the external eye muscles (3rd, 4th, and 6th cranial nerves) causing a slowly increasing inability to move the eyes.

exophthalmic o. Ophthalmoplegia due to thickening and white blood cell infiltration of the eye muscles; degeneration of some muscle fibers may also occur; thought to be caused by an autoimmune reaction.

external o. General term for inability to move the eyes normally as a result of a lesion in the brain involving nuclei of the 3rd, 4th, or 6th cranial nerves, which supply the external eye muscles.

migrainous o. Brief condition accompanying an attack of migraine, marked by unilateral paralysis of the 3rd cranial nerve, which causes lateral deviation of the affected eye and drooping of the eyelid.

ophthalmoplegic (of-thal-mo-ple´jik) **1.** Relating to ophthalmoplagia. **2.** An agent causing such an effect.

ophthalmorrhagia (of-thal-mo-ra´je-ă) Bleeding from the eye.

ophthalmorrhea (of-thal-mo-re´ă) Abnormal discharge from the eye.

ophthalmorrhexis (of-thal-mo-rek´sis) Rupture of the eyeball.

ophthalmoscope (of-thal´mŏ-skōp) Instrument for inspecting the interior of the eyeball.

ophthalmoscopy (of-thal-mos´kŏ-pe) Examination of the interior of the eye with an ophthalmoscope.

opthalmotrope (of-thal´mo-trōp) A teaching model of the two eyes designed to demonstrate the action of the extrinsic eye muscles.

ophthalmoxerosis (of-thal-mo-ze-ro´sis) See xerophthalmia.

opiate (o´pe-āt) Any preparation derived from opium.

opioid (o´pe-oid) Natural or synthetic compounds that have morphine-like pharmacologic activity.

opisthion (o-pis´the-on) The middle point on the posterior margin of the foramen magnum of the occipital bone of the skull.

opisthocheilia (o-pis-tho-ki´lē-ă) Receding lips.

opisthocranium (o-pis-tho-kra´ne-um) The area in the midline of the cranium that protrudes farthest backward.

opisthorchiasis (o-pis-thor-ki´ă-sis) Infection with Asiatic flukes (especially *Opisthorchis viverrini*), aquired by eating raw or undercooked infected fish.

Opisthorchis (o-pis-thor´kis) A genus of flukes (family Opisthorchiidae) that have testes at the posterior end of a lancet-shaped body; found in the gallbladder or bile ducts of fish-eating mammals, birds, and fish.

o. felineus The cat liver fluke from Eastern Europe and Asia, measuring from 7 to 12 by 2 to 3 mm; humans are frequently infected by eating raw or undercooked infected fish.

o. sinensis See *Clonorchis sinensis*, under *Clonorchis*.

opisthotonos (o-pis-thot´ŏ-nus) A muscle spasm causing rigidity of the neck and back and arching of the back with convexity forward, as in acute cases of tetanus or meningitis.

opium (o´pe-um) Drug prepared from the dried gummy juice of unripe pods of a poppy, *Papaver somniferum*; used as an analgesic; habitual use causes addiction, excessive use is fatal.

Oppenheim's sign (op´en-hīmz sīn) Dorsal extension of the big toe elicited by stroking the medial side of the tibia; seen in pyramidal tract disease.

Oppenheim's syndrome (op´en-hīmz sin´drōm) See amyotonia congenita, under amyotonia.

opponens (o-po´nenz) Opposing; descriptive term for several muscles of the hand and foot that pull the lateral digits across the palm or sole.

opportunistic (op-or-too-nis´tik) **1.** Denoting a disease that occurs in people whose immune system is impaired by other infections or by ongoing chemotherapy. **2.** Denoting the organisms causing such a disease, and which do not cause disease (or cause only mild infections) in healthy people.

opposure (op´pō-shur) The approximation of tissues for suturing.

opsin (op´sin) The protein constituent of the rhodopsin molecule (a retinal pigment).

opsoclonus (op-so-klo´nus) Abnormal condition characterized by rapid, multidirectional, nonrhythmic movement of the eyes. Popularly called dancing eyes.

opsonin (op´sŏ-nin) A substance capable of binding to bacteria or other cells and rendering them susceptible to phagocytosis; may be antibody or fragments of complement components.

opsonization (op-sŏ-nī-za´shun) The process by which antigen (i.e., bacteria and other cells) are modified, usually by antibody and/or complement, to make them more readily engulfed and destroyed (phagocytized) by white blood cells.

opsonize (op´sŏ-nīz) To sensitize microorganisms with specific opsonin.

opsonocytophagic (op-sŏ-no-si-to-faj´ik) Denoting the increased phagocytic activity of leukocytes in blood containing specific opsonin.

optesthesia (op-tĕs-the´zhă) The ability to perceive a light stimulus.

optic (op´tik) Pertaining to the eye.

optical (op´tĭ-kal) Relating to vision.

optician (op-tish´an) **1.** One who makes or sells lenses, eyeglasses, or other optical instruments. **2.** A person who adjusts eyeglasses after a prescription furnished by an ophthalmologist or optometrist.

opticociliary (op-tĭ-ko-sil´ē-ar-ē) Relating to the optic and ciliary nerves.

opticocinerea (op-ti-ko-sĭ-nĕr´e-ă) The gray substance of the optic nerve.

optics (op´tiks) The science concerned with the study of light and refracting media, especially of the eye.

optimum (op´tĭ-mum) Denoting the most favorable conditions.

O

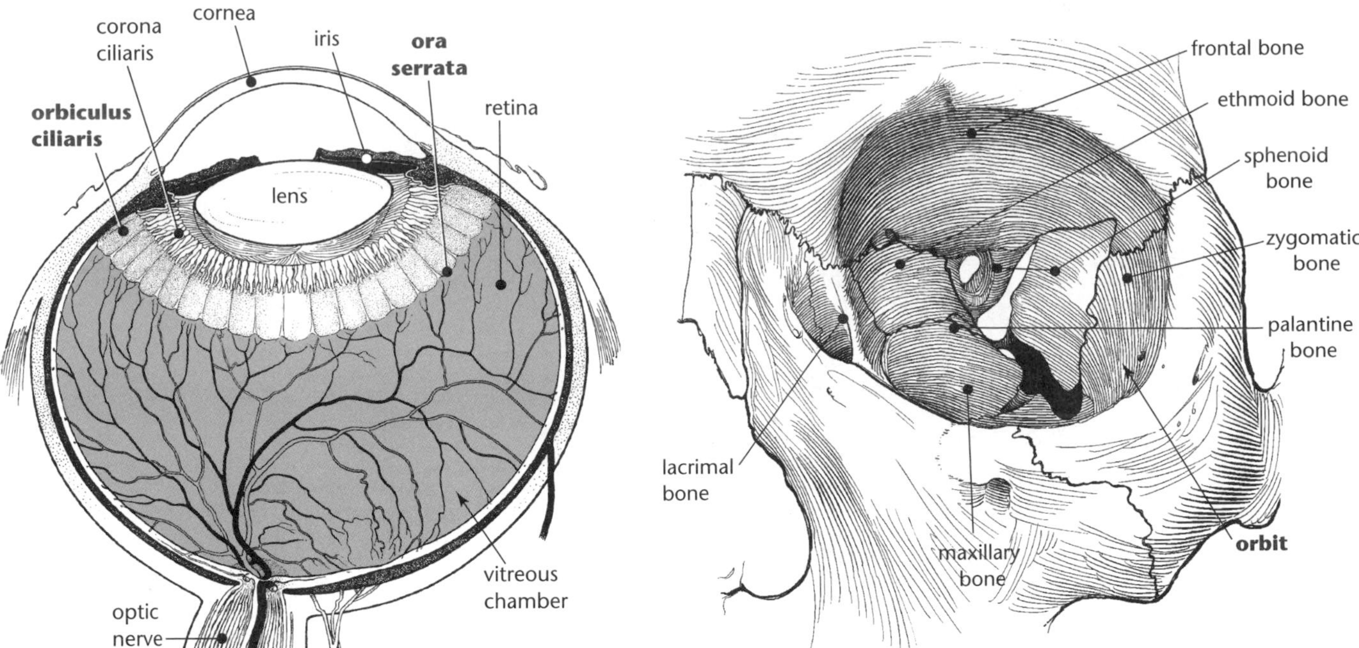

optometer (op-tom´ĕ-ter) Any of several devices for measuring the refractive state of the eye.

optometrist (op-tom´ĕ-trist) A person trained to examine the eyes to assess visual acuity and to prescribe, supply, and adjust eyeglasses or contact lenses.

optometry (op-tom´ĕ-tre) The measuring of visual acuity and correction of visual defects by means of eyeglasses or contact lenses.

optomyometer (op-to-mi-om´ĕ-ter) Device for determining the relative strength of the extrinsic eye muscles.

ora (o´ră), *pl.* **orae** A border.

o. serrata The serrated margin of the retina, within the anterior portion of the eyeball.

orad (o´rad) Toward the mouth.

oral (or´al) Relating to the mouth.

orality (o-ral´ĭ-te) In psychoanalysis, relating to the oral or earliest stage of sexual development.

orange (or´ĭnj) An edible fruit, *Aurantii fructus*; its rind contains numerous oil glands and is used in producing pharmaceutical preparations.

orbicular (or-bik´u-lar) Circular.

orbiculus ciliaris (or-bĭk´u-lus sil-ē-ā´ris) The dark zone within the eye along the circumference of the ora serrata.

orbit (or´bit) One of two cavities in the skull containing the eyeball and its associated structures; formed by portions of seven bones: frontal, maxillary, zygomatic, lacrimal, sphenoid, palatine, and ethmoid. Commonly called eye socket.

orbital (or´bĭ-tal) Relating to the orbit.

orbitography (or-bĭ-tog´ră-fe) The making of x-ray films of the orbit after infusion of a radiopaque substance over the orbit floor; a diagnostic technique used when a blow-out fracture is suspected.

orbitonometer (or-bĭ-to-nom´ĕ-ter) Instrument for measuring the degree of resistance offered by the eyeball when pressed into the socket.

orbitotomy (or-bĭ-tot´ŏ-me) Surgical incision into the orbit.

orcein (or-se´in) A purple dye used in the study of cells (cytology).

orchialgia (or-ke-al´jă) Pain in a testis. Also called orchiodynia; testalgia.

orchichorea (or-ke-ko-re´ă) Involuntary twitching of the testis.

orchidorrhaphy (or-kĭ-dor´ă-fe) See orchiopexy.

orchiectomy, orchidectomy (or-ke-ek´tŏ-me, or-kĭ-dek´tŏ-me) Removal of one or both testes. Popularly called castration.

orchiepididymitis (or-ke-ep-ĭ-did-ĭ-mi´tis) Inflammation of a testis and epididymis.

orchiocele (or´ke-o-sēl) A tumor of the testis.

orchiodynia (or-ke-o-din´e-ă) See orchialgia.

orchioncus (or-ke-ong´kus) A neoplasm or tumor of the testis.

orchiopathy (or-ke-op´ă-the) Any disease of the testes.

orchiopexy (or-ke-o-pek´se) Suturing of a testis to the scrotum as in the correction of an undescended testis. Also called orchidorrhaphy; orchiorrhaphy.

orchioplasty (or´ke-o-plas-te) Reparative surgery of the testes.

orchiorrhaphy (or-ke-or´ă-fe) See orchiopexy.

orchioscirrhus (or-ke-o-skir´us) Abnormal hardening of the testis.

orchiotomy (or-ke-ot´ŏ-me) Surgical incision into a testis.

orchis (or´kis) Greek for testis.

orchitis (or-ki´tis) Inflammation of the testis. Also called testitis.

order (or´der) A biologic taxonomic category ranking just below class and above family.

orderly (or´der-le) An attendant in a hospital ward whose responsibilities do not require professional training.

ordinate (or´dĭ-năt) The vertical coordinate that, together with a horizontal one (abscissa), forms a frame of reference for the plotting of data.

orexigenic (o-rek-sĭ-jen´ik) Stimulating the appetite.

orf (orf) A viral disease of sheep occasionally transmitted to the skin of man, especially to butchers and veterinarians; the chancre-type lesions appear most frequently on the hands and face. Also called contagious ecthyma.

organ (or´gan) A differentiated structure of the body that performs some specific function.

acoustic o. See spiral organ of Corti.

o. of Corti See spiral organ of Corti.

end o. (a) The expanded termination of a nerve fibril as found in muscle tissue, skin, mucous membrane, or glands. (b) The site of ultimate damage by a disease process (e.g., kidney damage secondary to hypertension).

Golgi tendon o. (GTO) Special bare nerve ending ramifying about bundles of collagen fibers of tendons, usually at the ends of muscles; the afferent fibers are among the largest fibers in peripheral nerve tissue. Also called Golgi corpuscle; neurotendinous organ; tendon spindle.

gustatory o. The organ concerned with the perception of taste, composed of taste buds (gustatory caliculi); most are located in the epithelial covering of the tongue; also of the soft palate, posterior surface of the epiglottis, and the back wall of the oropharynx (oral part of the pharynx).

neurotendinous o. See Golgi tendon organ.

o. of Rosenmüller See epoophoron.

sense o. Any organ of special sense, such as the eye, and the accessory structures associated with it.

spiral o. of Corti The sensory receptors for hearing, contained in the cochlear duct of the inner ear. Also called organ of Corti.

target o. The organ that is stimulated by a hormone.

o.'s of Zuckerkandl Small masses of chromaffin tissue located along the abdominal aorta; they are most prominent in the fetus.

organelle (or-gă-nel´) A specialized cytoplasmic structure of a cell performing a specific function (e.g., a mitochondrion).

organic (or-gan´ik) **1.** Relating to the organs of the body. **2.** Relating to living organisms. **3.** Organized; structural.

organic brain syndrome (or-gan´ik brān sin´drōm) (OBS), **organic mental syndrome** (OMS) A syndrome resulting from diffuse or local impairment of brain tissue function, manifested by alteration of orientation, memory, comprehension, and judgment.

acute o.b.s. Acute confusional state characterized by a sudden onset and a high degree of reversibility.

chronic o.b.s. Disorder marked by an insidious onset, a progressive course, and a high degree of irreversibility; always due to focal or diffuse brain lesions.

psychotic o.b.s. Acute or chronic organic brain syndrome associated with psychiatric symptoms.

organism (or´gă-niz-m) Any living entity, plant or animal.

organization (or-gă-ni-za´shun) **1.** An arrangement of distinct but dependent parts with varied functions that contribute to the whole; the organic structure of an organism. **2.** The process of forming into organs.

organizer (or´gă-nīz-er) **1.** A group of cells on the dorsal lip of the blastopore that stimulates differentiation of cells in the embryo. **2.** Any group of cells having such an ability.

organogenesis (or-gă-no-jen´ĕ-sis) The formation of organs.

organoid (or´gă-noid) **1.** Resembling an organ. **2.** Composed of the cellular elements of an organ.

organoleptic (or-gă-no-lep´tik) **1.** Stimulating a sense organ. **2.** Capable of receiving sensory stimuli.

organophosphates (or-gă-no-fos´fāts) A group of phosphorus-containing compounds used in pesticides; a common cause of acute pesticide poisoning. Have been used in war gases.

organotropism (or-gă-not´rŏ-piz-m) The predilection of microorganisms and chemicals for certain organs or tissues (e.g., viruses infecting primarily the central nervous tissue).

orgasm (or´gaz-m) The intense sensation experienced at the culmination of sexual intercourse or stimulation of the sex organs; it is accompanied in the male by ejaculation of semen and in the female

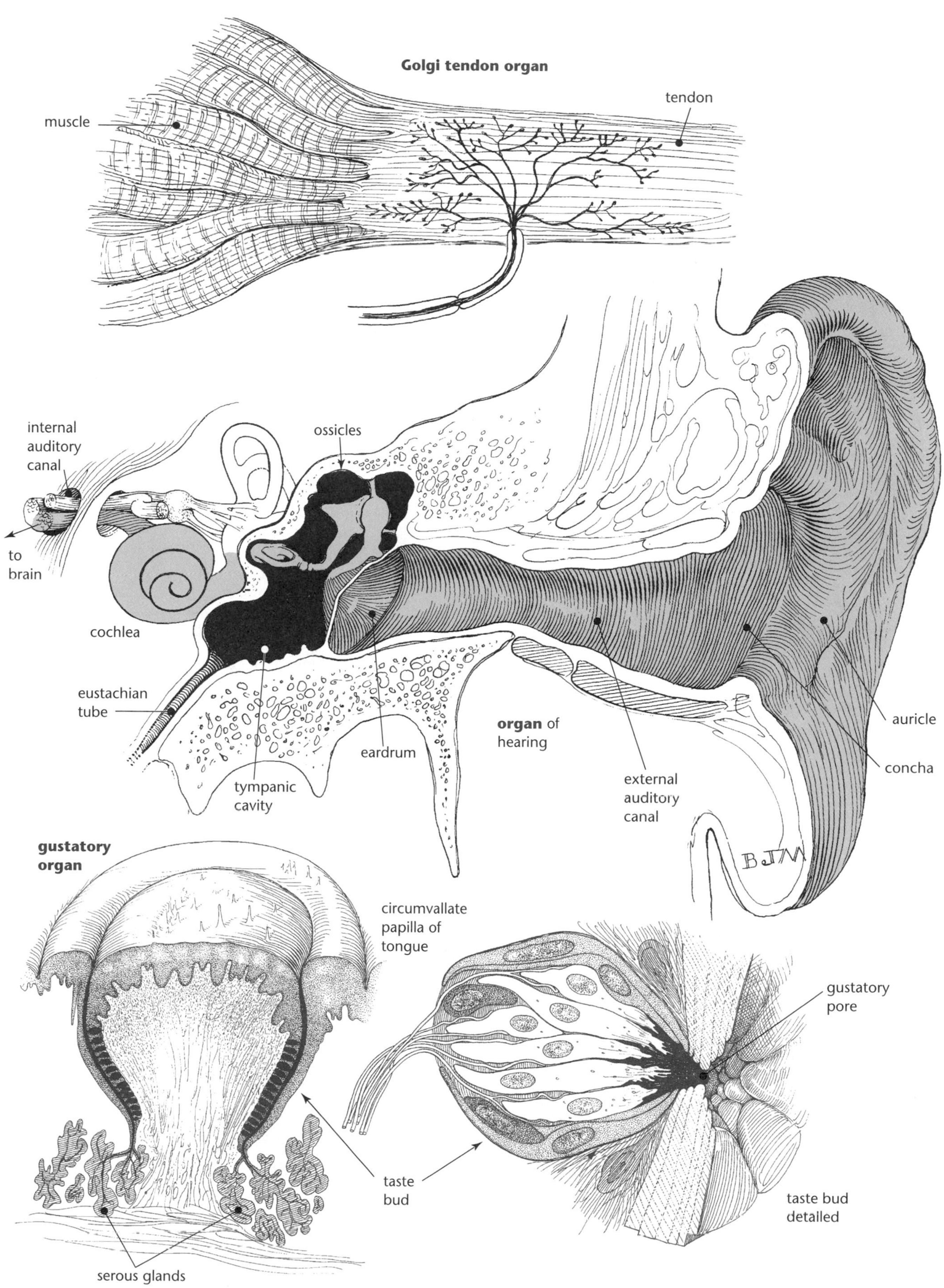

Golgi tendon organ
muscle
tendon
internal
auditory
canal
to
brain
ossicles
cochlea
eustachian
tube
tympanic
cavity
eardrum
organ of
hearing
external
auditory
canal
auricle
concha
BJM
gustatory
organ
circumvallate
papilla of
tongue
gustatory
pore
taste
bud
taste bud
detailed
serous glands

O

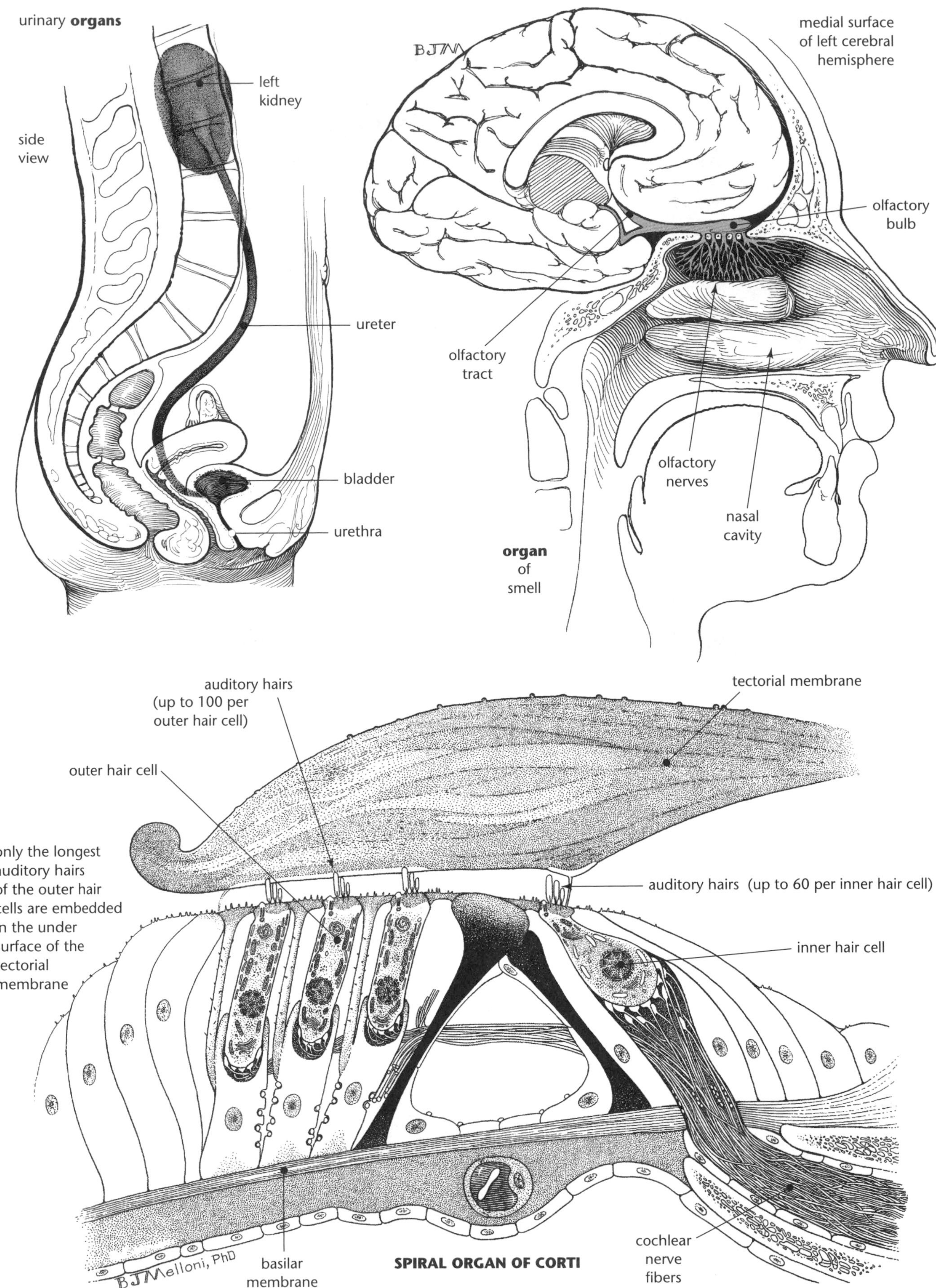
urinary **organs**
left
kidney
side
view
ureter
bladder
urethra
medial surface
of left cerebral
hemisphere
BJM
olfactory
bulb
olfactory
tract
olfactory
nerves
nasal
cavity
organ
of
smell
auditory hairs
(up to 100 per
outer hair cell)
tectorial membrane
outer hair cell
only the longest
auditory hairs
of the outer hair
cells are embedded
in the under
surface of the
tectorial
membrane
auditory hairs (up to 60 per inner hair cell)
inner hair cell
cochlear
nerve
fibers
basilar
membrane
BJMelloni, PhD

SPIRAL ORGAN OF CORTI

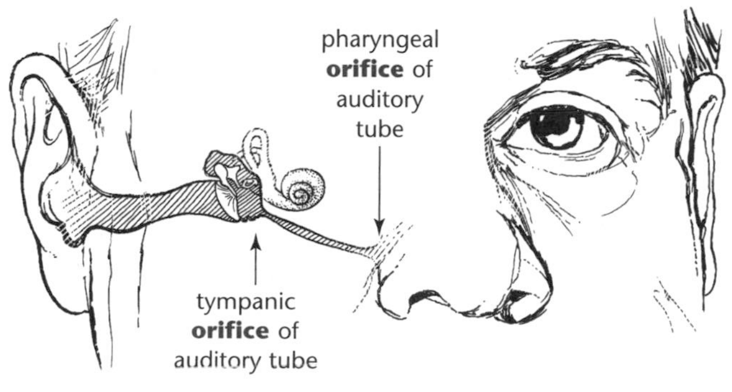

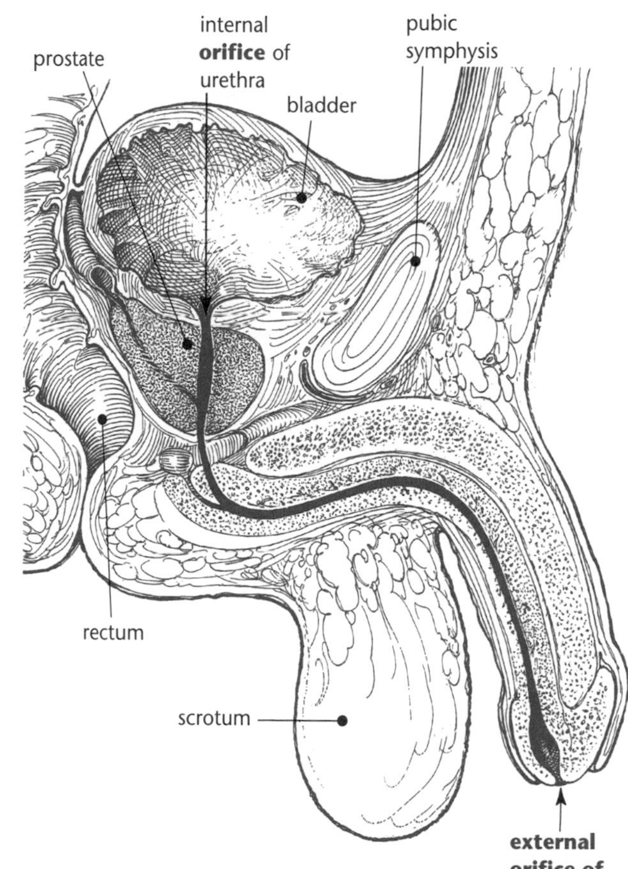

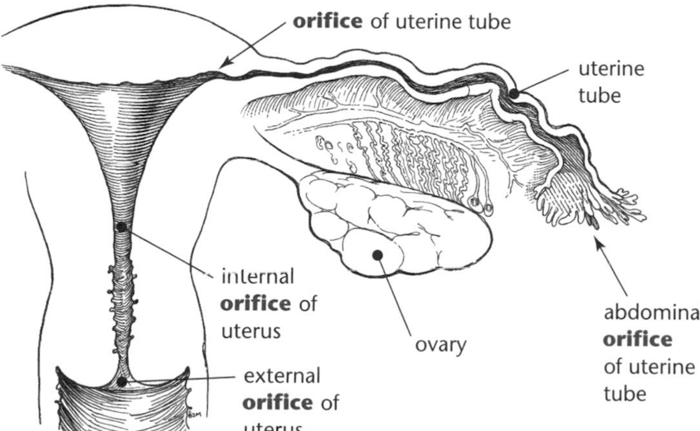

by involuntary contractions of the vagina.

orientation (or-e-en-ta´shun) **1.** Awareness of oneself in reference to time, place, and other individuals; the act of finding one's bearings. **2.** The relative position of atoms in a compound.

orifice (or´ĭ-fis) An opening.

cardiac o. The opening between the esophagus and adjacent portion of the stomach (cardia). Also called esophagogastric orifice.

esophagogastric o. See cardiac orifice.

external o. of urethra The external opening of the urethra, situated between the clitoris and vaginal opening in the female and at the end of the penis in the male.

origin (or´ĭ-jin) **1.** The site of attachment of a muscle to a bone that is less movable than the one to which it is inserted. **2.** The starting point or beginning of a nerve.

ornithine (or´nĭ-thēn) $NH_2(CH_2)_3CHCH_2COOH$; an amino acid formed when urea is removed from arginine; an important intermediate in urea biosynthesis, possessing one less carbon than its homolog lysine.

Ornithodoros (or-nĭ-thod´ŏ-ros) Genus of ticks (family Argasidae) some of which transmit the agents of relapsing fevers.

Ornithonyssus sylviarum (or-nĭ-tho-nis´sus sil-vea´rum) A species of mites parasitic on many domestic and wild fowl; they also infest man, producing a pruritic dermatitis. Also called northern fowl mite.

ornithosis (or-nĭ-tho´sis) Infectious disease of birds caused by *Chlamydia psittaci*; it is occasionally transmitted to humans, causing an influenza-like condition or pneumonia; when transmitted by parrots or other psittacine birds, the disease is known as psittacosis.

orolingual (or-o ling´gwal) Relating to the mouth and tongue.

oronasal (or-o-na´sal) Relating to the mouth and the nose.

oropharynx (or-o-far´ingks) The central portion of the pharynx directly behind the oral cavity, extending from the inferior border of the soft palate to the lingual surface of the epiglottis; it contains the palatine tonsils and the posterior faucial pillars.

orotic acid (ŏ-rot´ik) An intermediate in the formation of pyrimidine nucleotides.

orphan (or´fan) See under product.

orphan disease (or´fan dĭ-zēz´) A disease for which no treatment has been formulated because not many people have been afflicted with it.

orthetics (or-thet´iks) See orthotics.

orthobiosis (or-tho-bi-o´sis) Living in a manner that promotes physical and mental health.

orthochromatic (or-tho-kro-mat´ik) Staining the color of the dye used; said of certain cells.

orthocrasia (or-tho-kra´zĭ-ă, or-tho-kra´zhă) Condition in which the body reacts normally to drugs.

orthodigita (or-tho-dij´ĭ-tă) Correction of malformed fingers or toes.

orthodontics (or-tho-don´tiks) A specialty of dentistry dealing with correction and prevention of irregularities of the teeth.

orthodontist (or-tho-don´tist) A dentist who specializes in orthodontics.

orthodromic (or-tho-drom´ik) Conducting impulses along a normal path.

orthogenics (or-tho-jen´iks) The study and treatment of defects (physical and mental).

orthognathic (or-thog-na´thik) Having straight jaws and a straight profile; having a face with no projection of the lower jaw, one with a gnathic index below 98.

orthograde (or´tho-grād) The erect posture of man; opposed to pronograde.

orthokinetics (or-tho-kĭ-net´iks) A method of treatment for hypertrophic osteoarthritis in which a muscular action is transferred from one set of muscles to another in order to protect the affected joint.

orthometer (or-thom´ĕ-ter) Instrument used to measure the degree of protrusion of the eyeballs.

Orthomyxoviridae (or-tho-mik-so-vir´ĭ-de) A family of viruses, filamentous or spherical (80 to 120 nm in diameter), that contains single-stranded RNA and multiply in cytoplasm; includes all viruses that cause influenza.

orthopaedics (or-tho-pe´diks) See orthopedics.

orthopedic (or-tho-pe´dik) Relating to orthopedics.

orthopedics (or-tho-pe´diks) The surgically oriented branch of medicine concerned with the preservation and restoration of functions of the skeletal system and associated structures. Also written orthopaedics.

orthopedist (or-tho-pe´dist) One who practices orthopedics.

orthopercussion (or-tho-pĕr-kush´un) Percussion in which the left middle finger is flexed at a right angle and the tip of the finger is placed on the chest wall; the flexed finger is then struck upon the knuckle.

orthophoria (or-tho-fo´re-ă) Condition in which the visual axes of the two eyes are free from a tendency to deviate.

orthophosphate (or-tho-fos´fāt) A salt of phosphoric acid (H_3PO_4).

orthopnea (or-thop-ne´ă) Difficulty in breathing except in an upright position.

orthopneic (or-thop-ne´ik) Relating to or afflicted with orthopnea.

orthopod (or´tho-pod) Slang for orthopedist.

Orthopoxvirus (or´tho-poks-vi-rŭs) Genus of the subfamily Chordopoxvirinae (family Poxviridae); includes the viruses causing smallpox, ectromelia, and vaccinia.

orthopsychiatry (or-tho-si-ki´ă-tre) The study and treatment of human behavior for the purpose of promoting healthy emotional development.

Orthoptera (or-thop´ter-ă) An order of insects that includes grasshoppers, cockroaches, locusts, etc.

orthoptics (or-thop´tiks) A method of therapy aimed at achieving coordinate function of the two eyes through a set of exercises; used particularly in treating the muscular imbalance of strabismus.

orthoptist (or-thop´tist) One who is trained to treat ocular muscle imbalance and faulty visual habits by means of specially designid eye exercises.

orthoscope (or´tho-skop) An instrument that eliminates the refracting power of the cornea by means of a layer of water in a glass container held in contact with the eye.

orthoscopic (or-tho-skop´ik) **1.** Relating to the orthoscope. **2.** Having normal vision. **3.** Giving a correct and proportioned image.

orthoscopy (or-thos´kŏ-pe) **1.** Examination of the eye with an orthoscope. **2.** The state of an optical

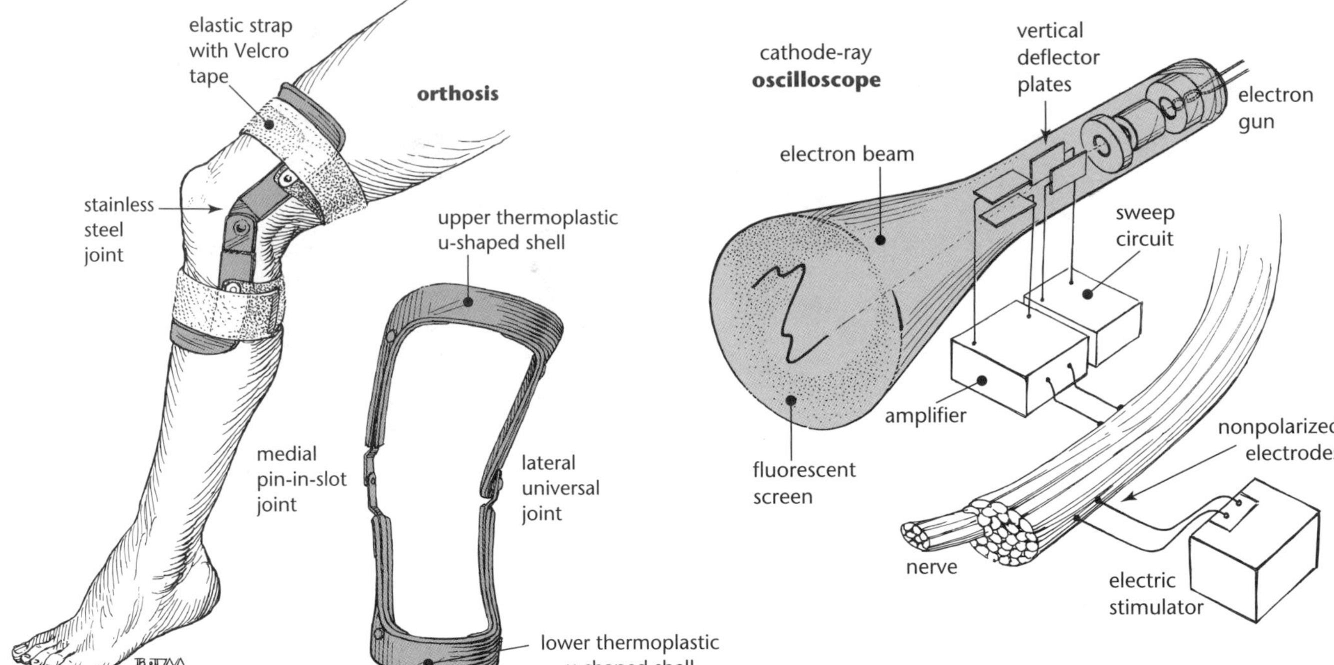

system that produces images free of distortion.

orthosis (or-tho′sis), *pl.* **ortho′ses** Any orthopedic mechanical device worn on the body to apply force to a part; used in the treatment of physical impairment (congenital or caused by disease or injury).

orthostatic (or-tho-stat′ik) Relating to or caused by the upright position.

orthothanasia (orth-o-thă-na′zhă) Natural death.

orthotics (or-thot′iks) The making and fitting of orthopedic appliances. Also called orthetics.

orthotist (or-thot′ist) One who makes and fits orthopedic appliances.

orthotonos, orthotonus (or-thot′ŏ-nos, or-thot′ŏ-nŭs) Tetanic spasm in which the head, body, and limbs are fixed rigidly in a straight line.

orthotopic (or-tho-top′ik) Occuring in the normal position.

O

orthotropic (or-tho-trop′ik) Growing or extending along a vertical axis.

orthovoltage (or-tho-vol′taj) Medium electromotive force, from 200 to 300 kilovolts; used in radiotherapy.

os (os), *pl.* **ora** Latin for mouth or orifice, as the os of the cervix.

os (os), *pl.* **ossa** Latin for bone.

oscheocele (os-ke-o-sēl) See inguinal hernia, under hernia.

oscheoplasty (os′ke-o-plas-te) See scrotoplasty.

oscillation (os-ĭ-la′shŭn) **1.** A backward and forward movement. **2.** A stage of inflammation in which leukocytes accumulate in small vessels, blocking the flow of blood and causing a to-and-fro movement with each cardiac contraction.

oscillogram (ŏ-sil′o-gram) A graphic record traced by an oscillograph.

oscillograph (ŏ-sil′o-graf) An apparatus for graphically recording the oscillations of an electric current.

oscillometer (os-ĭ-lom′ĕ-tĕr) An instrument used to measure variations in blood pressure.

oscillopsia (os-ĭ-lop′se-ă) A state in which observed objects seem to oscillate.

oscilloscope (ŏ-sil′o-skōp) An electronic instrument that temporarily displays the variations of a fluctuating electrical quantity on the fluorescent screen of a cathode-ray tube.

oscitate (os′ĭ-tāt) To gape; to yawn.

osculum (os′koo-lum), *pl.* **oscula** A tiny opening.

Osgood-Schlatter disease (oz′good-shlăt-er dĭ-zēz′) See traumatic tibial epiphysitis, under epiphysitis.

Osiander's sign (ōze-an′derz sīn) Pulsation of the vagina in early pregnancy.

Osler's disease (ōs-lerz dĭ-zēz′) See hereditary hemorrhagic telangiectasia, under telangiectasia.

Osler's sign (ōs-lerz sīn) Small painful swellings in the skin and subcutaneous tissues of the hands and feet occuring in endocarditis.

Osler-Weber-Rendu syndrome (ōs-ler-web′er-ron-doo′sin′drōm) See hereditary hemorrhagic telangiectasia, under telangiectasia.

osmatic (oz-mat′ik) See olfactory.

osmidrosis (oz-mĭ-dro′sis) Condition marked by a fetid odor of sweat. Also called bromidrosis.

osmiophilic (os-me-o-fil′ik) Easily fixed with osmium tetroxide.

osmium (oz′me-um) Metallic element; symbol Os, atomic number 76, atomic weight 190.2.

o. tetroxide OsO_4; a crystalline compound commonly used as a tissue fixative for electron microscopy; has an irritating odor.

osmoceptor (oz′mo-sep-tor) See osmoreceptor.

osmolality (oz-mo-lal′ĭ-te) The osmotic concentration of a solution, expressed as osmoles of dissolved substance per kilogram of water (solvent); normal serum osmolality is 280 to 300 mOsm/kg.

osmolar (oz-mo′lar) See osmotic.

osmolarity (oz-mo-lar′ĭ-te) The osmotic concentration of a solution expressed as osmoles of the dissolved substance per liter of solution.

osmole (oz′mōl) (Osm) Molecular weight (MW) of a substance in solution, in grams, divided by the number of particles that one molecule provides when it enters solution, e.g., glucose (MW 180), 1 Osm = (180 g / 1) = 180 g; sodium chloride (MW 58.5), 1 Osm = (58.5 g / 2) = 29.75 g; one osmol provides Avogadro's number (6.023×10^{23}).

osmometer (os-mom′ĕ-ter) Instrument for determining osmolality of a liquid (e.g., urine) by measuring the freezing point depression.

osmometry (oz-mom′ĕ-tre) The measure of concentration of solute per kilogram of water (solvent); serum osmolality is normally from 280 to 300 mOsm/kg.

osmophil, osmophilic (oz′mo-fil, oz-mo-fil′ik) Thriving in a solution of high osmotic pressure.

osmophore (oz′mo-for) An atomic group whose presence causes the particular odor in a compound.

osmoreceptor (oz-mo-re-sep′tor) **1.** A specialized sensory nerve ending in the hypothalamus that responds to increases in the osmotic pressure of the blood by stimulating the secretion of the neurohypophyseal antidiuretic hormone (ADH). **2.** A receptor that responds to the sensation of odors (olfactory stimuli). Also called osmoceptor.

osmoregulatory (oz-mo-reg′u-lă-tor-e) Influencing osmosis.

osmosis (oz-mo′sis, os-mo′sis) The passage of liquid from a concentrated solution to a diluted one through a semipermeable membrane that separates them.

osmotic (oz-mot′ik) Relating to osmosis. Also called osmolar. See also osmotic pressure, under pressure.

osseointegration (os-e-o-in-tĕ-gra′shun) The growing of bone onto an implanted metal device, such as one that serves as a base for a tooth implant.

osseous (os′e-us) Bony.

ossicle (os′ĭ-kl) A small bone.

auditory o.'s The three tiny bones (malleus, incus, and stapes) in the middle ear chamber secured to the chamber walls by ligaments; together they form a bony chain across the chamber for the conduction of sound waves from the tympanic membrane (eardrum) to the oval window (adjoining the inner ear).

ossicular (ŏ-sik′u-lar) Relating to an ossicle.

ossiculectomy (ŏ-sik-u-lek′tŏ-me) Surgical removal of one or more ossicles of the middle ear.

ossiculotomy (ŏ-sik-u-lot′ŏ-me) Surgical incision of one of the ossicles of the middle ear or of adhesions that prevent their movements.

ossification (os-ĭ-fĭ-kā′shun) The replacement of cartilage by bone.

ossify (os′ĭ-fi) To change into bone.

ostealgia, ostalgia (os-te-al′jă, os-tal′jă) Pain in a bone.

osteitis (os-te-i′tis) Inflammation of bone.

o. deformans See Paget's disease.

o. fibrosa cystica Disease characterized chiefly by softening and resorption of bone and replacement with fibrous tissue; caused by excessive secretion of hormone from the parathyroid glands. Also called Recklinghausen's disease of bone.

osteoarthritis (os-te-o-ar-thri′tis) (OA) Common form of chronic joint disease affecting middle-aged and elderly people; marked by degeneration of articular cartilage, thickening of underlying bone with formation of spurs near the joint margins, and stiffness of affected joints; may occur at an early age secondary to traumatic, congenital, or systemic disorders. Also called degenerative arthritis; hypertrophic arthritis; degenerative joint disease (DJD).

osteoarthropathy (os-te-o-ar-throp′ă-the) Disorder affecting the bones and joints almost always associated with disease elsewhere in the body.

hypertrophic o. Painful swelling and periosteal deposition of new bone in the long bones of the extremities, clubbing of the fingers, and swelling and tenderness of joints; occurs most commonly in association with pulmonary disease, especially pulmonary neoplasm; also seen with cyanotic heart disease, ulcerative colitis, regional enteritis, and liver disorders.

idiopathic hypertrophic o. Osteoarthropathy that does not occur secondary to any disease.

osteoblast (os′te-o-blast) A bone-forming cell; it

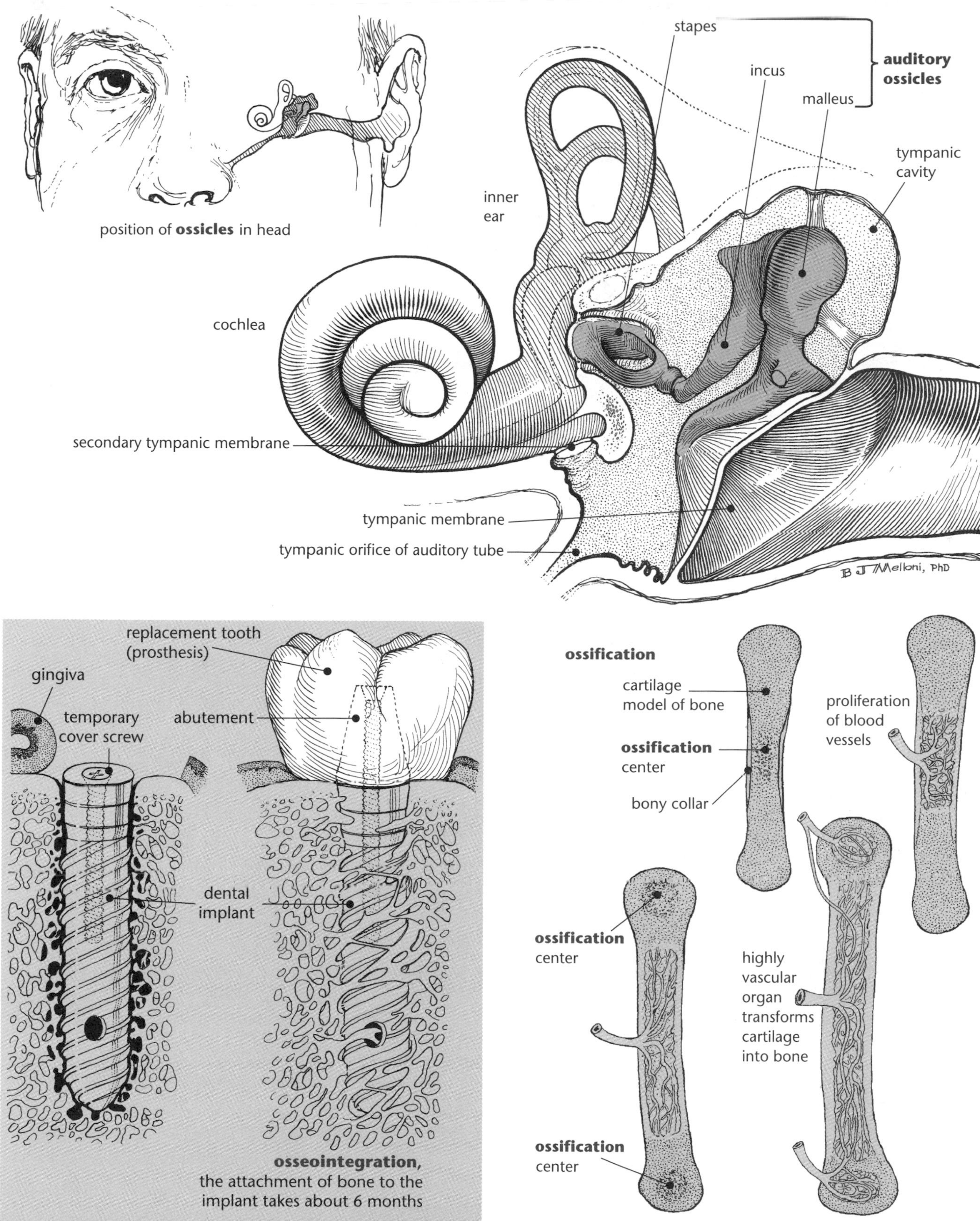

arises from a fibroblast and is responsible for the formation of bone matrix; found on the advancing surface of developing bone.

osteoblastoma (os-te-o-blas-to´mă) A benign tumor derived from primitive bone tissue; occurs most frequently on the spine of young individuals. Also called giant osteoid osteoma.

osteochondritis (os-te-o-kon-dri´tis) Inflammation of both bone and its cartilage.

osteochondrodysplasia (os-te-o-kon-dro-dis-pla´zhă) See camptomelic syndrome.

osteochondrodystrophy (os-te-o-kon-dro-dis-trŏ-fe) See chondro-osteodystrophy.

osteochondroma (os-te-o-kon-dro´mă) A single benign bony outgrowth capped by growing cartilage; most frequently occurring near the end of long bones of individuals between 10 and 25 years of age. Also called solitary osteocartilagenous exostosis.

osteochondromatosis (os-te-o-kon-dro-mă-to´sis) See multiple hereditary exostosis, under exostosis.

osteochondrosarcoma (os-te-o-kon-dro-sar-ko´mă) A malignant tumor of cartilaginous tissue usually arising from a benign bone tumor.

osteochondrosis (os-te-o-kon-dro´sis) Any disorder of the ossification centers in the bones of children; characterized by death of tissues in the absence of infection.

osteoclasis, osteoclasia (os-te-ok´lă-sis, os-te-o-kla´zhă) Surgical or manual fracture or refracture of a deformed bone for the purpose of resetting it in a more normal position.

osteoclast (os´te-o-klast) A large multinucleated

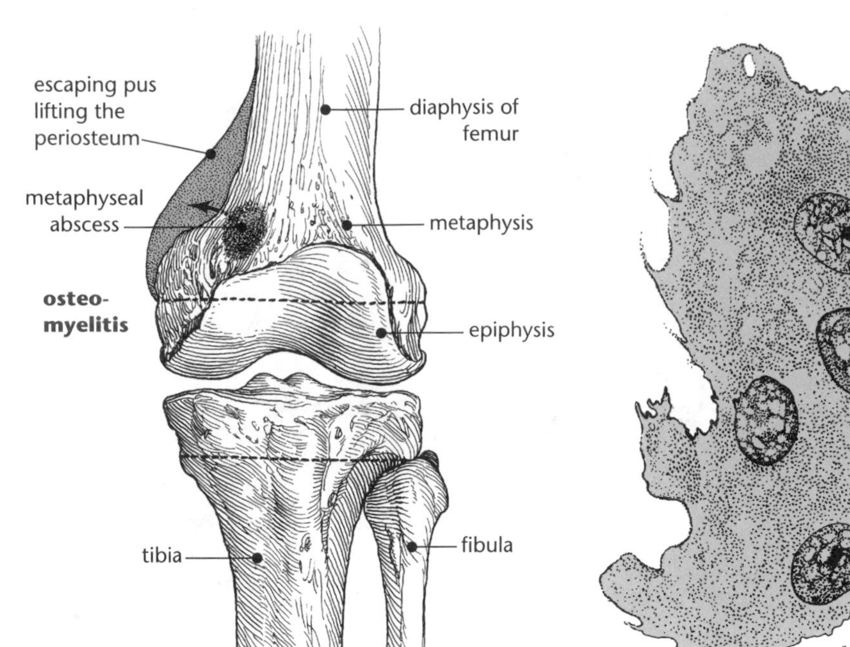

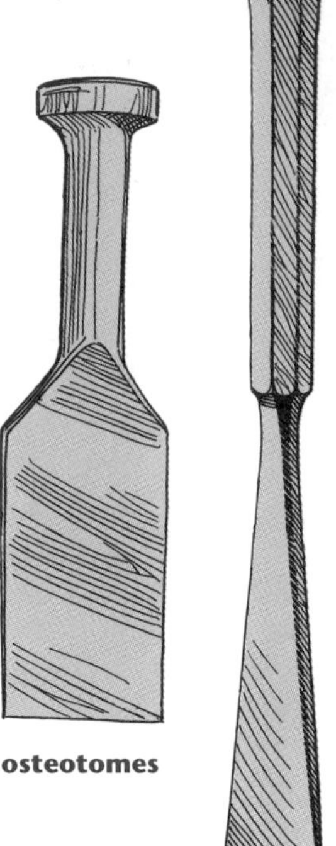

cell that is formed in bone marrow and absorbs bone tissue.

osteoclastoma (os-te-o-klas-to´mă) See giant cell tumor of bone, under tumor.

osteocranium (os-te-o-kra´ne-um) The fetal cranium after ossification has begun.

osteocystoma (os-te-o-sis-to´mă) See solitary bone cyst, under cyst.

osteocyte (os´te-o-sīt) One of numerous flattened, nucleated bone cells arising from osteoblasts by modulation; it plays a role in maintaining the constituents of intercellular bone matrix at normal levels; each is contained in a space (lacuna) and its processes extend through openings of the lacuna into minute canals within the bone tissue.

osteodentin (os-te-o-den´tin) A hard substance, structurally intermediate between dentin and bone, that partially fills the pulp cavity of teeth of elderly people.

osteodermia (os-te-o-der´me-ă) The presence of bony deposits on the skin.

osteodesmosis (os-te-o-des-mo´sis) The conversion of tendons into bone.

osteodynia (os-te-o-din´e-ă) See ostealgia.

osteodystrophy (os-te-o-dis´trŏ-fe) Defective bone formation.

renal o. Generalized bone changes consisting of a mixture of osteosclerosis, osteomalacia, and osteitis fibrosa cystica occuring in patients with chronic kidney failure.

osteofibroma (os-te-o-fi-bro´mă) A benign tumor-like lesion composed chiefly of bone and fibrous connective tissue.

osteogen (os´te-o-jen) The inner layer of periosteum from which new bone is formed.

osteogenesis (os-te-o-jen´ĕ-sis) The formation of bone.

o. imperfecta (OI) A group of genetic disorders characterized by bone fragility and susceptibility to fractures; may also include (depending on degree of genetic defect) deformity of long bones, laxness of ligaments, blueness of scleras, and deafness due to otosclerosis. A rare autosomal recessive variant causes multiple fractures starting at birth; death occurs in the first year of life. Also called brittle bones disease; brittle bones.

osteogenic, osteogenetic (os-te-o-jen´ik, os-te-o-je-net´ik) **1.** Relating to bone formation. **2.** Derived from bone.

osteoid (os´te-oid) Resembling bone; usually refers to the soft part of intercellular bone matrix preceding mineralization.

osteology (os-te-ol´ŏ-je) The study of the structure of bones.

osteolysis (os-te-ol´ĭ-sis) Destruction of bone.

osteoma (os-te-o´mă) A benign tumor composed of bone tissue; it may develop on a bone (homoplastic osteoma) or on other structures (heteroplastic osteoma).

dental o. Osteoma projecting from the root of a tooth.

giant osteoid o. See osteoblastoma.

osteomalacia (os-te-o-mă-la´shă) A disease marked by softening of the bones due to faulty calcification; characterized by increased amounts of osteoid or bone matrix which either fails to calcify or does so slowly; similar to rickets in children.

osteomere (os´te-o-mēr) One of a series of bony structures, such as the vertebrae.

osteometry (os-te-om´ĕ-tre) The branch of anthropology concerned with the relative size of human bones.

osteomyelitis (os-te-o-mi-ĕ-li´tis) Infection of bone, affecting the metaphyseal regions of the long bones; caused by bacteria, especially *Staphyloccus aureus*; salmonella infections are found in individuals with sickle cell disease; spinal lesions are commonly caused by tuberculosis or gram-negative organisms.

osteomyelodysplasia (os-te-o-mi-ĕ-lo-dis-pla´zhă) Disease characterized by enlargement of the bone marrow cavities, thinning of the osseous tissue, and associated leukopenia and fever.

osteomyelofibrotic syndrome (os-te-o-mi-ĕ-lo-fi-brot´ik sin´drōm) See myelofibrosis.

osteomyelography (os-te-o-mi-ĕ-log´ră-fe) X-ray examination of bone marrow.

osteon (os´te-on) The basic unit of compact bone; consists of a central canal (conveying blood vessels and nerve endings) and several layers of bony tissue around the canal. Also called haversian system.

osteonecrosis (os-te-o-nĕ-kro´sis) Death of bone tissue, occuring most commonly in the head of the femur, less frequently in the medial femoral condyle, and occasionally in the head of the humerus.

osteopath (os´te-o-path) A practitioner of osteopathy.

osteopathology (os-te-o-pă-thol´ŏ-je) The study of bone diseases.

osteopathy (os-te-op´ă-the) **1.** Disease of bones. **2.** Medical practice based on the concept that all body systems operate in unison and are capable of acting against disease; therapeutic measures consist mainly of manipulative procedures, although surgical, medicinal, and hygienic methods are used when indicated.

osteopenia (os-te-o-pe´ne-ă) Reduced bone mass or density; may or may not be due to deficient bone formation.

osteoperiostitis (os-te-o-per-e-os-ti´tis) Inflammation of a bone and its periosteum.

osteopetrosis (os-te-o-pe-tro´sis) An uncommon hereditary disorder transmitted as an autosomal recessive trait and characterized principally by overgrowth and denseness of bones and narrowing of the marrow, with resulting anemia, visual disturbances, deafness, and delayed tooth eruption; seen most frequently in children. Also called Albers-Schönberg disease; marble bone disease.

osteophlebitis (os-te-o-flĕ-bi´tis) Inflammation of the veins of a bone.

osteophony (os-tĕ-of´ŏ-ne) Conduction of sound by bone.

osteophyte (os´te-o-fīt) A bony outgrowth.

osteoplasty (os´te-o-plas-te) Plastic surgery of bones, such as bone grafting.

osteopontin (os-te-o-pon´tin) A hormone-like protein produced by a variety of cell types; involved in bone formation; frequently associated with mineralization processes; found in urine, plasma, milk, and bile and in lung specimens from tuberculosis and silicosis patients.

urinary o. See uropontin.

osteoporosis (os-te-o-pŏ-ro´sis) Disease that appears to be the result of increased resorption of bone and slowing of bone formation, seen most frequently in the elderly of both sexes, especially postmenopausal women; symptoms include bone pain, reduced height, deformity, and susceptibility to fractures; may be associated with other disorders or may be caused by certain drug therapies.

posttraumatic o. See Sudeck's atrophy, under atrophy.

osteoradionecrosis (os-te-o-ra-de-o-nĕ-kro´sis) Death and degeneration of bone tissue caused by radiation.

osteorrhagia (os-te-o-ra´jă) Bleeding from bone.

osteorrhaphy (os-te-or´ă-fe) Wiring of a broken bone. Also called osteosuture.

osteosarcoma (os-te-o-săr-ko´mă) Bone cancer, usually occuring in the shaft at either end of a long bone.

osteosarcomatous (os-te-o-săr-ko´mă-tus) Relating to or causing bone cancer.

osteosclerosis (os-te-o-sklĕ-ro´sis) Abnormally increased density or hardness of bone.

osteosuture (os´te-o-soo-chur) See osteorrhaphy.

osteosynthesis (os-te-o-sin´thĕ-sis) Fastening the ends of a fractured bone.

osteotabes (os-te-o-ta´bēz) Degeneration of bone marrow.

osteotome (os´te-o-tōm) Chisel used for cutting bone.

osteotomy (os-te-ot´ŏ-me) Cutting a bone, usually with a saw or chisel.

ostial (os´te-al) Relating to an orifice (ostium).

ostium (os´te-um), *pl.* **os´tia** A small opening into a hollow structure.

o. primum See interatrial foramen primum, under

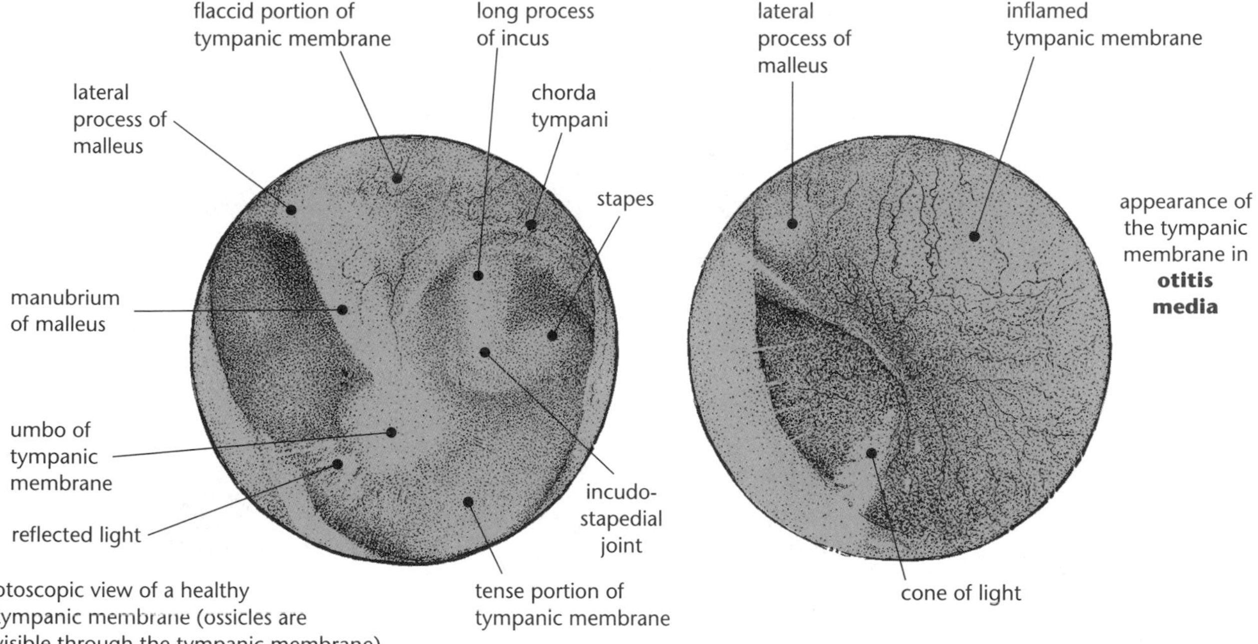

otoscopic view of a healthy tympanic membrane (ossicles are visible through the tympanic membrane)

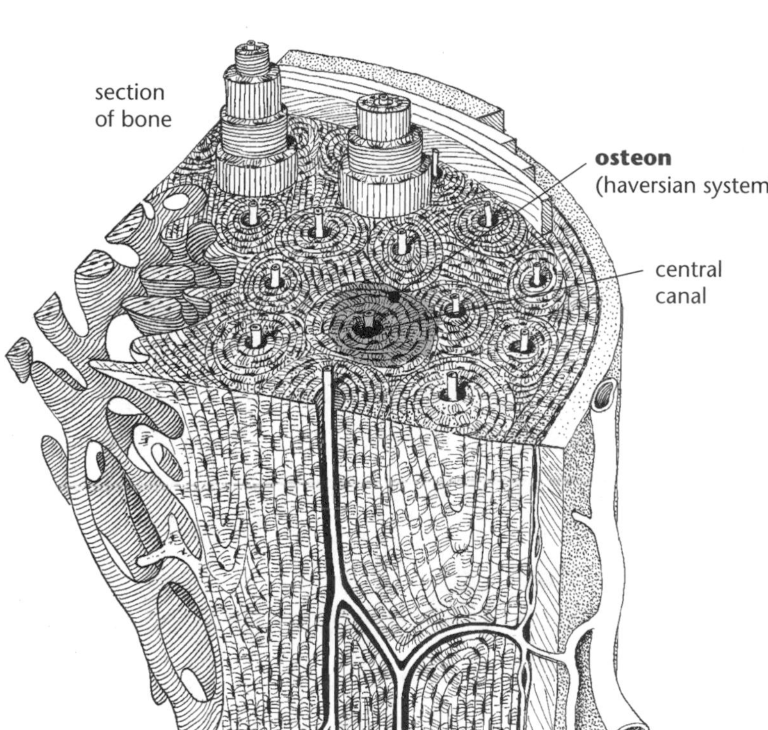

osteoporosis

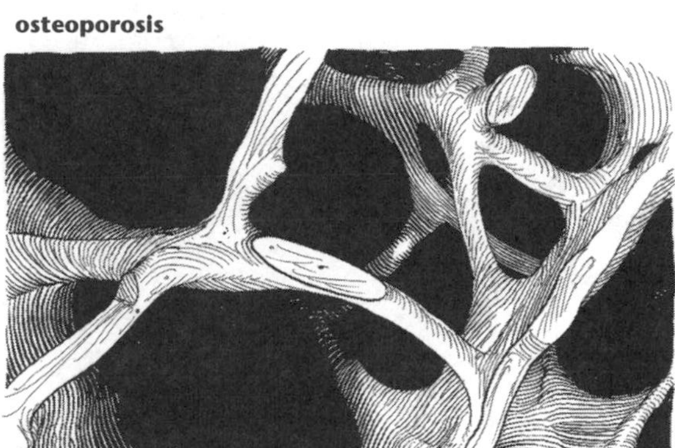

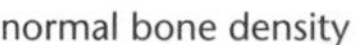
normal bone density

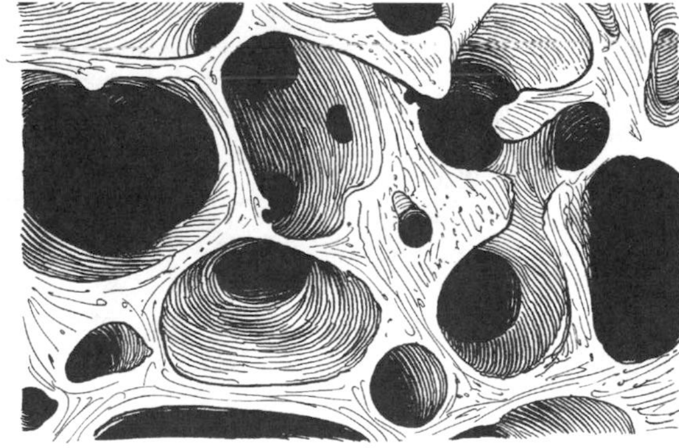

O

foramen.
o. secundum See interatrial foramen secundum, under foramen.
ostomy (os-´tŏ-me) General term for an artificial opening created surgically.
otalgia (o-tal´jă) See earache.
otalgic (o-tal´jik) **1.** Relating to earache. **2.** Any remedy for an earache.
otic (o´tik) Of or relating to the ear.
otitic (o-tit´ik) Relating to inflammation of the ear.
otitis (o-ti´tis) Inflammation of the ear.
chronic suppurative o. media Inflammation of the middle ear attended by a thick mucopurulent discharge from the mucous membrane; the infection may progress to involve the bone.
o. externa Inflammation of the external auditory canal due to the presence of any of a variety of infections.
o. interna See labyrinthitis.
o. media Infection of the middle ear, usually secondary to upper respiratory infections, generally transmitted to the middle ear through the auditory (eustachian) tube.
otoantritis (o-to-an-tri´tis) Inflammation of the mastoid antrum.
otocephaly (o-to-sef´ă-le) Defect characterized by extreme smallness of the chin and approximation of the ears toward the front of the neck.
otocerebritis (o-to-ser ĕ-bri´tis) See otoencephalitis.
otocleisis (o-to-klī´sis) **1.** Abnormal closure of the auditory (eustachian) tube. **2.** Obstruction of the external auditory canal.
otoconia (o-to-ko´ne-ă), *sing.* **otoco´nium** See statoconia.
otodecanoic acid (o-to-dek-ă-no´ik as´id) See stearic acid.
otodynia (o-to-din´e-ă) Earache.
otoencephalitis (o-to-en-sef-ă-lī´tis) Inflammation of the brain, secondary to inflammation of the middle ear and mastoid cells. Also called otocerebritis.
otoganglion (o-to-gang´gle-on) See otic ganglion, under ganglion.
otolaryngologist(o-to-lar-ing-gol´ŏ-jist) A specialist in otolaryngology.
otolaryngology (o-to-lar-ing-gol´ŏ-je) The branch of medicine concerned with the study of the ear and the upper respiratory tract and the diagnosis and

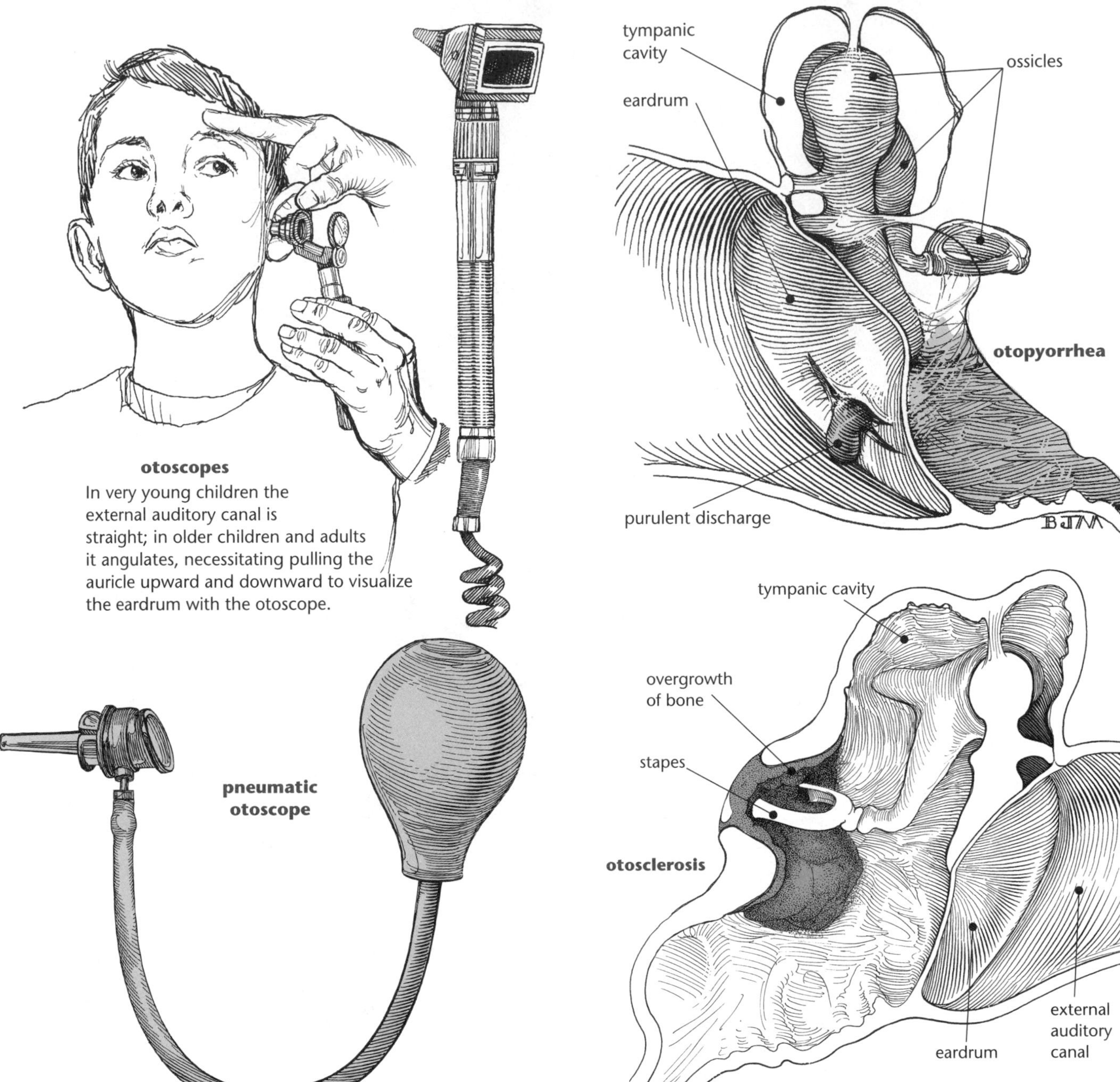

O

treatment of their diseases.

otoliths (o′to-lith) See statoconia.

otologic (o-to-loj′ik) Relating to otology.

otologist (o-tol′ŏ-jist) A specialist in ear diseases.

otology (o-tol′ŏ-je) The branch of medicine concerned with diseases of the ear.

otomycosis (o-to-mi-ko′sis) Fungal infection of the external auditory canal.

otoneuralgia (o-to-nōō-ral′jă) Neuralgic earache.

otopathy (o-top′ă-the) Any disease of the ear.

otoplasty (o′to-plas-te) Plastic surgery of the auricle on the ear.

otopyorrhea (o-to-pi-o-re′ă) Purulent discharge from the middle ear through a perforated tympanic membrane (eardrum).

otorhinolaryngology (o-to-ri-no-lar-in-gol′ŏ-je) The branch of medicine concerned with the ear, nose, and larynx, and their diseases.

otorhinology (o-to-ri-nol′ŏ-je) Study of the ear and the nose.

otorrhagia (o-to-ra′jă) Bleeding from the ear.

otorrhea (o-to-re′ă) Discharge from the ear.

otosclerosis (o-to-skle-ro′sis) Immobilization of the stapes by an overgrowth of spongy bone along the medial wall of the middle ear; it interferes with sound wave conduction, leading to hearing loss.

otoscope (o′to-skōp) An instrument for examining the ear.

pneumatic o. An otoscope that provides alternate positive and negative pressure, permitting observation of eardrum movement.

otoscopy (o-tos′kŏ-pe) Examination of the tympanic membrane (eardrum) with an otoscope.

ototomy (o-tot′ŏ-me) **1.** Dissection of the ear. **2.** See myringotomy.

ototoxic (o-to-tok′sik) Having a harmful effect upon the ear.

ototoxicity (o-to-tok-sis′ĭ-te) The quality of being ototoxic.

ouabain (wă-ba′in) A rapidly acting cardiac glycoside from the seeds of *Strophanthus gratus*; a constituent of African arrow poison.

ounce (ouns) (oz.) **1.** An avoirdupois unit of weight equal to one sixteenth of a pound (28.3495 g). **2.** An apothecaries' unit of weight equal to one twelfth of a pound (31.103 g).

fluid o. (fl.oz.) An apothecaries' unit of fluid measure, the equivalent of 29.57 milliliters.

outlay (out′lā) A graft on the surface of a bone.

outlet (out′let) A passage or exit.

pelvic o. The lower aperture of the pelvis, bounded by the pubic arch, the ischial tuberosities, the sacrotuberous ligaments, and the tip of the coccyx.

outbreak (out′brak) The sudden occurrence of a disease in several members of a community; may or may not spread sufficiently to become an epidemic.

outpatient (out′pa-shent) A patient treated in a hospital or clinic without being hospitalized.

output (out′poot) **1.** The quantity of a substance produced by or eliminated from the body during a given span of time. **2.** The measure of performance by an organ or a system.

cardiac o. The quantity of blood pumped by the heart per unit of time, usually per minute; the product of stroke volume and cardiac rate.

minute o. The quantity of blood pumped by the heart during one minute, normally 4 to 5 liters at rest in an average-sized person.

stroke o. The quantity of blood ejected with a single heartbeat.

urinary o. The quantity of urine excreted by the kidneys per unit time.

outtoed (out′tod) Foot position in which the toes are turned outward to a marked degree.

ova (o′va) Plural of ovum.

ovalbumin (ov-ăl-bu′min) Albumin from egg whites.

ovalocytosis (o-val-o-si-to′sis) See elliptocytosis.

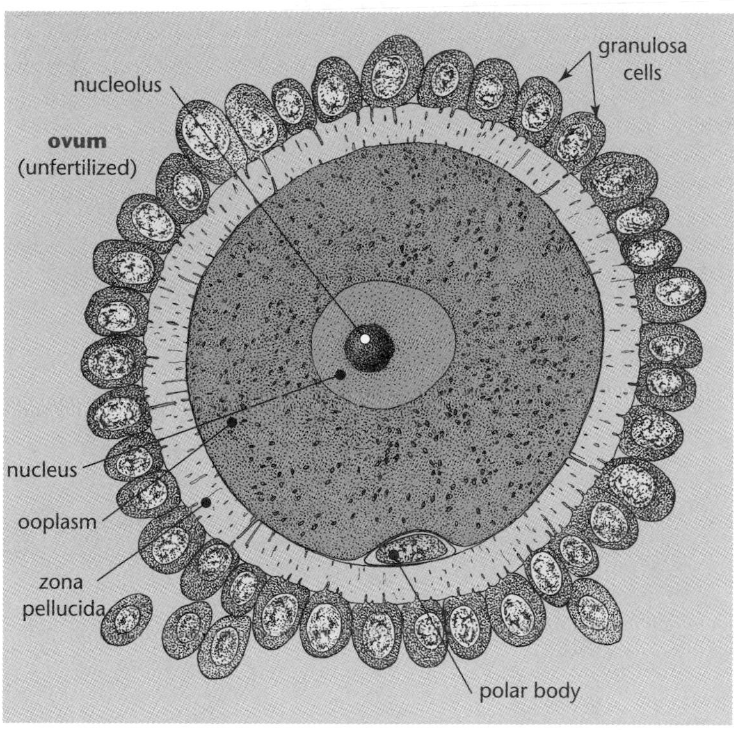

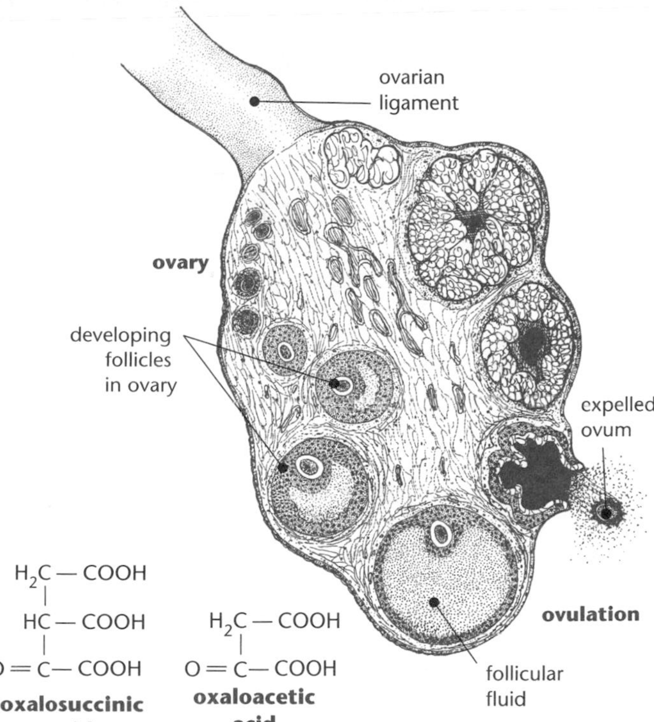

$$\begin{array}{l} H_2C-COOH \\ \quad | \\ HC-COOH \\ \quad | \\ O=C-COOH \end{array}$$

oxalosuccinic acid

$$\begin{array}{l} H_2C-COOH \\ \quad | \\ O=C-COOH \end{array}$$

oxaloacetic acid

ovarian (o-va′re-an) Relating to the ovary.

ovariectomy (o-va-re-ek′tŏ-me) See oophorectomy.

ovariocentesis (o-va-re-o-sen-te′sis) Puncture of an ovarian cyst.

ovariocyesis (o-va-re-o-si-e′sis) See ovarian pregnancy, under pregnancy.

ovariohysterectomy (o-va-re-o-his-ter-ek′tŏ-me) Surgical removal of the ovaries and uterus.

ovariolysis (o-var-e-o-lī′sis) The cutting away of adhesions preventing the normal mobility of the ovary; used in the treatment of certain cases of female infertility.

ovariopathy (o-var-e-op′ă-the) Disease of the ovary.

ovariopexy (o-var-e-o-pek′se) The suturing of an ovary to the abdominal wall.

ovariorrhexis (o-va-re-o-rek′sis) Rupture of an ovary.

ovariosalpingitis (o-va-re-o-sal-pin-jī′tis) Inflammation of one or both ovaries and uterine (fallopian) tubes.

ovarium (o-va′re-um) Latin for ovary.

ovary (o′vă-re) One of the paired sexual glands in which the ova are formed; situated on either side of the uterus, near the free end of each uterine (fallopian) tube; produces the hormones progesterone and estrogen; the female gonad.

large white o. See polycystic ovary.

oyster o. See polycystic ovary.

polycystic o. A diseased, usually enlarged ovary associated with infertility; it contains multiple cysts and is covered with a thick, pearly white capsule; seen in conditions such as Stein-Leventhal syndrome, abnormal bleeding, and virilism. Also called oyster ovary; commonly called large white ovary.

third o. An accessory ovary.

overbite (o′ver-bīt) See vertical overlap, under overlap.

overclosure (o-ver-klo′zhur) Condition in which the mandible rises too far before the teeth make contact, resulting in a shortened face length; may be due to changed shape of teeth (through grinding), or drifting or loss of teeth. Also called reduced interarch distance.

overcompensation (o′ver-kom-pen-sa′shun) Behavior in which an overwhelming feeling of inadequacy inspires exaggerated correction (e.g., overaggressiveness).

overdetermination (o-ver-de-ter-mĭ-na′shun) The multiple causation of a single event, behavior, or emotional symptom.

overdose (o′ver-dōs) **1.** An excessive dose. **2.** (O.D.) To poison with an excessive dose.

barbiturate o. An overdose of barbiturates causing severe poisoning, a common mode of suicide.

narcotic o. An excessive dose of a narcotic drug producing the clinical triad of stupor (or coma), respiratory depression, and pinpoint pupils (miosis); treatment generally consists of ventilatory and circulatory care and administration of narcotic antagonists.

overhang (o′ver-hang) The portion of a dental filling extending over the normal tooth contour. Also called gingival margin excess.

overhydration (o-ver-hi-dra ′shun) See hyperhydra-tion.

overjet, overjut (o′ver-jet, o′ver-jut) See horizontal overlap, under overlap.

overlap (o′ver-lap) A projection of one tissue or structure over another.

horizontal o. Excessive projection of the upper anterior and/or posterior teeth beyond their antagonists of the lower jaw in a horizontal direction. Also called overjet; overjut; buck teeth.

vertical o. The overlapping of the lower incisors by the upper incisors when the posterior teeth are in normal contact. Also called overbite.

overlay (o′ver-lā) Any condition that is superimposed on an existing one.

emotional o. An emotional disturbance resulting from, or added to, an organic disease.

overnutrition (o-ver-noo-trish′un) Overeating; excessive caloric intake.

overriding (o-ver-rīd′ing) The slipping of one fragment of a broken bone alongside the other.

over-the-counter (o′vĕr-thĕ-koun′tĕr) (OTC) Denoting a medication not requiring a prescription for purchase.

overventilation (o′ver-ven-tĭ-la′shun) See hyperventilation.

ovicidal (o-vĭ-si′dal) Causing destruction of the ovum.

oviduct (o′vĭ-dukt) See uterine tube, under tube.

oviferous (o-vif′ĕr-us) Containing or conveying eggs.

ovigenesis (o-vĭ-jen′ĕ-sis) See oogenesis.

ovine (o′vīn) Relating to sheep.

oviparous (o-vip′ă-rus) Egg-laying; producing eggs that hatch outside the body of the maternal organism. COMPARE: ovoviviparous; viviparous.

oviposit (o-vĭ-poz′it) To lay egg, especially with the aid of an ovipositor characteristic of insects.

oviposition (o-vĭ-po-zi′shun) The act of laying or depositing eggs; said especially of insects.

ovipositor (o-vĭ-pos′ĭ-tor) A specialized tubular structure at the end of the abdomen of many female insects for boring holes to house their eggs.

ovoid (o′void) Egg-shaped.

ovomucoid (o-vo-mu′koid) Mucoprotein of egg white.

ovotestis (o-vo-tes′tis) A gonad in which both testicular and ovarian tissues are present.

ovoviviparous (o-vo-vi-vip′ă-rus) Bearing young that develop from eggs retained within the maternal body (e.g., reptiles, certain fish, insects).

ovulation (ov-u-la′shun) The discharge of an ovum from the mature (vesicular) follicle of the ovary.

ovule (o′vūl) **1.** The ovum in the ovarian follicle. **2.** Any small egg-shaped structure.

ovulocyclic (o-vu-lo-sī′klik) Denoting any periodic occurrence that is associated with, or occurring within, the ovulatory cycle.

ovum (o′vum), *pl.* **ova** The female reproductive cell that, when fused with the male cell (spermatozoon), forms the zygote. Commonly called egg.

oxalate (ok′să-lāt) A salt of oxalic acid.

oxalic acid (ok-sal′ik as′id) A compound produced by oxidation of glyoxylate; present in excessive amounts in persons afflicted with primary hyperoxaluria.

oxaloacetic acid (ok-să-lo-ă-se′tik as′id) An intermediate in the tricarboxylic acid cycle. Also called ketosuccinic acid.

oxalosis (ok-să-lo′sis) Accumulation of calcium oxalate crystals in the kidneys, bones, arteries, and heart muscle; a feature of primary hyperoxaluria, usually leading to death by kidney failure.

oxalosuccinic acid (ok-să-lo-suk-sin′ik as′id) An intermediate in the tricarboxylic acid cycle.

oxaluria (ok-săl-u′re-ă) The presence of abnormally large quantities of calcium oxalate in the urine.

oxazepam (ok-saz′ĕ-pam) A benzodiazepine tranquilizer; Serax®.

oxazolidine (ok-saz-o-lid′īn) A class of synthetic antibiotics that act by preventing protein formation within bacteria.

oxazolidinones (ok-să-zo-lid′ĭ-nōnz) A class of synthetic antibiotics effective against gram-positive organisms; they act by disrupting the initiation of bacterial protein synthesis to block bacterial growth.

oxidase (ok′sĭ-dās) One of a group of oxidizing enzymes that promote either the addition of oxygen to a metabolite or the removal of hydrogen or of electrons.

oxidation (ok-sĭ-da′shun) **1.** A chemical reaction in which electrons from one reactant (the reducing agent) are transferred to the other reactant (the oxidizing agent); the atoms in the element losing electrons increase their valence correspondingly. COMPARE: reduction. **2.** The combination of a substance with oxygen.

oxidation-reduction (ok-sĭ-da′shun-re-duk′shun) Any chemical reaction in which electrons are transferred from one atom or molecule to another. Also called redox.

oxide (ok′sīd) A binary compound of oxygen with

O

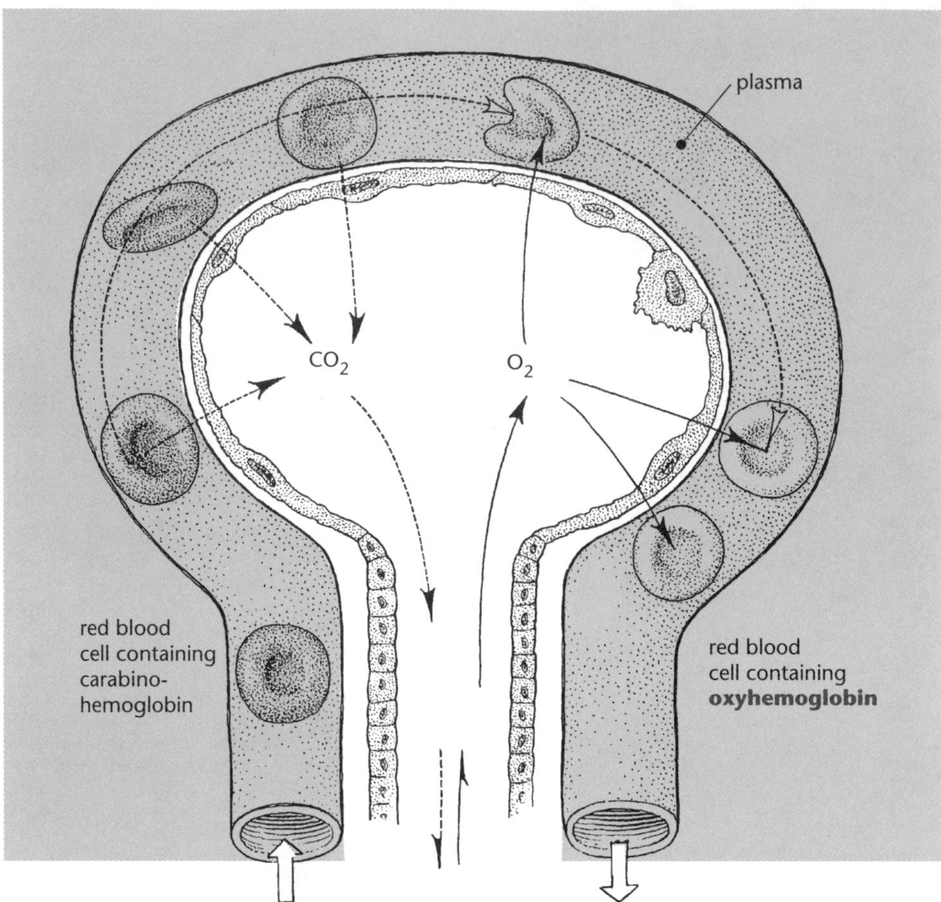

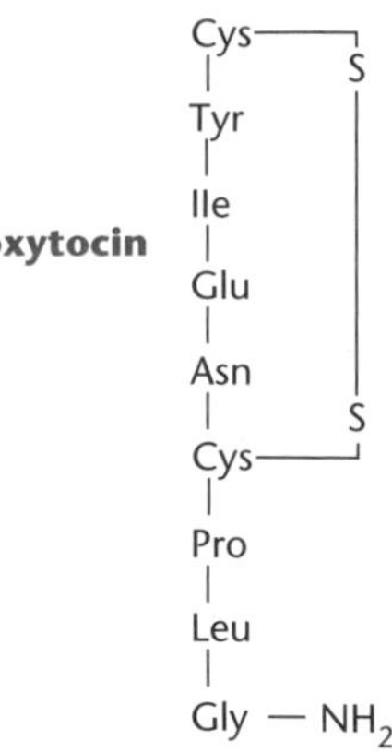

another element or radical (e.g., mercuric oxide).

acid o. An oxygen compound of nonmetals (e.g., SO_2).

basic o. An oxygen compound of metals (e.g., Al_2O_3).

oxidize (ok´sĭ-dīz) To combine or to cause combination with oxygen.

oxidoreductase (ok-sĭ-do-re-duk´tās) An enzyme that promotes an oxidation-reduction reaction.

oxime, oxim (ok´sim) A condensation product of the action of hydroxylamine on a ketone or an aldehyde.

oximeter (ok-sim´ĕ-ter) Instrument for measuring photoelectrically the degree of oxygen saturation in the blood.

pulse o. A monitor used in anesthetized patients, without pricking their skin, to measure oxygen saturation in the blood (i.e., the percentage of red blood cells that have oxygen attached to them). The monitor provides a continuous record of the oxygen level in the blood and sounds an alarm if the level falls too low.

oxyacid (ok-se-as´id) An acid containing oxygen. Also called oxacid.

oxycellulose (ok-se-sel´u-lōs) Cellulose in which all or most of the glucose residues have been converted to glucuronic acid residues.

oxycephaly (ok-se-sef´ă-le) Peaked, conical skull. Commonly called tower skull.

oxychromatic (ok-se-kro-mat´ik) Staining brightly with eosin and other acid dyes.

oxychromatin (ok-se-kro´mă-tin) Chromatin that stains with acid dyes. Also called oxyphil chromatin.

oxygen (ok´sĭ-jen) An odorless and colorless gas, symbol O, atomic number 8, atomic weight 16; it constitutes about one-fifth of the earth's atmosphere.

oxygen debt (ok´sĭ-jen det) The extra oxygen consumed by the body, above its resting needs, occurring at the end of intensive work or exercise.

oxygenase (ok´sĭ-jĕn-ās) One of several enzymes catalyzing the activation of molecular oxygen and the subsequent incorporation of both atoms of the oxygen molecule into the substrate.

oxygenate (ok sĭ-jĕn-āt) To saturate or infuse with oxygen.

oxygenation (ok-sĭ-jĕ-na shun) **1.** The combination of oxygen with the blood pigment hemoglobin. **2.** The supplying of oxygen to a tissue or individual.

apneic o. See diffusion respiration, under respiration.

oxygenator (ok-sĭ-jĕ-na tor) Device for the mechanical oxygenation of venous blood.

oxygen debt (ok´´sĭ-jĕn dĕt) The extra oxygen consumed by the body, above its resting needs, occurring at the end of intensive work or exercise.

oxygenize (ok´sĭ-jĕn-īz) To oxidize.

oxyhemoglobin (ok-se-he-mo-glo´bin) (HbO_2) Hemoglobin combined with oxygen, present in arterial blood. Also called oxygenated hemoglobin.

oxylalia (ok-se-la´le-ă) Abnormally rapid speech.

oxyphil, oxyphile (ok´se-fil, ok´se-fīl) See eosinophilic leukocyte, under leukocyte.

oxyphonia (ok-se-fo´ne-ă) Abnormal shrillness of voice.

oxypurine (ok-se-pu´rin) An oxygen-containing purine (e.g., uric acid and xanthine).

17-oxysteroid (ok-se-ster´oid) 17-Ketosteroid.

oxytetracycline (ok-se-tet-ră-si´klēn) Antibiotic produced by *Streptomyces rimosus*; Terramycin®.

oxytocia (ok-se-to se-ă) Rapid childbirth.

oxytocic (ok-se-to´sik) **1.** Relating to oxytocia. **2.** Hastening the childbirth process by stimulating uterine contractions.

oxytocin (ok-se-to´sin) (OXT) Hormone formed in the hypothalamus (at the base of the brain) and stored in the posterior lobe of the pituitary prior to its release into the circulation; it stimulates smooth muscle contraction; causes strong contraction of the pregnant uterus and ejection of milk from the lactating breast (distinguished from prolactin, which stimulates milk production).

oxyuriasis (ok-se-u-ri´ă-sis) Infection with pinworms.

oxyuricide (ok-se-u´rĭ-sīd) **1.** An agent that kills pinworms. **2.** Destructive to pinworms.

oxyurid (ok-se-u´rid) Any member of the superfamily Oxyuroidea.

ozena (o-ze´nă) See atrophic rhinitis, under rhinitis.

ozone (o´zōn) (O_3) A blue, poisonous, gaseous triatomic form of oxygen formed naturally from an electric discharge through oxygen or by exposure of oxygen to ultraviolet radiation; made commercially by passing oxygen over 10,000 volt charged aluminum plates; used chiefly as an antiseptic, disinfectant, and bleaching agent.

ozonometer (o-zo-nom´ĕ-ter) An apparatus that estimates the amount of ozone in the atmosphere by the use of a series of test papers.

ozostomia (o-zo-sto´me-ă) Bad breath.

P

p 53 A gene that is a global regulator of cell growth with a prominent role in a wide variety of cancers (e.g., its mutation or loss is the most common genetic alteration found in cancer of the breast, ovary, cervix, lung, liver).
pablum (pab´lum) A precooked food, usually for infants, made from wheat, oat, and corn meals, wheat embryo, alfalfa leaves, brewers' yeast, iron, and salt.
pabulum (pab´u-lum) Any nourishing substance.
pacchionian granulations (pak-e-o´ne-an gran-u-la´shuns) See arachnoid granulations, under granulation.
pacemaker (pās´mā-ker) **1.** Any bodily structure that serves to establish and maintain a rhythmic pace, such as the sinoatrial node of the heart that regulates the heartbeat. **2.** A substance whose rate of reaction regulates a series of chain or related reactions.
artificial cardiac p. Any of several miniaturized and surgically implanted electronic devices that substitute for the normal cardiac pacemaker and regulate the heartbeat; used in treating individuals with chronic heart block who have the following manifestations: episodes of syncope or convulsions owing to ventricular bradycardia, cardiac failure secondary to the bradycardia, and unstable ventricular rhythms associated with the heart block.
brain p. A pacemaker implanted on the surface of the cerebellum that is primarily used to bring intractable epilepsy under control. Also called cerebellar electrical stimulator.
demand p. A pacemaker in which the stimulus is only fired when the ventricular contraction does not occur within a specified period of time; a signal from the heart's previous ventricular depolarization inhibits the pulse generator from firing for an additional second.
ectopic p. Any cardiac pacemaker other than the sinus node.
external p. Artificial pacemaker with electrodes placed externally on the chest wall.
fixed-rate p. An artificial pacemaker that discharges electrical stimuli at a uniform and uninterrupted rate.
shifting p. See wandering pacemaker.
wandering p. Phenomenon in which the point of origin of the heart beat shifts back and forth from one center to another, usually between the sinus and A-V nodes. Also called shifting pacemaker.
pachy- Prefix meaning thick.
pachyblepharon (pak-e-blef´ă-ron) Thickening of the border of an eyelid.
pachycephaly, pachycephalia (pak-e-sef´ă-le, pak-e-sĕ-fa´le-ă) An abnormal thickening of the skull.
pachycholia (pak-e-ko´le-ă) Abnormal viscosity of the bile.
pachychromatic (pak-e-kro-mat´ik) Having a thick chromatin network.
pachydactyly (pak-e-dak´tĭ-le) Abnormal enlargement of the fingers or toes.
pachyderma (pak-e-der´mă) Abnormally thick skin.
p. laryngis A form of chronic laryngitis, marked by the formation of warty thickening of the epithelium, usually on the vocal cords; it is caused by chronic irritation.
pachydermatocele (pak-e-der-mat´o-sēl) **1.** Congenital looseness of the skin, which hangs in folds. Also called cutis laxa. **2.** A large neurofibroma.
pachydermatosis (pak-e-der-mă-to´sis) Pachyderma of long duration.
pachydermatous (pak-e-der´mă-tus) Characterized by pachyderma.
pachydermoperiostosis (pak-e-der-mo-per-e-os-to´sis) Inherited condition marked by osteoarthropathy, coarseness of facial features with thickening and oiliness of the skin, excessive sebaceous gland secretion, and enlargement of hands with clubbing of fingers.
pachygyria (pak-e-ji´re-ă) Abnormally thick convolutions of the cerebral cortex.
pachyleptomeningitis (pak-e-lep-to-men-in-ji´tis) Inflammation of the membranes of the brain and spinal cord.

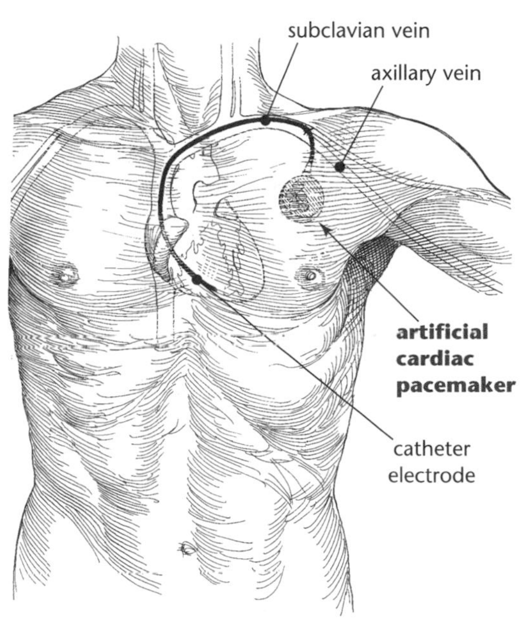

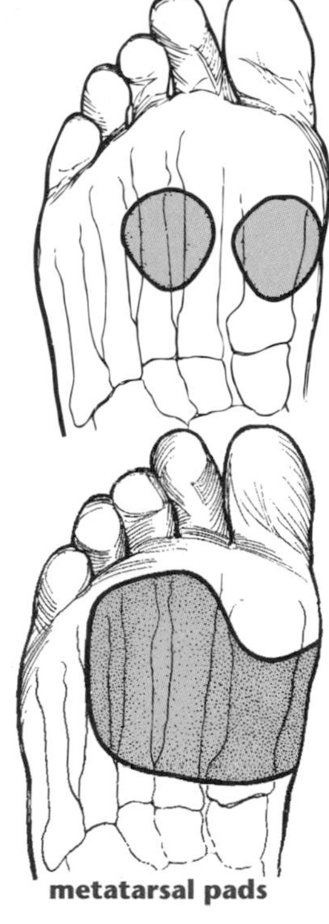

pachylosis (pak-e-lo´sis) A dry, thickened, scaly state of the skin, especially on the lower extremities.
pachymeningitis (pak-e-men-in-ji´tis) Inflammation and thickening of the dura mater.
pachymeningopathy (pak-e-men-in-gop´ă-the) Any disease of the dura mater.
pachymeter (pă-kim´ĕ-ter) Instrument used to measure the thickness of membranes or thin plates.
pachyonychia (pak-e-o-nik´e-ă) Excessive thickness of the fingernails or toenails.
p. congenita A congenital deformity characterized by abnormalities of the skin (bullae and papular hyperkeratoses) and mucous membranes (leukokeratoses) and excessively thick nails.
pachyperiostitis (pak-e-per-e-os-tī´tis) Proliferative thickening of the membrane enveloping bones due to inflammation.
pachyperitonitis (pak-e-per-ĭ-to-ni´tis) Inflammation and thickening of the peritoneum.
pachypleuritis (pak-e-ploo-rī´tis) Inflammation of the pleura accompanied by thickening of the membrane. Also called productive pleurisy.
pachysalpingitis (pak-e-sal-pin-ji´tis) Chronic interstitial inflammation of the muscular layer of the uterine (fallopian) tube, producing thickening. Also called chronic parenchymatous salpingitis.
pachysomia (pak-e-so´me-ă) Abnormal thickening of the soft parts of the body, as in acromegaly.
pachytene (pak´e-tēn) The stage of prophase in meiosis in which each paired chromosome separates into its two component sister chromatids, so that each homologous chromosome pair becomes a set of four intertwined chromatids called a bivalent.
pack (pak) **1.** To fill or stuff. **2.** To wrap a patient in hot, cold, wet, or dry blankets or sheets. **3.** The blankets or sheets so used. **4.** In dentistry, the application of a dressing to a surgical site. **5.** The dressing so used.
packer (pak´er) Instrument for inserting an absorbent dressing or tampon into a bodily cavity, such as the vagina.
packing (pak´ing) The material used to fill a cavity or a wound, such as gauze, sponge, etc.
paclitaxel (pak-lĭ-tak´sel) Antitumor drug used to treat metastatic ovarian cancer; Taxol®.
pad (pad) A cushion of soft material.
abdominal p. A large pad used for absorbing discharges from surgical abdominal wounds.
buccal fat p. An encapsulated mass of fat on the outer side of the cheek situated superficial to the buccinator muscle and pierced by the parotid duct; in infants it is prominent and is called sucking or suctorial pad because it is thought to help prevent the cheeks from being sucked inward while nursing.
fat p. A circumscribed cushion-like mass of fat.
infrapatellar fat p. A large pad of fat which separates the patellar ligament and part of the patella (kneecap) from the synovial membrane of the knee joint.
ischiorectal fat p. A pad of fat in the anal region extending upward on both sides of the anus; it contains many fibrous septa that support the anal canal.
metatarsal p. One of various shaped pads worn inside the shoe under the metatarsal bones to shield painful weight-bearing areas from pressure.
Passavant's p. See Passavant's ridge, under ridge.
retropubic fat p. A large quantity of fat in the U-shaped retropubic space located between the pubic symphysis and the bladder and extending backward on each side of the bladder; it is limited above by the peritoneum.
Paget's disease (paj´ets dĭ-zēz´) A bone disease of unknown cause; characterized by localized areas of bone destruction followed by replacement with overdeveloped, light, soft, porous bone and associated with deformities, such as thickening of portions of the skull and bending of weight-bearing bones; Beethoven is believed to have been afflicted with this disease. Also called osteitis deformans.
pagophagia (pa-go-fa´jă) The ingestion of abnormally large quantities of ice.
pain (pān) A physical or mental sensation of distress or suffering.
bearing-down p. One accompanying the contractions of the uterus during the second stage of labor.
false p.'s Those resembling true labor pains.
girdle p. A painful sensation encircling the waist like a tight belt, occurring in some diseases of the spinal cord.
growing p.'s Pains in the limbs of children, usually felt at night and resembling rheumatism; attributed to growth, faulty posture, or fatigue.
intermenstrual p. Mild pelvic pain occurring midway between two menstruations, associated with ejection of the ovum from the ovary. Also called mittelschmerz.
labor p.'s Rhythmic pains of increasing severity, frequency, and duration, caused by contraction of the uterus during childbirth.
phantom limb p. The sensation of pain felt in a limb, although that limb has been amputated.
referred p. Pain felt in an area other than the site of origin, such as the pain near the shoulder associated with biliary disease.
sympathetically maintained p. (SMP) Pain that begins with an injury, grows in severity out of proportion to the injury, and recurs intermittently for months or even years after the injury heals.

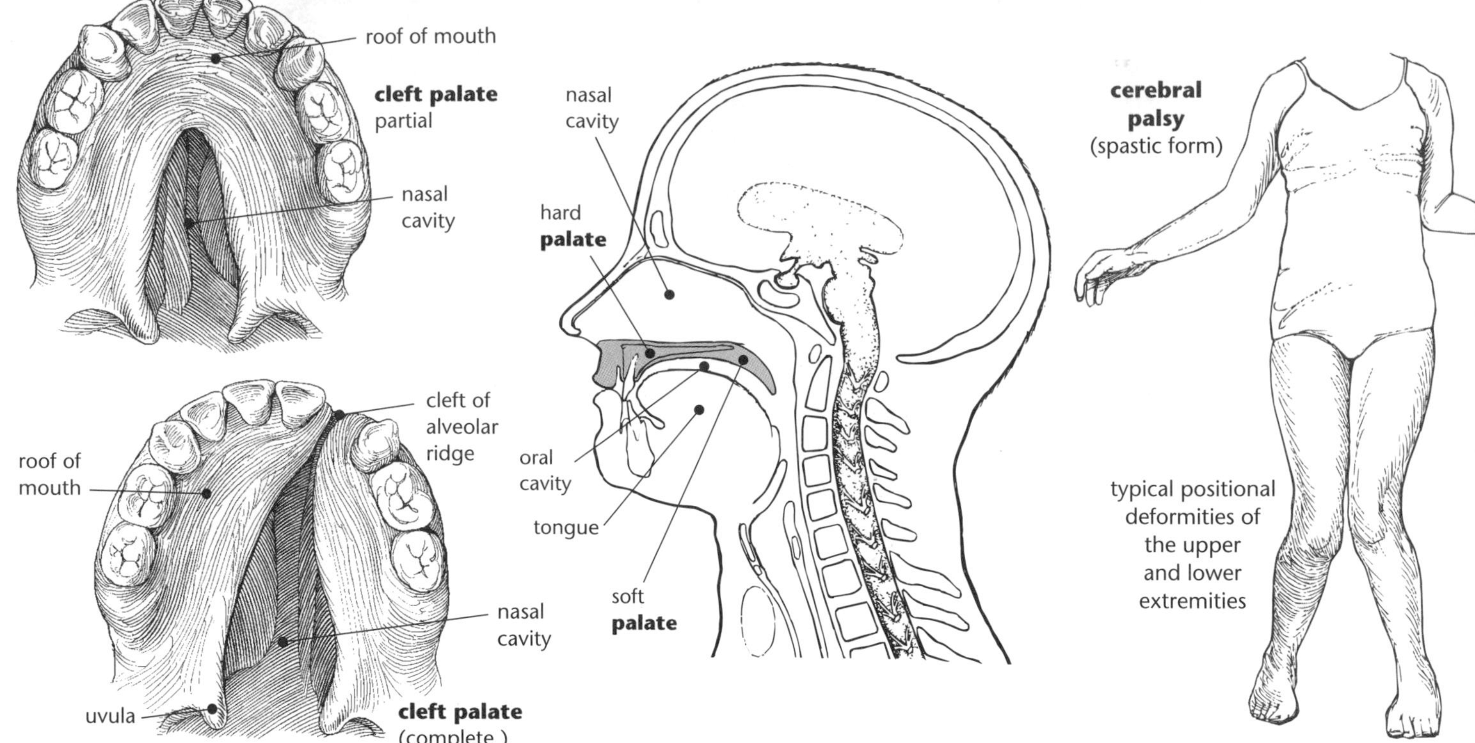

pair (pār) Two similar, identical, or associated things.
base p. Either of the two pairs of nucleic acid bases (one a purine and the other a pyrimidine), joined by hydrogen bonds, that make up the DNA molecule. Also called nucleotide or nucleoside pair.
pairing (pār´ing) Side by side attachment of two homologous chromosomes prior to their exchanging genetic material (crossing over) during meiosis.
palatal (pal´ă-tal) Relating to the palate.
palate (pal´at) It consists of a bony anterior part (hard palate) and a soft muscular posterior portion (soft palate). Also called roof of the mouth.
cleft p. Congenitally malformed palate, with a fissure along the midline; may be restricted to the soft and hard palate or extend forward through the dental arch, on either or both sides of the midline; often associated with a cleft lip.
primary p. The embryonic shelf separating the oral and nasal cavities of the early embryo. Also called primitive palate.
secondary p. The embryonic palate that eventually forms the hard palate by fusion of the lateral palatine processes.
palatiform (pă-lat´i-form) Resembling the palate or roof of the mouth.
palatine (pal´ă-tīn) Relating to the palate or roof of the mouth.
palatoglossal (pal-ă-to-glos´al) Relating to the palate and the tongue.
palatograph (pal´ă-to-graf) Instrument for recording the movements of the soft palate during speech and respiration. Also called palate myograph; palatomyograph.
palatopharyngeal (pal-ă-to-fă-rin´je-al) Relating to the palate and the pharynx.
palatopharyngoplasty (pal-ă-to-fă-rin´go-plaste) Operative procedure to correct a shortened soft palate (sometimes necessary in plastic repair of a cleft palate). Also called uvulopalatoplasty.
palatoplasty (pal´ă-to-plas-te) Reparative surgery of the palate, especially a cleft palate.
palatoplegia (pal-ă-to-ple´jă) Paralysis of the muscles of the soft palate.
palatoschisis (pal-ă-tos´kĭ-sis) See cleft palate, under palate.
paleencephalon (pa-le-en-sef´ă-lon) The phylogenetically older part of the brain that includes all of it except the cerebral cortex and closely related parts.
paleobiology (pa-le-o-bi-ol´ŏ-je) The study of evolution of life from a non-oxygen dominated environment.
paleocerebellum (pa-le-o-ser-ĕ-bel´um) The earlier developed parts of the cerebellum (i.e., vermis and flocculus).
paleocortex (pă-le-o-kor´teks) The earlier developed parts of the cerebral cortex (i.e., the olfactory cortex).
paleokinetic (pa-le-o-ki-net´ik) Denoting the primitive nervous motor mechanism concerned with automatic movements.
paleopathology (pa-le-o-pă-thol´ŏ-je) The study of disease of ancient man as revealed in mummies, bones, and art forms (e.g., paintings, statues).
palilalia (pal-ĭ-la´le-ă) See palinphrasia.
palindrome (pal´in-drōm) **1.** A word or sentence that reads the same forwards or backwards. **2.** In molecular biology, a length of DNA in which identical (or almost identical) base sequences in the two strands of the double helix run in opposite directions so that the compound reads the same forward or backward (e.g., ACB-BCA).
palindromia (pal-in-dro´me-ă) Recurrence of a pathologic condition.
palindromic (pal-in-dro´mik) Recurring.
palingenesis (pal-in-jen´ĕ-sis) The reappearance of ancestral structural features.
palinphrasia (pal-in-fra´zhă) The involuntary repetition of phrases in speaking; may be caused by encephalitis. Also called palilalia.
palladium (pă-la´de-um) Metallic element resembling platinum; symbol Pd, atomic number 46, atomic weight 106.4.
pallesthesia (pal-es-the´zhă) The perception of vibration, especially through bones. Also called vibratory sensibility.
palliate (pal´e-āt) To mitigate.
palliative (pal´e-a-tiv) **1.** Alleviating. **2.** A medicine or treatment that affords temporary relief but does not effect a cure.
pallidectomy (pal-ĭ-dek´tŏ-me) Surgical removal or destruction of the globus pallidus.
pallidotomy (pal-ĭ-dot´ŏ-me) Cutting of nerve fibers from the globus pallidus in the brain for the relief of pathologic involuntary movements.
pallium (pal´ĭ-dum) The cerebral cortex and subadjacent white substance.
pallor (pal´or) Paleness; lack of color.
palm (palm) The anterior or inner surface of the hand.
palmar (pal´mar) Relating to the palm of the hand.
palmitic acid (pal-mit´ik as´id) A saturated fatty acid found in various fats and oils. Also called hexadecanoic acid.
palpable (pal´pă-bl) Perceptible by palpation; tangible.
palpate (pal´pāt) To examine by touching or pressing with the fingers or the palms of the hands.
palpation (pal-pa´shun) Examination by touch or pressure of the hand, over an organ or area of the body, as a diagnostic aid.
palpebra (pal´pē-bră), *pl.* **pal´pebrae** Latin for eyelid.
palpebral (pal´pē-bral) Of or relating to the eyelids.
palpitation (pal-pĭ-ta´shun) Rapid or forceful heartbeat, of which the patient is conscious.
palsy (pawl´ze) Paralysis.
ataxic cerebral p. Cerebral palsy characterized by inability to coordinate voluntary muscular movements.
Bell's p. Term used for an abrupt unilateral facial nerve paralysis due to involvement of the facial (VII cranial) nerve when no specific cause is determined; a similar condition may be caused by viruses and Lyme disease.
cerebral p. Impairment of voluntary motor function caused by damage to the brain's motor control centers; marked primarily by spastic paralysis or impairment of control or coordination over voluntary muscles; often accompanied by mental retardation, seizures, and disorders of vision and communication; may be either congenital or acquired.
dyskinetic cerebral p. Cerebral palsy characterized by uncontrolled and purposeless movements that disappear during sleep.
Erb-Duchenne p. See Erb-Duchenne paralysis, under paralysis.
facial nerve p. Paralysis of the muscles on one side of the face caused by a lesion of the facial (VII cranial) nerve. See also Bell's palsy.
Klumpke's p. See Klumpke's paralysis, under paralysis.
obstetric p. See obstetric paralysis, under paralysis.
progressive bulbar p. Paralysis and atrophy increasingly involving the muscles of the lips, tongue, pharynx, and larynx due to lesions of motor neurons primarily in the brainstem.
shaking p., trembling p. See parkinsonism.
spastic cerebral p. Cerebral palsy characterized by increased muscle tension and exaggerated reflex activity in an arm and a leg of the same side (hemiplegia) or arms and legs on both sides (tetraplegia or quadriplegia).
paludism (pal´u-diz-m) Malaria.
panacea (pan-ă-se´ă) A remedy which is supposed to cure all diseases; a cure-all.
panagglutinin (pan-ă-gloo´tĭ-nin) An agglutinin that reacts with all human erythrocytes.
panangiitis (pan-an-je-i´tis) Inflammation of all layers of a blood vessel.
panarthritis (pan-ar-thri´tis) **1.** Inflammation of an entire joint. **2.** Inflammation of all the body joints.
panatrophy (pan-at´ro-fe) A generalized wasting away of the body.
pancarditis (pan-kar-di´tis) Inflammation of all layers of the heart (i.e., myocarditis, endocarditis,

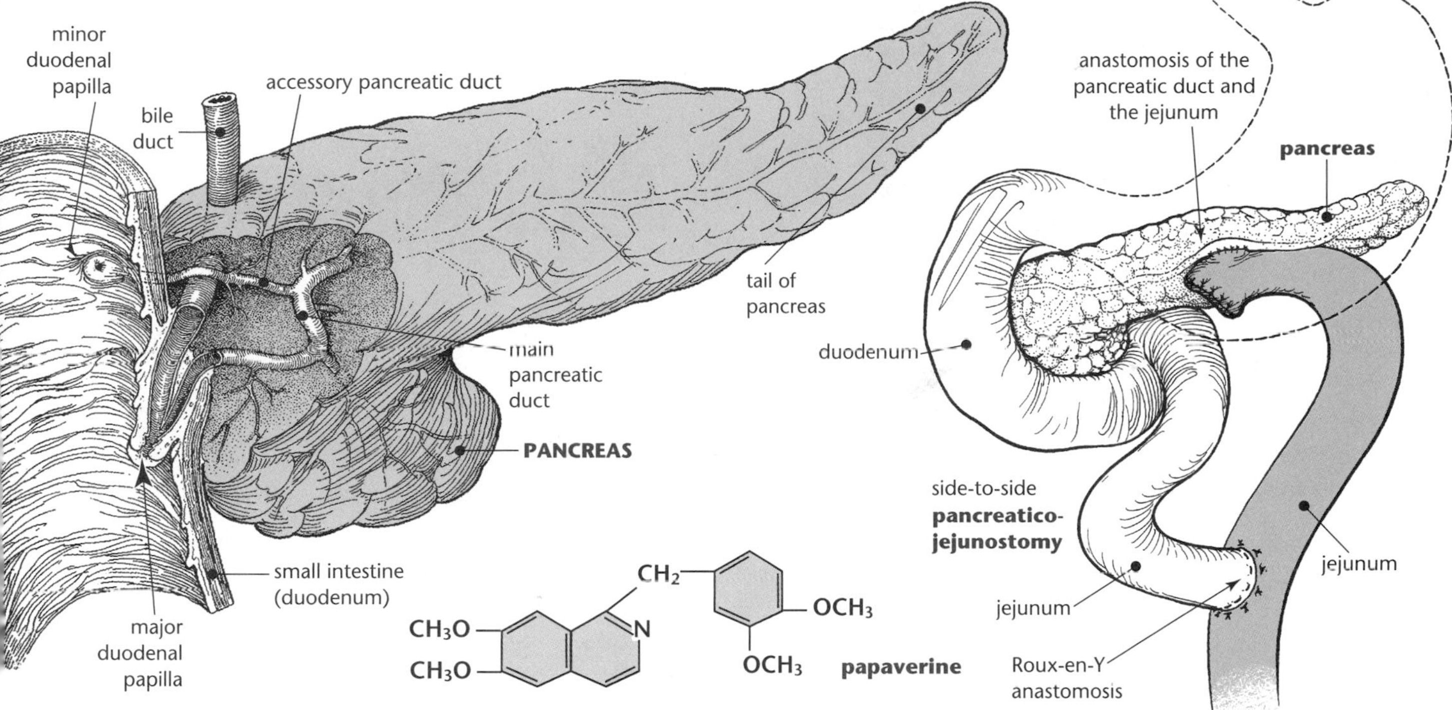

and pericarditis).

Pancoast's syndrome (pan´kōsts sin´drōm) Carcinoma of the apex of the lung or upper mediastinum (Pancoast's tumor) invading the brachial plexus and the cervical sympathetic chain and resulting in pain, weakness, and atrophy of the arm and hand muscles. Also called superior pulmonary sulcus syndrome; Ciuffini-Pancoast syndrome; Horner's syndrome.

pancolectomy (pan-ko-lek´tŏ-me) The removal of the entire colon.

pancreas (pan´kre-as) A soft gland, 10 to 15 cm long, lying behind the stomach and extending transversely from the concavity of the duodenum to the spleen; it secretes enzymes (amylase, lipase), which aid in digestion of food, into the small intestine; it also produces hormones (glucagon, insulin) which, when taken up by the bloodstream, help regulate carbohydrate metabolism by controlling blood sugar levels.

pancreatectomy (pan-kre-ă-tek´tŏ-me) Surgical removal of the pancreas.

pancreaticoduodenostomy (pan-kre-at-ĭ-ko-du-od-ĕ-nos´tŏ-me) Surgical joining of the pancreatic duct into the duodenum.

pancreaticogastrostomy (pan-kre-at-ĭ-ko-gas-tros´tŏ-me) The surgical anastomosis of the pancreatic duct to the stomach.

pancreaticojejunostomy (pan-kre-at-ĭ-ko-je-joo-nos´tŏ-me) Surgical implantation of the pancreatic duct into the jejunum.

pancreatin (pan´kre-ă-tin) A mixture of pancreatic enzymes extracted from hogs or cattle; used as a digestive aid.

pancreatitis (pan-kre-ă-ti´tis) Inflammation of the pancreas.

pancreatoduodenectomy (pan-kre-ă-to-du-od-ĕ-nek´tŏ-me) Surgical removal of the pancreas and the adjacent portion of the duodenum.

pancreatogenous (pan-kre-ă-toj´ĕ-nus) Originating in the pancreas.

pancreatography (pan-kre-ă-tog´ră-fe) The making of x-ray films of the pancreas.

pancreatolith (pan-kre-at´o-lith) A pancreatic stone. Also called pancreolith.

pancreatolithectomy (pan-kre-ă-to-lĭ-thek´tŏ-me) Surgical removal of pancreatic stones.

pancreatolithiasis (pan-kre-ă-to-lĭ-thi´ă-sis) Stones in the pancreas.

pancreatolithotomy (pan-kre-ă-to-lĭ-thot´o-me) Incision of the pancreas for the removal of a stone. Also called pancreolithotomy.

pancreatomy (pan-kre-at´ŏ-me) See pancreatotomy.

pancreatotomy (pan-kre-ă-tot´ŏ-me) Incision of the pancreas. Also called pancreatomy.

pancreatropic (pan-kre-ă-to-trop´ik) Exerting an effect on the pancreas.

pancreolith (pan´kre-o-lith) See pancreatolith.

pancreolithotomy (pan-kre-o-lĭ-thot´ŏ-me) See pancreatolithotomy.

pancreozymin (pan´kre-o-zi-min) A hormone secreted by the mucosa of the small intestine, that stimulates the secretion of pancreatic enzymes.

pancytopenia (pan-si-to-pe´ne-ă) Reduction of all the cell components of the blood (red blood cells, white blood cells, and blood platelets).

pandemic (pan-dem´ik) Denoting an epidemic that affects the population of a wide geographic area.

panencephalitis (pan-en-sef-ă-li´tis) Diffuse inflammation of the brain.

subacute sclerosing p. (SSPE) An uncommon progressive encephalitis caused by the measles virus; usually affects children and young adults who had the measles before the age of two years; characterized by a gradual progression of psychoneurologic deterioration, ending in death, usually within three years.

panendoscope (pan-en´dŏ-skōp) A cystoscope which offers a wide view of the interior of the urinary bladder.

panendoscopy (pan-en´dos-kō-pe) **1.** Endoscopic examination of more than one structure, e.g., of the esophagus, stomach, and duodenum. **2.** Visual examination of the interior of the bladder using a panendoscope.

panesthesia (pan-es-the´zhă) The sum of all sensations experienced at one time.

panhypopituitarism (pan-hi-po-pĭ-tu´ĭ-tar-iz-m) Condition characterized by absence of all the recognized anterior pituitary hormones. Also called Simmond's disease.

panhysterectomy (pan-his-ter-ek´tŏ-me) Surgical removal of the entire uterus, including the cervix.

panhysterosalpingectomy (pan-his-ter-o-sal-pin-jek´tŏ-me) The removal of the entire uterus and uterine tubes (the ovaries are left intact).

panhysterosalpingo-oophorectomy (pan-his-ter-o-sal-pin´go o-of-ŏ-rek´tŏ-me) Removal of the entire uterus, uterine tubes, and ovaries.

panic (pan´ik) A sudden, overpowering anxiety and fear.

panmixis (pan-mik´sis) See random mating, under mating.

panniculitis (pă-nik-u-li´tis) Inflammation of the subcutaneous layer of connective tissue and fat (superficial fascia) of the abdominal wall.

relapsing febrile nodular nonsuppurative p. A disease of unknown cause marked by recurring fever and formation of subcutaneous nodules and plaques with atrophy of subcutaneous fat; the thighs and trunk are most frequently affected. Also called Weber-Christian disease.

panniculus (pă-nik´u-lus) A layer of membranous tissue.

p. adiposus The subcutaneous layer of connective tissue and fat (superficial fascia).

pannus (pan´us) **1.** Superficial infiltration of the cornea with blood vessels; may progress to include a membrane-like granulation tissue; may occur in several degrees of denseness and cover part of or all the cornea; a common complication of trachoma. **2.** An inflammatory secretion covering the articular surfaces of affected joints in rheumatoid arthritis and related disorders.

panophthalmitis, panophthalmia (pan-of-thal-mi´tis, pan-of-thal´me-ă) Generalized infection and inflammation of the eyeball.

Panorex (pan´ŏ-reks) In dentistry, a radiography machine that rotates the film holder and x-ray tube around the patient's head and also shifts the patient to change the axis of rotation of the tube-film assembly relative to his head.

P

panosteitis, panostitis (pan-os-te-i´tis, pan-os-ti´tis) Inflammation of a bone in its entirety.

panotitis (pan-o-ti´tis) General inflammation of the ear.

pansinusitis (pan-si-nu-si´tis) Inflammation of all the paranasal sinuses.

pansystolic (pan-sis-tol´ik) Occurring throughout systole, from first to second heart sound.

pantothenic acid (pan-to-the´nik as´id) $HOCH_2$-$C(CH_3)_2$-CHOH-CO-NH-I-CH_2-CH_2-COOH; a colorless liquid component of the vitamin B complex, widely distributed in plant and animal tissues, especially the liver; part of coenzyme A.

pap (pap) Any soft or semiliquid food, such as bread soaked in milk.

papain (pă-pa´in) A proteolytic enzyme obtained from the unripe fruit of the papaya; used as a meat tenderizer and also in medicine as a protein digestant.

papaverine (pă-pav´er-in) A non-narcotic alkaloid of opium which has vasodilator properties.

paper (pa´per) A thin sheet substance made of the cellulose pulp of wood or other fibrous material; used for writing, filtering, medicating, and testing.

biuret p. A strip of filter paper dipped in biuret reagent and allowed to dry.

filter p. Porous unsized paper suitable for filtering solutions.

litmus p. White blotting paper impregnated with litmus; used as an acid-base indicator; it turns red in a slightly acidic solution and blue in an alkaline one.

paper point (pa´per point) In dentistry, a cone of absorbent paper that can be inserted into the entire

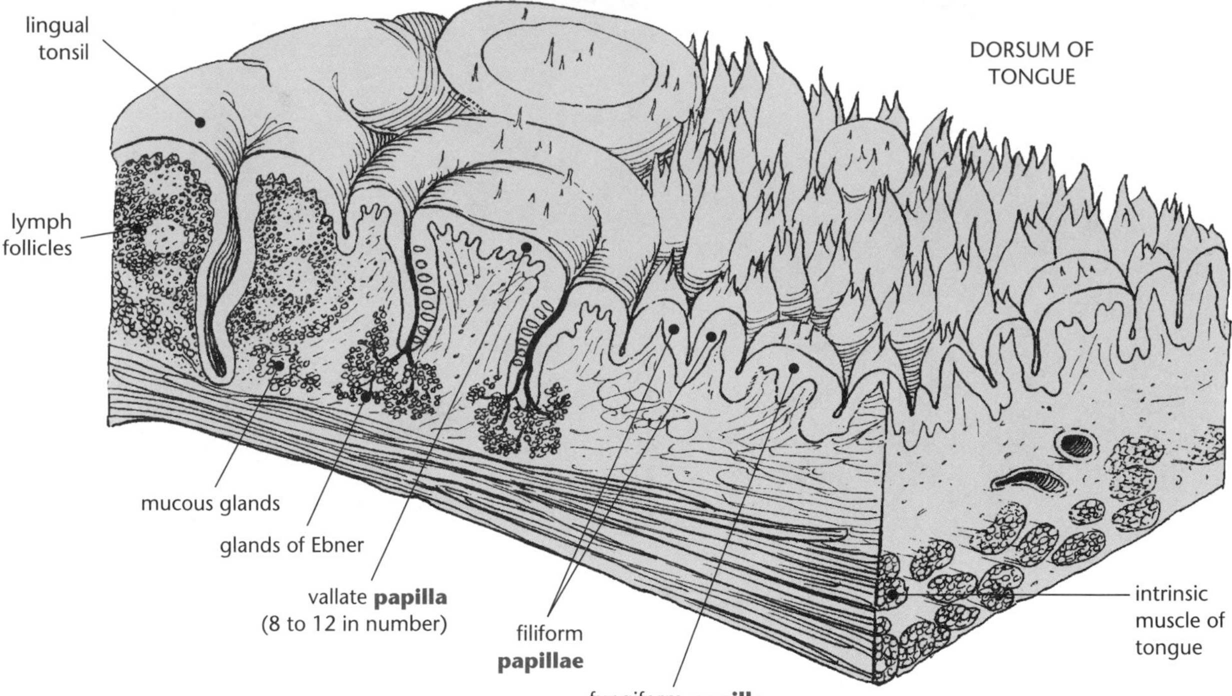

length of a root canal of a tooth; used to medicate the canal or to absorb fluid.

papilla (pă-pil′ă) A small, nipple-like protrusion.

papillary (pap′ĭ-ler-e) Relating to or resembling a papilla or nipple.

papillectomy (pap-ĭ-lek′tŏ-me) Surgical removal of any papilla.

papilledema (pap-il-ĕ-de′mă) Swelling of the optic nerve head caused by increased intracranial pressure.

papilliferous (pap-ĭ-lif′er-us) Containing papillae.

papilliform (pă-pil′ĭ-form) Resembling a papilla.

papillitis (pap-ĭ-li′tis) Inflammation of the optic nerve head. Also called neuropapillitis; intraocular optic neuritis.

necrotizing p. See renal papillary necrosis, under necrosis.

papilloadenocystoma (pă-pil-o-ad-ĕ-no-sis-to′mă) A lobulated benign tumor derived from epithelium, characterized by glands or glandlike structures, formation of cysts, and

P

finger-like projections of neoplastic cells enveloping a core of fibrous connective tissue.

papillocarcinoma (pă-pil-o-kar-sĭ-no′mă) **1.** A malignant tumor originating from a papilloma. **2.** A malignant tumor with papillary projections.

papilloma (pap-ĭ-lo′mă) An overgrowth of the papillae of the skin or mucous membrane. Also called papillary tumor; villoma.

hard p. One derived from squamous epithelium, such as corns or warts.

villous p. One composed of numerous slender outgrowths, usually found in the bladder, within the mammary gland, or arising from the choroid plexus in the lateral ventricle of the brain.

papillomatosis (pap-ĭ-lo-mă-to′sis) Development of several papillomas.

papillomatous (pap-ĭ-lo′mă-tus) Relating to papilloma.

Papillomavirus (pap-ĭ-lo-mă-vi′rus) Genus of DNA viruses (family Papovaviridae) that includes those causing papillomas and warts; some have been associated with cancer.

papillomavirus (pap-ĭ-lo-mă-vi′rus) Any member of the genus *Papillomavirus*.

human p. (hPV) A species with several serotypes; types 1 and 2 cause common and plantar warts; types 6, 11, 16, 18, and 31 cause genital warts.

papilloretinitis (pă-pil-o-ret-ĭ-ni′tis) Inflammation of the optic disk and neighboring parts of the retina. Also called retinopapillitis.

Papovaviridae (pap-o-vă-vir′ĭ-de) Family of viruses (45 to 55 nm in diameter) which contain double-stranded DNA and replicate in nuclei of vertebrate cells; may be transmitted through contact or (mechanically) by arthropods; includes viruses causing warts and papillomas. Also called papovavirus group.

Pap smear (pap smēr) See Pap test, under test.

papula (pap′u-la) Papule.

papular (pap′u-lar) Relating to papules.

papulation (pap-u-la′shun) The formation of papules.

papule (pap′ul) A superficial solid elevation on the skin, ranging in size up to 1 cm.

papulopustular (pap-u-lo-pus′tu-lar) Denoting an eruption composed of papules (small elevations on the skin) and pustules (elevations on the skin containing pus).

papulosis (pap-u-lo′sis) The occurrence of numerous papules, usually widespread.

papulosquamous (pap-u-lo-skwa′mus) Denoting a skin eruption composed of small elevations (papules) and loose scaly lesions.

papulovesicular (pap-u-lo-ve-sik′u-lar) Having both papules and vesicles.

para (par′ă) Denoting a woman's past pregnancies that have reached the period of viability, regardless of whether the infant is dead or alive at the time of delivery; used in conjunction with numerals to designate the number of pregnancies (e.g., para I, para II). The term refers to pregnancies, not fetuses; thus, a woman who gives birth to twins at the end of her first pregnancy is still para I.

parabiosis (par-ă-bi-o′sis) **1.** Union of two organisms, either natural (e.g., conjoined twins) or artificially produced. **2.** Temporary loss of conductivity of a nerve.

parablepsia, parablepsis (par-ă-blep′se-ă, par-ă-blep′sis) False vision, as in visual illusion or hallucination.

paracasein (par-ă-ka′sen) Compound produced when the enzyme rennin acts upon casein (the protein of milk); it reacts with calcium, resulting in the curdling of milk.

paracentesis (par-ă-sen-te′sis) The surgical puncture of a cavity for the purpose of removing fluid.

abdominal p. Paracentesis of the abdomen.

paracentral (par-ă-sen′tral) Located near a central structure.

paracetamol (par-as-et-am′ol) See acetaminophen.

parachordal (par-ă-kor′dal) In embryology, located near and anterior to the notochord.

parachromatopsia (par-ă-kro′mă-top′se-ă) See dichromatism.

paracoccidioidomycosis (par-ă-kok-sid-e-oi-do-mi-ko′sis) A chronic systemic fungal disease caused by a yeastlike fungus (*Paracoccidioides brasiliensis*), characteristically causing gastrointestinal symptoms, painful ulcers of the mouth and nose, and inflammation and suppuration of the lymph nodes of the neck; the infection disseminates to the skin and other organs. Also called South American blastomycosis.

paracolpium (par-ă-kol′pe-um) Tissues near the vagina.

paracusis (par-ă-ku′sis) **1.** Impaired hearing. **2.** Auditory hallucination.

paracyesis (par-ă-si-e′sis) Extrauterine pregnancy.

paracystic (par-ă-sis′ik) Near the bladder.

paradental (par-ă-den′tal) Periodontal.

paradidymis (par-ă-did′ĭ-mis) A small body made up of a few convoluted tubules attached to the lower part of the spermatic cord above the head of the epididymis; considered to be a remnant of the mesonephros (wolffian body). Also called parepididymis; organ of Giraldès.

paradipsia (par-ă-dip′se-ă) Abnormal craving for fluids.

paraffin (par′ă-fin) **1.** A waxy, somewhat transparent purified mixture of solid hydrocarbons derived from petroleum. Also called paraffin wax. **2.** One of the methane or alkane series of saturated aliphatic hydrocarbons having the general formula C_nH_{2n+2}.

soft p. See petrolatum.

paraformaldehyde (par-ă-for-mal′de-hīd) A water-soluble, white, crystalline polymer of formaldehyde; used in treating various skin disorders.

paraganglia (par-ă-gang′gle-ă), *sing.* **paragang′lion** Collection of chromaffin cells forming globular or ovoid bodies present about the ganglia of the sympathetic chain. Also called chromaffin bodies.

paraganglioma (par-ă-gang-gle-o′mă) A tumor composed of chromaffin tissue in a paraganglion or the medulla of the adrenal gland. Also called chromaffinoma.

paragene (par′ă-jen) Any extrachromosomal replicating unit or hereditary determinant. Also called plasmid.

parageusia (par-ă-gu′se-ă) Any abnormality in the sense of taste.

paragglutination (par-ă-gloo-tĭ-na′shun) See group agglutination, under agglutination.

paraglobulin (par-ă-glob′u-lin) A globulin present in blood plasma and lymph.

paragonimiasis (par-ă-gon-ĭ-mi′ă-sis) Infection with a worm of the genus *Paragonimus*, especially the lung fluke species *Paragonimus westermani*.

Paragonimus (par-ă-gon′ĭ-mus) A genus of trematode worms that includes the lung worms of man and animals.

parahepatic (par-ă-he-pat′ik) Located near the liver.

parakeratosis (par-ă-ker-ă-to′sis) The retention of nuclei in the cells of the stratum corneum of the epithelium, as seen in psoriasis.

parakinesia, parakinesis (par-ă-ki-ne′shă, par-

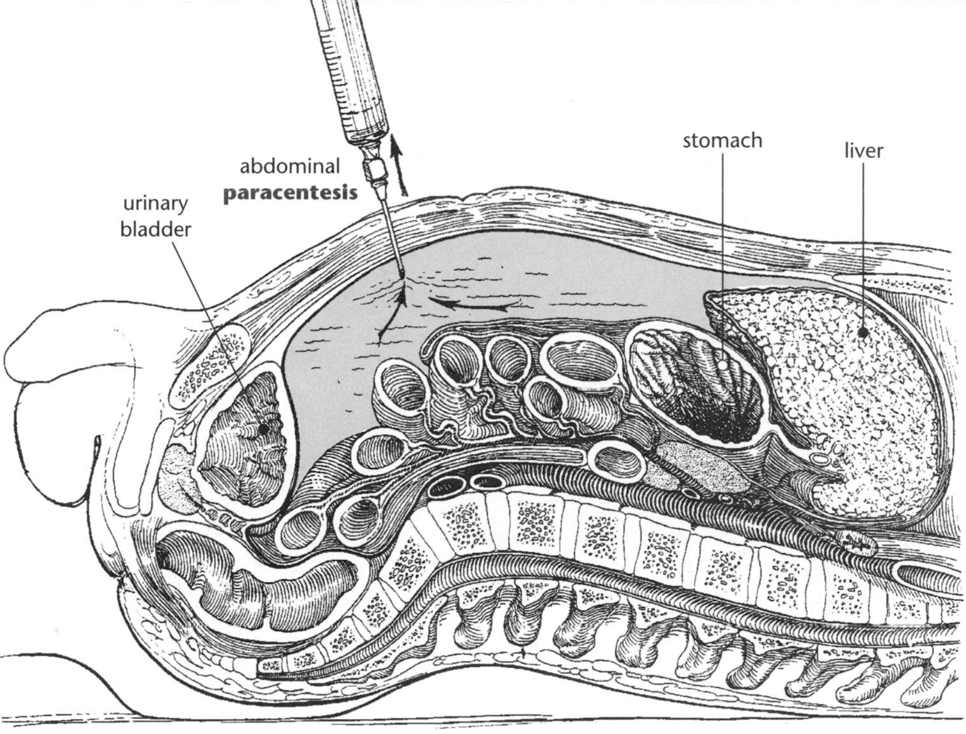

ă-ki-ne´sis) Any abnormality of motor function.

paralalia (par-ă-la´le-ă) Speech defect in which one letter is substituted for another.

paralbumin (par-al-bu´min) Albuminous substance usually present in ovarian cysts and ascites.

paralgesia (par-al-je´shă) Any abnormal painful sensation.

parallax (par´ă-laks) The apparent displacement of an object caused by a change in the observation position.

paralysis (pă-ral´ĭ-sis) **1.** Loss of voluntary muscular function. **2.** Loss of sensation. **3.** Loss of any organic function.

acute ascending p. Paralysis, often fatal, beginning in the lower limbs and ascending rapidly to the trunk, arms, and neck. Also called Landry's paralysis.

p. agitans See Parkinson's disease.

ascending p. Paralysis progressing from the periphery to a nerve center or from the lower limbs upward.

Brown-Séquard p. See Brown-Séquard syndrome.

congenital oculofacial p. See Möbius' syndrome.

crutch p. Paralysis of the arm muscles due to compression of a nerve at the armpit (axilla) by a crutch.

Duchenne's p. See Duchenne's muscular dystrophy, under dystrophy.

Erb-Duchenne p. Paralysis of the upper musculature of an infant's arm (deltoid, biceps, anterior brachial, and long supinator muscles); caused by trauma to the brachial plexus or to the roots of the fifth and sixth cervical nerves during birth. Also called Erb-Duchenne palsy.

global p. Paralysis affecting both sides of the body completely.

hyperkalemic p. Periodic paralysis associated with abnormally high serum potassium levels; attacks start in infancy, are frequent, mild, and last a few minutes to a few hours; autosomal dominant inheritance.

hypokalemic p. Periodic paralysis associated with a fall of serum potassium levels; attacks start in late childhood or adolescence, are relatively severe, and last from hours to days; may be precipitated by consumption of a high carbohydrate meal or alcohol, or by exposure to cold temperatures; autosomal dominant inheritance.

jake p. A form induced by drinking Jamaica ginger (jake). Also called ginger paralysis.

Klumpke's p. Paralysis of the small muscles of the hand resulting from a traction injury to the lower portion of the brachial plexus; most commonly seen in newborns, usually caused by traction during delivery.

Landry's p. See acute ascending paralysis.

obstetric p. Paralysis of the dorsiflexor and evertor muscles of the foot, causing dropfoot, as a result of injury to the common peroneal nerve during childbirth secondary to the position of the patient's legs in the stirrups of the delivery table.

periodic p. Recurrent abrupt episodes of paralysis or extreme muscular weakness lasting from a few minutes to a few days, occurring in otherwise healthy individuals.

postictal p. See Todd's paralysis.

progressive bulbar p. Progressive paralysis and atrophy of the muscles of the tongue, lips, palate, larynx, and pharynx, due to degeneration of the motor nerves innervating them.

pseudobulbar p. Paralysis of the tongue and lips, resulting in speech and swallowing difficulties, often accompanied by spasmodic laughter; caused by brain lesions in the upper motor neurons.

tick p. A rapidly progressive, usually symmetrical paralysis following a tick bite; symptoms include numbness of the extremities, throat, and face, progressing quickly to inability to stand, paralysis of the extremities and trunk, slurred speech, and impaired vision.

Todd's p. Temporary paralysis sometimes following an epileptic seizure and usually lasting from several minutes to several hours after the seizure. Also called postictal paralysis.

vasomotor p. See vasoparalysis.

wasting p. See progressive muscular atrophy, under atrophy.

paralytic (par-ă-lit´ik) **1.** Relating to paralysis. **2.** A person afflicted with paralysis.

paramecium (par-ă-me´she-um) Any of many ciliate protozoans of the genus *Paramecium*, usually slipper-shaped with an oral groove for feeding.

paramedian (par-ă-me´de-an) Near the midline.

paramedic (par-ă-med´ik) A person trained to provide initial medical care in emergency situations.

paramedical (par-ă-med´ĭ-kal) Adjunctive to or relating indirectly to the practice of medicine.

paramenia (par-ă-me´ne-ă) Any disorder or irregularity of menstruation.

parameter (pă-ram´ĕ-ter) In statistics, a characteristic of the population.

parametritis (par-ă-mĕ-tri´tis) Inflammation of the connective tissue adjacent to the uterus and the veins and lymphatics contained in it. Also called pelvic cellulitis.

parametrium (par-ă-me´tre-um) The connective tissue near the uterine cervix, extending upward along the sides of the uterus, between the two layers of the broad ligaments.

paramyloidosis (par-am-ĭ-loi-do´sis) Accumulation of the protein amyloid in lymph nodes; seen in some chronic nonspecific inflammations.

paramyotonia (par-ă-mi-o-to´ne-ă) An atypical form of myotonia, abnormal muscular tonicity and spasms.

Paramyxoviridae (par-ă-mik-so-vir´ĭ-de) Family of viruses that have a variety of shapes but are usually spherical (150 to 300 nm in diameter); contain single-stranded RNA, replicate in cytoplasm, produce cytoplasmic inclusion bodies, and cause cell fusion and hemadsorption; includes viruses causing measles, mumps, and Newcastle disease.

Paramyxovirus (par-ă-mik-so-vi´rus) Genus of viruses (family Paramyxoviridae), which includes the mumps and Newcastle disease viruses. Also called paramyxovirus group.

paranasal (par-ă-na´zal) Located near the nose.

paranoia (par-ă-noi´ă) Mental condition marked by the gradual development of an intricate, sometimes delusionary, system of thinking based on misinterpretation of remarks or events; unlike a paranoid personality disorder, paranoia is limited in scope and does not interfere with other areas of thinking or personality.

paranoiac (par-ă-noi´ak) Relating to or suffering from paranoia.

paranoid (par´ă-noid) Resembling paranoia; overly suspicious.

paranuclear (par-ă-nu´kle-ar) Located near the nucleus.

paranucleus (par-ă-nu´kle-us) An accessory nucleus or a small chromatin body resembling a nucleus, sometimes seen in the cell protoplasm lying just outside of the nucleus.

paraparesis (par-ă-par´ĕ-sis) Slight or partial paralysis of both lower limbs.

paraperitoneal (par-ă-per-ĭ-to-ne´al) Near or alongside the peritoneum.

paraphasia (par-ă-fa´zhă) A disturbance of speech marked by substitution of words and disorganized sentence formation; a mild form of aphasia.

literal p. Substitution of words that are similar in sound to the correct one.

verbal p. Substitution of words that are similar in meaning to the correct one.

paraphimosis (par-ă-fi-mo´sis) Tightness of the prepuce or foreskin, which when retracted behind the glans penis cannot be returned to its normal position.

p. palpebrae A turning outward of the margin of an eyelid (usually the upper one) due to spastic contraction of the orbicularis oculi muscle; usually it is of short duration.

P

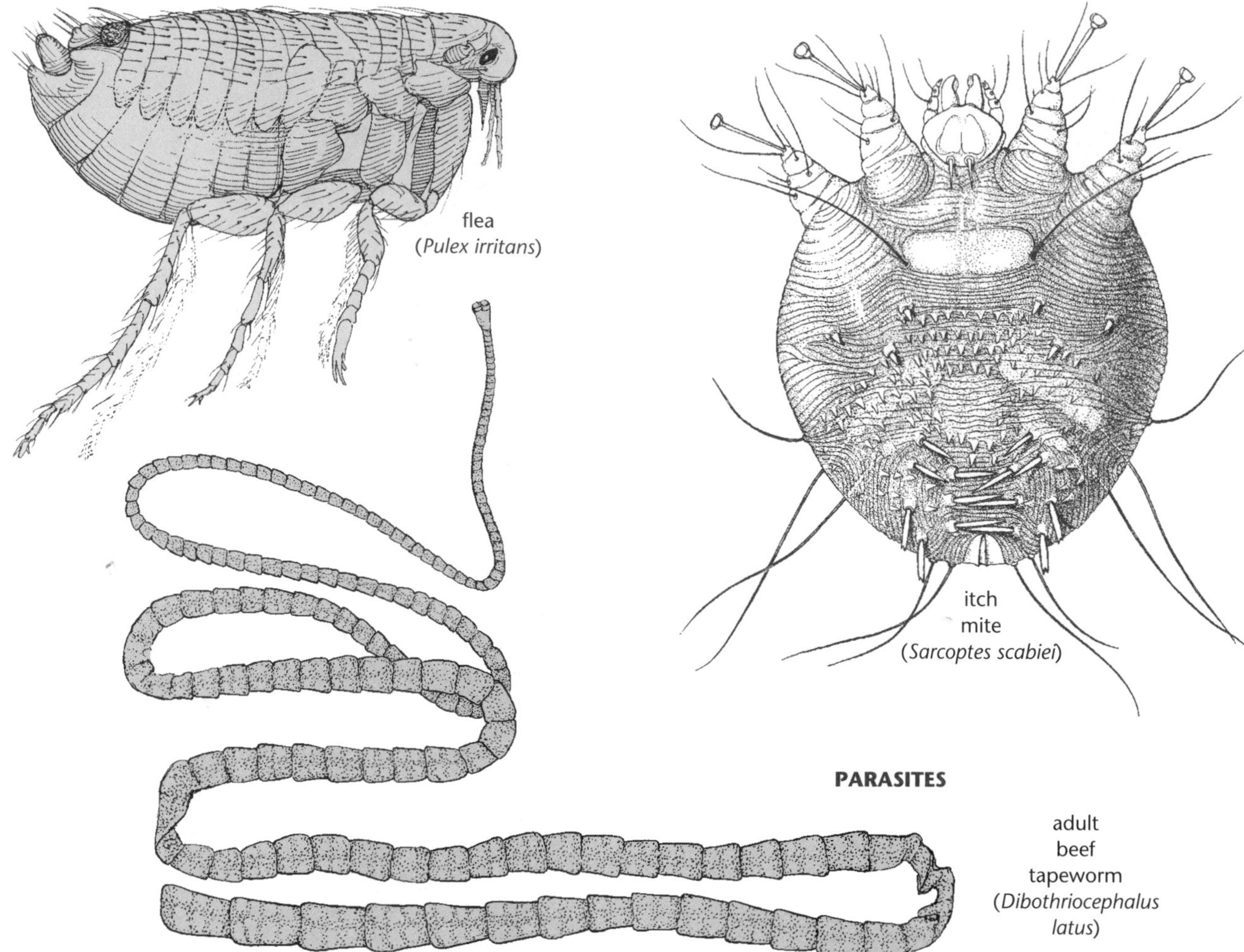

PARASITES

P

paraplegia (par-ă-plē´jă) Paralysis of both legs and, sometimes, the lower trunk.
paraproctitis (par-ă-prok-tī´tis) Inflammation of the tissues surrounding the rectum and anus.
paraprotein (par-ă-pro´ten) An abnormal serum protein, such as a macroglobulin, cryoglobulin, and myeloma protein, characterized by a well defined peak on electrophoresis.
paraproteinemia (par-ă-pro-ten-e´me-ă) A disorder marked by the presence of abnormal proteins in the blood as seen in multiple myeloma.
parapsychology (par-ă-si-kol´ŏ-je) The study of extrasensory phenomena.
paraquat (par´a-kwat) A dipyridilium compound used as a herbicide to eradicate marijuana fields and, in farming, to clear fields instead of "plowing under." A small quantity ingested or absorbed through the skin may cause kidney and liver failure and pulmonary insufficiency.
parasalpingitis (par-ă-sal-pin-jī´tis) Inflammation of the tissues surrounding a uterine tube.
parasite (par´ă-sīt) Any organism that feeds and lives on or in another organism.
parasitic (par-ă-sit´ik) Relating to parasites.
parasiticide (par-ă-sit´ĭ-sīd) Any agent that destroys parasites.
parasitism (par´ă-si-tiz-m) **1.** The mode of existence between a parasite and its host. **2.** An abnormal condition resulting from infestation with parasites.
parasitize (par´ă-si-tīz) To invade and live as a parasite.
parasitology (par-ă-si-tol´ŏ-je) The scientific study of parasites and parasitism; a branch of microbiology.
parasitosis (par-ă-si-to´sis) Infestation with parasites.
paraspadias (par-ă-spa´de-as) Developmental defect of the penis in which the urethral opening is on the side of the normal location.
parasympathetic (par-ă-sim-pă-thet´ik) Relating to the part of the autonomic nervous system concerned with conserving and restoring energy, as by slowing the heart rate.
parasympathomimetic (par-ă-sim-pă-tho-mĭ-met´ik) Producing effects similar to those caused by stimulation of the parasympathetic system.
parasystole (par-ă-sis´to-le) A second automatic cardiac rhythm existing simultaneously with normal sinus rhythm and firing at a regular and uninterrupted rate.
intermittent p. A parasystolic rhythm that is interrupted and subsequently resumes.
parathion (par´ă-thī´on) A highly poisonous organic phosphate insecticide; an inhibitor of cholinesterase.
parathormone (par-ă-thor´mōn) See parathyroid hormone, under hormone.
parathyroid (par-ă-thi´roid) **1.** Located beside the thyroid gland. **2.** See parathyroid gland, under gland.
parathyroidectomy (par-ă-thi-roi-dek´tŏ-me) Surgical removal of one or more parathyroid glands.
parathyrotropic, parathyrotrophic (par-ă-thi-ro-trop´ik, par-ă-thi-ro-trof´ik) Having an effect on the parathyroid glands.
paratope (par´ă-tōp) The region of the surface of an antibody that combines with an antigen. COMPARE: epitope.
paratrichosis (par-ă-tri-ko´sis) Any disorder affecting hair growth.
paratyphlitis (par-ă-tif-li´tis) Inflammation of tissues surrounding the cecum. Sometimes called epityphlitis.
paratyphoid (par-ă-ti´foid) Resembling typhoid (fever or bacillus).
paraumbilical (par-ă-um-bil´ĭ-kal) Situated near the navel (umbilicus).
paraungual (par-ă-ung´gwal) Alongside or near a fingernail or toenail.
paravaginal (par-ă-vaj´ĭ-nal) Near or next to the vagina.
paravertebral (par-ă-ver´tē-bral) Alongside the vertebral column.
parectasis, parectasia (par-ek´tă-sis, par-ek´ta´shă) Excessive distention of a part or organ.
paregoric (par-ĕ-gor´ik) An antiperistaltic compound consisting of powdered opium, anise oil, benzoic acid, camphor, and glycerin in diluted alcohol; principally used in relieving abdominal cramps and diarrhea. Also called camphorated opium tincture.
parencephalon (par-en-sef´ă-lon) The cerebellum.
parenchyma (pă-reng´kĭ-mă) The characteristic tissue of an organ or gland, as distinguished from connective tissue.
parenchymal, parenchymatous (pă-reng´kĭ-mal, par-eng-kim´ă-tus) Relating to the parenchyma.
parenteral (pă-ren´ter-al) **1.** Situated outside the alimentary tract. **2.** Taken into the body in a way other than through the alimentary canal, as by intravenous or intramuscular injection.
paresis (pă-re´sis) **1.** Partial paralysis; weakness. **2.** Neuromuscular disturbances progressing to generalized paralysis occurring 10 to 20 years after initial infection with syphilis.
paresthesia (par-es-the´zhă) Abnormal sensation (e.g., burning, tingling, numbness) perceived without an apparent stimulus.
paresthetic (par-es-thet´ik) Characterized by paresthesia.
paretic (pă-ret´ik) Relating to or suffering from paresis.
pareunia (par-u´ne-ă) See coitus.
paries (par´e-ēz), *pl.* **par´ietes** A wall of a body cavity, as of the chest.
parietal (pă-rī´ĕ-tal) Pertaining to the wall of a cavity.
parieto-occipital (pă-rī´ĕ-to ok-sip´ĭ-tal) Relating

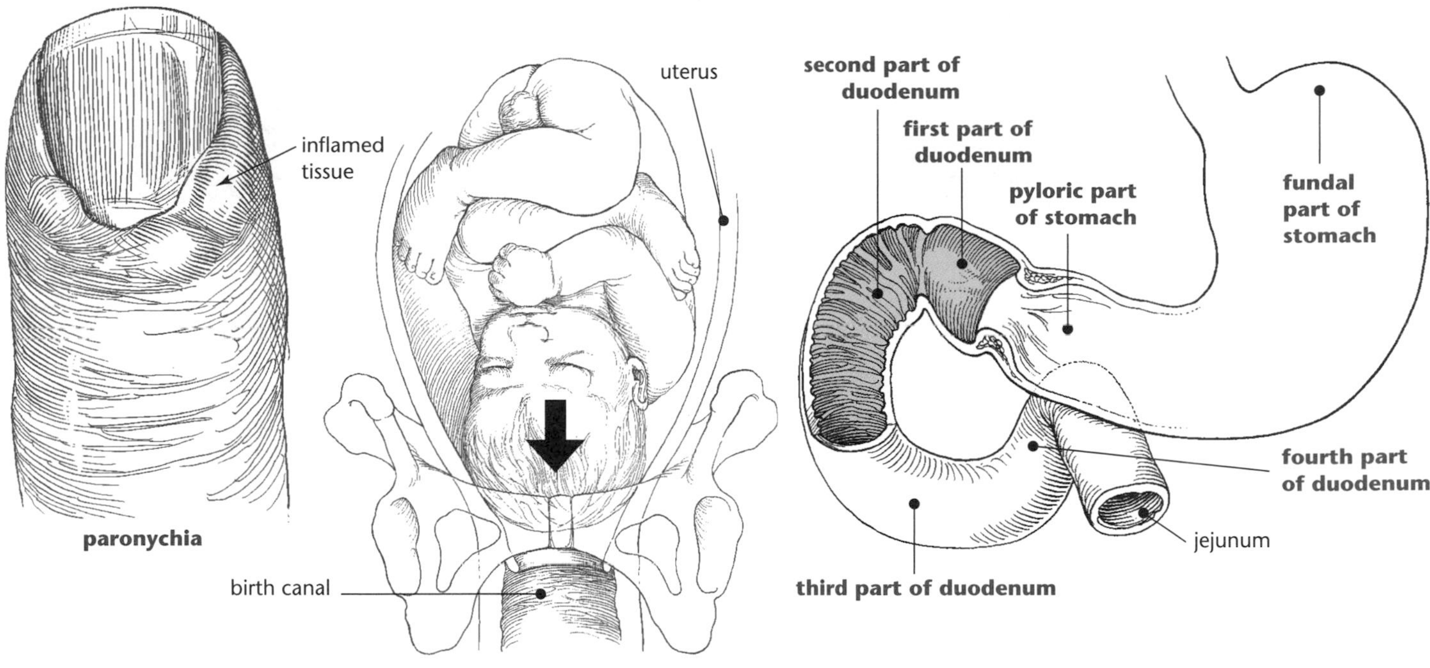

to the parietal and occipital bones of the skull or lobes of the cerebrum.

Paris green (par′is grēn) An insecticide composed of copper acetate and copper meta-arsenite.

parity (par′ĭ-te) The state of a woman in respect to having given birth to children.

parkinsonian (par-kin-sōn′e-an) Relating to Parkinson's disease.

parkinsonism (par′kin-sun-izm) Disturbance of motor function marked by muscular rigidity, stooped posture, tremors, and a progressively shortened accelerated gait; seen in conditions that damage the dopaminergic nerve cells of the substantia nigra (in the brain), principally Parkinson's disease; also seen in carbon monoxide poisoning, heavy metal toxicity, and sometimes after use of neurologic drugs. Also called shaking palsy; trembling palsy.

Parkinson's disease (par′kin-sunz dĭ-zēz′) A slowly progressing disease in which pigmented cells of the brainstem deteriorate and there is a deficiency of the neurotransmitter dopamine; marked by increased rigidity of muscles, resting tremors, slowness of movement, stooped walking posture, and a quick shuffling gait; cause is unknown; onset usually occurs after 50 years of age. Also called idiopathic Parkinson's disease; paralysis agitans.

paroniria (par-o-nī′re-ă) Terrifying dreams causing sleep disturbance. Also called morbid dreaming.

p. ambulans Morbid dreaming while sleep-walking.

paronychia (par-o-nik′e-ă) Inflammation of the tissues around a nail. Also called whitlow.

paroophoron (par-o-of′ŏ-ron) Embryonic remnants of the excretory portion of the mesonephros; consist of a group of coiled tubules in the broad ligament, between the epoophoron and the uterus; best seen in the child.

parosmia (par-oz′me-ă) Any disorder of the sense of smell, especially a perverted sense of smell as may occur in some cases of schizophrenia, uncinate gyrus lesions, and hysterias.

parotid (pă-rot′id) Situated near the ear, as the parotid salivary gland.

parotidectomy (pă-rot-ĭ-dek′to-me) Surgical removal of the parotid gland.

parotitis, parotiditis (par-o-tī′tis, pă-rot-ĭ-dī′tis) Inflammation of a parotid gland.

epidemic p. See mumps.

parous (par′us) Having borne one or more children.

parovarian (par-o-va′re-an) Situated near an ovary.

paroxysm (par′ok-siz-m) **1.** A sudden onset or recurrence of symptoms of a disease. **2.** A convulsion.

paroxysmal (par-ok-siz′mal) Occurring in or of the nature of paroxysms.

pars (parz), *pl.* **partes** A particular portion of a structure; a part.

p. flaccida The upper, flaccid portion of the eardrum (tympanic membrane).

p. infundibularis See pars tuberalis.

p. tensa The lower, taut portion of the eardrum (tympanic membrane).

p. tuberalis The upward expansion of the adenohypophysis that wraps around the infundibular stalk. Also called pars infundibularis.

part (part) A portion.

abdominal p. of esophagus The portion of the esophagus between the diaphragm and the stomach.

alveolar p. of mandible The upper part of the body of the mandible containing sockets for the roots of the lower teeth.

alveolar p. of maxilla The lower part of the maxilla containing sockets for the roots of the upper teeth.

bony p. of nasal septum The nasal septum composed of the perpendicular plate of the ethmoid bone and the vomer.

cardiac p. of stomach The part of the stomach that includes and immediately follows the gastric (cardiac) opening of the esophagus.

cervical p. of esophagus The part of the esophagus in the neck extending from the downward continuation of the pharynx (at the lower border of the cricoid cartilage) to the level of the first ribs.

first p. of duodenum The shortest part of the duodenum adjacent to the pylorus of the stomach; it contains the duodenal ampulla and forms the superior flexure of the duodenum.

flaccid p. of eardrum See pars flaccida, under pars.

fourth p. of duodenum The ascending terminal part of the duodenum extending from the third part of the duodenum to the beginning of the jejunum at the duodenojejunal flexure.

fundal p. of stomach The part of the stomach to the left of and above the cardiac orifice.

membranous p. of interventricular septum The small rounded upper part of the septum separating the ventricles of the heart.

membranous p. of male urethra The shortest and narrowest part of the male urethra, extending through the urogenital diaphragm, from the apex of the prostate to the bulb of the penis.

membranous p. of nasal septum The thickened skin and subcutaneous tissue of the nasal septum at the apex of the nose, immediately under the cartilaginous part of the septum.

muscular p. of interventricular septum The thick muscular part comprising most of the septum separating the ventricles of the heart.

presenting p. In obstetrics, the portion of the fetus closest to the birth canal and which is felt through the cervix on vaginal examination; the presenting part indicates the position of the fetus in the uterus during labor.

prostatic p. of male urethra The portion of the male urethra within the prostate gland; it is the widest and most dilatable part of the urethra.

pyloric p. of stomach The distal part of the stomach consisting of the pyloric antrum, pyloric canal, and pyloric valve (sphincter); the notch on the lesser curvature of the stomach marks the boundary between the pyloric part and body of the stomach.

second p. of duodenum The descending part of the duodenum extending from the superior flexure to the inferior flexure; it receives secretions from the bile and pancreatic ducts.

spongy p. of male urethra The portion of the urethra within the corpus spongiosum of the penis; extends from the end of the membranous urethra to the end of the penis; has two dilatations, one near the membranous urethra (intrabulbar fossa), the other near its external urethral orifice (navicular fossa).

tense p. of eardrum See pars tensa, under pars.

third p. of duodenum The horizontal part of the duodenum extending from the inferior duodenal flexure to the ascending fourth part of the duodenum.

partes aequales (par′tēz e-kwa′lēs) (part. aeq.) Latin for equal parts.

parthenogenesis (par-thĕ-no-jen′ĕ-sis) Reproduction of organisms in which the female reproduces without fecundation by the male.

particle (par′tĭ-kl) **1.** An extremely small part, portion, or division of matter. **2.** One of the minute subdivisions of matter (e.g., an electron).

alpha p. A positively charged particle ejected from the nucleus of a radioactive atom and consisting of two neutrons and two protons (helium nucleus).

beta p. An electron, either positively (positron) or negatively (negatron) charged, which is emitted from an atomic nucleus during beta decay of a radionuclide.

Dane p. A double-shelled particle about 42 nm in diameter constituting the intact virion of hepatitis B. Composed of a DNA-containing core (28 nm in diameter) and a lipoprotein outer coat (7 nm thick); the antigen on the surface is termed hepatitis B surface antigen (HBs Ag) and that in its core is hepatitis B core antigen (HBc Ag).

elementary p. 1. See platelet. **2.** One of many knoblike repeating units attached to the matrix side of the inner membrane of the mitochondrion; it has a 90 Å spherical head, spaced at approximately 100 Å intervals, and is connected by a 50 Å-long stalklike structure to a baseplate in the membrane itself. Also

P

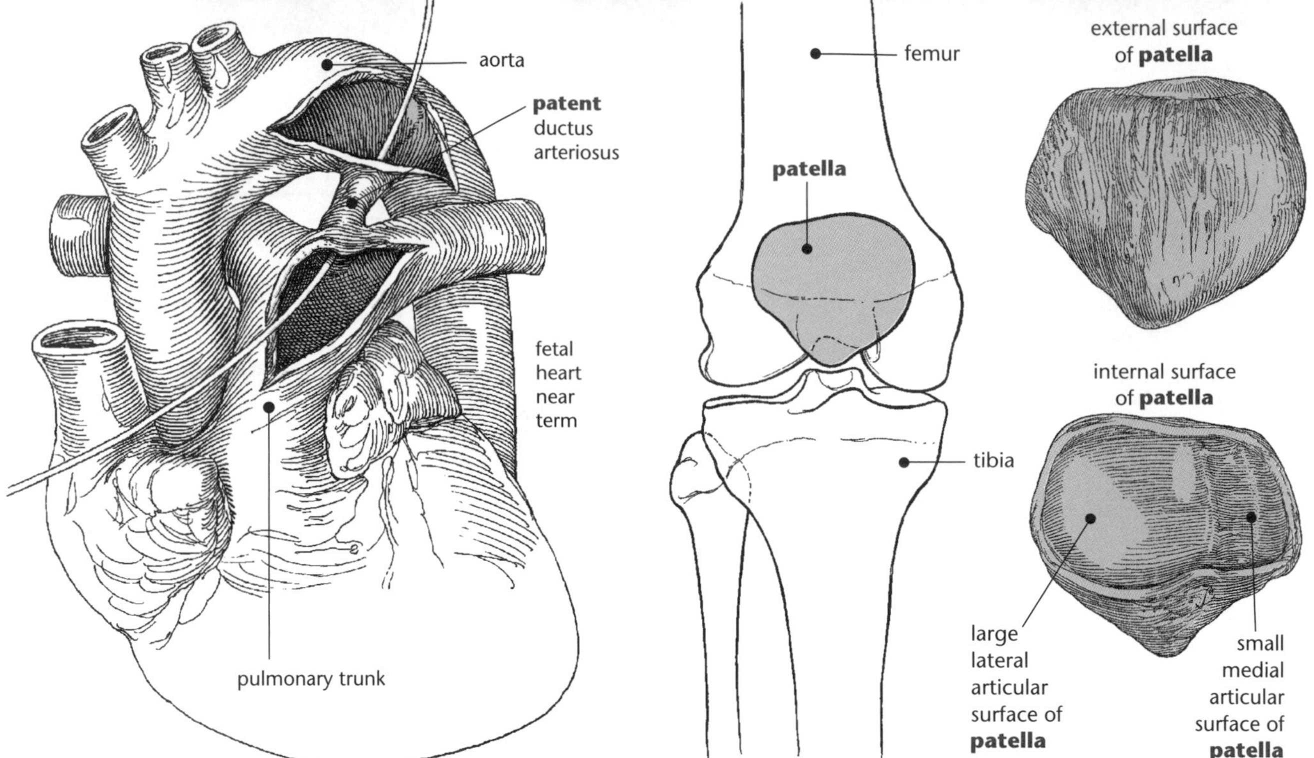

called elementary body.

particulate (par-tik′u-lāt) Relating to, or composed of, fine particles.

parturient (par-tu′re-ent) Relating to childbirth.

parturifacient (par-tu-re-fa′shent) Inducing labor.

parturition (par-tu-rish′un) The process of giving birth; childbirth.

partus (par′tus) Parturition.

parvicellular (par-vĭ-sel′u-lar) Pertaining to or composed of exceptionally small cells.

Parvovirus (par-vo-vi′rus) Genus of DNA viruses (family Parvoviridae) which includes the virus causing erythema infectiosum (fifth disease).

pascal (pas-kal) (Pa) The SI unit of pressure; a force of 1 newton per square meter.

passage (pas′ij) **1.** The act of passing. **2.** A channel, opening, or path along which something may pass. **3.** A discharge (e.g., of urine or feces).

nasopharyngeal p. The passage in the posterior part of the nasal cavity from the back part of the turbinates to the choanae. Also called nasopharyngeal meatus.

P

Passavant's cushion (pas′ă-vants koosh′un) See Passavant's ridge, under ridge.

passive (pas′iv) Submissive; inert; not initiating.

passivity (pă-siv′ĭ-te) **1.** The inertness exhibited by certain metals under conditions in which chemical activity should take place, due to the formation of a coating of peroxide, oxygen, or salt. **2.** In dentistry, the state of inactivity of the oral structures when a removable partial denture is in place but not used in mastication. **3.** Passivism, a passive or submissive attitude or behavior.

paste (pāst) A soft semisolid substance.

dermatologic p. Pharmaceutical preparation composed of starch, sulfur, dextrin, zinc oxide, or calcium carbonate mixed with glycerin, petrolatum, or soft soap and containing antiseptics for external use.

resorcinol p., mild A bactericidal and fungicidal paste composed of 10% resorcinol, 25% zinc oxide, 25% starch, and 40% light liquid petrolatum. Also called Lassar's mild resorcin paste.

zinc oxide p. with salicylic acid Mixture of 2% salicylic acid in paste of zinc oxide; used as an antiseptic and soothing agent. Also called Lassar's zinc paste with salicylic acid.

Pasteurella (pas-tĕ-rel′ă) A genus (family Pasteurellaceae) of round, ellipsoidal, or rod-shaped gram-negative bacteria that usually occur singly.

P. pestis See *Yersinia pestis*.

P. tularensis See *Francisella tularensis*.

pasteurellosis (pas-ter-ĕ-lo′sis) Infection with bacteria of the genus *Pasteurella*; it includes hemorrhagic septicemia, tularemia, plague, and pseudotuberculosis.

pasteurization (pas-ter-ĭ-za′shun) The process of destroying or retarding the growth of bacteria in milk and other liquids, without destroying the flavor of the product, by heating the liquid to a moderate degree (60–70°C) for a sustained period of time (30 minutes) rather than by boiling it quickly.

pasteurize (pas′ter-īz) To subject milk or other liquids to pasteurization.

past-pointing (past-poin-ting) Incoordination of voluntary movements characterized by inability to place a finger on some designated site (the finger overshoots its target).

patch (pach) A small area or section of a surface differing from or contrasting with the whole.

cotton wool p.'s Coagulated exudates from the retinal capillaries, appearing as white fluffy areas on the retina. Also called cotton-wool spots.

herald p. A solitary large lesion appearing before (sometimes days or weeks) the general eruption of pityriasis rosea.

mucous p. A moist, yellowish lesion on the mucous membrane of the mouth or external genitalia, usually seen in secondary syphilis.

Peyer's p.'s Small whitish masses of lymphoid tissue situated in the mucous and submucous layers of the small intestine.

smoker's p. See leukoplakia.

patella (pă-tel′ă) A flat, triangular bone embedded in the combined tendons of the extensor muscles of the leg, at the front of the knee joint; the largest sesamoid bone of the body. Also called kneecap.

patellapexy (pă-tel-ă-pek′se) The surgical fixation of the patella to the distal end of the femur.

patellar (pă-tel′ar) Relating to the patella.

patellectomy (pat-ĕ-lek′tŏ-me) Surgical removal of the patella.

patency (pa′ten-se) The state of being open.

patent (pa′tent) **1.** Open; unobstructed. **2.** Apparent.

path (path) The course taken by a nerve impulse.

pathfinder (path′fīnd-er) A thin cylindrical instrument (bougie) for locating strictures in tubular structures.

pathogen (path′ŏ-jen) Any microorganism or substance capable of causing disease.

pathogenesis (path-o-jen′ĕ-sis) The origin and development of disease. Formerly called nosogenesis.

pathogenic, pathogenetic (path-o-jen′ik) Causing disease.

pathogenicity (path-o-jĕ-nis′ĭ-te) Disease-producing capability.

pathogenism (path-o-jen′iz-m) The relationship between a pathogen and its host.

pathognomonic (path-og-no-mon′ik) A special characteristic of a disease; denoting one or more typical symptoms of a disease.

pathologic (path-o-loj′ik) Relating to disease.

pathologist (pă-thol′ŏ-jist) A specialist in pathology.

speech p. A professional with specialized training in speech pathology.

pathology (pă-thol′ŏ-je) The branch of medicine concerned with the study of disease in all its aspects (its nature, causes, development, and consequences).

anatomic p. The study of diseased or injured tissues. Also called pathologic anatomy.

speech p. The study of all aspects of functional and organic speech and language disorders, with particular reference to the underlying cause, evaluation, and treatment.

pathomimesis (path-o-mi-me′sis) Imitation of disease, whether intentional or unconscious.

pathoneurosis (path-o-nu-ro′sis) Abnormal preoccupation with disease.

pathophobia (path-o-fo′be-ă) An abnormal fear of disease.

pathophysiology (path-o-fiz-e-ol′ŏ-je) The study of pathologic alteration in bodily function, as distinguished from structural defects.

pathopsychology (path-o-si-kol′ŏ-je) The study of abnormal psychic processes from the point of view of general psychology.

pathway (path′wa) **1.** In neurology, the linked neurons through which an impulse is conducted to the cerebral cortex (afferent pathway), or from the brain to the skeletal musculature (efferent pathways). **2.** The series of metabolic reactions that convert one biochemical substance into another.

direct oxidative p. See pentose phosphate pathway.

Embden-Meyerhof p. In carbohydrate metabolism, the series of anaerobic reactions that convert glucose or glycogen to pyruvate and lactate, releasing energy in the form of adenosine triphosphate (ATP).

pentose phosphate p. In carbohydrate metabolism, a pathway of hexose oxidation whereby glucose 6-phosphate generates five-carbon sugars; plays major role in the production of NADPH for reductive biosyntheses (e.g., of fatty acids). Also called pentose shunt; monophosphate shunt; direct oxidative pathway.

patient (pa′shent) (pt) A person who is under medical treatment.

patrilineal (pat-rĭ-lin′e-al) Inherited through the paternal line; derived from the father.

patten (pat′ĭn) A support worn under one shoe to equalize the length of both legs.

pattern (pat′ern) **1.** An arrangement or design. **2.** In dentistry, a form used to develop a mold from which

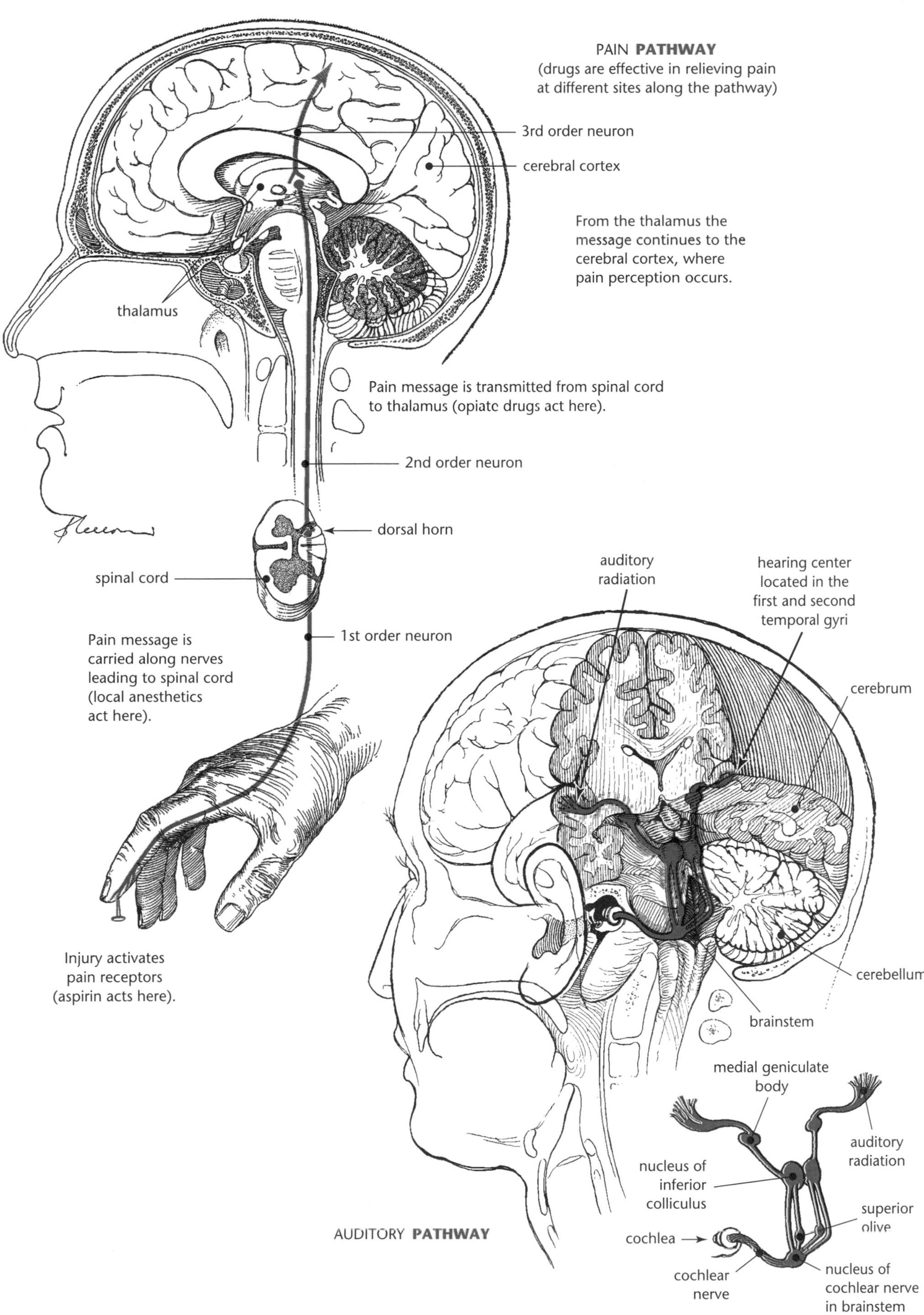
PAIN PATHWAY
(drugs are effective in relieving pain at different sites along the pathway)
3rd order neuron
cerebral cortex
From the thalamus the message continues to the cerebral cortex, where pain perception occurs.
thalamus
Pain message is transmitted from spinal cord to thalamus (opiate drugs act here).
2nd order neuron
dorsal horn
spinal cord
1st order neuron
Pain message is carried along nerves leading to spinal cord (local anesthetics act here).
Injury activates pain receptors (aspirin acts here).
auditory radiation
hearing center located in the first and second temporal gyri
cerebrum
cerebellum
brainstem
medial geniculate body
auditory radiation
nucleus of inferior colliculus
superior olive
cochlea
cochlear nerve
nucleus of cochlear nerve in brainstem
AUDITORY PATHWAY

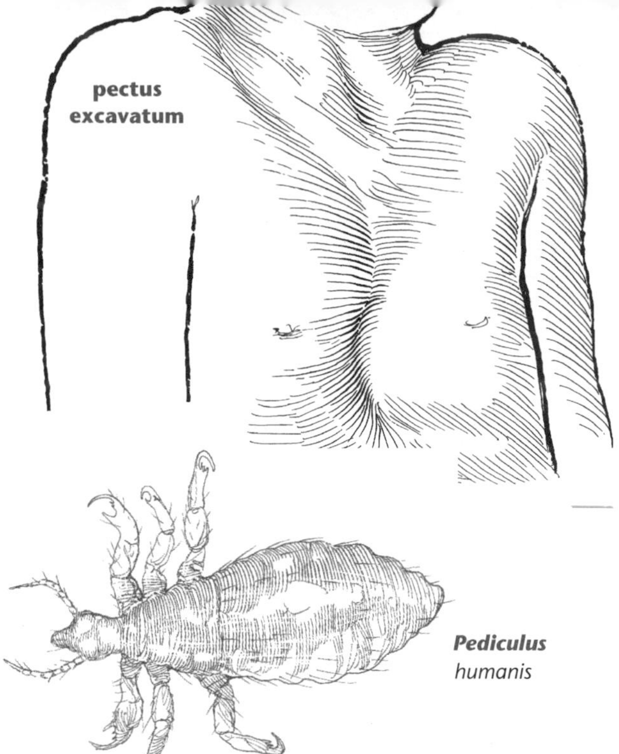

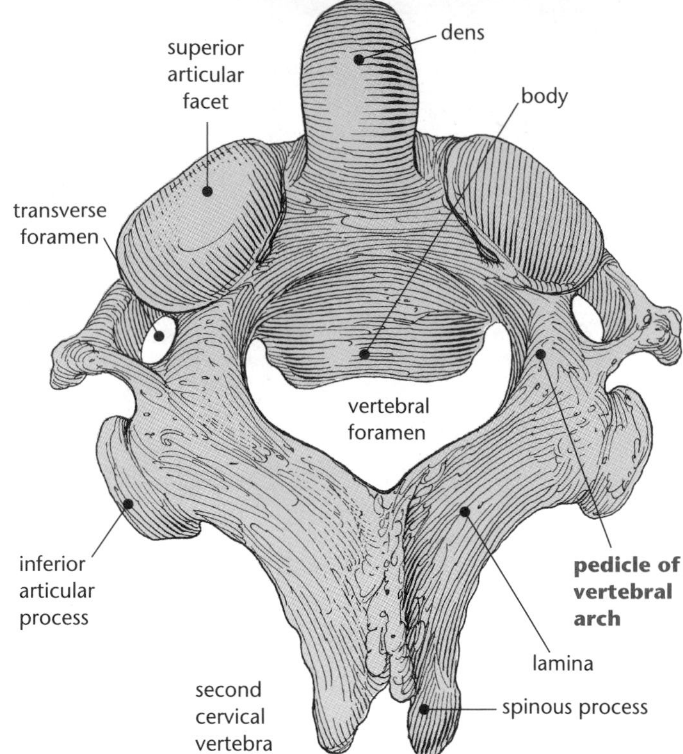

a restoration is produced, such as an inlay or denture.

butterfly p. Pattern seen on chest x-ray films; consists of symmetrical opacities on both lungs, sparing their periphery; usually caused by pulmonary edema.

honeycomb p. Pattern seen on x-ray films or computed tomography (CT) images of the chest; consists of dense, round shadows, usually at the base of the lung; associated with progressive fibrosis of lung tissue.

juvenile p. Precordial T-wave inversion in the electrocardiogram; a persistent juvenile pattern sometimes seen in healthy adults.

miliary p. Chest x-ray pattern consisting of minute round opacities, typical of blood-disseminated tuberculosis.

reticulonodular p. Chest x-ray pattern consisting of a netlike mesh with tiny masses at the fiber intersections.

wax p. An exact wax model of lost tooth structure which, when invested and burned out, will produce a mold in which a casting may be made.

patulous (pat´u-lus) Widely open; spread widely apart.

pause (pawz) A temporary stop.

compensatory p. In cardiology, the pause following a premature beat, usually a ventricular extrasystole; its duration compensates for the short interval preceding the heartbeat, so that the total heart rate is unchanged.

sinus p. In cardiology, spontaneous interruption in the regular sinus rhythm of the heart marked by a long-lasting absence of sinus P waves; thought to result from a high degree of S-A block or sinus arrest.

pearl (perl) **1.** A small hard mass. **2.** A small firm mass of mucus seen in the sputum of patients undergoing an attack of asthma.

enamel p. See enameloma.

epithelial p.'s See keratin pearls.

Epstein's p.'s Minute white masses of epithelium normally seen on the palate of newborns.

gouty p. Sodium urate concretion, seen on the ear cartilage of individuals with gout.

keratin p.'s Small aggregations of neoplastic tissue composed of compressed polygonal cells, frequently seen in squamous cell carcinoma. Also called epithelial pearls.

peau (po´) French for skin.

p. d'orange A dimpled appearance of the skin, like that of an orange; seen in some forms of breast cancer.

pecten (pek´ten) **1.** Any anatomic structure resembling a comb. **2.** A narrow area in the middle of the anal canal.

pectin (pek´tin) A vegetable mucilage found in abundance in certain fruits and roots; a purified form is used in pharmaceutical preparations.

pectinate (pek´tĭ-nāt) Comb-shaped.

pectineal (pek-tin´e-al) Relating to any comb-shaped structure.

pectoral (pek´tŏ-ral) Pertaining to the chest.

pectoralgia (pek-to-ral´jhă) Pain in the chest.

pectoriloquy (pek-to-ril´o-kwe) Transmission of the voice through the chest wall, audible through a stethoscope; commonly indicative of consolidation of underlying lung tissue (e.g., in pneumonia). Also called pectorophony.

pectorophony (pek-to-rof´o-ne) See pectoriloquy.

pectus (pek´tus), *pl.* **pec´tora** The chest; especially the anterior wall.

p. carinatum Deformity of the anterior chest wall marked by protrusion of the sternum (breastbone), thought to be due to unbalanced or excessive growth of the cartilages. Also called pigeon breast; keel breast; keel chest.

p. excavatum Depression of the sternum (breastbone) and rib cartilages; believed to be caused by a short central tendon and muscular imbalance of the diaphragm. Also called funnel chest.

pedal (ped´al) Relating to the feet.

pederasty (ped´ĕr-as-te) Homosexual anal intercourse, especially when practiced on a boy.

pediatric (pe-de-at´rik) Relating to the study and treatment of children's diseases.

pediatrician (pe-de-ă-trĭ-shun) A physician who specializes in pediatrics.

pediatrics (pe-de-at´riks) (Ped) The branch of medicine concerned with the care and development of children and the treatment of their diseases.

pedicel (ped´ĭ-sel) The secondary process of a podocyte that helps form the visceral capsule of a renal corpuscle. Also called foot process; foot plate.

pedicle (ped´ĭ-kl) **1.** A stalk attaching a tumor to healthy tissue. **2.** A tubular skin graft left temporarily attached to the donor site, through which the graft receives its blood supply. **3.** An anatomic structure resembling a short stem.

p. of vertebral arch One of two bars of bone extending backward from the bodies of each vertebra and forming the arch surrounding the spinal cord.

pedicular (pe-dik´u-lar) Relating to lice.

pediculicide (pe-dik´u-lĭ-sīd) Any agent or chemical capable of destroying lice.

pediculosis (pe-dik-u-lo´sis) The state of being infested with lice.

p. capitis Infestation of the scalp with lice.

p. corporis The presence of lice on the body or clothing (where they usually remain until feeding time).

p. pubis The presence of lice on the pubic hair or neighboring parts of the body; the infesting louse is usually a species of *Phthirus* (crab louse), not *Pediculus*; therefore, the condition is more correctly termed phthiriasis pubis.

Pediculus (pe-dik´u-lus) Genus of lice of the family Pediculidae. Includes: *P. humanus*, a blood sucking species infesting humans; vector of relapsing fever, trench fever, and typhus. *P. humanus capitis*, a species that infests the scalp of humans and attaches its eggs (nits) to hairs. Also called head louse. *P. humanus corporis*, a species that infests the body of humans (as distinguished from the head and limbs). Also called body louse.

P. pubis See *Phthirus pubis*, under *Phthirus*.

pediculus (pe-dik´u-lus), *pl.* **pedic´uli** **1.** Parasite of the genus *Pediculus*. Also called louse. **2.** Pedicle; stalk.

pedicure (ped´ĭ-kūr) **1.** Care and treatment of the feet. **2.** Cosmetic care of the feet, especially of the toenails.

pedigree (ped´ĭ-gre) **1.** In genetics, a diagram setting forth an individual's ancestral history. Also called family tree. **2.** In medical genetics, a graphic representation of a family history, indicating family members affected with the disease of concern and their relationship to the affected member (proband) who first drew attention to the family for study of the trait.

pedodontics (pe-do-don´tiks) The branch of dentistry dealing with the preventive care and treatment of children's teeth.

pedodontist (pe-do-don´tist) A specialist in pedodontics.

pedology (pe-dol´ŏ-je) A branch of biology and of sociology that studies the behavior and development of children.

pedophilia (pe-do-fil´e-ă) Engaging in sexual fantasies and activities with children as a repeatedly preferred or exclusive method by an adult.

peduncle (pē-dung´kl) **1.** A large stalklike mass of nerve fibers connecting a suprasegmental structure to other portions of the nervous system. **2.** The narrow part of a structure serving as support or attachment.

cerebellar p.'s Three pairs of thick bundles of nerve fibers interconnecting each side of the cerebellum with the brainstem (medulla oblongata, pons, and midbrain): *Inferior cerebellar p.'s*, a thick bundle of largely afferent nerve fibers of the medulla oblongata that interconnect the cerebellum with the medulla oblongata. Also called restiform body. *Middle cerebellar p.*, the largest of the three cerebellar peduncles; it interconnects the cerebellum with the dorsolateral region of the pons. Also called pontine cerebellar peduncle. *Superior cerebellar p.*, a large, flat bundle of chiefly efferent nerve fibers inter-

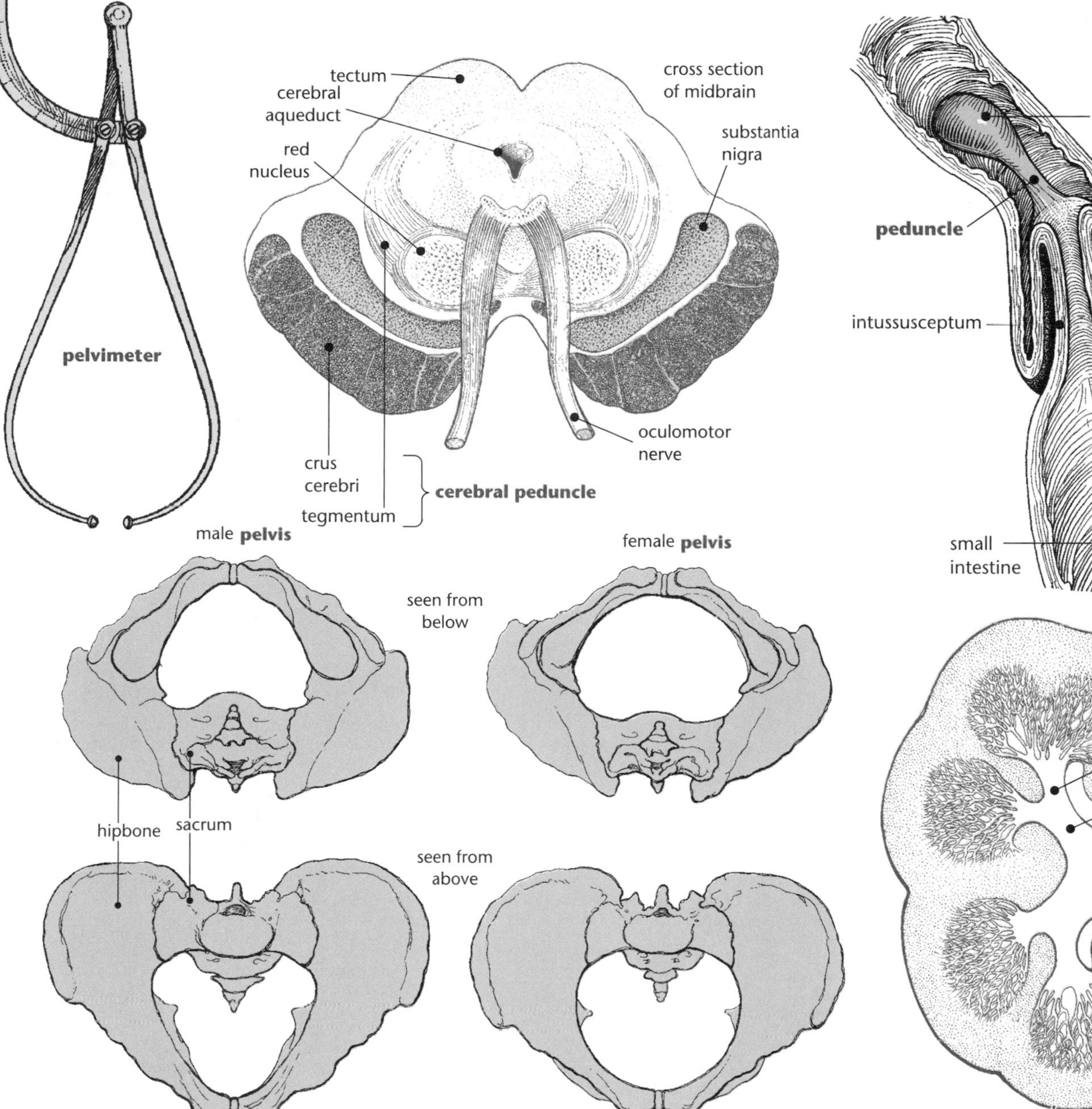

connecting the cerebellar hemisphere with the midbrain and thalamus. Also called cranial cerebellar peduncle.

cerebral p. The part of the midbrain in front of the cerebral aqueduct, composed of the tegmentum (dorsal part) and crus cerebri (ventral part).

cranial cerebellar p. See cerebellar peduncle, superior.

p. of the pineal body The dorsal stalk of the pineal body. Also called habenula.

pontine cerebellar p. See cerebellar peduncle, middle.

thalamic p. The fibers passing between the thalamus and cerebral cortex (subdivided into anterior, posterior, superior, and inferior peduncles).

pedunculate, pedunculated (pē-dung´ku-lāt, pē-dung´ku-lāt-ed) Having a stalk or peduncle.

pedunculotomy (pē-dung-ku-lot´ŏ-me) Surgical incision of the cerebral peduncle.

peel (pēl) To remove.

face p. Removal of facial blemishes with a chemical agent.

peliosis (pe-le-o´sis) See purpura.

pellagra (pĕ-lag´ră) Nutritional disorder caused by niacin deficiency; marked by skin lesions, diarrhea, and mental disorders or abnormalities.

pellagroid (pĕ-lag´roid) Resembling pellagra.

pellagrous (pĕ-lag´rus) Relating to pellagra.

pellicle (pel´ĭ-kl) **1.** Thin membrane or cuticle. **2.** A film on the surface of a liquid. **3.** A firm mass formed by some fungi on the surface of a liquid medium.

pelvic (pel´vik) Relating to the pelvis.

pelvicephalometry (pel-vĭ-sef-ă-lom´ĕ-tre) Measurement of the diameters of the fetal head in relation to those of the mother's pelvis.

pelvic inflammatory disease (pel´vik in-flam´ă-to-re dĭ-zēz´) (PID) Inflammation of the female reproductive organs and associated structures, often caused by sexually transmitted diseases; may also occur after abortion, miscarriage, or childbirth.

pelvilithotomy (pel-ve-lĭ-thot´ŏ-me) See pyelolithotomy.

pelvimeter (pel-vim´ĕ-ter) A caliper-type instrument for measuring the diameters of the pelvis.

pelvimetry (pel-vim´ĕ-tre) The measurement of the pelvic diameters.

x-ray p. Pelvimetry performed by application of a grid to roentgenograms of the pelvic bones.

pelviotomy (pel-ve-ot´ŏ-me) **1.** Surgical division of the pubic joint. **2.** Incision into the pelvis of the kidney.

pelvis (pel´vis), *pl.* **pel´ves** **1.** A basin-shaped skeletal structure formed by the two hipbones, the sacrum, and the coccyx; it supports the spinal column and rests on the lower limbs. **2.** A funnel-like dilatation (e.g., pelvis of the kidney).

android p. Female pelvis with characteristics of a typical male pelvis. Also called funnel-shaped pelvis; brachypellic pelvis.

brachypellic p. See android pelvis.

contracted p. Pelvis with diminished diameters of the inlet, outlet, or midpelvis, or a combination of the three.

false p. See major pelvis.

funnel-shaped p. See android pelvis.

greater p. See major pelvis.

gynecoid p. The average female pelvis, having a rounded oval shape.

lesser p. See minor pelvis.

major p. The expanded portion of the pelvis above and in front of the pelvic brim. Also called false pelvis; greater pelvis.

minor p. The portion of the pelvis situated below and behind the pelvic brim. Also called true pelvis.

renal p. The funnel-shaped dilatation formed by the junction of the calices of the kidney through which urine passes into the ureter. Also called pelvis of kidney; pelvis of ureter.

p. of kidney See renal pelvis.

true p. See minor pelvis.

p. of ureter See renal pelvis.

pelvisacral (pel-vĭ-sa´kral) Relating to the pelvis and the sacrum.

pelviscope (pel´vĭ-skōp) An illuminated instrument for examining the interior of the pelvis.

pelvospondylitis ossificans (pel-vo-spon-dĭ-li´tis o-sif´ĭ-kanz) The presence of bony deposits between the sacrum and lumbar vertebrae.

pemphigoid (pem´fĭ-goid) An eruption of soft blebs resembling those of pemphigus vulgaris.

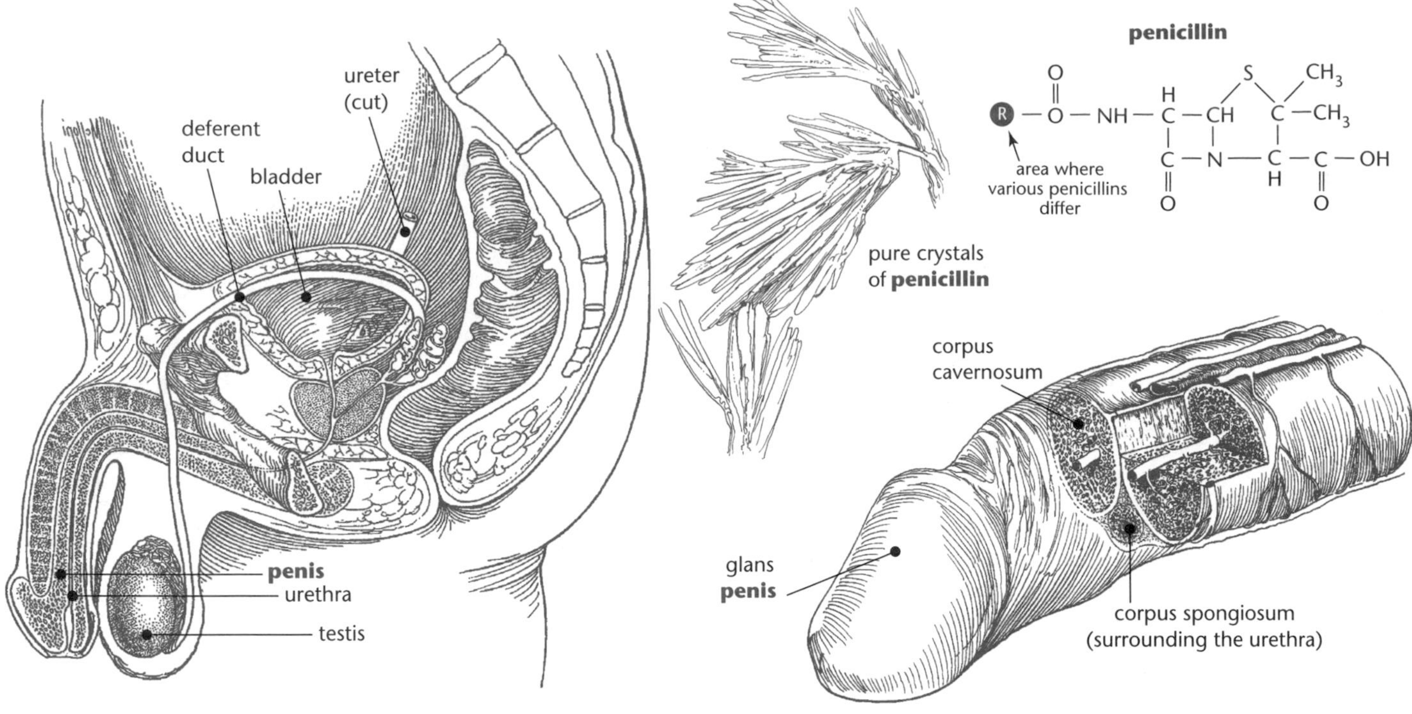

bullous p. (BP) Autoimmune skin disease typically affecting elderly people; marked by large blisters (4–8 cm in diameter) on the inner thighs, forearms, and lower abdomen; caused by circulating antibodies depositing along the deepest layer of the skin.

pemphigus (pem´fĭ-gus) **1.** A group of autoimmune skin diseases typically affecting people 40 to 60 years of age; characterized by blister formation due to the presence of circulating antibody reacting against certain tissue components of the skin. **2.** Pemphigus vulgaris.

p. erythematosus A localized mild form of pemphigus foliaceus typically affecting the sides of the face. Also called Senear-Usher syndrome.

familial benign chronic p. A blistering dermatosis; recurrent eruption of blisters that become scaling and crusted lesions with vesicular borders, predominantly on the neck, groin, and axillary regions; autosomal dominant inheritance.

p. foliaceus (PF) A mild form affecting primarily the face, scalp, and upper trunk; marked by formation of extremely superficial blisters that typically leave only slight redness and crusting after rupturing.

p. vegetans A rare form characterized by development of large, moist, rough plaques studded with pustules over erupted blisters.

p. vulgaris (PV) A chronic, severe, potentially fatal disease, marked by formation of large, flaccid, superficial blisters in the oral mucosa, scalp, face, trunk, and pressure points; the easily ruptured blisters leave shallow, crusted erosions.

Pendred's syndrome (pen´dredz sin´drōm) Congenital deafness and goiter with or without hypothyroidism; an autosomal recessive inheritance.

penectomy (pe-nek´tŏ-me) Surgical removal of the penis. Also called phallectomy.

penetrance (pen´ĕ-trans) In genetics, the frequency with which a heritable trait is manifested in individuals known to carry the gene for the trait.

penetrometer (pen-ĕ-trom´ĕ-ter) Device for measuring the penetrating power of x rays.

penicillamine (pen-ĭ-sil-a´mēn) A degradation product of penicillin; a chelating agent used in the treatment of hepatolenticular degeneration (Wilson's disease) and lead poisoning.

penicillin (pen-ĭ-sil´in) Antibiotic compound derived from the fungus *Penicillium notatum* (natural penicillin) or produced synthetically; it suppresses synthesis of bacterial cell walls, which results in eventual death to the cell when the penicillin-poisoned bacterium outgrows its cell wall.

benzathine p. G suspension Aqueous suspension of a salt formed by 1 mol of an ammonium base and 2 mol of penicillin G. Administered intramuscularly, it is very slowly absorbed and provides sustained blood levels of penicillin up to one month; Bicillin®.

p. V Oral semisynthetic penicillin; it is absorbed from the gastrointestinal tract. Also called phenoxymethyl penicillin.

penicillinase (pen-ĭ-sil´ĭ-nās) Enzyme produced by certain bacteria (e.g., some strains of staphylococcus) that renders penicillin inactive.

penicillus (pen-ĭ-sil´us), *pl.* **penicil´li** A small brushlike structure; a tuft.

Penicillium (pen-ĭ-sil´e-um) A genus of fungi; a saprophytic mold that yields several antibiotic substances.

P. notatum An ascomycete fungus from which penicillin and notatin are derived.

penile (pe´nīl) Relating to the penis.

penis (pe´nis) The male organ of copulation and urination; composed of three columns of erectile tissue, two dorsolateral (corpora cavernosa) and one medial (corpus spongiosum) which contains the urethra and forms the glans penis at the end.

pennate (pen´āt) Resembling a feather. Also called penniform.

penniform (pen´ĭ-form) See pennate.

pentabasic (pen-tă-ba´sik) Denoting an acid that has five hydrogen atoms replaceable by a metal or radical.

pentamidine isethionate (pen-tam´ĭ-dēn i-se-thi´o-nāt) Drug used to treat trypanosomiasis, leishmaniasis, and pneumonia caused by *Pneumocystis carinii*.

pentatomic (pen-tă-tom´ik) **1.** Denoting a molecule composed of five atoms. **2.** Denoting a compound possessing five atoms in a ring. **3.** Denoting a chemical with five replaceable hydrogen atoms. **4.** Denoting an alcohol containing five hydroxyl groups.

pentobarbital (pen-to-bar´bĭ-tal) Short-acting barbiturate, $C_{11}H_{12}N_2O_3$, generally used for sleep induction; Nembutal®.

pentose (pen´tōs) Any one of a class of monosaccharides containing five carbon atoms in the molecule (e.g., arabinose, lyxose, ribose, and xylose).

pentosuria (pen-to-su´re-ă) The presence of pentose in the urine.

pepsin (pep´sin) Enzyme present in gastric juice; it converts proteins into peptones and proteoses.

pepsinogen (pep-sin´ŏ-jen) The precursor of pepsin produced by the stomach lining; an inert substance that is converted into pepsin during digestion by the action of hydrochloric acid.

pepsinogenous (pep-sin-ŏ-jen´us) Producing pepsin.

pepsinuria (pep-sĭ-nu´re-ă) The presence of pepsin in the urine.

peptic (pep´tik) **1.** Relating to digestion. **2.** Relating to pepsin.

peptidase (pep´tĭ-dās) Enzyme that promotes the breakdown of peptide bonds in a protein molecule.

peptide (pep´tīd) Any of various compounds consisting of two or more amino acid residues.

atrial natriuretic p. (ANP) Hormone produced in the walls of the atria of the heart and released into the circulation in response to atrial dilatation or increased intravascular fluid volume; it is involved in renal salt and water excretion and in regulating blood pressure.

C p. A peptide chain in the proinsulin molecule that connects the A chain and B chain; it splits off as residue during conversion of proinsulin to insulin.

calcitonin gene-related p. (CGRP) A gene-encoded, 37-amino acid polypeptide present in the nervous system, adrenal medulla, and gastrointestinal tract; it dilates blood vessels.

defensin p.'s Naturally occurring antimicrobial peptides containing 29 to 35 amino acids; they act against bacteria (both gram-positive and gram-negative), fungi, and viruses.

gastric stimulating p. Any peptide that promotes or inhibits secretion from the stomach lining or stimulates gastric motility.

vasoactive intestinal p. (VIP) A substance found in the intestinal tract, especially the distal small bowel and colon, capable of suppressing acid secretion by the stomach and stimulating secretion in the small intestine and colon; may be responsible for the watery diarrhea syndrome associated with pancreatic islet cell tumor; causes hyperglycemia and hypercalcemia; also found in the brain.

peptidyl-dipeptidase A (pep´tĭ-dil-dī-pep´tĭ-dās ā) Enzyme that promotes the splitting of an angiotensin I to form the activated angiotensin II. Also called dipeptidyl carboxypeptidase.

peptidyltransferase (pep-tĭ-dil-trans´fer-ās) Enzyme responsible for development of peptide bonds on ribosomes during protein production in the body.

peptize (pep´tīz) To transform a gel into a sol.

peptolysis (pep-tol´ĭ-sis) The hydrolysis or splitting up of peptones.

peptone (pep´tōn) Any of various protein derivatives obtained by the action of enzymes on protein.

peptonemia (pep-to-ne´me-ă) The presence of peptone in the blood.

peptonize (pep´to-nīz) To convert protein into peptone.

peptonuria (pep-to-nu´re-ă) The presence of peptones in the urine.

Peptostreptococcus (pep-to-strep-to-kok´us) A

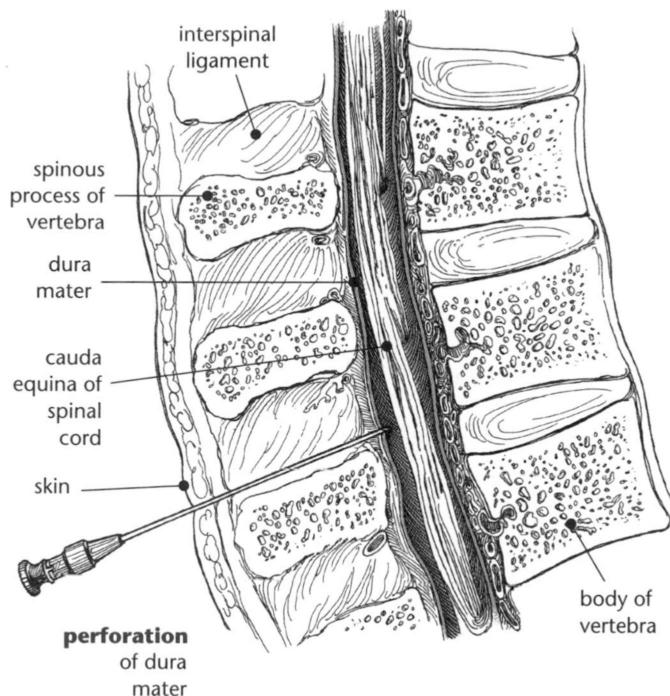

perforation of dura mater

electrocardiogram in **pericarditis**

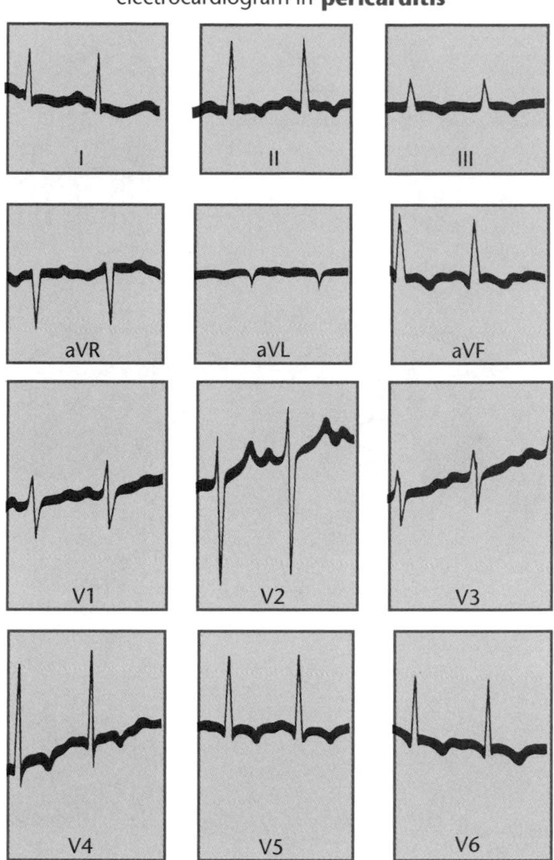

genus of spherical gram-positive, nonmotile bacteria found normally in the intestinal, respiratory, and female genital tracts, oral cavity, and certain pyogenic infections.

per anum (per an´um) Latin for through the anus.

percept (per´sept) A mental impression of something perceived by the senses.

perception (per-sep´shun) The mental process of becoming aware of something through any of the senses.

depth p. The ability to detect by sight the three-dimensional quality of objects and their position in space; perception of the third dimension. Also called stereoscopic vision.

extrasensory p. (ESP) Perception through other than the five senses.

perceptivity (per-sep-tiv´ĭ-te) The ability or faculty of perception.

perchloride (per-klo´rīd) A chloride having the largest possible amount of chlorine.

percolation (per-ko-la´shun) Extraction of the soluble parts of a solid mixture by passing a liquid solvent slowly through it.

percuss (per-kus´) To perform percussion.

percussion (per-kush´un) The act of tapping the body, especially the chest, back, and abdomen, to determine the condition of underlying structures by the sounds produced.

auscultatory p. Auscultation for the purpose of listening to sounds produced by percussion.

bimanual p. The tapping of a finger (placed on the patient's body) with a finger of the other hand.

palpatory p. Percussion combined with palpation in order to perceive tactile as well as auditory impressions.

percussor (per-kus´or) See plessor.

percutaneous (per-ku-ta´ne-us) **1.** Having the ability to pass through unbroken skin, as in absorption by inunction. **2.** Denoting procedures such as biopsies or intravenous or intra-arterial catheterizations performed with needle puncture without incision.

perflation (per-fla´shun) The forceful blowing of air into a cavity or canal to expel contained material.

perforation (per-fŏ-ra´shun) **1.** A hole in a tissue or organ resulting from injury or disease. **2.** The act of piercing.

perforin (per´fŏr-in) A protein present in granules of cytotoxic T lymphocytes; when released, it forms pores in the target cell membrane.

perfusate (per-fu´zāt) A fluid that has been poured over an organ or a special surface (e.g., a charged plate), or through a membrane.

perfusion (per-fu´zhun) The passage of a fluid through an organ or tissue by way of the blood vessels.

periadenitis (per-e-ad-ĕ-ni´tis) Inflammation of the tissues around a gland.

perianal (per-e-a´nal) Adjacent to or around the anus. Also called circumanal.

periangiitis, periangitis (per-e-an-je-i´tis, per-e-an-ji´tis) Inflammation of tissues surrounding blood vessels or lymph vessels.

periantritis (per-e-an-tri´tis) See type B gastritis, under gastritis.

periaortic (per-e-a-or´tik) Surrounding or located near the aorta.

periaortitis (per-e-a-or-ti´tis) Inflammation of tissues around the aorta.

periapical (per-e-ap´ĭ-kal) Surrounding the tip of a dental root, including the alveolar bone.

periappendicitis (per-e-ă-pen-dĭ-si´tis) Inflammation of tissues around the vermiform appendix.

periarterial (per-e-ar-te´re-al) Surrounding an artery.

periarteritis (per-e-ar-tĕ-ri´tis) Inflammation of the outer coat of an artery.

p. nodosa See polyarteritis nodosa.

periarthritis (per-e-ar-thri´tis) Inflammation of tissues around a joint.

peribronchial (per-ĭ-brong´ke-al) Surrounding a bronchus or bronchi.

peribuccal (per´ĭ-buk-al) Around the cheek.

peribulbar (per-ĭ-bul´bar) Surrounding any anatomic bulb, especially of the eye and the urethra.

peribursal (per-ĭ-ber´sal) Around a bursa.

pericardectomy (per-ĭ-kar-dek´tŏ-me) See pericardiectomy.

pericardial, pericardiac (per-ĭ-kar´de-al, per-ĭ-kar´de-ak) **1.** Around the heart. **2.** Relating to the pericardium.

pericardiectomy (per-ĭ-kar-de-ek´to-me) Surgical removal of a portion of the pericardium. Also called pericardectomy.

pericardiocentesis, pericardicentesis (per-ĭ-kar-de-o-sen-te´sis, per-ĭ-kar-de-sen-te´sis) Needle aspiration of fluid accumulated within the pericardium.

pericardiophrenic (per-ĭ-kar-de-o-fren´ik) Relating to the pericardium and the diaphragm.

pericardiorrhaphy (per-ĭ-kar-de-or´ă-fe) Suturing of a wound in the pericardium.

pericardiostomy (per-ĭ-kar-de-os´tŏ-me) The making of an opening into the pericardium.

pericardiotomy (per-ĭ-kar-de-ot´ŏ-me) Surgical incision of the pericardium. Also called pericardotomy.

pericarditis (per-ĭ-kar-di´tis) Inflammation of the pericardium, usually occurring secondary to disorders of adjacent structures.

acute p. Pericarditis marked by chest pain, sometimes resembling a heart attack (myocardial infarction) but relieved by leaning forward; palpitations and fever may also occur; causes include infection (especially viral), chronic kidney failure, and connective tissue diseases.

chronic adhesive p. Fibrous bands between the two layers of pericardium, between pericardium and heart, or between pericardium and adjacent structures; formed during healing of previous pericarditis.

chronic constrictive p. A rare form in which the pericardium becomes thick, dense, and fibrous, limiting heart muscle function; results from healing and scar formation of previous pericarditis.

pericardium (pre-ĭ-kar´de-um) The thin, double-layered, membranous sac that encloses the heart; the layers are separated by a small amount of fluid which lubricates the constantly rubbing surfaces; the layers fuse as they attach to the great vessels and diaphragm.

pericardotomy (per-ĭ-kar-dot´ŏ-me) See pericardiotomy.

pericecal (per-ĭ-se´kal) Surrounding the cecum.

pericellular (per-ĭ-sel´u-lar) Surrounding a cell.

pericementitis (per-ĭ-se-men-ti´tis) See periodontitis.

pericholangitis (per-ĭ-ko-lan-ji´tis) Inflammation of tissues around the bile ducts; frequently associated with inflammatory bowel disease.

perichondral, perichondrial (per-ĭ-kon´dral, per-ĭ-kon´dre-al) Relating to the perichondrium.

perichondritis (per-ĭ-kon-dri´tis) Inflammation of the perichondrium.

perichondrium (per-ĭ-kon´dre-um) A fibrous membrane that covers cartilage except at joint

P

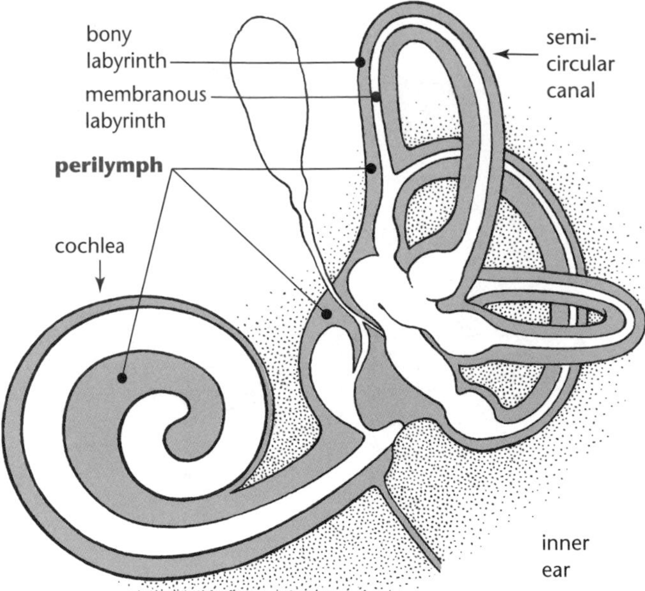

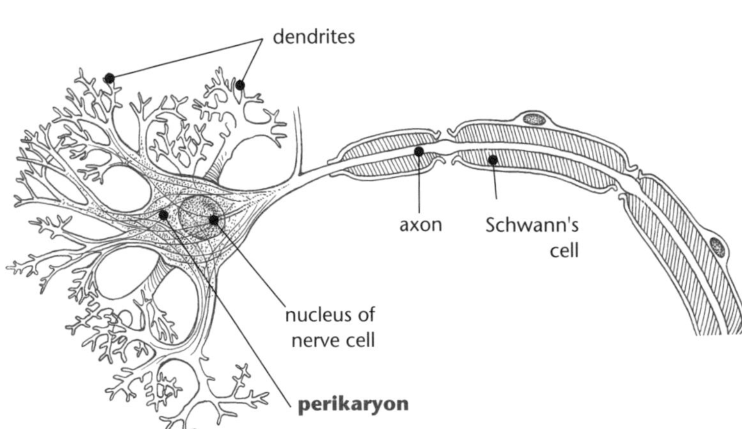

INCUBATION **PERIODS** OF VARIOUS DISEASES

disease	incubation period	rash
gastroenteritis	6–24 hours	–
diphtheria	2–5 days	–
scarlet fever	1–5 days	1st day
measles	10–15 days	4th day
rubella	14–21 days	1st day
chickenpox	14–21 days	1st day
mumps	7–26 days	–
smallpox	7–16 days	3rd day
whooping cough	2–21 days	–
poliomyelitis	7–21 days	–
virus influenza	1–4 days	–
gonorrhea	1–8 days	–
typhus	8–16 days	5th day
yellow fever	3–6 days	–
viral hepatitis A	15–35 days	–
viral hepatitis non A, non B	25–160 days	–
viral hepatitis B	30–180 days	–
brucellosis	7–14 days	–
typhoid fever	3–38 days	–
syphilis	1–6 weeks	6 weeks

GESTATION **PERIODS** OF SOME ANIMALS

Species	Range
mouse	18–20 days
rabbit	3–32 days
cat	56–65 days
dog	58–63 days
swine	111–116 days
cow	273–291 days
horse	329–346 days

P

endings, composed of an outer dense irregular connective tissue and an inner layer that is responsible for production of new cartilage.

perichord (per´ĭ-kord) The sheath covering the notochord.

pericolpitis (per-ĭ-kol-pi´tis) Inflammation of tissues surrounding the vagina.

pericoronal (per-ĭ-kor´o-nal) Surrounding the crown of a tooth.

pericoronitis (per-ĭ-kor-o-ni´tis) Inflammation of the gums around a partially erupted tooth.

pericranial (per-ĭ-kra´ne-al) Relating to the fibrous membrane covering the skull.

pericranium (per-ĭ-kra´ne-um) The fibrous membrane covering the skull. Also called periosteum of the skull.

pericystic (per-ĭ-sis´tik) **1.** Surrounding the urinary bladder. **2.** Around the gallbladder. **3.** Surrounding a cyst.

pericyte (per´ĭ-sīt) One of the contractile cells in the connective tissue layer around capillaries.

peridental (per-ĭ-den´tal) See periodontal.

peridesmic (per-ĭ-dez´mik) Surrounding a ligament. Also called periligamentous.

peridesmitis (per-ĭ-dez-mi´tis) Inflammation of the peridemium.

peridesmium (per-ĭ-dez´me-um) The connective tissue covering a ligament.

periesophageal (per-e-ĕ-sof´ă-je-al) Surrounding the esophagus.

periesophagitis (per-e-ĕ-sof-ă-ji´tis) Inflammation of tissues around the esophagus.

periganglionic (per-ĭ-gang-gle-on´ik) Surrounding a nerve ganglion.

perigastric (per-ĭ-gas´trik) Surrounding the stomach.

perihepatic (per-ĭ-he-pat´ik) Around the liver.

perihepatitis (per-ĭ-hep-ă-ti´tis) Inflammation of the covering membrane of the liver and surrounding tissues; in women, it may result from spread of pelvic organ infection (e.g., chlamydial, gonococcal) or trauma. Also called Fitz-Hugh-Curtis syndrome.

perikaryon (per-ĭ-kar´e-on) The cytoplasm surrounding the nucleus of a nerve cell; it is crowded with granular organelles including neurofibrils, chromidial substance (Nissl bodies), Golgi apparatus, mitochondria, and a centrosome.

periligamentous (per-ĭ-lig-ă-men´tus) See peridesmic.

perilymph (per´ĭ-limf) The fluid in the bony labyrinth of the inner ear surrounding the membranous labyrinth.

perilymphatic (per-ĭ-lim-fat´ik) **1.** Relating to the perilymph. **2.** Surrounding a lymph vessel.

perimenopause (per-ĭ-men´ŏ-pawz) The period encompassing the time before, during, and after the menopause; usually begins between the mid- and late-forties.

perimeter (pĕ-rim´ĕ-ter) Device for determining the extent and characteristics of the visual field.

perimetric (per-ĭ-met´rik) **1.** Relating to a perimeter or to measurement of the visual field. **2.** Surrounding the uterus.

perimetritis (per-ĭ-mĕ-tri´tis) Inflammation of the perimetrium.

perimetrium (per-ĭ-me´tre-um) The serous, outer layer of the uterine wall.

perimetry (per-im´ĕ-tre) Measurement of the visual field, usually performed to diagnose lesions of the visual pathways.

perimysial (per-ĭ-mis´e-al) Relating to the perimysium.

perimysium (per-ĭ-mis´e-um) Connective tissue separating adjacent bundles of skeletal muscle fibers.

perinatal (per-ĭ-na´tal) Relating to the period of time preceding and following birth; applied to the time that starts from completion of 20 weeks of gestation through the 28th day after birth.

perinatology (per-ĭ-na-tol´ŏ-je) A subspecialty concerned with the care of mother and baby during the last stage of pregnancy and early days after birth. Also called perinatal medicine.

perineal (per-ĭ-né al) Relating to the perineum.

perineoplasty (per-ĭ-ne´o-plas-te) Reparative surgery of the perineum (e.g., to correct a relaxed condition of the musculature).

perineorrhaphy (per-ĭ-ne-or´ă-fe) Suture of the perineum to repair lacerations or other injuries.

perinephric (per-ĭ-nef´rik) Surrounding the kidney. Also called perirenal.

perinephrium (per-ĭ-nef´re-um) The connective tissue and fat around the kidney.

perineum (per-ĭ-ne´um) **1.** The area bounded by the pubis, the coccyx, and the thighs. **2.** The area between the external genitalia and the anus.

perineural (per-ĭ-nu´ral) Surrounding a nerve.

perineuritis (per-ĭ-nu-ri´tis) Inflammation of the perineurium.

perineurium (per-ĭ-nu´re-um) A layer of connective tissue surrounding and supporting each separate bundle of nerve fibers in a peripheral nerve; it consists of a variable number of layers of squamous epithelial cells.

perinuclear (per-ĭ-nu´kle-ar) Surrounding or situated near a nucleus.

period (pe´re-od) **1.** An interval of time. **2.** An occurrence of menstruation.

absolute refractory p. 1. The period in the cardiac cycle when the heart muscle does not respond to even a high-intensity stimulus; it corresponds to the contraction phase. **2.** The time immediately

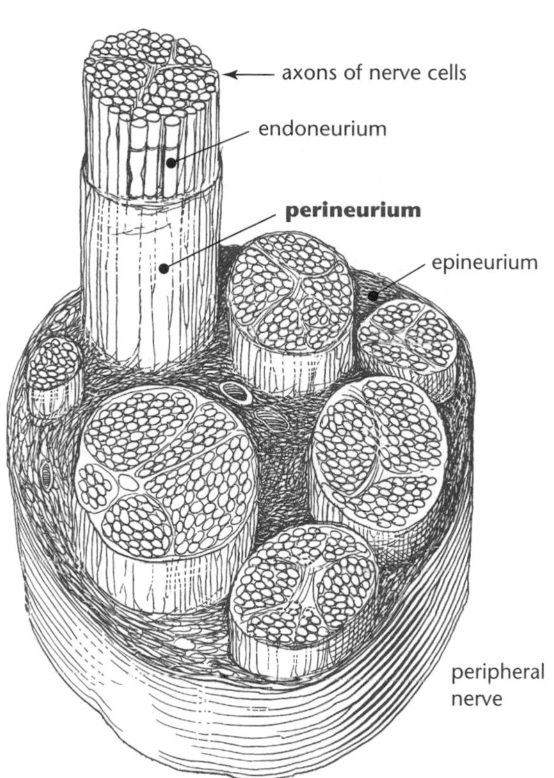

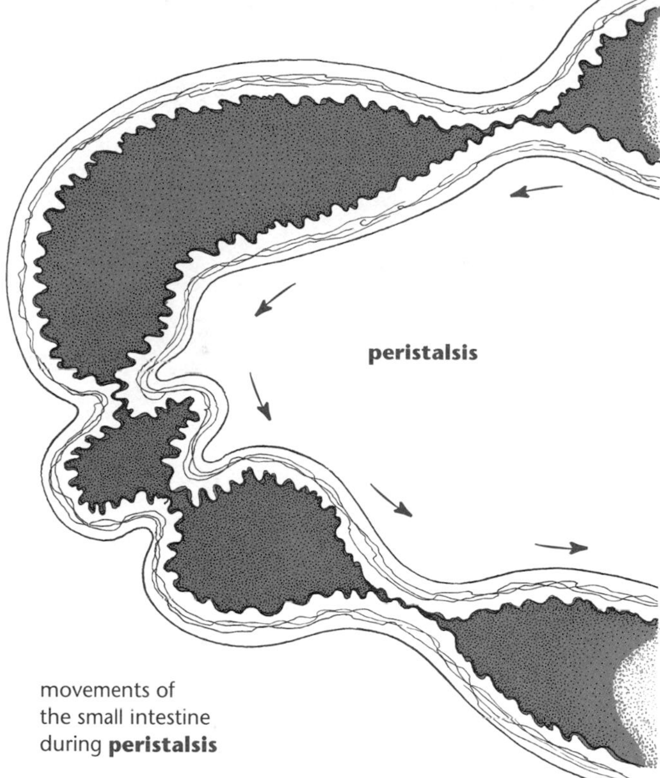

following the passage of an impulse through a nerve.

fertile p. The time in the midportion of the menstrual cycle when ovulation takes place and conception is most likely to occur; usually 10 to 18 days after the first day of the last menstruation.

gestation p. Time between fertilization of the ovum and parturition; period of pregnancy.

incubation p. Time between infection with a pathogenic microorganism and appearance of first symptoms of the disease. Also called incubative stage; latent period.

latent p. (a) An apparently inactive period (e.g., time elapsed between exposure to an injurious agent, such as radiation or poisons, and manifestation of effects, or between the application of a stimulus and a response to the stimulus). Also called latent stage. (b) See incubation period.

missed p. Failure of menstruation to occur in any given month.

neonatal p. The first 30 days of infant life.

perinatal p. The period of life from the 20th week of completed gestation through the 28th day after birth.

prodromal p. The time during which a disease has begun to develop but is not yet clinically apparent.

puerperal p. Period beginning just after childbirth and ending at the return of the uterus to its original state; usually lasts about 6 weeks.

relative refractory p. (a) Time during relaxation of heart muscle in which a stronger than ordinary stimulus is required to elicit a response. (b) Time following the absolute refractory period of a nerve, in which a stronger than ordinary stimulus is necessary to transmit an impulse.

safe p. The interval during the menstrual cycle when conception is least likely to occur; usually lasts from about 10 days before to 10 days after the first day of menstruation.

vulnerable p. The brief period after contraction of the cardiac ventricle when a stimulus applied to it is likely to precipitate fibrillation; occurs approximately at the peak of the T wave on the electrocardiogram.

Wenckebach p. The progressively lengthened P-R interval in successive cardiac cycles preceding a dropped beat, due to an atrioventricular (A-V) block.

periodic (pe-re-od′ik) Recurring at regular intervals (e.g., the paroxysms and fever of malaria).

periodic acid (pe-re-od′ik as′id) A colorless, water soluble, inorganic acid, $HIO_4 \cdot 2H_2O$, resulting from the action of concentrated hydrochloric acid on iodine.

periodical (per-e-od′ĭ-kal) A journal published at regular intervals.

periodicity (pe-re-o-dis′ĭ-te) The state of being periodic.

periodontal (per-e-o-don′tal) Surrounding a tooth. Also called peridental.

periodontal disease (per-e-o-don′tal dĭ-zēz′) Any disease of the tissues surrounding and supporting the teeth; may involve the gingiva only (gingivitis) or include the deeper structures (periodontitis).

periodontics (per-e-o-don′tiks) The branch of dentistry concerned with the study of the tissues surrounding the teeth and with the treatment of their diseases.

periodontist (per-e-o-don′tist) A specialist in periodontics.

periodontitis (per-e-o-don-ti′tis) A disease of the periodontium manifested by inflammation of the gums, loss of bone tissue around the teeth, degeneration of the peridontal membrane or ligament, and the formation of pockets between the teeth and the surrounding bone. Also called pyorrhea.

periodontium (per-e-o-don′she-um) The tissues surrounding and supporting the teeth, including the cementum, periodontal membrane or ligament, alveolar bone, and gingiva (gums). Also called peridentium.

periodontosis (per-e-o-don-to′sis) A rare condition of unknown cause marked by noninflammatory degeneration of the periodontal tissues, resulting in premature tooth loss.

periomphalic (per-e-om-fal′ik) See periumbilical.

perioral (per-e-or′al) Situated about the mouth.

periorbita (per-e-or′bĭ-tă) Periosteum lining the interior of the orbit.

periorbital (per-e-or′bĭ-tal) Related to the orbit.

periorchitis (per-e-or-ki′tis) Inflammation of the tunica vaginalis testis.

periosteal (per-e-os′te-al) Relating to the periosteum.

periosteoma (per-e-os-te-o′mă) A tumor derived from the periosteum.

periosteomyelitis (per-e-os-te-o-mi-ĕ-li′tis) Inflammation of the entire bone and the surrounding periosteum.

periosteotomy, periostotomy (per-e-os-te-ot′ŏ-me) A surgical incision into the periosteum.

periosteum (per-e-os′te-um) A thick fibrous membrane covering the surface of bones except at points of articulation; it consists, in adults, of two layers: the external layer of dense connective tissue conveying blood vessels and nerves to the bone, and the internal layer of loose connective tissue.

periostitis (per-e-os-ti′tis) Inflammation of the periosteum.

periostoma (per-e-os-to′mă) See periosteoma.

periostotomy (per-e-os-tot′ŏ-me) See periosteotomy.

peripapillary (per-ĭ-pap′ĭ-ler-e) Surrounding the optic disk.

peripheral (pĕ-rif′er-al) Relating to the periphery.

periphery (pĕ-rif′er-e) The area of the body away from the center; the outer surface of the body.

periproctitis (per-ĭ-prok-ti′tis) Inflammation of tissues around the rectum and anus.

perirectal (per-ĭ-rek′tal) Around the rectum.

perirenal (per-ĭ-re′nal) See perinephric.

perisplenitis (per-ĭ-splĕ-ni′tis) Inflammation of the peritoneum covering the spleen and surrounding structures.

peristalsis (per-ĭ-stal′sis) The alternate contraction and relaxation of the walls of a tubular structure (e.g., intestinal tract, ureter) by means of which its contents are moved onward.

peristole (pĕ-ris′to-le) Tonic contraction of the stomach wall about its contents. Distinguished from its peristaltic contractions.

perisynovial (per-ĭ-sĭ-no′ve-al) Around the lining (synovial membrane) of a joint cavity.

peritectomy (per-ĭ-tek′tŏ-me) Removal of a small portion of conjunctiva near the cornea.

peritendinitis (per-ĭ-ten-dĭ-ni′tis) Inflammation of the sheath around a tendon.

perithelioma (per-ĭ-the-le-o′mă) See hemangiopericytoma.

perithelium (per-ĭ-thel′le-um) Thin layer of connective tissue surrounding the small vessels.

peritomy (pĕ-rit′ŏ-me) The cutting of the conjunctiva at the edge of the cornea; a preliminary step in various surgical procedures.

peritoneal (per-ĭ-to-ne′al) Relating to the peritoneum.

peritoneocentesis (per-ĭ-to-ne-o-sen-te′sis) Aspiration of fluid from the abdominal cavity with a fine needle or any other hollow instrument. Also called abdominocentesis.

peritoneoclysis (per-ĭ-to-ne-o-klĭ′sis) Irrigation of the peritoneal cavity.

peritoneoscope (per-ĭ-to′ne-ŏ-skōp) See laparoscope.

peritoneoscopy (per-ĭ-to-ne-os′kŏ-pe) See laparoscopy.

peritoneotomy (per-ĭ-to-ne-ot′ŏ-me) See

P

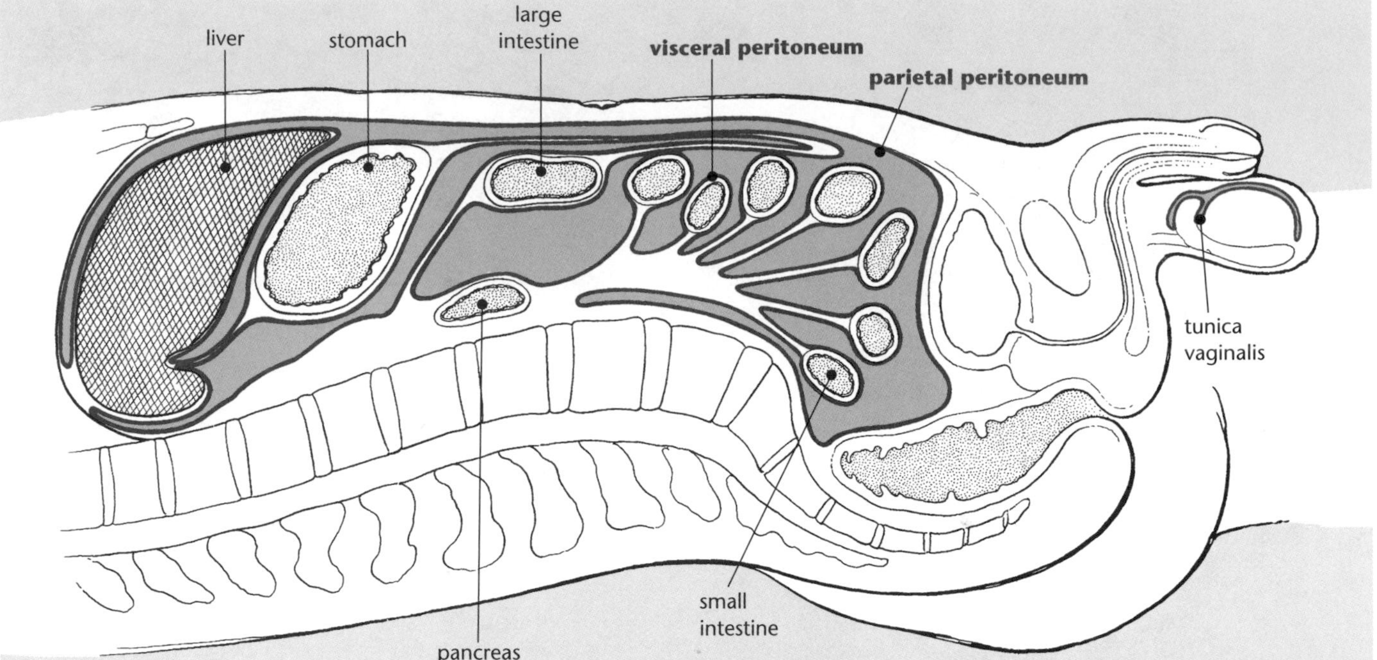

laparotomy.

peritoneum (per-ĭ-to-ne´um) The serous membrane lining the walls of the abdominal and pelvic cavities and enclosing the viscera.

parietal p. The layer of peritoneum lining the walls of the abdominal and pelvic cavities.

visceral p. The layer of peritoneum investing the abdominal and pelvic organs.

peritonitis (per-ĭ-to-ni´tis) Inflammation of the peritoneum, marked by pain, fever, constipation, and vomiting; may be caused by bacterial infection (e.g., from a ruptured appendix) or by chemical irritation (e.g., escaped bile or leaking pancreatic enzymes).

benign paroxysmal p. Periodic abdominalgia; see under abdominalgia.

peritonize (per´ĭ-to-nīz) To cover with peritoneum.

peritonsillar (per-ĭ-ton´sĭ-lar) Around a tonsil.

peritonsillitis (per-ĭ-ton-sĭ-li´tis) Inflammation of the peritonsillar tissues.

peritracheal (per-ĭ-tra´ke-al) Surrounding the trachea.

peritrichous (pĕ-rit´rĭ-kus) **1.** Relating to fine surface projections (cilia or flagella); applied to bacteria. **2.** Having modified cilia arranged in a spiral fashion around the mouth opening; said of certain protozoa.

periumbilical (per-ĭ-um-bil´ĭ-kal) Around the navel (umbilicus). Also called periomphalic.

periungual (per-e-ung´gwal) Around a nail.

periureteral, periureteric (per-ĭ-u-re´ter-al, per-ĭ-u-re-ter´ik) Around one or both ureters.

periureteritis (per-ĭ-u-re-ter-ĭ´tis) Inflammation of tissues around the ureter.

periurethritis (per-ĭ-u-re-thri´tis) Inflammation of tissues around the urethra.

perivascular (per-ĭ-vas´ku-lar) Around a vessel.

periwinkle (per´ĭ-wing-kl) Any of several evergreen shrubs or small trees with glossy blue-green leaves and fragrant flowers of the genus *Vinca*, especially *Vinca minor* and *Vinca rosea*; they contain active dimeric alkaloids, including vinblastine, vincristine, vinleurosine, and vinrosidine. Also called myrtle.

perlèche (per-lesh´) Inflammation with cracks and erosion at the corners of the mouth; may be caused by a primary or a superimposed infection with any of various microorganisms, including *Candida albicans* and streptococci; occurs mainly among undernourished children, especially those who have a habit of licking the angles of the mouth.

permanganate (per-man´gă-nāt) Any of the salts of permanganic acid.

permanganic acid (per-mang-gan´ik as´id) An unstable inorganic acid, $HMnO_4$, derived from manganese.

permeability (per-me-ă-bil´ĭ-te) The condition of being permeable.

permeable (per´me-ă-bl) Allowing passage (e.g., of fluid through a membrane). Also called pervious.

permeant (per´me-ant) Able to penetrate or pass through.

permease (per´me-ās) A specific protein in the cell membrane of microorganisms that facilitates passage of nutrients, such as sugar, across the membrane in the direction of the concentration gradient.

pernicious (per-nish´us) Highly destructive; tending to cause death.

pernio (per´ne-o) See chilblains.

peromelia (per-o-me´le-ă) Severe congenital malformation of the extremities, including absence of a hand or a foot.

peroneal (per-o-ne´al) **1.** Relating to the lateral portion of the leg. **2.** Fibular.

peroneus (per-o-ne´us) See table of muscles.

peroral (per-or´al) Via the mouth.

per os (per os) (p.o.) Latin for by mouth.

peroxidase (pe-rok´si-dās) Enzyme found in plant and animal tissues; it stimulates dehydrogenation (oxidation) of various substances using hydrogen peroxide as hydrogen acceptor (oxidant).

peroxide (pĕ-rok´sīd) The oxide of a series containing the greatest number of oxygen atoms.

hydrogen p. Hydrogen dioxide, H_2O_2; an unstable compound, used in solution as an antiseptic, bleaching agent, and oxidizing agent.

peroxisome (pĕ-roks´ĭ-sōm) A membrane bounded organelle (about 0.5 µm in diameter) that contains oxidase and peroxidase; a parenchymal cell contains approximately 200 peroxisomes. Formerly called microbody.

peroxyacetyl nitrate (per-ok-se-ă-se´til ni´trāt) The main pollutant of smog, responsible for eye irritation and respiratory distress.

per rectum (per rek´tum) (p.r.) By way of the rectum.

PERRLA Acronym for pupils equal, round, reactive to light and accommodation. A normal finding in neurologic examination.

persalt (per´sawlt) In chemistry, any salt containing the maximum amount of the acid radical.

perseveration (per-sev-er-a´shun) **1.** The pathologic, involuntary repetition of a single response to various questions, or the continuation of an activity no longer relevant or appropriate; seen in organic brain disease. **2.** The duration of a mental image.

personality (per-sŭ-nal´ĭ-te) The sum total of an individual's deeply ingrained patterns of thinking, perceiving, and reacting.

p. disorders See under disorder.

psychopathic p. See antisocial personality disorder, under disorder.

person-years (per´son yirs) In epidemiological studies, method of measuring incidence (e.g., of a disease) over extended and variable time periods; equal to the sum of the number of years each person in the study has been exposed to, or afflicted with, the disease of interest.

perspiration (per-spĭ-ra´shun) **1.** The process of sweating. **2.** Sweat.

persuasion (per-swa´zhun) In psychiatry, a therapeutic approach directed toward influencing the mind of another by authority, argument, reason, or entreaty.

pertechnetate (per-tek´nĕ-tāt) ($^{99m}TcO_4$) A negatively-charged form of the radioactive element technetium, used in nuclear scanning.

pertussis (per-tus´is) Acute respiratory illness of infants and young children caused by the bacterium *Bordetella pertussis*; marked by inflammation of the larynx, trachea, and bronchi and a typical paroxysmal coughing with a terminal whoop; a pertussis vaccine is available and is generally administered to infants together with diphtheria and tetanus toxoids. Also called whooping cough.

pervaporation (per-vap-o-ra´shun) The concentration of a colloidal solution by placing the solution in a bag of semipermeable material and suspending it over a hot plate; only the colloid remains in the bag while the rest of the substances pass through.

perversion (per-ver´shun) Deviation from what is considered normal.

pervert (per´vert) A person who practices perversions.

pervious (per´ve-us) See permeable.

pes (pes) **1.** Latin for foot. **2.** Any footlike or basal body structure.

p. anserinus (a) See parotid plexus, under plexus. (b) The combined insertions of the tendons of the sartorius, gracilis, and semitendinosus muscles at the medial border of the tibial tuberosity.

p. calcaneus See talipes calcaneous, under talipes.

p. cavus See clawfoot.

p. equinus See talipes equinus, under talipes.

p. planovalgus See talipes planovalgus, under talipes.

p. planus See flatfoot.

p. pronatus See talipes valgus, under talipes.

p. valgus See talipes valgus, under talipes.

p. varus See talipes varus, under talipes.

pessary (pes´ă-re) A device used to support a displaced uterus when surgery is contraindicated.

diaphragm p. See contraceptive diaphragm, under diaphragm.

donut p., doughnut p. An inflatable pessary shaped like a doughnut; formerly made of red rubber,

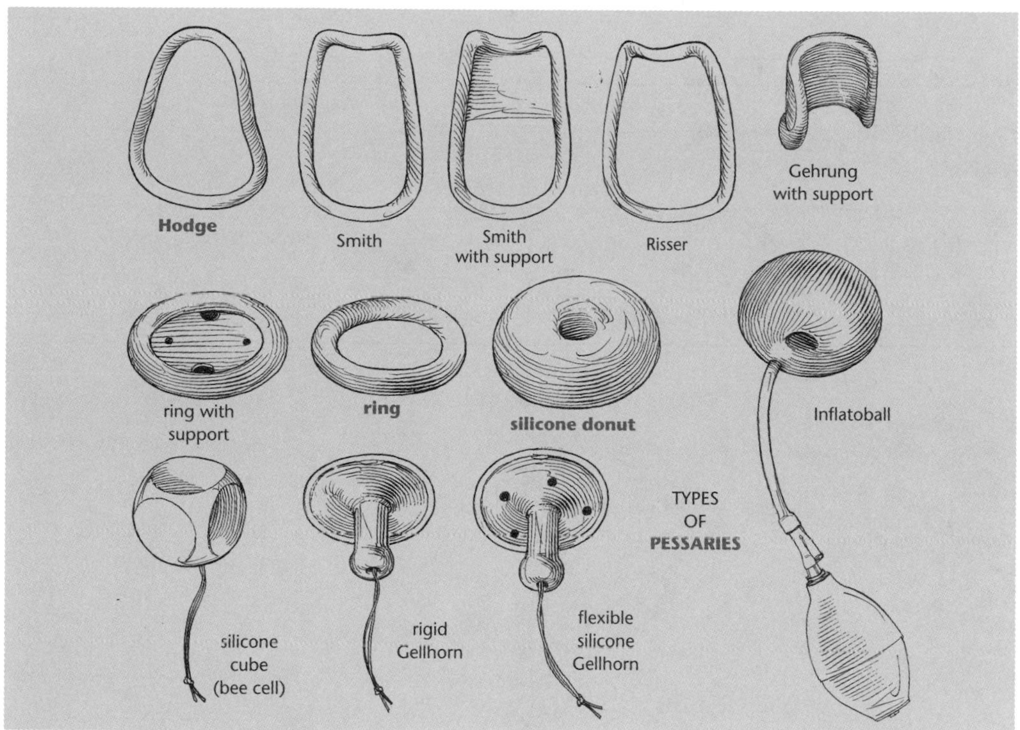

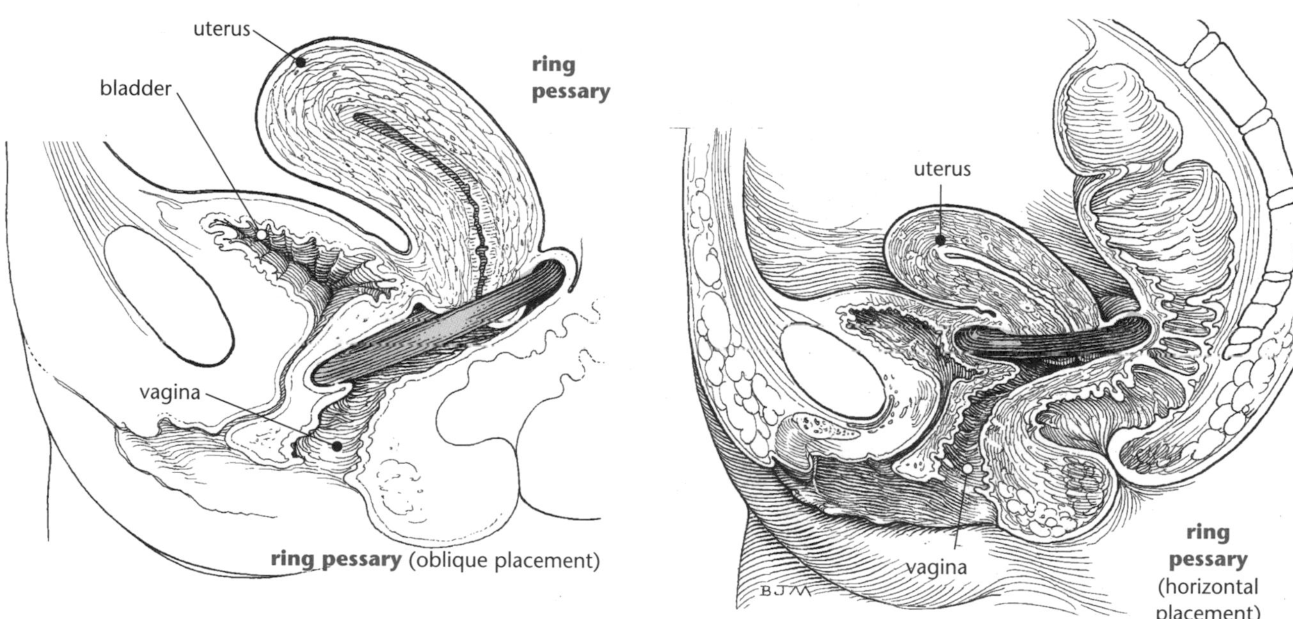

P

currently made of silicone; its use is much like that of the ring pessary.

Hodge p. A pessary used to hold the retroposed uterus in anteposition after it has been manually brought forward to its normal position. Also called Smith-Hodge pessary.

inflatable p. A ring-shaped pessary made of soft rubber that, once in place, is inflated with air.

ring p. A ring used to support the uterus in cases of slight prolapse.

Smith-Hodge p. See Hodge pessary.

pesticide (pes´tĭ-sīd) Any agent that is used to destroy pests, especially insects, rodents, and fungi.

pestilence (pes´tĭ-lens) An epidemic of a usually deadly disease, especially of the bubonic plague.

pestis (pes´tis) Latin for plague.

pestle (pes´l) A club-shaped tool, used for breaking and grinding substances in a mortar.

petechia (pe-te´ke-ă), *pl.* **pete´chiae** A nonraised, purplish red spot of the skin, nail beds, or mucous membranes resulting from subcutaneors bleeding.

petiole (pet´e-ōl) A slender stalk-like structure; a stem or pedicle. Also called petiolus.

epiglottic p. The pointed lower end of the epiglottic cartilage that is connected by the thyroepiglottic ligament to the back of the thyroid cartilage.

petiolus (pĕ-ti´o-lus) See petiole.

petit mal (pĕ-te´ mahl) See childhood absence epilepsy, under epilepsy.

Petri dish (pe´tre dish) A shallow circular container made of glass or plastic with a loose-fitting cover, used for the cultivation of microorganisms. Also called Petri plate.

petrifaction (pet-rĭ-fak´shun) The conversion of an organic substance into stone; fossilization.

pétrissage (pa-trĭ-săzh´) A kneading of the muscles in massage.

petrolatum (pet-ro-la´tum) A semisolid mixture of hydrocarbons obtained from petroleum; used as a soothing and lubricant agent and in the preparation of ointments. Also called petroleum jelly; soft paraffin; Vaseline®.

hydrophilic p. A mixture of cholesterol, stearyl alcohol, and white wax.

liquid p. See mineral oil, under oil.

white p. White, purified, and deodorized petrolatum.

petrosal (pĕ-tro´sal) Relating to the petrous part of the temporal bone.

petrositis (pet-ro-si´tis) Inflammation of the petrous portion of the temporal bone.

petrous (pet´rus) **1.** Denoting hardness. **2.** Relating to the petrous portion of the temporal bone.

Peutz-Jeghers syndrome (pertz-ja´gerz sin´drōm) A familial disorder characterized chiefly by the presence of numerous polyps in the intestinal tract, especially the jejunum, and dark brown spots on the lips, oral mucosa, and fingers.

peyote, peyotl (pa-o´te, pa-o´tl) A small gray-brown cactus, *Lophophora williamsii*, with a carrot-shaped root and a small mushroomlike spineless head ("button"); it has hallucinatory properties.

Peyronie's disease (pa-ron-ēz´ dĭ-zez´) The formation of dense fibrous tissue in the corpus cavernosum of the penis causing painful erection;

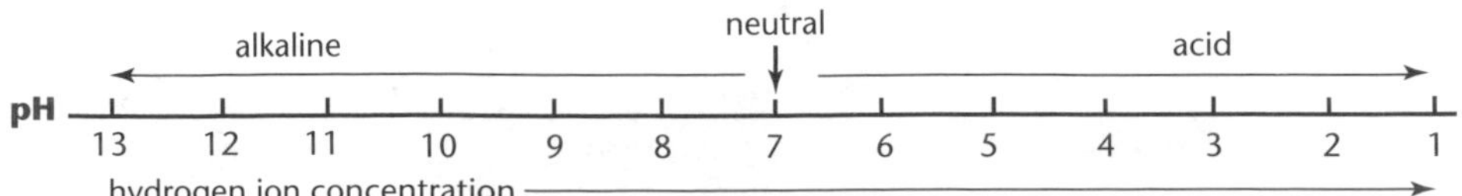

pH of some fluids

gastric juice	1.6	urine	5–8	blood plasma	7.4
lemon juice	2.3	saliva	6.5	interstitial fluid	7.4
tomato juice	4.3	cow's milk	6.6	pancreatic juice	7.9

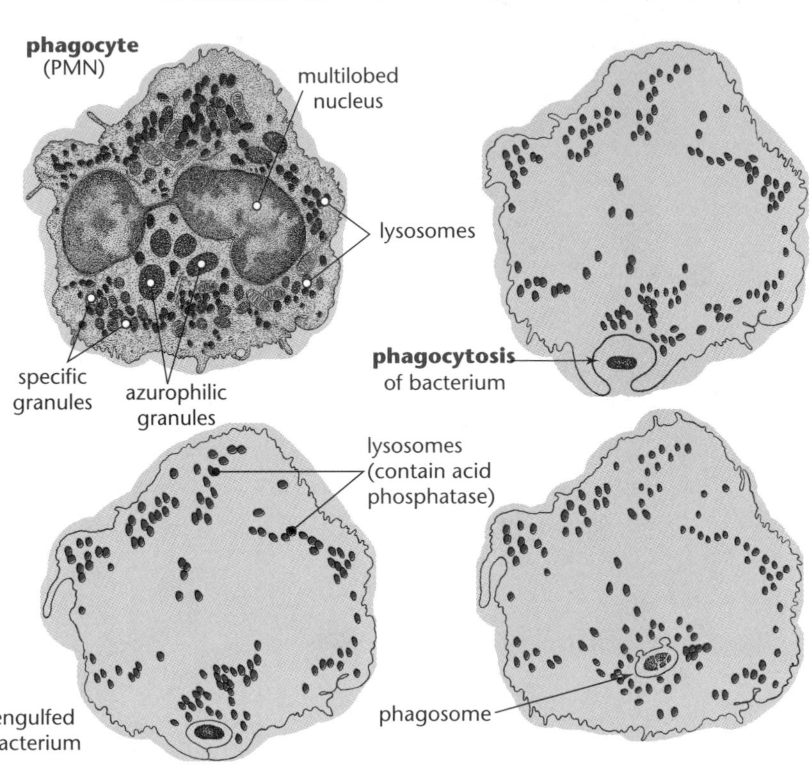

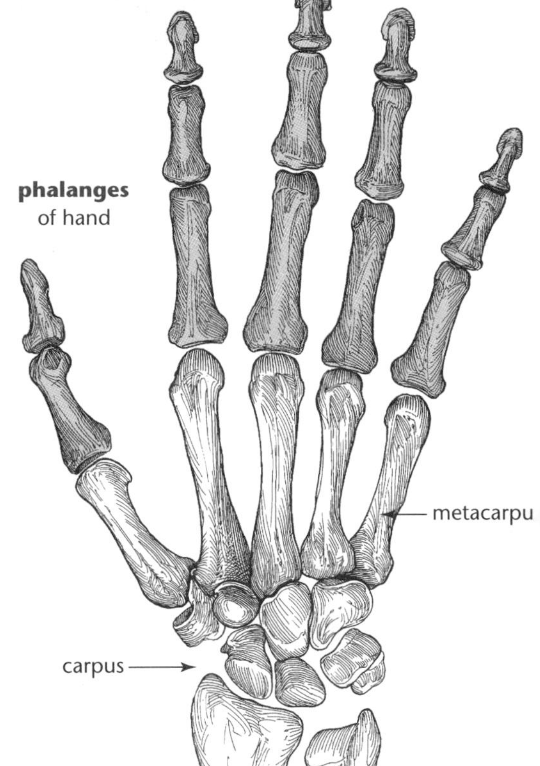

associated with sclerosis of other parts of the body. Also called fibrous cavernitis.

pH Symbol expressing the degree of alkalinity or acidity of a solution; it denotes the negative logarithm to the base 10 of the hydrogen ion concentration (e.g., a solution with a hydrogen ion concentration of 1×10^{-3} would have a pH of 3.0). A pH of 7.0 is considered neutral; a lower pH is acid and a higher pH alkaline. The normal pH of blood serum is approximately 7.4.

phacitis (fă-si´tis) Inflammation of the eye.

phacoanaphylaxis (fak-o-an-ă-fi-lak´sis) Intraocular inflammation due to hypersensitivity to protein of the lens of the eye induced by escape of lens material; may occur after cataract extraction of one eye.

phacocele (fak´o-sēl) Hernia of the eye lens, as through a ruptured sclera.

phacocyst (fak´o-sist) Capsule enclosing the eye lens.

phacocystectomy (fak-o-sis-tek´tŏ-me) Partial removal of the capsule of the eye lens.

phacocystitis (fak-o-sis-ti´tis) Inflammation of the capsule of the eye lens.

phacoemulsification (fak-o-e-mul-sĭ-fĭ-ka´shun) Cataract removal by emulsifying the diseased lens with low frequency ultrasonic vibrations, followed by aspiration with a needle.

phacoerysis (fak-o-er-e´sis) Removal of the eye lens by suction.

phacofragmentation (fak-o-frag-men-ta´shun) Cataract extraction by breaking up and irrigating the diseased eye lens.

phacoid (fak´oid) Lentil-shaped.

phacolysis (fă-kol´ĭ-sis) **1.** Liquefaction of the eye. **2.** Operative procedure to allow liquefaction and absorption of the lens.

phacomalacia (fak-o-mă-la´shă) Softening of the eye lens, as may occur in a soft cataract.

phacoscope (fak´o-skōp) Instrument for observing the eye lens, especially its changes during accommodation.

phage (fāj) See bacteriophage.

phagocyte (fag´ŏ-sīt) A white blood cell (neutrophil or macrophage) that ingests bacteria, foreign particles, and cellular debris. Also called scavenger cell.

alveolar p. See alveolar macrophage, under macrophage.

phagocytic (fag-o-sit´ik) Pertaining to phagocytes or phagocytosis.

phagocytin (fag-o-si´tin) Protein found in neutrophils that plays a role in the intracellular destruction of phagocytosed bacteria.

phagocytize (fag´o-sit´īz) See phagocytose.

phagocytoblast (fag-o-si´to-blast) Primitive cell that develops into a phagocyte.

phagocytolysis (fag-o-si-tol´ĭ-sis) Destruction of phagocytes.

phagocytose (fag-o-si´tōs) To engulf and digest; the function of phagocytes. Also called phagocytize.

phagocytosis (fag-o-si-to´sis) Process in which a substance is engulfed and then held or digested by certain white blood cells (neutrophils and macrophages), as the leukocyte engulfs and destroys pathogens; phagocytosis plays a nutritive and defensive role in cell function.

phagolysosome (fag-o-li´so-sōm) In phagocytosis, a phagocytic entity formed within certain white blood cells (e.g., neutrophils) by the fusion of a phagocytic vesicle (phagosome) and a cytoplasmic granule (lysosome), from which the phagosome receives an enzyme for digestion of the engulfed particle.

phagomania (fag-o-ma´ne-ă) A morbid compulsion to eat.

phagosome (fag´o-sōm) In phagocytosis, an intracellular vesicle formed within certain white blood cells (e.g., neutrophils) by invagination of the cytoplasmic membrane of the cell around an ingested particle; the vesicle then fuses with a cytoplasmic granule (lysosome) to form the phagolysosome.

phagotherapy (fag-o-ther´ă-pe) **1.** Treatment of infectious disease by a bacteriophage. **2.** Treatment by feeding, especially overfeeding.

phagotype (fag´o-tīp) In microbiology, a strain of bacteria that differs from other strains of the same species by its vulnerability to the action of a specific virus (bacteriophage).

phalangeal (fă-lan´je-al) Relating to a phalanx.

phalangectomy (fal-an-jek´tŏ-me) **1.** Amputation of a finger. **2.** Removal of one or more phalanges of a finger or toe.

phalanx (fa´lanks), *pl.* **pha´langes** Any bone of a finger or toe.

ungual p. The bone at the end of each digit.

phallectomy (fal-ek´tŏ-me) See penectomy.

phallic (fal´ik) Relating to the penis.

phallicism, phallism (fal´ĭ-sizm, fal´izm) Worship of the male genital.

phallocampsis (fal-o-kamp´sis) Any curvature of the penis during erection.

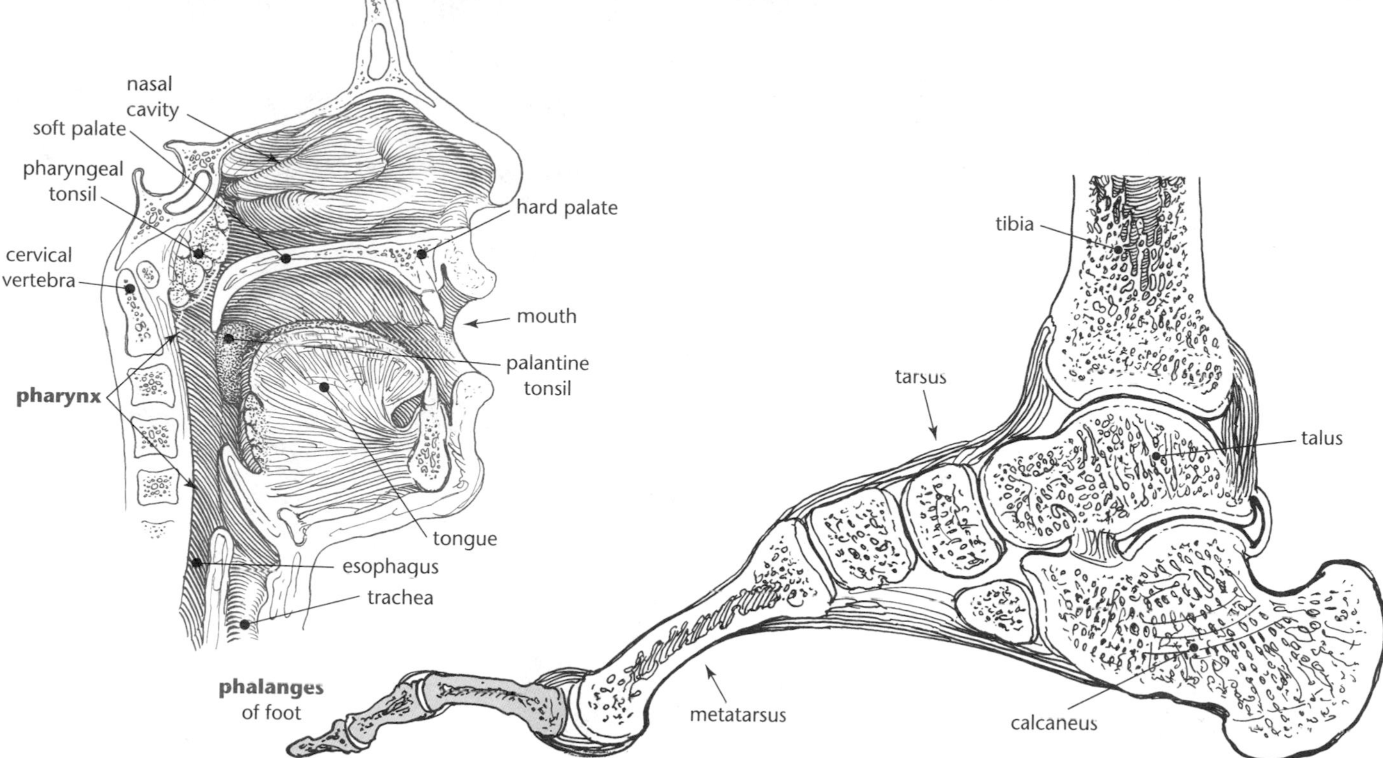

phallodynia (fal-o-din´e-ă) Pain in the penis.

phalloplasty (fal´o-plas-te) Reparative surgery of the penis.

phallotoxin (fal-o-tok´sin) One of the chief poisons present in the mushroom *Amanita phalloides.*

phallus (fal´us) Penis.

phanerosis (fan-er-o´sis) The process of becoming visible.

phantasm (fan´taz-m) The perception of an image; considered a pseudo-hallucination because it is usually recognized as imaginary by the person who sees it.

phantom (fan´tom) **1.** A teaching model of a body part (e.g., one of the female pelvis for demonstrating childbirth). **2.** A sensation that is felt, but has no physical origin (e.g., pain seemingly originating from an amputated limb).

phantosmia (fan-tos´me-ă) The intermittent or persistent odor, pleasant or unpleasant, perceived when no apparent odorant is inhaled.

pharmaceutic (fahr-mă-soo´tik) Relating to pharmacy.

pharmaceutical (fahr-mă-soo´tĭ-kal) **1.** Relating to pharmaceutics. **2.** Relating to medicinal drugs. **3.** A medicinal drug.

pharmaceutics (fahr-mă-soo´tiks) The branch of science concerned with the preparation and dosage of medicinal products.

pharmacist (fahr´mă-sist) One who is trained and licensed to prepare and dispense medicinal drugs and who is knowledgeable about their properties.

pharmacodiagnosis (făr-mă-ko-di-ag-no´sis) The use of drugs for diagnostic purposes.

pharmacodynamic (fahr-mă-ko-di-nam´ik) Relating to the action of drugs.

pharmacodynamics (fahr-mă-ko-di-nam´iks) The study of the effects of drugs on the body and the mechanism by which they act.

pharmacoepidemiology (fahr-mă-ko-epĭ-de-me-ol´o-je) The application of the principles of epidemiology to the study and determination of the effects of drugs in large populations.

pharmacogenetics (fahr-mă-ko-je-net´iks) The study of the genetic basis for differences in response to drugs.

pharmacognosist (fahr-mă-kog-nŏ´sist) A practitioner of pharmacognosy.

pharmacognosy, phermacognostics (fahr-mă-kog´no-se, fahr-mă-kog-nos´tiks) The study of medicinal chemicals in their natural, crude state.

pharmacography (fahr-mă kog´ră-fe) A description of drugs in their crude state.

pharmacokinetics (fahr-mă-ko-ki-net´iks) The study of the passage of drugs through the body, including their absorption, distribution, localization in tissues, metabolism, and excretion.

pharmacologic (fahr-mă-ko-loj´ik) Relating to pharmacology.

pharmacologist (fahr-mă-kol´ŏ-jist) A specialist in pharmacology.

pharmacology (fahr-mă-kol´ŏ-je) The science concerned with the study of all aspects of drugs, their interactions and their effects on living organisms.

clinical p. The branch of pharmacology concerned with therapeutic drugs and their effects on humans.

pharmacomania (fahr-mă-ko-ma´ne-ă) A morbid impulse to take drugs.

pharmacopedia (fahr-mă-ko-pe´de-ă) The total knowledge of crude drugs and medicinal preparations.

pharmacopeia, pharmacopoeia (fahr-mă-ko-pe-ă) (P) A book containing a list of medicinal drugs, description of their preparation and use, and chemical tests for identifying them and for determining their purity.

pharmacophobia (fahr-mă-ko-fo´be-ă) Abnormal fear of taking medicines.

pharmacotherapeutics (fahr-mă-ko-ther-ă-pu´tiks) The administration of drugs in the prevention or treatment of disease and their use in planned alteration of normal function.

pharmacy (fahr´mă-se) **1.** The science and practice of preparing and dispensing medicinal drugs. **2.** A drugstore or the department of a medical facility responsible for providing medications.

pharyngalgia (far-in-gal´jhă) Pain in the pharynx. Also called pharyngodynia.

pharyngeal (fă-rin´je-al) Relating to the pharynx.

pharyngectomy (far-in-jek´tŏ-me) Surgical removal of a portion of the pharynx.

pharyngismus (far-in-jiz´mus) See pharyngospasm.

pharyngitis (far-in-ji´tis) Inflammation of tissues lining the pharynx.

acute streptococcal p. Respiratory infection characterzed by some or all of the following symptoms: abrupt sore throat, headache, fever, malaise, and enlarged lymph nodes at the neck; children may additionally experience nausea, vomiting, and abdominal pain; caused by species of *Streptococcus*, especially group A, occasionally groups C or G. Commonly called strep throat.

fusospirochetal p. Sore throat, foul breath, and pharyngeal ulcers covered with a gray film, occasionally accompanied by fever. Also called Vincent's angina.

gonococcal p. Sexually transmitted infection of the pharynx; may be cause of sore throat, discomfort in swallowing and, rarely, a mucopurulent discharge with swelling of the uvula; caused by *Neisseria gonorrhoeae* acquired through orogenital contact with a gonorrhea infected individual. Also called pharyngeal gonorrhea.

granular p. Pharyngitis with enlargement of the lymphoid follicles of the mucous membrane, which appears granular. Also called clergyman's sore throat.

membranous p. Pharyngitis with a fibrous exudate forming a false membrane.

pharyngocele (fă-ring´go-sēl) Hernial protrusion of the pharyngeal wall into the pharynx.

pharyngodynia (fă-ring-go-din´e-ă) See pharyngalgia.

pharyngoesophageal (fă-ring-go-e-sof´ă-je-al) Relating to the pharynx and the esophagus.

pharyngoglossal (fă-ring-go-glos´al) Relating to the pharynx and the tongue.

pharyngolaryngeal (fă-ring-go-lă-rin´je-al) Relating to the pharynx and the larynx.

pharyngolaryngitis (fă-ring-go-lar-in-ji´tis) Inflammation of the pharynx and the larynx.

pharyngomycosis (fă-ring-go-mi-ko´sis) Fungal invasion of the mucous membrane of the pharynx.

pharyngopalatine (fă-ring-go-pal´ă-tīn) Referring to the pharynx and the palate.

pharyngoplasty (fă-ring´go-plas-te) Plastic surgery of the pharynx.

pharyngoplegia (fă-ring-go-ple´jhă) Paralysis of the muscles of the pharynx.

pharyngorhinoscopy (fă-ring-go-ri-nos´ko-pe) Inspection of the back of the nasal cavity by means of an instrument (rhinoscope).

pharyngoscleroma (fă-ring-go-skle-ro´mă) A circumscribed area of abnormal hard tissue in the mucous membrane of the pharynx.

pharyngoscope (fă-ring´go-skōp) An instrument for inspecting the pharynx.

pharyngoscopy (far-ing-gos´kŏ-pe) Visual examination of the pharynx with a pharyngoscope.

pharyngospasm (fă-ring´go-spaz-m) Sudden involuntary contractions of the pharyngeal muscles. Also called pharyngismus.

pharyngostenosis (fă-ring-go-ste-no´sis) Constriction of the pharynx.

pharyngotomy (far-ing-got´ŏ-me) Surgical incision of the pharynx.

pharyngotonsillitis (fă-ring-go-ton-sĭ-li´tis) Inflammation of the pharynx and tonsils.

pharynx (far´inks) A musculomembranous cavity, lined with mucous membrane, extending from the back of the nasal and oral cavities to the beginning of the trachea, esophagus, and larynx. The part of the pharynx above the soft palate is the nasopharynx; the portion that lies directly posterior to the mouth is

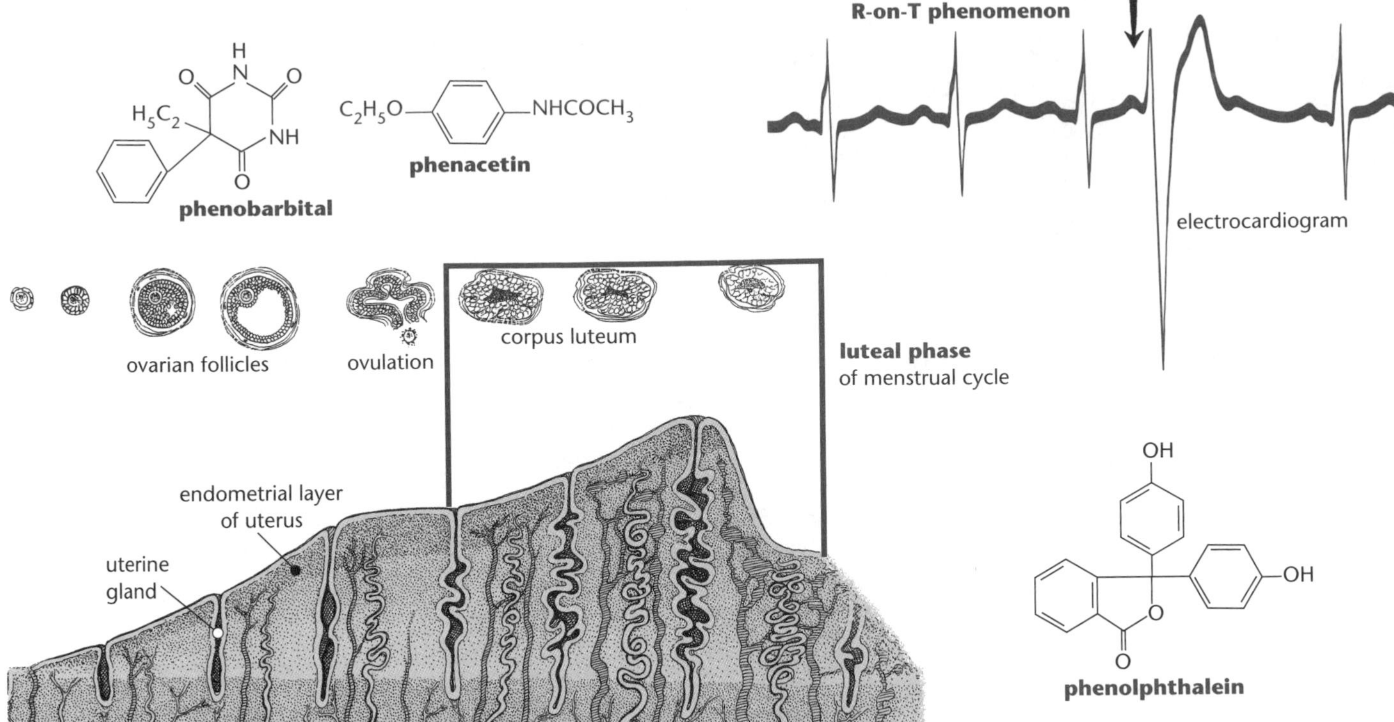

the oropharynx; and the portion behind the larynx and continuous with the esophagus is the laryngopharynx.

phase (fāz) **1.** A stage; relatively distinct part of a development or cycle. **2.** A homogeneous substance (solid, liquid, or gaseous), physically distinct and mechanically separable, present in a heterogeneous chemical system (e.g., the components of an emulsion) that is physically distinct and mechanically separable.

anal p. See anal stage, under stage.

aqueous p. The water portion of a mixture of water and an immiscible liquid.

continuous p. The surrounding or dispersion medium in a heterogeneous mixture. Also called external phase; dispersion phase.

dispersed p. The insoluble particles in a colloidal solution. Also called internal phase; enclosed phase.

dispersion p. See continuous phase.

enclosed p. See dispersed phase.

external p. See continuous phase.

internal p. See dispersed phase.

lag p. The period in the growth of a bacterial culture following inoculation into a medium; there is no increase in cell numbers and very little increase in cell size.

logarithmic p. Period in the development of a bacterial culture in which there is most rapid multiplication.

luteal p. Interval of the menstrual cycle from formation of the corpus luteum to beginning of the menstrual flow; lasts 12 to 14 days. Also called secretory phase.

meiotic p. Stage during formation of sexual cells in which the number of chromosomes per cell is halved. Also called reduction phase.

oedipal p. See oedipal stage, under stage.

oral p. See oral stage, under stage.

reduction p. See meiotic phase.

secretory p. See luteal phase.

supernormal recovery p. Interval during recovery of heart muscle following excitation, corresponding to the U wave of the electrocardiogram.

phasmid (faz′mid) **1.** One of a pair of minute caudal chemoreceptors present in roundworms of the class Phasmidia. **2.** A roundworm possessing such organs.

phenacetin (fĕ-nas′ĕ-tin) A bitter compound used to reduce pain and fever; when combined in a preparation with aspirin and caffeine, it is commonly known as APC (aspirin, phenacetin, and caffeine). Also called acetophenetidin.

phenanthrene (fe-nan′thrēn) Compound derived from coal; used in the manufacture of dyes and drugs.

phencyclidine (fen-si′klĭ-dēn) (PCP) A hallucinogenic drug that has a pressor effect upon the cardiovascular system and can produce profound psychological disturbances; toxicity includes necrosis of muscle and liver and severe hypertension. Commonly called angel's dust; peace pill.

pheniramine maleate (fen-ir′ă-mēn mal′e-āt) An antihistaminic agent.

phenobarbital (fe-no-bar′bi-tal) Phenylethylbarbituric acid; a barbiturate drug formerly used as a sedative and hypnotic; currently used mainly as an anticonvulsant agent.

phenocopy (fe′no-kop-e) Condition that resembles a genetic disorder but is not inherited; it results from environmental influences.

phenol (fe′nol) A caustic crystalline compound, C_6H_5OH, derived from coal tar; used as an anesthetic and disinfectant. Also called carbolic acid.

phenol red (fe′nol red) See phenolsulfonphthalein.

phenolphthalein (fe-nol-thal′e-in) A colorless, crystalline compound, slightly soluble in water; derived from heating phenol with phthalic anhydride in the presence of concentrated sulfuric acid; used as a hydrogen ion indicator and as a laxative.

phenolsulfonphthalein (fe-nol-sul-fōn-thal′e-in) (PSP) A dye used as an indicator, being yellow at pH 6.8 and red at pH 8.4; formerly used as a test for kidney function. Also called phenol red.

phenomenology (fe-nom-ĕ-nol′ŏ-je) The study, description, and classification of all possible phenomena in human experience, without attempting to explain or interpret them.

phenomenon (fĕ-nom′ĕ-non), *pl.* **phenom′ena** An event, manifestation, or fact that is perceptible by the senses.

Arthus p. An inflammatory and, eventually, necrotic lesion produced on the skin of a sensitized animal by the injection of antigen into the skin.

Bell's p. A unilateral upward and outward rolling of the eyeball on attempting to close the eyelids; seen in Bell's palsy.

Bordet-Gengou p. The removal of complement from fresh serum, when the serum is incubated with red blood cells or bacteria that have been sensitized with specific lysin.

declamping p. Shock occurring after the removal of clamps from a large blood vessel (e.g., aorta). Also called declamping shock.

déjà vu p. The feeling that an experience, occurring for the first time, has been experienced before.

dawn p. The abrupt increase of blood sugar (glucose) levels between 5 and 9 a.m., occurring in diabetic persons receiving insulin therapy.

Donath-Landsteiner p. Destruction of red blood cells occurring when a sample of blood from a person affected with paroxysmal cold hemoglobinuria is cooled to about 5°C and then returned to about 37°C.

Doppler p. See Doppler effect, under effect.

escape p. (a) The increase in excretion of sodium and water that occurs after two or three days of excessive mineralocorticoid activity (endogenous, as in primary aldosteronism, or due to administration of exogenous mineralocorticoid); after the initial phase of sodium and fluid retention there is an "escape" from the sodium-retaining effects and a new equilibrium is established. (b) After initial constriction, failure of the pupil of an eye to constrict upon repeated and alternate stimulation of both eyes; seen in retrobulbar neuritis.

Gunn's p. See jaw-winking syndrome.

immune adherence p. Adherence of a cell (platelet, red blood cell, leukocyte, or microorganism), that is coated with antibody and complement, to normal cells (platelets, etc.), resulting in agglutination. Also called immune adherence.

Pheiffer's p. Destruction of bacteria when introduced into the peritoneal cavity of an immunized guinea pig, or into that of a normal guinea pig when immune serum is introduced at the same time.

Raynaud's p. Numbness and pallor of the fingers, toes, and/or nose occurring secondary to another disease.

R-on-T p. In electrocardiography, a premature ventricular complex (QRS) of the electrocardiogram interrupting the T wave of the preceding heartbeat, associated with increased risk of disordered contractions of the ventricles.

Schultz-Charlton p. See Schultz-Charlton reaction, under reaction.

Shwartzman p. A reaction elicited when: (a) Two small subcutaneous doses of endotoxin are given 24 hours apart to an experimental animal; the second injection will cause a localized hemorrhagic necrosis and inflammation of blood vessels. Also called localized Shwartzman phenomenon. (b) If the injections are given intravenously, widespread hemorrhages and bilateral necrosis of kidney cortex will occur; the animal dies within 24 hours. Also called generalized Shwartzman phenomenon.

Wenckebach p. Increasing lengthening of the A-V (atrioventricular) conduction time (P-R interval) in successive cycles of the heart rhythm until a beat is skipped.

phenothiazine (fe-no-thi′ă-zēn) One of a group of

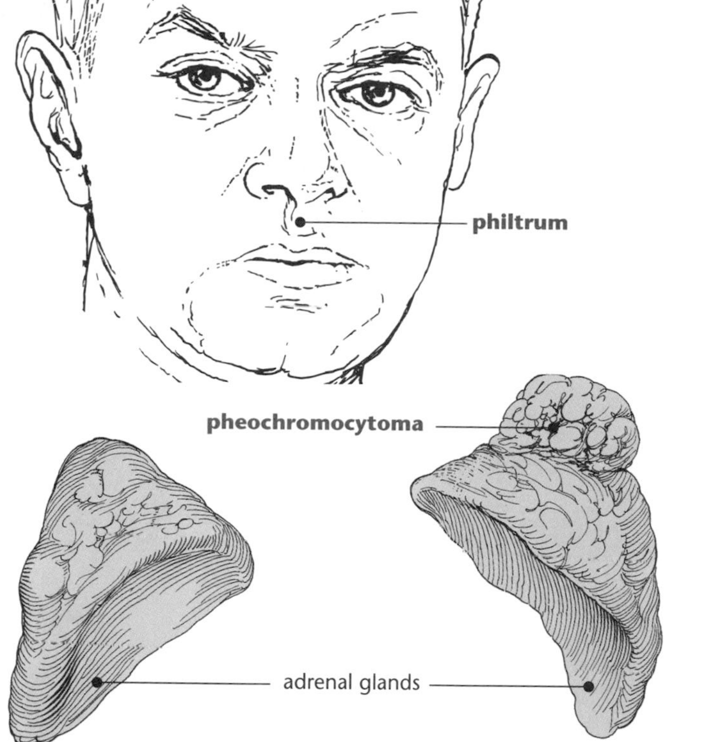

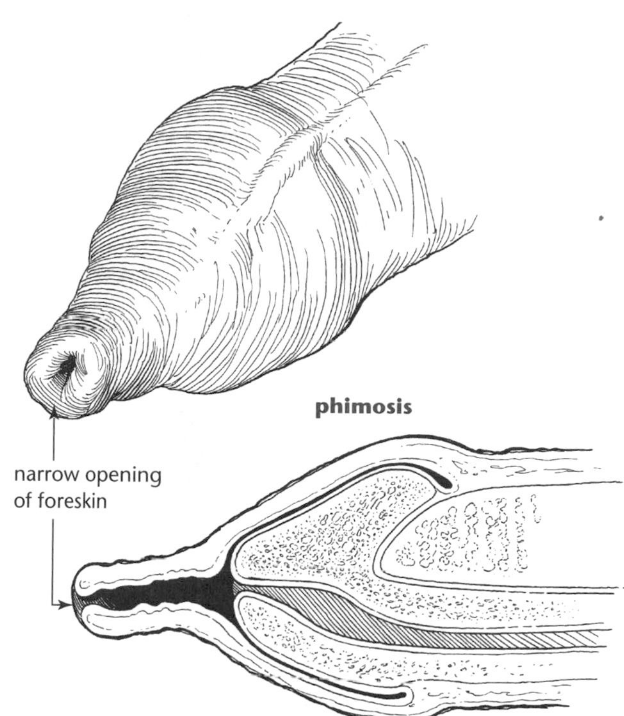

drugs used for antipsychotic effect (e.g., chlorpromazine and promethazine) and for antiemetic and antihistaminic activity.

phenotype (fe´no-tīp) In genetics, the visible appearance of an organism, produced by the interaction of its genetic constitution with the environment.

phenotypic (fe-no-tip´ik) Relating to a phenotype.

phenoxybenzamine hydrochloride (fĕ-nok-se-ben´ză-mēn hi-dro-klo´rīd) An alpha-adrenergic blocking agent that blocks the response of smooth muscle and endocrine glands to the alpha-adrenergic action of epinephrine and norepinephrine; used to treat pheochromocytoma symptoms; Dibenzyline®.

phentolamine hydrochloride (fen-tol´ă-mēn hi-dro-klo´rīd) An alpha-adrenergic blocking agent used in the diagnosis of pheochromocytoma; Regitine®.

phenyl (fen´il, fe´nil) (Ph) The univalent radical derived from benzene, $C_6H_5^-$

phenylalanine (fen-il-al´ă-nīn) (Phe) An essential amino acid occurring as a constituent of many proteins.

phenylalanine hydroxylase (fen-il-al´ă-nīn hi-drok´sĭ-lās) An enzyme that, with NAD (nicotine adenine dinucleotide) as coenzyme, promotes the oxidation of phenylalanine to tyrosine; absence of this enzyme produces phenylketonuria.

phenylbutazone (fen-il-bu´tă-zōn) A derivative of pyrazoline, used primarily to relieve pain in musculoskeletal disorders; an anti-inflammation agent.

phenylephrine hydrochloride (fen-il-ef´rin hi-dro-klo´rīd) A sympathomimetic amine closely related chemically to epinephrine; a powerful vasoconstrictor of sustained action, used as a nasal decongestant, as a mydriatic, and in preventing hypotension during spinal anesthesia; Neo-Synephrine®.

phenylethanolamine-*N*-methyltransferase (fen-il-eth-ă-nol´ă-mēn meth-il-trans´fer-ās) En-zyme that promotes the conversion of norepinephrine to epinephrine.

phenylethylbarbituric acid (fen-il-eth-il-bahr-bĭ-tu´rik as´id) See phenobarbital.

phenylglycolic acid (fen-il-gli-ko´lik as´id) See mandelic acid.

phenylhydrazine (fen-il-hi´dră-zin) Colorless liquid used in the detection of sugars, aldehydes, and ketones.

phenylketonuria (fen-il-ke-to-nu´re-ă) (PKU) Condition in which metabolism of the amino acid phenylalanine (Phe) is deficient, producing increased phenylalanine in the body with resulting nerve and brain cell damage and severe mental retardation. Formerly called phenylpyruvic oligophrenia.

phenylpropanolamine hydrochloride (fen-il-pro-pă-nol´ă-mēn hi-dro-klo´rīd) Preparation used as a nasal decongestant and bronchodilator.

phenylpyruvic acid (fen-il-pi-roo´vik as´id) A metabolism product of phenylalanine (an essential amino acid); present in excess in the urine of individuals with phenylketonuria.

phenylthiocarbamide (fen-il-thi-o-kar-bam´id) See phenylthiourea.

phenylthiourea (fen-il-thi-o-u-re´ă) A substance that is tasteless to those individuals (taste-blind) who are homozygous for an autosomal recessive gene, but tastes bitter to those individuals (tasters) who carry the dominant allele. Also called phenylthio-carbamide.

pheochrome (fe´o-krōm) Staining a brownish yellow with chromic salts.

pheochromoblast (fe-o-kro´mo-blast) A young chromaffin (one of the cells forming the medulla of the adrenal gland).

pheochromocyte (fe-o-kro´mo-sīt) A chromaffin cell forming the medulla of an adrenal gland, a sympathetic paraganglion, or a pheochromocytoma.

pheochromocytoma (fe-o-kro-mo-si-to´mă) A catecholamine-producing tumor of the chromaffin cells of the sympathoadrenal system, usually the adrenal medulla; the symptoms are due to increased secretion of epinephrine and norepinephrine and consist of headache, palpitation, tachycardia, and constant or paroxysmal hypertension of moderate to severe grade.

pheresis (fĕ-re´sis) See apheresis.

pheromones (fer´o-mōns) Substances secreted externally by an organism that influences the behavior of other organisms of the same species.

phial (fi´al) Vial.

philtrum (fil´trum) The middle vertical groove of the upper lip, below the nose.

phimosis (fi-mo´sis) Tightness of the foreskin, so that it cannot be retracted over the glans penis.

phlebalgia (flĕ-bal´jhă) Pain originating in a venule or vein.

phlebarteriectasia (fleb-ar-te-re-ek-ta´zhă) General dilatation of the veins and arteries.

phlebectasia (fleb-ek-ta´zhă) Dilatation of the veins.

phlebectomy (fle-bek´tŏ-me) Surgical removal of a vein or segment of a vein. Also called venectomy.

phlebitis (flĕ-bi´is) Inflammation of a vein.

phleboclysis (flĕ-bok´lĭ-sis) Injection of medicinal liquids into a vein.

phlebogram (fleb´o-gram) A tracing of the venous (usually jugular) pulse made by the phlebograph.

phlebograph (fleb´o-graf) A device for recording venous pulsations.

phlebography (flĕ-bog´ră-fe) The recording of a venous pulse.

phlebolith (fleb´o-lith) A concretion in a vein resulting from the calcification of an old thrombus. Also called vein stone.

phleboplasty (fleb´o-plas-te) Reparative operation on a vein.

phleborrhagia (fleb-o-ra´jhă) Bleeding from a vein.

phleborrhaphy (flĕ-bor´ă-fe) Suture of a vein. Also called venisuture.

phleborrhexis (fleb-o-rek´sis) Rupture of a vein.

phlebosclerosis (fleb-o-skle-ro´sis) Fibrous hardening of the walls of veins, especially the inner layer.

phlebostasis (flĕ-bos´tă-sis) Slow circulation through the veins due either to pathologic venous distention or to application of a tourniquet. Also called venostasis.

phlebothrombosis (fleb-o-throm-bo´sis) Blood clotting within a vein without inflammation of its walls. COMPARE: thrombophlebitis.

phlebotomize (fle-bot´o-mīz) To perform a phlebotomy.

Phlebotomus (flĕ-bot´ŏ-mus) Genus of blood-sucking sandflies of the family Psychodidae.

P. papatasii The species that is the vector of sandfly fever (phlebotomus or pappataci fever) and of the protozoan agents causing cutaneous leishmaniasis.

phlebotomy (flĕ-bot´ŏ-me) Withdrawal of blood from a vein. Also called venesection.

phlegm (flem) **1.** Mucus secreted by the mucosa of the respiratory tract. **2.** According to ancient Greek physiology, one of the four humors of the body.

phlegmasia (fleg-ma´zhă, fleg-ma´ze-ă) Inflammation.

p. alba dolens See puerperal thrombophlebitis, under thrombophlebitis.

p. cerulea dolens Severe pain, swelling, and cyanosis of a limb, followed by circulatory collapse and shock, due to thrombosis of the limb.

phlegmatic (fleg-mat´ik) Apathetic; calm.

phlegmon (fleg´mon) Acute inflammation of the subcutaneous connective tissue.

phlegmonous (fleg´mon-us) Relating to inflammation of subcutaneous tissues.

phlogiston (flo-jis´ton) A hypothetical substance of negative mass which, before the discovery of oxygen, was believed to be given off by substances undergoing combustion.

phlorizin (flo-ri´zin) Substance extracted from the roots of apple, pear, plum, and cherry trees; injected into experimental animals to produce glycosuria by

P

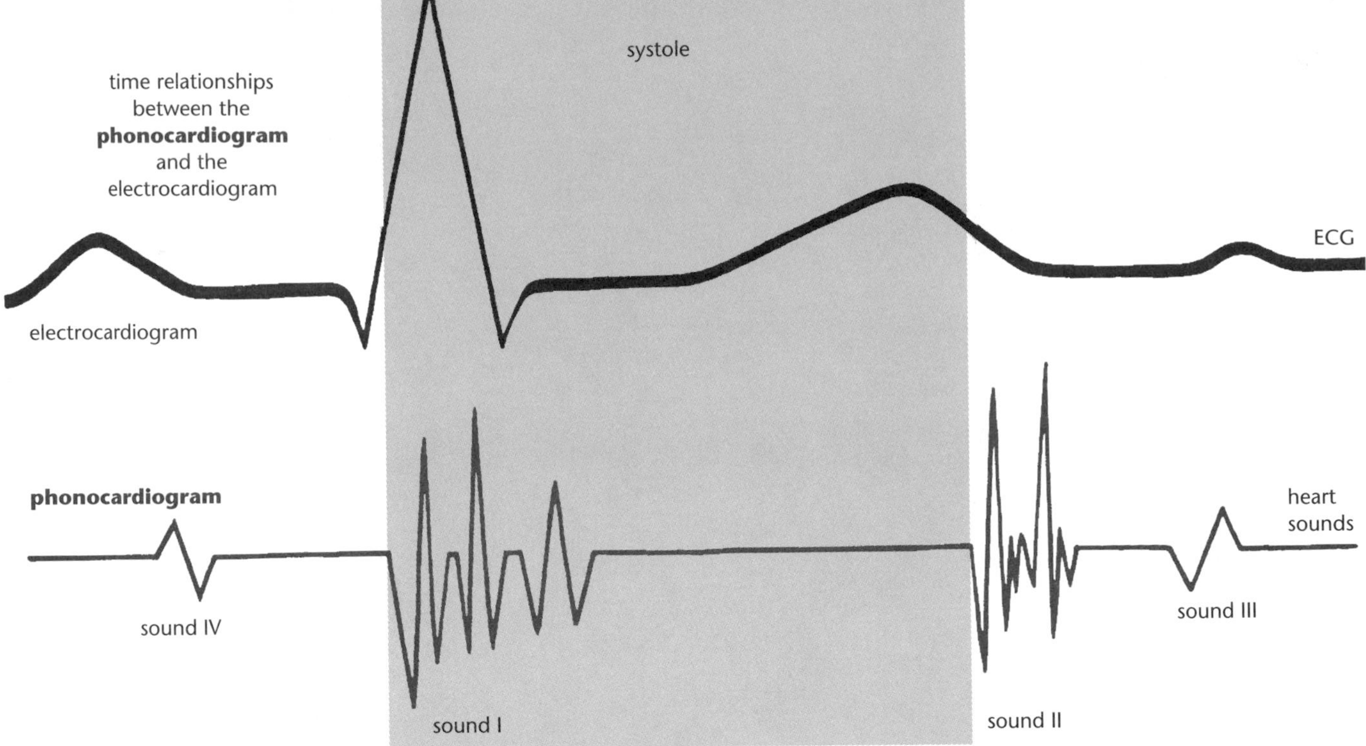

inhibiting the renal tubular reabsorption of glucose.

phlyctenule (flik´ten-ūl) A minute red nodular pustule occurring in the transparent covering of the eyeball (conjunctiva) or cornea.

phobia (fo´be-ă) Any abnormal, irrational fear.

phobic (fo´bik) Relating to abnormal fear.

phobism (fo´biz-m) The state of being affected by a phobia.

phocomelia (fo-ko-me´le-ă) Gross underdevelopment of extremities, particularly the arms; the hands and feet are attached close to the body.

phocomelus (fo-kom´ĕ-lus) An individual with phocomelia.

phonal (fo´nal) Related to sounds.

phonasthenia (fo-nas-the´ne-ă) Difficult or abnormal production of the voice.

phonation (fo-na´shun) The utterance of vocal sounds that are culturally appropriate for human communication.

phonatory (fo´nă-to-re) Relating to phonation.

phoneme (fo´nēm) The smallest sound of speech.

phonemic (fo-nē´mik) Relating to phoneme.

phonetic (fo-net´ik) Relating to speech sounds.

phonetics (fo-net´iks) The branch of linguistics concerned with the study of all aspects of speech sounds (their production, combination, and representation by written symbols). Also called phonology.

phoniatrics (fo-ne-at´riks) The study and treatment of speech defects.

phonic (fon´ik) Relating to sound or to the voice.

phonism (fo´niz-m) See auditory synesthesia, under synesthesia.

phonoangiography (fo-no-an-je-og´ră-fe) The recording and subsequent analysis of sound produced by the blood passing through an artery; useful in determining the extent of narrowing of the lumen by atherosclerosis.

phonocardiogram (fo-no-kar´de-ŏ-gram) (PCG) A graphic representation of the heart sounds made with the phonocardiograph.

phonocardiograph (fo-no-kar´de-ŏ-graf) An instrument that makes graphic records of the heart sounds.

phonocardiography (fo-no-kar-de-og´ră-fe) The recording of the sounds produced by the action of the heart.

phonocatheter (fo-no-kath´ĕ-ter) A catheter-microphone combination for recording cardiac sounds from within the heart and great vessels.

phonoelectrocardioscope (fo-no-e-lek-tro-kar´de-o-skōp) A dual-beam oscilloscope that displays both heart sounds and electrocardiographic tracings.

phonogram (fo´no-gram) A symbol representing a sound (e.g., a letter or a syllable in a phonetic alphabet).

phonology (fo-nol´ŏ-je) See phonetics.

phonometor (fo-nom´ĕ-ter) Apparatus used to measure the intensity and pitch of sounds.

phonopathy (fo-nop´ă-thē) Any disease of the organs involved in speech.

phonophore (fo´no-for) A funnel- or bell-shaped stethoscope.

phonophotography (fo-no-fo-tog´ră-fe) The photographic recording of sound-vibration curves.

phonopsia (fo-nop´se-ă) Subjective visual sensations, as of color, induced by the hearing of certain sounds.

phonoreceptor (fo-no-re-sep´ter) A receptor for sound stimuli.

phonosurgery (fo-no-ser´jer-ē) Surgical procedures upon the larynx, especially the vocal folds, designed for voice preservation, restoration, or enhancement.

phoria (for´e-ă) A tendency of the two eyes to deviate. The direction of the deviation is usually indicated by an appropriate prefix (e.g., exophoria, esophoria, hypophoria, hyperphoria).

phorometer (fo-rom´ĕ-ter) An instrument for detecting the presence and degree of imbalance of the eye muscles (heterophoria).

phoropter (fo-rop´tor) Instrument for determining the refractive state of the eyes, phorias, amplitude of accommodation, etc.

phose (fōz) A subjective visual sensation, as of a bright light or color.

phosgene (fos´jēn) Carbonyl chloride, $COCl_2$; a colorless gas that condenses to a liquid at temperatures below 8°C. Highly poisonous, primarily because of lung damage.

phosgenic (fos-jen´ik) Light-producing.

phosis (fo´sis) Any condition that produces subjective visual sensations.

phosphagenic (fos-fă-jen´ik) Phosphate-producing.

phosphatase (fos´fă-tās) Any of a group of enzymes that promote the hydrolysis of phosphoric esters.

acid p. A phosphatase that is most effective in an acid milieu (pH 5.4); present in relatively high concentrations in the prostate.

alkaline p. A phosphatase most effective in an alkaline milieu (pH 8.6); present in bone, blood, kidneys, and other tissues.

phosphate (fos´fāt) Any salt of phosphoric acid, present in the body combined with calcium or sodium.

phosphated (fos´fāt-ed) Containing phosphates.

phosphatic (fos-fat´ik) Relating to phosphates.

phosphatidic acid (fos-fă-tid´ic as´id) An acid that results from the partial hydrolysis of a phospholipid and that on hydrolysis yields two fatty acid molecules and one molecule each of glycerol and phosphoric acid.

phosphatidylcholine (fos-fă-ti-dil-ko´lēn) (PC) A phospholipid compound resulting from condensation of phosphatidic acid and choline. Also called lecithin.

phosphatidylethanolamine (fos-fă-ti-dil-eth-ă-nol´ă-mēn) A phospholipid, the product of condensation of phosphatidic acid and ethanolamine. Also called cephalin.

phosphatidylinositol 4,5-biphosphate (fos-fă-ti-dil-ĭ-no´sĭ-tol bi-fos´fāt) (PIP_2) A constituent of cell membrane phospholipids involved in calcium-mediated response to hormones.

phosphaturia (fos-fă-tu´re-ă) The presence of a high percentage of phosphates in the urine.

phosphene (fos´fēn) A sensation of light experienced upon pressure on, or electrical stimulation of, the eyeball.

phosphide (fos´fīd) A compound containing trivalent phosphorus (e.g., sodium phosphide, Na_3P).

phosphine (fos´fēn) PH_3; a colorless, poisonous gas of characteristic odor. Also called hydrogen phosphide; phosphorated hydrogen.

phosphite (fos´fīt) A salt of phosphorous acid.

phosphoarginine (fos-fo-ar´jĭ-nin) Compound serving as a store of energy for muscle contraction in invertebrates; it corresponds to phosphocreatine in muscles of vertebrates.

phosphocreatine (fos-fo-kre´ă-tin) See creatine phosphate, under creatine.

phosphodiester (fos-fo-di-es´ter) A diesterified orthophosphoric acid; $RO–(PO_2H)–OR'$, as in the nucleic acids.

phosphodiesterase (fos-fo-di-es´ter-ās) One of a group of enzymes that split phosphodiester bonds, as those between nucleotides.

phosphoenolpyruvic acid (fos-fo-e-nol-pi´roo-vik as´id) A high-energy compound, intermediate in the conversion of glucose to pyruvic acid.

phosphofructokinase (fos-fo-fruk-to-kĭ´nās) An essential enzyme in the cycle of glucose metabolism; it promotes the formation of fructose 1,6-bisphosphate from fructose

6-phosphate and adenosine triphosphate (ATP).

phosphoglucomutase (fos-fo-gloo-ko-mu´tās) Enzyme that promotes the reaction

glucose-6-phosphate↔glucose-1-phosphate.

phosphokinase (fos-fo-kĭ´nās) See phosphotransferase.

phospholipase (fos-fo-lip´ās) Any enzyme that promotes the hydrolysis of a phospholipid. Also called lecithinase.

phospholipid (fos-fo-lip´id) Any of several waxy

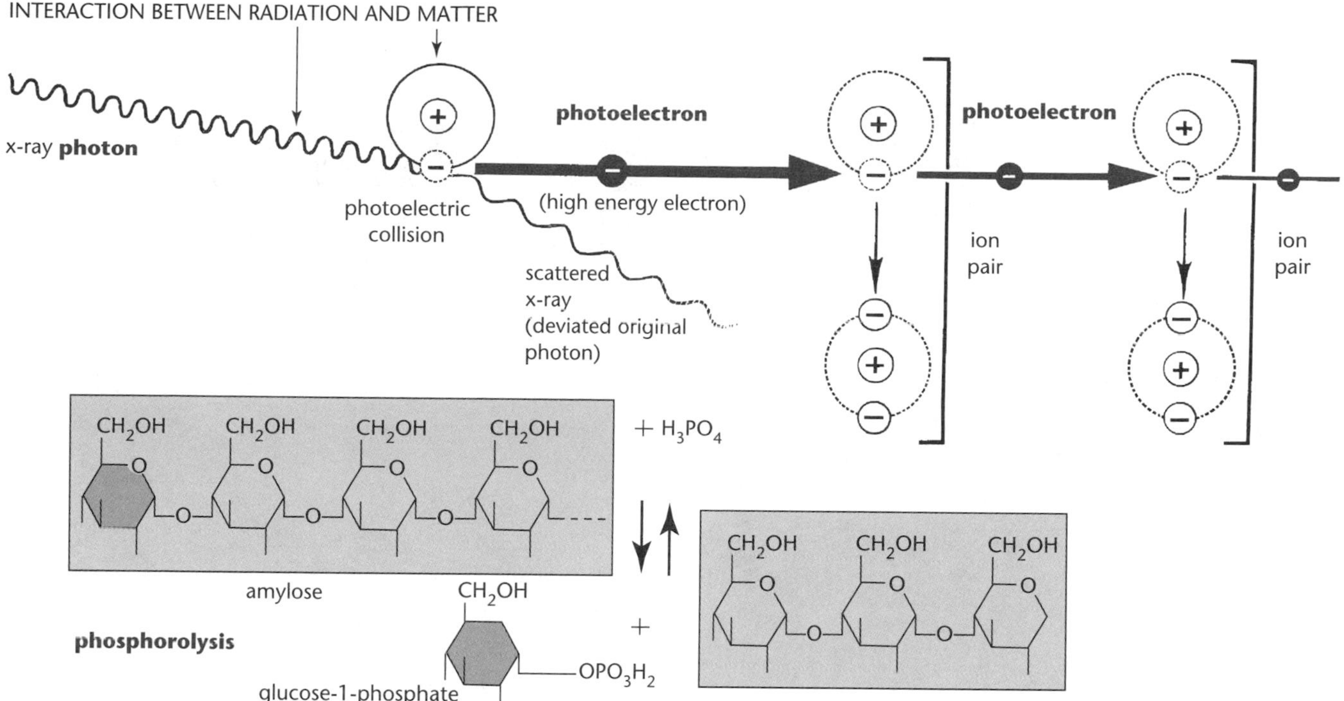

or greasy compounds containing phosphoric acid (e.g., phosphatidylcholine, phosphatidylethanolamine, sphingomyelin) present in plant and animal tissues, especially in membranes, such as red blood cell membranes and the myelin sheath of nerve cells.

phosphoprotein (fos-fo-pro´tēn) One of a group of conjugated proteins containing a simple protein combined with a phosphorous compound (e.g., casein).

phosphor (fos´fōr) A substance that glows when stimulated by external radiation; used in the detection of radioactivity.

phosphorated (fos´fo-rāt-ed) Combined with phosphorus.

phosphorescence (fos-fo-res´ens) **1.** The afterglow or continuous emission of light from a substance without temperature rise after exposure to light, heat, or electric current; distinguished from fluorescence, in which light is emitted essentially only when the exciting source is present. **2.** The faint greenish glow of white phosphorus in the presence of air, due to slow oxidation. **3.** The luminescence of certain living organisms such as fire flies.

phosphorescent (fos-fo-res´ent) Having the capacity to glow, especially in the dark.

phosphoribosyltransferase (fos-fo-ri-bo-sil-trans´fer-ās) Any of a group of enzymes (important in nucleotide biosynthesis) that transfer ribose 5-phosphate from 5-phospho-α-D-ribosyl 1-pyrophosphate to a purine, pyrimidine, or pyridine acceptor.

phosphoric acid (fos-for´ik as´id) H_3PO_4; colorless crystals that are soluble in water and important as a source of phosphate groups in metabolism; the principal component of silicate and zinc phosphate dental cement liquids.

phosphorism (fos´fo-riz-m) Chronic poisoning with phosphorus.

phosphorized (fos´fo-rīzd) Phosphorated.

phosphorolysis (fos-fo-rol´ĭ-sis) A reaction analogous to hydrolysis in which the elements of phosphoric acid, rather than of water, are added in the course of splitting a bond; the conversion of glycogen to glucose 1-phosphate is an example.

phosphorous (fos´fo-rus) **1.** Relating to phosphorus. **2.** Phosphorescent.

phosphorus (fos´fo-rus) A poisonous nonmetallic element, symbol P, atomic number 15, atomic weight 30.974; it occurs in nature always in combined form, as inorganic phosphates in minerals and water and as organic phosphates in all living cells.

phosphorus-32 (^{32}P) A beta-emitting radioactive phosphorus isotope with atomic weight 32 and with a half-life of 14.3 days; used in brain, eye, skin, and stomach tumor localization, as a tracer to study metabolism, and in the treatment of certain bone and blood-forming disorders.

phosphorylase (fos-for´ĭ-lās) Enzyme that triggers the splitting of the glycogen molecule to form glucose.

phosphorylation (fos-for-ĭ-la´shun) The addition of phosphate to an organic compound through the action of a phosphorylase.

phosphotransferase (fos-fo-trans´fer-ās) An enzyme that catalyzes the transfer of phosphorous-containing groups. Also called phosphokinase.

phosphotungstic acid (fos-fo-tung´stik as´id) Green crystals, soluble in water, used as a reagent for alkaloids and for albumin.

phot (fōt) A unit of illumination equal to 1 lumen per square centimeter of surface.

photalgia (fo-tal´jă) Pain in the eyes caused by light. Also called photodynia.

photesthesis (fo-tes-the´sis) Ability to perceive light.

photic (fo´tik) Relating to light.

photism (fo´tiz-m) Production of a visual sensation by stimulation of another sense organ.

photoablation (fo-to-ab-la´shun) Destruction of tissue with a laser beam.

photoactinic (fo-to-ak-tin´ik) Producing luminous and chemical effects, said of radiation.

photoallergy (fo-to-al´er-je) See photosensitization.

photobiology (fo-to-bi-ol´ŏ-je) The study of the effect of light on living organisms (plants or animals).

photobiotic (fo-to-bi-ot´ik) Capable of living only in the light.

photocatalyst (fo-to-kat´ă-list) A substance that brings about a light-stimulated reaction (e.g., chlorophyll).

photoceptor (fo-to-sep´tor) See photoreceptor.

photochemistry (fo-to-kem´is-tre) The branch of chemistry concerned with chemical changes caused by light.

photochemotherapy (fo-to-ke-mo-ther´ă-pe) See photoradiation.

photochromogens (fo-to-kro´mo-jens) See group I mycobacteria, under mycobacteria.

photocoagulation (fo-to-ko-ag-u-la´shun) The use of an intense beam of light (carbon arc or laser) focused to a fine point to destroy tissue or to create adhesive scars; used especially in intraocular surgery to bond a detached retina, to seal leaking blood vessels, or to reduce abnormal blood vessel growth.

photocoagulator (fo-to-ko-ag´u-la-tor) Apparatus used in photocoagulation.

laser p. A laser device used to stop minute spots of bleeding.

photodermatitis (fo-to-der-mă-ti´tis) Development of skin lesions in areas exposed to sunlight; may be due to extreme sensitivity, or to photosensitizing factors (e.g., certain drugs or diseases).

photodisintegration (fo-to-dis-in-tĕ-gra´shun) Nuclear deterioration due to absorption of high-energy radiation.

photodynamic (fo-to-di-nam´ik) Relating to the energy-producing effects of light.

photodynia (fo-to-din´e-ă) See photalgia.

photoelectricity (fo-to-e-lek-tris´ĭ-te) Electricity resulting from the action of light.

photoelectrometer (fo-to-e-lek-trom´ĕ-ter) Device for measuring concentration of substances in solution by means of a photoelectric cell.

photoelectron (fo-to-e-lek´tron) An electron that has been set free (ejected from its orbit) by collision with a high energy photon.

photoemulsification (fo-to-e-mul-sĭ-fĭ-ka´shun) Cataract removal by fragmenting the opaque lens of the eye with sound vibrations (ultrasonic energy) and simultaneously irrigating and aspirating the lens material.

P

photogen (fo´to-jen) A bacterium producing luminescence.

photogenesis (fo-to-jen´ĕ-sis) The production of light.

photogenic, photogenous (fo-to-jen´ik, fo-to-jen´us) **1.** Induced by exposure to light. **2.** Producing light.

photokinesis (fo-to-ki-ne´sis) In biology, movement in response to light.

photoluminescent (fo-to-lu-mĭ-nes´ent) Having the ability to emit light at room temperature after exposure to radiant energy of a different wavelength.

photolysis (fo-tol´ĭ-sis) Chemical decomposition of a compound by the action of radiant energy, especially light.

photolyte (fo´to-līt) A product of chemical decomposition caused by light.

photomacrography (fo-to-mă-krog´ră-fe) The photographic recording of images of gross specimens at low magnification using photomacro lenses mounted on a camera.

photometer (fo-tom´ĕ-ter) Instrument for measuring the intensity of light.

photometry (fo-tom´ĕ-tre) The measurement of the intensity of light.

photomicrograph (fo-to-mi´kro-graf) Photograph of an object as viewed through the microscope.

photomicrography (fo-to-mi-krog´ră-fe) The photographic recording of images seen through a microscope.

photon (fo´ton) A unit or quantum of energy of a light wave or other electromagnetic wave, regarded as a minute particle of no electric charge and zero

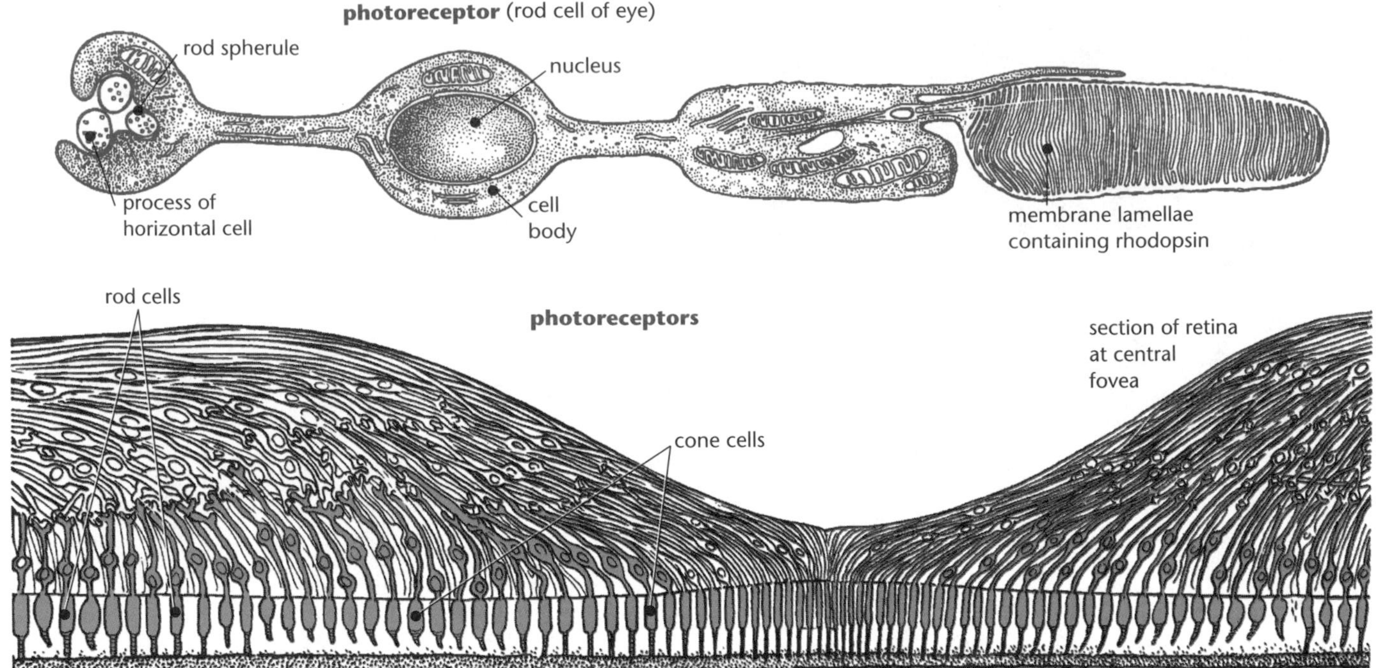

mass.

photoperceptive (fo-to-per-sep´tiv) See photoreceptive.

photoperiod (fo-to-pēr´e-od) The varying length of exposure of a living organism to light.

photoperiodism (fo-to-pe´re-od-iz-m) The physiologic, biomedical, and behavioral changes occurring in living organisms in response to varying periods of exposure to light (photoperiod).

photophobia (fo-to-fo´be-ă) Abnormal visual sensitivity to light.

photophobic (fo-to-fo´bik) Relating to photophobia.

photophthalmia (fo-to-of-thal´me-ă) Inflammation of the eyes caused by exposure to intense light, as in snow blindness.

photopsia, photopsy (fo-top´se-ă, fo-top´se) A subjective sensation of flashing light and sparks experienced with certain diseases of the retina, optic nerve, or brain.

P

photopsin (fo-top´sin) The protein constituent (opsin) of the pigment (iodopsin) in the retinal cones.

photoradiation (fo-to-ra-de-a´shun) Treatment of cancer by intravenous injection of a photosensitizing substance, such as hematoporphyrin (which concentrates on tumor cells and renders them hypersensitive to light), followed by exposure to red laser light if the tumor is superficial, or a fiberoptic probe if it is a deep one; a photochemical reaction is thus produced, with consequent destruction of cancerous tissue. Also called photochemotherapy.

photoreactivation (fo-to-re-ak-tĭ-va´shun) The reversal of a photochemical reaction by exposure to light (e.g., reversal of the effect of ultraviolet rays on cells by exposure to visible light rays).

photoreceptive (fo-to-re-sep´tiv) Capable of perceiving light rays. Also called photoperceptive.

photoreceptor (fo-to-re-sep´tor) A nerve end-organ capable of being stimulated by light, as the rods and cones of the retina. Also called photoceptor.

photoretinitis (fo-to-ret-ĭ-ni´tis) Inflammation of the retina caused by exposure to intense light.

photoscan (fo´to-skan) A photograph of the distribution and concentration of an internally administered radiopaque substance.

photosensitivity (fo-to-sen-sĭ-tiv´ĭ-te) Excessive sensitivity to light.

photosensitization (fo-to-sen-sĭ-ti-za´shun) Hypersensitization of skin to sunlight or ultraviolet rays; caused by ingestion of certain plants or drugs. Also called photoallergy.

photostable (fo´to-sta-bl) Unchanged upon exposure to light.

photosynthesis (fo-to-sin´thĕ-sis) The process by which green plants, using chlorophyll and the energy of sunlight, turn carbon dioxide and water into food substance (carbohydrate); molecular oxygen is liberated in the process.

phototaxis (fo-to-tak´sis) Movement of an organism (as a whole) toward or away from a light source. COMPARE: phototropism.

phototherapy (fo-to-ther´ă-pe) Treatment of disease with light.

photothermal (fo-to-ther´mal) **1.** Relating to both light and heat. **2.** Relating to heat produced by light.

phototoxic (fo-to-tok´sik) Relating to an injurious effect produced or promoted by overexposure to light, ultraviolet rays, or x rays.

phototropism (fo-tot´ro-piz-m) Movement of parts of an organism toward or away from a light source. COMPARE: phototaxis.

phren (fren) **1.** Greek for diaphragm. **2.** The mind.

phrenectomy (fre-nek´tŏ-me) See phrenicectomy.

phrenemphraxis (fren-em-frak´sis) See phreniclasia.

phrenic (fren´ik) **1.** Relating to the diaphragm. **2.** Relating to the mind.

phrenicectomy (fren-ĭ-sek´tŏ-me) Surgical removal of a portion of the phrenic nerve. Also called phrenectomy.

phreniclasia (fren-ĭ-kla´zhă, fren-ĭ-kla´ze-ă) The crushing of a small portion of the phrenic nerve. Also called phrenemphraxis.

phrenicotomy (fren-ĭ-kot´ŏ-me) Division of a phrenic nerve in order to paralyze one-half of the diaphragm.

phrenocolic (fren-o-kol´ik) Relating to the diaphragm and the colon.

phrenogastric (fren-o-gas´trik) Relating to the diaphragm and the stomach.

phrenohepatic (fren-o-hĕ-pat´ik) Relating to the diaphragm and the liver.

phrenology (frĕ-nol´ŏ-je) An obsolete doctrine concerned with the study of mental capacity and traits of character based upon the external configuration of the skull.

phrenoplegia (fren-o-ple´je-ă) Paralysis of the diaphragm.

phrenosin (fren´o-sin) A cerebroside present in the white matter of the brain. Also called cerebron.

phrenospasm (fren´o-spazm) Spasm of the diaphragm.

phrenotropic (fren-o-trop´ik) Exerting its foremost effect upon the mind or brain.

phrynoderma (fren-o-der´mă) A dry eruption of the skin thought to be due to vitamin A deficiency.

phthalein (thal´e-in) Any of various dyes, such as phenolphthalein, derived from the condensation of phthalic anhydride with the phenols; some are used as indicators and occasionally as purgatives.

phthiriasis (thir-i´ă-sis) Infestation with the crab louse (*Phthirus pubis).*

Phthirus (thir´us) A genus of sucking lice of the order Anoplura.

P. pubis A parasite of humans infesting areas of coarse hair, particularly in the pubic region, but also the hair of the chest, axillae, eyebrows, and eyelashes. Also called pubic louse; crab louse.

phthisic (thi´sik) Relating to or afflicted with phthisis.

phthisiology (thi-ze-ol´ŏ-je) The study and treatment of pulmonary tuberculosis.

phthisis (thi´sis) **1.** A wasting away of tissue. **2.** Obsolete term for tuberculosis.

black p., miners' p. See anthracosis.

p. bulbi Collapse and shrinking of the eyeball associated with an untreated bacterial infection of all structures of the eye.

marble cutters' p. See calcicosis.

potters' p. See silicosis.

stonecutters' p. See pneumoconiosis.

phycomycosis (fi-ko-mi-ko´sis) General term for acute and chronic systemic diseases caused by fungi of the class Phycomycetes, usually occurring in debilitated individuals.

phylaxis (fi-lak´sis) Protection against infection.

phylogenesis (fi-lo-jen´ĕ-sis) The evolutionary development or racial history of the species; distinguished from ontogenesis. Also called phylogeny.

phylogeny (fi-loj´ĕ-ne) See phylogenesis.

phylum (fi´lum), *pl.* **phy´la** A taxonomic division of animals and vegetables; below kingdom and above class.

phyma (fi´mă) A small skin tumor.

phymatosis (fi-mă-to´sis) Disorder marked by the presence of small skin nodules (phymas).

physiatrics (fiz-e-at´riks) See physical medicine and rehabilitation, under medicine.

physiatrist (fiz-e-at´rist) A physician who specializes in physical medicine and rehabilitation.

physic (fiz´ik) Any medicine, especially a cathartic.

physical (fiz´e-kal) Relating to the body.

physician (fĭ-zish´un) A doctor of medicine; an individual trained and licensed to treat the ill and injured.

attending p. Physician to whose service a patient is admitted to a hospital; a physician who cares for patients in the facility. Commonly called the attending.

admitting p. The physician responsible for a patient after the patient is admitted to a hospital or other inpatient health facility; it may be the attending physician or someone else who is acting for the attending.

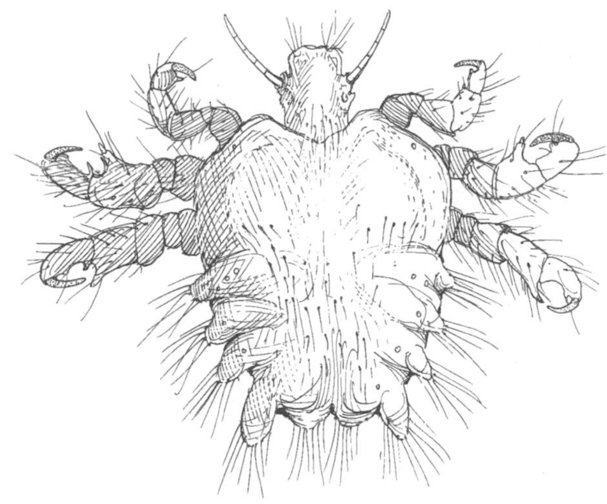

Phthirus pubis

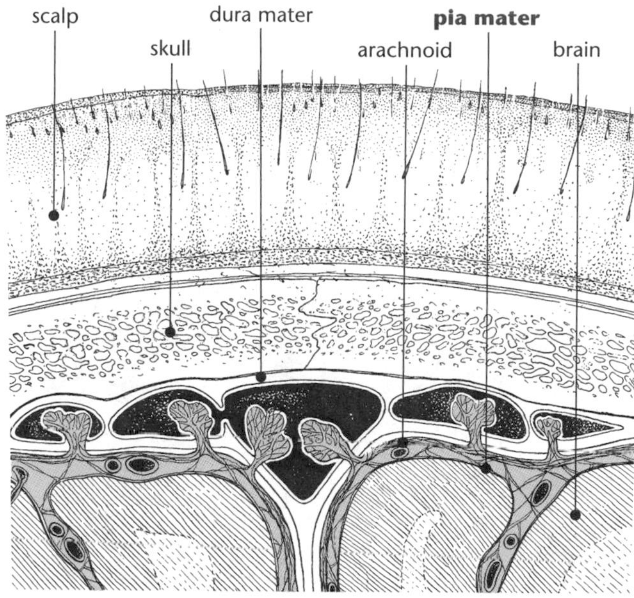

family p. A specialist in family practice (i.e., one who provides comprehensive health care for the whole family); generally must complete a three-year residency in family practice to qualify for board certification by the American Academy of Family Physicians. COMPARE: general practitioner, under practitioner.

osteopathic p. A practitioner of osteopathy.

primary care p. (PCP) A generalist in internal medicine, family practice, or pediatrics to whom the patient reports, except in emergency situations.

resident p. See resident.

physician assistant (fĭ-zish´un ă-sis´tant) (P.A.) An individual who has been trained in primary care medicine and is licensed to practice (in the United States) under the supervision of a physician.

physicochemical (fiz-ĭ-ko-kem´ĭ-kal) Relating to both physics and chemistry.

physics (fiz´iks) The science concerned with the study of matter and energy and the interactions between the two.

physiogenic (fiz-e-o-jen´ik) Caused by physical activity.

physiognomy (fiz-e-og´no-me) **1.** The art of judging human character and mental qualities from facial features and general bodily carriage. **2.** The countenance, especially regarded as an indication of the character.

physiologic, physiological (fiz-e-o-loj´ik, fiz-e-o-loj´ĭ-kal) **1.** Relating to physiology. **2.** Denoting the various normal processes of a living organism.

physiologist (fiz-e-ol´ŏ-jist) A specialist in physiology.

physiology (fiz-e-ol´ŏ-je) The science concerned with the normal functions and activities of the living organism.

physiotherapy (fiz-e-o-ther´a-pe) See physical therapy, under therapy.

physique (fĭ-zēk´) The structure of the body with reference to its proportions, muscular development, and appearance.

physohematometra (fi-so-hem-ă-to-me´tră) Distention of the uterine cavity with gas and blood.

physostigmine (fi-so-stig´mēn) A crystalline compound extracted from the Calabar bean; it is a reversible inhibitor of the cholinesterases and prevents destruction of acetylcholine. Also called eserine.

p. salicylate Used topically to reduce intraocular tension in glaucoma; also used to overcome excessive cholinergic activity. Also called eserine salicylate.

phytin (fi´tin) The mixed magnesium-calcium salt of phytic acid; used as a dietary supplement to provide calcium and phosphorus.

phytoagglutinin (fi-to-ă-gloo-tĭ-na´shun) See lectin.

phytobezoar (fi-to-be´zōr) An undigested concretion remaining in the stomach over a long period, composed mostly of vegetable fibers, seeds and skins of fruits, and sometimes starch granules and fat globules.

phytoestrogen (fi-to-es´tro-gen) Estrogen found in herbs (e.g., dong quai, black cohosh, damiana, and licorice) or other plant sources (e.g., soybeans and yams).

phytohemagglutinin (fi-to-hem-ă-gloo´tĭ-nin) (PHA) An extract derived from the stringbean; originally used as a red blood cell agglutinating reagent; it stimulates human lymphoid cells to divide, replicate their DNA, and transcribe RNA.

phytoid (fi´toid) Resembling a plant.

phytol (fi´tol) An unsaturated alcohol fragment obtained from hydrolysis of chlorophyll; an open-chain terpene used for the synthesis of vitamins E and K_1.

phytopathology (fi-to-pă-thol´ŏ-je) The study of plant diseases.

phytotoxic (fi-to-tok´sik) Having a poisonous effect on plant life; inhibiting plant growth.

phytotoxin (fi-to-tok´sin) A toxin produced by certain higher plants.

pia-arachnoid (pe´ă-ă-rak´noid) See leptomeninges.

pial (pe´al) Relating to the pia mater.

pia mater (pe-ă ma´ter) A delicate membrane, innermost of the three membranes enveloping the brain and spinal cord.

pian (pe-ăn) See yaws.

piarachnoid (pe´ar-ak´noid) See leptomeninges.

pica (pi´kă) Compulsive eating of unnatural food or substances.

pickling (pĭk´ling) In dentistry, the method of removing impurities and oxides from the surface of metals by immersion in acid.

pickwickian syndrome (pik-wik´e-an sin´drōm) See obesity-hypoventilation syndrome.

picogram (pi´ko-gram) (pg) A unit of weight equal to one-trillionth (10^{-12}) of a gram. Formerly called micromicrogram (μμg).

picometer (pi-kom´ĕ-ter) Unit of length equal to one-trillionth (10^{-12}) of a meter. Formerly called micromicron.

Picornaviridae (pi-kor-nă-vir´ĭ-de) A large family of viruses that contain single-stranded RNA and multiply in cytoplasm; represents the smallest known viruses (20 to 30 nm in diameter) and includes viruses causing poliomyelitis, meningitis, myocarditis, hepatitis type A, and the common cold.

picornavirus (pi-kor-nă-vi´rus) Any RNA infectious virus of the family Picornaviridae.

picrate (pik´rāt) A salt of picric acid.

picric acid (pik´rik as´id) Crystalline compound used as a reagent and in dyes and antiseptics. Also called trinitrophenol; carbazotic acid.

picrocarmine (pik-ro-kar´min) Solution containing ammonia and picric acid, used to stain tissues in histology.

picroformol (pik-ro-fōr´mol) Substance containing formalin and picric acid; used as a fixative.

picrotoxin (pik-ro-tok´sin) The bitter powder obtained from the fruit of *Anamirta cocculus*; a central nervous system stimulant formerly used as an antidote for barbiturate poisoning.

piebaldness (pi´bawld-nes) Localized areas of depigmented scalp and hair. Also called albinismus conscriptus.

piedra (pe-a´dră) Spanish for stone; a fungal disease of the hair characterized by formation of numerous small, hard, waxy concretions on extruded hairshafts. Also called trichosporosis.

Pierre Robin syndrome (pe-yair´ro-bă´ sin´drōm) A syndrome characterized by respiratory obstruction in infants with a receding jaw and glossoptosis; frequently accompanied by cleft palate. Also called primary micrognathia; Robin syndrome.

piesesthesia (pi-e-zes-the´zhă, pi-e-zes-the´ze-ă) Sensitivity to different degrees of pressure. Also called pressure sense.

piezochemistry (pi-e´zo-kem-is-tre) The study of the effects of extremely high pressures on chemical reactions.

piezoelectricity (pi-e-zo-e-lek-tris´ĭ-te) Electricity generated by pressure applied to certain crystals.

pigeon-toe (pij´ĕn-tō) See intoe.

pigment (pig´ment) **1.** Any colored material present in skin, whether deposited in the tissue proper or present in the blood passing through the skin. **2.** Any substance that produces a characteristic color in tissue (e.g., hemoglobin).

bile p. One of several substances derived from catabolism of a blood pigment, giving bile its characteristic color (e.g., bilirubin and biliverdin).

blood p. See hemoglobin.

malarial p. Denatured hemoglobin products, in rods or granules within the malarial parasite.

melanotic p. See melanin.

visual p. The photosensitive pigment in the rod and cone cells of the retina that initiates vision by the absorption of light.

pigmentation (pig-men-ta´shun) Coloration by deposition of pigment.

pigmentum nigrum (pig-men´tum ni´grum) The dark pigment lining the choroid layer of the eye.

piitis (pi-i´tis) Inflammation of the pia mater.

pilar, pilary (pi´lar, pil´ă-re) Pertaining to or covered

P

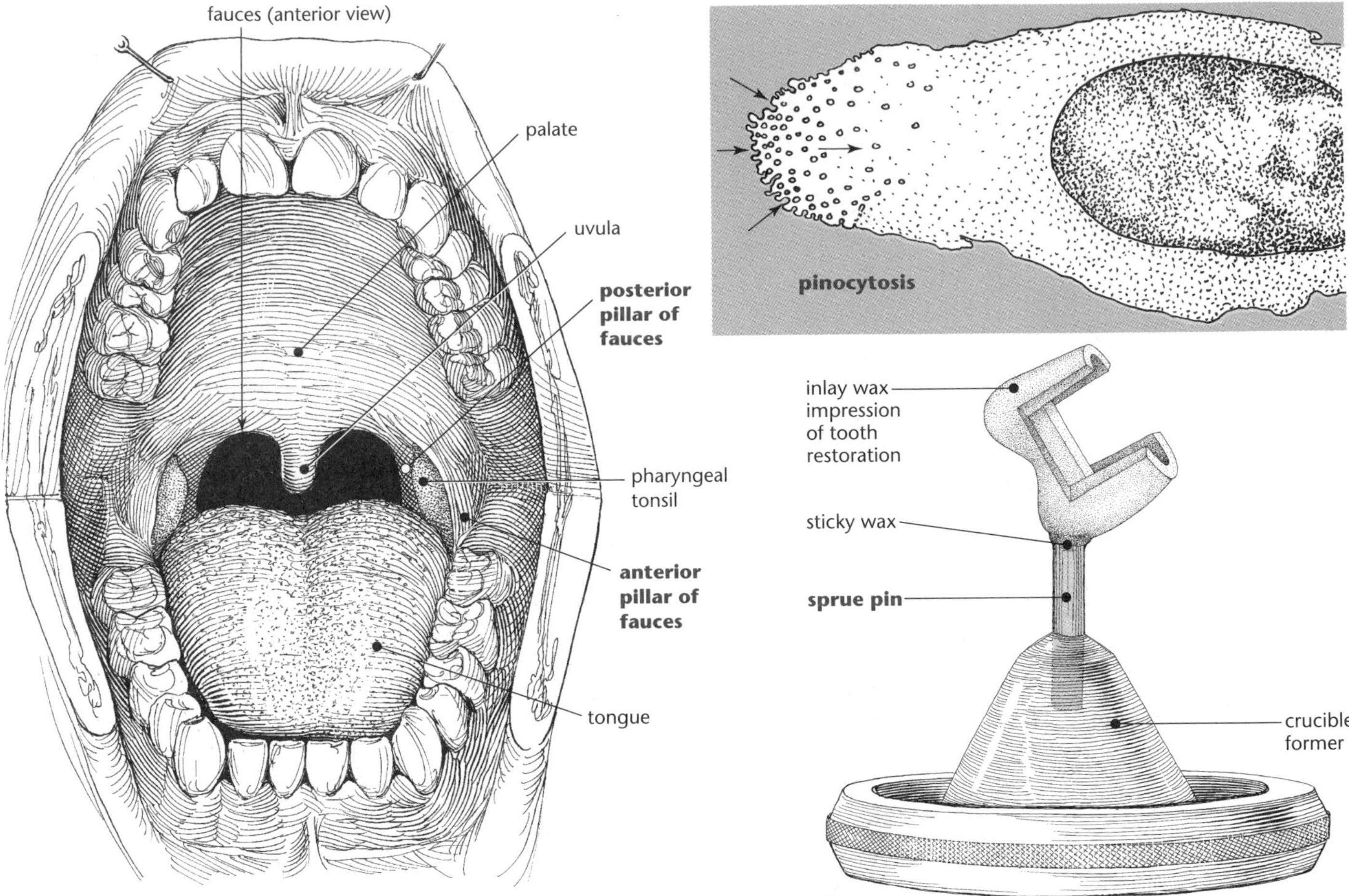

with hair.

pilaster (pi-las´ter) An abnormally prominent linea aspera on the femur, resulting in a backward concavity.

pile (pīl) **1.** A hemorrhoid. **2.** A vertical series of alternate plates of two different metals separated by layers of cloth or paper moistened with a dilute acid solution for producing a current of electricity. Also called voltaic or Volta's pile. **3.** A battery consisting of cells similarly constructed.

atomic p. Apparatus containing alternate layers of uranium and graphite in which a chain reaction is initiated and controlled, for the production of heat for power or for the production of plutonium. Also called nuclear reactor; atomic furnace.

sentinel p. A hemorrhoid-like tag at the end of an anal fissure.

volta's p.'s See pile (2).

piles (pīlz) Hemorrhoids.

pileous (po´le-us) Hairy.

pileus (pi´le-us) A cap; a caul.

p. ventriculi The first portion of the duodenum as seen in an x-ray picture. Also called duodenal cap.

pili (pi´li) Plural of pilus.

pill (pil) **1.** A small tablet of medicine. **2.** An oral contraceptive commonly referred to as *the pill*.

birth-control p. See oral contraceptive, under contraceptive.

bread p. A placebo made of bread.

enteric coated p. A pill coated with a substance, such as salol, that prevents its disintegration until it has reached the intestine.

morning-after p. See postcoital contraceptive, under contraceptive.

pep p. Colloquialism for an amphetamine or a related pharmaceutical with a pronounced stimulant effect on the central nervous system.

postcoital p. See postcoital contraceptive, under contraceptive.

pillar (pil´ar) Any vertical anatomic structure somewhat resembling a supporting column.

Corti's p.'s The pillars forming the center and inner walls of the tunnel in the spiral organ of Corti.

p. of fauces, anterior See palatoglossal arch, under arch.

p. of fauces, posterior See palatopharyngeal arch, under arch.

pill-rolling (pil-rōl-ing) The circular motion of the tips of the thumb and index finger, characteristic of Parkinson's disease.

pilocarpine (pi-lo-kar´pēn) An alkaloid obtained from the leaves of the jaborandi tree; a parasympathomimetic agent used to induce sweating or to increase salivary secretion; also acts topically to contract the pupils and reduce intraocular pressure.

Pilocarpus (pi-lo-kar´pus) A small genus of shrubs (family Rutaceae) native to the West Indies and tropical America; source of the alkaloid pilocarpine.

pilocystic (pi-lo-sis´tik) Denoting a cyst, usually dermoid, containing hair.

piloerection (pi-lo-e-rek´shun) Erection of hairs.

pilomatricoma (pi-lo-ma-trĭ-ko´mă) A benign tumor of the skin arising from the hair matrix. Also called Malherbe's calcifying epithelioma.

pilomotor (pi-lo-mo´tor) Relating to muscles or nerves in the skin that control the movement of hairs (in the formation of goose pimples).

pilonidal (pi-lo-ni´dal) Denoting the presence of hairs in a dermoid cyst, or ingrown hairs in the deep layers of skin.

pilose (pi´lōs) Covered with hair.

pilosebaceous (pi-lo-sĕ-ba´shus) Relating to a sebaceous gland and the hair follicle into which it opens, considered as a unit.

pilosia (pi-lo´se-ă) See hirsutism.

pilus (pĭ´lus), *pl.* **pĭ´li** **1.** One of the fine hairs covering the body except the palms and soles. **2.** A fine, strawlike filamentous appendage of some bacteria that serves to anchor the bacterial cell to the substrate on which it is growing; pili are shorter, straighter, and more numerous than flagella. Also called fimbria.

pi-meson (pi-mes´on) See pion.

pimple (pim´pl) Popular name for a papule or small pustule.

pin (pin) A short, straight, cyclindrical piece of metal.

retention p.'s Small griplike pegs extending from a metal casting into the tooth's dentin.

sprue p. A short metal pin used to attach a dental wax pattern to the crucible former; it provides the entrance through the investment, permitting the molten metal to flow into the mold.

Steinman's p. A firm metal pin used for the internal fixation of fractured bones.

pincement (pans-maw´) In massage, a gentle nipping or pinching of the skin.

pineal (pin´e-al) **1.** Shaped like a pine cone. **2.** Relating to the pineal body.

pinealectomy (pin-e-al-ek´tŏ-me) Surgical removal of the pineal body.

pinealocyte (pin´e-ă-lo-sīt) One of the cells forming the substance of the pineal body.

pineoblastoma (pin-e-o-blas-to´mă) A primitive undifferentiated tumor of the pineal body; found mainly in children.

pineocytoma (pin-e-o-si-to´mă) A rare tumor of the pineal body; found mainly in children.

pinguecula (ping-gwek´u-lă) A small, slightly raised, yellowish, nonfatty thickening of the conjunctiva of the eye near the sclerocorneal junction, usually on the nasal side.

piniform (pin´ĭ-form) See pineal (1).

pink disease (pink dī-zēz´) See acrodynia.

pinkeye (pink´ī) See acute contagious conjunctivitis, under conjunctivitis.

pin-lay (pin-lā) In dentistry, a veneer containing parallel pins for retention.

pinledge (pin´lej) In dentistry, vertical parallel pins placed in a tooth or teeth to aid in retention of a restoration.

pinna (pin´nă) See auricle.

pinocyte (pi-no-sīt) A cell that engulfs liquids in a way that resembles the engulfment of solid particles by a phagocyte.

pinocytosis (pi-no-si-to´sis) The engulfment of liquid droplets by a cell through minute invaginations formed on the surface, which close to form fluid-filled vacuoles (vesicles); by this process, protein is reabsorbed from the filtrate by tubular cells of the

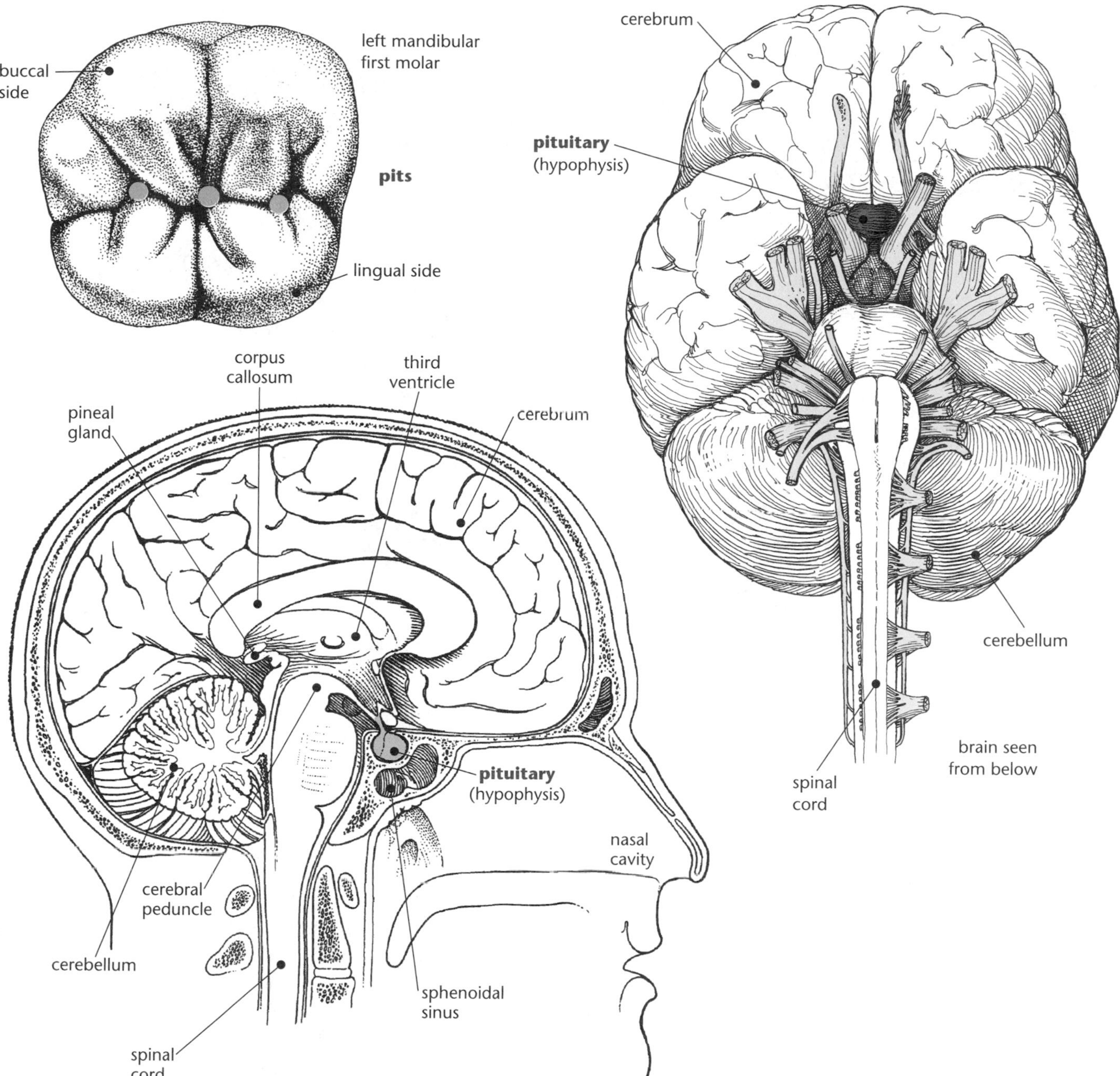

kidney; the phenomenon is similar to phagocytosis (the engulfing of solid particles).

pinosome (pi′no-sōm) A fluid-filled vesicle within a cell, formed during pinocytosis.

Pins' sign (pins sīn) See Ewart's sign.

pint (pīnt) (pt) A unit of liquid measure equal to 16 fluid ounces; 28.875 cubic inches; 473.1765 cc.

imperial p. A British unit of liquid equal to 20 fluid ounces; 34.67743 cubic inches; 568.2615 cc.

pinta (pēn′tă) A nonvenereal infection caused by the spirochete *Treponema carateum*; marked by patches of pronounced changes in skin color.

pinworm (pin′werm) A nematode worm, *Enterobius vermicularis*, that infests the intestines, especially in children. Also called seatworm (because it may cause pruritus ani); threadworm.

pion (pi′on) A small particle found in the nuclei of atoms; it constitutes the force that holds neutrons and protons together. Also called pi-meson.

piperazine (pi′per-ă-zēn) Compound used against pinworms and roundworms (intestinal parasites).

pipette, pipet (pi-pet′) A calibrated glass tube, open at both ends, used for transferring and/or measuring small quantities of liquids in laboratory work.

automatic p. An instrument for transferring small amounts of liquid repetitively and automatically.

piriform (pir′ĭ-form) Pear-shaped.

pisiform (pi′sĭ-form) Pea-shaped or pea-sized (e.g., one of the carpal bones).

pit (pit) **1.** Any natural depression on the surface of the body. **2.** A pockmark. **3.** A pointed depression in dental enamel at the junction of two or more developmental grooves (e.g., in the occlusal and buccal surfaces of molars).

pitch (pich) One of three important properties of sound (others are intensity and quality) denoting the function of the number of vibrations of sound waves per second; the greater the number of vibrations per unit time, the higher the pitch. Commonly called tone.

pitchblende (pich′blend) A brownish black mineral containing uranium oxide and products of radioactive breakdown; it is the principal source of uranium and radium.

pith (pith) **1.** The center of a hair. **2.** To pierce the medulla of a laboratory animal, usually by the insertion of a needle or a knife at the base of the skull, to render the animal nonfeeling.

pituicyte (pĭ-tu′ĭ-sīt) The dominant type of cell (fusiform) of the posterior lobe of the pituitary gland.

pituitary (pĭ-tu′ĭ-tar-e) Relating to the pituitary (hypophysis). Also called hypophyseal.

pityriasis (pit-ĭ-ri′ă-sis) A skin disease marked by fine scaly desquamation.

p. rosea (PR) A skin eruption of scaly papules (believed to be caused by herpesvirus 7) usually involving the trunk and extremities; begins as an oval patch (herald patch) 6 to 8 cm in diameter, followed in a few days by a generalized eruption that disappears spontaneously in one to two months; the disorder is benign and exposure to the sun is thought to accelerate clearing.

pityroid (pit′ĭ-roid) Scaly.

Pityrosporum (pit-ĭ-ros′po-rum) A genus of nonpathogenic, yeast-like fungi that produce extremely fine spores and no mycelium; generally found in dandruff and seborrheic dermatitis.

pivot (piv′ut) A part about which a related structure rotates or swings.

placebo (plă-se′bo) An inert substance containing no medication but prescribed as medicine, given especially to satisfy a patient; also used in controlled

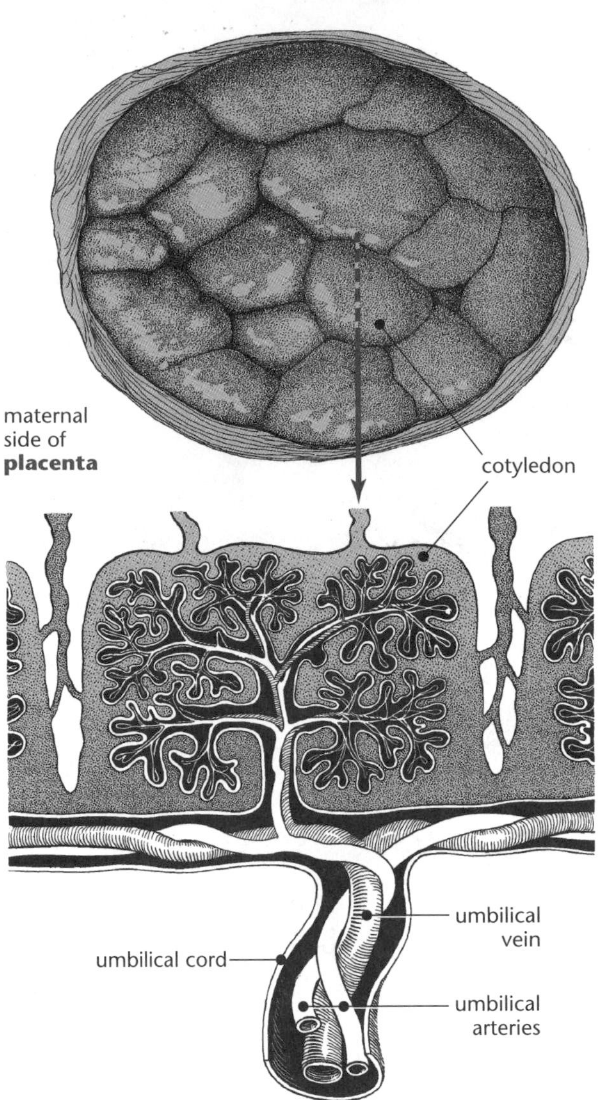

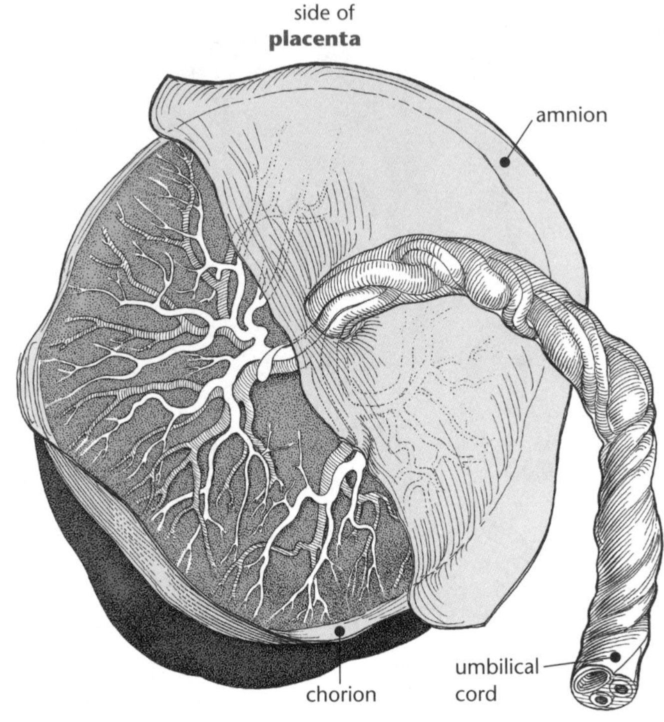

P

studies to determine the efficacy of drugs.

placenta (plă-sen´tă) The organ within the pregnant uterus through which the fetus derives its nourishment; at term it averages one-sixth the weight of the fetus; it is disk-shaped, about 2.5 cm thick, and 17.5 cm in diameter.

accessory p. One or more lobes of placental tissue that often have vascular connections of fetal origin and are developed in the membranes distant from the primary placenta. Also called succenturiate placenta.

p. accreta An abnormally adherent placenta; may be implanted directly on the muscular layer (myometrium) of the uterine wall. Based on the degree of penetration of the wall by placental tissue, it is classified as: *placenta acreta vera* (superficial but exceptional adherence), *placenta increta* (invasion of myometrium), and *placenta percreta* (full thickness penetration of uterine wall).

fundal p. A placenta that is implanted in the fundus of the uterus, the usual site.

p. previa Condition in which the placenta is implanted in the lower segment of the uterus and covers the cervical opening, partly or completely. Also called placental presentation.

retained p. Placental tissue that remains attached to the uterine wall after delivery.

succenturiate p. See accessory placenta.

placental (plă-sen´tal) Relating to the placenta.

placentation (plas-en-ta´shun) The development of the placenta and its structural relationship to maternal and fetal structures.

placentitis (plas-en-ti´tis) Inflammation of the placenta; usually caused by a bacterial infection ascending from the birth canal.

placentography (plas-en-tog´ră-fe) The making of roentgenograms of the placenta following injection of a radiopaque substance.

placode (plak´ōd) An ectodermal thickening in the early embryo from which a sense organ or a structure develops (e.g., lens placode).

pladaroma, pladarosis (pla-da-ro´ma, pla-da-ro´sis) A soft, wartlike tumor on the eyelid.

plagiocephaly (pla-je-o-sef´ă-le) Malformation of the skull in which one side is more developed anteriorly and the other side posteriorly.

plague (plāg) **1.** Any widespread disease or one causing excessive mortality. **2.** Acute infectious disease caused by *Yersinia pestis* (transmitted to humans by fleas that have bitten infected rodents); marked by high fever, prostration, glandular swelling, or pneumonia.

bubonic p. A form marked by buboes (inflammatory enlargement of lymphatic glands).

hemorrhagic p. Bubonic plague in which bleeding may occur into an organ or from the nose and alimentary, respiratory, or urinary tracts.

pneumonic p. A fatal form accompanied by pneumonia with abundant bloodstained sputum.

septicemic p. A variant of bubonic plague leading to death so quickly that localized lesions do not become clinically apparent.

sylvatic p. Bubonic plague in wild animals, especially rodents.

planchet (plan´chet) A flat metal disk container on which a radioactive sample is placed while its activity is measured.

plane (plān) **1.** A flat or level surface. **2.** An imaginary surface formed by extension through two points or an axis. **3.** A particular level (e.g., a stage in surgical anesthesia).

coronal p. A vertical plane that passes from side to side at right angles to the median plane, dividing the head into anterior and posterior portions; often used interchangeably with frontal plane.

frontal p. A vertical plane passing at right angles to the median plane, dividing the body into anterior and posterior portions. COMPARE: coronal plane.

p. of greatest pelvic dimension Plane passing through the roomiest portion of the pelvic cavity; extends from the middle of the posterior surface of the pubic symphysis to the junction of the second and third sacral vertebrae, passing laterally through the ischial bone over the middle of the acetabulum.

guide p. In dentistry, plane formed in the occlusal surfaces of occlusion rims to position the lower jaw in centric relation.

horizontal p. See transverse plane.

intercristal p. A horizontal plane passing through the highest points of the iliac crests; it lies at the level of the fourth lumbar vertebra.

interspinal p. A horizontal plane transecting the body at the level of the anterior superior iliac spines.

intertubercular p. A horizontal plane passing through the tubercles of the iliac crests; it lies at the level of the fifth lumbar vertebra.

p. of least pelvic dimension Plane extending from the lower margin of the pubic symphysis through the ischial spines to the sacrum.

median p. A vertical plane that divides the body into right and left halves. Also called midsagittal plane.

p. of midpelvis See plane of least pelvic dimension.

midsagittal p. See median plane.

occlusal p., p. of occlusion The plane formed by the contacting (occlusal) surfaces of the upper and lower teeth when the jaws are closed.

parasagittal p. Any vertical plane parallel to the median plane.

pelvic p. of inlet The rounded upper opening of the minor pelvis (between the minor and major pelves), bounded anteriorly by the pubic bone, laterally by the iliopectineal lines, and posteriorly

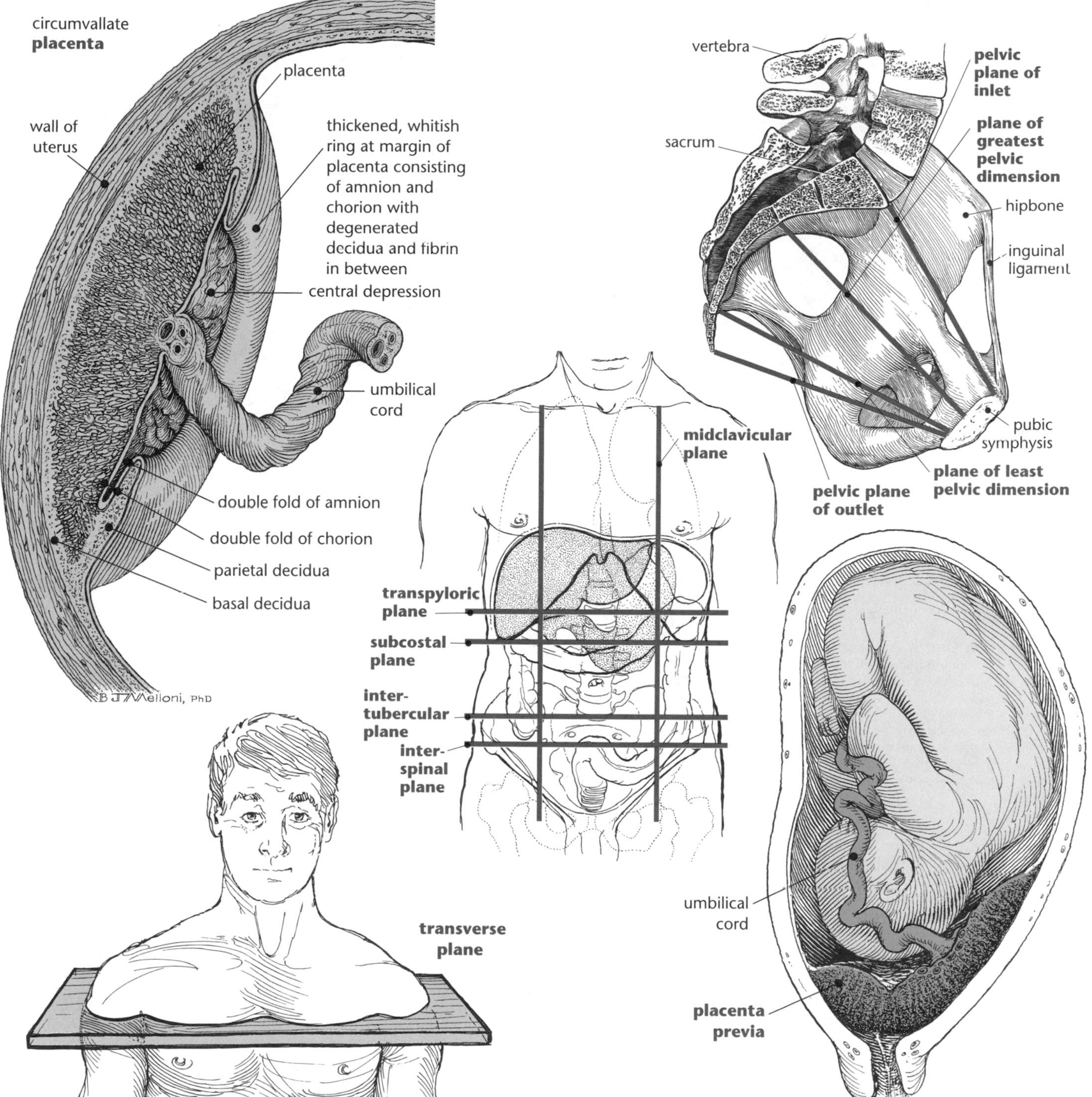

by the sacral promontory. Also called superior aperture of minor pelvis; superior pelvis strait.

pelvic p. of outlet Plane across the lower opening of the minor (true) pelvis, bounded anteriorly by the pubic arch, laterally by the ischial tubrosities, and posteriorly by the tip of the coccyx. Also called inferior aperture of minor pelvis; inferior pelvic strait.

p.'s of reference Planes that serve as a guide for the location of other planes.

sagittal p. In general, a vertical plane extending in an anteroposterior direction, parallel to the median plane.

subcostal p. A horizontal plane passing through the lowest point of the costal margin on each side, generally the inferior border of the tenth costal cartilage.

transpyloric p. A horizontal plane between the superior borders of the breastbone (sternum) and the pubic symphysis.

transverse p. A plane across the body at right angles to the coronal and sagittal planes. Also called horizontal plane.

planigraphy (plă-nig′ră-fe) Tomography.

planimeter (pla-nim′ĕ-ter) A device that measures the area of any surface by tracing its boundaries with a mechanically coupled pointer.

plano (pla′no) Having a flat surface; said of an afocal lens (i.e., one without refractive power).

planoconcave (pla-no-kon′kāv) Flat on one side and curved inward on the other; denoting a lens of that shape.

planoconvex (pla-no-kon′veks) Flat on one side and curved outward on the other; denoting a lens of that shape.

planta (plan′tă), *pl.* **plan′tae** Latin for the sole of the foot.

plantago Plan-ta′go) Any plant of the genus *Plantago.*

Plantago (plan-ta′go) A large genus of herbs (family Plantaginaceae) composed chiefly of roadside weeds.

P. psyllium A species producing seeds that are used as a mild laxative. See also psyllium.

plantain (plan′tan) **1.** Any plant of the genus *Plantago.* **2.** A type of banana plant (*Musa paradisiaca*). **3.** The starchy fruit of such a plant, resembling a large banana; a staple food in tropical regions.

plantalgia (plan-tal′jă, plan-tal′je-ă) Pain in the sole of the foot.

plantar (plan′tar) Relating to the sole of the foot.

plaque (plak) A small flat growth.

atheromatous p. A yellow-white fibrofatty deposit on the inner surface of arterial walls and protruding into the vessel lumen.

bacteriophage p. A clear ring surrounding a bacterial culture, indicative of peripheral destruction of the culture by bacterial viruses.

dental p. A deposit of bacteria and other materials bound to the surface of teeth; contributes to tooth decay and periodontal disease.

neuritic p. A cluster of nerve endings surrounding a core of extracellular amyloid (abnormal complex substance); commonly found in the cerebral cortex of individuals with Alzheimer's disease. Also called senile plaque.

senile p. See neuritic plaque.

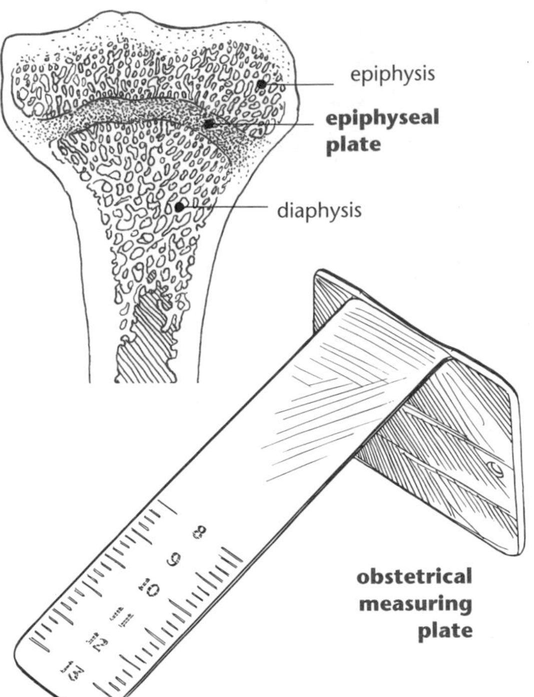

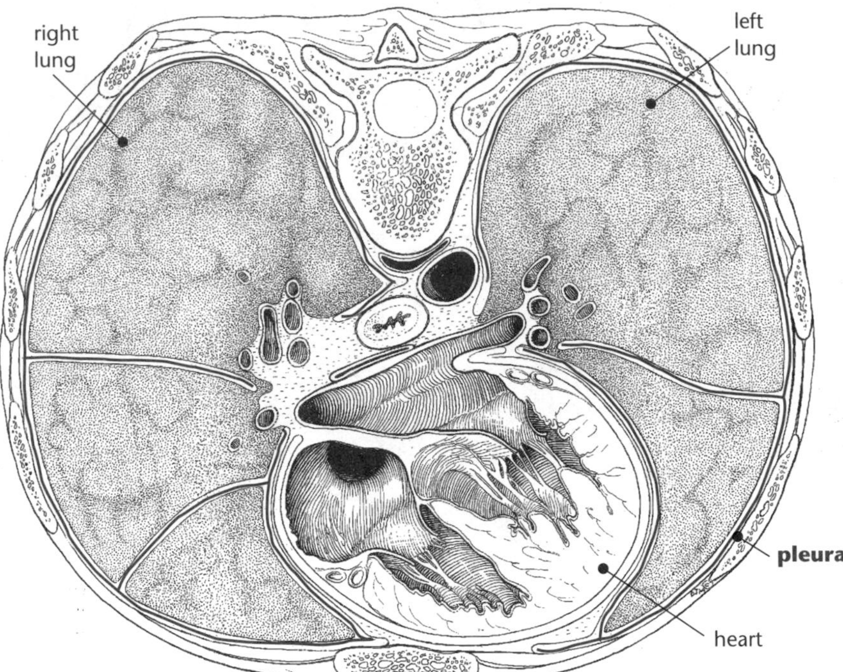

plasma (plaz´mă) **1.** The clear fluid of blood in which cells are suspended. Distinguished from serum. Also called blood plasma. **2.** The fluid component of lymph.

antihemophilic human p. Human plasma in which the antihemophilic components have been preserved; used for the temporary arrest of bleeding in hemophilic patients.

blood p. See plasma (1).

dried p. Preparation consisting of vacuum-dried frozen plasma which contains no added dextrose; it may be preserved at room temperature almost indefinitely, but usually is provided with a five-year expiration date.

fresh-frozen p. (FFP) Plasma that has been frozen within six hours of withdrawal from donor and stored at a constant temperature of –18°C or below; usually provided with a five-year expiration date.

liquid p. Preparation made by adding 5% dextrose to normal plasma and preserved at temperatures between 15° and 30°C; usually provided with a two-year expiration date.

plasmablast (plaz´mă-blast) The precursor of the plasma cell.

plasmacyte (plaz´mă-sīt) See plasma cell, under cell.

plasmacytoma (plaz-mă-si-to´mă) A malignant plasma cell tumor within bone marrow; it may also occur in other parts of the body.

multiple p. See multiple myeloma, under myeloma.

plasmacytosis (plaz-mă-si-to´sis) Abnormally large percentage of plasma cells in the tissues.

plasma expander (plaz´mă ek-span´der) See plasma substitute, under substitute.

plasmalemma (plaz-mă-lem´ă) See cell membrane, under membrane.

plasmalogen (plaz-mal´o-jen) One of a group of phospholipids present in the brain and muscle.

plasmapheresis (plaz-mă-fĕ-re´sis) A method of obtaining plasma without waste of blood components; blood is drawn, plasma is separated, and the blood cells are returned to the donor suspended in a suitable medium (e.g., Ringer's solution). Also called plasmopheresis.

plasmid (plaz´mid) See paragene.

plasmin (plaz´min) A proteolytic enzyme derived from plasminogen; essential in blood clot dissolution (fibrinolysis).

plasminogen (plaz-min´o-jen) A globulin present in tissues, body fluids, circulating blood, and within clots; the inactive precursor of plasmin.

plasminogen activator inhibitor 1 (plaz-min ´o-jen ak´tĭ-va-tor in-hib´ĭ-tor wun) (PAI-1) The chief inhibitor of tissue plasminogen activator (tPA), an activator that converts an inert protein to a clot- and fibrin-dissolving enzyme. Elevated blood levels of PAI-1 have been found in several diseases.

plasmocyte (plaz´mo-sīt) See plasma cell, under cell.

Plasmodium (plaz-mo´de-um) Genus of the class Sporozoa; some species cause malaria. See also malaria.

P. falciparum Species causing falciparum (malignant tertian) malaria, with fever recurring irregularly every 36 to 48 hours; it invades mature red blood cells that retain normal size and frequently contain basophilic granules and cytoplasmic precipitates (Maurer's dots); reproduction takes place in the visceral capillaries; except in severe fatal cases, only very young forms are seen in peripheral blood; multiple infection of red blood cells is extremely frequent.

P. malariae Species causing quartan malaria, with fever recurring every 72 hours; invades mature red blood cells and never fills the cell completely; infected cells occasionally show fine granules (Ziemann's dots).

P. ovale Species that rarely parasitizes humans, causing ovale (benign tertian) malaria, with fever recurring every 48 hours; infected cells are irregular and fimbriated with abundant acidophilic granules (Schüffner's dots).

P. vivax Species causing vivax (benign tertian) malaria, with fever recurring every 48 hours; invades young red blood cells; young forms are ameboid and one-third the size of the cell; mature forms almost fill the distended cell; infected cell appears enlarged, is deficient in hemoglobin, and contains acidophilic granules (Schüffner's dots).

plasmodium (plaz-mo´de-um), *pl.* **plasmo´dia** A mass of protoplasm with multiple nuclei.

plasmogen (plaz´mo-jen) See protoplasm.

plasmolysis (plaz-mol´ĭ-sis) Process in which the cytoplasm of a bacterial cell shrinks away from the cell wall when the cell is immersed in a hypertonic solution.

plasmopheresis (plaz-mo-fĕ-re´sis) See plasmapheresis.

plasmorrhexis (plaz-mo-rek´sis) The bursting of a cell due to increased internal pressure.

plaster (plas´ter) **1.** A white powder, essentially gypsum, that forms a paste when mixed with water and sets to a smooth solid; used for immobilization and impressions of bodily parts. **2.** A pastelike material for application to the surface of the body.

adhesive p. A pressure-sensitive, sticky mixture of rubber, resins, and waxes with an absorbent powder filler, spread upon a cotton fabric.

mustard p. A pastelike mixture of powdered mustard seed, flour, and water, spread on cloth and applied to the skin as a poultice; it exerts an emollient, relaxing effect upon the skin and underlying tissues.

p. of Paris Gypsum or calcium sulfate from which water of crystallization has been calcined or expelled by heat in the open air.

plastic (plas´tik) **1.** Capable of being reshaped or molded. **2.** In dentistry, a restorative substance that is soft enough to be molded, after which it will harden or set. **3.** Any of a large group of synthetic or semisynthetic organic compounds of high molecular weight produced by polymerization or by chemical treatment and which can be molded, cast, or laminated. **4.** Serving to reshape (e.g., certain surgical procedures).

plasticity (plas-tis´ĭ-te) The property of being plastic.

plastid (plas´tid) A self-replicating organelle in the cytoplasm of plant cells and in some plantlike organisms that serves as a center of special physiologic activities.

plate (plāt) **1.** In anatomy, any flat, relatively thin structure. **2.** In dentistry, an artificial denture, especially the portion to which artificial teeth are anchored. **3.** In microbiology, a glass culture container such as the Petri dish. **4.** A smooth, flat device of uniform thickness.

axial p. The primitive streak of an embryo.

bone p. A metal bar with perforations for immobilization of fractured bones.

chorionic p. Placental tissue on the fetal side of the placenta, giving rise to the chorionic villi; it is the primordium of the chorion frondosum.

cribriform p. of ethmoid bone The bony plate that forms part of the roof of the nasal cavity and is traversed by the filaments of the olfactory nerve.

epiphyseal p. The plate or disk of cartilage between the shaft and the epiphysis of a long bone during its growth. Also called growth plate; epiphyseal disk.

growth p. See epiphyseal plate.

Ishihara p.'s A series of plates designed as tests for color blindness; they consist of numbers made of primary colored dots printed on a background of many dots of various sizes and in confusing colors; individuals who are color blind are unable to read the numbers.

lateral pterygoid p. The lateral lamina of the pterygoid process projecting downward from the roots of the greater wings of the sphenoid bone; its lateral surface forms part of the medial wall of the infratemporal fossa; its medial surface forms part of the pterygoid fossa. Also called lateral lamina of pterygoid plate.

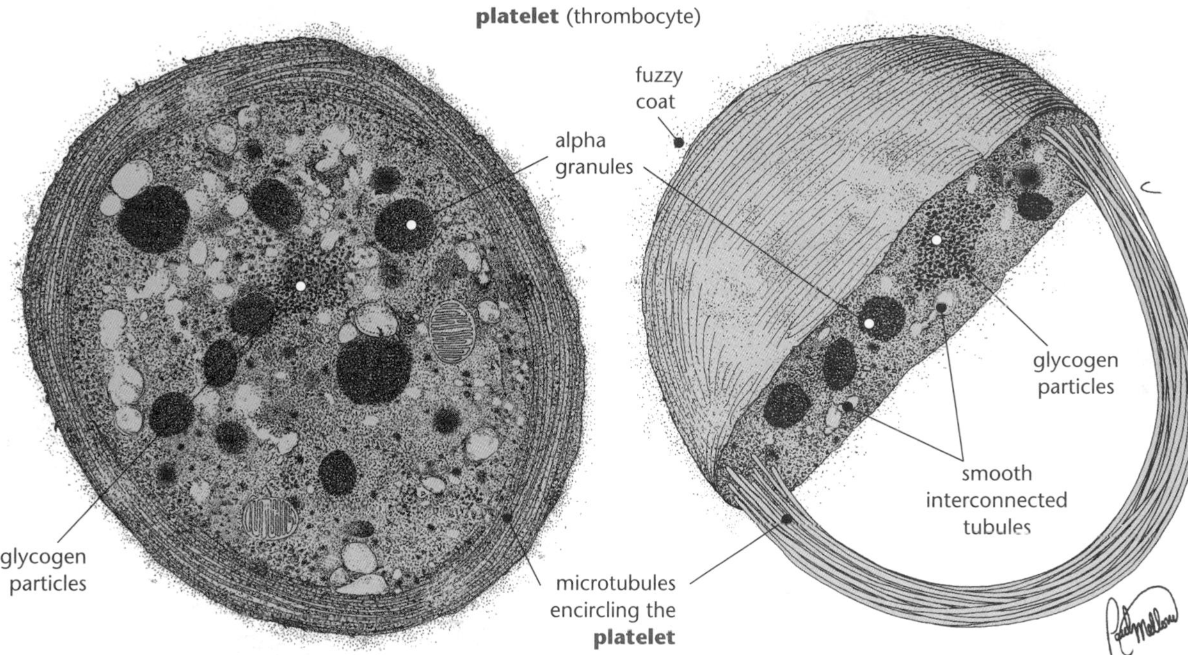

medial pterygoid p. The medial lamina of the pterygoid process projecting downward from the roots of the greater wings of the sphenoid bone, forming the most posterior part of the lateral wall of the nasal cavity; it curves laterally at its inferior extremity into a hooklike process, the pterygoid hamulus. Also called medial lamina of pterygoid plate.
medullary p. See neural plate.
motor p. A motor end-plate.
neural p. The middle ectodermal thickening in the embryo from which the neural tube develops; the anlage of the central nervous system. Also called medullary plate.
obstetrical measuring p. Plate for calculating the digital measurements of pelvic conjugates without a pelvimeter.
occlusal plane p. In dentistry, a metal plate used to establish the occlusal plane of the teeth.
pterygoid p.'s A short, broad lateral plate and a long, narrow medial plate that project inferiorly from the sphenoid bone; the pterygoid fossa lies between them.
skull p. A thin perforated plate, generally round or oval, that is screwed to the cranium to replace missing bone fragments.
platelet (plāt´let) A disk-shaped, colorless protoplasmic structure without a nucleus, derived from a megakaryocyte, and present in abundance in the blood of all mammals; it is smaller than a red blood cell (from 2 to 4 µm in diameter) and plays an important role in blood coagulation. Normal level in human blood is150,000 to 300,000 platelets per mm^3.
plateletpheresis (plāt-let-fĕ-re´sis) The removal of platelets from the drawn blood of a healthy donor, thereby permitting the transfusion of this blood fraction to individuals who have platelet deficiency disorders; the remainder of the blood (white and red blood cells and plasma) is immediately returned to the donor.
plating (plāt´ing) **1.** The planting or streaking of bacteria in a Petri dish or similar container. **2.** The application of a metal strip to the fractured ends of a bone to keep them in place. **3.** The electrolytic deposition of a metal.
platinum (plat´ĭ-num) A silver-white metallic element, symbol Pt, atomic number 78, and atomic weight 195.09.
platybasia (plat-e-ba´se-ă) Developmental deformity in which the floor of the occipital bone of the skull bulges inward, especially around the foramen magnum.
platycephalous, platycephalic (plat-e-sĕ-fal´us, plat-e-sĕ-fal´ik) Having a wide flat head with a vertical cranial index below 70.
platyhelminth (plat-e-hel´minth) Common name for a worm of the phylum Platyhelminthes; any tapeworm or fluke.
Platyhelminthes (plat-e-hel-min´thēz) A phylum of flatworms characterized by bilaterally symmetrical, flat bodies without a true body cavity; some are parasitic, such as tapeworms and flukes.
platyhieric (plat-e-hi-er´ik) Having a broad sacral bone with an index greater than 100.
platypellic, platypelloid (plat-e-pel´ik, plat-e-pel´oid) Having a broad, flat pelvis with a pelvic inlet index of less than 90.
platyrrhine (plat´e-rīn) **1.** Having a broad nose, generally with nostrils directed to the sides. **2.** Denoting a skull with a nasal index greater than 53.
platysma (plă-tiz´mă) See table of muscles.
platyspondylisis, platyspondylia (plat-e-spon-dil´ĭ-sis, plat-e-spon dil´e-ă) Having broad, flat vertebral bodies.
pledget (plej´et) A small, flattened tuft, usually of cotton or gauze.
pleiotropic (pli-o-trop´ik) In genetics, producing many effects; having several phenotypic expressions.
pleiotropy, pleiotropism (pli-ot´ro-pe, pli-ot´ro-piz-m) Phenomenon in which a single gene is responsible for several distinct and apparently unrelated observable effects, such as a hereditary syndrome.
pleochromatism (ple-o-kro´mă-tiz-m) The property of crystals by which they show different colors when illuminated from different angles.
pleocytosis (ple-o-si-to´sis) An increase in the number of leukocytes, especially lymphocytes, in the body; usually the term is applied to an increase in the number of lymphocytes in the spinal fluid.
pleomastia (ple-o-mas´te-ă) See polymastia.
pleomorphic (ple-o-mor´fik) See polymorphic.
pleomorphism (ple-o-mor´fiz-m) See polymorphism.
pleoptics (ple-op´tiks) Any type of orthoptic method of treating amblyopia (dimness of vision).
plerocercoid (ple-ro-ser´koid) The larval stage of a tapeworm, occurring in an intermediate host.
plessor (ples´or) A small rubber-headed hammer used in percussion. Also called plexor.
plethoric (ple-thor´ik) **1.** Overabundant; excessive. **2.** Denoting a ruddy complexion.
plethysmograph (ple-thiz´mo-graf) Device for measuring variation in size of a part or organ.
plethysmography (pleth-iz-mog´ră-fe) The recording of the variation in the size of a part produced by changes in the circulation of the blood within it.
plethysmometry (pleth iz mom´e-tre) Measurement of the fullness of a hollow structure such as a blood vessel.
pleura (ploor´ă) The serous membrane enveloping the lungs and lining the walls of the chest cavity.
parietal p. The layer lining the walls of the chest cavity.
visceral p. The layer covering the lungs.
pleuracotomy (ploor-ă-kot´ŏ-me) Incision into the pleural cavity, as for the introduction of a drainage tube.
pleuralgia (ploor-al´je-ă) Pain in the pleura.
pleurisy (ploor´ĭ-se) See pleuritis.
pleuritis (ploo-ri´tis) Inflammation of the pleura. Also called pleurisy.
hemorrhagic p. Pleuritis marked by a bloody secretion caused by bleeding disorders, tumors, or infarctions secondary to pulmonary emboli.
serofibrinous p. Pleuritis marked by a fibrinous secretion and accumulation of fluid caused by an inflammatory process in the lung (e.g., pneumonia, tuberculosis, abscesses) or by systemic diseases (e.g., rheumatoid arthritis, uremia).
suppurative p. Pleuritis marked by accumulation of pus in the pleural cavity caused by infection within the pleural space; may become chronic, leading to fibrinous adhesions and hindrance of lung expansion. Also called empyema.
pleurocentesis (ploor-o-sen-te´sis) Puncture and drainage of the pleural cavity.
pleurodynia (ploor-o-din´e-ă) Pain in the intercostal muscles, usually affecting one side only.
epidemic p. Acute infectious disease caused by the Coxsackie B virus; characterized chiefly by seizures of chest pain made worse by deep breathing and by movement. Also called devil's grip; benign dry pleurisy; Bornholm disease.
pleurogenic, pleurogenous (ploor-o-jen´ik, ploor-oj´ĕ-nus) Originating in the pleura.
pleurography (ploo-rog´ră-fe) Roentgenography of the pleura and lungs.
pleurolith (ploor´o-lith) A calculus in the pleural cavity.
pleuropericarditis (ploor-o-per-ĭ-kar-di´tis) Inflammation of the membranes enveloping the lungs and the heart.
pleuropulmonary (ploor-o-pul´mo-ner-e) Relating to the pleura and the lungs.
pleurotomy (ploor-ot´ŏ-me) Incision into the pleural cavity.
plexal (plek´sal) Relating to a plexus.
plexectomy (plek-sek´to-me) Surgical removal of a plexus.
plexiform (plek´sĭ-form) Resembling or forming a network of nerves, veins, or lymphatics.
plexor (plek´sor) See plessor.

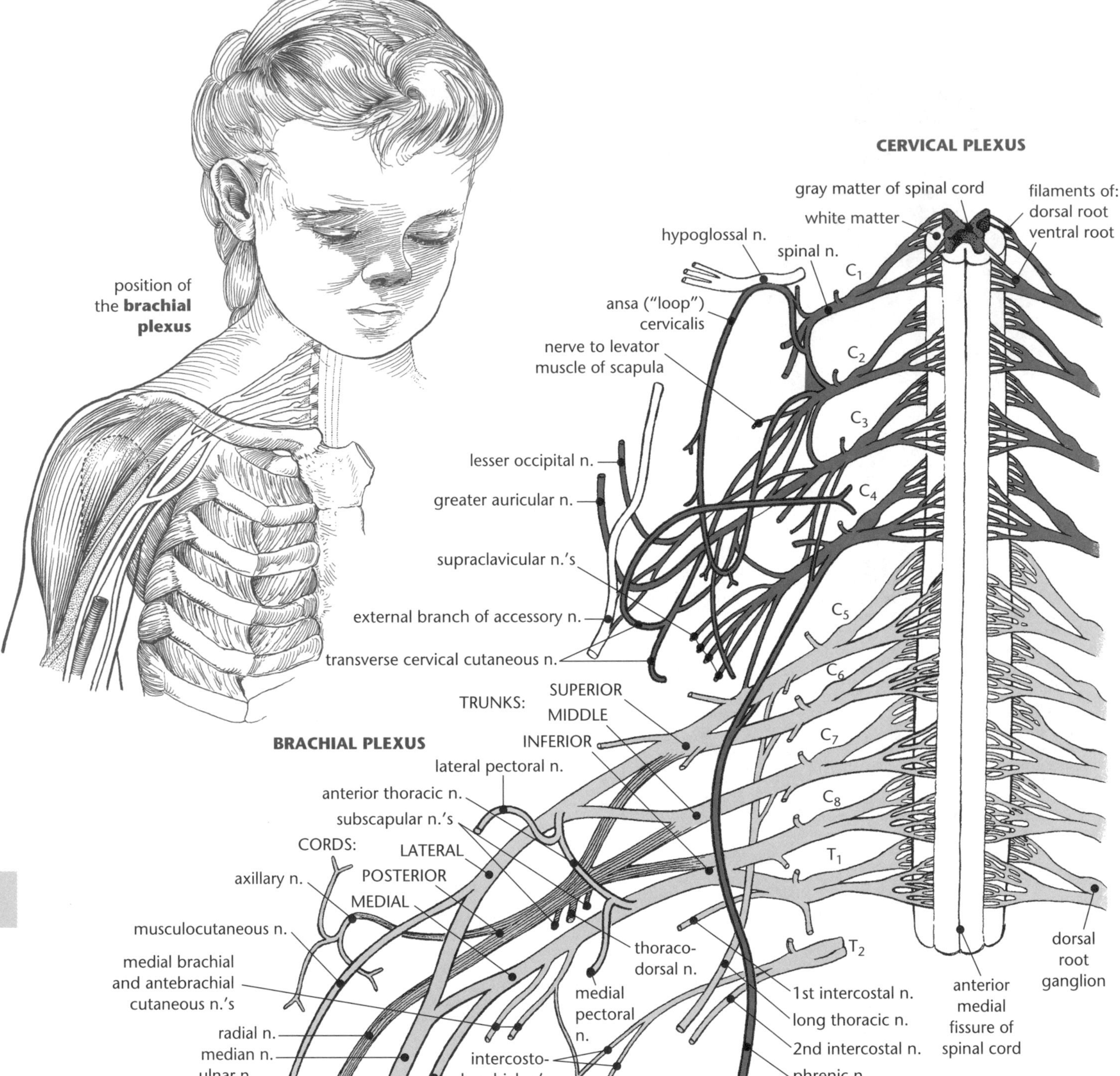

plexus (plek´sus), *pl.* **plex´uses** A network of nerves, veins, or lymphatics.

anococcygeal p. See coccygeal plexus.

aortic p., abdominal A plexus of nerve fibers around, but mainly in front of, the abdominal aorta which arises from the celiac and superior mesenteric plexuses; below the bifurcation of the aorta, it becomes the superior hypogastric plexus.

aortic p., thoracic A plexus of nerve fibers around the thoracic aorta formed by filaments from the sympathetic ganglia and vagus nerves.

Auerbach's p. See myenteric plexus.

brachial p. A plexus of the ventral primary divisions of the fifth to eighth cervical and the first thoracic nerves; it lies in the lateral part of the neck and extends into the axilla, supplying nerves to the upper limb.

celiac p. A large plexus of sympathetic nerves and ganglia located in the peritoneal cavity at the level of the first lumbar vertebra; it contains two large ganglionic masses and a dense network of fibers surrounding the roots of the celiac and superior mesenteric arteries; it supplies nerves to the abdominal viscera. Also called solar plexus.

cervical p. A plexus of the ventral primary divisions of the first four cervical nerves that sends out numerous cutaneous, muscular, and communicating branches.

choroid p. A vascular proliferation in a cerebral ventricle which regulates the intraventricular pressure by secretion or absorption of cerebrospinal fluid.

coccygeal p. A small plexus formed by the anterior branches of the fifth sacral and coccygeal nerves, supplemented by some fibers from the anterior branch of the fourth sacral nerve; forms a small trunk that pierces the coccygeal muscle to enter the pelvis; anococcygeal nerves arise from the plexus to innervate the skin around the coccyx. Also called anococcygeal plexus.

coronary p. of heart, anterior See coronary plexus of heart, right.

coronary p. of heart, left Autonomic nerve fibers derived chiefly from filaments of the deep part of the cardiac plexus (left half); accompanies the left coronary artery and distributes branches to the left atrium and left ventricle of the heart. Also called posterior coronary plexus of heart.

coronary p. of heart, posterior See coronary plexus of heart, left.

coronary p. of heart, right Autonomic nerve fibers derived from the superficial part of the cardiac plexus and partly from the deep part of the cardiac plexus (right side); it accompanies the right coronary artery, and distributes branches to the right atrium and right ventricle. Also called anterior coronary plexus of heart.

hypogastric p.'s Plexuses of autonomic nerve fibers located in the pelvis just below the bifurcation of the aorta: *Inferior hypogastric p.'s*, two networks of nerves located in front of the lower sacrum; innervate pelvic organs and blood vessels. *Superior hypogastric p.*, a network of nerves located between the bifurcation of the aorta and the promontory of the sacrum; innervates pelvic organs and blood vessels.

lumbar p. A plexus of the ventral primary divisions of the first three and the larger portion of the fourth lumbar nerves; located ventral to the transverse processes of the lumbar vertebrae.

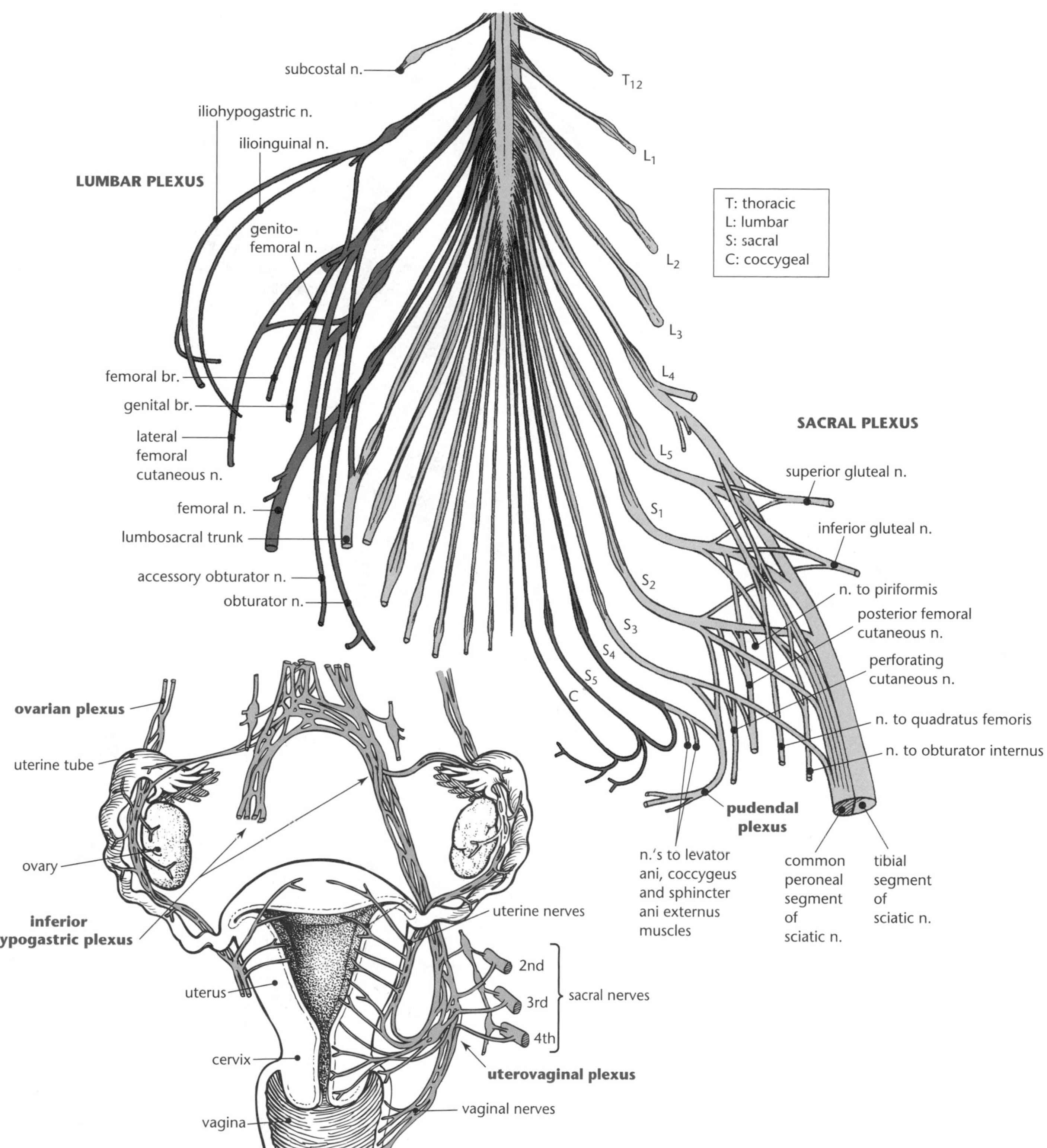

lumbosacral p. The combined lumbar, sacral, and pudendal plexuses.

lymphatic p. Any plexus of interconnecting lymph channels that absorb colloidal material and transport it to larger vessels for drainage into lymph nodes.

mammary arterial p. A network of anastomosing branches of the lateral and internal thoracic arteries, and intercostal arteries; they form a circular plexus around the areola, and a deeper plexus in the region of the acinar structures of the female breast.

mammary lymphatic p. A network of lymph vessels divided into two planes: superficial (subareolar) and deep (fascial); both originate in the interlobular spaces and in the wall of the lactiferous ducts, collecting lymph from the central parts of the gland, the skin, areola, and nipple; most of the superficial plexus drains laterally to the axillary lymph nodes; most of the deep fascial plexus drains medially to the internal mammary and mediastinal lymph nodes.

mammary venous p. A circular venous plexus draining the area around the nipple and areola into the axillary vein by way of the lateral thoracic vein.

Meissner's p. See submucosal plexus.

myenteric p. A network of nerves and ganglia situated between the circular and longitudinal muscular fibers of the esophagus, stomach, and intestines. Also called Auerbach's plexus.

ovarian p. A network of autonomic nerve fibers distributed to the ovary and fallopian (uterine) tube; formed by branches from the renal and aortic plexuses and reinforced below by branches from the superior and inferior hypogastric plexuses.

pampiniform p. In the female, a venous plexus in the broad ligament draining the ovary and fallopian (uterine) tube; it empties into the ovarian vein and communicates with the uterine plexus. In the male, a venous plexus in the spermatic cord draining the testis and emptying into the testicular vein.

parotid p. A plexus of nerves formed by the terminal branches of the facial (7th cranial) nerve, passing through the parotid gland; it innervates the muscles of facial expression.

prostatic p. Autonomic nerve plexus adjacent to

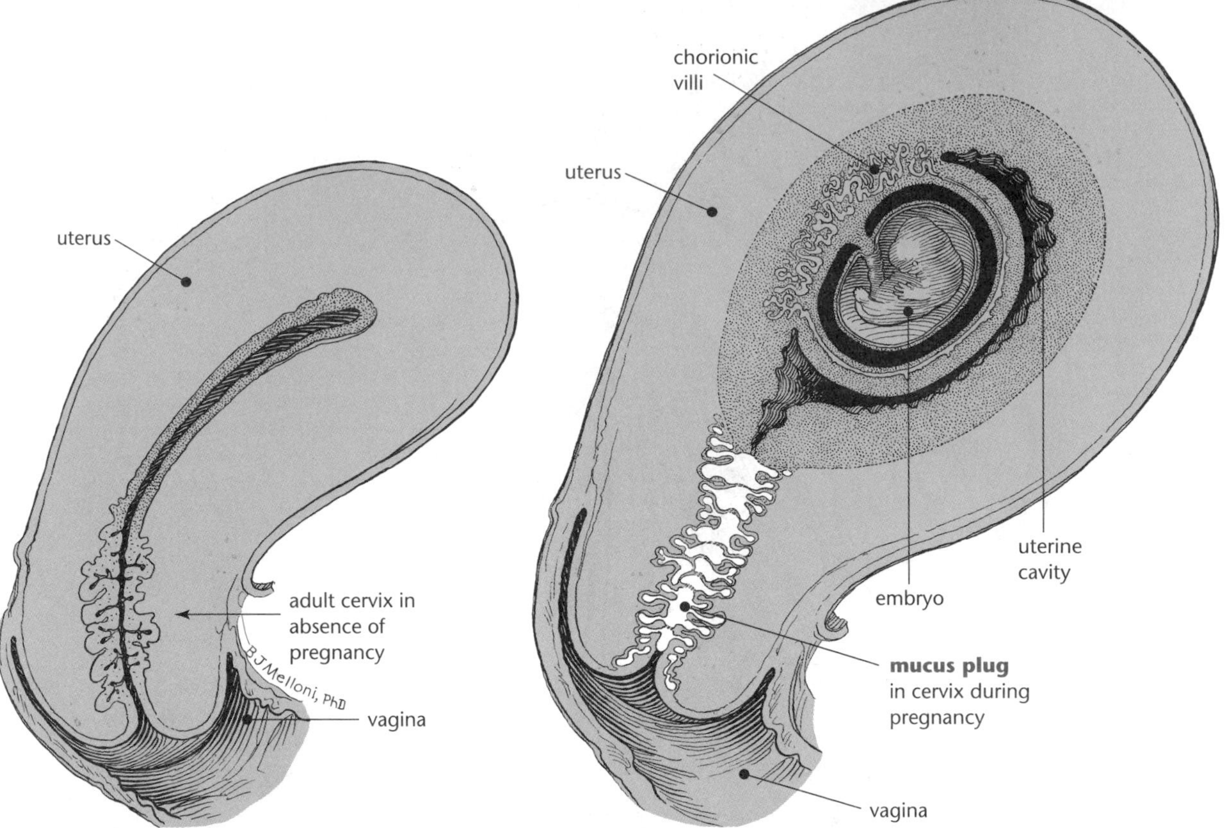

the prostate, an extension of the inferior hypogastric plexus; it innervates the prostate, seminal vesicles, urethra, and erectile tissue of the penis (corpora cavernosa and corpus spongiosum).

prostatic venous p. Network of veins between the pubic symphysis and the front of the prostate; drains into the vesical and internal iliac veins.

pudendal p. Plexus formed from the ventral branches of the second and third sacral nerves and all of the fourth sacral nerve; considered by some to be part of the sacral plexus.

rectal venous p. A network of veins surrounding the rectum; in the female it communicates with the vaginal and uterine plexuses, in the male with the vesical plexus. Consists of two divisions: *Internal rectal venous p.*, situated beneath the epithelium of the rectum and anal canal; drains chiefly into the superior rectal vein. *External rectal venous p.*, situated outside the muscular layers of the rectum; drains into the superior, middle, and inferior rectal veins.

sacral p. A plexus of the ventral primary divisions of the fourth lumbar to the third sacral nerves; it lies on the posterior wall of the pelvis and supplies the buttocks, perineum, lower extremities, and pelvic viscera.

solar p. See celiac plexus.

spermatic p. See testicular plexus.

submucosal p. Plexus of autonomic nerve fibers that ramifies in the submucosal coat of the intestine; it also has ganglia from which nerve fibers pass to the muscles and mucous membrane of the intestine. Also called Meissner's plexus.

testicular p. A network of autonomic nerve fibers distributed to the testis, epididymis, and deferent duct; formed by branches from the renal and aortic plexuses and reinforced by branches from the superior and inferior hypogastric plexuses. Also called spermatic plexus.

tympanic p. Plexus of nerves on the promontory of the middle ear chamber that supplies the mucous membrane of the middle ear, mastoid air cells, and the auditory tube; it also gives off a small branch to the otic ganglion.

uterine venous p. Venous plexus on both sides of the uterus within the broad ligament, closely associated with the vaginal and ovarian plexuses; drained by the uterine veins into the internal iliac vein.

uterovaginal p. Plexus of nerves in the base of the broad ligament, derived from the inferior hypogastric plexus; sends fibers to the vagina, cervix, and the uterine body.

vaginal venous p. Venous plexus around the vagina that is closely associated with the uterine, vesical, and rectal venous plexuses; drained by vaginal veins into the internal iliac vein.

vesical p. An autonomic nerve plexus along the side of the bladder; an extension of the inferior hypogastric plexus.

vesical venous p. Network of veins surrounding the base of the bladder, linked below with the vaginal plexus in the female and with the prostatic plexus in the male; drained by vesical veins into the internal iliac vein.

plica (pli´kă), *pl.* **pli´cae** **1.** A fold, as of skin or membrane. **2.** A matted state of the hair, resulting from filth and parasites.

p. circularis One of the transverse folds of mucous membrane of the small intestine. Also called circular fold; valve of Kerckring.

p. semilunaris conjunctivae The crescent-shaped fold formed by the conjunctiva at the inner angle of the eye.

p. triangularis A fold of mucous membrane covering the anteroinferior part of the palatine tonsil and projecting from the glossopalatine arch. Also called triangular fold.

plicate (pli´kāt) Arranged in folds; folded.

plication (pli-ka´shun) The surgical folding of a muscle or of the wall of a hollow organ to reduce its size.

plicotomy (pli-kot´ŏ-me) Surgical section of the posterior fold of the tympanic membrane (eardrum).

pliers (pli´erz) Any of several tools of varying shapes used in dentistry and orthopedic surgery for bending, cutting, contouring, etc.

ploidy (ploi´de) The number of chromosome sets present in a cell nucleus.

plombage (plom-bazh´) The surgical filling of a bodily space with inert material.

plosive (plo´siv) Designating a speech sound whose articulation requires retaining the air stream for a moment and then suddenly releasing it.

plot (plot) **1.** A graph. **2.** To represent graphically.

Scatchard p. A method for analyzing the reaction between a receptor and a ligand. The ratio of bound ligand (B) to the ligand (F) is plotted on the ordinate against the amount of bound ligand. The X intercept is the maximal velocity of the reaction and the slope is the affinity.

plug (plug) **1.** Any mass that occludes a passage or opening. **2.** A lumpy mass.

cervical p. See mucus plug.

epithelial p. A mass of epithelial cells that temporarily closes the external nares of the fetus.

mucus p. A thick, viscous mass of accumulated endocervical secretions filling the cervical canal during pregnancy and providing a mechanical and antibacterial barrier to the uterine cavity. Also called cervical plug.

plugger (plug´er) An instrument used to compress or condense filling material, such as amalgam, in a tooth cavity.

root canal p. A fine-tapered instrument with a blunt tip, used for packing dental material, such as gutta percha, into a root canal.

plumbic (plum´bik) Relating to lead.

plumbism (plum´biz-m) See lead poisoning, under poisoning.

plumbum (plum´bum) Latin for lead.

Plummer's disease (plum´erz dĭ-zēz´) Hyperthyroidism resulting from toxic adenoma of the thyroid gland.

Plummer-Vinson syndrome (plum´er-vin´son sin´drōm) Postcricoid esophageal web usually seen in middle-aged women with severe iron deficiency and associated with atrophy of the oral and pharyngeal mucosa, inflammation of the lips, spoon-shaped nails, and splenomegaly; symptoms usually include difficult swallowing, sore tongue, and dry mouth. Also called sideropenic dysphagia; Paterson-Kelly syndrome.

plumose (plu´mōs) Feathery.

pluricausal (ploor-ĭ-kaw´zal) Having two or more causes; applied to a disease that develops in the presence of two or more causative factors.

pluriglandular (ploor-ĭ-glan´du-lar) Denoting several glands. Also called polyglandular.

pluripara (ploo-rip´ă-ră) Multipara.

pluriparity (ploor-ĭ-par´ĭ-te) Multiparity.

pluripotent (ploo-rip´o-tent) **1.** Capable of affecting more than one organ. **2.** Denoting embryonic cells that can mature into any of several cell types.

plutonium (ploo-to´ne-um) A transuranian radioactive element having 15 isotopes with half-lives from 20 minutes to 76 million years; symbol Pu,

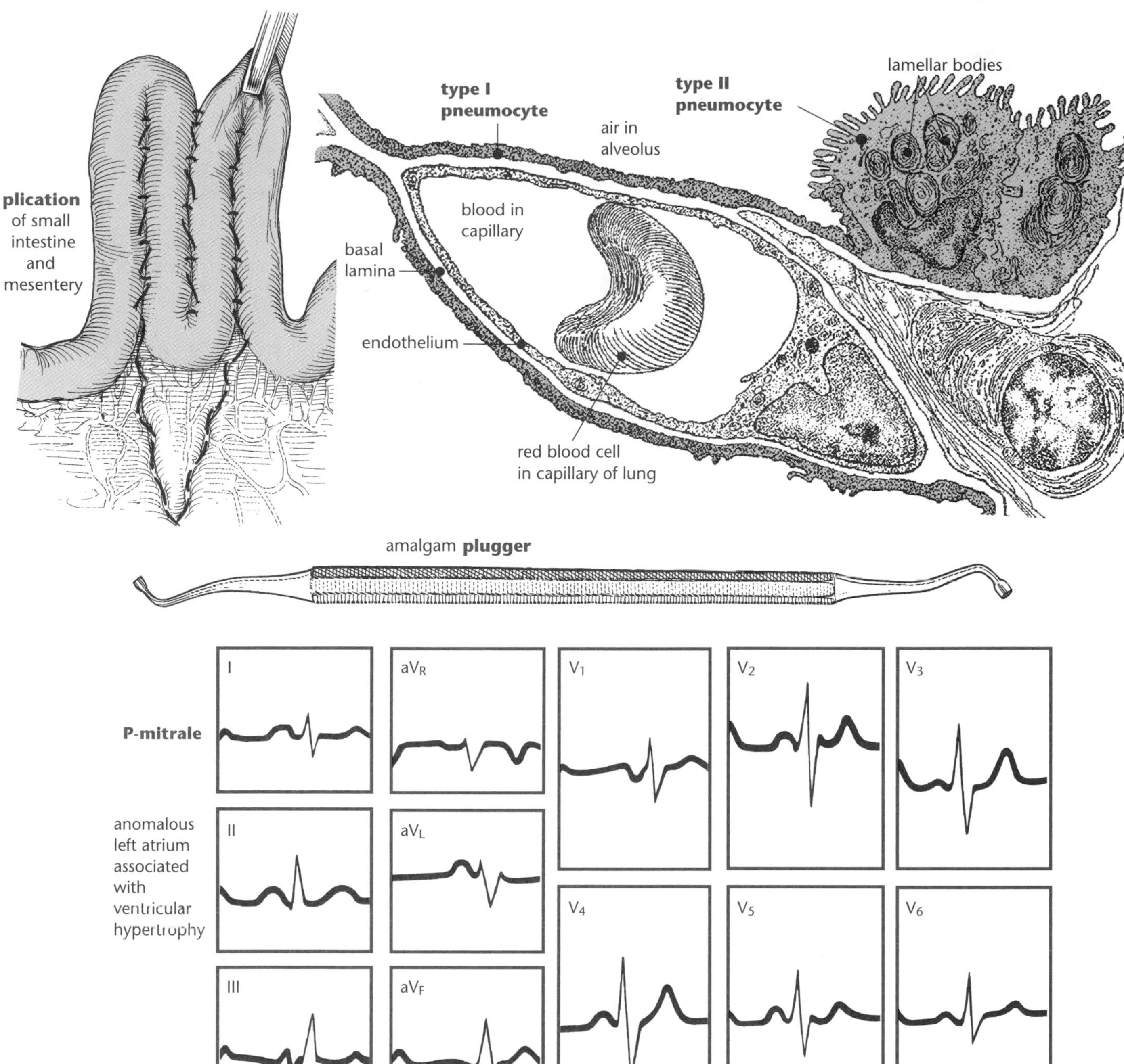

atomic number 94, atomic weight (chemical scale) 242.

P-mitrale (pē-mi-tral´e) A pattern in the electrocardiogram consisting of wide, notched P waves in leads I and II, with flat, inverted P waves in III, occurring in mitral (left atrioventricular) valve disease.

pneuma (nu´mă) In ancient Greek philosophy and medicine: A life-giving principle (now identified as oxygen); the soul or spirit of God.

pneumarthrosis (nu-mar-thro´sis) Air in a joint.

pneumatic (nu-mat´ik) **1.** Relating to air. **2.** Relating to breathing.

pneumatization (nu-mă-ti-za´shun) The development of air cells or cavities, especially those of the temporal and ethmoid bones.

pneumatocele (nu-mat´o-sēl) **1.** An air-filled cyst in the lung, characteristic of staphylococcal pneumonia. **2.** An air-containing hernia in the scrotum. Also called gas tumor. **3.** Herniation of lung tissue. Also called pneumonocele.

pneumatorrhachis (nu-mă-tor´ă-kis) See pneumorrhachis.

pneumaturia (nu-mă-tu´re-ă) The passage of gas through the urethra during urination, usually due to the entrance of air into the bladder from the bowel through a vesicocolic fistula.

pneumoarthrography (nu-mo-ar-throg´ră-fe) The making of an x-ray film of a joint after injection of air.

pneumocele (nu´mo-sēl) See pneumatocele.

pneumocephalus (nu-mo-sef´ă-lus) The presence of air within the skull.

pneumocholecystitis (nu-mo-ko-le-sis-ti´tis) Inflammation of the gallbladder with gas-producing organisms.

pneumococcemia (nu-mo-kok-se´me-ă) The presence of pneumococci in the blood.

pneumococci (nu-mo-kok´si) Collective name for the many serologic types of the bacterium *Streptococcus pneumoniae*.

pneumoconiosis (nu-mo-ko-ne-o´sis), *pl.* **pneumoconio´ses** Fibrosis of the lungs caused by prolonged inhalation of foreign material, particularly silica, coal, and asbestos, as occurs in coal mining and stone cutting; main symptoms are chronic dry cough and shortness of breath. Specific forms are named according to the offending agent (e.g., silicosis, asbestosis, anthracosis).

Pneumocystis carinii (nu mo-sis´tis kar-in´e) A parasitic, basophilic microorganism measuring one micrometer or less in diameter, occurring singly or in aggregates within a cystlike structure; the causative agent of *Pneumocystis carinii* pneumonia.

pneumocystosis (noo-mo-sis-to´sis) See *Pneumocystis carinii* pneumonia, under pneumonia.

pneumocyte, pneumonocyte (nu-mo-sīt´, nu-mon´o-sīt) Any of the alveolar epithelial cells of the lungs.

granular p. Type II pneumocyte.

membranous p. Type I pneumocyte.

type I p. A thin squamous epithelial cell lining the inside of the pulmonary alveolar wall; it has a large attenuated cytoplasm that may extend up to 100 µm. Also called alveolar cell; membranous pneumocyte; respiratory cell; type I cell.

type II p. A secretory cuboidal epithelial cell in the niches of the pulmonary alveolar wall; it possesses large, oval lamellar bodies thought to store surfactant, a surface-active phospholipid, which when secreted reduces the surface tension of the alveoli. Also called granular pneumocyte; great alveolar cell, septal cell, type II cell.

pneumodynamics (nu-mo-di-nam´iks) The mechanism of respiration.

pneumoencephalography (nu-mo-en-sef-ă-log´ră-fe) The making of x ray images of the subarachnoid spaces and ventricles of the brain after

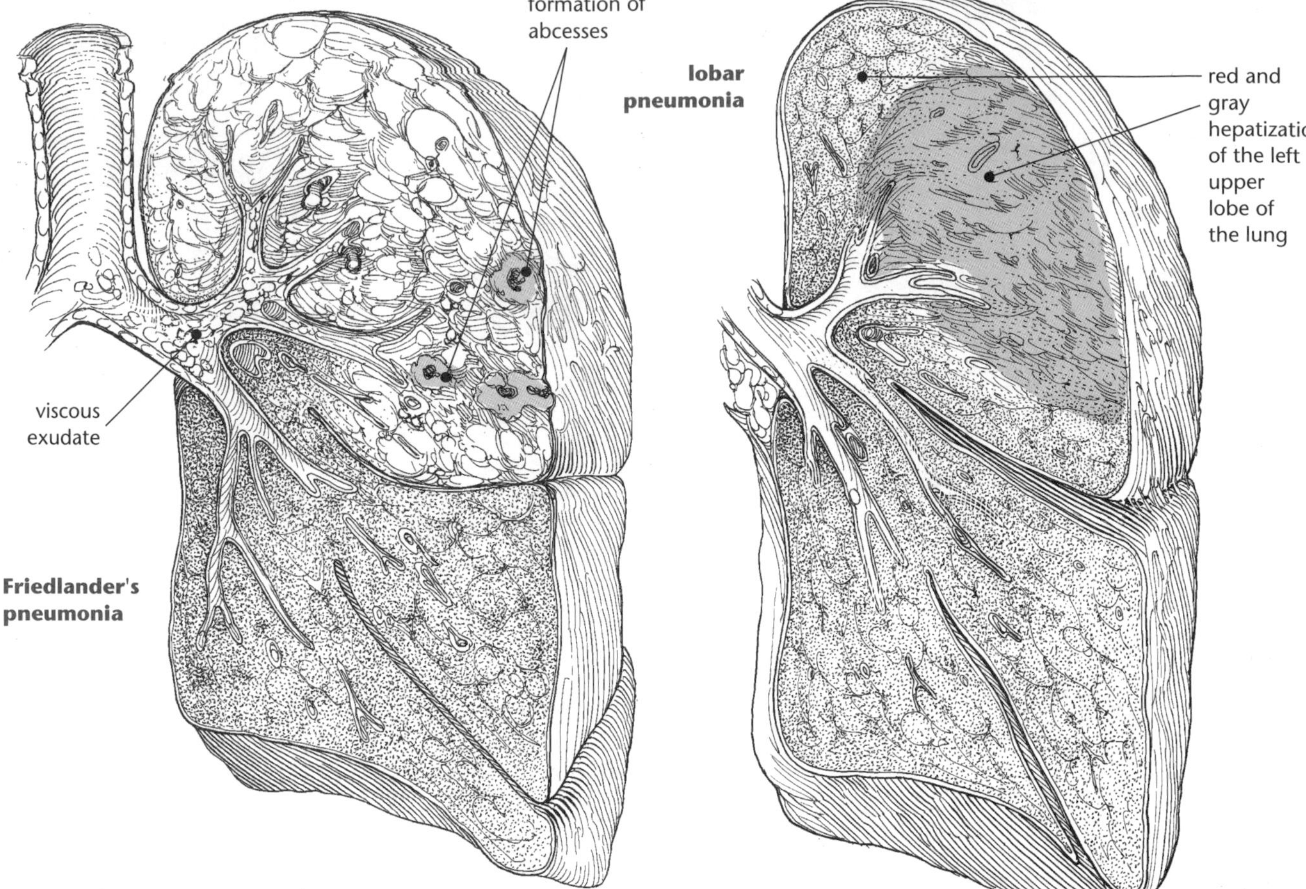

injecting a gas via a lumbar puncture.

pneumogram (nu′mo-gram) **1.** Tracing made by a pneumograph. **2.** X-ray image made in pneumoencephalography.

pneumograph (nu ′mo-graf) Instrument for recording the movements of respiration.

pneumography (nu-mog′ră-fe) Roentgenography of any body cavity after injection of air.

retroperitoneal p. Roentgenography of the retroperitoneal space after injecting gas into it to increase the contrast between a retroperitoneal organ (e.g., kidney) and the surrounding tissues.

pneumohemopericardium (nu-mo-he-mo-per-ĭ-kar′de-um) See hemopneumopericardium.

pneumohemothorax (nu-mo-he-mo-tho′raks) See hemopneumothorax.

pneumohydrometra (nu-mo-hi-dro-me′tră) The presence of gas and fluid in the uterine cavity.

pneumohydrothorax (nu-mo-hi-dro-tho′raks) See hydropneumothorax.

pneumolith (nu′mo-lith) A calculus in a lung.

pneumology (nu-mol′ŏ-je) Study of the lungs.

pneumolysis (nu-mol′ĭ-sis) Surgical separation of the pleura from the chest wall to allow the lung to collapse.

pneumomediastinum (nu-mo-me-de-as-ti′num) (PM) Accumulation of air in the mediastinum (the central space of the chest containing all the thoracic organs except the lungs).

pneumonectomy (nu-mo-nek′tŏ-me) Surgical removal of a lung or a portion of it. Also called pulmonectomy.

pneumonia (nu-mōn-yă, nu-mo′ne-ă) Inflammation of the lungs, caused by viruses, bacteria, or chemical and physical agents.

aspiration p. Pneumonia resulting from aspiration of food particles, vomit, water, or infected material from the upper respiratory tract.

bacterial p. Disease of sudden onset caused by a variety of bacterial agents (pneumococcus being the most common); high fever, chills, stabbing chest pains, cough, and rusty sputum are typical findings.

bronchial p. See bronchopneumonia.

chemical p. Pneumonia caused by inhalation of an extremely poisonous gas such as phosgene; characterized by swelling and hemorrhage of the lungs.

chlamydial p. Pneumonia caused by *Chlamydia trachomatis*; seen in infants during the first 3 to11weeks of life, usually acquired during vaginal delivery through the infected maternal cervix.

desquamative interstitial p. (DIP) Diffuse proliferation of alveolar lining cells, which desquamate into the air sacs, producing a gradual onset of breathing difficulties and nonproductive cough, with roentgenographic changes.

eosinophilic p. Disorder characterized by excessive eosinophils in peripheral blood, infiltration of eosinophils in the lung air spaces, and focal consolidation of lung tissue. Cause is unknown.

double p. Lobar pneumonia involving both lungs.

Eaton agent p. See mycoplasmal pneumonia.

Friedländer's p. A severe form of lobar pneumonia caused by infection with *Klebsiella pneumoniae* (Friedländer's bacillus); marked by much swelling of the affected pulmonary lobe.

hypostatic p. Infection occurring in poorly ventilated areas of the lung in the aged or in ill individuals who lie in the same position for long periods of time.

lipid p., lipoid p. Condition caused by aspiration of oily or fatty substances. Also called oil pneumonia.

lobar p. Acute pneumonia usually caused by a type of pneumococcus bacteria; marked by fever, chest pains, cough, and blood-stained sputum, with inflammation and consolidation of one or more lobes of the lungs.

mycoplasmal p. A pulmonary inflammation caused by *Mycoplasma pneumoniae* (Eaton agent); marked predominantly by severe cough, tracheal tenderness, pharyngitis with ear involvement, and occasionally blood-specked sputum; it may produce a bronchopneumonia, interstitial, or lobar pneumonia; mild forms are commonly called "walking pneu-monia". Also called primary atypical pneumonia; Eaton agent pneumonia.

oil p. See lipid pneumonia.

pneumococcal p. Acute lobar pneumonia caused by the pneumococcus organism.

***Pneumocystis carinii* p.** (PCP) An opportunistic pneumonia caused by *Pneumocystis carinii,* which invades and multiplies in the walls of the alveoli; occurs in premature and debilitated infants, children with primary immunodeficiency diseases, individuals receiving chemotherapy, and those in the last stage of an HIV infection (AIDS). Also called pneumocystosis.

primary atypical p. See mycoplasmal pneumonia.

secondary p. Inflammation of the lungs occurring as a complication of another disease.

staphylococcal p. Bacterial pneumonia caused by *Staphylococcus aureus*; it frequently occurs as a complication of viral influenza.

walking p. See mycoplasmal pneumonia.

wool-sorter's p. See pulmonary anthrax, under anthrax.

viral p. Acute systemic disease, caused by a variety of viruses (e.g., adenoviruses), with involvement of the lungs.

pneumonic (nu-mon′ik) **1.** Relating to the lungs. **2.** Relating to pneumonia.

pneumonitis (nu-mo-ni′tis) Inflammation of the lungs.

hypersensitivity p. Chronic progressive condition marked by wheezing and difficult breathing; diffuse infiltrates are seen in x-ray films of the lungs; results from long-term exposure to any of various substances (e.g., in occupational exposures).

pneumonocele (nu-mon′ŏ-sēl) See pneumatocele (3).

pneumonocyte (nu-mon-ŏ-sīt) See pneumocyte.

pneumonotomy (nu-mo-not′ŏ-me) Incision into the lungs. Also called pneumotomy.

pneumopericardium (nu-mo-per-ĭ-kar′de-um) The presence of air in the double-layered sac encasing the heart.

pneumoperitoneum (nu-mo-per-ĭ-to-ne′um) Abnormal collection of air in the peritoneal cavity; may be due to perforation of an abdominal organ or to a pulmonary air leak.

artificial p. Deliberate introduction of air into the peritoneal cavity for therapeutic purposes.

pneumoperitonitis (nu-mo-per-ĭ-to-ni′tis) Inflammation of the peritoneum with accumulation of air or gas in the peritoneal cavity.

pneumopyothorax (nu-mo-pi-o-tho′raks) See pyopneumothorax.

pneumoroentgenography (nu-mo-rent-gen-og′ră-fe) See pneumography.

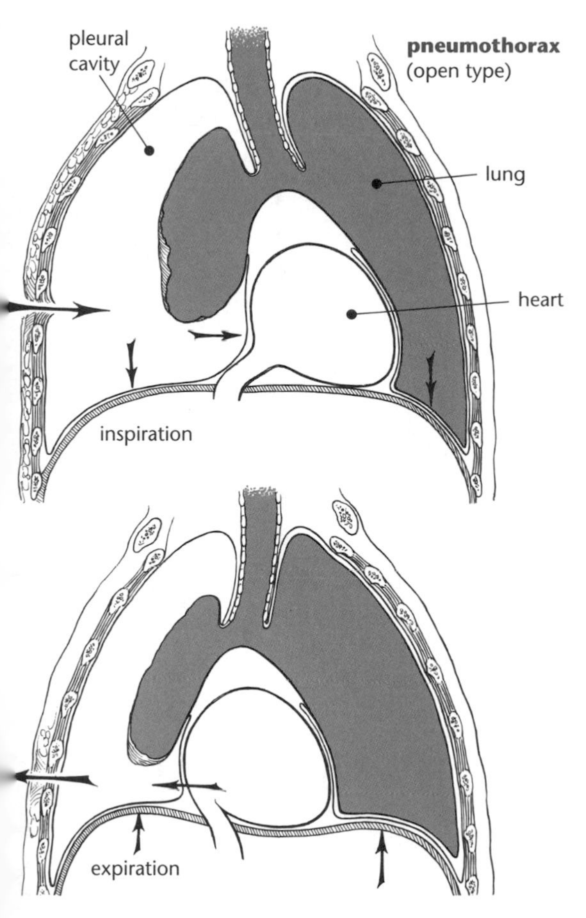

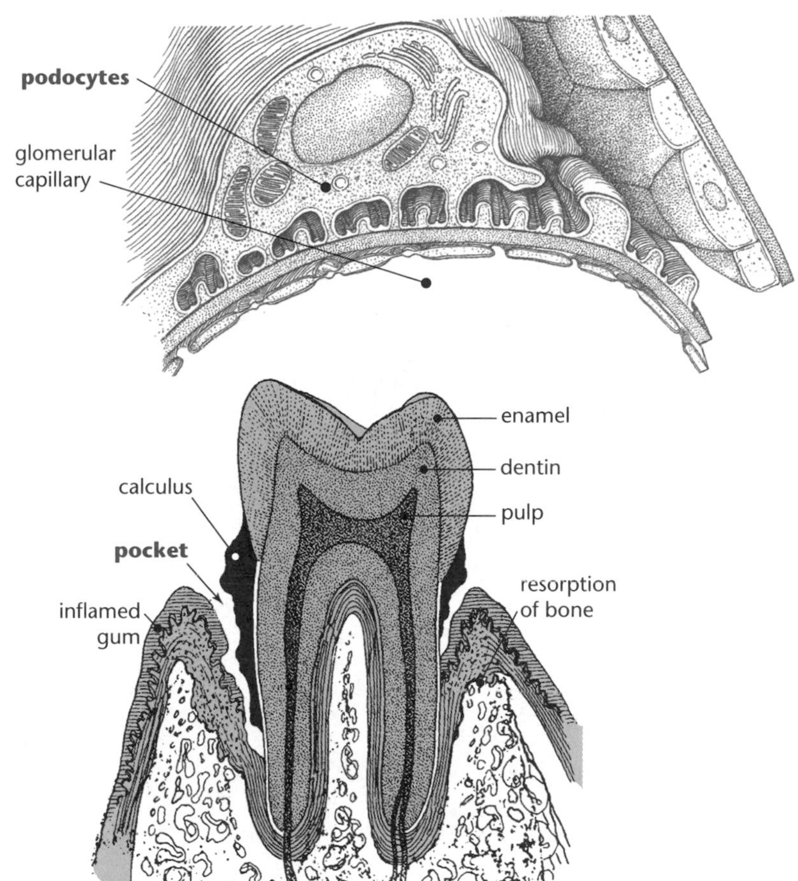

pneumorrhachis (nu-mor´ā-kis) Abnormal presence of gas in the spinal canal. Also called pneumatorrhachis.

pneumorrhagia (nu-mo-ra´je-ă) Bleeding from or into the lung.

pneumothorax (nu-mo-tho´raks) The presence of air or gas between the two layers of the pleura (pleural space).

spontaneous p. Pneumothorax secondary to disease of lung tissue.

tension p. A life-threatening condition occurring when lungs and heart are compressed by accumulated air in the pleural space.

pneumotomy (nu-mot´ŏ-me) See pneumonotomy.

Pneumovirus (nu-mo-vi´rus) Genus of viruses (family Paramyxoviridae) that are intermediate in size between other Paramyxoviridae and the Orthomyxoviridae; includes the respiratory syncytial virus, which causes bronchiolitis and pneumonia in infants.

pock (pok) A pustule caused by an eruptive disease, especially smallpox.

pocket (pok´et) **1.** A saclike cavity. **2.** A pathologically increased space between a tooth and the inflamed gum. **3.** To enclose the pedicle of a tumor (after its removal) within the edges of the wound.

pockmark (pok´mark) The scar left on the skin after the healing of a smallpox pustule.

podagra (po-dag´ră) Gout of the metatarsophalangeal joint of the big toe.

podagral, podagric, podagrous (pod´ă-gral, po-dag´rik, pod´ă-grus) Relating to gout.

podalgia (po-dal´jă) Pain in the foot.

podalic (po-dal´ik) Relating to feet.

podarthritis (pod-ar-thri´tis) Inflammation of the foot joints.

podiatrist (po-di´ă-trist) A specialist in podiatry. Formerly called chiropodist.

podiatry (po-di´ă-tre) The study and treatment of foot diseases, injuries, and defects. Formerly called chiropody.

poditis (po-di´tis) An inflammatory disorder of the foot.

podobromidrosis (pod-o-bro-mĭ-dro´sis) Sweating of the feet with a strong, offensive odor.

podocyte (pod´o-sīt) An epithelial cell of the renal glomerulus that squats upon the glomerular basement membrane, spreading thin cytoplasmic projections over the membrane; the outer surface of the engorged cell projects into the glomerular (Bowman's) space, where it is bathed by the glomerular ultrafiltrate.

pododynamometer (pod-o-di-nă-mom´ĕ-ter) Device for measuring the strength of the foot or leg muscles.

podophyllin (pod-o-fil´in) See podophyllum resin, under resin.

podophyllotoxin (pod-o-fil-o-tok´sin) The active principle of podophyllum resin; it has laxative properties.

podophyllum (pod-o-fil´um) The rhizome of the mayapple (*Podophyllum peltatum*), used as a bulk-forming laxative.

pogonion (po-go´ne-on) The most anterior midpoint of the chin. Also called mental point.

-poietin Suffix indicating a stimulatory effect on growth or multiplication of cells.

poikilocyte (poi´kĭ-lo-sīt) A red blood cell assuming an abnormal and often bizarre shape; it could be pear-shaped, racquet-shaped, or pessary-shaped; characteristically found in severe hemolytic anemias.

poikilocythemia (poi-kil-o-si-the´me-ă) See poikilocytosis.

poikilocytosis (poi-kĭ-lo-si-to´sis) The presence of poikilocytes in the blood. Also called poikilocythemia.

poikiloderma (poi-kĭ-lo-der´mă) Atrophic condition of the skin marked by streaks, patches of too much or too little pigmentation, and clustes of dilated capillaries.

poikilotherm (poi-kil´o-therm) An animal having a temperature that varies with the environment.

point (point) **1.** A minute spot or area. **2.** The sharp or tapered end of an object. **3.** A specific condition or degree.

alveolar p. See prosthion.

boiling p. (b.p.) The temperature at which a liquid boils; the vapor pressure of the liquid equals the atmospheric pressure.

contact p. The small area of the proximal surface of a tooth that touches the adjacent tooth. Also called contact area.

craniometric p. Any one of many fixed points on the skull used as landmarks for skull measurements.

critical p. The temperature at or above which it is not possible to liquefy a gas, regardless of the pressure applied.

cutoff p. In test interpretation, the value used to separate positive from negative results.

dew p. Temperature at which the moisture of the air condenses.

end p. In volumetric analysis of a solution, the point at which a reaction is completed.

p. of fixation The retinal point on which an image is formed; in normal vision it is the fovea.

focal p. Point at which light rays meet when deflected by refraction or reflection.

freezing p. Temperature at which a liquid changes to a solid state.

heat-rigor p. Temperature at which cell death occurs, usually due to coagulation of cell protoplasm.

isoelectric p. (IP) The pH at which an amphoteric electrolyte (e.g., an amino acid or protein) is electrically neutral owing to equality of ionization; above or below this pH, it acts as an acid or base, respectively.

J p. See J junction, under junction.

jugal p. The point where the zygomatic arch meets with the frontal process of the zygomatic bone.

p. of maximum impulse The point on the chest wall where the beat of the left ventricle of the heart is felt most intensely; normally felt in the left fifth intercostal space, at the midclavicular line.

McBurney's p. A point on the lateral third of a line between the navel and the anterior superior spine of the right ilium; it is especially tender in acute appendicitis.

melting p. (mp) Temperature at which a solid changes into a liquid state.

mental p. See pogonion.

mid-inguinal p. The point on the inguinal ligament halfway between the pubic symphysis and the anterior superior iliac spine.

nasal p. See nasion.

pressure p. (a) A point on the body at which pressure can be exerted to control hemorrhage from an arterial injury. (b) A point on the skin surface that is extremely sensitive to pressure.

P

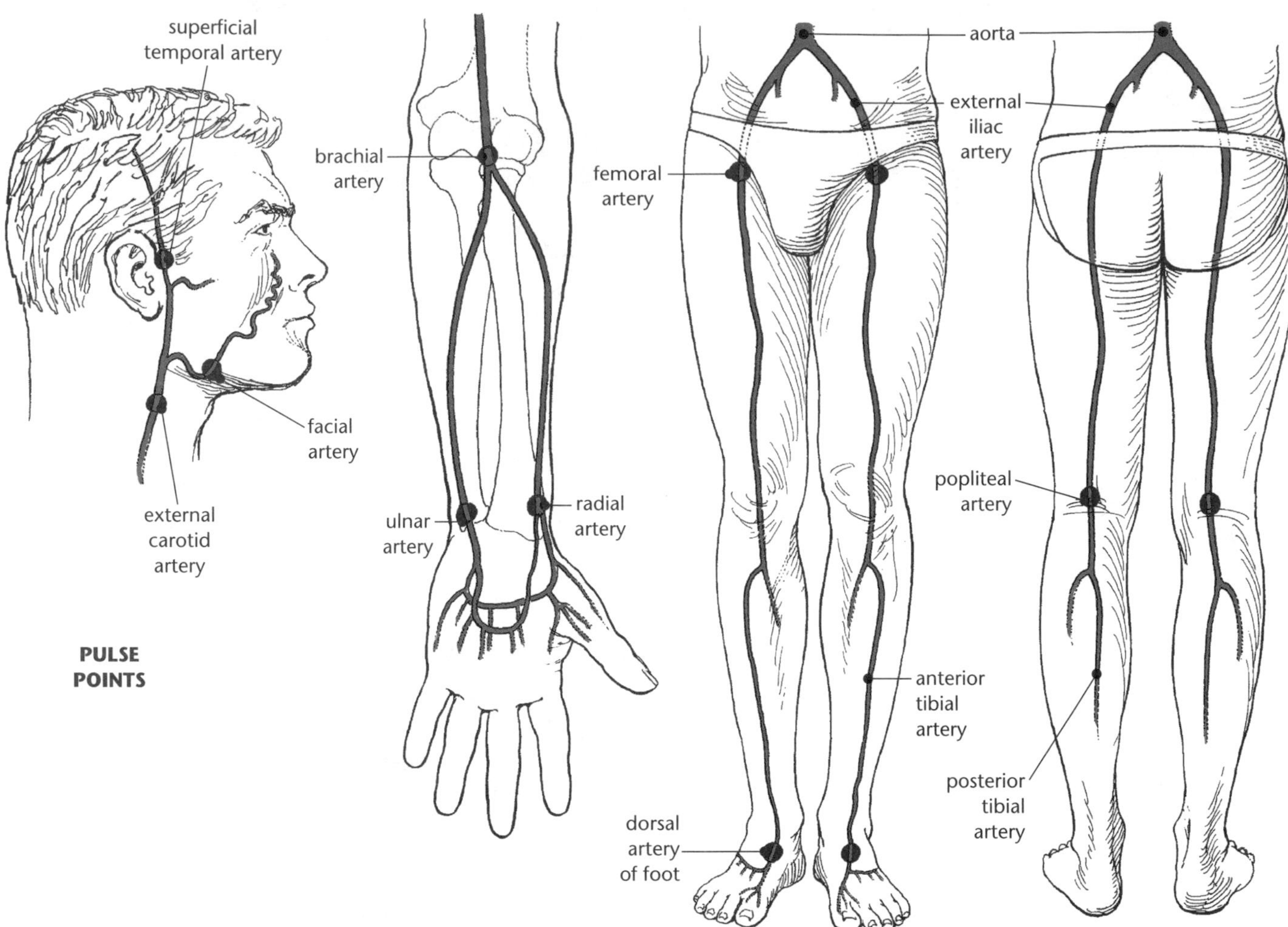

pulse p.'s Sites on the body where the rhythmic expansion of an artery can be readily felt with the finger.

thermal death p. The temperature required to heat kill microorganisms in a standard aqueous culture when exposed for 10 minutes.

trigger p. A spot on the body that, when touched or pressed, initiates pain in adjacent or distant parts.

pointing (point′ing) The process of reaching a point.

p. of an abscess An abscess or boil that is about to open spontaneously.

point-of-service (POS) **plan** A health care plan that offers its members coverage for care provided outside the plan (for additional out-of-pocket payment), but provides more extensive coverage for care provided by a designated primary care physician.

point source (point sōrs) In photometry, the source of light from which light radiates in straight lines in all directions.

poise (poiz) The unit of dynamic viscosity of a liquid equal to 1 dyne-second per square centimeter.

poison (poi′zn) Any substance that is injurious to health or causes death, either taken internally or applied externally.

"purse" p. Medication carried in the purse for personal use that results in poisoning of the curious child seeking candy or chewing gum and finding attractive multicolored pills and tablets.

poison ash (poi′zn ash) See *Rhus vernix*, under *Rhus*.

poison dogwood (poi′zn dog′wood) See *Rhus vernix*, under *Rhus*.

poison elder (poi′zn el′der) See *Rhus vernix*, under *Rhus*.

poison ivy, poison oak, poison sumac (poi′zn ī′ve, ōk, soo′mak) **1.** Shrubs of the genus *Rhus* with foliage that contains an irritating substance (urushiol). See *Rhus*. **2.** The itchy, vesicular skin eruption and inflammation caused by contact with the urushiol of such plants.

poisoning (poi′zŭ-ning) The condition produced by a poison.

arsenic p. Poisoning caused by ingestion of arsenic-containing compounds, usually insecticides or rodenticides; arsenic reacts with sulfhydryl groups to disrupt vital enzyme systems; symptoms of chronic poisoning include skin changes and peripheral neuropathy; headache and confusion may be seen in both acute and chronic forms.

blood p. A vague colloquial term; see septicemia and bacteremia.

carbon monoxide p. Acute (potentially fatal) poisoning with various degrees of severity, caused by inhalation of carbon monoxide; severe headache is usually an early symptom; subsequently nausea, weakness, and exertional breathing difficulty may develop; collapse and coma may supervene.

carbon tetrachloride p. Liver and kidney necrosis caused by ingestion, inhalation, or absorption of carbon tetrachloride, an industrial solvent.

cyanide p. Poisoning caused by inhalation or ingestion of compounds of cyanide; death may occur in minutes; cyanides combine with iron-containing enzymes such as cytochromes and catalase to block energy-releasing metabolism and cause tissue asphyxia; most common sources are fungicides and insecticides.

ergot p. See ergotism.

food p. Acute gastrointestinal illness or neurologic manifestations; resulting from ingestion of foods that have become contaminated with microorganisms, may contain harmful chemicals, or may themselves be poisonous.

heavy metal p. Poisoning caused by such metals as antimony, arsenic, bismuth, cadmium, copper, gold, lead, mercury, silver, and thallium; BAL and EDTA are used to treat many of these disorders.

lead p. Acute or chronic intoxication with lead or its salts, causing gastrointestinal and mental disturbances, anemia, basophilic stippling of red blood cells, and a bluish "lead line" on the gums; most commonly seen in young children who eat paint scales; other sources include lead toys, motor fuel, and lead water pipes. Also called plumbism.

mercury p. Poisoning caused by ingestion of soluble mercury salts such as mercuric chloride ($HgCl_2$), producing corrosive damage to the gastrointestinal tract and destruction of the kidney tubules; repeated inhalation of mercury vapor or ingestion of small amounts of mercury salts may lead to chronic mercury poisoning, characterized by mental symptoms, renal damage, and stomatitis.

***Salmonella* food p.** Inflammation of the gastrointestinal tract caused by ingestion of food contaminated with any of several strains of *Salmonella*; symptoms usually appear within 8 to 24 hours and include abdominal pain, nausea, diarrhea, vomiting and fever.

scombroid p. Poisoning caused by ingestion of a toxin produced by inadequately preserved fish of the order Scombroidea (tuna, mackerel, bonito); symptoms include pain above the stomach, nausea, vomiting, headache, and rash.

***Staphylococcus* food p.** Inflammation of the intestines caused by a toxin, specific for intestinal mucosa, produced by staphylococci; symptoms appear a few hours after ingestion of contaminated food and include severe vomiting and diarrhea.

polar (po′lar) **1.** Relating to poles. **2.** Having poles; said of certain nerve cells.

polarimeter (po-lă-rim′ĕ-ter) Instrument used to determine the amount of polarization of light or the rotation of the plane of polarization.

polarimetry (po-lă-rim′ĕ-tre) The process of using the polarimeter.

polariscope (po-lar′ĭ-skōp) Instrument used to study the properties of polarized light.

polarity (po-lar′ĭ-te) **1.** Having two opposite poles. **2.** Manifesting two opposite tendencies or attributes.

polarization (po-lar-i-za′shun) **1.** In optics, the process of altering the transverse wave motion of a light ray, whereby the vibrations of the wave occur in one plane only. **2.** In electricity, the deposition of gas in one or both electrodes of an electric cell, whereby the action of the battery is impeded. **3.** The development of ions of opposite charges (i.e., differences in potential) in two points of living tissue, as on both sides of a cell membrane.

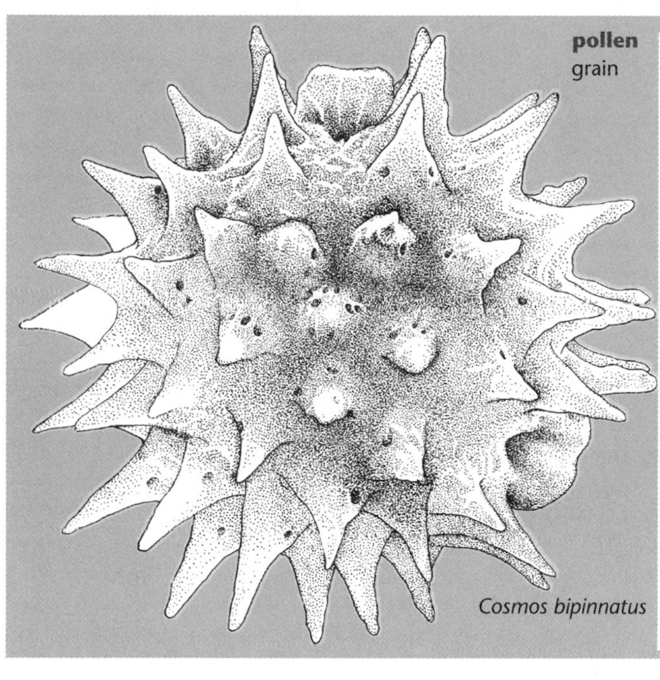

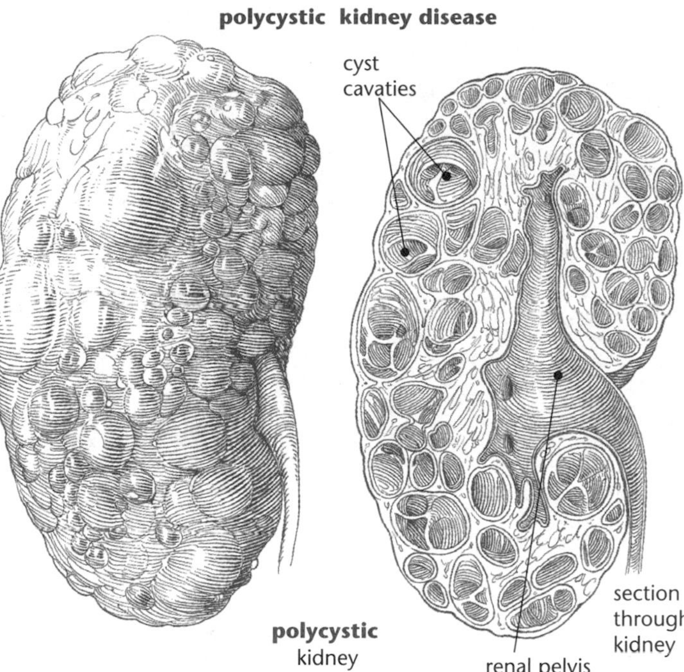

polarize (po'lar-īz) To induce polarization.
polarizer (po'lă-rīz-er) The part of a polarimeter or polariscope that receives and polarizes the light.
polarography (po-lar-og'ră-fe) In qualitative or quantitative microanalysis, the recording of the relationship between an increasing current flowing through a solution being analyzed and the increasing voltage used to produce the current.
pole (pōl) **1.** Either end of an axis. **2.** Either of two points having opposite physical properties (e.g., terminals of an electric cell or battery).
animal p. The site in the early ovum near the nucleus where most of the protoplasm is concentrated, and from which the polar bodies are pinched off. Also called germinal pole.
antigerminal p. See vegetal pole.
germinal p. See animal pole.
negative p. See cathode.
positive p. See anode.
vegetal p., vegetative p. The pole of an ovum where the bulk of the yolk is located, opposite to the germinal disk. Also called vitelline pole; antigerminal pole.
vitelline p. See vegetal pole.
polio (po'le-o) Colloquial term for poliomyelitis.
poliodystrophy (po-le-o-dis-tro'fe) Wasting of the gray substance of the nervous system.
polioencephalitis (po-le-o-en-sef-ă-li'tis) Inflammation of the gray substance of the brain.
poliomyelitis (po-le-o-mi-e-li'tis) A highly contagious, infectious disease caused by a poliovirus (genus *Enterovirus*, family Picornaviridae); occurs most commonly in children; in its acute form it involves the spinal cord, causing paralysis, atrophy, and permanent deformity of one or more muscular groups. Also called polio.
bulbar p. A form that involves nerve cells in the medulla oblongata and may cause respiratory paralysis and death.
poliomyelopathy (po-le-o-mi-ĕ-lop'ă-the) Any disease principally affecting the gray matter of the spinal cord and medulla oblongata.
poliovirus (po-le-o-vi'rus) The virus (genus *Enterovirus*, family Picornaviridae) causing poliomyelitis in humans; serologic types 1, 2, 3, and 4 are recognized.
pollen (pol'en) The powder-like microspores (male fertilizing elements) produced by the anthers of flowering plants that are carried by wind or insects and play a major role in the etiology of hay fever and some cases of asthma.
pollex (pol'eks) The thumb.
pollinosis, pollenosis (pol-i-no'sis, pol-ĕ-no'sis) Hay fever induced by certain airborne pollens.
pollutant (po-lū't'nt) A substance that contaminates; especially one that contaminates the air, water, or food.
pollute (po-lūt') To make impure; to contaminate.
pollution (po-lū'shun) The act or process of contaminating (e.g., discharge of noxious substances into the atmosphere or into a body of water).
polonium (po-lo'ne-um) A radioactive metallic element; symbol Po, atomic number 84, atomic weight 210; one of the rarest naturally occurring elements, a product of radium disintegration; discovered by Pierre and Marie Curie and named after Mme. Curie's native land, Poland.
polonium-210 (^{210}Po) A 138.4-day alpha-emitter isotope of polonium that is a member of the uranium natural radioactive decay series.
polyacid (pol-e-as'id) An acid that yields more than one hydrogen ion per molecule.
polyadenitis (pol-e-ad-ĕ-ni'tis) Inflammation of several lymph nodes.
poly (pol'e) Colloquial term for polymorphonoclear leukocyte.
polyamine (pol-e-am'ēn) Any of a group of substances (e.g., putrescine, cadaverine, spermidine, spermine) that are widely distributed in small quantities in living forms; they are essential growth factors for a number of microorganisms (e.g., *Hemophilus parainfluenzae),* and serve to stabilize membranous structures.
polyarteritis (pol-e-ar-tĕ-ri'tis) Simultaneous inflammation of several arteries.
p. nodosa (PAN) Polyarteritis with formation of numerous nodules within the walls of small- to medium-sized arteries anywhere in the body except in the lungs; it affects mostly young adults, especially males, and is frequently associated with hepatitis B antigens; symptoms depend on the organs involved; generally, they include fever, malaise, and weight loss. Also called periarteritis nodosa.
polyarthritis (pol-e-ar-thri'tis) Inflammation of several joints.
polybasic (pol-e-ba'sik) An acid that has more than one replaceable hydrogen atom.
polycholia (pol-e-ko'le-ă) Excessive production and flow of bile.
polychondritis (pol-e-kon-dri'tis) A rare syndrome marked by a widespread inflammatory and degenerative process in cartilaginous structures, such as those in the nose, ear, joints, and tracheobronchial tree; destruction of cartilage leaves deformities, such as saddle nose or floppy ear; death may occur from suffocation due to loss of stability in the tracheobronchial tree.
polychromasia, polychromatia (pol-e-kro-ma'ze-ă, pol-e-kro-ma'she-ă) Polychromatophilia.
polychromatic (pol-e-kro-mat'ik) Multicolored; exhibiting many colors.
polychromatophil (pol-e-kro-mat'o-fil) **1.** A cell or other element that stains readily with both acidic and basic dyes, especially certain red blood cells. **2.** A young or degenerating red blood cell that manifests acidic and basic staining affinities.
polychromatophilia (pol-e-kro-mă-to-fil'e-ă) **1.** Tendency to stain with basic and acid stains. **2.** Condition marked by the presence of an excessive number of red blood cells that stain with basic, acid, and neutral dyes.
polyclinic (pol-e-klin'ik) A clinic, dispensary, or hospital that treats any disease or injury.
polycystic (pol-e-sis'tik) Made up of several cysts.
polycystic kidney disease (pol-e-sis'tik kid'ne dĭ-zēz') (PCKD) An inherited kidney disease marked by formation of multiple enlarging cysts causing eventual degeneration of structure and function of the kidney. Occurs in two forms: The adult-onset form is an autosomal dominant inheritance; often causes uremia (blood in the urine) and hypertension and may be accompanied by microaneurysms in the brain. The less common form is an autosomal recessive inheritance; appears early in life (perinatal, neonatal, infantile, and juvenile ages) and is often associated with cysts and proliferating bile ducts in the liver.
polycystic liver disease (pol-e-sis'tik liv'er dĭ-zēz) Condition marked by development of multiple cysts in the liver, frequently associated with polycystic kidney disease. Also called polycystic liver.
polycystic ovary syndrome (pol-e-sis'tik o'vă-re sin'drōm) (PCOS) Disorder affecting young women characterized by bilaterally enlarged ovaries with multiple cysts, chronic failure to release ova, secondary absent or scanty menstruation (amenorrhea or oligomenorrhea), and infertility. Also called polycystic ovary disease.
polycythemia (pol-e-si-the'me-ă) Condition in which there is an increased concentration of erythrocytes in the blood. Also called erythrocythemia; eryhrocytosis.
absolute p. The result of an increase in red blood cell numbers. May be *primary absolute p.*, due to intrinsic abnormality of the immature red blood cell (as occurs in polycythemia vera); or *secondary absolute p.*, due to a response to another condition (e.g., chronic tissue hypoxia of advanced pulmonary disease).
primary p. See polycythemia vera.
relative p. An increase in the number of red blood cells per unit volume of blood (without an increase of red blod cell mass) due to a decrease in the total plasma of the body.

P

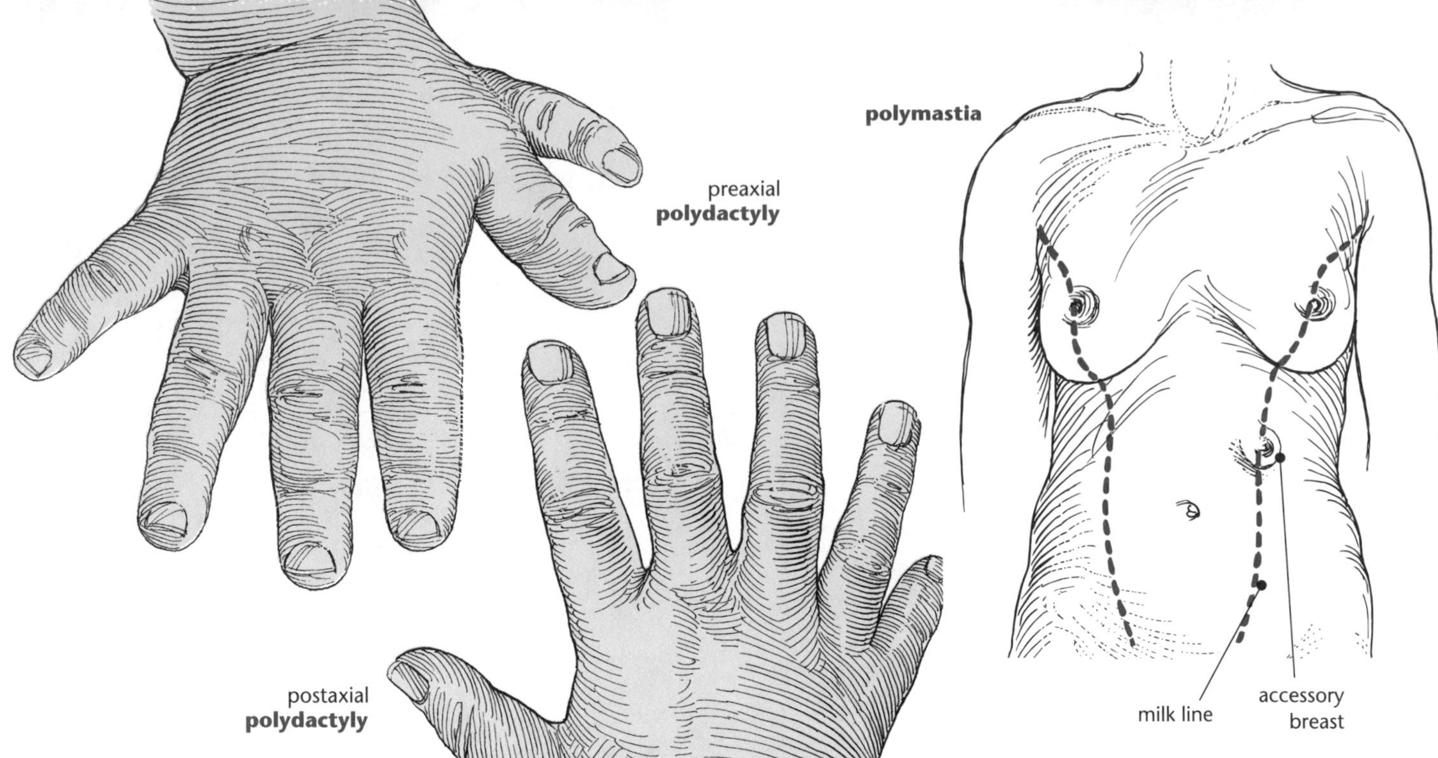

p. rubra vera See polycythemia vera.

p. vera (PV) Disease of unknown cause marked by proliferation of all the cellular elements of bone marrow and increased total number of red blood cells in the body, usually associated with abnormal increase of white blood cells and platelets (leukocytosis and thrombocytosis); it appears insidiously in people 40 to 60 years of age. Also called polycythemia rubra vera; primary polycythemia; erythremia.

polydactyly (pol-e-dak′tĭ-le) The presence of more than ten fingers or toes. Also called polydactylia; polydactylism.

polydipsia (pol-e-dip′se-ă) Insatiable thirst.

polydysplasia (pol-e-dis-pla′zhă, pol-e-dis-pla′ze-ă) Condition marked by multiple developmental abnormalities of tissues, organs, or systems.

polyene (pol-e′ēn) A chemical compound containing many conjugated (alternating) double bonds (e.g., carotenoids).

polyenoic acid (pol-e-e-no′ik as′id) Polyunsaturated fatty acid, essential in the diet, with more than one double bond in the carbon chain (e.g., linoleic acid with two double bonds, linolenic acid with three double bonds).

polyethylene (pol-e-eth′ĭ-lēn) Resin produced by the polymerization of ethylene under high pressure; a straight-chain paraffin hydrocarbon of high molecular weight.

p. glycol A condensation product of ethylene oxide and water.

polygen (pol′e-jen) A chemical element with two or more valences.

polygene (pol′e-jēn) One of a group of genes that, acting together, control a recognizable characteristic (phenotype), although the effect of each gene is not discernible.

polygenic (pol-e-jen′ik) Resulting from the action of a group of genes.

polyglandular (pol-e-glan′ju-lar) See pluriglandular.

polygraph (pol-ĕ-graf) An instrument for simultaneously recording changes in such physiologic processes as blood pressure, respiratory movements, and galvanic skin resistance; sometimes used to detect emotional reactions, as in lie detection. Also called lie detector.

polyhedral (pol-e-he′dral) Having many faces.

polyhydramnios (pol-e-hi-dram′nĭ-os) An excess volume of amniotic fluid in pregnancy, usually greater than 2000 ml.

polyhydric (pol-e-hi′drik) Containing more than one hydroxyl group.

polyhypermenorrhea (pol-e-hi-per-men-o-re′ă) Frequent menstruation accompanied by excessive flow.

polyhypomenorrhea (pol-e-hi-po-men-o-re′ă) Frequent menstruation accompanied by a scanty flow.

polyleptic (pol-e-lep′tik) Having many relapsing phases; said of a disease.

polylogia (pol-e-lo′je-ă) Garrulity or talkativeness (often incoherent) caused by a mental disorder.

polymastia (pol-e-mas′ti-ă) The presence of more than two breasts in the human. Also called accessory breasts; supernumerary breasts; multimammae; pleomastia.

polymer (pol′ĭ-mer) A complex compound made up of a chain of simple molecules (e.g., polyethylene, formed from many ethylene molecules).

addition p. A large molecule formed by a chain of small molecules (monomers) without the formation of any other product.

condensation p. A large molecule formed by a chain of small molecules, involving the elimination of water or some other simple compound.

polymerase (pol-im′er-ās) Any enzyme that promotes polymerization.

DNA p. An enzyme capable of synthesizing a new DNA strand, using a previously synthesized DNA strand as a template.

RNA p. An enzyme that synthesizes RNA on a DNA template from a ribonucleoside triphosphate precursor.

polymerization (pol-ĭ-mer-ĭ-za′shun) The chemical joining of similar monomers to form a compound of high molecular weight.

polymethylmethacrylate (pol-e-meth-il-meth-ak′rĭ-lāt) The principal base resin employed in making dentures; it is transparent and can be tinted to any shade of translucence; also used as bone cement.

polymicrolipomatosis (pol-e-mi-kro-lip-o-mă-to′sis) A condition marked by the presence of a number of small, nodular, fairly discrete masses of lipid (lipomata) in the subcutaneous connective tissue.

polymorph (pol′e-morf) Colloquial term for polymorphonuclear leukocyte (PMN).

polymorphic, polymorphous (pol-e-mor′fik, pol-e-mor′fus) Occurring in many forms.

polymorphism (pol-e-mor′fiz-m) **1.** Occurring in various forms, either during development or as adults within a single species. **2.** The presence of two or more recognizable characteristics (phenotypes) within a species.

polymorphonuclear (pol-e-mor-fo-nu′kle-ar) Having nuclei of varied shapes, or so deeply lobulated that they appear to be multiple; said of a variety of leukocytes (PMNs).

polymyalgia (pol-e-mi-al′je-ă) Pain in several muscles.

p. rheumatica (PMR) Syndrome occurring in the elderly; characterized by muscle aches, markedly elevated erythrocyte sedimentation rate, and fever; often associated with temporal arteritis.

polymyositis (pol-e-mi-o-si′tis) A painful inflammation of the muscles that may also involve skin and subcutaneous tissue; the muscles most affected are those of the pelvic and shoulder girdles and pharynx; when skin changes are prominent, the disorder is often called dermatomyositis; in 15 to 20 percent of cases it is associated with an occult malignant tumor.

polymyxin (pol-e-mik′sin) Any of a group of antibiotic substances derived from strains of the soil bacterium *Bacillus polymyxa*; they are polypeptides containing various amino acids and a branched fatty acid, (+)-6-methyloctanoic acid; there are five different types, designated A, B, C, D, and E.

polyneuritis (pol-e-nu-ri′tis) Inflammation of several peripheral nerves at the same time, characterized by widespread sensory and motor disturbances.

idiopathic p. See Guillain-Barré syndrome.

polyneuropathy (pol-e-nu-rop′ă-the) A disease affecting several peripheral nerves and occurring as a result of other disorders.

diabetic p. Polyneuropathy, usually bilateral, occurring as a complication of diabetes mellitus, affecting primarily the lower limbs; symptoms range from numbness to pain.

polyneuroradiculitis (pol-e-nu-ro-ră-dik-u-li′tis) Inflammation involving nerve roots and peripheral nerves.

polynuclear (pol-e-nu′kle-ar) See multinuclear.

polynucleotidase (pol-e-nu-kle-o′ti-dās) A class of enzymes that help to hydrolyze or split up nucleic acids of high molecular weight into their constituent mononucleotide units.

polynucleotide (pol-e-nu′kle-o-tīd) Compound containing many nucleotides; a nucleic acid.

polyol (pol′e-ol) General term for an alcohol that contains more than one hydroxyl group in the molecule.

polyopia (pol-e-o′pe-ă) Condition in which a person perceives more than one image of the same object; multiple vision. Also called polyopsia; polyopy.

p. monophthalmica Polyopia affecting only one eye.

polyorchidism, polyorchism (pol-e-or′kĭ-diz-m) The presence of more than two testes.

polyostotic (pol-e-os-tot′ik) Affecting several bones.

polyp (pol′ip) A growth of tissue arising from the mucous membrane of a hollow structure (e.g., uterus, colon, nose, bladder) and protruding into the lumen;

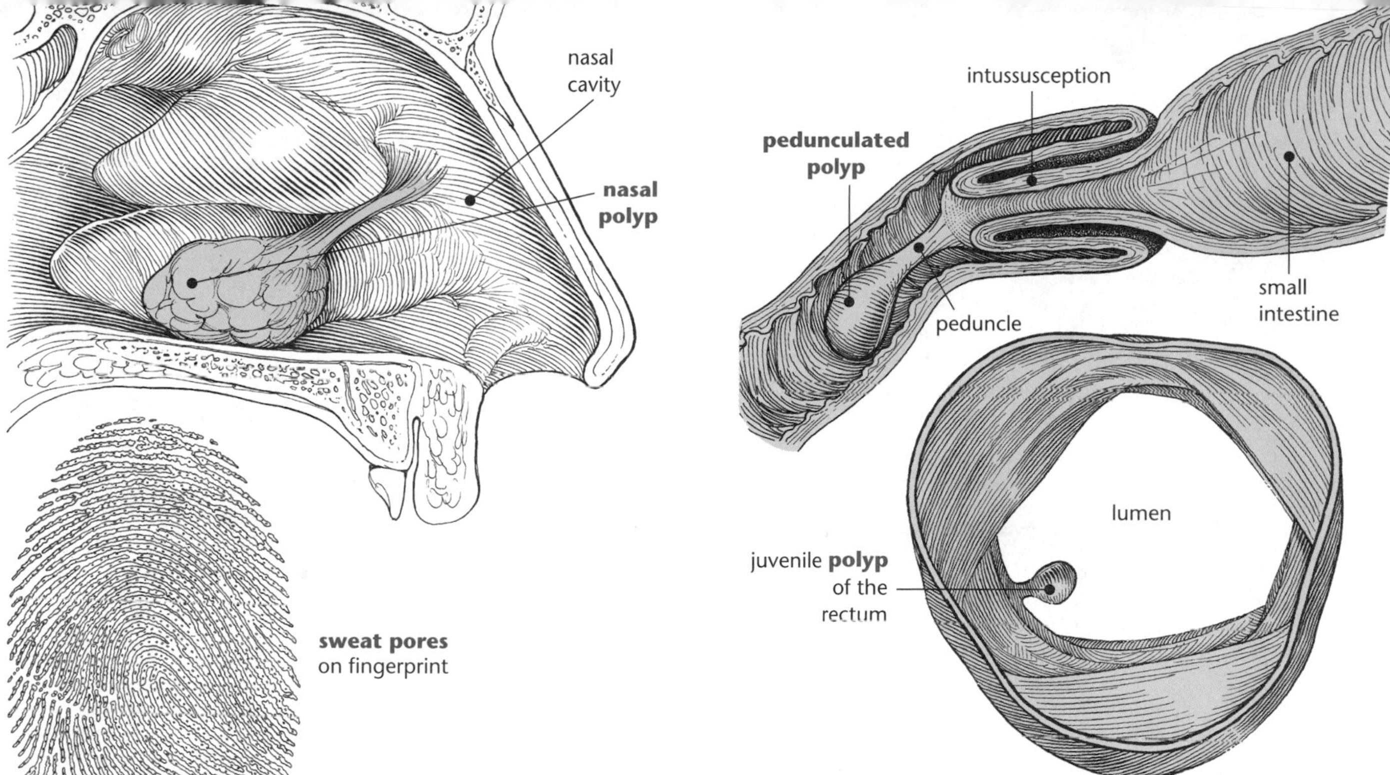

can be benign or malignant.

adenomatous p. Benign polyp composed of glandular tissue; may be pedunculated or sessile.

cervical p. A relatively common, usually benign polyp, most frequently seen in women over 20 years of age; some may cause intermenstrual or post-intercourse bleeding; a few may undergo malignant change.

ectocervical p. A pale, smooth cervical polyp arising from the surface of the vaginal cervix (i.e., the portion of the cervix protruding into the vagina).

endocervical p. A soft, fragile, pedunculated or sessile cervical polyp originating within the cervical canal and frequently protruding into the vagina.

endometrial p. Small benign mass composed of tissue from the lining of the uterine cavity (endometrium) and protruding into the cavity of the uterus.

fleshy p. Polyp composed of smooth muscle tissue.

hyperplastic p. A benign, sessile polyp, usually no larger than 5 mm in diameter, lying on top of a mucosal fold (e.g., of the large intestine) and producing no symptoms.

inflammatory p. See pseudopolyp.

juvenile p. A large (up to 2 cm in diameter), pedunculated, benign polyp composed of dilated mucosal glands of the rectum; occurs in young adults and children, especially under 5 years of age; may cause painless bleeding after defecation. Also called retention polyp.

nasal p. A focal inflammatory swelling of the lining of the nasal cavity or sinuses.

neoplastic p. A polyp composed of cells that develop the capacity for uncontrolled proliferation, which results in a cancerous process.

pedunculated p. Polyp that is attached to the mucosa by a slender stalk or pedicle.

retention p. See juvenile polyp.

sessile p. Polyp that has a broad base.

polypectomy (pol-ĭ-pek´tŏ-me) Surgical removal of a polyp.

polypeptide (pol-e-pep´tīd) A compound containing two or more amino acids united by peptide linkage; the ribosome is the site of polypeptide synthesis in the cytoplasm.

polypeptidemia (pol-e-pep-tĭ-de´me-ă) The presence of polypeptides in the blood.

polyphagia (pol-e-fa´jă, pol-e-fa´je-ă) Pathologic overeating.

polypharmacy (pol-e-fahr´mă-se) Concomitant administration or ingestion of many drugs.

polyplastic (pol-e-plas´tik) Capable of taking many forms.

polyplegia (pol-e-ple´jă, pol-e-ple´je-ă) Paralysis of several muscles.

polyploidy (pol´e-ploĭ-de) The state of having a chromosome number that is a multiple of the normal diploid number; results from the replication of chromosome sets without subsequent division of the nucleus (e.g., tetraploid = 92 chromosomes, triploid = 69 chromosomes).

polypoid (pol´e-poid) Having the outward appearance of a polyp.

polyposis (pol-e-po´sis) The presence of numerous polyps.

familial p. coli (FPC) The presence of numerous polyps in the colon causing intestinal bleeding and a 100% chance of developing cancer of the colon and rectum. An autosomal dominalt inheritance with defect on chromosome 5.

polypotome (po-lip´ŏ-tōm) A cutting instrument for excising polyps.

polypous (pol´e-pus) Relating to or characterized by the presence of polyps.

polyribosome (pol-e-ri´bo-sōm) A multiple structure composed of two or more ribosomes held together by a molecule of messenger RNA. Also called polysome.

polys (pol´ez) A colloquial term for polymorphonuclear leukocytes.

polysaccharide (pol-e-sak´ă-rīd) A carbohydrate containing a large number of saccharide units, such as starch and glycogen.

polyserositis (pol-e-se-ro-si´tis) Inflammation of several serous membranes. Also called multiple serositis.

polysome (pol´e-sōm) See polyribosome.

polysomy (pol-e-so´me) The state of a cell nucleus in which some but not all of the chromosomes of a set are reduplicated beyond the normal diploid number.

polysorbate 80 (pol-e-sor´bāt ā´tē) Polyoxyethylene sorbitan mono-oleate; a yellow, bitter oil, used as an emulsifier in the preparation of ointments; Tween 80®.

polyspermia (pol-e-sper´me-ă) Excessive secretion of semen.

polyspermy (pol-e-sper´me) The entry of more than one sperm into an ovum during fertilization.

polytetrafluoroethylene (pol-e-tet-ră-floor-ō-eth´ĭ-lēn) A waxy synthetic fabric that resists clotting of blood on its surface; used for surgical implantation; Teflon®.

polythelia (pol-e-the´le-ă) The presence of more than two nipples. Also called hyperthelia.

polytrichia (pol-e-trik´e-ă) The presence of excessive hair.

polyunsaturated (pol-e-un-sach´ĕ-ra-ted) Having two or more unsaturated (double) bonds; said of certain long-chain carbon compounds, especially fats and oils.

polyuria (pol-e-u´re-ă) Passage of abnormally large quantity of urine.

polyvalent (pol-e-va´lent) See multivalent.

polyvinylpyrrolidone (pol-e-vi-nil-pir-rol´ĭ-dōn) (PVP) See povidone.

Pompe's disease (pom´pĕz dĭ-zēz´) See type II glycogenosis, under glycogenosis.

pompholyx (pom´fo-liks) See dyshidrosis (2).

pomphus (pom´fus) A blister or a wheal.

pons (ponz) **1.** The part of the brain located between the cerebral peduncle above and the medulla oblongata below. **2.** Any bridgelike structure connecting two parts of an organ.

pontic (pon´tik) An artificial tooth on a fixed partial denture that replaces the missing natural tooth.

pontile, pontine (pon´tīl, pon´tīn) Relating to a pons, especially of the brain (pons varolii).

pontomedullary (pon-to-med´u-lār-e) Relating to the pons and medulla oblongata of the central nervous system.

pool (pōōl) **1.** An accumulation, as of blood. **2.** Combined resources.

gene p. The total collection of genes available for inheritance among members of a given population who are capable of sexual reproduction.

vaginal p. The secretions accumulated in the upper posterior area of the vagina, used as a specimen for hormonal evaluation and cancer detection.

poples (pop´lez) The back of the knee.

popliteal (pop-lĭ-te´al, pop-lit´e-al) Relating to the back of the knee.

porcelain (pōr´sĕ-lin, pōrs´lin) A fine ceramic powder (composed of clay, quartz, and flux) mixed with water to form a paste; used in the manufacture of artificial teeth, inlays, jacket crowns, and dentures.

porcine (por´sīn) Relating to pigs.

pore (pōr) A minute opening on a surface, as of a sweat gland on the skin.

gustatory p. A minute surface opening of a taste bud.

slit p. The linear ultraminute space between the footlike processes (pedicles) of the podocytes that cover the outside of the capillary of the renal corpuscle.

sweat p. The surface opening of a sweat gland.

porencephaly (po-ren-sef´ă-le) Congenital malformation of the brain characterized by a cystic outpouching of the ventricular system.

porokeratosis (po-ro-ker-ă-to´sis) A rare skin disease marked by cornification around pores and progressive centrifugal atrophy.

porphin (por´fin) $C_{20}H_{14}N_4$; a fundamental substance that contains four pyrrole-like rings linked by four

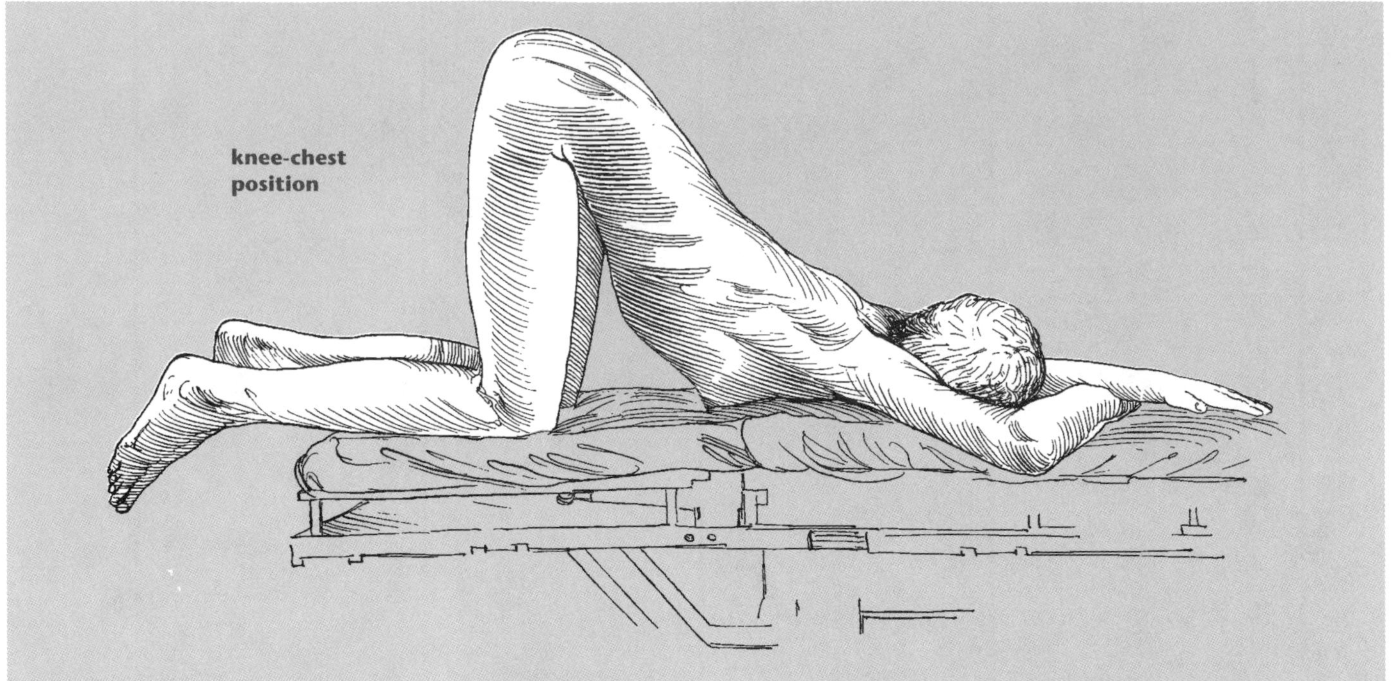

CH groups in a ring system; the unsubstituted tetrapyrrole nucleus of the porphyrins.

porphobilinogen (por-fo-bi-lin´o-jen) Organic compound present in large quantities in the urine of individuals with acute or congenital porphyria.

porphyria (por-fe´re-ă) Any disorder of blood pigment metabolism in which there is a marked increase in the formation, accumulation, and excretion of porphyrins.

congenital erythropoietic p. (CEP) Rare genetic disorder transmitted as an autosomal recessive trait in which excessive porphyrin is produced in the normoblasts of bone marrow; marked by excretion of excessive amounts of porphyrin in the urine, abnormal cutaneous sensitivity to sunlight, hemolytic anemia, and enlargement of the spleen. Also called Gunther's disease.

p. cutanea tarda, symptomatic p. (PCT) Hereditary disorder expressed only in the presence of liver dysfunction; marked by bullous skin rashes upon exposure to sunlight with scarring and pigmentation of the skin and by excessive porphyrin in the urine.

intermittent acute p. (IAP) Genetic disorder transmitted as an autosomal dominant trait; marked by neuropsychiatric symptoms, abdominal pain, and dark urine containing excessive amounts of aminolevulinic acid and porphobilinogen; attacks may be induced by certain drugs (e.g., barbiturates, oral contraceptives, alcohol).

varigate p. (VP) Genetic disorder transmitted as an autosomal dominant trait; marked by light sensitivity, skin fragility, and increased excretion of protoporphyrin and coproporphyrin in feces.

porphyrin (por´fĭ-rin) Any of various organic compounds present in protoplasm, forming the foundation structure for hemoglobin, chlorophyll, and other respiratory pigments; they are capable of combining with metals such as iron, magnesium, copper, etc. (metalloporphyrins), and with nitrogenous substances.

porphyrinuria, porphyruria (por-fĭ-rĭ-nu´re-ă, por-fir-u´re-ă) Presence of porphyrin in the urine in excess of the normal amount.

porta (por´tă) The point at which vessels, nerves, and excretory ducts enter and leave an organ.

p. hepatis The fissure on the under surface of the liver through which the portal vein, the hepatic artery, and the hepatic ducts pass.

portacaval (por-tă-ka´val) Relating to the portal vein and the inferior vena cava.

portal (por´tal) Relating to any entrance; specifically, to the porta hepatis.

portio (por´she-o), *pl.* **portio´nes** Latin for part.

portogram (por´to-gram) An x-ray film of the portal vein.

portography (por-tog´ră-fe) Splenic photography, a roentgenographic technique in which the splenic and portal veins and their tributaries are visualized after injection with a radiopaque material; widely used as a diagnostic and prognostic tool in cirrhosis.

porus (por´us), *pl.* **po´ri** Latin for pore; an orifice.

position (pŏ-zish´un) **1.** The placement of the body in a special way to facilitate specific diagnostic or therapeutic procedures. **2.** The particular arrangement of body parts. **3.** In obstetrics, the relationship of a designated point on the presenting part of the fetus to a designated point in the maternal pelvis. **4.** The place occupied. **5.** To place the body in a particular way.

anatomic p. Position in which the body is erect with the arms and hands turned forward.

centric p. The position of the mandible in its most retruded relation to the maxilla; the position in which an individual normally closes his jaws.

eccentric p. Any position of the mandible other than the centric position.

Fowler's p. An inclined position obtained by raising the head of the bed about 50 cm.

frog leg p. Lying on the back with both thighs acutely extended and knees flexed, as seen in infants with scurvy. Also called pithed frog position.

genupectoral p. See knee-chest position.

jackknife p. Position in which the individual is on his back with shoulders elevated and thighs at right angles to the abdomen, used to facilitate urethral instrumentation.

knee-chest p. A prone posture resting on the knees and chest with forearms supporting the head; assumed for rectal examinations. Also called genupectoral position.

lateral recumbent p., left See Sims' position.

lithotomy p. The individual lies on his back with buttocks at the end of the examining or operating table, the hips and knees being fully flexed with feet supported by slings or mechanical braces.

obstetric p. See Sims' position.

occlusal p. The relation of the mandible to the maxilla when the jaws are closed and the teeth are in contact.

orthopneic p. A sitting position with the individual's head and arms resting on an overbed table or on the arms of a chair.

pithed frog position See frog leg position.

prone p. Lying face down.

recovery p. Position in which an unconscious but breathing person is placed when no neck injury is suspected; the body is placed on its side; the arm under the body is flexed with the hand placed under the chin; the other arm is extended toward the back; and the upper, free leg is partially flexed.

recumbent p. A restful position in which the individual is on his back with legs slightly extended and flexed.

semiprone p. See Sims' position.

Sims' p. Position in which the individual lies on the left side with the right thigh acutely flexed; the left thigh slightly flexed; the left arm is behind the body. Used to facilitate certain procedures (e.g., vaginal and rectal examinations, curettement of uterus, intrauterine irrigation after labor, tamponade of vagina). Also called semiprone position; lateral recumbent position; obstetric position.

supine p. Lying on the back with the face up.

Trendelenburg's p. Position in which the individual lies on his back on an operating table, inclined at an angle of 45° with the head lower than the rest of the body; the legs and feet hang over the end of the table. Also called high pelvic position.

positive (poz´ĭ-tiv) **1.** Having a value opposite another (negative). **2.** Indicating the presence of a condition (especially one being tested) or the occurrence of a response. **3.** Having a value greater than zero.

positron (poz´ĭ-tron) A subatomic particle of the same mass as the electron and of equal but opposite (positive) charge.

postcardiotomy syndrome (post-kar-de-ot´ŏ-me sin´drōm) See postpericardiotomy syndrome.

postcholecystectomy syndrome (post-ko-le-sis-tek´tŏ-me sin´drōm) A group of symptoms suggestive of biliary disease, such as right upper quadrant pain, indigestion, and food intolerance, which persist after removal of the gallbladder (cholecystectomy).

postcibal (post-si´bal) After meals; after eating.

post cibum (post si´bum) (p.c.) Latin for after meals.

postclaviclar (post-klă-vik´u-lar) Situated in back of the clavicle (collarbone).

postclimacteric (post-kli-mak´ter-ik) Following the termination of the reproductive period.

postcoitus (pōst-ko´ĭ-tus) The time immediately following coitus (sexual intercourse).

postcommissurotomy syndrome (post-kom-ĭ-shūr-ot´ŏ-me sin´drōm) Fever, chest pains, and inflammation of the pericardium and pleura, occurring suddenly, within a few weeks, in patients who have undergone surgery of the heart valves.

postencephalitic (post-en-sef-ă-lit´ik) Occurring after encephalitis.

posterior (pos-ter´e-or) **1.** Located behind a structure. **2.** Relating to the back or dorsal side of the human body.

posterior inferior cerebellar artery

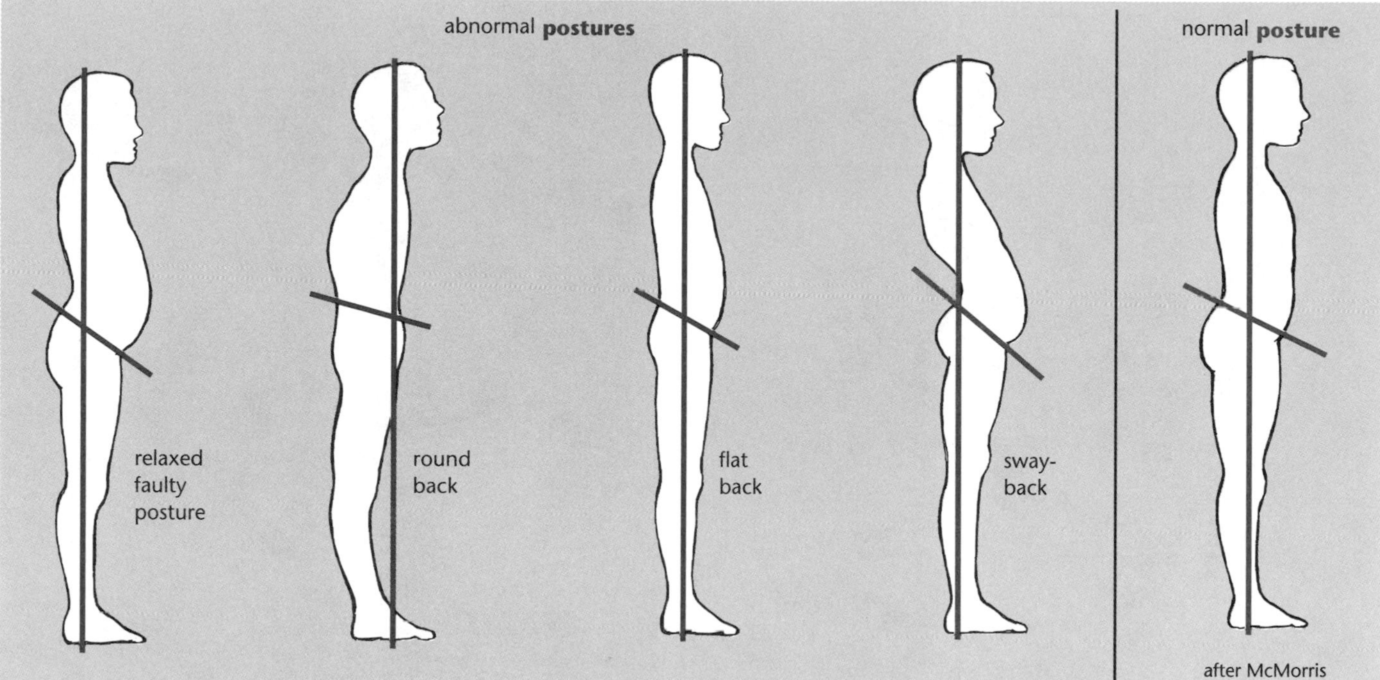

occlusion syndrome (pos-ter´e-or in-fer´e-or ser-ĕ-bel´ar ar´ter-e o-kloo´zhun sin´drōm) Syndrome occurring in occlusion of the posterior inferior cerebellar artery; symptoms include muscular weakness and loss of pain and temperature senses of the face, soft palate, pharynx, and larynx on the same side as the lesion, associated with loss of pain and temperature sensations of the extremities and trunk on the side opposite the lesion. Also called Wallenberg's syndrome.

posteroanterior (po-ster-o-an-tēr´e-or) From the back to the front.

posterolateral (po-ster-o-lat´er-al) Behind and to the outer side.

posteromedial (po-ster-o-me´de-al) Behind and to the inner side.

postganglionic (post-gang-gle-on´ik) Situated behind or distal to a ganglion.

postgastrectomy syndrome (post-gas-trek´tŏ-me sin´drōm) See dumping syndrome.

posthioplasty (pos´the-o-plas-te) Plastic surgery of the prepuce.

posthitis (pos-thi´tis) Inflammation of the prepuce. Also called acrobystitis.

postictal (post-ik´tal) Following a convulsion.

postmature (pōst-mă-tur´) See postterm.

postmenopausal (pōst-men-o-paw´zal) Relating to the period after the menopause.

postmortem (post-mor´tem) Pertaining to or occurring after death.

postmyocardial infarction syndrome (post-mi-o-kar´de-al in-fark´shun sin´drōm) Fever and pericarditis often accompanied by pleuritis occurring a week or more after a myocardial infarction. Also called Dressler's syndrome.

postnasal (pōst-na´zal) Behind the nasal cavity.

postnatal (pōst-na´tal) After birth.

postoperative (pōst-op´er-ă-tiv) Occurring after a surgical operation.

postpartum (pōst-par´tum) Occurring after childbirth.

postpericardiotomy (pōst-per-ĭ-kar-de-ot´ŏ-me) Occurring after surgery that involved cutting through the pericardium (two-layer membrane enveloping the heart).

postpericardiotomy syndrome (pōst-per-ĭ-kar-de-ot´ŏ-me sin´drōm) A complication of open-heart surgery occurring one or more weeks after the operation; appears to be a delayed autoimmune reaction characterized by inflammation of the membranes covering the heart and lungs, fever, chest pain, and raised erythrocyte sedimentation. Also called postcardiotomy syndrome.

postphlebitic syndrome (pōst-flĕ-bit´ik sin´drōm) Chronic swelling of leg, pain, and dermatitis secondary to stagnation of blood in the veins after phlebitis.

postpolio syndrome (pōst-po´le-o sin´drōm) Recurrence, 20 to 30 years later, of weakness and atrophy of muscle groups that had regained function after an attack of poliomyelitis (polio); thought to be due to overuse of motor nerves supplying the muscles rather than a recurrence of the disease. Also called postpolio atrophy; postpoliomyelitis neuromuscular atrophy.

postprandial (pōst-pran´de-al) After a meal.

postpubertal (pōst-pu´ber-tal) Of, or occurring during, the period immediately after puberty.

postsynaptic (pōst-sĭ-nap´tik) **1.** The time immediately following the transmission of an impulse from one neuron to another; occurring right after the crossing of a synapse. **2.** Situated distal to a synapse.

postterm (pōst´term) Denoting a fetus that remains in the uterus beyond 42 weeks of gestation.

posttraumatic (pōst-traw-mat´ik) Occurring after an injury or resulting from it.

posttraumatic syndrome (pōst-traw-mat´ik sin´drōm) A group of symptoms following head injury (with or without concussion) and persisting from weeks to a year or longer; they include: persistent headache, irritability, giddiness, fatigue, difficulty in concentration, disturbance of sleep, anxiety, and depression. Also called postconcussion syndrome; traumatic neurasthenia.

postulate (pos´tu-lit) An unproved assertion.

Koch's p.'s. To prove that a microorganism is the cause of a specific disease, it must be present in all cases of the disease, inoculations of its pure culture must produce the same disease in animals, and from these it must be obtained in pure cultures and propagated.

posture (pos´chur) Way of bearing one's body.

postvaccinal (pōst-vak´sĭ-nal) After vaccination.

pot (pot) A shortened version of the Mexican Indian word *potaguaya* meaning marijuana.

potable (po´tă-bl) Fit to drink; drinkable.

potassium (po-tas´e-um) A soft alkaline metallic element; symbol K (kalium), atomic number 19, atomic weight 39.10. It plays an important physiologic role in muscular contraction, conduction of nerve impulses, enzyme action, and cell membrane function. Normal potassium concentration of extracellular fluid is between 3.5 and 5 mEq/liter; normal potassium concentration of intracellular fluid is approximately 150 mEq/liter.

p. chloride A colorless crystalline solid or powder, KCl; used in the treatment of potassium deficiency.

p. iodide A crystalline powder, KI; soluble in water and used medicinally as an expectorant and antifungal agent.

p. nitrate KNO_3; a translucent, crystalline compound with diuretic properties. Also called niter; saltpeter.

p. permanganate A dark purple crystalline compound, $KMnO_4$, used as an antiseptic and deodorizing agent. Also called purple salt.

potassium-42 (^{42}K) An artificial isotope used as a tracer in studies of potassium distribution in body fluid compartments.

potency (po´ten-se) **1.** The quality of being potent; strength. **2.** The comparative expression of drug activity relating to the dose required to produce a specific effect of given intensity as compared to a standard of reference. COMPARE: selectivity. **3.** Inherent ability for growth and development.

sexual p. Ability to achieve and maintain adequate penile erection during sexual intercourse.

potent (pō´nt) **1.** Powerful. **2.** Capable of producing a particular physiologic or chemical effect of strong intensity. **3.** Possessing sexual potency.

potentia (po-ten´she-ă) Latin for potency.

potential (po-ten´shal) **1.** Existing in a state with a strong possibility for changing or developing. **2.** The force necessary to drive a unit positive charge from one point in an electrical field to another; the electromotive force that drives a current from one point to another.

action p. The electric current developed in a nerve, muscle, or other excitable tissue during its activity.

dark p. of the eye See resting potential of the eye.

demarcation p. The voltage difference between intact nerve or muscle fibers and the injured ends of the same fibers. Also called injury potential.

evoked p. See evoked response, under response.

excitatory postsynaptic p. (EPSP) The change in electrical potential occurring in the membrane of a postsynaptic nerve cell when an impulse that has an excitatory influence arrives at the synapse.

inhibitory postsynaptic p. (IPSP) The change in electrical potential occurring in the membrane of a postsynaptic nerve cell when an impulse that has an inhibitory influence arrives at the synapse.

injury p. See demarcation potential.

membrane p. The voltage difference between the two sides of a cell membrane; in the resting stage, the outside is positive and the inside negative.

oxidation-reduction p. (E_0^+, E^0) The relative potential, in volts, exerted by an inert (nonreacting) metallic electrode in a solution, as measured against that exerted by a normal hydrogen electrode at absolute temperature; the potential difference between an inert electrode and a reversible oxidation-

P

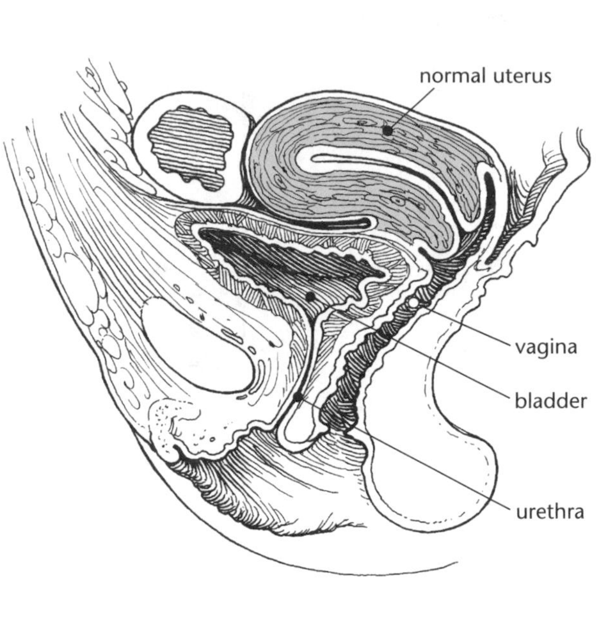

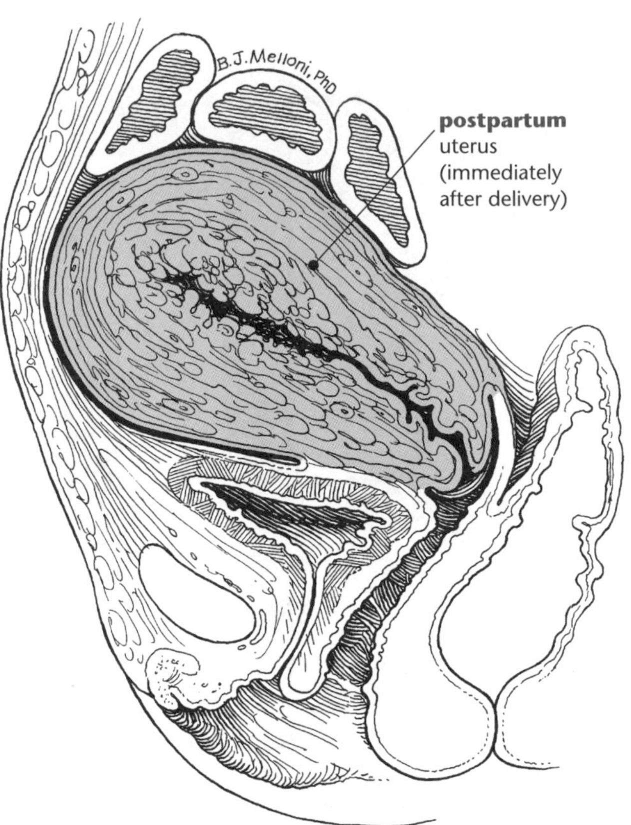

record of the extracellular **action potential** of a nerve fiber
(each number of the wave curve represents the membrane potential at the time the impulse passes by the registering electrode)

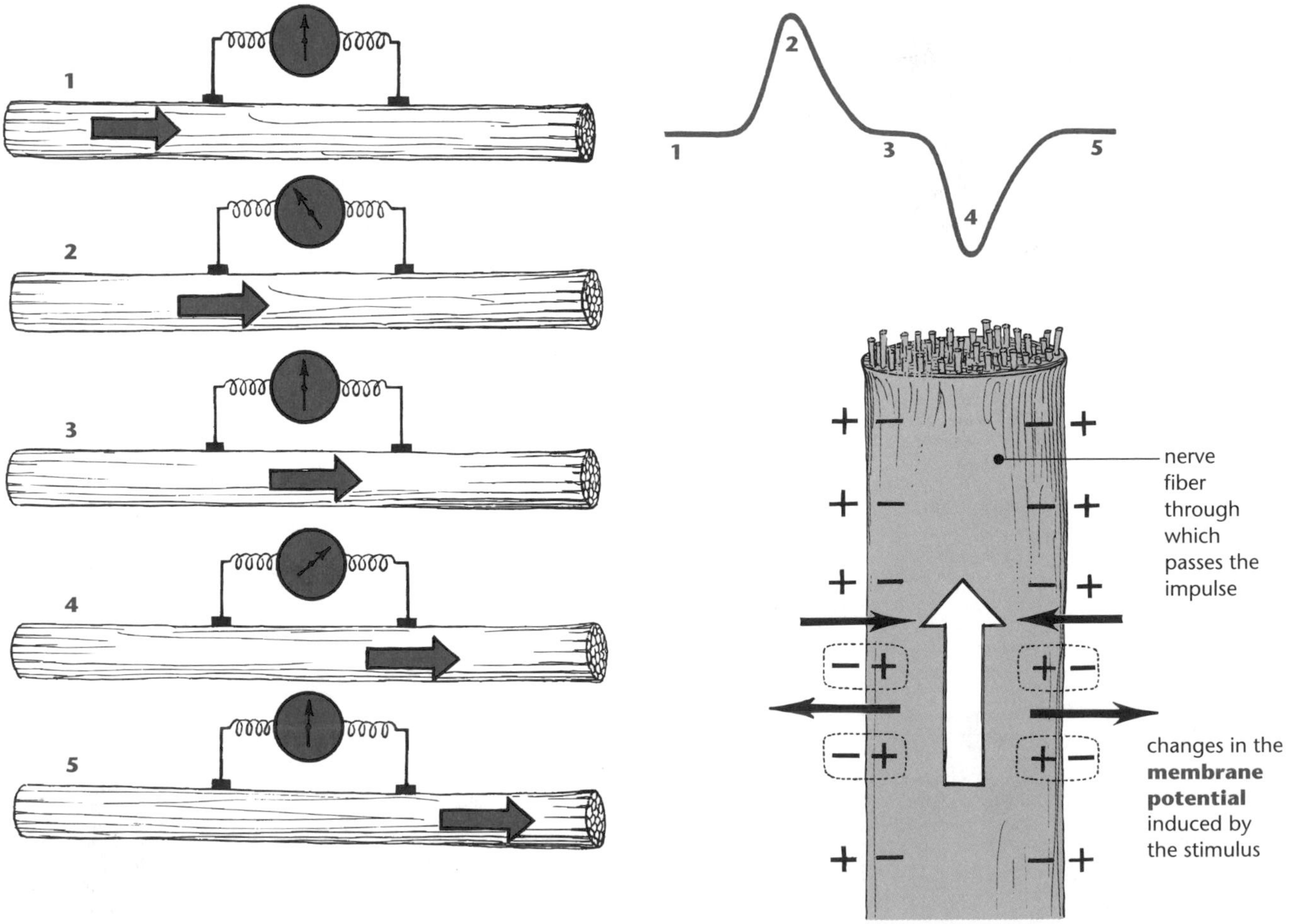

1

2

3

4

5

1 2 3 4 5

nerve fiber through which passes the impulse

changes in the **membrane potential** induced by the stimulus

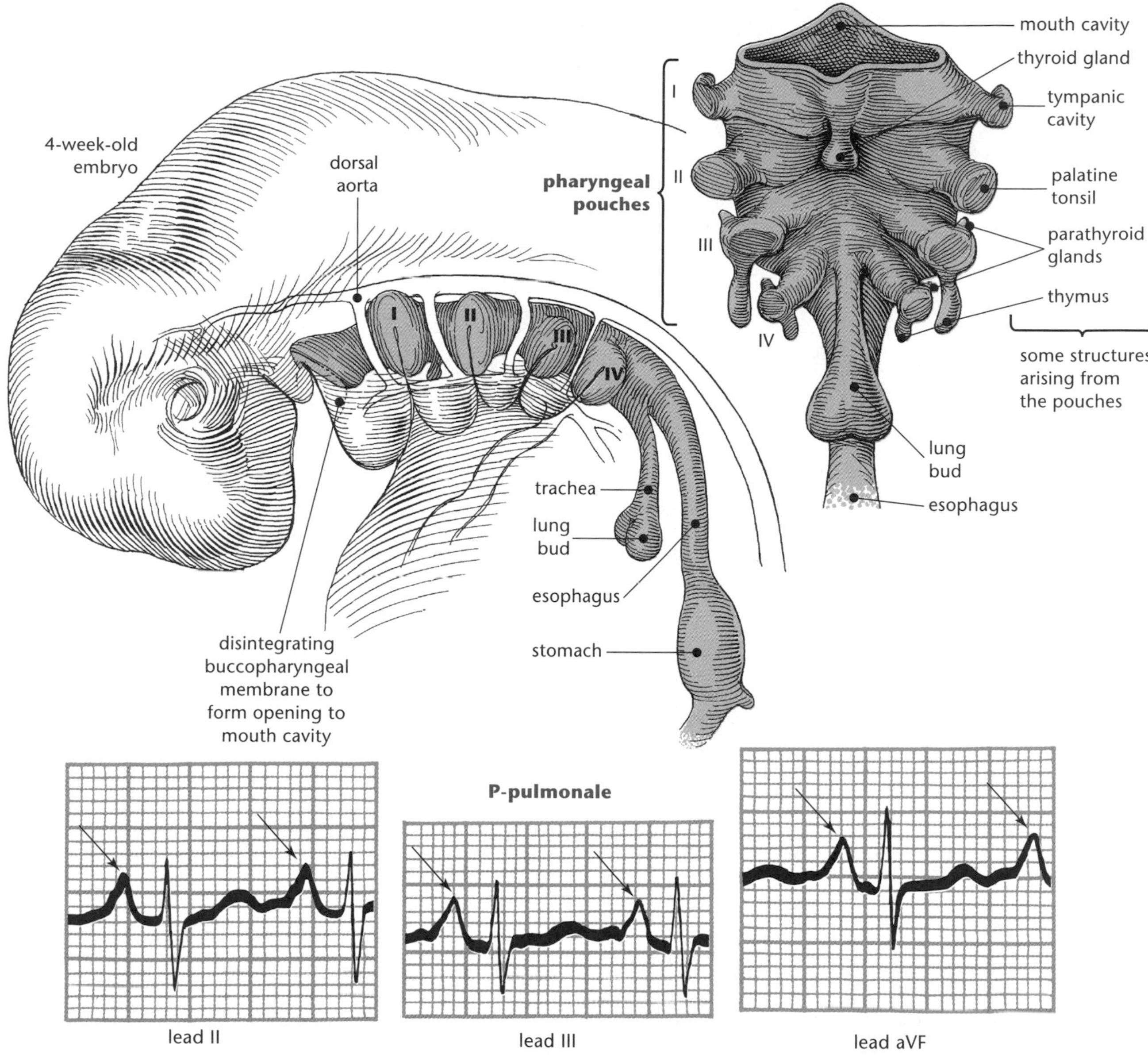

reduction system in which it is submerged. Also called redox potential.

redox p. See oxidation-reduction potential.

resting p. of the eye The direct current potential difference between the anterior pole of the eye (cornea) and the posterior one (retina); usually expressed in millivolts. Also called dark potential of the eye.

visual evoked p. The voltage fluctuations, recorded with an electroencephalograph from the scalp overlying the back of the head, resulting from retinal stimulation by a flashing light.

potentiation (po-ten-she-a´shun) The increase in the power of an activity, such as in the force of the contraction of a muscle; the term is frequently used improperly in reference to drug interaction as a synonym of synergism.

potentiometer (po-ten-she-om´ĕ-ter) Instrument for measuring electromotive forces precisely.

potion (po´shun) A large liquid dose, especially of medicine.

Pott's disease (pots dĭ-zēz´) See tuberculous spondylitis, under spondylitis.

pouch (pouch) A sac or pocket-like space.

craniobuccal p. See Rathke's pouch.

Douglas' p. See rectouterine pouch.

Hartmann's p. A dilatation at the neck of the gallbladder.

Heidenhain p. A small pouch made for the experimental study of gastric secretions; an isolated part of the stomach, with the nervous supply interrupted, is opened to the outside through the abdominal wall for drainage.

neurobuccal p. See Rathke's pouch.

Pavlov p. A small pouch made for the study of gastric secretions; an isolated part of the stomach, with the nervous supply left intact, is opened to the outside through an opening in the abdominal wall for drainage.

pharyngeal p.'s Paired lateral pouches of the embryonic pharynx; each pouch is in close relationship to an aortic arch and is situated opposite a branchial cleft.

Rathke's p. In embryology, the outpocketing of the stomodeum (embryonic mouth) occurring when the embryo is about three weeks old and subsequently forming the anterior (glandular) lobe of the hypophysis. Also called craniobuccal pouch; neurobuccal pouch.

rectouterine p. The pouch between the uterus and the rectum. Also called Douglas' pouch.

rectovesical p. The pouch between the rectum and the bladder in the male.

uterovesical p. The pouch between the bladder and the uterus.

vaginal p. See female condom, under condom.

pouchitis (pouch-i´tis) Acute inflammation of the intestinal pouch surgically created for collection of intestinal contents after removal of the colon.

poudrage (poo-drahzh´) The application of powder between two surfaces to promote their fusion (e.g., between the visceral and parietal layers of the pericardium or pleura).

poultice (pōl´tis) A hot, moist, soft mass of bread meal, linseed, or any other cohesive substance, applied to the skin between two pieces of muslin to soothe, relax, or stimulate an aching or inflamed part of the body.

pound (pound) A unit of weight equal to 16 ounces (avoirdupois weight) or 12 ounces (apothecaries' weight).

povidone (po´vĭ-dōn) A synthetic polymer used as a dispersing and suspending medium. Formerly called polyvinylpyrrolidone (PVP).

povidone-iodine (po´vĭ-dōn-i´o-dīn) Topical antiseptic formed by reacting povidone with iodine.

powder (pou´der) **1.** In pharmaceutics, a mixture of dry, fine particles. **2.** A single dose of such a powder, enclosed in paper.

Seidlitz p.'s A mild laxative composed of sodium bicarbonate, tartaric acid, and potassium sodium tartrate.

talcum p. A fine, soft toilet powder of perfumed talc.

power (pou´er) In optics, the refractive vergence of a lens.

back vertex p. The vergence power of a lens as measured from surface toward eye; standard for measurement of ophthalmic lenses.

focal p. See vergence power.

refractive p. The vergence power of a refracting optical system.

resolving p. A measure of the ability of a lens to image closely spaced objects so that they are recognized as separate objects; calculated by dividing the wavelength of the light used by twice the

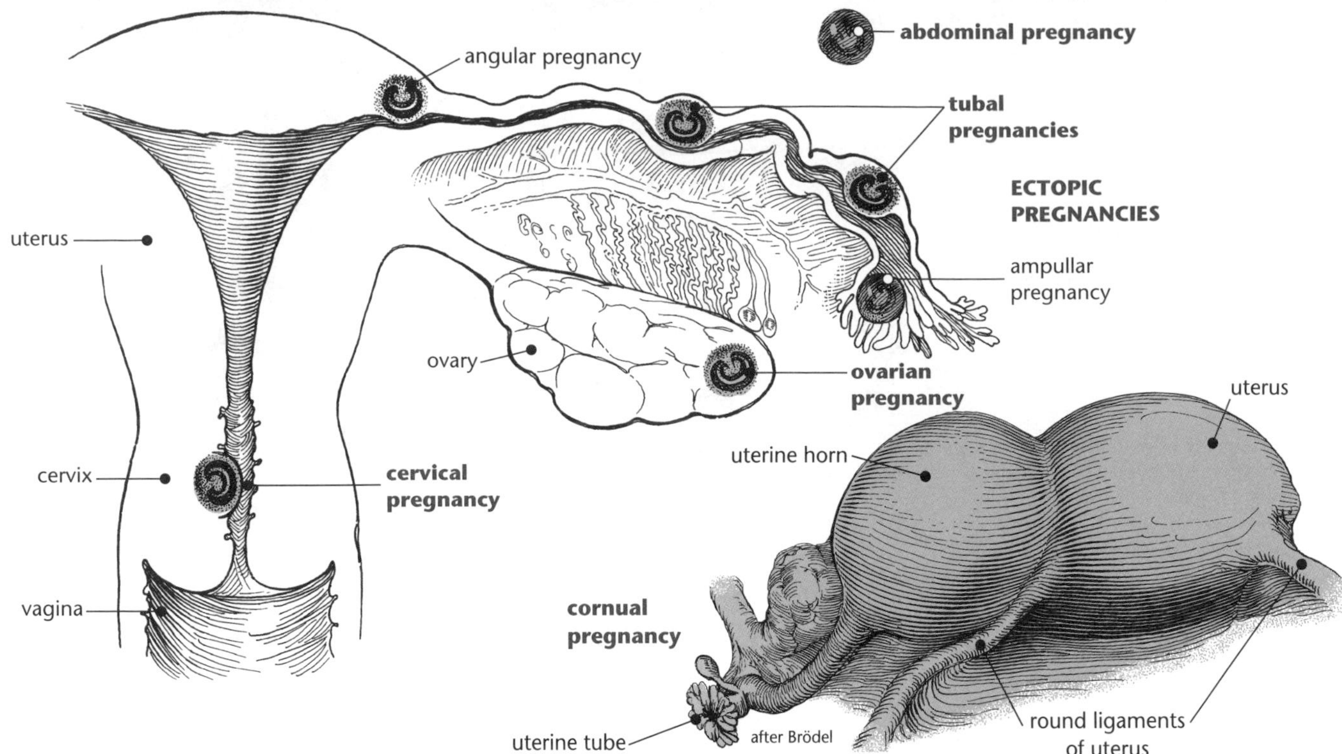

numerical aperture of the objective.

vergence p. The capability of an optical system to change the vergence of a cylinder of rays. Also called focal power.

pox (poks) **1.** Any disease characterized by purulent eruptions on the skin. **2.** Obsolete term for syphilis.

Poxviridae (poks-vir´ĭ-de) Family of large ovoid or brick-shaped viruses (300 to 450 nm × 170 to 260 nm) that contain a single molecule of double-stranded DNA and, unlike other DNA-containing viruses, multiply in cytoplasm; classified into two subfamilies of which only one (Chordopoxirinae) contains members infectious to humans; includes viruses causing smallpox, vaccinia, and orf.

poxvirus (poks-vi´rus) Any virus of the family Poxviridae.

PPO See preferred provider organization.

P-pulmonale (pē-pul-mo-nal´e) In electrocardiography, the P-wave pattern characteristic of cor pulmonale; a tall peaked P wave, usually seen in leads II, III, and AVF.

P

practice (prak´tis) **1.** The exercise of a profession or occupation. **2.** To engage in, especially as a profession. **3.** Collective term for the patients of a physician.

practitioner (prak-tish´un-er) One who exercises a profession.

general p. (GP) A physician who, after receiving an MD or DO degree, has trained at a hospital for at least one year but has not specialized in any field and usually provides primary care for the whole family. COMPARE: family physician, under physician.

pragmatagnosia (prag-mat-ag-no´ze-ă) Loss of the ability to recognize objects formerly known to the person.

praseodymium (pra-ze-o-dim´e-um) A soft, silvery, rare-earth element; symbol Pr, atomic number 59, atomic weight 140.907.

praxiology (prak-se-ol´ŏ-je) The study of behavior or conduct.

preagonal, preagonic (pre-ag´o-nal, pre-ag´o-nik) Just before death.

prealbumin (pre-al-bu´min) A protein constituent of plasma, so named because its mobility is greater than that of albumin (at the alkaline pH values used for electrophoresis).

thyroxine-binding p. One of the three carrier proteins of thyroxine in plasma.

preanal (pre-a´nal) In front of the anus.

preanesthetic (pre-an-es-thet´ik) Before anesthesia, a medication administered to facilitate the subsequent induction of general anesthesia.

preauricular (pre-aw-rik´u-lar) Situated in front of the auricle of the ear.

precancerous (pre-kan´ser-us) Denoting a lesion that precedes, develops into, or has a high risk of becoming a cancer. Also called premalignant.

precipitant (pre-sip´ĭ-tant) Anything that causes the chemical separation of a solid from a solution.

precipitate (pre-sip´ĭ-tāt) **1.** To cause a substance in solution to separate and form a solid deposit. **2.** (ppt) The solid deposit thus formed. **3.** Occurring abnormally fast (e.g., a precipitate labor).

precipitation (pre-sip-ĭ-ta´shun) **1.** The act of separating a solid held in suspension or solution. **2.** The clumping of protein in serum caused by the action of a specific precipitin.

precipitin (pre-sip´ĭ-tin) An antibody that reacts specifically with a soluble antigen to cause a precipitate.

precision (pre-sizh´un) The state of being sharply defined.

preclinical (pre-klin´ĭ-kal) **1.** Occurring before the onset of disease; referring to the stage of a disorder before clinical symptoms can be recognized and diagnosed. **2.** Occurring before clinical work; referring to medical training that usually takes place during the first two years.

precocious (pre-ko´shus) Characterized by unusually early physical or mental maturity.

precocity (pre-kos´ĭ-te) Unusually early development, physical, or mental.

sexual p. See precocious puberty, under puberty.

precognition (pre-kog-nish´un) Extrasensory perception of an event not yet experienced.

preconscious (pre-kon´shus) In psychoanalysis, thoughts and ideas that can be recalled by conscious effort.

preconvulsive (pre-kon-vul´siv) Preceding a convulsion.

precordial (pre-kor´de-al) Relating to the area of the chest over the heart.

precordium (pre-kor´de-um) The area of the chest wall that corresponds to the location of the heart. Also called antecardium.

precuneus (pre-ku´ne-us) A lobule on the medial surface of each cerebral hemisphere located between the posterior portion of the occipital lobe (cuneus) and paracentral lobule.

precursor (pre´kur-sor) Anything in the course of a process that is the forerunner or precedes a later stage, as a premalignant lesion, or as a physiologically inactive substance that is converted to an active substance such as a hormone or enzyme.

prediabetes An early stage in the course of diabetes before recognizable impairment of carbohydrate metabolism.

prediastole (pre-di-as´tŏ-le) The interval in the cardiac rhythm cycle just preceding the diastole. Also called late systole.

predigestion (pre-di-jes´chun) Artificial initiation of the digestive process in protein and starch before they are used therapeutically as food.

predispose (pre-dis-pōz´) To render susceptible or liable.

predisposition (pre-dis-po-zish´un) The state of being predisposed or susceptible to a disease; a special tendency or inclination toward a disease.

prednisolone (pred-nis´o-lōn) A synthetic glucocorticoid; white bitter crystals, insoluble in water; used as a cortisone substitute.

prednisone (pred´nĭ-sōn) A synthetic glucocorticoid with anti-inflammatory properties; used as a cortisone substitute, as it causes less water retention.

predormitum, predormition (pre-dor´mĭ-tum, pre-dor´mish-un) The state of waning consciousness that precedes sound sleep.

preeclampsia (pre-e-klam´se-ă) Disorder of the last trimester of pregnancy marked by hypertension, edema, and proteinuria; most common in first pregnancies. Formerly called toxemia of pregnancy.

preemy, preemie (pre´me) Informal term for premature infant.

preexcitation (pre-ek-si-ta´shun) Premature activation of the ventricular myocardium by a supraventricular impulse that bypasses the normal A-V conduction pathway; an intrinsic part of the Wolff-Parkinson-White syndrome.

preexcitation syndrome (pre-ek-si-ta´shun sin´drōm) See Wolff-Parkinson-White syndrome.

preferred provider organization (pre-fur´ed pro-vīd´er or-ga-nĭ-zā´shun) (PPO) A health plan that offers enrollees access to a panel of physicians and hospitals that have contracted with the carrier and accepted the fee schedule and conditions imposed by the carrier.

prefrontal (pre-fron´tal) Located in the anterior part of the frontal lobe or region of the brain.

preganglionic (pre-gang-gle-on´ik) Situated before or proximal to a ganglion.

pregnancy (preg´nan-se) Condition of the female from conception to delivery of the fetus or embryo. A full-term duration of human pregnancy is 40 weeks. Also called gestation.

abdominal p. Implantation of a fertilized ovum on a surface within the abdominal cavity resulting from an early rupture or expulsion of a tubal pregnancy.

cervical p. Rare ectopic pregnancy in which the fertilized ovum implants in the lining of the cervical canal.

cornual p. Rare ectopic pregnancy occurring in women with a double uterus; the fertilized ovum implants in a (usually rudimentary) uterine horn.

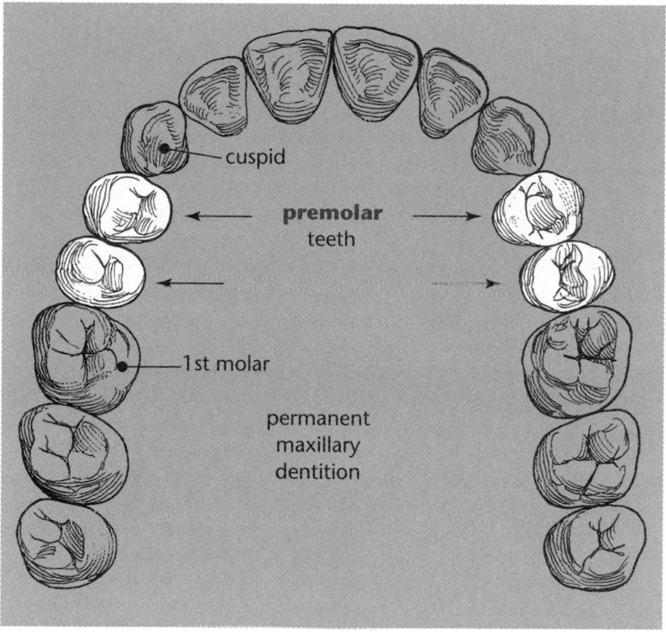

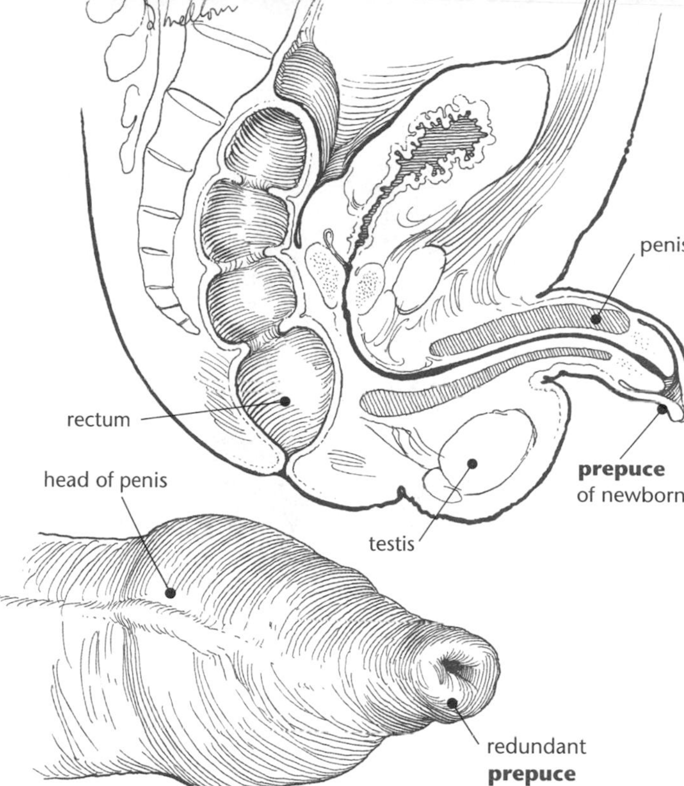

ectopic p. Implantation of the fertilized ovum outside of the uterine cavity (e.g., abdominal cavity, cervix, a uterine tube, an ovary). Also called eccyesis; extrauterine pregnancy; metacyesis. Popularly, simply called ectopic.
extrauterine p. See ectopic pregnancy.
fallopian p. See tubal pregnancy.
false p. See pseudocyesis.
high risk p. Pregnancy in which the mother, fetus, or newborn is or will be at increased risk of having a disease or of dying before or after delivery due to a variety of contributing factors (e.g., poor nutrition, absence of prenatal care, genetic disorders, abruptio placentae, preeclampsia-eclampsia).
interstitial p. See tubo-uterine pregnancy.
intramural p. See tubo-uterine pregnancy.
molar p. See hydatidiform mole, under mole.
multiple p. The simultaneous presence of two or more developing fetuses.
ovarian p. A rare form of ectopic pregnancy in which the fertilized ovum implants on an ovary. Also called oocyesis.
phantom p. See pseudocyesis.
postterm p. See prolonged pregnancy.
prolonged p. Pregnancy that has reached 42 weeks of gestation from the first day of the last menstrual period. Also called postterm pregnancy.
spurious p. See pseudocyesis.
tubal p. Ectopic pregnancy that occurs in a uterine tube. Also called fallopian pregnancy; salpingocyesis.
tubo-uterine p. An uncommon type of ectopic pregnancy in which the fertilized ovum implants in the interstitial portion of the uterine tube (i.e., the portion located within the uterine wall). Also called interstitial pregnancy; intramural pregnancy.

pregnane (preg´nān) A saturated steroid hydrocarbon, derivative of cholane; a precursor of progesterone and several adrenocortical hormones.

pregnanediol (preg-nān-di´ol) $C_{21}H_{36}O_2$; the main metabolic end product of progesterone; its concentration in the urine is an indicator of the status of corpus luteum function.

pregnanetriol (preg-nān-tri´ol) A precursor in the biosynthesis of the hormone hydrocortisone.

pregnanolone (preg-na´no-lon) A pregnane found in the urine of pregnant women; it has sedative, anesthetic, and hypnotic properties.

pregnant (preg´nant) Carrying a developing offspring within the body. Also called gravid.

pregnene (preg´nēn) An unsaturated steroid derivative of pregnane.

prehensile (pre-hen´sil) Adapted for grasping.

prehormone (pre-hor´mōn) An inactive glandular secretion capable of being converted into an active hormone.

preictal (pre-ik´tal) Before a convulsion or stroke.

preinfarction syndrome (pre-in-fark´shun sin´drōm) The sudden onset or worsening of angina pectoris prior to myocardial infarction.

preleukemia (pre-lu-ke´me-ă) A defect of cellular differentiation and maturation that precedes the onset of diagnosable acute leukemia as a primary maturational disturbance.

preload (pre´lod) The stretch imposed upon a muscle before its contraction; in terms of the left ventricle of the heart, it refers to the degree of cardiac return or filling.

preluxation (pre-luk-sa´shun) Forward dislocation.

premalignant (pre-mă-lig´nant) See precancerous.

premature (pre-mă-chōōr´) Occurring before the expected, usual, or normal time.

prematurity (pre-mă chōōr´ĭ-te) The state of being premature.

premed (prē´med) Popular term for a college student preparing to apply to medical school.

premedication (pre-med-ĭ-ka´shun) A drug or drugs administered before a general anesthetic to allay apprehension and produce sedation.

premelanosome (pre-mel´ă-no-sōm) The precursor of a melanin-containing cell (melanosome).

premenarchal (pre-mĕ-nar´kal) Relating to premenarche.

premenarche (pre-mĕ-nar´ke) The period before menstruation is established (i.e., before the menarche).

premenopause (pre-men´o-pawz) The transitional period of marked menstrual irregularity occurring prior to the permanent cessation of ovarian function and menstruation; represents the irregular maturation of ovarian follicles, with or without ovulation.

premenstrual (pre-men´stroo-al) Denoting the time of the month prior to the menstrual flow.

premenstrual syndrome (pre-men´stroo-al sin´drōm) (PMS) The occurrence of all or some of the following symptoms during the week before onset of the menstrual flow: lumbar and low abdominal pain, nervous irritability, headache, tenderness of the breasts, and pelvic congestion.

premolar (pre-mo´lar) A bicuspid tooth.

premunition (pre-mu-nish´un) Immunity established against a particular microorganism by infection (in a chronic form) with another related organism.

prenaris (pre-na´ris), *pl.* **prena´res** Nostril.

prenatal (pre-na´tal) Prior to birth. Also called antenatal.

preoperative (pre-op´er-ă-tiv) Before an operation.

prepallium (pre-pal´e-um) The cerebral cortex in front of the central sulcus (fissure of Rolando).

preparation (prep-ă-ra´shun) **1.** Readiness. **2.** Something that has been made ready for use (e.g., a pharmaceutical agent). **3.** The reduction of a natural tooth prior to enserting a prosthesis (e.g., a crown).
cavity p. The removal of caries from a tooth and the establishment of a cavity that is able to receive and retain a restoration.
depot p. A drug whose physical state is altered so that it can be absorbed over an extended period of time (e.g., special microcrystalline suspensions of penicillin).
spermicidal p. Any of various vaginal creams, gels, suppositories, and foams that kill sperm; it also acts as a mechanical barrier to the entry of sperm into the cervical canal.

preprandial (pre-pran´de-al) Before a meal.

prepatellar (pre-pă-tel´ă) In front of the kneecap (patella).

prepuberty (pre-pu´ber-te) The phase immediately preceding puberty.

prepuce (pre´pūs) The loose fold of skin that partly or completely covers the glans penis; the tissue removed by circumcision. Also called foreskin.
p. of clitoris A fold of tissue overlying the clitoris; the fused upper divisions of the opposing labia minora.

preputiotomy (pre-pu-she-ot´ŏ-me) Surgical incision of the prepuce (foreskin) of the penis, usually to relieve tightness (phimosis).

prepyloric (pre-pi-lor´ik) Located in the stomach, adjacent to the pylorus.

prerenal (pre-re´nal) In front of a kidney.

presbycusis (pres-bĕ-ku´sis) Progressive loss of hearing occurring in old age.

presbyopia (pres-be-o´pe-ă) (Pr) Diminution of accommodation power of the eye lens due to advancing age. Commonly called old sight.

prescribe (pre-skrīb´) To recommend a remedy for use in the treatment of a disorder.

prescribed occupation (pre-skrīb´d ok-u-pā´shun) A therapeutic activity recommended by a physician for a particular patient.

prescription (pre-skrip´shun) A written instruction by a licensed health science practitioner for the preparation and administration of any remedy (e.g., medication, corrective lenses).
shotgun p. A drug prescription containing many ingredients, given with the hope that one or more of them may be effective.

presenility (pre-sĕ-nil´ĭ-te) Premature old age.

present (pre-zent´) To appear first; said of the part of the fetus that is felt by the examining finger.

presentation (pre-zen-ta´shun) The position of the fetus in the uterus in relation to the birth canal during labor.
anterior parietal p. See anterior asynclitism,

P

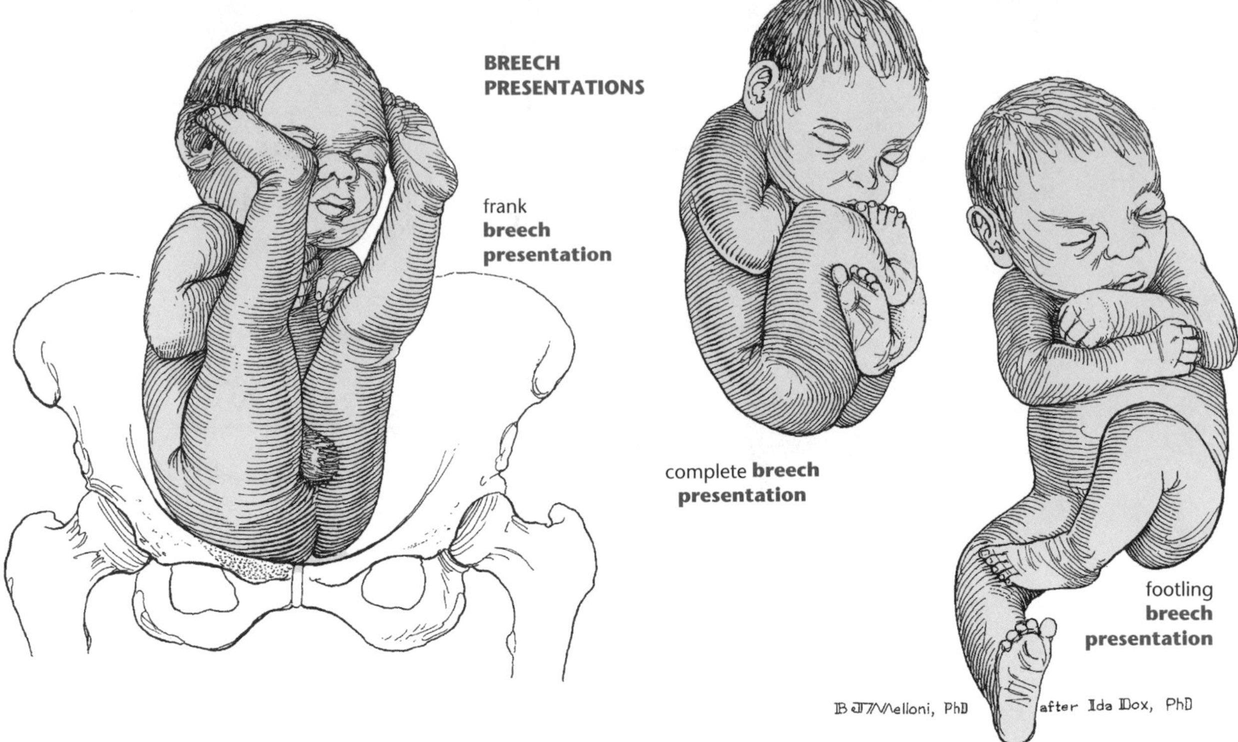

under asynclitism.

breech p. Presentation of the fetal pelvis; called *frank breech p.* when the legs of the fetus extend fully over the anterior surface of its body; *complete breech p.* when both thighs and legs are flexed; *footling breech p.* when one or both legs are extended below the level of the fetal buttocks.

cephalic p. Presentation in which the head is the presenting part; called *bregma p., vertex p.* when the occipital portion of the head is the presenting part, the head is flexed and the chin and thorax in contact; *sinciput p.* when the large fontanel is the presenting part; *brow p.* when the brow is the presenting part; *face p.* when the face is the presenting part, the head is sharply extended with the occipital portion in contact with the fetal back. Also called head presentation.

head p. See cephalic presentation.

placental p. See placenta previa, under placenta.

posterior parietal p. See posterior asynclitism, under asynclitism.

shoulder p. Presentation in which the long axis of the fetus lies transversely with the maternal long axis and a shoulder is the presenting part.

preservative (pre-zer′vă-tiv) **1.** A substance added to food products, such as fatty acids, for inhibiting the growth of food-spoiling bacteria. **2.** Capable of preserving.

presomite (pre-so′mīt) In embryology, before the appearance of somites.

pressor (pres′or) Causing constriction of blood vessels and a rise in blood pressure; said of certain substances and nerve fibers.

pressoreceptor (pres-o-re-sep′tor) See baroreceptor.

pressure (presh′ur) A force exerted or acting against resistance.

atmospheric p. The pressure exerted by the atmosphere; approximately 15 pounds per square inch at sea level, capable of supporting a column of mercury 760 millimeters high.

back p. Pressure exerted in the circulatory system resulting from obstruction to flow.

blood p. The pressure of the circulating blood on the walls of the arteries, primarily maintained by the contraction of the left ventricle, the resistance of the arterioles and capillaries, the elasticity of the arterial walls, and the volume and viscosity of the blood; the maximum or systolic blood pressure occurs at the moment of systole of the left ventricle of the heart; the minimum or diastolic blood pressure occurs during diastole of the ventricle; the upper limits of normal in adults are generally set at 140/90 mmHg.

central venous p. (CVP) Pressure of blood in the superior or inferior vena cava.

cerebrospinal p. Tension of the cerebrospinal fluid, normally 100 to150 mm of water (measured by lumbar puncture).

continuous positive airway p. (CPAP) Respiratory therapy in which pressure within the lung airways is mechanically maintained above atmospheric pressure throughout the respiratory cycle to prevent collapse of the airways.

critical p. The pressure required to condense or liquefy a gas at the critical temperature.

diastolic p. Arterial pressure during diastole; see blood pressure.

effective osmotic p. The portion of the total osmotic pressure of a solution that regulates the tendency of its solvent to pass through a boundary, such as a semipermeable membrane.

hydrostatic p. In a closed fluid system at rest, the pressure exerted at any level by the weight of the fluid above it.

hyperbaric p. Pressure higher than normal atmospheric pressure; used in therapy for shock, carbon dioxide poisoning, clostridial infections, and for some operations.

intracranial p. (ICP) Pressure within the skull.

intraocular p. (IOP) Pressure of the fluid within the eye, measured by a tonometer, usually in millimeters of mercury (mmHg). Also called intraocular tension; ocular tension.

negative p. A pressure lower than that of ambient atmosphere.

occlusal p. Any force exerted upon the occlusal surfaces of teeth.

oncotic p. Osmotic pressure exerted by colloids in solution.

osmotic p. Pressure or stress exerted by dissolved substances on a semipermeable membrane that separates a solution from the pure solvent.

partial p. The portion of the total pressure exerted by each component of a gas mixture, expressed in millimeters of mercury (mmHg).

positive end-expiratory p. (PEEP) Technique used in respiratory therapy to increase the amount of gases remaining in the lungs after expiration by maintaining pressure within the airways.

pulmonary p. Pressure in the pulmonary artery.

pulmonary capillary wedge p. Pressure obtained by wedging the tip of a cathether in a small pulmonary artery; blocking blood flow provides an indirect measure of the pressure in the left atrium of the heart.

pulse p. The difference between the systolic (maximum) and diastolic (minimum) blood pressures within an artery during the cardiac cycle; it normally varies between 30 and 50 mmHg.

systolic p. Arterial pressure during systole; see blood pressure.

vapor p. The pressure exerted by the molecules of a vapor in equilibrium with its solid or liquid phase.

presynaptic (pre-sĭ-nap′tik) **1.** Existing or taking place before a synapse is crossed. **2.** Situated proximal to a synapse.

presystole (pre-sis′to-le) The interval immediately preceding the systole.

pretibial (pre-tib′e-al) Pertaining to the front of the leg, especially that portion in front of the tibia.

prevalence (prev′ă-lens) The number of people with a specific condition in a given population.

preventive (pre-ven′tiv) Acting to ward off or hinder the occurrence of something such as a disease.

prevertebral (pre-ver′te-bral) In front of a vertebra or of the vertebral column.

prevesical (pre-ves′ ĭ-kal) In front of the bladder.

Prevotella melaninogenica A species of nonmotile, gram-negative bacteria (genus *Prevotella*) found in the oral cavity; feces; and infections of the intestinal, respiratory and genitourinary tracts. Implicated in periodontal disease. Also called *Bacteroides melaninogenicus.*

priapism (prī′ă-piz-m) A continuous and pathologic erection of the penis without sexual desire; usually associated with certain diseases, especially sickle cell disease.

primacy (prī′mă-sē) The state of being primary.

primaquine phosphate (prim′ă-kwin fos′fāt) Bitter, orange crystals, soluble in water; used in the treatment of malaria.

primary (prī′mer-e) **1.** Occurring first; not secondary. **2.** First in a sequence or importance. **3.** The simplest or most primitive form.

primate (prī′māt) A member of the order Primates.

Primates (pri-ma′tēz) The highest order of mammals, including man and such animals as apes, monkeys, and lemurs.

primigravida (pri-mĭ-grav′ ĭ-dă) A woman who has been pregnant only once. Also called gravida I.

primipara (pri-mip′ă-ră) A woman who has completed one pregnancy to the stage of viability, regardless of whether it was a single or multiple birth, or whether the fetus was live or stillborn. Also called para I.

primiparous (pri-mip′ă-rus) Denoting a primipara.

primitive (prim′ ĭ-tiv) Primary; embryonic.

primordial (pri-mor′de-al) **1.** Relating to the embryonic group of cells that develops into an organ or structure. **2.** Formed during the early stage of development.

primordium (pri-mor′de-um) The earliest cells forming an organ or structure in the embryo; usually denoting a theoretical stage later than anlage.

principle (prin′sĭ-pl) **1.** A fundamental concept. **2.**

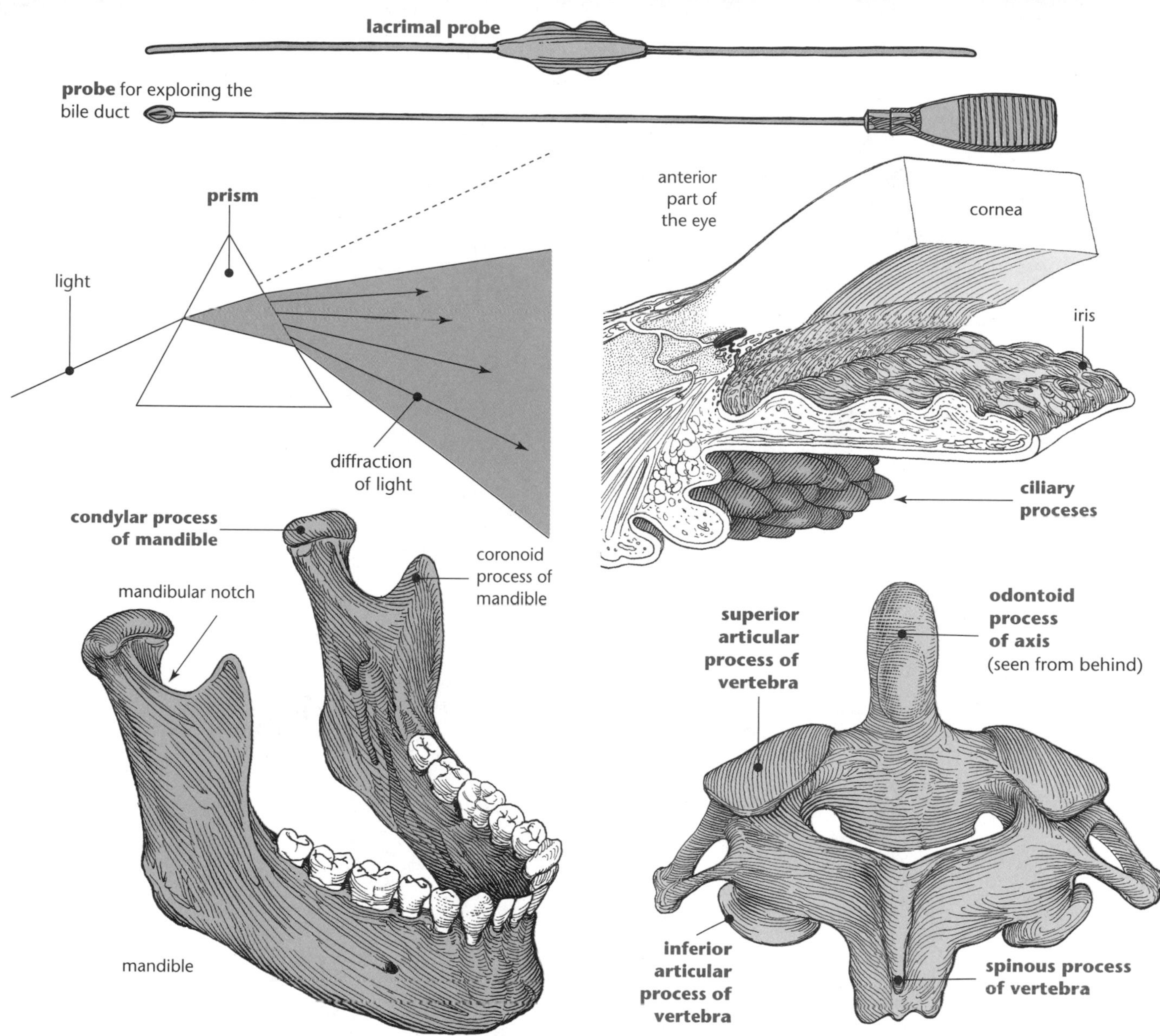

A drug ingredient that confers the chief pharmaceutical properties to the drug.

active p. The constituent of a drug to which its physiologic effect is due.

antianemic p. Substance (chiefly found in liver) that stimulates remission of symptoms in pernicious anemia.

Fick p. Principle used in measurement of cardiac output and blood flow to some organs.

hematinic p. Vitamin B_{12}.

pain-pleasure p. In psychoanalytic theory, the concept that humans instinctively avoid pain and discomfort and seek gratification and pleasure. Also called pleasure principle.

pleasure p. See pain-pleasure principle.

reality p. In psychoanalytic theory, the concept that the pleasure principle is normally modified in personality development by the demands of the external world (e.g., postponement of gratification to a more appropriate time).

Starling p. The principle that the exchange of fluids across capillary membranes is governed by the net difference between the hydrostatic and osmotic pressures.

prion (pri´on) A small (MW 27000–30000) proteinaceous infectious particle, resistant to inactivation by procedures that modify nucleic acids (DNA and RNA); contains no DNA or RNA; causes Creutzfeldt-Jakob disease.

prism (priz´m) A transparent body, usually made of optical glass or crystalline material, with at least two polished plane faces inclined toward each other from which light is reflected or through which light is refracted.

proarrhythmia (pro-ă-rith´me-ă) Drug-induced worsening of arrhythmia.

probability (prob-ă-bil´ĭ-te) The ratio of the likelihood of occurrence of a specific event to total events.

proband (pro´band) The member of a family in whom a particular trait is first observed and through whom the rest of the family is brought under observation to study the hereditary characteristics of the trait. Also called propositus; index case. COMPARE: consultand; relative of interest.

probang (pro´bang) A long, slender, flexible rod with a tuft of sponge or some other soft material at the end; used chiefly for removing obstructions from the esophagus or the larynx, or to apply medication.

probe (prōb) **1.** A slender metal rod with a blunt tip, used to explore bodily cavities or wounds. **2.** In genetics, a reagent capable of recognizing the clone of concern in a complex mixture of many DNA or RNA sequences. **3.** To explore.

lacrimal p. A probe, usually made of silver, that can be passed into the upper and lower puncta of the eyelids, through the upper and lower canaliculi, and down the nasolacrimal duct into the nose.

probenecid (pro-ben´ĕ-sid) An agent that enhances the excretion of uric acid by inhibiting its reabsorption by the kidney; also inhibits excretion of penicillin by the kidney; Benemid®.

problem (prob´lem) **1.** Any situation that presents difficulty or uncertainty. **2.** In psychiatry, term often used to denote a person whose behavior deviates from the norm (e.g., problem child); sometimes used in preference to the term mental disorder.

proboscis (pro-bos´is) A tubular structure located near the oral cavity of certain insects and worms, often associated with feeding and used as a means of attachment.

procainamide hydrochloride (pro-kān´ă-mīd hi-dro-klo´rīd) White crystals, soluble in water; a cardiac depressant used in treating ventricular arrhythmias.

procaine hydrochloride (pro´kān hi-dro-klo´rīd) A frequently used local anesthetic, $C_{13}H_{20}O_2N_2 \cdot HCl$; Novocaine®.

procaryote (pro-kar´e-ōt) See prokaryote.

procedure (pro-se´jur) A manner of effecting something.

cataract operative p. Any of several operations to remove a cataractous lens.

Irving's p. See Irving's operation, under operation.

loop electrosurgical excision p. (LEEP) A method of removing tissue (e.g., from the uterine cervix) for biopsy or therapeutic purposes, using an electrosurgical unit that supplies low levels of electrical current for cutting or coagulation with a thin (0.2 mm) stainless steel or tungsten wire. Also called loop excision; loop resection.

Madlener's p. See Madlener's operation, under operation.

Pomeroy's p. See Pomeroy's operation, under operation.

procercoid (pro-ser´koid) The larval stage of certain tapeworms, occurring in the intermediate host.

process (pros´es) **1.** A marked prominence extending from an anatomic structure, usually for the attachment of muscles and ligaments. **2.** A series of actions that attain a result.

articular p. of vertebra One of the small

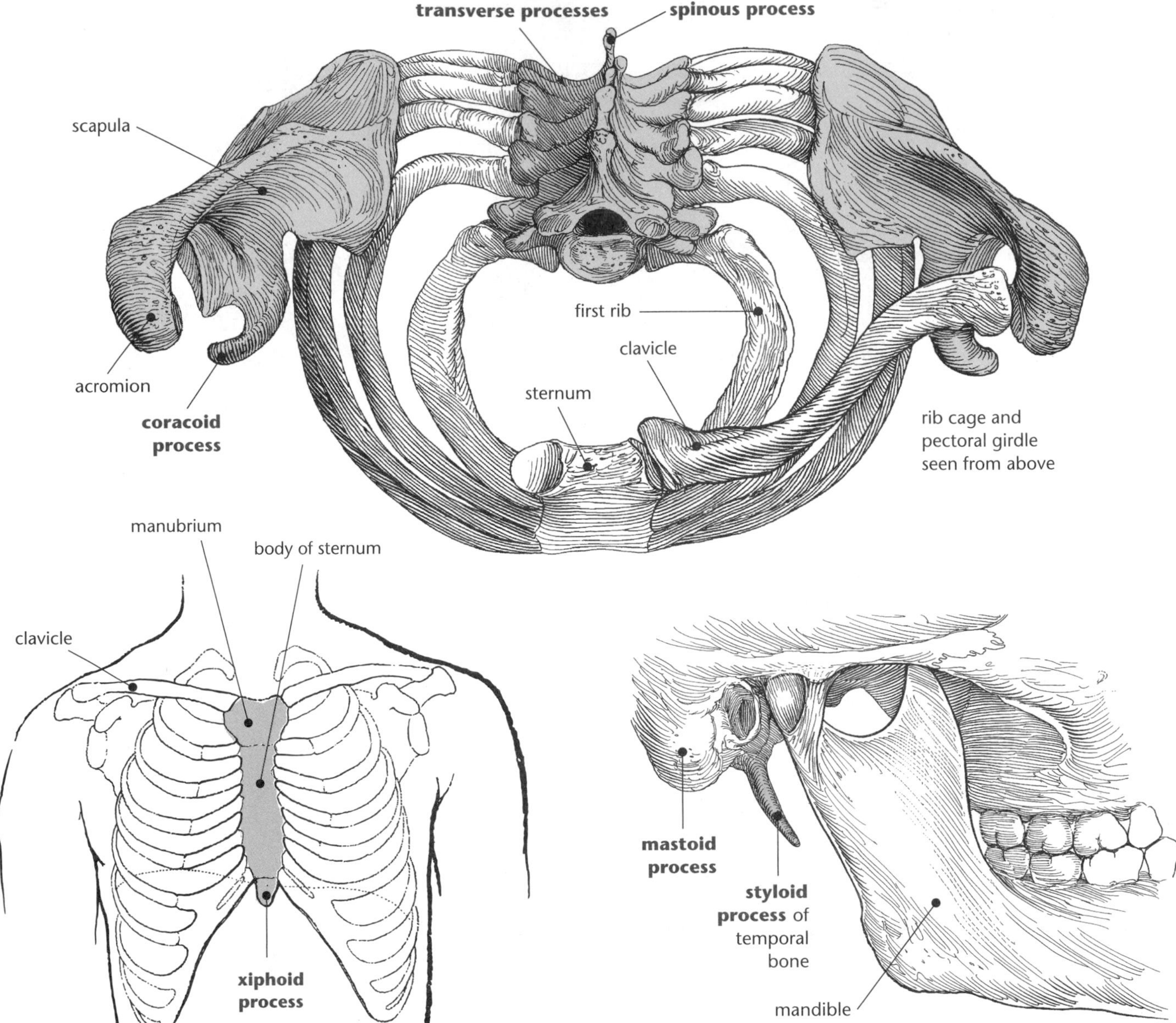

projections on the upper and lower surfaces of the vertebra, forming the vertebral joint; the surface is coated with hyaline cartilage.

ciliary p.'s Radiating pigmented ridges (70 to 80 in number) on the inner surface of the ciliary body of the eye; formed by the inward folding of the various layers of the choroid.

clinoid p. One of three pairs of extensions from the sphenoid bone of the skull.

condylar p. of the mandible The articular process of the ramus of the mandible and the constricted portion (neck) that supports it.

coracoid p. A thick, curved projection from the scapula (shoulder blade) overhanging the glenoid fossa.

dendritic p. See dendrite.

lenticular p. A right angle extension of the long limb of the incus bone of the middle ear; it articulates with the stapes.

mastoid p. A conical downward projection of the mastoid part of the temporal bone of the skull situated behind the ear with the apex on a level with the lobe of the auricle; it serves for the attachment of the sternocleidomastoid muscle, the splenius muscle of the head, and the longissimus muscle of the head.

odontoid p. A toothlike process of the second cervical vertebra (axis); articulates with the first cervical vertebra (atlas).

primary p. A type of thinking marked by the lack of any sense of time, and the use of allusion, analogy, and symbolic representation.

pterygoid p. A long process extending downward from the junction of the body and great wing of the sphenoid bone on either side; it consists of a medial and lateral plate, the upper parts of which are fused together.

secondary p. A type of thinking controlled by the laws that govern conscious (or preconscious) mental activity.

spinous p. of vertebra The process extending backward from the junction of the laminae of the vertebral arch. See also vertebral spine, under spine.

styloid p. A slender, pointed projection extending downward and slightly forward from the petrous portion of the temporal bone; it gives attachment to the styloglossus, stylohyoid, and stylopharyngetis muscles, and the stylohyoid and stylomandibular ligaments.

transverse p. A lateral projection present on each side of a vertebra.

trochlear p. A projection from the lateral side of the calcaneus bone of the foot between the tendons of the long and short peroneal muscles.

xiphoid p. The small and pointed process connected with the lower end of the body of the sternum (breastbone); it is cartilaginous in youth, ossifies with passing age.

zygomatic p. of frontal bone The thick prolongation of the supraorbital margin of the frontal bone; articulates with the frontal process of the zygomatic bone to form the lateral margin of the orbit.

zygomatic p. of maxilla A rough triangular projection from the maxilla; articulates with the zygomatic bone.

zygomatic p. of temporal bone A long arch projecting from the temporal bone; articulates with the temporal process of the zygomatic bone to form the zygomatic arch.

prochlorperazine (pro-klōr-per´ă-zēn) A phenothiazine compound used as a tranquilizer and to relieve nausea and vomiting; Compazine®.

prochondral (pro-kon´dral) Relating to the stage preceding the development of cartilage.

prochordal (pro-kor´dal) Anterior to the notochord.

procidentia (pro-sĭ-den´she-ă) Complete prolapse of an organ.

procollagen (pro-kol´ă-jen) A precursor of collagen.

proconvertin (pro-kon-ver´tin) See factor VII, under factor.

procreate (pro´kre-āt) To produce offspring.

proctalgia (prok-tal´jă, prok-tal´je-ă) Pain in the rectum or in and around the anus. Also called proctodynia.

p. fuga Acute spasmodic pain of only a few minutes duration in the rectum; occurring in young men usually at night.

proctatresia (prok-tă-tre´zhă, prok-tă-tre´ze-ă) Imperforation of the anus.

proctectasia (prok-tek-ta´zhă, prok-tek-ta´ze-ă) Dilatation of the anus or rectum.

proctectomy (prok-tek´to-me) Removal of the rectum.

proctencleisis (prok-ten-kli´sis) See proctostenosis.

proctitis (prok-ti´tis) Inflammation of the rectum.

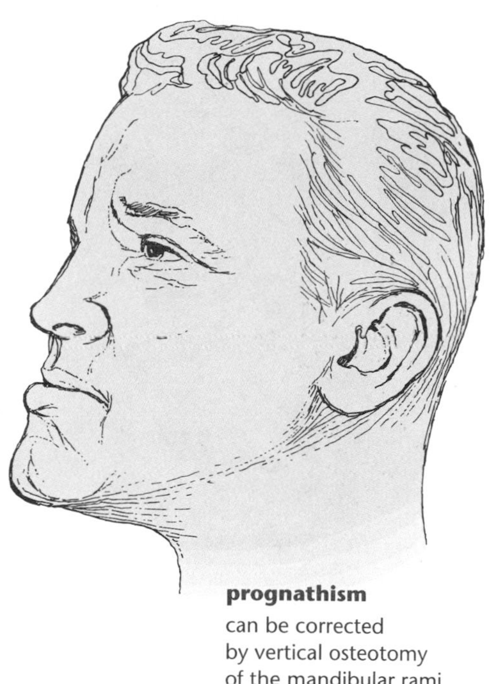

prognathism
can be corrected by vertical osteotomy of the mandibular rami

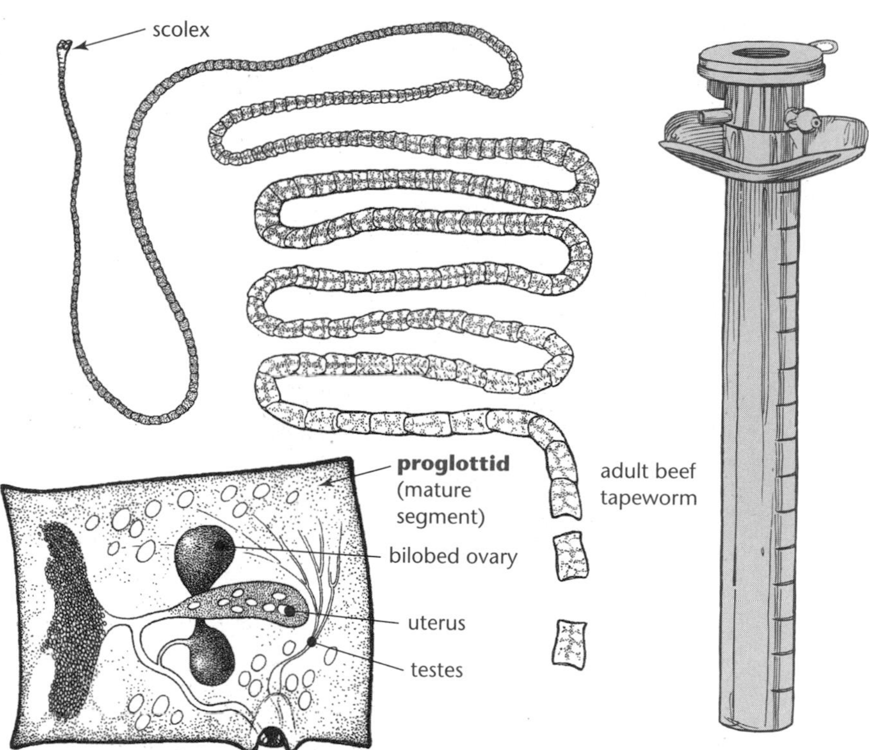

proctoscope

proctocele (prok´to-sēl) See rectocele.
proctoclysis (prok-tok´lĭ-sis) Continuous, slow infusion of saline solution into the rectum and sigmoid colon. Also called rectoclysis.
proctocolitis (prok-to-ko-li´tis) See coloproctitis.
proctocolonoscopy (prok-to-ko-lon-os´kŏ-pe) Examination of the rectum and colon.
proctocolpoplasty (prok-to-kol´po-plas-te) Surgical closure of a rectovaginal fistula.
proctocystocele (prok-to-sis´to-sēl) Bulging of the bladder into the rectum.
proctocystotomy (prok-to-sis-tot´ŏ-me) The incising of the bladder from the rectum.
proctodeum (prok-to-de´um) The hollowed ectodermal surface located beneath the tail of the embryo; it rapidly depresses toward the cloaca and comes in contact with the outer surface of the cloacal wall. Also called anal pit.
proctodynia (prok-to-din´e-ă) See proctalgia.
proctologic (prok-to-loj´ik) Relating to proctology.
proctologist (prok-tol´o-jist) A specialist in proctology.
proctology (prok-tol´ŏ-je) The branch of medicine concerned with the study and treatment of diseases of the rectum and anus.
proctoparalysis (prok-to-pă-ral´ĭ-sis) Paralysis of the anus, resulting in fecal incontinence.
proctoperineoplasty (prok-to-per-ĭ-ne´o-plas-te) Plastic surgery of the anus and perineum. Also called rectoperineorrhaphy.
proctopexy (prok´to-pek-se) Surgical fixation of a prolapsed rectum by suturing to another part. Also called rectopexy.
proctoplasty (prok´to-plas-te) Plastic surgery of the anus or rectum. Also called rectoplasty.
proctoplegia (prok-to-ple´je-ă) Paralysis of the muscles of the rectum and anus.
proctoptosis (prok-top-to´sis) Prolapse of the rectum and anus.
proctorrhagia (prok-to-ra´jă, prok-to-ra´je-ă) Bloody discharge from the rectum.
proctorrhaphy (prok-tor´ă-fe) Suturing of a lacerated rectum or anus.
proctorrhea (prok-to-re´ă) Mucous discharge from the rectum.
proctoscope (prok´to-skōp) Instrument for inspecting the rectum; a speculum. Also called rectoscope.
proctoscopy (prok-tos´ko-pe) Examination of the rectum with a proctoscope.
proctosigmoidectomy (prok-to-sig-moi-dek´tŏ-me) Removal of the rectum and sigmoid colon.
proctosigmoiditis (prok-to-sig-moi-di´tis) Inflammation of the rectum and sigmoid colon.
proctosigmoidoscopy (prok-to-sig-moi-dos´ko-pe) Examination of the interior of the rectum and sigmoid by means of a sigmoidoscope.
proctospasm (prok´to-spas-m) Spasmodic contraction of the rectum or anus.
proctostat (prok´to-stat) A tube containing radium for insertion into the rectum (through the anus) for the treatment of rectal cancer.
proctostenosis (prok-to-stĕ-no´sis) Abnormal narrowing of the rectum or anus. Also called rectostenosis; proctencleisis; proctenclisia.
proctostomy (prok-tos´tŏ-me) Surgical formation of a permanent opening into the rectum.
proctotomy (prok-tot´ŏ-me) Incision into the anus or rectum.
proctovalvotomy (prok-to-val-vot´ŏ-me) Incision into rectal valves.
procumbent (pro-kum´bent) Lying face down.
prodromal (pro-dro´mal) Relating to prodrome.
prodrome (pro´drōm) An early symptom of a disease.
product (prod´ukt) Any substance resulting from a natural process, or that is synthetically manufactured.
cleavage p. A substance produced by the splitting of large, complex molecules into simpler ones.
double p. A measure of heart work load, equal to the product of systolic blood pressure multiplied by the heartbeat frequency (or heart rate).
end p. The product at the end of a metabolic process.
fibrin/fibrinogen p. Any of several small peptides formed in the breakdown of the proteins fibrin and fibrinogen. Also called fibrin-split product; split product.
fibrin-fibrinogen degradation p. Any small peptide (X, Y, D, or E) produced by the action of plasmin on fibrinogen and fibrin during the fibrinolytic process.
fission p. Atomic species resulting from the splitting of large atoms.
gene p. A protein that was formed through gene management (i.e., encoded by a gene).
orphan p. Drugs, biologicals (e.g., sera, vaccines, antitoxins), tests, or medical devices that, although proven useful, are not manufactured because they are not considered commercially profitable, usually because of very limited application.
productive (pro-duk´tiv) **1.** Denoting an inflammatory condition leading to the formation of new tissue. **2.** Bringing forth (e.g., a cough that brings forth mucus).
proencephalon (pro-en-sef´ă-lon) See prosencephalon.
proenzyme (pro-en´zīm) The inactive precursor of an enzyme that requires some change to render it active (e.g., profibrolysin). Also called zymogen.
proerythroblast (pro-ĕ-rith´ro-blast) See pronormoblast.
proerythrocyte (pro-ĕ-rith´ro-sīt) An immature red blood cell; unlike the mature red cell, it has a nucleus.
profundus (pro-fun´dus), *fem.* **profun´da** Latin for deep; applied to certain anatomic structures.
progenital (pro-jen´ĭ-tal) On the exposed surface of the external genitalia.
progeria (pro-je´re-ă) Rare condition affecting adults and children in which affected persons undergo accelerated aging, independent of disease or environmental factors.
progestational (pro-jes-ta´shun-al) **1.** Conducive to pregnancy. **2.** Having effects similar to those of progesterone.
progesterone (pro-jes´tĕ-rōn) Hormone produced in the ovary by the corpus luteum; it stimulates changes in the uterine wall in preparation for implantation of the fertilized ovum.
progestin (pro-jes´tin) General term for a synthetic or natural drug that acts on the uterine lining.
progestogen (pro-jes´to-jen) An agent that produces effects similar to those of progesterone.
proglossis (pro-glos´is) The tip of the tongue.
proglottid (pro-glot´id) One of the segments of the tapeworm that contains both male and female reproductive organs; in a mature proglottid, ovules are produced and fertilized hermaphroditically.
prognathic (prog-na´thik) See prognathous.
prognathism (prog´nă-thiz-m) Abnormal forward projection of the lower jaw.
prognathous (prog´nă-thus) Having a projecting lower jaw. Also called prognathic.
prognose (prog-nōs´) See prognosticate.
prognosis (prog-no´sis) A prediction of the outcome of a disease.
prognosticate (prog-nos´tĭ-kāt) To give a prognosis. Also called prognose.
program (pro´gram) A plan of action toward a desired goal.
quality assurance p. A program designed to insure the quality of patient care in a health facility; peer groups monitor the care given to a patient; necessary changes are brought about through continuing education.
progranulocyte (pro-gran´u-lo-sīt) See promyelocyte.
progressive (pro-gres´iv) Denoting the unfavorable course of a disease, as from bad to worse. Also called advancing.
prohormone (pro-hor´mōn) Any precursor of a hormone (e.g., proinsulin).
proinsulin (pro-in´su-lin) A single chain precursor of insulin; formed in the endoplasmic reticulum of

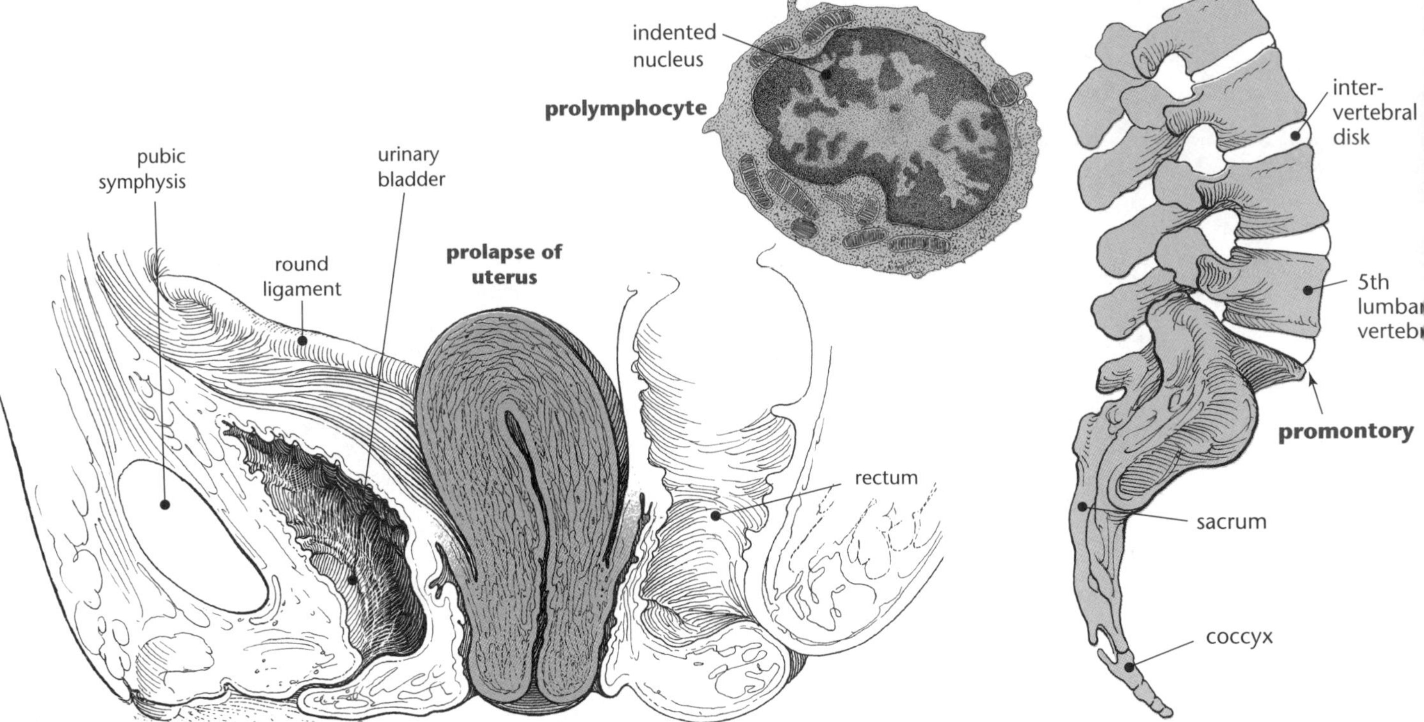

the beta cell of the pancreas and transferred to the Golgi apparatus where the connecting peptide (C-peptide) is removed enzymatically, resulting in the formation of insulin.

projection (pro-jek´shun) **1.** A prominence; a part that juts out. **2.** The referring of sensations from the sense organs to the source of the stimulus. **3.** The connection between the sense organs and the cerebral cortex. **4.** An unconscious psychological defense mechanism in which ideas, affects, or traits that are unacceptable to the self are attributed to another person. **5.** The application of x rays to a body part in a particular direction as it relates to the x-ray tube, e.g., anteroposterior (AP), posteroanterior (PA), right anterior oblique (RAO), right posterior oblique (RPO), left anterior oblique (LAO), left posterior oblique (LPO). Also called view.

Caldwell p. Radiographic projection obtained by placing the face against the cassette and the x-ray tube 15° caudad in a posterior-anterior plane; permits unobstructed viewing of orbital structures.

Towne p. Radiographic projection obtained by placing the back of the head against the cassette and the x-ray tube 30° caudad in an anterior-posterior plane, permits viewing of occipital bone, foramen magnum, dorsum sellae, and petrous ridges.

Waters' p. A radiographic projection of the skull in a posteroanterior plane; permits viewing of facial bones and maxillary sinuses.

prokaryosis (pro-kar-e-o´sis) A state in which the nuclear substance of a primitive cell is mixed or is in direct contact with the rest of the protoplasm, due to not having a nuclear envelope.

prokaryote (pro-kar´e-ōt) Any simple unicellular organism that does not have a nuclear membrane, membrane-bound organelles, and characteristic ribosomes (e.g., bacteria and blue-green algae). Also spelled procaryote.

prolactin (pro-lak´tin) (PRL) Hormone produced by the anterior lobe of the pituitary gland that stimulates milk secretion.

prolactinoma (pro-lak-tĭ-no-mă) A benign, prolactin-producing pituitary tumor.

prolapse (pro-laps´) The downward displacement of a body part or organ.

mitral valve p. Posterior displacement of the posterior (occasionally the anterior) leaflet of the mitral valve, occurring in mid or late systole, and often producing a click that may be followed by a late systolic murmur; may cause back flow (regurgitation) of blood through the valve.

p. of rectum Protrusion of the inner surface of the rectum through the anus.

p. of uterus Falling of the uterus into the vagina due to stretching and laxity of its supporting structures. Commonly called falling of the womb.

proliferation (pro-lif-ĕ-ra´shun) Multiplication of similar cells.

atypical melanotic p. See melanoma *in situ*, under melanoma.

pagetoid melanotic p. See melanoma *in situ*, under melanoma.

prolific (pro-lif´ik) **1.** Copiously productive. **2.** Bearing offspring in great abundance. Also called fertile.

proline (pro´lin) (Pro) Amino acid present in collagen.

prolymphocyte (pro-lim´fo-sīt) A cell midway in maturity between the lymphoblast and the lymphocyte; it has the capacity to divide, and may serve as a reservoir of immunologically uncommitted cells.

promastigote (pro-mas´tĭ-gōt) The flagellate stage of a trypanosomatid microorganism.

promazine hydrochloride (pro´mă-zēn hi-dro-klo´rīd) Phenothiazine compound used as a tranquilizer and antiemetic; Sparine®.

promegaloblast (pro-meg´ă-lo-blast) A large nucleated red blood cell; an early stage in the maturation of the megaloblast.

prometaphase (pro-met´ă-fāz) A stage of mitosis, between prophase and metaphase, marked by the disintegration of the nuclear membrane and formation of the spindle.

promethazine hydrochloride (pro-meth´ă-zēn hi-dro-klo´rīd) An antihistaminic compound used also as an adjuvant with narcotics; Phenergan®.

promethium (pro-me´the-um) A radioactive rare-earth element; symbol Pm; atomic number 61; atomic weight 147 (best-known isotope); half-life 2.6 years, used as a source of beta-rays.

prominence (prom´ĭ-nens) A projection.

laryngeal p. The projection in front of the neck produced by the thyroid cartilage. Also called Adam's apple.

promontory (prom´on-tor-e) A projection or elevation.

promoter (pro-mo´ter) **1.** A substance that increases the activity of a catalyst. **2.** The area on DNA in which RNA polymerase binds and initiates transcription of genetic code information.

promyelocyte (pro-mi´ĕ-lo-sīt) The developmental stage of a granular leukocyte, between a myeloblast and myelocyte; contains large ovoid or irregularly spherical granules; nucleoli are often present. Also called progranulocyte.

pronate (pro´nāt) To assume, or to be placed in, a face-down position.

pronation (pro-na´shun) **1.** The act of lying face downward. **2.** Rotation of the forearm so that the palm of the hand is turned backward or downward.

pronation sign (pro-na´shun sīn) In hemiplegia, when the paralized arm is placed in supination, it spontaneously turns to a pronated position. Also called Babinski's sign.

prone (prōn) Lying with the face downward.

pronephros (pro-nef´ros), *pl.* **proneph´roi** The primitive excretory organ of the embryo, consisting of a series of rudimentary tubules; it is replaced by the transitory mesonephros which forms caudally to it.

pronograde (pro´no-grād) The horizontal position of the body of a quadruped; opposed to orthograde.

pronometer (pro-nom´ĕ-ter) Instrument for determining the degree of pronation or supination of the forearm.

pronormoblast (pro-nor´mo-blast) The earliest red blood cell precursor, generally 12 to 19 µm in diameter; characterized by scanty, basophilic cytoplasm without hemoglobin, and a nucleus containing fine chromatin. Also called proerythroblast; rubriblast.

pronucleus (pro-noo´kle-us) One of two nuclei (haploid nuclei) undergoing fusion, as of an egg or sperm at the time of fertilization.

proof spirit (proof spir´it) A mixture of alcohol and water or a beverage containing 50% (100 proof) of ethyl alcohol by volume at 60°F.

pro-opiomelanocortin (pro-o´pe-o-mel-ă-no-kor´tin) (POMC) A large peptide molecule produced by the action of a single messenger RNA (mRNA) at a variety of sites in the body; it is the precursor of adrenocorticotropic hormone (ACTH), melanocyte-stimulating hormone (MSH), lipoprotein, and endorphin.

propagation (prop-ă-ga´shun) **1.** Reproduction. **2.** The continuance of an impulse along a nerve fiber.

proparacaine hydrochloride (pro-par´ă-kān hi-dro-klo´rīd) An effective surface anesthetic derived from aminobenzoic acid; used principally in ophthalmology; Ophthaine®.

propenyl (pro-pe´nil) The radical $-CH{=}CH{-}CH_3$.

properdin (pro´per-din) Natural euglobulin protein in human blood serum; molecular weight approximately eight times that of gamma globulins; acts in conjunction with complement and magnesium ions and plays a role in providing immunity from infectious diseases and possibly in initiating other immune processes.

properitoneal (pro-per-ĭ-to-ne´al) Situated in front of the peritoneum (i.e., between the parietal peritoneum and the abdominal wall).

prophage (pro´fāj) A bacteriophage incorporated into the entire genetic composition of a bacterial cell and replicating along with the bacterial genes. It does

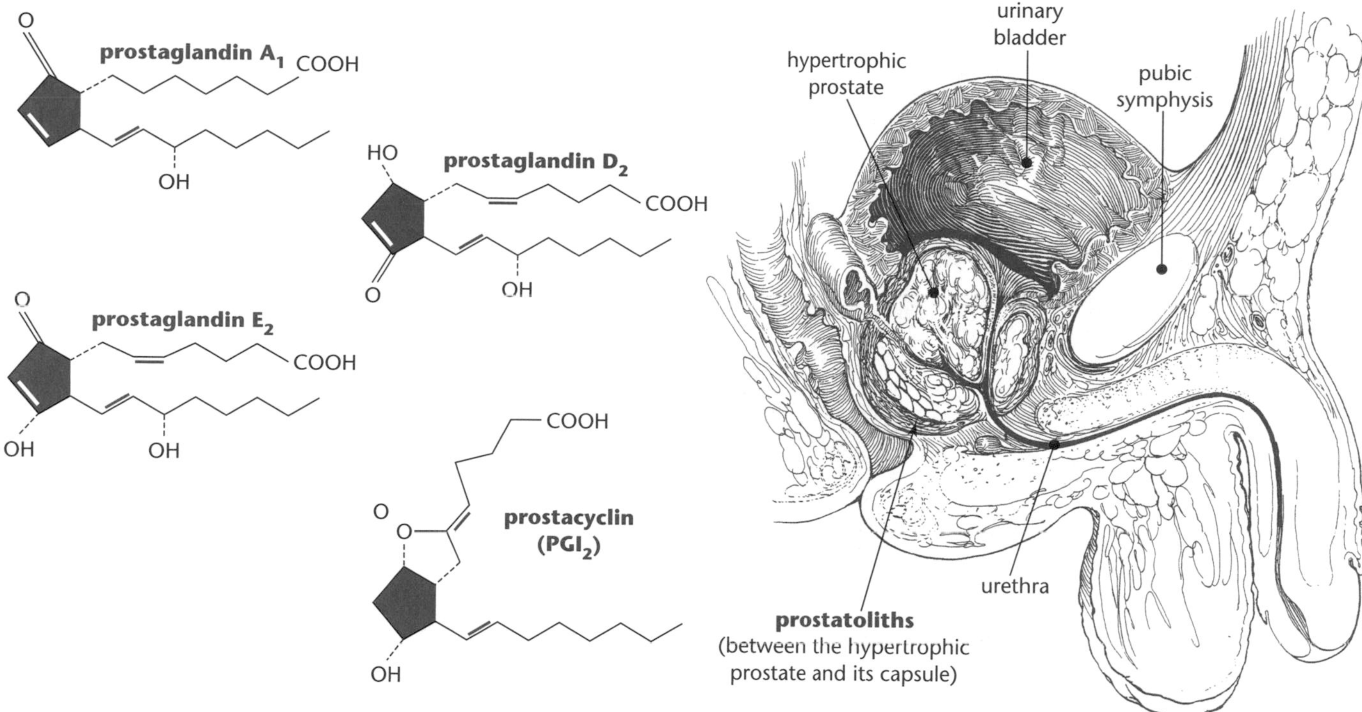

not destroy the cell. Also called probacteriophage.

prophase (pro´fāz) The first stage of cell division by mitosis, during which chromatin collects into a chromosomal thread that breaks up into pairs of rod-shaped chromosomes; each chromosome then splits longitudinally into chromatids.

prophylactic (pro-fĭ-lak´tik) **1.** Relating to the prevention of disease. **2.** An agent that wards off disease. **3.** Common name for a condom.

prophylaxis (pro-f ĭ-lak´sis) **1.** Precautions taken to prevent a disease; preventive treatment. **2.** In dentistry, cleaning of the teeth.

propositus (pro-poz´ĭ-tus) See proband.

propoxyphene hydrochloride (pro-pok´se-kān hi-dro-klo´rīd) A mild analgesic; Darvon®.

propranolol hydrochloride (pro-pran´o-lōl hi-dro-klo´rīd) An adrenergic beta-receptor blocking agent that diminishes the rate and contractile force of the heart, causing a fall in cardiac output and cardiac work; used in the treatment of arrhythmias, angina, and hypertension and for prevention of migraine.

proprioception (pro-pre-o-sep´shun) Position sense; awareness of position of the body.

proprioceptor (pro-pre-o-sep´tor) A sensory nerve ending, primarily located within the muscles and tendons, which receives stimuli pertaining to movements and position of the body.

muscle p. See neuromuscular spindle, under spindle.

proptometer (pro-tom´ĕ-ter) See exophthalmometer.

proptosis (prop-to´sis) Bulging or protrusion of an organ, as of the eyeball.

propulsion (pro-pul´shun) Displacement of the center of gravity producing a tendency to lean forward, seen in persons suffering from Parkinson's disease.

propyl (pro´pil) The radical of propyl alcohol or propane.

propyl alcohol (pro´pil al´ko-hol) A clear colorless fluid, $CH_3CH_2CH_2OH$, more toxic than ethyl alcohol and widely used as a solvent.

propylene (prop´ĭ-lēn) A flammable colorless gas soluble in water $CH_2 = CHCH_3$.

propylparaben (pro-pil-par´ă-ben) Any of several compounds used as preservatives in a number of pharmaceutical preparations; known to cause contact dermatitis when used in skin creams, lotions, etc.

propylthiouracil (pro-pil-thi-o-u´ră-sil) Compound used in the treatment of hyperthyroidism.

pro re nata (pro re na´ta) (p.r.n.) Latin for when necessary.

prorubricyte (pro-roo´brĭ-sīt) See basophilic normoblast, under normoblast.

prosection (pro-sek´shun) An anatomic dissection made specifically for demonstration or for exhibition.

prosector (pro-sek´tor) One who prepares or dissects anatomic structures for demonstration.

prosectorium (pro-sek-tor´e-um) A dissecting room; an anatomy laboratory.

prosencephalon (pros-en-sef´ă-lon) The part of the embryonic brain developed from the most anterior portion of the neural tube; later it forms the telencephalon and the diencephalon. Also called forebrain; proencephalon.

prosodemic (pros-o-dem´ik) Denoting a disease that is spread directly from one individual to another; an outbreak of a disease arising in this manner, in contrast to an epidemic.

prosody (pros´o-de) The variations in the stress and intonation patterns of speech by which different shades of meaning are communicated.

prosopagnosia (pros-o-pag-no´se-ă) A form of visual agnosia in which the person is unable to recognize, or has great difficulty recognizing, familiar faces.

prosopoplegia (pros-o-po-ple´jhă, pros-o-po-ple´je-ă) See facial nerve palsy, under palsy.

prostacyclin (pros-tă-si´klin) A prostaglandin produced by endothelial cells of the cardiovascular system; it inhibits platelet aggregation and helps maintain the integrity of the endothelial cells. Also called prostaglandin I_2.

prostaglandin (pros-tă-glan´din) (PG) Any of a group of hormone-like, lipid-soluble, acidic compounds derived from long-chain polyunsaturated fatty acids; occur in nearly all body tissues and fluids (including cerebrospinal and amniotic fluids), and have a multitude of physiologic actions (e.g., suppress gastric acid secretions, dilate peripheral blood vessels, increase renal blood flow, and dilate bronchial tubes); classified by chemical structure, using letters to designate ring substitution (e.g., PGA, PGB) and numerical subscripts to denote number of unsaturated bonds (e.g., PGA_1); their production is inhibited by nonsteroidal anti-inflammatory drugs (e.g., aspirin, indomethacin, phenylbutazone); discovered in semen and first believed to originate from the prostate, hence the name prostaglandin. See also eicosanoid; leukotriene; thromboxane.

p. I_2 (PGI_2) See prostacyclin.

prostaglandin endoperoxide synthase (pros-tă-glan´din en-do-pĕ-rok´sīd sin´thās) See cyclo-oxygenase.

prostanoic acid (pros-ta-no´ik as´id) The 20-carbon molecular skeleton of prostaglandins.

prostanoid (pros´tă-noid) Any derivative of prostanoic acid (e.g., prostaglandins, thromboxanes).

prostatalgia (pros-tă-tal´jă, pros-tă-tal´je-ă) Pain in the prostate.

prostate (pros´tāt) A chestnut-shaped body in the male consisting of glandular and muscular tissue that surrounds the urethra immediately below the bladder; it secretes a milky fluid that is discharged by excretory ducts into the urethra at the time of ejaculation.

prostatectomy (pros-tă-tek´tŏ-me) Surgical removal of the prostate, or a portion of it.

suprapubic p. Prostatectomy performed through an incision just above the pubic bone.

transurethral p. Removal of prostatic tissue with a viewing instrument equipped with a cutting tip (resectoscope) introduced through the urethra; performed in the treatment of noncancerous enlargement of the prostate (benign prostatic hypertrophy, BPH). Also called transurethral resection of prostate (TURP).

prostatic (pros-tat´ik) Relating to the prostate.

prostatism (pros´tă-tiz-m) Any condition caused by hypertrophy or other disease of the prostate; usually refers to symptoms of obstructive disease of the urinary tract caused by prostatic hypertrophy.

prostatitis (pros-tă-ti´tis) Inflammation of the prostate.

prostatocystitis (pros-ta-to-sis-ti´tis) Inflammation of the prostate and the bladder.

prostatolith (pros-tat´o-lith) A stone of the prostate.

prostatolithotomy (pros-tat-o-lĭ-thot´ŏ-me) Incision of prostate for removal of a calculus.

prostatomyomectomy (pros-tat-o-mi-o-mek´to-me) Removal of a myomatous or hypertrophied prostate.

prostatorrhea (pros-tă-to-re´ă) Abnormal discharge from the prostate.

prostatotomy (pros-tă-tot´ŏ-me) Incision into the prostate.

prostatovesiculectomy (pros-tă-to-ve-sik-u-lek´tŏ-me) Removal of the prostate and seminal vesicles.

prostatovesiculitis (pros-tă-to-ve-sik-u-li´tis) Inflammation of the prostate and the seminal vesicles.

prosthesis (pros-the´sis) An artificial replacement for a missing or dysfunctional part.

cleft palate p. Appliance used to correct a congenital structural deficiency in the roof of the mouth.

dental p. Artificial replacement of one or more teeth and/or related structures.

discoid valve p. An artificial heart valve consisting of a free disc in an open cage.

ocular p. An artificial eye.

P

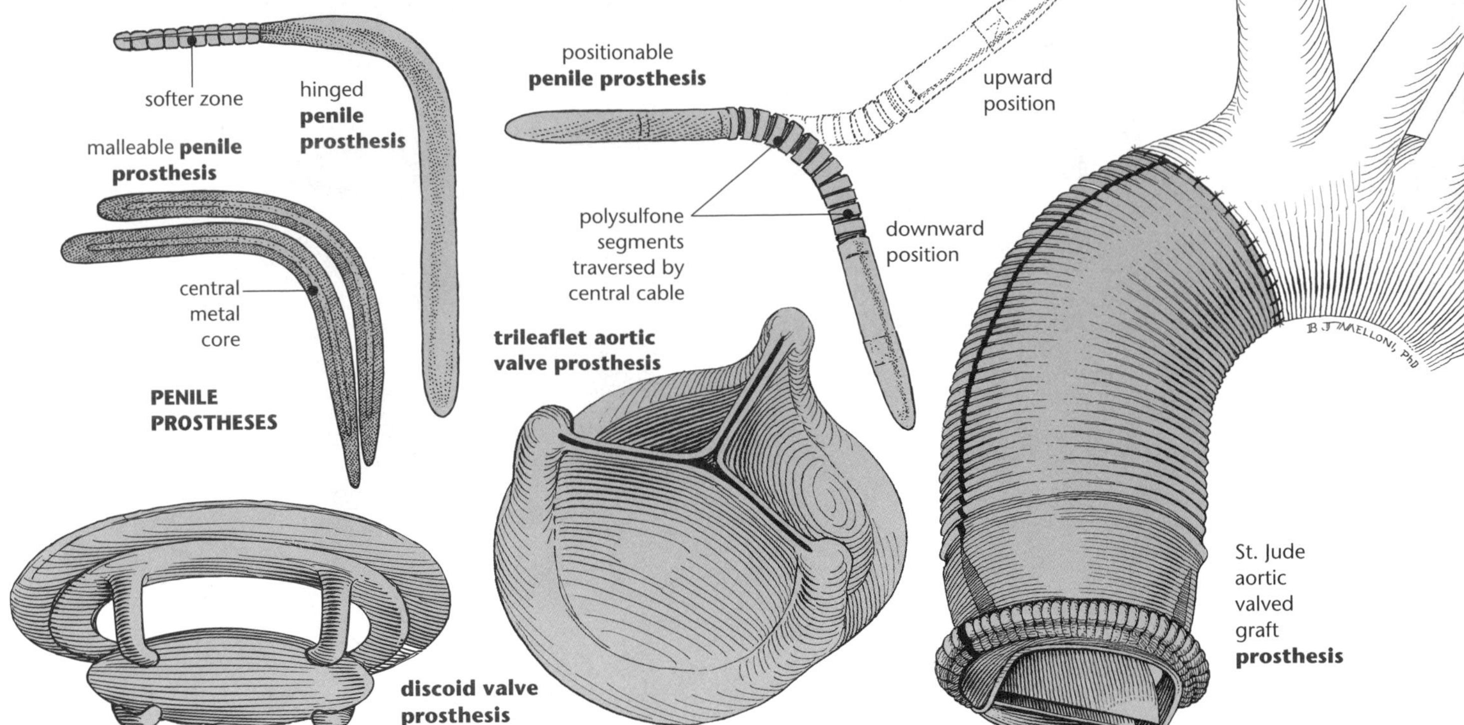

penile p. A device implanted within a penis to permit adequate rigidity for coitus; it could be a semirigid rod, or a two-cylinder inflatable device.

trileaflet aortic valve p. A one-piece trileaflet artificial heart valve that permits a full central flow pattern similar to that of the normal valve.

prosthetic (pros-thet´ik) Relating to an artificial part of the body.

prosthetics (pros-thet´iks) The making and adjusting of artificial parts of the body.

dental p. See prosthodontics.

prosthion (pros´the-on) A craniometric point situated on the maxillary alveolar process that projects most anteriorly in the midline; used in measuring facial depth. Also called alveolar point.

prosthodontics (pros-tho-don´tiks) The branch of dentistry pertaining to the restoration and maintenance of oral function by the replacement of missing teeth and associated structures by artificial appliances. Also called dental prosthetics.

prosthodontist (pros-tho-don´tist) A specialist in prosthodontics.

prosthokeratoplasty (pros-tho-ker´ă-to-plas-te) Replacement of diseased corneal tissue by a transparent implant.

prostration (pros-tra´shun) A state of extreme exhaustion.

protactinium (pro-tak-tin´e-um) A rare radioactive element, symbol Pa, atomic number 91, atomic weight 231; similar to uranium.

protaminase (pro-tam´ĭ-nās) An enzyme of the proteinase class that normally splits up protamines to peptides in the intestine. Also called carboxypeptidase B.

protamine (pro´tă-min) Any of a group of simple, highly basic proteins, rich in arginine and soluble in water; they neutralize the anticoagulant action of heparin.

p. sulfate A heparin antagonist used to neutralize excessive amounts of heparin in certain bleeding disorders.

protanopia (pro-tă-no´pe-ă) Inability to differentiate red, orange, yellow, and green.

protean (pro´te-an) Having the capacity to readily assume different shapes or forms.

protease (pro´te-ās) Any enzyme that splits the peptide bonds of proteins and peptides; a proteolytic enzyme.

protein (pro´tēn) Any of a group of complex nitrogenous substances of high molecular weight that contain amino acids as their fundamental structural units, are present in the cells of all animals and plants, and function in all phases of chemical and physical activity of the cells.

p27 p. An inhibitor of the enzyme cyclin-kinase; decreased levels of p27 protein are associated with an increased probability of prostate cancer recurrence.

Alzheimer's disease associated p. (ADAP) Protein found in the brain and spinal fluid of people afflicted with Alzheimer's disease.

Bence Jones p. Protein found in the urine of people with multiple myeloma; when the urine is heated, a precipitate forms at 50 to 60°C which dissolves when the temperature is raised to near boiling point. Also called Bence Jones albumin.

p. C A protein constituent of blood plasma that prevents coagulation of blood. Deficiency of protein C causes recurrent blood clots and vein inflammation (thrombophlebitis).

p. Ca The activated form of protein C.

conjugated p. Compound formed by the combination of a protein with a nonprotein (prosthetic) group.

C-reactive p. Abnormal protein found in the blood serum of persons in acute stages of inflammatory diseases such as rheumatic fever.

denatured p. One that has undergone a change, so that its characteristic properties are lost.

foreign p. One that differs from those normally found in the blood, lymph, or body tissues.

G p. Any of several proteins acting as mediators between activated cell receptors and their enzymes (i.e., they relay signals initiated by photons, odorants, and various hormones and neurotransmitters); *Gs* proteins stimulate and *Gi* proteins inhibit an enzyme target. Mutations altering G protein activation cause a variety of disorders, such as those of excessive transmission (e.g., adenomas) and deficient transmission (e.g., pseudoparathyroidism).

p. hydrolysate (intravenous) A product of protein hydrolysis used after surgery of the intestinal tract and certain severe illnesses. Also called casein hydrolysate 5%; Amigen®.

native p. Protein in its natural state.

plasma p.'s Proteins present in blood plasma (e.g., albumin, globulins, fibrinogen).

plasma p. fraction Selected proteins from blood plasma of adult human donors, used as a blood volume supporter.

receptor p. An intracellular protein with specific affinity for binding a given stimulant of cellular activity.

p. S A blood plasma protein needed as a cofactor for the functions of protein C.

simple p. Protein that yields only amino acids upon hydrolysis.

proteinaceous (pro-tēn-a´shus) Relating to a protein.

proteinase (pro´tēn-ās) Any enzyme that hydrolyzes native protein or polypeptides (e.g., pepsin).

protein kinase (pro´tēn ki´nās) Enzyme that promotes the phosphorylation of amino acids.

proteinosis (pro-tēn-o´sis) Condition marked by an increase in proteins in the tissues, especially abnormal proteins.

pulmonary alveolar p. Chronic progressive disease of the lungs affecting adults, marked by accumulation of a homogeneous granular substance in the alveoli (air sacs); cause is unknown.

protein sequencer (pro´tēn se-kwen´ser) An instrument that sequentially removes amino acids from the parent protein chain to determine the composition and structure of the protein.

proteinuria (pro-te-nu´re-ă) Excretion of protein in the urine in excess of the normal daily amount; an average-size healthy person normally excretes up to 100 mg of protein per day.

heavy p. Excretion of more than 4 g of protein daily, usually caused by renal disorders that greatly increase glomerular permeability.

orthostatic p. See postural proteinuria.

postural p. Excessive excretion of protein in the urine, usually mild, in healthy adolescents and young adults, occurring when the individual is upright, and disappearing during recumbency. Also called orthostatic proteinuria.

transient p. Proteinuria that may occur with febrile disorders, abdominal crises, heart disease, severe anemia, and emotional stress. Also called intermittent or functional proteinuria.

proteoglycan (pro-te-o-gli´kan) (PG) Glycoprotein of high molecular weight; a component of connective tissue, responsible for the stiffness of articular cartilage and its ability to withstand load.

proteolysis (pro-te-ol´ĭ-sis) The breaking down (hydrolysis) of proteins into simpler, soluble forms by the action of enzymes, as in digestion.

proteolytic (pro-te-o-lit´ik) Causing proteolysis.

proteose (pro´te-ōs) One of the intermediate products of protein digestion, between a protein and a peptone.

Proteus (pro´te-us) A genus of gram-negative bacteria, motile only at 25°C; most commonly associated with urinary tract and wound infections; may also be seen in diarrhea and gastroenteritis.

P. mirabilis A species found in putrid meat, effusions, and abscesses; thought to be a cause of gastroenteritis.

P. morgenii Species that is a common inhabitant of the gastrointestinal tract; seen in normal and diarrheal stools.

P. vulgaris Species found in putrefying tissues and abscesses; certain strains are agglutinated by typhus serum (Weil-Felix reaction) and therefore are used

P

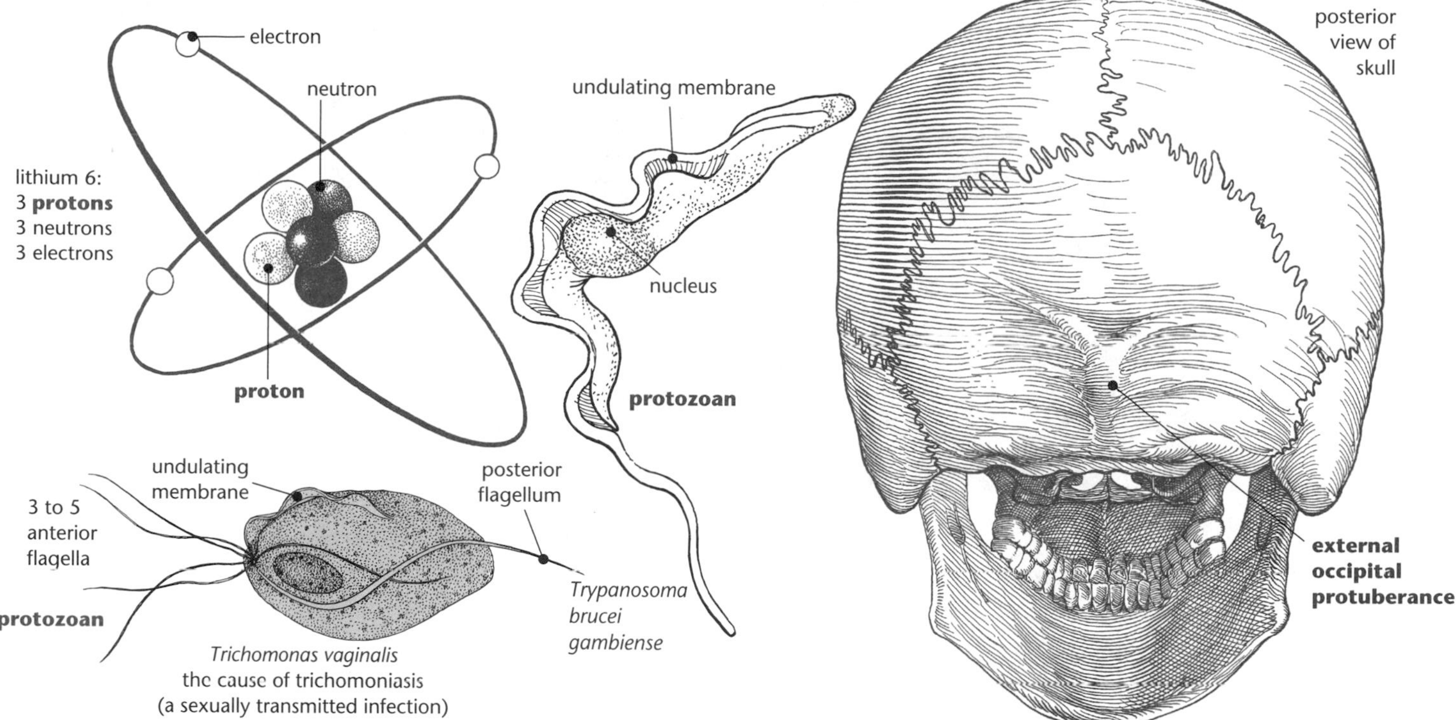

in diagnosing the disease.

Proteus syndrome (pro´te-us sin´drōm) Abnormally large hands, feet, and head, and abnormal growth. Also called elephant man disease.

prothrombin (pro-throm´bin) A plasma protein that is converted into thrombin during the second stage of blood coagulation; an enzymically inactive precursor of thrombin. Formerly called thrombinogen. Also called factor II.

Protista (pro-tis´tă) A third kingdom or division of living things composed of unicellular organisms such as bacteria, protozoa, and many fungi and algae.

protium (pro´te-um) See hydrogen-1.

protodiastolic (pro-to-di-ă-stol´ik) Relating to the initial one-third of a cardiac diastole or the period immediately following the second heart sound.

proton (pro´ton) (p) A particle in the nuclei of the atoms of all elements (in the case of the hydrogen atom, it forms the whole nucleus); has a positive charge equal numerically to the negative charge of an electron.

proto-oncogene (pro-to ong´ko-jēn) A normal gene involved in some aspects of cell division or proliferation, but capable of becoming a tumor forming gene (oncogene) if rearranged, mutated, or picked up by a retrovirus. See also oncogene.

protoplasm (pro´to-plaz-m) The essential substance of which all living cells, vegetable and animal, are made.

protoporphyria (pro-to-por-fir´e-ă) Condition marked by high concentrations of protoporphyrin in red blood cells, plasma, and feces.

protoporphyrin type III (pro-to-por´fĭ-rin tīp thrē) A porphyrin that, linked with iron, forms the heme of hemoglobin and the prosthetic groups of myoglobin, catalase, cytochromes, etc.

prototroph (pro´to-trōf) The nutritionally independent, wild-type strain of any organism. COMPARE: auxotroph.

prototype (pro´to-tīp) The primitive or ancestral species from which others develop or to which they conform.

Protozoa (pro-to-zo´ă) A subkingdom of the animal kingdom that includes all unicellular organisms; most are free-living, some form aggregates. Some are of medical interest.

protozoa (pro-to-zo´ă) Plural of protozoon.

protozoal (pro-to-zo´al) See protozoan (2).

protozoan (pro-to-zo´an) **1.** Any animal consisting of a single functional cell (e.g., *Trichomonas vaginalis, Pneumocystis carinii*). Also called protozoon. **2.** Relating to a protozoan.

protozoiasis (pro-to-zo-i´ă-sis) Any disease caused by protozoa.

protozoicide (pro-to-zo´ĭ-sīd) An agent capable of destroying protozoa.

protozoology (pro-to-zo-ol´ŏ-je) The biological study of the simplest or most primitive forms of animal life (protozoa).

protozoon (pro-to-zo´on), *pl.* **protozo´a** See protozoan (1).

protozoophage (pro-to-zo´o-fāj) A cell that ingests protozoa.

protraction (pro-trak´shun) In dentistry, condition in which teeth or other maxillary or mandibular structures are located anterior to their normal position.

protractor (pro-trak´tor) **1.** Instrument for extracting a foreign object (e.g., a bullet) from a deep wound. **2.** A muscle that extends a limb; an extensor muscle.

protrusion (pro-troo´zhun) In dentistry, position of the mandible forward or laterally forward from the centric position.

protuberance (pro-too´ber-ans) An eminence, projection, or bulge.

external occipital p. A prominence at the center of the outer surface of the occipital bone.

internal occipital p. A prominence at the midpoint of the inner surface of the occipital bone.

mental p. A triangular elevation on the lower portion of the outer surface of the mandible, at the midline, that helps to form the chin.

Providencia (prŏ-vĭ-den´se-ă) Genus of gram-negative bacteria found in human feces and urine. Some species are associated with diarrhea and urinary tract infections.

provirus (pro-vi´rus) The DNA sequence of a virus that has become an integral part of the DNA of the host cell and is transmitted from one cell generation to the next without destroying the host cell.

provitamin (pro-vi´tă-min) A substance that can be converted into a vitamin.

proximal (prok´sĭ-mal) **1.** Nearest the center, midline, point of attachment, or point of origin; opposite of distal. **2.** In dentistry, the surface of a tooth, either mesial or distal, which is nearest an adjacent tooth.

proximate (prok´sĭ-māt) Nearest; immediate.

proximoataxia (prok-sĭ-mo-ă-tak´se-ă) Lack of muscular coordination of the proximal parts of the limbs.

prune (proon) The partially dried fruit of the common plum *Prunus domestica*; used as a mild laxative.

prune-belly syndrome (proon-bĕl´ē sin´drōm) Congenital absence of the medial and lower muscles of the abdominal wall, associated with urinary tract abnormalities and undescended testicles; males are affected almost exclusively; cause is unknown.

prurient (proor´e-ent) Denoting morbid interest in aberrant matter, especially of a sexual nature.

pruriginous (proo-rij´ĭ-nus) Relating to prurigo.

prurigo (proo-ri´go) An itchy skin eruption of papules.

pruritic (proo-rit´ik) Itchy.

pruritus (proo-ri´tus) Persistent and severe itching of clinically normal skin; may be due to a systemic disease.

p. ani Intense itching at the anus; may be caused by infections, hemorrhoids, or allergy; fecal soiling of the perianal skin may play an important role, inducing a chemical dermatosis.

p. gravidarum Generalized pruritus occurring during pregnancy, usually the third trimester; thought to be a sign of reduced liver function resulting from impedance of bile flow within the liver.

prussiate (prus´e-āt) **1.** A salt of hydrocyanic acid; a cyanide. **2.** A ferricyanide or ferrocyanide.

prussic acid (prus´ik as´id) See hydrogen cyanide, under hydrogen.

pseudarthrosis (soo-do-ar-thro´sis) A false joint formed on the shaft of a long bone, at the site of a fracture that failed to fuse. Also called neoarthrosis.

pseudesthesia (soo-des-the´ză, soo-des-the´ze-ă) Subjective sensation without an external stimulus (e.g., one felt from an amputated limb). Also called pseudoesthesia.

pseudoankylosis (soo-do-an-kĭ-lo´sis) See fibrous ankylosis, under ankylosis.

pseudoaneurysm (soo-do-an´u-riz-m) Dilatation of an artery resembling an aneurysm.

pseudocoarctation (soo-do-ko-ark-ta´shun) An elongated and tortuous condition of the aortic arch in the area of the ligamentum arteriosum without occlusion of the vessel.

pseudochromesthesia (soo-do-kro-mes-the´ziă) See color hearing, under hearing.

pseudocroup (soo-do-kroop´) See laryngismus stridulus.

pseudocryptorchism (soo-do-krip-tor´kiz-m) Condition in which the testes occasionally move high into the inguinal canal.

pseudocyesis (soo-do-si-e´sis) Development of pregnancy symptoms in a nonpregnant woman (e.g., menstrual abnormalities, abdominal enlargement, and breast changes). Also called false pregnancy; phantom pregnancy; spurious pregnancy.

pseudocyst (soo´do-sist) **1.** Accumulation of fluid without an enclosing membrane. **2.** An aggregation of *Toxoplasma* parasites within a host cell.

pseudodementia (soo-do-de-men´she-ă) Reversible condition secondary to other disorders (e.g., depression); it resembles (and is often confused with) true dementia.

pseudoesthesia (soo-do-es-the´ze-ă) See pseud-

P

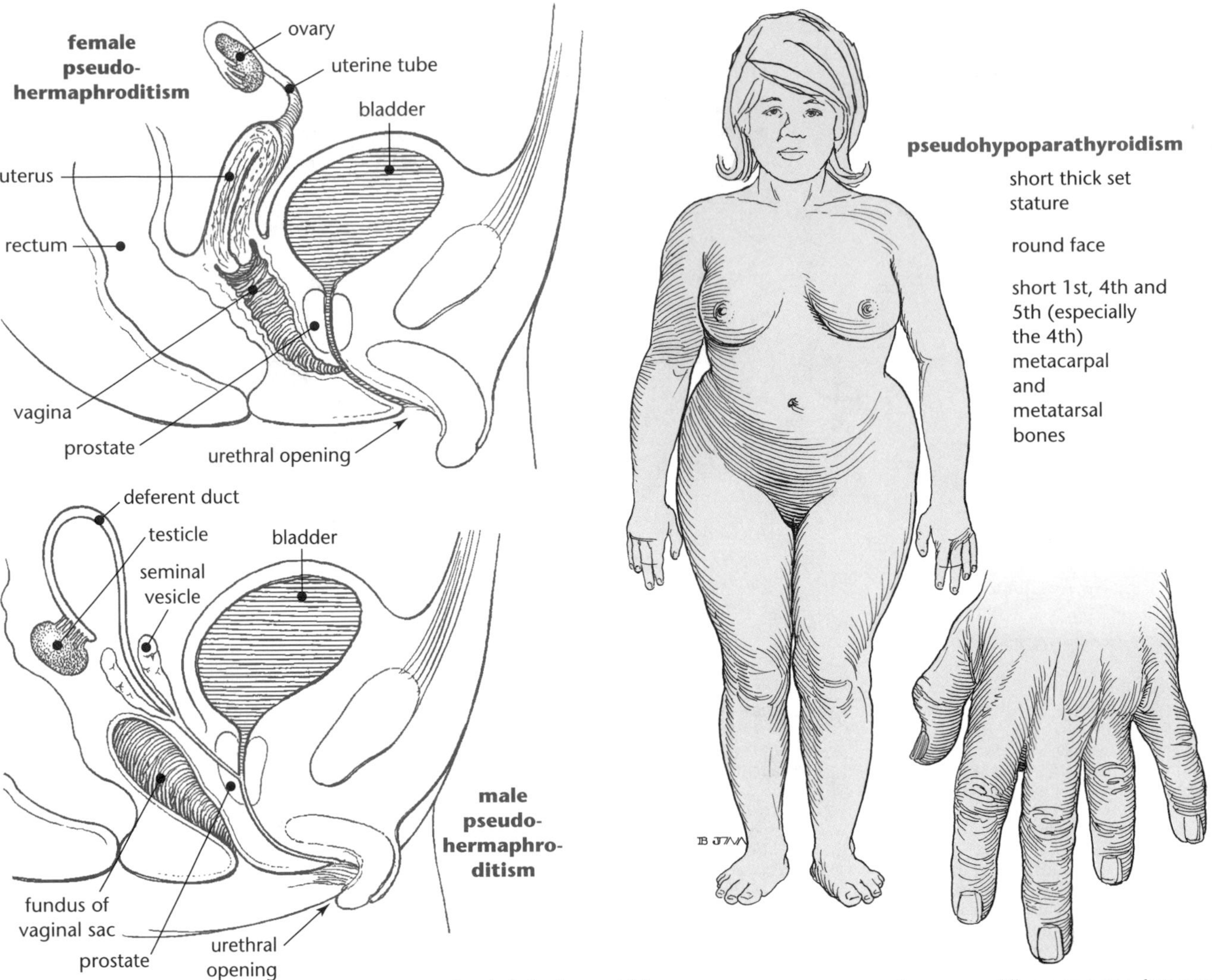

esthesia.

pseudofracture (soo-do-frak′tūr) New bone tissue and thickening of periosteum formed at the site of an injury; resembles an incomplete fracture on x-ray images.

pseudoganglion (soo-do-gang′gle-on) Localized thickening of a nerve trunk simulating a ganglion.

pseudoglaucoma (soo-do-glaw-ko′mă) Abnormality of the optic disk resembling glaucoma, due to conditions other than pressure within the eyeball.

pseudogout (soo′do-gowt) A form of chondrocalcinosis caused by urate-free deposits of calcium pyrophosphate in articular cartilage, leading to goutlike attacks of pain, swelling, stiffness, local warmth, and joint tenderness; the knee is the joint predominantly affected.

pseudohemophilia (soo-do-he-mo-fil′e-ă) An acquired condition resembling hemophilia but caused by another disorder.

pseudohemoptysis (soo-do-he-mop′tĭ-sis) Spitting of blood from a source other than the lungs or bronchi.

pseudohermaphrodite (soo-do-her-maf′ro-dīt) An individual having the characteristics of pseudohermaphroditism.

pseudohermaphroditism (soo-do-her-maf′ro-dit-izm) Condition in which the individual has internal sex organs that are distinctly of one sex but has superficial sex characteristics that are either ambiguous or of the opposite sex. Erroneously called hermaphroditism.

female p. Condition in which an individual has ovaries and the genetic make-up of a female but whose external genitalia are those of a male.

male p. Condition in which an individual has testes and the genetic make-up of a male but whose external genitalia are morphologically those of a female.

pseudohernia (soo-do-her′ne-ă) A swelling resembling a hernia, caused by inflammation of an inguinal gland or scrotal tissue.

pseudohypha (soo-do-hi′fă) A structure of many fungi that is formed by budding, is composed of a chain of cells, and resembles a hypha.

pseudohypoparathyroidism (soo-do-hi-po-par-ă-thi′roi-diz-m) (PHP) Genetic disorder resembling hypoparathyroidism but with normal or elevated levels of parathyroid hormone; marked primarily by renal unresponsiveness to parathyroid hormone; affected persons usually have short stature, round face, and short metacarpal and metatarsal bones, associated with high levels of phosphates and low levels of calcium in the blood; an X-linked dominant inheritance.

pseudomembrane (soo-do-mem′brān) See false membrane, under membrane.

Pseudomonas (soo-do-mo′nas) A genus of gram-negative motile bacteria with polar flagella, occurring in soil, water, sewage, and air.

P. aeruginosa Species found in human feces and skin; causes blue pus infections of wounds and burns and may cause infections in other parts of the body through the use of contaminated instruments (e.g., in the urinary tract, or in the subarachnoid space through lumbar puncture); some strains produce a blue compound soluble in chloroform (pyocyanin); others produce a greenish compound soluble in water (fluorescin).

P. mallei Former name for *Burkholderia mallei.* See under *Burkholderia.*

P. pseudomallei Former name for *Burkholderia pseudomallei.* See under *Burkholderia.*

pseudomucin (soo-do-mu′sin) Gelatinous substance similar to mucin.

pseudomycelium (soo-do-mi-se′le-um) A group of pseudohyphae.

pseudomyopia (soo-do-mi-o′pe-ă) Eye condition resulting from spasm of the ciliary muscle, causing the same focusing defect as myopia.

pseudomyxoma (soo-do-mik-so′ma) A gelatinous tumor resembling a myxoma, but composed of epithelial mucus.

pseudoneoplasm (soo-do-ne′o-plaz-m) See pseudotumor.

pseudoparalysis (soo-do-pă-ral′ĭ-sis) Apparent loss of power of voluntary movement.

pseudoparaplegia (soo-do-par-ă-ple′jă, soo-do-par-ă-ple′je-ă) Apparent loss of power of voluntary movement of the lower extremities.

pseudopodium (soo-do-po′de-um), *pl.* **pseudopodia** **1.** A cytoplasmic process used by certain protozoa (e.g., amebae) for locomotion and feeding. **2.** A small cytoplasmic extension from a cell.

pseudopolyp (soo-do-pol′ip) A protruding mass in the colon, composed of edematous mucosa, granulation tissue, or inflamed epithelium; commonly associated with ulcerative colitis. Also called inflammatory polyp.

pseudopregnancy (soo-do-preg′nan-se) See pseudocyesis.

pseudohypoparathyroidism (soo-do-soo-do-hi-po-par-ă-thi′roid-iz-m) (PPHP) Heritable disorder that has the constitutional features of pseudohypoparathyroidism (round face, short stature, obesity, abnormally short hands and feet) but lacks the chemical findings.

pseudopterygium (soo-do-ter-ij′e-um) A superficial adhesion of the cornea to the conjunctiva resulting from injury. Also called scar pterygium.

pseudosmia (soo-doz′me-ă) Sensation of an odor that is not present.

pseudotubercle (soo-do-tu′ber-kl) A nodule resembling a tuberculous granuloma, but not caused by the tubercle bacillus.

pseudotumor (soo-do-too′mor) The occurrence of symptoms and signs indicating the presence of a tumor in the absence of one, with subsequent spontaneous recovery. Also called pseudoneoplasm.

p. cerebri Increased intracranial pressure suggesting the presence of an intracranial tumor but

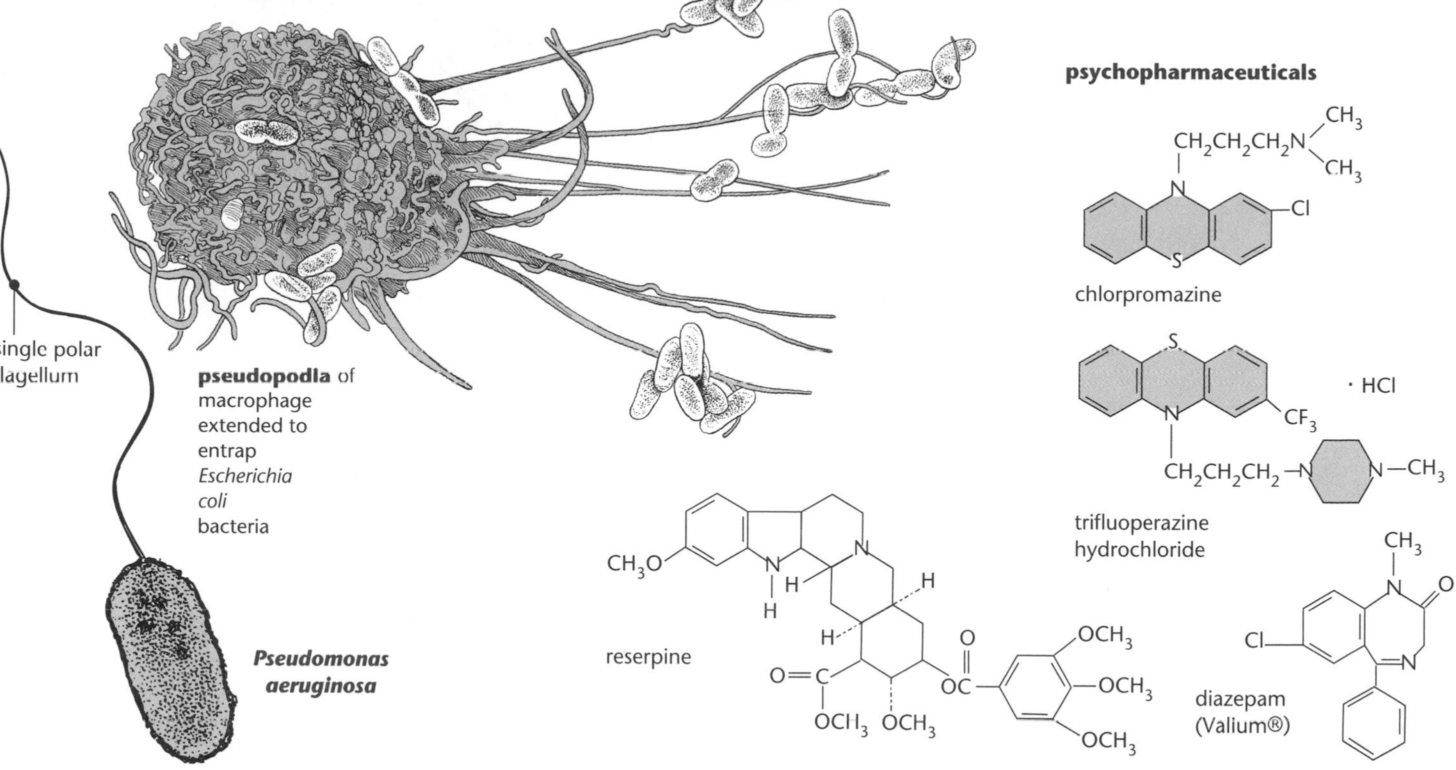

due to other causes. Also called benign intracranial hypertension.

pseudoxanthoma elasticum (soo-do-zan-tho´mă e-las´tĭ-kum) (PXE) Inherited condition marked by slightly elevated papules or plaques on the skin that, as yellowish aggregates, resemble xanthomas; the lesions usually appear on the neck, axillae, abdomen, and thighs, and are due to degenerated elastic tissue; angioid streaks occur in the retina; premature arterial degeneration is common and internal hemorrhage occurs in 10% of cases.

Psilocybe mexicana (si-lo-si´be mek´sĭ-kan-ă) A species of mushrooms (family Agaricaceae) containing the hallucinogenic substance psilocybin. Commonly known as the Mexican magic mushroom.

psilocybin (si-lo-si´bin) A hallucinogenic substance obtained from *Psilocybe mexicana*.

psilosis (si´lo-sis) Loss of hair.

psittacosis (sit-ă-ko´sis) A disease of birds caused by *Chlamydia psittaci*, transmitted to humans by parrots or parakeets through inhalation of infective material; in humans, the disease is characterized by fever, chills, headache, sore throat, and cough. See also ornithosis.

psoas (so´as) See table of muscles.

psoralen (sor´ă-len) A drug that promotes a sunburn effect on the skin; used in combination with ultraviolet light (PUVA, photochemical therapy) to treat severe cases of psoriasis and vitiligo.

psoriasiform (so-re-as´ĭ-form) Resembling psoriasis.

psoriasis (sŏ-ri´ă-sis) A chronic skin disease characterized by reddish patches covered with silvery scales, occurring mostly on the knees, elbows, scalp, and trunk.

psoriatic (so-re-at´ik) Relating to psoriasis.

psyche (si´ke) The mind as distinguished from the body.

psychedelic (si-kĕ-del´ik) Relating to drugs that cause hallucinations, distortions of perception and, sometimes, conditions resembling psychosis.

psychiatric (si-ke-at´rik) Relating to psychiatry.

psychiatrist (si-ki´ă-trist) A specialist in psychiatry.

psychiatry (si-ki´ă-tre) The branch of medicine concerned with the study, diagnosis, and treatment of mental disorders.

social p. The field of psychiatry concerned with the cultural and sociologic factors that cause, intensify, or prolong mental disorders.

psychic (si´kik) **1.** Relating to the mind. **2.** One who supposedly has extraordinary mental or spiritual abilities (e.g., mental telepathy; extrasensory perception).

psycho (si´ko) Street term for a psychopath.

psychoanalysis (si-ko-ă-nal´ĭ-sis) **1.** Psychotherapy that uses dream interpretation, free association, and analysis of manifestations to bring into consciousness repressed feelings and experiences causing the emotional problems. **2.** A theory of mental functioning and human psychosocial development.

psychoanalyst (si-ko-an´a-list) Psychotherapist trained in the techniques of psychoanalytic therapy. Also called analyst.

psychobiology (si-ko-bi-ol´o-je) **1.** The branch of biology dealing with the interrelationship of the brain and the mental processes. **2.** The school of thought that focuses on the individual as a biologic unit in relation to the environment. Also called objective psychobiology.

objective p. See psychobiology (2).

psychodiagnosis (si-ko-di-ag-no´sis) The use of psychological tests and interviews to determine the extent and nature of a person's psychopathology, his characteristic defense style, and the strengths and weaknesses of his ego.

psychodrama (si-ko-dram´ă) A method of group psychotherapy that involves a structured, directed, and dramatized acting out of the patient's emotional problems.

psychodynamics (si-ko-di-nam´iks) The science of human behavior and its unconscious motivation.

psychogenesis (si-ko-jen´ĕ-sis) Origination or causation by mental or psychic factors rather than organic (somatic) ones.

psychogenic, psychogenetic (si-ko-jen´ik, si-ko-je-net´ik) Due to mental or emotional factors rather than detectable organic (somatic) causes.

psychogeriatrics (si-ko-jer-e-at´riks) The study of old age as it relates to psychological problems and mental illnesses.

psychokinesis (si-ko-ki-ne´sis) (PK) In parapsychology, the influence on motion, especially of distant inanimate objects, through concentrated directed thought.

psycholagny (si´ko-lag-ne) Sexual excitement and satisfaction from mental imagery.

psychologic, psychological (si-ko-loj´ik, si-ko-loj´e-kal) Relating to mental processes, emotions, and behavior.

psychologist (si-kol´ŏ-jist) One who is trained to perform psychological evaluation, therapy, or research on mental functioning.

clinical p. One who holds a doctoral degree from an accredited clinical psychology program and is licensed or certified at the independent practice level by the state in which he practices.

psychology (si-kol´ŏ-je) The science concerned with the processes of the mind, especially as they are manifested in behavior.

clinical p. Psychology concerned with the study, assessment, treatment, and prevention of emotional or behavioral disorders.

community p. The practical application of social psychology.

counseling p. Psychology that focuses on healthy adaptation to life situations, generally using brief therapy and educative methods.

forensic p. Psychology concerned with the relationship between the law and disorders manifesting themselves in behaviors that adversely affect society; it is important in such matters as determining competence in contract actions, responsibility for torts and crimes, competence to testify, ability to give informed consent to treatment, and particularly competence to stand trial.

industrial p. See occupational psychology.

medical p. Psychology concerned with the collaboration between physicians and psychologists for managing certain medical problems.

occupational p. Utilization of methods, principles, and theories of psychology for solution of problems arising in industrial settings. Also called industrial psychology.

social p. Psychology concerned with cultural and sociologic factors that cause, intensify, or prolong mental disorders. The body of knowledge upon which community psychology is based.

psychometry (si-kom´ĕ-tre) The measuring of mental efficiency, functioning, and potential.

psychomotor (si-ko-mo´tor) Relating to the mental origin of muscular activity (e.g., compulsive movements).

psychoneurosis (si-ko-nu-ro´sis) See neurosis.

psychoneurotic (si-ko-nu-rot´ik) See neurotic.

psychopath (si´ko-path) An individual who manifests the characteristics of antisocial personality disorder.

psychopathology (si-ko-pă-thol´ŏ-je) **1.** The study of mental disorders. **2.** Manifestation of a mental disorder.

psychopathy (si-kop´ă-the) See antisocial personality disorder, under disorder.

psychopharmaceuticals (si-ko-fahr-mă-su´tĭ-kal) A class of drugs used in the treatment of emotional disorders.

psychopharmacologist (si-ko-fahr-mă-kol´o-jist) A psychiatrist who treats mental disorders with drugs (e.g., antidepressant drugs).

psychopharmacology (si-ko-fahr-ma-kol´ŏ-je) The study of the action of drugs on the mind and emotions.

psychophysical Relating to mental responses evoked by physical stimuli.

psychophysics (si-ko-fiz´iks) The relationship

P

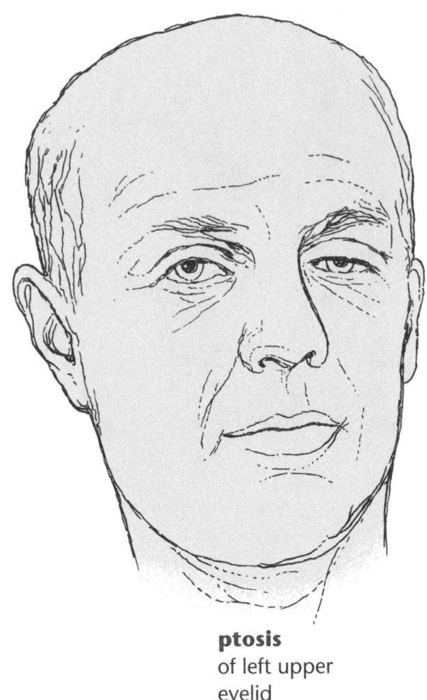

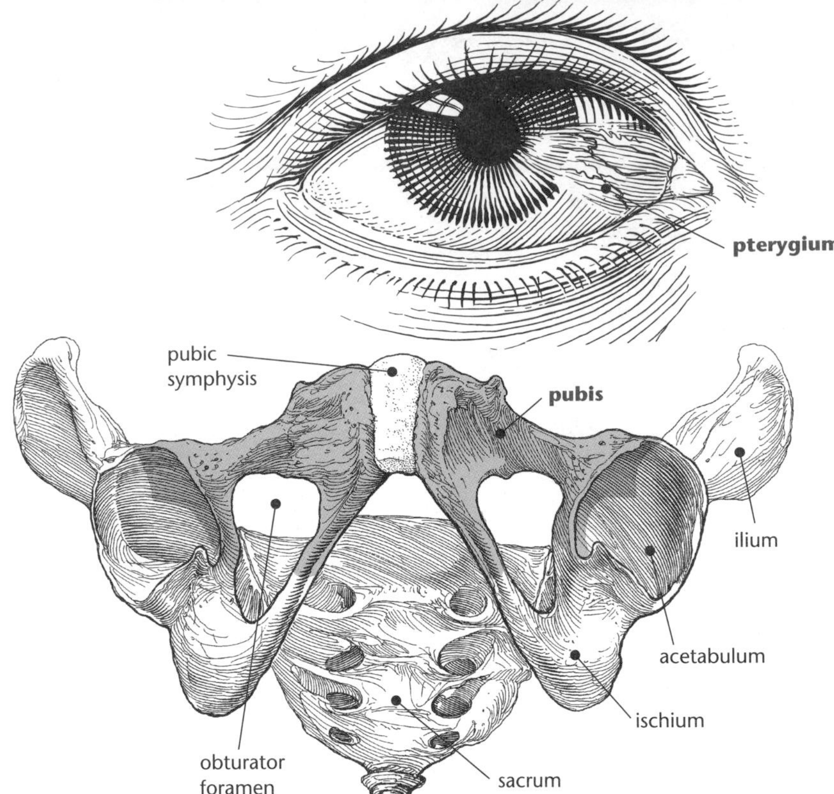

between the physical attributes of a stimulus (e.g., a changing sound) and the measured sensory perception of that stimulus.

psychophysiologic (si-ko-fiz-e-o-loj´ik) **1.** Relating to psychophysiology. **2.** See psychosomatic.

psychophysiology (si-ko-fiz-e-ol´ŏ-je) The study of interactions between psychologic and physiologic processes.

psychosensory (si-ko-sen´so-re) Relating to the perception and interpretation of sensory stimuli.

psychosexual (si-ko-seks´u-al) Relating to the emotional aspects of sex.

psychosis (si-ko´sis), *pl.* **psychoses** A severe mental disorder of organic and/or emotional origin, marked by impairment of the ability to think, communicate, respond emotionally, and interpret reality; the person is unable to meet the ordinary demands of life and frequently undergoes regressive behavior, delusions, and hallucinations.

alcoholic p. Mental disorders caused by alcoholism.

Korsakoffs p. See Korsakoff's syndrome.

manic-depressive p. See bipolar disorder, under disorder.

reactive p. A brief (less than 2 weeks) psychosis following a traumatic psychosocial experience.

schizoaffective p. Psychosis in which both affective and schizophrenic symptoms are present, but the affective symptoms are particularly pronounced in the early stages.

psychosocial (si-ko-so´shal) Involving psychologic and social factors.

psychosomatic (si-ko-so-mat´ik) Referring to the interaction of the mind and the body; applied commonly to physical symptoms that have, at least partially, an emotional cause.

psychosomimetic (si-ko-so-mi-met´ik) See psychotomimetic.

psychostimulant (si-ko-stim´u-lant) Any agent that has mood-elevating properties.

psychosurgery (si-ko-ser´jer-e) Surgical destruction or removal of brain tissue for the treatment of severe mental disorders or to relieve intractable pain.

psychotherapeutic (si-ko-ther-ă-pu´tik) Relating to psychotherapy.

psychotherapist (si-ko-ther´ă-pist) An individual, usually a psychiatrist or a clinical psychologist, trained in psychotherapy.

psychotherapy (si-ko-ther´ă-pe) Treatment of behavioral, emotional, and mental disorders or distress conducted by a variety of psychological methods involving communication between a trained therapist and an individual, couple, family, or group. See under therapy for definitions of various psychotherapeutic approaches.

psychotic (si-kot´ik) Relating to, afflicted with, or caused by a psychosis.

psychotogen (si-kot´o-jen) A drug that produces psychotic symptoms.

psychotomimetic (si-kot-o-mi-met´ik) Denoting the effect of certain drugs (e.g., LSD), which simulate psychotic states. Also called psychosomimetic.

psychotropic (si-ko-tro´pik) Affecting the mind; applied to certain drugs used in treating mental disorders.

psychrometer (si-krom´ĕ-ter) Device used to calculate the relative humidity of the atmosphere; consists of two thermometers, one with a bulb that is kept wet to cause evaporation and the other with a dry bulb.

psychrometry (si-krom´ĕ-tre) **1.** The science of the physical laws controlling air and water mixture. **2.** Estimation of the relative humidity of the air by means of a psychrometer.

psychrophilic (si-kro-fil´lik) Thriving in cold temperature; said of some bacteria.

psychrophobia (si-kro-fo´be-ă) **1.** Extreme sensitivity to cold. **2.** Abnormal fear of cold temperatures.

psyllium (sil´e-um) **1.** A plant of the genus *Plantago*. **2.** The seeds of *Plantago psyllium*, which, when moist, swell and become gelatinous; useful in treating simple constipation.

ptarmic (tar´mik) An agent that causes sneezing.

pterion (te´re-on) A craniometric point on either side of the skull at the junction of the frontal, sphenoid, parietal, and temporal bones.

pteroylmonoglutamic acid (ter-o-il-mon-o-glootam´ik as´id) See folic acid.

pterygium (tĕ-rij´e-um) A slowly advancing triangular growth of the transparent covering of the eyeball (bulbar conjunctiva), usually extending from the inner canthus to the border of the cornea or beyond; believed to be caused by ultraviolet radiation.

scar p. See pseudopterygium.

pterygoid (ter´ĭ-goid) Wing-shaped.

pterygopalatine (ter-ĭ-go-pal´ă-tin) Relating to the pterygoid process of the sphenoid bone and the bony palate.

ptilosis (ti-lo´sis) Loss of eyelashes.

ptomaine (to´mān) Vague term denoting a poisonous substance.

ptosed (tōst) Prolapsed.

ptosis (to´sis) **1.** A prolapse or sinking of an organ. **2.** Drooping of an upper eyelid when the eyes are open.

ptotic (tot´ik) Relating to prolapse.

ptyalin (tí´ă-lin) Enzyme present in saliva; it partially digest carbohydrates.

ptyalolith (ti´ă-lo-lith) See sialolith.

ptyalolithiasis (ti-ă-lo-lĭ-thi´ă-sis) See sialolithiasis.

ptyalolithotomy (ti-ă-lo-lĭ-thi´ă-sis) See sialolithotomy.

pubarche (pu-bar´ke) The growth of pubic hair at the beginning of puberty.

pubertal, puberal (pu´ber-tal, pu´ber-al) Relating to the onset of puberty.

pubertas (pu-ber´tas) Puberty.

p. precox See precocious puberty, under puberty.

puberty (pu´ber-te) The span of time during which, under the influence of hormones, secondary sexual characteristics develop and reproductive function is attained. Onset of puberty varies with health, genetic, and socioeconomic factors; usually, in boys it extends between the ages of 8 and 16 years, in girls between 10 and 17 years (beginning with development of breast buds and culminating with establishment of cyclic menstruation).

precocious p. Sexual maturation occurring at an abnormally early age (before 8 years of age in girls, 9 years in boys); may be caused by a variety of disease processes (e.g., brain lesions; disorders of the adrenal glands, testes, and ovaries). Also called pubertas praecox.

pubescence (pu-bes´ens) The beginning of sexual maturity.

pubescent (pu-bes´ent) One who is reaching the age of sexual maturity.

pubic (pu´bik) Relating to the pubic bone or area.

pubis (pu´bis), *pl.* **pub´es** **1.** The pubic bone. **2.** The region over the pubic bone. **3.** The hair of the pubic region.

pubomadesis (pu-bo-mă-de´sis) Loss or absence of pubic hair.

pubovesical (pu-bo-ves´ĭ-kal) Relating to the pubic bone and the bladder.

pubovesicocervical (pu-bo-ves-ĭ-ko-ser´vĭ-kal) Relating to the pubic symphysis, bladder, and uterine cervix.

pudendal (pu-den´dal) Relating to the genitals.

pudendum (pu-den´dum), *pl.* **puden´da** External genitals, especially the female genitals; the vulva.

puericulture (pu´er-ĭ-kul-chur) The care of the unborn child through attention to the health of the pregnant woman.

puerile (pu´er-il) **1.** Relating to childhood. **2.** Childish.

puerilism (pu´er-ĭ-liz-m) Second childhood.

puerpera (pu-er´per-ă) A woman who has just given

P

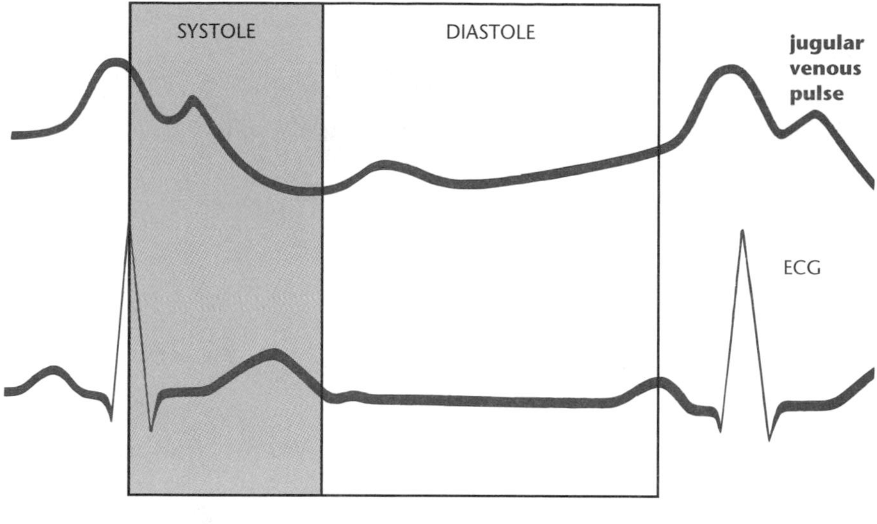

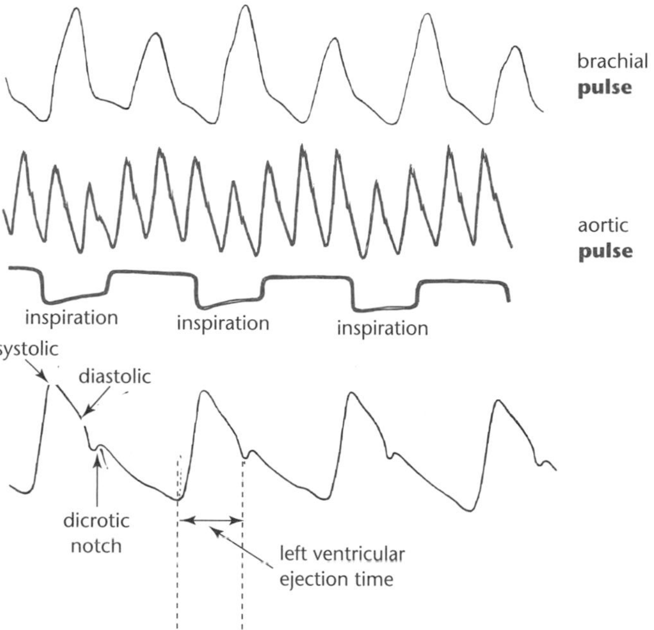

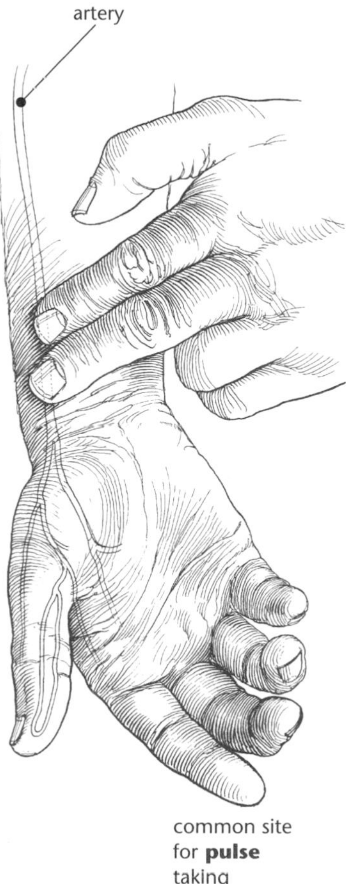

birth.

puerperal (pu-er´per-al) Relating to the first few weeks following childbirth.

puerperalism (pu-er´per-al-izm) Any disease associated with the puerperium.

puerperium (pu-er-pe´re-um) The postpartum period, from the end of labor to return of the uterus to normal size, usually from 3 to 6 weeks.

puffer (puf´er) One who exhales forcibly.

pink p. Informal term for describing the appearance of a patient with emphysema. The patient is able to maintain an adequate supply of oxygen in the bloodstream (hence the pink complexion) by constantly taking forceful short breaths (puffing). COMPARE: blue bloater, under bloater.

Pulex (pu´leks) A genus of fleas.

P. irritans The species commonly infecting and parasitizing humans and various animals; its bite produces itching.

pulicicide, pulicide (pu-lis´ĭ-sīd, pu´li-sīd) Any agent that destroys fleas.

pullulation (pul-u-la´shun) Sprouting; budding.

pulmo (pul´mo), *pl.* **pulmones** Latin for lung.

pulmonary (pul´mo-ner-e) Relating to the lungs. Also called pulmonic.

pulmonectomy (pul-mo-nek´to-me) See pneumonectomy.

pulmonic (pul-mon´ik) See pulmonary.

pulp (pulp) Any soft, moist tissue.

dental p. The vascular and innervated connective tissue contained in the pulp cavity of a tooth.

pulpal (pul´pal) Relating to the pulp or the pulp cavity of a tooth.

pulpectomy (pul-pek´to-me) Removal of the pulp tissue from the entire tooth, including the pulp in the root canals.

pulpifaction (pul-pi-fak´shun) The act of reducing to pulp.

pulpitis (pul-pi´tis) Inflammation of the pulp of a tooth.

pulpless (pulp´les) Denoting a dead or nonvital tooth, or a dental pulp that has been replaced with an inert substance.

pulpotomy (pul-pot´ŏ-me) Partial removal of the pulp from a tooth, usually the coronal portion.

pulpy (pul´pe) The condition of a solid when it is soft and moist.

pulsate (pul´sāt) To expand and contract rhythmically (e.g., the heart); to throb.

pulsatile (pul´să-tĭl) Throbbing; pulsating.

pulsation (pul-sa´shun) **1.** The act of pulsating. **2.** A single throb, as of the heart.

pulse (puls) (p) The rhythmic increase in pressure within a blood vessel produced by the increased volume of blood forced through the vessel with each contraction of the heart.

alternating p. Pulse with alternating weak and strong beats; seen in severe left ventricle dysfunction. Also called pulsus alternans.

anacrotic p., anadicrotic p. A pulse (usually palpable in the carotid arteries) in which the ascending limb of the pulse tracing has a secondary notch.

bisferious p. A pulse with two peaks, the second stronger than the first; seen in aortic regurgitation and hypertrophic cardiomyopathy. Also called pulsus bisferiens.

bigeminal p. A pulse in which two beats occur in rapid succession followed by a pause. Also called coupled pulse.

capillary p. Rhythmic blanching and reddening of capillary areas (under the nail); seen in aortic regurgitation. Also called Quincke's pulse; Quincke's sign.

Corrigan's p. Pulse with an abrupt rise followed by a rapid collapse; seen in aortic regurgitation. Also called water-hammer pulse.

coupled p. See bigeminal pulse.

jugular venous p. (JVP), jugular p. Pulsation observed in a jugular vein.

paradoxical p. A pulse that diminishes during inspiration; seen in pericardial effusion and constriction (tamponade) and in obstructive lung disease. Also called pulsus paradoxus.

plateau p. Pulse with a slowly rising pressure and sustained peak.

Quincke's p. See capillary pulse.

thready p. A small-volume pulse that is difficult to perceive.

trigeminal p. Pulse occurring in groups of three.

twice-beating p. See coupled pulse.

venous p. Pulse occurring in the veins.

water-hammer p. See Corrigan's pulse.

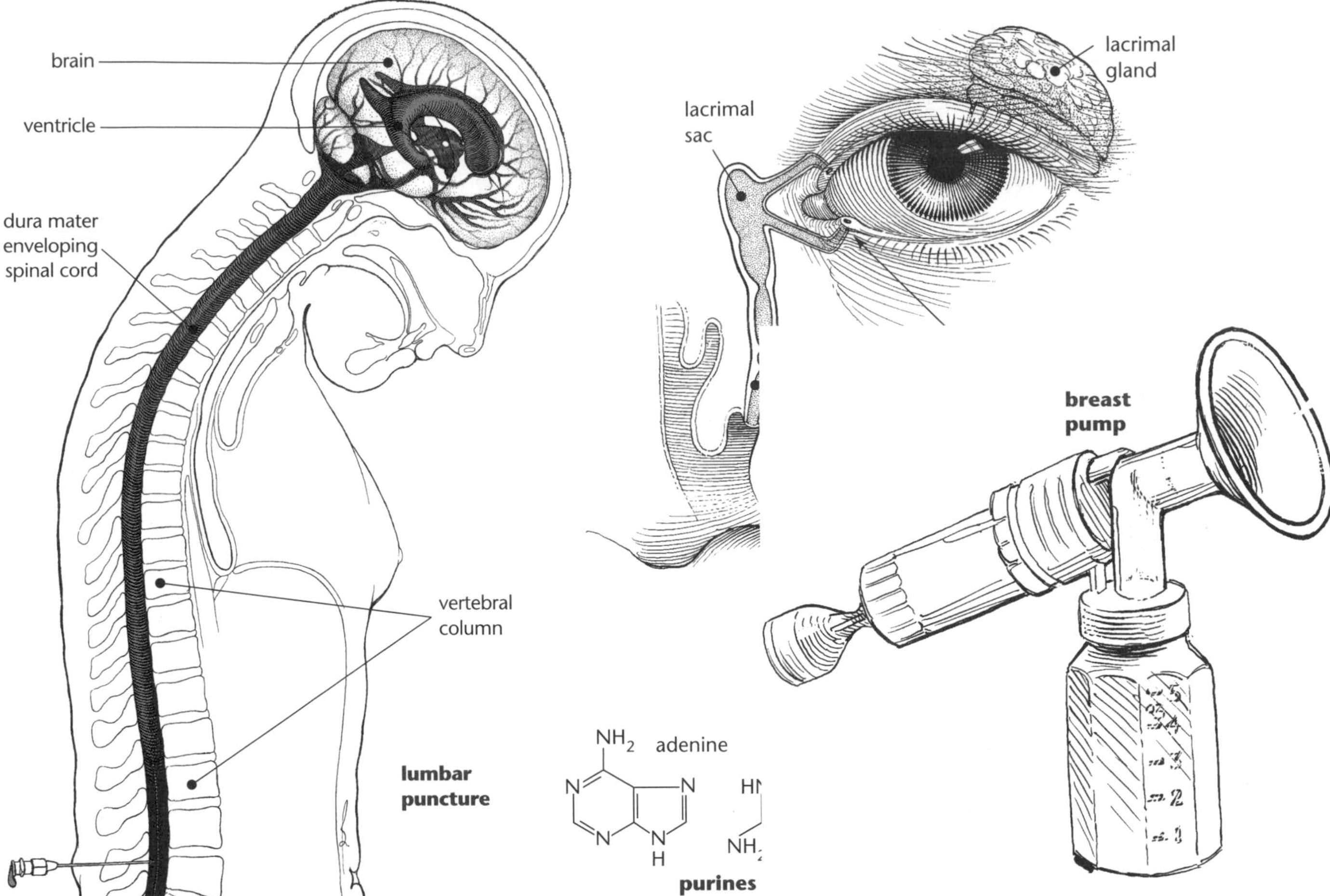

P

pulseless disease (puls´les dī-zēz´) See Takayasu's arteritis, under arteritis.
pulsimeter (pul-sim´ĕ-ter) Instrument used to measure the force and frequency of the pulse.
pulsion (pul´shun) A swelling.
pulsus (pul´sus) Latin for pulse.
p. alternans See alterating pulse, under pulse.
p. bisferiens See bisferious pulse, under pulse.
p. paradoxus See paradoxical pulse, under pulse.
p. paritus A small pulse.
p. tardus A pulse with a delayed rise and fall, as seen in aortic stenosis.
pulvinar (pul-vi´nar) The angular prominence constituting the posteromedial portion of the thalamus.
pumice (pum´is) A porous volcanic substance; in dentistry, used in powdered form to polish teeth and dentures.
pump (pump) An apparatus for transferring a liquid or gas through tubes from or to any part.
breast p. A suction pump for withdrawing milk from the breast.
Carrel-Lindbergh p. A perfusion pump by means of which an organ taken out of the body may be kept functioning. Also called Lindbergh pump.
coronary-sucker p. A pump for aspirating the small quantity of blood that enters the heart while the heart-lung machine is used during open-heart surgery.
counterpulsation p. See intra-aortic balloon pump.
hydrogen p. Molecular system for transporting protons across the cell membrane; in the stomach, it provides the hydrogen ion (H^+) to make gastric acid (HCl); in the kidney, it provides a way of removing acid from the blood. Also called proton pump.
insulin p. Battery-powered pump for infusing a continuous subcutaneous dose of insulin in the management of diabetes mellitus.
intra-aortic balloon p. (IAPB) A pump connected to a balloon that is introduced into the descending aorta to produce counterpulsation. The balloon inflates during diastole and deflates during systole, thereby increasing blood flow to coronary and peripheral vessels and diminishing impedance to left ventricular ejection. Also called counterpulsation pump.
ion p. A protein complex in the cell membrane that, using energy from the metabolic activities of the cell, transports a solute from an area of relatively low to one of higher chemical concentration.
proton p. See hydrogen pump.
stomach p. A suction pump with a flexible tube for removing the contents of the stomach in an emergency, as in a case of poisoning.
pump-oxygenator (pump´ok-sĭ-jĕ-na´tor) A mechanical apparatus that facilitates open heart surgery by temporarily substituting for both the heart (pump) and the lungs (oxygenator).
punchdrunk syndrome (punch´drunk sin´drōm) Condition seen in some boxers and alcoholics supposedly caused by repeated concussions or brief loss of consciousness; characterized by slurred speech, hand tremors, impaired concentration, and slowed thought processes.
punctate (pungk´tāt) Marked with minute dots.
punctiform (punk´tĭ-form) Of the size and shape of a very small point, usually having a diameter of less than one millimeter; used principally to describe minute colonies of bacteria.
punctum (punk´tum), *pl.* **punc´ta** A point or a spot.
lacrimal p. The minute opening of the lacrimal duct on the margin of each eyelid at the inner canthus.
puncture (pungk´chur) **1.** To pierce with a pointed instrument. **2.** A small hole made with a needle.
lumbar p. Insertion of a hollow needle into the subarachnoid space, between two of the lower lumbar vertebrae, to remove cerebrospinal fluid for diagnostic purposes, or to inject an anesthetic solution. Also called spinal puncture; spinal tap.
spinal p. See lumbar puncture.
pupil (pu´pil) (p) The circular opening in the center of the iris, through which light enters the eye.
Argyll-Robertson p. A pupil characterized by the loss of response to light, with retention of a normal response to convergence accommodation.
fixed p. One that is unresponsive to all stimuli.
tonic p. A larger than normal pupil that contracts slowly, or not completely, in response to light stimulation; associated with loss of tendon reflexes due to degeneration of postganglionic nerve fibers, which supply the sphincter muscle of the iris.
pupillary (pu´pĭ-ler-e) Relating to the pupil.
pupillography (pu-pi-log´ră-fe) The recording of pupillary reactions to light stimuli.
pupillometer (pu-pĭ-lom´ĕ-ter) An instrument for measuring the diameter of the pupil.
pupillometry (pu-pil-lom´ĕ-tre) Measurement of the pupil of the eye.
pupillomotor (pu-pĭ-lo-mo´tor) Relating to motor activity affecting the size of the pupil; specifically, denoting the motor nerve fibers supplying the iris.
pupilloplegia (pu-pĭ-lo-ple´jă, pu-pĭ-lo-ple´je-ă) Slow or absent response of the pupil to a light stimulus.
pupillostatometer (pu-pĭ-lo-stă-tom´ĕ-ter) Instrument for measuring the distance between the pupils of the eyes.
pure (pūr) Free from contamination; unadulterated.
purebred (pūr´brĕd) An animal derived from a line subjected to inbreeding.
purgation (pur-ga´shun) Vigorous evacuation of the bowels effected by a cathartic medicine (purgative). Also called catharsis.
purgative (pur´gă-tiv) See cathartic.
purge (purj) **1.** To induce evacuation of the bowels. **2.** Any agent having such properties. **3.** To eliminate subpopulations of cells from bone marrow after it has been removed for transplantation.
purine (pu´rin) The base of a group of organic compounds (uric acid compounds), known as purines or purine bases; when synthetically produced, it is a colorless crystalline compound; it is not known to exist as such in nature.
purpura (pur´pu-ră) Spontaneous bleeding in the subcutaneous tissues, mucous membranes or serous lining of intestinal organs appearing as purple patches on the surface.
anaphylactoid p. See Henoch-Schönlein purpura.
annular telangiectatic p. Purpura marked by lesions (usually limited to the lower extremities) appearing as circular pigmented areas with a yellowish necrosed center. Also called Majocchi's

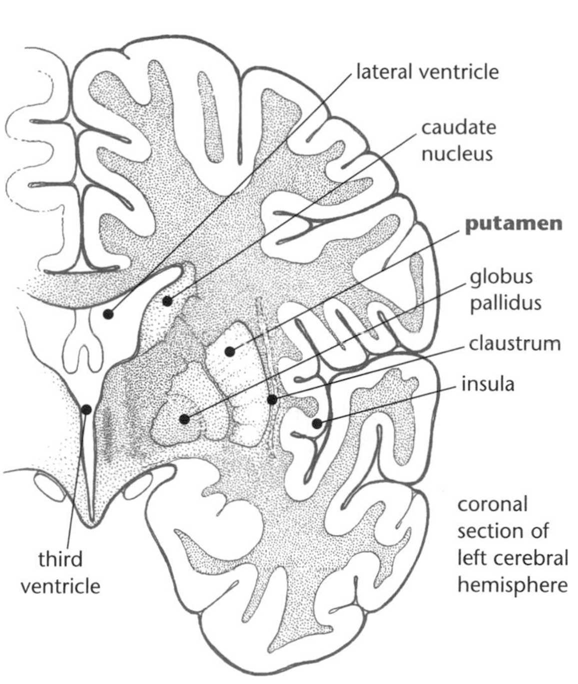

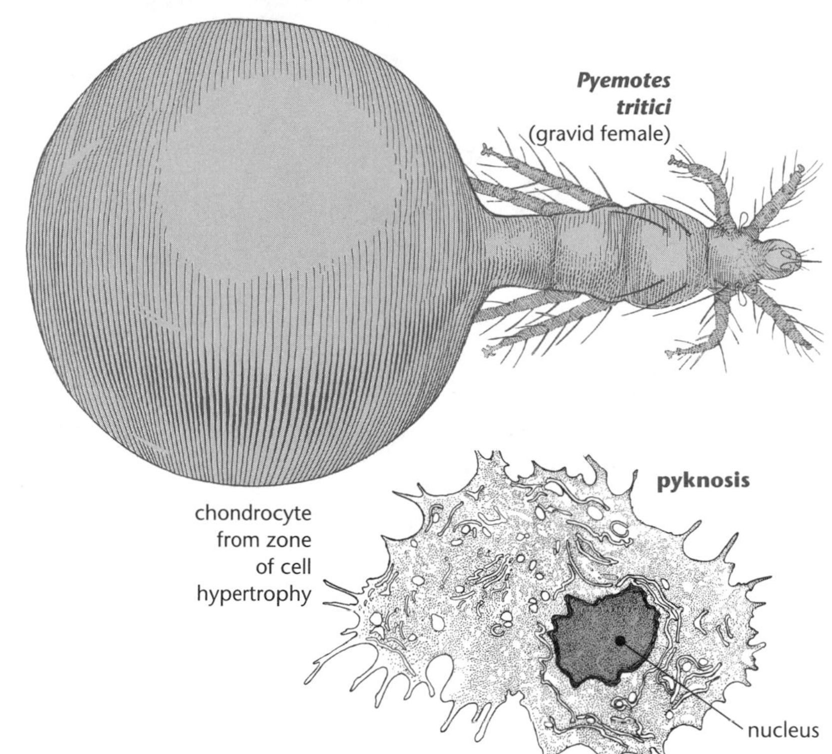

disease.

Henoch-Schönlein p. Purpura, seen especially in children and young adults, associated with gastrointestinal symptoms, joint pains, and acute glomerulonephritis; the appearance of cutaneous lesions (most common on the extremities) is preceded by a pinprick itchy sensation. Also called Schönlein's disease; anaphylactoid purpura; rheumatic purpura.

idiopathic thrombocytopenic p. (ITP) Purpura associated with immune destruction of blood platelets. *Acute idiopathic thrombocytopenic p.*, a self-limited disorder seen mainly in children after a viral infection (e.g., rubella, infectious mononucleosis). *Chronic idiopathic thrombocytopenic p.*, a long-standing disorder with multiple relapses and remissions seen in adults, mostly women of childbearing age. Also called thrombocytopenic purpura.

rheumatic p. See Henoch-Schönlein purpura.

thrombocytopenic p. See idiopathic thrombocytopenic purpura.

thrombotic thrombocytopenic p. (TTP) A severe and frequently fatal disorder characterized by a low platelet count in the blood and blood clot formation in the terminal arterioles and capillaries of many organs; other findings may include azotemia, hemolytic anemia, hypertension, and central nervous system symptoms.

purpuric (pur-pu′rik) Relating to purpura.

purpuriferous (pur-pu-rif′er-us) Forming the visual purple or rhodopsin.

purulence, purulency (pu′roo-lens, pu′roo-len-se) The condition of being purulent.

purulent (pu′roo-lent) Containing or producing pus.

pus (pus) A thick, viscous, yellowish fluid, product of inflammation, composed chiefly of dead white blood cells (leukocytes) and a thin liquid (liquor puris), and often the microbiologic agent responsible for the inflammation.

cheesy p. The thick, nearly solid pus of a tuberculous abscess.

pustular (pus′chū-lar) Characterized by pustules.

pustulation (pus-chū-la′shun) Formation of pustules.

pustule (pus′chūl) A small elevation of the skin containing pus.

malignant p. See cutaneous anthrax, under anthrax.

pustuliform (pus′chū-li-form) Resembling a pustule.

pustulosis (pus-chū-lo′sis) A pustular eruption.

putamen (pu-ta′men) A thick, convex, dark gray mass in the brain between the insular cortex laterally and the globus pallidus and the internal capsule medially.

putrefaction (pu-trĕ-fak′shun) **1.** Decomposition of organic matter, especially proteins, by the action of bacteria, resulting in the formation of foul-smelling compounds. **2.** Decomposed matter.

putrefactive (pu-trĕ-fak′tiv) Causing decomposition of organic matter.

putrefy (pu′trĕ-fi) To decompose or decay.

putrescence (pu-tres′ens) Rottenness.

putrid (pu′trid) Decayed; rotten.

PUVA Acronym for oral administration of psoralen followed by long wavelength ultraviolet light (UVA); a form of photochemotherapy for the treatment of psoriasis.

pyarthrosis (pi-ar-thro′sis) The presence of pus in a joint cavity.

pycnidium (pik-nid′e-um), *pl.* **pycnid′ia** A flask-shaped or round spore fruit of various imperfect fungi; it contains conidia.

pyelectasis (pi-ĕ-lak′tă-sis) Dilatation of the kidney pelvis.

pyelectomy (pi-ĕ-lek′tō-me) Surgical removal of the redundant portion of a greatly distended kidney pelvis.

pyelitis (pi-ĕ-li′tis) Outmoded term for pyelonephritis.

pyelocaliectasis (pi-ĕ-lo-kal-e-ek′tă-sis) See caliectasis.

pyelocaliceal (pi-ĕ-lo-kal-ĭ-se′al) Relating to the kidney pelvis and calices. Also spelled pyelocalyceal.

pyelocystitis (pi-ĕ-lo-sis-tī′tis) Inflammation of the kidney pelvis and the bladder.

pyelogram (pi′e-lo-gram) An x-ray image of the kidney pelvis and the ureter.

pyelography (pi-ĕ-log′ră-fe) The making of x-ray images of the ureter and the kidney pelvis.

antegrade p. See antegrade urography, under urography.

intravenous p. (IVP) See intravenous urography, under urography.

retrograde p. See retrograde urography, under urography.

pyelolithotomy (pi-ĕ-lo-lĭ-thot′ŏ-me) Surgical removal of a stone from the pelvis of the kidney.

pyeloneostomy (pi-ĕ-lo-ne-os′tŏ-me) The division and reimplantation of a ureter for the improvement of kidney drainage.

pyelonephritis (pi-ĕ-lo-nĕ-fri′tis) Inflammation of the kidney, especially of the kidney pelvis and calices. Formerly called pyelitis.

acute p. Active pyogenic infection of the kidney.

chronic p. Disease of the kidney thought to result from scarring from previous bacterial infections.

xanthogranulomatous p. A rare form of chronic pyelonephritis in which the kidney shows xanthogranulomas with lipid-containing foam cells, multinucleated giant cells, lymphocytes, and plasma cells.

pyelonephrolithotomy (pi-ĕ-lo-nĕ-fro-lĭ-thot′ŏ-me) The removal of kidney stones by combining an incision in the kidney pelvis with one in the cortex.

pyeloplasty (pi′ĕ-lo-plas-te) Plastic repair of the kidney pelvis either to improve drainage or to reduce its size.

pyeloplication (pi-ĕ-lo-pli-ka′shun) An outmoded operation for reducing the size of the kidney pelvis when abnormally dilated.

pyeloscopy (pi-ĕ-los′ko-pe) Fluoroscopic examination of the kidney pelvis after introduction of a radiopaque solution through the ureter or intravenously.

pyelostomy (pi-ĕ-los′tŏ-me) Surgical formation of an opening into the pelvis of the kidney.

pyelotomy (pi-ĕ-lot′ŏ-me) Incision into the kidney pelvis.

pyeloureterectasis (pi-ĕ-lo-u-re-ter-ek′tă-sis) Dilatation of kidney pelvis and ureter.

pyemesis (pi-em′ĕ-sis) The vomiting of pus-containing material.

pyemia (pi-e′me-ă) A form of septicemia in which there is a general secondary infection with formation of multiple abscesses in several areas of the body. Also called metastatic infection.

pyemic (pi-e′mik) Afflicted with pyemia.

Pyemotes tritici (pi-ĕ-mo′tez tri-tī′kī) A soft bodied mite that is a common parasite of insect larvae in stored grain, straw, or hay; it frequently burrows in the skin of people who are in contact with such products, causing an itchy skin rash. The young female has an elongated body that becomes greatly distended when gravid; the fertilized eggs are retained in her abdomen where they hatch and mature, and are then discharged. Also called hay mite; grain itch mite.

pyesis (pi-e′sis) Suppuration.

pygmyism (pig′me-izm) See primordial dwarfism, under dwarfism.

pyknic (pik′nik) Having a short, stocky, well rounded body build with ample body cavities.

pyknomorphous (pik-no-mor′fus) Having the stainable elements closely packed; said of a cell.

pyknosis (pik-no′sis) Condensation and shrinking of a cell nucleus, e.g., during maturation of a red blood cell prior to ejection of the nucleus from the cell, and in any cell necrosis.

pyla (pi′lă) The opening between the third ventricle of the brain and the cerebral aqueduct (aqueduct of Sylvius).

pylemphraxis (pi-lem-frak′sis) Obstruction of the portal vein.

P

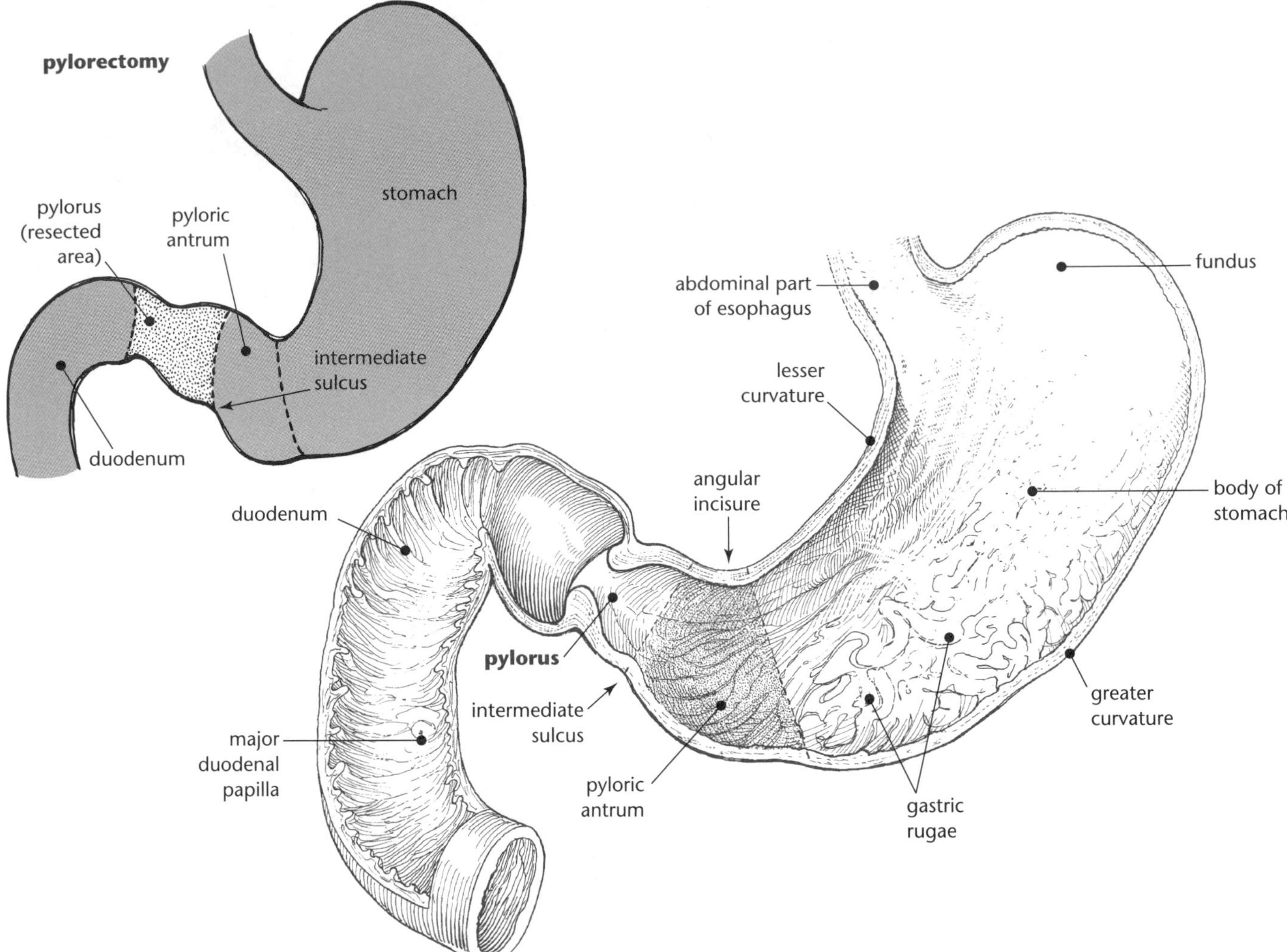

pylephlebectasia (pi-le-fle-bek´tă-sis) Dilatation of the portal vein.
pylephlebitis (pi-le-fle-bi´tis) Inflammation of the portal vein or its branches.
pylethrombophlebitis (pi-le-throm-bo-fle-bi´tis) Inflammation and thrombosis of the portal vein.
pylethrombosis (pi-le-throm-bo´sis) Thrombosis of the portal vein or its branches.
pylic (pi´lik) Relating to the portal vein.
pylon (pi´lon) A temporary artificial leg.
pyloralgia (pi-lo-ral´je-ă) Pain in the pyloric area of the stomach.
pylorectomy (pi-lo-rek´to-me) Removal of the pylorus.
pyloric (pi-lor´ik) Relating to the pylorus.
pyloric-channel syndrome (pi-lor´ik-chan´el sin´drōm) A syndrome characterized by inflammation of the pylorus and the prepyloric region with muscle hypertrophy and narrowing of the pyloric canal, resulting in pyloric obstruction.
pyloristenosis (pi-lor-e-stĕ-no´sis) See pyloric stenosis, under stenosis.
pyloritis (pi-lo-ri´tis) Inflammation of the pyloric area of the stomach.
pylorogastrectomy (pi-lo-ro-gas-trek´tŏ-me) Removal of the pyloric portion of the stomach.
pyloromyotomy (pi-lo-ro-mi-ot´ŏ-me) Surgical splitting of the pyloric muscle for the treatment of pyloric stenosis, a condition occasionally seen in the newborn.
pyloroplasty (pi-lor´o-plas-te) Longitudinal incision of the pylorus and a transverse closure, performed especially to enlarge a constricted pylorus due to peptic ulcers.
pylorospasm (pi-lor´o-spaz-m) Spasm of the pylorus or the pyloric area of the stomach; in adults, usually associated with nearby duodenal or gastric ulcer or severe gastritis.
pylorotomy (pi-lo-rot´ŏ-me) Surgical incision of the pylorus.
pylorus (pi-lor´us) The opening between the stomach and duodenum.
pyocele (pi´o-sēl) Distention of a body cavity due to accumulation of pus.
pyocephalus (pi-o-sef´ă-lus) The presence of a purulent fluid within the skull.
pyochezia (pi-o-ke´ze-ă) Discharge of pus with the stools.
pyococcus (pi-o-kok´us) A pus-producing microorganism (e.g., *Streptococcus pyogenes*).
pyocolpos (pi-o-kol´pos) Accumulation of pus in the vagina.
pyocyanic (pi-o-si-an´ik) Relating to blue pus or to the bacillus that produces it (*Pseudomonas aeruginosa*).
pyocyanin (pi-o-si´ă-nin) An antibiotic substance obtained from the bacillus *Pseudomonas aeruginosa*.
pyocyst (pi´o-sist) A pus-containing cyst.
pyoderma, pyodermia (pi-o-der´mă, pi-o-der´me-ă) Any pus-producing skin disease.
p. gangrenosum Chronic ulcerations associated with a variety of systemic diseases (e.g., ulcerative colitis, rheumatoid arthritis).
pyogen (pi´o-jen) Anything that causes pus formation.
pyogenesis (pi-o-jen´ĕ-sis) The formation of pus. Also called pyopoiesis.
pyogenic (pi-o-jen´ik) Producing pus.
pyohemothorax (pi-o-he-mo-tho´raks) The presence of pus and blood in the pleural cavity.
pyoid (pi´oid) Resembling pus. Also called puriform.
pyometra (pi-o-me´tră) Accumulation of pus in the uterus.
pyometritis (pi-o-me-tri´tis) Inflammation of the wall of the uterus with accumulation of pus in the uterine cavity.
pyomyositis (pi-o-mi-o-si´tis) Condition marked by the formation of single or multiple deep-seated abscesses in voluntary muscles; usually caused by *Staphylococcus aureus*.
pyonephrolithiasis (pi-o-nef-ro-lĭ-thi´ă-sis) The presence of pus and stones in the kidney.
pyonephrosis (pi-o-nĕ-fro´sis) Distention of the calices and pelvis of the kidney with pus.
pyo-ovarium (pi´o o-va´re-um) An ovarian abscess.
pyopericarditis (pi-o-per-ĭ-kar-di´tis) Suppurative inflammation of the sac enveloping the heart (pericardium).
pyopericardium (pi-o-per-ĭ-kar´de-um) Accumulation of pus in the sac enveloping the heart (pericardium).
pyoperitonitis (pi-o-per-ĭ-to-ni´tis) Suppurative inflammation of the peritoneum.
pyophthalmia, pyophthalmitis (pi-of-thal´me-ă, pi-of-thal-mi´tis) Suppurative inflammation of the eye, especially the conjunctiva.
pyophysometra (pi-o-fi-so-me´tră) Accumulation of gas and pus in the uterine cavity.
pyopneumocholocystitis (pi-o-nu-mo-ko-le-sis-ti´tis) Distention of an inflamed gallbladder with gas and pus; caused by gas-producing organisms or by entry of air from the intestine through the biliary tree.
pyopneumopericardium (pi-o-nu-mo-per-ĭ-kar´de-um) The presence of pus and gas in the sac enveloping the heart (pericardium).
pyopneumoperitoneum (pi-o-nu-mo-per-ĭ-to-ne´um) The presence of pus and gas in the peritoneal cavity.
pyopneumothorax (pi-o-nu-mo-tho´raks) The presence of pus and air between the two layers of the pleura (pleural cavity). Also called pneumopyothorax.
pyopoiesis (pi-o-poi-e´sis) Formation of pus. Also called pyogenesis.
pyopoietic (pi-o-poi-et´ik) Pus-producing.
pyoptysis (pi-op´tĭ-sis) Spitting of pus.
pyorrhea (pi-o-re´ă) See periodontitis.
pyosalpingitis (pi-o-sal-pin-ji´tis) Suppurative inflammation of a uterine tube.
pyosalpingo-oophoritis (pi-o-sal-ping´go o-of-

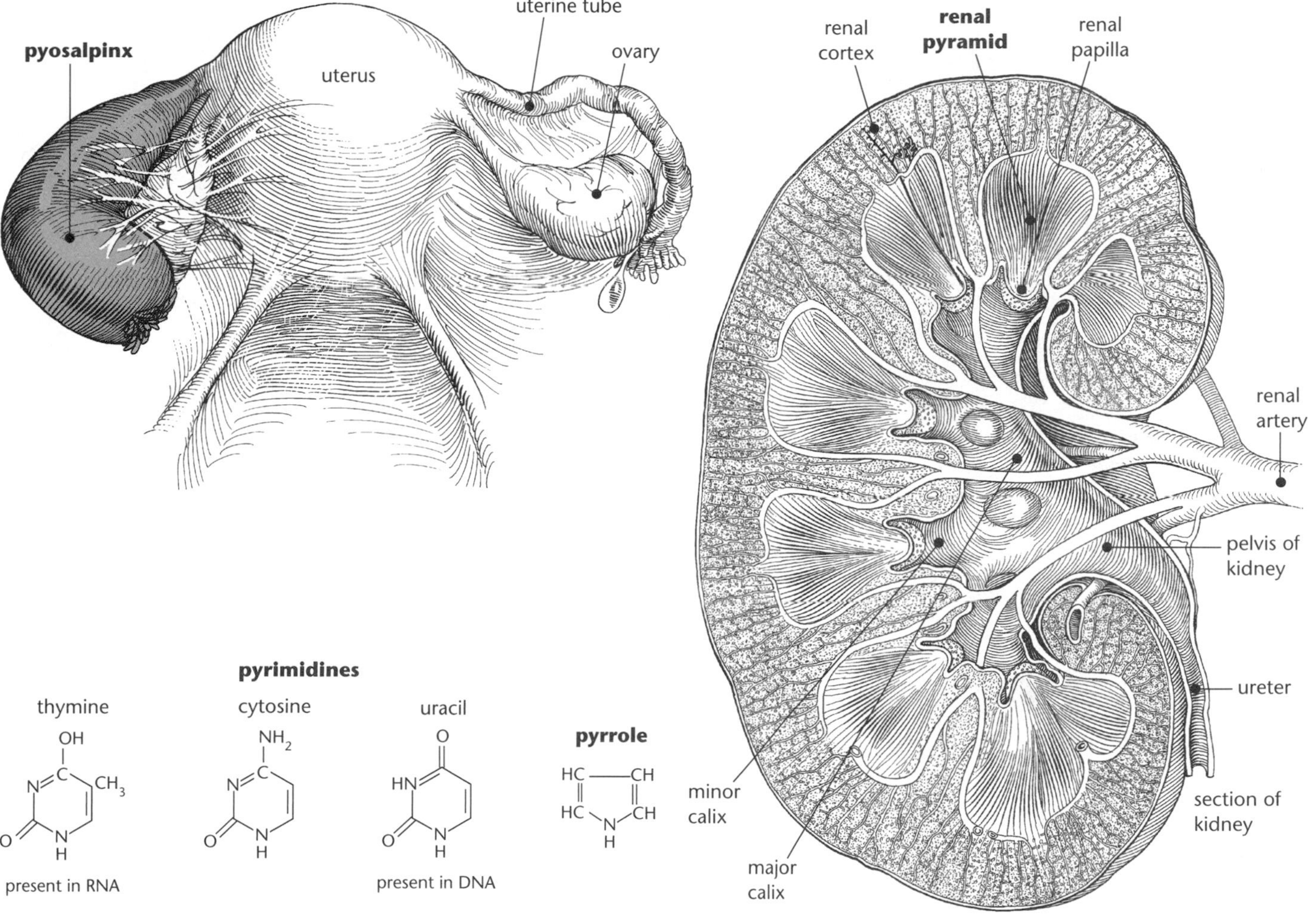

P

ŏ-ri´tis) Suppurative inflammation of a fallopian (uterine) tube and the adjacent ovary.
pyosalpinx (pi-o-sal´pinks) Accumulation of pus in the fallopian (uterine) tube.
pyosis (pi´o-sis) Suppuration.
pyostatic (pi-o-stat´ik) Denoting an agent that arrests the formation of pus.
pyoureter (pi-o-u-re´ter) Pus in a ureter.
pyramid (pēr´ă-mid) Any of numerous anatomic structures that are pyramidal or cone-shaped.
cerebellar p. The central portion of the inferior vermis of the cerebellum between the uvula and tuber. Also called pyramid of vermis.
p. of kidney See renal pyramid.
p. of light See cone of light, under cone.
malpighian p. See renal pyramid.
p. of medulla oblongata Either of two wedge-shaped prominences of longitudinal nerve fibers on the anterior surface of the medulla oblongata, on either side of the anterior median fissure.
renal p. One of a number of pyramidal masses formed by the medullary substance of the kidney, containing part of the secreting and collecting tubules; the apex projects into the minor calix. Also called malpighian pyramid; pyramid of kidney.
p. of thyroid gland See pyramidal lobe of thyroid gland, under lobe.
p. of vermis See cerebellar pyramid.
pyramidal (pĭ-ram´ĭ-dal) Relating to or having the shape of a pyramid; said of certain anatomic structures.
pyrectic (pi-rek´tik) Relating to or causing fever.
pyretogenesis (pi-rĕ-to-jen´ĕ-sis) The causation of fever.
pyretogenetic (pi-rĕ-to-jĕ-net´ik) Relating to pyretogenesis.
pyretotherapy (pi-rĕ-to-ther´ă-pe) See fever therapy, under therapy.
pyrexia (pi-rek´se-ă) See fever.
pyridine (pēr´ĭ-dēn) A colorless, flammable liquid, C_5H_5N, used in the preparation of vitamins and drugs, as a solvent, and as a denaturant of alcohol.
pyridoxal phosphate (pēr-ĭ-dok´sal fos´fāt) A vitamin derivative or coenzyme essential to many reactions of amino acid metabolism (e.g., transamination, decarboxylation, racemization).
pyridoxine (pēr-ĭ-dok´sēn) One of the active forms of vitamin B_6. Deficiency occurs in alcoholism, in pregnancy, and when taking certain drugs (e.g., oral contraceptives).
pyrimethamine (pēr-ĭ-meth´ă-mēn) An antimalarial agent.
pyrimidine (pĭ-rim´ĭ-dēn) The fundamental substance of several organic bases, some of which are components of nucleic acid.
pyrogallol (pi-ro-gal´ol) Pyrogallic acid, $C_6H_3(OH)_3$; used in the treatment of skin disorders (e.g., psoriasis, ringworm).
pyrogen (pi´ro-jen) A fever-producing agent.
pyrogenic (pi-ro-jen´ik) **1.** Causing fever. **2.** Generating heat.
pyroligneous (pi-ro-lig´ne-us) Relating to or obtained from the destructive distillation of wood.
pyrolysis (pi-rol´ĭ-sis) Chemical change induced by heat.
pyromania (pi-ro-ma´ne-ă) Compulsion to set fires.
pyrometer (pi-rom´ĕ-ter) An electric thermometer for measuring extremely high temperatures.
pyronin (pi´ro-nin) A basic red dye used in histologic stains.
pyrophobia (pi-ro-fo´be-ă) Abnormal fear of fire.
pyrophosphatase (pi-ro-fos´fă-tās) Any enzyme that splits pyrophosphates.
pyrophosphate (pi-ro-fos´fāt) (PP) A salt of pyrophosphoric acid.
pyrophosphoric acid (pi-ro-fos-for´ik as´id) A water-soluble, crystalline substance, $H_4P_2O_7$, obtained by heating phosphoric acid.
pyrosis (pi-ro´sis) See heartburn.
pyrotherapy (pi-ro-ther´ă-pe) See fever therapy, under therapy.
pyrotic (pi-rot´ik) **1.** Relating to heartburn. **2.** Caustic.
pyrrole (pēr´ol) A toxic heterocyclic compound with an odor suggestive of chloroform; the parent of many biologically important natural compounds (e.g., bile pigments, porphyrins, chlorophyll).
pyruvate (pi´roo-vāt) A salt or ester of pyruvic acid.
p. kinase (PK) Enzyme that promotes the transfer of phosphate from phosphoenolpyruvate to ADP, forming ATP and pyruvate. Deficiency of pyruvate kinase in red blood cells is the cause of an autosomal recessive hemolytic anemia.
pyruvic acid (pi-roo´vik as´id) A colorless liquid, $CH_3COCOOH$, with an odor similar to that of acetic acid; an intermediate product in the metabolism of carbohydrate.
pyrvinium pamoate (pir-vin´e-um pam´o-āt) Compound used in treating pinworm infections.
pyuria (pi-u´re-ă) The presence of pus in the urine.

Q

quack (kwak) One who fraudulently claims to have medical or dental capability to diagnose and treat disease and who generally makes extravagant claims as to the effects achieved by the worthless treatment he provides; a charlatan.
quackery (kwak´er-e) The practice of a quack.
quadrant (kwod´rant) (Q) **1.** One-quarter of a circle. **2.** In anatomy, one of the four regions into which roughly circular areas of the body are divided for descriptive purposes (e.g., tympanic membrane, fundus of the eye, abdomen).
quadrantal (kwod-ran´tal) Relating to a quadrant.
quadrantanopsia (kwod-rant-ă-nop´se-ă) Blindness in approximately a quarter of the visual field. Also called quadrantic hemianopsia.
crossed binasal q. Blindness of the lower nasal quarter of the visual field of one eye and the upper nasal of the other eye.
crossed temporal q. Blindness of the lower temporal quarter of the visual field of one eye and the upper temporal of the other eye.
lower heteronymous q. Blindness of either both lower nasal or both lower temporal quarters of the visual fields.
upper heteronymous q. Blindness of both upper nasal or both upper temporal quarters of the nasal fields.
quadrantectomy (kwod-ran-tek´to-me) Removal of one quarter of an organ, especially a breast, as a treatment for a tumor.
quadrate (kwod´rāt) Square; four-sided.
quadratus (kwod-ra´tus) Denoting certain muscles that have a roughly square shape.
quadribasic (kwod-rĭ-ba´sik) Referring to an acid that has four replaceable hydrogen atoms.
quadriceps (kwod´rĭ-seps) Having four heads, as some muscles.
quadrigeminal (kwod-rĭ-jem´ĭ-nal) Occurring in a group of four; fourfold; having four parts.
quadrilocular (kwod-rĭ-lok´u-lar) Having four cavities or chambers.
quadripara (kwod-rip´ă-ră) A woman who has given birth to four children.
quadriplegia (kwod-rĭ-ple´jă, kwod-rĭ-ple´je-ă) Paralysis of all four extremities. Also called tetraplegia.
quadriplegic (kwod-rĭ-ple´jik) One whose four limbs are paralyzed.
quadrivalent (kwod-rĭ-va´lent) Having the combining ability of four hydrogen atoms. Also called tetravalent.
quadruplet (kwod´rup-let) One of four offspring born at one birth.
quanta (kwon´tă) Plural of quantum.
quantimeter (kwon-tim´ĕ-ter) Device for measuring the quantity of x rays generated by a tube such as a Coolidge tube.
quantitative (kwon´tĭ-ta-tiv) Expressible as a quantity; involving the constituent portions of a compound.
quantity (kwon´tĭ-te) **1.** An indefinite amount. **2.** The duration, intensity, and frequency of a speech sound as distinct from its individual quality. **3.** The length of time vocal organs remain in specific positions for the production of a particular sound.
quantum (kwon´tum), *pl.* **quan´ta** **1.** A unit of radiant energy. **2.** A specified amount.
q. libet (q.l.) Latin for as much as desired.
q. sufficit (q.s.) Latin for sufficient amount or as much as suffices.
q. vis (q.v.) Latin for as much as you want.
quaque (kwa´ke) (q.) Latin for each; every.
q. die (q.d.) Latin for every day.
q. quarta hora (q.q.h.) Latin for every four hours.
quarantine (kwor´an-tēn) **1.** Restriction of freedom of movement of persons or animals that have been exposed to a communicable disease; originally the period of restriction was 40 days. **2.** Isolation of a person afflicted with a communicable disease.
quart (kwort) (qt) **1.** A measure of fluid capacity equal to two pints; one-fourth of a gallon; 32 ounces; 0.9468 liter. **2.** A unit of volume in dry measure equal to 1.201 liters.
quartan (kwor´tan) Recurring every four days, as a malarial fever; actually, the attack occurs on day one and day four, so that there is really only an interval of two days.

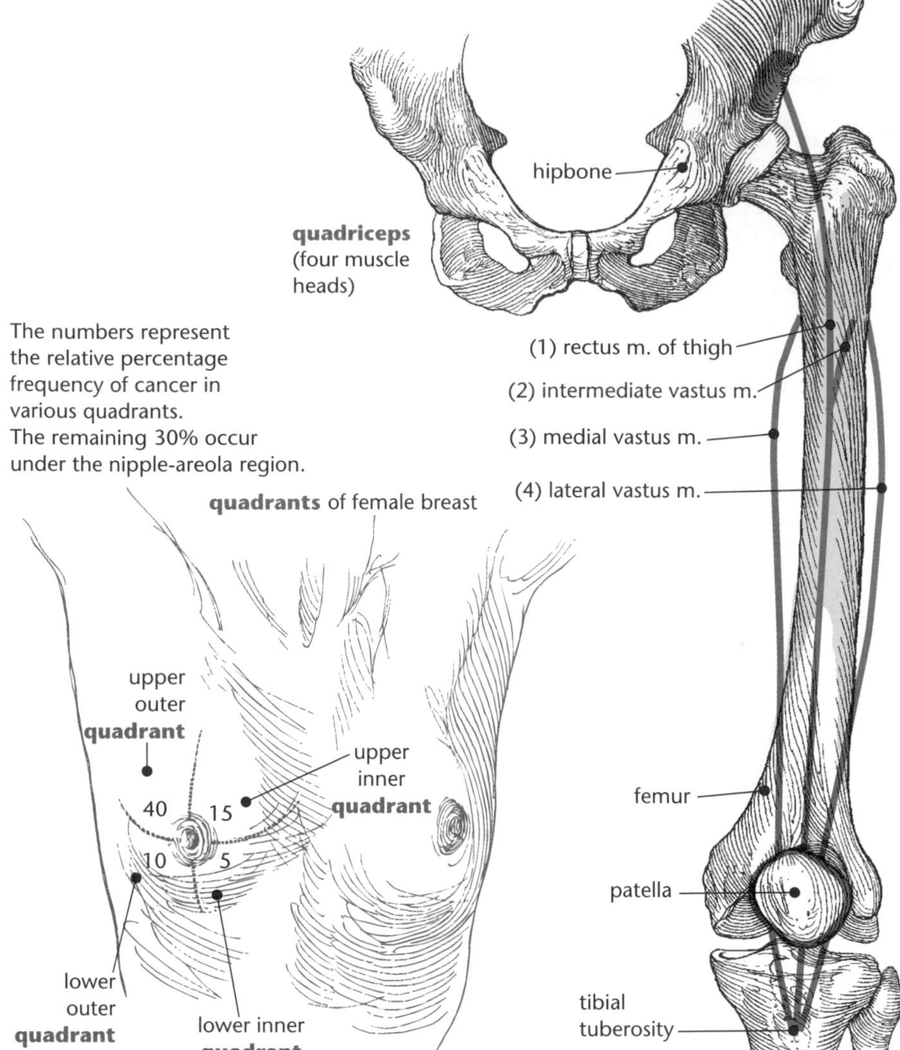

quartile (kwort´tīl) The middle of each half of a set of variables.
quartz (kwōrts) A form of silica, used in dentistry as one of three main ingredients of dental porcelain.
quasidominance (kwa-zi-dom´ĭ-nans) Direct transmission, from generation to generation, of a recessive trait occurring in inbreeding populations; it results from the mating of a homozygous affected person with a heterozygous carrier of the same recessive gene; the pedigree pattern superficially resembles that of a dominant trait, hence the name.
quater in die (q.i.d.) Latin for four times a day.
quaternary (kwă´ter-ner-e) **1.** The member of a series that is fourth in order. **2.** A chemical compound containing four different elements (e.g., $NaHSO_4$).
quenching (kwench´ing) **1.** The extinguishing or suppressing of an energy emission (e.g., heat, electrical discharge). **2.** In liquid scintillation counting, the lowering of the amount of energy recorded from the sample container.
quick (kwik) A sensitive part, painful to the touch.
quickening (kwik´en-ing) The sensation caused by the movement of the fetus within the uterus, felt by the mother for the first time about the fourth or fifth month of pregnancy.
quicksilver (kwik´sil-ver) See mercury.
quin-2 (kwin-tōō) Fluorescent compound that binds to calcium; injected into cells to measure moment-to-moment variations in intracellular calcium concentration.
quinacrine (kwin´ă-krin) A bright yellow antimalarial drug with a biologic half-life of 10 days; Atabrine®.
Quincke's sign (kwink´ez sīn) See capillary pulse, under pulse.
quinhydrone (kwin-hi´dron) A compound of equimolecular quantities of quinone and hydroquinone; $C_6H_4O_2.C_6H_4(OH)_2$; used in pH determinations.
quinidine (kwin´ĭ-din) An alkaloid from cinchona bark; used to control cardiac arrhythmias.
quinine (kwi´nīn) A white, crystalline, bitter alkaloid obtained from the bark of the cinchona tree; used in the treatment of malaria.
quininism (kwin´ĭ-niz-m) See cinchonism.
quinolones (kwin´o-lōnz) A class of broad-spectrum antibiotics used to treat a variety of bacterial infections.
quinquina (kwin-kwi´nă, kin-ke´nă) Cinchona bark from which quinine is extracted.
quinsy (kwin´ze) See peritonsillar abscess, under abscess.
quintuplet (kwin-tup´let) One of five children born of a single birth.
quod vide (kwod vī´de) (q.v.) Latin for which see; usually placed in parentheses after a cross-reference.
quotidian (kwo-tid´e-an) Recurring every day (e.g., a fever).
quotient (kwo´shent) The number of times a quantity is contained in another.
blood q. See color index, under index.
intelligence q. (IQ) The ratio of a person's attained score on a standardized test of intelligence to the expected mean score for his age, multiplied by 100.
respiratory q. (RQ) The ratio between the volume of carbon dioxide expired and the volume of oxygen consumed; it varies with the diet, but normally is about 0.82.

R

rabid (rab´id) Relating to rabies.
rabies (ra´bēz) A viral encephalitis transmitted through saliva of an infected animal; the incubation period varies from 10 days to several months; invariably fatal in man unless preventive treatment is administered. Also called hydrophobia.
racemic (ra-se´mik) **1.** Composed of clustered parts; said of glands. **2.** Denoting a chemical compound composed of equal parts of dextrorotatory and levorotatory substances, therefore incapable of rotating the plane of polarized light.
racemization (ra-sĕ-mĭ-za´shun) The chemical conversion of an optically active substance into another that is relatively, or completely, inactive.
racemose (ras´ĕ-mōs) Resembling a bunch of grapes.
rachial (ra´ke-al) Spinal.
rachicentesis (ra-ke-sen-te´sis) See lumbar puncture, under puncture.
rachidian (ra-kid´e-an) Spinal.
rachiocampsis (ra-ke-o-kamp´sis) See spinal curvature, under curvature.
rachiocentesis (ra-ke-o-sen-te´sis) See spinal puncture, under puncture.
rachiopathy (ra-ke-op´ă-the) See spondylopathy.
rachiotome (ra´ke-o-tōm) A surgical bone-cutting instrument for dividing the vertebral laminae.
rachiotomy (ra-ke-ot´ŏ-me) The operative procedure of cutting into the vertebral column.
rachischisis (ra-kis´kĭ-sis) See spondyloschisis.
rachitic (ra-kit´ik) Relating rickets.
rachitogenic (ră-kit-o-jen´ik) Causing rickets (e.g., a vitamin D-deficient diet).
rachitome (rak´i-tōm) See rachiotome.
rad (rad) Acronym for radiation absorbed dose; unit of radiation exposure expressing the absorbed dose; 1 rad represents absorption of 100 ergs of energy per gram of tissue, and is roughly equivalent to 1 roentgen.
radectomy (ra-dek´tŏ-me) Removal of the root of a tooth, or a portion of it.
radial (ra´de-al) **1.** Relating to the radius (a bone in the forearm), or to any radius. **2.** Diverging in various directions from a central point.
radial-immunodiffusion (ra´de-al-im-u-no-dĭ-fu´zhun) A method of quantifying immunoglobulins; plates of agar impregnated with various antisera to specific immunoglobulins are used as receptacles for the plasma to be tested; as the test sample immunoglobulin diffuses into the agar, a circle of precipitation forms, the diameter of which is proportional to the amount of immunoglobulin in the test sample.
radiant (ra´de-ant) **1.** Emitting heat or light rays. **2.** A central point from which rays diverge. **3.** Emitted as radiation.
radiate (ra´de-āt) **1.** To expose to radiation. **2.** To emit radiation. **3.** To diverge in all directions from a center.
radiation (ra-de-a´shun) **1.** High-speed emission and projection of energy (waves or particles). **2.** A bundle of white fibers in the brain.
background r. The measured radioactivity in a given location from sources other than the source of interest.
Cerenkov r. Light produced when high energy particles travel through a clear liquid at a velocity greater than the speed of light in that liquid.
corpuscular r. Subatomic particles of specific masses that travel in streams at various speeds (e.g., protons, electrons, neutrons, and alpha or beta particles). COMPARE: electromagnetic radiation.
electromagnetic r. Forms of energy that have no mass and travel in waves at the speed of light; they differ in wavelengths (from 10^{17} to 10^{-6} Å), frequency, and photon energy (e.g., x and gamma rays, radio and infrared waves, visible light, and ultraviolet or cosmic radiation). COMPARE: corpuscular radiation.
external r. Radiation therapy in which the radiation source (e.g., a standard orthovoltage x-ray machine) is located at a distance from the body.
"hard" r. Short wavelength radiation having high energy and the ability to penetrate deeply.

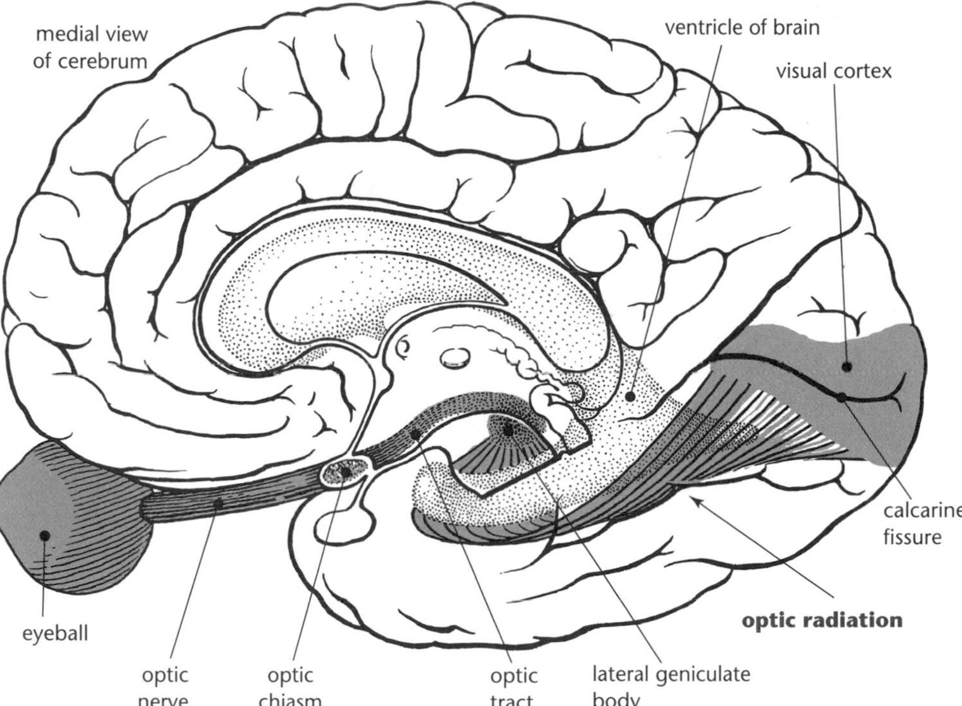

interstitial r. Local radiation in which the radiation source is placed within the tissue under treatment, usually in the form of pellets or needles.
intracavitary r. Local radiation in which the radiation source is placed in a body cavity.
intraperitoneal r. Instillation of a radioactive colloid, such as radiophosphorus (^{32}P), into the peritoneal cavity.
ionizing r. Electromagnetic radiation (e.g., x rays, gamma rays) or corpuscular radiation (e.g., protons, electrons) capable of producing electrically charged atoms (ions).
local r. Therapeutic radiation from a source in direct proximity to the tissues under treatment. See also brachytherapy.
optic r. A band of fibers in the brain passing from the lateral geniculate body of the thalamus to the cortex of the occipital lobe.
postoperative r. Radiation applied after surgery to destroy cancerous cells that may remain in the area.
preoperative r. Radiation of a cancerous growth before surgery (e.g., to shrink a large tumor to facilitate its removal.
scattered r. The change in direction of the x-ray photon as a result of collision with matter. Also called secondary radiation.
secondary r. See scattered radiation.
"soft" r. Long wavelength radiation of low penetrability.
radical (rad´ĭ-kal) **1.** A group of atoms that can pass from one compound to another without changing and that forms one of the basic parts of a molecule; in chemical formulas it is enclosed in parentheses. **2.** Treatment marked by extreme, extensive, or innovative measures.
acid r. A radical formed by an acid by loss of one or more hydrogen ions.
free r. A chemical group that has unshared electrons available for reaction (e.g., as CH_3).
radiculalgia (ră-dik-u-lal´jă, ră-dik-u-lal´je-ă) Neuralgia of the sensory root of a spinal nerve, usually due to an irritation.
radicular (ră-dik´u-lar) Relating to a root, especially a nerve or a tooth root.
radiculectomy (ră-dik-u-lek´tŏ-me) See rhizotomy.
radiculitis (ră-dik-u-li´tis) Inflammation of the portion of a spinal nerve root within the dura mater.
radiculomeningomyelitis (ră-dik-u-lo-mĕ-ning-go-mi-ĕ-li´tis) See rhizomeningomyelitis.
radiculomyelopathy (ră-dik-u-lo-mi-ĕ-lop´ă-the) See myeloradiculopathy.
radiculoneuropathy (ră-dik-u-lo-nu-rop´ă-the) Disease of the spinal nerve roots and nerves.
radiculopathy (ră-dik-u-lop´ă-the) Disease of the spinal nerve roots.

radioactive (ra-de-o-ak´tiv) Relating to radioactivity.
radioactivity (ra-de-o-ak-tiv´ĭ-te) The property, possessed by certain elements of high atomic weight, of emitting rays and subatomic particles, either due to unstable atomic nuclei or as a result of nuclear reaction.
radioautograph (ra-de-o-aw´to-graf) See autoradiograph.
radiobiology (ra-de-o-bi-ol´ŏ-je) The branch of science concerned with the effects of radiation on living tissues and with the use of radioactive isotopes.
radiocalcium (ra-de-o-kal´se-um) (^{45}Ca) Radioisotope of calcium, usually used in bone tumor localization and bone metabolism studies.
radiocarbon (ra-de-o-kar´bon) (^{14}C) Radioactive isotope of carbon used as a tracer in metabolic studies.
radiocarpal (ra-de-o-kar´pal) Relating to the radius and the carpal bones, especially the joint between the radius and the proximal row of carpal bones.
radiochemistry (ra-de-o-kem´is-tre) The study of chemical reactions of radioactive elements.
radiocinematography (ra-de-o-sin-ĕ-ma-tog´ră-fe) The technique of making motion pictures of the passage of a radiopaque substance through the internal organs as seen on x-ray examination.
radiocurable (ra-de-o-kūr´ă-bl) Susceptible to cure by irradiation; said of some cancer cells.
radiodermatitis (ra-de-o-der-mă-ti´tis) Inflammation of the skin caused by excessive exposure to x or gamma rays.
radiodontics (ra-de-o-don´tiks) The branch of dentistry that specializes in the taking and interpreting of roentgenograms of teeth and related structures.
radioelectrophysiolograph (ra-de-o-e-lek-tro-fis-ĭ-ol´o-graf) An apparatus by means of which changes in the electrical potential of brain or heart are radiotransmitted and recorded at some other site; the apparatus is carried by the patient under unrestricted movements.
radioelement (ra-de-o-el´ĕ-ment) Any radioactive element.
radioepidermitis (ra-de-o-ep-ĭ-der-mi´tis) Inflammation of the superficial layer of the skin caused by exposure to ionizing radiation.
radiofrequency (ra-de-o-fre´kwen-se) A frequency of electromagnetic radiation in the range between audio frequencies and infrared frequencies.
radiogenesis (ra-de-o-jen´ĕ-sis) The production of radioactivity.
radiogenic (ra-de-o-jen´ik) **1.** Producing rays. **2.** Produced by radioactivity.
radiogram (ra´de-o-gram) Radiograph.
radiograph (ra´de-o-graf) A processed photographic film produced by radiography. Commonly

R

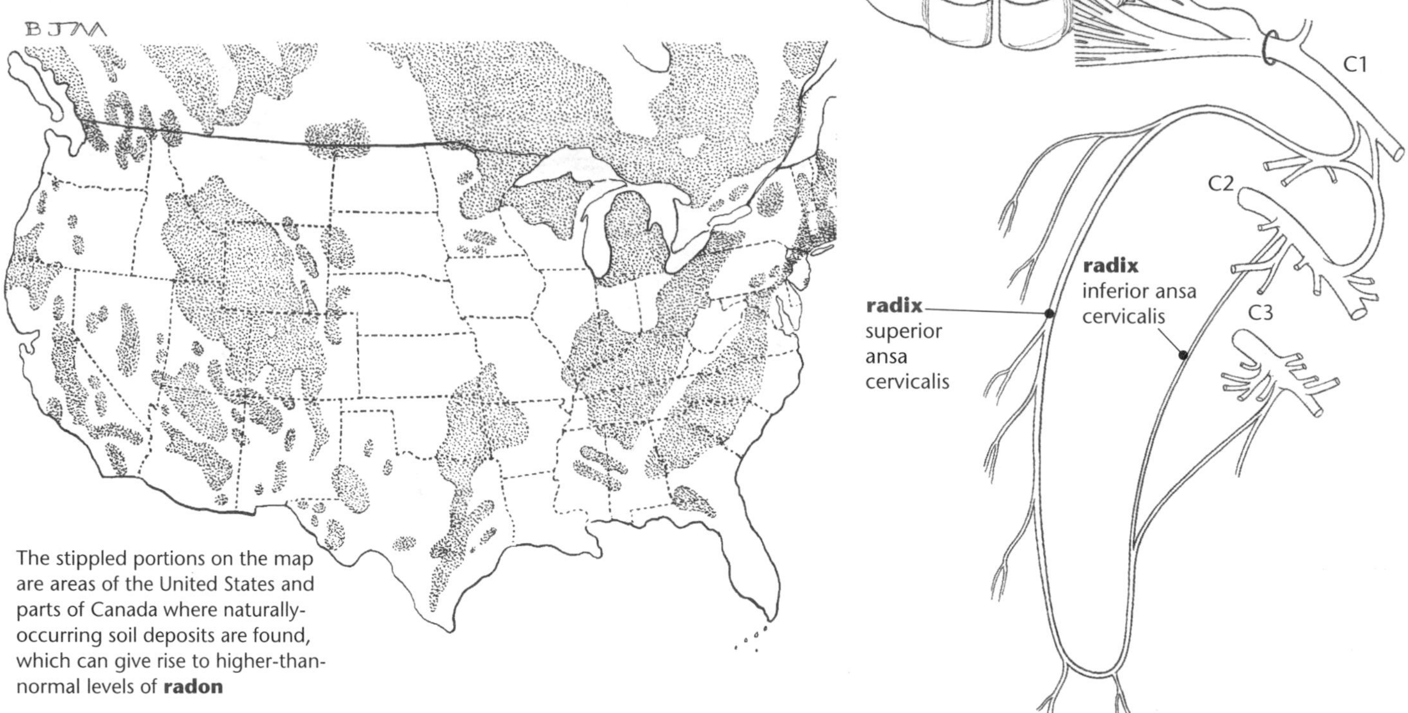

The stippled portions on the map are areas of the United States and parts of Canada where naturally-occurring soil deposits are found, which can give rise to higher-than-normal levels of **radon**

called an x-ray.

bitewing r. X-ray film adapted to show the crown and cervical third of the roots of both upper and lower teeth and the dental arches.

body-section r. See tomography.

cephalometric r. X-ray picture of the skull, including the mandible, for taking measurements.

mucosal relief r. Radiography of the lining of the rectum, made after a barium enema has been evacuated and the rectum has been distended with air; the small amount of barium remaining on the intestinal wall reveals fine details. Also called air-contrast study.

panoramic r. A radiograph showing all the teeth in one film as if the curved dental arches had been straightened into one flat plane.

sectional r. See tomography.

spot-film r. The making of several localized x-ray pictures during a fluoroscopic examination.

radiography (ra-de-og´ră-fe) The making of an image of internal structures of the body by transmitting radioactive energy (x or gamma rays) through it onto a sensitized film. Formerly called roentgenography.

radiologist (ra-de-ol´ŏ-jist) A specialist in the use of x rays and other forms of radiation in the diagnosis and treatment of disease.

radiology (ra-de-ol´ŏ-je) **1.** The science dealing with radioactive substances and radiant energy and the effects of such radiation. **2.** The medical specialty concerned with the diagnosis and treatment of disease by means of ionizing and nonionizing radiation.

radiohumeral (ra-de-o-hu´mer-al) Relating to the radius and the humerus.

radioimmunoassay (ra-de-o-im-u-no-as´a) (RIA) A method of analysis, such as determination of the concentration of substances in blood plasma, through the use of radioactive reagents.

radioimmunodiffusion (ra-de-o-im-u-no-dif-fu´zhun) The study of antigen-antibody reactions by gel diffusion using radioisotope-labeled antigen or antibody.

radioimmunoelectrophoresis (ra-de-o-im-u-no-e-lek-tro-fo-re´sis) Immunoelectrophoresis using radioisotope-labeled antigen or antibody.

radioiodinated (ra-de-o-i´o-din-a-ted) Combined or treated with radioiodine.

radioiodine (ra-de-o-i´o-dīn) A radioactive isotope of iodine; about two dozen are known, the most commonly used at present being ^{131}I and ^{125}I; used diagnostically and therapeutically in thyroid disease.

radioiron (ra-de-o-i´ern) A radioactive isotope of iron.

radioisotope (ra-de-o-i´so-tōp) An isotope of an element that is naturally or artificially radioactive.

radioligand (ra-de-o-li´gand) A radioactive-labeled substance.

radiologist (ra-de-ol´o-jist) A physician with specific training in radiology.

radiology (ra-de-ol´o-je) The science concerned with radiant energy (x rays and radioactive isotopes) and its use for the diagnosis and treatment of disease.

interventional r. The use of fluoroscopy, ultrasonography, or computed tomography (CT) as a guide to the performance of procedures carried out via catheters or needles introduced into a blood vessel or directly through the skin.

radiolucency (ra-de-o-loo´sen-se) The state of being moderately permeable to x rays or other forms of radiation.

radiometer (ra-de-om´ĕ-ter) Device for detecting and measuring radiant energy.

radiomimetic (ra-de-o-mi-met´ik) Denoting a chemical that has a destructive effect on tissues similar to that of high energy radiation (e.g., sulfur mustards, nitrogen mustards).

radionecrosis (ra-de-o-nĕ-kro´sis) Destruction of tissues by radiation.

radionuclide (ra-de-o-nu´klīd) A radioactive nuclide; a species of a nuclide with an unstable nucleus which disintegrates emitting radiant energy; may be found in a natural state or in a chemical element made radioactive by artificial means.

radiopacity (ra-de-o-pas´ĭ-te) The state of being radiopaque.

radiopaque (ra-de-o-pāk´) Impenetrable by x rays or other forms of radiation.

radiopathology (ra-de-o-pă-thol´ŏ-je) The study and treatment of conditions caused by radiation.

radiopelvimetry (ra-de-o-pel-vim´ĕ-tre) An x-ray procedure for determining the size and shape of the pelvis.

radiopharmaceutical (ra-de-o-fahr-mă-su´tĭ-kal) A radioactive pharmaceutical preparation used for diagnostic or therapeutic purposes.

radio-pharmacy (ra-de-o-fahr´mă-se) The branch of pharmacy dealing with the preparation and dispensing of radioactive drugs utilizing short-lived radioisotopes.

radioreaction (ra-de-o-re-ak´shun) A body reaction to radiation, especially of the skin.

radioreceptor (ra-de-o-re-sep´tor) A receptor on a cell surface capable of responding to such radiant energy as light or heat.

radioresistance (ra-de-o-re-zis´tans) The relative resistance of cells or organisms to the injurious action of radiation.

radioscopy (ra-de-os´ko-pe) See fluoroscopy.

radiosensitivity (ra-de-o-sen-sĭ-tiv´ĭ-te) Relative susceptibility of biologic tissues or substances to the action of radiation.

radiostereoscopy (ra-de-o-ster-e-os´ko-pe) Simultaneous observation of two x-ray pictures taken at slightly different angles, so that the viewed area appears three-dimensional.

radiotherapist (ra-de-o-ther´ă-pist) A physician who specializes in radiotherapy.

radiotherapy (ra-de-o-ther´ă-pe) See radiation therapy, under therapy.

radiothermy (ra-de-o-ther´me) Therapeutic use of heat from radiant sources.

radiotoxemia (ra-de-o-tok-se´me-ă) See radiation sickness, under sickness.

radiotransparent (ra-de-o-trans-par´ent) Allowing the passage of radiant energy.

radioulnar (ra-de-o-ul´nar) Relating to the radius and the ulna.

radium (ra´de-um) A radioactive metallic element that emits alpha, beta, and gamma radiation and a radioactive gas called radon; it has a half-life of 1,590 years; symbol Ra, atomic number 88, atomic weight 226.05; in medicine, it is used in the treatment of some malignancies.

radius (ra´de-us), *pl.* **ra´dii** (r) **1.** The smaller of the two bones of the forearm, on the side of the thumb. **2.** A straight line extending from the center to the periphery of a circle.

radix (ra´diks), *pl.* **ra´dices** Latin for root; applied to the beginning or primary portion of a structure (e.g., of a nerve at its origin from the spinal cord).

radon (ra´don) A colorless gas emanating from radium, with a half-life of about four days; it is a natural isotope produced during the radioactive decay of radium; symbol Rn, atomic number 86, atomic weight 222.

raffinose (raf´ĭ-nōs) $C_{18}H_3O_{16}.5H_2O$; a sugar occurring in cottonseed meal and in sugar beets, composed of D-galactose, D-glucose, and D-fructose. Also called melitose.

rage (rāj) Intense, violent anger.

sham r. An outburst of motor activity in an animal whose cerebral hemispheres have been removed, characterized by manifestations of fear and anger on slight provocation and accompanied by struggling, piloerection, dilatation of pupils, and increase in blood pressure.

ragweed (rag´wēd) Weed of the genus *Ambrosia*; some species produce abundant pollen that is a hazard to many hay fever sufferers, especially the species

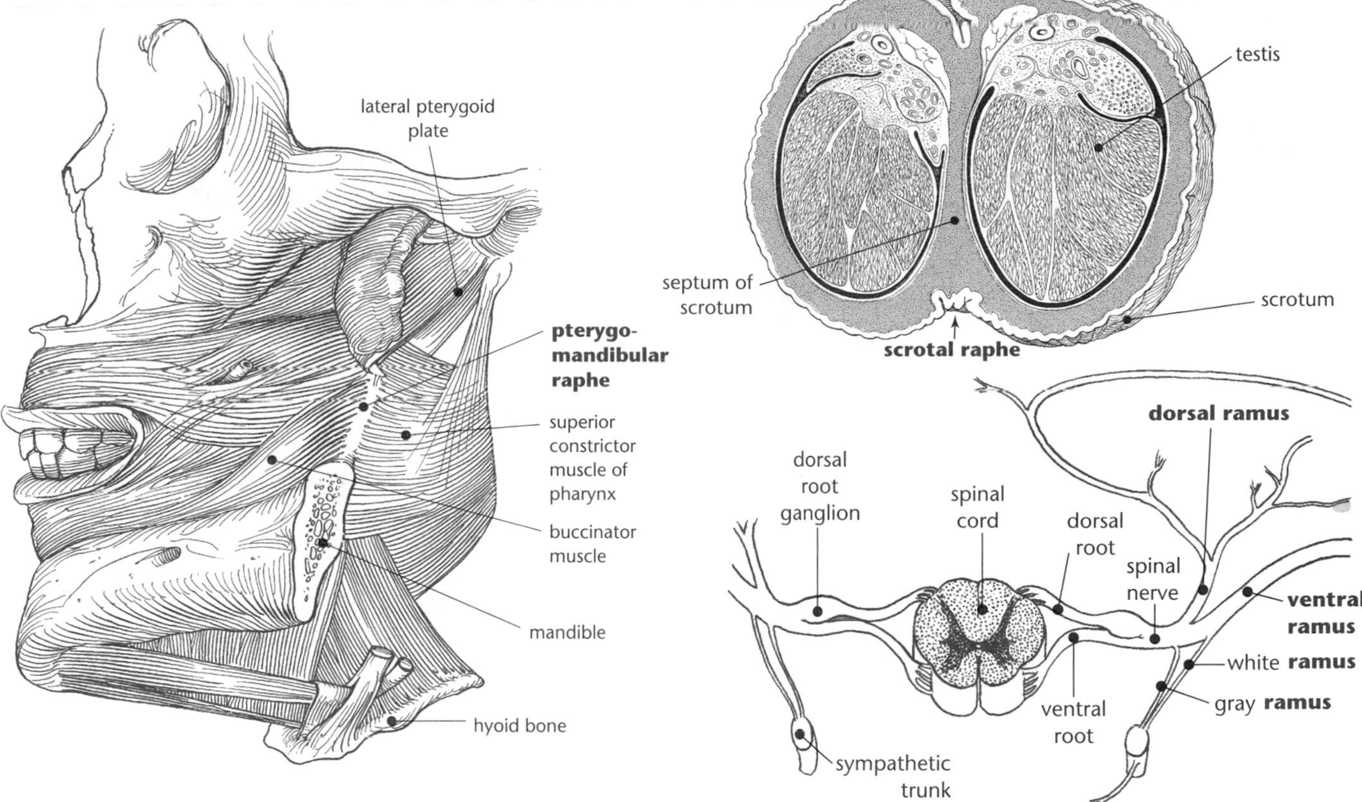

A. artemisiifolia (common ragweed), *A. trifida* (giant ragweed) or *A. psilostachya* (Western ragweed).

rale (rahl) Abnormal sound heard on auscultation of the chest, originating in the pulmonary airway, and usually indicating disease of the small bronchi of the lungs.

atelectatic r. A crackling sound that disappears upon deep breathing or coughing, associated with collapse of part of a lung; often noted postoperatively.

coarse r. See rhonchus.

crepitant r. A fine sound resembling the rubbing of hair between the fingers, produced by a thin secretion in the bronchioles.

dry r. A whistling or squeaking sound produced by the presence of thick, sticky secretions in the bronchial tubes or by spastic constriction of the tubes, as heard in bronchitis and asthma.

fine r. Short, high-pitched sound originating in the alveoli and terminal bronchi; the sound is simulated by rubbing hair between one's fingers close to the ear.

medium r. A rale having a pitch that is lower than that of a fine rale.

moist r. A rale produced by accumulation of relatively liquid secretions in the airways, as occurs in saccular dilatations of the bronchi (bronchiectasis), especially in the lower portions of the lungs.

ramose, ramous (ra´mōs, ra´mus) Branching.

ramulus (ram´u-lus) A minute terminal branch.

ramus (ra´mus), *pl.* **ra´mi** A branchlike part of a nerve, artery, or vein, especially a primary division.

dorsal r. of spinal nerve A bundle of nerve fibers given off by a spinal nerve immediately after the union of its dorsal and ventral roots; it innervates the structures of the back.

r. communicans A bundle of nerve fibers connecting two nerves or a nerve to a ganglion.

ventral r. of spinal nerve The continuation of a spinal nerve soon after it emerges from the intervertebral foramen, dividing ultimately into the lateral and anterior divisions; it innervates the limbs and the anterolateral parts of the body wall; the major plexuses (cervical, brachial, and lumbosacral) are formed by the ventral rami of spinal nerves.

random (ran´dom) Governed by chance; not completely determined by other circumstances.

randomization (ran-dom ĭ za´shun) Allocation of subjects to experimental and control groups by chance.

range (rānj) The interval in which the largest and smallest values lie in a distribution.

therapeutic r. A range expected to achieve a desired curative effect; applied to dosages (e.g., of a drug or radiation).

ranine (ra´nīn) Pertaining to the undersurface of the tongue.

RANTES An interleukin-8 that is a chemoattractant for memory T lymphocytes and monocytes.

ranula (ran´u-lă) A cystic tumor occurring on the floor of the mouth or the undersurface of the tongue. Also called sublingual cyst.

rape (rāp) An illegal, nonconsensual act of sexual penetration of any body orifice, usually carried out by force or other forms of duress, including intimidation, deceit, impairment of the victim's senses (by any means), or any other method used to overcome the physical and psychological resistance of the victim. Also called aggravated sexual assault; criminal sexual conduct; sexual assault; sexual battery.

statutory r. The act of sexual penetration usually by an adult with a minor. May also include two minors if the age difference between the two is significant.

raphe (ra´fe) A ridge or line marking the union of two similar structures.

pterygomandibular r. A line of interlacing tendinous fibers stretching from the hamulus of the medial pterygoid plate to the inner surface of the mandible at the level of the third molar; the superior pharyngeal constrictor and buccinator muscles attach to it.

r. of medulla oblongata The line between the right and left halves of the medulla oblongata.

scrotal r. A line extending from the anus to the base of the penis; it marks the attachment of the scrotal septum which separates the testes.

raptus (rap´tus) Any sudden seizure.

rarefaction (rār-ĕ-fak´shun) The process of becoming less dense.

rarefy (rār´ĕ-fi) To make light, less dense, or less compact.

rash (rash) Any eruption on the skin.

heat r. See prickly heat, under heat.

morbilliform r. Condition of the skin resembling the eruption of measles.

nettle r. See urticaria.

raspatory (ras´pă-tor-e) Instrument for scraping bone.

rat (rat) Any of various long-tailed rodents of the genus *Rattus*; many are vectors of disease-causing organisms.

albino r. White rat used extensively in laboratory experiments.

black r. English black rat, *Rattus rattus*, that harbors the flea *Zenopsylla cheopis*, responsible for transmitting plague to humans.

brown r. Large brownish gray rat, *Rattus norvegicus*, with short ears and a smaller than usual tail.

inbred r.'s Genetically identical rats developed usually from brother and sister matings that have occurred for twenty or more generations.

inbred BB r.'s A strain that is used as a model for spontaneous diabetes mellitus.

nude r.'s A mutant strain of rats that are devoid of hair and a thymus and have diminished or absent T cell function.

spontaneously hypertensive r. (SHR) A strain of rats prone to develop hypertension without recourse to special diets or hormones; originally developed in Japan. Useful in hypertension research.

Sprague-Dawley r. Genetically similar, inbred strain of rats developed by the Sprague-Dawley Company.

transgenic r. A rat genetically engineered to study the effect of changing (adding, deleting, altering) a particular gene; often done to develop disease models that mimic human diseases.

Wistar r. A white rat extensively used in experimental biology and medicine; strain developed at the Wistar Institute.

R

rat-bite disease (rat-bīt dĭ-zēz´) See rat-bite fever, under fever.

rate (rāt) Strictly, a measured quantity, or a counted value, per unit time in which there is a distinct relationship between the two (i.e., between the quantity or value and the unit of time). The term is often used less strictly in epidemiologic and demographic studies to express values or quantities that are dimensionless in time.

basal metabolic r. (BMR) See basal metabolism, under metabolism.

birth r. The number of births in a given population per year or any other unit of time.

death r. See mortality rate.

erythrocyte sedimentation r. (ESR) The rate (in millimeters per hour) of settling of red blood cells when anticoagulated blood is allowed to stand under standard conditions in a vertical glass column; the two standard methods commonly used are those of Wintrobe and Westergren (see under method). Also called sedimentation rate.

fetal death r. The number of stillbirths occurring in one year per 1000 infants born (including live births and stillbirths) in that same year. Also called stillbirth rate.

fetal heart r. (FHR) The number of fetal heartbeats per minute, normally ranging from 120 to

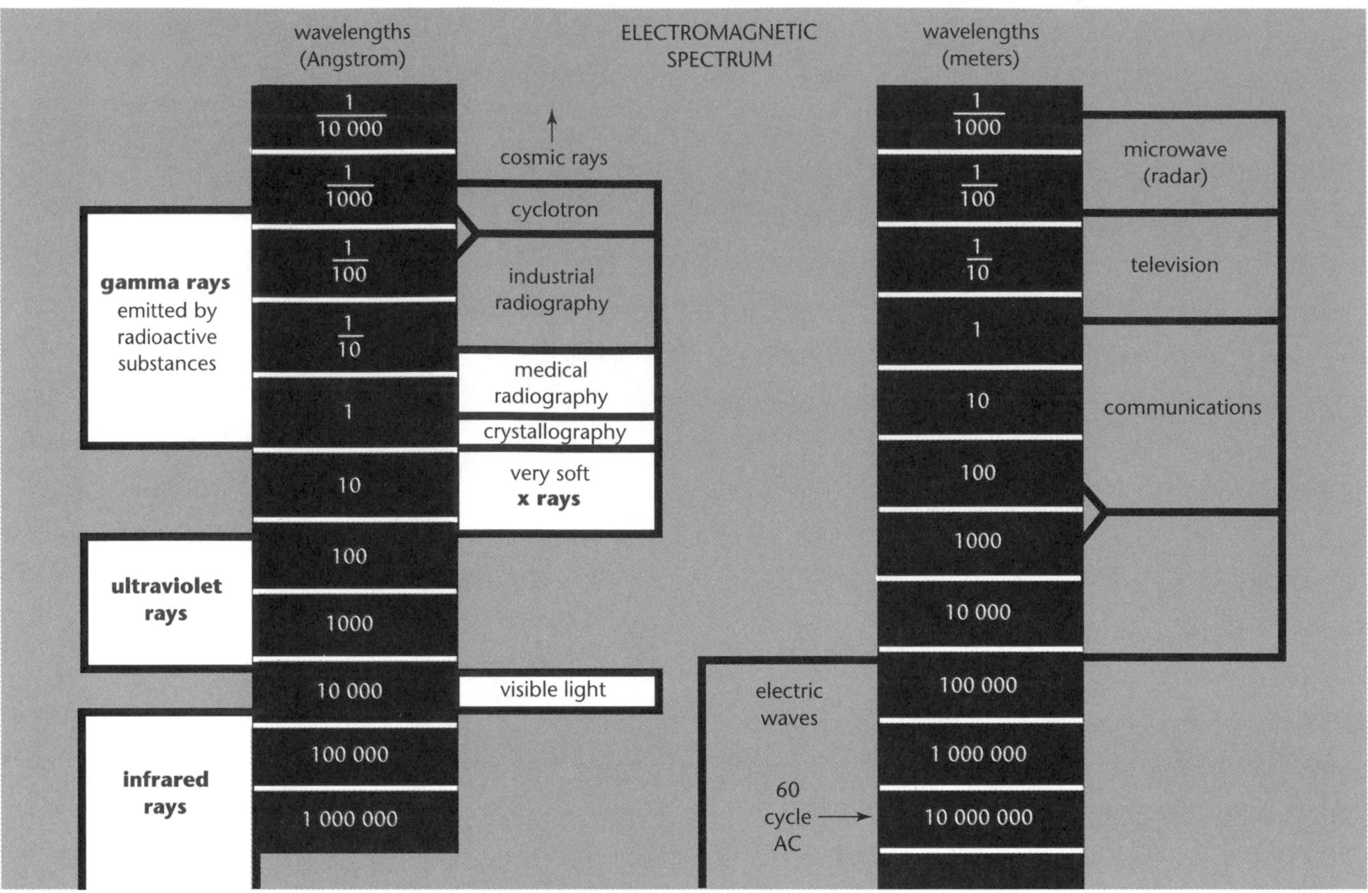

160.

glomerular filtration r. (GFR) The volume of plasma filtered through the glomerular capillary membranes of the kidney in one minute.

growth r. Absolute or relative growth increase, expressed in units of time.

infant mortality r. The relation of the number of deaths in the first year of life to the total number of live births in the same population during the same period of time.

morbidity r. The number of persons with a particular disease in a specified time per given unit of the total population.

mortality r. The relation between the number of registered deaths in a specified area and the total population during a given period, usually one year. Also called death rate.

neonatal mortality r. The number of deaths in infants under 28 days of age in a given year per 1000 live births of that same year.

peak expiratory flow r. (PEFR) The maximal rate of airflow out of the lungs during forced expiration beginning with lungs fully inflated.

perinatal mortality r. The number of deaths in infants less than 7 days of age plus the number of fetal deaths after 28 weeks of gestation in a year per 1000 live births of that same year.

pulse r. The number of beats per minute of a peripheral arterial pulse.

respiratory r., r. of respiration The rate of breathing; the number of inspirations (breaths) per minute.

sedimentation r. See erythrocyte sedimentation rate.

stillbirth r. See fetal death rate.

ratio (ra´she-o) (r) A proportion; the relation that one thing bears to another relating to magnitude or quantity.

albumin-globulin r., A/G r. See systolic/diastolic ratio.

body-weight r. Body weight in grams divided by the height in centimeters.

cardiothoracic r. The ratio of the transverse diameter of the heart to the internal diameter of the thoracic cage at its widest point. A ratio greater than 0.5 indicates an enlarged heart.

extraction r. (E) The fraction of a substance removed from the blood flowing through the kidney.

lecithin-sphingomyelin r. (L/S r.) The ratio of lecithin to sphingomyelin in amniotic fluid; used to determine the degree of maturity of the fetal lungs and thus predict respiratory problems.

mendelian r. The ratio in which the offspring, or later generations, show the characteristics of their parents, in accordance with genetic principles.

nucleocytoplasmic r. The ratio of the volumes of nucleus and cytoplasm within a given cell; the ratio is generally constant for a particular cell type, and is usually increased in malignant neoplasms. Also called nucleoplasmic ratio.

nucleoplasmic r. See nucleocytoplasmic ratio.

segregation r. Ratio of the various segregating genotypes among offspring.

systolic/diastolic r. A quantitative assessment of velocities of umbilical artery flow; often used to assess the fetal condition.

therapeutic r. The ratio of the maximally tolerated dose of a drug to the minimal effective dose; the higher the ratio the safer the drug.

urea reduction r. (URR) The ratio of urea concentration in blood before and after hemodialysis, measured as urea in blood urea nitrogen (BUN).

rational (rash´un-al) **1.** In possession of reasoning abilities. **2.** Based on reason.

rationalization (rash-un-al-i-za´shun) A plausible explanation provided to justify an act that is prompted by factors other than reason.

rauwolfia (raw-wul´fe-ă) An alkaloid derived from a number of tropical trees and shrubs of the genus *Rauwolfia*.

r. serpentina The dried root of *Rauwolfia serpentina*; a source of drugs (e.g., reserpine) with tranquilizing and antihypertensive properties.

ray (ra) **1.** A narrow beam of electromagnetic radiation (e.g., light, heat). **2.** A linear anatomic structure.

actinic r. A ray at the violet and ultraviolet end of the spectrum, capable of producing chemical changes; a photochemically active radiation.

alpha (α) **r.** Ray composed of a stream of high-velocity, positively charged particles (alpha particles) ejected from radioactive substances.

Becquerel r.'s Alpha, beta, and gamma rays emitted from uranium, radium, and other radioactive substances.

beta (β) **r.** Ray composed of streams of high-velocity, negatively charged particles (beta particles), especially electrons, ejected from radioactive substances that have greater velocity and penetrative power than that of the alpha rays.

borderline r.'s Grenz rays.

cathode r.'s A stream of electrons emitted by the negative electrode (cathode) in a vacuum tube (Crookes' tube); their bombardment against the glass wall of the tube or against the anode gives rise to x rays (roentgen rays).

cosmic r.'s High energy particles that bombard the earth from outer space.

gamma (γ) **r.** A stream of photons emitted by the nucleus of an atom during the radioactive decay process; analogous to the x ray but of shorter wavelength.

grenz r.'s Very soft x rays, greater in length than one Å; closely allied to the ultraviolet rays in their wavelength and in their biologic action upon tissue; used in x-raying soft tissues.

hard r. X ray of short wavelength and great penetrability; produced by a high-voltage tube.

hertzian r.'s See radio waves, under wave.

incident r. A ray of radiant energy striking a surface before reflection.

infrared r.'s Rays with wavelengths greater than 7700 Å, beyond the red end of the spectrum.

medullary r. The center of the renal lobe, which has the shape of a small steep pyramid, consisting of straight ascending and descending limbs of the nephronic loop and collecting ducts.

reflected r. A ray of radiant energy thrown back after striking a nonabsorbent surface.

roentgen r. See x ray.

soft r. A ray of long wavelength and slight penetrability.

ultraviolet r. An electromagnetic, invisible ray with wavelength between 4000 and 40 Å, between the violet end of the visible spectrum and the x-ray region of the electromagnetic spectrum.

vital ultraviolet r.'s Rays of wavelengths between 3200 and 2900 Å necessary for normal

R

COMMON MANIFESTATIONS OF **ADVERSE REACTIONS** TO SOME DRUGS

MANIFESTATIONS		DRUGS
dermatologic	urticaria (hives)	penicillin aspirin barbiturates sulfonamides
	exfoliative dermatitis (loss of superficial skin layers)	penicillin barbiturates
respiratory	apnea (difficulty in breathing)	local anesthetics
	inflammation of mucus membranes of nose	reserpine
	pulmonary infection	antineoplastic-immuno-suppressive drugs
cardiovascular	hypotension (fall in blood pressure)	imipramine amitriptyline
	arrhythmia (abnormal rhythm of heart beat)	thyroid hormone sympathomimetic amines
gastrointestinal	swollen or hairy tongue	tetracycline
	discoloration of dental enamel	tetracycline (in children)
	peptic ulceration hemorrhage	aspirin

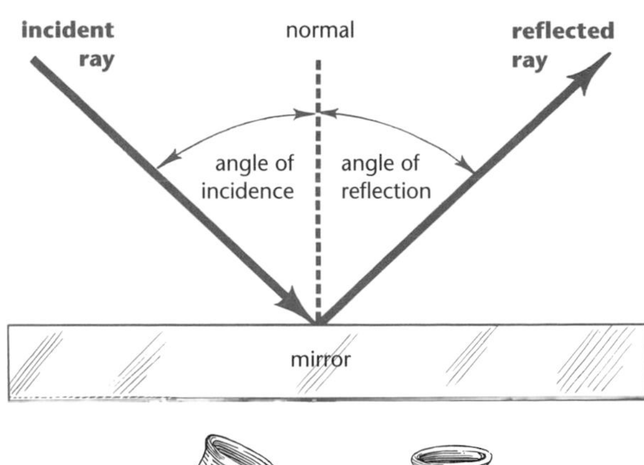

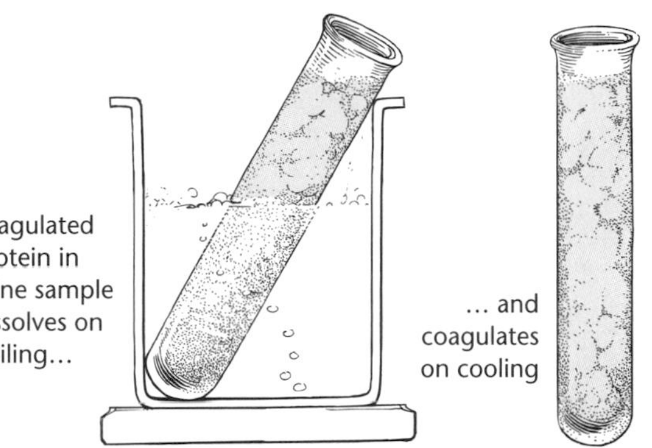

growth; they promote calcium metabolism.

x r. An electromagnetic radiation (high energy photon) with a very short wavelength (0.05 to 100 Å), generated at the point of impact of a stream of high-speed cathode electrons on the target of an x-ray tube; x rays, because of their penetrating power, are used to record on film shadows of the varying densities within a portion of the body. Also called roentgen ray.

Raynaud's disease (ra-nōz´ dĭ-zēz´) Bilateral cyanosis of the digits due to spasmodic contraction of the peripheral arteries, usually precipitated by cold or by emotion.

Raynaud's phenomenon (ra-nōz´ fĕ-nom´ĕ-non) See under phenomenon.

reabsorption (re-ab-sorp´shun) The process of reabsorbing or the state of being reabsorbed.

active r. Reabsorption requiring the expenditure of energy.

passive r. Reabsorption requiring no energy expenditure; the substances are reabsorbed along a concentration gradient.

tubular r. Selective reabsorption of extracellular fluid by the kidney tubules; it helps restore essential components to the body.

reactance (re-ak´tans) (X) Opposition to the flow of an alternating electric current, by passage through a coil of wire or a condenser.

reactant (re-ak´tant) Any substance that takes part in a chemical reaction.

reaction (re-ak´shun) **1.** A force produced by and opposing an acting force. **2.** Any response to a stimulus. **3.** The transformation of molecules into others. **4.** The observable color change in, or produced by, indicators or reagents in chemical analysis.

acid r. A positive test indicating the presence of hydrogen ions in a solution (e.g., the reddening of blue litmus).

adverse r. An undesirable and sometimes life-threatening response to a therapeutic drug.

alarm r. (AR) The body's response to a sudden exposure to a violent or stressful stimulus.

alkaline r. A positive test indicating the presence of hydroxyl ions in a solution (e.g., the bluing of red litmus).

allergic r. A reaction stimulated by exposure to a substance (allergen) to which the individual has become sensitized.

amphoteric r. The reaction of a substance that is capable of reacting chemically both as an acid and as a base.

anamnestic r. See secondary response, under response.

anaphylactic r. See anaphylaxis.

antigen-antibody r. The specific binding of an antibody with the same type of antigen that activated the formation of the antibody, resulting in precipitation, agglutination, or neutralization of exotoxin.

anxiety r. An uncontrollable apprehension out of proportion to any apparent external cause.

arousal r. Change in the brain wave pattern of an individual when suddenly awakened.

Arthus r. A severe local sensitivity reaction produced at the site of injection of antigen into an animal possessing specific precipitating serum antibodies.

Bence Jones r. Coagulation of Bence Jones protein when a urine sample from a patient with Bence Jones proteinuria is heated, followed by its redissolving on boiling, and coagulation again on cooling.

biuret r. See biuret test, under test.

cell-mediated r. Delayed allergic reaction involving T lymphocytes.

chain r. A series of chemical reactions, each one initiated by the one preceding.

complement fixation r. See complement fixation, under fixation.

consensual r. Constriction of the pupil of one eye when a light is flashed into the other eye. Also called consensual response.

conversion r. See conversion disorder, under disorder.

cross r. Reaction occurring between an antibody and an antigen of a type different from, but related to, the one that stimulated the production of the antibody.

cytotoxic r. Reaction that results in damage to or destruction of cells.

delayed r. See delayed-type hypersensitivity, under hypersensitivity.

dissociative r. A reaction marked by dissociated behavior (e.g., amnesia, sleepwalking).

false-negative r. An erroneous negative reaction; a test that wrongly indicates that the individual does not have the condition for which the test is conducted.

false-positive r. An erroneous positive reaction; a test that wrongly indicates that the individual has the condition for which the test is conducted.

first-order r. Reaction in which the rate is proportional to the concentration of the substance undergoing chemical change.

graft versus host r. (GVHR) Pathologic conditions in a transplantation patient occurring as a reaction of the immunocompetent cells in the donor's graft against cells of the immunodeficient and incompatible patient.

Herxheimer's r. See Jarisch-Herxheimer reaction.

id r. A skin eruption occurring in an area of the body other than that of the infection (e.g., on the hands during acute tinea infection of the feet); most commonly follows fungus infections of the feet or the scalp, severe contact dermatitis of the hands, and varicose ulcers; considered to be an allergic reaction.

immediate hypersensitivity r. An antibody-mediated immunologic sensitivity manifested by histamine release and tissue swelling within minutes after a second exposure to an antigen.

immune r. See immune response, under response.

Jarisch-Herxheimer r. Inflammatory condition sometimes occurring 2 to 8 hours after instituting antibiotic therapy for syphilis; believed to be due to rapid release of treponemal antigen. Also called Herxheimer's reaction.

leukemoid r. Condition marked by the presence of increased white blood cells in the blood; similar to, but not associated with, leukemia; seen in certain infectious diseases and some malignant tumors.

ninhydrin r. The production of violet color by proteins, peptones, peptides, and amino acids having a free carboxyl and an alpha-amino group, when boiled with ninhydrin.

normal lymphocyte transfer r., NLT r. Reaction resulting from the injection of allogeneic lymphocytes into the skin.

nuclear r. Reaction in which an atomic nucleus changes its atomic number (number of protons) or its mass number (number of nucleons), as a result of natural or artificial radioactivity, or through direct nuclear bombardment.

Pándy's r. The change occurring in a mixture of cerebrospinal fluid (CSF) and a test solution, indicating the abnormal presence of protein in the CSF; the change may range from a slight turbidity to a milky appearance, depending on the amount of protein present. Also called Pándy's test.

polymerase chain r. (PCR) A method of amplifying a short stretch of DNA; applications include genetic testing, detection of difficult-to-isolate pathogens, mutation analysis, DNA sequencing, diagnosis of disease, and analyzing evolutionary relationships.

Prausnitz-Küstner r. Reaction occurring when blood serum from an allergic person is injected into the skin of a nonallergic individual, followed (48 hours later) by injection of antigens to which the donor is allergic; a wheal appears at the site of injection. Also called Prausnitz-Küstner test; P-K test.

quellung r. See Neufeld capsular swelling, under swelling.

Schultz-Charlton r. Blanching of scarlatinal rash

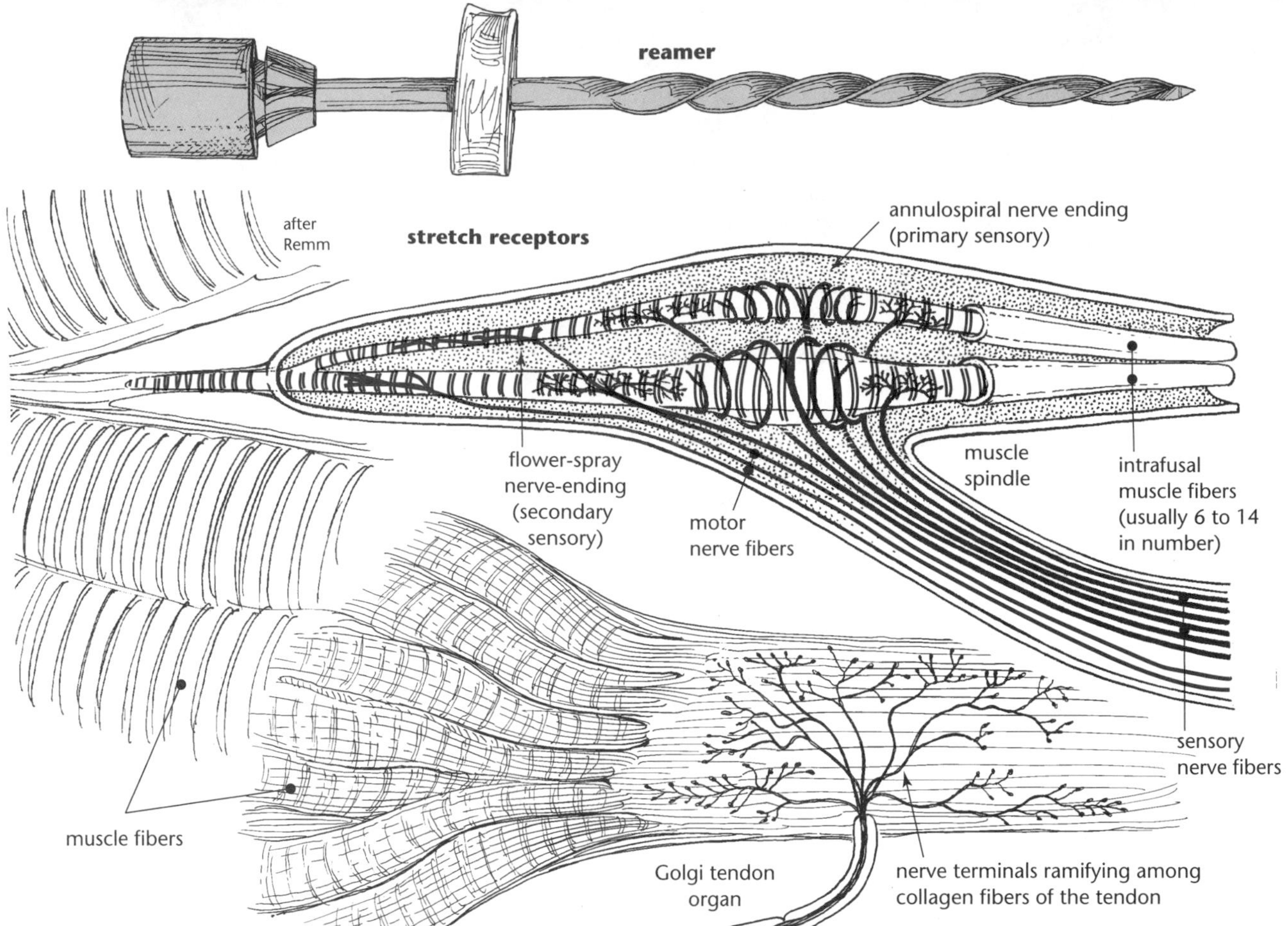

at site of intracutaneous injection of scarlatina antiserum. Also called Schultz-Charlton phenomenon.

Schultz-Dale r. Smooth muscle contraction produced *in vitro* when antigen is applied to the excised muscle of a sensitive animal.

Wassermann r. (WR) See Wassermann test, under test.

wheal-flare r. A skin sensitivity reaction due to histamine, characterized by an edematous elevation and erythematous flare.

white-graft r. A reaction to a tissue graft in which the graft fails to vascularize and is quickly rejected.

Widal's r. Agglutination reaction used in the diagnosis of typhoid.

zero-order r. A reaction that, regardless of the concentration of the reactants, proceeds at a definite rate.

R

reactivate (re-ak′tĭ-vāt) To restore activity, as in an inactivated immune serum to which normal serum is added.

reactivity (re-ak-tiv′ĭ-te) The ability to react.

reagent (re-a′jent) Any substance, added to a solution, that participates in a chemical reaction, especially one employed in chemical analysis for the detection of biologic constituents.

Benedict-Hopkins-Cole r. Magnesium glyoxalate, made by adding a saturated solution of oxalic acid to powdered magnesium; used for testing proteins for the presence of tryptophan.

biuret r. An alkaline solution of copper sulfate.

diazo r. Reagent consisting of two solutions, sodium nitrate and acidified sulfanilic acid; used to bring about diazotization.

Esbach's r. Reagent consisting of a 1% aqueous solution of picric acid mixed with a 2% solution of citric acid; used in estimating the quantity of albumin in urine.

Nessler's r. Reagent used to determine the level of urea nitrogen in blood and urine.

reagin (re′ă-jin) **1.** Antibody involved in immediate hypersensitivity reactions; the human IgE antibody. **2.** Obsolete term for antibodies detected by the Wassermann test for syphilis.

reaginic (re-ă-jin′ik) Relating to a reagin.

reality (re-al′ĭ-te) The sum of all things that have an objective existence.

reality testing (re-al′ĭ-te test-ing) In psychiatry and psychology, ability to evaluate the outside world and to adequately comprehend one's relationship to it.

reamer (re′mer) Dental instrument used to enlarge root canals.

rebase (re-bās′) To replace or add to the base material of a denture without changing the occlusal relations of the teeth.

rebound (re′bownd) **1.** In anesthesia, new reflex activity following the withdrawal of a stimulus. **2.** Reappearance of a condition often with greater force than originally, after the effect of a therapeutic agent has worn off (e.g., when the effect of a vasoconstrictor, such as nose drops, wears off and there is subsequently increased vasocongestion).

recall (re′kol, rĕ-kol′) The process of summoning back a memory into consciousness; to remember; often used to describe the recollection of events in the immediate past.

recanalization (re-kan-ăl-ĭ-zā′shun) Formation of a canal through the obstructed lumen of an tubular structure (e.g., of a blood vessel obstructed with a clot, or of a deferent duct after a vasectomy).

receiver (re-sēv′er) **1.** An electronic device capable of receiving incoming electromagnetic signals and converting them to perceptible forms. **2.** In chemistry, a container attached to a condenser for collecting distillation products.

receptaculum (re-sep-tak′u-lum) A pouchlike structure.

r. chyli See cisterna chyli, under cisterna.

receptor (re-sep′tor) **1.** A molecule on the surface of a cell membrane that binds selectively to a specific substance (protein or peptide), producing a biologic effect that is specific to that binding. **2.** The sensory end organ; the small structure in which a sensory nerve fiber terminates; it receives stimuli and converts them into nervous impulses.

adrenergic r.'s Constituents of effector tissues innervated by adrenergic postganglionic fibers of the sympathetic nervous system. Also called adrenoceptors.

alpha-adrenergic r.'s Adrenergic receptors that mediate such actions as constriction of blood vessels and dilatation of the pupils; they respond to stimulation by norepinephrine and are blocked by the action of such compounds as phenoxybenzamine and phentolamine.

B cell antigen r.'s Immunoglobulins attached to the cell membrane that, with T cell help, trigger B cell activity upon contact with antigens.

beta-adrenergic r.'s Adrenergic receptors that are stimulated by epinephrine and respond to the blocking action of such compounds as propranolol; there are two kinds: *beta$_1$adrenergic r.'s*, responsible for acceleration of the heartbeat and lipolysis;

beta$_2$adrenergic r.'s, responsible for dilatation of bronchi and blood vessels.

histamine r.'s Receptors that respond to histamine; vascular dilatation of histamine is mediated by receptors of both H_1 and H_2 types; (a) H_1 receptors, when stimulated, cause bronchoconstriction and contraction of the intestines; blocked by antihistamines; (b) H_2 receptors, when stimulated, cause gastric secretion; blocked by substances such as cimetidine.

muscarinic (M) **r.'s** Membrane proteins on autonomic effector cells; stimulated by muscarine (an alkaloid) or acetylcholine.

nicotinic r.'s Receptors on cells within autonomic ganglia, medulla of adrenal gland, and striated muscle cells; stimulated by nicotine (an alkaloid) or acetylcholine.

opiate r.'s Receptors in specific tissues of the brain (e.g., along the cerebral aqueduct) that have the capacity to combine with morphine or endorphins.

stretch r. Receptor (e.g., the muscle spindle and the Golgi tendon organ) whose function is to detect elongation.

T cell antigen r. (TCR) The characteristic marker for T lymphocytes; interacts simultaneously with foreign (nonself) antigens and the (self) antigens of the major histocompatibility complex (MHC).

recess (re′ses) A shallow cavity.

piriform r. A recess in the pharynx on each side of the opening of the larynx.

recession (resesh′un) The process of withdrawing.

gingival r. Displacement of gingiva with resulting added exposure of tooth surface.

tendon r. Posterior surgical displacement of the insertion of an eye muscle.

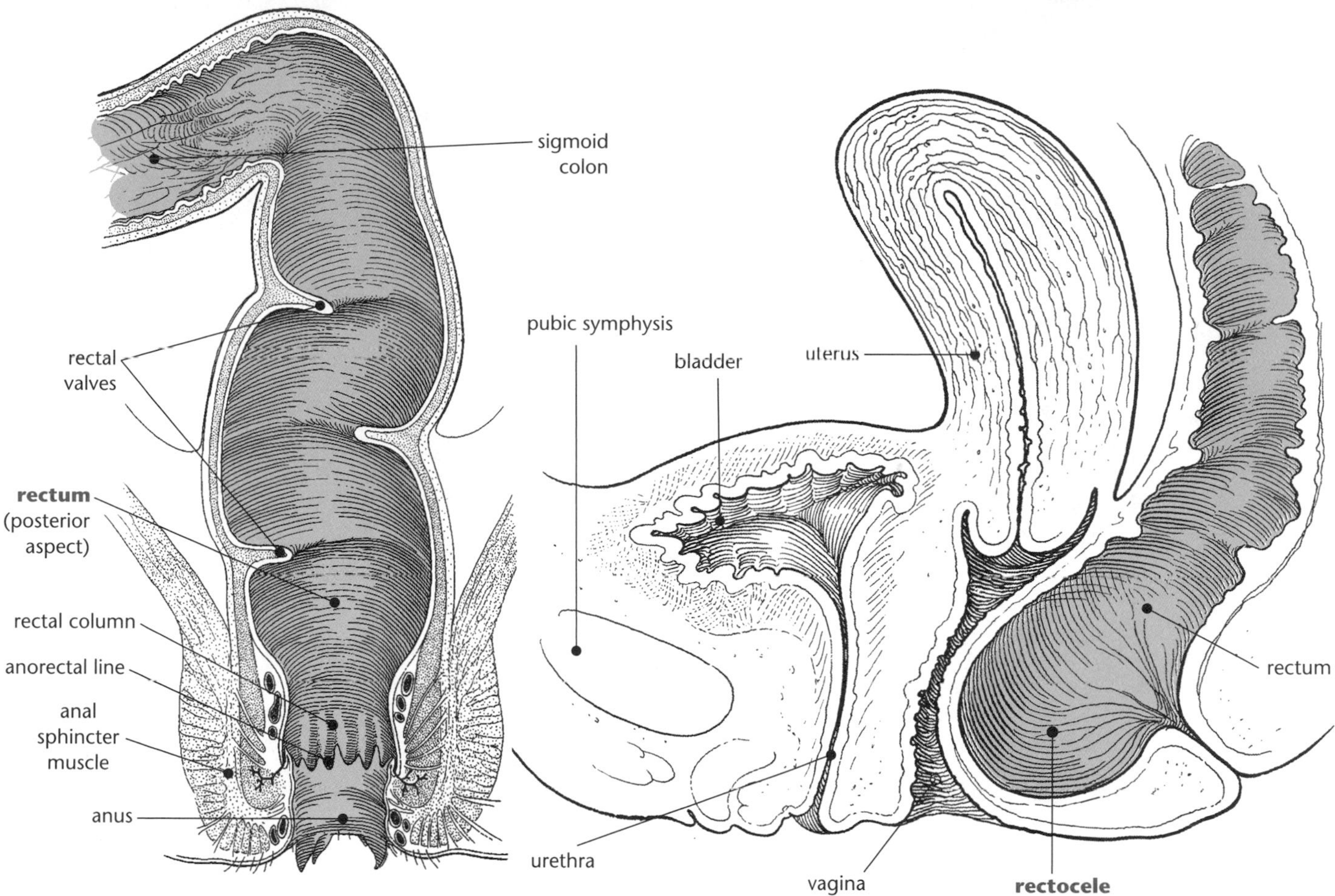

recessive (re-ses´iv) **1.** Receding. **2.** In genetics, not expressed unless present in both sets of chromosomes, homozygous or heterozygous.
recidivation (re-sid-ĭ-va´shun) Reappearance of a disease, symptom, or pattern of behavior.
recidivism (re-sid´ĭ-viz-m) The tendency of an individual to relapse into a previous mode of behavior, especially a tendency to return to criminal or delinquent habits.
recidivist (re-sid´ĭ-vist) A person who tends to relapse into a previous pattern of bad behavior after rehabilitation (e.g., a habitual criminal).
recipe (res´ĭ-pe) **1.** Latin for take, usually represented by the symbol R_x; used as the heading (superscription) of a physician's prescription. **2.** The prescription itself.
recipiomotor (re-sip-e-o-mo´tor) The recipient of a motor stimulus.
Recklinghausen's disease (rek´ling-how-zenz dĭ-zēz´) See neurofibromatosis I.
Recklinghausen's disease of bone (rek´ling-how-zenz dĭ-zēz´ ŭv bōn) See osteitis fibrosa cystica, under osteitis.
recombinant (re-kom´bĭ-nant) Organism, chromosome, or DNA that has resulted from the introduction of genetic material from an outside source.
recombination (re-kom-bĭ-na´shun) The formation of gene combinations in the offspring that were not present in either parent, caused by the exchange of genes between homologous chromsomes (crossing over).
recon (re´kon) In genetics, the smallest unit of a single DNA nucleotide capable of recombination.
reconduction (re-kon-duk´shun) See retrograde conduction, under conduction.
reconstitution (re-kon-stĭ-tu´shun) **1.** Restoration to original form, as of a substance previously altered for preservation. **2.** Regeneration of a lost bodily part.
record (rek´ord) Information preserved in an enduring form.
interocclusal r. A record of the positional relations of teeth or jaws to each other. Also called checkbite.
maxillomandibular r. Maxillomandibular registration, a record of any positional relations of the maxilla to the mandible.
medical r. A confidential record that documents a patient's medical history and history of medical care, including illness, diagnoses, treatment, and results of treatment.
problem oriented r. (POR) A system of recording medical information about a patient, characterized by a defined universe of information for the data base, a complete up-to-date problem list, and numbered and titled plans and progress notes that preserve the course of action of the physicians and other medical personnel; it is adaptable for the computer. Also called problem oriented medical record (POMR).
problem oriented medical r. (POMR) See problem oriented record (POR).
source oriented medical r. The traditional method of recording medical information about a patient as it happens.
recording (re-kord´ing) Preserving, in writing or any other permanent form, the results of a study.
recrement (rek´rĕ-ment) Any body secretion (e.g., saliva, bile) that is reabsorbed after having performed its function.
recrudescence (re-kroo-des´ens) A return of a disease process after a dormant or inactive period.
recruitment (re-kro͞ot´ment) **1.** In the testing of hearing, the abnormally rapid increase in loudness experienced by a patient when a sound stimulus is gradually increased. **2.** A gradual increase in response to a stimulus that has a constant intensity but prolonged duration.
rectal (rek´tal) Relating to the rectum.
rectalgia (rek-tal´jă, rek-tal´je-ă) See proctalgia.
rectify (rek´tĭ-fī) **1.** To purify a liquid through redistillation. **2.** To transform an alternating current into a direct one. **3.** To correct.
rectoabdominal (rek-to-ab-dom´ĭ-nal) Relating to the rectum and abdomen, especially a method of examination in which one hand is placed on the abdomen, and a finger of the other hand is inserted into the rectum.
rectocele (rek´to-sēl) Hernial protrusion of the rectum into the posterior vaginal wall; caused by disruption of the connective tissue (rectovaginal fascia) between the rectum and vagina, which weakens the wall. Also called proctocele.
rectocolitis (rek-to-ko-ki´tis) See coloproctitis.
rectoperineorrhaphy (rek-to-per-ĭ-ne-or´ă-fe) See proctoperineoplasty.
rectopexy (rek´to-pek-se) See proctopexy.
rectoplasty (rek´to-plas-te) See proctoplasty.
rectoscope (rek´to-skōp) See proctoscope.
rectosigmoid (rek-to-sig´moid) The portion of the intestinal tract adjacent to the junction of the rectum and the sigmoid colon, on both sides.
rectostenosis (rek-to-stĕ-no´sis) See proctostenosis.
rectourethral (rek-to-u-re´thral) Relating to the rectum and urethra.
rectouterine (rek-to-u´ter-ĭn) Relating to the rectum and uterus.
rectovaginal (rek-to-vaj´ĭ-nal) Relating to the rectum and vagina.
rectovesical (rek-to-ves´ĭ-kal) Relating to the rectum and bladder.
rectum (rek´tum) The terminal portion of the intestinal tract extending from the sigmoid colon to the anus.
rectus (rek´tus) Straight; describes muscles that run a straight course (e.g., the abdominal rectus muscle).
recumbent (re-kum´bent) Lying down; reclining.
recuperate (re-ku´per-āt) To recover.
recurrence (re-kur´ens) **1.** A return of symptoms occurring as a natural course of certain diseases. **2.** The return of a morbid state after a period of improvement.
recurrent (re-kur´ent) Returning after abatement or disappearance.
recurvation (re-kur-va´shun) A backward bending or curving.
Red Cross (red kros) **1.** Red Cross Society; an international organization established for the caring for the injured and homeless during wartime and natural disasters. **2.** The emblem of the Red Cross Society, a red Geneva cross or red Greek cross on a white background; a sign of neutrality.
redia (re´de-ă), *pl.* **re´diae** The larval stage in the life cycle of a trematode.
redox (red´oks) In chemistry, a combined shortened version of the term reduction-oxidation.
reduce (re-do͞os´) **1.** To return a part to its normal position (e.g., the ends of a fractured bone). **2.** To

R

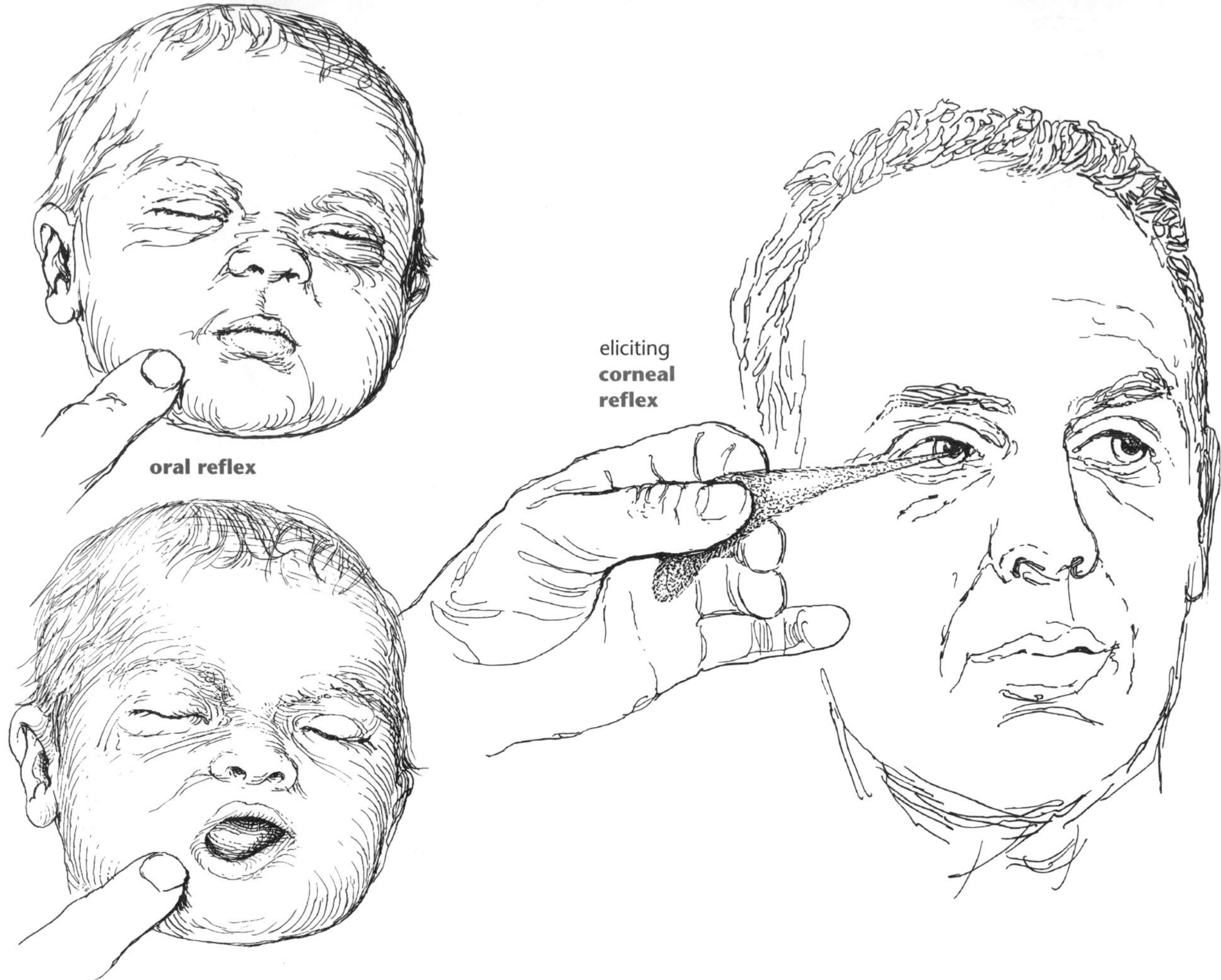

decrease the valence number of an atom by adding electrons. **3.** To diminish in size, amount, or number.

reducible (re-doo´sĭ-bl Capable of being reduced.

reductant (re-duk´tant) The donor of electrons in an oxidation-reduction reaction.

reductase (re-duk´tās) The reducing enzyme in an oxidation-reduction reaction.

reduction (re-duk´shun) **1.** The correction, through surgical or manipulative methods, of a hernia, a fracture, or a dislocation. **2.** In chemistry, the removal of oxygen from a substance or the addition of hydrogen; the reverse of oxidation.

selective r. In reproductive medicine, the destruction of one or more embryos in a multiple gestation resulting from *in vitro* fertilization.

R

reduplication (re-doo-plĭ-ka´shun) A doubling.

reefing (rēf´ing) The act of folding, such as the surgical folding and suturing of a tissue to reduce its size.

reentry (re-en´tre) The return of an impulse to an area of heart muscle that it has recently stimulated, as occurs in reciprocal heart rhythms.

refine (re-fin´) To purify.

reflect (re-flekt´) **1.** To bend back from a surface (e.g., light rays). **2.** To move aside (e.g., to expose an underlying structure). **3.** To meditate.

reflection (re-flek´shun) **1.** The return of light from an optical surface into the same medium from which it came. **2.** A bending back.

reflector (re-flek´tor) A surface that reflects light, heat, or sound waves.

reflex (re´fleks) **1.** An involuntary and immediate response to a stimulus. **2.** Turned backward; reflected.

abdominal r. Contraction of the muscles of the abdominal wall upon stroking of the overlying skin.

accommodation r. The increase in convexity of the lens of the eye when the eyes are directed from a distant to a near object, in order to bring the image into focus; initiated by an out-of-focus image on the retina; effected by contraction of the ciliary muscle and relaxation of the suspensory ligament of the lens.

Achilles r., Achilles tendon r. Contraction of the calf muscles with resulting plantar flexion of the foot on striking of the calcaneal (Achilles) tendon. Also called ankle jerk; ankle reflex; calcaneal tendon reflex.

acquired r. See conditioned reflex.

anal r. Contraction of the anal sphincter muscle upon irritation of the perianal area, or upon insertion of a finger into the rectum.

ankle r. See Achilles reflex.

attitudinal r. See statotonic reflex.

Babinski's r. See extensor plantar reflex.

Bainbridge r. Acceleration of the heartbeat caused by a rise in pressure in the great veins at the entrance to the right atrium.

biceps r. Flexion of the forearm when the tendon of the biceps is struck.

bladder r. See micturition reflex.

brachioradial r. Flexion of the forearm upon tapping of the brachioradial muscle at its attachment to the lower end of the radius.

calcaneal tendon r. See Achilles reflex.

carotid sinus r. See carotid sinus syndrome.

ciliospinal r. See pupillary-skin reflex.

conditioned r. A reflex that is developed through association with, and repetition of, a stimulus. Also called acquired reflex; trained reflex.

conjunctival r. Closure of the eyelids upon touching of the conjunctiva with a fine wisp of cotton.

coordinated r. A reflex in which several muscles take part.

corneal r. Blinking induced by touching of the cornea with a fine wisp of cotton while the patient looks in the direction opposite to the approaching cotton.

cremasteric r. Retraction of the testicle upon gentle scratching of the inner aspect of the upper thigh of the same side.

crossed r. Movement on one side of the body when the opposite side is stimulated.

crossed adductor r. Inward rotation of the leg upon tapping of the sole.

crossed extension r. Response elicited from a newborn infant, indicating spinal cord integrity; placing the child in the supine position, the examiner extends and presses down on one of the child's legs and stimulates the sole of the foot; this causes the free leg to flex, adduct, and then extend.

deep r., deep tendon r. Contraction of a muscle upon tapping of its tendon. Also called tendon reflex.

diving r. Slowing of heartbeat and constriction of peripheral blood vessels brought about by immersing the face or body in (especially cold) water.

elbow r. See triceps reflex.

extensor plantar r. Extension of the large toe with fanning of the small toes upon scratching the sole of the foot; an abnormal reflex after 6 months of age. Also called Babinski reflex; Babinski sign.

fundus r. The red glow seen in the pupil during inspection of the interior of the eyeball, produced by reflection of light from the choroid.

gag r. Gagging initiated by introduction of a foreign body into the pharynx. Also called pharyngeal reflex.

gastrocolic r. The wavelike contraction of the colon, propelling its contents onward, initiated by introduction of food into the empty stomach.

Gordon r. Extension of the big toe upon firm squeezing of the calf.

grasp r. The immediate grasping of an object placed in the hand; occurring normally only in infants.

Hering-Breuer r. The effects of afferent impulses from the vagus nerves and sensory receptors in the lungs and airways in the control of respiration (e.g., deflation of the lungs brings on inspiration).

Hoffmann's r. See Hoffmann's sign.

hung-up r. Prolonged relaxation time of the deep tendon reflexes (particularly the ankle jerks in hypothyroidism).

knee jerk r. See patellar reflex.

light r. See pupillary reflex.

magnet r. Normal response elicited from a newborn infant; with the baby in the supine position with legs semiflexed, the examiner's thumbs press against the soles of the infant's feet, causing extension of the legs.

micturition r. Any of the reflexes controlling effortless urination and the subconscious ability to retain urine within the bladder. Also called bladder reflex; urinary reflex; vesical reflex.

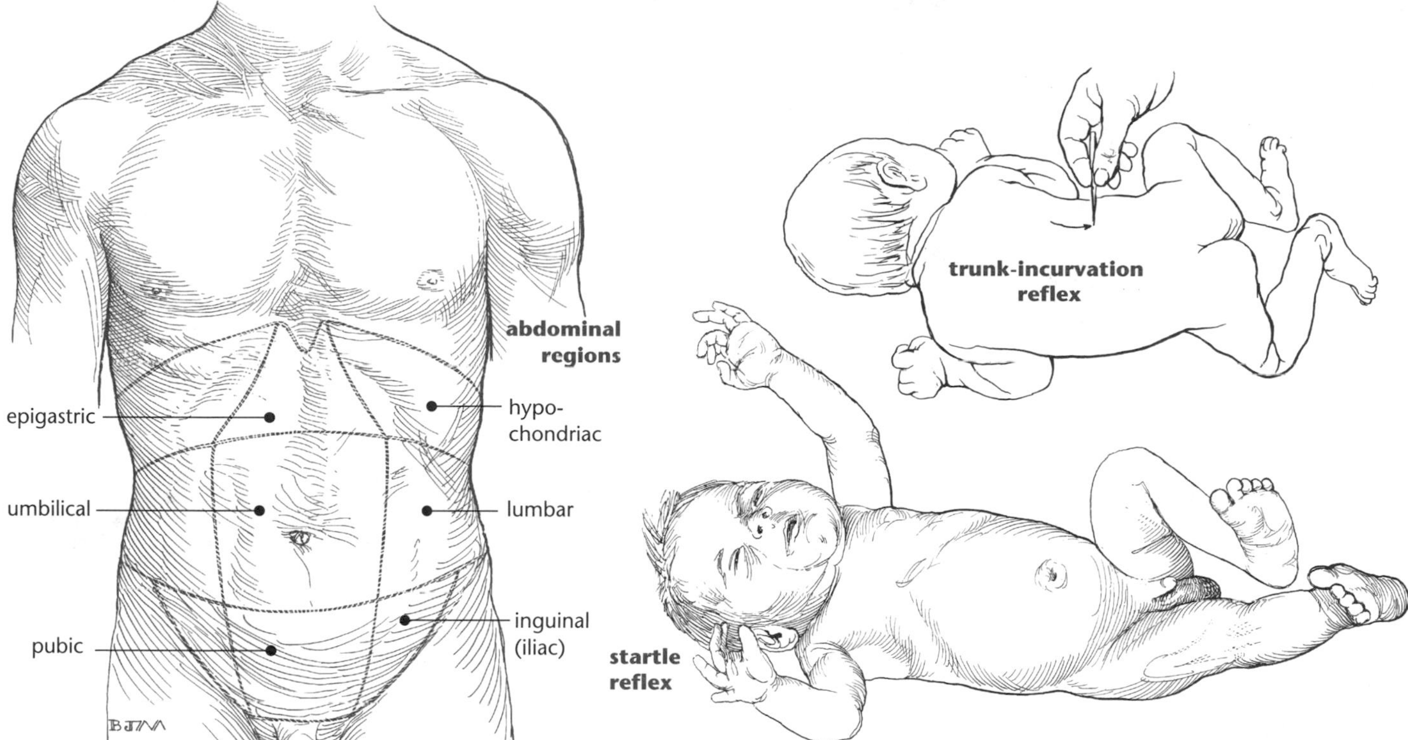

milk-ejection r. Release of milk from the breast upon stimulation of the nipple.
Moro's r. See startle reflex.
myotatic r. Contraction of a muscle in response to a passive stretching force. Also called stretch reflex.
Oppenheim's r. Extension of the toes elicited by pressing down firmly on the shin from the knee to the ankle; an abnormal reflex.
oral r. Normal reflex elicited from a newborn infant; when one corner of the infant's mouth is touched, the bottom lip lowers on the same side and the tongue moves forward and toward the examiner's finger.
orbicularis pupillary r. Unilateral contraction of the pupil while trying to close the eyelids, which are forcibly held open. Also called Westphal's pupillary reflex.
palmomental r. Unilateral twitching of the chin upon scratching of the palm of the hand of the same side. Also called palm-chin reflex.
patellar r. Extension of the leg upon tapping of the patellar tendon while the leg hangs loosely at right angles to the thigh. Also called knee jerk reflex; patellar tendon reflex; quadriceps reflex.
patellar tendon r. See patellar reflex.
pharyngeal r. See gag reflex.
pilomotor r. Formation of goose flesh on lightly touching the skin, or on exposure to cold or emotional stimuli.
plantar r. Flexion of the toes on scratching of the sole of the foot; a normal reflex. Also called sole reflex.
primitive r.'s Reflexes occurring naturally in the newborn infant; an indication of normal neuromuscular development; occur in the adult only in certain disorders.
proprioceptive r. Any of various reflexes brought about by stimulation of proprioceptors (e.g., labyrinth, carotid sinus).
pupillary r. Any change in the size of the pupils, especially in response to a light stimulus.
pupillary-skin r. Dilatation of the pupil upon scratching of the neck. Also called ciliospinal reflex.
quadriceps r. See patellar reflex.
radial r. Flexion of the forearm upon tapping of the end of the radius.
rectal r. Desire to defecate stimulated by accumulation of feces in the rectum.
rooting r. Response elicited from a newborn infant; when the cheek is lightly touched, the infant's head turns in the direction of the touch and his lips purse in preparation for sucking.
startle r. Response of the newborn to loud noises or sudden changes in position; characterized by tensing of muscles, a wide embracing motion of the arms, and extension of the thighs, legs, and fingers (except the thumb and index, which remain in a "C" position). Also called Moro's reflex.
statotonic r. Any of several reflexes stimulated by changes of position of the body in space. Also called attitudinal reflex.
stretch r. See myotatic reflex.
superficial r. Any reflex elicited by stimulation of the skin or mucous membranes.
tendon r. See deep reflex.
trained r. See conditioned reflex.
triceps r. A sudden extension of the forearm on tapping of the triceps tendon at the elbow while the forearm hangs loosely at a right angle to the arm. Also called elbow reflex; elbow jerk.
trunk-incurvation r. Reflex occurring in a newborn infant with normal spinal cord; while the baby is in the prone position, the examiner's finger, running along one side of the spine, causes the infant's body to curve in the direction of the stimulus.
tympanic r. Percussion sound heard over a hollow structure.
urinary r. See micturition reflex.
vagovagal r. A cardiac reflex elicited by irritation of the respiratory tract.
vesical r. See micturition reflex.
Westphal's pupillary r. See orbicularis pupillary reflex.

reflexograph (re-flek´so-graf) An apparatus for graphically recording a reflex.

reflux (re´fluks) Backward flow.
gastroesophageal r. (GER) Reflux of stomach contents into the esophagus.
hepatojugular r., abdominojugular r. Distention of the jugular veins induced by pressing firmly upon the liver; indicative of congestive heart failure.
vesicoureteral r. Flow of urine from the bladder back into a ureter during urination.

refract (re-frakt´) **1.** To change the direction of a propagating wave, as of light. **2.** To measure the refractive and muscular state of the eyes.

refraction (re-frak´shun) (R) **1.** The measurement and/or correction of refractive errors of the eye. **2.** The deflection of a ray of light as a result of passing obliquely from one medium to another of different optical density.
double r. The splitting of light in two slightly different directions to form two rays. Also called birefringence.

refractive (re-frak´tiv) Relating to refraction.

refractometer (re-frak-tom´ĕ-ter) An instrument that measures indices of refraction in translucent substances.

refractoriness (re-frak´tor-e-nes) The inability of nerve cells to respond to a second stimulus delivered immediately after the first stimulus.

refractory (re-frak´to-re) Not responsive or yielding to treatment.

refracture (re-frak´chur) The breaking again of a bone that was improperly set.

refrigerant (re-frij´er-ant) An agent that produces a sensation of coolness.

Refsum's disease (ref´soomz dĭ-zēz´) A hereditary (autosomal recessive) disorder marked by cerebellar ataxia, chronic polyneuritis, pigmentary degeneration of the retina, and night blindness; death is commonly due to degenerative heart disease at an early age. Also called heredopathia atactica polyneuritiformis.

refusion (re-fu´zhun) The return of the circulation of blood after its temporary removal from the same individual.

regeneration (re-jen-er-a´shun) **1.** Replacement of a lost or damaged part by the growth of new tissue. **2.** A form of asexual reproduction.

regimen (rej´ĭ-men) A systematic procedure or regulation of an activity (exercise, diet) designed to achieve certain ends, usually hygienic or therapeutic in nature.

regio (re´je-o), *pl.* **regiones** Latin for region.

region (re´jun) **1.** Any large segment of a body surface with more or less definite boundaries. **2.** A body part with a special nerve or blood supply. **3.** A portion of any structure in the body having a special function.
abdominal r.'s The nine regions into which the abdomen is divided by four imaginary planes, namely the right and left hypochondriac, lumbar, and inguinal (iliac) regions and the epigastric, umbilical, and pubic regions.
chromosomal r.'s Defined areas along both the long and short arms of a chromosome, numerically designated in either direction, starting from the centromere.
hinge r. A short sequence of amino acids present in the three-lobed, Y-shaped immunoglobulin molecule; it is situated between the two short arms of the "Y", which allows movement when necessary (e.g., when binding to an antigen, the Y-shape changes to a taut T-shape).

registration (rej-ĭ-stra´shun) In dentistry, a record of jaw relations.

regression (re-gresh´un) **1.** A relapse. **2.** An unconscious psychological defense mechanism in which there is a partial return to an earlier pattern of behavior or level of adaptation.

regulation (reg-u-la´shun) **1.** A law or rule designed to control details of procedure. **2.** In experimental embryology, the power of a very young embryo to

R

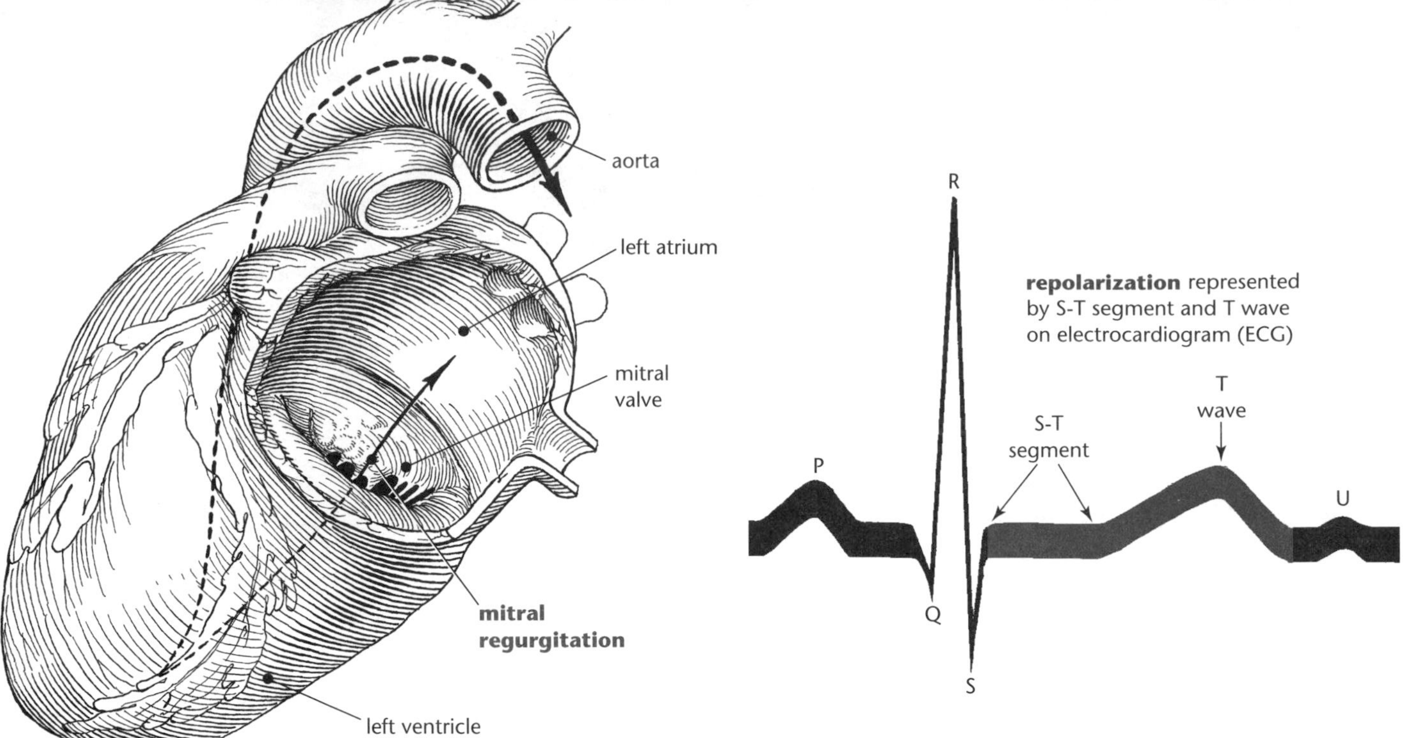

regenerate and continue its development in spite of experimental interference.

regurgitation (re-gur-jĭ-ta´shun) A backward flow (e.g., the return of stomach contents).

aortic r. Regurgitation of blood through an incompetent aortic valve into the left ventricle during ventricular relaxation (diastole).

mitral r. Back flow of blood, from the left ventricle to the left atrium, through an incompetent mitral (left atrioventricular) valve.

rehabilitation (re-hă-bil-ĭ-ta´shun) **1.** Restoration of form and function following illness or injury. **2.** Restoration of an individual's capability to achieve the fullest possible life compatible with his abilities and disabilities.

mouth r. The restoration of all lost tooth structure.

Reifenstein's syndrome (rī´fen-stīnz sin´drōm) An X-linked recessive inheritance; a form of male pseudohermaphrodism associated with hypospadias, small testes, sterility, absence of beard, short stature, and often enlarged breasts. Also called hereditary familial hypogonadism.

reimplantation (re-im-plan-ta´shun) Replacement of a body structure to its natural position, as a tooth to the socket from which it was previously removed. Also called replantation.

reinfection (re-in-fek´shun) A second infection by the same agent following recovery or during the course of the primary infection.

reinforcement (re-in-fors´ment) **1.** Added force or strength, such as the increased reflex response when the person performs some mental or physical work while the reflex is being elicited. **2.** A structural addition to strengthen a denture.

reinnervation (re-in-er-va´shun) The restoration of a damaged nerve either by grafting of a live nerve or by spontaneous regrowth of nerve fibers.

reintegration (re-in-te-gra´shun) In psychiatry, the resumption of normal functioning after a mental disorder.

Reiter's syndrome (ri´terz sin´drōm) (RS) A symptom complex consisting of urethritis, conjunctivitis, arthritis, and mucocutaneous lesions; recurrences or chronicity occur in more than one-half of the patients; cause is unknown.

rejection (re-jek´shun) Immune response against transplanted tissue (graft) that is antigenically incompatible with the host's body, leading to failure of function of the graft.

chronic allograft r. Gradual immunologic damage to a kidney transplant, marked by diffuse fibrosis of the glomerulus, fibrosis of blood vessel walls, and tubular atrophy and loss of tubular structures.

hyperacute r. (a) Rejection of a graft within one hour of implantation. (b) Diffuse clot formation throughout a transplanted organ.

second-set graft r. Accelerated rejection of a second graft due to immunity developed to a primary graft.

relapse (re-laps´) The return of a disease after apparent recovery or improvement.

relation (re-la´shun) The position of one object when considered in association with another.

centric r. The most posterior position of the mandible from which lateral jaw movements can be made at any given degree of jaw separation.

eccentric r. Any deviation from the centric relation.

rest r. The relation of the mandible to the maxilla when the person is resting in an upright position and the jaws are not in contact.

relationship (re-la´shun-ship) An association; a kinship.

coefficient of r. See under coefficient.

object r. The emotional bonds existing between two people or groups.

relative biologic effectiveness (re-la´tiv bi-o-loj´ik ĕ-fek´tiv-nes) (RBE) A measure of the capacity of absorbed doses of various types of radiation (x rays, neutrons, alpha particles, etc.) to produce a specific biologic effect; it may vary with the kind and degree of biologic effect considered, the duration of the exposure, and other factors.

relative of interest (re-la´tiv ŭv in´trĭst) In genetic counseling, anyone who seeks counsel about recurrence of a disease in a family. COMPARE: proband; consultand.

relax (re-laks´) To loosen or slacken; to make less tense.

relaxant (re-lak´sant) **1.** A drug or therapeutic treatment that produces relaxation by relieving muscular or nervous tension. **2.** Tending to reduce tension.

relaxation (re-lak-sa´shun) **1.** Loosening. **2.** The lengthening of muscle fibers.

relaxin (re-lak´sin) Ovarian hormone, produced by the corpus luteum, that relaxes the pubic symphysis and other pelvic joints and softens and dilates the uterine cervix during labor.

relief (re-lēf´) **1.** The lessening of pain or distress, physical or mental. **2.** In dentistry, the removal of pressure from a specific area under a denture base.

relieve (re-lēv´) **1.** To free wholly or partly (e.g., from pain, discomfort, anxiety, fear). **2.** Colloquially, to eliminate body waste.

reline (re-līn´) To resurface the tissue side of a denture with new base material in order to make it fit better.

rem (rem) Acronym for roentgen-equivalent-man. A unit of radiation dose equal to the amount of absorbed ionizing radiation that is required to produce a biologic effect equivalent to the absorption of 1 rad of x rays or γ rays; 1 rem = 1 rad × RBE (relative biologic effectiveness).

remediable (re-me´de-ă-bl) Capable of being cured. Also called curable.

remedial (re-me´de-al) Able to correct a deficiency, especially a reading deficiency.

remedy (rem´ĕ-de) **1.** A drug or a therapy that cures or palliates disease, or corrects a disorder. **2.** To effect a cure.

remineralization (re-min-er-al-ĭ-za´shun) Restoration of mineral elements to the body, especially of calcium salts to bone.

remission (re-mish´un) Abatement of the symptoms of a disease.

remit (re-mit´) To temporarily abate in severity without absolutely ceasing; to diminish.

remittent (re-mit´ent) Characterized by alternating periods of abatement and returning of symptoms.

renal (re´nal) Relating to the kidneys. Also called nephric.

renaturation (re-nā-chur-a´shun) The return of denatured protein to its normal characteristic biologic activity, accompanied by the return of its native form. Also called refolding; annealing.

Rendu-Osler-Weber syndrome (ron-dur´-ōs-ler-web´er sin´drōm) See hereditary hemorrhagic telangiectasia, under telangiectasia.

reniform (ren´ĭ-form) Kidney-shaped.

renin (re´nin) Enzyme formed in the kidneys and released into the bloodstream; it has an important role in the formation of angiotensin (a potent pressor agent) thereby in the regulation of blood pressure.

rennet (ren´et) A dry extract containing rennin, obtained from the lining of the fourth stomach of the calf; used in curdling milk.

rennin (ren´in) A milk-curdling enzyme obtained from rennet, used in making cheese. Also called chymosin.

renogram, radioactive (re´no-gram, ra-de-o-ak´tiv) A graphic record produced by the continuous recording of radioactivity of the kidney after injection of a radiopharmaceutical; an aid in the clinical evaluation of kidney function.

renography (re-nog´ră-fe) Roentgenography of the kidney.

renomegaly (re-no-meg´ă-le) Abnormal enlargement of the kidney.

renoprival (re-no-pri´val) Resulting from removal of kidneys or total absence of kidney function.

renotrophic (re-no-trof´ik) Affecting the growth of the kidney. Also called nephrotropic.

renotrophin (re-no-trof´in) An agent that affects the growth of the kidney.

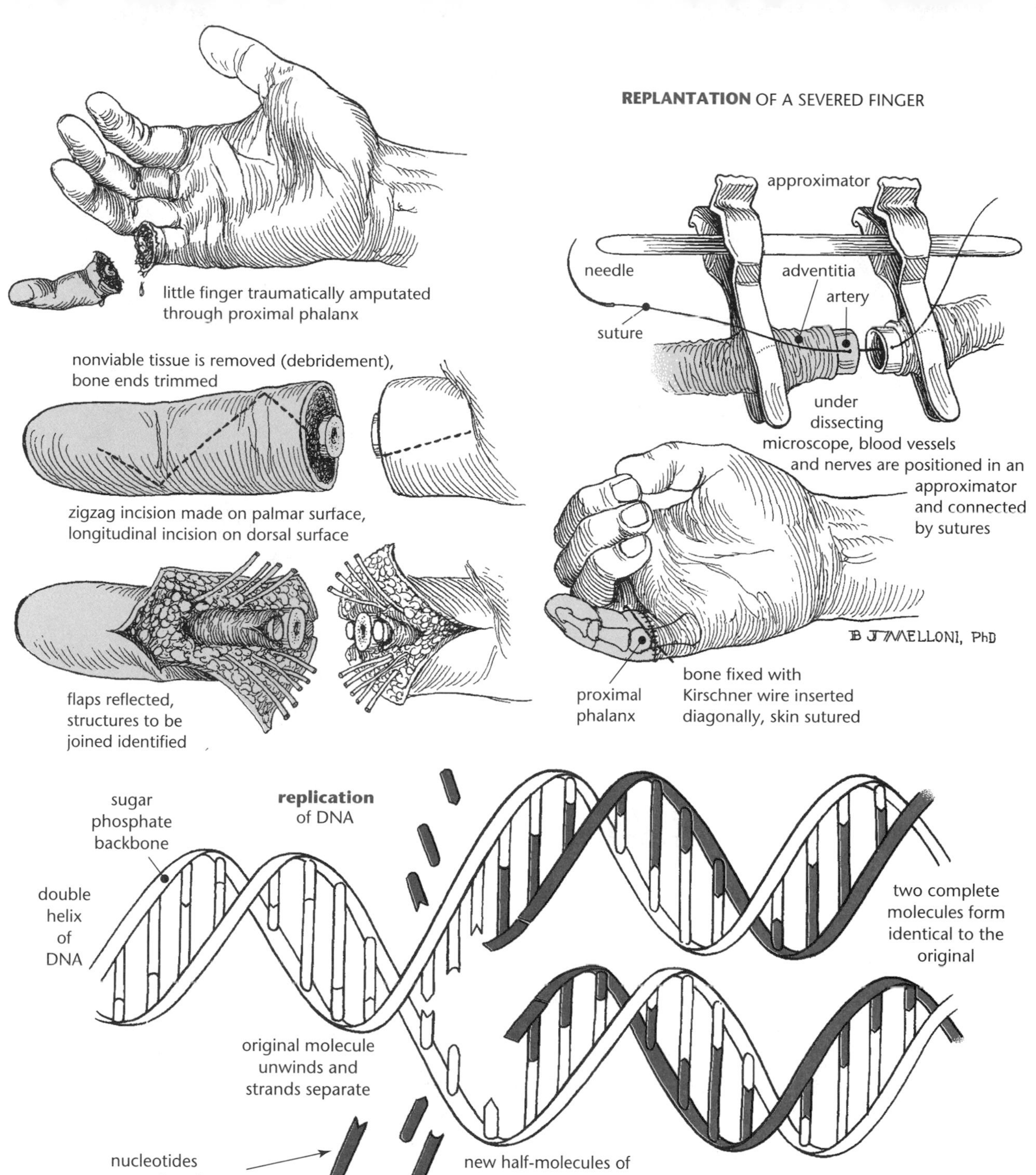
REPLANTATION OF A SEVERED FINGER
little finger traumatically amputated through proximal phalanx
nonviable tissue is removed (debridement), bone ends trimmed
zigzag incision made on palmar surface, longitudinal incision on dorsal surface
flaps reflected, structures to be joined identified
approximator
needle
adventitia
artery
suture
under dissecting microscope, blood vessels and nerves are positioned in an approximator and connected by sutures
B J MELLONI, PhD
proximal phalanx
bone fixed with Kirschner wire inserted diagonally, skin sutured
replication of DNA
sugar phosphate backbone
double helix of DNA
two complete molecules form identical to the original
original molecule unwinds and strands separate
nucleotides present in cells
new half-molecules of DNA formed on old halves

renovascular (re-no-vas´ku-lar) Referring to the blood vessels of the kidneys.

reoviruses (re-o-vi´rus-ēz) An RNA group of viruses (genus *Reovirus*) replicating in the cytoplasm; associated with sporadic upper respiratory infections, skin rashes, and certain types of pneumonia and encephalitis.

repellent (re-pel´ent) **1.** Capable of causing aversion. **2.** Any agent that repels something, especially one that repels insects.

replantation (re-plan-ta´shun) Replacement of a body part to its natural position, as the reinsertion of a dislodged tooth into its original socket, or the reattachment of a severed finger. Also called reimplantation.

replicase (rep´lĭ-kās) Any enzyme that promotes RNA replication; associated with replication of RNA viruses.

replication (rep-lĭ-ka´shun) The process of duplicating something (e.g., the repeated formation of the same molecule, as of DNA). Also called autoreproduction.

repolarization (re-pol-lar-ĭ-za´shun) A process, immediately following depolarization of the cell, in which the surface of the cell membrane is polarized again by the gradual restoration of the positive charges on the outer and negative charges on the inner surface of the membrane; for cardiac muscle, graphically shown on the electrocardiogram by the S-T segment and T wave.

repositor (re-poz´ĭ-tor) An instrument for replacing a prolapsed or dislocated organ, especially the uterus.

repositioning (re-pŏ-zish´un-ing) See reduction (1).

repression (re-presh´un) **1.** A defense mechanism by which unacceptable ideas, impulses, or feelings are forced into the unconscious and kept out of conscious awareness. **2.** The prevention of the formation of an enzyme as programmed by a structural gene in the presence of a small corepressor molecule.

repressor (re-pres´or) The product of a regulatory gene, capable of combining with a corepressor to form an active complex, or with an inducer to form an inactive complex.

reproduction (re-pro-duk´shun) The process of producing offspring.
asexual r. Reproduction without the union of male and female sex cells.
assisted r. Reproduction achieved with the aid of any of several technologies involved in direct retrieval of oocytes from the ovary (e.g., *in vitro* fertilization [IVF], gamete intrafallopian transfer [GIFT], tubal embryo transfer [TET]).
sexual r. Reproduction by the union of male and female sex cells.
somatic r. Reproduction by splitting or budding of cells other than sex cells.

Reptilia (rep-til´e-ă) A class of cold-blooded, usually egg laying, vertebrates that includes snakes, lizards, turtles, and crocodiles.

repulsion (re-pul´shun) **1.** The act of repelling, or the condition of being repelled. **2.** Extreme dislike.

reradiation (re-ra-de-a´shun) Radiation emanating from a substance as a result of its absorbing radiation.

research (re-serch´) Investigation or experimenta-

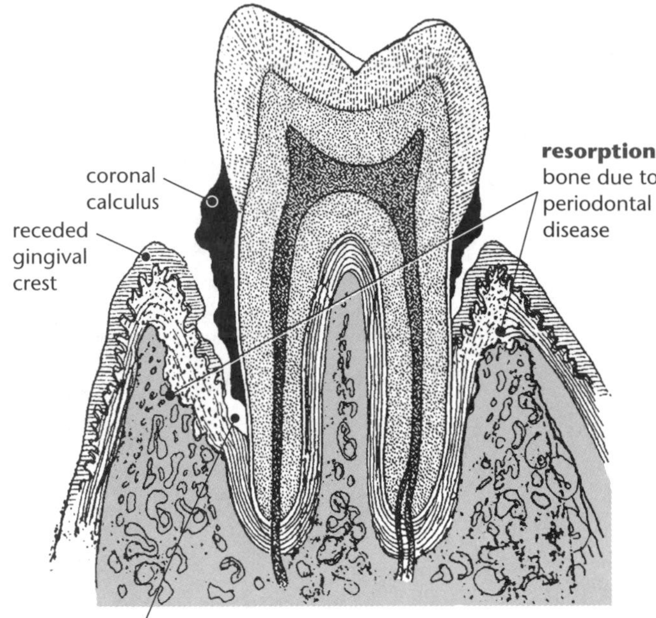

patterns of **respiration**

one minute

normal **respiration**

ataxic respiration

Cheyne-Stokes respiration

tion.

resect (re-sekt´) To cut off.

resectable (re-sek´tă-bl) Amenable to surgical removal; capable of being cut off.

resection (re-sek´shun) The surgical removal of a portion of any part.

loop r. See loop electrosurgical excision procedure (LEEP), under procedure.

transurethral r. of prostate (TURP) Removal of obstructive prostatic tissue with an instrument introduced through the urethra.

resectoscope (re-sek´tŏ-skōp) An instrument for removing prostate gland tissue through the urethra.

reserpine (re-ser´pēn) An alkaloid, $C_{33}H_{40}N_2O_9$, isolated from the roots of certain species of *Rauwolfia*; used to reduce blood pressure in hypertension and as a tranquilizer.

reserve (re-zerv´) Something stored and available for future use.

cardiac r. The work that the heart is capable of performing beyond ordinary requirements.

reset (re´set) To set again, as a broken bone.

resident (rez´ĭ-dent) A house officer in a hospital receiving clinical training in a specialized field of medicine. Also called resident physician.

postgraduate year 1 r. See intern.

residual (re-zid´u-al) Relating to the quantity remaining or left behind at the end of a process; left over.

residue (rez´ĭ-doo) **1.** Material remaining after the completion of an abstractive physical or chemical process. Also called residuum. **2.** An amino acid unit in a polypeptide chain.

residuum (re-zid´u-um) See residue.

resilience (re-zil´yĕns) Elasticity.

resin (rez´in) **1.** Any of various viscous substances of plant origin, such as amber and rosin, that are usually transparent or translucent; used in synthetic plastics, adhesives, and pharmaceuticals. **2.** Any of various polymerized synthetics, such as polyethylene, epoxies and silicones, that are used with other components to form plastics. **3.** In dentistry, a plastic filling material having good esthetic appearance.

acrylic r. A thermoplastic resinous material of the various esters of acrylic acid; the principal ingredient of many plastics used in dentistry.

autopolymer r. A resin that can be polymerized by an activator and a catalyst rather than by the application of heat; it sets at room or body temperature. Also called cold-curing resin; quick-curing resin; self-curing resin.

cold-curing r. See autopolymer resin.

cholestyramine r. An insoluble chloride salt of a basic anion exchange resin that binds bile acids in the intestine and prevents their reabsorption; the reduced levels of bile acids increase the rate of conversion of cholesterol to bile acids in the liver; used in treatment of hyperlipoproteinemia; Cuemid®; Questran®.

dental r. A synthetic acrylic resin widely used in dentistry.

epoxy r. Any thermosetting resin that is a condensation polymer of epichlorohydrin and bisphenol and forms a tight cross-linked structure that exhibits strong adhesion and chemical resistance, used in surface coatings, adhesives, and as embedding medium for electron microscopy.

ion-exchange r. An insoluble, porous solid material of high molecular weight containing an active electrolyte; it contains either acidic groups (cation-active) or basic groups (anion-active); one type is used to lower the potassium content of the body in the treatment of hyperkalemia.

methyl methacrylate r. A stable, transparent resin that is liquid at room temperature and is polymerized by the use of a chemical initiator; widely used in medical and dental appliances.

podophyllum r. A bitter-tasting resin derived from the dried rhizome and root of the May apple (*Podophyllum peltatum*); used as a cathartic and topical caustic.

quick-curing r. See autopolymer resin.

quinine carbacrylic r. A quinine salt of a resin containing about 2% quininium ion; used in testing deficiency of acids in the gastric juice, especially of hydrochloric acid.

self-curing r. See autopolymer resin.

thermoplastic r. A synthetic resin that becomes soft when heated and hard when cooled.

resinous (rez´ĭ-nus) Relating to a resin.

resistance (re-zis´tans) **1.** Any force that opposes and/or retards motion. **2.** (R) In electricity, the opposition to the passage of electric current. **3.** In psychiatry, an individual's psychologic defense against recalling repressed or unpleasant experiences.

drug r. A state of decreased response to drugs that ordinarily inhibit cell growth or cause cell death.

expiratory r. Resistance in the air passages to the flow of air out of the lungs.

peripheral r. See total peripheral resistance.

total peripheral r. The sum of resistance to the flow of blood through the blood vessels; MAP/CO (mean arterial pressure/cardiac output). Also called peripheral resistance.

resolution (rez-o-loo´shun) **1.** The return of tissues to their normal state at the end of an acute morbid condition (e.g., inflammation). **2.** The ability to perceive two separate adjacent objects as two; visual resolution.

resolve (re-zolv´) To return to normal after an inflammatory process.

resolvent (re-zol´vent) **1.** Causing or capable of causing resolution of a tumor or swelling. **2.** Any substance that promotes the dissipation of a pathologic growth or reduces an inflammation. **3.** Promoting the separation into constituents.

resonance (rez´o-nans) **1.** The sound heard on percussion. **2.** In chemistry, the property of a substance whereby two or more structural forms of the substance are simultaneously present.

amphoric r. Sound resembling that produced by blowing over the mouth of an empty bottle.

electron spin r. (ESR) In spectrometry, resonance arising from electron spin, related to the extent of activity of free radicals in an organic reaction.

nuclear magnetic r. (NMR) A measure of the dipole moment of atomic nuclei (i.e., the ratio of the maximum torque applied to the nuclei in a magnetic field to the induction of the field); used in studies of covalent bonds involved in organic reactions; also used for diagnostic imaging. See also imaging.

tympanic r. Percussion sound heard over a hollow structure.

vesicular r. Sound heard on percussion of normal lungs.

vocal r. (VR) Voice sounds heard on auscultation of the chest.

resonator (rez´o-na-ter) An apparatus designed to create an electric current of very high potential and small volume.

resorcinol (rĕ-zor´sĭ-nol) A keratolytic compound, $C_6H_4(OH)_2$; in concentrations of 2 to 10%, it is used in treating acne by causing a mild irritation that produces some peeling.

resorption (re-sorp´shun) **1.** Assimilation of excreted material. **2.** Dissolution of tissue by physiologic or pathologic means, as of the gums or of the bones surrounding the teeth.

respirable (rĕ-spīr´ă-bl) Fit for breathing.

respiration (res-pĭ-ra´shun) (R) **1.** The physical and chemical processes through which an organism acquires oxygen and releases carbon dioxide. **2.** The act of breathing.

abdominal r. Respiration effected mainly by the abdominal muscles.

aerobic r. Respiration effected in the presence of air through the consumption of free oxygen.

anaerobic r. Respiration that is carried on in the absence, or near absence, of air, without involving free oxygen.

apneustic r. Breathing characterized by inspiratory spasms of varying duration, often lasting several seconds; seen in persons with lesions of the lower pons.

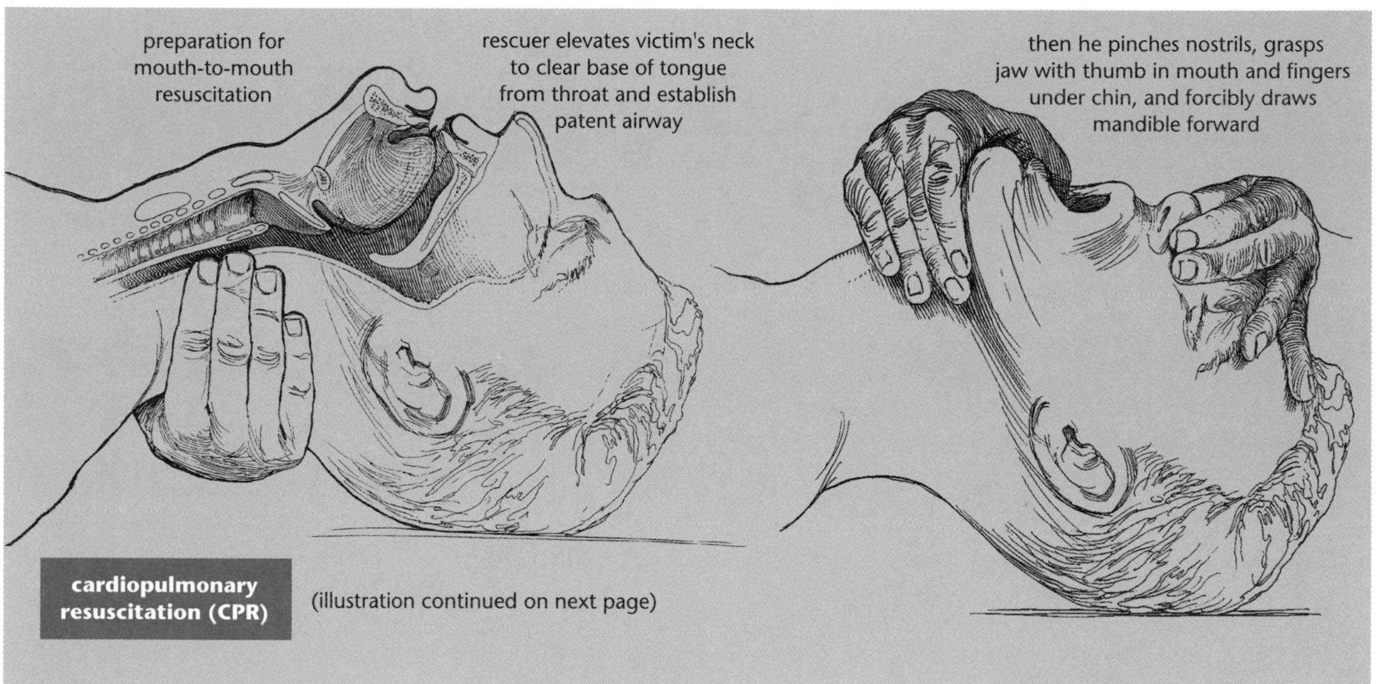
preparation for
mouth-to-mouth
resuscitation
rescuer elevates victim's neck
to clear base of tongue
from throat and establish
patent airway
then he pinches nostrils, grasps
jaw with thumb in mouth and fingers
under chin, and forcibly draws
mandible forward
cardiopulmonary
resuscitation (CPR)
(illustration continued on next page)

artificial r. See artificial ventilation, under ventilation.

assisted r. See assisted ventilation, under ventilation.

ataxic r. Gasping, irregular (in rate and depth) breathing; seen in individuals with medullary lesions. Also called Biot's breathing.

Cheyne-Stokes r. A rhythmic increase and decrease in the depth of respiration.

controlled r. See controlled ventilation, under ventilation.

diffusion r. Introduction of oxygen into the lungs through a catheter. Also called apneic oxygenation.

external r. The interchange of gases in the lungs.

forced r. Voluntary increase in the rate and depth of breathing.

internal r. See tissue respiration.

Kussmaul r. Respiration marked by deep sighing; characteristic of diabetic acidosis.

mouth-to-mouth r. See mouth-to-mouth breathing, under breathing.

positive pressure r. See continuous positive pressure ventilation and intermittent positive pressure ventilation, under ventilation.

tissue r. The exchange of gases between tissue cells and blood. Also called internal respiration.

respirator (res´pĭ-ra-tor) **1.** An apparatus used to administer artificial respiration. **2.** A screenlike device fitted over the nose and mouth to protect the respiratory passages.

Drinker r. An airtight metal tank designed to enclose the body (except the head) and provide artificial respiration by exerting intermittent negative air pressure on the chest. Its use has decreased in favor of less cumbersome equipment. Also called iron lung; tank respirator.

pressure-controlled r. A respirator that supplies a predetermined pressure to gases during inhalation; the volume of gas delivered varies, depending upon resistance.

tank r. See Drinker respirator.

volume-controlled r. A respirator that supplies a predetermined volume of gases during inhalation; the pressure needed to move the gases varies, depending upon resistance.

respiratory (re-spī´ră-tor-e) Relating to respiration.

respiratory distress syndrome (RDS) of newborn (re-spi´ră-tor-e dĭ-stres´ sin´drōm ŭv noo´born) Acute difficult breathing and bluish coloration of the skin commonly occurring as a complication of premature birth; also seen in infants born to diabetic mothers and in those delivered by cesarean section; caused by deficient fetal production of surfactant. Also called hyaline membrane disease of newborn.

respire (rĕ-spīr´) To breathe.

respirometer (res-pĭ-rom´ĕ-ter) See spirometer.

response (re-spons´) A reaction to a specific stimulus.

autoimmune r. An immune response in which the action of an autoantibody is directed to a "self" antigen; distinguished from autoimmune disease, with which it may or may not be associated.

biphasic r. (a) Two responses separated by time. (b) Immediate reaction to a substance (antigen) and recurrence after a symptom-free period.

consensual r. See consensual reaction, under reaction.

evoked r. A change in the electrical activity of the nervous system resulting from an incoming sensory stimulus. Also called evoked potential.

galvanic skin r. The change in skin resistance in response to a stimulus.

immune r. A specific response resulting in immunity, which includes an afferent phase during which responsive cells are primed by antigen, a central response during which antibodies are formed, and an efferent response in which immunity is effected by antibodies.

primary r. The immune response resulting from an initial encounter with a particular antigen; it may be cellular or humoral.

secondary r. The increased and more rapid production of antibodies upon a second and subsequent exposure to a particular antigen; an immune response. Also called anamnestic reaction.

triple r. The three degrees of reaction of the skin to injury; i.e., a red line, a flare around the red line, and a wheal surrounded by the flare.

rest (rest) **1.** Repose. **2.** A portion of displaced embryonic tissue that becomes embedded in other structures. **3.** In dentistry, an extension from a prosthesis that aids in supporting a restoration.

adrenal r. An accessory adrenal (suprarenal) gland.

restenosis (re-stĕ-no´sis) Recurrence of stenosis, after corrective surgery of the primary condition.

restiform (res´tĭ-form) Shaped like a rope, as the ropelike restiform body (inferior peduncle) connecting the cerebellum to the medulla oblongata.

restitution (res-tĭ-tu´shun) See external rotation, under rotation.

restless legs syndrome (rest´les legs sin´drōm) A feeling of creepiness, twitching, and restlessness deep in the legs, usually occurring in the elderly upon lying down; cause is unknown.

restoration (res-to ra´shun) **1.** The process of returning to a healthy state. **2.** In dentistry, a prosthetic device or appliance designed to replace lost teeth or oral tissues.

restorative (res-stōr´ă-tiv) Tending to renew health.

restraint (re-strānt´) **1.** Any device for controlling or preventing the free movement of an excited or violent patient who may cause harm to himself or to others. **2.** Any device (excluding splints and casts) used to stabilize or prevent motion of the body or a body part.

resuscitate (re-sus´ĭ-tāt) To restore from a state of apparent or potential death.

resuscitation (re-sus-ĭ-ta´shun) The act of resuscitating or the state of being resuscitated.

cardiopulmonary r. (CPR) Restoration of respiration and cardiac contraction by following three basic steps: establishing a patent airway, mouth-to-mouth breathing, and external cardiac compression (the ABCs of CPR).

mouth-to-mouth r. See mouth-to-mouth breathing, under breathing.

resuscitator (re-sus´ĭ-ta-tor) An apparatus that forces gas, usually oxygen, into the lungs to initiate respiration as in asphyxia.

retainer (re-ta´ner) **1.** Device for maintaining teeth in proper alignment after orthodontic treatment. **2.** The part of a fixed denture (dental bridge) attaching the prosthesis to the supporting natural tooth; may be an inlay, partial-veneer, or complete crown. **3.** Any device (e.g., a clasp) used for stabilizing a prosthesis.

continuous bar r. A metal bar placed in contact with the lingual surfaces of teeth to aid in stabilizing the teeth or in retaining a partial denture.

direct r. A clasp or attachment placed on a supporting tooth to maintain a removable appliance in position.

indirect r. An attachment of a removable partial denture that assists the direct retainers in preventing displacement of free-end denture bases.

retardate (re-tar´dāt) A mentally retarded person.

retardation (re-tar-da´shun) Slow or diminished development.

mental r. Subnormal intellectual functioning originating during the individual's developmental period, often associated with impairment of adjustment (social and learning) or maturation, or both; an IQ score of 69 or below on a standardized intelligence test. Also called mental deficiency.

rete (re´te), *pl.* **retia** A network, as of nerve fibers or minute blood vessels.

retention (re-ten´shun) **1.** The act of holding food and drink in the stomach. **2.** The holding back of body wastes that are normally discharged. **3.** The ability to remember. **4.** Maintaining in position.

denture r. The means by which a denture is maintained in proper position in the mouth.

direct r. Retention of a removable partial denture

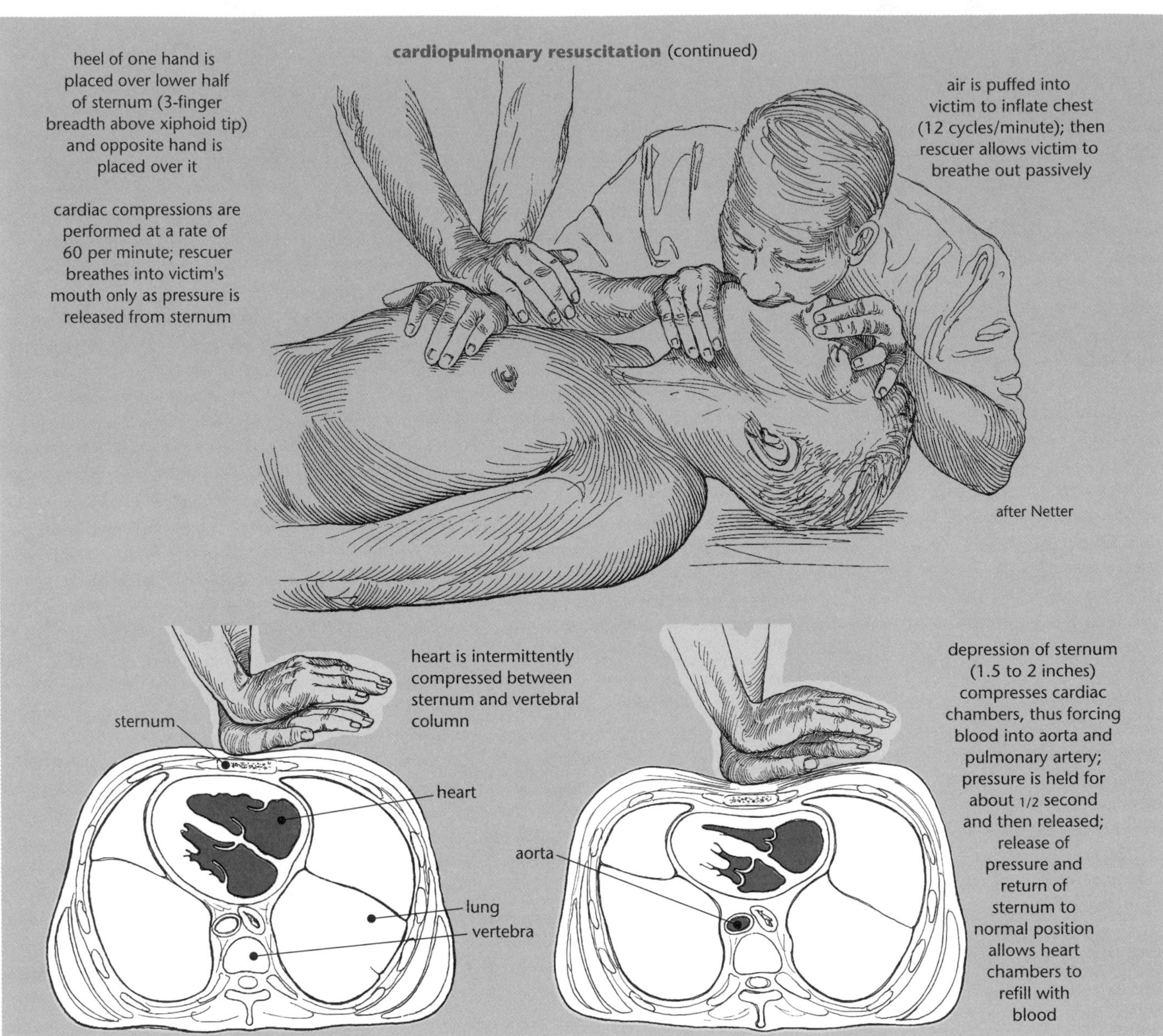
cardiopulmonary resuscitation (continued)
heel of one hand is placed over lower half of sternum (3-finger breadth above xiphoid tip) and opposite hand is placed over it
cardiac compressions are performed at a rate of 60 per minute; rescuer breathes into victim's mouth only as pressure is released from sternum
air is puffed into victim to inflate chest (12 cycles/minute); then rescuer allows victim to breathe out passively
after Netter
heart is intermittently compressed between sternum and vertebral column
sternum
heart
aorta
lung
vertebra
depression of sternum (1.5 to 2 inches) compresses cardiac chambers, thus forcing blood into aorta and pulmonary artery; pressure is held for about 1/2 second and then released; release of pressure and return of sternum to normal position allows heart chambers to refill with blood

by means of clasps attached to the anchoring teeth.

indirect r. Retention of a removable partial denture by means of an attachment used in conjunction with a direct retainer.

retention lug (re-ten′shun lug) A metal attachment soldered to either an orthodontic band or an artificial crown to insure stabilization of a dental prosthesis.

reticular (rĕ-tik′u-lar) Netlike; pertaining to a reticulum.

reticulin (rĕ-tik′u-lin) A scleroprotein present in the connective fibers of reticular or lymphatic tissues.

reticulocyte (rĕ-tik′u-lo-sīt) The youngest red blood cell in the circulating blood; it constitutes 1% of the red blood cell population. When supravitally stained with cresyl blue, the scattered ribosomes of the cell clump together, giving it a reticulated appearance.

reticulocytopenia (rĕ-tik-u-lo-si-to-pe′ne-ă) Diminution of reticulocytes in the blood.

reticulocytosis (rĕ-tik-u-lo-si-to′sis) The abnormal increase in the percentage of reticulocytes in the blood.

reticuloendothelial (rĕ-tik-u-lo-en-do-the′le-al) Relating to the reticuloendothelium (i.e., to tissues having both reticular and endothelial properties).

reticuloendothelioma (rĕ-tik-u-lo-en-do-the-le-o′mă) A localized neoplasm (e.g., malignant lymphoma) derived from reticuloendothelial tissue.

reticuloendotheliosis (rĕ-tik-u-lo-en-do-the-le-o′sis) Abnormal conditions, especially hyperplasia, of the reticuloendothelium in any of the organs or tissues.

reticuloendothelium (rĕ-tik-u-lo-en-do-the′le-um) A widely dispersed body system of morphologically varied cells concerned with phagocytosis; present in the thymus, spleen, lymph nodes, etc.

reticulosis (rĕ-tik-u-lo′sis) A short version of the term for reticuloendotheliosis.

reticulum (rĕ-tik′u-lum) A fine network, especially one formed of protoplasmic material within a cell.

agranular endoplasmic r. (AER) Endoplasmic reticulum that is free of ribosomal granules. Also called smooth endoplasmic reticulum (SER).

endoplasmic r. (ER) An extensive network of fine folded membranes interspersed throughout the cytoplasm of the cell; it is continuous with the outer portion of the nuclear membrane and with the Golgi apparatus; depending on the cell type in which it is located, it can play a role in detoxification of certain drugs, lipid and cholesterol metabolism, production of steroid hormones, and other biologic processes.

granular endoplasmic r. (GER) Endoplasmic reticulum with numerous ribosomal granules on its surface. Also called rough endoplasmic reticulum (RER); ergastoplasm.

rough endoplasmic r. (RER) See granular endoplasmic reticulum.

smooth endoplasmic r. (SER) See agranular endoplasmic reticulum.

retina (ret′ĭ-nă) The innermost of the three tunics of the eyeball, consisting of an outer pigmented layer and an inner nervous layer or retina proper which, in turn, is composed of eight microscopic layers, named from within outward as follows: nerve fiber layer, ganglionic layer, inner plexiform layer, inner nuclear layer, outer plexiform layer, outer nuclear layer, layer of rods and cones, and pigment layer.

retinaculum (rĕt-ĭ-nak′u-lum), *pl.* **retina′cula** A retaining bandlike ligament, as seen in the wrist and ankle.

retinal (ret′ĭ-nal) **1.** Pertaining to the retina. **2.** See retinaldehyde.

retinaldehyde (ret-ĭ-nal′dĕ-hīd) The aldehyde of retinol present in the visual pigments of the retina; one isomer (11-*cis*-retinal) occurs in rhodopsin in combination with the protein group opsin; another (all-*trans*-retinal) is the yellow pigment resulting from the bleaching of rhodopsin by light. Also called retinal.

retinitis (ret-ĭ-ni′tis) Inflammation of the retina (the innermost layer of the eyeball).

r. pigmentosa (RP) Hereditary degeneration and atrophy of the retina, usually with migration of pigment, causing gradual reduction of peripheral vision; its first symptom, night blindness, is usually seen in children and adolescents; an autosomal dominant inheritance.

retinoblastoma (ret-ĭ-no-blas-to′mă) A congenital malignant tumor of the retina, composed of embryonic retinal cells; usually observed before the age of four.

retinochoroiditis (ret-ĭ-no-ko-roi-di′tis) See chorioretinitis.

retinoic acid (ret′in-o′ik as′id) Acid derived from

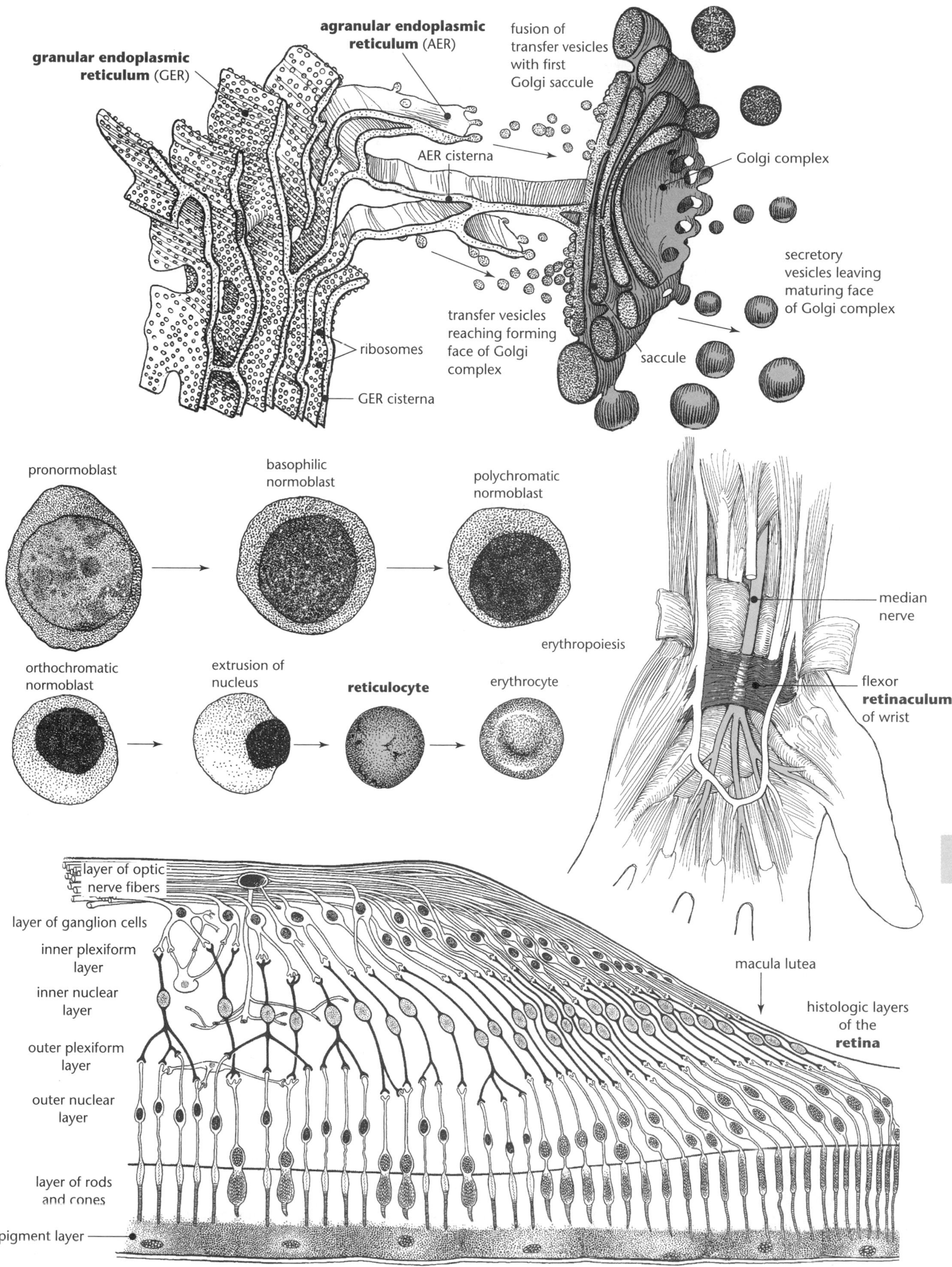
agranular endoplasmic reticulum (AER)
fusion of transfer vesicles with first Golgi saccule
granular endoplasmic reticulum (GER)
AER cisterna
Golgi complex
secretory vesicles leaving maturing face of Golgi complex
transfer vesicles reaching forming face of Golgi complex
ribosomes
saccule
GER cisterna
pronormoblast
basophilic normoblast
polychromatic normoblast
median nerve
erythropoiesis
orthochromatic normoblast
extrusion of nucleus
reticulocyte
erythrocyte
flexor retinaculum of wrist
layer of optic nerve fibers
layer of ganglion cells
inner plexiform layer
inner nuclear layer
macula lutea
histologic layers of the retina
outer plexiform layer
outer nuclear layer
layer of rods and cones
pigment layer

R

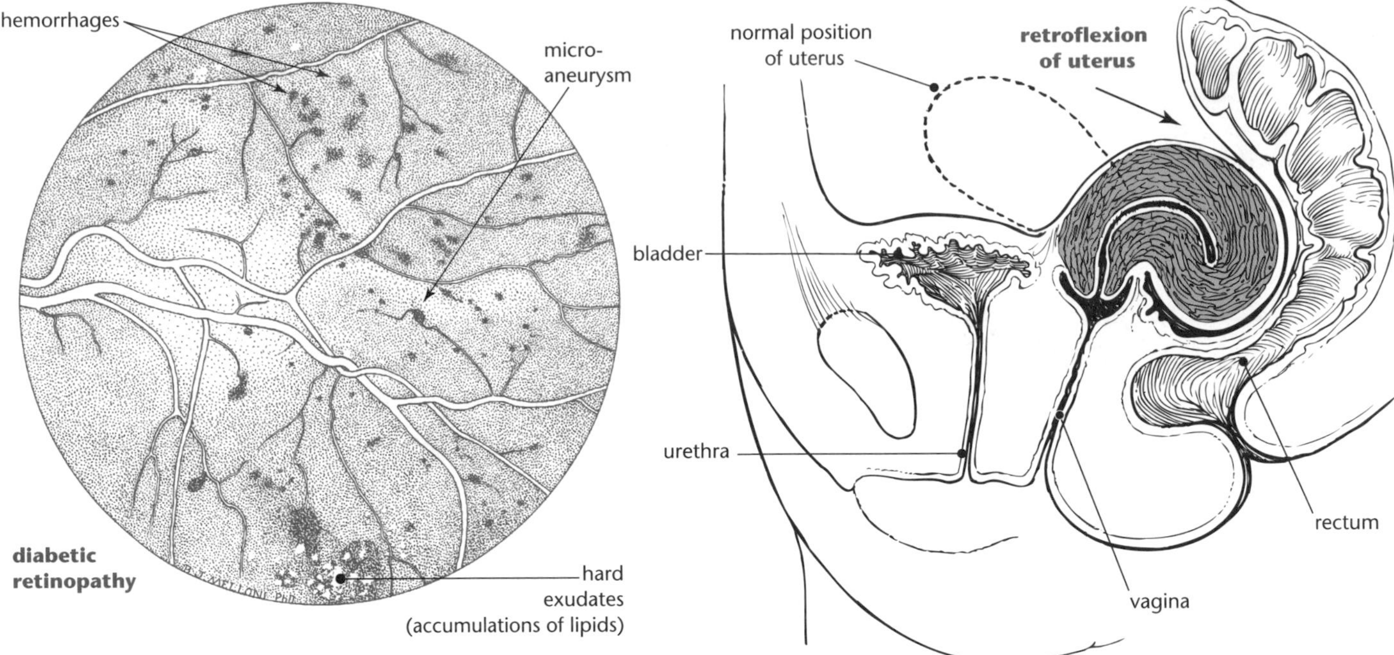

oxidation of the alcohol group of retinol (vitamin A) to an aldehyde and carboxyl; used topically to treat acne.

retinoid (ret´ĭ-noid) **1.** Resembling a resin. **2.** Resembling the retina.

retinoids (ret´ĭ-noids) Compounds derived from retinoic acid; used to treat severe acne and psoriasis.

retinol (ret´ĭ-nol) A 20-carbon alcohol. Also called vitamin A_1.

retinomalacia (ret-ĭ-no-mă-la´she-ă) Degeneration of the retina.

retinopapillitis (ret-ĭ-no-pap-ĭ-li´tis) See papilloretinitis.

retinopathy (ret-ĭ-nop´ă-the) Any degenerative noninflammatory disease of the retina.

arteriosclerotic r. Changes in the fundus of the eye associated with arteriosclerosis and benign hypertension; blood vessels show variations in caliber, increased tortuosity, and compression of veins at arteriovenous crossings.

diabetic r. Progressive disease of the blood vessels in the retina, occurring as a complication of diabetes of long duration; usually includes capillary hemorrhages, waxy and cottonlike deposits, microaneurysms, and development of new blood vessels; it may lead to severe visual disability.

R

hypertensive r. Disease of the blood vessels in the retina occurring as a complication of hypertension; the initial change is narrowing of the arterioles caused by spasm; in later stages hemorrhages and exudates are seen; papilledema may appear in extreme cases associated with hypertensive encephalopathy.

macular r. See maculopathy.

r. of prematurity (ROP) Eye condition of premature infants, associated with exposure to high concentrations of oxygen; marked by constriction and obliteration of retinal capillaries, followed by new blood vessel formation, retinal hemorrhages, fibrosis, and retinal detachment; it is usually reversible before fibrosis occurs. Formerly called retrolental fibroplasia.

retinopiesis (ret-ĭ-no-pi-e´sis) The pressing of a detached retina back into its normal position, as by air, intravitreal silicone, saline, etc.

retinoscope (ret´ĭ-no-skōp) An optical instrument for examining the refractive state of the eye.

retinoscopy (ret-ĭ-nos´ko-pe) Ophthalmologic examination with a retinoscope to determine the objective measurements of the refractive properties of the eyes. Also called shadow test; skiametry; skiascopy.

retort (re-tort´) A closed, long-necked laboratory vessel resembling a flask; used in distillation.

retract (re-trakt´) **1.** To shrink back. **2.** To pull back.

retractile (re-trak´til) Capable of being drawn back.

retraction (re-trak´shun) **1.** Drawing back. **2.** A shrinking.

gingival r. Retraction of the gums from the tooth surface due to an underlying inflammation.

retractor (re-trak´tor) A surgical instrument used to draw apart the edges of a wound.

retrad (re´trad) Directed toward the back.

retrobulbar (ret-ro-bul´bar) Behind the eyeball.

retrocecal (ret-ro-se´kal) Behind the cecum.

retrocervical (ret-ro-ser´ve-kal) Behind the uterine cervix.

retrocolic (ret-ro-kol´ik) Behind the colon.

retrodisplacement (ret-ro-dis-plās´ment) Backward displacement of an organ.

retroflexion (ret-ro-flek´shun) The backward bending of an organ.

r. of uterus Extreme backward bending of the body of the uterus while the cervix remains in its normal position.

retrognathia (ret-ro-nath´e-ă) Condition characterized by a retruded position of the lower jaw without diminution of its size.

retrograde (ret´ro-grād) Moving backward retracing original course.

retrogression (ret-ro-gresh´un) **1.** A return to an earlier or more primitive condition. **2.** Degeneration of tissues.

retroillumination (ret-ro-ĭ-lu-mĭ-na´shun) The technique of examining transparent or semitransparent tissues (e.g., the cornea) by reflecting light from posteriorly located tissues.

retrolental (ret-ro-len´tal) Located behind the eye lens.

retromandibular (ret-ro-man-dib´u-lar) Behind the lower jaw.

retroperitoneal (ret-ro-per-ĭ-to-ne´al) Behind the peritoneum.

retroperitoneum (ret-ro-per-ĭ-to-ne-um) The retroperitoneal space between the parietal peritoneum and the posterior body wall.

retroperitonitis (ret-ro-per-ĭ-to-ni´tis) Inflammation of tissues behind the peritoneum.

idiopathic fibrous r. See sclerosing retroperitonitis.

sclerosing r. An inflammatory fibrous overgrowth of retroperitoneal tissues beginning in the area of the sacral promontory; may encircle the lower abdominal aorta or extend laterally, encroaching on and obstructing the ureters; cause is unknown. Also called retroperitoneal fibromatosis; idiopathic fibrous retroperitonitis; retroperitoneal fibrosis; idiopathic retroperitoneal fibrosis.

retropharyngeal (ret-ro-fă-rin´je-al) Behind the pharynx.

retroplasia (ret-ro-pla´zhă, ret-ro-pla´se-ă) The state of decreased or retrogressive activity in a tissue.

retroposition (ret-ro-pŏ-zish´un) Backward displacement of an organ without retroflexion or retroversion.

adherent r. of uterus A fixed retroposition of the uterus caused by adhesions; seen in a variety of pelvic inflammatory conditions (e.g., sexually transmitted infections, endometriosis, pyosalpinx, hydrosalpinx).

retropulsion (ret-ro-pul´shun) An involuntary walking or falling backward.

retrospondylolisthesis (ret-ro-spon-dĭ-lo-lis-the´sis) Posterior displacement of a vertebra, bringing it out of alignment with the other vertebrae.

retrosternal (ret-ro-ster´nal) Behind the sternum (breastbone).

retrouterine (ret-ro-u´ter-in) Behind the uterus.

retroversion (ret-ro-ver´zhun) The backward tilting of an entire organ.

r. of uterus The leaning backward of the entire uterus with the cervix pointing forward.

retroverted (ret-ro-vert´ed) Inclined backward.

Retroviridae (ret-ro-vir´ĭ-de) Family of viruses (100 nm in diameter) that have RNA-dependent DNA polymerases (reverse transcriptases); includes the tumor viruses.

retrovirus (ret-ro-vi´rus) Any virus of the family Retroviridae. Retroviruses are named for their ability to convert RNA into DNA and thus use genetic material of the cells they infect to make the proteins they need to survive, causing several diseases in the process. Retroviruses include the cancer-causing virus HTLV (human T cell leukemia/lymphoma virus) and HIV (human immunodeficiency virus), the cause of AIDS (acquired immune deficiency syndrome); these viruses have a tropism for T4 (helper) lymphocytes and contain a Mg^{++}-dependent reverse transcriptase.

retrusion (re-troo´zhun) The backward displacement of the lower jaw.

reunient (re-u´ne-ent) Connecting; denoting the ductus reuniens that connects the saccule to the cochlear duct in the inner ear.

revascularization (re-vas-ku-lar-ĭ-za´shun) Reestablishment of blood supply to a part of the body by blood vessel grafting, or by development of collateral channels.

reversal (re-ver´sal) A turning in the opposite direction.

sex r. The apparent change to the opposite sex, as in certain pseudohermaphroditic individuals.

reversible (re-ver´sĭ-bl) Capable of returning to the original form or state.

reversion (re-ver´shun) **1.** Reverse mutation; the restoration in a mutant gene of its ability to produce

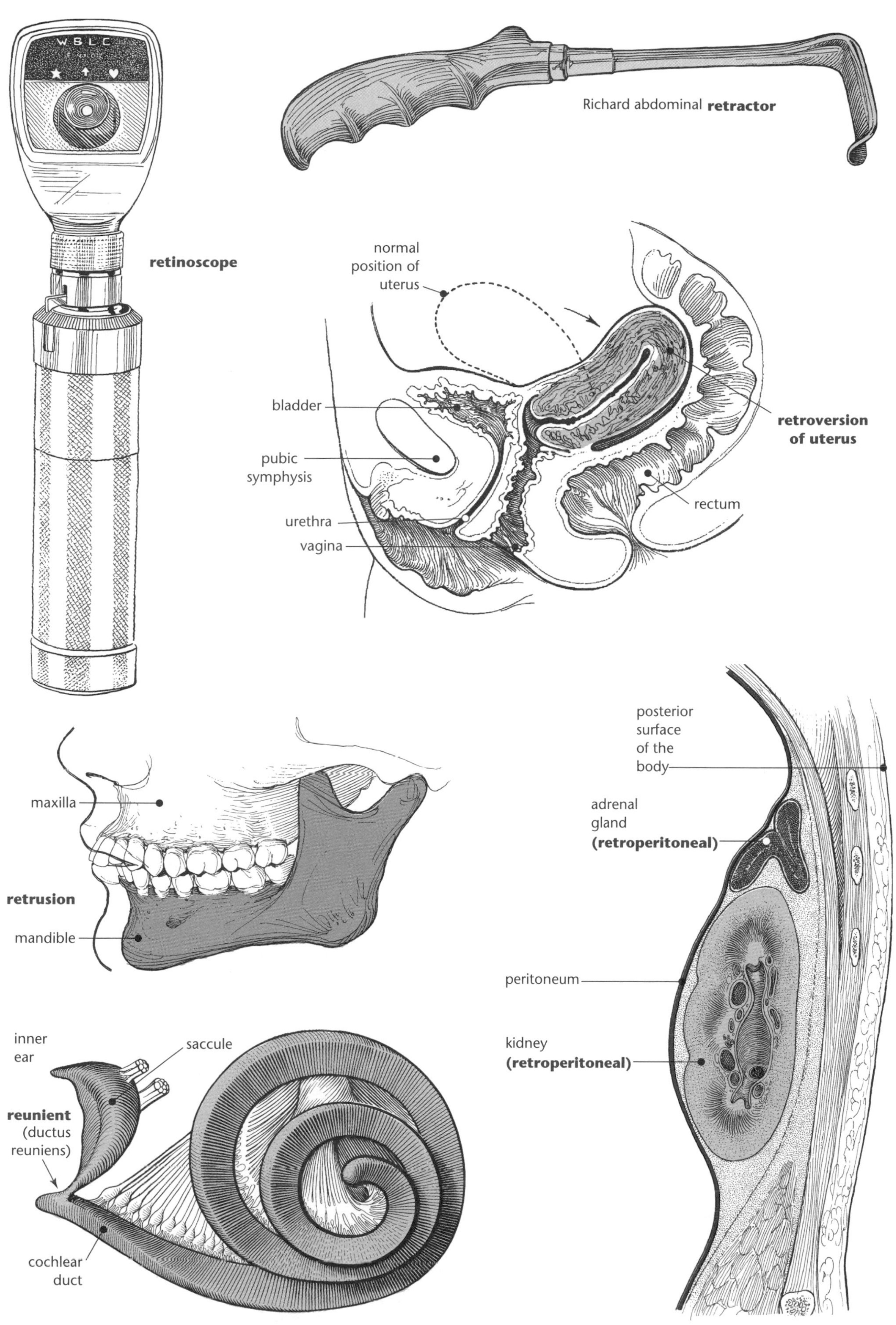
Richard abdominal **retractor**
retinoscope
normal
position of
uterus
bladder
pubic
symphysis
urethra
vagina
retroversion
of uterus
rectum
maxilla
retrusion
mandible
posterior
surface
of the
body
adrenal
gland
(retroperitoneal)
peritoneum
kidney
(retroperitoneal)
inner
ear
saccule
reunient
(ductus
reuniens)
cochlear
duct
R

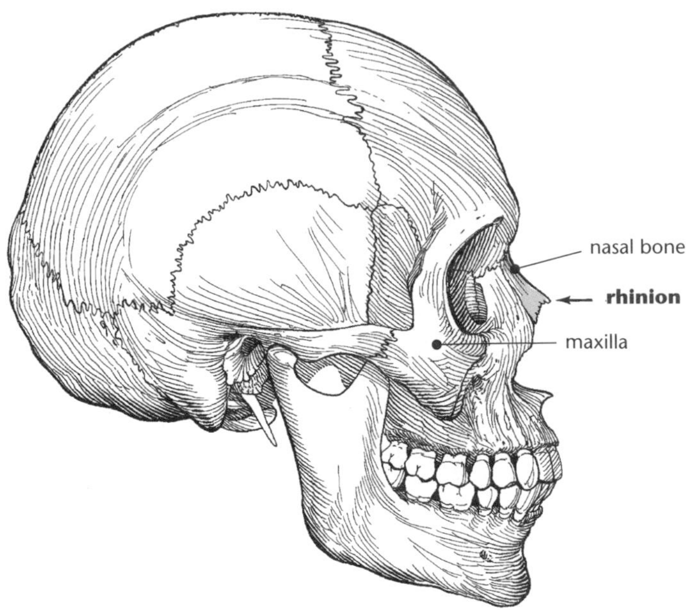

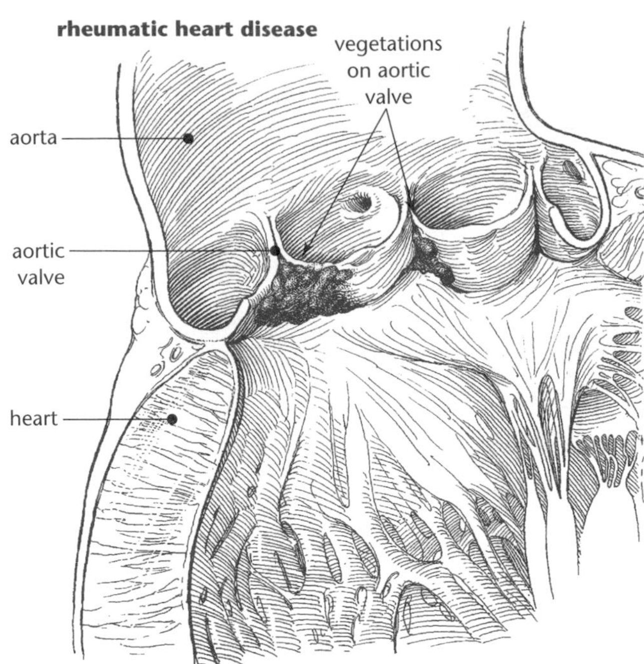

a functional protein. **2.** The appearance in an individual of a characteristic that has been absent for several generations.

revivification **1.** Renewal of life. **2.** Refreshing the edges of a wound to promote healing.

Reye's syndrome (rīz sin´drōm) An acute and frequently fatal childhood syndrome marked by encephalopathy, hepatitis, and fatty accumulations in the viscera; follows a viral infection such as influenza or varicella; epidemiologically related to administration of salicylates during infection and rarely seen since avoidance of salicylates has become standard practice.

Rhabditis (rab-di´tis) Genus of small phasmid nematode worms; some are parasitic in humans.

rhabdoid (rab´doid) Rod-shaped.

rhabdomyolysis (rab-do-mi-ol´ĭ-sis) Acute, fulminating, potentially fatal disorder characterized by disintegration of skeletal muscle and urine excretion of the muscle pigment myoglobin. Also called paroxysmal idiopathic myoglobulinuria.

rhabdomyoma (rab-do-mi-o´mă) Benign tumor occurring most commonly in the hearts of children.

rhabdomyosarcoma (rab-do-mi-o-sar-ko´ma) Malignant soft-tissue tumor occurring most frequently in children under 10 years of age.

R

Rhabdoviridae (rab-do-vir´ĭ-de) Family of large rod-shaped viruses that contain single-stranded RNA and replicate in cytoplasm. Includes the rabies virus.

rhagades (rag´ă-dēz) Cracks or fissures in the skin, especially around body openings; seen in congenital syphilis and in vitamin deficiencies.

rhagadiform (ra-gad´ĭ-form) Fissurelike.

rhe (re) The absolute unit of fluidity; the reciprocal of the unit of viscosity.

rhenium (re´ne-um) A rare, silver-white metallic element with a melting point exceeded only by tungsten and carbon; symbol Re, atomic number 75, atomic weight 186.2.

rheobase (re´o-bās) The minimal strength of an electric stimulus required to excite a tissue if allowed to flow through it for an adequate time.

rheoencephalography (re-o-en-sef-ă-log´ră-fe) The measurement of blood flow in the brain.

rheology (re-ol´o-je) The study of the deformation and flow of liquids and semisolids (e.g., the flow of blood through the heart and blood vessels).

rheometer (re-om´ĕ-ter) **1.** A device for measuring the velocity of viscous liquids such as blood. **2.** A galvanometer.

rheometry (re-om´ĕ-tre) The measurement of a flow or current.

rheostat (re´o-stat) Appliance for regulating the current entering an electric circuit; it consists of a continuously variable electrical resistor.

rheotaxis (re-o-tak´sis) The movement of an organism in response to the direction of fluid flow.

negative r. Rheotaxis in which the organism moves in the same direction as that of fluid flow.

positive r. Rheotaxis in which the organism moves in the opposite direction from that of fluid flow.

rhesus monkey (rē´sus mung´kē) A light brown monkey, *Macaca mulatta*, of India and China; used in medical research.

rheum (rōōm) Any abnormal watery discharge from the nose or eyes.

rheumatic (roo-mat´ik) Relating to rheumatism.

rheumatic heart disease (roo-mat´ik hart dĭ-zēz´) (RHD) A manifestation of rheumatic fever consisting of inflammatory changes (carditis) and/or damaged heart valves.

rheumatid (roo´mă-tid) A skin eruption sometimes accompanying disorders of the musculoskeletal system.

rheumatism (roo´mă-tiz-m) A general term applied to various diseases that cause pain in the muscles, joints, and fibrous tissues, including minor aches as well as diseases such as rheumatoid arthritis and osteoarthritis.

rheumatoid (roo´mă-toid) **1.** Resembling rheumatism. **2.** Associated with rheumatoid arthritis.

rheumatology (roo-mă-tol´ŏ-je) The study of the diagnosis and treatment of rheumatic conditions.

rhexis (rek´sis) Rupture of a vessel or an organ.

rhinal (ri´nal) Relating to the nose.

rhinalgia (ri-nal´jă, ri-nal´je-ă) Pain in the nose.

rhinedema (ri-nĕ-de´mă) Swelling of the nasal mucous membrane.

rhinencephalon (ri-nen-sef´ă-lon) The region of the forebrain involved with the function of olfaction (smell), consisting of the olfactory bulb and peduncle, parolfactory area, subcallosal gyrus, and anterior perforated substance.

rhinion (rin´e-on) A craniometric point; the lower end of the suture between the nasal bones.

rhinitis (ri-ni´tis) Inflammation of the mucous membrane of the nose accompanied by excessive mucus discharge.

acute r. Infection of the upper respiratory tract; may be caused by a variety of viruses, most commonly by the rhinovirus, influenza virus, myxovirus, paramyxovirus, and adenovirus; characterized by acute inflammation of the nasal mucosa with a copious watery discharge, and sometimes sore throat, fever, and muscle ache. Also called coryza.

allergic r. Pale boggy swelling of nasal mucosa associated with sneezing and watery discharge, occasionally producing skin eruptions, due to hypersensitivity to foreign substances (e.g., pollens, dust).

atrophic r. Chronic rhinitis causing thinning of the mucous membrane; often associated with crusts and foul-smelling discharge. Also called ozena.

hypertrophic r. Chronic rhinitis marked by thickening of mucous membrane.

seasonal allergic r. See hay fever, under fever.

vasomotor r. Rhinitis without infection.

rhinoantritis (ri-no-an-tri´tis) Inflammation of the mucous membrane of the nasal cavity and maxillary sinuses.

rhinocanthectomy (ri-no-kan-thek´to-me) Surgical removal of the inner canthus of the eye.

rhinocheiloplasty, rhinochiloplasty (ri-no-ki´lo-plas-te) Reparative surgery of the nose and lip.

rhinocleisis (ri-no-klī´sis) Obstruction of the nasal passages.

rhinodacryolith (ri-no-dak´re-o-lith) A concretion in the nasolacrimal duct.

rhinogenous (ri-noj´ĕ-nus) Originating in the nose.

rhinokyphosis (ri-no-ki-fo´sis) Deformity of the nose characterized by an abnormal hump in the ridge.

rhinolalia (ri-no-la´le-ă) Nasal speech due to disease or defect of the nasal passages.

rhinolith (ri´no-lith) A stone in the nasal cavity formed in layers, usually around a foreign body.

rhinolithiasis (ri-no-lĭ-thi´ă-sis) The presence of calculi in the nose.

rhinology (ri-nol´ŏ-je) The study of the nose and its diseases.

rhinomanometer (ri-no-mă-nom´ĕ-ter) Instrument for determining the amount of nasal obstruction.

rhinometer (ri-nom´ĕ-ter) Instrument for measuring the nasal passages.

rhinomycosis (ri-no-mi-ko´sis) Fungus infection of the mucous membrane of the nose.

rhinopathy (ri-nop´ă-the) Any disease of the nose.

rhinopharyngitis ri-no-far-in-ji´tis) Inflammation of the mucous membrane of the nasopharynx.

r. mutilans See gangosa.

rhinopharynx (ri-no-far´inks) See nasopharynx.

rhinophyma (ri-no-fī´mă) Acne rosacea of the nose, causing the skin to become coarsened, purplish, and thickened with nodulation and pitted scars.

rhinoplasty (ri´no-plas-te) **1.** Plastic surgery of the nose. **2.** Surgical reconstruction of the nose, frequently with tissue taken from another site.

rhinorrhagia (ri-no-ra´je-ă) Nosebleed.

rhinorrhaphy (ri-nor´ă-fe) Operation for the relief of epicanthus, in which a piece of skin is removed from the bridge of the nose and the edges of the wound are sutured together.

rhinorrhea (ri-no-re´ă) A profuse, watery nasal discharge.

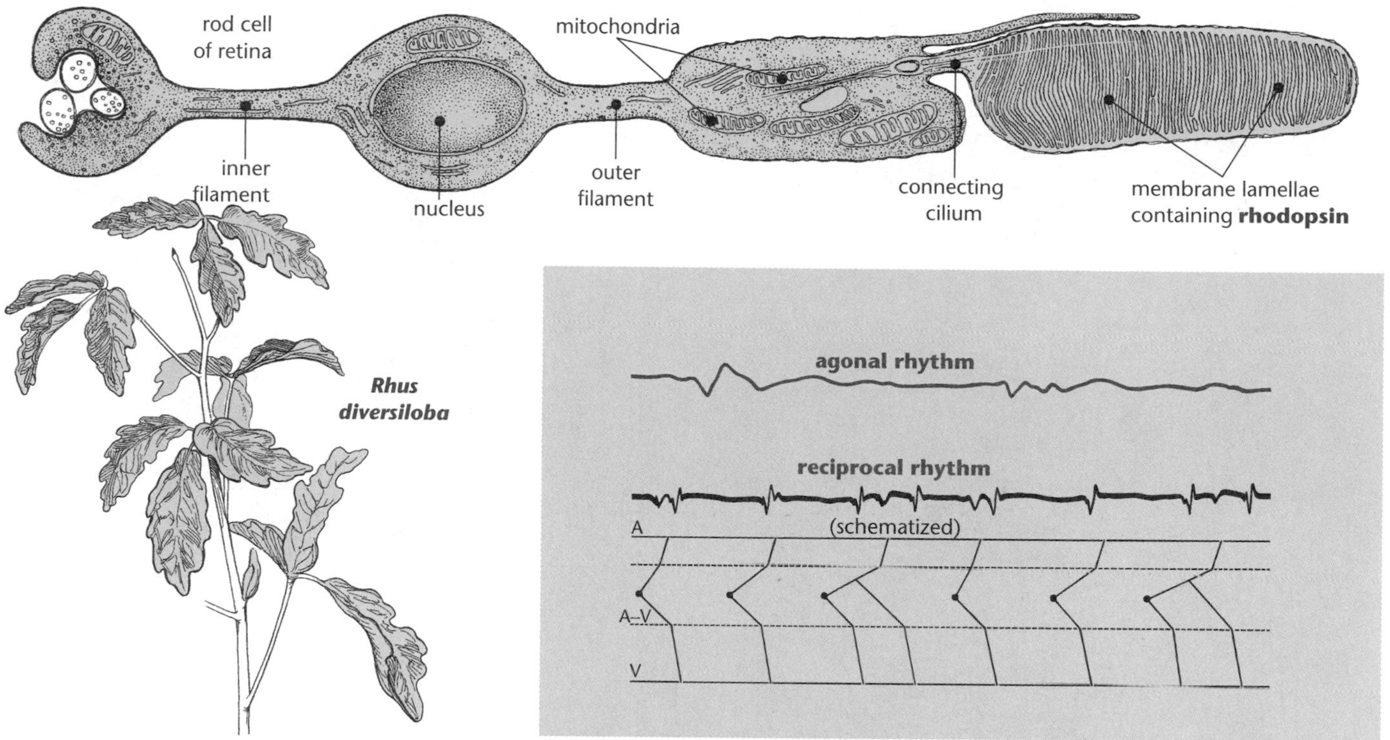

rhinosalpingitis (ri-no-sal-pin-jī´tis) Inflammation of the mucous membranes of the nasal cavity and eustachian (auditory) tube or tubes.

rhinoscleroma (ri-no-skle-ro´mă) Chronic disease involving the nose and upper respiratory tract, marked by the formation of hard nodules, sometimes leading to deformity.

rhinoscope (rī´no-skōp) Instrument for inspecting the back of the nasal cavity; a speculum. Also called nasoscope.

rhinoscopy (ri-nos´ko-pe) Visual examination of the back of the nasal cavity with a rhinoscope.

median r. Inspection of the nasal cavity and the openings of the ethmoid cells and sphenoidal sinus with a long nasal speculum.

rhinostenosis (ri-no-stě-no´sis) Abnormal narrowing of the nasal passage; nasal obstruction.

rhinotomy (ri-not´ŏ-me) Operative incision on the nose.

Rhinovirus (ri-no-vi´rus) Genus of viruses (family Picornaviridae) that includes those causing the common cold in humans and foot-and-mouth disease in cattle; over 100 antigenic types have been identified.

rhinovirus (ri-no-vi´rus) Any member of the genus *Rhinovirus*.

rhizome (ri´zōm) A horizontal rootlike stem, growing under or along the ground, which gives off roots from its lower side and leafy shoots or buds from its upper side.

rhizomeningomyelitis (ri-zo-mě-nin-go-mi-ě-li´tis) Inflammation of the nerve roots, the meninges, and the spinal cord. Also called radiculomeningomyelitis.

rhizoplast (ri´zo-plast) A fine fibril connecting the flagellum to the nucleus of certain flagellate organisms.

Rhizopoda (ri-zop´o-dă) Subclass of protozoa (class Sarcodina) that have rootlike pseudopodia.

rhizotomy (ri-zot´o-me) Surgical division of a nerve root for the relief of pain. Also called radicotomy; radiculectomy; root section.

posterior r. Division of posterior (sensory) spinal nerve roots.

trigeminal r. Surgical interruption of the preganglionic root of the trigeminal (5th cranial) nerve for the relief of spasmodic facial neuralgia (tic douloureux). Also called retrogasserian neurotomy.

rhodium (ro´de-um) A hard metallic element of the platinum group; symbol Rh, atomic number 45, atomic weight 102.91.

Rhodococcus (ro-do-kok´us) Genus of rod-shaped, aerobic, gram-positive bacteria usually found in soil and the intestinal tract of farm animals. Some species cause disease in animals and people.

R. equi Species that causes bronchopneumonia in foals and can be responsible for infection in humans whose immune system is compromised (e.g., by immunosuppressive drugs, lymphoma, AIDS).

rhodopsin (ro-dop´sin) A purplish red, light-sensitive pigment found in the membrane of the outer segments of the rod-shaped photoreceptor cells of the retina; composed of a vitamin A derivative (11-*cis*-retinal) and a protein group (opsin); when light is absorbed by rhodopsin, it is transformed and separated into all-*trans*-retinal and opsin, but regenerates in the dark (the all-*trans*-retinal reverts back to 11-*cis*-retinal, which combines with opsin to form rhodopsin); this unique property makes possible the transformation of light energy into visual perception. Also called visual purple.

rhombencephalon (rom-ben-sef´ă-lon) The embryonic hindbrain; the third cephalic dilatation of the neural tube that divides into the metencephalon (anterior portion), which later forms the pons and cerebellum, and the myelencephalon (posterior portion), which develops into the medulla oblongata.

rhombocele (rom´bo-sēl) See rhomboidal sinus, under sinus.

rhonchal, rhonchial (rong´kal, rong´ke-al) Relating to a rhonchus.

rhonchus (rong´kus), *pl.* **rhon´chi** A loud rale or snoring sound produced in the bronchial tubes or the trachea. Also called coarse rale.

Rhus (rus) Genus of the family Anacardiaceae; contains plants that produce pruritic skin lesions on contact; the irritating substance is urushiol, a catechol present in the sap.

R. diversiloba A shrub of the North American Pacific states; has varied leaflets, often with three to seven subacute lobes resembling oak leaves; the species growing in the Atlantic states is known as *Rhus toxicodendron*. Also called poison oak.

R. radicans A shrub or vine growing abundantly throughout the United States and parts of southern Canada; has smooth glossy leaflets in groups of three, with margins varying from crenate or serrate to deeply lobate. Also called poison ivy.

R. toxicodendron See *Rhus diversiloba*.

R. vernix A swamp shrub that grows in marshy areas of eastern North America; has compound leaves with branches of 7 to 13 elongated leaflets. Also called poison ash; poison dogwood; poison elder; poison sumac; swamp sumac.

rhythm (rith´m) The pattern of recurrence of a biologic cycle (e.g., the heartbeat and sexual cycle).

agonal r. A rhythm appearing in the electrocardiogram as wide distorted ventricular complexes, often seen in dying patients.

alpha (α) **r.** See alpha waves, under wave.

A-V nodal r. Heart rhythm originating in the atrioventricular (A-V) node; resulting from anything that suppresses sinus node activity, or from anything that enhances A-V node automaticity. Also called nodal rhythm; junctional rhythm.

beta (β) **r.** See beta waves, under wave.

bigeminal r. Heart rhythm in which every beat is followed by a weak premature beat and then a pause, so that the beats appear coupled. Also called coupling.

cantering r. See gallop.

circadian r. See circadian.

circus r. See circus movement, under movement.

coronary nodal r. Term, not uniformly accepted, for rhythm appearing in the electrocardiogram with normal upright P waves in leads I and II with a short P-R interval. Occasionally called short P-R interval.

coronary sinus r. Heart rhythm appearing in the electrocardiogram with inverted P waves in inferior leads with a normal P-R interval; thought to originate in the coronary sinus.

delta (δ) **r.** See delta waves (a), under wave.

ectopic r. Heart rhythm originating from any focus other than the sinus node.

gallop r. See gallop.

idionodal r. A slow independent heart rhythm arising in the atrioventricular (A-V) junction and controlling only the ventricles.

idioventricular r. A slow independent heart rhythm arising in an ectopic center in the ventricles and controlling only the ventricles.

infradian r. See infradian.

junctional r. See A-V nodal rhythm.

nodal r. See A-V nodal rhythm.

quadruple r. A quadruple cadence of the heart sounds, not heard in normal hearts.

reciprocal r. Phenomenon in which the impulse arises in the A-V junction and travels both downward to the ventricles and upward to the atria; before reaching the atria, it is reflected and descends to reactivate the ventricles. Also called reciprocal beating.

reciprocating r. A variation of the reciprocal rhythm in which the impulse circulates around the A-V junction and gives off two daughter impulses, one to the atria and one to the ventricles.

sinus r. The normal heart rhythm, originating in the sinoatrial node.

theta (θ) **r.** See theta wave, under wave.

trigeminal r. Rhythm in which the heartbeats are grouped in three; either two premature beats follow each normal beat, or two normal beats are followed by a premature beat. Also called trigeminy.

triple r. A triple cadence to the heart sounds, generally caused by the presence of a third (diastolic) or fourth (presystolic) heart sound or gallop in

R

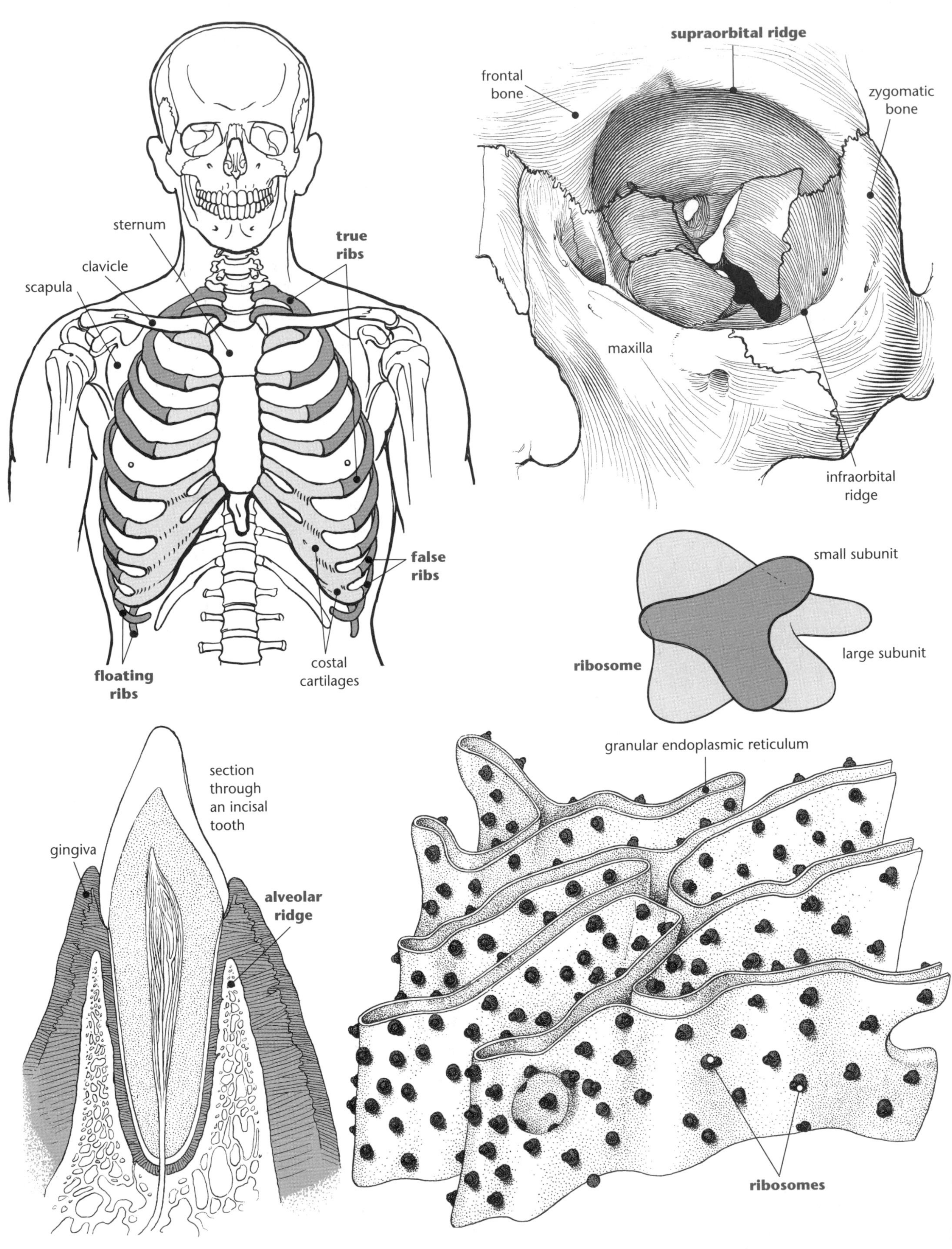
sternum
true ribs
clavicle
scapula
false ribs
floating ribs
costal cartilages
supraorbital ridge
frontal bone
zygomatic bone
maxilla
infraorbital ridge
small subunit
ribosome
large subunit
section through an incisal tooth
gingiva
alveolar ridge
granular endoplasmic reticulum
ribosomes

R

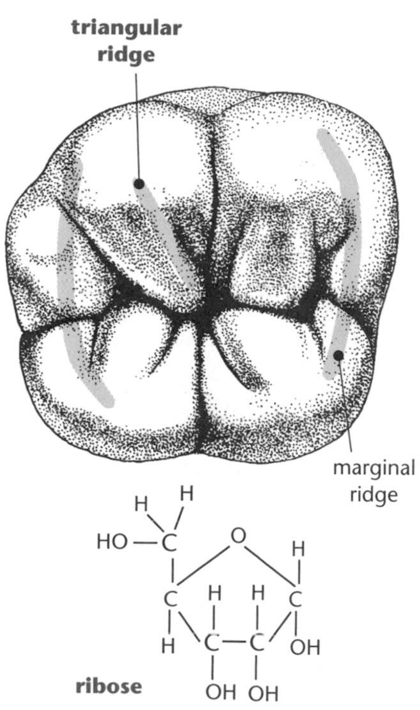

ribose

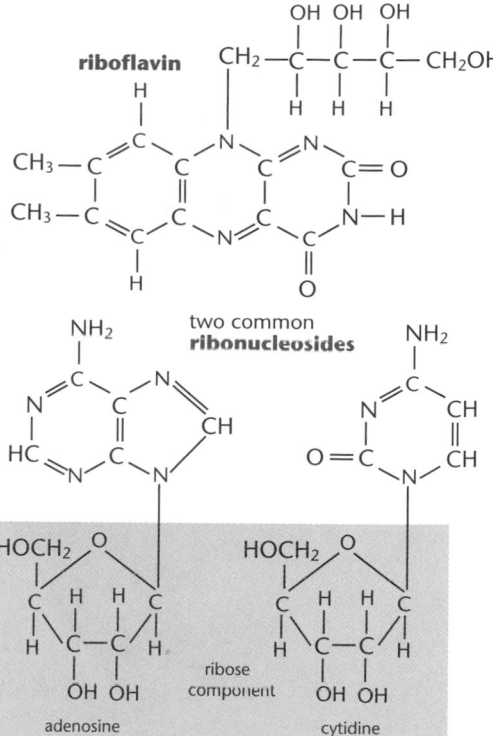

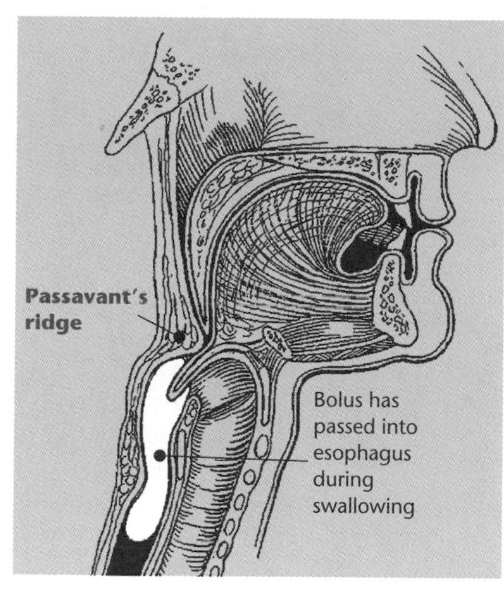

riboflavin

two common **ribonucleosides**

ribose component

adenosine

cytidine

addition to the usual first and second heart sounds.

ultradian r. See ultradian.

rhytidectomy (rit-ĭ-dek´to-me) A face-lift; surgical elimination of wrinkles and sagging skin from the facial area; the excess skin is removed so that the remaining skin may be tightened, thus smoothing out the wrinkles. Also called face-lift; rhytidoplasty.

rhytidoplasty (rit-ĭ-do-plas-te) See rhytidectomy.

rhytidosis (rit-ĭ-do´sis) **1.** Premature wrinkling of the face. **2.** Wrinkling of the cornea.

rib (rib) One of a series of long, thin, rather elastic, curved bones that articulates posteriorly with a thoracic vertebra and extends anteriorly toward the sternum; normally there are 12 ribs on each side.

cervical r. An extra rib similar to, but independent of, the first dorsal rib; usually attached to the seventh cervical vertebra.

false r. One of the five lower pairs of ribs that is not directly connected anteriorly, through the costal cartilage, to the sternum. Also called vertebrochondral rib.

floating r. One of the two lower pairs of false ribs that is free at the anterior end. Also called vertebral rib.

slipping r. Recurrent dislocation of a rib's costal cartilage.

sternal r. See true rib.

true r. One of the seven upper pairs of ribs that is connected anteriorly, through the costal cartilage, to the sternum. Also called sternal rib.

vertebral r. See floating rib.

vertebrochondral r. See false rib.

riboflavin (ri-bo-fla´vin) A yellow, crystalline pigment present in milk, egg yolk, and fresh meat, and produced synthetically; it acts as coenzyme for hydrogen transfer in reactions catalyzed by flavoproteins. Formerly called vitamin B_2.

ribonuclease (ri-bo-noo´kle-ās) (RNase) Enzyme responsible for the breakdown of ribonucleic acid.

ribonucleic acid (ri-bo-noo-kle´ik as´id) (RNA) Any of a family of polynucleotides, component of all living cells, especially the cytoplasm and nucleolus, that are characterized by their constituent sugar (*d*-ribose) and single-stranded molecules.

chromosomal RNA Segments of RNA associated with a chromosome that may have a role in transferring genetic code information.

messenger RNA (mRNA) An RNA fraction with a base ratio that corresponds to the DNA of the same organism; it carries information from DNA to the protein-forming areas of the cell. Also called template RNA.

ribosomal RNA (rRNA) The RNA ribosomes and polyribosomes.

soluble RNA (sRNA) See transfer RNA.

template RNA See messenger RNA.

transfer RNA (tRNA) An RNA molecule that transfers an amino acid to a growing polypeptide chain; the smallest biologically active nucleic acid known, present in cells in at least 20 varieties. Also called soluble RNA.

ribonucleoprotein (ri-bo-noo-kle-o-pro´tēn) (RNP) A complex macromolecule containing ribonucleic acid (RNA) and protein.

ribonucleoside (ri-bo-noo´kle-o-sīd) A nucleoside (purine or pyrimidine attached to a sugar) in which the sugar component is ribose (e.g., adenosine, cytidine, guanosine, uridine).

ribonucleotide (ri-bo-noo´kle-o-tīd) A compound consisting of a purine or pyrimidine base bonded to the sugar component ribose, which in turn is esterified with a phosphate group; the most common ribonucleotides are adenylic, guanylic, cytidylic, and uridylic acids.

ribose (ri´bōs) A five-carbon sugar present in ribonucleic acid (RNA); an aldopentose.

riboside (ri´bo-sīd) A glycoside that, on hydrolysis, yields ribose.

ribosome (ri´bo-sōm) One of the minute granules free in the cytoplasm or attached to the endoplasmic reticulum of a cell, containing a high concentration of RNA; it plays an important role in protein synthesis, ranges in size from 100 to 150 Å in diameter, and is assembled from two subunits produced in the nucleolus.

ribosuria (ri-bo-su´re-ă) Excessive excretion of ribose in the urine; seen in muscular dystrophy.

ribosyl (ri´bo-sil) The radical formed from ribose, $C_5H_9O_4$.

riboviruses (ri-bo-vi´rus-es) See RNA viruses, under virus.

rib-spreader (rib spred´er) Surgical instrument for widening and maintaining space between ribs during intrathoracic operations.

ricin (ri´sin) A highly toxic protein occurring in the castor-oil bean; used as a biochemical reagent.

rickets (rik´ets) Disease of infants and young children caused by deficiency of vitamin D, resulting in defective bone growth.

renal r. A form of rickets occurring in children due to chronic disease of the kidneys.

vitamin D-resistant r. A severe form of rickets that is not relieved by the administration of vitamin D; is caused by a congenital defect of the kidneys; seen most frequently in males.

Rickettsia (rĭ-ket´se-ă) Genus of gram-negative, pathogenic, intracellular parasitic bacteria that are transmitted to humans through the bites of infected fleas, ticks, mites, and lice.

R. akari Species causing rickettsialpox; transmitted to humans by the mouse-infecting mite *Liponyssoides sanguineus.*

R. prowazekii Species causing epidemic typhus and Brill-Zinsser disease (a carrier or latent type of typhus); transmitted by body lice.

R. rickettsii Species causing Rocky Mountain spotted fever; transmitted through the bites of infected ticks, especially *Dermacentor andersoni* and *Dermacentor variabilis.*

R. tsutsugamushi Species causing tsutsugamushi disease (scrub typhus); transmitted by mites.

R. typhi Species causing endemic flea-borne typhus (murine typhus); transmitted by rat fleas.

rickettsialpox (rĭ-ket´se-al-poks) An acute, mite-borne disease of several days' duration, characterized by an initial cutaneous lesion followed by a rash, fever, backache, and headache; caused by *Rickettsia akari.*

rickettsiosis (rĭ-ket-se-o´sis) Any disease caused by a species of *Rickettsia* (e.g., Rocky Mountain spotted fever, typhus, rickettsialpox, Q fever).

ridge (rij) A linear elevation on a bone or a tooth.

alveolar r. The bony ridge of the jaw containing the sockets (alveoli) in which the roots of the teeth fit.

dental r. Any linear elevation on the surface of a tooth forming the border of a cusp or the margin of a crown.

lateral supracondylar r. A curved ridge on the lateral surface of the humerus to which two of the dorsal muscles of the forearm attach.

medial supracondylar r. A curved ridge on the medial surface of the humerus to which two of the muscles of the arm attach.

oblique r. A variable ridge (formed by the union of two triangular ridges) crossing obliquely the occlusal surface of an upper molar.

palatine r. One of four or six transverse ridges on the anterior portion of the hard palate.

Passavant's r. The prominence formed in the posterior wall of the pharynx by the contraction of the superior constrictor muscle during the act of swallowing. Also called Passavant's bar; Passavant's cushion; Passavant's pad.

supraorbital r. The curved elevation of the frontal bone forming the upper border of the orbit.

transverse r. A ridge (formed by the union of two triangular ridges) crossing transversely the occlusal surface of a posterior tooth.

triangular r. The ridge that runs from the tip of the cusp toward the central part of the occlusal surface of a posterior tooth.

rifampin (rif´am-pin) Antibiotic drug used to treat tuberculosis and other bacterial infections.

rigidity (rĭ-jid´ĭ-te) **1.** Abnormal stiffness. **2.** In

R

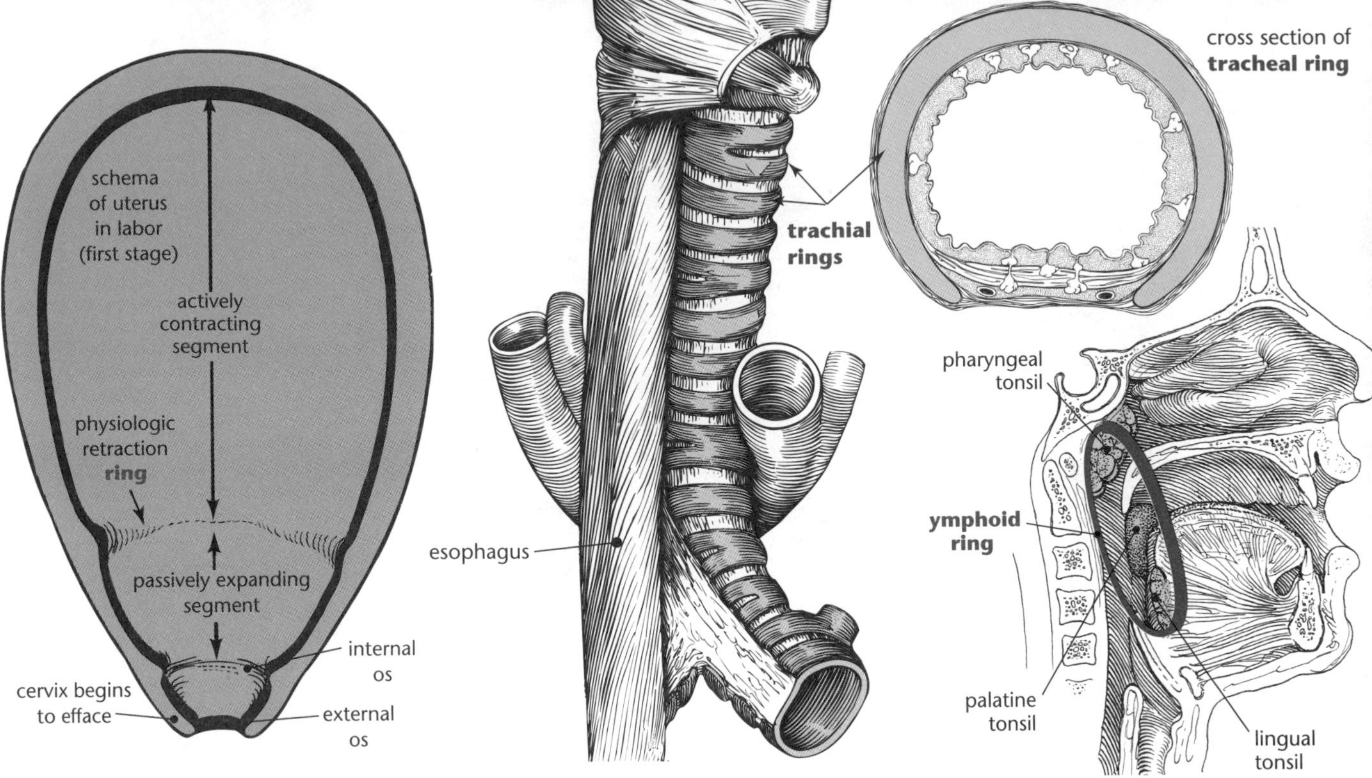

psychiatry, an individual's excessive resistance to change.

cerebellar r. Stiffness of the body and limbs due to an injury or lesion of the veins of the cerebellum.

clasp-knife r. See clasp-knife spasticity, under spasticity.

cogwheel r. Rigidity of a muscle which, when passively stretched, gives way to a series of small jerks, as seen in Parkinson's disease.

decerebrate r. (a) Rigid extension of the extremities of an experimental animal following transsection of the brain between the red nucleus and the vestibular nuclei; lesions of the upper part of the brainstem produce similar effects in humans. (b) In humans, rigidity caused by an extensive, usually bilateral lesion above the brainstem, which results in separation of the vestibular nuclei from brainstem control; characterized by extension of all extremities, or of one arm and leg on the same side of a unilateral lesion, and backward bending of the spine.

lead-pipe r. Diffuse tonic contraction of muscles seen in Parkinson's disease.

pathologic r. Rigidity of the uterine cervix in labor due to fibrosis, cancer, or other diseases.

postmortem r. See rigor mortis.

R

rigor (rig´or) **1.** Rigidity; stiffness. **2.** A chill.

r. mortis Stiffening of the muscles of a dead body generally detectable 2 to4 hours after death, reaching completion after 6 to 12 hours, and disappearing after 24 to 28 hours; caused by coagulation of the muscle plasma. Also called postmortem rigidity.

Riley-Day syndrome (ri´le-da sin´drōm) See familial dysautonomia, under dysautonomia.

rim (rim) An outer edge, border, or margin, generally circular in form.

bite r. See occlusion rim.

occlusion r. Occluding surface built on denture bases for recording maxillomandibular relation and for arranging teeth. Also called record rim; bite rim.

record r. See occlusion rim.

rima (ri´ma) A slit or elongated opening.

r. glottidis The opening between the true vocal cords.

r. oris The longitudinal aperture of the mouth.

r. palpebrarum The slit between the lids of the closed eye.

rimantadine (ri-man´tă-dēn) Antiviral drug used to treat influenza.

ring (ring) **1.** A circular or oval object with a vacant center. **2.** In anatomy, any circular band surrounding an opening. **3.** In chemistry, a group of atoms bound in a manner graphically representable as a circle.

abdominal r. See deep inguinal ring.

anterior limiting r. of eye A ridgelike ring composed of collagenous fibers marking the peripheral edge of Descemet's membrane and the anterior border of the trabecular meshwork, as seen by gonioscopy. Also called Schwalbe's ring; Schwalbe's annular line.

benzene r. The hexagonal ring arrangement of carbon and hydrogen atoms in the benzene molecule. Also called benzene nucleus.

casting r. See refractory flask, under flask.

common tendinous r. See common annular tendon, under tendon.

deep inguinal r. The oval orifice in the transverse fascia of the external oblique muscle marking the deep opening of the inguinal canal. Also called abdominal ring; internal inguinal ring.

external inguinal r. See superficial inguinal ring.

Falope r. A nonreactive rubber band used for occluding each fallopian (uterine) tube as a procedure for sterilization; the ring is placed around a 2.5 cm loop of the tube, at the junction of its proximal and middle thirds. Also called silastic band; silastic ring; Yoon ring.

femoral r. The abdominal or superior oval opening of the conical femoral canal underlying the inguinal ligament at the groin; it is bounded posteriorly by the pectineus muscle, medially by the lacunar ligament and laterally by the femoral vein. It is normally filled with extraperitoneal fatty and lymphoid tissues and is a potential site of hernia.

fibrous r. of intervertebral disk The outer fibrocartilaginous ring surrounding the softer center of the pads between vertebrae (intervertebral disks).

inguinal r.'s The two openings (superficial and deep) of the inguinal canal through which pass the spermatic cord in males or round ligament in females. See superficial inguinal ring; deep inguinal ring.

internal inguinal r. See deep inguinal ring.

Kayser-Fleischer r. A brownish ring, about 1 to 3 mm wide, in the periphery of the cornea; seen in Wilson's disease.

lower esophageal r. Annular fibrous narrowing of the esophagus occurring 1 to 4 cm above the hiatus (diaphragmatic opening); may be asymptomatic or may cause attacks of difficult swallowing precipitated by hasty swallowing of improperly chewed solid foods; may also be asymptomatic. Also called Schatzki's ring.

lymphoid r. A mass of lymphoid tissue, encircling the entrance to the pharynx, that includes the palatine, pharyngeal, and lingual tonsils and the small lymph follicles on the posterior oropharyngeal wall. Also called Waldeyer's ring; tonsillar ring.

signet r. An early trophozoite of the malaria parasite (plasmodium), appearing as a small hyaline disk with a nucleus on one side.

Schatzki's r. See lower esophageal ring.

Schwalbe's r. See anterior limiting ring of eye.

silastic r. See Falope ring.

subcutaneous inguinal r. See superficial inguinal ring.

superficial inguinal r. The orifice in the aponeurosis of the external oblique muscle forming the external opening of the inguinal canal. Also called external inguinal ring; subcutaneous inguinal ring.

teething r. A ring, usually of hard rubber or plastic, designed for a teething baby to bite on.

tonsillar r. See lymphoid ring.

tracheal r. One of the cartilages forming the trachea. Also called tracheal cartilage.

umbilical r. The opening in the linea alba of the fetus through which the umbilical vessels pass.

Yoon r. See Falope ring.

Waldeyer's r. See lymphoid ring.

ringworm (ring´werm) A superficial infectious condition of the skin marked primarily by ring-shaped or oval itchy lesions; caused by any of a number of fungi, chiefly of the genera *Trichophyton*, *Microsporum*, and *Epidermophyton*. See also tinea.

risk (risk) **1.** The probability of suffering harm or a loss. **2.** In medical statistics, the probability that a disease will occur during a specified time period; it is equal to the number of individuals who develop the disease during the period, divided by the number of disease-free people at the beginning of the period.

relative r. (RR) In epidemiology, the ratio of the incidence rate of a disease among people exposed to a particular risk factor to the incidence of the disease among people unexposed to the risk factor.

ristocetin (ris-to-se´tin) Antibiotic produced by *Nocardia lurida*; used against staphylococcic and enterococcic infections.

risus (ri´sus) A laugh.

r. caninus, r. sardonicus A peculiar grin caused by spasm of the facial muscles, occurring in tetanus. Also called sardonic grin.

ritual (rich´u-al) In psychiatry, any psychomotor behavior or activity performed compulsively and repeatedly to relieve or forestall anxiety; seen in obsessive-compulsive neurosis.

riziform (riz´ĭ-form) Resembling rice grains.

Robin syndrome (ro-ba´ sin´drōm) See Pierre Robin syndrome.

robust (ro-bust´) In statistics, denoting a procedure that is relatively insensitive to departures from the statistical assumptions on which it is based.

Rocher's sign (ro-shārz sīn) See drawer sign.

rod (rod) **1.** Any slender, cylindrical structure or formation. **2.** One of the cells forming, with the cones, the layer of rods and cones of the retina.

rodenticide (ro-den´tĭ-sīd) An agent lethal to rodents.

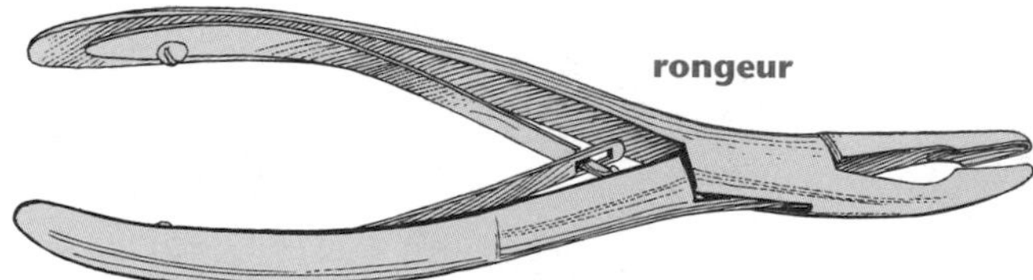

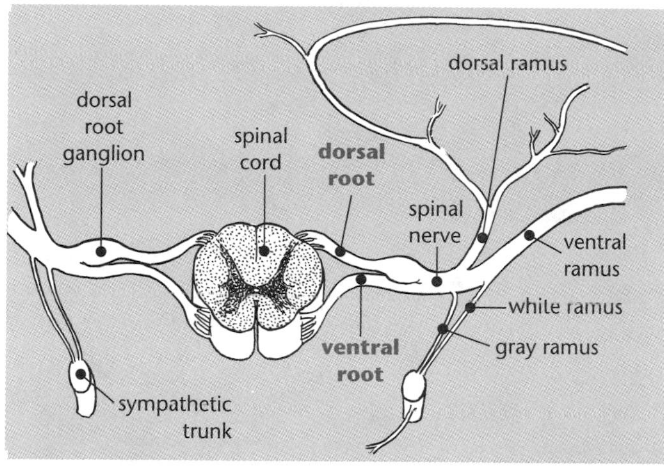

MANDIBULAR TEETH	LENGTH OF ROOT OF TOOTH	LENGTH OF CROWN OF TOOTH
central incisor	12.5 mm	9.0 mm
lateral incisor	13.0 mm	9.5 mm
cuspid	13.0 mm	11.0 mm
first bicuspid	14.0 mm	8.5 mm
second bicuspid	14.5 mm	8.5 mm
first molar	14.0 mm	8.0 mm
second molar	13.0 mm	7.5 mm
third molar	11.5 mm	7.0 mm
MAXILLARY TEETH		
central incisor	13.0 mm	10.5 mm
lateral incisor	12.0 mm	9.5 mm
cuspid	17.0 mm	11.0 mm
first bicuspid	14.0 mm	8.5 mm
second bicuspid	14.0 mm	8.5 mm
first molar	12.5 mm	7.5 mm
second molar	11.5 mm	7.0 mm
third molar	10.5 mm	6.5 mm

roentgen (rent′gen) (R, r) A unit of x-ray or gamma-ray dosage, equal to the quantity of ionizing radiation that can produce 1 electrostatic unit of electricity in 1 cubic centimeter of dry air at 0°C and standard atmospheric pressure.

roentgen-equivalent-man (rent′gen-e-kwiv′ă-lent-man) See rem.

roentgen-equivalent-physical (rent′gen-e-kwiv′ă-lent-fiz′e-kal) (rep) The amount of ionizing radiation which, upon absorption by living tissue, produces an energy gain per gram of tissue equivalent to that produced by 1 roentgen of x rays or gamma rays.

roentgenkymograph (rent-gen-ki′mo-graf) Apparatus for graphically recording the movements of the heart and great vessels on a single x-ray film.

roentgenogram (rent-gen′o-gram) See radiograph.

roentgenography (rent-gen-og′ră-fe) See radiography.

roentgenologist (rent-gĕ-nol′ŏ-jist) See radiologist.

roentgenology (rent-gĕ-nol′ŏ-je) See radiology.

roentgenometry (rent-gĕ-nom′e-tre) **1.** Measurement of the therapeutic dosage of x rays. **2.** Measurement of the penetrating power of x rays.

roentgenoscopy (rent-gĕ-nos′kŏ-pe) See fluoroscopy.

Roger's disease (ro-zhārz′ dĭ-zēz′) Congenital heart anomaly consisting of a small hole in the interventricular septum. Also called maladie de Roger.

role (rōl) **1.** The pattern of social behavior that a person develops, influenced by what others expect or demand of him. **2.** A part played by an individual in relation to a group.

role-playing (rōl-plā′ing) A method of treating emotional conflicts by having the person assume various roles.

Romberg's disease (rom′bergz dĭ-zēz′) See facial hemiatrophy, under hemiatrophy.

Romberg's sign (rom′bergz sīn) Swaying and loss of balance when standing with feet together and eyes closed; indicates a loss of proprioceptive control; occurs in disease of the posterior columns of the spinal cord.

Romberg's syndrome (rom′bergz sin′drōm) See facial hemiatrophy, under hemiatrophy.

rongeur (rawn-zhur′) Instrument used to cut bone.

roof (ro͞of) A top covering structure.

r. of fourth ventricle The upper structure of the fourth ventricle of the brain; formed by the superior and inferior medullary vela and by the epithelial lining, the tela choroidea. Also called tegmen ventricule quarti.

r. of mouth See palate.

room (ro͞om) An area in a building surrounded by walls.

anechoic r. A room that is devoid of echo; used in acoustical testing.

birthing r. A hospital room in which women undergo both labor and delivery; it is provided with infant warmers and resuscitation equipment. See also birth center, under center.

delivery r. Hospital room to which women in labor are taken for delivery.

emergency r. (ER) Area in a hospital where immediate attention is given by trained personnel to people brought in with sudden and unexpected medical problems, such as acute illness, trauma, etc. Also called accident ward.

first recovery r. See recovery room.

labor r. (LBR) A hospital room in which women in labor are monitored prior to delivery. Also called predelivery room.

operating r. (OR) An area in a hospital equipped for performing surgical procedures.

postanesthesia r. See recovery room.

predelivery r. Hospital room in which a woman is placed during the first stage of labor. Also called labor room.

recovery r. (RR) Hospital room provided for the immediate care of postoperative patients.

rooming-in (ro͞om′ing in) The practice of allowing a newborn to stay in the mother's hospital room, in a bassinet, instead of the nursery during the hospital stay.

root (ro͞ot) **1.** The embedded part of a structure, as of a tooth, hair, or nail. **2.** The origin of a structure (e.g., the proximal end of a nerve).

anatomic r. The root of a tooth extending from the cervical line to its apical extremity and contained in the bony socket of the jaw.

anterior r.'s See ventral roots.

r. of aorta The origin of the ascending aorta from the left ventricle.

clinical r. The portion of the tooth below the gingival crevice.

dorsal r.'s The nerve roots that carry impulses from bodily parts to the back of the spinal cord; they are attached along the dorsal lateral sulcus of the cord by six to eight rootlets. Also called sensory or posterior roots.

r. of hair The proximal part of hair embedded in the bulbous portion of the hair follicle.

inferior r. ansae cervicalis. Fibers from the second and third cervical nerves that form the inferior portion of the cervical loop (ansa cervicalis).

r. of lung All the structures entering or emerging at the hilus of the lung, forming a pedicle.

motor r.'s See ventral roots.

r. of nail The proximal end of the nail, underlying a fold of skin (cuticle).

nerve r.'s The two bundles of nerve fibers (dorsal and ventral) emerging from the spinal cord and joining to form a single spinal nerve.

r. of penis The proximal part of the penis, including the two crura of the corpora cavernosa and the bulb.

posterior r.'s See dorsal roots.

sensory r.'s See dorsal roots.

r. of tongue The posterior attached part of the tongue.

superior r. ansa cervicalis Fibers from the first and second cervical nerves that form the superior portion of the cervical loop (ansa cervicalis).

r. of tooth The part of the tooth below the neck which is normally embedded in the alveolar process and covered with cementum.

ventral r.'s The nerve roots that carry impulses from the anterior part of the spinal cord out to muscles and other structures; they are attached along the ventral lateral sulcus in two or three irregular rows of rootlets. Also called motor roots; anterior roots.

rootlet (ro͞ot′let) A filament-like root.

nerve r.'s See radicular fila, under filum.

rosacea (ro-za′she-ă) Chronic inflammatory disorder superficially resembling acne; occurring most often in middle-aged people; characterized by papules, pustules, and dilatation of capillaries on the cheeks and nose, and sometimes the forehead and chin. Sometimes called acne rosacea.

rosanilin (ro-zan′ĭ-lin) Red needle-like crystals, soluble in water; a component of the stain fuchsin.

rosary (ro′ză-re) An arrangement resembling a string of beads.

rachitic r. A row of nodules at the junction of the ribs with their cartilages, sometimes seen in rachitic children. Also called beading of the ribs.

Rosenbach's sign (ro′zen-bahks sīn) **1.** Fine tremor of gently closed eyelids occurring in exophthalmic goiter. **2.** Loss of abdominal reflexes seen in acute inflammation of the abdominal organs.

roseola (ro-ze′o-lă) A reddish rash.

r. infantum See exanthem subitum.

rosette (ro-zet′) A spherical group of fine red vacuoles surrounding the cytocentrum of a monocyte.

rostellum (ros-tel′um) The anterior, hook-bearing portion of a tapeworm.

rostral, rostrad (ros′tral, ros′trad) **1.** Directed toward the front end of the body. **2.** Relating to any beaklike structure.

rostrum (ros′trum) Any beak-shaped structure.

rot (rot) **1.** To decay. **2.** The process of decomposition.

rotameter (ro-tam′ĕ-ter) A flow rate meter used to

R

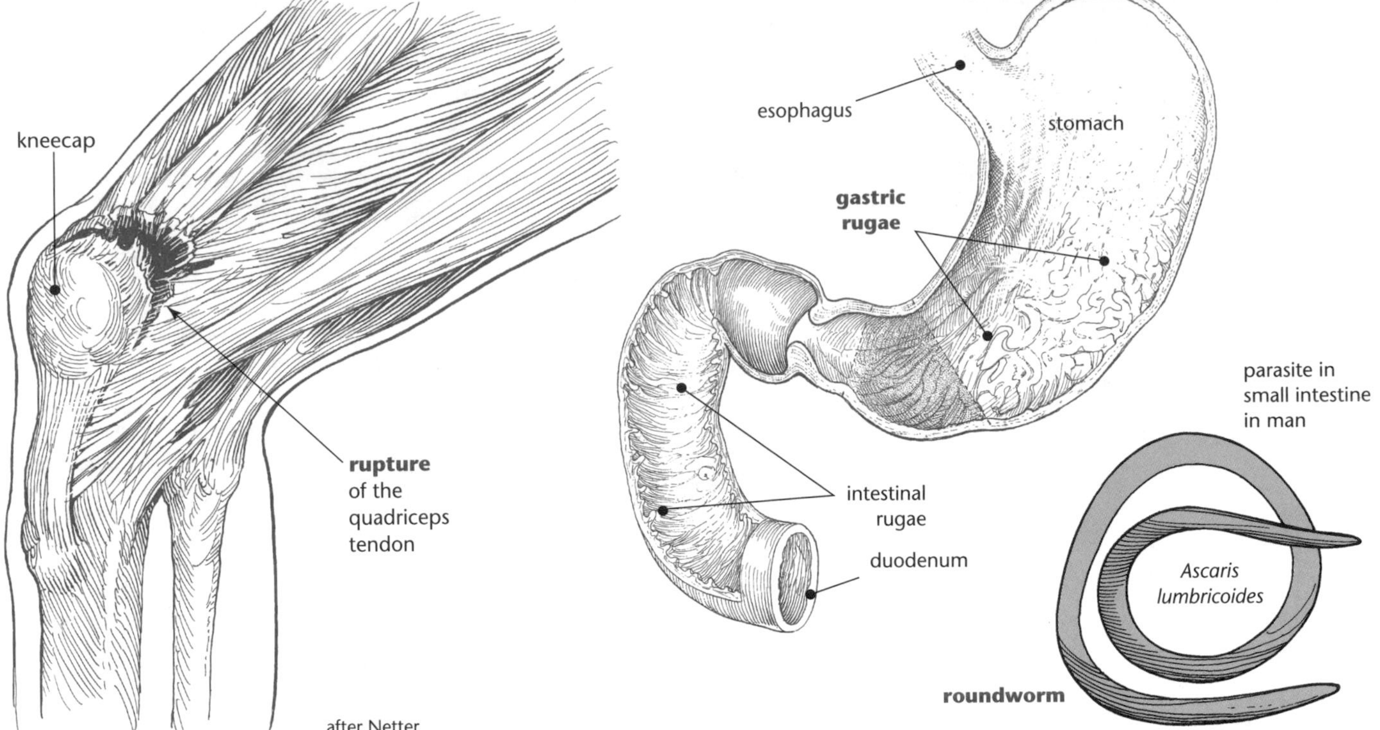

measure gases during administration of anesthesia.

rotation (ro-ta′shun) Motion around an internal axis.

external r. The spontaneous turning of the fetal head when it reaches the level of the ischial spines during labor; the back of the head (occiput) may turn either anteriorly toward the pubic symphysis or posteriorly toward the sacrum. Also called restitution.

internal r. The return of the rotated infant's head to its natural alignment with the shoulders, after the head's complete emergence from the maternal vulva.

rotator (ro-ta′tōr) A muscle that rotates a part, as one of several muscles that rotate the vertebral column.

Rotavirus (ro′tă-vi-rus) Genus of wheel-shaped RNA viruses (family Rotaviridae) including the human gastroenteritis virus; the most important cause of severe dehydration, diarrhea, vomiting, and low-grade fever in children under three years of age.

Rothmund's syndrome (rot′mundz sin′drōm) Syndrome transmitted as an autosomal recessive trait, characterized by juvenile cataracts, saddle nose, premature graying and loss of hair, and wasting of muscles. Also called Rothmund-Thomson syndrome; congenital poikiloderma-juvenile cataract syndrome.

rouge (ro͞ozh) A fine red powder of iron oxide; used as a final polishing agent for dental restorations made of gold and precious metal alloys.

R

rough (ruf) Denoting the granular surface of certain bacterial colonies.

roughage (ruf′ij) Indigestible material in the diet (coarse vegetable fibers and cellulose) that serves to stimulate peristalsis of the bowel.

roughing (ruf′ing) The grinding of lenses with a coarse abrasive.

rouleau (roo-lo′), *pl.* **rouleaux** Red blood cells aggregated like a stack of coins.

roundworm (round′werm) A member of the phylum Nemathelminthes.

rub (rub) **1.** To apply pressure and friction on a surface. **2.** Friction encountered in moving a structure against another.

friction r. Auscultatory sound produced by the rubbing together of two serous surfaces roughened by an inflammatory exudate. Also called friction sound.

pericardial r. A friction or scraping sound produced by the rubbing together of inflamed pericardial surfaces during each heartbeat.

pleuritic r. Grating sound produced by the rubbing together of the inflamed surfaces of the costal and visceral pleurae during breathing.

rubber-dam (rub′er-dam) See dam.

rubedo (roo-be′do) Temporary redness of the skin.

rubefacient (roo-bĕ-fa′shent) Causing redness and irritation of the skin.

rubella (roo-bel′ă) Contagious exanthematous disease of short duration, caused by a virus (genus *Rubivirus,* family Togaviridae); capable of causing congenital defects in infants born of mothers who acquire the disease during the first three months of pregnancy; incubation period is usually two to three weeks. Also called German measles; three-day measles.

rubeola (roo-be-o′lă) See measles.

rubeosis (roo-be-o′sis) Redness.

r. iridis Formation of numerous new blood vessels on the anterior surface of the iris; most frequently associated with diabetes; occasionally seen in other conditions.

rubescent (roo-bes′ent) Reddening.

rubidium (roo-bid′e-um) Chemical element; symbol Rb, atomic number 37, atomic weight 85.47.

Rubivirus (roo-bĭ-vi′rus) Genus of viruses (family Togaviridae) that, unlike other members of Togaviridae, are not transmitted by arthropods; humans are the only vertebrate host; includes the rubella (German measles) virus.

rubor (roo′bor) Latin for redness.

rubriblast (roo′brĭ-blast) See pronormoblast.

rubricyte (roo′brĭ-sīt) See polychromatic normoblast, under normoblast.

rubrospinal (roo-bro-spi′nal) Relating to the red nucleus and the spinal cord.

rudiment (roo′dĭ-ment) An incompletely developed structure.

rudimentary (roo-dĭ-men′tă-re) Incompletely developed.

Ruffini's corpuscle (roo-fe′nēz kor′pus′l) See Ruffini's nerve ending, under ending.

ruffling (ruf′ling) The method by which a cell moves (perambulates) across a surface; characterized by the extension of thin, veil-like folds (ruffles) sprouting upward, extending out like an arm, and then dropping to the surface; when this "arm" adheres to the surface the cell flows into it as if it were pulling itself along.

ruga, (roo′gă) *pl.* **ru′gae** A fold or wrinkle.

gastric r. One of the folds in the lining of the stomach.

r. palatina One of several transverse ridges on the anterior portion of the palate.

r. of vagina One of several transverse folds of the vaginal mucosa.

rugal (roo′gal) Creased; wrinkled; corrugated.

rugitus (roo′ji-tus) Intestinal rumbling.

rugose (roo′gōs) Marked by rugae or ridges; wrinkled.

rugosity (roo-gos′ĭ-te) **1.** The state of having folds or ridges. **2.** A fold or ridge (ruga).

rule (ro͞ol) A guide.

American Law Institute r. A 1962 American rule stating, "a person is not responsible for criminal conduct if at the time of such conduct as a result of mental disease or defect he lacks substantial capacity either to appreciate the wrongfulness of his conduct or to conform his conduct to the requirements of law."

Durham r. A 1954 American test of criminal responsibility stating, "an accused is not criminally responsible if his unlawful act was the product of mental disease or mental defect." This test was repudiated in 1966 (Brawner vs. U.S.) by the court that originated it.

M'Naghten r., McNaughton r. A British test of criminal responsibility stating, "it must be shown that, at the time of committing the act, the accused was acting under such defect of reason from a diseased mind as not to know the nature and quality of the act or if he knew this, that he did not know that what he was doing was wrong."

Nägele's r. Estimation of the day of birth by counting back 3 months from the first day of the last menstrual period and adding 7 days.

ruminant (roo′mi-nant) Any of various hoofed, usually horned, animals (cattle, goats, etc.) that have a stomach with four compartments and that regurgitate and chew partially digested food (cud).

rumination (roo-mi-nā′shun) **1.** The process of chewing cud. **2.** The recurring of thoughts.

rump (rump) Buttocks or gluteal region.

rupture (rup′chur) **1.** The bursting or tearing of a part. Distinguished from dehiscence. **2.** Popular term for a hernia.

premature follicular r. Rupture of an immature ovarian follicle with release of an ovum that is too immature for fertilization.

r. of uterus Rupture of the uterine wall; classified as *complete*, when the tear traverses the whole thickness of the wall and *incomplete,* when the peritoneal covering of the uterus remains intact. May occur during childbirth under certain predisposing conditions (e.g., abnormally adherent placenta, fibroids), by misuse of forceps, application of strong pressure on the uterine fundus, or extensive use of uterine stimulants (e.g., oxytocin, prostaglandins, ergot infusions); or by factors not associated with labor (e.g., uterine cancer, invasive hydatidiform mole).

rut (rut) A period of sexual desire in the males of certain species of mammals; corresponds to heat or estrus in the female.

ruthenium (roo-the′ne-um) A rare, brittle, metallic element; symbol Ru, atomic number 44, atomic weight 101.1.

rutherford (ruth′er-ford) Unit of radioactivity, equal to the amount of radioactive material that undergoes 1 million disintegrations per second.

rypophobia (re-po-fo′be-ă) A morbid fear of dirt.

S

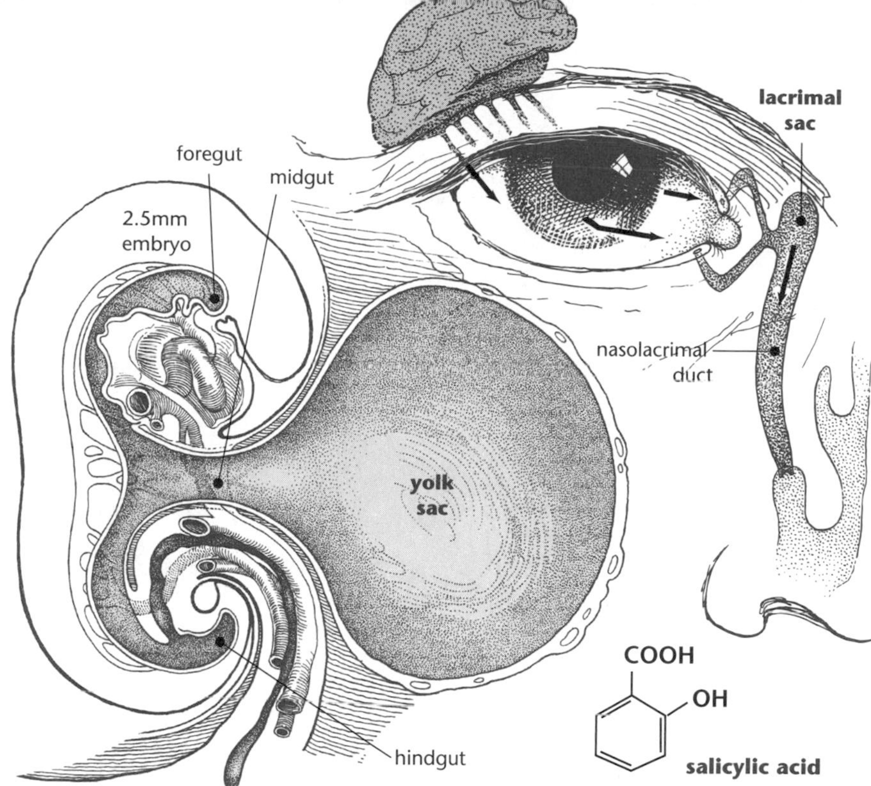

sabulous (sab´u-lus) Sandy; gritty.
sac (sak) A bag or pouchlike anatomic structure.
abdominal s. The part of the embryonic celom that develops into the abdominal cavity.
air s. See pulmonary alveolus, under alveolus.
allantoic s. The dilated distal part of the allantois.
aneurysmal s. The dilated wall of an artery in a saccular aneurysm.
dental s. See dental follicle, under follicle.
dural s. The continuation of the dura mater below the inferior end of the spinal cord.
endolymphatic s. The blind extremity of the endolymphatic duct of the inner ear.
greater s. of peritoneum The main part of the peritoneal cavity; it extends across the whole breadth of the abdomen, and from the diaphragm to the pelvis.
heart s. See pericardium.
hernial s. The peritoneal envelope of a hernia.
lacrimal s. The slightly dilated upper part of the nasolacrimal duct situated in the lacrimal fossa. Also called tear sac.
lesser s. of the peritoneum The smaller part of the peritoneal cavity; a diverticulum of the greater sac of the peritoneum, situated behind the lesser omentum; it extends upward as far as the diaphragm, extends downward between the layers of the greater omentum, and opens through the epiploic foramen. Also called omental bursa.
lymphatic s. See cisterna chyli, under cisterna.
omental s. A recess of the lesser sac of the peritoneum situated between the layers of the greater omentum.
pleural s. A closed sac enveloping each lung, composed of a double-layered membrane (pleura).
synovial s. A closed sac formed by the synovial membrane; it contains a thick, viscous, lubricating fluid (similar to the white of an egg) that facilitates movement of joints.
tear s. See lacrimal sac.
vitelline s. See yolk sac.
yolk s. The vascular umbilical vesicle enveloping the nutritive yolk of an embryo; attached to the embryo's midgut. Also called vitelline sac.
saccades (să-kāds´) Quick; jerky; sudden; said of certain movements of the eye.
saccadic (să-kad´ik) Relating to saccades.
saccate (sak´āt) Pouched.
saccharate (sak´ă-rāt) A salt of saccharic acid.
saccharated (sak´ă-rāt-ed) Sweetened; sugary.
saccharic (să-kar´ik) Relating to sugar.
saccharic acid (să-kar´ik as´id) A white crystalline compound obtained by oxidation of glucose or its derivatives.
saccharide (sak´ă-rid) Any of a series of compounds containing carbon, hydrogen, and oxygen in which the ratio of hydrogen to oxygen is 2:1.
sacchariferous (sak-ă-rif´er-us) Containing or producing sugar.
saccharimeter (sak-ă-rim´ĕ-ter) Device for measuring the amount of sugar in a solution.
saccharin (sak´ă-rin) A white crystalline powder, $C_6H_4COSO_2NH$; used as a sugar substitute.
saccharine (sak´ă-rīn) Sweet.
saccharometabolism (sak-ă-ro-mĕ-tab´ŏ-liz-m) Utilization of sugar by the tissues.
Saccharomyces (sak-ă-ro-mi´sēz) Genus of yeast fungi containing species that ferment sugar.
S. cerevisiae The beer, wine, and bread yeast. Also called brewer's yeast; baker's yeast; wine yeast.
saccharose (sak´ă-rōs) See sucrose.
saccharum (sak´ă-rum) Latin for sucrose.
sacciform, saccular (sak´sĭ-form, sak´u-lar) Baglike.
sacculated (sak´u-lāt-ed) Formed of or divided into a series of pouches.
sacculation (sak-u-la´shun) The presence or the formation of sacs.
saccule, sacculus (sak´ūl, sak´u-lus) **1.** A small sac. **2.** The smaller of the two sacs of the membranous labyrinth in the vestibule of the inner ear.
sacrad (sak´rad) Toward the sacrum.
sacral (sa´kral) Relating to the sacrum.
sacralgia (sa-kral´jă) Pain in the sacral area. Also called sacrodynia.
sacralization (sa-kral-ĭ-za´shun) A bony anomaly in which one or both (usually both) transverse processes of the fifth lumbar vertebra are wing-shaped and long, and articulate with the sacrum or ilium, or both.
sacrectomy (sa-krek´tŏ-me) Surgical removal of a portion of the sacrum.
sacrococcygeal (sa-kro-kok-sij´e-al) Relating to the sacrum and coccyx.
sacrodynia (sa-kro-din´e-ă) See sacralgia.
sacroiliac (sa-kro-il´e-ak) Relating to the sacrum and ilium.
sacroiliitis (sa-kro-il-e-i´tis) Inflammation of the joint between the sacrum and the back of the hipbone on either side.
sacrosciatic (sa-kro-si-at´ik) Relating to the sacrum and ischium.
sacrospinal (sa-kro-spi´nal) Relating to the sacrum and the rest of the vertebral column above it.
sacrovertebral (sa-kro-ver´te-bral) Relating to the sacrum and the vertebrae above it.
sacrum (sa´krum) A slightly curved, triangular bone comprising five fused vertebrae, wedged dorsally between the two hipbones, and forming the posterior section of the pelvis. Articulates with the fifth lumbar vertebra above, and the coccyx below.
saddle (sad´l) See denture base, under base.
sadism (sa´diz-m) Derivation of pleasure from inflicting physical or psychological pain on others, in both social and sexual relationships.
sadist (săd´ist) A person who practices sadism.
sadomasochism (sa-do-mas´ŏ-kizm) The simultaneous existence of submissive (masochistic) and aggressive (sadistic) attitudes in an individual, in both social and sexual relationships.
safflower (saf´lou-er) *Carthamus tinctorius*, a plant having seeds from which safflower oil is extracted.
safranin O (saf´ră-nin ō) A red basic dye used in biologic stains.
safranophile (saf´ră-no-fīl) Staining readily with safranin.
sagittal (saj´ĭ-tal) In an anteroposterior direction.
sal (sal) Latin for salt.
salicin (sal´i-sin) A glucoside obtained from the bark of willow and poplar trees; used as a bitter tonic.
salicylamide (sal-i-sil´ă-mīd, sal-ĭ-sil-am´īd) A white, crystalline compound with analgesic properties.
salicylate (să-lis´i-lāt) A salt of salicylic acid.
methyl s. Oil of wintergreen.
salicylazosulfapyridine (sal-ĭ-sil-ă-zo-sul-fă-pir´ĭ-dēn) A sulfonamide used in the treatment of ulcerative colitis.
salicylic acid (sal-ĭ-sil´ik as´id) $C_7H_6O_3$; a white crystalline powder derived from phenol; used externally for the local treatment of corns and warts.
salicylism (sal´ĭ-sil-iz-m) Poisoning by salicylic acid or its salts.
salicyluric acid (sal-ĭ-sil-ūr´ik as´id) $C_9H_9NO_4$; an acid found in the urine after administration of salicylic acid or some of its derivatives.
salient (sāl´yent) Projecting; protruding.
salify (sal´ĭ-fi) To convert into a salt.
salimeter (să-lim´ĕ-ter) Instrument used to determine the concentration of saline solutions.
saline (sa´lēn) Relating to or containing salt.
saliva (să-li´vă) The fluid mixture of secretions from the parotid, sublingual, and submandibular glands and the mucous glands of the oral cavity; contains an enzyme (ptyalin) that partially digests carbohydrates.
salivant (sal´ĭ-vant) **1.** Increasing the flow of saliva. **2.** An agent having such an effect.
salivary (sal´ĭ-ver-e) Relating to saliva.
salivary gland virus disease (sal´ĭ-ver-e gland vi´rus dĭ-zēz´) See cytomegalic inclusion disease.
salivate (sal´ĭ-vāt) To produce excessive secretion of saliva.
salivation (sal-ĭ-va´shun) The secretion of saliva.
Salmonella (sal-mo-nel´ă) A genus of gram-negative, rod-shaped, motile bacteria, some species of which cause acute intestinal inflammation.
S. typhi Species that is the causative agent of typhoid fever. Formerly called *Salmonella typhosa*.
S. typhimurium Species causing food poisoning in humans.
S. typhosa Former name for *Salmonella typhi*.
salmonellosis (sal-mo-nel-o´sis) Infection with bacteria of the genus *Salmonella*, usually marked by severe diarrhea.
salpingectomy (sal-pin-jek´tŏ-me) Surgical removal of a uterine (fallopian) tube. Also called tubectomy.
salpingemphraxis (sal-pin-jem-frak´sis) Obstruction of a uterine (fallopian) or an auditory (eustachian) tube.
salpingian (sal-pin´je-an) Relating to the uterine (fallopian) or to the auditory (eustachian) tubes.
salpingitis (sal-pin-ji´tis) Inflammation of a fallopian (uterine) tube.
salpingitis isthmica nodosa (sal-pin-ji´tis ith´mĭ-că no-do´să) (SIN) Noninflammatory condition of the narrowest portion of a uterine tube in which the epithelial lining of the tubal lumen extends deeper into the tube's muscular layer, forming a tiny pouch (diverticulum); may be associated with (not necessarily the cause of) tubal ectopic pregnancy.
salpingocele (sal-ping´go-sēl) Hernia of a uterine (fallopian) tube.
salpingocentesis (sal-ping-go-sen-te´sis) Aspi-

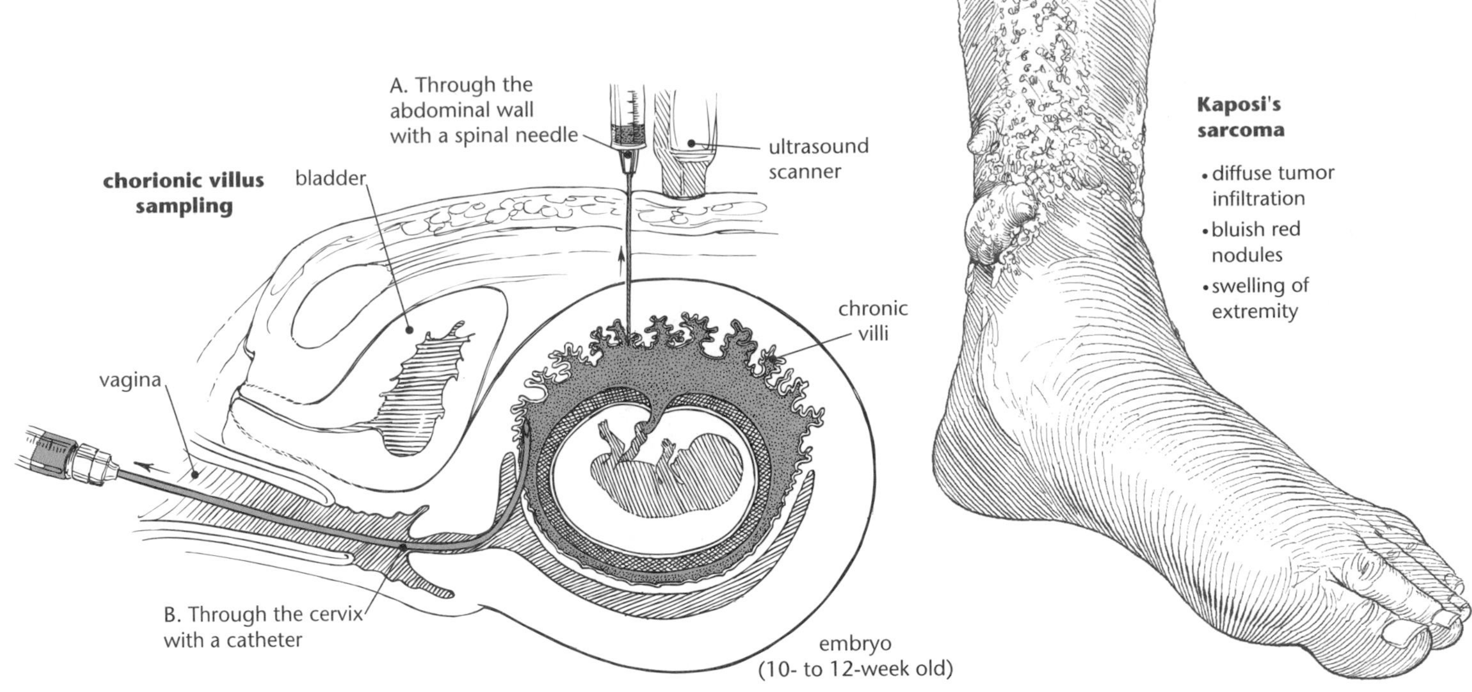

ration of amniotic fluid from an ectopic pregnancy in a uterine tube, followed by injection of a chemical agent.

salpingocyesis (sal-ping-go-si-e´sis) See tubal pregnancy, under pregnancy.

salpingography (sal-ping-gog´ră-fe) Radiography of a uterine tube after the injection of a radiopaque compound.

salpingolysis (sal-ping-gol´ ĭ-sis) The release of adhesions about a uterine (fallopian) tube or its fringed end.

salpingo-oophorectomy (sal-ping´go o-of-ŏ-rek´tŏ-me) Removal of an ovary and its corresponding fallopian (uterine) tube. Also called salpingo-ovariectomy; tubo-ovariectomy.

salpingo-oophoritis (sal-ping´go o-of-ō-ri´tis) Inflammation of a uterine tube and ovary. Also called tubo-ovaritis.

salpingo-ovariolysis (sal-ping-go-o-va-re-ol´ĭ-sis) Removal of adhesions from a uterine tube and ovary.

salpingoperitonitis (sal-ping´go-per-i-tō-ni´tis) Inflammation of a uterine (fallopian) tube and adjacent peritoneum.

salpingopharyngeal (sal-ping´go-fă-rin´je-al) Relating to an auditory (eustachian) tube and the pharynx.

salpingoplasty (sal-ping´go-plas-te) Reparative operation on a uterine tube. Also called tuboplasty.

salpingorrhaphy (sal-ping-gor´ă-fe) Stitching of a uterine (fallopian) tube.

salpingoscopy (sal-ping-gos´kŏ-pe) Endoscopic inspection of the lumen of a uterine tube at its wide (ampullary) portion.

salpingostomy (sal-ping-gos´tŏ-me) The making of an artificial opening in a uterine tube when the fringed end of the tube is occluded; an operative treatment for sterility.

salpingotomy (sal-ping-got´ŏ-me) Surgical incision into a uterine tube.

salpinx (sal´pinks) A tube; especially, a uterine (fallopian) tube or an auditory (eustachian) tube.

salt (sawlt) **1.** Compound produced by the reaction between an acid and a base in which all or part of the hydrogen ions of the acid are replaced by one or more radicals of the base. **2.** Table salt (sodium chloride).

acid s. A salt containing unreplaced hydrogen atoms from the acid (e.g., $NaHSO_4$).

basic s. A salt containing unreplaced hydroxyl radicals from the base (e.g., $Bi(OH)Cl_2$).

binary s. A salt containing only two elements.

effervescent s. One of several preparations containing sodium bicarbonate, tartaric and citric acids, and an active salt; when mixed with water, the acids break up the sodium bicarbonate, releasing the carbonic acid gas.

Epsom s. See magnesium sulfate.

iodized s. Table salt containing one part sodium or potassium iodide to 10,000 parts sodium chloride.

smelling s. A preparation of ammonium carbonate with any of several aromatic oils, sniffed as a restorative.

salt-abrasion (sawlt-ă-bra´zhun) Technique of superficially rubbing away the skin with salt to a uniform depth; used to remove tatoos.

saltation (sal-ta´shun) Leaping, as in certain nervous disorders.

salting out (sawl´ting out) The separation of a protein from its solution by the addition of a neutral salt such as sodium chloride.

saltpeter (sawlt-pe´ter) See potassium nitrate.

salubrious (să-lu´bre-us) Healthful.

saluresis (sal-u-re´sis) Excretion of sodium in the urine.

saluretic (sal-u-ret´ik) Promoting excretion of sodium.

salutary (sal´u-ta-re) Healthful.

salve (sav) **1.** An ointment. **2.** Anything that soothes or heals.

samarium (să-ma´re-um) A rare earth element; symbol Sm, atomic number 62, atomic weight 150.35.

sample (sam´pl) **1.** A representative segment of the whole. **2.** In biostatistics, the portion of the population being studied. **3.** A specimen.

random s. Sample made in such a way that each member of the population from which the sample is derived has an equal chance of being selected.

sampling (sam´pling) Selection and examination of a sample.

chorionic villus s. (CVS) Sampling of placental tissue (chorionic villi) of a 10 to 12 week old fetus to detect chromosomal defects.

percutaneous umbilical blood s. (PUBS) Sampling of fetal blood from the umbilical cord by transabdominal aspiration under ultrasound guidance. Also called cordocentesis.

sanative, sanatory (san´ă-tiv san´ă-to-re) Curative.

sanatorium (san-ă-to´re-um) Institution for treating long term illnesses, such as tuberculosis and mental disorders.

sand (sand) Granules of disintegrated rock.

brain s. See brain sand granules, under granules.

sandfly (sand´flī) A tiny, long-legged fly (genus *Phlebotomus* or *Lutzomyia*); vector of leishmaniasis.

sane (sān) Relating to sanity or to one who is of sound mind.

Sanfilippo's syndrome (san-fĭ-lip´ō sin´drōm) A form of mucopolysaccharidosis characterized by severe mental retardation and excretion of heparan sulfate in the urine; skeleton may be normal or exhibit slight dwarfism; inherited as an autosomal recessive trait. Also called mucopolysaccharidosis III.

sanguiferous (sang-gwif´er-us) Conveying blood.

sanguineous (sang-gwin´e-us) Relating to or containing blood.

sanguinolent (sang-gwin´ō-lent) Blood-tinged.

sanguinopurulent (sang-gwĭ-no-pu´roo-lent) Containing blood and pus.

sanguis (sang´gwis) Latin for blood.

sanguivorous (sang-gwiv´o-rus) Blood-sucking, as certain animals.

saniopurulent (sa-ne-o-pu´roo-lent) Denoting a blood-tinged discharge with pus.

sanioserous (sa-ne-o-se´rus) Denoting a blood-tinged serum.

sanitarium (san-ĭ-ta´re-um) A health resort. COMPARE: sanatorium.

sanitary (san´ĭ-ta-re) Relating to or conducive to health.

sanitation (san-ĭ-ta´shun) Application of measures to create environmental conditions conducive to health.

sanity (san´ĭ-te) Soundness of mind.

santonin (san´to-nin) The bitter principle of santonica (dried flower heads of the plant *Artemicia cina*); sometimes used to effect expulsion of roundworms.

saphenectomy (saf-ĕ-nek´tŏ-me) Surgical removal of a saphenous vein.

saphenous (să-fe´nus) **1.** Relating to either of two large superficial veins of the leg (saphena) that carry blood from the toes upward. **2.** Denoting various structures in the leg.

sapid (sap´id) Affecting the organs of taste.

saponaceous (sa-po-na´shus) Soapy; resembling soap.

saponification (să-pon-ĭ-fi-ka´shun) The formation of a soap by the hydrolytic action of an alkali upon fat.

saponify (să-pon´ĭ-fī) To convert fat into soap.

saponin (sap´o-nin) Any of a group of vegetable substances possessing the property of making suds.

sapphism (saf´iz-m) Lesbianism.

saprogen (sap´ro-jen) An organism that causes decay of organic matter.

saprogenic (sap-ro-jen´ik) Causing decay.

saprogenous (să-proj´ĕ-nus) Resulting from decay.

saprophilous (să-prof´ĭ-lus) Thriving on decaying matter.

saprophyte (sap´ro-fīt) A plant, such as a bacterium or fungus, that lives on and derives nourishment from dead or decaying organic matter. Also called necro-

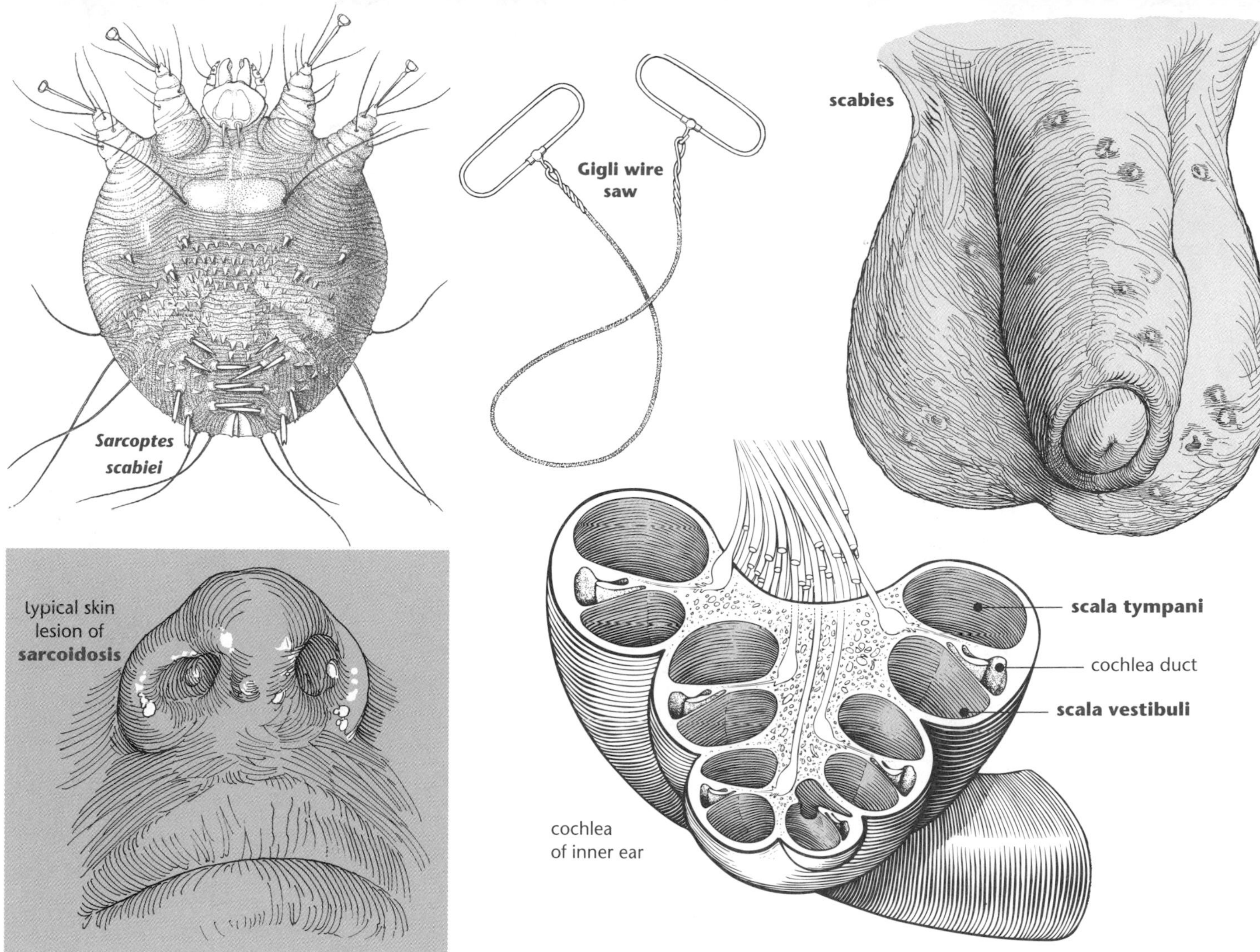

parasite.

saprophytic (sap-ro-fit´ik) Thriving on dead organic matter.

saprozoic (sap-ro-zo´ik) Relating to animals (e.g., protozoa) that thrive on decaying organic material.

sarcoid (sar´koid) **1.** See sarcoidosis. **2.** Resembling flesh.

sarcoidosis (sar-koi-do´sis) Multiple benign nodular lesions involving any tissue of the body, especially the lungs; a systemic granulomatous disease of undetermined etiology. Also called Boeck's sarcoid.

sarcolemma (sar-ko-lem´ă) The delicate plasma membrane that invests every striated muscle fiber.

sarcoma (sar-ko´mă) A malignant tumor composed of connective tissue.

Ewing's s. A rapidly growing malignant tumor arising from medullary tissue within a single bone, usually the long bones; occurring most frequently in individuals between the ages of 10 and 25 years; symptoms include fever, pain, and leukocytosis. Also called Ewing's tumor.

Kaposi's s. (KS) Malignant skin tumor occurring on multiple sites, especially lower extremities; spreads to lymph nodes and internal organs; initial lesions are small red papules which enlarge and fuse to form purple to brown spongy nodules; usually a slowly progressive disease, its course is much more aggressive when associated with AIDS.

Rous s. A sarcoma-like growth of fowl; shown in 1910 by Peyton Rous to be caused by a virus.

synovial s. A highly malignant tumor arising from synovial epithelial cells. Also called malignant synovioma.

sarcomatoid (sar-ko´mă-toid) Resembling a sarcoma.

sarcomatous (sar-ko´mă-tus) Pertaining to or of the nature of sarcoma.

sarcomere (sar´ko-mēr) One of a series of repeated segments of a muscle fibril that comprises the fundamental units of contraction; the area between two Z lines, composed of overlapping thick and thin myofilaments.

sarcoplasm (sar´ko-plaz-m) The interfibrillary cytoplasm of a muscle fiber; the substance in which the muscle fibrils are embedded.

sarcopoietic (sar-ko-poi-et´ik) Forming muscle.

Sarcoptes scabiei (sar-kop´tēz skā´bē-ī) The species of itch mite that causes the parasitic skin disorder scabies; the fertilized female tunnels intradermally and deposits eggs and excreta; the male mites generally do not burrow, but remain on the surface of the skin searching for unfertilized females. Also called itch mite.

sarcosome (sar´ko-sōm) A mitochondrion of muscle; in cardiac muscle, sarcosomes are large, numerous, and usually aligned in columns between the myofibrils.

sarcostosis (sar-kos-to´sis) Ossification of muscle tissue.

sarcotubules (sar-ko-tu´būlz) A system of membranous tubules surrounding each fibril of striated muscle.

sardonic grin (sar-don´ik grin) See risus caninus, under risus.

satellite (sat´e-līt) In genetics, a small globoid chromatin mass attached to the end of the chromosome by a slender secondary constriction, usually associated with the short arm of an acrocentric chromosome.

satellitosis (sat-ĕ-li-to´sis) Phenomenon in which interstitial brain cells of a certain type (oligodendroglia), normally found as satellites about nerve cells, increase in number about a damaged nerve cell.

saturate (sach´ĕr-āt) **1.** To impregnate completely. **2.** To neutralize.

saturated (sach´ĕr-āt-ed) **1.** Denoting a solution in which the addition of any more of a solute will cause precipitation. **2.** Neutral (i.e., having all chemical affinities satisfied).

saturnine (sat´ur-nīn) Relating to lead.

saturnism (sat´ur-niz-m) Lead poisoning.

satyriasis (sat-ĭ-rī´a-sĭs) Excessive sexual desire in the male.

saucerization (saw-ser-ĭ-za´shun) **1.** A flat, disk-shaped defect formed along the shaft of a long bone; it contains microscopic calcifications and is considered typical of a fibrosarcoma with bone involvement. **2.** Excavation of tissue to form a shallow depression, intended to facilitate drainage from infected areas.

sauriasis (saw-rī´ă-sis) See ichthyosis.

saw (saw) A cutting instrument with a serrated edge, used to cut bone.

Gigli wire s. A wire with saw teeth.

Stryker s. A saw designed for cutting hard material such as bone or plastic casts.

scab (skab) **1.** The crust formed on the surface of an ulcer or a superficial wound, composed of dried pus, lymph, or blood. **2.** To develop a scab.

scabicide (skā´bĭ-sīd) Destructive to itch mites.

scabies (skā´bēz) Skin disorder caused by the mite *Sarcoptes scabiei*; the female mite excavates tunnels in the superficial layers of the skin and deposits eggs and irritating excreta, causing red lesions, itching, and swelling of the skin surface along the elevated tracts; the most common sites of entry are between the fingers, the hands, and wrists; the infection can persist for months or years in untreated individuals, hence the colloquial term seven-year itch. Also called sarcoptic acariasis.

scabrites (skā-brish´ēz) Rough, scaly skin.

scala (skā´lă) One of the spiral canals of the cochlea.

s. media See cochlear duct, under duct.

s. tympani The spiral canal of the cochlea located below the bony spiral lamina. Also called tympanic canal.

s. vestibuli The spiral canal of the cochlea located above the bony spiral lamina. Also called vestibular

S

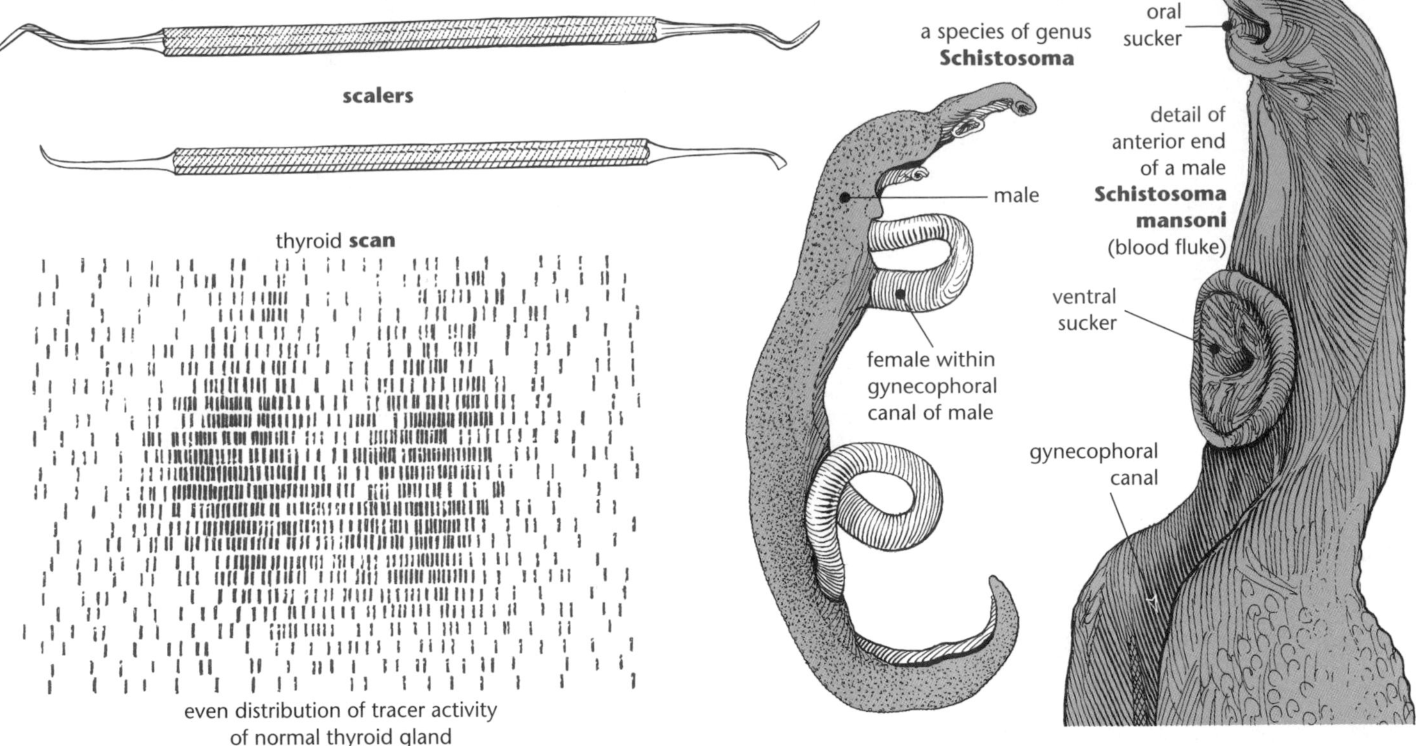

canal.

scald (skawld) **1.** To burn with a hot liquid or vapor. **2.** The lesion produced in such a manner. **3.** Any crusty lesion of the scalp.

scale (skāl) **1.** A small thin piece of epithelium shed from the skin. **2.** To shed such material. **3.** In dentistry, to scrape tartar off the teeth. **4.** A system of marks at regular intervals serving as a standard of measurement. **5.** An instrument having such marks.
absolute s. A temperature scale with its zero point at absolute zero (approximately –273.16°C). Also called Kelvin scale.
activities of daily living s. Scale to assess the state of physical capabilities, based on answers to questions regarding self care, mobility, etc.
Celsius s. A temperature scale in which 0° represents the freezing point of water and 100° its boiling point, at sea level; the normal human body temperature is recorded at 37°; named after Anders Celsius, the Swedish astronomer who invented it. Also called centigrade scale.
centigrade s. See Celsius scale.
Fahrenheit s. Temperature scale that records the freezing point of water at 32°, the boiling point of water at 212°, and the normal human body temperature at 98.6° under standard atmospheric pressure; named after the German physicist Gabriel D. Fahrenheit.
Glasgow coma s. A numerical scale for assessing levels of consciousness (e.g., following a head injury), based on precise clinical criteria, i.e., the patient's ability to respond to three tests of neurologic function: eye opening, with a score ranging from 0 to 4; best motor response, 0 to 5; and best verbal response, 0 to 5. The sum of the three scores provides the level of consciousness.
Kelvin s. See absolute scale.

S

scalded skin syndrome (skawld-ed skin sin´drōm) See staphylococcal scalded skin syndrome.

scalene (ska´lēn) Having three sides of unequal length; said of a triangle or a muscle of such proportions.

scalenectomy (ska-lĕ-nek´tŏ-me) Surgical removal of a scalene muscle, or a portion of it.

scalenus-anticus syndrome (ska-le´nus-an-ti´kus sin´drōm) Pain in the shoulder, often radiating to the arm and back of the neck, caused by compression of nerves and vessels between the first thoracic rib and a hypertonic anterior scalene muscle.

scaler (ska´ler) An instrument designed to be used in removing deposits, especially tartar, from the teeth.

scaling (skāl´ing) Removal of calculus from the exposed surfaces of the teeth and the area under the margin of the gums by use of special instruments called scalers.

scalp (skalp) The skin covering the cranium.

scalpel (skal´pel) A thin surgical knife, usually with a removable blade.

scalpriform (skal´prĭ-form) Resembling a chisel.

scaly (ska´le) **1.** Flaking. **2.** Covered with scales or flakes.

scan (skan) **1.** To survey by a continuous sweep of a sensing device. **2.** A graphic record of an area so obtained (e.g., the distribution of a specific radioactive element within an organ).
brain s. One of the essential methods of cerebrospinal diagnosis; it entails injection or inhalation of radioisotopes and production of pictures by radiation detectors. Also called radioisotopic brain scan.
radioisotopic brain s. See brain scan.

scandium (skan´de-um) A light, silvery-white metallic element that reacts rapidly with acids; symbol Sc, atomic number 21, atomic weight 44.956; present in the earth's crust in a concentration of about 5 parts per million.

scanner (skan´er) **1.** Apparatus used to determine radioactivity distribution within an organ; it consists of a sensitive, collimated detector that is mechanically coupled to a recorder. **2.** Any sensing device that scans a region point by point in a continuous, systematic manner.
CT s. A machine for performing computed tomography. Also called CAT scanner.

scanning (skan´ning) The act of surveying an area by a continuous sweep of a sensing device.
bone s. A sensitive technique of scanning bone for detecting lesions usually employing a radioactive material; a valuable aid in the diagnosis, treatment, and prognosis of a variety of benign and malignant skeletal disorders.

scapha (ska´fă) The long longitudinal depression or furrow between the helix and the antihelix of the auricle.

scaphocephalic (skaf-o-sĕ-fal´ik) Characterized by scaphocephaly.

scaphocephalism (skaf-o-sef´ă-liz-m) See scaphocephaly.

scaphocephaly (skaf-o-sef´ă-le) A deformity in which the skull is abnormally long and narrow (high vertex, bulging forehead, lateral flattening, and increased anteroposterior diameter), due to the premature closure of the sagittal suture. Also called scaphocephalism.

scaphoid (skaf´oid) Boat-shaped; sunken; hollowed.

scapula (skap´u-lă) Either of two large, flat, triangular bones overlying the upper portion of the ribs, and forming the back of the shoulder; articulates with the clavicle and the humerus. Also called shoulder blade.

scapular (skap´u-lar) Relating to the scapula (shoulder blade).

scar (skahr) The fibrous tissue formed during the healing of a wound. Also called cicatrix.

scarification (skar-ĭ-fĭ-ka´shun) The making of several superficial scratches on the skin, as when vaccinating.

scarlatina (skahr-lă-te´nă) See scarlet fever, under fever.

scarlatiniform (skahr-lă-tin´ĭ-form) Resembling scarlet fever, said of a rash.

scatology (skă-tol´ŏ-je) The scientific study and analysis of feces for diagnostic and physiologic purposes.

scatoma (skă-to´mă) An inspissated fecal mass in the colon or rectum resembling, on palpation, an abdominal tumor.

scatophagy (skă-tof´ă-je) See coprophagia.

scatoscopy (skă-tos´ko-pe) Examination or inspection of the feces for diagnostic purposes.

scattergram (skat´er-gram) A graph showing distribution of paired observations of two variables; used to determine whether there is a correlation between the two.

scattering (skat´er-ing) The change in direction or dispersal of a beam of particles or radiation as a result of physical interaction, as the dispersal of electrons by the specimen in the electron microscope.

Scheie's syndrome (shāz sin´drōm) A type of mucopolysaccharidosis considered to be a variant of Hurler's syndrome; characterized by progressive corneal clouding, stiff joints, hirsutism, aortic valvular disease, and excretion of the mucopolysaccharide heparan sulfate in the urine; an autosomal recessive inheritance. Also called mucopolysaccharidosis IS; formerly called mucopolysaccharoidosis V.

schema (ske´mă) An arrangement or plan.

schistocelia (shis-to-se´le-ă) Congenital furrow of the abdominal wall.

schistocystis (shis-to-sis´tis) Fissure or exstrophy of the bladder; a congenital gap in the anterior wall of the bladder and the abdominal wall in front of it, with the posterior wall of the bladder presenting through the opening.

schistocyte, schizocyte (shis´to-sīt, skiz´ŏ-sīt) A fragment of a red blood cell; it can assume a variety of sizes and shapes.

schistocytosis (shis-to-si-to´sis) The occurrence of many red blood fragments (schistocytes) in the blood.

schistoglossia (shis-to-glos´se-ă) Congenital cleft of the tongue.

Schistosoma (shist-to-so´mă) A genus of blood flukes (class Trematoda); some species are parasitic

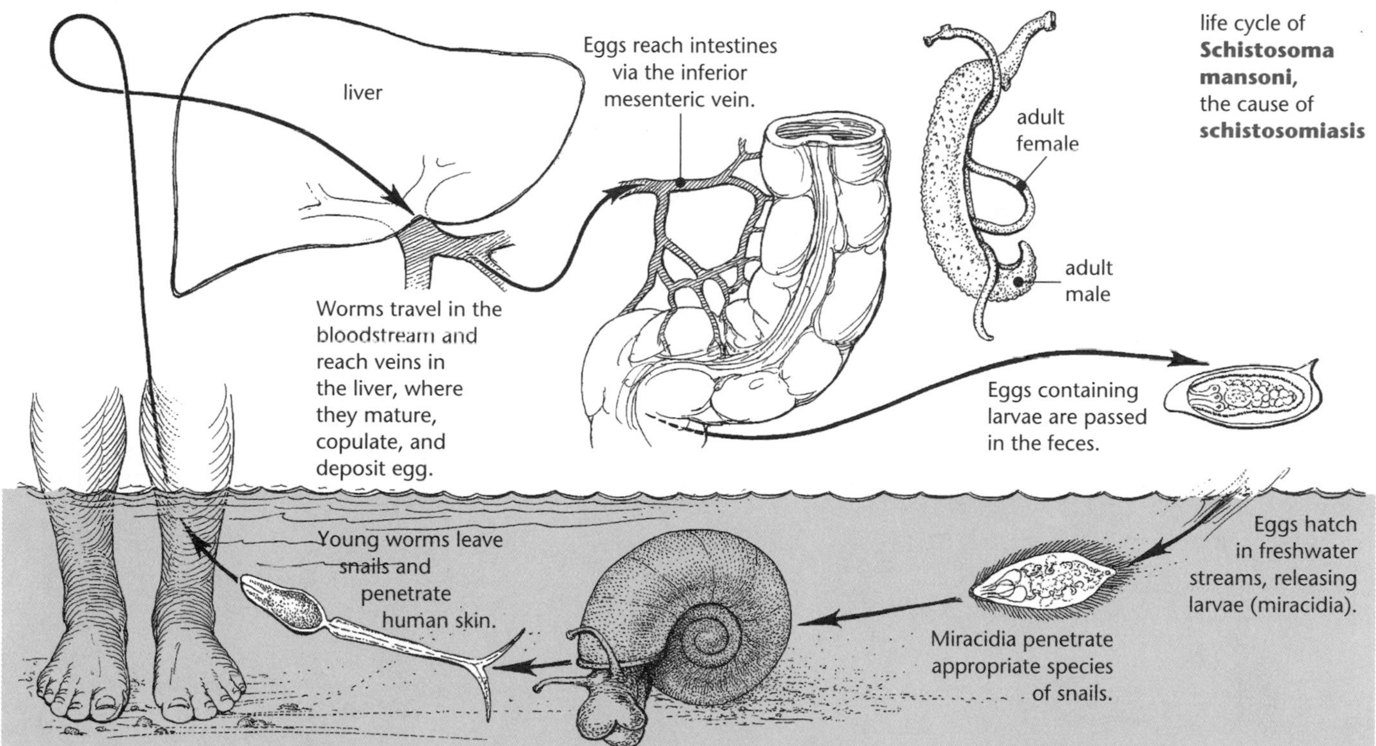
life cycle of
Schistosoma mansoni,
the cause of
schistosomiasis
liver
Eggs reach intestines via the inferior mesenteric vein.
adult female
adult male
Worms travel in the bloodstream and reach veins in the liver, where they mature, copulate, and deposit egg.
Eggs containing larvae are passed in the feces.
Young worms leave snails and penetrate human skin.
Eggs hatch in freshwater streams, releasing larvae (miracidia).
Miracidia penetrate appropriate species of snails.

in humans, causing debilitating illnesses over wide geographical areas of the world; parasites penetrate the skin of persons who come in contact with infested waters.

S. haematobium Species found in the Middle East, large areas of Africa, and small areas of India; invertebrate host is a snail of the genus *Bulinus*; adult worms live exclusively in humans, within the veins of the bladder, causing symptoms of the urinary tract and, to a lesser degree, of the intestines.

S. japonicum Species found in the Far East; invertebrate host is a snail of the genus *Oncomelania*; adult worm infests rodents, domestic animals, and humans; in humans, it lives within the venules of the small intestine and, because of the large number of eggs it deposits, causes the most serious of blood fluke diseases, with intestinal, hepatic, and pulmonary symptoms.

S. mansoni Species found mainly in northeastern Brazil and the Caribbean islands; invertebrate host is a snail of the genus *Biomphalaria*; in humans, it lives within veins of the large intestine; disease is similar to that caused by *Schistosoma japonicum* but milder.

schistosome (shis´to-sōm) A fluke of the genus *Schistosoma*.

schistosomiasis (shis-to-so-mi´ă-sis) Infection with schistosomes (blood flukes); involves mainly the intestinal tract, liver, or bladder. Also called bilharziasis; bilharziosis.

s. japonica, Japanese s. Infection with *Schistosoma japonicum;* manifestations include enlargement of liver and spleen, fluid accumulation in tissues, anemia, and brain lesions.

s. mansoni, Manson's s. Infection with *Schistosoma mansoni* that may last for several decades, leading to enlargement of liver and spleen, liver fibrosis, portal hypertension, and central nervous system involvement.

pulmonary s. Manifestations of *Schistosoma* infections, usually a cough, as the organisms travel in the bloodstream to the digestive system through the lungs.

schizogony (skĭ-zog´ŏ-ne) A stage in the asexual cycle of the malarial parasite occurring in the red blood cells of man. Also called multiple fission.

schizoid (skiz´oid), skit´soid) See schizoid personality disorder, under disorder.

Schizomycetes (skiz-o-mi-se´tēz) A class of microorganisms containing all bacteria.

schizont (skiz´ont) The adult asexual form of the malarial parasite in man, following the trophozoite, with two or more divisions of its nucleus; it eventually divides, producing merozoites.

schizophasia (skiz-o-fa´zhă) The disordered, incomprehensible speech of the schizophrenic individual. Commonly called "word-salad" speech.

schizophrenia (skiz-o-fre´ne-ă) A category of severe emotional disorders with onset before age 45; marked by disturbances of thinking including misinterpretation of reality and sometimes delusions and hallucinations; there are associated changes in mood and behavior, particularly withdrawal from people. Formerly called dementia praecox.

schizophrenic (skiz-o-fren´ik) Relating to schizophrenia.

schizotrichia (skiz-o-trik´e-ă) A splitting of the hairs at their ends. Also called scissura pilorum.

Schmidt's syndrome (shmits sin´drōm) **1.** Primary hypothyroidism and adrenal insufficiency; organ-specific antibodies against the adrenal and thyroid glands may be present; diabetes mellitus may also be present. **2.** Unilateral paralysis of the vocal folds, the palate, and the trapezius and sternocleidomastoid muscles.

Schönlein's disease (shern´līnz dĭ-zēz´) See Henoch-Schönlein purpura, under purpura.

Schüffner's dots (shĕf´nĕrz dotz) The dots or stipples appearing in red blood cells infected with malarial parasites (especially *Plasmodium vivax*), due to accumulation of granules. Also called Schüffner's granules.

Schüller disease (shĕl´ĕr dĭ-zēz´) See multifocal Langerhans-cell histiocytosis, under histiocytosis.

schwannoma (shwă-no´mă) A slowly growing, typically single, noncancerous tumor originating from Schwann cells; commonly occurs in relation to sensory cranial nerves and the sensory root of spinal nerves.

vestibular s. Schwannoma typically involving the vestibular division of the vestibulocochlear (8th cranial) nerve of one ear; rate of growth varies; symptoms include progressive sensory hearing loss, ringing in the ear, vertigo, and poor balance. Also called acoustic neuroma; acoustic neurinoma; acoustic neurilemoma; acoustic nerve schwannoma.

acoustic nerve s. See vestibular schwannoma.

sciatic (si-at´ik) Relating to the hip or to the ischium.

sciatica (si-at´ĭ-kă) Any condition characterized by pain along the course of the sciatic nerve; usually a neuritis and generally caused by mechanical compression or irritation of the fifth lumbar spinal root.

scinticisternography (sin-tĭ-sis-ter-nog´ră-fe) A test for diagnosing hydrocephalus and for studying the dynamics of cerebrospinal fluid movement, by use of a radioactive tracer.

scintigraphy (sin-tĭg´ră-fe) Injection of a radioactive substance and determination of its distribution in the tissues with the aid of a scintiscanner.

scintillation (sin-tĭ-la´shun) A flash of light produced in a chemical crystal by absorption of an ionizing photon; the minuscule flash of light seen on a fluorescent screen results from the spontaneous emission of charged alpha particles across the sensitized surface.

scintillator (sin-tĭ-la´tor) A substance that emits light when hit by a subatomic particle, x radiation, or gamma radiation.

scintiphotography (sin-tĭ-fo-tog´ră-fe) The process of recording on photographic film the distribution of an internally administered radioactive substance. Also called scintography.

scintiscan (sin´tĭ-skan) A graphic pattern recorded on paper of pulses derived from a radioactive isotope, revealing its concentration in a specific organ or tissue; it serves to outline the tissue or organ or its actively metabolizing portion.

scintiscanner (sin-tĭ-skan´er) A directional scintillation counter that automatically scans a region of the body to record the concentration of a gamma-ray-emitting isotope in tissue.

scintography (sin-tog´ră-fe) See scintiphotography.

scirrhous (skir´us) Relating to a scirrhus; hard.

scirrhus (skir´us) A hard cancerous tumor composed chiefly of fibrous connective tissue.

scissors (siz´ĕrz) A double-bladed cutting instrument.

sclera (skler´ă) The tough, white, membranous, outermost coat of the eye; covers the eyeball surface except the anterior portion, which is occupied by the cornea. Commonly called white of the eye.

scleradenitis (skler-ad-ĕ-ni´tis) Hardening of a gland due to infection.

scleral (skler´ăl) Relating to the sclera.

scleral buckling (sklĕr´al buk´ling) Technique for repair of detachment of the retina in which the deep sclera and the choroid are infolded over the retinal tear to promote adherence of the retina to the choroid layer of the eye.

sclerectasia (skler-ĕk-ta´zhă) Outward bulging of a small area of the sclera.

sclerectomy (sklĕ-rek´tŏ-me) Surgical removal of a small portion of the sclera (e.g., for the treatment of glaucoma).

scleredema (skler-ĕ-de´mă) Disease of unknown cause marked by induration and swelling of the skin and subcutaneous tissues.

sclerema (sklĕ-re´mă) Hardening of the skin and underlying tissues.

scleritis (sklĕ-ri´tis) Inflammation of the sclera.

annular s. Ring-shaped scleritis that extends around the limbus of the cornea.

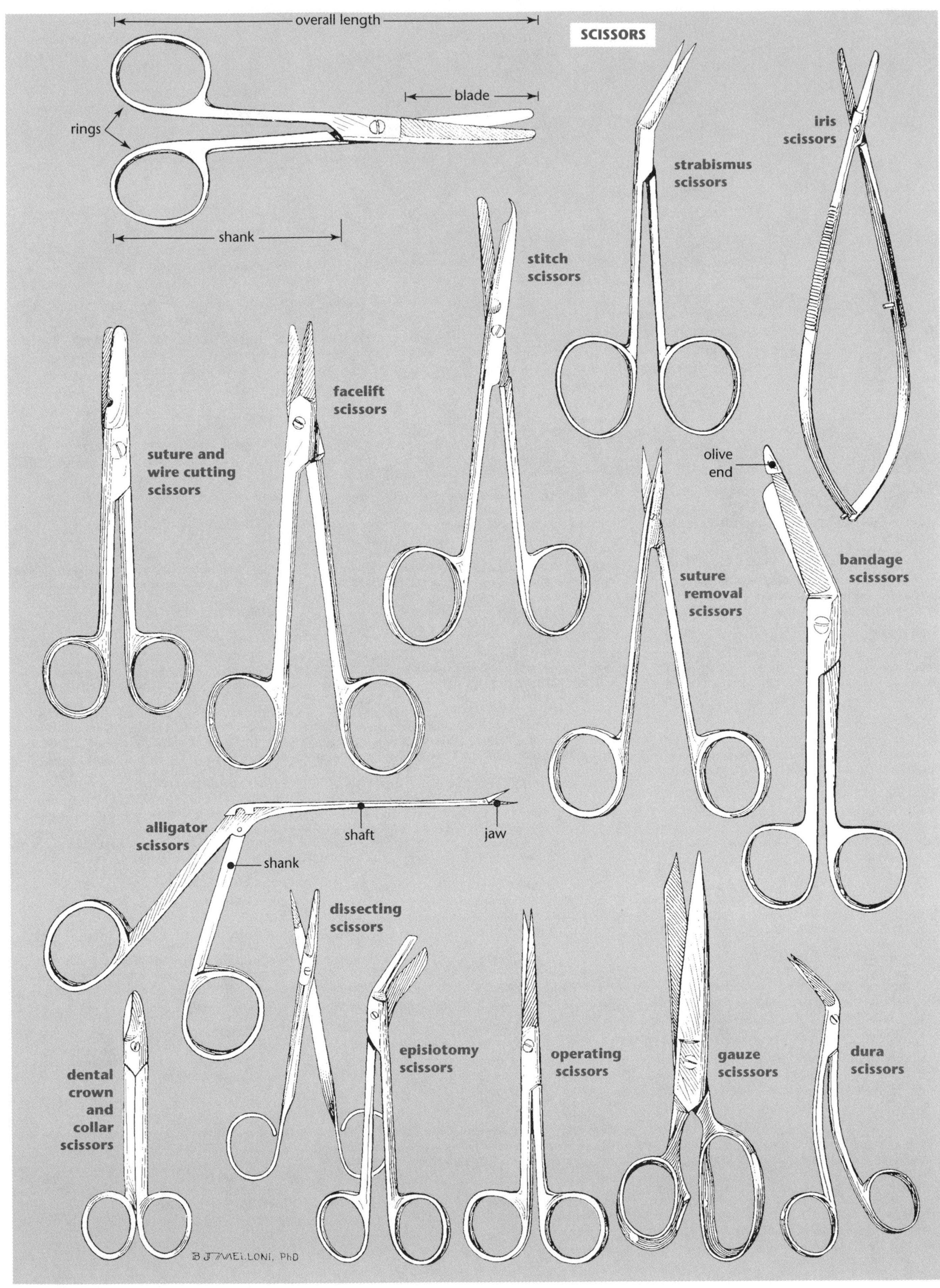
SCISSORS
overall length
blade
rings
shank
strabismus scissors
iris scissors
stitch scissors
facelift scissors
suture and wire cutting scissors
olive end
bandage scisssors
suture removal scissors
alligator scissors
shaft
jaw
shank
dissecting scissors
episiotomy scissors
operating scissors
gauze scisssors
dura scissors
dental crown and collar scissors
B J MELLONI, PhD

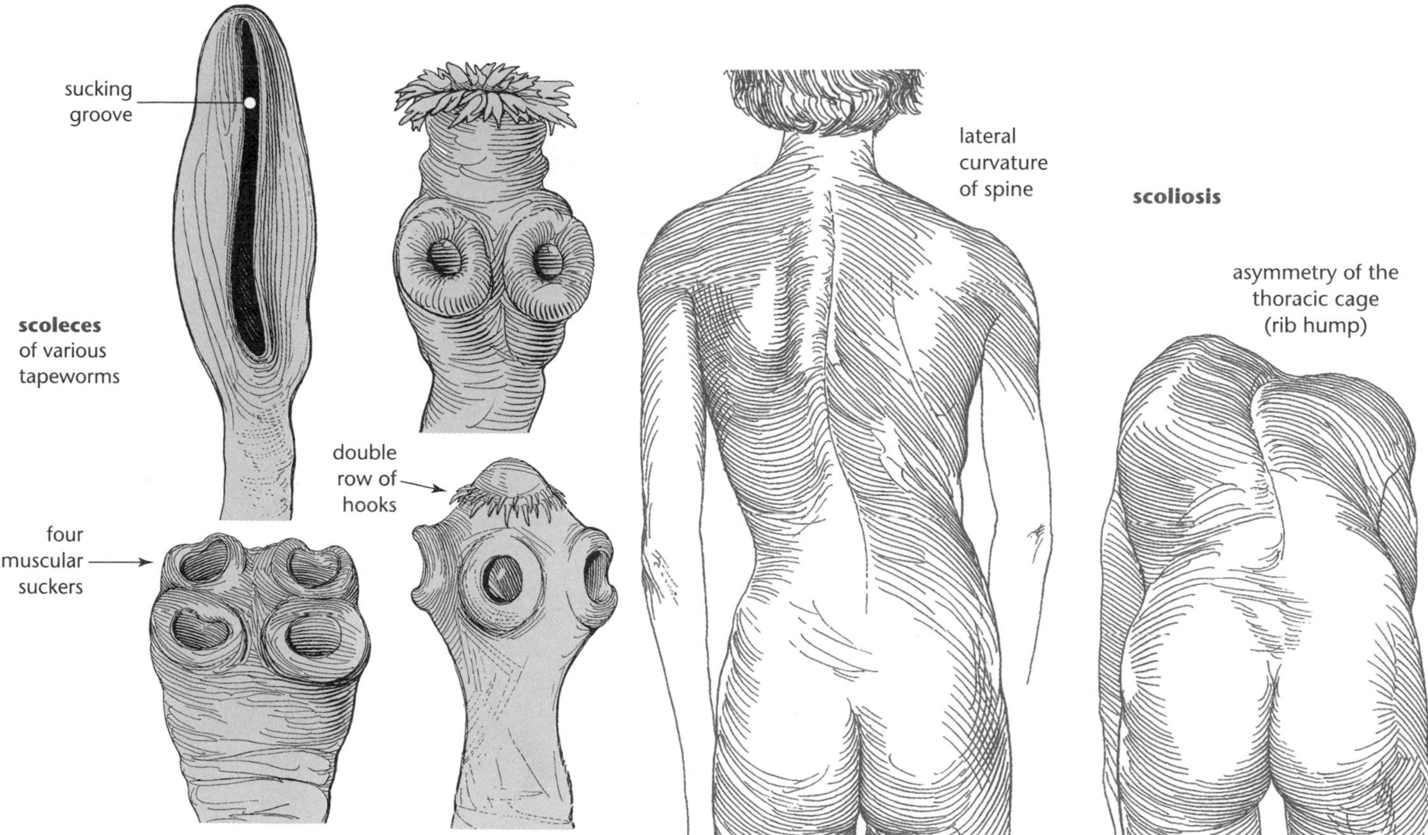

anterior s. Scleritis of the exposed, visible part of the sclera.
brawny s. Annular scleritis with thickening of the episcleral tissues adjoining the cornea.
herpetic s. Herpes zoster involving the sclera.
posterior s. Inflammation of the sclera at the back of the eyeball, near the optic nerve; may also involve the underlying choroid and retina; usually associated with severe rheumatoid arthritis.

sclerochoroidal (skler-o-ko-roi´al) Relating to both the sclera and choroid, the outer and middle layers of the eyeball.

scleroconjunctival (skler-o-kon-junk-ti´val) Relating to the sclera and the conjunctiva.

sclerocornea (skler-o-kor´ne-ă) The sclera and cornea considered as a unit.

sclerodactyly (skler-o-dak´tĭ-le) Scleroderma affecting the fingers or toes.

scleroderma (skler-o-der´mă) See progressive systemic sclerosis, under sclerosis.

sclerodermatitis, sclerodermitis (skler-o-der-mă-tī´tis, skler-o-der-mī´tis) Inflammation, thickening, and hardening of the skin.

sclerogenous, sclerogenic (sklĕ-roj´ĕ-nus, sklĕ-ro-jen´ik) Producing a hard tissue or substance; causing sclerosis.

scleroiritis (skler-o-i-ri´tis) Inflammation of the sclera and iris.

scleroma (sklĕ-ro´mă) A circumscribed area of hard or granulation tissue in the skin or mucous membrane.

scleromalacia (skler-o-mă-la´shă) Extreme thinning of the sclera, usually occurring in patients with rheumatoid arthritis.

scleronychia (skler-o-nik´e-ă) Excessively hardened and thickened condition of the nails.

sclero-oophoritis (sklĕ-ro-o-of-ŏ-ri´tis) Inflammatory hardening of the ovary.

sclerophthalmia (skler-of-thal´me-ă) Rare congenital condition in which scleral tissue encroaches on the cornea, with only a small central area remaining clear.

scleroplasty (skler-o-plas´te) Reparative surgery of the sclera.

scleroprotein (skler-o-pro´tēn) A hard fibrous protein resembling albumin. Also called albuminoid.

sclerose (sklĕ-rōs´) To harden or to become sclerotic.

sclerosis (sklĕ-ro´sis) Hardening of tissues due to proliferation of connective tissue, usually originating in chronic inflammation.
amyotrophic lateral s. (ALS) Disease characterized by degeneration of the lateral motor tracts of the spinal cord, causing twitching of muscle fibers, exaggerated reflexes, and progressive muscular atrophy. Commonly called Lou Gehrig's disease.
arterial s. See arteriosclerosis.
arteriolar s. See arteriolosclerosis.
endocardial s. See endomyocardial fibroelastosis, under fibroelastosis.
Mönckeberg's s. See Mönckeberg's arteriosclerosis, under arteriosclerosis.
medial calcific s. See Mönckeberg's arteriosclerosis, under arteriosclerosis.
multiple s. (MS) Disease of the brain and spinal cord affecting mostly young adults and characterized by loss of the fatty sheaths (myelin) that surround nerve fibers; its name is derived from the plaques or patches of scarred (sclerosed) nervous fibers that dot the central nervous system; symptoms vary with distribution of the sclerotic patches, but the most frequently seen are weakness, incoordination, scanning (halting, monosyllabic) speech, involuntary oscillation of the eyeballs (nystagmus), and coarse tremors.
progressive systemic s. (PSSc) Multisystem disorder marked by progressive thickening and hardening of the skin, eventually involving the blood vessels, kidneys, heart, lungs, and gastrointestinal tract. Also called scleroderma.
systemic s. (SSc) Multisystem disorder marked by progressive thickening and hardening of the skin, blood vessels, and visceral organs (kidneys, heart, lungs, and gastrointestinal tract). Also called scleroderma.
tuberous s. An autosomal dominant inherited disease marked by progressive mental deterioration, epileptic convulsions, and sometimes sebaceous adenomas on the skin. Also called epiloia; Bourneville's disease.

sclerostomy (sklĕ-ros´tŏ-me) Operative creation of a fistulous opening in the sclera, as for the relief of glaucoma.

sclerotherapy (skler-o-ther´ă-pe) Injection of a chemical into a vein to obliterate its lumen; a method of treating varicose veins.

sclerotic (sklĕ-rot´ik) **1.** Relating to or characterized by sclerosis. **2.** Relating to the outer layer of the eyeball (sclera).

sclerotome (skler´o-tōm) In embryology, the cells that break off from the somite, surround the notochord and spinal cord, later differentiate into cartilage, and eventually form the vertebrae.

sclerotomy (sklĕ-rot´ŏ-me) Surgical incision of the sclera.

sclerous (skler´us) Hardened.

scoleces (sko´lĕ-sēz) Plural of scolex.

scolecology (sko-lĕ-kol´ŏ-je) See helminthology.

scolex (sko´leks), *pl.* **sco´leces** The head of a tapeworm by which it attaches to the mucosa of the small intestine; it is connected by a short and narrow neck to a large number of proglottids (segments).

scoliosis (sko-le-o´sis) A rotary lateral curvature of the spine.
congenital s. Scoliosis resulting from malformation of the spine or chest.
idiopathic s. Scoliosis of unknown cause.
myopathic s. Scoliosis due to weakness of the spinal muscles.
neuromuscular s. Scoliosis caused by any of various diseases affecting the motor nerve cells.
osteopathic s. Lateral curvature resulting from pathologic conditions of the vertebrae, such as tuberculosis, rickets, osteomalacia, and tumors.
static s. Scoliosis due to difference in the length of the legs.

scoliotic (sko-le-ot´ik) Relating to scoliosis.

scopolamine (sko-pol´ă-mēn) A nonbarbiturate hypnotic alkaloid found in the leaves and seeds of *Hyoscyamus niger* (henbane), *Scopola carniolica*, *Atropa belladonna*, and other solanaceous plants; used to prevent motion sickness; in toxic doses, it can cause excitation, hallucinations, delirium, and other peculiar mental effects; because of its amnestic qualities, is used with morphine to produce "twilight sleep"; formerly used extensively in obstetrics.

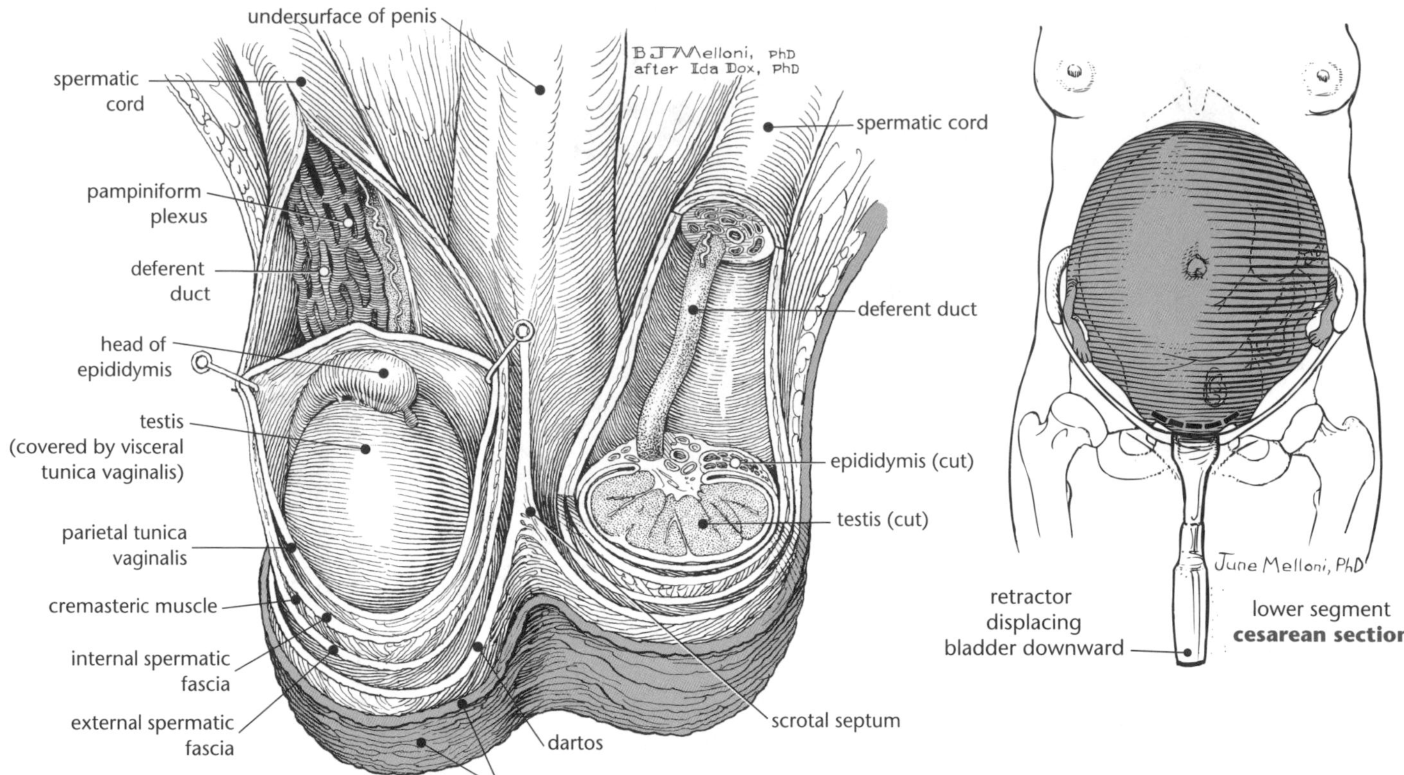

scorbutic (skōr-bu´tik) Relating to scurvy.
scorbutus (skor-bu´tus) See scurvy.
score (skor) An evaluative record, usually expressed numerically.
APACHE s. Acronym for acute physiology and chronic health evaluation. A method of determining the severity of illness in acutely ill patients in intensive care units.
Apgar s. A numerical expression of the condition of a newborn infant on a scale of 0 to 10. Numerical values are assigned to the status of skin color, heart rate, respiratory effort, muscle tone, and reflex irritability; usually recorded at 1 and 5 minutes after delivery and become a permanent part of the child's health record.
Gleason's s. See Gleason's grading system, under system.
symptom s. A scoring system devised by the American Urologic Association to quantitate the degree of prostatic obstruction. There are 7 questions, graded from 0 to 5 points, each depending on severity. The symptoms relate to nocturia, incomplete emptying, frequency, intermittency, urgency, weak stream, and straining. A score of 7 or less needs watchful waiting. Scores of 8 to 20 (moderate) and greater than 20 (severe) require treatment to avoid complications.
scorpion (skōr´pe-on) A member of the order Scorpionida having a segmented body and an erectile tail that contains a venomous sting.
scotochromogens (sko-to-kro´mo-jenz) See group II mycobacteria, under mycobacteria.
scotoma (sko-to´mă) **1.** An abnormal blind spot; an area in the visual field in which vision is absent or greatly diminished. **2.** In psychiatry, a figurative blind spot in an individual's psychologic awareness characterized by an absence of insight into or inability to grasp a mental problem.
scotomatous (sko-tom´ă-tus) Relating to an area of absent or depressed vision (scotoma) in the visual field.
scotometer (sko-tom´ĕ-ter) Instrument used to plot and measure an isolated area of absent or depressed vision (scotoma) in the visual field.
scotopia (sko-to´pe-ă) See scotopic vision, under vision.
scotopic (sko-top´ik) **1.** Relating to vision that is adapted to low levels of illumination. **2.** Denoting the low levels of illumination to which the eye's sensitivity to light becomes greatly increased when it is dark-adapted.
screen (skrēn) **1.** A thin sheet of any material used as a shield. **2.** To conduct a screening.
fluorescent s. A screen coated with calcium tungstate, which produces light when exposed to x rays; used in fluoroscopy.
tangent s. A large, usually black screen used in the clinical measurement of the central field of vision.
screening (skrēn´ing) **1.** The process of examining large groups of people for a given disease. **2.** Survey of a specimen for a variety of substances (e.g., a narcotic screen of a urine sample).
genetic s. Any method of identifying individuals in a given population at high risk of having, or transmitting, a specific genetic disorder.
scrofula (skrof´u-lă) Tuberculous inflammation of lymph nodes of the neck.
scrotal (skro´tal) Relating to the scrotum.
scrotectomy (skro-tek´tŏ-me) Surgical removal of part of the scrotum.
scrotitis (skro-ti´tis) Inflammation of the scrotum.
scrotocele (skro´to-sēl) See inguinal hernia, under hernia.
scrotoplasty (skro´to-plas-te) Reparative surgery of the scrotum. Also called oscheoplasty.
scrotum (skro´tum) The two-layered sac enclosing the testes and lower part of spermatic cords; composed of skin, muscles, and fascia, and divided on its surface into two portions by a ridge (raphe).
scruff (skrŭf) Nape.
scruple (skroo´pl) A unit of apothecary weight equal to 20 grains or one-third of a dram.
scurvy (skur´ve) A nutritional deficiency disease resulting from a lack of vitamin C (ascorbic acid), characterized by spongy, swollen, and bleeding gums, hemorrhages, and extreme weakness. Also called scorbutus.
scute (skyo͞ot) A thin lamina or plate, such as the thin bony plate separating the upper part of the middle ear from the mastoid cells.
scybalous (sib´ă-lus) Of the nature of a scybalum.
scybalum (sib´ă-lum) An abnormally hard mass of feces in the intestine.
Scyphozoa (si-fo-zo´ă) A class of marine animals (phylum Coelenterata) that includes the jellyfishes.
seal (sēl) **1.** To effect an airtight closure. **2.** Any agent used to prevent seepage of air or moisture.
seasickness (sē´sik´nes) Nausea, pallor, sweating, and vomiting provoked by the motion of a vessel at sea.
seatworm (sēt´werm) See pinworm.
sebaceous (sĕ-ba´shus) Relating to or secreting fatty material (sebum).
seborrhea (seb-o-re´ă) See seborrheic dermatitis, under dermatitis.
sebum (se´bum) The secretion of a sebaceous gland.
secobarbital (se-ko-bar´bĭ-tal) A short-acting, fast-onset sedative and hypnotic; Seconal®.
secondary (sek´un-der-e) **1.** Dependent on the occurrence of another event (e.g., a complication). **2.** Second in a sequence or importance.
secreta (se-kre´ă) Secretions.
secretagogue, secretogogue (se-krēt´ă-gog, se-krē´tŏ-gog) **1.** A substance that promotes secretion, as of the stomach. **2.** Stimulating secretion.
secrete (se-krēt´) To produce cell products and deliver them into the blood or bodily cavity either through a duct or by direct diffusion.
secretin (se-kre´tin) An intestinal hormone released primarily by the mucosa of the duodenum during digestion; it stimulates the secretion of water and bicarbonate by the pancreas.
secretion (se-kre´shun) **1.** The production of a substance by a cell or a gland. **2.** The substance produced.
secretomotor, secretomotory (se-kre-to-mo´tor, se-kre-to-mo´tor-e) Stimulating glandular secretion; said of certain nerves.
secretor (se-kre´tor) A person whose saliva and other body fluids contain water-soluble forms of the ABO blood group antigens. An autosomal dominant inheritance.
secretory (se-kre-tor´e) Relating to secretion.
sectile (sek´tīl) Capable of being cut.
section (sek´shun) **1.** The act of cutting. **2.** One of several component segments of a structure. **3.** A thin slice of tissue suitable for examination under the microscope. **4.** A cut surface.
abdominal s. See laparatomy.
C s. See cesarean section.
cesarean s., C s. (CS) Incision through the walls of the abdomen and uterus for delivery of the fetus. Also called C section; abdominal delivery.
coronal s. A section parallel to the coronal suture of the skull, at right angles to the sagittal section.
cross s. A section at right angles to the long axis.
frozen s. A section cut by a microtome from tissue preserved by freezing; often used in microscopic diagnosis.
histologic s. See section (3).

APGAR SCORE

Criteria	Score		
	0	1	2
skin color	pale blue	pink body blue extremities	all pink
heart rate	absent	<100	>100
respiratory effort	absent	irregular; slow	good; crying
muscle tone	limp	some flexion of extremities	active
reflex response to nose catheter	no response	grimace	sneeze; cough

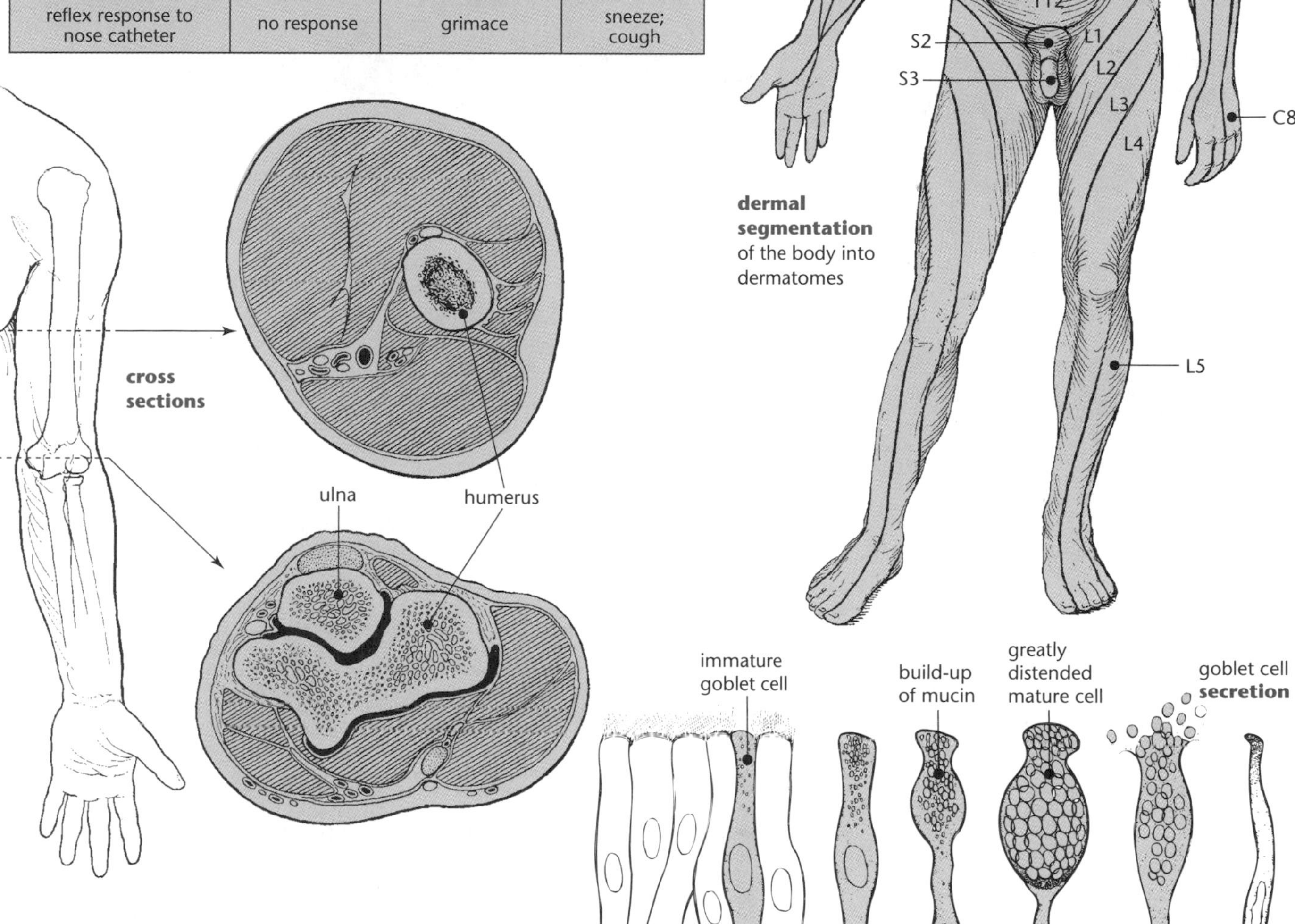

cross sections

dermal segmentation of the body into dermatomes

goblet cell **secretion**

longitudinal s. Any section along the long axis of a structure or the body.
paraffin s. A histologic section cut with a microtome from tissue embedded in paraffin wax.
root s. See rhizotomy.
sagittal s. An anteroposterior section which divides the body into more or less equal right and left parts.
serial s. One of several consecutive histologic sections of a structure (e.g., spinal cord) for the purpose of microscopic examination.
trigeminal root s. See trigeminal rhizotomy, under rhizotomy.

secundigravida (sĕ-kun-dĭ-grav´ĭ-dă) A woman who has been pregnant twice.

secundines (se-kun´dinz) See afterbirth.

secundipara (se-kun-dip´ă-ră) A woman who has given birth twice. Also called para-II; formerly called bipara.

sedate (sĕ-dāt´) **1.** To bring under the influence of a sedative. **2.** To administer a sedative to an individual.

sedation (sĕ-da´shun) The reduction of anxiety or stress by the administration of a sedative drug.

sedative (sed´ă-tiv) Any agent that slows down nervous activity.

sediment (sed´ĭ-ment) The insoluble material that settles to the bottom of a liquid. Also called hypostasis (what rises to the surface is called epistasis).
urinary s. The solid matter that sinks to the bottom after urine has been allowed to stand for some time or has been centrifuged; microscopic examination of urine is usually performed on sediment resuspended in a few drops of the supernatant urine.

sedimentation (sed-ĭ-men-ta´shun) The formation of a deposit of insoluble materials at the bottom of a liquid.

sedimentator (sed-ĭ-men-ta´tor) Centrifuge.

seed (sēd) In bacteriology, to introduce a microorganism into a culture medium.

segment (seg´ment) **1.** One of the parts into which a structure can be divided. **2.** A differentiated subdivision of an organism or part, such as a metamere.
anonymous DNA s. A piece of DNA of unknown gene content that has been localized to a chromosome.

segmentation (seg-men-ta´shun) **1.** Differentiation into similar parts. **2.** Cleavage, as of the fertilized ovum.
cutaneous s. See dermal segmentation.
dermal s. The division of the skin into segments (dermatomes) according to the different nervous innervation of each segment. Also called cutaneous segmentation.

segregation (seg-re-ga´shun) In meiosis, the separating of two alleles of a pair of allelic genes so that they can pass to different gametes (ovum or sperm).

seizure (se´zhur) **1.** An attack or sudden onset of a disease. **2.** An epileptic attack. See also epilepsy.
absence s. A brief (10 to 30 seconds) break of consciousness of thought or activity.
clonic s. Rhythmic jerking of all or part of the body.

S

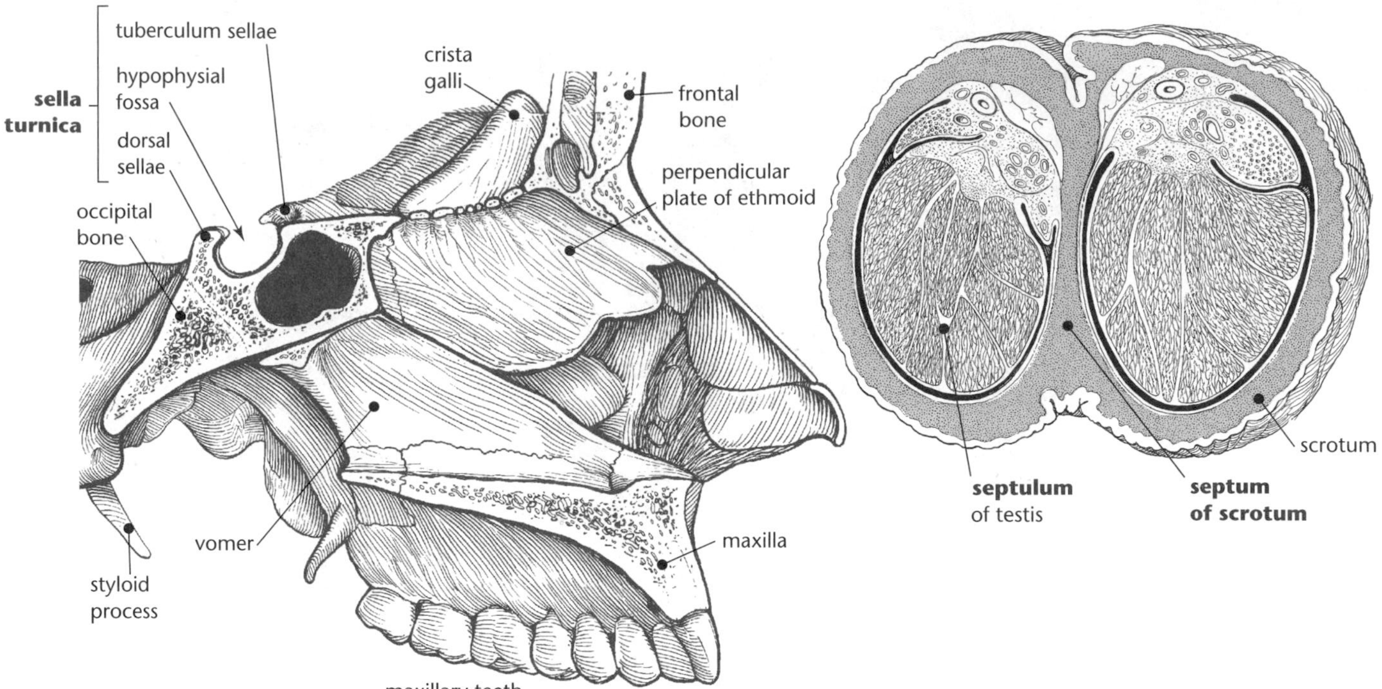

focal motor s. Seizure involving motor activities restricted to isolated areas of the body.

generalized-onset s. Seizure arising from simultaneous involvement of all or large parts of both cerebral hemispheres from the start.

generalized tonic-clonic s. Sustained (tonic) muscular contractions, followed by jerking (clonic) movements.

grand mal s. See generalized tonic-clonic seizure.

myoclonic s. Seizure characterized by jerky muscular contractions.

partial s., focal s. Seizure arising in an area of one cerebral hemisphere; may be: *Simple partial s.,* in which consciousness is preserved; or *Complex partial s.,* with impairment or cloudiness of consciousness.

tonic s. Seizure characterized by muscle contractions.

selectin (sĕ-lek´tin) Glycoproteins on the surface of lymphocytes or endothelial cells; some are implicated in the adhesion of white blood cells to the inner lining of blood vessels.

selection (sĕ-lek´shun) In population genetics, the biologic process through which some individuals survive while others do not, with the result that the frequency of particular genes in the population is altered.

artificial s. The purposeful interference by man with natural selection to produce organisms with a desired trait; e.g., breeding of specific strains of cows for the abundant production of milk.

natural s. The biologic process that causes survival and reproduction of those organisms best adjusted to the conditions under which they live.

sexual s. A form of natural selection through which male and female members of a species are attracted by certain traits, thus ensuring the passing of those traits to subsequent generations.

selectivity (sĕ-lek-tiv´ĭ-te) In pharmacology, a comparative measure of the tendency of one drug to produce several effects; the relationship between the desired and undesired effects of a drug. COMPARE: potency (2).

selenium (sĕ-lĕ´ne-um) An element; symbol Se, atomic number 34, atomic weight 78.96; it resembles sulfur.

self (self) **1.** The totality of a person's body and mental processes. **2.** A person's awareness of his own being. **3.** In immunology, applied to cell components (antigens) that are normal constituents of the body of an individual and against which immunologic responses are suppressed.

self-accusation (self-ak-yoo-za´shun) Condemning oneself to misery, often because of some trivial error; a psychiatric symptom seen frequently in the depressive phase of manic-depressive psychosis.

self-commitment (self-ko-mit´ment) Voluntary confinement to a mental hospital.

self-digestion (self-di-jest´yun) See autodigestion.

self-hypnosis (self-hip-no´sis) See autohypnosis.

self-infection (self-in-fek´shun) See autoinfection.

self-limited (self-lim´it-ed) Denoting a disease that runs a definite course in a specific time, limited by its own characteristics rather than external factors.

self-poisoning (self-poi´zŏn-ing) **1.** The intentional or accidental taking of a substance that causes illness or death, especially by chemical means. **2.** See autointoxication.

sella turcica (se´lă tur´sĭ-kă) A depression with two prominences (anterior and posterior) on the upper surface of the spheroid bone at the base of the skull, resembling a Turkish saddle and housing the pituitary gland.

semeiography (se-mi-og´ră-fe) See semiography.

semeiology (se-mi-ol´ŏ-je) See symptomatology (2).

semelincident (sem-el-in´sĭ-dent) Occurring only once; said of certain diseases.

semen (se´men) A viscous whitish secretion of the male reproductive organs; composed chiefly of sperm, fructose-rich secretions from the seminal vesicles, and secretion from the prostate gland (sperm usually comprises about 10% of the semen). Also called seminal fluid.

semenuria (se-mĕ-nu´re-ă) The discharge of seminal fluid with the passage of urine. Also called seminuria; spermaturia.

semicoma (sem-e-ko´mă) A state of impaired responses to stimuli which is not profound and from which a person can be aroused.

semicomatose (sem-e-ko´mă-tōs) In a state of unconsciousness or stupor from which one can be aroused.

semiconscious (sem-e-kon´shus) Partly conscious.

semiflexion (sem-e-flek´shun) The position of an extremity midway between extension and flexion.

semilunar (sem-e-lu´nar) Shaped like a half-moon.

semimembranous (sem-e-mem´bră-nus) Consisting partly of membrane or fascia.

seminal (sem´ĭ-nal) Relating to the semen.

semination (sem-ĭ-na´shun) See insemination.

seminiferous (se-mĭ-nif´er-us) Conveying semen.

seminoma (se-mĭ-no´mă) A malignant testicular neoplasm made up of large cells resembling spermatogonia; it usually metastasizes to paraortic lymph nodes.

ovarian s. See dysgerminoma.

seminormal (sem-e-nor´mal) (0.5N, N/2) Denoting a solution containing one-half the standard (normal) strength.

seminuria (se-mĭ-nu´re-ă) See semenuria.

semiography (se-me-og´ră-fe) A description of the symptoms of a disease. Also written semeiography.

semiology (se-me-ol´o-je) See symptomatology (2).

semipenniform (sem-e-pen´ĭ-form) Shaped like a feather on only one side; said of certain muscles.

semipermeable (sem-e-per´me-ă-bl) Relating to a membrane that allows some molecules in a solution to pass through but not others.

semiprone (sem-e-prōn) About three-quarters prone, between the midposition and pronation.

semis (se´mis) (ss, s) Latin for one half, in prescriptions, it follows the sign indicating the measure.

semisulcus (sem-e-sul´kus) A slight groove on the edge of a structure which, when united with a similar groove of an adjoining structure, forms a complete sulcus.

semisupination (sem-e-su-pĭ-na´shun) A position midway between supination and pronation.

semisupine (sem-e-su´pīn) Lying in semisupination.

semisynthetic (sem-e-sin-thet´ik) Made from chemical reactions in which a naturally occurring substance was used as a starting material.

semitendinous (sem-e-ten´dĭ-nus) Partly tendinous, applied to certain muscles.

Senear-Usher syndrome (se-nēr´ush´ĕr sin´drōm) See pemphigus erythematosus, under pemphigus.

senescence (se-nes´ens) The process of aging or growing old.

senescent (se-nes´ent) Aging; growing old.

senile (se´nīl) **1.** Characteristic of or resulting from old age. **2.** Exhibiting mental deterioration with old age.

senility (sĕ-nil´ĭ-te) **1.** The condition of being senile. **2.** The physical and mental changes associated with old age.

senna (sen´ă) Preparation made from the dried leaves of the plants *Cassia acutifolia* or *Cassia angustifolia*; a laxative.

senopia (se-no´pe-ă) See second sight, under sight.

sensate (sen´sāt) **1.** To perceive through a sense, especially the sense of touch. **2.** One who is so able; referring to a patient who regains sensation after partial paralysis.

sensation (sen-sa´shun) The conscious perception of a stimulus acting on any of the organs of sense.

sense (sens) **1.** The power of perceiving any stimulus. **2.** Any of the special functions of sight, hearing, touch, taste, or smell.

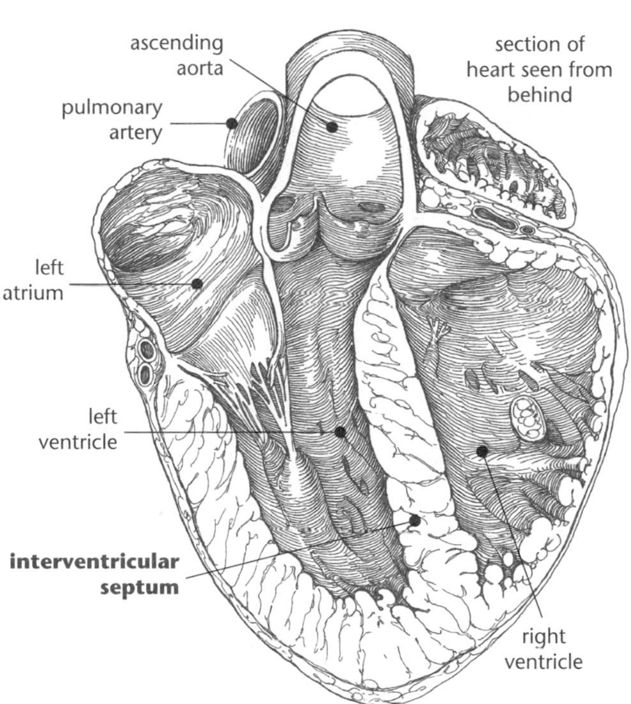

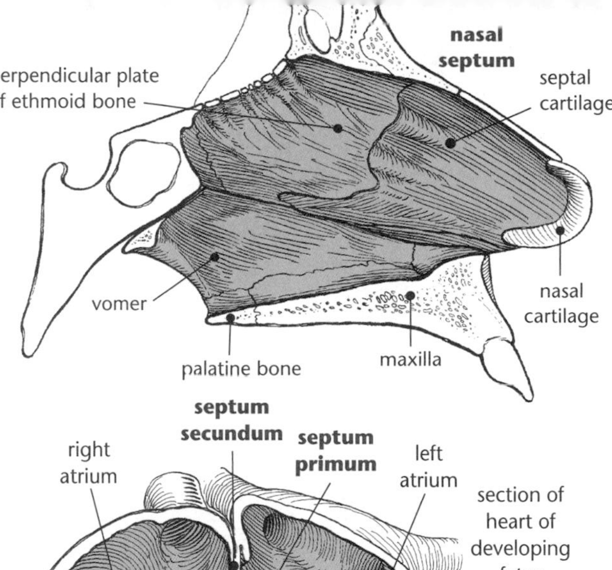

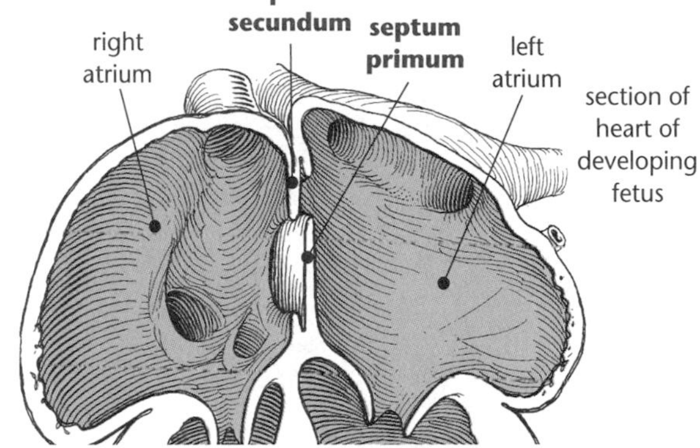

sensibility (sen-sĭ-bil´ĭ-te) The capability of perceiving sensations.

sensible (sen´sĭ-bl) **1.** Perceptible by the senses. **2.** Able to feel.

sensimeter (sen-sim´ĕ-ter) An instrument for measuring degrees of cutaneous sensation, as in anesthetized areas.

sensitive (sen´sĭ-tiv) **1.** A state of increased capacity to respond specifically to an antigen or hapten. **2.** Responsive to external stimulation. **3.** Easily irritated or altered by the action of some agents. **4.** Susceptible (e.g., to the action of an antibiotic).

sensitivity (sen-sĭ-tĭ-vĭ-te) **1.** The state of being sensitive; often implying a keen perception of, or responsiveness to, a stimulus. **2.** Applied to a screening test: the proportion of persons who truly have a disease in a screened population, and who are identified as such by the screening test.

disk s. A measurement of the susceptibility of a bacterial species to a variety of antibiotics placed on the culture medium in the form of disks; the sensitivity is measured by the area of inhibition of growth produced by the antibiotic disk.

sensitization (sen-sĭ-tĭ-za´shun) The process of increasing the reactivity of a subject, usually to specific antibodies or immune cells.

sensitize (sen´sĭ-tīz) To render sensitive; to increase the specific reactivity of a subject to an agent.

sensorimotor (sen-so-re-mo´tor) Both sensory and motor; said of certain nerves.

sensorium (sen-sor´e-um) **1.** A sense organ. **2.** In psychiatry, the state of mental clarity and consciousness at a given time.

sensory (sen´sŏ-re) Relating to sensation; said of a nerve.

sentiment (sen´tĭ-ment) An attitude, thought, or judgment based on feeling instead of reason.

sentinel loop sign (sen-tĭ-nel loop sīn) In radiology, a dilated segment of intestine, indicative of a nearby inflammatory obstruction.

separator (sep´ă-ra-tor) **1.** Instrument used to separate two teeth, so as to gain access to adjacent surfaces. **2.** A substance applied to a surface to prevent other material from adhering to that surface.

Sephadex (sef´ă deks) Proprietary name for gel particles composed of cross-linked dextrans; used as molecular sieves in gel filtration.

sepsis (sep´sis) The systemic response to infection, characterized by (but not limited to) two or more of the following features: elevation of body temperature, heart rate, respiratory rate, and white blood cell count.

septa (sep´tă) Plural of septum.

septal (sep´tal) Relating to a septum.

septate (sep´tāt) Divided into compartments by a septum.

septation (sep-ta´shun) The formation of thin dividing walls or septa.

septectomy (sep-tek´tŏ-me) Surgical removal of part of the nasal septum.

septic (sep´tik) Relating to sepsis.

septicemia (sep-tĭ-se´me-ă) Generalized infection caused by microorganisms or their toxins and spread throughout the body via the bloodstream. Also called hematosepsis; popularly called blood poisoning.

septicemic (sep-tĭ-se´mik) Relating to septicemia.

septivalent (sep-tĭ-va´lent) Having a valency of seven.

septomarginal (sep-to-mar´jĭ-nal) Relating to the margin of a partition or septum.

septonasal (sep-to-na´zal) Relating to the nasal septum.

septoplasty (sep-to-plas´te) Reparative operation on a septum.

septotome (sep´to-tōm) An instrument for incising the nasal septum.

septotomy (sep-tot´ŏ-me) Surgical incision of a septum.

septulum (sep´tu-lum), *pl.* **sep´tula** Latin for a minute partition or septum.

septum (sep´tum), *pl.* **sep´ta** A thin wall dividing two bodily cavities or masses of soft tissue.

atrial s. See interatrial septum.

interalveolar s. One of the bony partitions between the tooth sockets.

interatrial s. The partition between the atria of the heart. Also called atrial septum.

interventricular s. The musculomembranous wall dividing the ventricles of the heart. Also called ventricular septum.

s. ludicum See septum pellucidum.

nasal s. The thin wall dividing the nasal cavities composed posteriorly of bone and anteriorly of cartilage.

s. pellucidum A thin triangular partition between the anterior portions of the lateral ventricles of the brain; it is composed of two laminae and is attached to the undersurface and reflected portion of the corpus callosum and to the fornix. Also called septum lucidum.

placental septa Incomplete partitions dividing the maternal surface of the placenta into 15 to 20 compartments (cotyledons).

s. primum In embryology, the sickle-shaped partition that initiates the division of the single atrial cavity of the embryonic heart into right and left chambers.

rectovesical s. The thin layer of fascia in the male separating the prostate and bladder from the anterior wall of the rectum.

rectovaginal s. The thin layer of fascia separating the vagina from the anterior wall of the rectum.

s. of scrotum The layer of fascia dividing the scrotum into two completely separate sacs, each containing a testis.

s. secundum The sickle-shaped partition appearing on the roof of the right atrium of the embryonic heart, adjacent to the septum primum; it remains open (forming the foramen ovale) until after birth, when pulmonary respiration begins.

sequel, sequela (se´kwĕl, se-kwe´lă), *pl.* **se´quels, seque´lae** Any abnormal condition following and caused by another disease.

sequence (se´kwens) **1.** A group of related elements. **2.** Order in which one event follows another.

coding s. See exon.

dysmorphic s. A "cascading" pattern of multiple secondary fetal anomalies caused by a single event. Distinguished from syndrome, in which the anomalies occur independently rather than sequentially, although originating from a single cause.

intervening s. See intron.

sequester (se-kwes´ter) **1.** To undergo sequestration. **2.** To detach, separate, or isolate.

sequestration (se-kwes-tra´shun) **1.** The formation of a sequestrum. **2.** The isolation of a person with a contagious disease. **3.** An increase in the quantity of blood within the blood vessels, occurring physiologically or produced artificially.

bronchopulmonary s. Congenital anomaly marked by the presence of an independent mass of lung tissue having its own bronchial branch and artery (a branch from the thoracic aorta).

sequestrectomy (se-kwes-trek´tŏ-me) The surgical removal of a dead bone fragment that has become separated from the surrounding healthy bone.

sequestrum (se-kwes´trum) A piece of dead tissue, especially bone that has become separated from, or is abnormally attached to, the surrounding healthy tissue.

sera (se´ră) Plural of serum.

series (sēr´ēz) A group of related events, objects, or compounds, arranged systematically.

aromatic s. Compounds derived from benzene.

erythrocytic s. The group of cells in various stages of development that ultimately form red blood cells.

fatty s. The series of saturated open-chain hydrocarbons, denoted by the suffix *-ane* (methane, ethane, propane, etc.). Also called methane series; paraffin series.

granulocytic s. The cells in various stages of development, culminating in the formation of granulocytes.

homologous s. A succession of organic

S

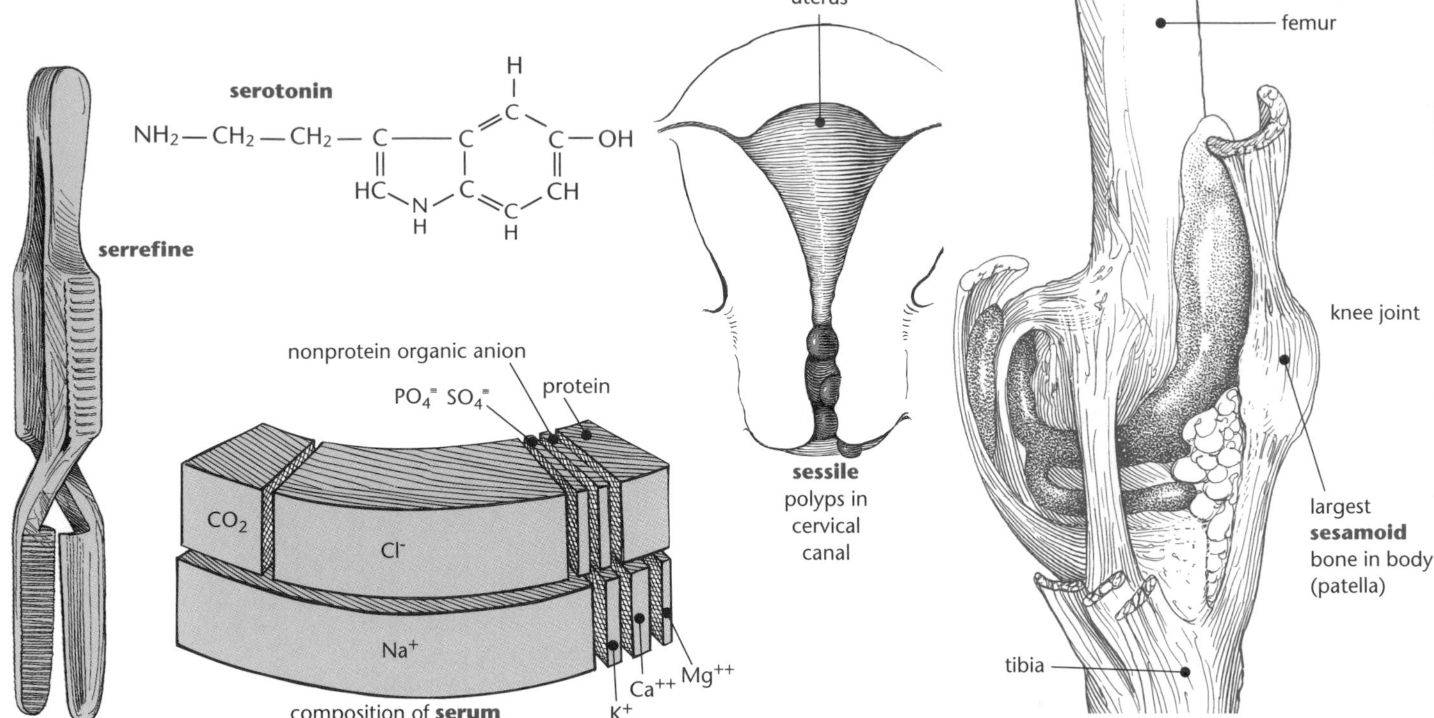

compounds, each one differing from the preceding one by a radical or atomic group such as CH_2.

lymphocytic s. Cells in different stages of development leading to the formation of mature lymphocytes.

methane s. See fatty series.

paraffin s. See fatty series.

small bowel s. A series of radiographic images of the small intestine obtained after oral administration of a contrast medium.

serine (sĕr´ēn) (Ser) A nonessential amino acid; one of the hydrolysis products of proteins.

seriograph (se´re-o-graf) Instrument for taking a series of six to eight radiographic exposures; used in radiography of the cerebral blood vessels.

seriscission (ser-ĭ-sizh´un) Division of soft tissue, such as the pedicle of a tumor, by a silk ligature.

seroconversion (sēr-o-kon-ver´zhun) A change in immunologic reactivity of the serum from negative to positive for a particular antibody; most commonly refers to one of the serologic tests for syphilis.

serocystic (sēr-o-sis´tik) Composed of, or relating to, serum-filled cysts.

serodiagnosis (sēr-o-di-ăg-no´sis) Diagnosis by means of reactions tested in the bloodstream.

seroenteritis (sēr-o-en-tĕ-ri´tis) Inflammation of the serous or peritoneal coat of the intestine.

serofibrinous (sēr-o-fi´brin-us) Containing serum and fibrin; said of a discharge or exudate.

serofibrous (sēr-o-fi´brus) Relating to both a serous membrane and a fibrous tissue.

seroimmunity (sēr-o-ĭ-mu´nĭ-te) See passive immunity, under immunity.

serologic (sēr-o-loj´ik) Relating to serology.

serology (sēr-ol´ŏ-je) The study of serum, especially with respect to immunity.

seroma (sēr-o´mă) A tumorlike mass formed by the collection of serum in the tissues, usually in a wound site.

seromembranous (sēr-o-mem´bră-nus) Relating to a serous membrane.

seromucous (sēr-o-mu´kus) Composed of serum and mucus.

seronegative (sēr-o-neg´ă-tiv) Lacking antibodies or any other specific immunologic marker for the microorganism of concern.

seropositive (sēr-o-poz´ĭ-tiv) Containing antibodies or any other specific immunologic marker for the microorganism under consideration, indicating a previous exposure or an ongoing infection.

seropurulent (sēr-o-pu´roo-lent) Containing serum and pus; said of a discharge.

seropus (sēr´o-pus) Serum mixed with pus.

serosa (sēr-o´sa) See serous membrane, under membrane.

serosanguinous (sēr-o-sang-gwin´us) Containing serum and blood; said of an exudate or discharge.

seroserous (sēr-o-sēr´us) Relating to two or more serous membranes.

serositis (sēr-o-si´tis) Inflammation of a serous membrane.

adhesive s. Serositis causing mobile organs to stick together.

multiple s. See polyserositis.

serosynovitis (sēr-o-sin-o-vi´tis) Inflammation of the synovial membrane of a joint with effusion of serum.

serotonin (ser-o-to´nin) 5-Hydroxytryptamine; $C_{10}H_{12}N_2O$; a substance occurring predominantly in the gastrointestinal mucosa, in small amounts in blood platelets, and in the brain; also found in carcinoid tumors; it stimulates smooth muscle contraction, constricts blood vessels, and inhibits stomach secretions.

serotype (sēr´o-tīp) See serovar.

serous (sēr´us) Relating to, resembling, secreting, or containing serum.

serovaccination (sēr-o-vak-sĭ-na´shun) Combination of injection of serum to produce passive immunity and vaccination to produce active immunity.

serovar (se´ro-var) A taxonomic subdivision of bacteria based on the antigenic characteristics of the microorganisms. Also called serotype; subtype.

serpiginous (ser-pij´ĭ-nus) Creeping; denoting an ulcer or skin lesion that heals at one margin while spreading on the opposite side.

serpigo (ser-pi´go) **1.** Ringworm. **2.** Herpes. **3.** Any creeping eruption.

serrate, serrated (ser´āt, sĕ-rā´tid) Notched.

Serratia (sĕ-ra´she-ă) Genus of motile gram-negative, rod-shaped bacteria (family Enterobacteriaceae) that thrive in decaying organic matter and produce a characteristic red pigment.

S. marcescens Species found in soil, water, and food; occasionally found in pathologic specimens in which the red pigment produced suggests erroneously the presence of blood (e.g., in sputum); a cause of hospital acquired infection, especially in patients with impaired immunity.

serration (sĕ-rā´shun) **1.** The state of having a sawlike edge. **2.** A series of toothlike projections.

serrefine (sār-fēn´) A fine clamp; a small surgical spring forceps, usually used for clamping blood vessels.

serrulate, serrulated (ser´u-lāt, ser-u-lā´ted) Having fine notches.

serum (se´rum), *pl.* **serums, sera** **1.** The clear fluid moistening serous membranes. **2.** Loosely used term denoting serum that contains antitoxins, used for therapeutic or laboratory diagnostic purposes. **3.** Blood serum.

anticomplementary s. A serum that destroys complement.

antilymphocyte s. (ALS) A serum used to inhibit rejection of grafts or organ transplants.

antitoxic s. Serum containing antibodies to the toxins of a disease-causing microorganism.

blood s. The clear, fluid portion of blood that is left after fibrinogen (a protein) and the cellular elements of blood are removed by coagulation; distinguished from plasma, which is the cell-free liquid portion of uncoagulated blood.

convalescent s. Blood serum from a person recovering from an infectious disease.

polyvalent s. A serum containing antibodies against more than one strain of a microorganism.

truth s. A name for certain chemicals (sodium amobarbital and sodium thiopental) administered intravenously to facilitate questioning of an individual who is unwilling or unable to answer queries; a misnomer since the subject's revelations elicited under the influence of the drug are not necessarily factually true.

servomechanism (ser-vo-mek´ă-niz-m) **1.** An automatic control device used to maintain the operation of a mechanical system. **2.** A self-regulatory biologic process.

sesamoid (ses´ă-moid) Resembling a grain of sesame seed; denoting a small bone that is embedded in a tendon or in a joint capsule; it is found mainly within tendons of the extremities; the patella (kneecap) is the largest such bone in the body.

sessile (ses´il) Attached by a broad base rather than by a peduncle; applied to certain polyps.

set (set) **1.** To put into a position that will restore function; said of a fractured bone. **2.** Denoting plastic material after it has hardened or jelled.

seta (se´tă) A short bristle-like hair or structure.

setaceous (se-ta´shus) **1.** Having bristles or setae. **2.** Resembling a bristle.

setting (set´ing) Hardening, as of plaster of Paris.

setup (set´up) The arrangement of artificial teeth on a trial denture base, preliminary to construction of an appliance.

sex (seks) The classification of organisms as male or female according to their reproductive characteristics.

chromosomal s. An individual's sex determined by the presence or absence of the Y chromosome in the spermatozoon at the time of its union with the ovum.

genetic s. Chromosomal sex.

morphologic s. Sex determined by the morphology of the external genitalia.

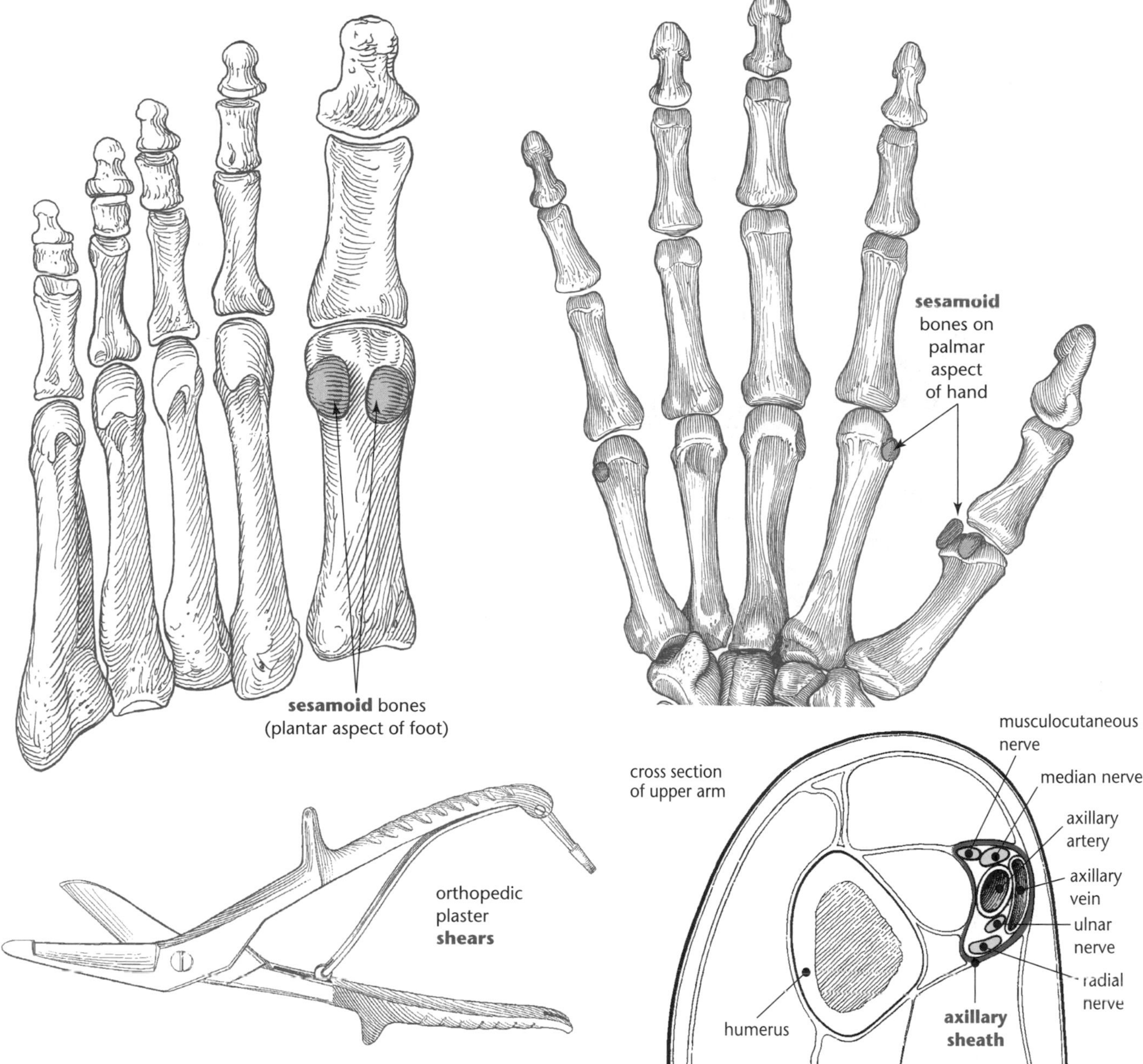

safe s. The use of condoms for sexual intercourse to reduce the spread of sexually transmitted diseases (STDs).

sex-influenced (seks-in´floo-ĕnst) Occurring predominantly in one sex, either male or female.

sexivalent (sek-siv´ă-lent) Having the combining power of six hydrogen atoms.

sex-limited (seks lim´it-ed) Occuring in one sex only, either male or female.

sex linkage (seks´lingk´ij) See under linkage.

sex-linked (seks´ linkt) See X-linked; Y-linked.

sexology (seks-ol´o-je) The study of the sexes and their relationship.

sextan (seks´tan) Denoting a malarial paroxysm recurring every sixth day.

sexual (sek´shoo-ăl) **1.** Relating to sex. **2.** Causing erotic desires.

sexuality (sek-shoo-al´ĭ-te) The state of having sexual characteristics, experiences, and behaviors.

infantile s. In psychoanalysis, the capacity of the infant and child to have experiences of a sexual nature.

Sézary syndrome (sa´ză-re sin´drōm) Erythroderma associated with infiltration of the skin by atypical cells, believed to be of T lymphocyte origin, which spill into the blood.

shadow-casting (shad´o kast´ing) A method of increasing the visibility of ultramicroscopic specimens under the microscope by coating them with a film of carbon, platinum, or chromium.

shaft (shaft) The rodlike portion of a structure, such as that of a long bone.

shakes (shāks) **1.** Colloquial term for severe chills, especially those of malarial fever. **2.** A popular name for the tremor associated with withdrawal from acute alcoholism.

shank (shangk) The anterior part of the human leg, from the knee to the ankle.

shears (shērz) Large double-bladed cutting instrument, similar to a pair of scissors.

sheath (shēth) An enveloping structure.

axillary s. A tubular, fibrous membrane encasing the large vessels and nerves of the arm (axillary artery and vein and brachial plexus); located between the clavicle (collarbone) and the first rib.

carotid s. A tubular sheath enclosing the carotid artery, internal jugular vein, and vagus nerve; extends from the base of the skull to the first rib and sternum (breastbone).

A taxonomic subdivision of bacteria based on the antigenic characteristics of the microorganisms.

crural s. See femoral sheath.

femoral s. A funnel shaped sheath located in the groin below the inguinal ligament and divided into three compartments by two vertical partitions; the lateral compartment contains the femoral artery, the middle one contains the femoral vein, and the medial one (femoral canal) contains lymphatic vessels and a lymph node. Also called crural sheath.

myelin s. The multiple-layered covering of many of the axons of both central and peripheral nerves; composed of lipid and protein molecules, and serving mainly to increase the velocity of conduction of nerve impulses.

s.'s of optic nerve The three sheaths (dura, arachnoid, and pia) surrounding the optic nerve; continuous with the membranes of the brain.

s. of Schwann See neurilemma.

synovial tendon s. A double-layered sheath forming a closed sac; one layer surrounds the tunnel through which the tendon passes, the other covers the surface of the tendon; serves to facilitate the gliding of tendons through fibrous and bony tunnels.

Sheehan's disease (she´anz dĭ-zēz´) Hypopituitarism due to postpartum pituitary necrosis, usually following hemorrhage and shock during delivery; results in failure to lactate, absence of menstrual function, loss of hair, cold intolerance, atrophy of sex organs, and wrinkling of the skin; a specific form of panhypopituitarism.

shelf (shelf) A structure in the body resembling a shelf.

Blumer's s. See rectal shelf.

rectal s. A shelf occurring in the rectum due to infiltration by neoplasm or inflammation. Also called Blumer's shelf.

shield (shēld) **1.** A means of protection, such as a lead rubber apron or sheet used to protect an individual from radiation. **2.** A dense substance enclosing radioisotopes to reduce the amount of radiation that escapes into the area. **3.** To protect from radiation or other toxic agents.

breast s. A rubber cap or dome, used to protect

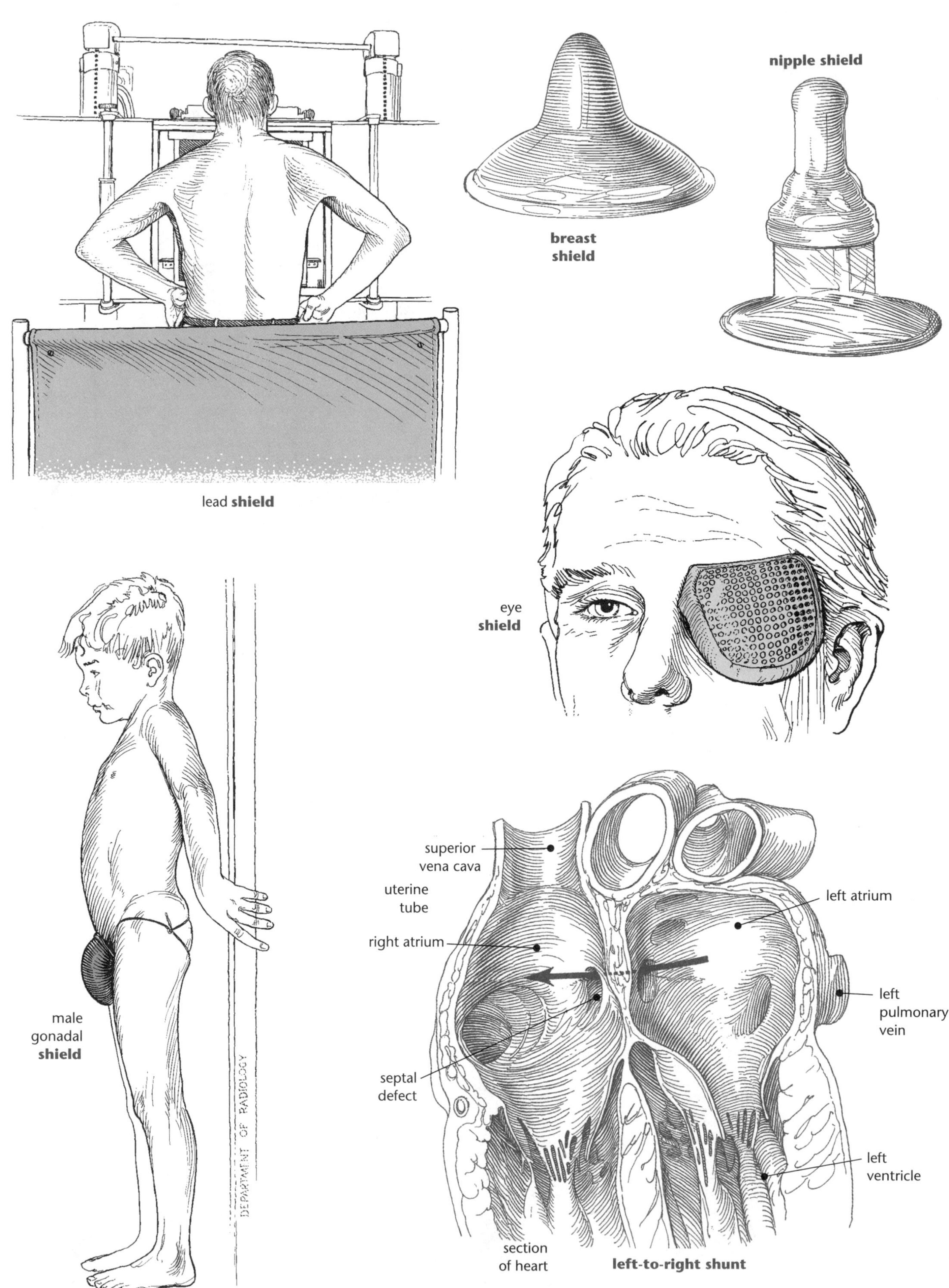

lead **shield**

breast shield

nipple shield

eye **shield**

male gonadal **shield**

left-to-right shunt

S

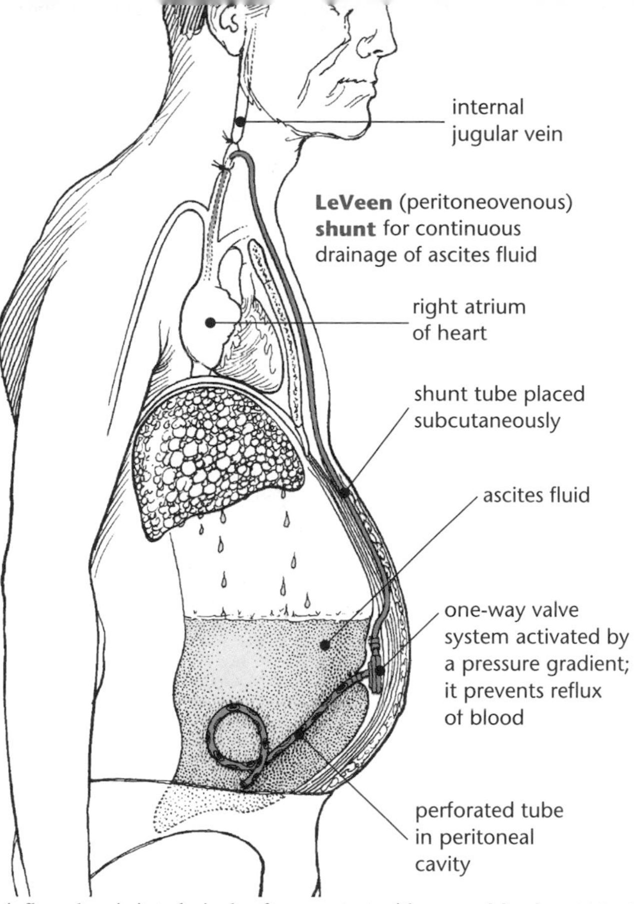

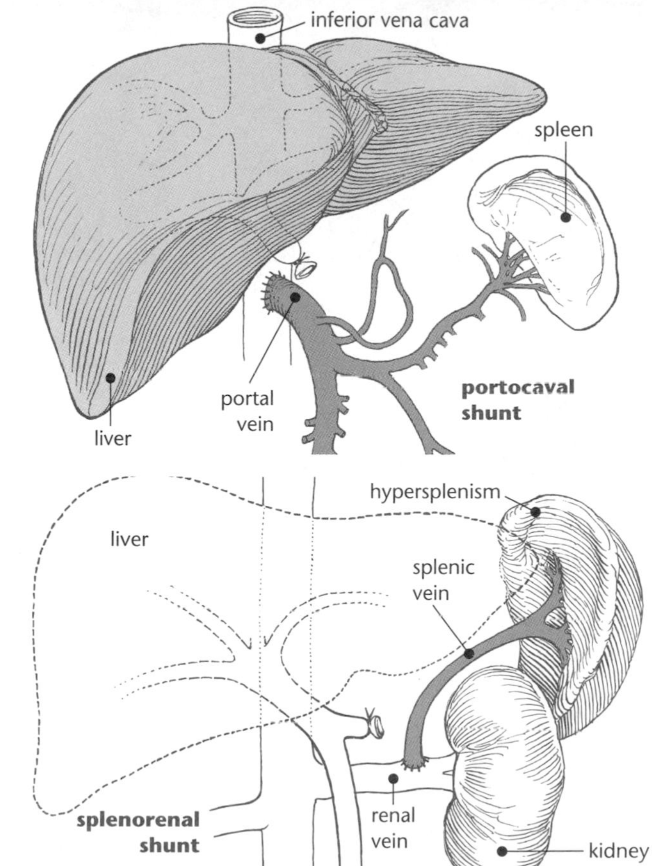

inflamed or irritated nipples from contact with clothing.

Buller's s. A watchglass in a frame of adhesive tape secured over the unaffected eye to protect it from the infected eye.

embryonic s. A swelling of the embryonic blastoderm within which the primitive streak appears.

eye s. A protective covering for the eye.

nipple s. A round glass or plastic plate with a short central projecting tube to which a rubber nipple is attached; used over sore nipples during nursing so that the pressure from the infant's mouth is attenuated by the resistance of the rubber nipple.

shift (shift) A change.

axis s. See axis deviation, under deviation.

Doppler s. The magnitude of the frequency change with the velocity of motion in the Doppler effect.

s. to the left Increased percentage of young neutrophils in the blood.

s. to the right Decreased percentage of young neutrophils in the blood.

threshold s. A deviation in decibels from an individual's previous audiogram, indicating loss of hearing.

Shigella (shĭ-gel´ă) A genus of nonmotile, gram-negative bacteria (family Enterobacteriaceae) that is the principal cause of human dysentery; divided into four major groups (A, B, C, and D) and subdivided serologically into different types.

S. dysenteriae Group A species, a particularly virulent form that causes dysentery in man; found in the excreta of infected individuals or convalescent carriers.

S. flexneri Group B species, one of the most common causes of dysentery epidemics and sometimes of infantile gastroenteritis.

S. sonnei Group D species, a cause of mild dysentery and summer diarrheal disorders in children.

shigellosis (shĭ gel-o´sis) Acute infection of the bowel with *Shigella* organisms, often occurring in epidemic patterns; characterized by frequent passage of stools containing blood, pus, and mucus and accompanied by cramps, tenesmus, and fever.

shim (shim) In magnetic resonance imaging (MRI), minute adjustments of the magnetic field made to improve uniformity.

shin (shin) The anterior portion of the leg below the knee.

shinbone (shin´bōn) See tibia.

shingles (shing´gilz) See herpes zoster, under herpes.

shin splints (shin splints) Irritation or inflammation of the extensor muscles of the lower lateral area of the legs caused by an unusually great adduction of the legs and aggravated by overexercise.

shistocyte (shis´to-sīt) An irregular, contracted, somewhat triangular erythrocyte; seen in microangiopathic anemia.

shiver (shiv´er) To shudder or shake, especially from a chill produced by fever-induced decreased skin temperature.

shock (shok) A severe physiologic reaction to bodily trauma characterized by pale clammy skin, diminished blood pressure, weak rapid pulse, and sometimes unconsciousness.

anaphylactic s. A severe, often fatal, reaction occurring upon a second exposure to an antigen against which the body has previously formed antibodies.

anaphylactoid s. Shock that resembles anaphylactic shock but is unrelated to antigen-antibody reactions.

cardiogenic s. Shock due to the sudden reduction of the cardiac output, as in myocardial infarction.

counter s. See countershock.

deferred s., delayed s. Shock occurring a number of hours after the injury.

electric s. The effects of the passage of an electric current through any part of the body.

endotoxin s., endotoxic s. Septic shock caused by toxins produced and released by bacteria.

histamine s. Shock produced by the injection of histamine.

hypovolemic s. Shock produced by reduction of blood volume, as in hemorrhage.

insulin s. Shock resulting from a sudden reduction of blood sugar caused by an overdose of insulin.

irreversible s. Shock that does not respond to any form of treatment.

neurogenic s. Shock due to the action of the nervous system immediately after injury.

primary s. Shock directly related to, and appearing immediately after, a severe injury, mainly due to anxiety or pain.

septic s. Shock due to severe infection, particularly with gram-negative bacilli.

spinal s. Loss of spinal reflexes after injury to the spinal cord, manifested in the muscles innervated by the nerves situated below the injury.

shoe (shoo) An outer covering for the human foot.

Scarpa's s. A metal brace that prevents plantar extension of the foot beyond a right angle; used in treating talipes equinus.

short bowel syndrome (short bow´el sin´drōm) Condition that occurs following removal of an extensive segment of small intestine, characterized by intractable diarrhea with impaired absorption of fats and other nutrients.

shortsightedness (short-sīt´ed-nes) See myopia.

shoulder (shōl´der) The region where arm and trunk meet.

shoulder blade (shōl´der blād) See scapula.

shoulder-hand syndrome (shōl´der-hand sin´drōm) See reflex sympathetic dystrophy, under dystrophy.

show (sho) The discharge from the vagina of bloodstained mucus indicating the onset of labor; it is caused by the expulsion of the mucus plug that has filled the cervical canal during pregnancy.

shunt (shunt) **1.** To bypass or divert. **2.** A passage between two natural channels; may be congenital, as a defect between the two atria of the heart, or a surgical anastomosis to divert blood from one part of the body to another or to divert intestinal contents from one portion of the intestinal tract to another.

arteriovenous s. A synthetic external or subcutaneous tube inserted into a vein and an artery, bypassing the capillary network, to provide repeated vascular access in renal dialysis or in chemotherapy; vessels most commonly used are the radial artery and cephalic vein in the forearm.

left-to-right s. Diversion of blood from the left to the right side of the heart (through a septal defect) or from the systemic to the pulmonary circulation (through a patent ductus arteriosus).

LeVeen s. (peritoneovenous) A device for restoring ascitic fluid to the circulation; plastic tubing, equipped with a valve, is inserted into the peritoneal cavity, tunneled under the skin and connected to a large vein in the neck. The Denver variation of the LeVeen shunt has a valved chamber that is manually compressible.

metabolic s. Catabolism of a substance by an alternate pathway.

monophosphate s. See pentose phosphate pathway, under pathway.

pentose s. See pentose phosphate pathway, under pathway.

portacaval s. Any communication between the

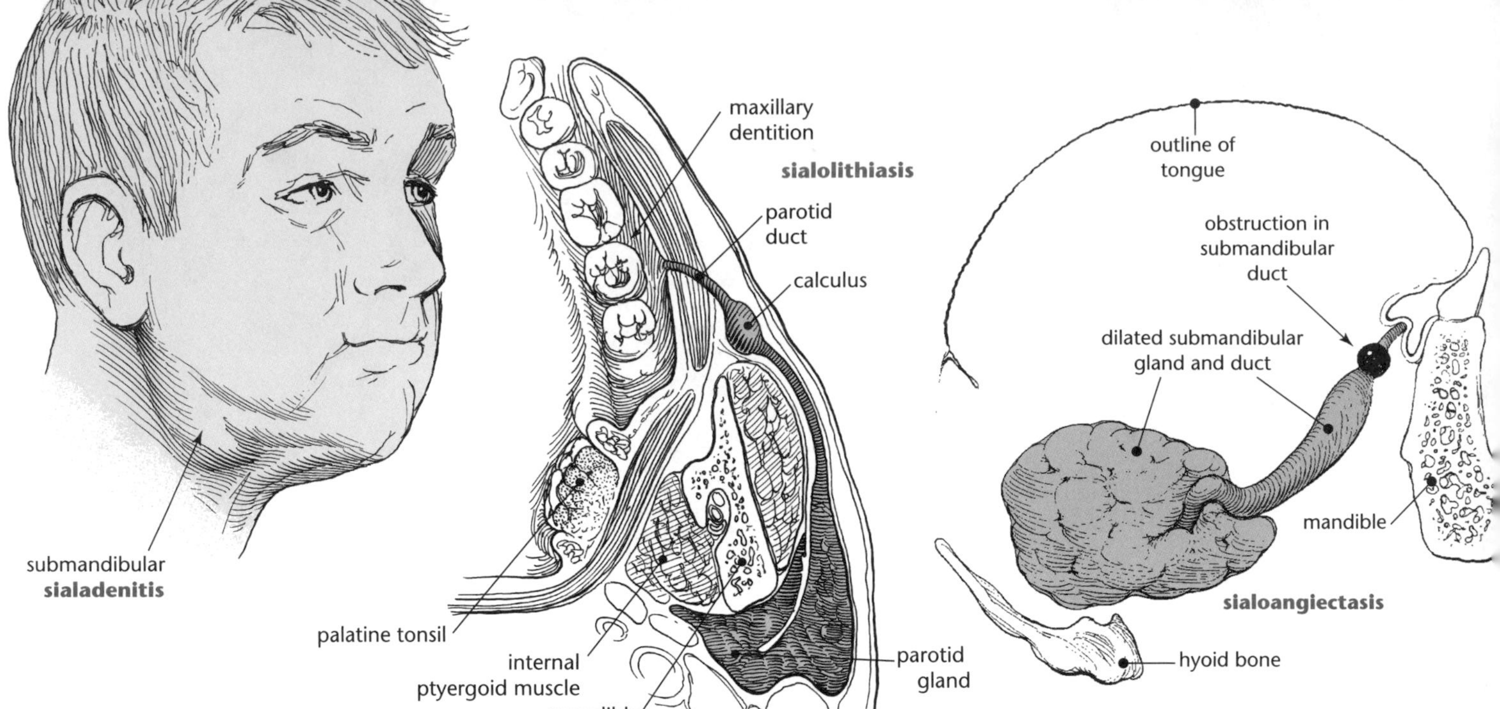

portal vein and the systemic veins; surgical anastomosis between the portal and caval veins.

portasystemic s. Any surgical communication established between the portal vein or its tributaries and those of the inferior vena cava.

reversed s. See right-to-left shunt.

right-to-left s. The passage of unoxygenated venous blood from the right heart into the arterial circulation without passing through the lungs. Also called reversed shunt.

splenorenal s. Surgical anastomosis between the splenic vein and the left renal vein.

Shy-Drager syndrome (shi-dra´ger sin´drōm) A rare condition, resembling parkinsonism, characterized by tremors, muscular wasting, atrophy of the iris, ocular palsies, and orthostatic hypotension.

sialaden (si-al´ă-den) A salivary gland.

sialadenitis (si-al-ad-ĕ-ni´tis) Inflammation of a salivary gland.

sialadenotropic (si-al-ad-ĕ-no-trop´ik) Influencing the activity of salivary glands.

sialagogue (si-al´ă-gog) Any agent that stimulates saliva secretion.

sialaporia (si-al-ă-po´re-ă) Deficient secretion of saliva.

sialectasis (si-al-ek-ta´sis) Dilatation of a salivary duct.

sialic (si-al´ik) Salivary.

S

sialic acids (si-al´ik as´ids) A group of naturally occurring derivatives of a 9-carbon, 3-deoxy-5-amino sugar acid; present in bacteria and in animal tissue as constituents of lipids, polysaccharides, and mucoproteins.

sialism, sialismus (si´al-iz-m, si´al-iz´mus) Excessive flow of saliva for any reason, including teething, mental retardation, ill-fitting dental appliances, mercurialism, periodontic disease, and acute inflammation of the mouth. Also called sialorrhea; sialosis.

sialoadenectomy (si-ă-lo-ad-ĕ-nek´tŏ-me) Surgical removal of a salivary gland.

sialoadenitis (si-ă-lo-ad-ĕ-ni´tis) See sialadenitis.

sialoadenotomy (si-ă-lo-ad-ĕ-not´ŏ-me) Incision of a salivary gland.

sialoangiectasis (si-ă-lo-an-je-ek´tă-sis) **1.** Condition in which a salivary duct is vastly dilated by stagnated saliva, usually resulting from an obstructive stone or ductal constriction. **2.** Dilatation of salivary ducts, usually by means of bougies.

sialoangiitis (si-ă-lo-an-je-i´tis) Inflammation of a salivary duct.

sialodochitis (si-ă-lo-do-ki´tis) Inflammation of the duct of a salivary gland.

sialodochoplasty (si-ă-lo-do´ko-plas-te) Repair of a salivary duct.

sialogenous (si-ă-loj´ĕ-nus) Producing saliva.

sialogogue (si-al´o-gog) See sialagogue.

sialogram (si-al´o-gram) An x-ray picture of a salivary gland and its ducts, produced by sialography. Also called sialograph.

sialograph (si-al´o-graf) See sialogram.

sialography (si-ă-log´ră-fe) The process of making x-ray pictures of the salivary glands and ducts after the injection of radiopaque material into the ducts; an invaluable technique for determining the presence and location of an obstruction in the ducts and the condition of the salivary acini.

sialolith (si-al´o-lith) A salivary calculus. Also called ptyalolith.

sialolithiasis (si-ă-lo-lĭ-thi´ă-sis) Presence of a calculus in the salivary gland or duct. Also called ptyalolithiasis.

sialolithotomy (si-ă-lo-lĭ-thot´ŏ-me) Surgical incision of a salivary duct or gland for the removal of a calculus. Also called ptyalolithotomy.

sialorrhea (si-ă-lo-re´ă) See sialism.

sialoschesis (si-ă-los´kĕ-sis) Suppression of the secretion of saliva.

sialosis (si-ă-lo´sis) See sialism.

sialostenosis (si-ă-lo-stĕ-no´sis) Stricture or stenosis of a salivary duct.

sib, sibling (sib, sib´ling) One of two or more children having one, but especially both, parents in common.

sibilant (sib´ĭ-lant) Hissing or whistling; said of a rale.

sibilus (sib´ĭ-lus) A hissing or whistling sound heard on auscultation.

sibship (sib´ship) A group of children of the same parents; occasionally used to denote all blood relatives.

sicca syndrome (sik´ă sin´drōm) See Sjögren's syndrome.

siccant (sik´ănt) Drying.

siccolabile (sik-o-la´bĭl) Destroyed by drying.

siccostabile (sik-o-sta´bĭl) Not destroyed by drying.

siccus (sik´us) Latin for dry.

sick (sik) **1.** Afflicted with a disease. **2.** Nauseated.

sickle cell disease (sik´l sel dĭ-zēz´) See sickle cell anemia, under anemia.

sickle cell C disease (sik´l sel se dĭ-zēz´) Hemolytic anemia present in patients who are heterozygous for hemoglobin S and C.

sickle form (sik´l form) See malarial crescent, under crescent.

sicklemia (sik-le´me-ă) Outmoded term, formerly used to denote any sickle cell disorder. See sickle cell anemia, under anemia.

sickling (sik´ling) The production of crescent-shaped red blood cells.

sickness (sik´nes) Disease.

African sleeping s. See African trypanosomiasis, under trypanosomiasis.

air s. Motion sickness occurring during travel in aircraft flying at low altitude where the atmosphere is most turbulent.

altitude s. Condition marked by giddiness, headache, difficult rapid breathing on exertion, insomnia, and nausea; experienced by some unacclimatized individuals within a few hours after exposure to high attitude. Also called mountain sickness.

car s. Motion sickness brought about by riding in any land vehicle (automobile, train, bus, motorcycle).

decompression s. A disorder occurring in divers, tunnel workers, or individuals exposed to increased atmospheric pressures; the high pressure causes the gases to dissolve in the blood and body tissues; when the individual returns too suddenly to normal pressure, the dissolved gases return to their original gaseous form and are trapped as bubbles within blood vessels and tissues; symptoms include pain in the joints, respiratory distress, and sometimes coma and death. Also called caisson disease.

falling s. See generalized tonic-clonic epilepsy, under epilepsy.

morning s. Nausea and/or vomiting sometimes occurring during early pregnancy.

motion s. A group of symptoms such as pallor, sweating, excessive salivation, nausea, and frequently vomiting induced by motion; caused by stimulation of the semicircular canals and/or certain psychic factors.

mountain s. See altitude sickness.

radiation s. Illness caused by excessive exposure to ionizing radiation; massive exposure usually causes symptoms occurring in four stages: (a) nausea, vomiting, and sometimes diarrhea and weakness; (b) a period of relative well being; (c) fever, loss of appetite, nausea, abdominal distention, bloody diarrhea, and loss of hair (death usually occurs during this stage); (d) those who survive experience temporary sterility and eventually develop cataracts. Also called radiotoxemia.

sea s. Seasickness.

serum s. An immune complex reaction following injection of an exogenous serum, marked by fever, skin eruptions, edema, and painful joints.

sleeping s. See trypanosomiasis.

sick-sinus syndrome (SSS) A syndrome caused by failure of the sinus node to maintain normal rhythmicity; characterized by chaotic atrial activity with continual changes in P wave contour, bradycardia interspersed with multiple and recurring

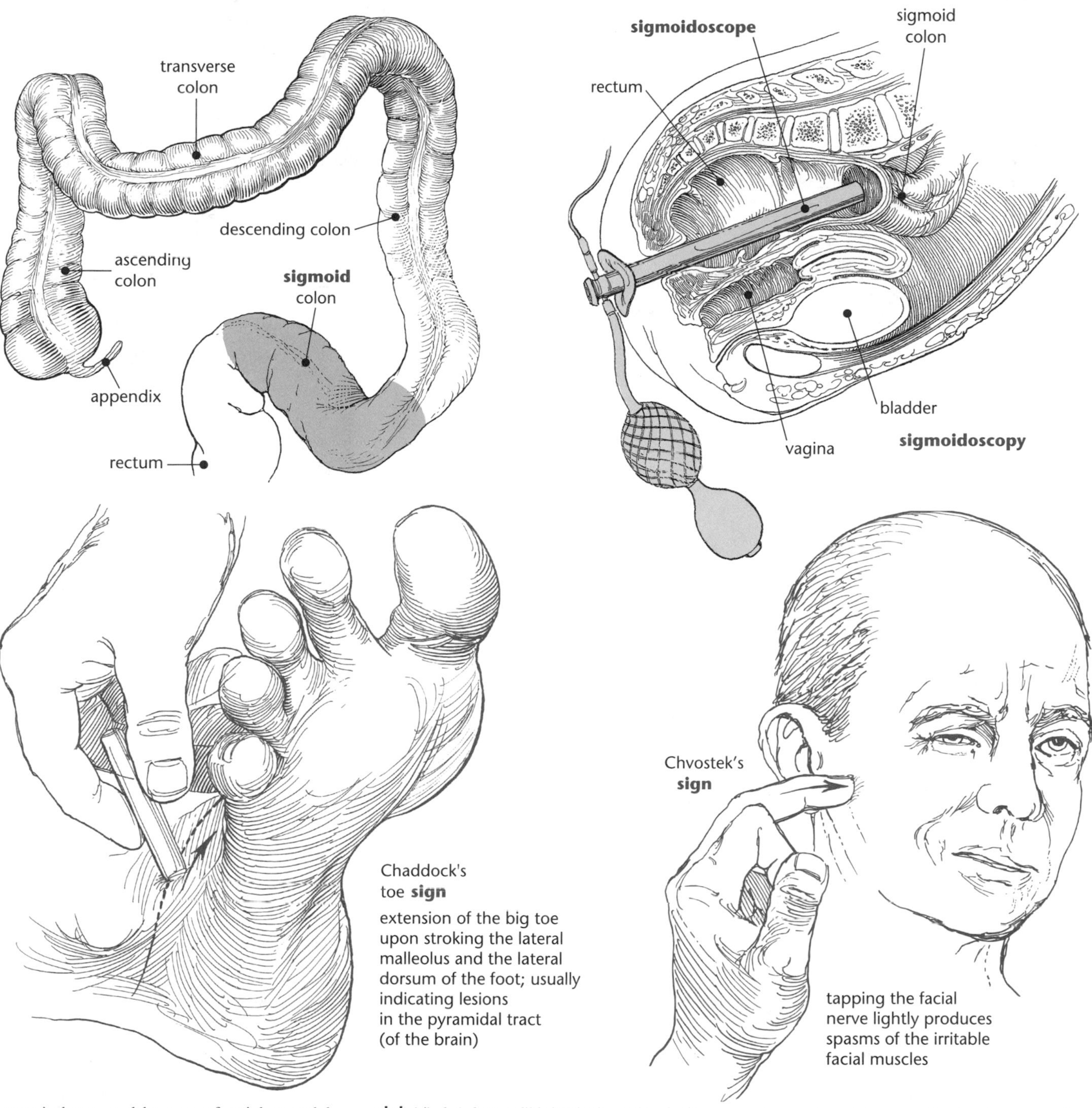

ectopic beats, and by runs of atrial or nodal tachycardia.

sideroblast (sid′ĕr-o-blast) An immature red blood cell containing granules of iron.

siderocyte (sid′ĕr-o-sīt) A red blood cell having iron-containing granules.

sideroderma (sid-ĕr-o-der′mă) Brownish discoloration of the skin, especially of the legs, caused by accumulation of hemosiderin deposits.

siderofibrosis (sid-ĕr-o-fi-bro′sis) Abnormal formation of fibrous tissue associated with multiple small deposits of iron.

sideropenia (sid-ĕr-o-pe′ne-ă) Iron deficiency, especially in the blood and bone marrow.

siderophil (sid′ĕr-o-fil) A cell or tissue that has an affinity for iron.

siderophilin (sid-ĕr-of′ĭ-lin) See transferrin.

siderosis (sid-ĕr-o′sis) Deposit of iron dust or particles in a tissue.

s. bulbi Rust coloration of the eyeball caused by the prolonged presence of an iron particle in the eye.

pulmonary s. A form of pneumoconiosis seen in welders, due to inhalation of fine iron dust, which causes a brick red discoloration of the lungs with little or no fibrosis.

sigh (si) **1.** A deep audible inspiration and expiration made involuntarily under the influence of some emotion or an anesthetic. **2.** To emit such a sound.

sight (sīt) The ability to see.

day s. See nyctalopia.

far s. See hyperopia.

near s. See myopia.

night s. See hemeralopia.

old s. See presbyopia.

second s. The unaided improvement of near vision in the aged; usually a sign of incipient cataract. Also called senopia; gerontopia.

sigmatism (sig′mă-tiz-m) Inability to pronounce sibilant (s, sh) sounds correctly; lisping.

sigmoid (sig′moid) Having the shape of the letter S; applied to the distal portion of the colon.

sigmoidectomy (sig-moi-dek′to-me) Surgical removal of part of the sigmoid colon; excision of the sigmoid flexure.

sigmoidopexy (sig-moi′do-pek-se) Suturing of the sigmoid colon to the abdominal wall for the correction of a prolapsed rectum.

sigmoidoscope (sig-moi′do-skōp) An instrument for inspecting the interior of the sigmoid colon.

sigmoidoscopy (sig-moi-dos′kŏ pe) Inspection of the interior of the sigmoid colon by means of an instrument (sigmoidoscope).

sigmoidotomy (sig-moi-dot′ŏ-me) Surgical incision of the sigmoid colon.

sign (sīn) **1.** Any objective evidence indicative of disease, perceptible to the examiner, as compared to subjective sensations (symptoms) of the patient. Some signs are deliberately elicited by means of tests for diagnostic purposes. For individual signs, see specific names. **2.** An indication of continued existence.

signa (sig′nă) (Sig. or S.) Latin for write, or set a mark upon; used in prescriptions to introduce the signature.

signature (sig′nă-chur) The part of a pharmaceutical prescription containing instruction to the patient for the use of the medication. Also called transcription. See also superscription, inscription, and subscription.

significant (sig-nif′ĭ-kant) In statistics, anything that is probably not the result of chance.

silica (sil′ĭ-kă) Silicon dioxide, SiO_2; a white or colorless crystalline compound; one of the three major ingredients of dental porcelain.

silicate (sil′ĭ-kāt) A salt of silicic acid.

siliceous, silicious (sĭ-lish′us) Containing silica.

drawer **sign** A sign of ruptured cruciate ligaments at the knee, elicited while the patient lies on his back, knee flexed at 90°; the examiner grasps the upper part of the patient's leg with both hands and pulls the head of the tibia; a forward movement indicates rupture of the anterior cruciate ligament; if the tibia can be pushed under the femoral condyle, the posterior cruciate ligament is ruptured. Also called Rocher's sign.

Heimlich **sign** The characteristic sudden gesture of distress of a person with an obstruction of the airway (e.g., with a piece of food or small object or toy); the person brings a hand to his throat with the thumb and index finger spread apart, forming a V

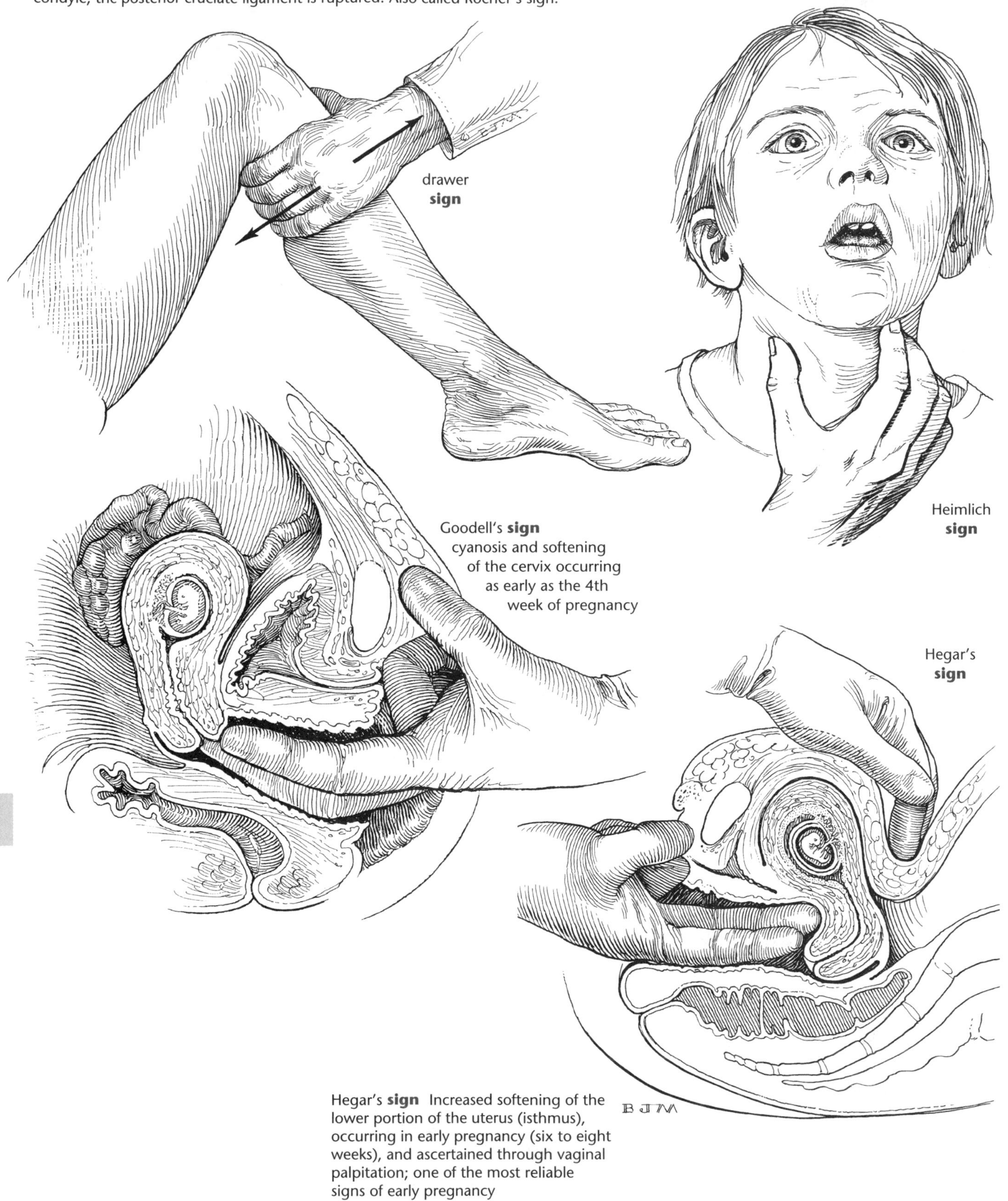

Hegar's **sign** Increased softening of the lower portion of the uterus (isthmus), occurring in early pregnancy (six to eight weeks), and ascertained through vaginal palpitation; one of the most reliable signs of early pregnancy

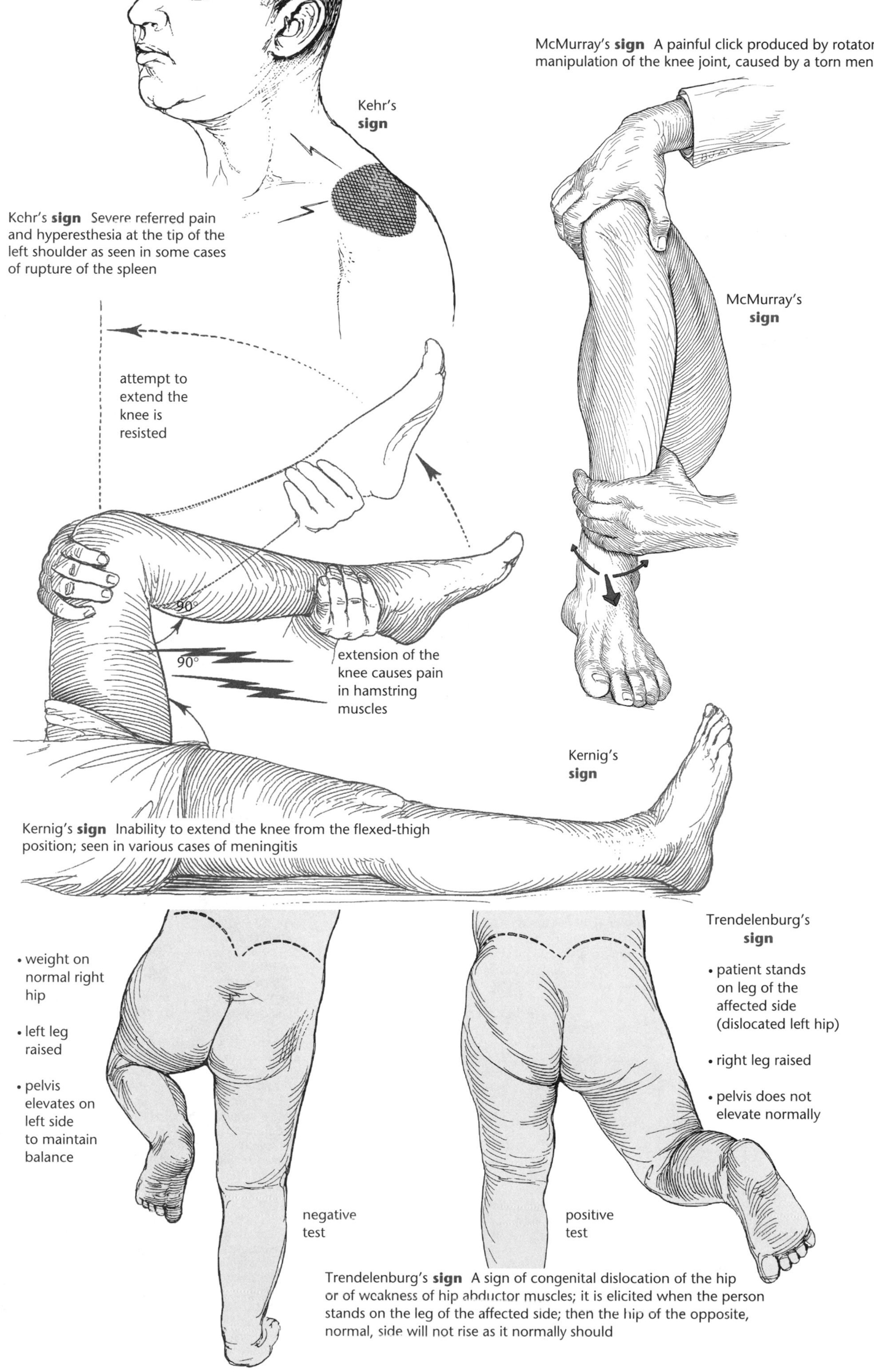

McMurray's **sign** A painful click produced by rotatory manipulation of the knee joint, caused by a torn meniscus
Kehr's **sign**
Kehr's **sign** Severe referred pain and hyperesthesia at the tip of the left shoulder as seen in some cases of rupture of the spleen
McMurray's **sign**
attempt to extend the knee is resisted
90°
90°
extension of the knee causes pain in hamstring muscles
Kernig's **sign**
Kernig's **sign** Inability to extend the knee from the flexed-thigh position; seen in various cases of meningitis
Trendelenburg's **sign**
• weight on normal right hip
• left leg raised
• pelvis elevates on left side to maintain balance
• patient stands on leg of the affected side (dislocated left hip)
• right leg raised
• pelvis does not elevate normally
negative test
positive test

Trendelenburg's **sign** A sign of congenital dislocation of the hip or of weakness of hip abductor muscles; it is elicited when the person stands on the leg of the affected side; then the hip of the opposite, normal, side will not rise as it normally should

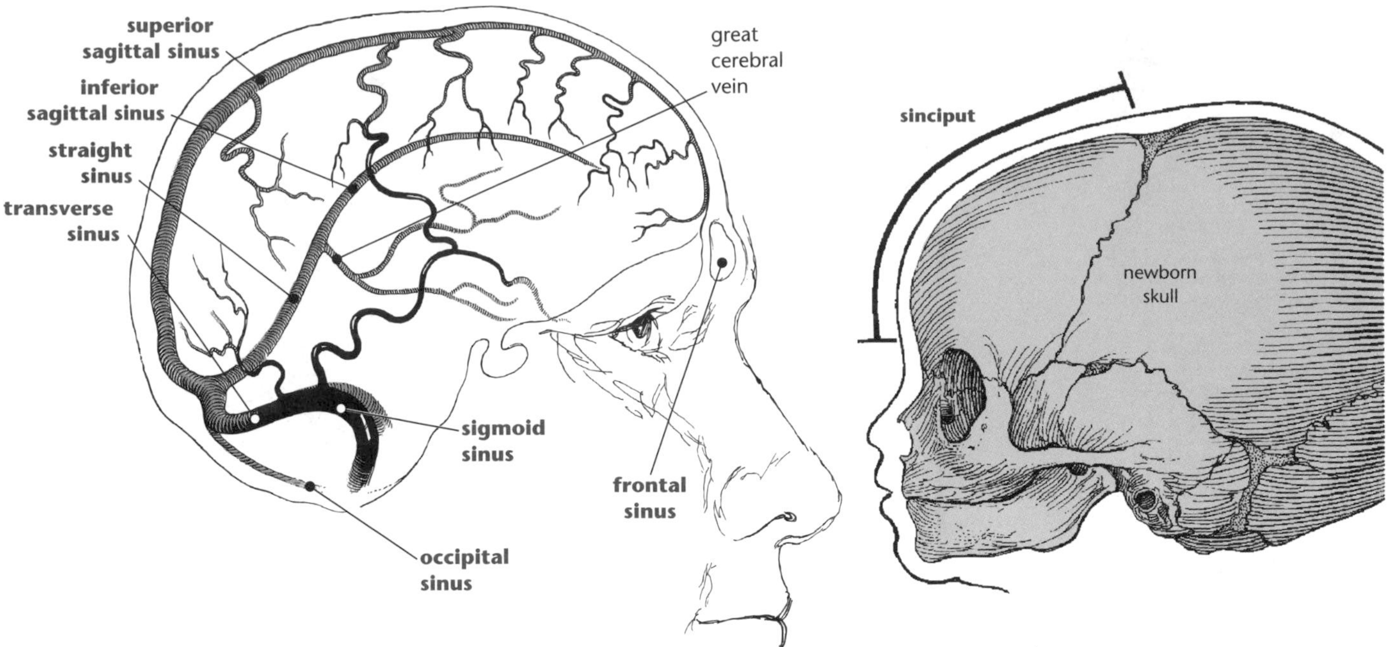

silicic acid (sĭ-lik´ik as´id) Generally, any acid containing silicon.
silicon (sil´ĭ-kon) A nonmetallic element abundantly present in the earth's crust in silica and silicates; symbol Si, atomic number 14, atomic weight 28.09.
silicone (sil´ĭ-kōn) Any of a group of semiorganic polymers marked by physiochemical inertness and a high degree of water repellence and lubricity; used in prosthetic replacement of bodily parts, protective coatings, and adhesives.
silicosis (sil-ĭ-ko´sis) Fibrosis of the lungs caused by prolonged inhalation of silica dust (stone dust, SiO_2); a pneumoconiosis. Also called stonemason's disease; potters' phthisis.
silicotuberculosis (sil-ĭ-ko-too-ber-ku-lo´sis) Silicosis associated with tuberculosis.
silk (silk) The fine lustrous fiber produced by the silkworm to make its cocoon.
surgical s. Thread used in surgical operations.
silver (sil´ver) A lustrous white, malleable, ductile metallic element; symbol Ag (from the Latin *argentum*), atomic number 47, atomic weight 107.87.
s. nitrate A caustic colorless crystalline compound, $AgNO_3$, with antiseptic properties; used in dressings for burns and wounds.
Simmond's disease (sim´ondz dĭ-zēz´) See panhypopituitarism.
simulation (sim-u-la´shun) **1.** Imitation; said of a disease or symptom that resembles or mimics another. **2.** A feigning or pretending, such as malingering.
simulator (sim-u-la´tor) A device designed to produce effects simulating or approximating actual conditions.
patient s. A functional replica of a body part used for teaching or training.
space s. A hermetically sealed chamber with human or animal subjects at ground level, used to study some of the physiologic effects of space traveling.
Simulium (si-mu´le-um) A genus of biting black gnats (family Simuliidae), some species of which transmit onchocerciasis.
sincipital (sin-sip´ĭ-tal) Relating to the forehead and upper part of the head.
sinciput (sin´sĭ-put) The upper anterior part of the head from the forehead to the crown.
sine (sīn) (s, s̄) Latin for without.
sine (sīn) A trigonometric ratio between parts of a triangle; in a right triangle, it is the side opposite an acute angle divided by the side opposite the right angle (hypotenuse); graphed with two coordinates, the values produce a sinusoid or sine curve with the equation y = sin x.
sinew (sin´u) A tendon.
singlet (sing´glit) A single member, as a single microtubule in the middle of a cilium.
singultation (sing-gul-ta´shun) Hiccupping.
singultous (sing-gul´tus) Relating to hiccups.
singultus (sing-gul´tus) A hiccup.
sinister (sin-is´ter) (s) Latin for left.
sinistral (sin´is-tral) **1.** Relating to the left side. **2.** Left-handed.
sinistrality (sin-is-tral´ĭ-te) Left-handedness.
sinistrocardia (sin-is-tro-kar´de-ă) Displacement of the heart toward the left, beyond its normal position.
sinistrocerebral (sin-is-tro-ser´ē-bral) Relating to the left hemisphere of the brain.
sinistrocular (sin-is-trok´u-lar) **1.** Having better vision in the left eye. **2.** Relating to dominance of the left eye.
sinistropedal (sin-is-trop´ĕ-dal) Using the left foot in preference to the right.
sinoatrial, sinoauricular (si-no-a´tre-al, si-no-aw-rik´u-lar) (S-A) Relating to the sinus venosus and the right atrium of the heart; especially the sinus (S-A) node.
sinus (sī´nus) **1.** An air-filled cavity within a cranial bone. **2.** A dilated channel for the passage of fluid (blood, lymph, aqueous humor) that lacks the coats of an ordinary vessel wall. **3.** A small pouchlike furrow. **4.** An abnormal fistula or tract.
anal s's. Small pouchlike furrows at the posterior upper end of the anal canal. Also called anal crypts; crypts of Morgagni.
aortic s. Any of the three slight dilatations of the aorta between each semilunar valve and the wall of the aorta. Also called sinus of Valsalva.
carotid s. A slight dilatation of the most proximal part of the internal carotid artery containing in its wall pressoreceptors which, when stimulated by changes in blood pressure, cause slowing of the heart, vasodilatation, and a fall in blood pressure. Also called carotid bulb.
cavernous s. A paired, irregularly shaped venous sinus in the dura mater on each side of the body of the sphenoid bone in the middle cranial fossa; it drains the superior ophthalmic vein, superficial middle cerebral vein, and sphenoparietal sinus; it empties by way of the petrosal sinuses into the transverse sinus and internal jugular vein.
cerebral s.'s See dura mater sinuses.
circular s. **1.** A venous ring around the hypophysis (pituitary gland) formed by the anterior and posterior intercavernous sinuses communicating with the cavernous sinus. **2.** The venous sinus at the periphery of the placenta. **3.** The scleral venous sinus of the eye.
coronary s. The short venous sinus receiving most of the veins of the heart, situated in the posterior part of the coronary sulcus between the left atrium and the ventricle; it opens into the right atrium between the inferior vena cava and the atrioventricular orifice.
dermal s. An abnormal, congenital sinus tract lined with skin and usually extending from the skin to the spinal canal.
dura mater s.'s The venous sinuses in the dura mater (e.g., cavernous, superior sagittal, and transverse). Also called cerebral sinuses.
epididymal s. A narrow slitlike recess between the upper part of the testis and the overlying epididymis; formed by the invagination of the tunica vaginalis.
ethmoidal s. Any of the air cells of the ethmoid bone.
frontal s. One of the paired paranasal sinuses in the lower part of the frontal bone; it communicates by way of the nasofrontal duct (infundibulum) with the nasal cavity of the same side.
jugular s.'s Two slight dilatations of the internal jugular vein; a superior one located at its origin near the base of the skull and an inferior one near its termination, just before it unites with the subclavian vein.
lactiferous duct s. The spindle-shaped dilated portion of the lactiferous duct of the mammary gland, just before it enters the nipple.
lymphatic s. Irregular, tortuous channels of a lymph node through which a continuous flow of lymph passes on its way to the efferent lymphatic vessels.
marginal s. of placenta A discontinuous, circumferential venous sinus at the margin of the placenta.
maxillary s. An air cavity in the body of the maxilla on either side, communicating with the middle meatus of the nasal cavity.
occipital s. The smallest of the sinuses of the dura mater, usually unpaired, that drains the area of the foramen magnum, ascends along the attached margin of the falx cerebelli, and terminates in the confluence of the sinuses near the internal occipital protuberance.
omphalomesenteric duct s. A sinus caused by persistent patency of the distal part of the embryonic omphalomesenteric (vitelline) duct.
paranasal s. Any of the air sinuses (frontal, ethmoid, sphenoid, maxillary) in the bones of the face that are lined with mucous membrane and open into the nasal cavity.
petrosal s., inferior A paired venous sinus passing along in the groove of the petro-occipital fissure connecting the cavernous sinus with the beginning of the internal jugular vein.

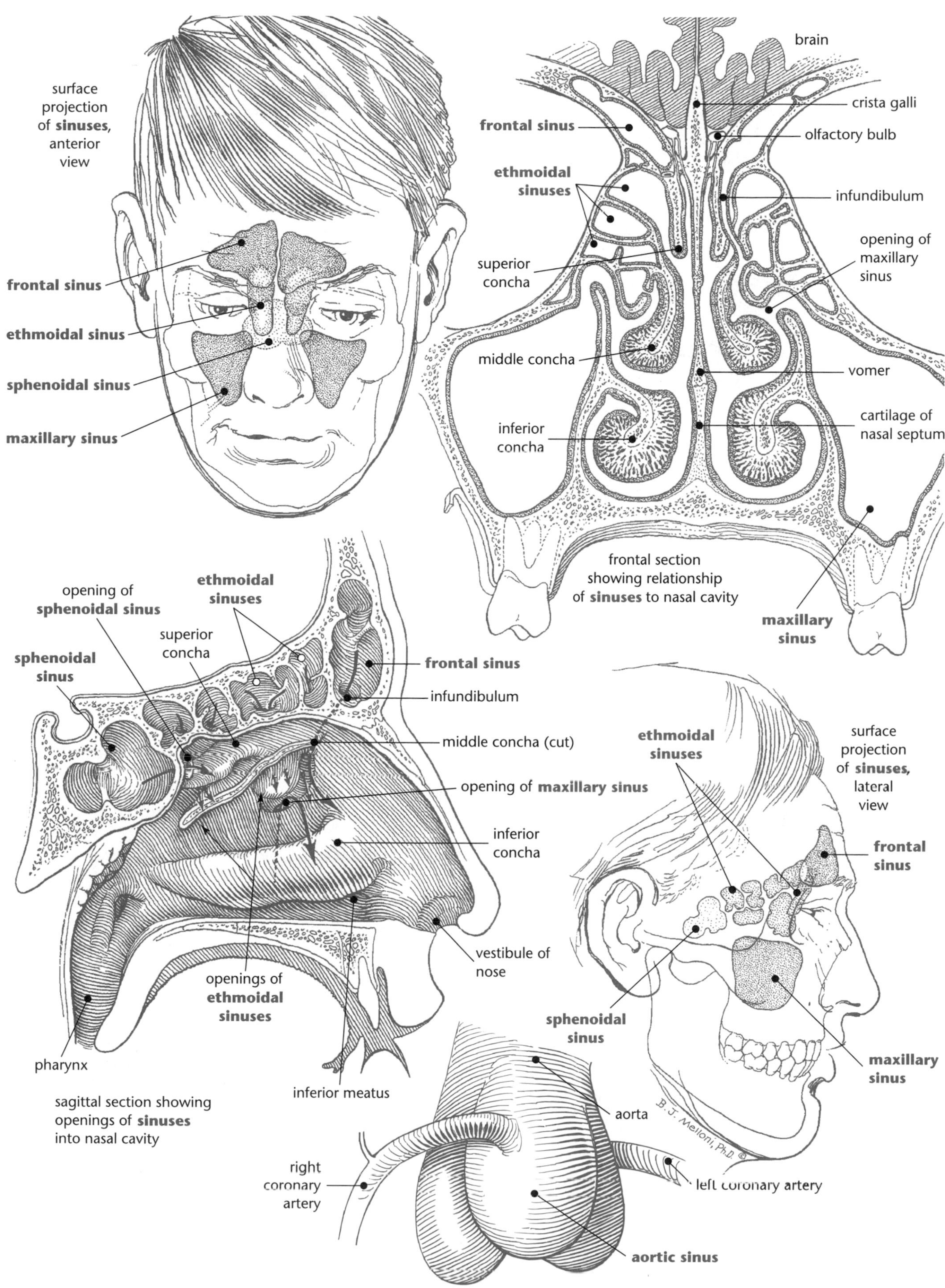
surface
projection
of sinuses,
anterior
view
frontal sinus
ethmoidal sinus
sphenoidal sinus
maxillary sinus
brain
crista galli
frontal sinus
olfactory bulb
ethmoidal
sinuses
infundibulum
opening of
maxillary
sinus
superior
concha
middle concha
vomer
inferior
concha
cartilage of
nasal septum
frontal section
showing relationship
of sinuses to nasal cavity
maxillary
sinus
opening of
sphenoidal sinus
ethmoidal
sinuses
superior
concha
sphenoidal
sinus
frontal sinus
infundibulum
middle concha (cut)
opening of maxillary sinus
inferior
concha
vestibule of
nose
openings of
ethmoidal
sinuses
pharynx
inferior meatus
sagittal section showing
openings of sinuses
into nasal cavity
ethmoidal
sinuses
surface
projection
of sinuses,
lateral
view
frontal
sinus
sphenoidal
sinus
maxillary
sinus
B. J. Melloni, Ph.D. ©
aorta
right
coronary
artery
left coronary artery
aortic sinus

S

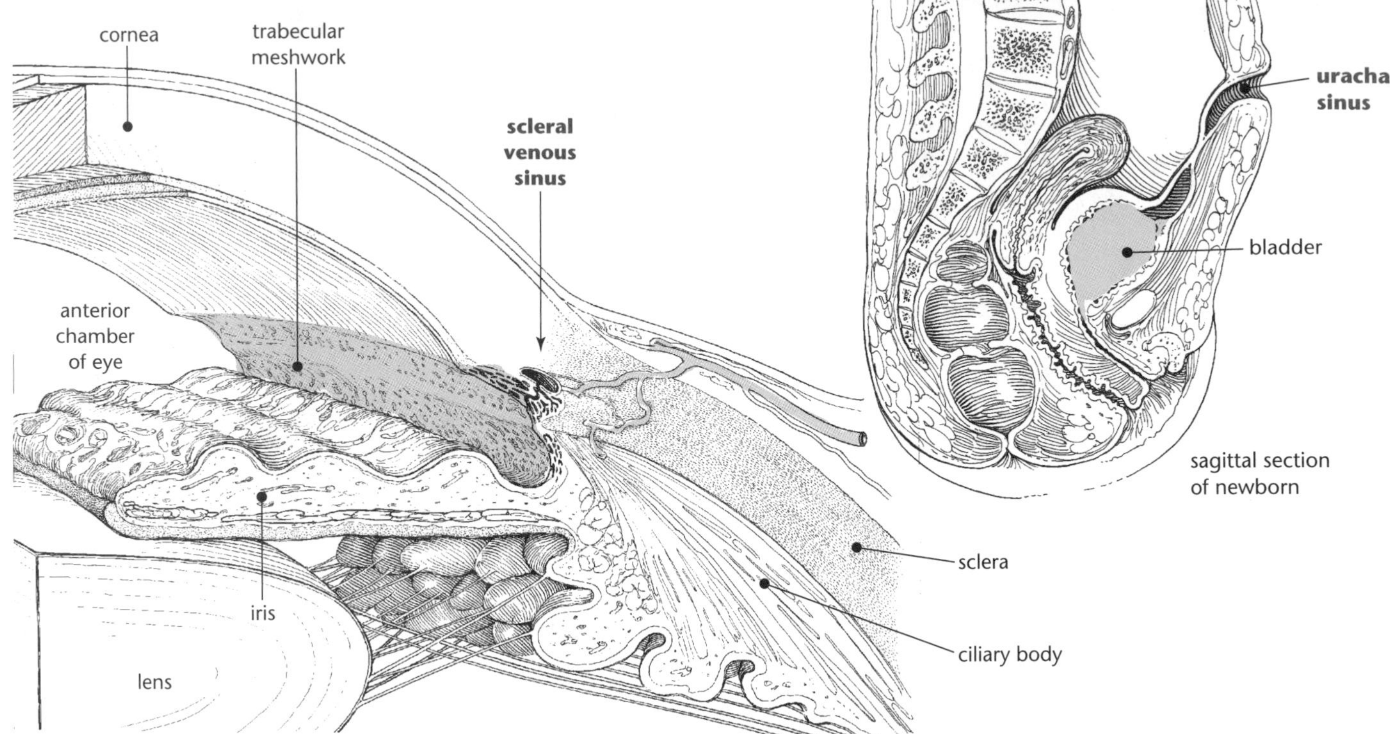

petrosal s., superior A paired venous sinus passing along the attached margin of the tentorium cerebelli connecting the cavernous sinus with the transverse sinus.

pilonidal s. A congenital sinus in the sacral region, leading to the exterior; often containing a tuft of hair and prone to suppuration.

piriform s. See piriform recess, under recess.

prostatic s. The sinus or recess on either side of the urethral crest in the prostatic part of the urethra.

rhomboidal s. A dilatation of the central canal of the spinal cord in the lumbar region. Also called rhombocele.

Rokitansky-Aschoff s. One of a number of small evaginations of the gallbladder extending through the lamina propria and muscular layer; may be seen in chronic cholecystitis.

sagittal s., inferior An unpaired venous sinus in the lower margin of the cerebral falx, running parallel to the superior sagittal sinus and emptying into the upper end of the straight sinus.

sagittal s., superior An unpaired venous sinus in the sagittal groove of the cranium, beginning near the crista galli and extending backward to empty into the confluence of the sinuses near the internal occipital protuberance; it is invaginated by arachnoid granulations.

scleral venous s. The ringlike sinus surrounding the cornea, at the junction of the cornea and sclera; it serves as a drain for the excess aqueous humor of the anterior chamber of the eye. Also called venous sinus of sclera; Schlemm's canal.

sigmoid s. The S-shaped continuation of the transverse sinus on either side, situated along the posterior surface of the petrous portion of the temporal bone to the jugular foramen where it joins the jugular vein.

sphenoidal s. One of the paired, asymmetrical, paranasal sinuses situated in the body of the sphenoid bone; it opens into the nasal cavity, of which it forms part of the roof.

sphenoparietal s. A small dural venous sinus along the lesser wing of the sphenoid bone; it empties into the cavernous sinus.

splenic s.'s Dilated venous sinusoids, lined with reticuloendothelial cells, that connect splenic capillaries with collecting venules and serve to convey blood through the spleen.

straight s. A triangular venous sinus formed by the union of the great cerebral vein and the inferior sagittal sinus; it receives the cerebellar veins before draining into the transverse sinus.

tonsillar s. See tonsillar fossa, under fossa.

transverse s. Either of two (right and left) large venous sinuses of the dura mater lying along the attached margin of the tentorium cerebelli; the right one is frequently the direct continuation of the superior sagittal sinus; the left, of the straight sinus; at their origin in the confluence, they communicate with each other; they drain via the sigmoid sinuses to the internal jugular veins.

urachal s. Congenital abnormality that occurs when the lumen of either end of the embryonic allantois (which extends from the navel to the bladder) fails to close.

urogenital s. In embryology, an elongated sac formed by the division of the cloaca below the entrance of the genital ducts; it develops into the lower part of the bladder in both sexes, the vestibule in the female, and most of the urethra in the male.

s. of Valsalva See aortic sinus.

s. venosus The common venous chamber of the embryonic heart into which the cardinal, vitelline, and umbilical veins drain.

venous s. of sclera See scleral venous sinus.

sinusitis (si-nŭ-si´tis) Inflammation of the mucous membrane of a sinus, especially of a paranasal sinus.

frontal s. Infection in the frontal sinuses.

sinusoid (si´nŭ-soid) **1.** Like a sinus. **2.** An irregular blood channel formed by anastomosing blood vessels; present in certain organs, such as the liver and spleen.

siphon (sī´fun) **1.** A U-shaped tube, used to transfer liquids or in draining wounds. **2.** The act of transferring a fluid by means of a siphon.

carotid s. The U-shaped bend of the intracranial portion of the internal carotid artery alongside the sella turcica.

Sipple syndrome (sip´l sin´drōm) See multiple endocrine neoplasia, type 2, under neoplasia.

site (sīt) A location.

active s. The area of an enzyme molecule that binds the substrate (substance that undergoes chemical change) and activates the reaction.

allosteric s. The part of an enzyme molecule that binds an effector (substance that does not undergo chemical change but either inhibits or accelerates the enzymatic reaction). Also called regulatory site.

ligand binding s. The site on a protein to which another, usually smaller molecule binds.

sitosterol (sī-tos´ter-ol) Any of several widely occurring plant sterols, or a mixture of such sterols.

situs (sī´tus) Position or location; especially normal location.

s. inversus Congenital anomaly in which internal organs are located on the side of the body opposite to their normal location.

Sjögren's syndrome (sho´grenz sin´drōm) Immunologic disorder marked by atrophic changes of lacrimal and salivary glands leading to scanty lacrimal and salivary secretions with dry eyes (keratoconjunctivitis sicca) and dry mouth (xerostomia); may occur in association with such diseases as rheumatoid arthritis, systemic lupus erythematosus, or scleroderma. Also called sicca syndrome.

skatole (skat´ōl) A crystalline compound formed in the intestine as a result of protein decomposition.

skein (skān) A length of coiled thread; said mainly of the coiled chromatin seen in the prophase stage of mitosis.

skeletal (skel´ĕ-tal) Relating to the skeleton.

skeletogenous (skel-ĕ-toj´ĕ-nus) Giving rise to bone formation.

skeleton (skel´ĕ-ton) The internal framework of vertebrates, composed of bones and cartilages and supporting the soft tissues.

skenitis (ske-nī´tis) Inflammation of Skene's glands of the female urethra.

skin (skin) The membranous covering of the body; the human skin is an integument composed of a thin outer layer (epidermis) and a thicker, deeper, connective tissue layer (dermis).

alligator s., fish s. See ichthyosis.

skin popping (skin pop´ing) Slang expression denoting the injection of a narcotic drug intradermally; often results in ulcerations.

skin writing (skin rīt´ing) See dermatographism.

skull (skul) The framework of the head composed of the bones encasing the brain and the bones of the face. Also called cranium.

tower s. See oxycephaly.

sleep (slēp) A natural, periodically recurring state of rest in which consciousness is temporarily interrupted.

non-rapid eye movement s. The dreamless period of sleep during which breathing is slow and deep, heart rate and blood pressure are low and regular, and brain waves are slow and of high voltage. Also called NREM sleep.

NREM s. See non-rapid eye movement sleep.

paroxysmal s. See narcolepsy.

rapid eye movement s. Phenomenon occurring at regular intervals during the dreaming phase of sleep, in which both eyes move rapidly and in unison under the closed eyelids; thought to represent the activated state of sleep, in which activity levels of many functions approach those occurring during wakefulness. Also called REM sleep.

REM s. See rapid eye movement sleep.

twilight s. State in which, although pain is felt, the memory of it is abolished, induced by injection of a mixture of morphine and scopolamine.

sleep apnea syndrome (slēp ap-ne´ă sin´drōm) Clinical manifestations resulting from recurring

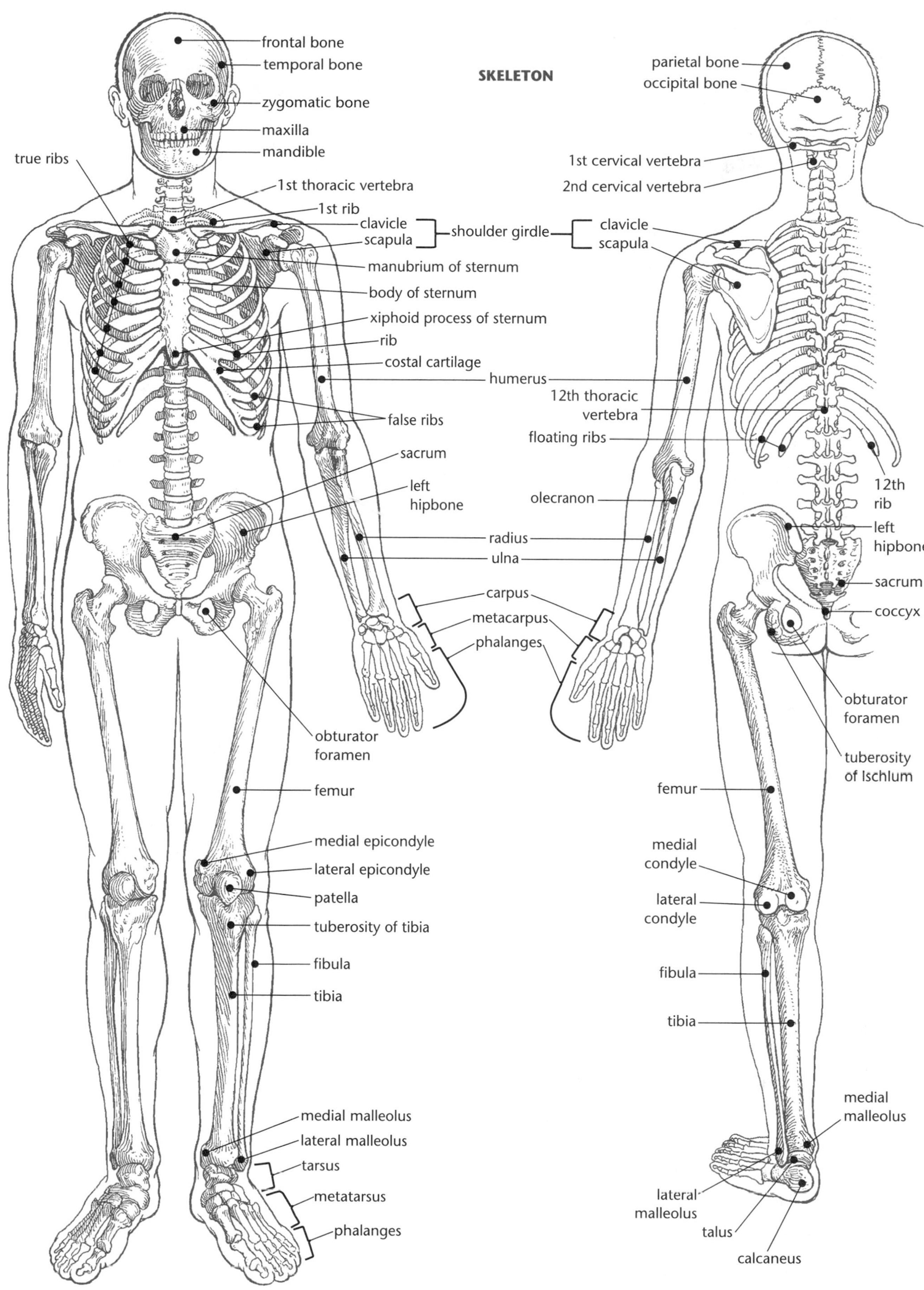
SKELETON
frontal bone
temporal bone
zygomatic bone
maxilla
mandible
true ribs
1st thoracic vertebra
1st rib
clavicle
scapula
shoulder girdle
manubrium of sternum
body of sternum
xiphoid process of sternum
rib
costal cartilage
humerus
false ribs
sacrum
left
hipbone
radius
ulna
carpus
metacarpus
phalanges
obturator
foramen
femur
medial epicondyle
lateral epicondyle
patella
tuberosity of tibia
fibula
tibia
medial malleolus
lateral malleolus
tarsus
metatarsus
phalanges
parietal bone
occipital bone
1st cervical vertebra
2nd cervical vertebra
clavicle
scapula
12th thoracic
vertebra
floating ribs
olecranon
12th
rib
left
hipbone
sacrum
coccyx
obturator
foramen
tuberosity
of Ischium
femur
medial
condyle
lateral
condyle
fibula
tibia
medial
malleolus
lateral
malleolus
talus
calcaneus

S

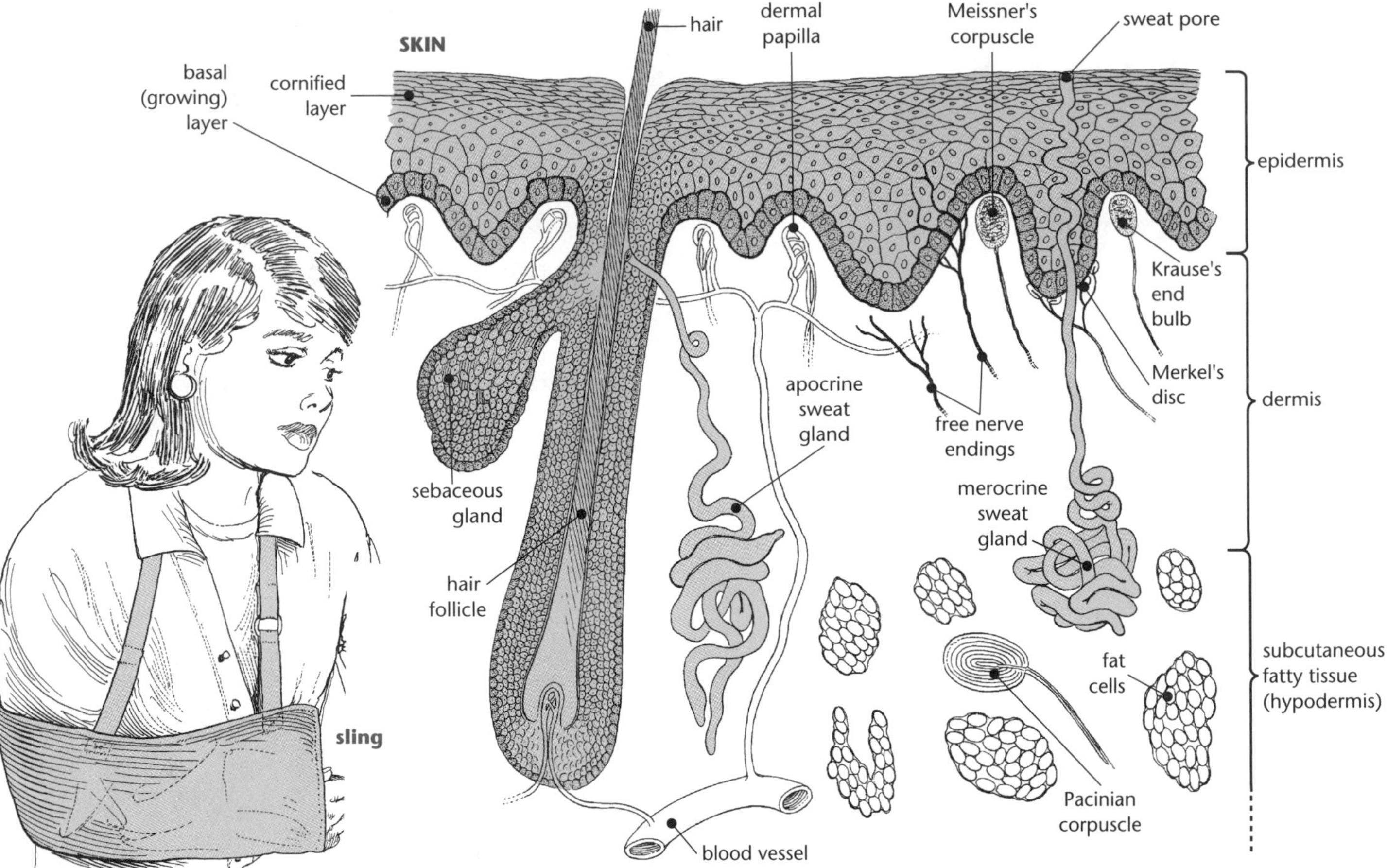

periods of cessation of breathing during sleep; symptoms include morning headaches, daytime sleepiness, personality changes, and sexual impotence.

sleeplessness (slēp′lis-nes) Insomnia.

sleeptalking (slēp′tawk-ing) Talking while asleep or while in a condition resembling sleep. Also called somniloquism.

sleepwalking (slēp′wawk-ing) Walking while asleep. Also called somnambulism.

slide (slīd) A glass plate for mounting specimens to be examined under the microscope.

dip s. A special plastic slide capable of holding an even thickness of culture medium on a molded grid; used to quantify the bacterial population of urine.

sling (sling) A band suspended from the neck, serving as a supporting bandage for an injured arm or hand.

slit (slit) A long, narrow opening, entrance, or cleft.

vulvar s. The cleft between the labia majora.

slitlamp (slit′lamp) A microscope equipped with a slitlike opening through which a beam of intense light is projected to examine the anterior structures of the eye. Also called biomicroscope.

slough (sluf) A mass of dead tissue separated from, or partially attached to, a living structure.

sludge (sluj) A muddy sediment.

smallpox (smawl′poks) Severe contagious disease caused by a poxvirus with incubation period of 14 to 17 days; begins with headache, fever, abdominal and muscular pain, and vomiting; after 3 or 4 days, these symptoms lessen and the eruptive stage begins, with ulcers in the oral mucosa, papules developing into vesicles and pustules throughout the body; after about 3 weeks, scabs form and upon falling leave permanent markings on the skin (pock marks); it remains infectious until scabs fall off. Also called variola.

smear (smēr) A specimen spread thinly on a slide for microscopic examination.

buccal s. Smear obtained by scraping the inside of the cheek.

cervical s. Smear obtained from the uterine cervix or cervical canal.

cytologic s. Smear made by spreading the specimen onto a glass slide, then fixing it and staining it. Also called cytosmear.

Pap s., Papanicolaou s. A smear of vaginal and cervical cells. See also Bethesda System of Classification, under system.

smegma (smĕr) The material that collects under the foreskin of the penis, consisting of sebaceous secretions of preputial glands mixed with desquamated epithelial cells.

smell (smel) **1.** To perceive the scent of a substance by means of the olfactory apparatus. **2.** To emit an odor.

smog (smog) A fog made heavier and darker by industrial gases, motor vehicle exhaust fumes, or smoke.

snap (snap) A sharp sound.

closing s. The accentuated first sound of the heart occurring during closure of the abnormal mitral valve in mitral stenosis.

opening s. A high-pitched click heard during diastole; caused by opening of the abnormal mitral valve in mitral stenosis.

snare (snār) A surgical instrument with a wire loop that is tightened about the pedicle of a tumor or polyp, in order to sever it; also used to remove an intrauterine device.

sneeze (snēz) The forceful, involuntary expulsion of air through the nose and mouth.

snore (snor) **1.** To breathe through the mouth and nose with a rattling noise produced by vibration of the soft palate. **2.** The noise produced while snoring.

snorting (snor′ting) Slang expression denoting the inhalation of a narcotic drug, especially heroin or cocaine.

snuff (snuf) **1.** To inhale forcibly through the nose; to sniff. **2.** Finely pulverized tobacco that is inhaled through the nostrils or applied to the gums. **3.** Any medicated powder that is inhaled through the nose.

snuffbox, anatomic (snuf′boks, an-ă-tom′ik) A somewhat triangular depression formed on the radial aspect of the wrist when the thumb is extended and abducted.

snuffles (snuf′ilz) Noisy breathing due to obstructed nasal passages; when occurring in the newborn, it may be caused by congenital syphilis.

soap (sōp) A cleansing agent; a salt formed by fatty acids with potassium or sodium.

insoluble s. A salt formed by fatty acids and metals other than sodium or potassium; insoluble in water and without detergent properties.

soapstone (sōp′stōn) A relatively soft stone having a soapy feel and composed mainly of talc and chlorite.

social psychiatry (so′shal si-ki′ă-tre) The application of psychiatric principles to the solutions of social problems and issues.

socioacusis (so-se-o-ă-ku′sis) Denoting a hearing loss caused by a noisy environment.

sociomedical (so-se-o-med′ĭ-kal) Pertaining to the interrelations of the practice of medicine and social welfare.

sociopath (so′se-o-path) Former designation for a person with an antisocial personality disorder.

socket (sok′et) A cavity into which another part fits, as the socket of the eye or of a joint.

dry s. A condition sometimes occurring after extraction of a tooth in which the blood clot in the socket disintegrates, leading to exposure of the bone and secondary infection.

eye s. See orbit.

tooth s. The cavity in the jaw in which a tooth fits. Also called alveolus.

soda (so′dă) General term commonly used to designate sodium bicarbonate, sodium carbonate, and sodium hydroxide.

baking s. See sodium bicarbonate.

benzoate s. See sodium benzoate.

bicarbonate s. See sodium bicarbonate.

caustic s. See sodium hydroxide.

sal s. See sodium carbonate.

washing s. See sodium carbonate.

sodium (so′de-um) A soft, silvery white metallic element; symbol Na, atomic number 11, atomic weight 22.99.

s. benzoate A white, crystalline, odorless powder, C_6H_5COONa; used as a food preservative and in the manufacture of pharmaceuticals. Also called benzoate of soda.

s. bicarbonate A white crystalline compound with a slight alkaline taste, $NaHCO_3$; used medicinally as a gastric antacid. Also called baking soda; bicarbonate of soda.

s. bisulfite White, water-soluble crystals, $NaHSO_3$; used as a preservative, a disinfectant, and

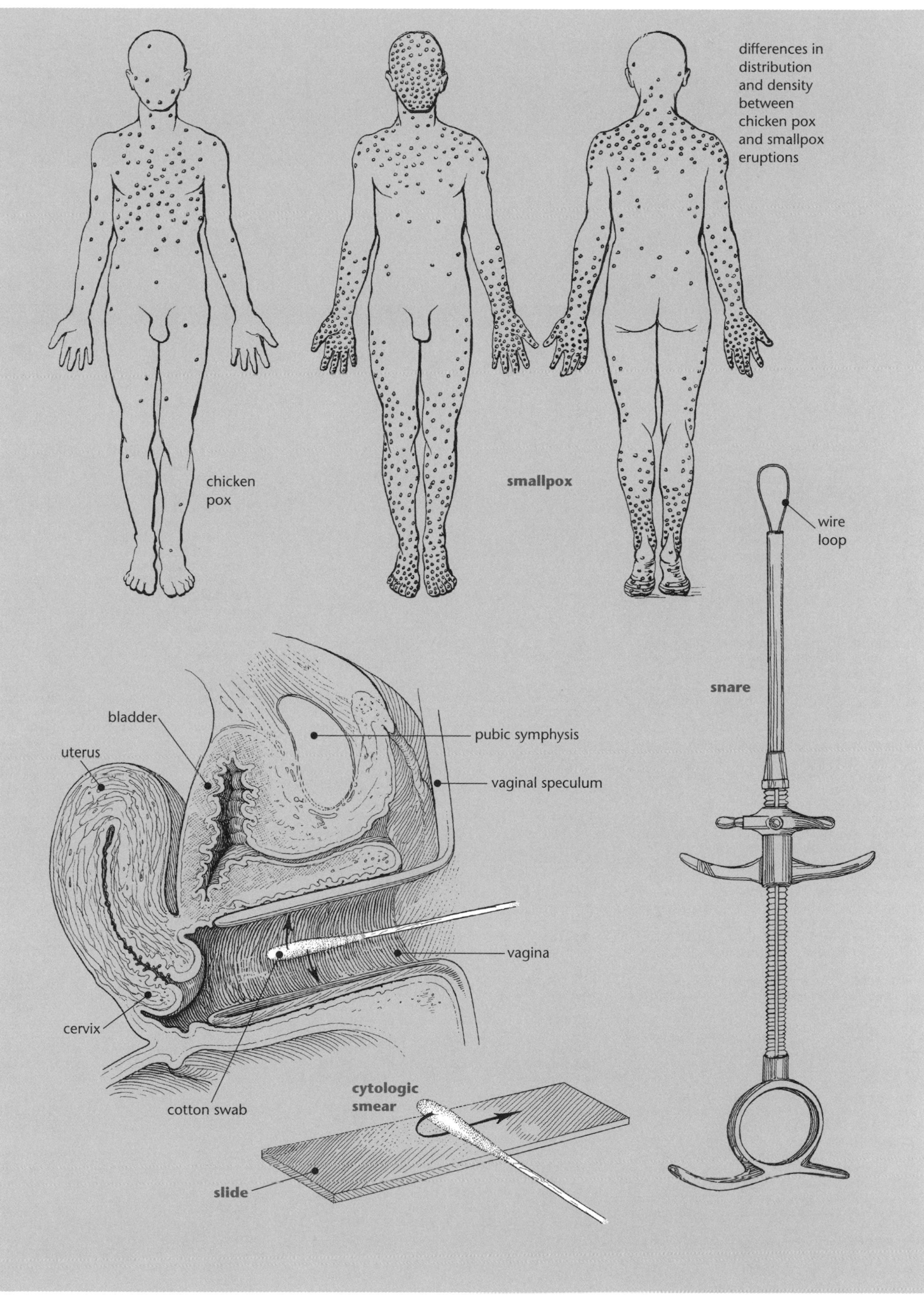
differences in distribution and density between chicken pox and smallpox eruptions
chicken pox
smallpox
wire loop
snare
bladder
uterus
pubic symphysis
vaginal speculum
vagina
cervix
cotton swab
cytologic smear
slide

S

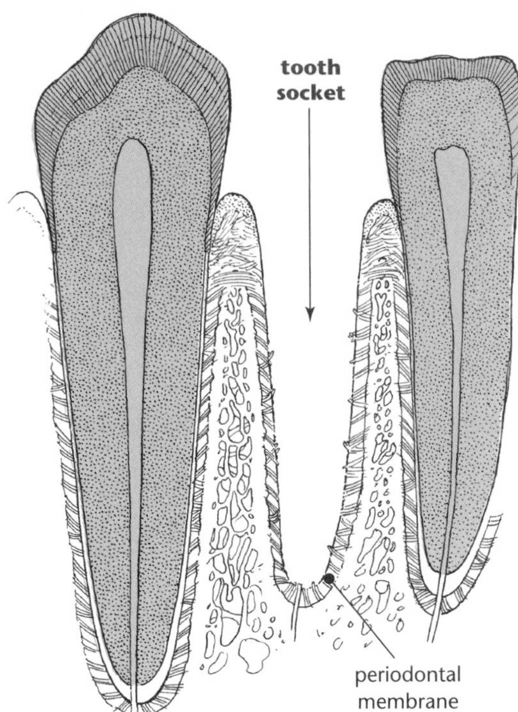

sole
of
newborn

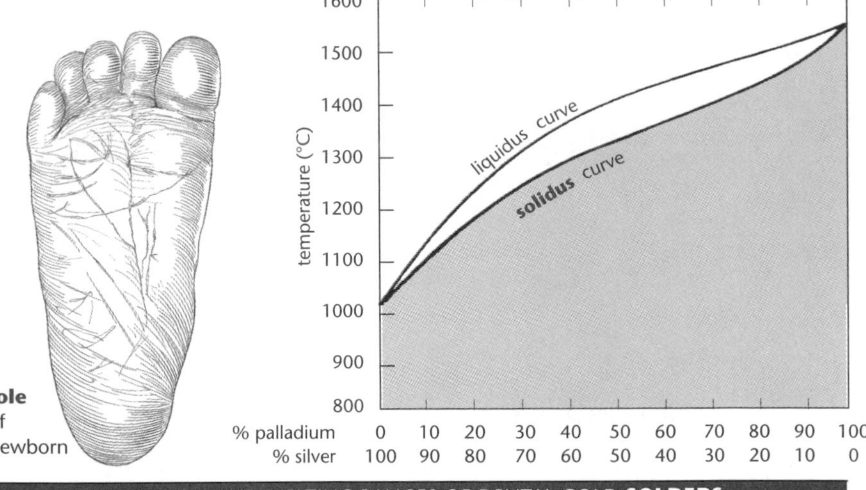

COMPOSITION AND MELTING RANGES OF DENTAL GOLD **SOLDERS**

Solder no.	Gold %	Silver %	Copper %	Zinc %	Tin %	Melting range °F	°C
A	65.4	15.4	12.4	3.9	3.1	1375–1445	745–785
B	66.1	12.4	16.4	3.4	2.0	1385–1480	750–805
C	65.0	16.3	13.1	3.9	1.7	1410–1470	765–800
D	72.9	12.1	10.0	3.0	2.0	1390–1535	755–835
E	80.9	8.1	6.8	2.1	2.0	1375–1595	745–870

an antioxidant in certain injections.

s. borate A colorless crystalline compound, $Na_2B_4O_7{\cdot}10\,H_2O$; used in dentistry as a retardant and in the manufacture of pharmaceuticals and detergents. Also called borax.

s. carbonate **1.** A white powdery compound, Na_2CO_3; used as a reagent and in water treatment. **2.** Any of several hydrated forms, such as $Na_2CO_3{\cdot}10\,H_2O$ (washing soda; sal soda).

s. chloride A crystalline compound, NaCl; used medicinally in solution. Also called table salt; common salt.

s. citrate A white, water-soluble, granular powder, $Na_3C_6H_5O_7{\cdot}2\,H_2O$; used as a blood anticoagulant.

s. cyclamate A water-soluble powder, used as an artificial sweetener.

s. diatrizoate A radiopaque, water-soluble powder, an organic compound of iodine, $C_{11}H_8O_4{\cdot}N_2I_3Na{\cdot}4H_2O$; used in excretory radiography of the urinary tract.

s. glutamate See monosodium glutamate.

s. hydroxide Alkaline, water-soluble compound, NaOH; used in the chemical and pharmaceutical industries. Also called caustic soda; lye.

s. iodide White crystalline powder, NaI; used as a source of iodine.

s. levothyroxine The sodium salt of the natural isomer of thyroxin; used in the treatment of thyroid deficiency conditions.

s. liothyronine The sodium salt of L-triiodothyronine; used in the treatment of thyroid deficiency.

s. nitrate White crystalline compound, $NaNO_3$; formerly used to treat dysentery. Also called Chile saltpeter; soda niter.

s. pentothal See thiopental sodium.

s. perborate A white odorless compound, $NaBO_2H_2O_2{\cdot}3H_2O$; used as an antiseptic.

s. peroxide A white or yellowish powder, Na_2O_2; used in the manufacture of pharmaceuticals.

s. phosphate A crystalline, water-soluble sodium salt of phosphoric acid, $Na_2HPO_4{\cdot}H_2O$; used as a laxative.

s. salicylate White scales, soluble in water, formerly used in the treatment of rheumatic fever.

s. thiosulfate A crystalline compound, $Na_2S_2O_3{\cdot}5H_2O$; used as an antidote in cyanide poisoning, to prevent ringworm infection, and as a photographic fixing agent. Also called hypo; hyposulfite.

sodium group (so´de-um gro͞op) The alkali metals: lithium, sodium, potassium, rubidium, and cesium.

sodoku (so´do-koo) See rat-bite fever, under fever.

sodomy (sod o-me) Sexual practice in which the penis is introduced into the anus or mouth of another person.

softening (sof´en-ing) The process of becoming soft. Also called malacia.

gray s. A stage in softening of the brain in which absorption of fat occurs, following yellow softening.

hemorrhagic s. Red softening.

red s. Softening of the brain with bleeding into the necrotic tissue.

white s. Softening of the brain caused by obstruction of blood supply.

yellow s. Late stage in softening of the brain in which fatty degeneration takes place.

sol (sol) A colloidal dispersion of a solid in a liquid.

Solanaceae (sōl-ă-na´se-e) A family of herbs, shrubs, and trees, including several poisonous species and some that are used medicinally.

solanaceous (sōl-ă-na´shus) Relating to the family Solanaceae.

solation (sol-a´shun) In chemistry, the conversion of a gel into a sol (e.g., by melting gelatin).

solder (sod´er) A fusible alloy of metals used to join metallic parts when applied in the melted state to the solid metal.

soldering (sod´er-ing) The joining of metals by the fusion of intermediate alloys which are of a lower melting point than that of the components to be connected.

sole (sōl) The plantar surface (undersurface) of the foot.

solid (sol´id) **1.** Of definite shape; not liquid or gaseous. **2.** Compact; firm.

solidus (sol´ĭ-dus) The temperature line on a constitution diagram below which the indicated metal element or alloy is in a solid state.

solubility (sol-u-bil´ĭ-te) The property of being soluble.

soluble (sol´u-bl) Capable of being dissolved.

solute (so´lūt) The substance dissolved in a solution.

solution (sŏ-loo´shun) (sol) **1.** A homogeneous substance formed by the mixture of a gaseous, liquid, or solid substance (solute) with a liquid or a noncrystalline solid (solvent), and from which the dissolved substance can be recovered. **2.** The process of making such a mixture.

alcoholic s. A solution in which alcohol is used as the solvent.

Benedict's s. A water solution of sodium citrate, sodium carbonate, and copper sulfate; used to detect the presence of reducing substances in the urine.

Burrow's s. A solution of aluminum acetate.

C3 s. Solution used for perfusion of tissues before freezing. Also called Collins solution.

Collins s. See C3 solution.

Dakin's s. A mixture of hypochlorite and perborate of sodium with hypochlorous and boric acids; an antiseptic. Also called Dakin's modified solution.

Dakin's modified s. See Dakin's solution.

gram-molecular s. Molar solution.

hyperbaric s. A solution possessing a higher specific gravity than a standard of reference; e.g., in spinal anesthesia, one having a specific gravity higher than that of the cerebrospinal fluid (CSF), thereby producing anesthesia below the level of injection due to its downward migration.

hypertonic s. A solution possessing a higher osmotic pressure than a standard of reference (e.g., a solution of sodium chloride having a higher osmotic pressure than that of blood plasma); often denotes a solution that, when surrounding a cell, causes a flow of water to leave the cell through the semipermeable cell membrane.

hypobaric s. A solution possessing a lower specific gravity than a standard of reference; e.g., in spinal anesthesia, one having a specific gravity lower than that of the cerebrospinal fluid (CSF), thereby producing anesthesia above the level of injection due to its upward migration.

hypotonic s. A solution possessing a lower specific gravity than a standard of reference (e.g., a solution of sodium chloride having a lower osmotic pressure than that of blood plasma); often denotes a solution that, when surrounding a cell, causes a flow of water to enter the cell through the semipermeable cell membrane.

iodine s. A solution containing approximately iodine 2%, sodium iodide 2.5%, and water; generally applied to superficial lacerations to prevent bacterial infections.

iodine s., strong See Lugol's iodine solution.

isotonic sodium chloride s. A solution of sodium chloride with the same osmotic pressure as plasma; 0.9% sodium chloride. Also called physiologic salt solution.

lactated Ringer's s. A solution containing sodium chloride 600 mg, sodium lactate 310 mg, calcium chloride 20 mg, and potassium chloride 30 mg in 100 ml of boiled distilled water; the ionic concentration of the solution is 130 mEq sodium, 4 mEq potassium, 4 mEq calcium, 111 mEq chloride, and 27 mEq lactate.

Locke's s. A solution consisting of sodium chloride 0.9 g, calcium chloride 0.024 g, potassium chloride 0.042 g, with sodium bicarbonate 0.01 to 0.03 g, glucose 0.1 g, and distilled water to make 100 ml; used for irrigation of tissues during laboratory experiments.

SELECTED **SOLVENTS**

NAME	MOLECULAR WEIGHT	MELTING POINT °C	BOILING POINT °C
water	18.02	0.0	100.0
methanol	32.04	–97.7	64.7
acetaldehyde	44.05	–123.0	20.4
ethanol	46.07	–114.1	78.3
acetone	58.05	-94.7	56.3
acetic acid	60.05	16.7	117.9
cyclopentane	70.13	–93.8	49.3
benzene	78.12	5.5	80.1
hexane	86.17	–95.3	68.7
pyruvic acid	88.06	13.6	165.0
toluene	92.14	–94.9	110.6
phenol	94.12	40.9	181.8
caprylic acid	144.22	16.5	239.9
engenol	164.20	9.2	255.0
oleic acid	282.47	13.4	360.0

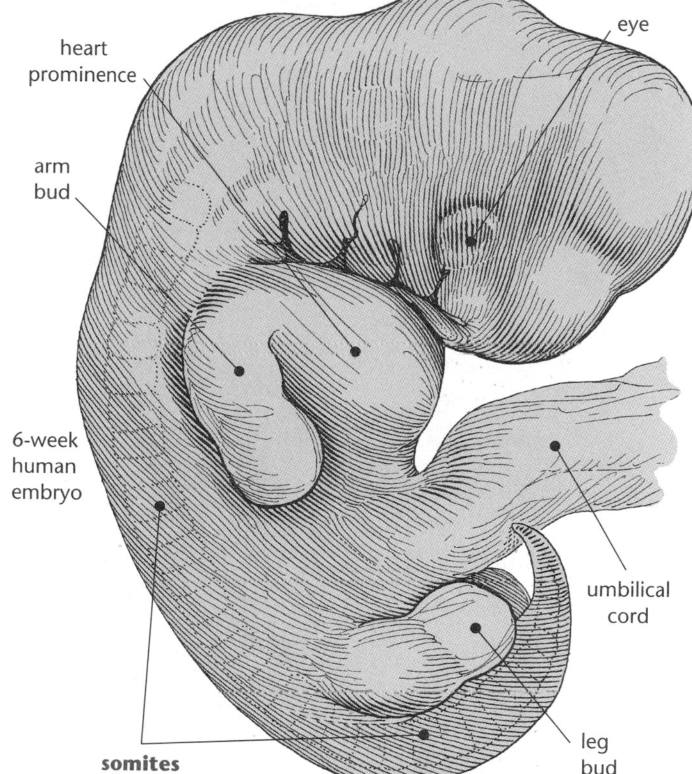

Locke-Ringer s. A solution containing sodium chloride 9 g, calcium chloride 0.24 g, potassium chloride 0.42 g, and magnesium chloride 0.2 g, with sodium bicarbonate 0.5 g, glucose 0.5 g, and water to make one liter; used for physiologic and pharmacologic experiments.

Lugol's iodine s. A deep brown solution containing iodine 5 g, potassium iodide 10 g, and enough distilled water to make 100 ml; used as a therapeutic source of iodine, as a fixative of histologic stains, and as a testing solution for cancer of the cervix and vaginal mucosa. Also called strong iodine solution.

normal s. A solution that contains one gram equivalent weight of the dissolved substance in each liter of solution.

ophthalmic s. A sterile solution for application onto the eye, containing a preservative and having an osmotic pressure and pH similar to that of normal tears.

physiologic salt s. See isotonic sodium chloride solution.

pickling s. An acid solution used to remove oxide and other impurities from dental casts; commonly made from one part of concentrated hydrochloric acid and one part water.

Ringer's s. A solution containing sodium chloride 8.6 g, potassium chloride 0.3 g, and calcium chloride 0.33 g in one liter of boiled distilled water; the ionic concentration of the solution is 147 mEq sodium, 4 mEq potassium, 5 mEq calcium and 156 mEq chloride; used locally for burns and wounds. Also called Ringer's mixture.

saline s. A solution of any salt, especially of sodium chloride. Commonly known as saline.

saturated s. A solution containing the maximum amount of solute that a given amount of solvent can dissolve.

sclerosing s. A solution that causes formation of fibrous tissue; used in oral surgery (e.g., to arrest bleeding, cauterize ulcers) and in sclerotherapy (e.g., to obliterate a varicose vein).

standard s. A solution of known concentration, used as a basis of comparison.

supersaturated s. A solution containing a greater amount of the solute than a given amount of solvent would dissolve at ordinary temperatures.

test s. Standard solution of specific substances, used in chemical analysis.

Tyrode's s. Solution containing sodium chloride 8 g, potassium chloride 0.2 g, calcium chloride 0.2 g, and magnesium chloride 0.1 g, with sodium biphosphate 0.05 g, sodium bicarbonate 1 g, glucose 1 g, and water to make one liter; used in irrigation of the peritoneal cavity and in laboratory work.

volumetric s. (VS) A standard solution containing a specific quantity of a substance dissolved in one liter of water.

solvate (sol´vāt) A compound formed by the loose combination of a solvent (the dissolving substance) and a solute (the substance dissolved).

solve (solv) Latin for dissolve.

solvent (sol´vent) Capable of dissolving another substance. Also called dissolvent.

soma (so´mă) **1.** An organism as a whole, exclusive of its germ cells. **2.** The body, distinguished from the mind. **3.** The body of a nerve cell.

somatesthesia (so-mat-es-the´zhă) Bodily awareness. Also called somesthesia.

somatic (so-mat´ik) **1.** Relating to the body. **2.** Parietal; relating to the wall of the body cavity.

somatization (so-mă-tĭ-za´shun) The unconscious conversion of anxiety into physical symptoms.

somatogenic (so-mă-to-jen´ik) Of bodily origin; originating in the body cells.

somatology (so-mă-tol´o-je) The study of the human body in relation to form and function.

somatomammotropin (so-mă-to-mam-o-tro´pin) See human placental lactogen, under lactogen.

human chorionic s. See human placental lactogen, under lactogen.

somatomedin (so-mă-to-me´din) See insulin-like growth factors, under factor.

somatometry (so-mă-tom´ĕ-tre) Measurement of the body.

somatoplasm so-mat´o-plas-m) The totality of protoplasm of all cells (except germ cells) that make up the body.

somatopsychic (so-mă-to-si´kik) Relating to the relationship of the body and mind; denoting the effects of the body on the mind.

somatopsychosis (so-mă-to-si-ko´sis) An emotional disorder associated with physical disease.

somatosexual (so-mă-to-sek´shoo-al) Relating to both physical and sexual characteristics; usually refers to physical manifestations of sexual development.

somatostatin (so-mă-to-stat´in) A peptide found in the central nervous system, stomach, small intestine, and islets of Langerhans; it inhibits the release of growth hormone, insulin, and glucagon; it may act as a neurotransmitter in the central nervous system. Also called somatotropin release-inhibiting factor.

somatotherapy (so-mă-to-ther´ă-pe) Treatment directed toward physical ailments, as opposed to psychiatric treatments.

somatotropic, somatotrophic (so-mă-to-trop´ik, so-mă-to-trōf´ik) Having a stimulating effect on body growth or an influence on the body.

somatotropin (so-mă-to-tro´pin) (STH) See growth hormone, under hormone.

somatotype (so-mat´o-tīp) Body type; the physical characteristics of the body.

somesthesia (so-mes-the´zhă) See somatesthesia.

somite (so´mīt) One of paired, segmented blocks of epithelioid cells on either side of the neural tube of the embryo, which in later stages of development give rise to connective tissue, bone, muscle, and the dermis and subcutaneous tissue of the skin; the size of the embryo may be expressed by the number of somites; usually 42 to 44 develop in man.

somnambulism (som-nam´bu-liz m) Walking while asleep without any recollection upon awakening; applied also to some states of hypnosis. Also called sleepwalking; noctambulism.

somnambulist (som-nam´bu-list) One who walks in his sleep.

somniloquism, somniloquence (som-nil´o-kwiz-m, som-nil´o-kwens) Talking while asleep or in a condition resembling sleep. Also called sleep-talking.

somniloquist (som-nil´o-kwist) A person who talks in his sleep.

somnolence, somnolency (som´no-lens, som´no-len-se) Drowsiness; sleepiness.

somnolent (som´no-lent) Drowsy.

somnus (som´nus) Latin for sleep.

sone (sōn) A subjective unit of loudness; the intensity of sound of a pure tone of 1000 cycles per second at 40 decibels above an individual's threshold of audibility.

sonic (son´ik) **1.** Pertaining to audible sound. **2.** Relating to the speed of sound in air (approximately 740 mph at sea level).

sonicate (son´ĭ-kāt) To expose to high frequency sound in order to break up a suspension of cells.

sonography (so-nog´ră-fe) See ultrasonography.

sopor (so´por) Unusually profound sleep.

soporific (so po-rif´ik) Producing sleep.

soporous (so´por-us) Relating to unusually deep sleep.

sorbefacient (sor-bĕ-fa´shent) Facilitating absorption.

sorbitan (sor´bĭ-tan) A general term for esters of sorbitol.

sorbitol (sor´bĭ-tol) A sweet crystalline substance occurring in mountain ash fruits and made synthetically by reduction of glucose; used in the

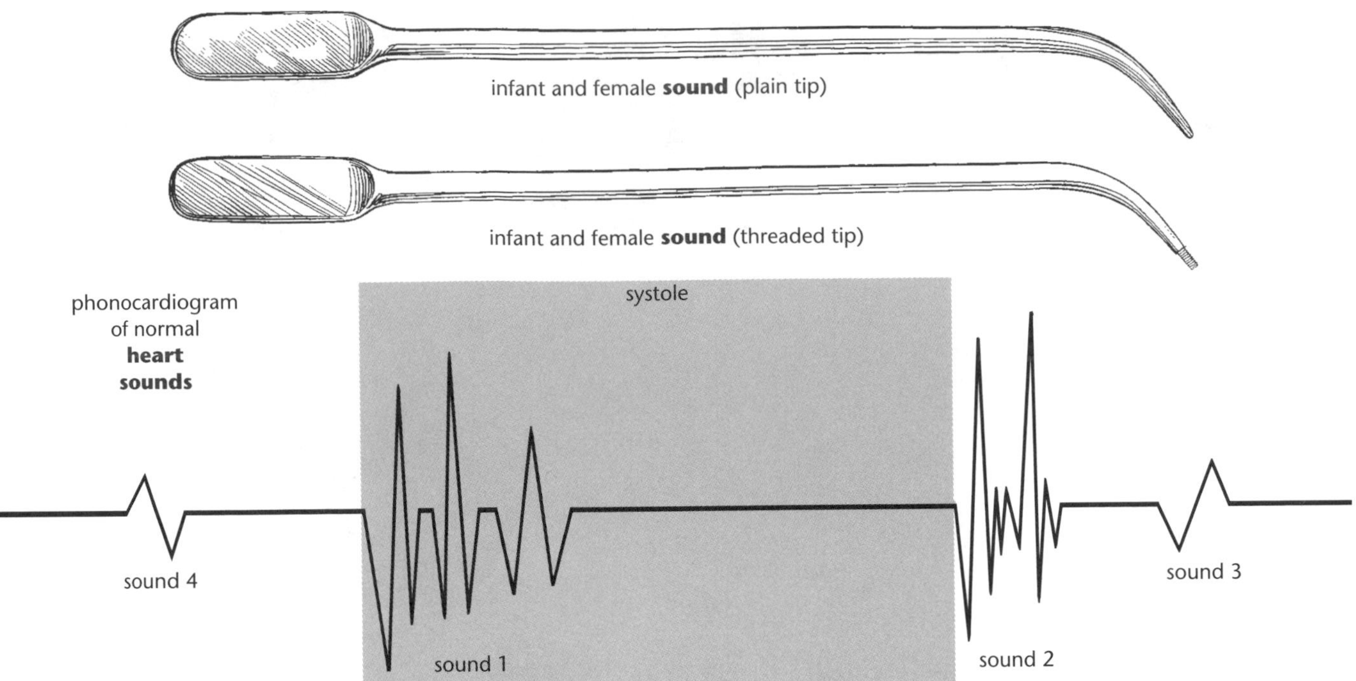

preparation of ascorbic acid and as a laxative, working by an osmotic effect.

sordes (sor´dēz) Foul brown or blackish crust formed about the lips and teeth of patients with some forms of prolonged low grade fever.

sore (sōr) Any open skin lesion.
canker s. See aphthous stomatitis, under stomatitis.
cold s. Popular mane for herpes febrilis. See under herpes.
hard s. See chancre.
oriental s. See cutaneous leishmaniasis, under leishmaniasis.
pressure s. See decubitus ulcer, under ulcer.
soft s. See chancroid.

souffle (soo´fl) A soft blowing sound heard on auscultation.
fetal s. A blowing, whistling sound synchronous with the fetal heartbeat, heard during late pregnancy; caused by blood rushing through the umbilical arteries when the umbilical cord is subject to torsion, tension, or pressure. Also called funic souffle; umbilical souffle.
funic s. See fetal souffle.
mammary s. A blowing murmur heard at the medial border of the breast during late pregnancy and lactation; attributed to a change of dynamics in blood flow through the internal thoracic (mammary) artery.
placental s. Uterine souffle.
splenic s. A soft blowing sound heard over the spleen in malaria.
umbilical s. Fetal souffle.
uterine s. A soft, blowing sound heard over the uterus in late pregnancy, synchronous with the maternal heartbeat; caused by blood flowing through engorged uterine vessels; also may be heard in nonpregnant women with large myomatous tumors of the uterus or with enlarged ovaries. Also called placental souffle.

sound (sownd) **1.** A noise. **2.** A cylindrical, usually curved metal instrument used for exploring bodily cavities or for dilating a canal such as the urethra. **3.** Healthy.
friction s. A grating sound heard on auscultation, produced by the rubbing of two inflamed surfaces. Also called friction rub.
heart s.'s Sounds heard on auscultation over the area of the heart: first heart sound (S_1) is caused by closure of the atrioventricular valves (mitral and tricuspid); second heart sound (S_2) results from closure of the semilunar valves (aortic and pulmonic); third heart sound (S_3) is audible sometimes during rapid filling of the ventricles; fourth heart sound (S_4) coincides with atrial contraction. The presence of a third or fourth heart sound generally indicates an abnormality. Also called cardiac sounds.

soya (soi´yă) The seed of the soybean plant.

soybean (soi´bēn) **1.** A leguminous, climbing Asiatic plant, *Glycine soya* or *Glycine hispida*. **2.** The seed of this plant, rich in protein and low in starch content; given to individuals who are allergic to cow's milk.

space (spās) Any body area or volume between specified boundaries; a delimited three-dimensional area.
anatomic dead s. See dead space (b).
antecubital s. See cubital fossa, under fossa.
Bowman's s. See capsular space.
capsular s. The space or sac between the parietal and visceral epithelium of the renal corpuscle; it receives the filtrate of the blood from the glomerular vessels. Also called Bowman's space; glomerular space; urinary space.
corneal s.'s The interlamellar spaces of the cornea; very small spaces between the lamellae of the corneal stroma that contain tissue fluid.
dead s. (a) A space or cavity left after improper closure of a surgical or other wound. (b) The portion of the respiratory tract from the nostrils to the terminal bronchioles where no gaseous interchange can take place. Also called anatomic dead space.
disk s. In radiology, the translucent space between two vertebrae, indicating the position of the cartilaginous intervertebral disk.
epidural s. The space between the dura mater and the periosteum of the skull and vertebrae; it contains loose areolar tissue and a plexus of veins.
epitympanic s. The upper portion of the middle ear cavity above the tympanic membrane; it contains the head of the malleus and the body of the incus.
freeway s. See interocclusal distance, under distance.
glomerular s. See capsular space.
intercostal s. (ICS, IS) The space or interval between two adjacent ribs; the breadth is greater between the upper ribs and on the ventral surface of the ribs.
interproximal s. The space between adjacent teeth in a dental arch.
interradicular s. The space between the roots of a multirooted tooth, occupied by a bony septum and the periodontal membrane.
intervillous s. The space in the placenta in which maternal blood bathes chorionic villi, thus allowing exchange of materials between the fetal and maternal circulations; it is bounded by the chorion on the fetal side and the decidua basalis on the maternal side.
medullary s. The central cavity and the cellular intervals between the trabeculae of marrow-containing bone.
palmar s. A large fascial space in the hand, divided by a fibrous septum, into the middle palmar space (toward the little finger) and the thenar space (toward the thumb).
pharyngeal s. The area within the pharynx.
physiologic dead s. The portion of the respiratory passage, at the end of inspiration, that is filled with air that has not mixed with alveolar air.
pleural s. The potential space between the parietal and visceral layers of the pleura. Also called cavum pleurae.
retroperitoneal s. The space between the parietal peritoneum and the structures of the posterior abdominal wall.
retropubic s. The extraperitoneal area of loose connective tissue separating the bladder from the pubis and anterior abdominal wall. Also called Retzius' space.
Retzius' s. See retropubic space.
s. 's of Fontana The spaces of the trabecular tissue that connect the anterior chamber of the eye to the venous sinus of the sclera (Schlemm's canal); involved with drainage of the aqueous humor.
subarachnoid s. The space or interval between the arachnoid and the pia mater; it is filled with a delicate meshwork of fibrous trabeculae and contains cerebrospinal fluid.
subdural s. The narrow space between the dura mater and the arachnoid; it contains only a small amount of fluid sufficient to moisten the opposing surfaces of the two membranes.
subphrenic s. The space between the diaphragm and the organs immediately below it.
subpodocytic s.'s Spaces beneath the cell body of the podocyte and its trabeculae; they contain numerous fine foot processes (pedicels) that support the trabeculae on the basement membrane of glomerular capillaries.
Traube's s. A space on the left side of the chest about 7.6 cm wide, bounded on the right by the sternum, above by the oblique line from the cartilage of the sixth rib to the ninth rib, and below by the inferior border of the rib cage.
urinary s. See capsular space.
Zang's s. See lesser supraclavicular fossa, under fossa.
zonular s. The circumlental space between the equator of the lens of the eye and the ciliary processes; it contains aqueous humor.

space maintainer (spās mān-tān´er) A dental appliance, either fixed or removable, used to preserve the space created by the premature loss of a tooth.

space obtainer (spās ob-tān´er) An orthodontic appliance that slowly increases space between teeth.

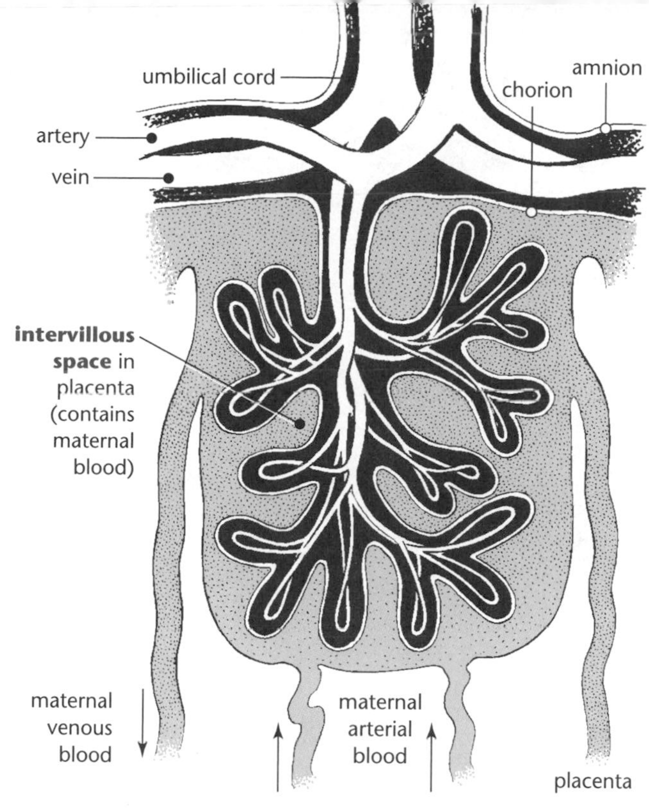

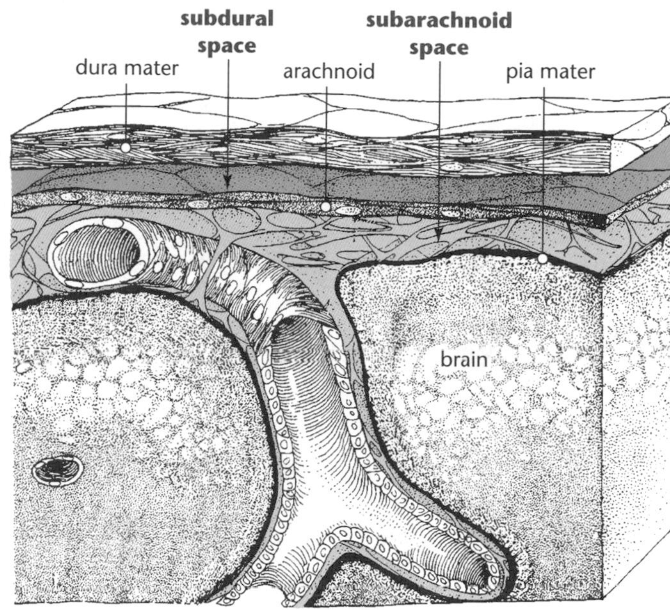

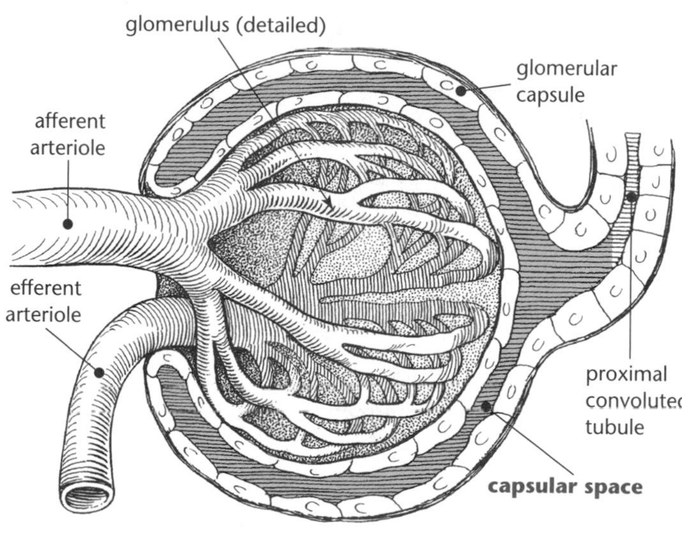

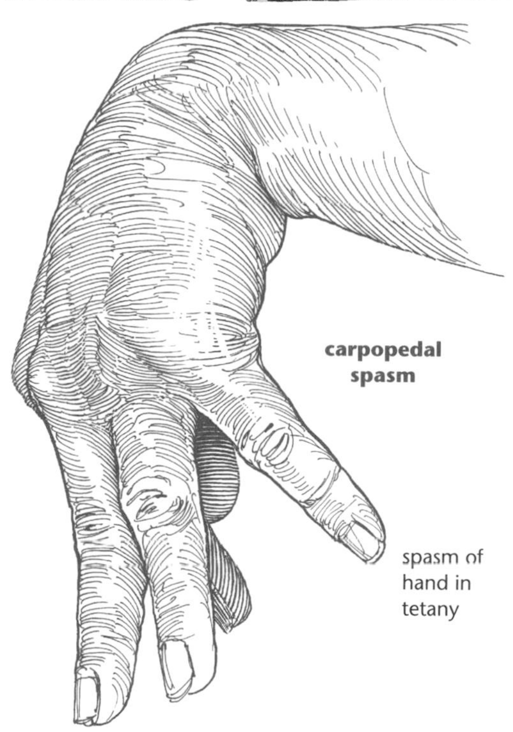

spallation (spaw-la´shun) **1.** A nuclear reaction in which nuclei eject a number of protons and alpha particles when bombarded by high energy particles. **2.** The process of breaking up or splintering into small fragments; applied to the breaking off of the coating from a catheter.

span (span) A full extent or reach.

auditory s. The number of words, letters, or digits that can be repeated after hearing them once; used to test immediate memory.

sparganosis (spar-gă-no´sis) Infection with tapeworm larva, usually of the genus *Spirometra.*

sparganum (spar-ga´num), *pl.* **sparga´na** The intramuscular parasitic larva of tapeworms of the genus *Spirometra.*

spasm (spaz´m) An involuntary, sudden, violent contraction of a muscle or a group of muscles.

carpopedal s. Spasm of the feet and hands occurring in tetany and other disorders.

clonic s. A spasm characterized by alternate rigidity and relaxation of the muscles.

diffused esophageal s. Spontaneous, nonpropulsive contractions of the esophagus causing pain and difficult swallowing.

intention s. A spasm occurring when voluntary movements are attempted.

nictitating s. Involuntary winking.

tonic s. A spasm in which the muscular contraction is persistent.

vasomotor s. Spasm of small arteries.

spasmodic (spaz-mod´ik) Relating to or characterized by spasm.

spasmogenic (spaz-mo-jen´ik) Causing spasms.

spasmolysis (spaz-mol´ĭ-sis) The arrest or elimination of spasm.

spasmolytic (spaz-mo-lit´ik) A drug that reduces spasm. Also called antispasmodic.

spastic (spas´tik) Convulsive.

spasticity (spas-tis´ĭ-te) Increased tone or rigidity of a muscle.

clasp-knife s. Spasticity of the extensor muscles induced by passive flexion of a joint which suddenly gives way on exertion of further pressure, allowing the joint to be easily flexed; the rigidity is due to an exaggeration of the stretch reflex. Also called clasp-knife rigidity.

spatula (spach´ū-lă) **1.** A thin, flat, blunt, blade-shaped instrument used especially for spreading or mixing substances such as dental impression materials. **2.** A device used for scraping tissue for biopsy.

Ayre wooden s. A spatula generally used for taking a smear from the cervix or fornix of the uterus.

Roux s. A small steel spatula for transferring bits of infected material to culture tubes.

spatulate (spach´ū-lāt) **1.** Shaped like a spatula, or having a flat blunt end. **2.** To mix substances by forced compression with a spatula.

spatulation (spach-ū-la´shun) The manipulation of two or more substances with a spatula in order to mix them into a homogeneous mass; usually done by repeatedly and forcefully smoothing out the mass on the side of a mixing bowl or on a flat surface.

spay (spa) To remove the ovaries of an animal.

specialist (spĕ´shal-ist) One whose training, practice, and/or research is devoted to one branch of knowledge. In the usual medical context, a physician who has received advanced training and is board-certified in a recognized field of medicine.

specialize (spĕ´shal-īz) To channel one's training or practice to a specific branch of a field of study or profession.

species (spe´shēz, spe´sēz) **1.** A taxonomic category between a genus and a variety, composed of individuals that bear common characteristics and are capable of interbreeding; a subdivision of a genus. **2.** A type of pharmaceutical preparation consisting of a mixture of crushed, but not pulverized, dried leaves used in making decoctions.

species-specific (spe´sēz-spĕ-sif´ik) Affecting a particular species in a characteristic manner; term applied to a drug or a virus.

specific (spĕ-sif´ik) **1.** Relating to a species. **2.** Relating to one disease only. **3.** A remedy intended

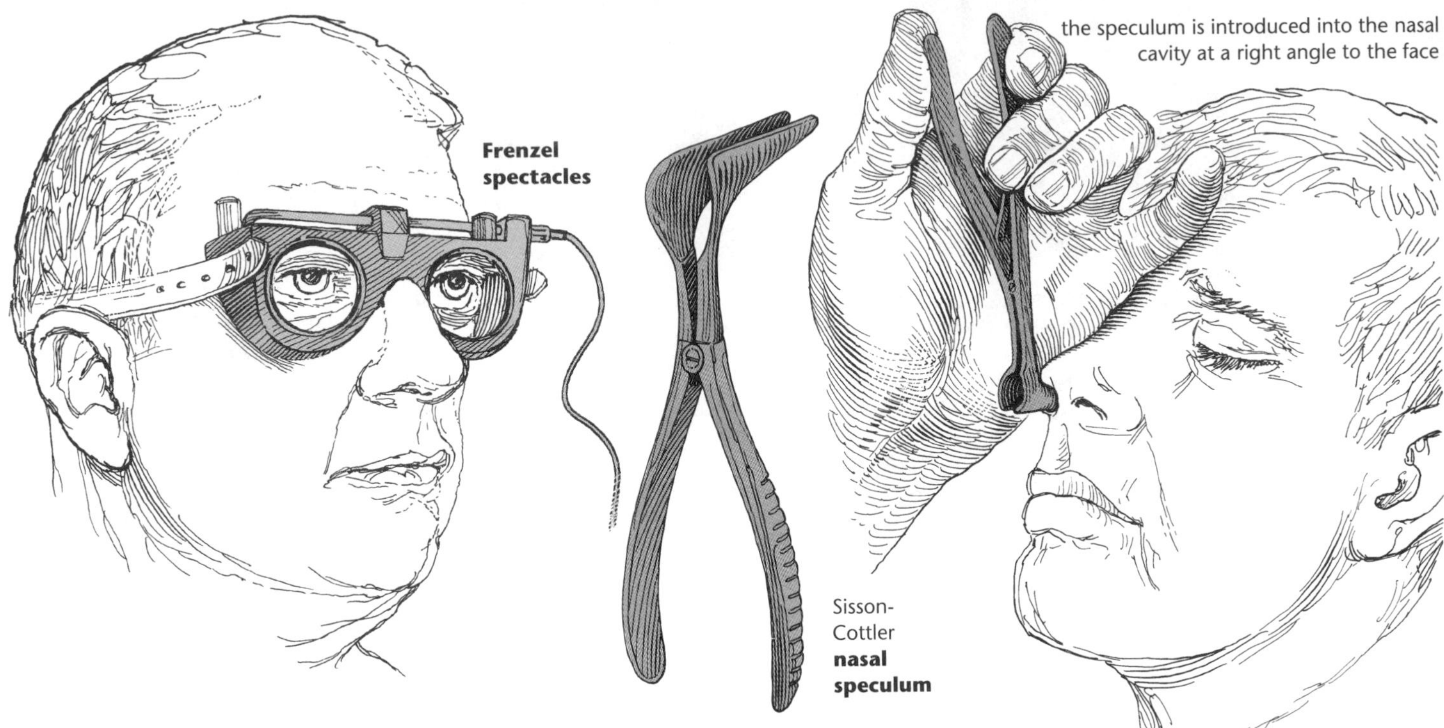

Frenzel spectacles
Sisson-Cottler nasal speculum
the speculum is introduced into the nasal cavity at a right angle to the face

for one particular disease.

specificity (spes-ĭ-fis´ ĭ-te) **1.** The state of being specific, having a fixed affinity, as the antigen-antibody relation. **2.** Applied to a screening test: The proportion of persons who are truly free of a disease in a screened population, and who are identified as such by the test.

specimen (spes´ĭ-men) A small part or sample of any substance, as tissue, blood, or urine, obtained for analysis and diagnosis.

spectacles (spek´tă-kĭlz) Eyeglasses.

clerical s. See half-glass spectacles.

Frenzel s. Plano spectacles with built-in illumination and 20-diopter lenses for the purpose of dazzling the eyes and preventing their fixation on an external object; used in a darkened room to observe and record nystagmus.

half-glass s. Eyeglasses used for reading in which the top halves of the lenses are removed so as not to affect distant vision. Also called clerical spectacles; pantoscopic spectacles.

lid crutch s. Spectacles with a ptosis crutch attachment (little offsets of smooth metal which engage below the upper eyelid to keep it raised above the pupil). Also called Masselon's spectacles.

Masselon's s. See lid crutch spectacles.

pantoscopic s. See half-glass spectacles.

stenopaic s. Spectacles having, in place of lenses, opaque disks with narrow slits or circular perforations allowing a minimum amount of light to enter.

spectrin (spek´trin) A protein attached to membrane proteins on the inner surface of the erythrocyte membrane; together, the proteins form a network that stiffens the membrane and enables the cell to regain its shape and dimension after passing through fine capillary lumens.

spectrochemistry (spek-tro-kem´is-tre) The study and analysis of chemical substances by the use of light waves (spectroscopy); the study of the spectra of substances.

spectrocolorimeter (spek-tro-kul-or-im´ĕ-ter) Instrument for detecting color blindness for one color through the use of a light source from a selected wavelength.

spectrogram (spek´tro-gram) **1.** A machine that translates sounds into a pattern on paper. **2.** A photograph, graph, or map of a spectrum.

spectrograph (spek´tro-graf) A spectroscope designed for photographic recording of a spectrum.

spectrometer (spek-trom´ĕ-ter) An instrument designed to break up light from a source into its constituent wavelengths and to indicate wavelength on its calibrated scale.

nuclear magnetic resonance s. Spectrometer that makes it possible to observe the magnetic properties of atoms in a molecule and provide description of their spatial relationships and movements.

spectrometry (spek-trom´ĕ-tre) Measuring of the wavelengths of rays of a spectrum with the spectrometer.

spectrophotofluorimetry (spek-tro-fo-to-floo-rim´ĕ-tre) The photometric measurement and analysis of the intensity and quality of fluorescence spectra.

spectrophotometer (spek-tro-fo-tom´ĕ-ter) An optical instrument for measuring photometrically the intensity of any particular wavelength range absorbed by a colored solution.

spectrophotometry (spek-tro-fo-tom´ĕ-tre) Analysis using a spectrophotometer.

spectropolarimeter (spek-tro-po-lar-im´ĕ-ter) An instrument for measuring optical rotation of different wavelengths of light passing through a solution or translucent solid; a combined spectroscope and polariscope.

spectroscope (spek´tro-skōp) Any one of several forms of optical instruments used for dispersion of light and visual observation of the resulting spectrum.

spectroscopy (spek-tros´ko-pe) The experimental observation and study of optical spectra.

spectrum (spek´trum) **1.** An orderly distribution of radiant energy presented when white light is dispersed into its constituent colors by passing through a prism or a diffraction grating; the colors, arranged according to the increasing frequency of molecular vibration or decreasing wavelength, are red, orange, yellow, green, blue, indigo, and violet. **2.** A range of activity of pathogenic microorganisms affected by an antibiotic or antibacterial agent.

antibacterial s. See spectrum (2).

s. of disease The complete range of manifestations of a disease.

speculum (spek´u-lum) An instrument used to dilate and hold open the orifice of a body cavity or canal to facilitate inspection of its interior.

duckbill s. See Graves vaginal speculum.

Graves vaginal s. A two-valved speculum for examination of the adult vagina. Also called duckbill speculum.

nasal s. A small, short-bladed speculum for inspecting the cavity of the nose; also used to inspect a child's vagina.

Sims s. A double-ended, retractor-like vaginal speculum.

weighted vaginal s. A single blade retractor-like vaginal speculum with a weighted element that frees both hands of the examiner or surgeon; frequently used on obese patients and patients that have borne many children.

speech (spēch) The production of articulate sounds to convey ideas.

esophageal s. Speech produced by swallowing air and regurgitating it; used by an individual who has had his larynx removed.

scanning s. Slow speech with pauses between syllables.

staccato s. Jerky, abrupt speech in which each syllable is pronounced separately.

telegraphic s. Sparse speech usually consisting mainly of nouns, important adjectives, and transitive verbs, omitting articles, prepositions, and conjunctions; seen in certain types of aphasia.

speed (spēd) Slang name for methamphetamine hydrochloride.

sperm (sperm) A mature reproductive cell of the male.

spermatic (sper-mat´ik) Relating to the sperm.

spermatid (sper´mă-tid) One of the four cells resulting from the division of a spermatocyte; it develops into a spermatozoon without further division.

spermatoblast (sper´mă-to-blast) See spermatogonium.

spermatocele (sper´mă-to-sēl) An intrascrotal, painless cyst containing sperm, usually less than 1 cm in diameter and occurring just above and posterior to the testis; caused by obstruction of the sperm-transporting tubules. Also called spermatocyst.

spermatocide (sper-mat´ŏ-sīd) See spermicide.

spermatocyst (sper´mă-to-sist) **1.** See seminal vesicle, under vesicle. **2.** See spermatocele.

spermatocystectomy (sper-mă-to-sis-tek´to-me) Surgical removal of the seminal vesicles.

spermatocyte (sper-mat´o-sīt) A cell originating from the division of a spermatogonium which in turn divides into four spermatids.

spermatogenesis (sper-mat-ŏ-jen´e-sis) The formation of spermatozoa.

spermatogenetic (sper-mat-ŏ-je-net´ik) Relating to spermatogenesis.

spermatogenic, spermatogenous (sper-mat-ŏ-jen´ik, sper-mă-toj´ĕ-nus) Producing sperm.

spermatogonium, spermatogone (sper-mat-ŏ-go´ne-um, sper´mă-to-gōn) An undifferentiated young cell located close to the basement membrane of the seminiferous tubules; it either gives rise to new spermatogonia (type A) or differentiates into a more developed primary spermatocyte (type B), which eventually becomes a sperm. Also called spermatoblast.

spermatoid (sper´mă-toid) Resembling semen.

spermatolysin (sper-mă-tol´ĭ-sin) A specific lysin of spermatozoa formed in the female body following

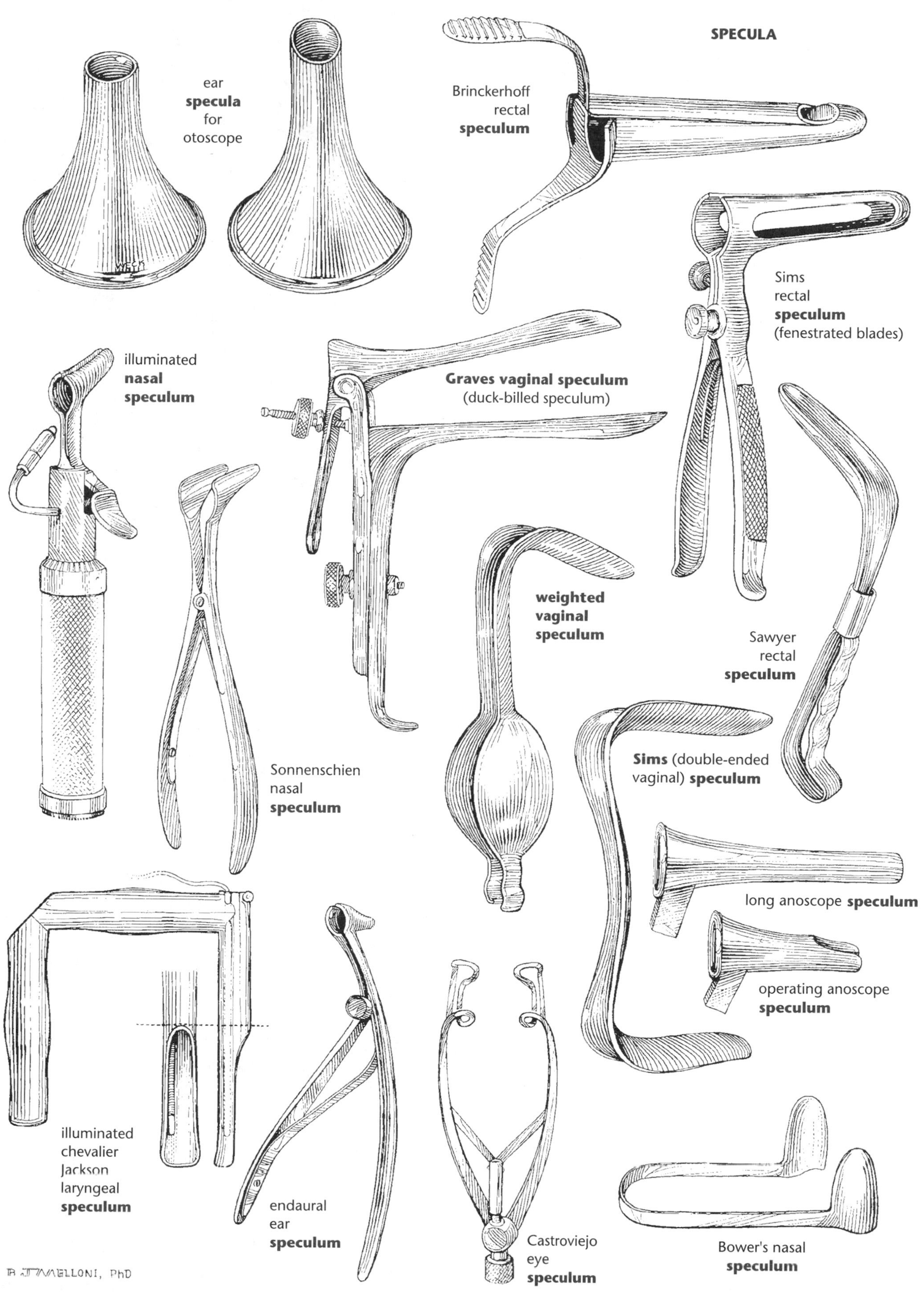
SPECULA
ear
specula
for
otoscope
Brinckerhoff
rectal
speculum
Sims
rectal
speculum
(fenestrated blades)
illuminated
nasal
speculum
Graves vaginal speculum
(duck-billed speculum)
weighted
vaginal
speculum
Sawyer
rectal
speculum
Sonnenschien
nasal
speculum
Sims (double-ended
vaginal) speculum
long anoscope speculum
operating anoscope
speculum
illuminated
chevalier
Jackson
laryngeal
speculum
endaural
ear
speculum
Castroviejo
eye
speculum
Bower's nasal
speculum
B. J. MELLONI, PhD

S

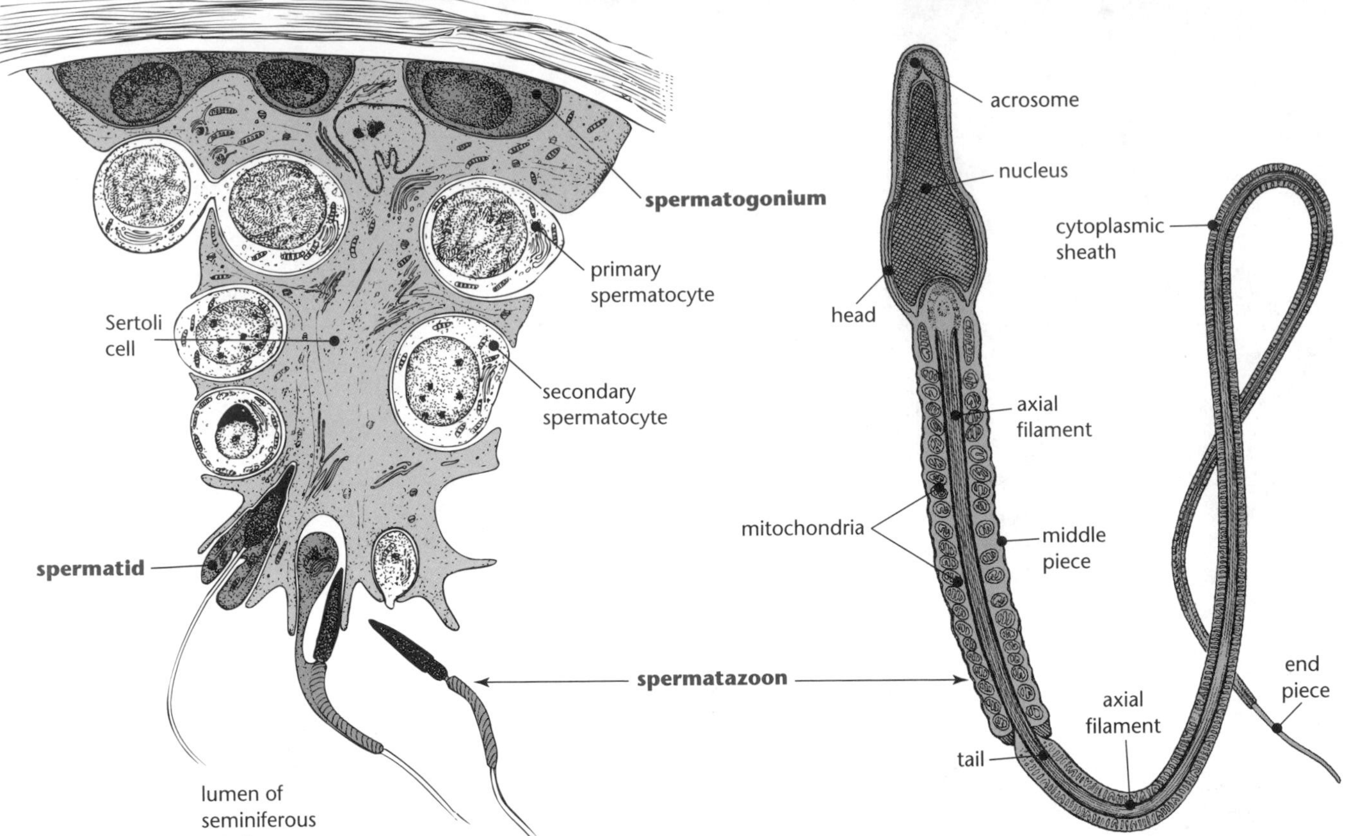

exposure to spermatozoa.

spermatolysis (sper-mă-tol′ĭ-sis) Destruction and dissolution of the spermatozoa.

spermatorrhea (sper-mă-to-re′ă) Abnormal involuntary discharge of semen without orgasm.

spermatoschesis (sper-mă-tos′kĕ-sis) Suppression of seminal discharge; nonsecretion of semen.

spermatotoxin (sper-mă-to-tok′sin) A cytotoxic antibody that destroys spermatozoa. Also called spermotoxin.

spermatozoa (sper-mă-to-zo′ă) Plural of spermatozoon.

spermatozoon (sper-mă-to-zo′on), *pl.* **spermatozo′a** The male sexual cell produced in the testes; a nucleated cell with a thin motile tail by means of which it migrates up the female reproductive passages where fertilization takes place.

spermaturia (sper-mă-tu′re-ă) See semenuria.

spermiation (sper-me-a′shun) The release of spermatozoa from the seminiferous epithelium.

spermicide (sper′mĭ-sīd) Any agent that destroys spermatozoa. Also called spermatocide.

spermiogenesis (sper-me-o-jen′ĕ-sis) The phase of spermatogenesis in which spermatids develop into spermatozoa.

spermolith (sper′mo-lith) A stone in the deferent (spermatic) duct.

spermotoxin (sper-mo-tok′sin) See spermatotoxin.

sphacelate (sfas′ĕ-lāt) To become gangrenous.

sphaceloderma (sfas-ĕ-lo-der′mă) Gangrene of the skin.

sphenion (sfe′ne-on) A craniometric point located at the tip of the sphenoid angle of the parietal bone.

sphenoid (sfe′noid) Wedge-shaped; denoting a large wedge-shaped bone at the base of the skull.

sphenoiditis (sfe-noi-di′tis) Inflammation of the sphenoid sinus.

sphenoidostomy (sfe-noi-dos′tŏ-me) Removal of a portion of the anterior wall of the sphenoid sinus.

sphenoidotomy (sfe-noi-dot′ŏ-me) Incision into the sphenoid sinus.

sphenopalatine (sfe-no-pal′ă-tin) Relating to the sphenoid and palatine bones.

sphenorbital (sfe-nor′bĭ-tal) Relating to the sphenoid bone and the orbit.

sphenosquamosal (sfe-no-skwa-mo′sal) Relating to the sphenoid bone and the thin portion of the temporal bone.

sphere (sfēr) A ball-shaped structure; a globular body.

attraction s. See astrosphere.

Morgagni's s.'s See Morgagni's globules, under globule.

spherocyte (sfēr-o-sīt) A red blood cell that appears spherical in the living state and has a diameter of less than 6 µm; it has a greater than normal density of hemoglobin and a decreased surface-to-volume ratio; characteristic of hereditary spherocytosis and certain other hemolytic anemias.

spherocytosis (sfēr-o-si-to′sis) The presence of red blood cells that are more spherical than biconcave, as in hemolytic anemia. Also called congenital spherocytic anemia.

spherule (sfēr′ūl) **1.** A small sphere. **2.** A minute, thick-walled, spherical structure containing many fungal spores; characteristic of the parasitic phase of *Coccidioides immitis.*

rod s. The miniature terminal part of the retinal rod cell that forms synaptic relationships with the processes of bipolar cells and horizontal cells of the retina.

sphincter (sfingk′ter) **1.** Any circular muscle that, when contracted, closes a natural body opening. **2.** A portion of a tubular structure that functions as a sphincter.

external anal s. A three-layered flat band of muscular fibers, elliptical in shape, surrounding the anal orifice; attached posteriorly to the coccyx and anteriorly to the central tendon of perineum.

internal anal s. A muscular ring surrounding about 2.5 cm of the anal canal; in contact with, but separate from, the external anal sphincter.

lower esophageal s. (LES) A high pressure zone in the distal portion of the esophagus where resting pressure is usually higher than pressure in the fundus of the stomach; acts as a barrier preventing the reflux of gastric contents; cannot be identified anatomically but its pressure can be measured and demonstrated; normally it straddles the diaphragm extending 1 to 3 cm below to 1 to 2 cm above the diaphragmatic hiatus.

pupillary s. A narrow circular band of muscle fibers, about 1 mm in width, in the pupillary margin of the iris.

pyloric s. A muscular ring formed by a thickening of the circular layer of the stomach at the pyloric orifice; it acts as a valve to close the pyloric lumen.

s. of bladder vesicular s., A thickening of the middle circular layer of the muscular fibers of the bladder, surrounding the internal urethral opening.

sphincteralgia (sfingk-ter-al′jă) Pain in a sphincter muscle, especially of the anus.

sphincteritis (sfingk-ter-i′tis) Inflammation of a sphincter, particularly the sphincter of the hepatopancreatic duct.

sphincterotomy (sfingk-ter-ot′ŏ-me) Surgical division of a sphincter muscle.

sphingolipid (sfing-go-lip′id) A group of lipids (e.g., ceramide, cerebroside, sphingomyelin, ganglioside) containing in their structure a long-chain, aliphatic base; found primarily in tissues of the central nervous system.

sphingolipidosis (sfing-go-lip-ĭ-do′sis) General term for a number of disorders marked by abnormal metabolism of sphingolipids.

cerebral s. Any of a group of inherited diseases caused by a disturbance of metabolism resulting in increased lipids in the brain and characterized by progressive decrease in vision leading to complete blindness (usually within two years), severe mental deterioration, retinal atrophy, convulsions, and paralysis; there are four types of the disorder: infantile (Tay-Sachs disease), early juvenile (Jansky-Bielschowsky disease), late juvenile (Spielmeyer-Vogt or Batten-Mayou disease), and adult (Kufs' disease).

sphingomyelin (sfing-go-mi′ĕ-lin) One of a group of phospholipids present in large quantities in brain and nerve tissue; on hydrolysis, it yields a fatty acid, phosphoric acid, choline, and the amino alcohol sphingosine.

sphingosine (sfing′go-sin) A complex amino alcohol; a constituent of cerebrosides.

sphygmic (sfig′mik) Relating to the pulse.

sphygmogram (sfig′mo-gram) A curve representing the arterial pulse, made with a sphygmograph.

sphygmograph (sfig′mo-graf) Instrument used to make a graphic representation (curve) of the arterial pulse.

sphygmography (sfig-mog′ră-fe) **1.** The graphic recording of the arterial pulse by means of the sphygmograph. **2.** A treatise on the pulse.

sphygmoid (sfig′moid) Resembling the pulse.

sphygmomanometer (sfig-mo-mă-nom′ĕ-ter) An instrument for measuring arterial blood pressure.

sphygmometer (sfig-mom′ĕ-ter) Sphygmomanometer.

sphygmophone (sfig′mo-fōn) An instrument for rendering audible the vibrations of each individual

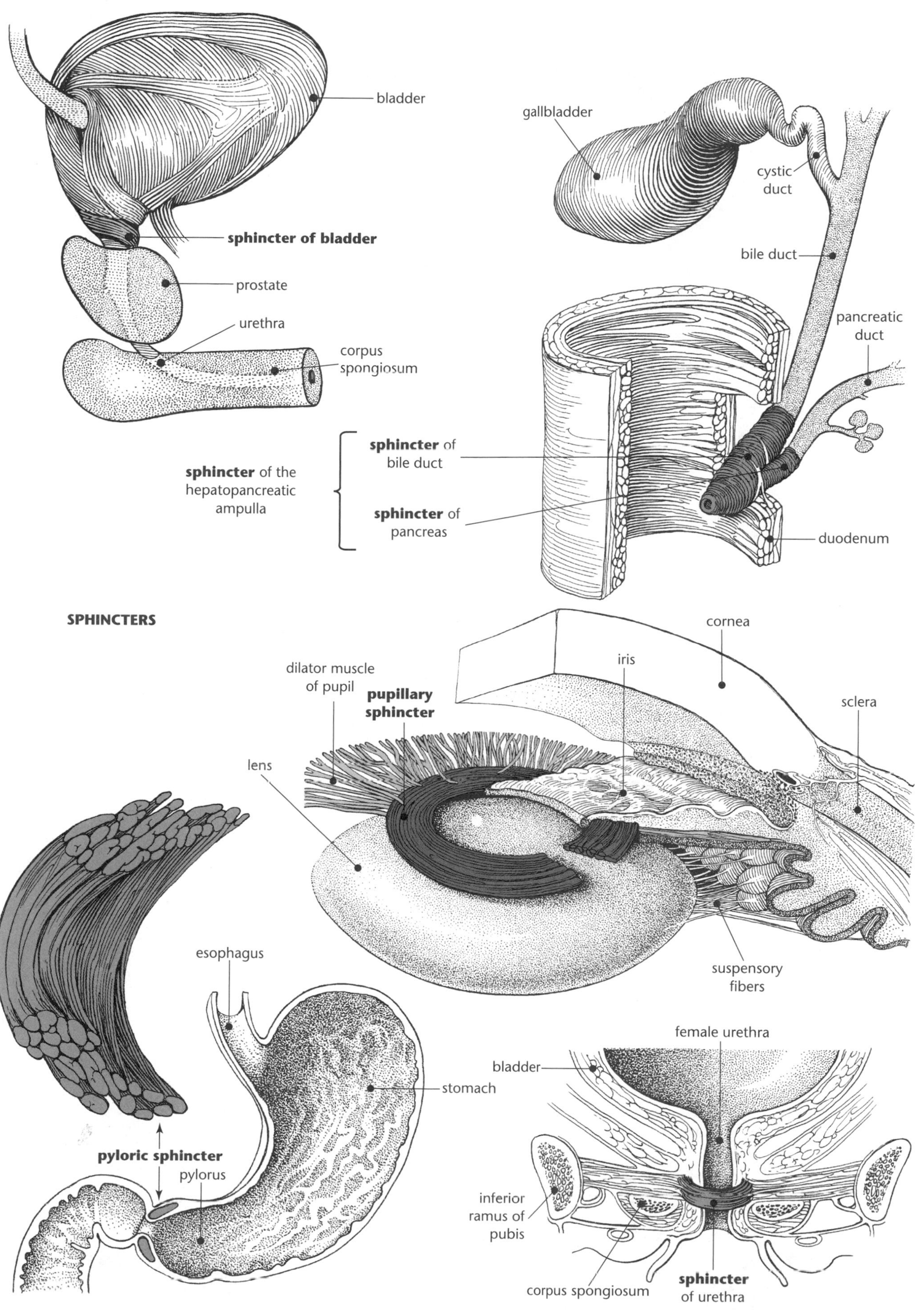
bladder
sphincter of bladder
prostate
urethra
corpus spongiosum
gallbladder
cystic duct
bile duct
pancreatic duct
sphincter of bile duct
sphincter of the hepatopancreatic ampulla
sphincter of pancreas
duodenum
SPHINCTERS
cornea
iris
dilator muscle of pupil
pupillary sphincter
sclera
lens
suspensory fibers
esophagus
stomach
pyloric sphincter
pylorus
female urethra
bladder
inferior ramus of pubis
corpus spongiosum
sphincter of urethra

S

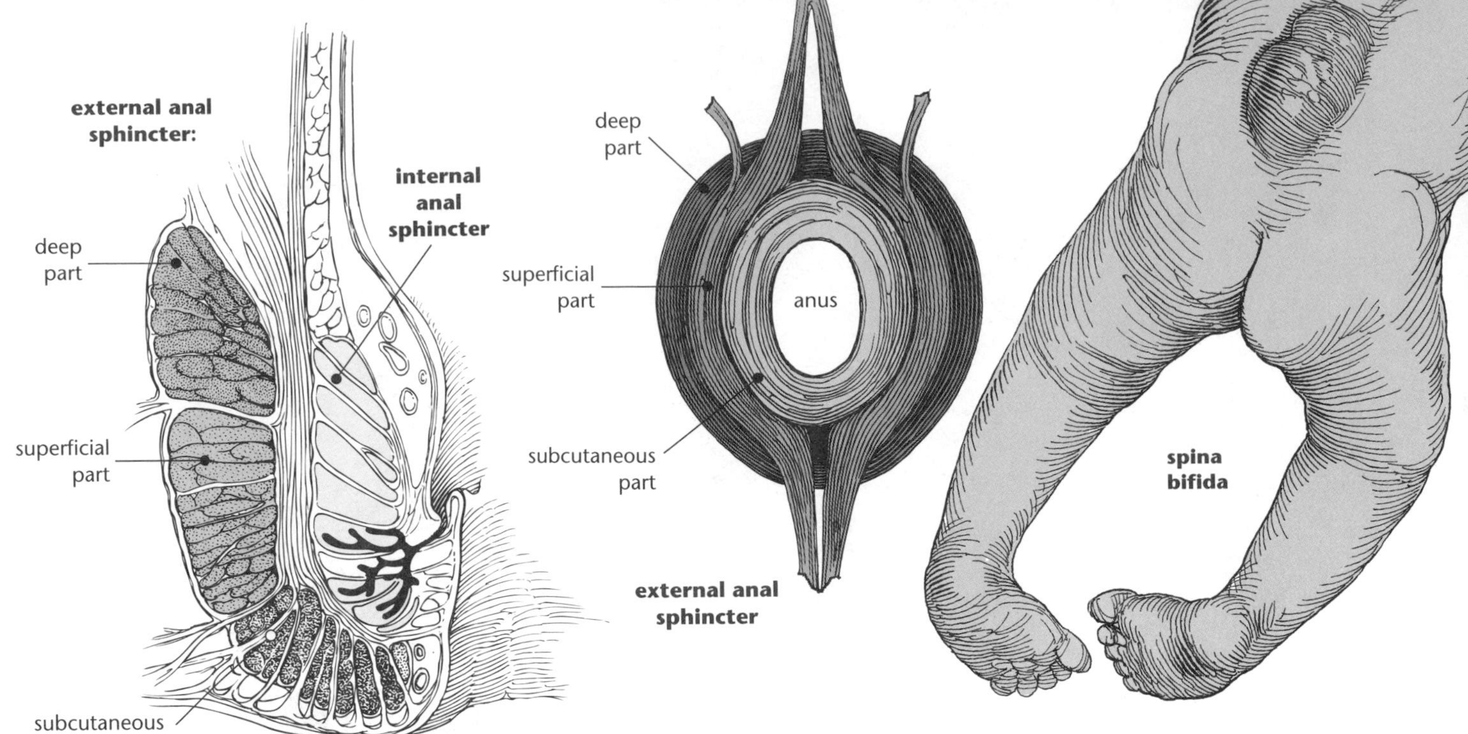

beat of the pulse.

sphygmoscope (sfig´mo-skōp) Instrument used to render the pulse beat visible.

spica (spi´kă) See spica bandage, under bandage.

spicule (spik´ūl) A small needle-shaped structure.

spider (spi´der) **1.** Any of numerous arachnids having four pairs of legs, usually eight eyes, a body divided into a cephalothorax and an abdomen, and a complex of web-spinning spinnerets that produce silk; some venomous spiders are the black widow (*Latrodectus mactans*), brown recluse (*Loxosceles reclusus*), Chilean brown (*Loxosceles laeta*), and red-legged widow (*Latrodectus bishopi*). **2.** Exhibiting a pattern suggestive of a spider or a spider's web.

arterial s. See spider telangiectasia, under telangiectasia.

Spielmeyer-Vogt disease (shpēl´mi-er-fōkt dĭ-zēz´) See cerebral sphingolipidosis, under sphingolipidosis.

spike (spīk) A brief electrical cerebral activity of 3 to 25 milliseconds' duration that is recorded on the electroencephalogram as a rising and falling vertical line.

spillway (spil´wa) The labial, buccal, and lingual embrasures or passageways through which food escapes from the occlusal surfaces of teeth during chewing.

spina (spī´na), *pl.* **spinae** **1.** The vertebral column. **2.** Any sharp projection.

S

s. bifida Congenital defect in which part of the vertebral column is absent; it allows the spinal membranes and sometimes the spinal cord to protrude.

s. bifida occulta Spina bifida without protrusion of the spinal cord or its membranes. Also called cryptomerorachischisis.

spinal (spī´nal) **1.** Relating to a spine. **2.** Relating to the vertebral column.

spindle (spin´dl) Any spindle-shaped or fusiform anatomic structure.

mitotic s. The fusiform figure characteristic of a dividing cell formed by protoplasmic fibers extending between the two asters, along which the chromosomes are distributed.

muscle s. Neuromuscular spindle.

neuromuscular s. Small bundle of delicate muscular fibers (intrafusal fibers) invested by a capsule within which the sensory nerve fibers terminate; they vary in length from 0.8 to 5 mm and have a fusiform appearance. Also called muscle proprioceptor.

tendon s. See Golgi tendon organ, under organ.

spine (spīn) **1.** A short projection of bone. **2.** See vertebral column, under column.

anterior nasal s. The anterior projection of the anterior crest of the maxilla.

bamboo s. The rigid spine typical of ankylosing spondilitis (ossification of spinal ligaments), so called because of the bamboo-shaped lipping of vertebral margins seen in x-ray films.

iliac s. One of the four spines of the ilium.

ischial s. A spine on the posterior aspect of the ischium near the posteroinferior border of the acetabulum.

mental s.'s See genial tubercles, under tubercle.

neural s. The middle spinous process of a typical vertebra.

vertebral s. See spinous process of vertebra, under process.

spinnbarkeit (spin´bar-kīt) A state of extreme stretchability of the cervical mucus which, when spread on a glass slide, dries in a fernlike pattern; indicative of ovulation; it peaks on the 14th day of the menstrual cycle. Also spelled spinnbarkheit.

spinobulbar (spi-no-bul´bar) Relating to the spine and the medulla oblongata.

spiradenoma (spīr-ad-ĕ-no´mă) A benign tumor or overdevelopment of sweat glands.

spiral (spī´ral) Circling around a fixed center; coiled.

Curschmann's s.'s Coiled masses of mucus sometimes found in the sputum of patients with bronchial asthma.

spirillosis (spi-rĭ-lo´sis) Any disease caused by bacteria of the family Spirillaceae.

Spirillum (spi-ril´um) A genus (family Spirillaceae) of flagellated spiral or corkscrew-shaped bacteria, found in fresh and salt waters that contain organic material.

spirit (spir´it) **1.** An alcohol solution of a volatile substance. **2.** Archaic term denoting any liquid produced by distillation. **3.** Used in the plural, an alcoholic beverage.

pyroxylic s. See methyl alcohol, under alcohol.

Spirochaeta (spi-ro-ke´tă) A genus of nonflagellated microorganisms with a slender wavy shape; found in sewage and stagnant water.

spirochete (spī´ro-kēt) Any organism of the genus *Spirochaeta.*

spirochetosis (spi-ro-ke-to´sis) Any infection caused by a spirochete, such as syphilis.

spirogram (spi´ro-gram) The tracing made by a spirometer.

spirograph (spi´ro-graf) A device for graphically recording the depth and rapidity of respiratory movements.

spirometer (spi-rom´ĕ-ter) Device for measuring the rate and volume of breathing; it records the volume of air and the time used to complete both inspiration and expiration.

spironolactone (sper-o-no-lak´tōn) A drug that acts directly on the renal tubules to block the action of aldosterone, producing sodium loss with potassium retention; used to minimize the lowering of potassium levels induced by the thiazides or other potassium-losing diuretics; Aldactone®.

spissated (spis´āt-ed) Thickened by evaporation or absorption of fluid.

spittle (spit´l) Saliva.

splanchnectopia (splank-nek-to´pe-ă) Malposition of any of the abdominal organs.

splanchnic (splank´nik) Pertaining to the viscera.

splanchnicectomy (splank-ne-sek´tŏ-me) Surgical resection of a portion of the greater splanchnic nerve.

splanchnicotomy (splank-ne-kot´ŏ-me) Surgical transection of a splanchnic nerve or nerves.

splanchnocele (splank´no-sēl) **1.** Hernia of an abdominal organ. **2.** The embryonic body cavity.

splanchnomegaly (splank-no-meg´ă-le) Abnormal largeness of abdominal organs.

splay (splā) **1.** To make a longitudinal cut through, and spread open, the end of a tubular structure to increase its diameter. **2.** The deviation between the expected and the observed performance of the renal tubules due to variations in individual nephrons (e.g., the appearance of glucose in the urine before the theoretical tubular maximum is reached).

splayfoot (splā´foot) See flatfoot.

spleen (splēn) A large vascular lymphatic organ situated in the abdominal cavity on the left side below the diaphragm; it is the sole lymphatic tissue specialized to filter blood; it removes effete or worn out cells from the circulatory system, converts hemoglobin to bilirubin, and releases iron into the blood for reuse. Also called lien.

accessory s. A mass of splenic tissue sometimes found attached to the spleen or in one of the peritoneal folds.

sago s. A spleen containing deposits of amyloid.

splenectomy (sple-nek´tŏ-me) Surgical removal of the spleen.

spleneolus (sple-ne´o-lus) Accessory spleen.

splenic (splen´ik) Relating to the spleen.

splenic flexure syndrome (splen´ik flek´sher sin´drōm) Painful discomfort in the upper left abdomen which may radiate to the area over the heart and to the left shoulder; believed to be due to distention or spasmodic contraction of the colon.

splenitis (sple-ni´tis) Inflammation of the spleen.

splenium (sple´ne-um) A body structure resembling a bandaged part.

s. of corpus callosum The round, thick, posterior part of the corpus callosum of the brain.

splenocele (sple´no-sēl) **1.** Hernial protrusion of the spleen. **2.** A splenic tumor.

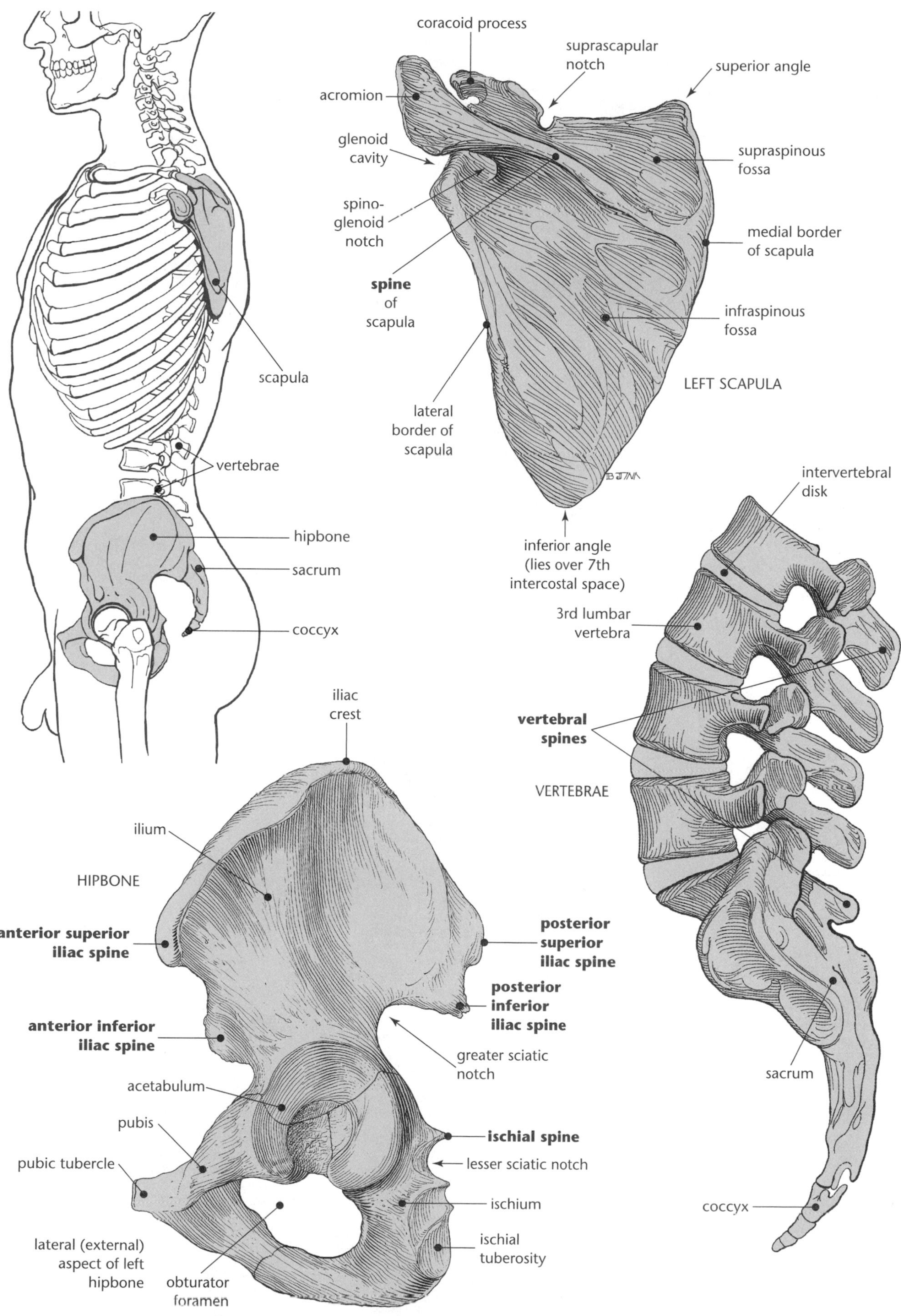

coracoid process
suprascapular notch
superior angle
acromion
glenoid cavity
supraspinous fossa
spino-glenoid notch
medial border of scapula
spine of scapula
infraspinous fossa
scapula
LEFT SCAPULA
lateral border of scapula
vertebrae
intervertebral disk
hipbone
inferior angle (lies over 7th intercostal space)
sacrum
3rd lumbar vertebra
coccyx
iliac crest
vertebral spines
VERTEBRAE
ilium
HIPBONE
anterior superior iliac spine
posterior superior iliac spine
posterior inferior iliac spine
anterior inferior iliac spine
greater sciatic notch
sacrum
acetabulum
pubis
ischial spine
pubic tubercle
lesser sciatic notch
ischium
coccyx
lateral (external) aspect of left hipbone
obturator foramen
ischial tuberosity

S

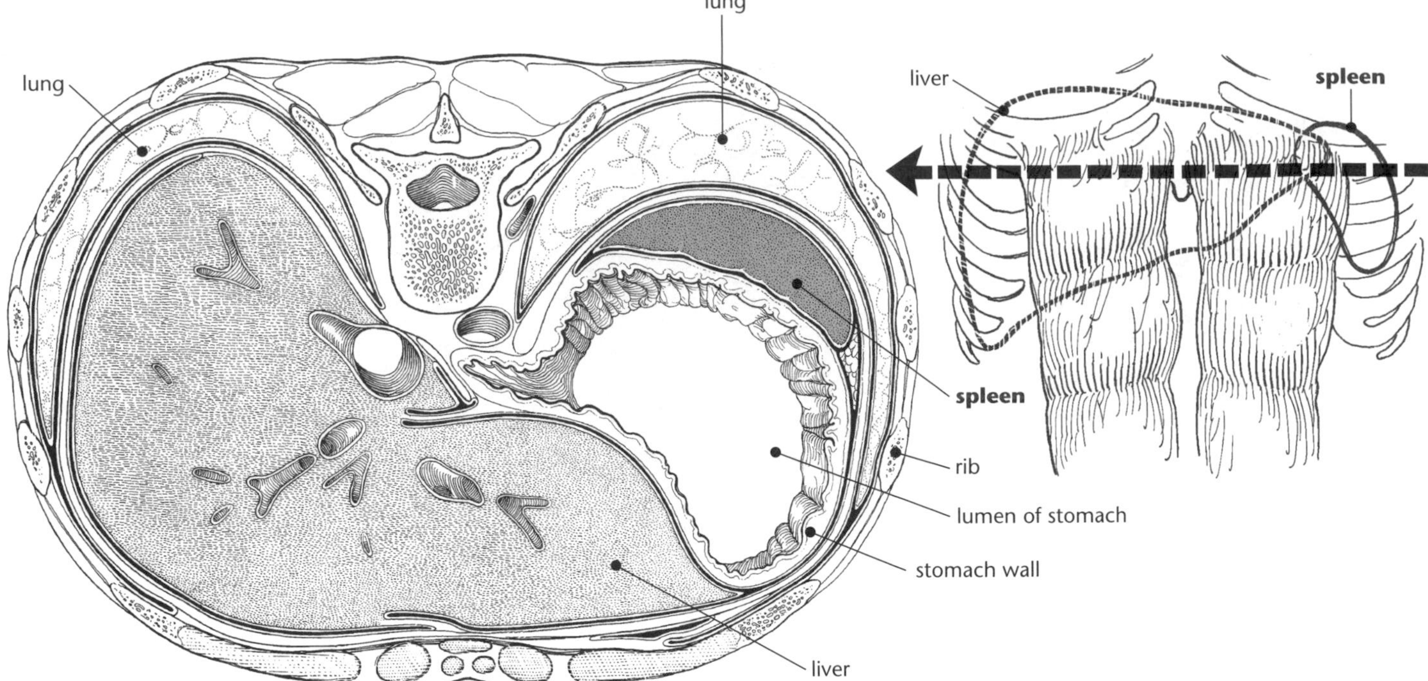

splenocolic (sple-no-kol′ik) Relating to the spleen and colon (e.g., the peritoneal fold connecting the two organs).

splenocyte (splen´o-sīt) A large, phagocytic, mononuclear white blood cell of the spleen; a splenic macrophage.

splenogram (sple´no-gram) A roentgenogram of the spleen.

splenogranulomatosis (sple-no-gran-u-lo-mă-to′sis) A granulomatous condition of the spleen with enlargement of the organ and thickening of the capsule.

splenohepatomegaly (sple-no-hep-ă-to-meg´ă-le) Abnormal enlargement of the spleen and the liver.

splenolysis (sple-nol´ĭ-sis) Destruction (lysis) of spleen tissue.

splenomalacia (sple-no-mă-la´shă) Pathologic softening of the spleen.

splenomegaly, splenomegalia (sple-no-meg′ă-le, sple-no-me-ga′le-ă) Enlargement of the spleen. Also called megalosplenia.

chronic congestive s. Disorder usually following hypertension of the portal vein, marked by splenic enlargement, anemia, and occasional gastrointestinal bleeding; leukopenia and thrombocytopenia may develop in some cases. Also called Banti's syndrome.

tropical s. See visceral leishmaniasis, under leishmaniasis.

S

splenonephric (sple-no-nef′rik) See splenorenal.

splenopancreatic (sple-no-pan-kre-at´ik) Relating or belonging to the spleen and the pancreas.

splenopathy (sple-nop´ă-the) Any disease or disorder of the spleen.

splenophrenic (sple-no-fren´ik) Relating to the spleen and the diaphragm.

splenoportogram (sple-no-por´to-gram) X-ray image of the splenic and portal veins obtained after injection of radiopaque material into the spleen.

splenoptosis sple-nop-to′sis) Abnormal mobility of the spleen resulting in downward displacement.

splenorenal (sple-no-re′nal) Relating to the spleen and the kidney. Also called splenonephric.

splenorrhagia (sple-no-ra´jă) Bleeding from a ruptured spleen.

splenosis (sple-no′sis) The presence of numerous nodules composed of splenic tissue throughout the peritoneal cavity. Distinguished from accessory spleen by the absence of elastic or smooth muscle fibers in their covering capsules.

splenotomy (sple-not´ŏ-me) Incision into the spleen.

splenotoxin (sple-no-tok′sin) A cytotoxin that has a particular affinity for the cells of the spleen.

splint (splint) A device used to immobilize, support, and correct injured, displaced, or deformed structures.

acrylic s. A splint covering only the labial and lingual (outside and inside) surfaces of teeth and connected around the last molar by continuous acrylic material or a wire; used only to anchor fractured jaws of children with deciduous teeth.

acrylic resin bite-guard s. An appliance used to eliminate movement of teeth.

airplane s. Splint designed to hold the arm in abduction at shoulder level.

Balkan s. See Balkan frame, under frame.

cast cap s. A one-piece metal appliance, cemented over the crowns of teeth to immobilize the fragments of a fractured jaw.

cervical s. Splint for supporting the head, thus taking some pressure off the cervical area.

Cramer's s. See ladder splint.

Denis Browne s. A splint used to correct clubfoot, consisting of two padded metal plates that are securely fastened to the infant's feet and connected by a metal crossbar.

Frejka s. A pillow splint used to correct dislocations of the hip in infants under the age of 12 months.

Hodgen's s. Splint designed for a fractured femur, essentially used to apply balanced traction.

ladder s. A flexible splint resembling a ladder; consists of two parallel wires connected with a series of fine wires. Also called Cramer's splint.

open-cap s. A cast cap splint that does not cover the occlusal surface of teeth.

palatal s. Splint applied to the palate and fastened to the upper teeth by clasps or wires; used to hold tissue flaps in place for 48 hours after removal of a maxillary bony growth (torus) from the hard palate; thereafter the splint is worn as a removable bandage until the wound heals.

plaster s. Splint made of gauze impregnated with plaster of Paris.

Thomas' s. Splint used to immobilize the leg, consisting of an iron ring that fits on the upper thigh (near the groin) connected to a continuous iron bar that has a W shape at the opposite end.

treatment s. Temporary artificial tooth or teeth that protect and hold in position the teeth adjacent to the space while the fixed partial denture is being constructed.

splinting (splint-ing) **1.** The application of a rigid device to a limb to prevent motion of a dislocated joint or the ends of a fractured bone. **2.** In dentistry, the linking of two or more teeth with a fixed restoration. **3.** Protection against pain by reducing motion of the painful part (e.g., the shallow breathing and fixed position assumed by a patient to reduce pain in his chest).

splitting (split′ing) In chemistry, the conversion of a complex substance into two or more simpler products.

spodogenous (spo-doj´ĕ-nus) Resulting from accumulation of waste material in an organ.

spodography (spo-dog′ra-fe) See microincineration.

spondylarthritis (spon-dil-ar-thri´tis) Inflammation of one or more intervertebral articulations.

spondylitis (spon-dĭ-li′tis) Inflammation of one or more vertebrae.

ankylosing s. Ossification of the ligaments of the spine with involvement of the hips and shoulders. Also called Marie-Strümpell disease; rheumatoid spondylitis.

rheumatoid s. See ankylosing spondylitis.

tuberculous s. Tuberculosis of the spine with anterior erosion of vertebral bodies and abscess formation. Also called Pott's disease.

spondylolisthesis (spon-dĭ-lo-lis´the-sis) Forward slippage of one vertebra over another, usually of a lumbar vertebra on the vertebra below it, or upon the sacrum. Also called spondyloptosis.

spondylolysis (spon-dĭ-lol´ĭ-sis) Breaking down or destruction of a vertebra.

spondylopathy (spon-dĭ-lop′ă-the) Any disorder of the vertebrae. Also called rachiopathy.

spondyloptosis (spon-dĭ-lop-to´sis) See spondylolisthesis.

spondylopyosis (spon-dĭ-lo-pi-o′sis) Suppurative inflammation of the body of a vertebra.

spondyloschisis (spon-dĭ-los′kĭ-sis) Congenital fissure of the vertebral column. Also called rachischisis.

spondylosis (spon-dĭ-lo′sis) Abnormal immobility and fixation of a vertebral joint.

sponge (spunj) **1.** The light fibrous skeleton of certain aquatic animals used as an absorbent. **2.** A folded piece of gauze or cotton.

absorbable gelatin s. A sterile, absorbable, water-insoluble gelatin-based sponge, used in surgery to control bleeding.

spongiform (spun′jĭ-form) Resembling a sponge.

spongioblast (spun′je-o-blast) An embryonic cell of the supportive (non-neuronal) component of the central nervous system.

spongioblastoma (spun-je-o-blas-to′mă) Tumor composed mainly of spongioblasts.

spongiocyte (spun´je-o-sīt) **1.** A cell of the supportive tissue of the central nervous system. **2.** One of the vacuolated cells situated in the cortex of the adrenal gland.

spongiositis (spun-je-o-si′tis) Inflammation of the corpus spongiosum of the penis.

spontaneous (spon-ta´ne-us) Arising without

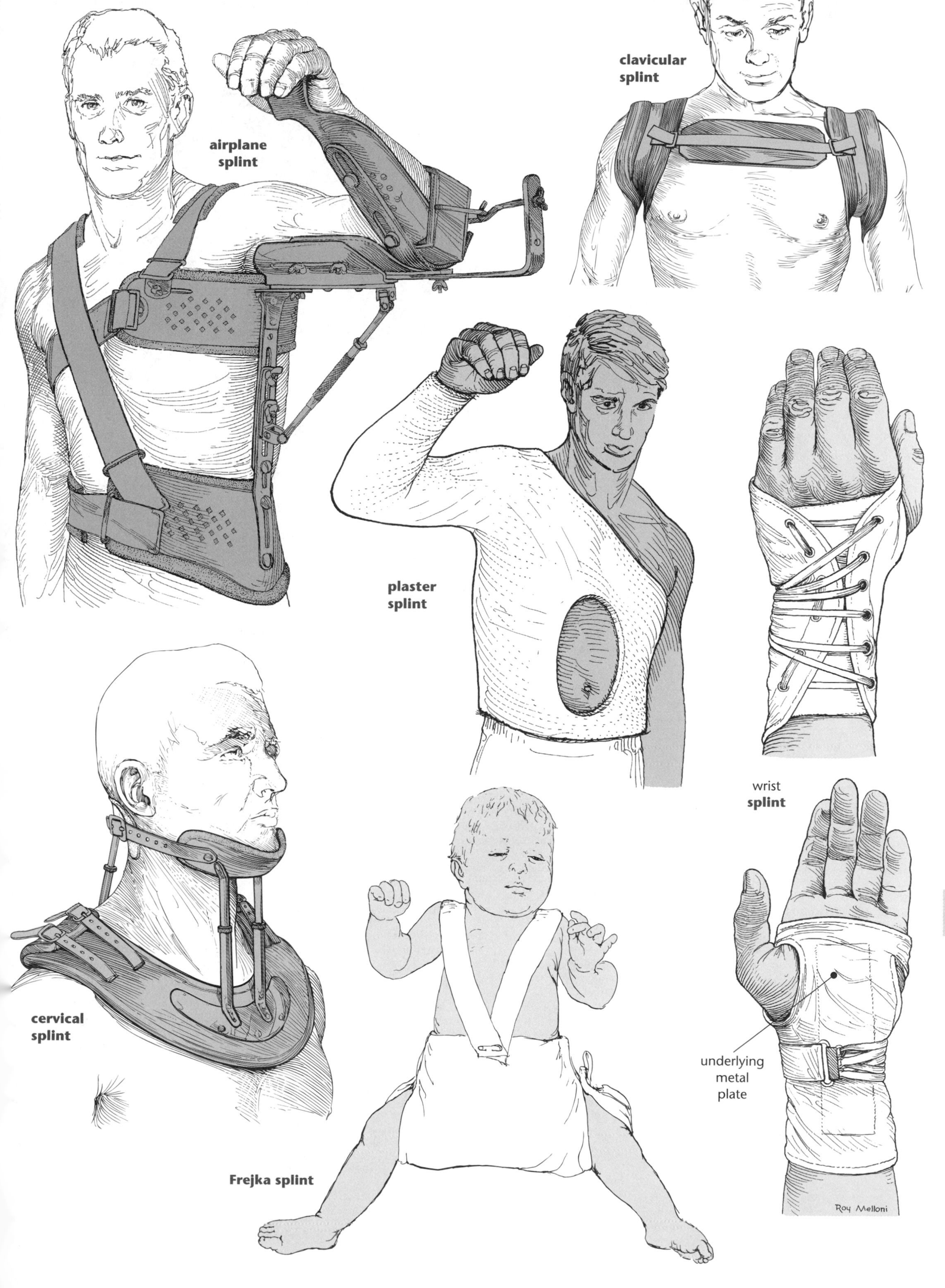

airplane splint
clavicular splint
plaster splint
wrist splint
cervical splint
Frejka splint
underlying metal plate
Roy Melloni

S

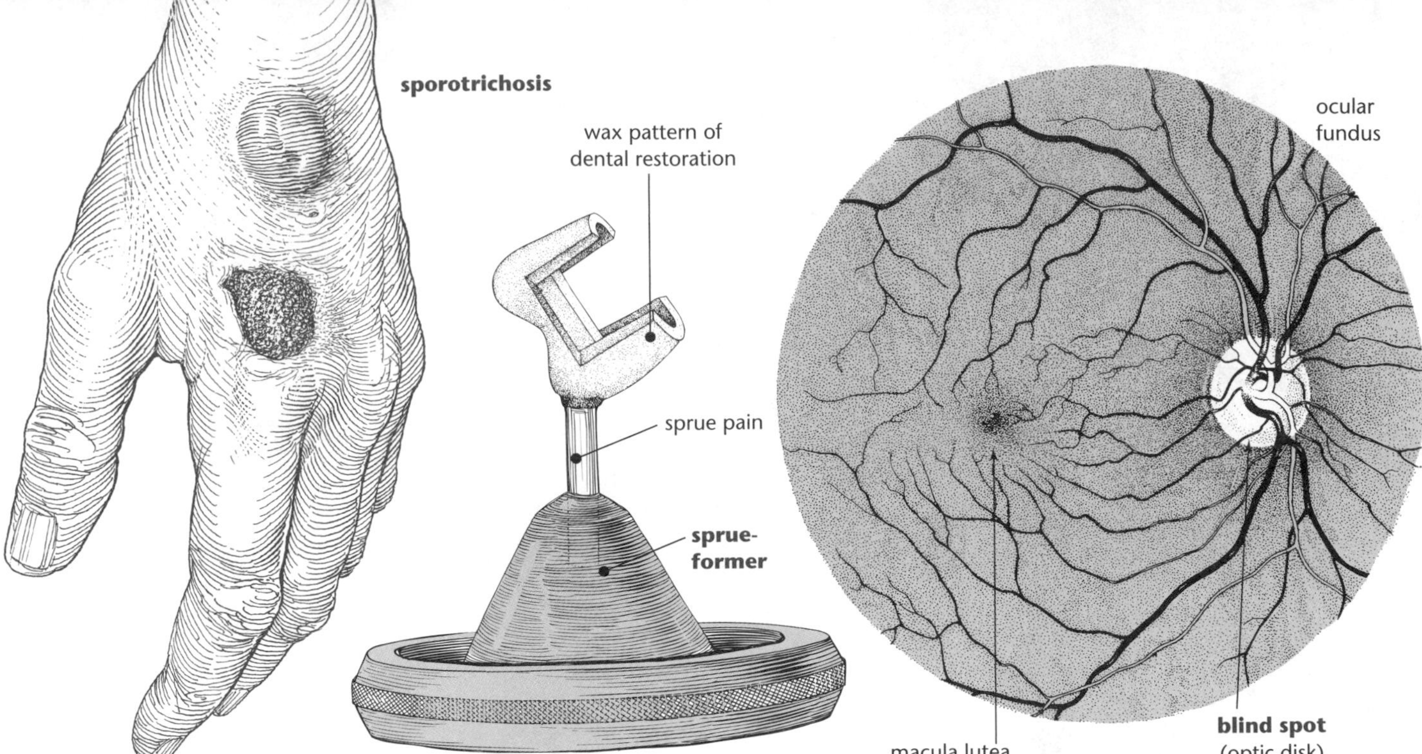

apparent cause.

spoon (spōōn) **1.** An implement consisting of a small, shallow, oval bowl on a handle. **2.** A slang expression for a measure of pure heroin, about 1/16 ounce.

cataract s. An instrument used for removing a cataractous lens from the eye.

sharp s. A sharp-edged spoon used for scraping away granulations, carious bone, or other diseased tissue.

sporadic (spo-rad´ik) **1.** Occurring infrequently or at irregular intervals. **2.** Not widespread.

sporangia (spo-ran´je-ă) Plural of sporangium.

sporangiophore (spo-ran´je-o-fōr) A fungal structure that bears one or more sporangia.

sporangium (spo-ran´je-um), *pl.* **sporangia** A capsule or encystment within a plant in which spores are produced.

spore (spōr) A primitive, thick walled, usually unicellular reproductive cell that is capable of giving rise to a new plant.

sporicide (spo´rĭ-sīd) A substance that destroys spores.

sporidium (spor´ĭ-de-um) The spore stage of a protozoan organism.

sporoblast (spor´o-blast) An early stage in the development of a sporocyst, from which sporozoites later develop.

sporocyst (spor´o-sist) A stage in the life cycle of many protozoa in which two or more parasites are enclosed within a common wall.

sporogenesis (spor-o-jen´ĕ-sis) The production of spores.

sporogony (spo-roj´ĕ-ne) A sexual cycle of certain protozoans in which spores are produced as a result of sexual fusion of gametes prior to multiple fission.

sporont (spo´ront) A sexually mature protozoan parasite.

sporotrichosis (spo-ro-tri-ko´sis) A fungal disease usually affecting cutaneous, subcutaneous, and lymphatic tissues; caused by *Sporotrichum schenkii*.

Sporotrichum (spo-rot´rĭ-kum) A genus of cigar-shaped parasitic fungi.

S. schenkii A species that is the cause of sporotrichosis in man and animals.

Sporozoa (spo-ro-zo´ă) A class of the phylum Protozoa that includes parasitic organisms that reproduce by spores.

sporozoan (spo-ro-zo´an) A member of the class Sporozoa.

sporozoite (spo-ro-zo´īt) The infectious stage in the life cycle of sporozoan organisms; one of the minute elongated bodies formed by division of the encysted zygote (oocyst); in malaria, forms of the plasmodium organism are concentrated in the salivary glands of mosquitoes and transferred to man in the act of feeding.

sporozoon (spo-ro-zo´on) See sporozoan.

sporulate (spor´u-lāt) To produce spores.

sporulation (spor-u-la´shun) Reproduction by spores.

sporule (spor´ūl) A minute spore.

spot (spot) **1.** A small area of discoloration. **2.** To discharge a small amount of blood from the vagina.

blind s. The area in the eye, insensitive to light, where the optic nerve leaves the retina. See also scotoma; optic disk, under disk.

café au lait s.'s Hyperpigmented light brown patches on the skin, as seen in neurofibromatosis.

cherry red s. See Tay's cherry red spot.

cotton-wool s. See cotton-wool patch, under patch.

Koplik's s.'s One of the signs of measles; minute bluish white lesions surrounded by a bright ring on the mucous membrane of the cheeks, occurring about two days before the appearance of the skin rash.

liver s.'s See senile lentigo, under lentigo.

mongolian s. A type of blue nevus of infants, appearing as a dark blue-to-brown spot 2 to 15 cm in diameter over the sacrum; usually disappears in childhood.

rose s.'s Pinkish spots on the abdomen, seen in the early stages of typhoid fever.

Roth's s.'s Round white spots sometimes seen in the retina of patients with bacterial endocarditis.

soft s. See fontanel.

Tay's cherry red s. The cherry red spot in the macular area of the retina, seen in patients with Tay-Sachs disease.

yellow s. See macula retinae.

sprain (sprān) The overstretching or partial tearing of a ligament connecting two bones of a joint.

spray (spra) **1.** A jet of liquid droplets. **2.** To sprinkle.

sprue (sproo) **1.** A malabsorptive disorder. **2.** In dentistry, the wax or metal used to form the opening through which a material such as gold or resin is poured into a mold to make a casting; also the waste piece of material that fills the opening.

celiac s. See celiac disease.

nontropical s. See celiac disease.

tropical s. Disease occurring in certain tropical areas, characterized by abnormal small bowel structure and malabsorption; unlike celiac disease, it is not associated with gluten intolerance but is caused by vitamin deficiencies and/or bacterial contamination of the intestines; it responds to treatment with folic acid, sometimes supplemented by antibiotics. COMPARE: celiac disease.

sprue-former (sproo-for´mer) In dentistry, the cone-shaped base to which the sprue pin is anchored while the wax pattern is being invested.

spur (spur) A spinelike projection from a bone or a horny outgrowth from the skin.

calcaneal s. A bony outgrowth from the plantar surface of the calcaneous (heel bone) which often causes pain when walking. Also called heel spur.

heel s. See calcaneal spur.

sputum (spu´tum) Matter ejected from the air passages. Also called expectoration.

squalene (skwa´lēn) An unsaturated terpene hydrocarbon found in shark liver oil and an intermediate in the biosynthesis of cholesterol; present in small amounts in blood plasma.

squama (skwa´mă), *pl.* **squa´mae** **1.** A thin plate of bone. **2.** A scalelike structure.

squamomastoid (skwa-mo-mas´toid) Relating to the squamous and mastoid portions of the temporal bone.

squamopetrosal (skwa-mo-pe-tro´sal) Relating to the squamous and petrous parts of the temporal bone.

squamosa (skwa-mo´să) The scalelike portion (squama) of the temporal bone.

squamous (skwa´mus) **1.** Scaly; covered with scales. **2.** Resembling scales.

squint (skwint) See strabismus.

$S_1S_2S_3$ syndrome (ĕs 1, ĕs 2, ĕs 3 sin´drōm) Prominent S waves in the three standard limb leads with a small R´ deflection in V_1 and a normal QRS interval; most commonly seen in young adults without heart disease, but may also be seen in right ventricular hypertrophy, and occasionally with acute myocardial infarction.

stab (stab) To pierce or wound with a pointed instrument or weapon.

stabile (sta´bīl, sta´bil) **1.** Fixed; immobile. **2.** Resistant to chemical change.

stability (stă-bil´ĭ-te) **1.** The condition of being resistant to change. **2.** The ability of a denture to resist displacement by functional forces.

dimensional s. The property of a material to retain its shape.

stabilizer (sta´bil-ī-zer) **1.** An instrument employed in an x-ray unit to render constant the milliamperage output of the x ray. **2.** Any substance used to maintain the equilibrium or velocity of a chemical reaction.

stable (sta´bl) Denoting a balanced condition, resisting alteration.

staff (staf) **1.** The professional personnel of an institution such as a hospital. **2.** See director (2).

attending s. Physicians who are members of a hospital staff and regularly see their patients at the hospital; may also supervise members of the house staff, fellows, and medical students.

consulting s. Specialists in a particular medical field, affiliated with a hospital, who serve in an

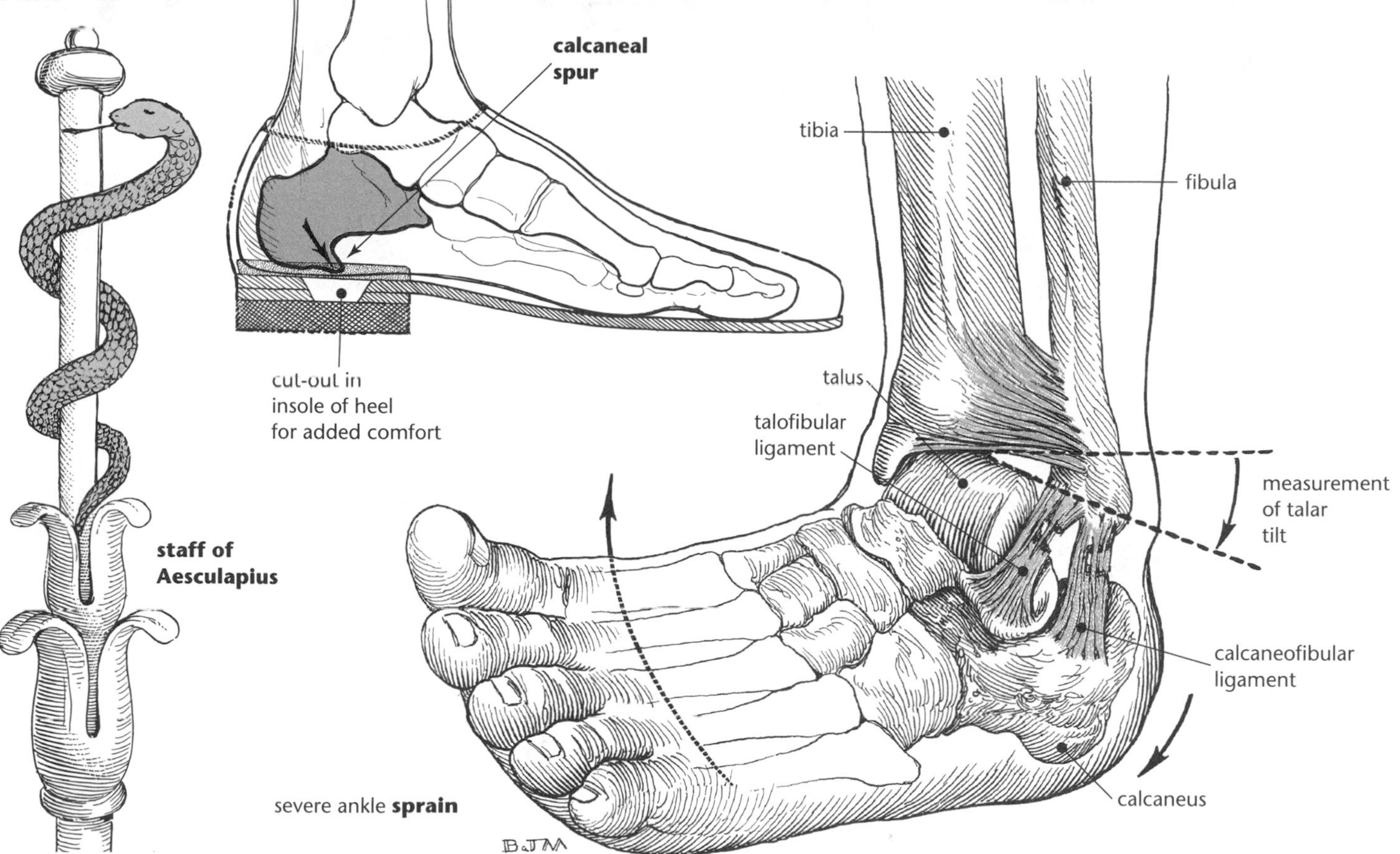

advisory role to the attending physician.

house s. The resident or junior physicians and surgeons of a hospital.

staff of Aesculapius (staf ŭv es-ku-la′pe-us) A rod encircled by a single snake (without wings); symbol of the medical profession and emblem of the American Medical Association.

stage (stāj) A phase in the course of a disease or the life cycle of an organism. **2.** The platform of a microscope on which the slide is placed for viewing.

anal s. Stage in infantile psychosexual development during which interest is focused on elimination and retention of feces. Also called anal phase.

exoerythrocytic s. Stage in the life cycle of the malarial parasite (*Plasmodium*) outside of the red blood cells of the host.

incubative s. See incubation period, under period.

latent s. See latent period (a), under period.

mechanical s. Device attached to, or built into, the stage of a microscope that permits moving of the specimen slide while holding it in the plane of focus.

Oedipal s. Stage in psychosexual development following the phallic stage in which the child has an erotic attachment to the parent of the opposite sex. Also called Oedipal phase.

oral s. Stage of infantile psychosexual development (from birth to approximately 12 months); divided into oral erotic, associated with the pleasurable sensation of sucking, and oral sadistic, related to aggressive biting. Also called oral phase.

phallic s. Stage in psychosexual development (usually between the ages of 3 and 6) during which the child becomes aware of his/her genital sexuality.

prodromal s. The early stage of a disease, following the incubation period, in which some clinical manifestations appear but before characteristic symptoms and signs of the disease are noted.

psychosexual s.'s Stages of development of infantile sexuality, as elaborated in psychoanalytic theory (oral, anal, phallic, Oedipal).

resting s. See interphase.

separation-individuation s. Stage in personality (around 18 months) when the child begins to develop his/her own sense of self as an autonomous person.

symbiotic s. Earliest stage in personality development during which the child just barely sees itself as separate from its environment and perceives the self and parent (usually mother) as a single omnipotent being.

s.'s of labor See under labor.

staging (sta′jing) A clinical method of providing an estimate of the gravity of a cancerous tumor, based on the size of the primary tumor and the extent of local and distant spread.

Breslow's s. See Breslow classification, under classification.

Clark's s. See Clark's classification, under classification.

Gleason's s. See Gleason's grading system, under system.

TNM (tumor-node-metastasis) s. An international system for staging tumors, used as a basis for treating cancer; it measures three basic parameters: T for the size and local invasion of the primary tumor, N for the number of involved lymph nodes, M for the presence of metastasis; each letter is followed by a number, from 0 through 4, to indicate the extent of involvement. Lowercase letters are sometimes added as a means of providing additional information: aTNM (autopsy staging), cTNM (clinical-diagnostic staging), pTNM (post-surgical pathologic staging), rTNM (retreatment staging), sTNM (surgical-evaluation staging).

stain (stān) **1.** Any dye used to render cells and tissues visible for microscopic study. **2.** To impart color to cells and tissues for microscopic examination. **3.** A superficial discoloration of the skin.

acid s. A dye salt whose acid radical combines with the basic (alkaline) components of cells; it stains mainly the protoplasm.

aldehyde fuchsin s. A stain containing potassium permanganate, sulfuric acid, sodium bisulfate, fuchsin, and paraldehyde; used to demonstrate elastic fibers, beta cells of islets of Langerhans, and basement membranes.

basic s. A dye salt whose basic (alkaline) radical combines with the acidic components of cells; it stains mainly the nuclei.

contrast s. See counterstain.

differential s. A dye that stains tissues nonselectively but can be extracted with a solvent at different rates to facilitate differentiation of elements in a specimen.

Giemsa s. A stain consisting of azure II eosin, azure II, and glycerin dissolved in methanol; used for staining blood cells, Negri bodies, and certain protozoan parasites, and for staining chromosomes to demonstrate characteristic banding patterns.

Golgi s. A heavy metal stain used to enhance the cytoarchitectural appearance of nervous tissue; usually the metal (silver or gold) becomes impregnated along the membranes or within neurons or neuroglia.

Gram's s., Gram's method Method used to classify bacteria, based on the ability of the organisms to retain a basic dye (crystal violet); those retaining the violet stain are gram- positive and those that do not retain it are gram-negative.

H&E s. See hematoxylin and eosin stain.

hematoxylin and eosin s. A water solution of hematoxylin and eosin; it stains cytoplasm pink and nuclei blue; used widely for routine examination of tissues. Also called H&E stain.

intravital s. A dye that is taken up by living cells after intravenous or subcutaneous administration.

Janus-green B s. A supravital stain used to demonstrate mitochondria.

Mallory's trichrome s. Stain suitable for demonstrating connective tissue.

metachromatic s. A stain that produces different colors in varied cell elements.

Nissl s. See Nissl's method, under method.

oil red O s. Oil red O in isopropyl alcohol; it stains lipid a cherry red color.

orcein s. A natural dye used to demonstrate elastic fibers and membranes.

osmic acid s. Aqueous solution of osmic acid (OsO_4) used in electron microscopy as a fixative and stain.

Papanicolaou s. Stain employed on smears of body secretions to detect the presence of malignancy; consists generally of aqueous hematoxylin with multiple counterstaining dyes in ethyl alcohol.

periodic acid-Schiff s., PAS s. A tissue stain for demonstration of polysaccharides and mucopolysaccharides of epithelial mucins, basement membranes, and connective tissue.

port-wine s. See nevus flammeus, under nevus.

potassium dichromate s. A stain used to demonstrate catecholamine granules of the adrenal medulla and paraganglionic cells.

silver and gold impregnation s. Solutions of silver and gold compounds used to demonstrate reticular fibers, collagenous connective tissue, Golgi

Stain	demonstrates
acid stain acid-fast stain	pancreatic alpha cells acid-free bacteria
alcian blue stain	mucoproteins
aldehyde fuchsin	elastic fibers basement membranes beta cells of islets of Langerhans neuro secretion mast cell granules thyrotrophs
azan stain	nuclei of cells muscle fibers collagen
basic stain	nuclei of cells
Best's carmine stain	glycogen
brilliant cresyl blue stain	platelets reticulocytes
Feulgen nuclear reaction stain	chromatin
Giemsa stain	blood, spleen, and bone marrow certain protozoan parasites
Golgi stain	nerve tissue
hematoxylin and eosin stain	cytoplasm and nuclei of cells muscle fibers collagen
Janus-green stain	mitochondria
Mallory's stain	collagen reticular fibers elastic fibers nuclei neuroglia
Nissl stain	cell bodies of neuron dendrites of neuron
oil red O stain	lipids
orcein stain	elastic fibers
osmic acid stain	lipids myelin Golgi apparatus
periodic acid-Schiff stain	glycoproteins glycogen basement membranes granules in some pituitary cells
picric acid and carmine stain	collagenous fibers epithelium muscle fibers
potassium dichromate stain	catecholamine granules of the adrenal medulla and paraganglionic cells
silver and gold impregnation stain	reticular fibers collagenous connective tissue Golgi apparatus neurofibrils
Sudan stain	lipids myelin
Toluidine blue stain	nucleic and cytoplasmic ribonucleic acid cartilage matrix mast cell granules basophilic granules Nissl bodies
van Gieson's stain	connective tissue
von Kossa's stain	calcium salts in bone
Weigert's stain	elastic fibers nerve fibers
Wright's stain	bone marrow erythrocytes eosinophils basophils neutrophils malarial parasites
Ziehl-Neelsen stain	tubercle bacilli

apparatus, and neurofibrils.

Sudan s.'s Oil-soluble compounds used for demonstrating lipids.

supravital s. A relatively nontoxic dye (neutral red) used to study living cells.

tumor s. In radioscopy, a dense area in an x-ray film indicating accumulation of contrast material in abnormal distorted blood vessels, thought to represent a tumor.

vital s. A dye introduced into a living organism.

von Kossa's s. A silver nitrate stain for calcium salts in bone.

Weigert's s. for myelin A ferric chloride and hematoxylin that stains intact myelin deep blue and degenerated myelin light yellow.

Wright's s. A stain commonly used for the demonstration of blood cells; consists of both acid (eosin) and basic (methylene blue, methylene azure, and methylene violet) dyes; also used to stain malarial parasites.

Ziehl-Neelsen s. Stain used in the identification of tubercle bacilli.

staining (stān´ing) **1.** The coloration of a microscopic specimen with a dye to improve the visibility of certain parts. **2.** In dentistry, modification of the color of teeth.

acid-fast s. Procedure for staining acid-free bacteria (those retaining Ziehl's solution even when decolorized with acid alcohol); after decolorization, a contrasting second stain (counterstain) is applied; the acid-fast cells remain red; others take the color of the counterstain.

negative s. Process of suspending bacteria in an opaque medium (e.g., India ink) that fails to penetrate the organism, thus providing contrast.

simple s. Staining with one dye only.

stalagmometer (stă-lag-mom´ĕ-ter) Device used to obtain and measure drops from a liquid at definite intervals to calculate the surface tension of the liquid.

stalk (stawk) A slender or elongated connection with a structure or organ.

allantoic s. A narrow connection between the urogenital sinus and the allantoic sac.

body s. A bridge of mesenchymal mass connecting the caudal end of the young embryo to the inner face of the chorionic vesicle; a precursor of the umbilical cord.

optic s. A slender structure connecting the optic vesicle to the forebrain of the early embryo.

yolk s. A narrowed passage connecting the midgut of the embryo with the yolk sac. Also called omphalomesenteric duct; vitelline duct.

stammering (stam´er-ing) A faltering manner of speaking marked by involuntary pauses and syllabic repetitions; distinguished from stuttering.

stanch (stanch) To arrest bleeding. Also called staunch.

standard (stan´dard) An established rule of comparison for qualitative or quantitative value.

s. of care A description of the conduct expected of a health care provider in a given situation regarding the care of a patient.

standardization (stan-dard-i-za´shun) **1.** The formulation of standards for any preparation or procedure. **2.** Making anything fit a standard.

stannic (stan´ik) Containing tin with a valence of four.

stannous (stan´us) Containing tin with a valence of two.

stannum (stan´um) Latin for tin.

stapedectomy (sta-pĕ-dek´tŏ-me) Surgical removal of the stapes from the middle ear chamber.

stapedial (stă-pe´de-al) Relating to the stapes of the middle ear.

stapediotenotomy (stă-pe-de-o-tĕ-not´ŏ-me) Surgical division of the stapedius muscle of the middle ear.

stapediovestibular (stă-pe-de-o-ves-tib´u-lar) Relating to both the stapes and the vestibule of the ear.

stapedius (sta´pe´de-us) See table of muscles.

stapes (sta´pēz) The smallest and innermost of the three ossicles of the middle ear and the smallest bone of the human body; it articulates by its head with the incus; its base (footplate) is inserted and attached to the margin of the oval window. Popularly called stirrup.

staphylectomy (staf-il-ek´to-me) Surgical removal of the uvula.

staphyline (staf´ĭ-lin) Resembling a bunch of grapes.

staphylion (stă-fil´e-on) A craniometric landmark; the midpoint of the posterior edge of the hard palate.

staphylococcal (staf-ĭ-lo-kok´al) Relating to staphylococci.

staphylococcal scalded skin syndrome (staf-ĭ-lo-kok´al skol´ded skin sin´drōm) (SSSS) Skin condition affecting infants, characterized by rapid blistering and peeling of large areas of the skin (resembling a second-degree burn) with little or no inflammation; caused by an exotoxin elaborated by *Staphylococcus aureus* in an upper respiratory infection. Also called Ritter's disease; Lyell's disease; scalded skin syndrome.

staphylococcemia (staf-ĭ-lo-kok-se´me-ă) The presence of staphylococci in the blood.

staphylococcus (staf-ĭ-lo-kok´us), *pl.* **staphylococ´ci** Any organism of the genus *Staphylococcus.*

Staphylococcus (staf-ĭ-lo-kok´us) A genus (family Micrococcaceae) of gram-positive, nonmotile, usually pathogenic bacteria that tend to aggregate in irregular grapelike clusters.

S. aureus Species containing the pigmented, coagulase-positive variety, often carried in the nasal cavity; causes boils, carbuncles, abscesses, and other suppurative infections.

S. epidermidis Species containing the nonpigmented, mannitol- and coagulase-negative nonpathogenic variety that causes stitch abscesses; normally present on skin.

staphyloderma (staf-ĭ-lo-der´mă) Pus-forming skin disorder caused by staphylococci.

staphylolysin (staf-ĭ-lol´ĭ-sin) **1.** A substance elaborated by a staphylococcus that causes destruction of red blood cells and liberation of hemoglobin. **2.** An antibody causing dissolution of staphylococci.

staphyloma (staf-ĭ-lo´mă) Localized protrusion of the cornea or sclera; usually lined with uveal tissue.

staphyloplasty (staf´ĭ-lo-plas-te) Surgical repair of the uvula and/or the soft palate.

staphyloptosia, staphyloptosis (staf-ĭ-lop-to´se-ă, staf-ĭ-lop-to´sis) Relaxation or lengthening of the uvula.

starch (starch) **1.** A carbohydrate with the general formula $(C_6H_{10}O_5)_n$; exists abundantly in the vegetable kingdom and is converted into dextrins and glucose by amylase enzyme action in saliva and pancreatic juice. **2.** A substance consisting of granules separated from the mature grain of *Zea mays* (Indian corn); used in pharmaceuticals and as a dusting powder.

stare (stār) To look intently with a steady, often wide-eyed, unblinking gaze.

postbasic s. An odd expression of the eyes marked by downward rolling of the eyeballs and retraction of the upper eyelids; seen in persons with posterior basic meningitis.

starvation (star-vā´shun) The condition of suffering from prolonged lack of food.

stasis (sta´sis) Stoppage of the flow of a fluid, especially of the blood.

venous s. Impairment of blood flow through the veins with accumulation of blood in a part, usually in the legs. Also called hypostatic congestion.

state (stāt) A condition.

carrier s. The condition of harboring pathogenic microorganisms without being affected by them.

central excitatory s. A condition of hyperexcitability of nerve cells produced by the storing up of subthreshold stimuli in a reflex center of the spinal cord.

convulsive s. See status epilepticus, under status.

dreamy s. A prolonged state of detachment or semiconscious condition associated with an attack

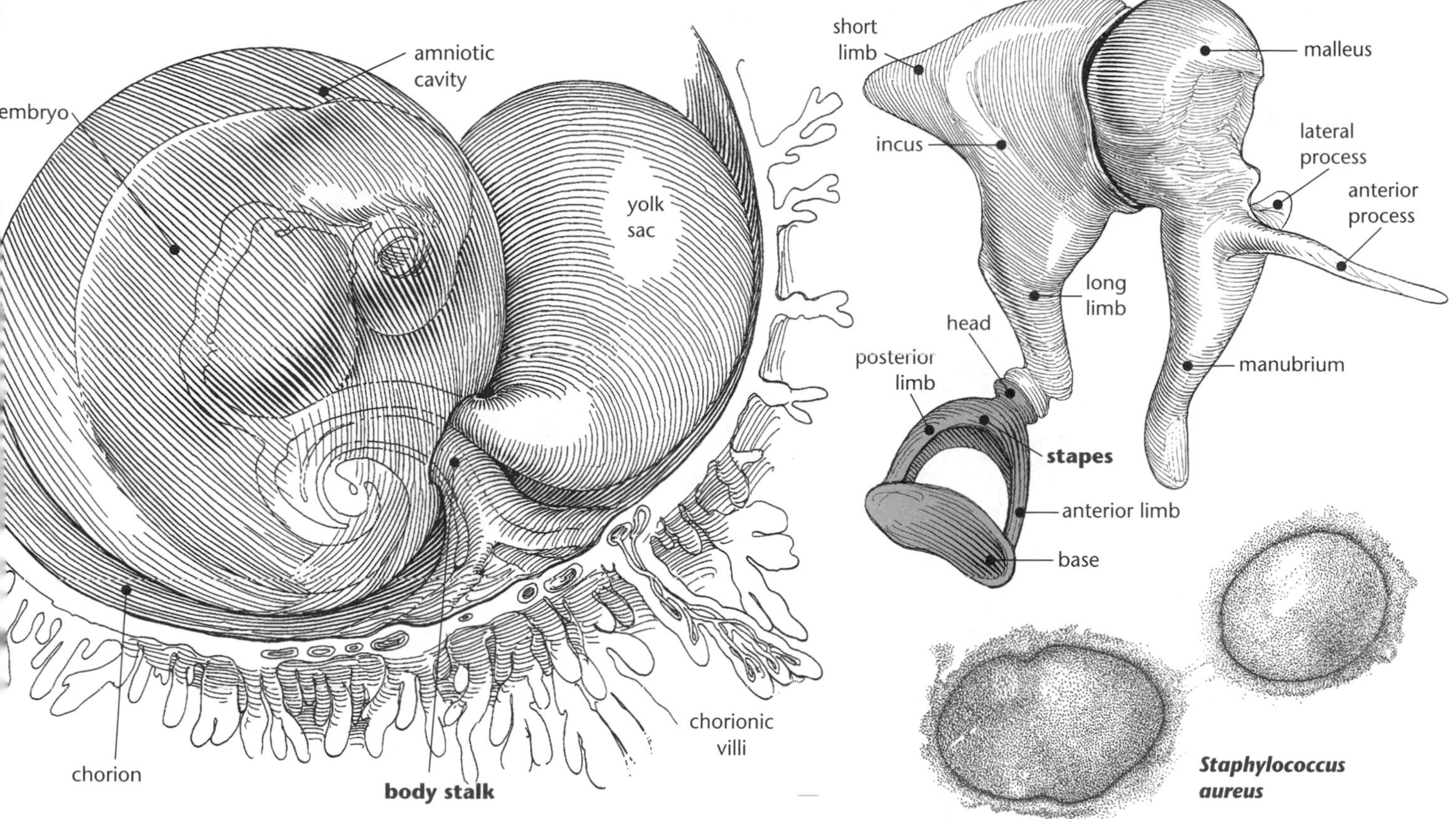

of epilepsy.

permanent vegetative s. A persistent vegetative state that has been diagnosed irreversible with a high degree of clinical certainty, based on probabilities (not absolutes). COMPARE: persistent vegetative state.

persistent vegetative s. (PVS) Irreversible brain damage, usually from trauma or insufficient supply of oxygen to the brain; characterized by a wakeful state but without signs of cognition or responsiveness; the brainstem maintains breathing movements; the patient requires nutritional support (parenteral or via a nasogastric tube) but does not require respiratory or circulatory assistance. Formerly called appallic syndrome.

refractory s. The reduced excitability of a nerve following a response to previous stimulation.

steady s. Any condition that remains constant because opposing forces or processes cancel each other's effects.

twilight s. Condition of impaired consciousness in which a person may perform elaborate purposeful acts and have no recollection of them afterward.

vegetative s. A condition in which self-awareness and all evidence of learned behavior has been lost. See permanent vegetative state; persistent vegetative state.

statim (sta′tim) (stat) Latin for at once, immediately.

statin (sta′tin) Term applied to any of a group of drugs that inhibit formation of cholesterol in the body (e.g., levostatin, pravostatin, simvastatin).

statistics (stă-tis′tiks) A collection of organized numerical data.

medical s. The branch of statistics concerned with quantitative information relating to the incidence, prevalence, course, and management of disease.

vital s. Tabulated information pertaining to human births, health, diseases, and deaths based on nationally recorded data.

statoconia (stat-o-ko′ne-ă) Granular particles composed of calcium carbonate and protein normally embedded in the gelatinous membrane of the macula within the utricle and saccule of the inner ear. Also called otoconia; otoliths.

stature (stach′oor) The natural height of a person.

status (sta′tus, stat′us) State; condition.

s. asthmaticus Asthma attack in which the airway obstruction persists for several days or weeks.

s. choleraicus The stage of shock and collapse in cholera, marked by cold skin, weak pulse, and lethargy.

s. epilepticus Prolonged or repetitive epileptic seizures without recovery between individual seizures. Also called convulsive state.

staunch (stawnch) See stanch.

steal (stēl) Diversion of blood from a vascular area to one deprived of circulation.

subclavian s. See subclavian steal syndrome.

stearate (ste-ă-rāt) A salt of stearic acid.

stearic acid (ste-ăr′ik as′id) A common fatty acid made by the hydrolysis of fats; used in pharmaceutical preparations.

steatocryptosis (ste-ă-to-krip-to′sis) Dysfunction of sebaceous glands.

steatocystoma multiplex (ste-ă-to-sis-to′mă mul′tĭ-pleks) Condition beginning in adolescent or early adult life, marked by the presence of numerous dermal cysts containing sebum; usually an autosomal dominant inheritance. Also called epidermal cystic disease; sebocystomatosis.

s. m. simplex A form developing only one or two small lesions.

steatogenous (ste-ă-toj′ĕ-nus) **1.** Causing fat degeneration. **2.** Producing any disease of the sebaceous glands.

steatolysis (ste-ă-tol′ĭ-sis) The hydrolysis or emulsion of fat preparatory to absorption.

steatoma (ste-ă-to′mă) **1.** A tumor composed chiefly of fatty tissue. **2.** A sebaceous cyst.

steatonecrosis (ste-ă-to-nĕ-kro′sis) See fat necrosis, under necrosis.

steatopygia (ste-ă-to-pij′e-ă) Excessively fat buttocks.

steatorrhea (ste-ă-to-re′ă) Excessive amount of fat in the feces; manifestation of a malabsorption syndrome.

steatosis (ste-ă-to′sis) **1.** Fatty degeneration. **2.** Any disease of the sebaceous glands.

stegnosis (steg-no′sis) **1.** Stoppage of secretions or excretions. **2.** Constriction.

steinstrasse (shtīn′shtră-sĕ) The x-ray appearance of stone fragments filling a portion of the ureter after a large kidney stone has been broken up by extracorporeal lithotripsy. Term means street of stone in German.

stellate (stel′āt) Having the shape of a star.

stellectomy (stel-lek′tŏ-me) Excision of the stellate ganglion; usually performed for the relief of intractable pain. Also called stellate ganglionectomy.

Stellwag's sign (shtel′vahgz sīn) Infrequent and incomplete blinking; seen in exophthalmic goiter.

stem cell renewal (stem sel rĭ-noo′ăl) A residual population of cells that retain the ability to divide.

stenion (sten′e-on) The craniometric point located at each end of the shortest transverse diameter of the skull in the temporal region.

stenochoria (sten-o-ko′re-ă) Constriction of a duct or orifice.

stenopeic (sten-o-pe′ik) Having a narrow opening.

stenosed (stĕ-nōzd′) Abnormally constricted.

stenosis (stĕ-no′sis), *pl.* **steno′ses** Abnormal constriction of a channel or orifice.

aortic s. (AS) Pathologic constriction of the orifice between the aorta and the left ventricle of the heart.

congenital pyloric s. See hypertrophic pyloric stenosis.

hypertrophic pyloric s. Overdevelopment of the pyloric sphincter muscle causing narrowing of the pyloric orifice and projectile vomiting, occurring in the second or third week of life. Also called congenital pyloric stenosis.

idiopathic hypertrophic subaortic s. (IHSS) Disease of the heart muscle marked by disproportionate hypertrophy of the interventricular septum and left ventricular wall which sometimes causes obstruction to the left outflow tract. Also called asymmetric septal hypertrophy (ASH).

infundibular pulmonic s. Obstruction of the infundibulum (outflow tract) of the right ventricle of the heart, usually caused by either or both of two conditions: a fibrous ring just below the pulmonic valve, or hypertrophy of heart muscle surrounding the infundibulum.

mitral s. Narrowing of the mitral valve opening (between the left atrium and the left ventricle).

pulmonary s. Constriction of the orifice between the pulmonary trunk and the right ventricle.

pyloric s. Constriction of the pyloric orifice of the stomach. Also called pyloristenosis.

subaortic s., subvalvular s. Obstruction of the outflow tract of the left ventricle of the heart; caused by a fibrous band, or by muscular hypertrophy just below the aortic valve.

supravalvular s. Constriction of the aorta just above the aortic valve, caused by a congenital fibrous ring around the vessel.

tricuspid s. Narrowing of the tricuspid valve opening (between the right atrium and right ventricle).

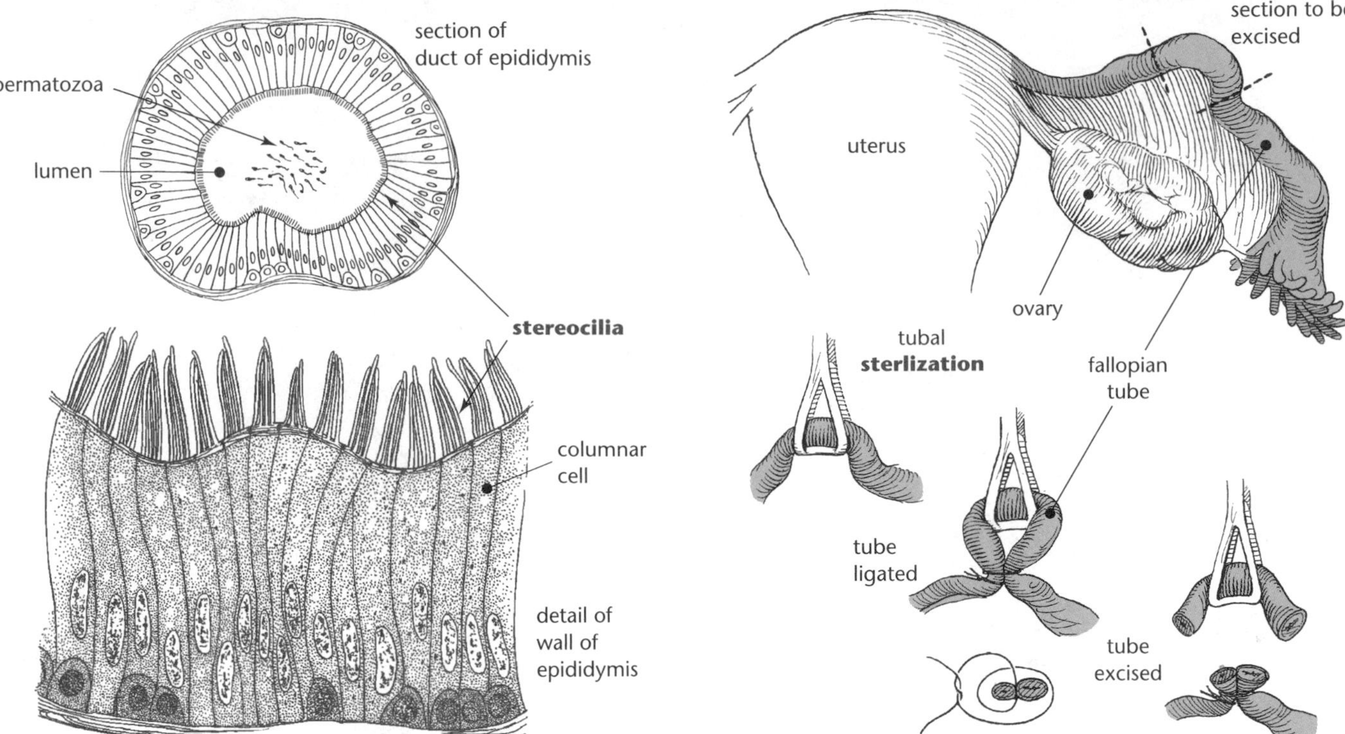

stenostenosis (stě-no-stě-no´sis) Constriction of the parotid duct.

stenostomia (stě-no-sto´me-ă) A narrow state of the oral cavity.

stenothermal (sten-o-ther´mal) Capable of withstanding only slight changes in temperature.

stenothorax (sten-o-tho´raks) An abnormally narrow chest.

stenotic (stě-not´ik) Narrowed abnormally; affected with stenosis.

stent (stent) **1.** A mold for holding a skin graft in place. **2.** A device for supporting tubular structures during surgical procedures (e.g., anastomosis). **3.** A device that maintains patency within tubular structures and prevents the passage of emboli.

steppage (step´ij, step-ahzh´) See high steppage gait, under gait.

stercobilin (ster-ko-bi´lin) A brown pigment present in the feces, derived from bile.

stercolith (ster´ko-lith) See coprolith.

stercoraceous (ster-ko-ra´shus) Fecal; relating to feces.

stere (stēr) A unit of volume equivalent to one cubic meter.

stereoanesthesia (ster-e-o-an-es-the´zhă) See tactile agnosia, under agnosia.

stereoarthrolysis (ster-e-o-ar-throl´ĭ-sis) Surgical creation of a movable joint.

S

stereocampimeter (ster-e-o-kam-pim´ĕ-ter) Instrument for examining the central visual field of each eye separately while both eyes fixate similar targets.

stereochemistry (ster-e-o-kem´is-tre) The branch of chemistry concerned with the spatial arrangement of atoms in a compound.

stereocilia (ster-e-o-sil´e-ă) Unusually long, slender, nonmotile microvilli on the free surface of epithelial cells; found primarily in parts of the male reproductive tract.

stereocinefluorography (ster-e-o-sin-ĕ-flo͞o-rog´ră-fe) Motion picture photography of x-ray images obtained by stereoscopic fluoroscopy, producing three-dimensional visualization.

stereognosis (ster-e-og-no´sis) The recognition of objects through the sense of touch.

stereoisomer (ster-e-o-i´so-mer) One of two compounds that contain the same chemical structure but which have different optical properties because the atoms in each have different spatial positions.

stereoisomerism (ster-e-o-i-som´er-iz-m) Isomerism in which two compounds have the same structural formula but the atoms are linked in a different order.

stereology (ster-e-ol´ŏ-je) A study of the three-dimensional aspects of morphology, especially ultrastructure.

stereo-orthopter (ster-e-o-or-thop´ter) A visual training instrument used to correct strabismus.

stereopsis (ster-e-op´sis) Visual depth perception produced by slight disparateness of images (i.e., when images fall on slightly disparate points of the retina). Also called stereoscopic vision.

stereoroentgenography (ster-e-o-rent-gen-og´ră-fe) The taking of an x-ray picture from two slightly different positions to produce a three-dimensional effect.

stereoscope (ster´e-o-skōp) Instrument that permits two different portions of the same picture (or two photographs of different views of the same object) to be viewed by the two eyes at the same time, resulting in a three-dimensional perception.

stereospecific (ster-e-o-spĭ-sif´ik) Denoting enzymes or synthetic organic reactions that act only with a given molecule or with a limited class of molecules.

stereotaxis (ster-e-o-tak´sis) **1.** The localization of the three-dimensional arrangement of body structures by means of coordinate landmarks. **2.** The movement of an organism toward, or away from, a rigid surface with which it comes in contact; applied to the organism as a whole.

stereotaxy (ster-e-o-tak´se) A method of inserting an electrode into a specific area of the brain by means of three-dimensional coordinates; used to destroy deep-seated nuclear masses and fiber tracts in the brain.

stereotropism (ster-e-ot´rŏ-piz-m) The movement of parts of an organism toward (positive stereotropism) or away from (negative stereotropism) a solid body with which it comes in contact.

stereotypy (ster´e-o-ti-pe) The persistent mechanical repetition of certain movements or gestures; common in schizophrenia.

oral s. See verbigeration.

steric (ste´rik) Relating to stereochemistry.

sterile (ster´il) **1.** Incapable of reproducing. **2.** Free from bacteria or other microorganisms. Also called aseptic.

sterility (stě-ril´ĭ-te) Absence or nonfunctioning of the organs of reproduction.

sterilization (ster-ĭ-lĭ-za´shun) **1.** A treatment that deprives living organisms of the ability to reproduce. **2.** The process of destroying or removing all living microorganisms.

sterilizer (ster´ĭ-līz-er) An apparatus for rendering anything germ-free.

sternal (ster´nal) Relating to the sternum (breastbone).

sternalgia (ster-nal´jă) Pain in the sternum or sternal area. Also called sternodynia.

sternoclavicular (ster-no-klă-vik´u-lar) Relating to the sternum and the clavicle.

sternocleidal (ster-no-kli´dal) Relating to the sternum and the clavicle.

sternocleidomastoid (ster-no-kli-do-mas´toid) Relating to the sternum, clavicle, and mastoid process; denoting the muscle that has its origin and insertion on these structures.

sternocostal (ster-no-kos´tal) Relating to the sternum and the ribs.

sternodynia (ster-no-din´e-ă) See sternalgia.

sternotomy (ster-not´ŏ-me) Cutting through the sternum.

sternum (ster´num) A long, flat bone forming the middle part of the anterior wall of the thoracic cage, articulating with the clavicles and the costal cartilages of the first seven pairs of ribs. Popularly called breastbone.

sternutatory (ster-nu´tă-tor-e) Causing sneezing.

steroid (ster´oid, ste´roid) **1.** One of a family of chemical substances characterized by four interlocking rings of carbon atoms; included are the adrenal steroids, corticosteroids, the male and female sex hormones, and the D vitamins; cholesterol is one of the main building blocks for the other steroids; examples include aldosterone, androsterone, cholecalciferol, cholesterol, cortisol, cortisone, estradiol, estriol, progesterone, and testosterone. **2.** A shortened form for an adrenal corticosteroid or a synthetic compound with similar actions.

anabolic s. Any of a group of synthetic drugs (derivatives of the male hormone testosterone) that have protein-building properties; they accelerate muscle recovery after injury and help strengthen bones. Adverse effects include acne, liver and adrenal gland damage, and infertility.

steroidogenesis (ste-roi-do-jen´ĕ-sis) The natural production of steroids.

steroid withdrawal syndrome (ster´oid with-draw´al sin´drōm) Weakness, nausea, fever, malaise, and slight hypotension experienced by persons upon withdrawal of steroid therapy to which they have been subjected for prolonged periods.

sterol (ster´ol) One of a group of unsaturated solid alcohols, a subdivision of the steroids, present in all animal and plant tissue except bacteria; the best known member of the group is cholesterol.

stertor (ster´tor) A snoring sound produced in breathing.

stertorous (ster´to-rus) Characterized by snoring.

stethograph (steth´o-graf) Apparatus used for recording the respiratory movements of the chest.

stethoscope (steth´o-skōp) Instrument for listening to sounds produced within the body, especially respiratory and vascular sounds; originally designed by René Laënnec.

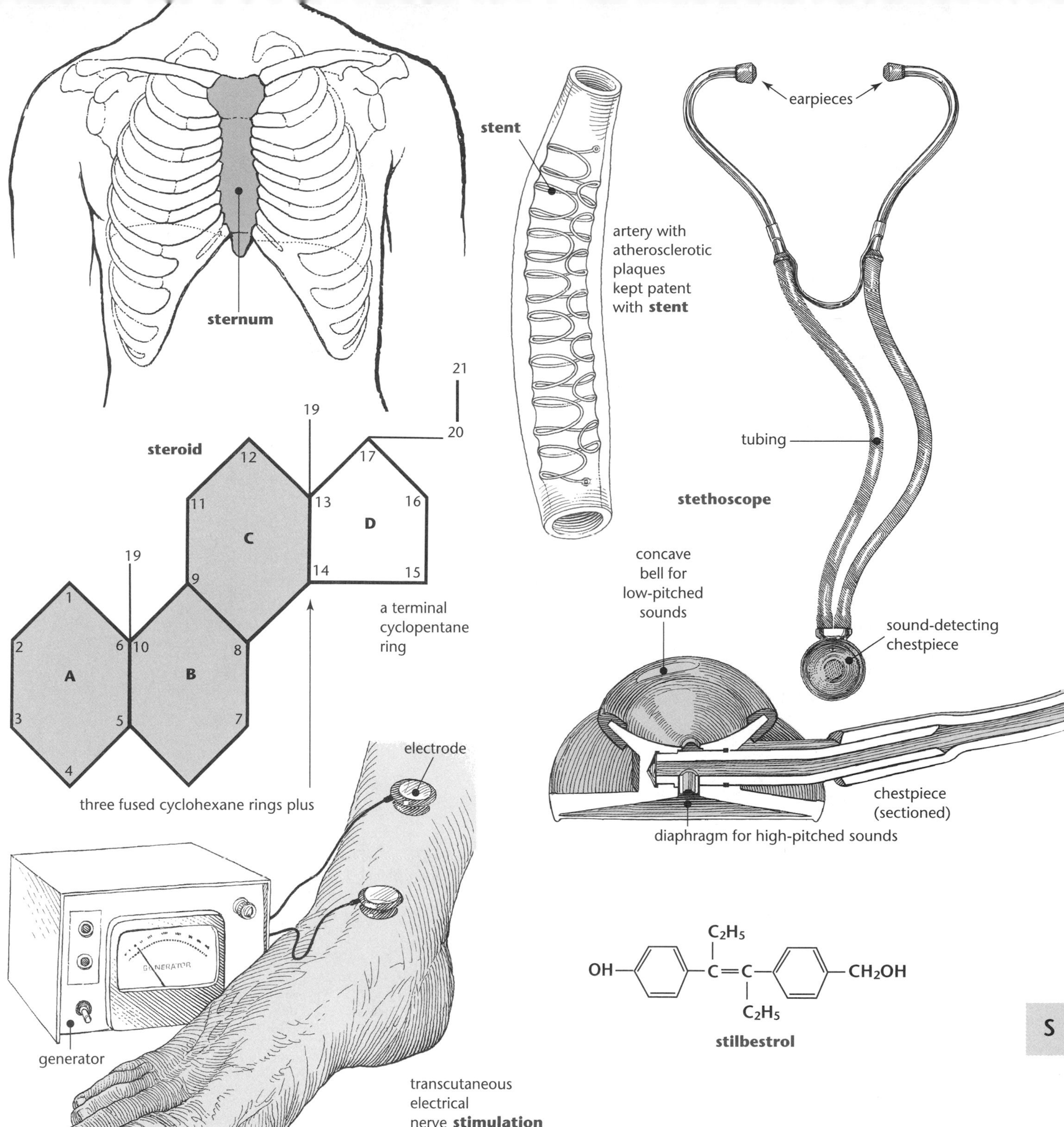

Stevens-Johnson syndrome (ste´venz-jon´son sin´drōm) See erythema multiforme exudativum, under erythema.
stibialism (stib´e-al-iz-m) Poisoning with antimony.
stiff-man syndrome (stif-man sin´drōm) A chronic disorder of unknown cause marked by fluctuating muscular rigidity and spasm that progresses to generalized stiffness involving the extremities, neck, and trunk; associated with severe muscle pains and disability, difficult swallowing, and weight loss.
stigma (stig´mă), *pl.* **stig´mata** **1.** Visible evidence characteristic of a disease (spot, blemish, symptom, sign, etc.). **2.** The pigmented eyespot of certain protozoa.
stilbestrol (stil-bes´trol) See diethylstilbestrol.
stillbirth (stil´birth) Delivery of an infant who has died while in the uterus.
stillborn (stil´born) An infant who is dead at delivery.
Still's disease (stils dĭ-zēz) See juvenile arthritis, under arthritis.
stilus (stī´lus) A pencil-shaped medicinal preparation for external application.
stimulant (stim´u-lant) Anything that accelerates organic activity.
stimulation (stim-u-la´shun) **1.** The process of exciting the body, or a part, to increased functional activity. **2.** The state of being stimulated.
photic s. The use of a flickering light to alter the pattern of the electroencephalogram.
stimulator (stim´u-la-tor) An agent that increases functional activity.
B lymphocyte s. (BLyS) A protein that incites the growth and activity of B lymphocytes.
cerebellar electrical s. See brain pacemaker, under pacemaker.
long-acting thyroid s. (LATS) Substance found in the blood of hyperthyroid patients, not elaborated in the pituitary gland, and having a prolonged stimulatory action on the thyroid gland.
stimulus (stim´u-lus), *pl.* **stim´uli** **1.** Anything causing a response. **2.** A stimulant; an agent or action that elicits a physiologic or psychologic activity.
conditioned s. (CS) A stimulus which prior to

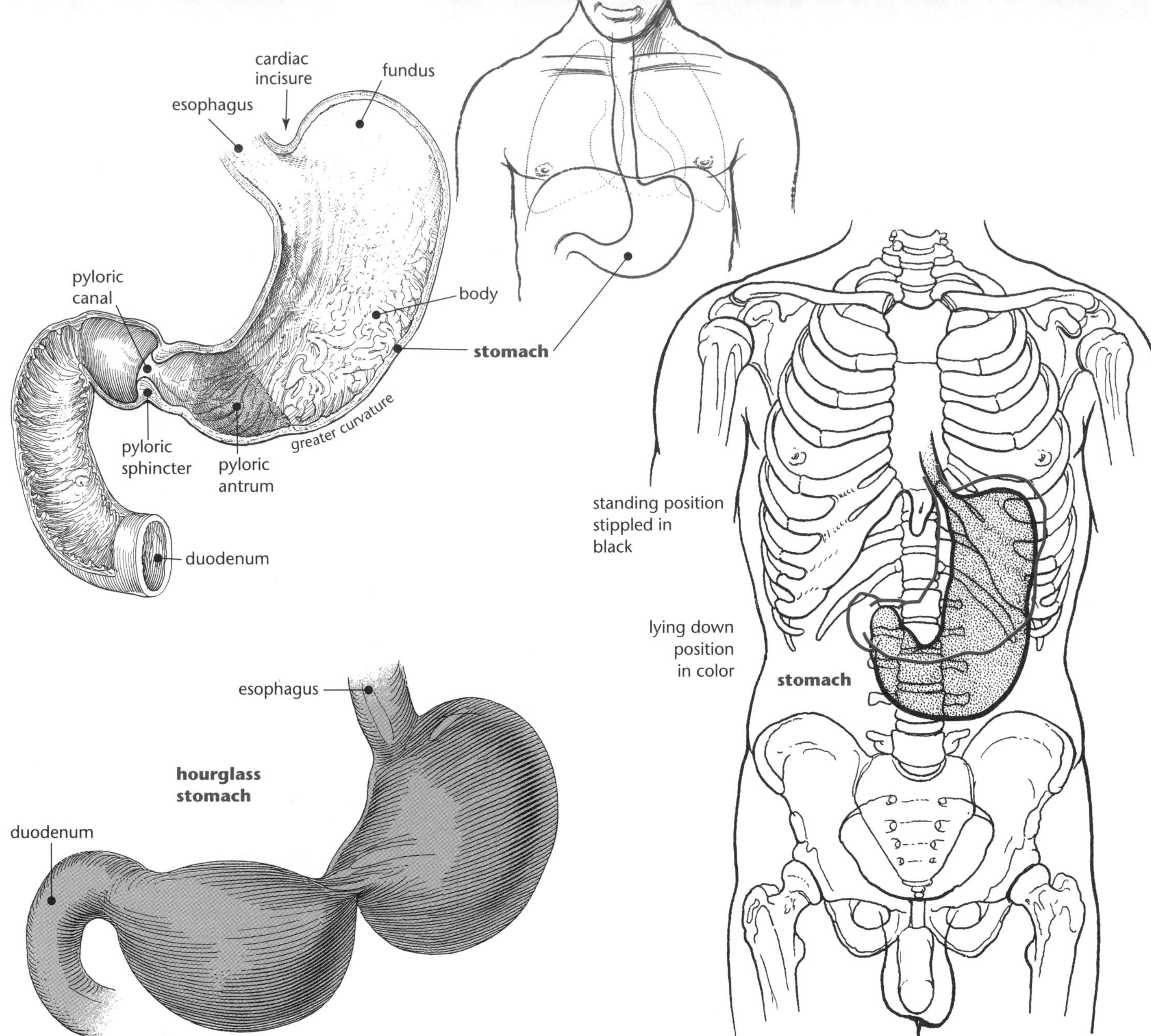

the procedure does not evoke the specific reflex or response under study.

unconditioned s. (UCS) A stimulus that normally evokes the particular response under study.

sting (sting) **1.** To pierce the skin with a sharp-pointed organ or part (e.g., the ovipositor of a wasp) and deposit venom. **2.** The sharp transitory pain produced by stinging.

stippling (stip´ling) In histology, the staining of basophilic granules in a cell protoplasm when exposed to the action of a basic stain.

Ziemann's s. Fine spots sometimes seen in red blood cells of persons with quartan malaria.

stirrup (stir´up) See stapes.

stitch (stich) **1.** A suture. **2.** A sudden, short sharp pain. **3.** The act of suturing.

stoichiometry (stoi-ke-om´ĕ-tre) The study of the combining proportions (by weight and volume) of elements participating in a chemical reaction.

Stokes-Adams syndrome (stōks-ad´ămz sin´drōm) See Adams-Stokes syndrome.

stoma (sto´mă) *pl.* **sto´mas, sto´mata** **1.** Any small opening. **2.** The mouth or an artificial opening between two cavities or channels or between any cavity or tube and the exterior.

stomach (stum´ăk) The enlarged, saclike portion of the digestive tract, between the esophagus and the small intestine, in which ingested food is acted on by the enzymes and hydrochloric acid of gastric juice, and then released into the duodenum by gastric peristalsis; the stomach is entirely covered with peritoneum and normally has a capacity of about 1 quart.

hourglass s. A stomach with a stricture at the midpoint.

leather bottle s. See linitis plastica, under linitis.

stomachache (stum´ăk-āk) Pain in the stomach or abdomen.

stomachal (stum´ā-kal) Relating to the stomach.

stomal (sto´mal) Pertaining to a stoma or small aperture.

stomata (sto´mă-tă) Alternative plural of stoma.

stomatalgia (sto-mă-tal´jă) Pain in the mouth, occurring in varying degrees of severity as a result of injury or disease. Also called stomatodynia.

stomatic (sto-mat´ik) **1.** Relating to the mouth. **2.** Relating to a stoma.

stomatitis (sto-mă-ti´tis) Inflammation of the mucous membrane of the mouth.

angular s. Superficial fissuring and inflammation at the angles of the mouth.

aphthous s. A chronically recurrent disease marked by the appearance of small, painful, single or multiple ulcers on the mucous membrane of the mouth. Also called canker, canker sore; ulcerative stomatitis.

gangrenous s. See noma.

herpetic s. A recurrent infection of the oral mucosa, caused by the herpes simplex virus, with painful vesicle and ulcer formation.

ulcerative s. See aphthous stomatitis.

stomatocyte (sto´mă-to-sīt) Red blood cell in which the central area appears as a slit rather than a biconcave circular area.

stomatodynia (sto-mă-to-din´e-ă) See stomatalgia.

stomatology (sto-mă-tol´ŏ-je) The study of the structures, functions, and diseases of the mouth.

stomatomalacia (sto-mă-to-mă-la´shă) Abnormal softening of structures in the mouth.

stomatomycosis (sto-mă-to-mi-ko´sis) Fungal disease of the mouth.

stomatopathy (sto-mă-top´ă-the) Any disorder of the oral cavity.

stomatorrhagia (sto-mă-to-ra´jă) Bleeding from any structure in the mouth.

stomodeum (sto-mo-de´um) A midline invagination or depression of the ectoderm of the embryo between the maxillary and mandibular processes which later develops into the mouth cavity.

stone (stōn) An abnormal concretion usually composed of mineral salts and formed most frequently in the cavities of the body which serve as reservoirs for fluids. Also called calculus.

bladder s. A stone lodged in the bladder; it may be either formed in the bladder or passed from the kidney or ureter. Also called vesical calculus.

dental s. Gypsum that has been calcined under

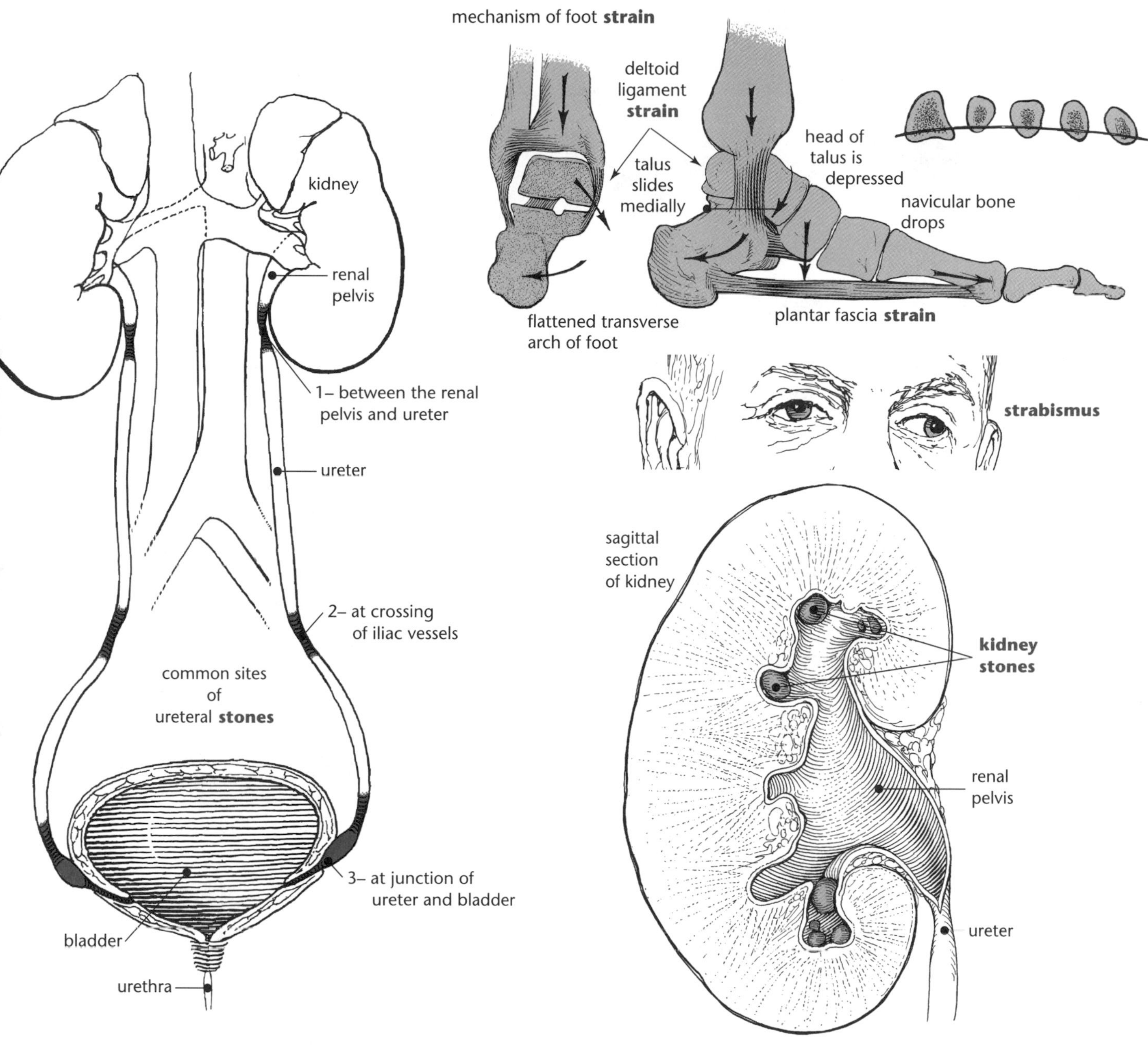

steam pressure to 130°C; used for making casts and models of the oral cavity.

gallbladder s. See gallstone.

kidney s. Stone in the kidney, most commonly made up of calcium oxalate, uric acid, or calcium phosphate. Also called nephrolith; renal calculus.

pulp s. The collection of calcified material in the pulp chamber of a tooth or a projection into the chamber from the cavity wall. Also called endolith; denticle.

tear s. See dacryolith.

urinary s. Concretion formed anywhere within the urinary tract (kidney, ureter, bladder, urethra); frequently causing obstruction, bleeding, and pain. Also called urinary calculus; urolith.

vein s. See phlebolith.

womb s. A calcified myoma of the uterus.

stonemason's disease (stōn´mā-sonz dĭ-zēz´) See silicosis.

stool (stool) **1.** A bowel movement. **2.** Feces.

tarry s. Bloody stool, especially one in which blood can be grossly recognized.

stopcock (stop´kok) A valve that stops or regulates the flow of a liquid through a tube or pipe.

strabismic, strabismal (stră-biz´mik, stră-biz´mal) Relating to or afflicted with strabismus.

strabismometer (stră-biz-mom´ĕ-ter) Instrument used to measure the angle of strabismus.

strabismus (stra-biz´mus) A visual disorder in which one eye cannot focus with the other. Also called heterotropia.

convergent s. See esotropia.

divergent s. See exotropia.

external s. See divergent strabismus.

internal s. See convergent strabismus.

strabotomy (stră-bot´ŏ-me) Division of one or more of the ocular muscles or their tendons in treatment of strabismus.

straight back syndrome (strāt băk sin´drōm) Loss of the physiologic dorsal kyphosis of the thoracic spine; this may result in the leftward shift of the heart or a "pancake" appearance; the close proximity of the outflow structures to the anterior chest wall results in an easily heard innocent systolic murmur.

straightjacket (strāt-jak´et) See straitjacket.

strain (strān) **1.** Partial tearing of a muscle or its tendon. **2.** To injure a part by misuse or excessive effort. **3.** In bacteriology, a group of microorganisms (e.g., bacteria) made up of descendants of a single isolation in pure culture. **5.** A measure of the deformation produced on a structure by an external force; used in reference to the elastic property of solids.

strait (strāt) A narrow space or passageway.

inferior pelvic s. See pelvic plane of outlet, under plane.

superior pelvic s. See pelvic plane of inlet, under plane.

straitjacket (strāt-jak´et) A longsleeved garment used to restrain a violent patient by securing the arms tightly against the body. Also called camisole.

stramonium (stră-mo´ne-um) The dried leaves of jimsonweed (*Datura stramonium*), formerly used in the treatment of asthma.

strand (strand) A single filamentlike structure.

antisense s. In molecular genetics, the strand of double-stranded DNA that serves as the template for the synthesis of mRNA (messenger RNA). Also called noncoding strand.

coding s. In molecular genetics, the nontranscribed strand of double-stranded DNA; it corresponds both in polarity and in base sequence to the antisense strand. Also called sense strand.

noncoding s. See antisense strand.

sense s. See coding strand.

strangle (strang´gl) To suffocate by compressing the trachea so as to prevent respiration; to choke.

strangulation (strang´gu-lā´shun) **1.** Constriction of the air passages that interferes with or terminates normal breathing. **2.** Compression that cuts off the blood supply to a part, specifically to a loop of intestine.

strangury (strang´gu-re) Difficult, slow, painful urination.

strap (strap) **1.** A strip of adhesive plaster. **2.** To bind with adhesive plaster.

S

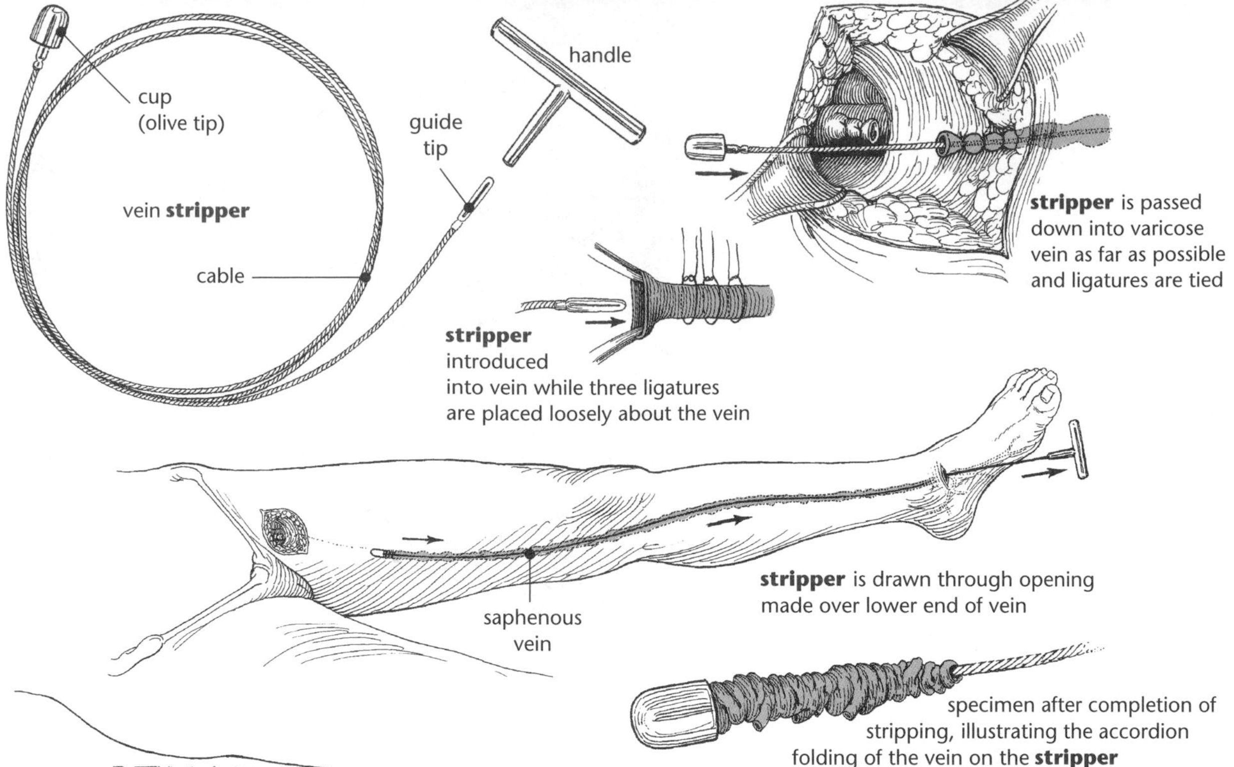
handle
cup
(olive tip)
guide
tip
vein **stripper**
cable
stripper is passed
down into varicose
vein as far as possible
and ligatures are tied
stripper
introduced
into vein while three ligatures
are placed loosely about the vein
stripper is drawn through opening
made over lower end of vein
saphenous
vein
specimen after completion of
stripping, illustrating the accordion
folding of the vein on the **stripper**
B J Melloni, PhD

stratified (strat´ĭ-fīd) Arranged in layers.
stratiform (strat´ĭ-form) Arranged in a series of superimposed layers.
stratum (stra´tum), *pl.* **stra´ta** Latin for layer, especially of differentiated tissue comprising one of several associated layers. See layer.
streak (strēk) **1.** A line or furrow. **2.** Inoculation of bacteria on a culture medium by a loop.
angioid s.'s Brownish red lines in the fundus of the eye radiating from the optic disk and resembling blood vessels; caused by breaks in the basal lamina of the choroid due to degeneration of elastic tissues. May occur in pseudoxanthoma, Paget's disease, and sickle cell anemia. Also called Knapp's streaks; Knapp's striae; elastosis dystrophica.
germinal s. Primitive streak.
Knapp's s.'s See angioid streaks.
medullary s. The embryonic neural groove, the closure of which forms the primordium of the brain and spinal cord.
primitive s. A midline narrow groove, with slightly bulging regions on either side, situated on the caudal end of the embryonic disk; site from which the mesodermal cells migrate from the surface to form the middle germ layer; clearly visible in a 15- to 16-day embryo and provides the earliest evidence of the cephalocaudal axis. Also called germinal streak.
strephosymbolia (stref-o-sim-bo´le-ă) A perception disorder, occurring mainly in children, in which certain letters or words are seen reversed, as if in a mirror.
strepitus (strep´ĭ-tus) A sound heard on auscultation. Rarely used term.
Streptobacillus (strep-to-bă-sil´us) A genus (family Bacteriodiaceae) of bacteria containing gram-negative rods; some species are pathogenic.
streptococcal (strep-to-kok´al) Relating to streptococcus.
streptococcemia (strep-to-kok-se´me-ă) The presence of streptococci in the blood.
streptococci (strep-to-kok´si) Plural of streptococcus.
streptococcosis (strep-to-kŏ-ko´sis) Any infection with streptococci.
Streptococcus (strep-to-kok´us) A genus of gram-positive, round or ovoid bacteria (family Streptococcaceae), occurring in pairs or chains. They are classified according to their hemolytic activity on blood agar as: *alpha streptococci,* which produce a zone of incomplete hemolysis and green discoloration adjacent to the colony; *beta streptococci,* which produce a clear zone of hemolysis around the colony; and *gamma streptococci,* which produce no hemolysis. Beta forms are classified into groups A through O according to the carbohydrate found in the cell wall; they are further subdivided by Arabic numerals into types based on the cell wall protein; group A strains are pathogenic for humans.
S. faecalis Former name for *Enterococcus faecalis.*
S. pneumoniae Species causing lobar pneumonia and other acute pus-forming conditions such as sinusitis, middle ear infections, and meningitis. Formerly called *Diplococcus pneumoniae*.
S. pyogenes Species causing several acute pyogenic infections such as scarlet fever, erysipelas, and septic sore throat. Has been isolated from skin lesions, blood inflammatory exudates, and upper respiratory tract of humans.
S. salivarius Species found in saliva and throughout the intestinal tract; generally nonpathogenic but has been implicated in contributing to the formation of dental caries.
streptococcus (strep-to-kok´us), *pl.* **streptococ´ci** Any member of the genus *Streptococcus.*
streptodermatitis (strep-to-der-mă-ti´tis) Inflammation of the skin caused by streptococci.
streptodornase (strep-to-dor´nās) (SD) Enzyme produced by hemolytic streptococci, capable of causing liquefaction of purulent exudates. Also called dornase.
streptogramins (strep-to-gra´mins) A family of polypeptide antibiotics active against the cell wall of bacteria.
streptokinase (strep-to-ki´nās) (SK) Enzyme released by hemolytic streptococci, capable of dissolving fibrin; used to dissolve blood clots and fibrinous adhesions.
streptolysin (strep-tol´ĭ-sin) A hemolysin produced by streptococci.
Streptomyces (strep-to-mi´sēz) A genus of bacteria (family Streptomycetacea) present in the soil; antibiotics have been obtained from cultures of some species.
S. antibioticus Species that yields actinomycin.
S. fradiae Species that yields neomycin.
S. griseus Species that yields streptomycin.
streptomycete (strep-to-mi´sēt) A member of the genus *Streptomyces.*
streptomycin (strep-to-mi´-sin) An antibiotic obtained from cultures of *Streptomyces griseus*; white granules or powder soluble in water, acid alcohol, and methyl alcohol; active against the tubercle bacillus, many gram-negative bacteria, and some gram-positive bacteria; excessive dosage leads to damage to the eighth cranial (vestibulocochlear) nerve, usually affecting the vestibular part first.
stress (stres) **1.** The internal force of a body generated to resist an external force tending to deform it. **2.** In dentistry, pressure against the teeth and their attachments exceeding that produced by normal function. **3.** Any physical or psychological condition that tends to disrupt normal functions of the body or mind.
stressbreaker (stres´brāk-er) An attachment in a removable partial denture that relieves the anchoring teeth of all or part of the pressure during mastication.
stretcher (strech´er) A canvas stretched over a frame, used to transport disabled or dead persons. Also called litter.
stria (stri´ă), *pl.* **striae** A thin stripe or band, especially one of several that are more or less parallel.
s. atrophica One of several glistening white bands in the skin of the abdomen, breasts, buttocks, and thighs, caused by overstretching and weakening of the elastic tissues; associated with pregnancy, obesity, rapid growth during puberty, Cushing's syndrome, and other conditions. Commonly called stretch mark.
Knapp's striae See angioid streaks, under streak.
striate, striated (strī´āt, strī´āt-ed) Marked by striae; striped.
striation (stri-a´shun) **1.** A stria. **2.** The state of having striae.
stricture (strik´chur) An abnormal narrowing of a tubular structure.
strident (strī´dent) Harsh, shrill, or grating, as certain sounds heard on auscultation.
stridor (stri´dor) A harsh, shrill respiratory sound, as in acute laryngeal obstruction.
stridulous (strid´u-lus) Having a harsh, shrill sound.
string sign (string sīn) In radiology, a stringlike configuration of contrast material (barium), seen in constriction of the canal between the esophagus and stomach, or in narrowed segments of the intestines.
strip (strip) **1.** To remove the contents of a tubular structure by gently running a finger along the structure; to milk. **2.** To excise a varicose vein of the leg with a stripper. **3.** Any narrow piece.
abrasive s. A piece of linen with an abrasive material bonded to one side; used to shape and polish proximal surfaces of artificial teeth.
lightning s. A metal strip with abrasive on one side; used to remove rough or improper points of contact between artificial teeth.
stripe (strīp) A streak.
Mees' s.'s See Mees' lines, under line.
stripper (strip´er) An instrument for the removal of a diseased vein; generally consists of a cable with a disk or cup at one end and a guide tip at the other.
strobila (stro-bi´lă), *pl.* **strobilae** The linear

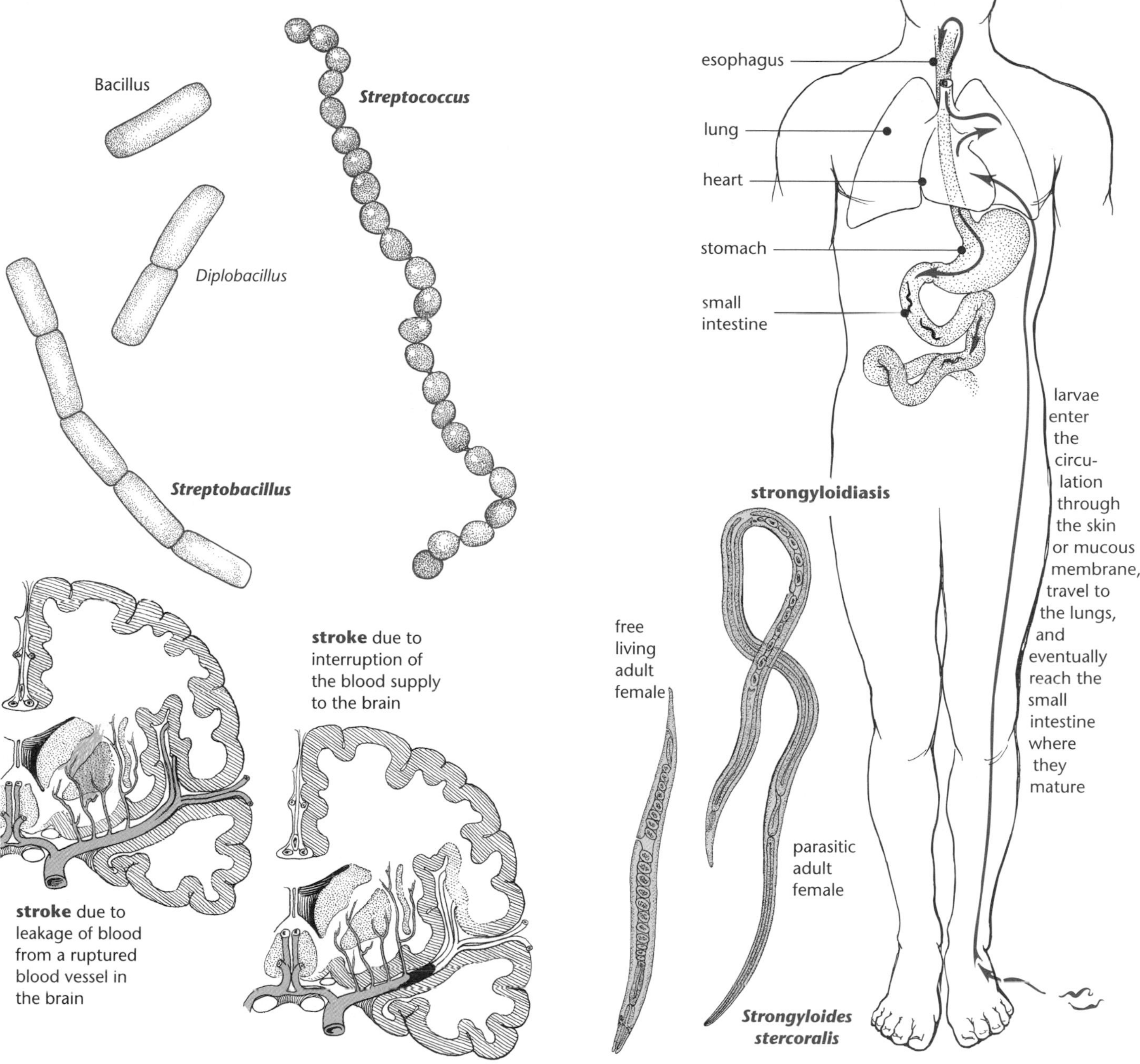
Bacillus
Streptococcus
Diplobacillus
Streptobacillus
esophagus
lung
heart
stomach
small intestine
larvae enter the circu-lation through the skin or mucous membrane, travel to the lungs, and eventually reach the small intestine where they mature
strongyloidiasis
free living adult female
parasitic adult female
Strongyloides stercoralis
stroke due to interruption of the blood supply to the brain
stroke due to leakage of blood from a ruptured blood vessel in the brain

collection of segments comprising the body of a tapeworm.

strobiloid (stro′bĭ-loid) Resembling the segmented body of a tapeworm.

strobolaryngoscope (stro-bo-lă-ring′go-skōp) A type of stroboscope used to observe in detail the vibratory motion of the vocal cords.

stroboscope (stro′bo-skōp) **1.** Instrument for observing moving objects by making them appear stationary through intermittently interrupted illumination. **2.** An electronic instrument that produces brief pulses of light at controllable frequency, used to alter electrical activity of the cerebral cortex.

stroke (strōk) **1.** Occlusion or rupture of a blood vessel in the brain. Also called cerebrovascular accident; cerebral vascular accident; brain attack. **2.** Any sudden, severe attack or seizure.

heat s. Condition caused by excessive exposure to high temperatures, marked by high fever, dry skin, and in severe cases, coma.

paralytic s. Sudden paralysis caused by injury to the brain.

stroma (stro′ma) The framework of an organ, usually composed of connective tissue, which supports the functional elements or cells.

stromuhr (stro′moor) Instrument used to measure the amount of blood flowing per unit of time through a blood vessel.

Strongyloides (stron-jĭ-loi′dēz) A genus of threadworms (class Nematoda); intestinal parasites of higher vertebrates, especially mammals.

S. stercoralis The causative agent of strongyloidiasis.

strongyloidiasis, strongyloidosis (stron-jĭ-loi-dĭ′ă-sis, stron-jĭ-loi-do′sis) Parasitic infection caused by a nematode, *Strongyloides stercoralis*; the threadlike worms enter the body through the skin or mucous membrane of the mouth, travel to the lungs, and eventually reach the small intestine where the female lays her eggs.

strontium (stron′she-um) A soft, easily oxidized metallic element similar to calcium in chemical properties; symbol Sr, atomic number 38, atomic weight 87.62.

strontium 90 A radioactive isotope which emits a high energy beta particle and has a half-life of 28 years; a product of atom bomb blasts that constitutes an important fallout hazard, since it is incorporated into bone tissue upon absorption.

Strophanthus (stro-fan′thus) A genus of African vines of the family Apocynaceae.

S. gratus Species containing ouabain, a cardiac glycoside.

S. kombe A species containing strophanthin, a cardiac glycoside.

structure (struk′chur) The configuration of the component parts of an entity.

brush heap s. The fibrils in a gel or hydrocolloid impression material.

denture-supporting s. The tissues, teeth, and/or residual ridges that serve as support for removable dentures (partial or complete).

fine s. See ultrastructure.

struma (stroo′mă) See goiter.

Hashimoto's s. See Hashimoto's thyroiditis, under thyroiditis.

s. lymphomatosa See Hashimoto's thyroiditis, under thyroiditis.

Riedel's s. See Riedel's thyroiditis, under thyroiditis.

strumitis (stroo-mi′tis) See thyroiditis.

strychnine (strik′nīn) An extremely poisonous alkaloid, derived from seeds of *Strychnos nux-vomica* and possessing an intensely bitter taste; formerly used as a stimulant of the central nervous system.

strychninism (strik′nin-iz-m) A toxic condition resulting from excessive use of strychnine.

Strychnos (strik′nos) A genus of tropical trees or shrubs (family Loganiaceae) that yield the alkaloids strychnine, curare, ignatia, and brucine.

study (stud′e) The pursuit and acquisition of information.

air-contrast s. See mucosal relief radiography, under radiography.

bioavailability s. See bioequivalence study.

bioequivalence s. The comparison of two or more different formulations of the same parent drug, one of which is an acceptable standard. Also called bioavailability study.

blind s. See blind trial, under trial.

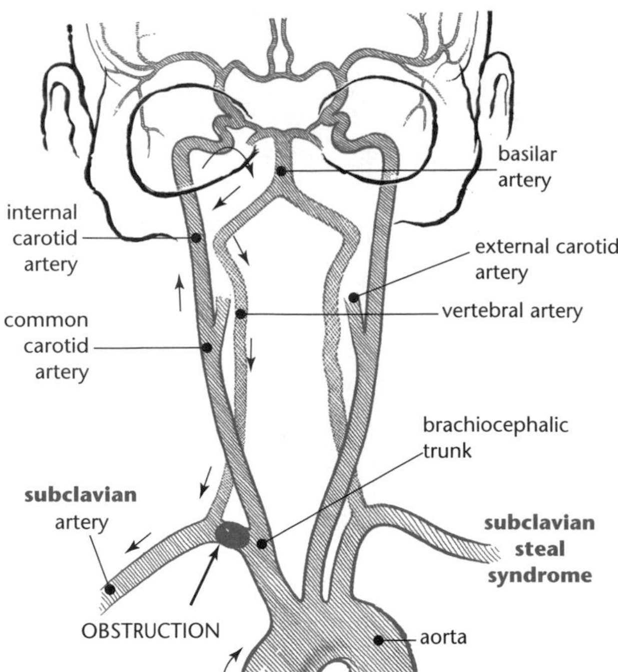

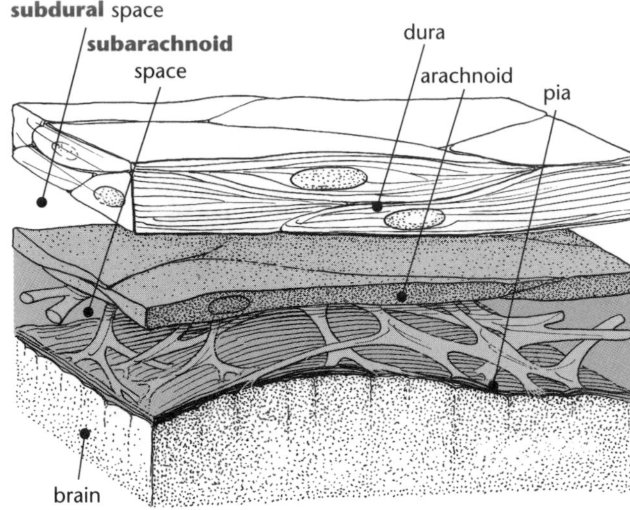

case comparison s. See case control study.
case control s. Epidemiological study that begins with identification of persons with the disease of interest, and a comparison (control) group of people without the disease; the relationship of a particulate attribute (e.g., sex, age, race) to the disease is examined by comparing the frequency with which the attribute appears in both groups. Also called case comparison study; case history study; case referent study.
case history s. See case control study.
case referent s. See case control study.
cohort s. An epidemiological study of a defined population with a statistical factor in common (e.g., smokers, recipients of a medication) that is supposed to influence the occurrence of a disease or other outcome; the study is conducted over a prolonged period (e.g., a year). Also called longitudinal study.
double-blind s. See double-blind trial, under trial.
longitudinal s. See cohort study.

stump (stump) **1.** The portion of a limb left after amputation. **2.** The pedicle remaining after removal of the tumor that was attached to it.
stun (stun) **1.** To daze or render senseless by a blow or other force. **2.** In cardiac muscle, to impair function markedly, but temporarily, as a result of an ischemic episode.
stupe (stoo̅p) A dampened, medicated, hot compress applied externally as a counterirritant.
stupefacient (stoo-pĕ-fa´shent) **1.** Causing stupor. **2.** Any agent that causes stupor, as a narcotic.
stupefaction (stoo-pĕ-fak´shun) The act of inducing stupor or narcosis.
stupefy (stoo´pĕ-fī) To make senseless; to induce a stupor.
stupor (stoo´por) A state of semiconsciousness.
stuporous (stoo´por-us) In a semiconscious state.
Sturge-Weber syndrome (sterj-web´er sin´drōm) An uncommon congenital condition marked by localized atrophy and calcification of the cerebral cortex, and an ipsilateral port-wine hemangioma on the face; often associated with mental retardation; attributed to faulty development of certain mesodermal and ectodermal elements.
stuttering (stut´er-ing) A speech disorder characterized by involuntary spasmodic hesitation and repetition of sounds.
St. Vitus' dance (sānt vīd-us dans) See acute chorea, under chorea.
stye, sty (sti) See hordeolum.
stylet, style (sti´let, stīl) A wire inserted into the lumen of a flexible catheter in order to stiffen it during passage.
styliform (sti´lĭ-form) See styloid.
styloglossus (sti-lo-glos´us) Relating to the styloid process of the temporal bone and the tongue.
styloid (sti´loid) Shaped like a peg; denoting certain bony processes. Also called styliform.
stylomastoid (sti-lo-mas´toid) Relating to the styloid and mastoid processes of the temporal bone.
stylostixis (sti-lo-stik´sis) See acupuncture.
stylus (sti´lus) **1.** A pencil-like device for applying medicines or caustics topically. **2.** A needle-like device for tracing a graphic recording on paper (e.g., in an electrocardiogram).
stype (stīp) A tampon; a plug or pledget of absorbent material.
stypsis (stip´sis) **1.** The action of an astringent or hemostatic agent. **2.** The application of an astringent.
styptic (stip´tik) An agent that contracts the tissues; an astringent.
subacromial (sub-ă-kro´me-al) Beneath the lateral extension (acromion) of the spine of the scapula (shoulder blade).
subacute (sub-ă-kūt´) A state between acute and chronic; applied to the intensity of a disease or toxicity of a chemical.
subalimentation (sub-al-ĭ-men-ta´shun) Insufficient nourishment.
subarachnoid (sub-ă-rak´noid) Beneath the arachnoid membrane of the brain or spinal cord.
subarcuate (sub-ar´ku-āt) Slightly bowed.
subareolar (sub-ă-re´o-lar) Beneath an areola, particularly of the nipple.
subatomic (sub-ă-tom´ik) Relating to the components of the atom.
subaural (sub-aw´ral) Below the ear.
subcapsular (sub-kap´su-lar) Situated beneath a capsule.
subcarbonate (sub-kar´bo-nāt) Any basic carbonate such as bismuth subcarbonate; a complex of a base and its carbonate.
subcartilaginous (sub-kar-tĭ-laj´ĭ-nus) **1.** Beneath a cartilage. **2.** Partly cartilaginous.
subchondral (sub-kon´dral) Beneath or just under the cartilages of the ribs.
subclavian (sub-kla´ve-an) **1.** Situated beneath the clavicle (collarbone). **2.** Relating to the subclavian artery.
subclavian steal syndrome (sub-kla´ve-an stēl sin´drōm) Reduced blood supply of the brainstem caused by obstruction of the subclavian artery proximal to the origin of the vertebral artery; blood flow through the vertebral artery is reversed and diverted from the brainstem to the arm, thus the subclavian "steals" cerebral blood.
subclavicular (sub-klă-vik´u-lar) Situated beneath the clavicle (collarbone).
subclinical (sub-klin´ĭ-kal) Denoting the phase of a disease prior to the manifestation of symptoms.
subconjunctival (sub-kon-junk-ti´val) Under the conjunctiva of the eye.
subconscious (sub-kon´shus) **1.** Less than fully conscious. **2.** In psychology, not fully in conscious awareness but easily accessible; distinguished from unconscious, which implies inaccessibility to awareness.
subcorneal (sub-kor´ne-al) Beneath or just under the cornified layer of the skin.
subcortex (sub-kor´teks) The portion of an organ immediately below the cortex, especially below the cerebral cortex.
subcostal (sub-kos´tal) Beneath the ribs.
subcranial (sub-kra´ne-al) Below the skull.
subculture (sub´kul-chur) A secondary culture of microorganisms, derived by inoculation from the primary culture.
subcutaneous (sub-ku-ta´ne-us) (SQ) Located beneath the skin. Also called hypodermic; subdermic.
subcuticular (sub-ku-tik´u-lar) Below the epidermis.
subcutis (sub-ku´tis) The loose fibrous tissue directly below the skin.
subdermic (sub-der´mik) See subcutaneous.
subdiaphragmatic (sub-di-ă-frag-mat´ik) Located beneath the diaphragm. Also called subphrenic.
subdural (sub-doo´ral) Located beneath the dura mater.
subendocardial (sub-en-do-kar´de-al) Under the membrane covering the heart (endocardium).
subfamily (sub-fam´ĭ-le) A taxonomic category between a family and a tribe.
subfertility (sub-fer-til´ĭ-te) Less than normal ability, in either the male or the female, to accomplish fertilization.
subgenus (sub-je´nus) A taxonomic classification ranking between a genus and a species.
subgingival (sub-jin´jĭ-val) At a level below the gingival margin.
subglottic (sub-glot´ik) Situated or occurring beneath the glottic opening between the vocal cords.
subhepatic (sub-hĕ-pat´ik) Situated below the liver.
subintimal (sub-in´tĭ-mal) Under the inner layer of a vessel wall (intima).
subinvolution (sub-in-vo-lu´shun) Failure of an organ to return to its normal size, as when the uterus remains abnormally large after childbirth.
subjacent (sub-ja´sent) Situated beneath or below.
subject (sub´jekt) **1.** A person or animal under treatment or experimentation. **2.** A cadaver used for dissection.
subjective (sub-jek´tiv) Perceived by the patient only and not by the examiner (e.g., discomfort or a sense of fatigue or malaise).

S

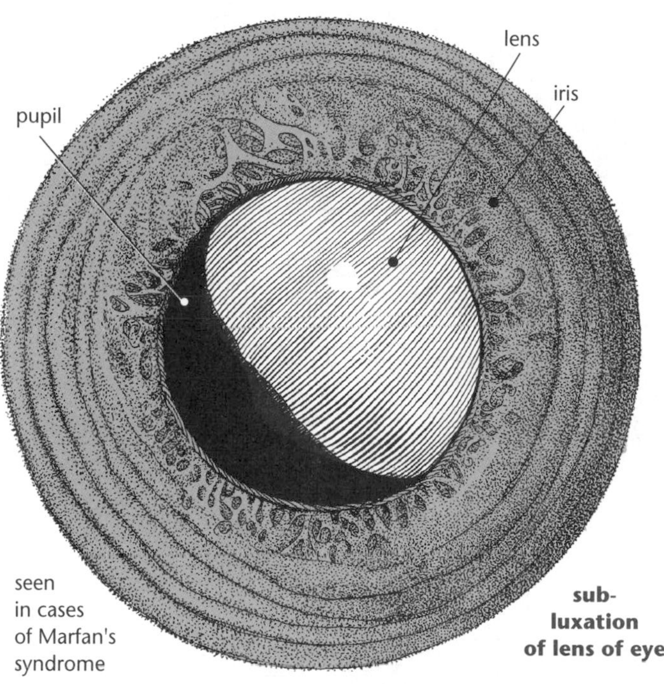

sub-luxation of lens of eye

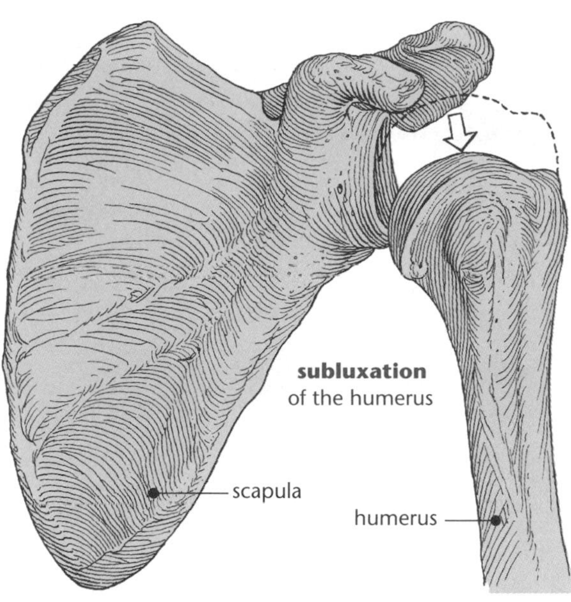

subluxation of the humerus

sublation (sub-la'shun) Detachment of a body part.
sublethal (sub-le'thal) Slightly less than lethal.
sublimate (sub'lĭ-māt) **1.** To convert a solid into a gas and back into a solid without passing through the liquid stage. **2.** A substance that has been subjected to sublimation. **3.** In psychoanalysis, to divert consciously unacceptable, instinctive drives into personally and socially acceptable channels; an unconscious process.
sublimation (sub-lĭ-ma´shun) The process of sublimating.
subliminal (sub-lim'ĭ-nal) Below the level of sensory perception.
sublimis (sub-li'mis) Latin for superficial.
sublingual (sub-ling´gwal) Located beneath the tongue.
subluxation (sub-luk-sa'shun) Partial dislocation.
s. of lens Incomplete dislocation of the lens of the eye.
submandibular (sub-man-dib´u-lar) Situated below the lower jaw.
submaxillary (sub-mak'sĭ-ler-e) Located beneath the upper jaw.
submental (sub-men'tal) Situated beneath the chin.
submicroscopic (sub-mi-kro-skop'ik) Too small to be seen through an ordinary light microscope.
submucosa (sub-mu-ko´să) The layer of tissue located beneath the mucous membrane.
subnormal (sub-nor'mal) Less than normal.
suboccipital (sub-ok-sip'ĭ-tal) Situated below the occipital bone or the back of the head (occiput).
suborbital (sub-or'bĭ-tal) Located beneath the orbit.
suborder (sub-or'der) A taxonomic classification ranking between an order and a family.
suboxide (sub-ok'sīd) An oxide of an element (e.g., carbon suboxide) containing the smallest proportion of oxygen. COMPARE: protoxide.
subphrenic (sub-fren'ik) See subdiaphragmatic.
subphylum (sub-fī'lum) A taxonomic classification ranking between a phylum and a class.
subscapular (sub-skap'u-lar) Located beneath or below the scapula (shoulder blade).
subscleral (sub-skle'ral) Beneath the sclera.
subscription (sub-skrip´shun) The part of a pharmaceutical prescription that contains directions to the pharmacist for the compounding of ingredients, or dispensing of medication, in a form suitable for use by the patient; it indicates the class of preparation (e.g., capsules) and the number of doses (e.g., 20). See also superscription, inscription, and signature.
subserous (sub-se'rus) Located beneath a serous membrane.
substage (sub'stāj) An attachment to a microscope, situated beneath the stage, by means of which accessories (mirror, diaphragm, condenser, or prism) are held in place.
substance (sub'stans) Matter; material.
alpha s. See reticular substance (a).
black s. See substantia nigra, under substantia.
gray s. See gray matter, under matter.
reticular s. (a) A mass of filaments seen in immature red blood cells after vital staining. Also called alpha substance; filar mass. (b) See reticular formation, under formation.
Rolando's s. See substantia gelatinosa of Rolando, under substantia.
slow-reacting s. (SRS SRS-A) Substance (possibly a leukotriene) released in anaphylactic shock, formed through the interaction of antigen with sensitized cells; produces a slow prolonged contraction of smooth muscle.
specific capsular s. A polysaccharide present in the capsule of many bacteria, believed to have a role in the transport of nutrients and protection against noxious agents. Also called specific soluble substance.
specific soluble s. (SSS) See specific capsular substance.
s. P A polypeptide found in the brain (concentrated in the substantia nigra) and elsewhere; a sensory transmitter that mediates pain perception; may also serve as a neurohormone.
white s. See white matter, under matter.
substantia (sub-stan'she-ă) Latin for substance.
s. gelatinosa of Rolando A mass of translucent gelatinous tissue, containing small nerve cells, on the posterior gray column of the spinal cord; appearing in cross-section as a crescentic cap over the horn.
s. nigra A layer of gray substance in the cerebral peduncles containing deeply pigmented nerve cells; it extends from the upper border of the pons into the subthalamic region; on cross-section it appears crescentic. Also called black substance.
substernal (sub-ster´nal) Situated beneath the sternum (breastbone).
substitute (sub'stĭ-tūt) A replacement.
blood s. Any of various fluid substances (human plasma, serum albumin, dextran solution, etc.) used for transfusion.
plasma s. Any sterile solution (usually saline, frequently with dextrans or serum albumins) administered intravenously as a substitute for plasma; used in dehydration, hemorrhage, and shock. Also called plasma expander.
salt s. Any low-sodium food additive (e.g., potassium chloride) used as a dietary alternative to table salt.
substitution (sub-stĭ-tu'shun) **1.** In chemistry, the replacement of one or more atoms of one element by those of another. **2.** An unconscious mechanism by which an unacceptable goal or emotion is replaced by a more acceptable one.
substrate (sub'strāt) Any substance upon which an enzyme acts.
renin s. See angiotensinogen.
substratum (sub-stra´tum) Any layer of tissue located beneath another layer.
substructure (sub´struk-chur) A structure or a dental appliance that is partly beneath the surface.
implant denture s. A metal framework embedded beneath soft tissue, in contact with bone, for supporting and stabilizing the superstructural portion of an implant denture.
subthalamic (sub-thă-lam'ik) **1.** Situated beneath the thalamus. **2.** Relating to the subthalamus.
subthalamus (sub-thal'ă-mus) The portion of the diencephalon lying immediately beneath the thalamus, between the tegmentum of the midbrain and the dorsal thalamus.
subtype (sub'tīp) See serovar.
subungual (sub-ung´gwal) Beneath the nail of a toe or finger. Also called hyponychial.
subunit (sub-u'nit) A secondary unit or part of a more comprehensive unit.
suburethral (sub-u-re'thral) Located beneath the urethra.
subvirile (sub-vĭr'il) Characterized by deficient potency or masculine vigor; lacking in virility.
subvitrinal (sub-vit´rĭ-nal) Beneath the vitreous body.
subvolution (sub-vo-lu´shun) The operative procedure of turning over a flap of mucous membrane to prevent adhesion.
succagogue (suk'ă-gog) **1.** Stimulating glandular secretion. **2.** An agent having such property.
succedaneum (suk-sĕ-da'ne-um) A substitute, as the permanent teeth that replace the deciduous teeth, or a drug with properties similar to those of another.
succenturiate (suk-sen-tu´re-āt) Supplemental; accessory.
succinate (suk'sĭ-nāt) A salt of succinic acid.
succinic acid (suk-sin'ik as'id) An intermediate in the metabolism of tricarboxylic acid.
succinylcholine chloride (suk-sĭ-nil-ko'lēn klor´rīd) Choline chloride succinate, a muscle-relaxing drug used as an adjunct during anesthesia.
succinyl-coenzyme A (suk-sĭ-nil ko-en´zīm ā) (succinyl-CoA) The condensation product of succinic acid and coenzyme A.
succorrhea (suk-o-re'ă) An excessive flow of a digestive fluid, such as saliva or gastric juice.
succussion (sŭ-kush´un) The act of shaking the body as a diagnostic procedure; a splashing sound is produced in the presence of fluid and gas in a body cavity.

S

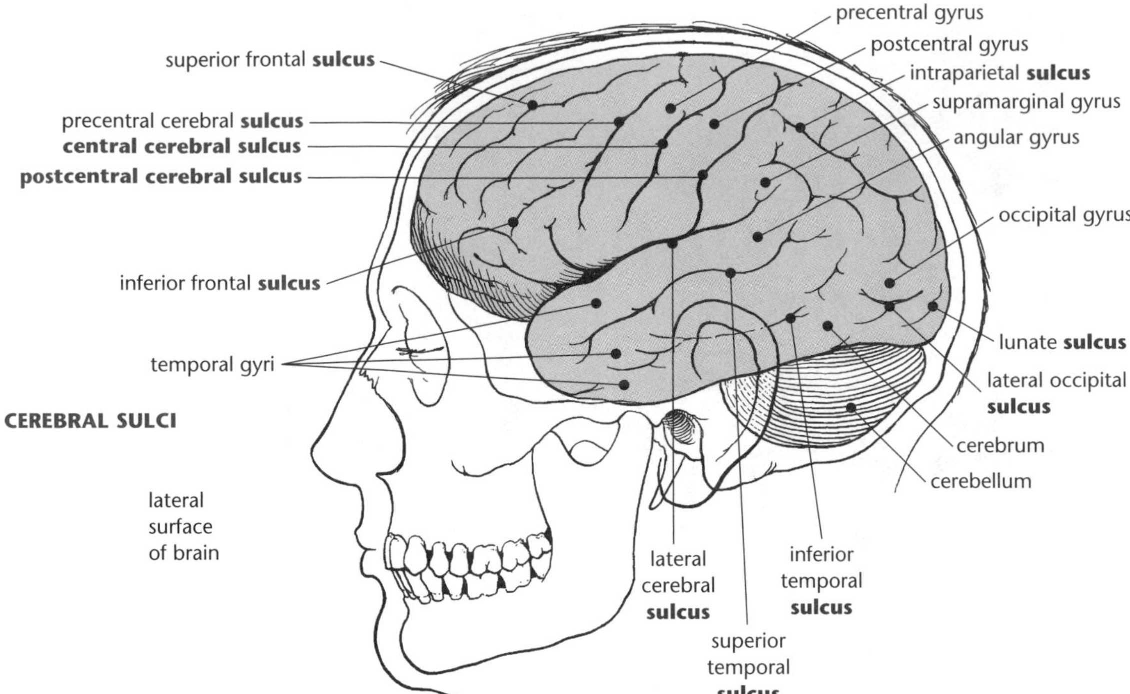

CEREBRAL SULCI

suck (suk) **1.** To draw fluid into the mouth. **2.** To draw fluid into a tube by establishing a partial vacuum.
sucrase (soo´krās) See invertase.
sucrose (soo´krōs) A disaccharide, $C_{12}H_{22}O_{11}$, which on hydrolysis yields glucose and fructose (monosaccharides); obtained chiefly from sugar cane, sugar beet, and maple; used as a sweetener and preservative. Also called cane sugar; saccharose.
suction (suk´shun) The process of aspirating or sucking.
sudamen (soo-da´men), *pl.* **sudamina** A minute vesicle formed by retention of sweat.
Sudan (soo-dan´) Name given to a series of histologic dyes. See under stain.
sudanophilia (soo-dan-o-fil´e-ă) Affinity for Sudan stain.
sudation (soo-da´shun) Sweating.
sudden infant death syndrome (sŭd´n in´fant deth sin´drōm) (SIDS) The sudden death of a baby caused by a disease which can be neither predicted nor prevented and that displays no specific symptoms; it is a major cause of death in infants after the first month of life. Also called crib death; cot death.
sudomotor (soo-do-mo´tor) Stimulating sweat glands.
sudor (soo´dor) Sweat.
sudoral (soo-dor´al) Relating to sweat.
sudoresis (soo-do-re´sis) Profuse sweating.
sudoriferous (soo-do-rif´er-us) Conveying sweat.
sudorific (soo-do-rif´ik) Causing sweat production.
sudoriparous (soo-do-rip´ă-rus) Producing sweat.
suet (soo´et) The fat within the abdomen or around the kidneys of sheep and cattle.
prepared s. Purified suet from sheep, used in pharmaceutical ointments.
suffocate (suf´ă-kāt) To impede respiration; to choke.
suffusion (sŭ-fu´zhun) **1.** Pouring of a fluid over the body. **2.** Flushing of the skin. **3.** Extravasation or spreading of a body fluid, such as blood, into surrounding tissues.
sugar (shoog´ar) A type of sweet carbohydrate.
amino s. A sugar containing an amino group (e.g., glucosamine).
blood s. See glucose.
brain s. See galactose.
cane s. See sucrose.
deoxy s. A sugar that contains fewer atoms of oxygen than of carbon (e.g., deoxyribose).
fruit s. See fructose.
grape s. See glucose.
hexose s. A simple sugar having six carbon atoms per molecule.
invert s. A mixture of equal parts of glucose and fructose, used in solution as a parenteral nutrient.
malt s. See maltose.
milk s. See lactose.
pentose s. A sugar that has five carbon atoms per molecule.
suggestion (sug-jes´chun) **1.** In psychiatry, the technique by which a therapist induces an idea or attitude that is adopted by the patient without questioning. **2.** Any idea or attitude so induced.
suicide (soo´ĭ-sīd) **1.** The act of taking one's own life voluntarily and intentionally. **2.** One who commits such an act.
suicidology (soo-ĭ-sīd-ol´ŏ-je) The study of the nature, causes, and control of suicide.
suit (so͞ot) An outer garment designed to be worn under particular environmental conditions.
antiblackout s. See anti-G suit.
anti-G s. A flight garment worn by pilots to increase their ability to withstand the effects of high acceleration (gravitational force or G) by exerting pressure on parts of the body below the chest; bladders (balloons) in the suit expand to apply external pressure to the abdomen and lower extremities during positive G maneuvers in flight, thereby preventing the pooling of blood in those areas. Also called antiblackout suit.
sulcate, sulcated (sul´kāt, sul-kā´ted) Furrowed.
sulculus (sul´ku-lus), *pl.* **sul´culi** A small groove.
sulcus (sul´kus), *pl.* **sul´ci** A groove or furrow.
alveolabial sulci The oral sulci between the anterior part of the jaws and the lips. Also called gingivolabial sulci.
alveololingual s. The sulcus at the floor of the mouth between the lower jaw and the tongue. Also called gingivolingual sulcus.
arterial sulci Grooves on the interior surface of the skull that house the meningeal arteries and their branches. Also called arterial grooves.
calcarine s. A deep arched sulcus on the medial surface of the occipital lobe; it separates the cuneus gyrus from the lingual gyrus. Also called calcarine fissure.
carpal s. A deep sulcus in the volar (front) side of the wrist formed by the carpal bones.
central cerebral s. A deep oblique sulcus on the lateral surface of each cerebral hemisphere between the parietal and frontal lobes of the brain. Also called central fissure; fissure of Rolando.
cerebral sulci The groves separating the convolutions (gyri) on the surface of the cerebral cortex. Also called cerebral fissures.
cingulate s. A sulcus on the medial surface of each cerebral hemisphere from the front of the corpus callosum to a point just behind the central sulcus; it separates the cingulate gyrus below from the medial frontal gyrus and the paracentral lobule above.
collateral s. A long sagittal sulcus on the inferior surface of the temporal lobe of each cerebral hemisphere; it separates the fusiform gyrus from the hippocampal and lingual gyri.
coronary s. Sulcus encircling the external surface of the heart between the atria and ventricles; occupied by arterial and venous vessels. Also called atrioventricular groove.
dorsal lateral s. of spinal cord A shallow longitudinal sulcus on either side of the dorsal median sulcus of the spinal cord; it marks the line of entrance of the posterior (dorsal) nerve roots.
dorsal median s. of spinal cord A shallow sulcus in the median line of the posterior (dorsal) surface of the spinal cord.
gingival s. The shallow groove between the free gingiva and the surface of a tooth.
gingivolabial s. See alveololabial sulci.
gingivolingual s. See alveololingual sulcus.
horizontal s. of cerebellum See horizontal fissure of cerebellum, under fissure.
lateral cerebral s. A deep oblique sulcus on the inferior and lateral surfaces of each cerebral hemisphere separating the temporal lobe below from the frontal and parietal lobes above; it divides into three branches: anterior horizontal, anterior ascending, and posterior branches. Also called sylvian sulcus; fissure of Sylvius; lateral cerebral fissure.
median s. of tongue A slight, median, longitudinal depression running forward on the dorsal surface of the tongue from the foramen cecum; it divides the tongue into symmetrical halves.
occlusal s. A sulcus on the occlusal surface of a tooth.
parietooccipital s. A sulcus on the medial surface of the occipital region of each cerebral hemisphere extending upward from the calcarine sulcus; it separates the parietal and occipital lobes.
postcentral cerebral s. A somewhat vertical sulcus on the lateral surface of the parietal lobe of the cerebrum, posterior and parallel to the central sulcus; it separates the postcentral gyrus from the rest of the parietal lobe.
postcentral s. of spinal cord A sulcus on the lateral surface of the parietal lobe of the cerebrum; it separates the postcentral gyrus from the remainder of the parietal lobe.
precentral s. of spinal cord An interrupted sulcus on the lateral surface of the frontal lobe, anterior and somewhat parallel to the central sulcus.
terminal s. of tongue A shallow V-shaped groove on the tongue running laterally and forward from the foramen cecum; it marks the separation

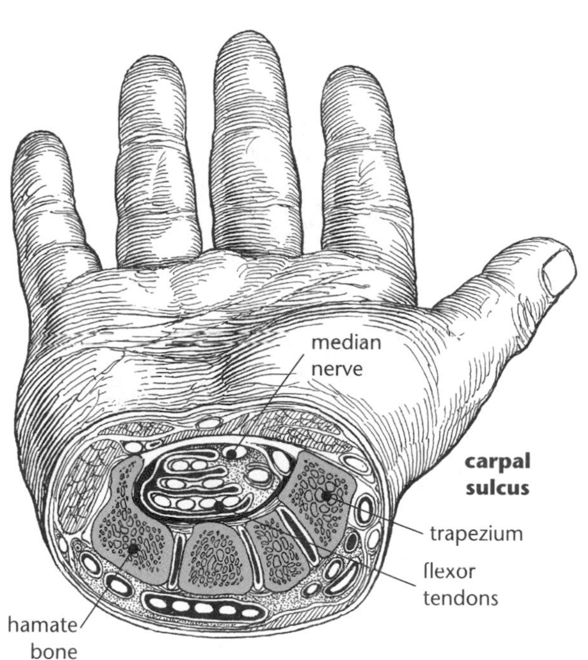

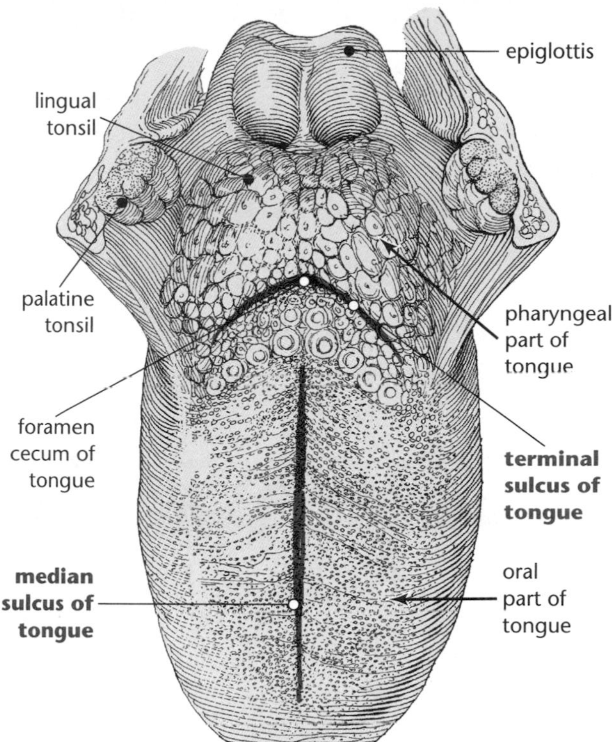

between the oral and pharyngeal parts of the tongue.

ventral lateral s. of spinal cord An indistinct sulcus on either side of the ventral median fissure of the spinal cord, marking the line of exit of the ventral nerve roots.

sulfa (sul´fă) Denoting any of the sulfa drugs chemically similar to sulfonamide, such as sulfisoxazole and sulfadiazine.

sulfanilamide (sul-fa-nil´ă-mīd) A potent antibacterial crystalline compound, $C_6H_8N_2SO_2$; first of the sulfonamides discovered and used in the treatment of bacterial infections.

sulfonamides (sul-fon´ă-mīdz) A group of synthetic antibacterial compounds effective against a wide range of gram-positive and gram-negative organisms; currently used only in specific circumstances. Commonly called sulfa drugs.

sulfate (sul´fāt) A salt of sulfuric acid; a compound containing the group SO_4.

sulfhemoglobin (sulf-he-mo-glo´bin) A compound derived from the action of hydrogen sulfide on hemoglobin.

sulfhemoglobinemia (sulf-he-mo-glo-bin-e´me-ă) Condition marked by persistent cyanosis, caused by the presence of sulfhemoglobin in the blood.

sulfide (sul´fīd) A compound of bivalent sulfur with a metal.

sulfisoxazole (sul-fī-sok´să-zōl) A sulfonamide (sulfa drug) used chiefly in the treatment of bacterial infections of the urinary tract; Gantrisin®.

sulfite (sul´fīt) A salt of sulfurous acid.

sulfmethemoglobin (sulf-met-he-mo-glo´bin) Compound formed by the combination of sulfide with the ferric ion of methemoglobin.

sulfobromophthalein sodium (sul-fo-bro-mo-thal´ēn so´de-ŭm) (BSP) A crystalline powder, soluble in water and used in testing liver function; Bromsulphalein®.

sulfonamides (sul-fon´ă-mids) General term for a group of antibacterial drugs containing the sulfanilamide group; commonly known as sulfa drugs.

sulfonate (sul´fo-nāt) **1.** A salt of sulfonic acid. **2.** To treat with sulfonic acid.

sulfone (sul´fōn) Any of various compounds containing the radical SO_2 and carbon.

sulfonic acid (sul-fon´ik as´id) Any of various acids containing one or more sulfonic groups ($-SO_3H$).

sulfonylurea compounds (sul-fo-nil-u-re´ă kom´ pounds) Derivative compounds of isopropylthiodiazylsulfanilamide; because of their hypoglycemic action, they are used in the treatment of certain cases of diabetes mellitus. Also called sulfonylureas.

sulfosalicylic acid (sul-fo-sal-i-sil´ik as´id) A soluble solid, $C_6H_3(OH)\cdot(COOH)\cdot SO_3H$, used as a reagent for albumin and ferric ion.

sulfur (sul´fur) A pale yellow nonmetallic element, symbol S, atomic number 16, atomic weight 32.06; used in the preparation of pharmaceuticals and insecticides.

sulfur-35 (^{35}S) A radioactive sulfur isotope; a beta emitter with a half-life of 87.1 days; used as a tracer in studying protein systems, since it can be taken up by proteins by way of the sulfur-containing amino acids.

sulfuric (sul-fūr´ik) Containing sulfur, especially with valence 6.

sulfuric acid (sul-fūr´ik as´id) A heavy, oily, highly corrosive liquid, H_2SO_4. Also called oil of vitriol.

sulfurize (sul´fu-rīz) To combine with sulfur.

sulfurous (sul-fūr´us) **1.** Containing or derived from sulfur; denoting compounds of sulfur with a low valence (+4). **2.** Having the characteristics of sulfur.

sulfurous acid (sul-fūr´us as´id) A solution of sulfur dioxide, H_2SO_3; used as a disinfectant and bleaching agent.

sumat (soo´mat) (sum) Latin for let him take.

sumendum (sum) Latin for to be taken.

summation (sum-ma´shun) **1.** Totality. **2.** The quality of two or more drugs whereby their combined effects are equal to the sum of their individual effects.

s. of stimuli Muscular or neural effects produced by the frequent repetition of slight stimuli, one of which alone might not excite a response.

sunburn (sun´bern) An inflammation or blistering of the skin caused by excessive exposure to ultraviolet rays of the sun.

sundowning (sun-dou´ning) Colloquialism for the exacerbation of symptoms in the evening with improvement during the day; seen in advanced stages of certain dementias (e.g., Alzheimer's disease).

sunstroke (sun´strōk) A state of extreme prostration and collapse caused by prolonged exposure to intense sunlight.

superacidity (soo-per-ă-sid´ĭ-te) An excess of acid, beyond the normal; particularly increased acidity of the gastric juice.

superacute (soo-per-ă-kūt´) Extremely acute; said of a disease.

superalimentation (soo-per-al-ĭ-men-ta´shun) The therapeutic administration of nutrients in excess of the patient's nutritional requirements for the treatment of certain wasting diseases.

superalkalinity (soo-per-al-kă-lin´ĭ-te) Excessive alkalinity, beyond the normal.

superciliary (soo-per-sil´e-ar-e) Relating to the area of the eyebrow.

supercilium (soo-per-sil´e-um) Eyebrow.

superego (soo-per-e´go) In psychoanalytical theory, the part of the personality structure associated with ethics and standards formed in early life through identification with important persons, particularly parents; the conscience.

superexcitation (soo-per-ek-si-ta´shun) Excessive stimulation.

superfamily (soo-per-fam´ĭ-le) A taxonomic category between an order and a family.

superfatted (soo-per-fat´ed) Containing additional fat; said of certain soaps.

superfecundation (soo-per-fe-kun-da´shun) The impregnation of two or more ova, liberated during the same ovulatory cycle but not at the same sexual act and not necessarily by the same man.

superficial (soo-per-fish´al) On or near the surface.

superinfection (soo-per-in-fek´shun) Appearance of a new infectious agent complicating an infection already under treatment.

superior (soo-pe´re-or) Above; higher.

superior cerebellar artery syndrome (soo-pe´re-or ser-ĕ-bel´ar ar´ter-e sin´drom) Syndrome occurring in occlusion of the superior cerebellar artery; consists of loss of pain and temperature sensations on the side of the face and body opposite to that of the lesion, with incoordination in executing skilled movements.

superior mesenteric artery syndrome (soo-pe´re-or mes-en-ter´ik ar´ter-e sin´drōm) Obstruction of the superior mesenteric artery, marked by vomiting, pain, and extreme abdominal distention.

superior vena cava syndrome (soo-pe´re-or vē´nă kā´vă sin´drōm) Edema of the face, neck, and/or upper arms caused by obstruction of the superior vena cava, usually by lung cancer or lymphoma invading the mediastinum.

supernatant (soo-per-na´tant) Floating on a surface; denoting the liquid floating above a precipitate.

supernumerary (soo-per-noo´mer-ar-e) **1.** Accessory. **2.** Exceeding a normal or fixed number.

superovulation (soo-per-ov-u-la´shun) The production of a greater than normal number of ova, usually resulting from administration of gonadotropins (hormones) for assisted fertilization procedures.

supersaturate (soo-per-sach´u-rāt) To add a substance beyond saturation.

superscription (soo-per-skrip´shun) The part of the pharmaceutical prescription that directs the pharmacist to take the drugs listed to prepare the medication; indicated by the symbol R (from the Latin term *recipe*, take). See also inscription; subscription; signature.

supersonic (soo-per-son´ik) **1.** Having a frequency above the level of audibility of the human ear. **2.** Relating to speeds greater than the speed of sound in air.

S

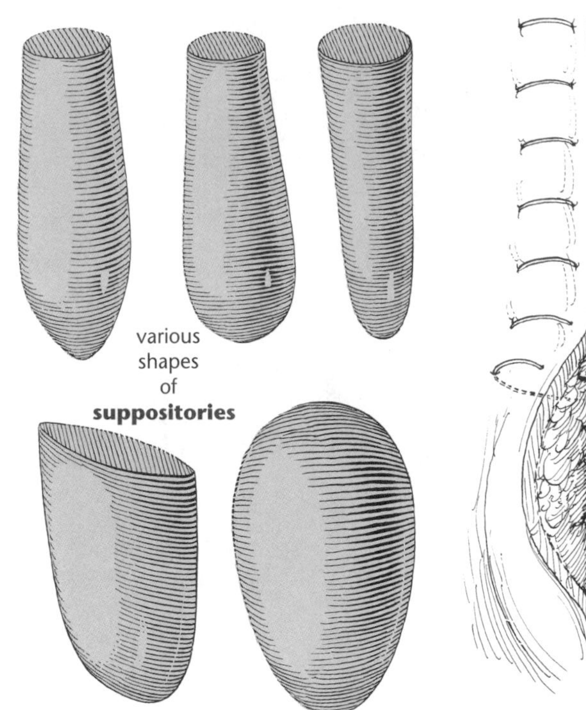

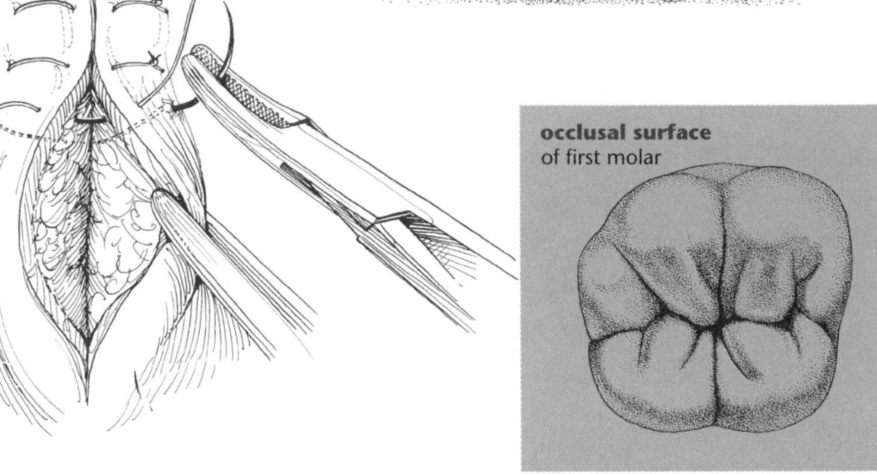

superstructure (soo-per-struk′chur) Any structure above a surface.

implant denture s. A dental prosthesis that is supported by a structure implanted beneath the oral soft tissues.

supervoltage (soo′per-vol-tij) A very high electromotive force, from 10 to 50 million electron volts; used in radiation therapy.

supination (soo-pĭ-na′shun) **1.** The act of lying on the back. **2.** Rotation of the forearm so that the palm of the hand is turned forward or upward.

supinator (soo′pĭ-na-tor) A muscle that supinates the forearm.

supine (soo′pīn) Lying on the back.

support (sŭ-port′) A device for holding a part in position.

suppository (sŭ-poz′ĭ-to-re) A solid medication designed for introduction into and dissolving within a body cavity other than the mouth.

suppression (sŭ-presh′un) **1.** The conscious exclusion from awareness of painful memories or feelings; distinguished from repression, which is unconscious. **2.** The cessation of a secretion; contrasted with retention, in which secretion occurs without discharge from the body.

immune s. Suppression of the immune response.

suppuration (sup-u-ra′shun) The production and discharge of pus.

suppurative (sup′u-ra-tiv) Pus-forming.

supra-anal (soo-pră-a′nal) Situated above the anus.

suprabuccal (soo-pră-buk′al) Above the cheek.

suprachoroid (soo-pră-kor′oid) The outer layer of the vascular (choroid) coat of the eye, consisting chiefly of pigmented, loose, connective tissue.

supraclavicular (soo-pră-klă-vik′u-lar) Located above a clavicle (collarbone).

supracondylar, supracondyloid (soo-pră-kon′dĭ-lar, soo-pră-kon′dĭ-loid) Situated above a condyle.

supracostal (soo-pră-kos′tal) Located above or over the ribs.

supradiaphragmatic (soo-pră-di-ă-frag-mat′ik) Above the diaphragm.

supraduction (soo-pră-duk′shun) In vertical divergence testing, upward movement of one eye when an ophthalmic prism is placed base down before it.

suprahepatic (soo-pră-he-pat′ik) Above the liver.

suprahyoid (soo-pră-hi′oid) Above the hyoid bone.

suprainguinal (soo-pră-in′gwi-nal) Above the groin.

supraliminal (soo-pră-lim′ĭ-nal) Above the threshold of sensory perception.

supralumbar (soo-pră-lum′bar) Above the lumbar region.

supramandibular (soo-pră-man-dib′u-lar) Above the mandible (lower jaw).

supramental (soo-pră-men′tal) Above the chin.

supranuclear (soo-pră-noo′kle-ar) Situated above a nucleus.

supraorbital (soo-pră-or′bĭ-tal) Above the orbit.

suprapubic (soo-pră-pu′bik) Above the pubic arch.

suprarenal (soo-pră-re′nal) **1.** Above or over the kidney. **2.** Pertaining to the adrenal (suprarenal) gland.

suprascapular (soo-pră-skap′u-lar) Situated above or in the upper part of the scapula (shoulder blade).

suprasellar (soo-pră-sel′ar) Above the sella turcica of the sphenoid bone.

supraspinal (soo-pră-spi′nal) Above or over a spine or spinal column.

supraspinatus syndrome (soo-pră-spi-na′tus sin′drōm) Pain and tenderness over the supraspinatus tendon upon abduction of the arm.

supraspinous (soo-pră-spi′nus) Situated above a spine, especially those of the vertebrae.

suprasternal (soo-pră-ster′nal) Above the sternum (breastbone).

supratympanic (soo-pră-tim-pan′ik) Above the middle ear.

supraventricular (soo-pră-ven-trik′u-lar) Above the ventricles.

supravergence (soo-pră-ver′jens) The upward movement of one eye while the other remains stationary. Also called sursumvergence.

supraversion (soo-pră-ver′zhun) **1.** Condition in which a tooth is abnormally elongated. **2.** The upward movement of both eyes.

sura (soo′ră) Latin for the calf of the leg.

surface (sur′fis) The outer boundary of an object.

buccal s. The surface of premolars and molars facing the cheek.

distal s. (a) The surface of a structure that is farther from a point of reference. (b) The surface of a tooth most distant from the median line.

dorsal s. (a) The surface of a structure that is directed toward the back of the human body. (b) The back of the human body.

facial s. The combined buccal and labial surfaces of anterior teeth.

incisal s. The cutting surface of incisors and cuspids.

labial s. The surface of incisors and cuspids facing the lips.

lingual s. The surface of a tooth facing the tongue.

mesial s. The proximal surface of a tooth facing the median line.

occlusal s. The grinding surface of a posterior tooth that comes in contact with one in the opposite jaw during occlusion.

proximal s. (a) A surface that is nearer to a point of reference. (b) The surface of a tooth that faces an adjoining tooth in the same dental arch.

ventral s. (a) The anterior or abdominal surface of the human body. (b) The surface of a structure that is directed toward the anterior side of the human body.

surface-active (sur′fis-ak′tiv) Altering the surface of a liquid, usually by reducing the surface tension.

surfactant (sur-fak′tant) A surface-active lipoprotein that normally serves to decrease the surface tension of fluids within the alveoli (air sacs) of the lungs; permits pulmonary tissues to expand during inspiration and prevents alveoli from collapsing and sticking together after each breath; in the fetus, it is largely produced after the 35th week of gestation.

surgeon (sur′jun) A health practitioner who specializes in surgery.

attending s. A member of the staff of a surgical department.

dental s. A dentist.

house s. A resident training in surgery in a hospital who acts under the orders of the attending surgeon.

oral s. A dental specialist concerned with the diagnosis and the surgical and adjunctive treatment of diseases, injuries, and defects of the jaws and associated structures.

surgeon general (sur′jun jen′er-al) The chief medical officer in the United States Army, Navy, Air Force, or Public Health Service.

surgery (sur′jer-e) The medical specialty concerned with the treatment of disease, injury, or deformity by means of manual and instrumental operations.

ambulatory s. Operative procedures performed on an outpatient basis; may be performed in a physician's office, a surgical center, or a hospital. Also called outpatient surgery.

cardiovascular s. Surgery performed on the heart and/or blood vessels.

elective s. Surgery of a nonemergency nature; although recommended, it can be scheduled in advance without affecting the health of the patient or the expected result of the procedure.

keratorefractive s. See refractive keratoplasty, under keratoplasty.

laparoscopic s. Operative procedure performed through a small incision with the aid of a tubular instrument (laparoscope), camera, light source, and various ancillary instruments. Also called operative laparoscopy.

laser s. The use of laser beams (e.g., carbon dioxide, argon, excimer) for thermal cutting, vaporizing, coagulation, or destruction of tissues.

Mohs' s. See Mohs' technique, under technique.

open heart s. Operative procedure performed on

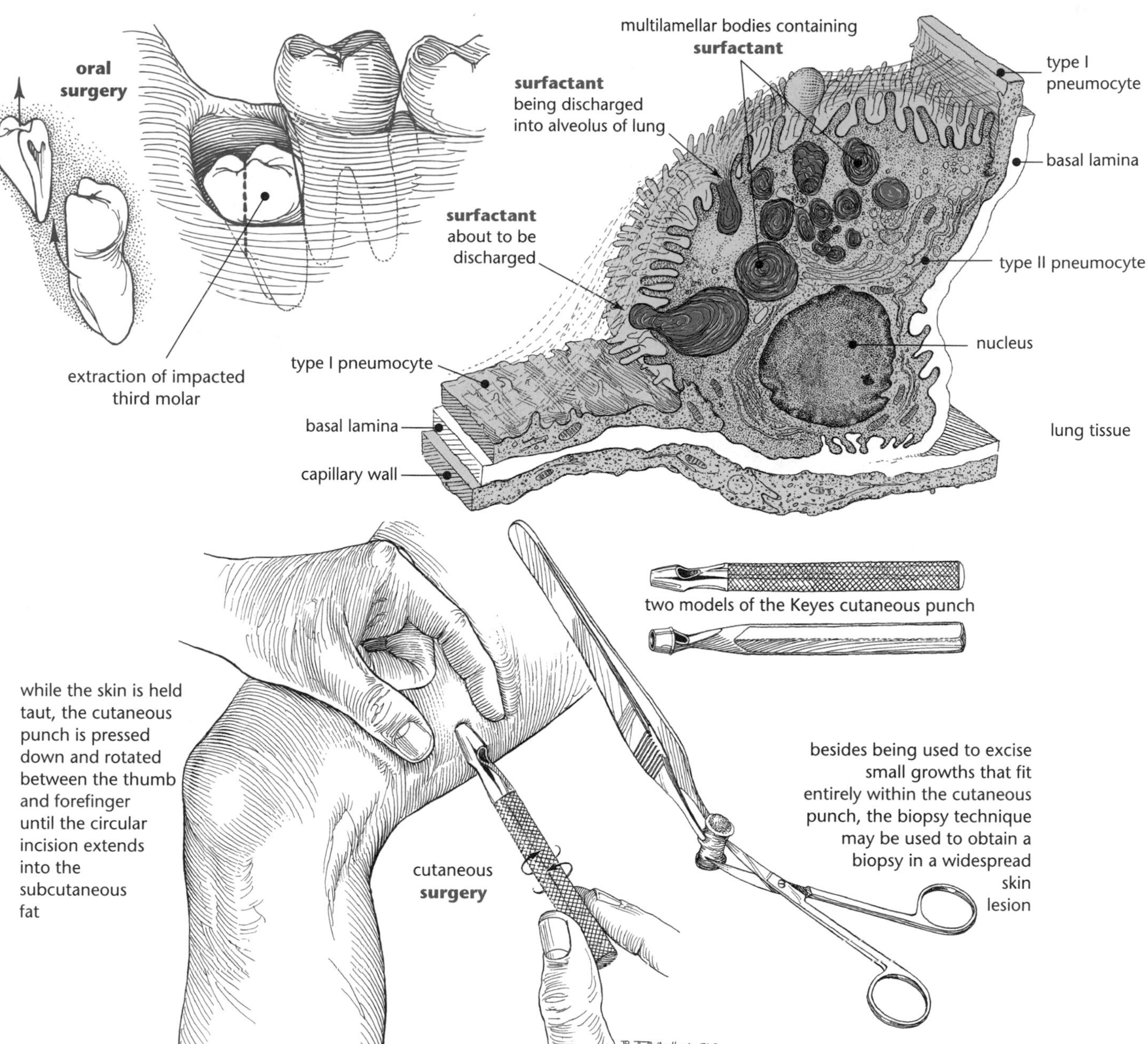

or within the exposed heart, usually to correct defects of the heart's interior through direct visualization.

oral s. The branch of dentistry dealing with the surgical treatment of disorders of the oral cavity.

orthopedic s. The branch of surgery specializing in the treatment of injuries and deformities of bones and chronic joint diseases.

plastic s. Surgery for the repair of physical defects or for the replacement of tissues lost through injury.

transsexual s. A series of major operations on the genitourinary tract designed to change a person's anatomic gender.

video-assisted thoracic s. (VATS) Operative procedure performed on the chest organs through a small incision with the aid of a video camera.

surrogate (sur´o-gāt) **1.** A person who substitutes for another. **2.** In psychiatry, a person who replaces a parent in the feelings of the patient.

mother s. One who replaces an individual's mother in his emotional feelings.

surveying (sur-vā´ing) In dentistry, studying the relative position of teeth and associated structures before designing a removable partial denture, in order to select a path of insertion and removal that will encounter the least interference.

susceptibility (sus-sep-tĭ-bil´ĭ-te) **1.** The state or quality of being sensitive or predisposed (e.g., to a familial disease). **2.** The state of lacking resistance to disease.

susceptible (sus-sep´tĭ-bl) **1.** Capable of being readily influenced or affected. **2.** Not immune to an infectious disease.

suspension (sus-pen´shun) **1.** The hanging of a body part from a support in order to subject it to traction. **2.** A noncolloidal dispersion of solid particles in a liquid.

suspensory (sus-pen´so-re) **1.** Denoting a structure (ligament or muscle) that aids in keeping an organ or part in place. **2.** Denoting a support for a dependent body part, such as a pouch attached to a body belt that provides support for the scrotum (used to relieve discomfort from such conditions as orchitis, varicocele, or epididymitis, or from scrotal surgery).

sustentacular (sus-ten-tak´u-lar) Supporting.

sustentaculum (sus-ten-tak´u-lum) A supporting structure.

s. tali A process that projects medially from the anterior end of the calcaneus and that serves to support the head of the talus bone of the foot.

Sutton-Rendu-Osler-Weber syndrome (sut´on-ron-duh´-ōs´ler-web´er sin´drōm) See hereditary hemorrhagic telangiectasia, under telangiectasia.

sutura (soo-tu´ră) Latin for suture.

suture (soo´chur) **1.** Stitch or stitches used in surgery to unite two surfaces. **2.** To apply a surgical stitch. **3.** The material used in closing a wound with stitches. **4.** A type of immovable fibrous joint uniting the bones of the cranium.

absorbable s. A sterile strand obtained from tissues of healthy animals that is capable of being gradually absorbed by living tissue; it may be treated to alter its absorbability, may be impregnated with antimicrobial substances, and may be treated with coloring materials.

blanket s. A continuous self-locking stitch. Also called lock-stitch suture.

button s. Suture in which the ends of the strand are passed through the eyes of a button and then tied.

catgut s. An absorbable suture obtained from the small intestine of sheep.

cobbler s. A suture made with a needle at each end of the strand.

continuous s. A suture running the length of the wound with only two anchoring knots, at the beginning and at the end.

Connell's s. Continuous suture in which the apposing edges are inverted.

coronal s. The articulation on top of the skull, between the posterior border of the frontal bone and the anterior borders of the two parietal bones.

cranial s. Any immovable fibrous articulation joining two bones of the skull.

Cushing s. A continuous inverting suture passed through the seromuscular layers of the gastrointestinal tract.

frontal s. The articulation between the two halves of the developing frontal bone.

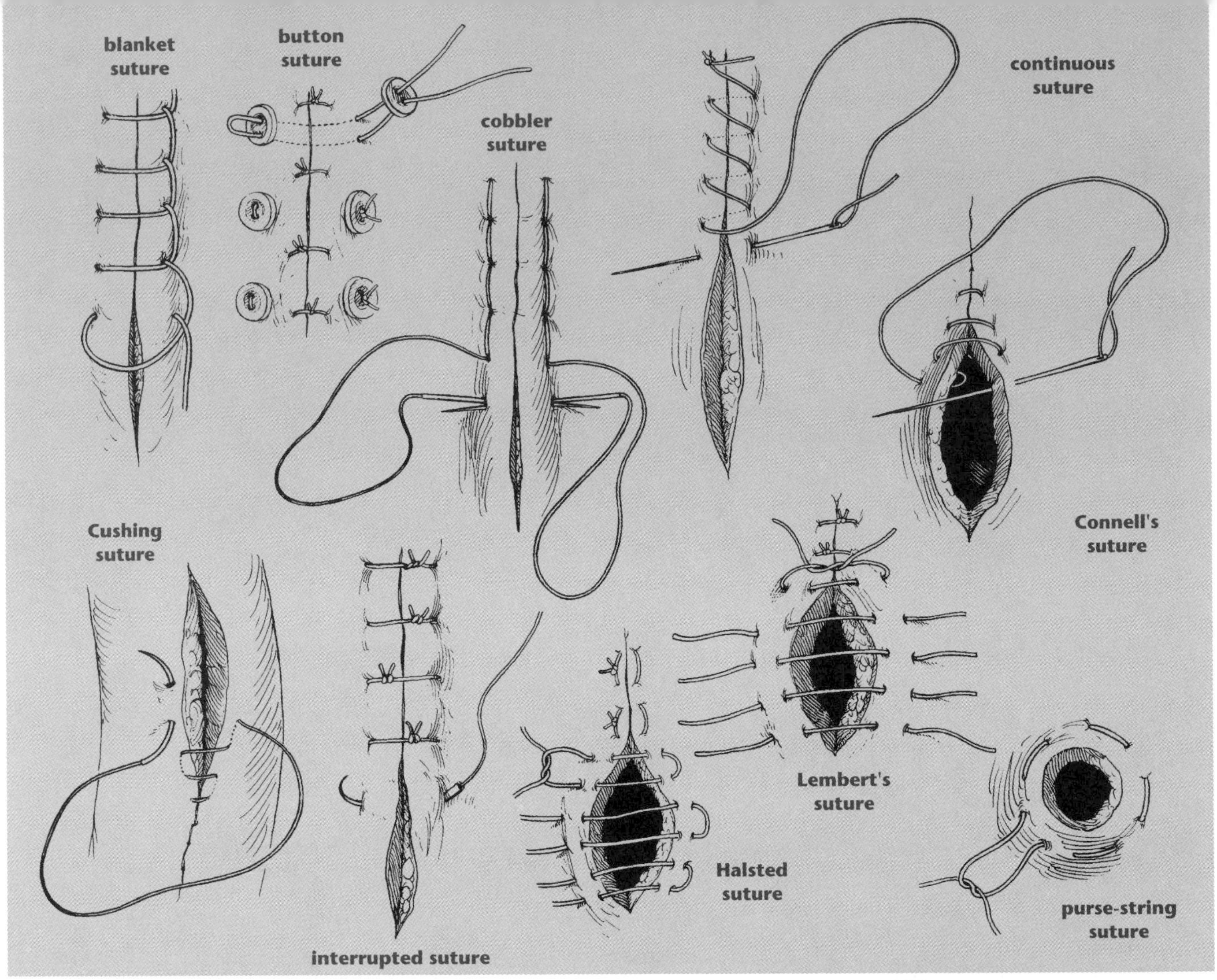

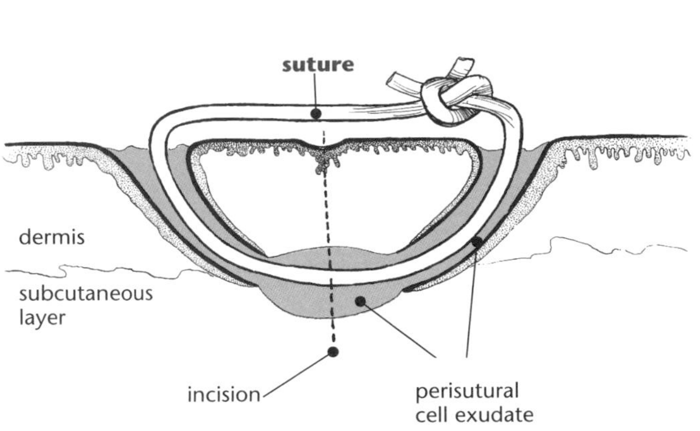

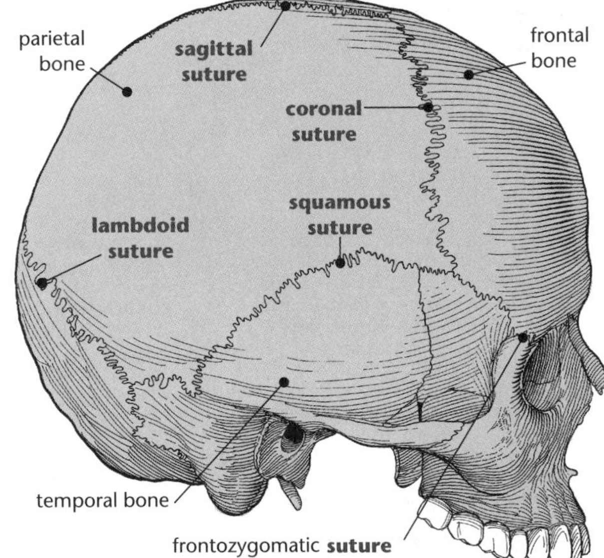

S

Halsted s. Interrupted inverting stitch, parallel to the wound and tied on one side.
interrupted s. A single stitch inverted and tied separately.
inverting s. A stitch that turns the apposing surfaces inward.
lambdoid s. The articulation at the back of the skull, between the occipital and parietal bones; it resembles the Greek letter lambda (λ). Also called parietooccipital suture.
Lembert s. An inverting suture, either continuous or interrupted, used to join two segments of intestine without entering the lumen.
lock-stitch s. See blanket suture.
mattress s. A suture that may be parallel to the wound (interrupted and continuous) or at right angles (interrupted on-end or vertical) and is inserted deep into the tissues.
metopic s. A frontal articulation occurring in some adult individuals; results from failure of the two frontal bones to fuse in childhood.
nonabsorbable s. A suture that is not absorbed by living tissues (e.g., silk, cotton, plastic, and alloy steel wire).
parietooccipital s. See lambdoid suture.
purse-string s. A continuous, circular inverting suture.
sagittal s. The articulation between the upper serrated margins of the two parietal bones, at the top of the skull.
squamous s. A type of articulation in which one bone margin overlaps its apposing bone margin, as the suture between the temporal and parietal bones on the side of the skull.
subcuticular s. Continuous suture inserted so as to approximate the tissues immediately under the skin, without penetrating the skin.
tension s. Large simple or mattress interrupted stitch used to prevent undue stress.

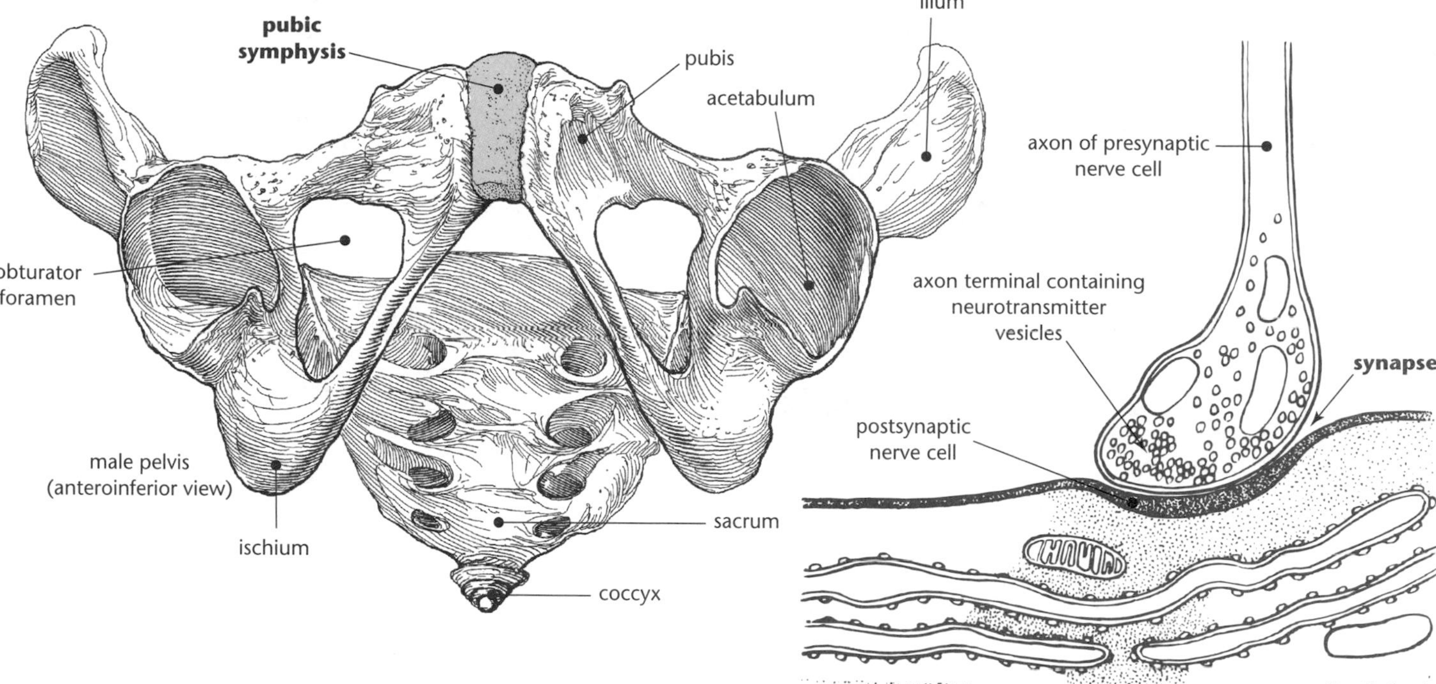

uninterrupted s. A continuous suture.

Svedberg (S) Unit of sedimentation, proportional to the rate of sedimentation of a molecule in a given centrifugal field; a sedimentation constant of 1×10^{-13} sec.

swab (swŏb) A small ball of cotton or gauze wrapped around the end of a stick or wire; used for cleansing, for applying medication, or for obtaining samples of material for bacteriologic examination.

swallow (swă´lo) To pass a substance from the mouth via the throat and the esophagus into the stomach; to perform deglutition.

swarming (swor´ming) Denoting the progressive spreading of motile bacteria, especially *Proteus* species, over the surface of the colony or solid culture medium.

sway-back (swa´bak) See lordosis.

sweat (swĕt) **1.** Perspiration. **2.** To perspire.

sweetbread (swēt´bred) The thymus or pancreas of a calf used for food.

swelling (swel´ing) **1.** A temporary enlargement that may or may not be inflammatory. **2.** In embryology, an elevation or protuberance indicating an early stage of development of certain structures.

Neufeld's capsular s. Swelling and opacity of the capsule of pneumococci when exposed to specific immune serum. Also called quellung reaction.

switch (swich) A change; transfer.

class s. Switch between C (constant) regions of heavy chains within a single immunoglobulin; results in a new class of antibody with the same binding site but a new heavy chain.

sycoma (si´ko-mă) **1.** A pendulous growth. **2.** A large soft wart.

sycosiform (si-ko´sĭ-form) Resembling sycosis.

sycosis (si-ko´sis) Disease involving the hair follicles of the beard, marked by pustules and crusting of the skin.

symbiont, symbiot (sim´bi-ont, sim´bi-ot) One of the organisms associated with another in a symbiotic relationship. Also called symbiote.

symbiosis (sim-bi-o´sis) **1.** The living together in intimate association of two dissimilar organisms. **2.** The mutually reinforcing dependency between two people.

symbiote (sim´bi-ōt) See symbiont.

symblepharon (sim-blef-ă-ron) Adhesion of the eyelid to the eyeball.

symblepharopterygium (sim-blef-ă-ro-ter-ij´e-um) Adhesion of the eyelid to the eyeball through a cicatricial band resembling a pterygium.

symbol (sim´bul) **1.** A mark or character representing a substance, quality, quantity, or relation. **2.** Something that represents something else.

chemical s. A symbol (letter or combination of letters) representing an atom or molecule of an element.

symbolization (sim-bol-ĭ-za´shun) An unconscious mental process whereby one object or idea stands for another through some aspect that both have in common.

symmetry (sim´ĕ-tre) Exact correspondence of constituent parts on opposite sides of a dividing plane or about an axis.

sympathectomy, sympathetectomy (sim-pă-thek´tŏ-me, sim-pă-thĕ-tek´tŏ-me) Surgical removal of a portion of a sympathetic nerve or of a sympathetic ganglion.

chemical s. Interruption of a sympathetic nervous pathway by means of a chemical.

sympathetic (sim-pă-thet´ik) **1.** Denoting the thoracolumbar autonomic nervous system. **2.** Relating sympathy.

sympathicotripsy (sim-path-ĭ-ko-trip´se) Therapeutic crushing of a ganglion of the sympathetic nervous system.

sympathicotropic (sim-path-ĭ-ko-trop´ik) Having an influence upon the sympathetic nervous system.

sympathoadrenal (sim-path-o-ă-dre´nal) Relating to the sympathetic nervous system and the hormones of the medulla of the adrenal gland (epinephrine and norepinephrine), which produce effects similar to those produced by sympathetic stimulation.

sympathoblast (sim-path´o-blast) One of the primitive undifferentiated cells that migrate from the embryonic neural crest and give rise to sympathetic ganglion cells and to the adrenal medulla.

sympathoblastoma (sim-pă-tho-blas-to´mă) See neuroblastoma.

sympathogonia (sim-pă-tho-go´ne-ă) The primitive ectodermal stem cells that migrate down from the neural crest to form the medulla of the adrenal (suprarenal) glands during embryologic development.

sympathogonioma (sim-pă-tho-go-ne-o´mă) See neuroblastoma.

sympatholytic (sim-pa-tho-lit´ik) Inhibiting the activity of the sympathetic nervous system. Also called sympathoparalytic.

sympathomimetic (sim-pă-tho-mĭ-met´ik) Producing effects similar to those caused by stimulation of the sympathetic nervous system.

sympathoparalytic (sim-pă-tho-par-ă-lit´ik) See sympatholytic.

sympathy (sim´pă-the) **1.** The physiologic or pathologic interrelationship between parts of the body. **2.** The capacity for understanding the feelings of another person.

symphyseal (sim-fiz´e-al) Relating to a symphysis.

symphysiorrhaphy (sim-fiz-e-or´ă-fe) Fastening of a divided symphysis.

symphysiotomy, symphyseotomy (sim-fiz-e-ot´ŏ-me) In obstetrics, division of the pubic symphysis with a wire saw to increase the capacity of a contracted pelvis and facilitate delivery.

symphysis (sim´fĭ-sis) **1.** Articulation in which the two opposing bone surfaces are covered with a thin layer of hyaline cartilage and united by a plate of fibrocartilage. **2.** In pathology, the abnormal fusion of two surfaces.

pubic s. The symphysis between the pubic bones at the anterior plane of the pelvis.

symport (sim´port) The simultaneous transport of two compounds across a cell membrane in the same direction by a common carrier mechanism.

symptom (simp´tum) Any manifestation of illness consciously experienced by a patient. For individual symptoms, see specific names.

cardinal s. A symptom that is of primary significance.

withdrawal s.'s A group of physiologic and psychic disturbances that follow the abrupt cessation of use of a psychoactive substance taken for a prolonged period of time. Also called withdrawal syndrome.

symptomatic (simp-to-mat´ik) Relating to a symptom.

symptomatology (simp-tom-ă-tol´ŏ-je) **1.** The group of symptoms of a disease. **2.** The study of the symptoms of a disease, their causes, and the information they furnish. Also called semiology; semeiology.

synalgia (sin-al´jă) See referred pain, under pain.

synapse (sin´aps) A gap (10–50 nm wide) through which a nerve impulse must pass to be transmitted from one nerve cell to another or from one nerve cell to a muscle or gland cell; accomplished by release of a special substance (neurotransmitter).

axodendritic s. The junction of the axon of a nerve cell with a dendrite of another nerve cell.

axosomatic s. The junction of the axon of a nerve cell with the cell body of another.

synapsis (sĭ-nap´sis) Process during the prophase stage of meiosis in which homologous chromosomes pair off and unite.

synaptic (sĭ-nap´tik) Relating to a synapse.

synarthrosis (sin-ar-thro´sis), *pl.* **synarthro´ses** A joint in which two bones are united by fibrous tissue permitting little or no movement between the bones. Also called synarthrodial joint.

syncanthus (sin-kan´thus) Adhesion of the eyeball to orbital structures.

synchondrosis (sin-kon-dro´sis), *pl.* **synchondro´ses** The union of two bones by cartilage; usually the cartilage is replaced by bone (e.g.,

S

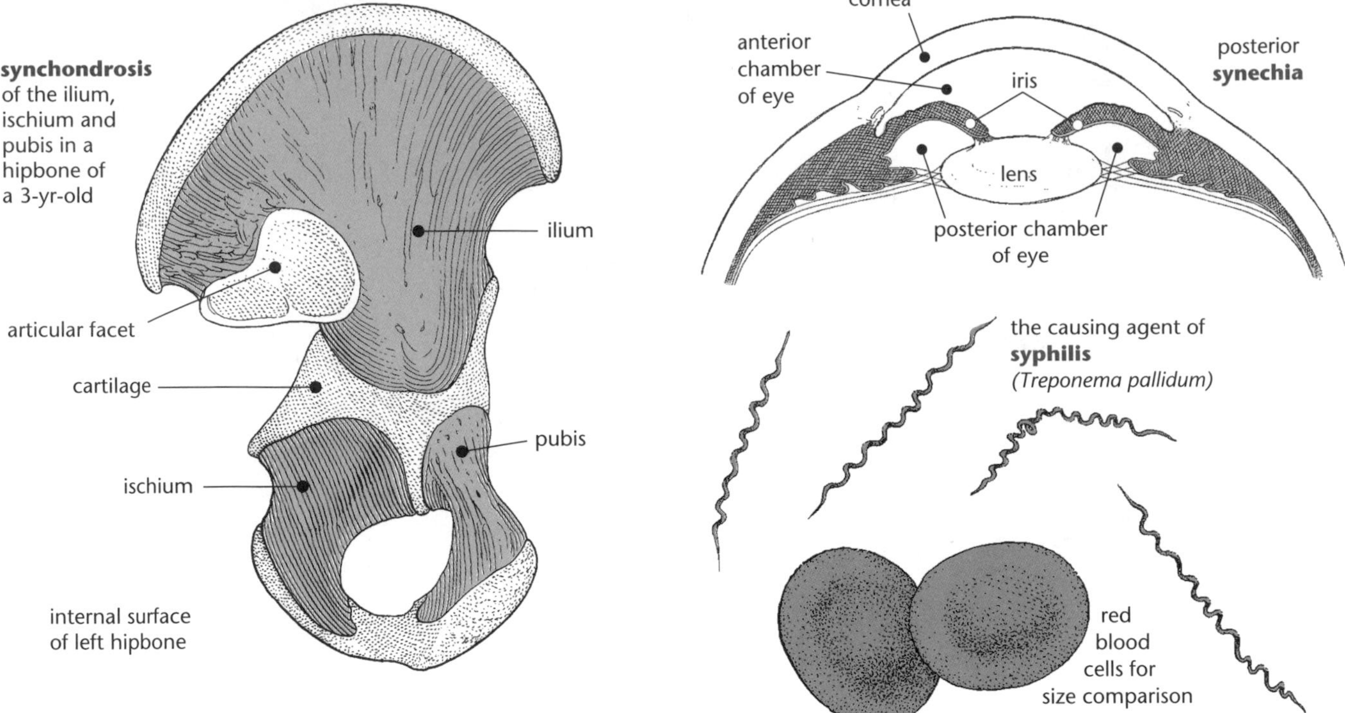

between the skull bones of the newborn).

synchronia (sin-kro´ne-ă) **1.** Synchronism. **2.** The formation and development of tissues at the normal time.

synchronism (sin´kro-niz-m) The simultaneous occurrence of two or more events.

synchrotron (sin´kro-tron) An accelerator for generating high speed electrons or protons around a fixed circular path by a radio-frequency potential.

synchysis (sin´kĭ-sis) Condition of the eye marked by liquefaction of the vitreous body.

s. scintillans The presence of numerous minute, glistening cholesterol crystals floating in a liquefied vitreous body. The person's vision is not affected.

synclitism (sin´klit-iz-m) The attitude of the fetal head in relation to the maternal pelvis as it descends into the pelvis; the head enters the pelvis with its sagittal suture in the transverse plane of the maternal pelvis, midway between the pubic bone and the sacrum. Formerly called obliquity.

syncopal (sin´ko-pal) Relating to fainting.

syncope (sin´ko-pe) A brief loss of consciousness; a faint.

syncytiotrophoblast (sin-sit-e-o-trof´o-blast) The peripheral part of the trophoblast, developed as a thick layer of syncytium from the single-layered trophoblast; it penetrates maternal tissues to attach the blastocyst to the uterus and eventually enters into the formation of the placenta. Also called syntrophoblast.

syncytium (sin-sish´e-um) A mass of protoplasm with many nuclei, seemingly resulting from the merging of several cells.

syndactyly, syndactylism (sin-dak´tĭ-le, sin-dak´tĭ-liz-m) Partial or total webbing or fusion of two or more fingers or toes.

syndesmitis (sin-des-mi´tis) Inflammation of a ligament.

syndesmectomy (sin-des-mek´tŏ-me) Excision of a section of a ligament.

syndesmopexy (sin-des-mo-pek´se) Operative fixation of a dislocation by reconstruction of the ligaments of the joint.

syndesmoplasty (sin-des-mo-plas´te) Reparative surgery of a ligament.

syndesmorrhaphy (sin-des-mor´ă-fe) Surgical suture or repair of a ligament.

syndesmosis (sin-des-mo´sis), *pl.* **syndesmo´ses** A type of fibrous articulation in which the fibrous tissue between the bones forms a membrane or ligament, as the tibiofibular articulation or the union of the footplate of the stapes to the oval window of the inner ear.

syndrome (sin´drōm) A set of signs and symptoms that appear together with reasonable consistency. For individual syndromes, see specific names.

syndrome of inappropriate secretion of antidiuretic hormone (sin´drōm ŭv in-ă-pro´pre-ĭt se-kre´shun ŭv an-tĭ-di-u-ret´ik hor´mōn) (SIADH) Persistent high levels of antidiuretic hormone, expanded extracellular volume, and low concentration of plasma sodium; osmolality of urine is greater than that of plasma despite low plasma osmolality.

syndromic (sin-drom´ik) Relating to a syndrome.

synechia (sĭ-nek´e-ă), *pl.* **synech´iae** Any adhesions; especially adhesion of the iris to the cornea or to the lens of the eye.

synechotomy (sin-ĕ-kot´ŏ-me) Division of the adhesions in synechia.

synechtenterotomy (sin-ĕk-ten-ter-ot´ŏ-me) Division of intestinal adhesions.

syneresis (sĭ-ner´ĕ-sis) The shrinking or contraction of gels upon prolonged standing, causing the solid components to become more concentrated and droplets of the liquid medium to form on the surface (e.g., the shrinkage of blood clots, agar culture media, custards).

synergism, synergy (sin´er-jiz-m, sin´er-je) **1.** Cooperation in action, as the coordinated action of two or more substances or organs to produce an effect of which each is individually incapable. **2.** In pharmacology, the quality of two drugs whereby their combined effects are greater than the algebraic sum of their individual effects.

synergist (sin´er-jist) Anything such as a drug or muscle, that acts in conjunction with another toward a common purpose.

synesthesia (sin-es-the´zhă) Condition in which, in addition to the normal sensation, a stimulus produces another unrelated sensation.

auditory s. Synesthesia in which the secondary sensation is that of a sound. Also called phonism.

synesthesialgia (sin-es-the-ze-al´jă) Condition in which a stimulus, in addition to exciting the normal sensation, produces pain somewhere else.

syngamy (sing´gă-me) Conjugation or union of the nuclei of two gametes in fertilization to produce a zygote nucleus.

syngeneic (sin-je-ne´ik) Relating to genetically identical (isogenic) or near-identical mammals (identical twins or highly inbred animals).

syngenesis (sin-jen´ĕ-sis) Sexual reproduction.

syngraft (sin´graft) See isograft.

synkaryon (sin-kar´e-on) The nucleus formed when the nuclei of two cells fuse during fertilization.

synkinesis (sin-ki-ne´sis) Involuntary motion of one part when another part is moved.

synoptophore (sin-op´to-fōr) A modified stereoscope used in training individuals afflicted with ocular muscle imbalance to use the two eyes together.

synorchidism, synorchism (sin-or´kĭ-diz-m) Congenital fusion of the testes.

synostosis (sin-os-to´sis) Abnormal fusion of bones forming a joint by proliferation of bone tissue. Also called true ankylosis; bony ankylosis.

synovectomy (sin-o-vek´tŏ-me) Surgical removal of a portion or all of a diseased synovial membrane of a joint.

synovia (sĭ-no´ve-ă) The clear, thick, lubricating fluid in a joint, bursa, or tendon sheath; it is secreted by the membrane lining the cavity or tendon sheath (synovial membrane).

synovial (sĭ-no´ve-al) Relating to synovia.

synovianalysis (sĭ-no-ve-ă-nal´ĭ-sis) The microscopic examination, identification, and cell count of joint fluid (synovia); five categories can be distinguished: normal, noninflammatory, inflammatory-immunologic, inflammatory-crystalline, and inflammatory-infectious.

synovin (sin´o-vin) Mucinous substance found in synovia.

synovioma (sĭ-no-ve-o´mă) Tumor of synovial origin.

synovitis (sin-o-vi´tis) Inflammation of the membranes lining a joint (synovial membranes).

pigmented villonodular s. Diffuse inflammation and nodular thickening of the synovial membrane of a joint, usually of the knee, often with orange-brown outgrowths containing hemosiderin pigment. Cause is unknown.

syntenic (sin-ten´ik) Relating to synteny.

synteny (sin´tĕ-ne) In genetics, the physical presence of two or more loci together on the same chromosome.

synthermal (sin-ther´mal) Of the same temperature.

synthesis (sin´thĕ-sis) A building up; especially the formation of a compound by the combination of simpler compounds or elements.

synthesize (sin-thĕ-sīz´) To combine so as to produce a complex compound from simpler compounds; to form by synthesis.

synthetase (sin´thĕ-tās) Trivial name for ligase.

synthetic (sin-thet´ik) Made by synthesis.

syntonic (sin-ton´ik) In balance.

syntrophism (sin´trōf-iz-m) Enhanced growth of a strain of bacteria resulting from admixture with or nearness of another strain.

syntrophoblast (sin-trof´o-blast) See syncytiotrophoblast.

syntrophus (sin´trō-fus) Any congenital disease.

syphilid (sif´ĭ-lid) Any of the skin lesions of syphilis. Also called syphiloderma.

syphilis (sif´ĭ-lis) An infectious venereal disease caused by *Treponema pallidum*, transmitted through

S

SYNOVIANALYSIS

DISEASE	APPEARANCE	MUCIN CLOT VISCOSITY	LEUKOCYTES PER ML (% polymorphonuclear leukocytes)	OTHER FEATURES
normal	clear, straw-colored	good	<200 (<25%)	sugar is 90% of serum level
GROUP I NONINFLAMMATORY				
osteoarthritis	clear, straw-colored	good	100–1000 (<25%)	
traumatic arthritis	clear to bloody	good	1000 (<25%)	red blood cells may be present
GROUP II INFLAMMATORY — IMMUNOLOGICAL				
systemic lupus erythematosus	clear to slightly cloudy	good to fair	2000–5000 (10–15%)	low complement + LE prep
rheumatoid arthritis	cloudy, light yellow	poor	8,000–20,000 (60–75%)	low complement, slightly low sugar
Reiter's syndrome	cloudy	poor	10,000–40,000 (60–90%)	high complement
GROUP III INFLAMMATORY — CRYSTALLINE				
gout	cloudy	poor	10,000–20,000 (60–95%)	sodium urate crystals (negatively birefringent)
pseudogout	cloudy	fair to poor	5000–40,000 (60–95%)	calcium pyrophosphate crystals (weakly positive birefringent)
GROUP IV INFLAMMATORY— INFECTIONS				
acute bacterial arthritis	cloudy, gray	poor	50,000+ (98%)	low sugar (less than 2/3 plasma level)
tuberculosis arthritis	cloudy, yellow or gray	poor	25,000 (50–90%)	low sugar (less than 1/2 plasma level)

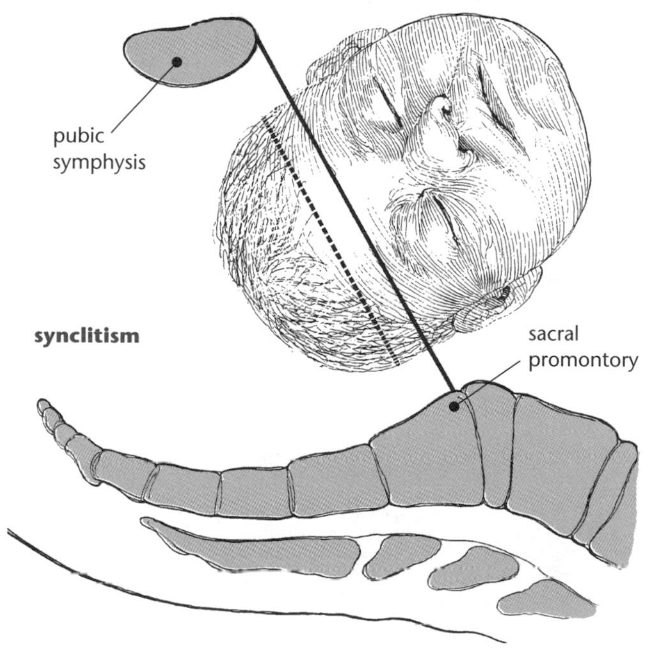

synclitism

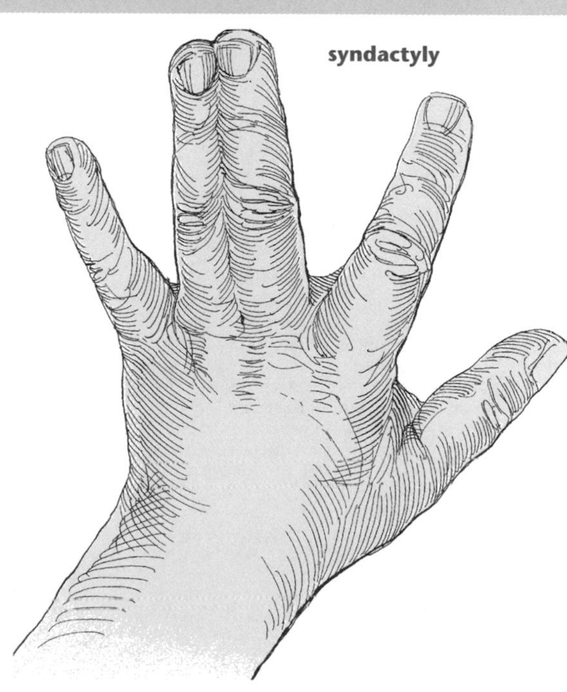
syndactyly

S

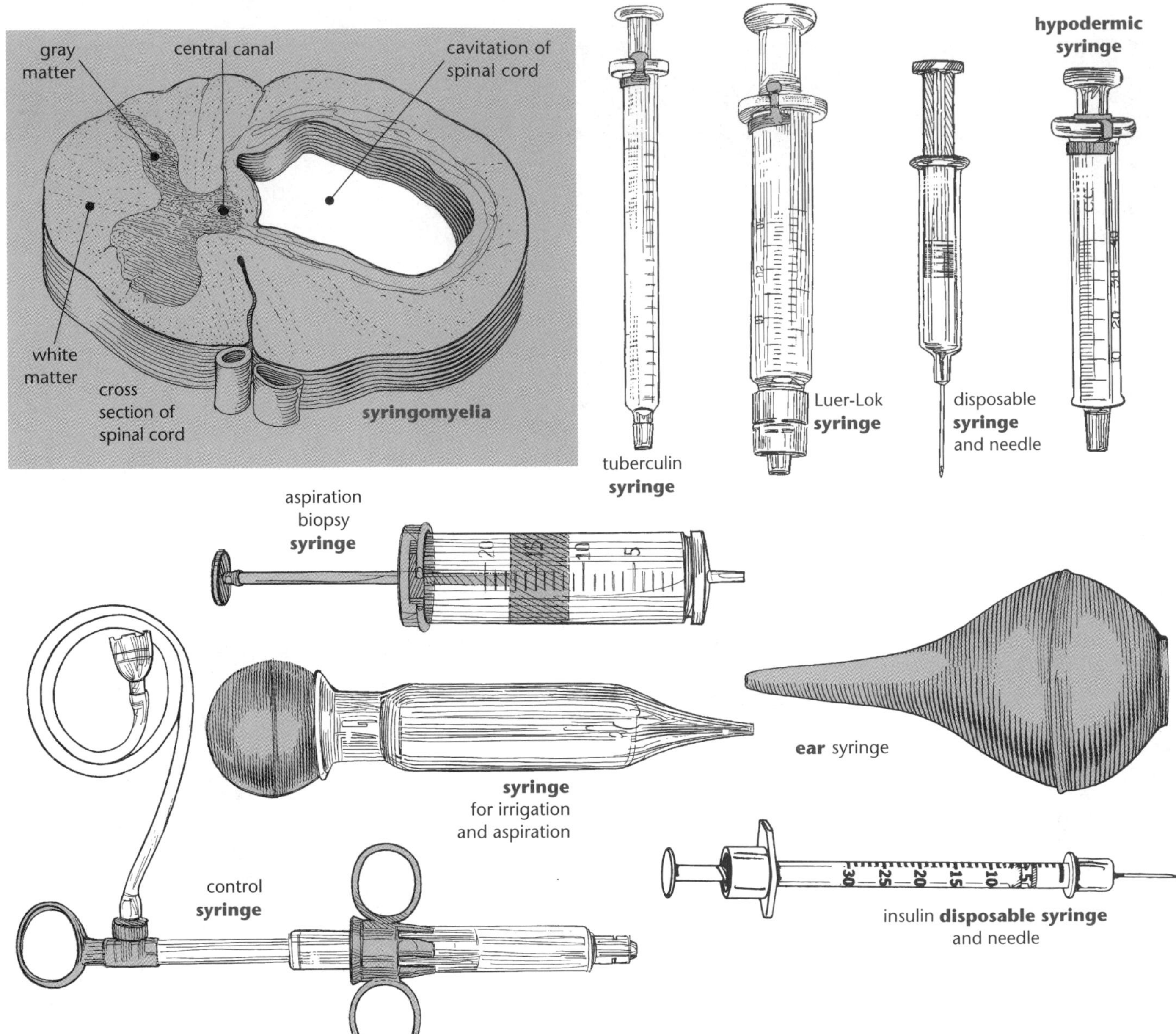

sexual intercourse or any direct contact; the first symptoms develop after an incubation period of 12 to 20 days. Nonvenereal infection with a treponeme very similar to *Treponema pallidum*; occurs mainly in arid climates. Also called bejel; nonvenereal syphilis.

congenital s. Syphilis present at birth.

endemic s. Nonvenereal infection with a treponeme similar to *Treponema pallidum*; occurs mainly in arid climates. Also called bejel; nonvenereal syphilis.

late latent s. A form of the disease in which there is serologic or historic evidence of syphilis of more than four years' duration; it is not detectable by physical examination, by examination of the cerebrospinal fluid, or by roentgenographic examination of the heart and aorta.

latent s. A phase of syphilis following the primary infection in which the organisms disappear from the skin and blood, and the foci of infection are beyond diagnostic reach; if evidence of infection is present in the cerebrospinal fluid the stage is designated as asymptomatic neurosyphilis.

primary s. The first stage of the disease, beginning with the appearance on the genitalia, and sometimes the oral cavity, of a small ulcer which develops into a chancre.

secondary s. The second stage of syphilis, beginning after healing of the initial chancre (between 6 and 12 weeks after its appearance) and lasting indefinitely; it is marked by infectious, copper-colored skin eruptions, mucous patches, fever, and other constitutional symptoms.

tertiary s. The final, noninfectious stage of the disease, beginning after a lapse of several months or years; marked by the development throughout the body of masses of granulomatous tissue (gummas); serious disorders of the nervous and vascular systems may occur.

syphilitic (sif-ĭ-lit′ik) Relating to or suffering from syphilis.

syphiloderma (sif-ĭ-lo-der′mă) See siphilid.

syphilogenesis (sif-ĭ-lo-jen′ĕ-sis) Origin of syphilis.

syphiloid (sif′ĭ-loid) Resembling or characteristic of syphilis.

syphilology (sif-ĭl-ol′ŏ-je) The medical study pertaining to the nature and treatment of syphilis.

syphiloma (sif-ĭ-lo′mă) A gumma; a syphilitic tumor.

syphilophobia (sif-ĭ-lo-fo′be-ă) An unwarranted fear of acquiring syphilis.

syringadenoma (sĭ-ring-gad-ĕ-no′mă) A benign sweat gland tumor. Also called syringoadenoma.

syringadenosus (sĭ-ring-gad-ĕ-no′sus) Relating to sweat glands.

syringe (sĭ-rinj′, sir′inj) A device used for injecting or withdrawing fluids.

fountain s. An apparatus consisting of a reservoir for holding water or special solutions, to the bottom of which is attached a tube with a nozzle at the end; used for enemas and vaginal irrigations (douches).

hypodermic s. A syringe for the introduction of liquid remedies through a hypodermic needle into subcutaneous tissues.

syringitis (sir-in-ji′tis) Inflammation of a tubular structure of the body (e.g., a uterine tube).

syringoadenoma (sĭ-ring-go-ad-ĕ-no′mă) See syringadenoma.

syringobulbia (sĭ-ring-go-bul′be-ă) The presence of abnormal cavities in the brainstem.

syringocystoma (sĭ-ring-go-sis-to′mă) Cystic tumor of a hair follicle.

syringoma (sir-ing-go′mă) A benign neoplasm of the tubular portion of a sweat gland.

syringomyelia (sĭ-ring-go-mi-e′le-ă) A disease marked by the presence of cavities in the gray matter adjacent to the central canal of the spinal cord, causing loss of the senses of pain and temperature with retention of the sense of touch; in advanced cases, it often causes paralysis of the extremities and scoliosis of the lumbar spine.

syringomyelitis (sĭ-ring-go-mi-ĕ-li′tis) Inflammation of the spinal cord with formation of cavities in its substance.

syringomyelocele (sĭ-ring-go-mi′ĕ-lo-sēl) Protrusion of the spinal cord, with the central canal greatly distended with cerebrospinal fluid, through an abnormal gap in the vertebral column.

syringotomy (sir-in-got′ŏ-me) See fistulotomy.

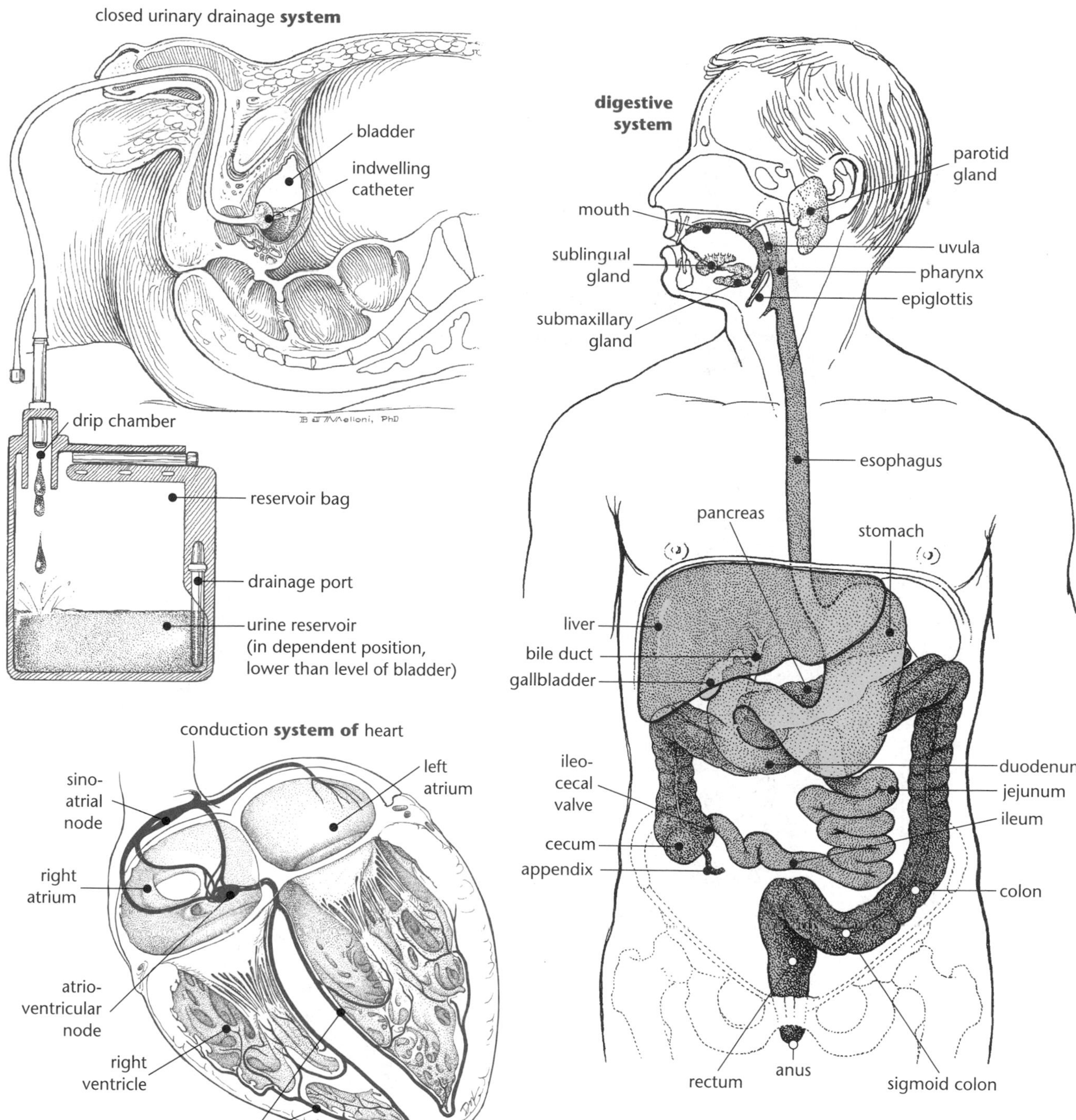

S

syrinx (sir´inks) A cavity in the brain or spinal cord caused by disease.

syrup (sir´up) In pharmacy, a solution of sugar in water used as a vehicle for active ingredients.

syssarcosis (sis-sar-ko´sis) A muscular articulation; the union of bones by muscular tissue, as in the connection between the hyoid bone and the mandible (lower jaw).

system (sis´tem) **1.** A functionally related group of parts or organs. **2.** An organized set of interrelated ideas, procedures, techniques, etc.

APUD s. See APUD.

autonomic nervous s. (ANS) The division of the nervous system that innervates the striated muscles of the heart and the smooth muscles and glands of the body; it is divided into the sympathetic (thoracolumbar) system and the parasympathetic (craniosacral) system.

Bethesda s. See Bethesda system of classification.

Bethesda s. of classification A system of classification used in cytopathology reports for describing results of the cytologic examination of a cervical/vaginal specimen (Pap smear). It is composed of three categories: *Specimen adequacy* (e.g., satisfactory; satisfactory but limited by ...; unsatisfactory); *General categorization* (e.g., within normal limits; benign cellular changes; epithelial cell abnormality); and *Descriptive diagnosis* (e.g., low grade squamous intraepithelial lesion [mild dysplasia]; high grade squamous intraepithelial lesion [severe dysplasia]; cancer [adenocarcinoma; squamous cell carcinoma; etc.]). Sometimes simply called Bethesda system.

cardiovascular s. (CVS) The heart and blood vessels.

centimeter-gram-second s. (CGS) A system of metric units in which the basic units of length, mass, and time are the centimeter, gram, and second.

central nervous s. (CNS) The brain and spinal cord.

complement s. (a) See complement. (b) See component of complement, under component.

digestive s. The alimentary canal from the mouth through the anus and the associated glands.

endocrine s. Collectively, all the ductless glands.

extrapyramidal s. A functional system of tracts in the brain which controls and coordinates motor activities, especially postural, static, and supportive.

female reproductive s. The genital organs in the female, consisting of the ovaries, uterine tubes, uterus, vagina, and external genitalia.

genitourinary s. The reproductive organs, kidneys, and urinary tract considered as a whole. Also called urogenital system.

Gleason's grading s. A widely used histologic system of grading cancer of the prostate; in this system, two numbers (from 1 to 5) are assigned to each area of prostatic cancer, based on a major and minor pattern of tissue differentiation in the area; a sum of 2-4 indicates a well differentiated cancer; 5-7, a moderately differentiated cancer; and 8-10, a poorly differentiated cancer. The Gleason's grading system provides a correlation between the histologic appearance and the prognosis of the tumor (most well differentiated cancers have a good prognosis). Also

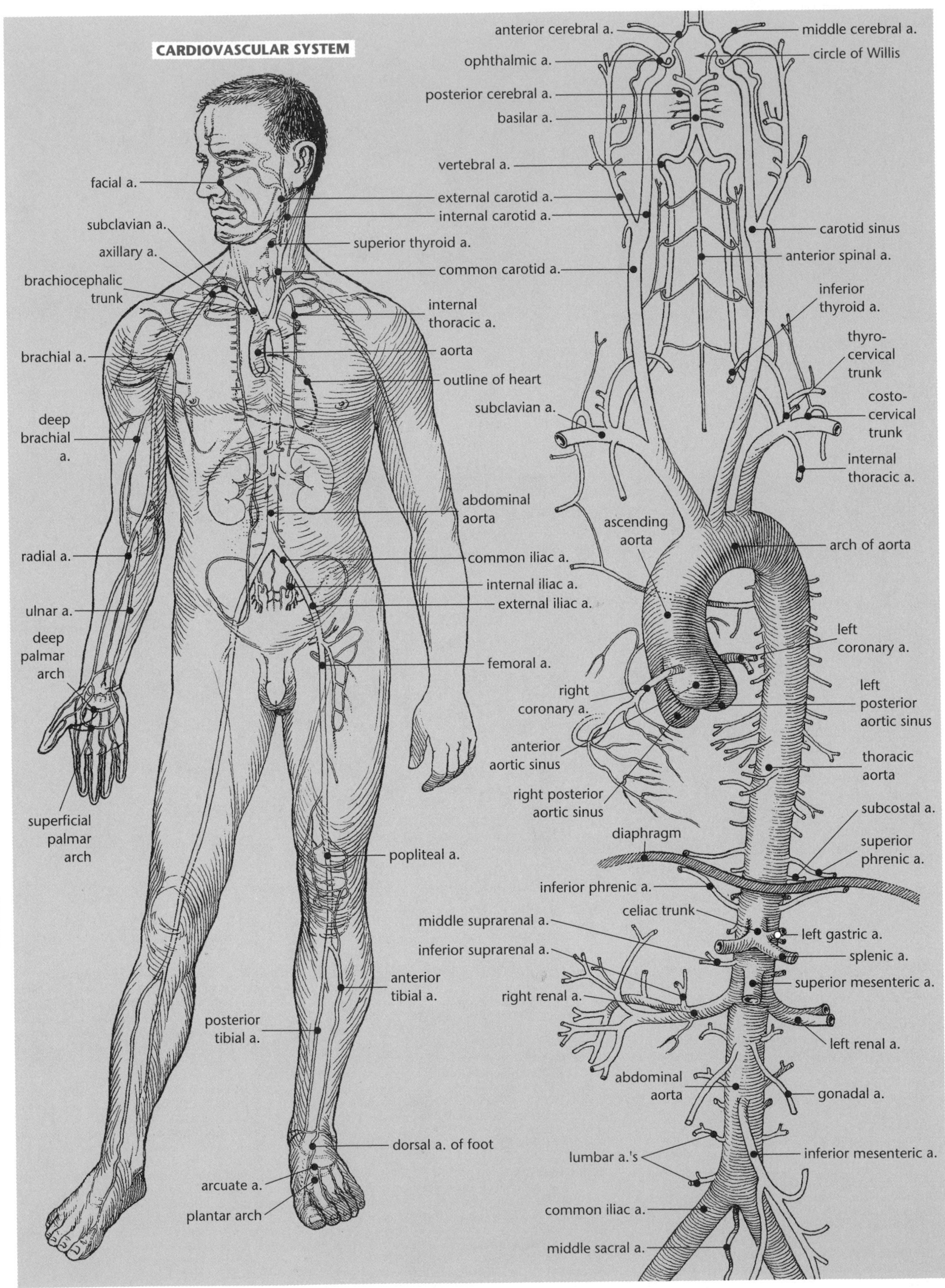

CARDIOVASCULAR SYSTEM
facial a.
subclavian a.
axillary a.
brachiocephalic trunk
brachial a.
deep brachial a.
radial a.
ulnar a.
deep palmar arch
superficial palmar arch
external carotid a.
internal carotid a.
superior thyroid a.
common carotid a.
internal thoracic a.
aorta
outline of heart
abdominal aorta
common iliac a.
internal iliac a.
external iliac a.
femoral a.
popliteal a.
anterior tibial a.
posterior tibial a.
dorsal a. of foot
arcuate a.
plantar arch
anterior cerebral a.
middle cerebral a.
ophthalmic a.
circle of Willis
posterior cerebral a.
basilar a.
vertebral a.
carotid sinus
anterior spinal a.
inferior thyroid a.
thyro-cervical trunk
costo-cervical trunk
subclavian a.
internal thoracic a.
ascending aorta
arch of aorta
left coronary a.
right coronary a.
left posterior aortic sinus
anterior aortic sinus
thoracic aorta
right posterior aortic sinus
subcostal a.
diaphragm
superior phrenic a.
inferior phrenic a.
celiac trunk
middle suprarenal a.
left gastric a.
inferior suprarenal a.
splenic a.
superior mesenteric a.
right renal a.
left renal a.
abdominal aorta
gonadal a.
lumbar a.'s
inferior mesenteric a.
common iliac a.
middle sacral a.

S

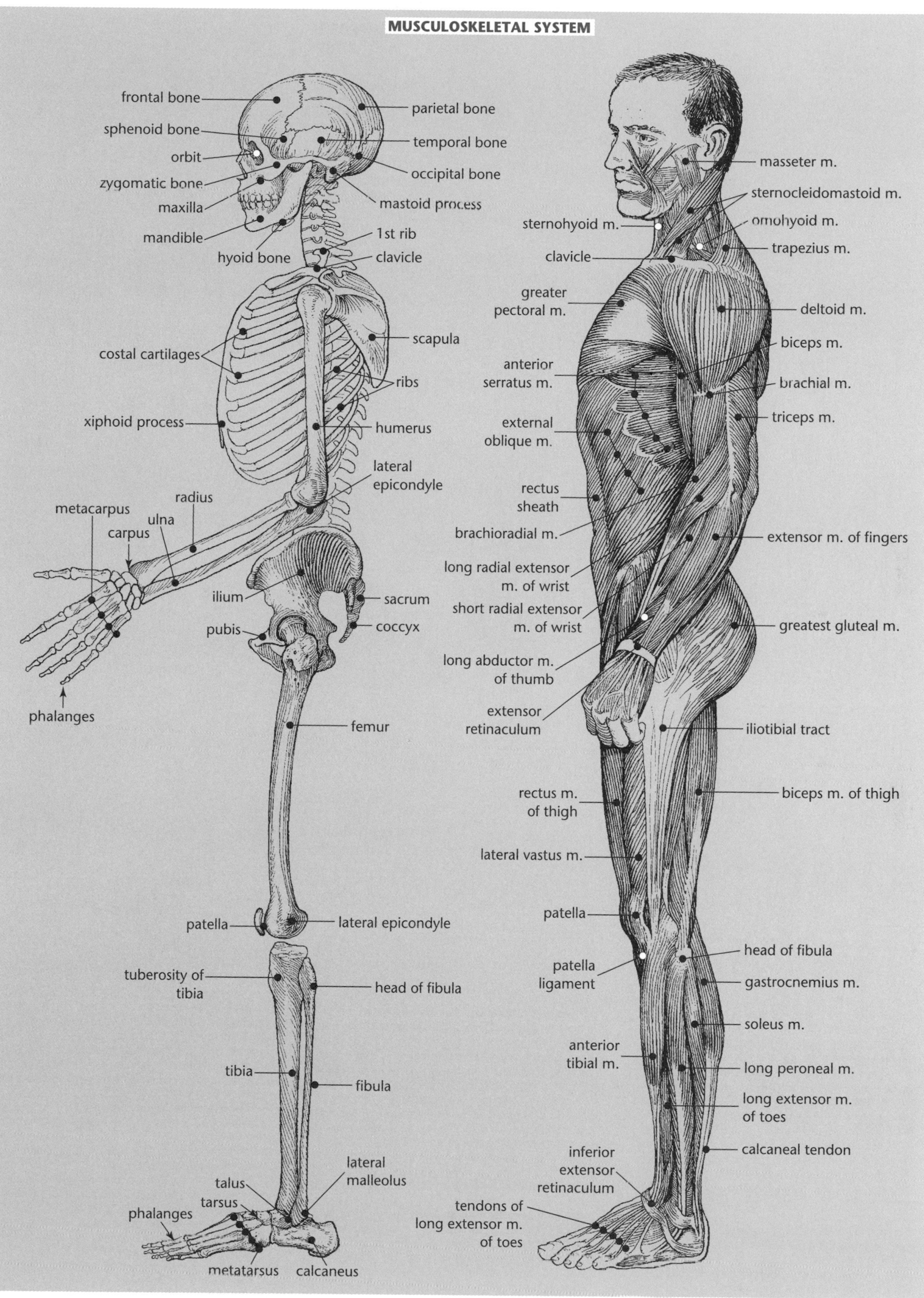
MUSCULOSKELETAL SYSTEM
frontal bone
parietal bone
sphenoid bone
temporal bone
orbit
occipital bone
zygomatic bone
maxilla
mastoid process
mandible
hyoid bone
1st rib
clavicle
scapula
costal cartilages
ribs
xiphoid process
humerus
lateral epicondyle
metacarpus
radius
ulna
carpus
ilium
sacrum
pubis
coccyx
phalanges
femur
patella
lateral epicondyle
tuberosity of tibia
head of fibula
tibia
fibula
talus
lateral malleolus
tarsus
phalanges
metatarsus
calcaneus
masseter m.
sternocleidomastoid m.
sternohyoid m.
omohyoid m.
trapezius m.
clavicle
greater pectoral m.
deltoid m.
biceps m.
anterior serratus m.
brachial m.
triceps m.
external oblique m.
rectus sheath
brachioradial m.
extensor m. of fingers
long radial extensor m. of wrist
short radial extensor m. of wrist
greatest gluteal m.
long abductor m. of thumb
extensor retinaculum
iliotibial tract
rectus m. of thigh
biceps m. of thigh
lateral vastus m.
patella
head of fibula
patella ligament
gastrocnemius m.
soleus m.
anterior tibial m.
long peroneal m.
long extensor m. of toes
calcaneal tendon
inferior extensor retinaculum
tendons of long extensor m. of toes
S

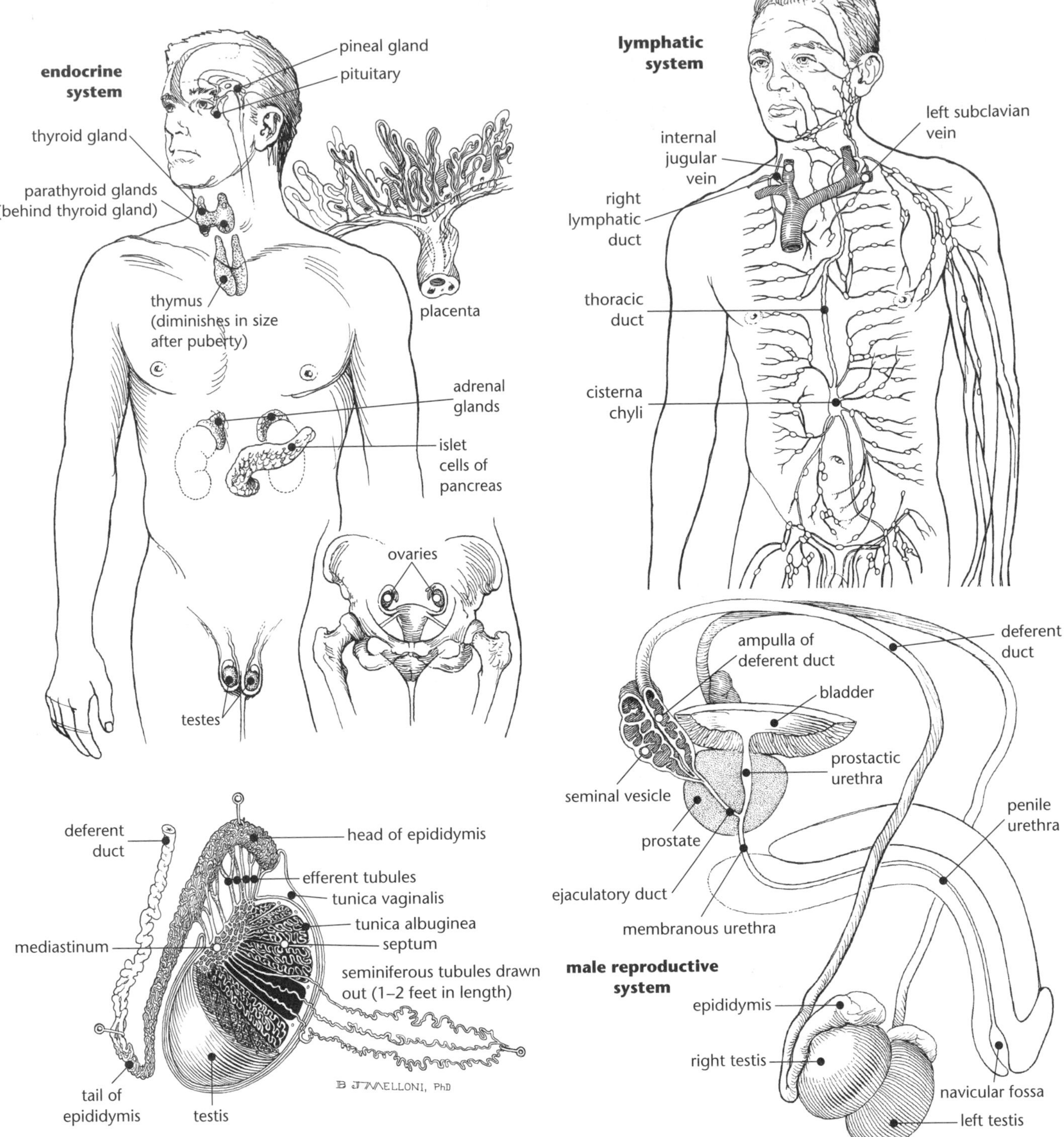

called Gleason's score; Gleason's staging.

haversian s. See osteon.

hematopoietic s. The blood-producing organs.

heterogeneous s. A combination of matter containing two or more distinct components that have definite boundaries; e.g., a suspension or an emulsion.

International S. of Units A system of units for the basic quantities of length, mass, time, electric current, temperature, luminous intensity, and amount of substance; the corresponding units are: meter, kilogram, second, ampere, kelvin, candela, and mole. In all languages it is abbreviated SI.

limbic s. Term loosely applied to the part of the nervous system that controls autonomic functions and the emotions.

lymphatic s. The lymphatic vessels, nodes, tonsils, spleen, thymus, and lymphoid or adenoid tissue.

lymphoreticular s. In immunology, a collection of cellular elements strategically distributed throughout the body; they can be activated by a variety of influences that are recognized as foreign by the host.

macrophage s. Phagocytic cells in bone marrow, spleen, liver, and lymph nodes where they free the blood or lymph of inert particles; includes all major phagocytic cell types, except the polymorphonuclear leukocytes. Also called mononuclear phagocyte system. Formerly called reticuloendothelial system.

meter-kilogram-second s. An absolute system of units; the system on which the International System of Units (SI) is based.

mononuclear phagocyte s. See macrophage system.

male reproductive s. The genital organs in the male, consisting of the testes, excretory ducts, seminal vesicles, prostate gland, and penis.

metric s. A system of measures and weights based upon the meter and the gram, respectively.

muscular s. The muscles of the body collectively.

musculoskeletal s. All the muscles and bones of the body and their connecting structures considered collectively.

nervous s. The brain and spinal cord (central nervous system), the cranial and spinal nerves (peripheral nervous system), and the autonomic nervous system.

neuroendocrine s. See APUD.

neuromuscular s. The nerves and the muscles they innervate.

oculomotor s. The part of the nervous system that controls eye movements.

oxidation-reduction s. A system in which the reversible oxidation-reduction reaction can take place (e.g., the enzyme systems of living cells).

parasympathetic nervous s. The smaller of the two divisions of the autonomic nervous system.

peripheral nervous s. (PNS) The nervous system that connects the central nervous system (CNS) to the rest of the body.

International System of Units (SI)

Quantity	Name	Symbol
SI base units:		
length	meter	m
mass	kilogram	kg
time	second	s
electric current	ampere	A
thermodynamic temperature	kelvin	K
amount of substance	mole	mol
luminous intensity	candela	cd
SI supplementary units:		
plane angle	radian	rad
solid angle	steradian	sr

Prefixes and their symbols used to designate decimal multiples and submultiples

Prefix	Symbol	Factor
tera	T	10^{12} = 1 000 000 000 000
giga	G	10^{9} = 1 000 000 000
mega	M	10^{6} = 1 000 000
kilo	k	10^{3} = 1 000
hecto	h	10^{2} = 100
deka	da	10^{1} = 10
deci	d	10^{-1} = 0.1
centi	c	10^{-2} = 0.01
milli	m	10^{-3} = 0.001
micro	μ	10^{-5} = 0.000 001
nano	n	10^{-9} = 0.000 000 001
pico	p	10^{-12} = 0.000 000 000 001
femto	f	10^{-15} = 0.000 000 000 000 001
atto	a	10^{-18} = 0.000 000 000 000 000 001

Examples of SI derived units expressed in terms of base units

Quantity	SI unit	Unit Symbol
area	square meter	m^2
volume	cubic meter	m^3
speed, velocity	meter per second	m/s
acceleration	meter per second squared	m/s^2
wave number	1 per meter	m^{-1}
density, mass density	kilogram per cubic meter	kg/m^3
current density	ampere per square meter	A/m^2
magnetic field strength	ampere per meter	A/m
concentration (of amount of substance)	mole per cubic meter	$mol/^3$
specific volume	cubic meter per kilogram	m^3/kg
luminance	candela per square meter	cd/m^2

SI derived units with special names

Quantity	Name	Symbol	Expression in terms of other units
frequency	hertz	Hz	s^{-1}
force	newton	N	$kg \cdot m/s^2$
pressure, stress	pascal	Pa	N/m^2
energy, work, quantity of heat	joule	J	N·m
power, radiant flux	watt	W	J/s
quantity of electricity, electric charge	coulomb	C	A·s
electric potential, potential difference, electromotive force	volt	V	W/A
capacitance	farad	F	C/V
electric resistance	ohm	ω	V/A
conductance	siemens	S	A/V
magnetic flux	weber	Wb	V·
magnetic flux density	tesla	T	Wb/m^2
inductance	henry	H	Wb/A
luminous flux	lumen	lm	cd·sr
illuminance	lux	lx	lm/m^2
activity (of a radionuclide)	becquerel	Bq	s^{-1}
absorbed dose	gray	Gy	J/kg

Recommended units

Quantity	Symbol	Dimension	Unit	Unit symbol	Recommended sub-units	Not recommended units
Length	l	L	meter	m	mm, μm, m	cm, μ, u, mμ, mu, A
Area	A	L^2	square meter	m^2	mm^2, μm^2	cm^2, μ^2
Volume	V	L^3	cubic meter liter	m^3 l	dm^3, cm^3, mm^3, μm^3 ml, μl, nl, pl, fl	cc, ccm, μ^3, u^3 L, λ, ul, μμl, uul
Mass	m	M	kilogram	kg	g, mg, μg, ng, pg	Kg, gr, γ, ug, mμg, mug, γγ, μμg, uug
Number	N	I	one	1	10^9, 10^6, 10^3, 10^{-3}	all other factors
Amount of substance	n	N	mol	mol	mmol, μmol, nmol	M, eq, val, g-mol, mM, meq, mval, μM μeq, μval, nM, neq, nval
Mass concentration		$K^{-3}m$	kilogram per liter	kg/l	g/l, mg/l, μg/l, ng/l	g/ml, %, g%, % (w/v), g/100 ml, g/dl, ‰, ‰, ‰(w/x), mg%, mg% (w/v), mg/100 ml, mg/dl, ppm, ppm (w/v), μg%, μg% (W/v), μg/100 ml,μ/dl, γl%, ppb, ppb (w/v), μμg/ml, uug/ml
Substance concentration	c	L^{-3} N	mol per liter	mol/l	mmol/l, Igmmol/l, nmol/l	M, eq/l, val/l, N, n, mM, meq/l, mval/l, μM, uM, μeq/l, nM, neq/l
Molality	m	M^{-1}N	mol per kilogram	mol/kg	mmol/kg, μmol/kg	m, mmol/g, μmol/mg, mm, μm, um

S

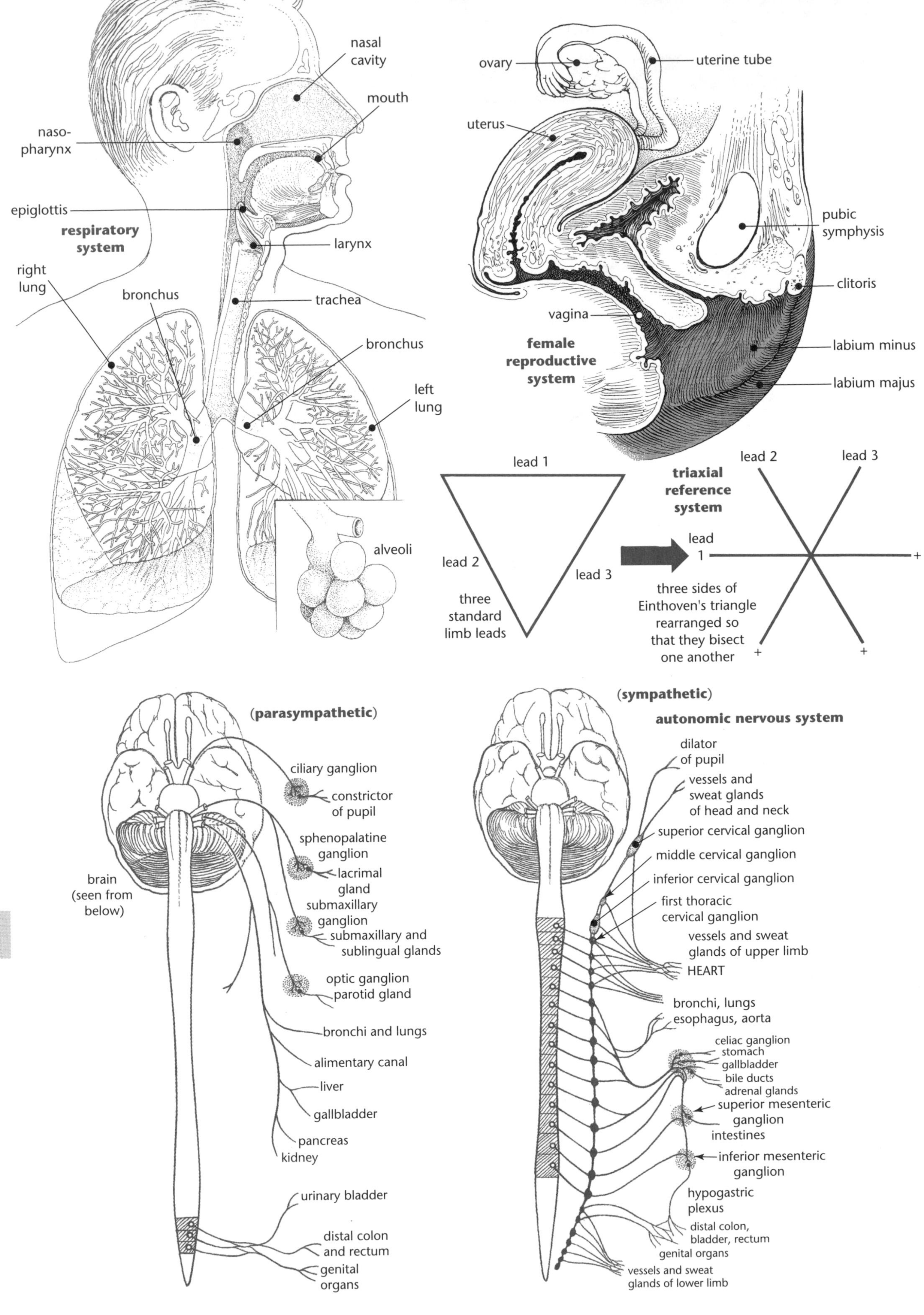

nasal cavity
mouth
naso-pharynx
epiglottis
respiratory system
larynx
right lung
bronchus
trachea
bronchus
left lung
alveoli
ovary
uterine tube
uterus
pubic symphysis
clitoris
vagina
female reproductive system
labium minus
labium majus
lead 1
lead 2
lead 3
triaxial reference system
lead 2
lead 3
lead 1
+
three standard limb leads
three sides of Einthoven's triangle rearranged so that they bisect one another
+
+
(parasympathetic)
ciliary ganglion
constrictor of pupil
sphenopalatine ganglion
lacrimal gland
submaxillary ganglion
submaxillary and sublingual glands
brain (seen from below)
optic ganglion
parotid gland
bronchi and lungs
alimentary canal
liver
gallbladder
pancreas
kidney
urinary bladder
distal colon and rectum
genital organs
(sympathetic)
autonomic nervous system
dilator of pupil
vessels and sweat glands of head and neck
superior cervical ganglion
middle cervical ganglion
inferior cervical ganglion
first thoracic cervical ganglion
vessels and sweat glands of upper limb
HEART
bronchi, lungs
esophagus, aorta
celiac ganglion
stomach
gallbladder
bile ducts
adrenal glands
superior mesenteric ganglion
intestines
inferior mesenteric ganglion
hypogastric plexus
distal colon, bladder, rectum
genital organs
vessels and sweat glands of lower limb

S

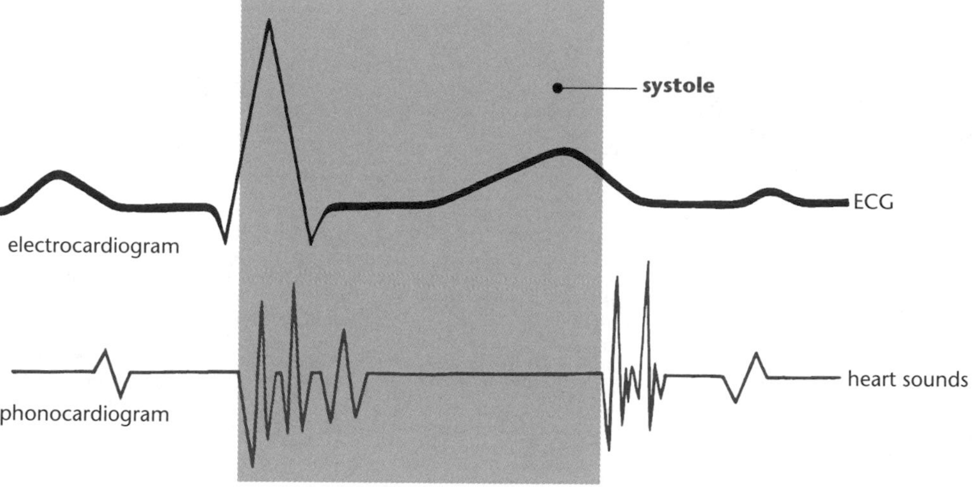

portal s. The arrangement of vessels and capillaries in the liver; the portal vein and its branches.
Purkinje s. The system of modified muscle fibers in the heart concerned with conduction of impulses.
renin-angiotensin-aldosterone s. A biochemical feedback system involving the kidneys that regulates sodium balance, fluid volume, and blood pressure.
respiratory s. The air passages, lungs, and the muscles of respiration.
reticular activating s. (RAS) The portion of the reticular formation of the brainstem that controls wakefulness, arousal from sleep, and focusing of attention.
reticuloendothelial s. (RES) Former name for the macrophage system.
sympathetic nervous s. The larger of the two divisions of the autonomic nervous system.
triaxial reference s. In electrocardiography, the figure resulting from rearranging the sides of the Einthoven triangle (which represent the three standard limb leads) so that they bisect one another.
urogenital s. See genitourinary system.
vascular s. The blood vessels.
vertebral-basilar s. The system composed of the two vertebral arteries as they join to form the basilar artery and their immediate branches.

systematic (sis-te-mat´ik) Relating to a system or arranged in accordance with a system.

systematization (sis-tem-ă-ti-za´shun) Formulation or arrangement of ideas in orderly sequence, according to a system.

systematized (sis´te-mă-tīzd) Denoting widespread pathology that has a significant pattern rather than haphazard distribution.

systemic (sis-tem´ik) Relating to or affecting the entire body.

systemic inflammatory response syndrome (sis-tem´ik in-flam´ă-to-re re-spons´ sin´drōm) (SIRS) Systemic changes occurring in response to a variety of severe clinical insults, representing an acute alteration from baseline without another known cause for the abnormalities; manifested by (but not limited to) two or more of the following: temperature greater than 38°C, or less than 30°C; heart rate greater than 90 beats/min; respiratory rate greater than 20 breaths/min, or arterial carbon dioxide less than 32 mmHg; and white blood cell count greater than 12000 cells/mm^3, less than 4000 cells/mm^3, or greater than 10% immature forms.

systole (sis´to-le) The rhythmic and synchronous contraction of the muscles of the heart chambers.
atrial s., auricular s. Atrial contraction giving impetus to the blood flowing from the atria into the ventricles; it has a duration of about 0.1 sec.
electrical s. The interval between the onset of the QRS complex on the electrocardiogram and the latest T wave.
ventricular s. Ventricular contraction immediately following atrial systole. It is divided into two phases: isometric contraction, occurring when the ventricular pressure firmly closes the atrioventricular valves; and the period of ejection, occurring when the pressure in the ventricles overcomes the diastolic pressure of the aorta and pulmonary trunk and the aortic and pulmonary valves open, forcefully ejecting the ventricular blood. The period of ejection lasts 0.3 sec in an individual with a heart rate of 70 beats per minute.

systolic (sis-tol´ik) Relating to or resulting from ventricular systole.

systremma (sis-trem´ă) A cramp in the muscles of the leg, chiefly of the bellies of the gastrocnemius and soleus muscles; may be associated with swimmer's cramp or a charleyhorse.

S

T

T-1824 Evans blue.

Tabanus (tă-ba´nus) A genus of biting flies, some species of which transmit anthrax, infectious equine anemia, and other diseases. Commonly called horseflies; gadflies; breezeflies.

tabefaction (ta-be-fak´shun) Atrophy or wasting of the body.

tabes (ta´bez) Progressive wasting away.

t. dorsalis A late manifestation of syphilis characterized by sclerosis of the sensory nerve roots and the posterior columns of the spinal cord; the usual symptoms are: shooting pains, muscular incoordination and atrophy, and functional disturbance of certain organs. Also called locomotor ataxia.

tabescent (tă-bes´ent) Wasting away progressively.

tabetic (tă-bet´ik) Afflicted with tabes.

tabetiform (tă-bet´ĭ-form) Resembling tabes dorsalis.

table (ta´bl) **1.** An orderly arrangement of written, typed, or printed data. **2.** A flat layer, as one of the two laminae, separated by the diploe, into which the cranial bones are divided. **3.** An article of furniture having a flat horizontal surface.

Aub-DuBois t. Table of rates of basal metabolism in calories per square meter of body surface per hour for all age groups.

examining t. Table on which the patient lies during a medical examination.

operating t. Table on which a patient is placed during a surgical procedure.

periodic t. An arrangement of chemical elements listed according to their atomic number; it demonstrates the recurrence of similar properties after certain intervals.

Reuss' color t.'s Diagrams in which colored letters are superimposed on colored backgrounds as a test for colorblindness.

tilt t. One with a top that tilts so that the patient lying on it can be brought toward an erect position.

vitreous t. The inner table of the cranial bones; it is denser than the outer table.

tablespoon (ta´bl-spo͞on) (tbsp) A large spoon used as a measure in the dosage of liquid medicines; equivalent to 15 milliliters, 4 liquid drams, one-half fluid ounce, or 3 teaspoons.

tablet (tab´let) A small disc containing measured amounts of medicinal substances.

buccal t. Tablet placed between the cheek and the gum where it dissolves quickly, permitting the medicinal substance to be absorbed through the mucosa.

compressed t. Tablet prepared by compressing granulated medicinal substances under several hundred kilograms of pressure per square centimeter.

enteric coated t. Tablet coated with material that does not disintegrate in stomach fluids; the medication is released in the intestines.

hypodermic t. A small water-soluble tablet, intended to be dissolved in the barrel of a hypodermic syringe prior to injection.

sublingual t. Tablet placed under the tongue to permit absorption of the medicinal ingredients through the mucosa.

taboparesis (ta-bo-pă-re´sis) Condition marked by symptoms of tabes dorsalis and general paresis.

tabular (tab´u-lar) **1.** Arranged as a table or list. **2.** Having a flat surface.

Tac A 55 kilodalton polypeptide, component of the interleukin 2 receptor.

tache (tahsh) A minute spot or blemish.

t. noir The crust-covered lesion produced by the bite of a tick.

tachistesthesia (tă-kis-tes-the´zhă) Perception of a flicker of light.

tachistoscope (tă-kis´to-skōp) Instrument that projects a slide for a brief period of time; used in experimental optics to measure the speed of conscious visual perception.

tachogram (tak´o-gram) The graphic record made by tachography.

tachography (tă-kog´ră-fe) The recording of the rate of arterial blood flow.

tachyarrhythmia (tak-e-ă-rith´me-ă) Heart rhythm with over 100 beats per minute.

tachycardia (tak-ĭ-kar´de-ă) An abnormally fast heart beat. Also called tachyrhythmia.

fetal t. Tachycardia of the fetus in which the heart rate is 160 beats per minute or more (normal rate is 120–160 beats per minute); causes may include maternal or fetal infection, fetal oxygen deficiency (hypoxia), or maternal use of certain drugs.

junctional t. Tachycardia starting at the atrioventricular junction.

paroxysmal atrial t. (PAT) Sudden onset of rapid heart action originating in the atria.

paroxysmal atrial t. with block PAT with a block in transmission of some of the beats from the atria to the ventricles so that the ventricular rate is less than the atrial.

supraventricular t. (SVT) Tachycardia in which the stimulating point is above the ventricles (e.g., sinus node elsewhere in an atrium or atrioventricular

periodic table

METALS | NON METALS

Group	I	II											III	IV	V	VI	VII	0
Period																		
1	H 1																	He 2
2	Li 3	Be 4											B 5	C 6	N 7	O 8	F 9	Ne 10
3	Na 11	Mg 12											Al 13	Si 14	P 15	S 16	Cl 17	Ar 18
4	K 19	Ca 20	Sc 21	Ti 22	V 23	Cr 24	Mn 25	Fe 26	Co 27	Ni 28	Cu 29	Zn 30	Ga 31	Ge 32	As 33	Se 34	Br 35	Kr 36
5	Rb 37	Sr 38	Y 39	Zr 40	Nb 41	Mo 42	Tc 43	Ru 44	Rh 45	Pd 46	Ag 47	Cd 48	In 49	Sn 50	Sb 51	Te 52	I 53	Xe 54
6	Cs 55	Ba 56	* 57–71	Hf 72	Ta 73	W 74	Re 75	Os 76	Ir 77	Pt 78	Au 79	Hg 80	Ti 81	Pb 82	Bi 83	Po 84	At 85	Rn 86
7	Fr 87	Ra 88	** 89–103	Rf 104	Ha 105													
*	lanthanide elements (rare earth)	La 57	Ce 58	Pr 59	Nd 60	Pm 61	Sm 62	Eu 63	Gd 64	Tb 65	Dy 66	Ho 67	Er 68	Tm 69	Yb 70	Lu 71		
**	actinide elements	Ac 89	Th 90	Pa 91	U 92	Np 93	Pu 94	Am 95	Cm 96	Bk 97	Cf 98	Es 99	Fm 100	Md 101	No 102	Lw 103		

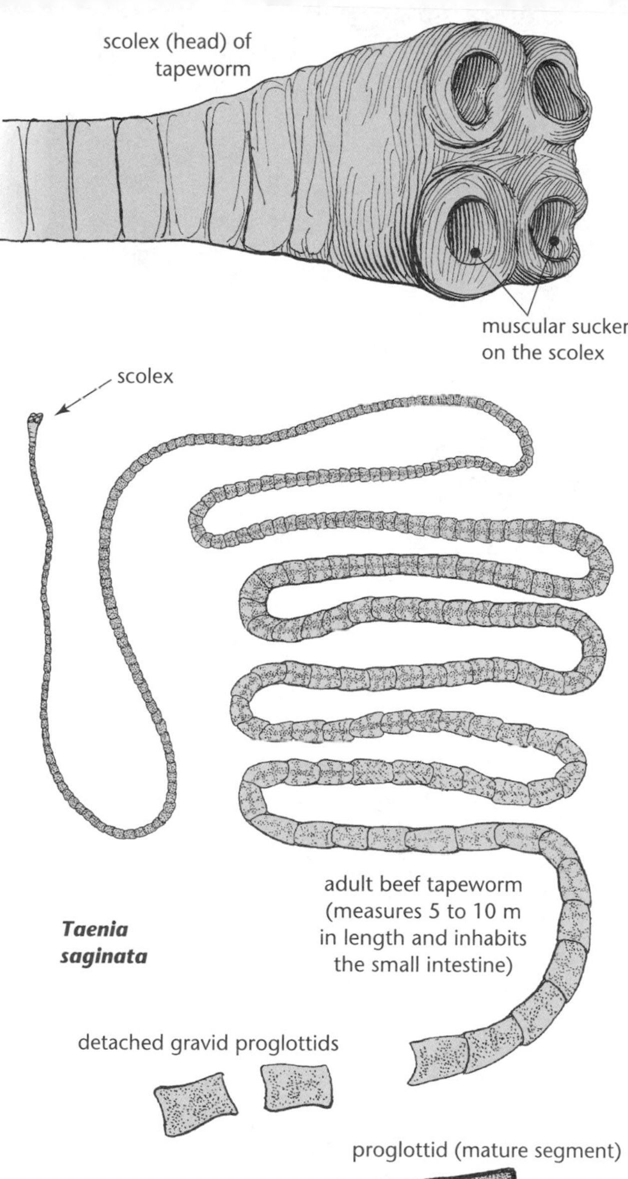

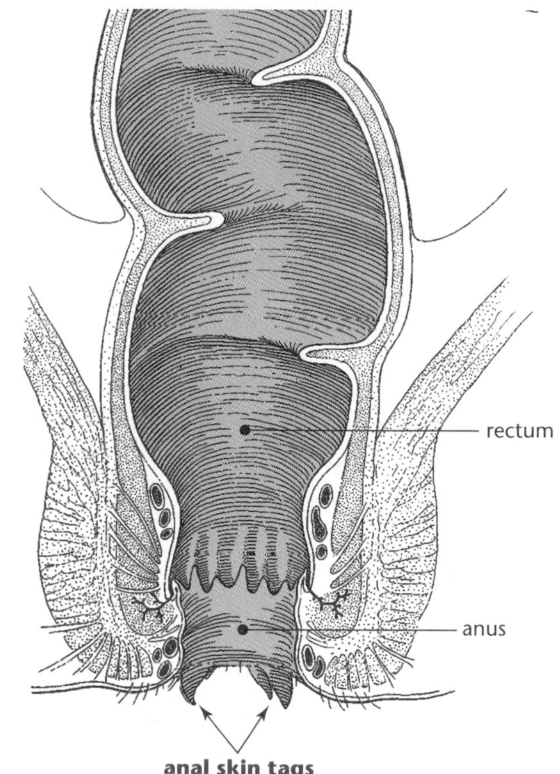

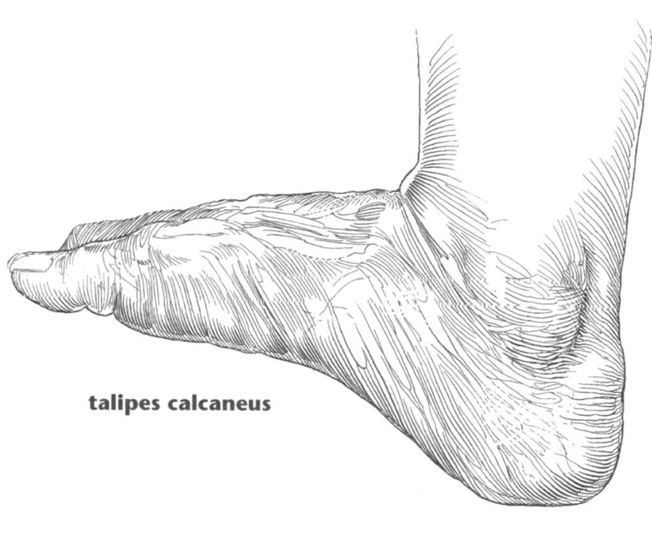

junction).

tachycardiac (tak-e-kar´de-ak) Relating to tachycardia.

tachycrotic (tak-e-krot´ik) Relating to a rapid pulse.

tachykinin (tak-e-ki´nin) One of a group of structurally related peptides involved in blood vessel dilatation, smooth muscle contraction, stimulation of saliva secretion, and neurotransmission of painful stimuli.

tachylalia (tak-e-la´le-ă) See tachylogia.

tachylogia (tak-e-lo´jĭ-ă) Rapid speech. Also called tachyphrasia.

tachyphagia (tak-ĭ-fa´je-ă) Abnormally rapid eating; bolting of food.

tachyphrasia (tak-ĭ-fra´zhă) See tachylogia.

tachyphylaxis (tak-e-fĭ-lak´sis) Rapid production of immune tolerance, as by repeated injections of small doses of a substance.

tachypnea (tak-ip-ne´ă) Abnormally rapid, shallow breathing.

tachyrhythmia (tak-e-rith´me-ă) See tachycardia.

tachysterol (tak-is´te-rol) A sterol produced by ultraviolet irradiation of ergosterol.

tachysystole (tak-ĭ-sis´to-lĭ) See tachycardia.

tacrolimus (ta-kro-lĭ´mus) Antibiotic isolated from the soil fungus *Streptomyces tsukubaensis;* used in organ transplants to prevent rejection. Also called FK-506.

tactile (tak´til) Relating to the sense of touch.

taction (tak´shun) **1.** An act of touching; a contact. **2.** The sense of touch.

tactometer (tak-tom´ĕ-ter) Instrument used to determine the condition of the sense of touch.

tactor (tak´tor) A sensory (tactile) end-organ.

tactus (tak´tus) Latin for touch; the sense of touch.

Taenia (te´ne-ă) A genus of tapeworms (family Taeniidae).

T. echinococcus *Echinococcus granulosus.*

T. saginata The common tapeworm transmitted to man by the ingestion of infected beef; the larvae exist in the muscles and organs of cattle; the adults, measuring from 5 to 10 m in length, are found in the human small intestine, attached to the mucosa by means of muscular suckers on the scolex (head). Also called beef tapeworm.

T. solium A species whose larval state exists in the muscles of the hog; the adult forms are found in the human intestine, to which they gain access by the ingestion of insufficiently cooked infested pork. Also called pork tapeworm; armed tapeworm because of the double row of hooks on its head.

tag (tag) **1.** To introduce a radioactive isotope to a substance. **2.** The radioactive material so used. **3.** A small outgrowth of flaplike appendage. **4.** To add an easily identifiable marker, such as a radioactive isotope.

anal skin t. A polypoid projection in the anus.

skin t. A small flesh-colored to brown polypoid growth. Also called acrochordon.

tagging (tag´ing) The process of using chemical or radioactive substances as a label or marker for diagnostic or experimental purposes. Also called labeling.

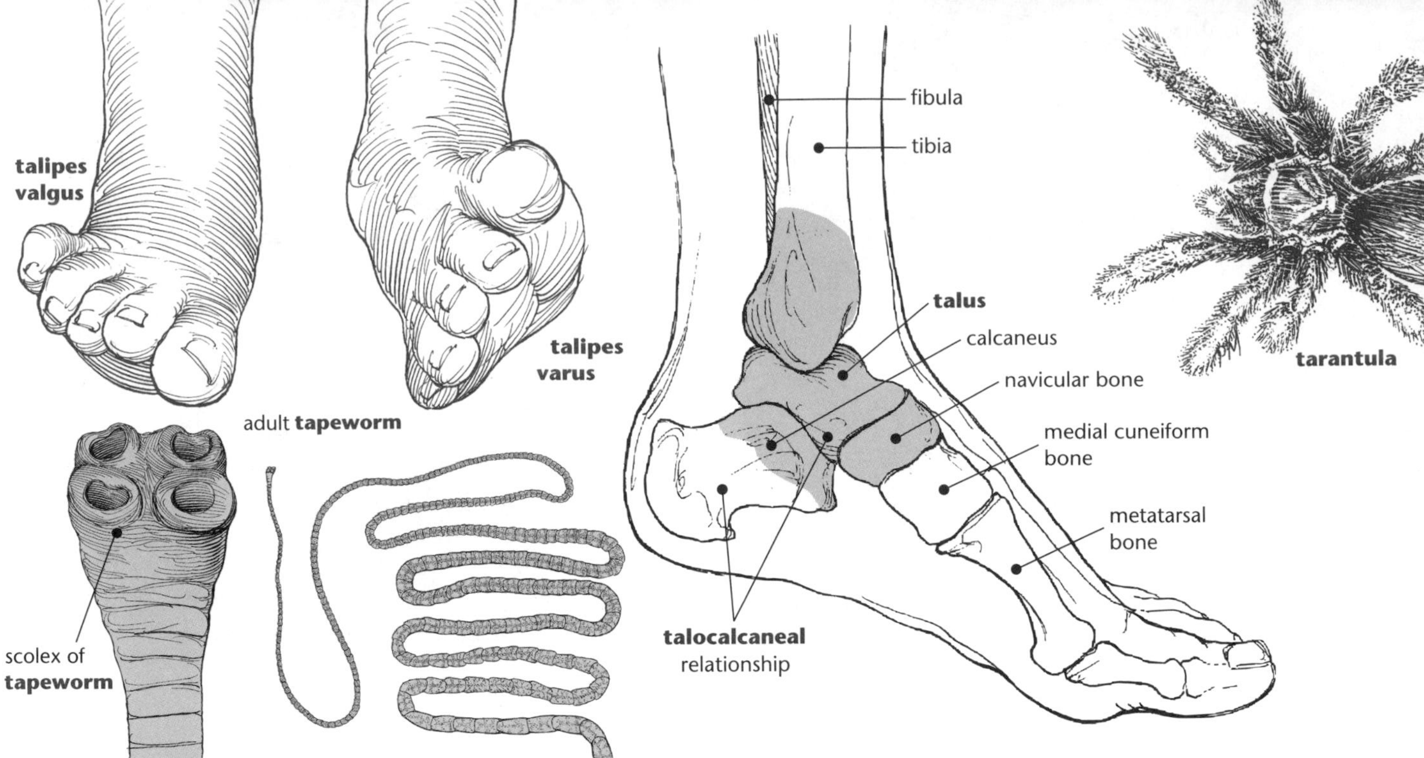

Takayasu's syndrome (tă-kă-yă´so͞oz sin´drōm) See Takayasu's arteritis, under arteritis.

take (tāk) A successful grafting procedure.

talalgia (tal-al´jă, tal-al´je-ă) Discomfort or pain in the heel or ankle.

talc, talcum (talk, tal´kum) A fine-grained hydrous magnesium silicate, having a soft texture; used in face and talcum powder, and in cosmetic and pharmaceutical preparations.

talcosis (tal-ko´sis) Disorder of the lungs produced by inhalation of talc.

taliped, talipedic (tal´ĭ-ped, tal-ĭ-pe´dik) Having a clubfoot; clubfooted.

talipes (tal´ĭ-pez) General term that denotes a deformity involving the talus (ankle bone) and the foot, which results in an abnormal shape and position.

t. arcuatus See talipes cavus.

t. calcaneovalgus A relatively common congenital disorder in which the ankle joint is dorsiflexed and the foot is everted; believed to be caused by the position of the fetus in the uterus; the opposite of clubfoot (talipes equinovarus).

t. calcaneovarus A deformity of the ankle and foot with combined features of talipes calcaneus and talipes varus.

t. calcaneus Foot deformity characterized by an elevated forefoot and a depressed heel, placing the weight of the body on the heel; generally the result of calf muscle paralysis. Also called pes calcaneus.

t. cavus Condition in which the longitudinal arch of the foot is exaggerated due to contraction of the plantar fascia or to a deformed bony arch. Also called talipes arcuatus.

t. equinovalgus Foot deformity in which the characteristics of talipes equinus and talipes valgus are present, with weight borne on the metatarsophalangeal joints; the heel is elevated and turned outward from the body's midline.

t. equinovarus One of the most common congenital deformities of the foot in which only the outer portion of the ball of the foot touches the ground; the ankle is plantar flexed, the foot is inverted, and the anterior half of the foot is directed toward the midline. Also called clubfoot.

t. equinus A deformity characterized by fixed plantar extension of the foot, causing the weight of the body to rest on the ball of the foot or the metatarsophalangeal joints; the ankle joint is plantar flexed. Also called tip foot; pes equinus.

t. planovalgus A deformity of the foot in which the characteristics of both talipes planus (flatfoot) and talipes valgus are present, with body weight distributed along the medial edge of the everted foot; the heel is turned outward and the foot's outer border is more elevated than the inner border; it may be congenital (permanent) or caused by reflex spasm of the muscles controlling the foot. Also called pes planovalgus.

t. planus See flatfoot.

t. valgus Outward turning of the foot, causing only the inner side of the sole to touch the ground; accompanied by flattening of the longitudinal arch. Also called pes valgus; pes pronatus.

t. varus Deformity considered to be an incomplete form of clubfoot (talipes equinovarus); characterized by a turning inward of the foot, causing only the outer part of the sole to touch the ground; accompanied by increased height of the longitudinal arch. Also called crossfoot; pes varus.

talocalcaneal (ta-lo-kal-ka´ne-al) Pertaining to the talus and calcaneus bones of the foot; denoting the joint between those bones and the ligaments attaching them.

talocrural (ta-lo-kroo´ral) Relating to the ankle joint.

talonavicular (ta-lo-nă-vik´u-lar) Relating to the talus and the navicular bone.

talus (ta´lus) The large bone articulating with the tibia and fibula to form the ankle joint. Also called ankle bone.

tambour (tam-boor´) A drum-shaped apparatus used to transmit and register slight movements.

tampon (tam´pon) A plug of any absorbent material placed in a canal or cavity to control hemorrhage or absorb secretions.

tamponade (tam- pon-ād´) The use of a tampon as a surgical aid. Also called tamponage.

cardiac t. Compression of the heart due to accumulation of blood in the pericardium, as in rupture of the heart or after penetrating wounds.

Tangier disease (tan-jēr´ dĭ-zēz´) An inherited disorder of lipid metabolism marked by deficiency of high density lipoproteins (HDLs), deposition of cholesterol esters in foam cells, enlargement of liver, spleen, and lymph nodes, enlarged orange-colored tonsils, and corneal opacity; the disease was named after Tangier Island, a geographically isolated community of the Chesapeake Bay, where the disease was first discovered. Also called analphalipoproteinemia.

tangle (tang´gl) A twisted interwoven mass.

neurofibrillary t. An accumulation of paired helical filaments within a cell body; commonly seen in areas of the cerebral cortex of individuals with Alzheimer's disease.

tannate (tan´āt) A salt of tannic acid.

tannic acid (tan´ik as´id) A lustrous brownish yellow substance, $C_{76}H_{52}O_{46}$, extracted from the bark and fruit of various plants and in tea leaves; used as an astringent and, formerly, to treat diarrhea; it is toxic to the liver. Also called tannin.

tannin (tan´in) See tannic acid.

tantalum (tan´tă-lum) A metallic noncorrosive element; symbol Ta, atomic number 73, atomic weight 180.95; used in surgical appliances and prostheses (e.g., skull plate, wire mesh in the abdominal wall).

tantrum (tan´trum) Unprovoked fit of bad temper; unreasoning anger that may be accompanied by violent acts or gestures.

tap (tap) **1.** To deliver a quick, gentle blow or blows, as when eliciting a tendon reflex. **2.** To strike lightly but audibly. **3.** To withdraw fluid from a body cavity.

spinal t. See lumbar puncture, under puncture.

tapetum (tă-pe´tum) **1.** The portions of the corpus callosum that border the posterior horns (laterally) of the lateral ventricles of the brain. **2.** The outer and posterior part of the choroid (the vascular layer of the eyeball).

tapeworm (tāp´werm) Any of several ribbonlike worms (class Cestoda) that infest the intestines of vertebrates, including humans; its body consists of a head or scolex with hooks for attachment to the intestinal wall and a series of segments or proglottids (from four to several thousand) containing the reproductive organs.

armed t. See *Taenia solium.*

beef t. See *Taenia saginata.*

fish t. See *Diphyllobothrium latum.*

dwarf t., dwarf mouse t. See *Hymenolepis nana.*

pork t. See *Taenia solium.*

tapinocephalic (tap-ĭ-no-se-fal´ik) Characterized by a flattened skull.

tapinocephaly (tap-ĭ-no-sef´ă-le) Deformity in which the skull is flattened.

tapotement (tă-pōt-maw´) Tapping with the side of the hand; a massage movement.

tar (tahr) A dark, semisolid substance obtained from the destructive distillation of various organic materials, such as wood or coal.

coal t. Tar obtained from bituminous coal; used in the preparation of certain drugs and dyes.

pine t. A dark, viscous syrup produced by the destructive distillation of pine wood; it contains resins, turpentine, and oils and is used as a disinfectant and antiseptic in the treatment of skin disorders such as eczema.

tarantula (tă-ran´cho͞o-lă) Any of several large, hairy, dark spiders (family Theraphosidae) capable of inflicting a painful but not significantly poisonous bite.

American t. *Eurypelma hentzii,* a large, greatly feared, although harmless spider; it causes a pinprick bite similar to a bee sting.

black t. *Sericopelma communis,* a large black tarantula of Panama, whose bite is poisonous

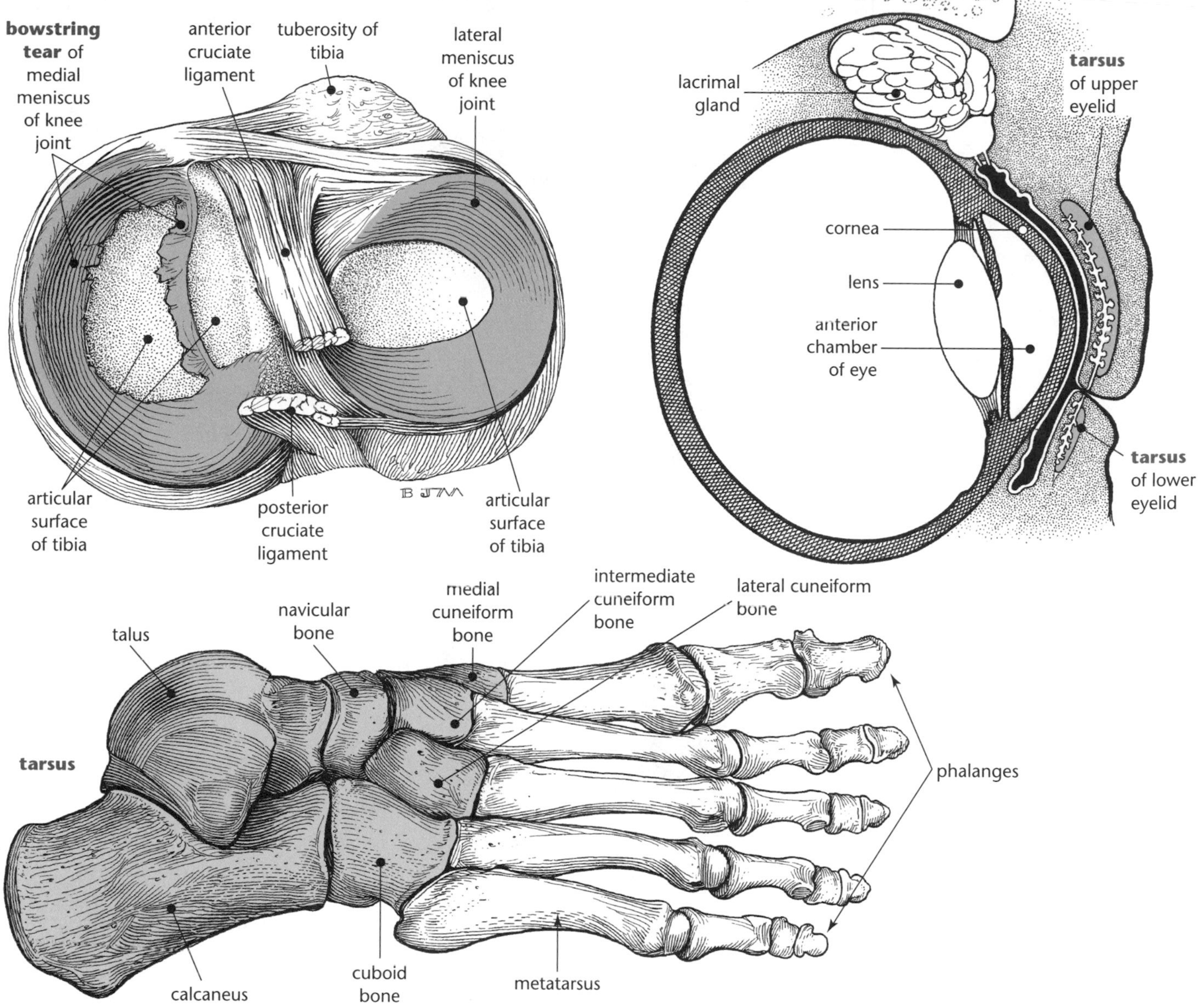

although the effect is localized.

tardive (tahr′div) Late; applied to the characteristic lesion of a disease that is late in appearing.

tare (tār) In chemistry, (1) the weight of an empty container; (2) a weight used to counterbalance the weight of the container holding the substance being weighed.

target (tahr′get) **1.** An object of fixation or observation used in vision training or testing. **2.** Denoting a cell or organ that is selectively affected by a hormone, drug, or infective organism.

targeting (tahr′get-ing) Process by which certain proteins are directed toward certain cellular locations.

tarsadenitis (tahr-sad-ĕ-ni′tis) Inflammation of the borders of the eyelids and the meibomian glands.

tarsal (tahr′sal) **1.** Relating to the small bones forming the posterior part of the foot (tarsus). **2.** Relating to the border of an eyelid.

tarsectomy (tahr-sek′tŏ-me) **1.** Surgical removal of the tarsus of the foot, or part of it. **2.** Surgical removal of the margin of an eyelid, or part of it.

tarsitis (tahr-si′tis) **1.** Inflammation of the margin of the eyelid. Also called marginal blepharitis. **2.** Inflammation of the tarsus of the foot.

tarsoclasis (tahr-sok′lă-sis) Surgical fracture of the tarsus, as for the correction of clubfoot.

tarsomalacia (tahr-so-mă-la′shă) Softening of the tarsal cartilage of an eyelid.

tarsometatarsal (tahr-so-met-ă-tahr′sal) Relating to the tarsus and metatarsus.

tarsorrhaphy (tahr-sor′ă-fe) A surgical procedure to close or to reduce the length of the palpebral fissure by suturing.

tarsotomy (tahr-sot′ŏ-me) Surgical incision of the eyelid.

tarsus (tahr′sus), *pl.* **tarsi** **1.** The part of the foot between the leg and the metatarsus formed by seven small bones. **2.** The fibrous tissue that strengthens and shapes the edge of the eyelid.

tartar (tahr′tar) Popular term for dental calculus. See under calculus.

tartaric acid (tahr-tar′ik as′id) A soluble white powder, a laxative and refrigerant, used in preparing Seidlitz powders and effervescing tablets.

tartrate (tahr′trāt) A salt of tartaric acid.

tartrated (tahr′trāt-ed) Containing tartar or tartaric acid.

taste (tāst) **1.** The special sense that distinguishes the different flavors of substances that come in contact with the taste buds in the mouth. **2.** To perceive such sensations.

tattoo (tă-too′) A permanent design made on the skin by ingraining an indelible pigment through punctures.

tau (tou) A protein that plays an important role in the transport of nutrients within nerve cells (neurons). Abnormal function of tau protein may be involved in the genesis of Alzheimer's disease.

taurine (taw′rēn) Water-soluble, colorless crystals produced by the decomposition of taurocholic acid.

taurocholate (taw-ro-ko′lāt) A salt of taurocholic acid.

taurocholic acid (taw-ro-ko′lik as′id) A bile acid; a compound of cholic acid and taurine. Also called cholytaurine.

taurodontism (taw-ro-don′tiz-m) Abnormal development of the molars of either or both primary or secondary dentition; the teeth have short roots, long crowns, and large pulp cavities.

Taussig-Bing syndrome (taw′sig-bing sin′drōm) Congenital malformation of the heart in which the aorta arises from the right ventricle (instead of the left) and the pulmonary artery arises from both ventricles, anterior to the aorta; a ventricular septal defect is also present.

tautomerism (taw-tom′er-iz-m) Phenomenon in which a chemical compound exists in a state of equilibrium between two isomeric forms and is able to react according to either.

taxis (tak′sis) **1.** Correction of a dislocation or reduction of a hernia by gentle pressure. **2.** The reaction of certain organisms to a stimulus, i.e., motion away from or toward the stimulus, or arrangement in a particular position relating to the stimulus; used with a prefix indicating the type of stimulus (e.g., chemotaxis, electrotaxis).

Taxol (tak′sol) Trade name for a preparation of paclitaxel; an anticancer agent used to treat cancer, especially ovarian cancer.

taxon (tak′son), *pl.* **taxa** A category in a systematic classification (e.g., genus, species).

taxonomy (tak-son′ŏ-me) The classification of living organisms into categories (taxa).

Tay-Sachs disease (ta-saks′ dĭ-zēz′) See cerebral sphingolipidosis, under sphingolipidosis.

tear (tēr) **1.** The clear saline liquid secreted by the lacrimal gland, serving to keep the cornea and conjunctiva moist and to facilitate movement of the eyelid. **2.** The act of secreting tears.

tear (tār) **1.** To pull apart or divide forcefully. **2.** To wound by lacerating.

bowstring t. A longitudinal split of a meniscus, a semilunar cartilage within the knee joint; the anterior and posterior portions of the cartilage remain attached to the joint capsule while the free inner

T

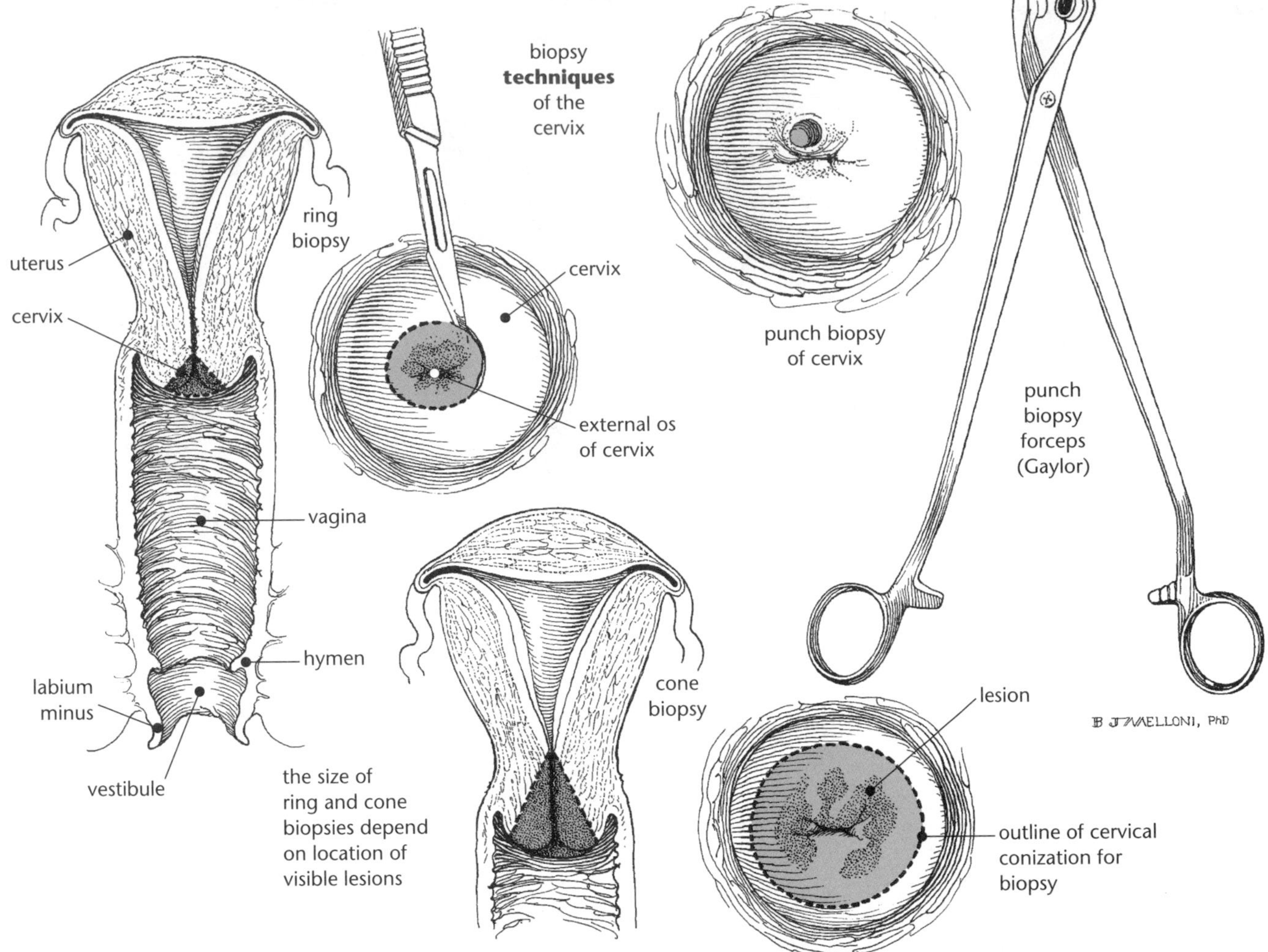

border becomes displaced across the joint like a bowstring. Also called bucket-handle tear.

bucket-handle t. See bowstring tear.

tease (tēz) To separate gently with a fine instrument, as the minute components of a tissue.

teaspoon (te´spōōn) (tsp) A small spoon used as a measure in the dosage of fluid medicines, equivalent to 5 ml.

teat (tēt) A nipple or breast.

technetium (tek-ne´she-um) Artificial radioactive element; symbol Tc, atomic number 43, atomic weight 99.

technetium-99m (tek-ne´she-um) (^{99m}Tc) A radioisotope with a half-life of 6 hours suitable for clinical and research purposes; used in the preparation of radiopharmaceuticals and as a radiotracer in determining blood flow and for tumor localization.

technical (tek´nĭ-kal) **1.** Relating to technique. **2.** Specialized.

T

technician (tek-nish´an) A person trained in the performance of special technical procedures.

dental laboratory t. A person trained in the making of dental appliances, such as dentures, crown and bridge work, restorations, and orthodontic appliances.

histologic t. One trained in fixing, embedding, sectioning, mounting, and staining tissues that have been removed from the body for microscopic examination.

medical laboratory t. A person who has an Associate Degree with special training in medical laboratory techniques (such as physical, chemical, and microscopic analysis of body fluids and tissues) and who works under appropriate supervision, such as that of a certified medical technologist. COMPARE: medical technologist, under technologist.

radiation therapy t. A person trained to assist the radiologist in treatment of disease by exposing specific areas of the patient's body to prescribed doses of x-ray or other forms of ionizing radiation.

x-ray t. A person trained to make x-ray films of a bodily part. Also called radiologic technologist.

technique (tek-nēk´) The systematic procedure by which a surgical operation, scientific experiment, or any complex act is accomplished.

fluorescent antibody t. An immunofluorescent technique used for detecting antigen in tissue sections by either: (a) *direct method*, in which immunoglobulin (antibody) treated with a fluorescent dye is added to the tissue, specific antigen in the tissue (e.g., microbe) combines with the fluorescent antibody, and the resulting antigen-antibody complex is then detected through fluorescence microscopy; or (b) *indirect method*, in which unlabeled immunoglobulin (antibody) is added to tissue, specific antigen in the tissue combines with the antibody resulting in an antigen-antibody complex, fluorescein-conjugated anti-immunoglobulin antibody is added, and the resulting triple complex is then located by fluorescence microscopy.

flush t. Technique for determining the systolic blood pressure in infants; the hand or foot is blanched by manual squeezing or application of an elastic bandage before applying the pressure cuff on the extremity; the flush of the extremity is observed as the cuff pressure is slowly reduced; used for detecting coarctation of the aorta when applied simultaneously to upper and lower extremities.

hydro-flow t. In dentistry, a method of cavity preparation in which the tooth being prepared is kept under a stream of water.

invasive t. Technique in which the skin of the patient is punctured or incised.

Irving's t. See Irving's operation, under operation.

Madlener's t. See Madlener's operation, under operation.

McDonald's t. In obstetrics, measurement of the uterus by placing a centimeter tape on the abdomen and following the curvature of the abdominal surface from the pubic bone margin to the top of the uterine mass; useful for detecting fetal growth retardation, especially in the third trimester. Also called McDonald's maneuver.

Mohs' t. A microscopically controlled surgical technique for removing broad-based but shallow skin tumors (especially basal and squamous cell carcinoma); the surface of the tumor plus 3 to 5 mm margin is fixed (coagulated) with dichloracetic acid, overlaid with zinc chloride paste, and covered with a dressing; after 24 to 48 hours, sections of the tissue are examined at the border of the lesion and the procedure continues until tumor-free margins are obtained. Also called microscopically controlled excision; Mohs' surgery.

non-invasive t. Technique in which the skin of the patient is not punctured or incised.

Ouchterlony t. A double diffusion method for performing a precipitin test.

Pastore t. In obstetrics, a method of delivering the placenta.

technologist (tek-nol´ŏ-jist) An individual who is a graduate of a four-year college with special training in a particular field and who is certified in that field.

medical t. (M.T.) Application of technology to the field of medicine, including a variety of diagnostic procedures and therapeutic and surgical methods and techniques. COMPARE: medical laboratory technician.

nuclear medicine t. A certified medical technologist or a registered nurse who has been trained in the use of radioactive materials for diagnostic purposes.

pharmaceutical laboratory t. Certified medical technologist in industry who analyzes and tests medications for strength and purity.

technology (tek-nol´o-je) The application of scientific knowledge to the practical purposes of any field, including methods, techniques, and instrumentation.

assisted reproductive t. (ART) The field of reproductive medicine involved with techniques for increasing fecundability by nonphysiologic methods that enhance the probability of fertilization. Includes *in vitro* fertilization (IVF), gamete intrafallopian transfer (GIFT), zygote intrafallopian transfer

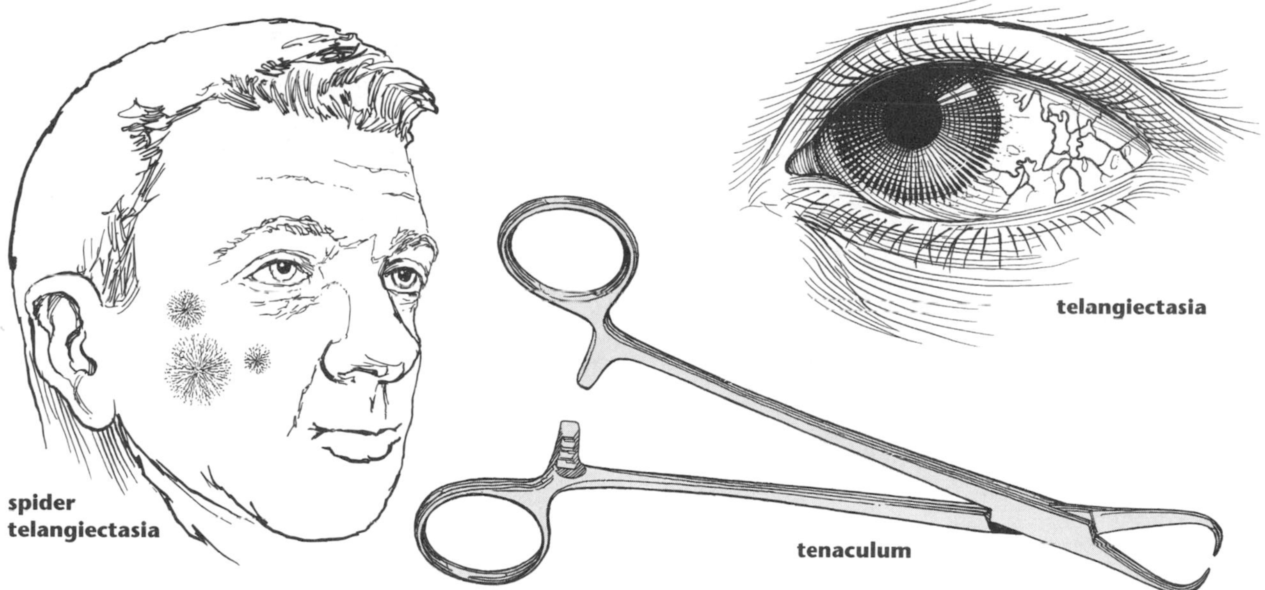

(ZIFT), tubal embryo transfer (TET), peritoneal oocyte and sperm transfer (POST), subzonal insertion of sperm by microinjection (SUZI), and intracytoplasmic sperm injection (ICSI).

tectiform (tek´tĭ-form) Shaped like a roof.

tectonic (tek´ton-ik) Relating to plastic surgery or grafting.

tectorial (tek-to´re-al) Relating to, or forming, a cover or roof.

tectorium (tek-to´re-um) Any rooflike structure.

tectum (tek´tum) Any anatomic covering or roofing structure, especially the roofplate of the midbrain; it is dorsal to the cerebral aqueduct and includes the superior and inferior colliculi, their brachii, and the tectal lamina.

teething (tēth´ing) The eruption of the primary or baby teeth into the oral cavity.

tegmen (teg´men) A rooflike structure over a part.

t. tympani Roof of the middle ear chamber formed by the thin plate of the petrous part of the temporal bone; it separates the middle ear chamber from the middle cranial fossa.

t. ventriculi quarti See roof of fourth ventricle, under roof.

tegmentum (teg-men´tum) The larger dorsal portion of the brainstem.

tegument (teg´u-ment) See integument.

tela (te´lă), *pl.* **te´lae** A thin, delicate, weblike membrane.

telalgia (tel-al´jă) Referred pain.

telangiectasia, telangiectasis (tel-an-je-ek-ta´zhă, tel-an-je-ek´tă-sis) Dilatation of a group of capillaries.

hereditary hemorrhagic t. Telangiectasia in the skin and mucous membranes, usually appearing after puberty; transmitted as a simple dominant trait. Also called Rendu-Osler-Weber syndrome.

spider t. A group of tiny dilated arterioles arranged in a radial pattern around a central core, occurring usually above the waist; seen in small numbers during pregnancy and estrogen therapy; a large number indicates a systemic disease (cirrhosis of the liver). They are also seen normally in children. Also called arterial spider; spider nevus; nevus araneus; spider angioma.

telangiectatic (tel-an-je-ek-tat´ik) Afflicted with telangiectasia.

telangioma (tel-an-je-o´ma) A tumor made up of dilated capillaries or arterioles.

telecardiogram (tel-ĕ-kar´de-o-gram) See telelectrocardiogram.

telecardiograph (tel-ĕ-kar-de-o-graf) See telelectrocardiograph.

telediagnosis (tel-ĕ-di-ag-no´sis) Diagnosis of disease in a patient located at some distance from the physician by evaluation of data transmitted to a receiving station.

telelectrocardiogram (tel-ĕ-lek-tro-kar´de-o-gram) An electrocardiogram recorded at some distance from the patient. Also called telecardiogram.

telelectrocardiograph (tel-ĕ-lek-tro-kar´de-o-graf) An apparatus for the transmission and remote reception of electrocardiograph signals. Also called telecardiograph.

telemetry (tĕ-lem´e-tre) The science and technology of remote sensing for monitoring living systems (e.g., blood pressure, heart rate) by use of radio transmitters placed in or on animal or human subjects.

cardiac t. Transmission of electrical signals from the heart to a receiving location where the electrocardiogram is displayed for monitoring.

telencephalon (tel-en-sef´ă-lon) The portion of the embryonic brain from which develop the cerebral hemispheres, the lateral ventricles, the anterior part of the third ventricle, and the olfactory lobes; together with the diencephalon it makes up the prosencephalon.

teleneuron (tel-ĕ-noor´on) A nerve ending.

teleology (tel-e-ol´o-je) Doctrine according to which all biologic events are directed toward some final purpose.

telepathy (tĕ-lep´ă-the) The phenomenon of communication of thought from one individual to another without the aid of physical means; since the means of extrasensory thought transference is unknown, it is generally not accepted as scientifically valid.

telereceptor (tel-ĕ-re-sep´tor) An organ that perceives sense stimuli from a distance (e.g., the eye).

teletherapy (tel-ĕ-ther´ă-pe) Radiotherapeutic treatment with an external radiation source many centimeters from the patient.

tellurium (tĕ-lu´re-um) A lustrous semimetallic element; symbol Te, atomic number 52, atomic weight 127.6.

telocentric (tel-o-sen´trik) Denoting a chromosome with its centromere at the end.

telodendron (tel-o-den´dron) The terminal branching of an axon.

telogen (tel´o-jen) The resting or final phase of a hair cycle; the period of time before a hair is shed.

telomere (tel´o-mēr) One of the two ends of a chromosome.

telophase (tel´o-fāz) The last stage of cell division by mitosis, beginning when the chromatids reach the poles of the cell and the nuclear membranes enclose each new set of chromosomes to complete the separation of two daughter cells.

temperament (tem´per-ă-ment) The unique natural predispositions of an individual that influence his manner of thinking, behaving, and reacting.

temperature (tem´per-ă-chur) (t) **1.** Intensity of heat as measured in any of several arbitrary scales. **2.** Popular term for fever.

absolute t. (T) Temperature measured on an absolute scale.

basal body t. (BBT) The lowest body temperature of a healthy person during waking hours under conditions of absolute rest.

critical t. Temperature above which a gas cannot be reduced to liquid form.

effective t. A comfort index that takes into consideration the temperature, movement, and moisture content of the air.

maximum t. Temperature above which bacteria will not grow.

neonate body t. The range of normal temperatures in a term newborn infant. Skin temperature: 36.0 to 36.5°C (96.9–97.7°F); core temperature, 36.5 to 37.5°C (97.7–99.5°F).

normal body t. The average oral temperature in healthy human adults (40 years or younger): 98.2°F (36.8°C), with upper limits ranging between an early morning temperature of 98.9°F (37.2°C) and an evening temperature of 99.9°F (37.7°C); other variables include exercise, eating and drinking, age and, in women, the time of the menstrual cycle.

template (tem´plāt) **1.** The macromolecular mold for the synthesis of complementary macromole-cules. **2.** In dentistry, a curved or flat plate used as an aid in setting teeth. Also called pattern.

wax t. A wax impression of the occlusion of the teeth.

temple (tem´pl) The lateral region on either side of the forehead above the zygomatic arch.

tempolabile (tem-po-la´bīl) Unstable over a period of time or changed or destroyed by time; said of a serum.

temporal (tem´pŏ-ral) Relating to the side of the head or temple.

temporomandibular (tem-po-ro-man-dib´u-lar) Relating to the temporal bone and mandible, as the articulation of the lower jaw (temporomandibular joint, TMJ).

temporo-occipital (tem-pŏ-ro ok-sip´-ĭ-tal) Relating to the temporal and occipital bones of the skull.

tempostabile, tempostable (tem-po-sta´bīl, tem-po-sta´bl) Not altered by the passage of time; said of certain chemicals.

tenacious (tĕ-na´shus) Sticky; adhesive.

tenacity (tĕ-nas´ĭ-te) The state of being adhesive or cohesive.

tenaculum (tĕ-nak´u-lum) A hooked surgical instrument for grasping and holding parts, such as the divided end of a blood vessel during an operation.

tenalgia (te-nal´jă) Pain in a tendon. Also called

T

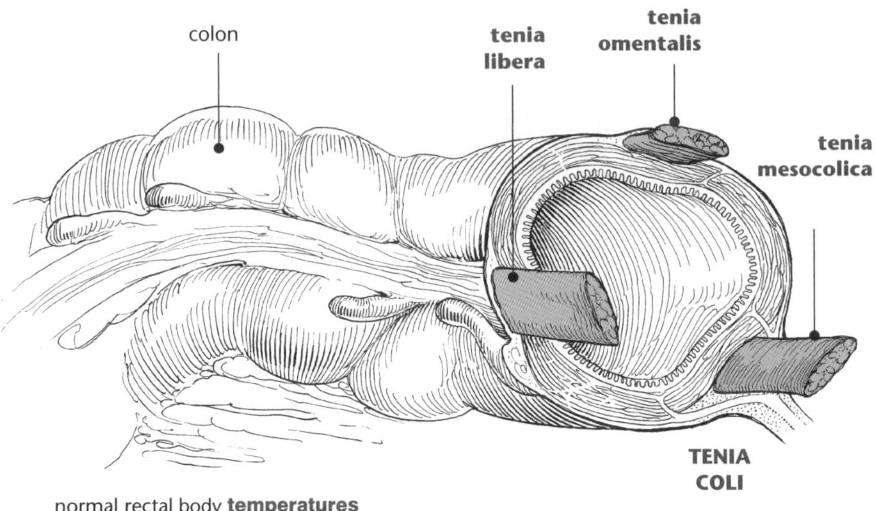

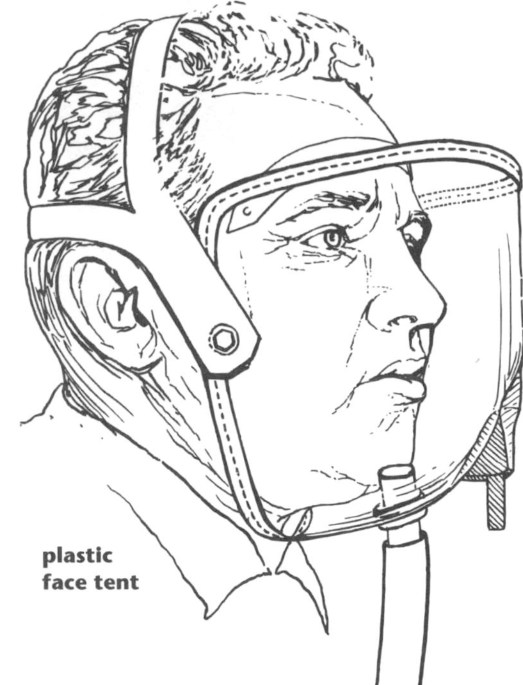

normal rectal body **temperatures**

Species	°F (±1°F)	°C (±0.5°C)
mouse	97	36
man	98.6	37.0
cat	101.5	38.5
dog	102	39
chicken	106.2	41.5

tenontodynia; tenodynia.

tender (ten´der) Painful on pressure; sensitive.

tenderness (ten´der-nes) Abnormal sensitivity to pressure or contact.

rebound t. Pain felt when pressure is released suddenly; in the abdomen it is characteristic of peritonitis.

tendinitis (ten-dĭ-ni´tis) See tendonitis.

tendinous (ten´dĭ-nus) Relating to a tendon.

tendo calcaneus (ten´do kal-ka´ne-us) See calcaneal tendon, under tendon.

tendolysis (ten-dol´ĭ-sis) The removal of adhesions from a tendon. Also called tenolysis.

tendon (ten´dun) A fibrous band that attaches a muscle to a bone.

Achilles t. See calcaneal tendon.

calcaneal t. The large common tendon that attaches the gastrocnemius and soleus muscles to the calcaneus (heel bone). Also called Achilles tendon; tendo calcaneus.

common annular t. A fibrous ring in the back of the eye socket (orbit) attached to the superior, inferior, and medial margins of the optic canal; it serves as origin for the four rectus muscles of the eye. Also called anulus tendineus communis; common tendinous ring; ligament of Zinn.

conjoined t. The fused tendons of the transversus abdominis and internal oblique muscles; it inserts onto the crest of the pubic bone and the pectineal line. Also called inguinal falx; conjoint tendon.

conjoint t. See conjoined tendon.

hamstring t. One of the two strong tendons at the back of the knee, on either side of the popliteal fossa, attaching the back muscles of the thigh to the bones of the leg: *lateral hamstring t.*, a tendon attaching the biceps muscle of the thigh to the fibula and *medial hamstring t.*, tendons attaching the semitendinous and the semimembranous muscles to the tibia.

tendonitis (ten-do-ni´tis) Inflammation of a tendon. Also called tendinitis; tenonitis.

tendoplasty (ten´do-plas-te) See tenoplasty.

tendotomy (ten-dot´ŏ-me) See tenotomy.

tenectomy (te-nek´tŏ-me) Surgical removal of part of a tendon.

tenesmic (te-nez´mik) Relating to tenesmus.

tenesmus (te-nes´mus) A painful, ineffectual straining to defecate or urinate.

tenia (te´ne-ă), *pl.* **teniae** **1.** Any narrow bandlike anatomic structure. **2.** The line of attachment of a choroid plexus. **3.** Any flatworm of the genus *Taenia*.

t. coli Any of three thickened bands of longitudinal muscular fibers about 6 mm broad, on the wall of the colon.

t. libera The tenia coli almost midway between the tenia mesocolica and tenia omentalis. Also called free band.

t. mesocolica The tenia coli situated along the attachment of the mesocolon to the colon.

t. omentalis The tenia coli of the transverse colon situated along the site of attachment of the greater omentum.

t. thalami The tenia, or line of attachment, of the choroid plexus that runs along the dorsomedial border of the thalamus; the lateral ventricles lie above it and the third ventricle lies below it. Also called tenia of thalamus; tenia of third ventricle.

t. of thalamus See tenia thalami.

t. of third ventricle See tenia thalami.

teniacide (te´ne-ă-sīd) Any agent that destroys tapeworms.

teniafuge (te´ne-ă-fūj´) An agent for expelling tapeworms.

tenial (te´ne-al) **1.** Relating to a tapeworm. **2.** Relating to a band of tissue (tenia).

teniasis (te-ni´ă-sis) Infestation with tapeworms in the intestine.

tenioid (te´ne-oid) **1.** Resembling a ribbon. **2.** Resembling a tapeworm.

tenodesis (ten-od´ĕ-sis) The transferring of the proximal end of a tendon to another site.

tenodynia (ten-o-din´e-ă) See tenalgia.

tenolysis (ten-ol´ĭ-sis) See tendolysis.

tenonectomy (ten-o-nek´tŏ-me) Surgical procedure for shortening a tendon in which a segment of the tendon is removed and the two remaining ends are joined.

tenonitis (ten-o-ni´tis) See tendonitis.

tenontodynia (ten-on-to-din´e-ă) See tenalgia.

tenontoplasty (tĕ-non´to-plas-te) See tenoplasty.

tenophyte (ten´o-fīt) A growth of cartilaginous or bony tissue attached to a tendon.

tenoplasty (ten´o-plas-te) Reparative surgery of the tendons. Also called tendonoplasty; tendoplasty; tenontoplasty.

tenorrhaphy (ten-or´ă-fe) The suturing of a divided tendon.

tenosynovectomy (ten-o-sin-o-vek´tŏ-me) Surgical removal of a tendon sheath.

tenosynovitis (ten-o-sin-o-vi´tis) Inflammation of the inner lining of a tendon sheath. Also called tenovaginitis.

t. crepitans Tenosynovitis that produces a crackling sound upon movement of the affected tendon.

nodular t. A sharply localized tenosynovitis involving usually peripheral joints, considered by some authorities to be a benign tumor (rather than an inflammatory condition) with a tendency to recur after surgical removal. Also called giant cell tumor of tendon sheath.

suppurative t. Tenosynovitis caused by direct invasion by pus-forming bacteria; organisms may gain entry into the tendon sheath cavity through a wound.

tenotomy (ten-ot´ŏ-me) The cutting of a tendon for corrective measures, as for clubfoot or strasbismus. Also called tendotomy.

tenovaginitis (ten-o-vaj-ĭ-ni´tis) See tenosynovitis.

tension (ten´shun) (T) **1.** The act of stretching or the condition of being taut or strained. **2.** A force tending to produce extension or expansion, as of a liquid or gas, when a confining force is removed. **3.** Emotional or mental strain.

arterial t. The pressure produced on the wall of an artery by the blood current at the peak of a pulse wave.

interfacial surface t. The resistance to separation offered by the film of liquid between two well adapted surfaces, as that of the thin film of saliva between a denture base and the tissues.

intraocular t. (Tn) See intraocular pressure, under pressure.

ocular t. See intraocular pressure, under pressure.

premenstrual t. See premenstrual syndrome.

surface t. The force that tends to pull together the molecules of a liquid surface when in contact with another substance.

tensor (ten´sor) A muscle that makes a part tense or firm.

tent (tent) **1.** A covering of canvas or plastic placed over a patient's bed for the administration of inhaled medications or oxygen. **2.** An expandable plug placed in an orifice to keep it open.

laminaria t. A sterile tent made of dried stems of the seaweed *Laminaria digitata*, measuring 1 to 2 mm in diameter and 5 to 7 mm in length, with a cord attached to one end to facilitate removal. The tent is inserted in the cervical canal and left in place 6 to 12 hours for gradual, atraumatic expansion of the cervix; employed as a preoperative procedure in first trimester abortion by suction aspiration or D&C, or during second trimester abortion as a supplement to other procedures; also used to soften and dilate an "unripe" cervix in preparation for induction of labor at or near term. See also *Laminaria digitata*.

oxygen t. Tent placed over a patient's bed into which oxygen is conducted.

plastic face t. One placed over a patient's face to facilitate the administration of gaseous medications.

steam t. Tent in which steam is provided.

tentorial (ten-to´re-al) Relating to the tentorium.

tentorium (ten-to´re-um) A membranous partition.

t. cerebelli A fold of dura mater separating the

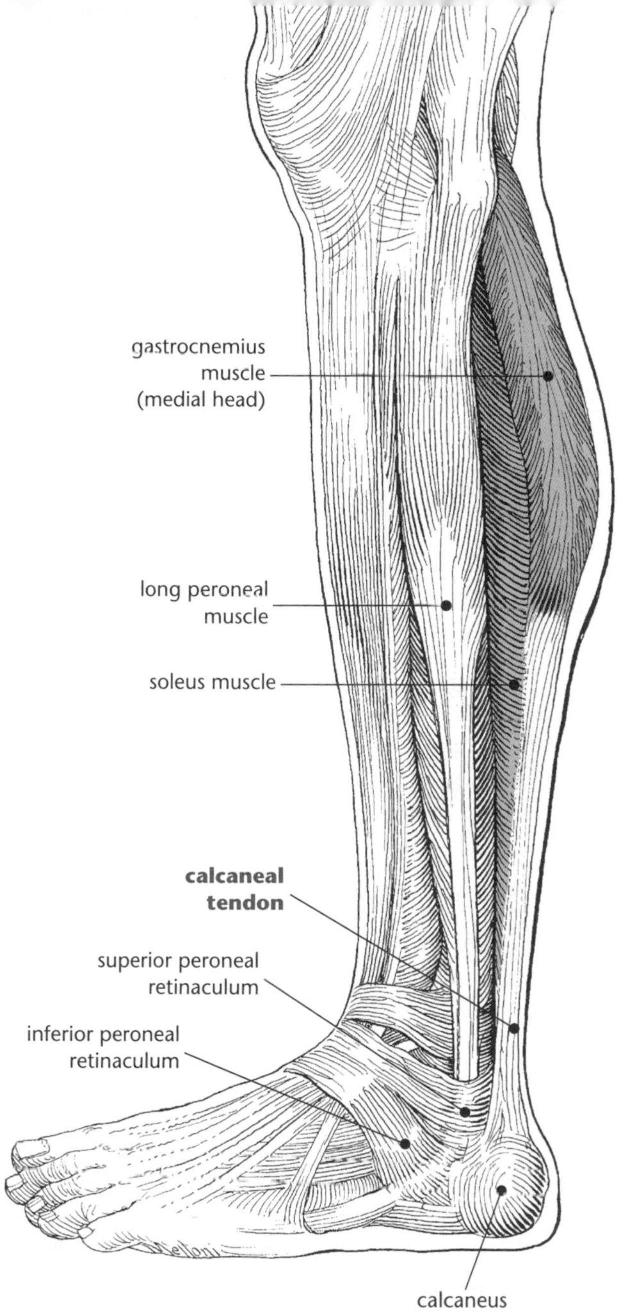

gastrocnemius
muscle
(medial head)
long peroneal
muscle
soleus muscle
**calcaneal
tendon**
superior peroneal
retinaculum
inferior peroneal
retinaculum
calcaneus

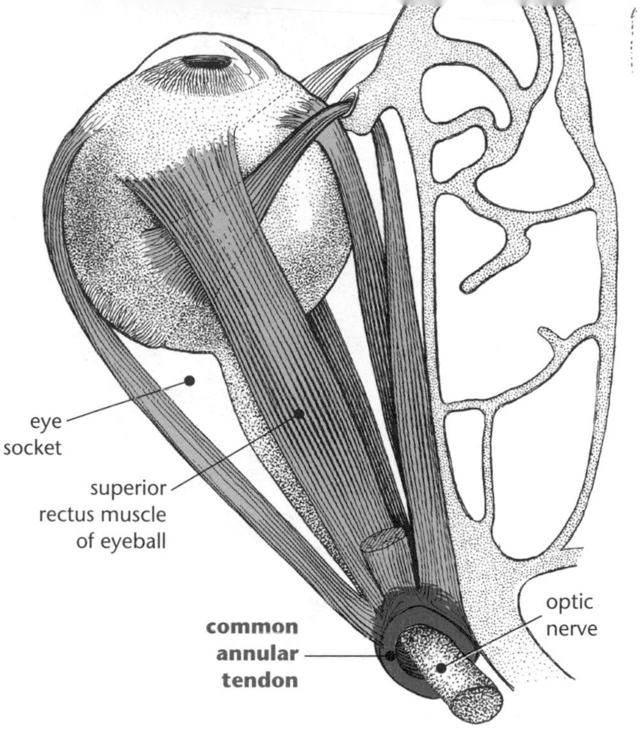

eye
socket
superior
rectus muscle
of eyeball
**common
annular
tendon**
optic
nerve

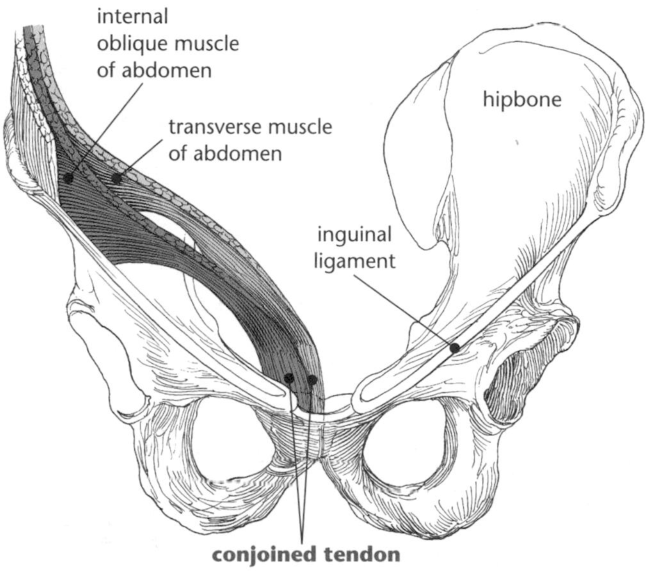

internal
oblique muscle
of abdomen
transverse muscle
of abdomen
hipbone
inguinal
ligament
conjoined tendon

tenoplasty
(stages in tendon repair)
after Lorraine

T

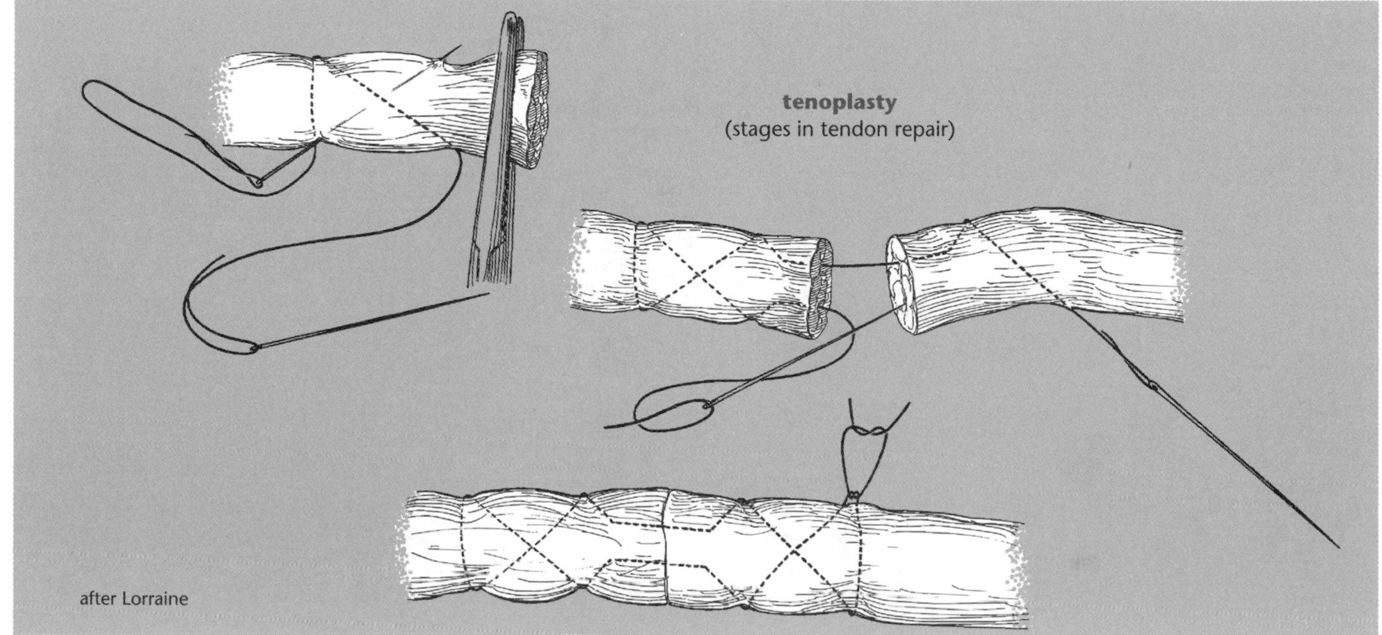

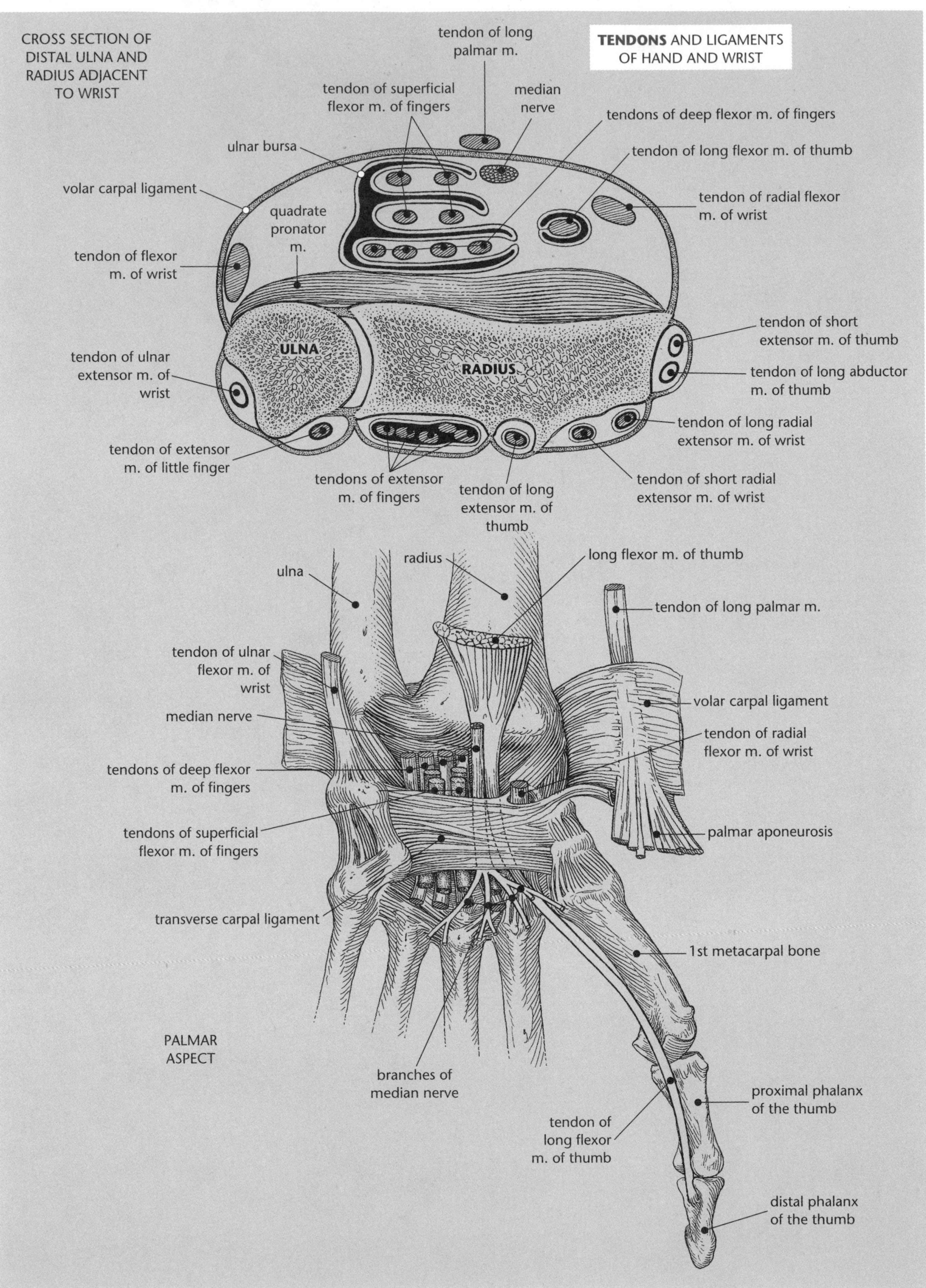

CROSS SECTION OF DISTAL ULNA AND RADIUS ADJACENT TO WRIST
TENDONS AND LIGAMENTS OF HAND AND WRIST
tendon of long palmar m.
tendon of superficial flexor m. of fingers
median nerve
tendons of deep flexor m. of fingers
ulnar bursa
tendon of long flexor m. of thumb
volar carpal ligament
quadrate pronator m.
tendon of radial flexor m. of wrist
tendon of flexor m. of wrist
ULNA
RADIUS
tendon of short extensor m. of thumb
tendon of ulnar extensor m. of wrist
tendon of long abductor m. of thumb
tendon of long radial extensor m. of wrist
tendon of extensor m. of little finger
tendons of extensor m. of fingers
tendon of long extensor m. of thumb
tendon of short radial extensor m. of wrist
radius
ulna
long flexor m. of thumb
tendon of long palmar m.
tendon of ulnar flexor m. of wrist
volar carpal ligament
median nerve
tendon of radial flexor m. of wrist
tendons of deep flexor m. of fingers
tendons of superficial flexor m. of fingers
palmar aponeurosis
transverse carpal ligament
1st metacarpal bone
PALMAR ASPECT
branches of median nerve
proximal phalanx of the thumb
tendon of long flexor m. of thumb
distal phalanx of the thumb

T

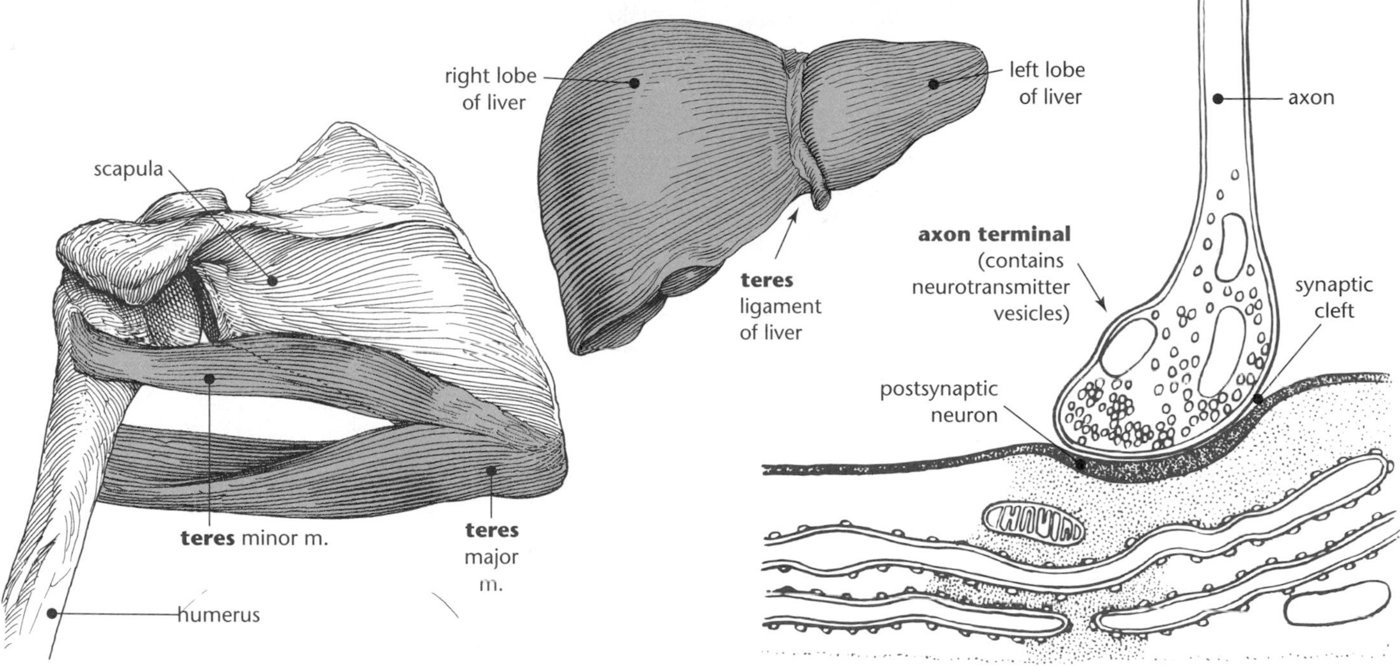

cerebellum and the posterior part of the cerebrum.

tephromalacia (tef-ro-mă-la´shă) Condition marked by softening of the gray substance of the brain and spinal cord.

ter (ter) Latin for three times.

t. die sumendum (t.d.s.) Latin for to be taken three times a day.

t. in die (t.i.d.) Latin for three times a day.

teratocarcinoma (ter-ă-to-kar-sĭ-no´mă) **1.** A malignant tumor composed of several types of tissues, usually occurring in the testis. **2.** A malignant epithelial tumor originating in a teratoma.

teratogen (ter´ă-to-jen) Any environmental or chemical agent that causes abnormal development of the fetus.

teratogenesis, teratogeny (ter-ă-to-jen´ĕ-sis, ter-ă-toj´ĕ-ne) The origin of congenital malformations.

teratogenic (ter-ă to-jen´ik) Causing physical abnormalities.

teratoid (ter´ă-toid) Resembling a malformed fetus.

teratology (ter-ă-tol´ŏ-je) The subspecialty of developmental anatomy that deals with abnormal development. Also called desmorphology.

teratoma (ter-ă-to´mă) Any of a group of tumors derived from cell types of the three germ layers (i.e., endoderm, mesoderm, and ectoderm); seen most commonly in the ovary and testis, also along the midline of the chest between the lungs; some are benign, others malignant; may occur at any age.

benign cystic t. See dermoid cyst, under cyst.

immature t. of ovary See malignant teratoma of ovary.

malignant t. of ovary An uncommon, bulky tumor, usually solid with areas of tissue degeneration and hemorrhage; it contains embryonic elements of all three germ layers (i.e., tissue elements differentiating toward cartilage, glands, muscle, bone, nerve); extraovarian spread depends on the predominant cell type present and degree of tissue immaturity; occurs most commonly unilaterally in adolescent and young women. Also called immature teratoma of ovary; solid teratoma of ovary.

mature benign t. See dermoid cyst, under cyst.

sacroccoxygeal t. Teratoma occurring usually as a large mass in the area of the sacrum and coccyx of newborn infants.

solid t. of ovary See malignant teratoma of ovary.

teratomatous (ter-ă-to´mă-tus) Relating to, or having, the characteristics of a teratoma.

teratophobia (ter-ă-to-fo´be-ă) Morbid fear of giving birth to a grossly deformed baby.

terbium (ter´be-um) A metallic element; symbol Th, atomic number 65, atomic weight 158.93.

teres (te´rēz) Round and elongated, such as certain ligaments and muscles.

term (term) A definite or limited period of time.

at t. At the normal time; at the end of a normal pregnancy or gestation period.

terminal (ter´mĭ-nal) **1.** Relating to an end. **2.** Relating to, situated at, or forming the extremity of any body part. **3.** The part of an electric circuit at which an electric connection is generally made.

axon t. The knoblike expansion of an axonal branch at the site of a synapse; it is in apposition either to other nerve cells (forming interneuronal zones), to muscles (forming neuromuscular junctions), or to glands (forming neuroglandular junctions). Also called bouton terminaux; terminal bouton; terminal button; end-foot; neuropodium.

ternary (ter´nă-re) Composed of three (e.g., a molecule containing three different types of atoms).

tertian (ter´shun) Recurring every third day, such as certain malarial fevers.

tertigravida (ter-tĭ-grav´ĭ-dă) A woman who is pregnant for the third time. Also called gravida III.

tertipara (ter-tip´ă-ră) A woman who has had three pregnancies reaching the period of viability. Also called para III.

test (test) **1.** An examination. **2.** A means to determine the presence and quantity of a substance. **3.** To perform such functions. **4.** A substance used in a test.

achievement t. A standardized educational test to measure the degree of knowledge or skills acquired after instruction in specific subjects. Distinguished from intelligence test.

acid perfusion t. Test to establish that a pain under the breastbone is due to reflux esophagitis; a weak hydrochloric acid solution is instilled into the lower esophagus through a nasogastric tube; pain disappears when the acid solution is replaced by saline solution. Also called Bernstein test.

ACTH t. See ACTH stimulation test.

ACTH stimulation t. Test for adrenal cortex function; limited or nonexistent increase of plasma cortisol after administration of ACTH indicates adrenal cortex insufficiency. Also called ACTH test.

Adson's t. A test for the detection of thoracic outlet syndrome; the patient sits with the palm of the hands on his knees, chin held high, head turned toward the side to be examined; if on deep inspiration the radial pulse diminishes or disappears on the affected side, it indicates temporary occlusion of the subclavian artery. Also called Adson's maneuver.

alkali denaturation t. Test to determine the concentration of fetal hemoglobin.

alpha-fetoprotein t., AFP t. A prenatal screening test based on detection of AFP (a fetal glycoprotein) in maternal serum; performed on pregnant women between 14 and 16 weeks of gestation, especially women over 35 years of age; abnormally high levels of AFP are usually associated with open neural-tube defects (e.g., spina bifida); abnormally low levels are usually indicative of Down syndrome (trisomy 21). Positive results may be followed by amniocentesis to determine AFP levels in amniotic fluid and final diagnosis. See also alpha-fetoprotein.

antibody screening t. See indirect Coombs' test.

antiglobulin t. See Coombs' test.

antistreptolysin-O t. See streptococcal antibody test.

aptitude t. A test that measures a person's skills, interests, talents and abilities; useful in vocational counseling.

ASLO t. See streptococcal antibody test.

ASO t. See streptococcal antibody test.

association t. A method for examining the content of the mind; the subject is required to respond as quickly as possible to a given stimulus word with the first word that comes to mind. Also called word association test.

Bárány's caloric t. Test for vestibular function of the ear; reduced or absent response (e.g., nystagmus or past pointing) after irrigation of external auditory canal with hot or cold water indicates vestibular disease. Also called nystagmus test.

Bender gestalt t. A test of visual motor function in which the subject is asked to copy nine standard designs; its chief application is to determine organic brain dysfunction in both children and adults and level of development of visual motor function in children; secondarily used to assess personality variables. Also called Bender visual-motor gestalt test.

Bender visual-motor gestalt t. See Bender-gestalt test.

benzidine t. Test to detect the presence of blood; a portion of the suspected sample is added to benzidine reagent (benzidine, glacial acetic acid, and hydrogen peroxide); a blue color develops in the presence of blood.

Bernstein t. See acid perfusion test.

Binet t., Stanford-Binet t. Test used to determine the mental age of a child; it consists of a series of questions standardized according to the mental capacity of normal children at different ages.

biuret t. Test used to determine the presence of proteins in body fluids; the sample is mixed with alkaline copper sulfate; a violet-pinkish color indicates a positive result. Also called biuret reaction.

CAGE t. A screening test for alcoholism. The patient is asked if he (she) ever cut down on drinking; felt annoyed by criticisms about drinking; had guilty

T

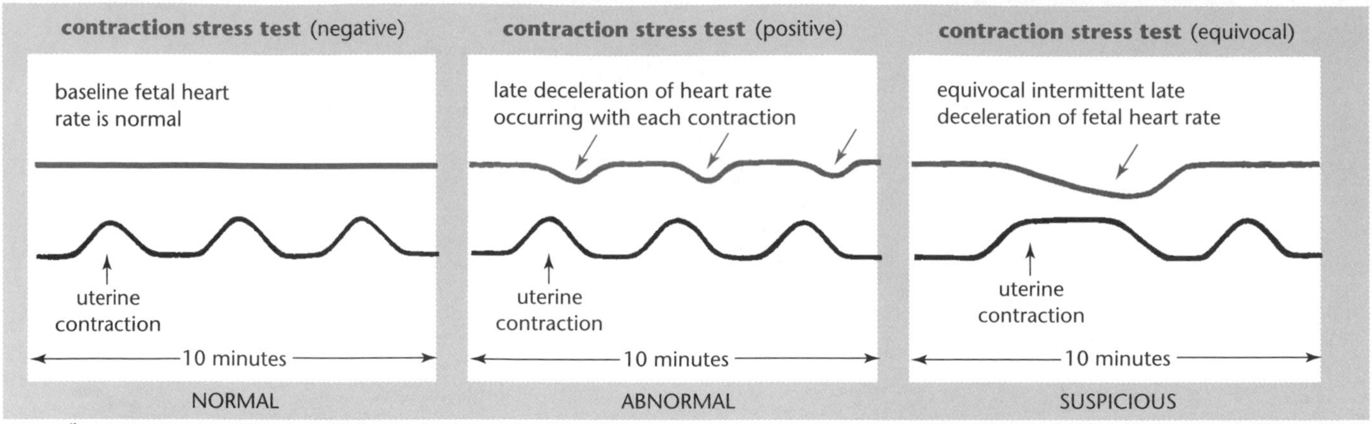

contraction stress test (negative)

baseline fetal heart rate is normal

uterine contraction

10 minutes

NORMAL

contraction stress test (positive)

late deceleration of heart rate occurring with each contraction

uterine contraction

10 minutes

ABNORMAL

contraction stress test (equivocal)

equivocal intermittent late deceleration of fetal heart rate

uterine contraction

10 minutes

SUSPICIOUS

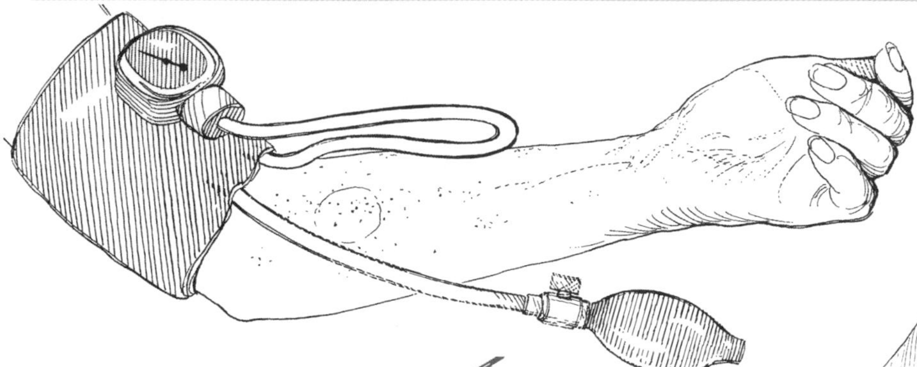

capillary fragility test

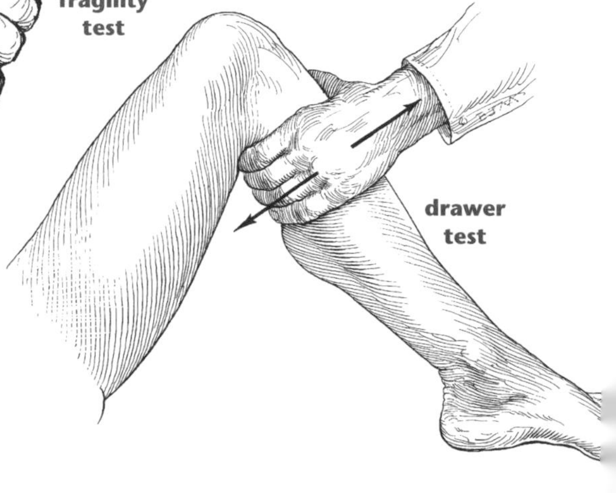

drawer test

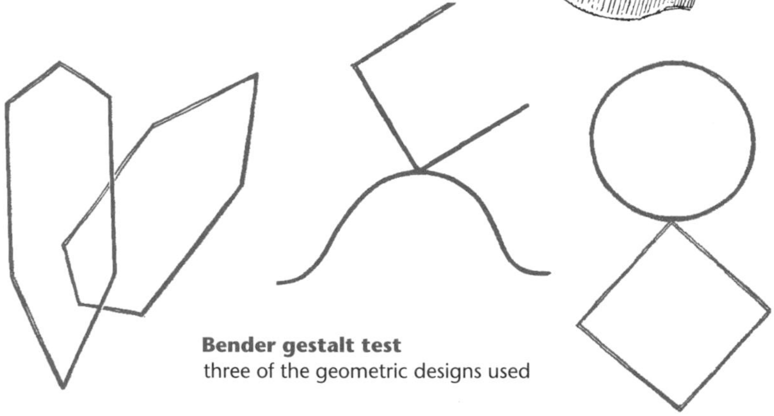

Bender gestalt test
three of the geometric designs used

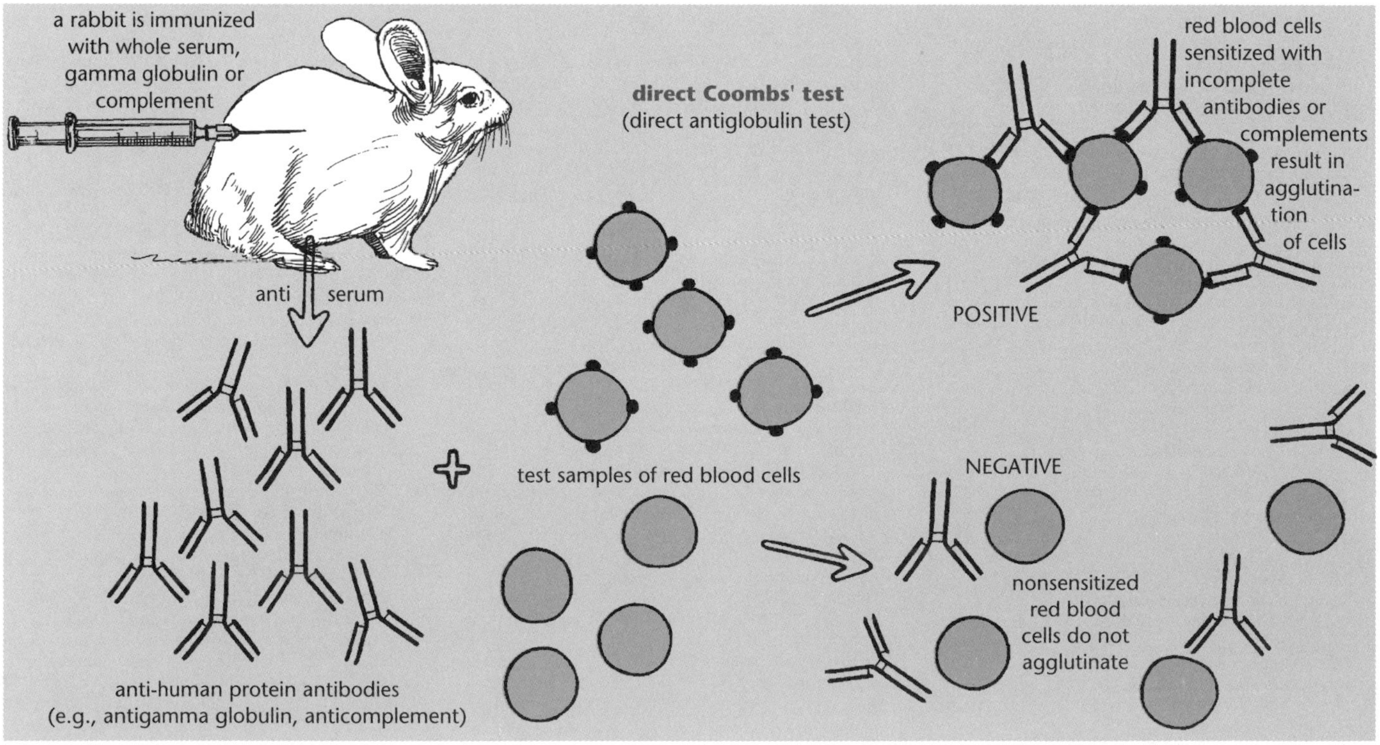

a rabbit is immunized with whole serum, gamma globulin or complement

anti serum

anti-human protein antibodies (e.g., antigamma globulin, anticomplement)

direct Coombs' test
(direct antiglobulin test)

test samples of red blood cells

POSITIVE

red blood cells sensitized with incomplete antibodies or complements result in agglutination of cells

NEGATIVE

nonsensitized red blood cells do not agglutinate

T

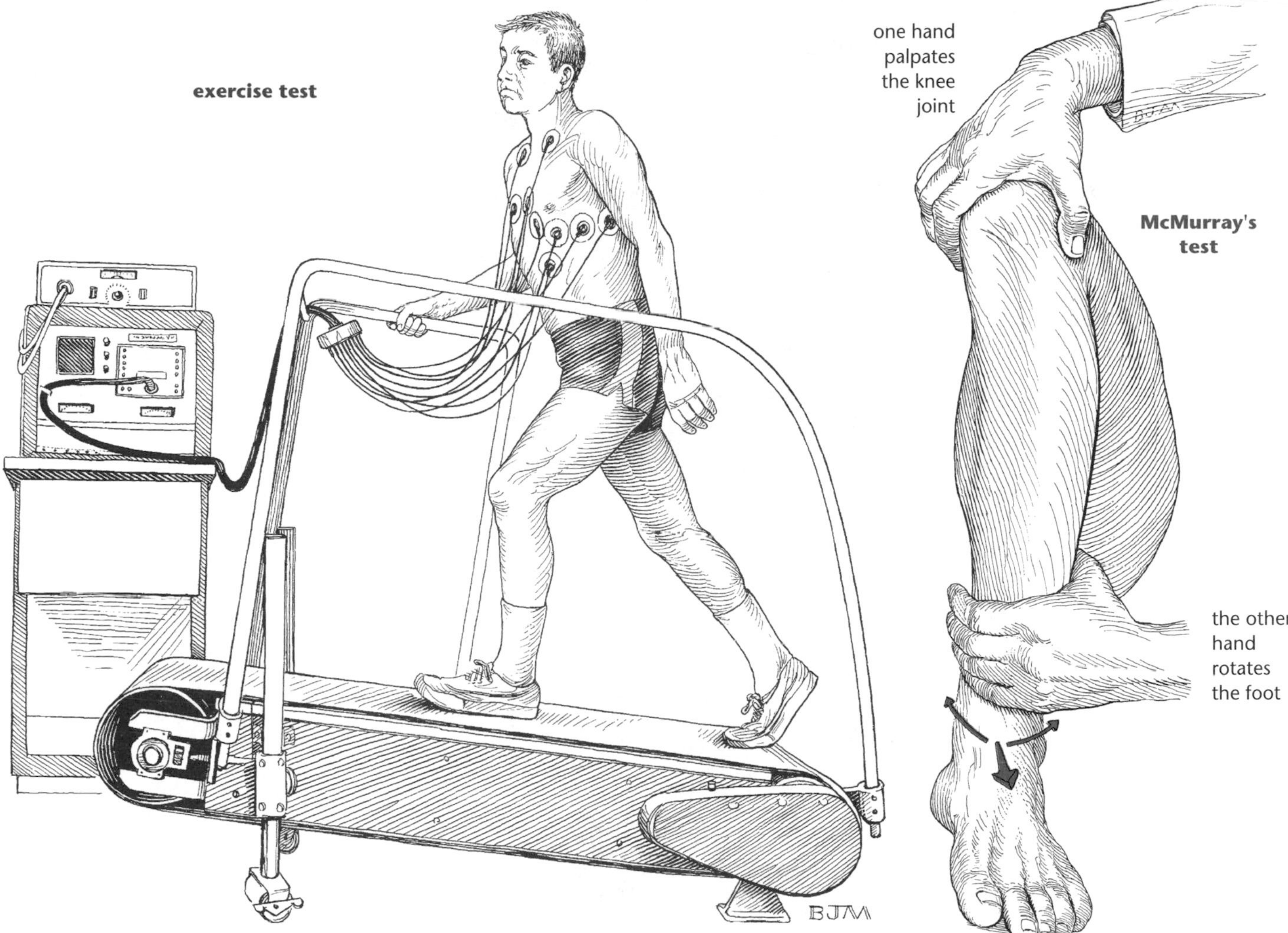
exercise test
one hand
palpates
the knee
joint
McMurray's
test
the other
hand
rotates
the foot
BJM

feelings about drinking; had an eye opener in the morning.

capillary fragility t. A tourniquet test to determine weakness of the capillary walls and to identify platelet deficiency; a circle 2.5 cm in diameter is drawn on the inner aspect of the forearm 4 cm below the crease of the elbow, and a blood pressure cuff is inflated above the elbow to the mean arterial pressure for 10 minutes; the petechiae (minute hemorrhagic spots) formed within the circle are counted; a number over 20 is abnormal. Also called Rumpel-Leede test; capillary resistance test; tourniquet test.

capillary resistance t. See capillary fragility test.

complement-fixation t. A widely used test to detect the presence of antibodies in serum; based on the fact that antibodies, when combined with their specific antigens, are able to fix or remove complement (thus making it undetectable in a subsequent test).

contraction stress t. (CST) Test for assessing a fetus at risk for compromised placental respiratory function (placental insufficiency). A monitoring device is placed on the maternal abdomen to continuously monitor the fetal heart rate and uterine contractions; contractions are induced by intermittent stimulation of the nipples or by intravenous infusion of dilute oxytocin until three (no more than five) contractions occur within 10 minutes; each contraction should last no longer than 40 to 60 seconds; uterine stimulation is then discontinued but the fetal heart rate is monitored until contractions have subsided. Interpretation of test results depends on the occurrence of late decelerations (i.e., when there is a fetal heart-rate decrease beginning at, or after, the peak of a uterine contraction and returning to baseline levels well after the contraction has ended).

Coombs' t. (CT) An agglutination test designed to detect the presence on cells of serum proteins (commonly functionally univalent antibodies) not usually identifiable by simple *in vitro* agglutination techniques; two methods may be used: *direct* (test for antibody on red blood cells) or *indirect* (test for antibody in serum). Also called antiglobulin test. See also direct Coombs' test; indirect Coombs' test.

cytotoxicity t., cytoxicity t. One used in testing for compatibility for organ transplant; living cells are mixed with antibody and complement; if antibody to a cell-bound antigen is present, cell death will occur in the presence of complement.

Denver Developmental Screening t., Revised Test for assessing general development of preschool children.

dexamethasone suppression t. A test for diagnosing Cushing's syndrome; administration of 1 mg of dexamethasone suppresses cortisol secretion to low levels in normal persons but not in those with Cushing's syndrome. Sometimes used to test for organic depression.

direct antiglobulin t. See direct Coombs' test.

direct Coombs' t. Test for detecting sensitized red blood cells in erythroblastosis fetalis and acquired hemolytic anemia; a sample of the patient's red blood cells is washed with saline and mixed with Coombs' antihuman globulin, then centrifuged; agglutination indicates a positive test. Also called direct antiglobulin test.

double-blind t. Test in which neither the person giving the test nor the one receiving it knows whether the drug used is active or inert.

draw-a-person t. In psychology, (a) a method of determining a child's level of intellectual development based upon the complexity of the subject's "best" drawing of a human figure. Also called Goodenough test. (b) A projective personality test requiring the subject to draw a person. Also called Machover test.

drawer t. A test to assess the state of the cruciate ligaments of the knee; with the knee bent at a 90° angle, if the tibia can be drawn forward on the lower femur, it indicates laxity or tear of the anterior cruciate ligament; if it can be drawn backward, it indicates laxity or tear of the posterior cruciate ligament.

Duke bleeding time t. Test conducted by puncturing the ear lobe and measuring the interval between the beginning and ending of bleeding.

erythrocyte fragility t. One that measures the osmotic fragility of red blood cells; cells are placed in a series of test tubes with saline of decreasing concentrations ranging from 0.85 to 0.10%; the red cells absorb water, swell to a spheroid shape, and rupture; in normal cells hemolysis begins at concentrations of 0.45 to 0.39%; and complete hemolysis occurs at 0.33 to 0.30%. Also called fragility test.

exercise t. A test to assess cardiovascular function through the use of exercise on a treadmill or pedaling a stationary bicycle (bicycle ergometer) while under continuous electrocardiographic monitoring; useful in detecting coronary artery disease.

ferric chloride t. Test for detecting phenylketonuria, which is indicated when a urine sample turns blue-green by addition of ferric chloride.

finger-nose t. Test of ability to coordinate voluntary movement of the arm; the person is asked to slowly touch the end of his nose with the tip of his extended index finger.

fluorescent treponemal antibody-absorption t., FTA-ABS t. A specific test for syphilis using a suspension of *Treponema pallidum* (Nichols strain).

fragility t. See erythrocyte fragility test.

genetic screening t. A test to identify individuals at risk of developing or passing on inherited illnesses.

gestational diabetes t. A screening glucose tolerance test routinely administered during 24 and 28 weeks of pregnancy for the detection of abnormal carbohydrate metabolism; the patient drinks 50 g of glucose solution or equivalent and a blood sample is drawn 1 hour later. Generally, a plasma value over 140 mg/dl is an indication for conducting an extended glucose tolerance test. See also gestational diabetes, under diabetes.

T

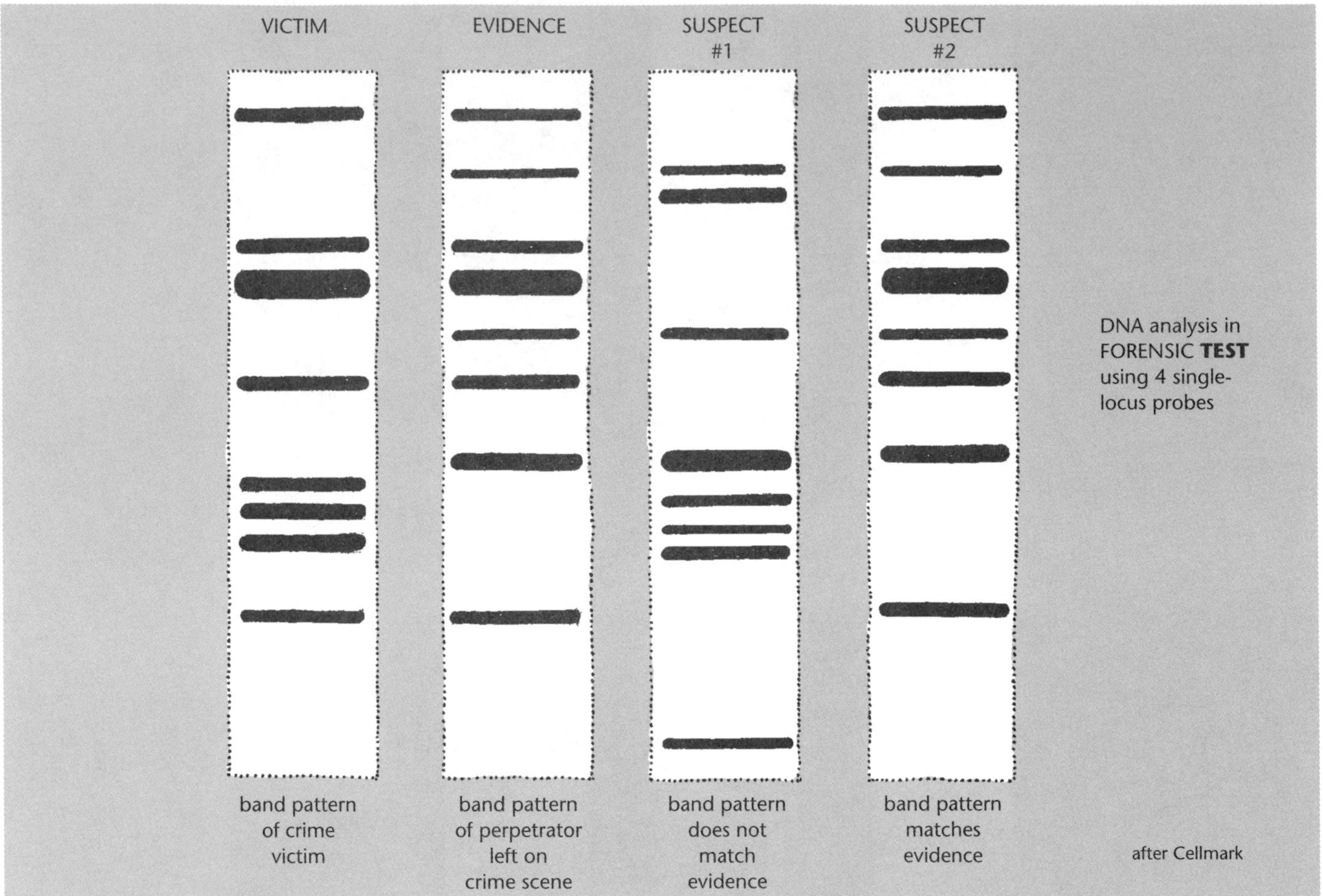

glucose tolerance t. (GTT) Any of a series of tests in which a measured amount of glucose is given orally or intravenously and the plasma glucose is measured at fixed intervals; it measures the ability of the liver to absorb and store excessive amounts of blood sugar (glucose) as glycogen. A fasting glucose level above 140 mg/dL on more than one occasion also establishes the diagnosis of diabetes mellitus. False-positive results may be caused by infection, severe emotional stress, diuretics, oral contraceptives, glucocorticoids, excess thyroxine, and some psychotropic drugs. In the intravenous test, a smaller dose of glucose (usually 25 g) is given; used in patients with gastrointestinal abnormalities (e.g., malabsorption).

Goodenough t. See draw-a-person test (a).

guaiac t. Test for detection of blood; specimen is mixed with glacial acetic acid and gum guaiac solution; blood is present if a blue color develops upon addition of hydrogen peroxide.

heel-to-shin t. A test to assess the coordinated movements of the lower extremities; the patient, while lying on his back, is instructed to touch the knee of one leg with the heel of the other, then move the heel slowly down the front of the shinbone (tibia) to the foot; the motion is then repeated with the other leg.

T

hemagglutination t. Test to measure certain antigens, antibodies, or viruses through their ability to agglutinate red blood cells.

Hickey-Hare t. Test for diabetes insipidus; hypertonic saline is infused intravenously after establishment of water diuresis; test is positive when antidiuresis is not produced; when the posterior pituitary is normal, the hypertonicity causes release of antidiuretic hormones, which concentrates the urine.

histamine t. (a) A test for determining the absence of gastric acidity; histamine phosphate is injected subcutaneously to stimulate secretion of gastric juice. (b) A provocative test for pheochromocytoma; histamine phosphate is injected intravenously; normally there is a prompt, slight fall in blood pressure, but if a lesion is present, a marked rise in blood pressure follows immediately after the fall.

HIV infection t.'s Tests for infection with HIV (human immunodeficiency virus, the cause of AIDS). Two tests are commonly used, ELISA (enzyme-linked immunosorbent assay) and Western blot analysis; both aim to detect HIV-specific antibody, a protein produced by the infected person's immune system in response to the presence of the HIV virus. In ELISA, the presence of antibody in a blood sample is indicated by a reaction-dependent color, which is then measured by spectrophotometry. The Western blot analysis gives information about particular antibodies among the several that HIV antigens may elicit; it uses electrophoresis and is thus more expensive and demanding of expertise than the ELISA. See also enzyme-linked immunosorbent assay (ELISA), under assay; Western blot analysis, under analysis.

home pregnancy t's Any do-it-yourself pregnancy test using commercial over-the-counter kits for detection of human chorionic gonadotropin (hCG) in a urine sample; detection of hCG in the sample indicates pregnancy since this hormone is not usually present in nonpregnant women.

immunologic pregnancy t. Test utilizing latex particles coated with human chorionic gonadotropin (hCG) as antigen, anti-hCG serum, and urine to be tested; if the latex particles do not clump, the woman is pregnant. Also called agglutination inhibition test for pregnancy.

indirect antiglobulin t. See indirect Coombs' test.

indirect Coombs' t. Test used in crossmatching of blood and transfusion reaction studies; the patient's serum is incubated with a suspension of donor red blood cells; after a washing with saline, Coombs' serum is added; clumping indicates that the cells had been coated or sensitized by antibodies present in the patient's serum. Also called antibody screening test.

indole t. Any test used to identify gram-negative bacilli of the family Enterobacteriaceae, based on their ability to produce indole from tryptophan.

intelligence t. Any test designed to measure the mental capacity of the subject.

Ishihara's t. A test for detection of color blindness, based on the ability to see patterns in a series of multicolored plates or cards (Ishihara plates).

131I uptake t. A test of thyroid function; ^{131}iodide is administered orally; 24 hours later the amount of uptake by the thyroid gland is measured at specific intervals and compared against normal values. A greater than normal uptake indicates hyperthyroidism; a lower than normal uptake indicates hypothyroidism but may also occur when the patient has received unlabeled iodine. Also called radioactive iodine uptake test; RAI test.

Kirby-Bauer t. Test for microbiological susceptibility; a standardized pure culture of the microorganism of interest is placed in a Petri dish containing Muller-Hinton agar; growth of the organisms is observed in the presence of disks containing antibiotics.

Kolmer's t. (a) A complement-fixation test for certain bacterial diseases. (b) A modified Wassermann test for syphilis.

Kveim t. Test for detection of sarcoidosis; a dose of ground sarcoid lymph nodes, tested for sterility and preserved in phenol, is injected intradermally; a papule appears; biopsy of the papule in a positive test shows giant cell formation.

latex t. See latex agglutination test.

latex agglutination t. Test for rheumatoid arthritis; minute spherical particles of latex in suspension are coated with antigen and incubated with the patient's serum; when rheumatoid factor is present in the serum, clumping of the latex particles occurs. Also called latex test; latex fixation test.

latex fixation t. See latex agglutination test.

LE cell t. A test for systemic lupus erythematosus; polymorphonuclear leukocytes engulf nuclear material from damaged white blood cells, forming LE cells, in blood or serum samples from patients with the disease.

lepromin t. Test for leprosy; a lepromin injection produces a papule in tuberculoid leprosy; no such reaction occurs in lepromatous leprosy.

McMurray's t. A test for tears of the posterior aspect of the meniscus in the knee joint. With the patient's knee fully flexed, the examiner palpates the knee with one hand and rotates the foot with the other;

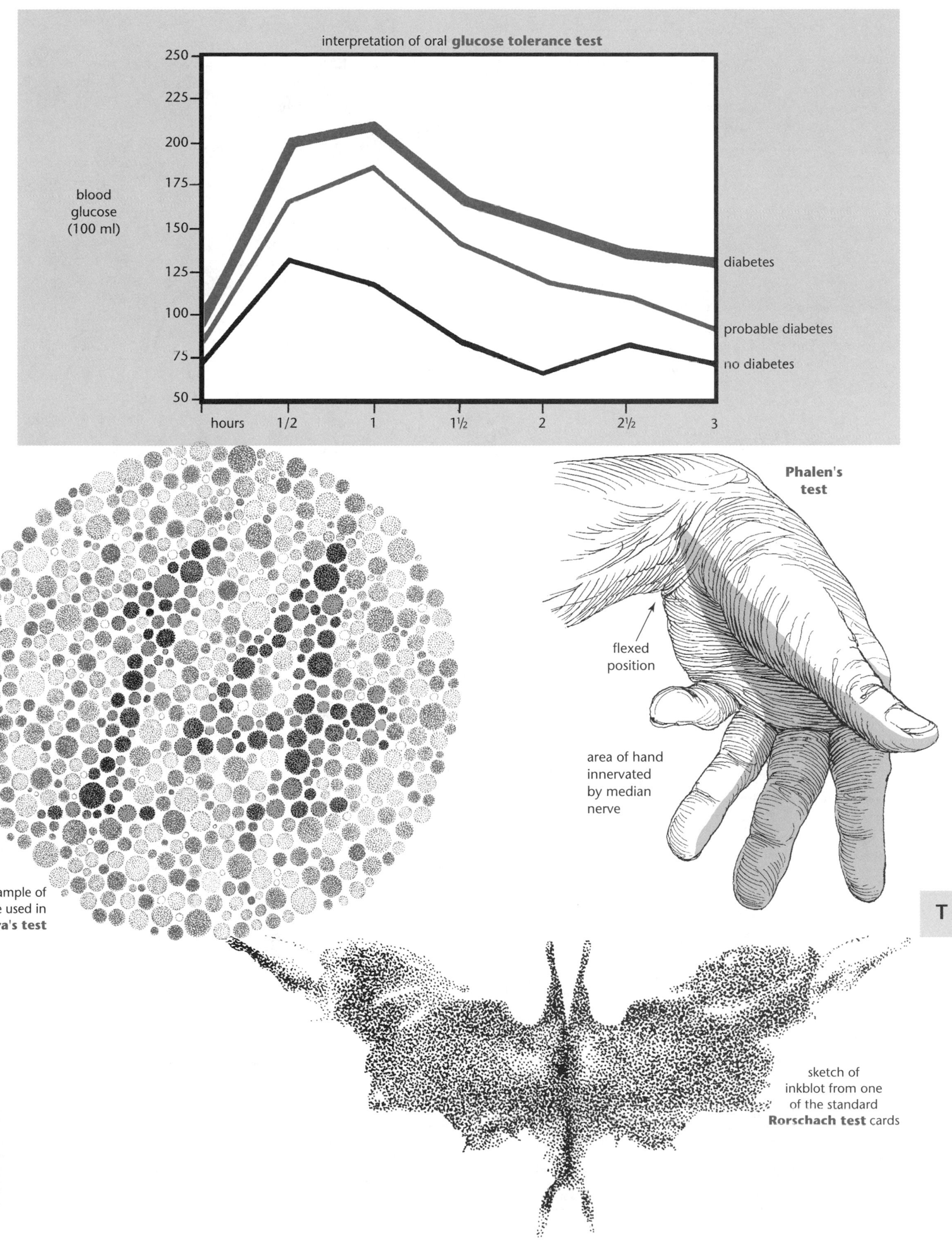

sample of
e used in
ra's test

sketch of inkblot from one of the standard **Rorschach test** cards

T

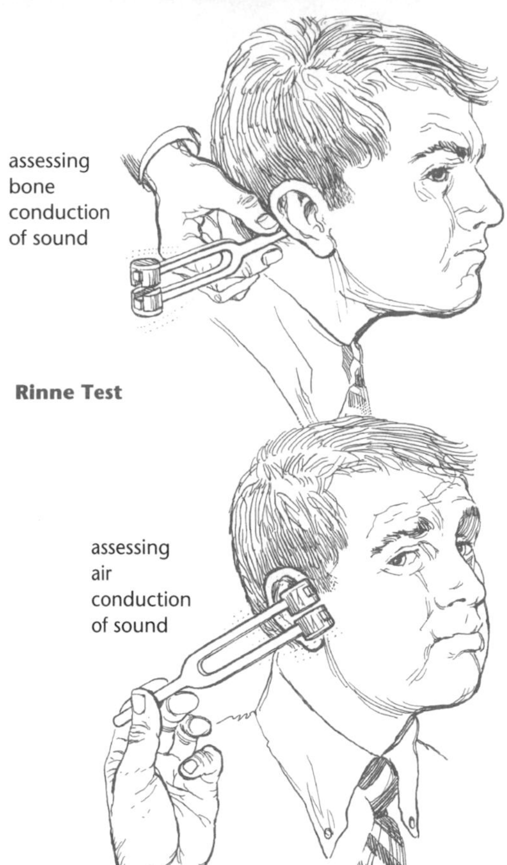
assessing
bone
conduction
of sound
Rinne Test
assessing
air
conduction
of sound

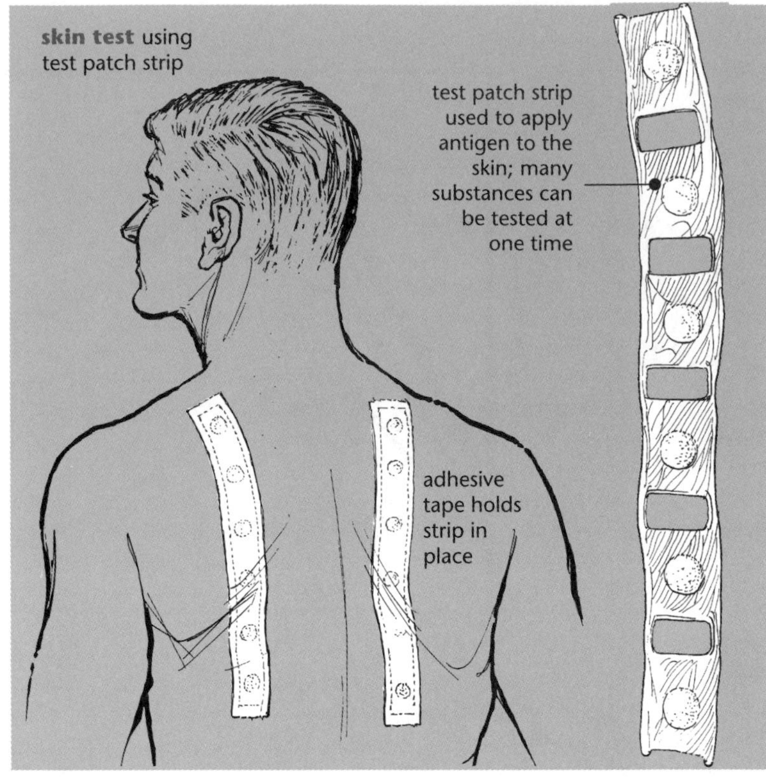
skin test using
test patch strip
test patch strip
used to apply
antigen to the
skin; many
substances can
be tested at
one time
adhesive
tape holds
strip in
place

a palpable painful click indicates a torn meniscus.

Machover t. See draw-a-person test (b).

Mantoux t. A tuberculin test in which a derivative of tuberculin, such as purified protein derivative (PPD), is injected intracutaneously; considered positive if redness and induration of 10 mm diameter occur.

migration inhibitory factor t. (MIF) *In vitro* test for delayed type sensitivity (cell mediated); when specific antigen is present, peritoneal exudate cells (macrophages) from a sensitized animal do not migrate from a chamber in the manner typical of those from a normal animal.

Minnesota multiphasic personality inventory (MMPI) **t.** Psychological test in the form of a questionnaire composed of 550 true-false statements; answers are scored by codes, standardized on different diagnostic groups and personality types.

mixed lymphocyte culture t., MLC t. Test to measure a person's ability to accept a tissue transplant; lymphocytes from donor and recipient are mixed in culture, whereupon the degree of incompatibility is measured by estimating the number of cells that have undergone transformation and mitosis, or by the amount of radioactive isotope-labeled thymidine that was incorporated.

multiple sleep latency t. Assessment of the propensity to fall asleep by the use of continuous monitoring of physiologic activity during multiple brief opportunities to sleep.

nitroblue tetrazolium (NBT) **t.** Test of neutrophil capacity to kill bacteria; normally, phagocytosis of bacterial cells is accompanied by NBT reduction to a blue formazan pigment; absence of NBT reduction indicates neutrophil defects.

nitroprusside t. Test to detect cystine in the urine; sodium cyanide is first added to the urine sample, then nitroprusside; a red-purple color develops if the cyanide has reduced to cysteine any cystine that was present in the urine.

nonstress t. (NST) Test for detecting oxygen deficiency in the fetus (fetal hypoxia) by evaluating fetal heart rate response to fetal movement with the aid of a recording system applied to the maternal abdomen.

oxytocin challenge t. (OTC) A contraction stress test using oxytocin to evoke uterine contractions.

Pap t., Papanicolaou t., Procedure in which cells from body secretions are fixed and stained and examined microscopically for abnormal cells; used in the detection of cancer (especially of the female genital tract, but also of the respiratory, urinary and gastrointestinal tracts) and for the evaluation of the hormonal state. Also called Pap smear; Pap smear test.

patch t. A test for allergic sensitivity made by placing filter paper or gauze saturated with a suspected allergen against the skin (usually on the forearm) under a small patch; on removal of the patch the reaction of the skin is observed; a positive reaction is indicated by reddening at the site; also used for tuberculin testing.

paternity t. A medicolegal test based upon genetic interpretation of blood groups of mother, child, and alleged father to exclude the possibility of paternity.

Paul-Bunnell t. A test to determine the presence of heterophil antibodies in the circulating blood; an elevated titer is found in infectious mononucleosis.

Phalen's t. A test for determining median nerve compression in the carpal tunnel of the wrist; the wrists are placed in a flexed position; if there is median nerve compression, paresthesias of the fingers usually occur after several seconds; most normal individuals develop paresthesias after a few minutes of acute wrist flexion.

phentolamine t. Test for pheochromocytoma in patients with sustained hypertension; administration of phentolamine produces a sustained fall in blood pressure in the presence of pheochromocytoma.

postprandial blood sugar t. A test utilizing a sample of blood drawn, usually two hours after the ingestion of a 100-gram carbohydrate meal, for the diagnosis of diabetes mellitus.

PPD t. See tuberculin test.

precipitin t. Any test in which a positive result is indicated by the formation of a precipitate. Also called precipitation test.

pregnancy t. Any test for pregnancy (e.g., Aschheim-Zondek test, immunologic pregnancy test).

prostate-specific antigen t., PSA t. Blood test for detection of prostatic cancer; it measures serum concentrations of a protein (antigen) produced exclusively by prostate epithelial cells; levels of up to 4 micrograms/liter are generally considered normal; increased levels may be caused by a very large gland or by inflammation (prostatitis); in the absence of inflammation, a rapid rate of increases, regardless of the level, may indicate cancer.

prothrombin t. Test that determines the amount of thrombin present in plasma, based on the clotting time of blood; used to measure blood coagulability and as a guide to anticoagulation with coumarin and related drugs.

provocative t. A test for pheochromocytoma performed on patients with normal blood pressure; the presence of pheochromocytoma causes a sudden rise in blood pressure immediately following the administration of histamine, tyramine, or glucagon.

PSA t. See prostate-specific antigen test.

psychological t. Any test dealing with mental phenomena.

pulp t. A test that measures the response of the dental pulp to various stimuli (thermal, electrical, or mechanical); it determines whether a pulp is alive, diseased, or dead. Also called vitality test.

Queckenstedt-Stookey t. When the jugular vein is compressed in a healthy person, there is rapid increase in the pressure of the cerebrospinal fluid (CSF), and an equally rapid return to normal when pressure is released; when there is a block in the vertebral canal, compression of the jugular vein causes little or no increase in pressure.

radioactive iodine uptake t. See ^{131}I uptake test.

radioallergosorbent t. (RAST) Test for detection of IgE-bound allergens causing tissue hypersensitivity; antigen is fixed in an insoluble medium, serum from the patient is added, and then a radiolabeled antigammaglobulin; if antibody to the allergen is present in the serum, it complexes to the allergen.

RAI t. See ^{131}I uptake test.

rapid plasma reagin t., RPR t. A test for syphilis using unheated serum and a standard antigen containing charcoal particles.

Rinne's t. Hearing test that compares bone conduction with air conduction by alternately holding a vibrating tuning fork in contact with the skull and in the air near the auditory orifice; in normal hearing, the vibrations are heard twice as long by air as by bone conduction; in conductive hearing loss, the ratio varies in favor of bone conduction.

Rorschach t. Projective psychological test for evaluating conscious and unconscious personality traits and emotional conflicts through the individual's associations to a set of inkblot patterns.

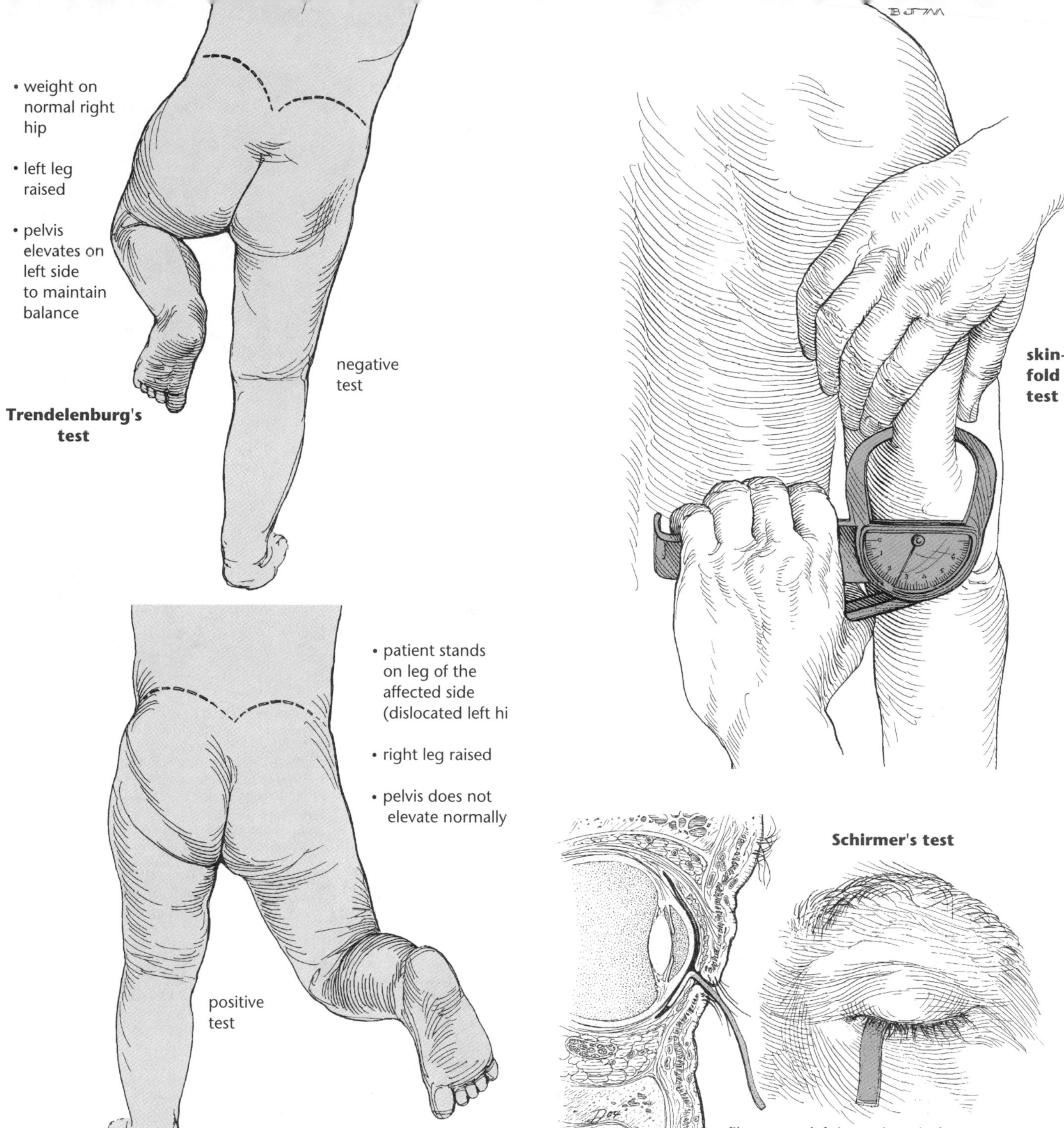
• weight on normal right hip
• left leg raised
• pelvis elevates on left side to maintain balance
negative test
Trendelenburg's test
• patient stands on leg of the affected side (dislocated left hi
• right leg raised
• pelvis does not elevate normally
positive test
skin-fold test
Schirmer's test
filter paper left in conjunctival sac for five minutes

T

Rumpol-Loode T. See capillary fragility test.

Sabin-Feldman dye t. One used to diagnose toxoplasmosis; heat-inactivated serum from the patient (in the presence of a nonspecific serum factor) kills *Toxoplasma* organisms; methylene blue fails to stain damaged organisms.

Schick t. A test to measure immunity to diphtheria; diphtheria toxin (one-fiftieth of a guinea pig median lethal dose) is injected intracutaneously; if the person does not have sufficient antitoxin to neutralize the dose of toxin, an inflammation appears at the site of injection, usually within 48 hours.

Schiller's t. A test for early squamous cell carcinoma of the cervix; the cervix is coated with an aqueous iodine solution; a normal cervix stains brown; any area that does not stain needs evaluation.

Schilling t. Test to determine ability to absorb vitamin B_{12}; cyanocobalamin is tagged with a cobalt radioisotope and administered orally; the amount of vitamin B_{12} absorbed by the body is determined by the amount of radioactive material excreted in the urine over the next 24 hours.

Schirmer's t. Test to measure the production of tears with a strip of filter paper.

scratch t. See skin test.

screening t. One devised to separate individuals or objects according to a fixed characteristic or property.

secretin t. Test for excretory function of the pancreas; secretion of pancreatic enzymes is stimulated for analysis by intravenous injection of the hormone secretin.

sickle cell t. See sickling test.

sickling t. Test to demonstrate the presence of abnormal sickle hemoglobin S in blood; when blood is mixed with sodium bisulfite, red blood cells containing the abnormal sickle hemoglobin (Hb S) assume a crescentic or elongated shape. Also called sickle cell test.

skin t. Any test for allergy or infectious disease in which the allergen or an extract of a disease-causing organism is injected intracutaneously or applied to the skin by means of a patch. Also called scratch test.

skinfold t. Measurement of skinfolds with special constant tension calipers to determine the degree of obesity.

sniff t. Test for assessing diaphragmatic function; the diaphragm is observed with the use of fluoroscopy, as the patient in a supine position sniffs vigorously; a paralyzed diaphragm (or half of it) will move cranially instead of caudally.

streptococcal antibody t. Serologic test to confirm an infection with beta-hemolytic streptococci, to help diagnose acute rheumatic fever and acute poststreptococcal glomerulonephritis, and to distinguish between rheumatic fever and rheumatoid arthritis when joint pains are present; measurements are made of the relative serum concentrations of the antibody to streptolysin O (an enzyme produced by

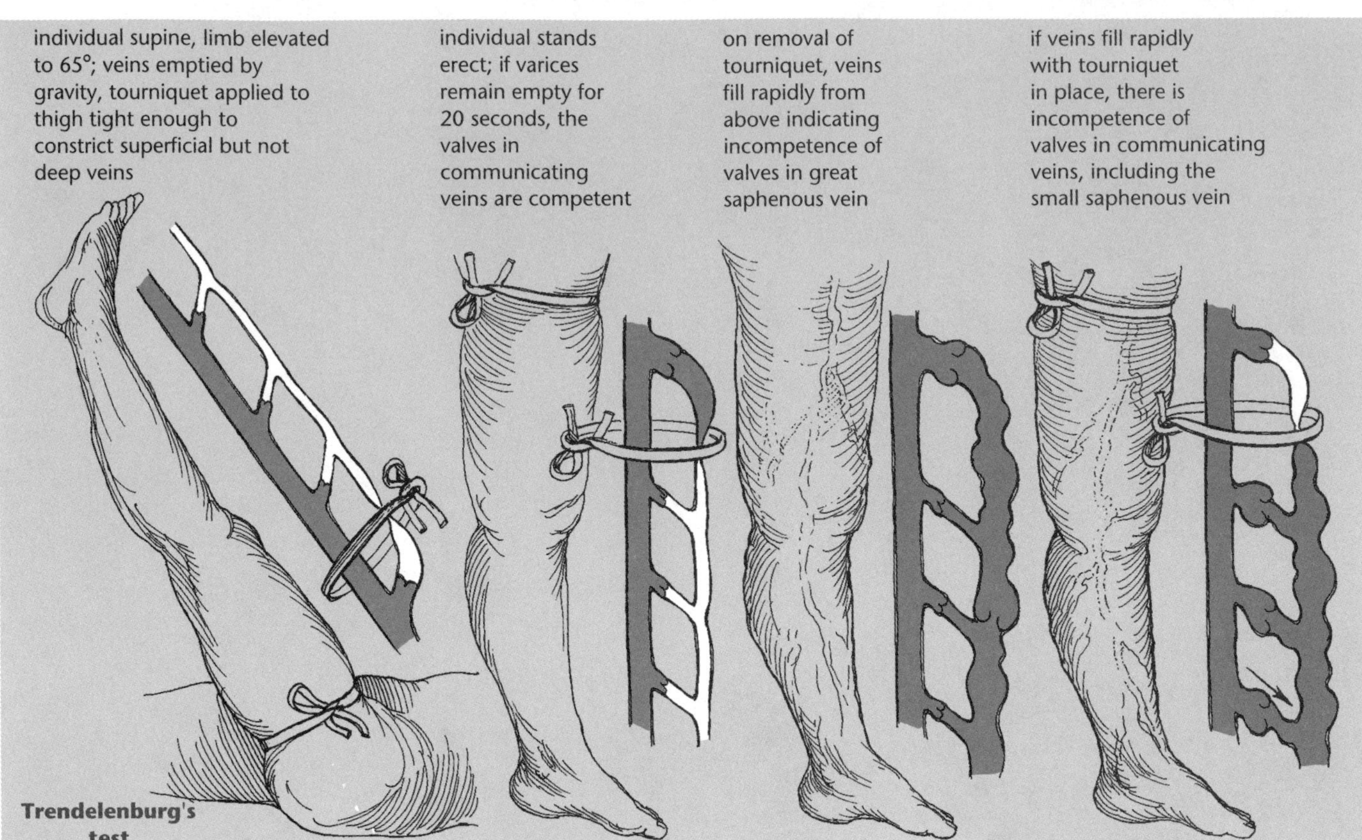
individual supine, limb elevated to 65°; veins emptied by gravity, tourniquet applied to thigh tight enough to constrict superficial but not deep veins
individual stands erect; if varices remain empty for 20 seconds, the valves in communicating veins are competent
on removal of tourniquet, veins fill rapidly from above indicating incompetence of valves in great saphenous vein
if veins fill rapidly with tourniquet in place, there is incompetence of valves in communicating veins, including the small saphenous vein
Trendelenburg's test

group A beta-hemolytic streptococci). Also called antistreptolysin-O test; ASO test; ASLO test.

stress t. Any test to assess cardiac function after subjecting the heart to a physical, pharmacologic, or mental challenge (usually an exercise) under monitored conditions, most commonly electrocardiography.

string t. Any of various tests to determine the approximate site of bleeding from the upper gastrointestinal tract, using a white string which is passed into the duodenum or beyond; the string is removed and checked along its length for blood; the blood-stained portion indicates the site of hemorrhage.

sweat t. Test for diagnosis of cystic fibrosis of the pancreas; high concentration of sodium chloride in the sweat is suggestive of the disease.

thematic apperception t. (TAT) Psychological test in which the subject is asked to tell stories about ambiguous pictures that may be interpreted in different ways according to the patient's personality.

three-glass t. Test for locating the site of inflammation of the male urinary tract; the patient urinates into three glass containers; the contents of each container reveal the approximate site; the urine in the first container has washings from the anterior urethra, that in the second from the bladder; after prostatic massage, the third has cells from the prostate, seminal vesicles and posterior urethra.

T

tilt t. (a) Test to measure predilection for fainting (syncope); excretion of urinary epinephrine and norepinephrine is measured during three consecutive intervals with the patient first in a horizontal and then in a nearly vertical position; a marked increase in the second period indicates a positive test. (b) A rise in pulse or drop in blood pressure as a patient is moved from the supine toward the upright position indicating a loss of extracellular fluid, as during hemorrhage or dehydration.

tine t. Test for skin sensitivity performed by pressing tines previously impregnated with antigens into the skin; used for tuberculin testing.

tourniquet t. See capillary fragility test.

Trendelenburg's t. (a) A test for hip abnormalities; with the subject standing, weight is borne on the normal side of the hip, the opposite side of the pelvis is elevated to maintain balance (negative test); when weight is borne on the dislocated side, the opposite side of the pelvis does not elevate (positive test), as seen in congenital dislocation of the hip, deformity of the femoral neck, or weakness of the hip abductor muscles. Also called Trendelenburg's sign. (b) A test for determining the presence of incompetent valves in the communicating veins between the superficial and deep vessels in patients with varicose veins in the lower extremity. The patient lies on his back with the leg elevated 65 degrees; after the veins empty of blood by gravity, a tourniquet is applied around the thigh tight enough to constrict superficial veins but not deep veins; the patient stands erect; if varices remain empty for 20 seconds, the valves in the communicating veins are competent; on removal of the tourniquet, veins fill rapidly from above indicating incompetence of valves in the great saphenous vein; if veins fill rapidly with the tourniquet in place, there is incompetence of valves in communicating veins, including the small saphenous vein. Also called Brodie-Trendelenburg test.

treponemal immobilization (TPI) t. Test for syphilis; serum from a syphilitic patient (in the presence of complement) immobilizes the actively motile *Treponema pallidum* obtained from testes of a syphilitic rabbit (antigen).

triiodothyronine (T_3) **uptake t.** An *in vitro* measurement using the patient's serum and radioactive triiodothyronine to determine the concentration of thyroxin-binding globulin present.

tuberculin t. Any test for tuberculosis in which tuberculin or its protein derivative (PPD) is introduced into the skin by means of a patch (patch test), multiple punctures (tine test), or injection (Mantoux test). Also called PPD test.

two-tail t. In statistics, test based on the assumption that data are distributed in both directions from a central point.

Tzanck t. Microscopic examination of fluid from vesicles or blisters to identify characteristic cells of certain vesicular diseases, such as herpes and pemphigus.

van den Bergh's t. Test to measure serum levels of bilirubin.

vanillylmandelic acid (VMA) **t.** Test for catecholamine-secreting tumors, such as a pheochromocytoma; levels of VMA (the major urinary metabolite of norepinephrine and epinephrine) are measured in a 24-hour urine specimen; normal VMA levels range from 0.7 to 6.8 mg/24 hours. Also called VMA test.

VDRL t. Flocculation test for syphilis developed by the Venereal Disease Research Laboratory of the United States Public Health Service.

vitality t. See pulp test.

VMA t. See vanillylmandelic acid test.

Wada t. A test to determine which cerebral hemisphere is dominant for language function; intracarotid injection of amobarbital temporarily abolishes the power of speech (transient aphasia) in the dominant cerebral hemisphere for language function, while it does not interfere with the power of speech in the nondominant cerebral hemisphere.

Wassermann t. The original (1906) effective serologic test for the diagnosis of syphilis. It was a complement-fixation test between the subject's serum and a known antigen. Also called Wassermann reaction.

Watson-Schwartz t. A test for diagnosing acute intermittent porphyria, based on the formation of red coloration upon addition of Ehrlich's aldehyde reagent to a urine specimen.

Weber hearing t. The application of a vibrating tuning fork to the midline of the forehead, bridge of the nose, and against the chin, for audiologic assessment; if the individual hears the tone in the middle of his head, he may have either normal hearing or deafness equal on both sides; if there is nerve deafness on one side, the tone will be heard better on the other side; when asymmetric conductive deafness is present, the tone is heard better in the poor ear.

Weil-Felix t. Test for the presence of typhus and other types of rickettsial infection, based on the agglutination of *Proteus* X bacteria in a patient's blood serum.

D-xylose absorption t. A test of gastrointestinal absorption; after fasting for 8 hours, a patient drinks a 25 g dose of D-xylose dissolved in 250 ml of water, followed immediately by another 250 ml of water; all urine voided during the following 5 hours is pooled; since poor renal function may affect the test, blood samples are tested; normally 16 to 33% of the ingested xylose should be excreted over the 5-hour period; less than this amount is indicative of intestinal malabsorption. Also called D-xylose tolerance test.

D-xylose tolerance t. See D-xylose absorption test.

testa (tes′tă) An outer shell.

testalgia (tes-tal′jă) See orchialgia.

testcross (test′kros) A way of determining an unknown genotype by crossing it with a homozygous

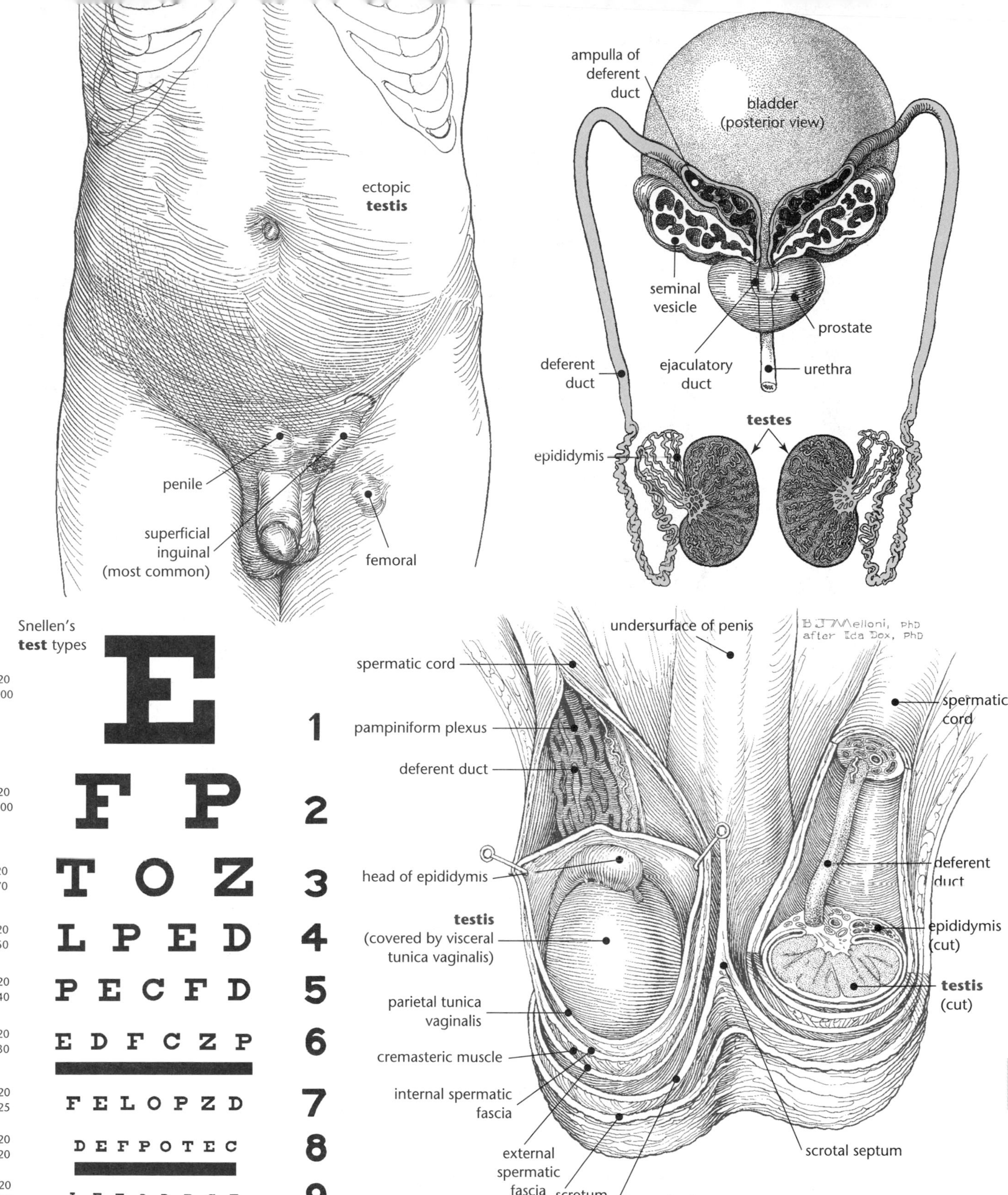

recessive.

testes (tes´tēz) Plural of testis.

testicle (tes´tĭ-kl) See testis.

undescended t. See cryptorchidism.

testicular (tes-tik´u lar) Of the testes.

testicular feminization syndrome (tes-tik´u-lar fem-ĭ-ni-za´shun sin´drōm) Familial male pseudohermaphroditism marked by female external genitalia with a short vaginal pouch and absent uterus, undescended or labial testes, and absent or sparse pubic and axillary hair; the karyotype is XY, but there is a lack of end organ response to testosterone.

testis (tes´tis), *pl.* **testes** One of the two egg-shaped glands which produce spermatozoa, normally situated in the scrotum. Also called testicle.

descent of the t. The gradual change of location of the testis, in the fetus and infant, from the abdominal cavity to the scrotum.

undescended t., retained t. See cryptorchidism.

testitis (tes-ti´tis) See orchitis.

testosterone (tes-tos´tĕ-rōn) A hormone produced by the testes, responsible for the development and maintenance of secondary sexual characteristics; the most potent of the naturally produced androgens, it is produced in the Leydig's cells under control of luteinizing (interstitial cell-stimulating) hormone.

test types (test tīps) Letters or figures printed on a card, used to test visual acuity.

Jaeger's t. t. Words and phrases printed in ordinary printer's type of varying sizes, used to test near vision.

Snellen's t. t. (a) Block letters of varying sizes printed on a white card. (b) A simplified chart that does not require the subject to understand letters; instead one must simply indicate which direction the three prongs of the letter E point.

tetanic (tĕ-tan´ik) Relating to tetanus or tetany.

tetaniform (tĕ-tan´ĭ-form) Resembling tetanus.

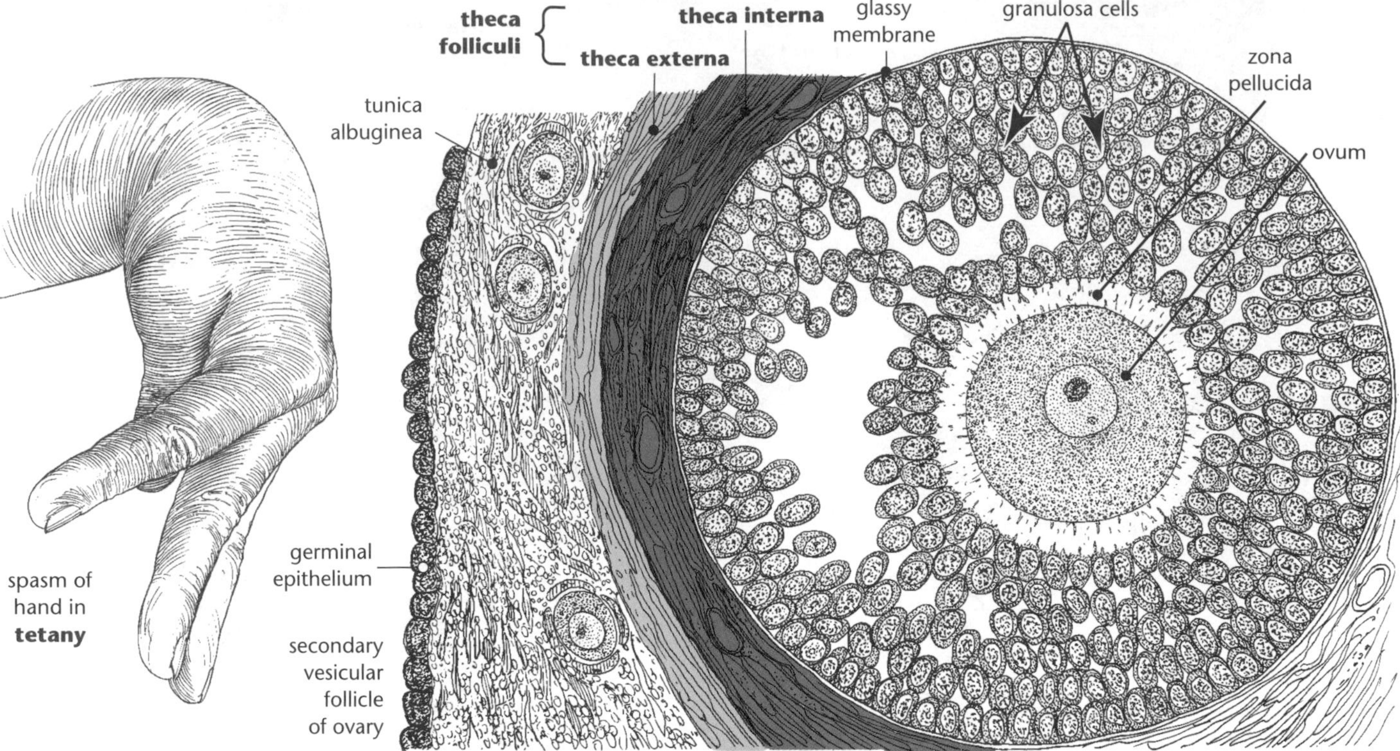

tetanize (tet´ă-nīz) To produce a sustained contraction of a muscle by the application of numerous stimuli in rapid succession.

tetanode (tet´ă-nōd) The quiet period between the muscle spasms in tetanus.

tetanoid (tet´ă-noid) **1.** Resembling tetanus. **2.** Resembling tetany.

tetanolysin (tet-ă-nol´ĭ-sin) A hemolysin produced by the tetanus bacillus (*Clostridium tetani*).

tetanospasmin (tet-ă-no-spaz´min) The neurotoxin produced by *Clostridium tetani*, the causative agent of tetanus; it interferes with neuromuscular transmission by inhibiting the release of acetylcholine from nerve terminals in muscles producing the characteristic symptoms of tetanus; sites of action include the motor end plates in skeletal muscles, spinal cord, brain, and sympathetic nervous system.

tetanotoxin (tet-ă-no-tok´sin) A filtrate of a culture of *Clostridium tetani* (the tetanus bacillus) containing the toxins tetanospasmin and tetanolysin.

tetanus (tet´ă-nus) **1.** Acute infectious disease caused by the toxin of *Clostridium tetani*, which affects the central nervous system; marked by painful muscular contraction, most commonly beginning in the jaws (trismus) and neck muscles; it results from deposition of spores of *Clostridium tetani* in an area of injury, often minor, where the devitalized tissue permits growth; incubation period is from three days to four weeks or longer; in generalized tetanus, mortality rate approximates 50 percent. **2.** Sustained or prolonged contraction of a muscle.

generalized t. Tetanus involving most of the muscles of the body.

local t. A mild form of tetanus that affects only the immediate area of the infected wound; may progress to the generalized form.

t. neonatorum Tetanus affecting newborn infants due to infection of the umbilical stump.

tetany (tet´ă-ne) A disorder marked by intermittent muscle spasms, usually beginning with sharp flexion of the wrists and ankles; may progress to involve other muscles and produce convulsions; occurs as a result of hypocalcemia, alkalosis, or hypokalemia.

hyperventilation t. Tetany caused by reduction of carbon dioxide in the blood, as in prolonged rapid breathing.

latent t. Tetany which is made apparent only by certain stimulating procedures.

neonatal t. A relatively continuous hypertonicity of muscles in newborn infants.

tetartanopsia (tet-ar-tă-nop´se-ă) Loss of vision in homonymous quadrants of the visual fields of both eyes (e.g., the lower nasal quadrant of one eye and lower temporal quadrant of the other eye).

tetracaine hydrochloride (tet´ră-kān hi-dro-klo´rīd) A white crystalline compound used as a local or spinal anesthetic.

tetrachloride (tet-ră-klo´rīd) Compound containing four atoms of chlorine per molecule.

tetracycline (tet-ră-si´klēn) A yellow crystalline compound produced synthetically or from certain species of *Streptomyces*; a broad-spectrum antibiotic.

tetrad (tet´rad) **1.** A set of four related things. **2.** In chemistry, an element that has the combining power of four. **3.** A group of four chromatids (chromosomal elements) that were formed during meiosis.

tetradactyl (tet-ră-dak´til) Having only four fingers or toes.

tetraethylammonium chloride (tet-ră-eth-il-ă-mo´ne-um klo´rīd) Compound of ammonium having a ganglionic blocking action of short duration.

tetrahydrocannabinol (tet-ră-hi-dro-kă-nab´ĭ-nol) (THC) The chief active ingredient in marijuana; it has no accepted medical use.

tetralogy (te-tral´ŏ-je) Any series of four related elements, such as four concurrent defects.

t. of Fallot Cyanotic congenital heart disease; the four abnormalities that constitute the deformity are: pulmonary stenosis (usually infundibular), right ventricular hypertrophy, ventricular septal defect, and overriding of the aorta; thought to be due to a single embryologic error whereby the conus septum is located in an abnormally anterior position.

tetraplegia (tet-ră-ple´jă) See quadriplegia.

tetraploid (tet´ră-ploid) A cell with four haploid sets of chromosomes in its nucleus.

tetravalent (tet´rav´ă-lent) See quadrivalent.

tetrose (tet´rōs) A four-carbon sugar; a monosaccharide containing four carbon atoms (e.g., threose and erythrose).

thalamic (thah-lam´ik) Relating to the thalamus.

thalamic syndrome (thah-lam´ik sin´drōm) Syndrome usually occurring during recovery from a lesion in the thalamus (lateral to the third ventricle of the brain), resulting from an arterial occlusion; characterized by loss of sensation in parts of the body on the opposite side of the lesion, followed by a severe burning pain. Also called Déjerine-Roussy syndrome.

thalamocortical (thal-ă-mo-kor´tĭ-kal) Relating to the thalamus and the cerebral cortex.

thalamolenticular (thal-ă-mo-len-tik´u-lar) Relating to the thalamus and the lentiform nucleus of the brain.

thalamomamillary (thal-ă-mo-mam´ĭ-ler-e) Relating to the thalamus and the mamillary bodies of the brain.

thalamotegmental (thal-ă-mo-teg-men´tal) Relating to the tegmentum of the brainstem and the thalamus.

thalamotomy (thal-ă-mot´ŏ-me) Operative destruction of a portion of the thalamus.

thalamus (thal´ă-mus), *pl.* **thal´ami** An ovoid gray mass about 4 cm in length, located on either side of the third ventricle of the cerebrum, which primarily serves as a relay center for sensory impulses in the cerebral cortex; it is also an important structure for the perception of some types of sensation.

thalassemia (thal-ă-se´me-ă) A group of hereditary disorders characterized by deficient or absent production of one of the polypeptide chains in the hemolytic molecule (in the red blood cell).

α t., alpha t. Disorder characterized by reduced formation of alpha-globin chains in erythrocyte precursor cells in bone marrow, caused by deletion of one or more of the four alpha-globin genes normally present in each cell. The number of deletions determines the severity of the disorder; lack of a single gene produces a silent carrier state, which has little or no effect on the blood and is completely asymptomatic; a lack of all four genes is incompatible with life. The condition caused by lack of three alpha-globin genes was formerly called hemoglobin H disease.

β t., beta t. Disorder characterized by a reduced quantity of hemoglobin in red blood cells (erythrocytes) due to diminished formation of the beta-globin chains in hemoglobin; may be beta° thalassemia, beta⁺ thalassemia, or beta⁺⁺ thalassemia depending on whether the mutant gene directs formation of no beta-globin, a small amount, or a moderate amount of beta-globin, respectively.

β t. major, beta t. major A generally severe form of thalassemia beginning in early childhood, usually the result of inheritance of genes for beta thalassemia from both parents (homozygous state); characterized by severe anemia, bone abnormalities, growth retardation, enlargement of spleen and liver, and jaundice. Death usually occurs before puberty. Also called Cooley's anemia.

β t. minor, beta t. minor Mild thalassemia due to inheritance of an alpha or a beta thalassemia gene from only one parent (thalassemia trait); may produce symptoms resembling those of iron deficiency anemia. Also called β-thalassemia trait.

thalidomide (thă-lid´o-mīd) A sedative and hypnotic drug, $C_{13}H_{10}N_2O_4$; produces fetal deformities of the limbs and other defects when taken by pregnant women.

thallium (thal´e-um) A rare metallic element, symbol Tl, atomic number 81, atomic weight 204.37; the lightest known element with naturally radioactive isotopes; used in scintillation scanning.

thallospore (thal´o-spōr) An organ of reproduction

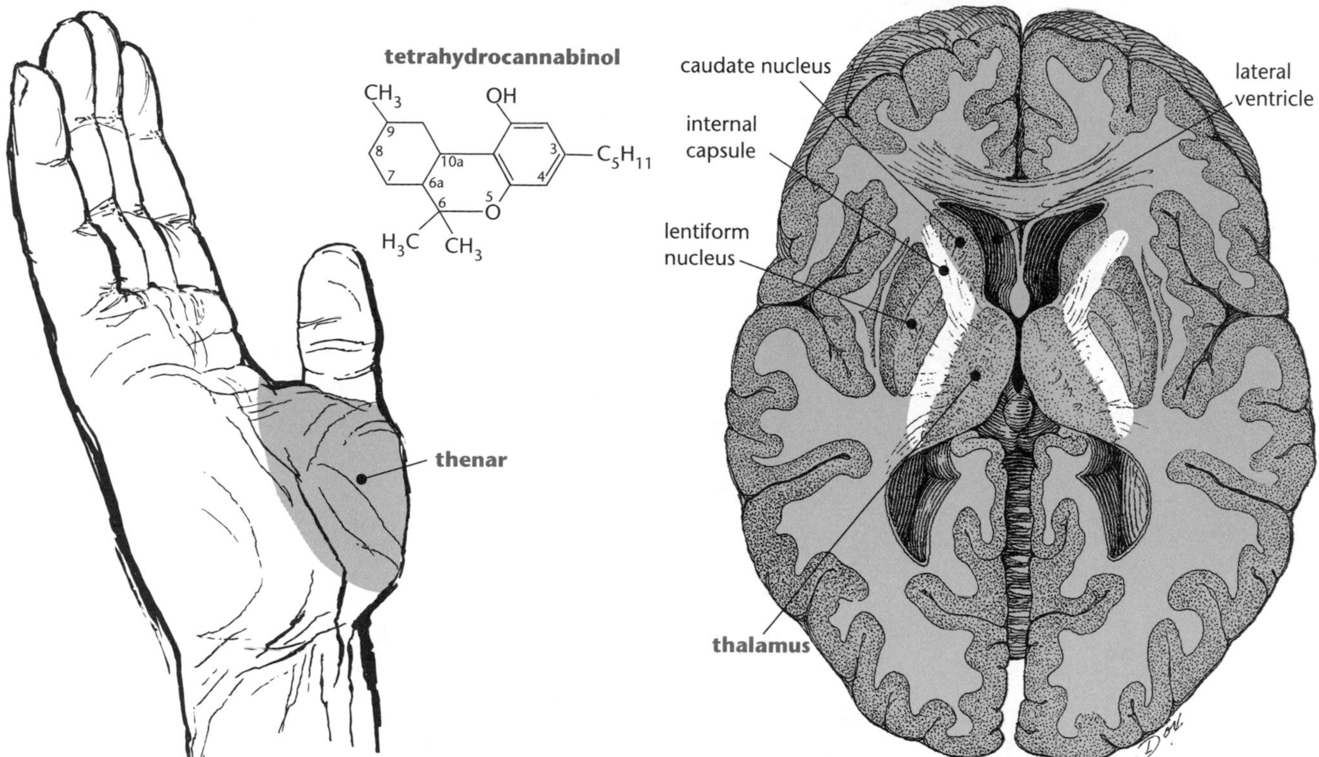

derived directly from the thallus or vegetative portion of certain fungi and algae.

thallotoxicosis (thal-o-tok-sĭ-ko´sis) Poisoning resulting from the intake (accidental or purposeful) of thallium salts (widely used as pesticides); clinical features include ptosis, ataxia, tremors, paresthesias, and a toxic encephalopathy.

thallus (thal´us) The vegetative plant body of certain fungi and algae, which is not differentiated into root, stem, and leaf.

thanatoid (than´ă-toid) **1.** Resembling death. **2.** Deadly.

thanatology (than-ă-tol´ŏ-je) The study of death in all its aspects.

thanatophobia (than-ă-to-fo´be-ă) Extreme fear of death.

thanatopsia, thanatopsy (than-ă-top´se-ă, than´ă-top´se) Autopsy.

theca (the´kă), *pl.* **thecae** A sheath, such as the one covering a tendon or a vesicular ovarian follicle.

t. externa The outer fibrous part of the theca folliculi; it is poorly vascularized.

t. folliculi An envelope of concentrically arranged hypertrophied stromal cells surrounding the vesicular ovarian follicle.

t. interna The inner secretory part of the theca folliculi; it is permeated by a rich capillary network.

thecitis (the-si´tis) Inflammation of a tendon sheath.

thecoma (the-ko´mă) A firm, yellow-to-orange benign tumor of the ovary; composed of theca cells with varying degrees of lipid content; found most commonly in the fifth to seventh decade of life; it has estrogenic activity. Also called theca cell tumor; theca lutein cell tumor.

thelarche (the-lar´ke) The beginning of breast development at puberty.

theleplasty (the´le-plas-te) See mamillaplasty.

thelerethism (thĕ-ler´ĕ-thizm) Erection of the nipple.

thelitis (the-li´tis) Inflammation of the nipple.

thelorrhagia (the-lo-ra´jă) Hemorrhage or bleeding from the nipple.

thenar (the´nar) The fleshy mass of the palm at the base of the thumb.

theophylline (the-of´ĭ-lin) Drug used to treat bronchial asthma.

theorem (the´o-rem) A proven proposition.

theory (the´o-re) A hypothetical concept given credibility by working experimentation but lacking absolute proof.

clonal selection t. Theory according to which certain predestined antibody-producing cells, when exposed to the host's own tissues during fetal life, were deleted or destroyed; thus there would be no "antiself" clones or colonies of cells to react against one's own tissues.

germ layer t. The concept that the embryo develops three primary germ layers (ectoderm, mesoderm, and endoderm) and that each layer gives rise to specific tissues and organs.

gestalt t. Theory claiming that mental phenomena are total configurations and cannot be analyzed into their component parts.

lamarckian t. The theory that acquired characteristics may be transmitted.

Planck's t. See quantum theory.

quantum t. Theory proposing that atoms emit and absorb energy discontinuously, in finite discrete amounts (quanta) in individual acts of emission and absorption, rather than in a continuous fashion. Also called Planck's theory.

reentry t. In cardiology, the concept that premature ectopic heartbeats arise because of reentry of the same impulse that initiated the preceding beat.

van't Hoff's t. The theory that substances in dilute solutions obey the gas laws.

Young-Helmholtz t. The theory that the perception of colors depends on three sets of receptors in the retina: for red, green, and violet.

therapeutic (ther-ă-pu´tik) **1.** Curative. **2.** Relating to the treatment of disease.

therapeutics (ther-ă-pu´tiks) The aspect of medicine concerned with the treatment of disease.

therapist (ther´ă-pist) A person trained to conduct of a specific therapy.

respiratory t. A graduate of an approved respiratory therapy program or registered by the National Board for Respiratory Care to provide respiratory care under the supervision of a physician.

rehabilitation t. A member of the health-care team (i.e., physical, occupational, and recreational therapists) engaged in restoring the injured, the disabled, and the physically or mentally sick to their rightful place in society.

therapy (ther´ă-pe) The treatment of disease or disability.

adjuvant t. Treatment used in addition to the primary therapy (e.g., radiation therapy in addition to surgery).

anticoagulant t. The use of drugs that prevent or arrest formation of blood clots in the cardiovascular system.

antisense t. Introduction of a noncoding (antisense) strand of DNA to inhibit translation of a specific gene product.

behavior modification t. See behavior modification, under modification.

chelation t. Treatment for heavy metal poisoning by administration of agents that sequester the metal from organs or tissues and bind it firmly within the chemical structure of a new compound that can be eliminated from the body.

cognitive t. Psychotherapeutic treatment that aims to alter a patient's distorted thinking process; based on the belief that the way a person perceives the world determines his feelings and behavior.

electroconvulsive t. (ECT) Treatment of certain psychiatric illnesses, especially severe depression, in which convulsive seizures are induced by passing an electric current through two electrodes placed on the patient's head. Also called electroshock therapy; shock therapy; shock treatment; electroshock treatment; electroconvulsive treatment.

electroshock t. (EST) See electroconvulsive therapy.

extracorporeal shock-wave t. See extracorporeal shock wave lithotripsy, under lithotripsy.

fever t. Treatment of disease by intermittent raising of body temperature. Also called pyretotherapy; pyrotherapy.

gene t. Introduction of a functional gene into an organism to replace or supplement the activity of a defective gene. Recipient cells may be zygote or early embryo cells (germline gene therapy), or somatic cells (somatic cell gene therapy).

gestalt t. Psychotherapeutic treatment that aims to develop a person's full potential through a growth process involving the whole person as he experiences and interacts with the environment.

hyperbaric oxygen t. The use of oxygen in a compression chamber at a prevailing pressure greater than one atmosphere.

inhalation t. Administration of gases, steam, or vaporized medications through inhalation.

interpersonal t. (IPT) Psychotherapeutic treatment that focuses on interpersonal behavior rather than intrapsychic phenomena, aiming to change the way the patient thinks, feels, and acts in current problematic relationships.

occupational t. (O.T.) (a) An adjunctive method of treatment for the sick or injured through purposeful and healthy activity. (b) The field of allied health concerned with that form of adjunct therapy.

oxygen t. Treatment with oxygen inhalation.

palliative t. A treatment that may relieve symptoms but does not cure the disease.

parenteral t. Administration of medications through routes other than the alimentary canal (e.g., intramuscular or intravenous).

photodynamic t. Treatment of cancer by intravenous injection of a photosensitizing substance, such as hematoporphyrin (which concentrates on tumor cells and renders them hypersensitive to light), followed by exposure to red laser light if the tumor is superficial, or a fiberoptic probe if it is a deep one.

T

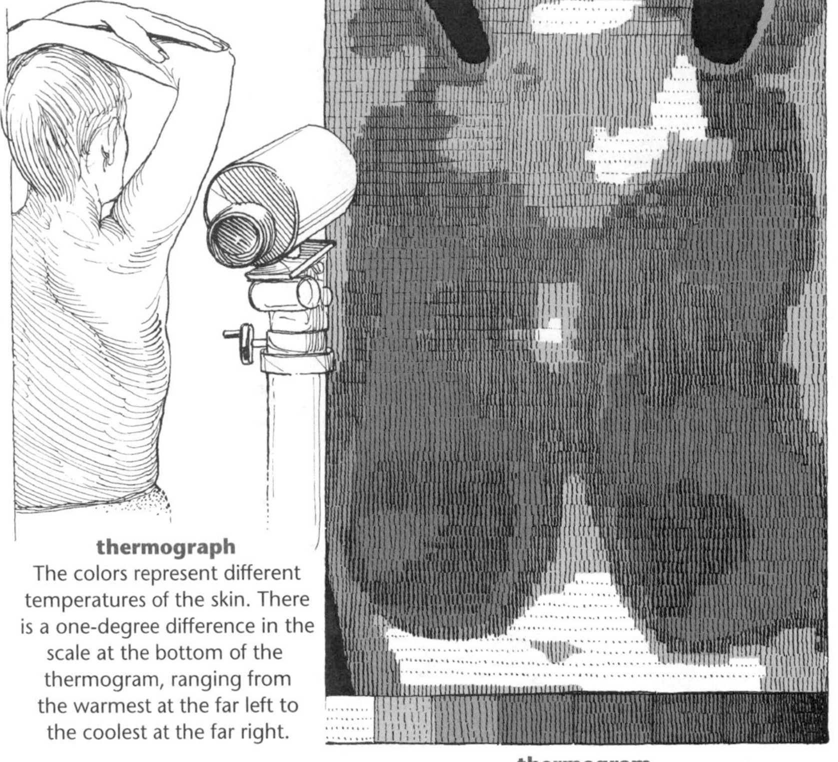

thermograph
The colors represent different temperatures of the skin. There is a one-degree difference in the scale at the bottom of the thermogram, ranging from the warmest at the far left to the coolest at the far right.

thermogram

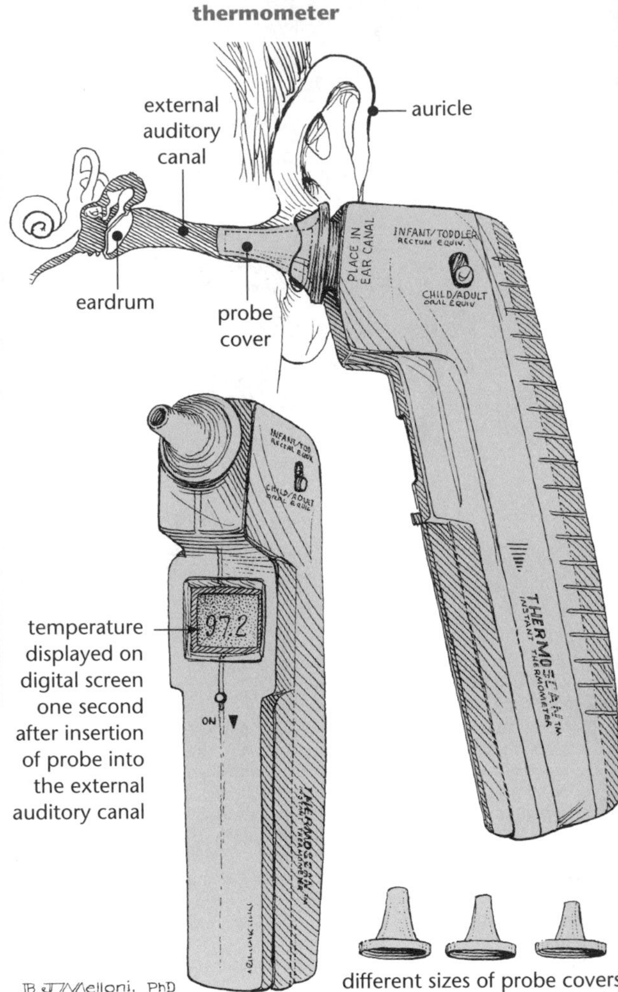

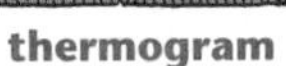

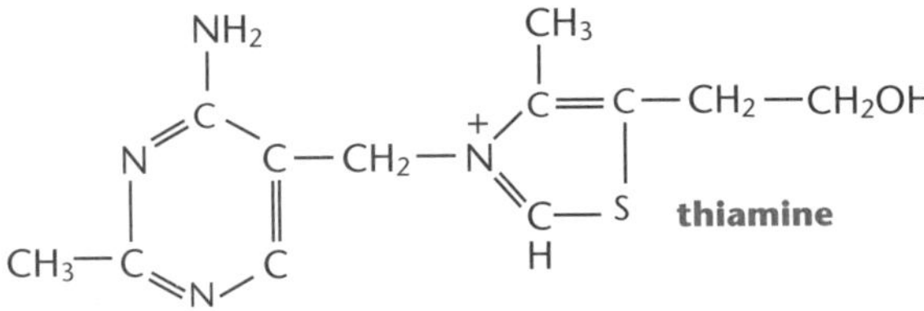

thiamine

electronic **thermometer**

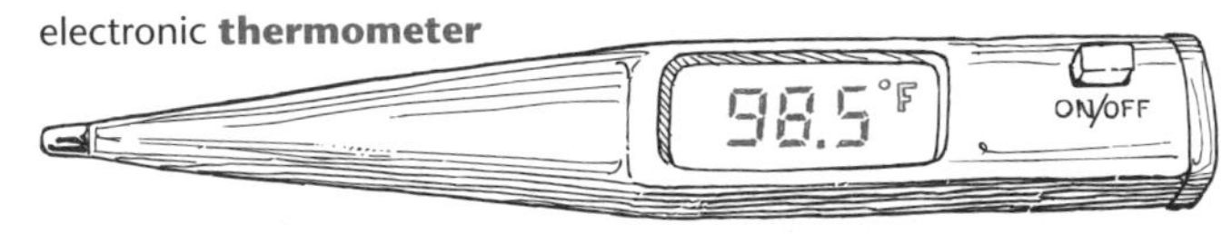

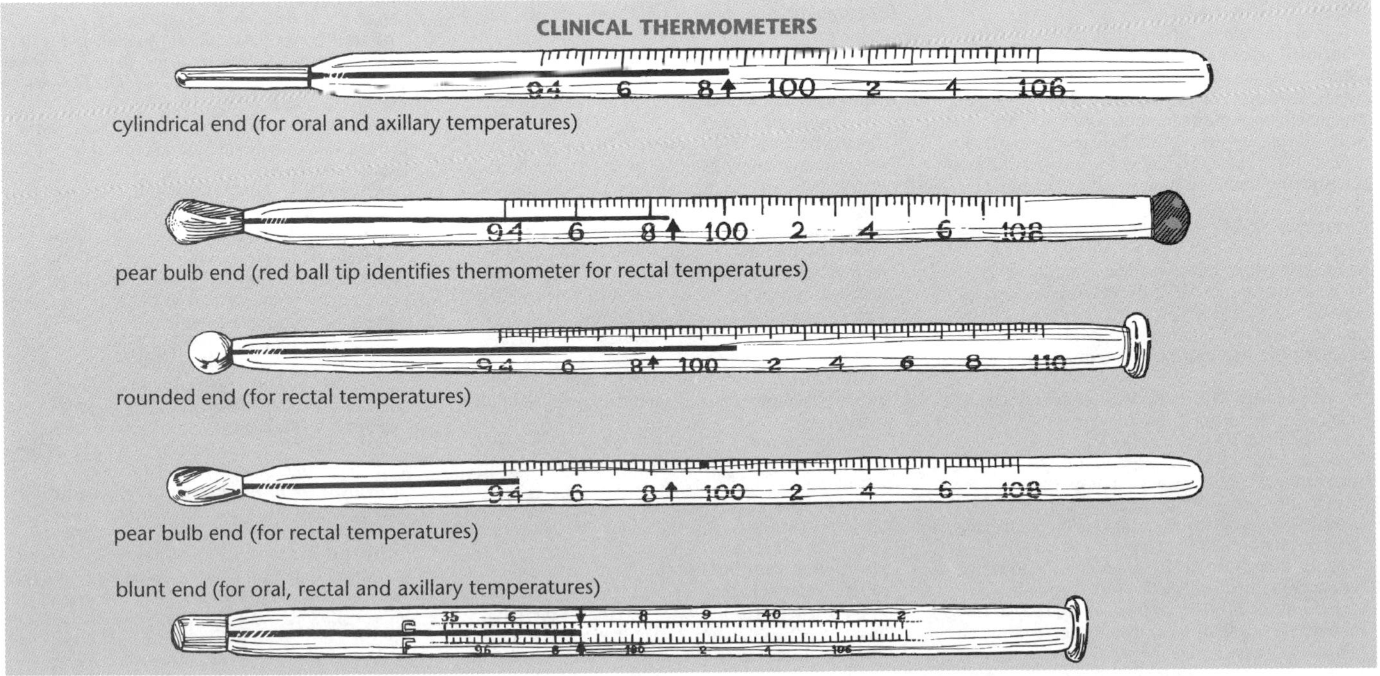

cylindrical end (for oral and axillary temperatures)

pear bulb end (red ball tip identifies thermometer for rectal temperatures)

rounded end (for rectal temperatures)

pear bulb end (for rectal temperatures)

blunt end (for oral, rectal and axillary temperatures)

T

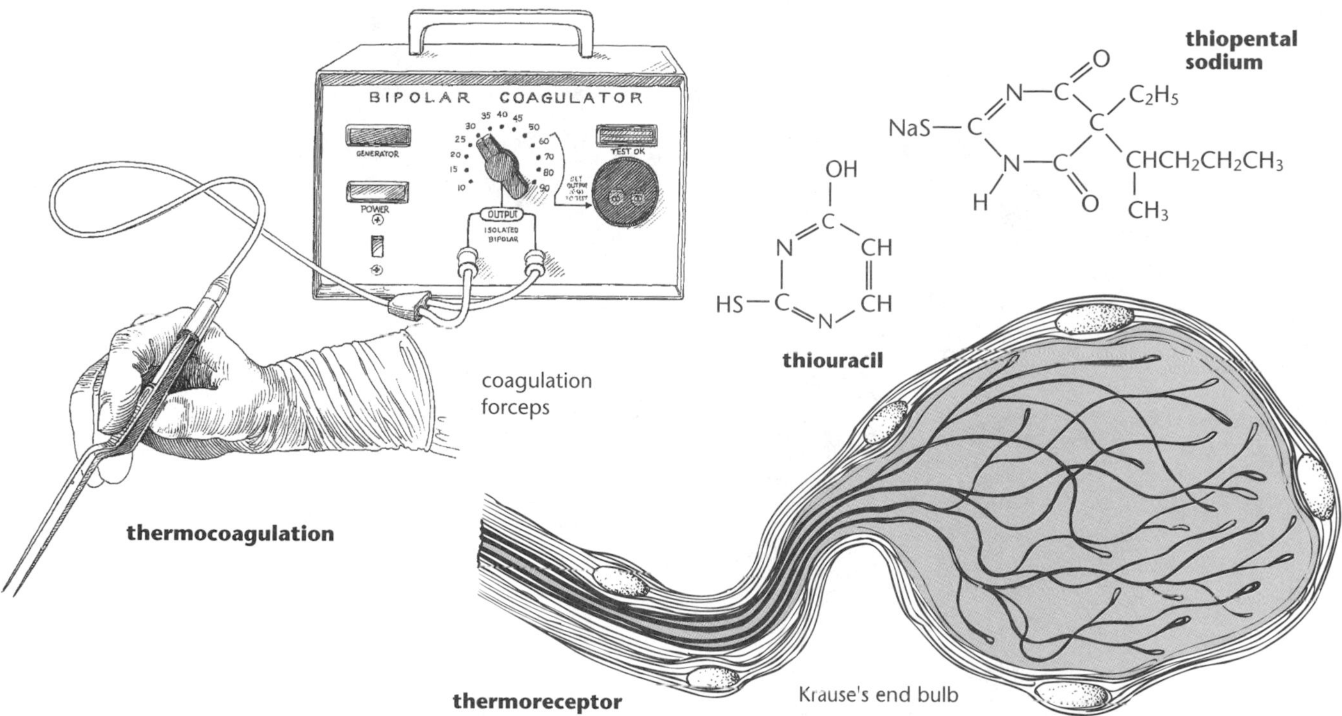

Also called photoradiation; photochemotherapy.

physical t. (PT) The use of physical agents (heat, massage, electricity, and exercise) to restore body functions. Also called physiotherapy.

play t. A method of psychotherapy for treating emotional disorders of children in which the child's play with toys, pictures, drawings, etc. is used as a communication medium between child and therapist.

psychoanalytical t. See psychoanalysis.

psychodynamic t. Psychotherapeutic treatment that focuses on intrapsychic conflict, aiming to help the patient gain insight into both conscious and unconscious factors affecting thoughts, feelings, and behavior.

radiation t. Treatment of disease with high-energy rays or subatomic particles, such as x rays, alpha and beta particles, gamma rays; radioactive materials include cobalt, radium, cesium, and iridium. Also called radiotherapy.

replacement t. Administration of natural body products, or synthetic substitutes to compensate for a deficiency.

sclerosing t. See sclerotherapy.

shock t. See electroconvulsive therapy.

speech t. The application of special techniques to correct speech disabilities.

therm (therm) General term for any of the following units of heat quantity: a small calorie; a large calorie; 1,000 large calories; 100,000 British thermal units.

thermal (ther′mal) Relating to heat.

thermalgesia (ther-mal-je′zhă) Extreme sensitivity to heat.

thermanalgesia (therm-an-al-je′zhă) See thermoanesthesia.

thermatology (ther-mă-tol′ŏ-je) The study of heat as applied to the treatment of disease.

thermelometer (ther-mel-om′ĕ-ter) An electric thermometer.

thermoanesthesia (ther-mo-an-es-the′zhă) Inability to distinguish between heat and cold or to feel variations in temperature. Also called thermanalgesia.

thermocautery (ther-mo-kaw′ter-e) The destruction of tissue (cauterization) with a heated wire.

thermochemistry (ther-mo-kem′is-tre) The branch of chemistry concerned with the relationship of heat and chemical reactions.

thermochrose (ther′mo-krōs) The property of heat rays which enables them to be reflected, refracted, and absorbed.

thermocoagulation (ther-mo-ko-ag-u-la′shun) Coagulation effected by the application of heat.

thermocouple (ther′mo-kup-l) Device for measuring slight temperature changes formed by the junction of two dissimilar metal conductors. Also called thermojunction.

thermodiffusion (ther-mo-dĭ-fu′zhun) Diffusion of a gas or a liquid through heat; the rise in temperature increases the molecular motion.

thermodilution (ther-mo-di-lu′shun) Change in temperature of a gas or a liquid occurring when it is added to a colder or warmer one; the volume of the latter can be calculated from the degree of change in its temperature. The principle is employed to measure the volume or the rate of flow through a chamber (e.g., ventricular volume, cardiac output, or renal blood flow).

thermodynamics (ther-mo-di-nam′iks) The branch of physics concerned with heat and its conversion to other forms of energy.

thermoesthesia (ther-mo-es-the′zhă) The ability to perceive changes in temperature.

thermogenesis (ther-mo-jen′ĕ-sis) The production of heat in the body; a physiologic process.

thermogram (ther′mo-gram) A colored photograph displaying the surface temperatures of the body; produced by infrared sensing devices.

thermograph (ther′mo-graf) Device used to make thermograms.

thermography (ther-mog′ră-fe) A process for measuring temperature by photographically recording infrared radiations emanating from the body surface; it can aid in diagnosing underlying pathology by indicating thermal variations.

thermohyperesthesia (ther-mo-hi-per-es-the′zhă) Extreme sensitivity to variations in temperature.

thermohypesthesia (ther-mo-hi-pes-the′zhă) Diminished sensitivity to temperature fluctuations. Also called thermohypoesthesia.

thermohypoesthesia (ther-mo-hi-po-es-the′zhă) See thermohypesthesia.

thermoinhibitory (ther-mo-in-hib′ĭ-tor-e) Preventing or arresting the production of heat.

thermolabile (ther-mo-la′bīl) Susceptible to alteration or destruction by heat.

thermolysis (ther-mol′ĭ-sis) **1.** The loss of body heat. **2.** The chemical decomposition of compounds by heat.

thermomassage (ther-mo-mă-sahzh′) The use of heat and massage in physical therapy.

thermometer (ther-mom′ĕ-ter) Instrument to measure temperature.

clinical t. A small scaled glass tube containing mercury, used to measure the maximum temperature in the mouth, axilla, or rectum.

digital t. A version of the clinical thermometer, equipped with a temperature-sensitive, electronic probe connected to a digital readout display.

surface t. A disposable skin thermometer consisting of a disk that contains heat-sensitive chemicals, which change color at specific temperatures; generally considered less accurate than the clinical or digital thermometers.

Thermoscan® instant t. A battery-operated device placed in the ear canal to measure body temperature in one second; it contains a temperature-sensitive probe, a mode switch to convert ear temperatures to familiar frame references (i.e., infant/toddler, child/adult), and a digital readout display.

thermometry (ther-mom′ĕ-tre) Measurement of temperature by direct contact.

thermophile (ther′mo-fīl) An organism that grows best at warm temperatures, usually from 40° to 70°C.

thermophore (ther′mo-fōr) An appliance for applying heat to the body.

thermoplacentography (ther-mo-plas-en-tog′ră-fe) Determination of the placental location by recording the increased temperature (due to large amounts of blood) with the thermograph.

thermoplastic (ther-mo-plas′tik) A type of material that can be made soft by heating and which rehardens upon cooling (without chemical change).

thermoplegia (ther-mo-ple′jă) Rarely used term for sunstroke.

thermoreceptor (ther-mo-re-sep′tor) A special nerve-ending (receptor) that is sensitive to change in temperature.

thermoregulation (ther-mo-reg-u-la′shun) The regulation of heat. Also called temperature control.

thermoset (ther′mo-set) A material that becomes rigid or hardened by a chemical reaction involving heat.

thermostabile, thermostable (ther-mo-sta′bĭl, ther-mo-sta′bl) Not changed or destroyed by moderate heat.

thermotaxis (ther-mo-tak′sis) **1.** Movement of an organism toward (positive thermotaxis) or away from (negative thermotaxis) a heat source. **2.** The adjustment of the body to temperature changes.

thermotherapy (ther-mo-ther′ă-pe) The use of heat as an aid in the treatment of disease.

thesaurosis (the-saw-ro′sis) Abnormal or excessive storage in the body, or in particular organs, of phosphatides, fats, heavy metals, or other material.

thesis (the′sis) An essay containing results of original research written by a candidate for an academic degree.

theta (thĕ′tă) **1.** The eighth letter of the Greek alphabet θ,Θ; used to denote the eighth in a series. **2.** In chemistry, the position on the eighth atom from the carboxyl or other functional group.

thiaminase (thi-am′ĭ-nās) A thiamine-splitting enzyme.

thiamine, thiamin (thi′ă-min) A vitamin of the B-complex, present in yeast, meat, and the bran coat of

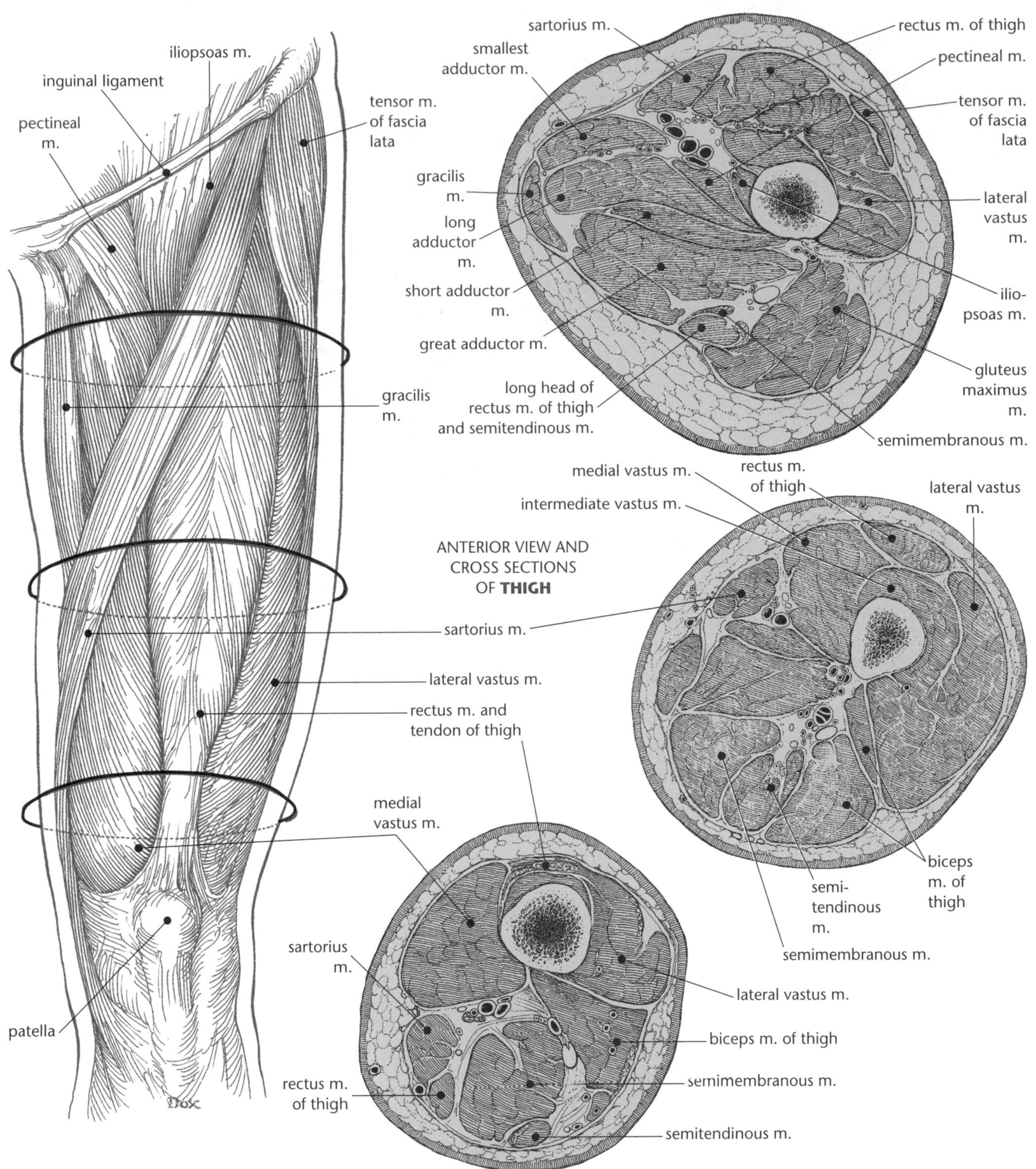

T

grains; essential in carbohydrate metabolism; lack of thiamine causes beriberi. Also called vitamin B_1.

t. pyrophosphate The diphosphoric ester of thiamine; a coenzyme that is a cofactor in decarboxylation. Also called cocarboxylase.

thiazides (thī´ă-zīds) A shortened term for the class of diuretics called benzothiadiazides; widely used in treating both edema and hypertension.

thickness (thik´nes) The dimension between two surfaces of an object.

Breslow's t. See Breslow classification, under classification.

thigh (thī) The portion of the upper leg between the knee and the hip.

driver's t. Inflammation of the sciatic nerve due to prolonged pressure on the nerve, as from the continued use of the accelerator pedal in long distance driving of an automobile.

thighbone (thī´bōn) The femur; see table of bones.

thigmesthesia (thig-mes-the´zhă) Sensitiveness to touch.

thigmotaxis (thig-mo-tak´sis) The response of animal or plant protoplasm to contact with a solid body.

thioguanine (thi-o-gwa´nĕn) An antineoplastic agent used in the treatment of some types of leukemia.

thiol (thi´ol) **1.** The univalent radical –SH. **2.** Any substance containing the radical –SH bound to carbon.

thionic (thi-on´ik) Relating to sulfur.

thionin (thi´o-nin) A greenish-black powder giving a violet color in solution; often used to stain the Nissl substance of nerve cells. Also called Lauth's violet.

thiopental sodium (thi-o-pen´tal sod´de-um) A rapid-acting, potent barbiturate capable of inducing anesthesia within 30 to 60 seconds after being administered intravenously or rectally. Also called sodium pentothal; Pentothal Sodium®.

thiosemicarbazone (thi-o-sem-e-kar´bă-zōn) One of several compounds containing the radical -N-NH-C(S)-NH_2, having an inhibitory effect on tuberculous infections.

thiosulfate (thi-o-sul´fāt) A salt of thiosulfuric acid.

thiosulfuric acid (thi-o-sul-fūr´ik as´id) A highly unstable acid, $H_2S_2O_3$, which decomposes readily to sulfur and sulfurous acid.

thiotepa (thi-o-tep´ă) A white crystalline compound $C_6H_{12}N_3PS$; an alkylating agent used as a palliative medication in malignant diseases.

thiouracil (thi-o-u´ră-sil) A compound that inhibits the formation of thyroid hormones.

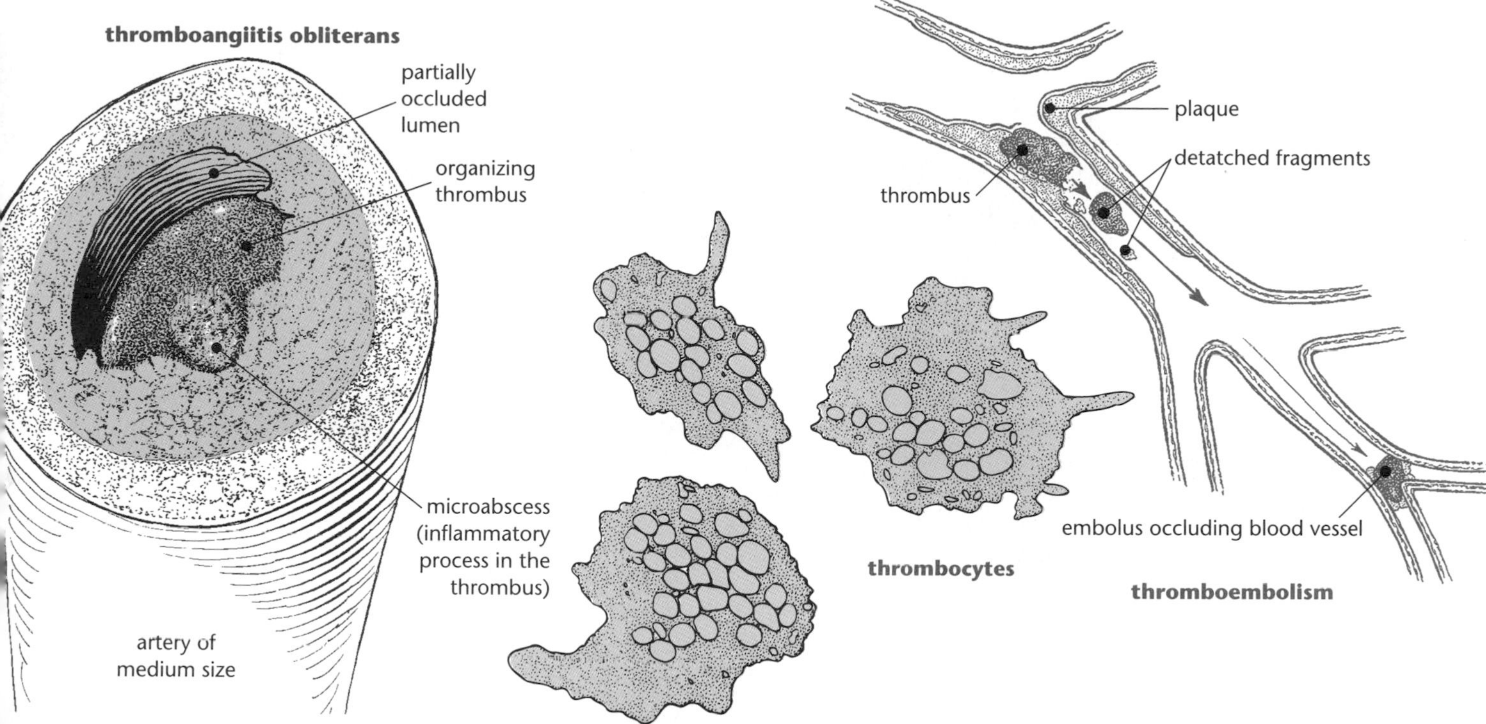

thiourea (thi-o-u′re-ă) An antithyroid substance of the thiocarbamide group.

thirst (thurst) A desire to drink, often associated with an uncomfortable sensation of dryness in the mouth and pharynx.

excessive t. See polydipsia.

Thoma's counting chamber (to′mahz kownt′ing chām′ber) See Thoma-Zeiss hemocytometer, under hemocytometer.

Thomsen's disease (tom′senz dĭ-zēz′) See myotonia congenica, under myotonia.

thoracectomy (tho-ră-sek′tŏ-me) Removal of part of a rib.

thoracentesis (tho-ră-sen-te′sis) The removal of fluid from the chest cavity by puncture. Also called thoracocentesis.

thoracic (tho-ras′ik) Relating to the thorax or chest.

thoracicoabdominal, thoracoabdominal (tho-ras-ĭ-ko-ab-dom′ĭ-nal, thor-ă-ko-ab-dom′ĭ-nal) Relating to the thorax and the abdomen.

thoracicoacromial (tho-ras-ĭ-ko-ă-kro′me-al) See acromiothoracic.

thoracic outlet syndrome (tho-ras′ik out′let sin′drōm) Abnormal sensations of fingers (numbness, burning, etc.) attributed to compression of the brachial plexus; similar symptoms also may be caused by cervical disk or carpal tunnel syndromes.

thoracoabdominal (tho-ră-ko-ab-dom′ĭ-nal) See thoracicoabdominal.

thoracocentesis (tho-ră-ko-sen-te′sis) See thoracentesis.

thoracolumbar (tho-ră-ko-lum′bar) Relating to the thoracic and lumbar regions of the spine.

thoracomyodynia (tho-ră-ko-mi-o-din′e-ă) Pain in the muscles of the chest.

thoracopathy (tho-ră-kop′ă-the) Any disease of the chest.

thoracoplasty (tho-ră-ko-plas′te) Plastic surgery or repair of defects of the chest.

thoracopneumoplasty (tho-ră-ko-noo′mo-plas-te) Reparative surgery of the lung and chest.

thoracoscopy (tho-ră-kos′ko-pe) Visual examination of the pleural cavity by means of an endoscope.

thoracostomy (tho-ră-kos′tŏ-me) The surgical creation of an opening into the chest wall.

thoracotomy (tho-ră-kot′ŏ-me) Surgical incision on the chest wall.

thorax (tho′raks) The upper part of the body between the neck and the diaphragm; it contains the chief organs of the circulatory and respiratory systems. Also called chest.

thorium (tho′re-um) A radioactive metallic element; symbol Th, atomic number 90, atomic weight 232.038.

threadworm (thred′werm) See pinworm.

threonine (thre′o-nin) (Thr) An amino acid present in most proteins; essential to the diet of man and other mammals.

threose (thre′ōs) A monosaccharide containing four carbon atoms; $C_4H_8O_4$; one of the two aldoses, the other being erythrose.

threshold (thres′hōld) The point where a stimulus just begins to produce a sensation the intensity below which a mental or physical stimulus cannot be perceived.

absolute t. The stimulus of least strength which will cause a response. Also called stimulus test.

auditory t. The intensity of the lowest perceptible sound.

t. of consciousness The lowest gradient of sensation that can be perceived.

galvanic t. See rheobase.

radiologic t. The level of radiation dose below which there may not be permanent injury to the body.

renal t. The level at which the kidney can no longer reabsorb a substance (e.g., sugar, ketones) and some of it appears in the urine.

stimulus t. See absolute threshold.

thrill (thril) A tremor or vibration associated with a vascular or cardiac murmur and discerned by palpation.

throat (thrōt) **1.** The back part of the mouth extending to the beginning of the esophagus; generally the area from the nasopharynx to the larynx. **2.** The front of the neck.

sore t. A throat condition characterized by discomfort, especially when swallowing, due to inflammation of the fauces, pharynx, tonsils, or larynx.

strep t. See streptococcal pharyngitis, under pharyngitis.

throb (throb) **1.** To pulsate. **2.** A pulsation.

throe (thro) A severe pang or seizure of pain, as experienced during childbirth.

thrombasthenia (throm-bas-the′ne-ă) Abnormality of the blood platelets in which they lack factors that are effective in blood coagulation. Also called Glanzmann's disease.

thrombectomy (throm-bek′tŏ-me) Surgical removal of a thrombus (blood clot).

thrombelastograph (throm-bel-as′tŏ-graf) Device for recording elastic variations of a thrombus during the process of coagulation.

thrombi (throm′bi) Plural of thrombus.

thrombin (throm′bin) An enzyme in the blood derived from factor II (prothrombin) that converts fibrinogen into fibrin, thus producing a blood clot.

thrombinogen (throm-bin′o-jen) Factor II (prothrombin).

thromboangiitis (throm-bo-an je-i′tis) Inflammation of the wall of a blood vessel with clot formation.

t. obliterans Disorder of the medium-sized arteries and veins, especially of the lower extremities; marked by inflammation of the wall of the vessel and surrounding connective tissue, resulting in tissue ischemia and gangrene. Also called Buerger's disease.

thrombocytasthenia (throm-bo-sĭ-tas-the′ne-ă) A disorder of platelet function characterized by abnormal adhesion and/or aggregation; congenital varieties are known, and acquired forms are seen, especially in uremia.

thrombocyte (throm′bo-sīt) A blood platelet.

thrombocythemia (throm-bo-si-the′me-ă) See thrombocytosis.

thrombocytopathy (throm-bo-si-top′ă-the) General term denoting any disorder involving faulty function of blood platelets. Also called thrombopathy.

thrombocytopenia (throm-bo-si-to-pe′ne-ă) Abnormally small number of platelets in the blood (less than 150,000 cells per microliter). Also called thrombopenia.

thrombocytosis (throm-bo-si-to′sis) Abnormally elevated number of platelets in the blood (above 600,000 cells per microliter). Also called thrombocythemia.

thromboembolectomy (throm-bo-em-bo-lek′tŏ-me) The removal of an embolism that obstructs the flow of blood through a vessel.

thromboembolism (throm-bo-em′bo-liz-m) Embolism (obstruction) in a blood vessel caused by a dislodged thrombus (clot).

thromboendarterectomy (throm-bo-end-ar-ter-ek′tŏ-me) The surgical removal of an obstructing blood clot together with the inner lining of the obstructed artery.

thrombogenic (throm-bo-jen′ik) Producing thrombosis or coagulation of the blood.

thrombolysis (throm-bol′ĭ-sis) The dissolving of blood clots within blood vessels.

thrombomodulin (throm-bo-mod′u-lin) Glycoprotein in the plasma membrane of endothelial cells that binds thrombin (enzyme that promotes blood clotting).

thrombopathy (throm-bo-path′e) See thrombocytopathy.

thrombopenia (throm-bo-pe′ne-ă) See thrombocytopenia.

thrombophlebitis (throm-bo-flĕ-bi′tis) Inflammation of the walls of a vein associated with formation of a thrombus (blood clot), causing tenderness and swelling along the involved vessel.

deep t. Thrombophlebitis of a deep vein,

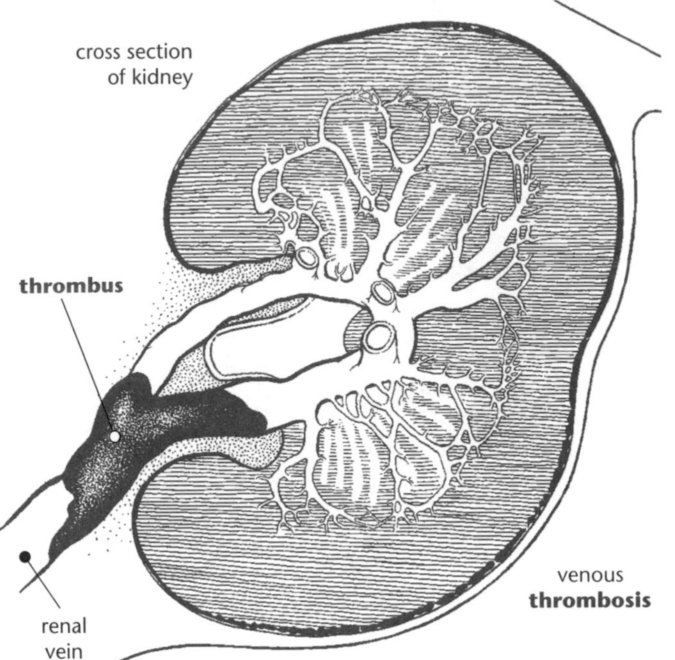

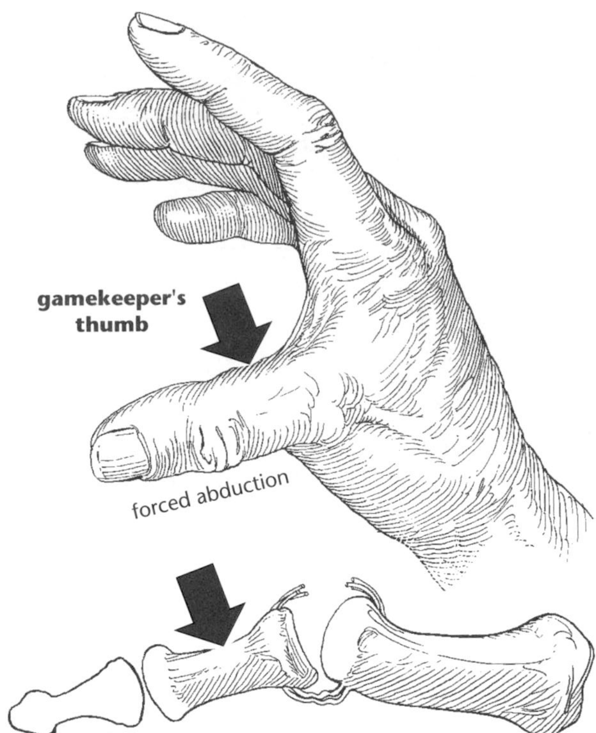

especially of the calf and thigh.

migratory t. Inflammation appearing first in one site, then another; associated with cancer, especially of internal organs. Also called Trousseau's syndrome.

puerperal t. Thrombophlebitis of a deep vein of the iliofemoral area occurring during late pregnancy and after delivery, caused by compression of the vein by the pregnant uterus and the hypercoagulability of pregnancy; marked by extreme swelling of the leg with severe pain, elevated temperature, and usually arterial spasm, which causes the leg to become pale and cold. Also called milk leg; painful white leg; phlegmasia alba dolens.

septic pelvic t. Thrombophlebitis of a pelvic vein caused by bacterial infection (usually by *Staphylococcus aureus*).

superficial p. The most common form of thrombophlebitis associated with pregnancy, usually involving a varicose superficial vein, particularly the long saphenous vein and its tributaries; marked by a painful, palpable, cordlike induration of the affected vein and redness of the overlying skin, usually without significant swelling of the limb as a whole.

thromboplastin (throm-bo-plas´tin) A protein complex that initiates the clotting of blood. Also called factor III.

plasma t. A complete thromboplastin capable of converting factor II (prothrombin) to thrombin directly.

tissue t. An incomplete thromboplastin requiring the presence of factor V, factor VII, and factor X to convert prothrombin to thrombin.

T

thrombopoiesis (throm-bo-poi-e´sis) **1.** The formation of a blood clot. **2.** The formation of blood platelets.

thrombosis (throm-bo´sis) The formation or presence of a blood clot.

cerebral t. Obstruction of a blood vessel of the brain by a thrombus; one of the causes of stroke.

coronary t. The presence of a blood clot in an artery that supplies the heart muscle; a cause of heart attack.

deep venous t. (DVT) Clotting of blood inside deep-seated veins, especially of the legs, often causing pain and tenderness in the thigh or calf; seen most commonly in people immobilized for long periods and those with chronic debilitating diseases, cancer, or after surgery. The condition is a common source of embolism, especially pulmonary embolism.

thrombospondin (throm-bo-spon´din) (TSP) A glycoprotein released from activated platelets and present in other types of cells involved in inflammation.

thromboxane (throm-bok´sān) A compound isolated from blood platelets (thrombocytes); it contains an oxane ring and is related to the prostaglandins; thromboxane exists in two forms, A_2 and B_2; the A_2 form appears to be much more potent than prostaglandin in some important biologic activities, such as smooth muscle contraction and platelet aggregation.

thrombus (throm´bus) A blood clot, usually one located at the point of its formation, in a blood vessel or a chamber of the heart.

thrush (thrush) Infection of the mouth with *Candida albicans*; marked by the appearance of white patches in the oral mucosa, which later become shallow ulcers; seen most commonly in infants or in patients receiving antibiotics or immunosuppressive drugs.

thulium (thoo´le-um) A metallic element of the lanthanide series, symbol Tm, atomic number 69, atomic weight 168.94.

thumb (thum) The first digit on the radial side of the hand, apposable to each of the other four digits.

gamekeeper's t. A subluxation of the metacarpophalangeal joint of the thumb.

tennis t. Tendonitis accompanied by calcification in the tendon of the long flexor muscle of the thumb due to activities in which the thumb is subject to great pressure and strain, as in tennis playing.

thumbprinting (thum´print-ing) A sign of submucosal edema of the bowel wall; the colon appears in the x-ray image as having a series of smooth depressions; seen in such disorders as Crohn's disease and ischemia.

thumb sign (thum´ sīn) When making a fist over the thumb, the thumb extends clearly beyond the ulnar margin of the hand, as seen in individuals with the Marfan syndrome.

thymectomy (thi-mek´tŏ-me) Surgical removal of the thymus.

thymic (thi´mik) Relating to the thymus.

thymic hypoplasia syndrome (thi´mik hi-po-pla´zhă sin´drōm) See DiGeorge syndrome.

thymidine (thi´mĭ-dēn) (dThd, dT) A condensation product of thymine with deoxyribose; a nucleoside in DNA.

thymidylic acid (thi-mĭ-dil´ik as´id) A constituent of DNA.

thymine (thi´min) (Thy) A component of DNA.

thymitis (thi-mi´tis) Inflammation of the thymus.

thymocyte (thi´mo-sīt) A lymphocyte that originates in the thymus.

thymogenic (thi-mo-jen´ik) **1.** Originating in the thymus. **2.** Of hysterical origin.

thymokinetic (thi-mo-ki-net´ik) Stimulating the thymus.

thymoma (thi-mo´mă) A tumor of the anterior mediastinum arising from the thymus; associated with a variety of diseases, including myasthenia gravis, agammaglobulinemia, and hematologic abnormalities; it may undergo malignant change.

thymopathy (thi-mop´ă-the) **1.** Any disease of the thymus. **2.** Any mental disorder.

thymosin (thi´mo-sin) An immunologically active thymic fraction of low molecular weight; believed to develop immunologic competency in T lymphocytes (thymus-dependent lymphocytes).

thymus (thi´mus) **1.** A ductless glandlike lymphoid structure located just behind the top of the sternum; it appears to be the master organ in immunogenesis in the young and is believed by some to monitor the total lymphoid system throughout life; it consists of two lobes surrounded by a thin capsule of connective tissue; it grows quickly until the age of 3 years, after which it grows very slowly until the age of about 13, at which time it begins to decrease in size; in old age, very little thymic tissue remains, having been replaced by fat and connective tissue. **2.** One of the organs of cattle called sweetbread.

thyroaplasia (thi-ro-ă-pla´zhă) Congenital defects associated with faulty thyroid functioning.

thyroarytenoid (thi-ro-ar-ĭ-te´noid) Relating to both the thyroid and arytenoid cartilages.

thyrocalcitonin (thi-ro-kal-sĭ-to´nin) See calcitonin.

thyrocricotomy (thi-ro-kri-kot´ŏ-me) Tracheostomy performed in extreme emergency conditions whereby the neck opening is made through the most superficial portion of the respiratory tract, the cricothyroid membrane. See also tracheostomy.

thyroglobulin (thi-ro-glob´u-lin) A protein produced and stored in the thyroid gland; a prohormone (precursor of hormone), which on hydrolysis yields iodinated tyrosines and thyroxin.

thyroglossal (thi-ro-glos´al) Relating to the thyroid cartilage and the tongue.

thyrohyoid (thi-ro-hi´oid) Relating to the thyroid cartilage and the hyoid bone.

thyroid (thi´roid) **1.** Pertaining to the thyroid gland; see under gland. **2.** Resembling a shield. **3.** A pharmaceutical preparation derived from the thyroid gland of certain domestic animals; used in the treatment of hypothyroid states.

thyroidectomy (thi-roi-dek´tŏ-me) Removal of the thyroid gland.

thyroiditis (thi-roi-di´tis) Inflammation of the thyroid gland.

de Quervain's t. See subacute granulomatous thyroiditis.

granulomatous t. See subacute granulomatous thyroiditis.

Hashimoto's t. Autoimmune inflammatory disorder responsible for most cases of primary

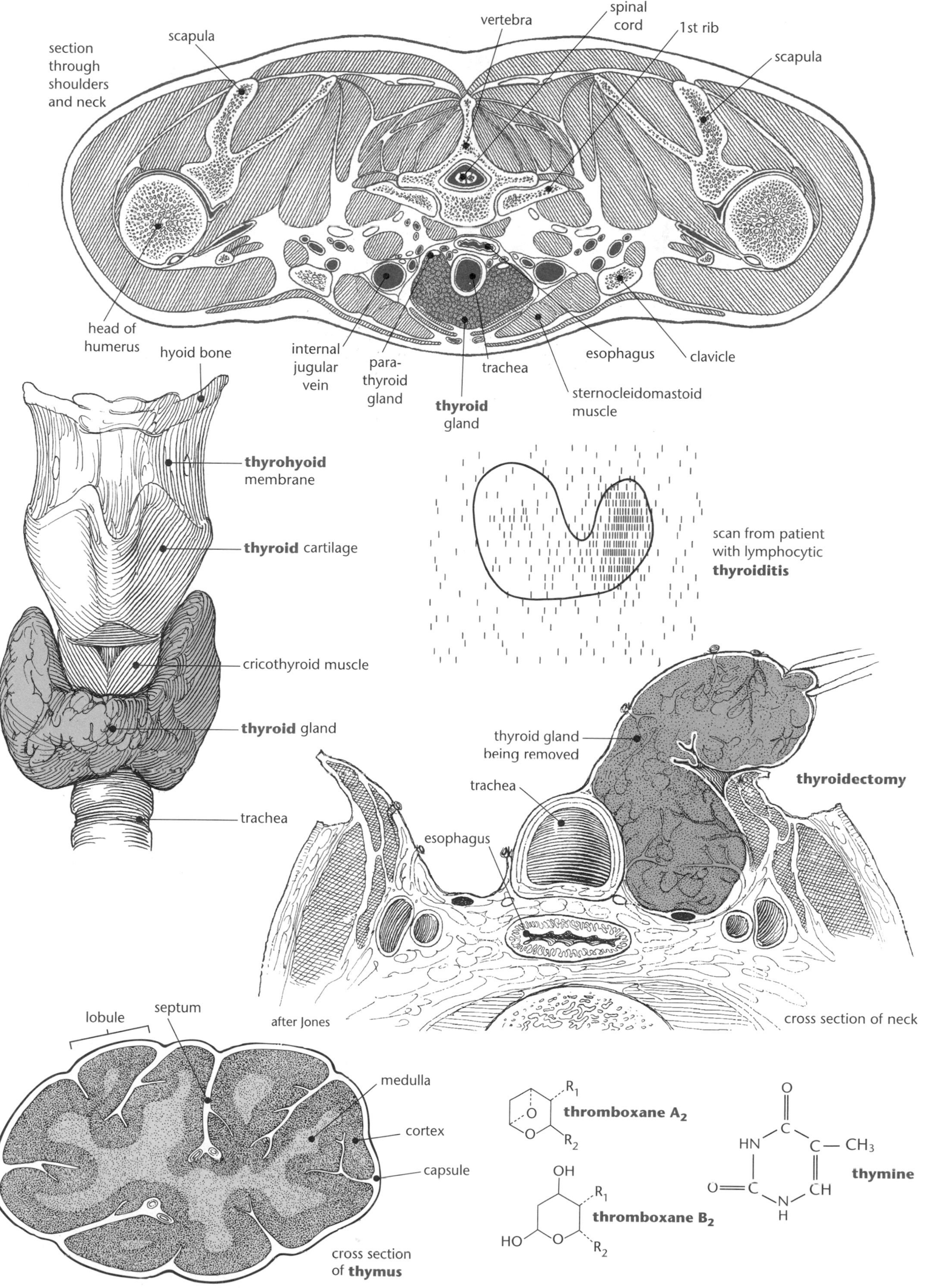
section through shoulders and neck
scapula
vertebra
spinal cord
1st rib
scapula
head of humerus
hyoid bone
internal jugular vein
para-thyroid gland
thyroid gland
trachea
esophagus
clavicle
sternocleidomastoid muscle
thyrohyoid membrane
thyroid cartilage
cricothyroid muscle
thyroid gland
trachea
scan from patient with lymphocytic thyroiditis
thyroid gland being removed
trachea
thyroidectomy
esophagus
after Jones
cross section of neck
lobule
septum
medulla
cortex
capsule
cross section of thymus
R1
O
O
R2
thromboxane A2
OH
R1
HO
O
R2
thromboxane B2
O
HN
C
C
CH3
O
C
N
H
CH
thymine

T

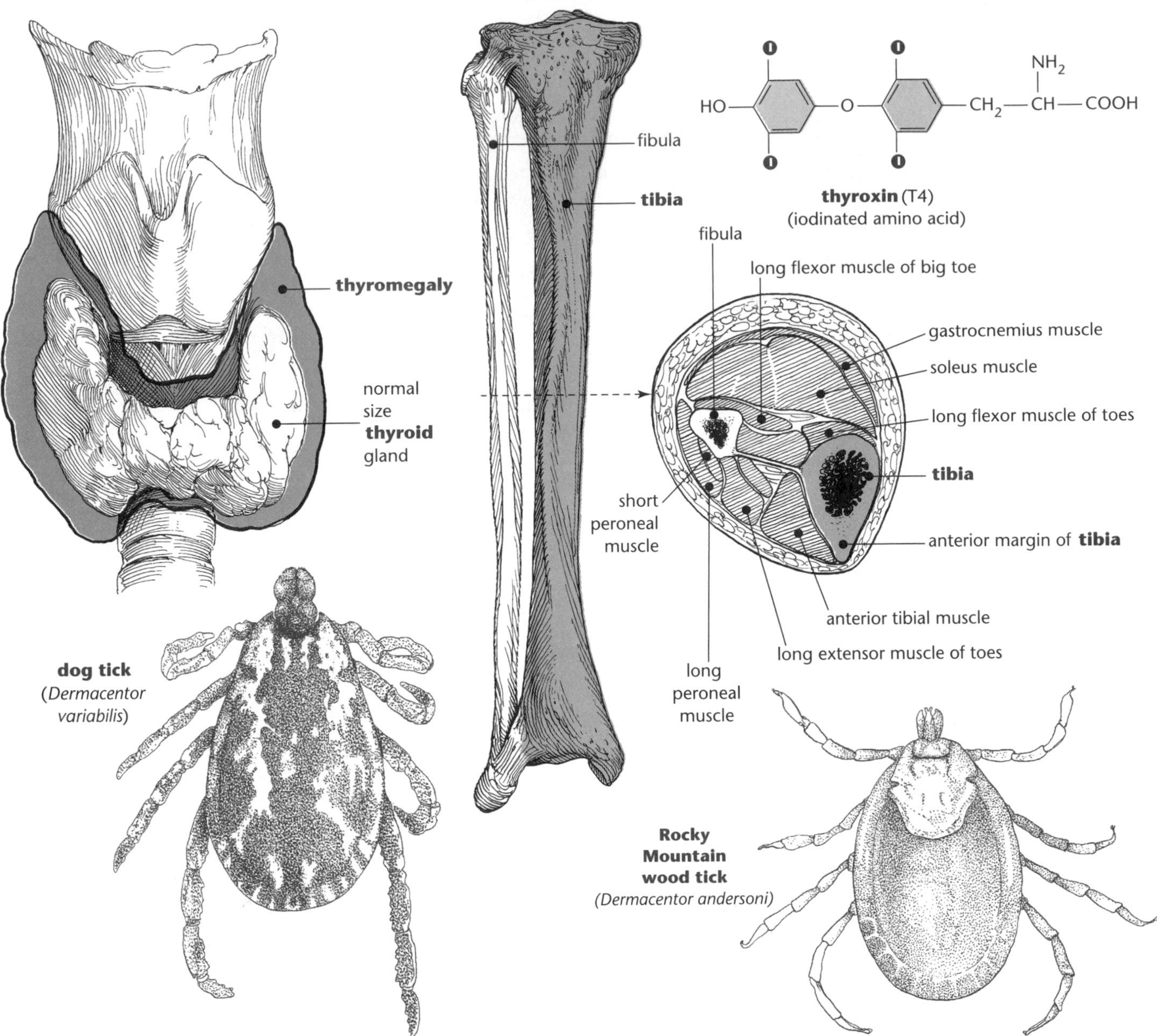

hypothyroidism; characterized by progressive, painless enlargement of the thyroid gland, which becomes firm and rubbery and then slowly diminishes in size, eventually becoming atrophic and fibrous; seen most commonly in women between 30 and 50 years old. Also called Hashimoto's disease; Hashimoto's struma; struma lymphomatosa.

Riedel's t. Uncommon condition in which the thyroid gland and adjacent structures are replaced by dense fibrotic tissue. Also called Riedel's struma.

subacute granulomatous t. Inflammation of the thyroid gland following viral infection, usually of the upper respiratory tract. Also called de Quervain's thyroiditis; granulomatous thyroiditis.

thyroid storm (thī′roid storm) See thyrotoxic crisis, under crisis.

thyromegaly (thi-ro-meg′ă-le) Abnormal enlargement of the thyroid gland.

thyronine (thi′ro-nēn) An amino acid present in proteins only as iodinated derivatives (iodothyronines).

thyroparathyroidectomy (thi-ro-par-ă-thi-roidek′tŏ-me) Surgical removal of the thyroid and parathyroid glands.

thyropathy (thi-rop′ă-the) Disease of the thyroid gland.

thyroprival (thi-ro-pri′val) Caused by removal of the thyroid gland or the arrest of its function.

thyroprotein (thi-ro-pro′tēn) **1.** See thyroglobulin. **2.** Preparation made by iodinating protein (such as casein), having a physiologic action similar to that of thyroxin.

thyrotomy (thi-rot′ŏ-me) **1.** Surgical division or cutting of the thyroid cartilage. **2.** Operative cutting of the thyroid gland.

thyrotoxicosis (thi-ro-tok-sĭ-ko′sis) Toxic condition caused by an excess of thyroid hormone.

thyrotropic, thyrotrophic (thi-ro-trop′ik, thi-ro-trof′ik) Stimulating the thyroid gland.

thyrotropin (thi-ro-tro′pin) Hormone of the anterior hypophysis (pituitary) that stimulates the growth and function of the thyroid gland. Also called thyrotrophic hormone; thyrotropic hormone; thyroid-stimulating hormone.

thyroxine, thyroxin (thi-rok′sin) (T_4) An active iodine-containing hormone, produced normally in the thyroid gland, that aids in regulating metabolism; produced synthetically or extracted from the thyroid gland in crystalline form for treatment of thyroid disorders such as hypothyroidism, cretinism, and myxedema.

tibia (tib′e-ă) The larger and medial of the two bones of the leg between the knee and the ankle. Commonly called shinbone. See table of bones.

tibiofibular (tib-e-o-fib′u-lar) Relating to both the tibia and fibula.

tic (tik) An involuntary, brief, and recurrent twitching of a group of muscles, most commonly involving the face, neck, and shoulders.

t. douloureux See trigeminal neuralgia, under neuralgia.

tick (tik) A mite of the families Ixodidae (hard shell ticks) and Argasidae (soft shell ticks), some of which are parasitic and the carriers of disease-causing microorganisms.

deer t. Either of two species of hard shell ticks, *Ixodes dammini* or *Ixodes pacificus*, that transmit Lyme disease.

dog t., American dog t. *Dermacentor variabilis*, a hard shell tick that can transmit Rocky Mountain spotted fever; found on the East Coast of the United States; usually in mountainous, heavily wooded, or sagebrush areas.

Rocky Mountain wood t. *Dermacentor andersoni*, a hard shell, reddish-brown tick of the Western United States; most important vector of Rocky Mountain spotted fever; also conveys tularemia, Colorado tick fever, and Q fever, and is a cause of tick paralysis.

tickle (tik′l) **1.** To feel a tingling or restless sensation. **2.** To excite the surface nerves by repeated light stimulation of the skin.

tide (tīd) An alternate rise and fall; a lapse of time.

alkaline t. Alkalinity of the urine following ingestion of food; a consequence of secretion of gastric juice. Also called alkaline wave.

Tietze's syndrome (tēt′sez sin′drōm) Pain and swelling of the junction of ribs with cartilage; the pain may mimic that of coronary artery disease.

timbre (tim′ber, tam′br) The characteristic quality of a sound whereby one may distinguish between two sounds of equal pitch and loudness.

time (tīm) A degree or measure of duration.

activated clotting t. (ACT) Measurement of whole blood clotting time; used in operative procedures that require extracorporeal blood circu-

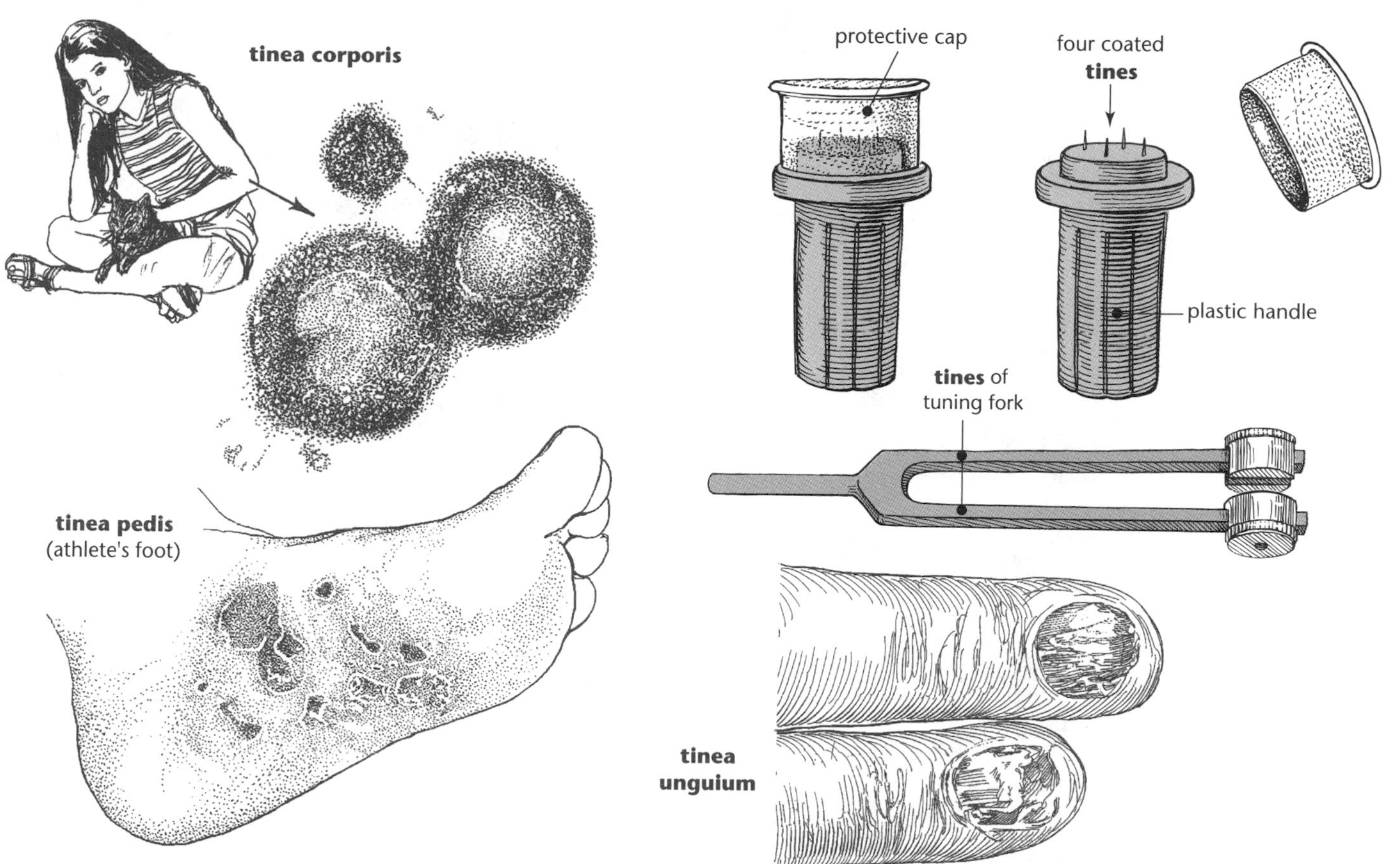

lation (e.g., cardiopulmonary bypass, hemodialysis, ultrafiltration). Also called automated coagulation time.

activated partial thromboplastin t. (aPTT) Time required for a fibrin clot to form after addition of calcium and phospholipid emulsion to a plasma sample; an activator (e.g., kaolin) is added to shorten clotting time. Used in preoperative screening for bleeding tendencies.

automated coagulation t. See activated clotting time.

bleeding t. The duration of bleeding (normally from 1 to 3 minutes) from a small puncture made on the skin.

circulation t. Time required for blood to flow once through a given circuit of the circulatory system.

clot retraction t. Time required for a blood clot to become firm and separated from the sides of the tube containing it; about 50 percent retraction is considered normal.

clotting t. Coagulation time.

coagulation t. Time required for blood to clot in a test tube.

doubling t. In microbiology, the time needed for a population of cells to double in number. Also called generation time.

generation t. See doubling time.

partial thromboplastin t. (PTT) See activated partial thromboplastin time.

prothrombin t. Time required for a clot to form when calcium and a preparation of thromboplastin (e.g., brain tissue) are added to plasma.

reaction t. Time elapsed between application of a stimulus and an observable response.

recognition t. Time elapsed between the application of a stimulus and the recognition of its nature.

survival t. (a) The duration of life after such events as onset of illness, therapeutic intervention, or an experimental procedure. (b) The life span of cells.

tin (tin) A malleable, silvery metallic element; symbol Sn (stannum), atontic number 50, atomic weight 118.69; a member of the subgroup containing carbon, silicon, germanium, and lead.

tinctorial (tink-to´re-al) Relating to staining.

tinctura (tink-tu´ră) Latin for tincture.

tincture (tink´chūr) (tr.) An alcohol or hydroalcohol solution of nonvolatile animal or vegetable drugs or chemical substances, prepared usually by a percolation or maceration process; the strength is usually 1 to 2 parts by weight of the dry drug to 10 parts by volume of the tincture (i.e., 1 to 2 g per 10 ml).

alcoholic t. One made with undiluted alcohol.

belladonna t. An anticholinergic, antispasmodic, alcoholic preparation containing between 27 and 33 mg of alkaloids of belladonna leaf to 100 ml of tincture.

iodine t. A simple 2% solution of iodine with 2.5% sodium iodide in water and 44 to 50% alcohol; used as an anti-infective on the skin (iodine solution is generally preferred to the tincture).

opium t. A tincture containing 10 mg of morphine per ml; used for the symptomatic treatment of diarrhea.

opium t, camphorated See paregoric.

tine (tīn) **1.** One of a set of slender prongs on a tuning fork. **2.** An instrument used for introducing an antigen, such as tuberculin, into the skin.

tinea (tin´e-ă) A superficial infectious condition of the skin caused by fungi belonging chiefly to the genera *Trichophyton*, *Microsporum*, and *Epidermophyton*; the fungi live on the dead horny layer of the skin and produce an enzyme that enables them to digest keratin, thus disintegrating hair, nails, and the keratinized cells of the skin. Also called ringworm.

t. barbae Tinea of the beard area; the lesions are dark red and dotted with perifollicular abscesses; it is prevalent in the United States, particularly in cattle-raising regions, where the usual causative organisms are *Trichophyton mentagrophytes* and *Trichophyton verrucosum*. Also called barber's itch; folliculitis barbae; tinea sycosis.

t. capitis Infection of the scalp and hair caused by species of *Microsporum* and *Trichophyton*, producing patches of round balding areas; likely sources of infection are hair clippers, theater seats, and domestic animals. Also called tinea of scalp; ringworm of scalp.

t. corporis A highly contagious form most commonly seen in children; caused by many species of *Microsporum* and *Trichophyton* and transmitted through contact with kittens, puppies, and other children; the typical lesion is round or oval, with a scaly center that usually tends to heal; the periphery of the lesion is an advancing circle of vesicles and papules. Also called tinea of smooth skin; ringworm of smooth skin.

t. cruris Tinea involving the groin, perineum, and perianal region; most frequently caused by *Epidermophyton floccosum*. Also called jock itch; tinea of groin; eczema marginatum.

t. of groin See tinea cruris.

t. pedis A common infection of the feet; the acute form, caused by *Trichophyton mentagrophytes*, is characterized by blisters on the soles and sides of the foot and/or between the toes; the chronic form is caused by *Trichophyton rubrum* and the lesions are dry and scaly. Also called athlete's foot; ringworm of foot.

t. of scalp See tenia capitis.

t. of smooth skin See tines corporis.

t. sycosis See tinea barbae.

t. unguium Infection of the nails, especially the toenails, usually caused by *Trichophyton mentagrophytes*, *Trichophyton ruhrum*, and *Epidermophyton floccosum*. Also called onychomycosis.

t. versicolor A mild, superficial infection of the skin, usually of the trunk, appearing as tan, irregularly shaped, scaly patches; caused by *Malassezia furfur*.

tinfoil (tin´foil) An extremely thin, pliable sheet of tin; a base metal foil used in dentistry as a separating material, as between a cast and denture-base material during flasking and curing procedures.

t. substitute An alginate solution that serves as a separating medium.

tingle (ting´gl) To have a peculiar pricking or stinging sensation, as from an emotional shock or striking a nerve, such as the "funny bone" sensation.

tinkle (tink´kl) A metallic sound sometimes heard on auscultation over large pulmonary cavities (e.g., pneumothorax), or over a distended loop of bowel as in an ileus.

tinnitus (tĭ-ni´tus) Noises in the ear, such as ringing, buzzing, roaring, etc.

tintometer (tin-tom´ĕ-ter) An apparatus containing a standard color scale for determining by comparison the relative proportion of coloring matter in a fluid, such as blood.

TIPS Acronym for transjugular intrahepatic portosystemic shunts; a procedure for lessening portal hypertension in chronic liver disease.

tissue (tish´oo) A mass of similar cells and the substances that surround them.

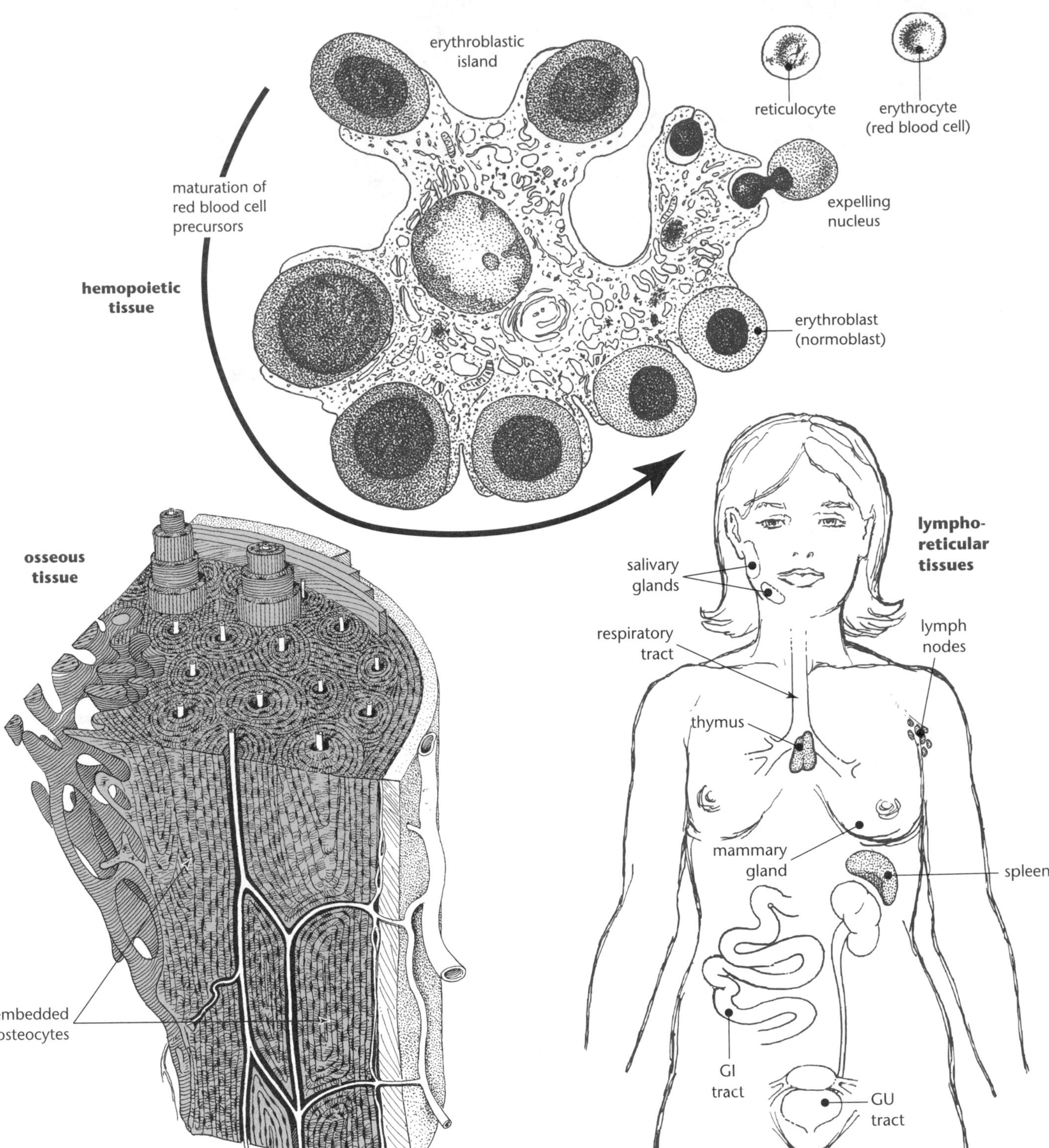

T

adipose t. Connective tissue composed of fat cells clumped together and surrounded by reticular fibers.
alveolar t. A loose, interlacing connective tissue with sparse collagenous, elastic, and reticular fibers in a protein polysaccharide ground substance; its extensibility permits adjacent structures some mobility.
areolar t. A type of connective tissue composed of loosely woven collagenous bundles and elastic fibers with comparatively wide interspaces that are filled with a mucopolysaccharide ground substance.
bone t. See osseous tissue.
cancellous t. A honeycomb arrangement of bone cells as seen in the center of some bones such as the clavicle, vertebrae, the end of long bones, etc.
cartilaginous t. Connective tissue with a solid, elastic matrix which may or may not have fibers embedded in it.
chondrogenic t. A connective tissue forming the inner layer of perichondrium, concerned with the formation of cartilagenous tissue.
chromaffin t. One composed mainly of chromaffin cells and a large supply of blood vessels and nerves; found in the adrenal medulla and the paraganglia.
connective t. (CT) A general term denoting any of the tissues that support and connect the various parts of the body except the nervous system. Also called interstitial tissue.
elastic t. Connective tissue composed chiefly of yellow elastic fibers; found in some ligaments and the walls of arteries and air passages.
epithelial t. See epithelium.
erectile t. Tissue containing an abundance of vascular spaces which, when distended with blood, render the part firm.
fibrous t. Connective tissue containing bundles of white fibers and a fluid ground substance; found in tendons, ligaments, aponeuroses, and such membranes as the dura mater.
granulation t. Tissue that appears in the early stages of wound healing; composed of different cell types and young blood vessels.
gut-associated lymphoid t. (GALT) Lymphoid tissue lining the gastrointestinal tract; configuration ranges from pinhead-sized solitary nodules, as in the jejunum, to large aggregates of ellipsoid nodules (Peyer's patches) confined to the ileum.
hemopoietic t. Tissue that is actively involved with the development of formed elements of the blood, as in the medulla of long bones.
interstitial t. See connective tissue.
lymphatic t. See lymphoid tissue.
lymphoid t. A network of fibers enclosing masses of lymphocytes. Also called lymphatic tissue.
lymphoreticular t. Tissue that carries out the functions of immunity through a variety of cell types,

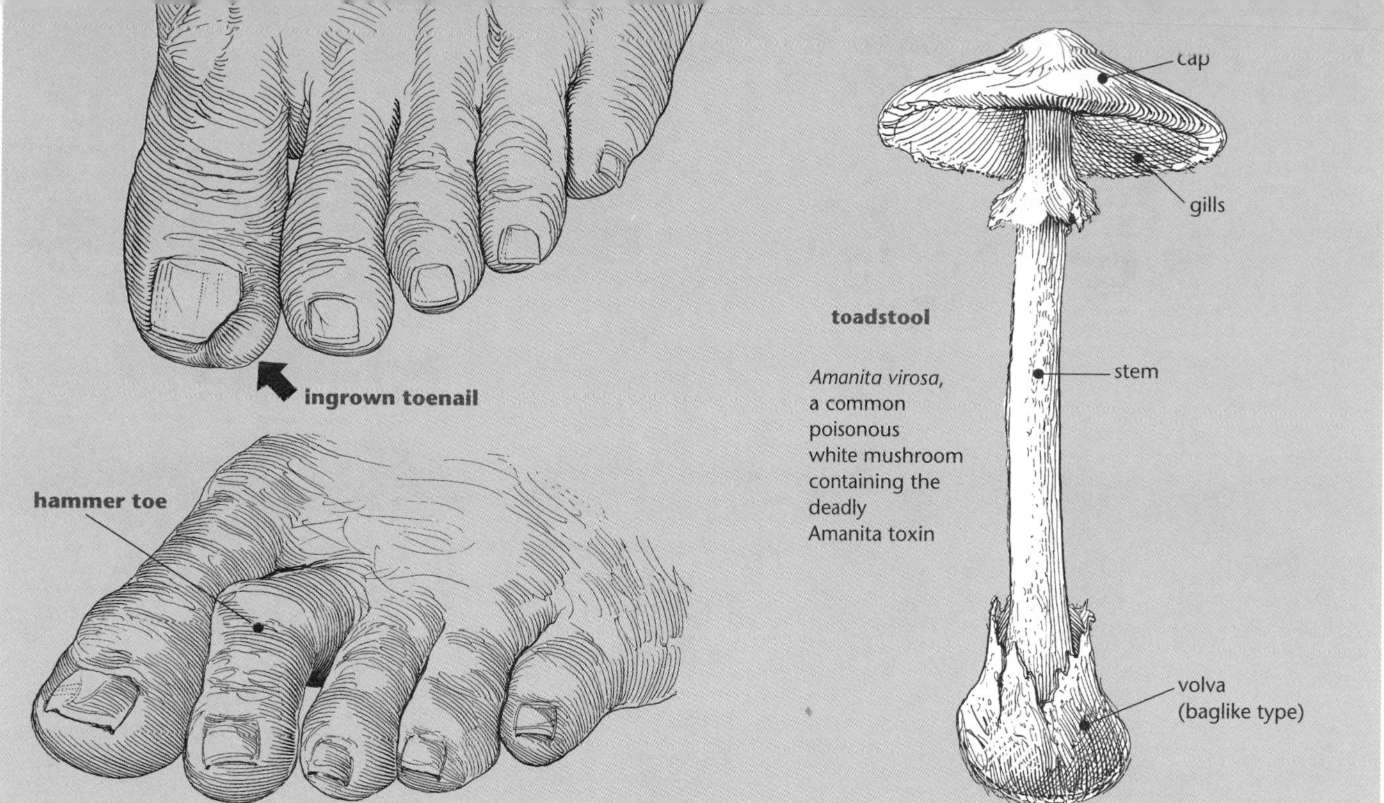

Amanita virosa, a common poisonous white mushroom containing the deadly Amanita toxin

each performing a specific function, either by direct cell action or through the elaboration of antibody.

mesenchymal t. See mesenchyme.

metanephrogenic t. Portion of the intermediate mesoderm that eventually forms the excretory tubules of the kidney.

mucoid t. A loose form of connective tissue in which the matrix is jellylike due to the presence of mucopolysaccharides, as seen in the umbilical cord (Wharton's jelly). Also called mucous tissue.

mucous t. See mucoid tissue.

muscular t. Tissue composed of threadlike fibers, either striated (skeletal) or nonstriated (smooth), which contract upon stimulation.

myeloid t. The red bone marrow that forms both red and white blood cells, consisting of the developmental and adult stages of erythrocytes, granulocytes, and megakaryocytes in a stroma of reticular cells and fibers.

nervous t. Tissue composed basically of nerve cells (neurons) supported by connective tissue (neuroglia).

osseous t. Connective tissue with a tough, rigid, fibrous matrix containing deposits of mineral salts. Also called bone tissue.

osteogenic t. A connective tissue forming the inner layer of periosteum, concerned with the formation of osseous tissue.

osteoid t. Bone matrix prior to calcification; uncalcified osseous tissue.

reticular t. The most delicate type of connective tissue, composed of a network of fine fibrils; it surrounds individual cells, the acini of glands, and muscle fibers.

t. at risk Tissue surrounding a cancerous lesion which, although healthy, is removed along with the cancer as a precautionary measure.

subcutaneous t. The loose, generally fatty tissue immediately beneath the skin, attached to the dermis by coarse fibers (retinacula cutis).

target t. In immunology, the tissue against which antibodies are formed.

titanium (ti-ta´ne-um) A low-density, amorphous metallic element of the carbon group, symbol Ti, atomic number 22, atomic weight 47.90.

t. dioxide An exceptionally opaque white powder, TiO_2, used in creams and powders as a protectant against external irritations and solar rays.

titer (ti´ter) **1.** In chemistry, the standard strength of a volumetric test solution determined by titration; assay value of an unknown measure by volumetric means. **2.** The highest dilution of a material (serum or other body fluids) that produces a reaction in an immunologic test system.

titrate (ti´trāt) To analyze the concentration of a solution by titration.

titration (ti-tra´shun) The process of estimating the quantity of a substance in solution by adding to it a measured amount of standard test solution until a reaction of known proportion is reached (shown by a color change in a suitable indicator, the development of turbidity, or the change in electrical state); from this the unknown concentration of the substance is calculated.

colorimetric t. Titration in which the end point is indicated by sudden change in color.

formol t. A process of titrating the amino group of amino acids by adding formaldehyde to the standard test solution (reagent).

potentiometer t. Titration in which the pH is constantly monitored, with a specific pH value serving as end point.

TM-mode (tē-ĕm-mod) See M-mode.

toadstool (tōd´stōōl) Popular name for an inedible, umbrella-shaped mushroom; a poisonous mushroom.

tobramycin (to-brā-mi´sin) Antibiotic substance produced by *Streptomyces tenebrarius*; active against several types of bacteria, especially *Pseudomonas aeruginosa*.

tocodynamometer (to-ko-di-nă-mom´ĕ-ter) A pressure sensor placed on the abdomen of a woman in labor to determine the frequency, duration, and strength of uterine contractions. It does not measure accurately the intensity of contractions or the resting tone of the uterus. Also called tocometer.

tocolysis (to-kol´ĭ-sis) Inhibition of uterine contractions.

tocolytic (to-ko-lit´ik) Relating to tocolysis.

tocometer (to-kom´ĕ-ter) See tocodynamometer.

tocopherol (to-kof´er-ol) See vitamin E.

α-tocopherol (al´fă-to-kof´er-ol) (α-T) A derivative of vitamin E; a light yellow, completely fat-soluble substance that occurs in the fatty portions of food; it is stored in the adipose tissue of humans and functions in all tissues in the stabilization of the lipids of the cell's membranes; believed to play an important role in cellular metabolism.

toe (tō) One of the digits of the feet.

clawing t.'s An exaggerated dorsal contraction of the toes resulting from imbalance of the short intrinsic musculature and causing the toes to appear clawlike.

great t. See hallux.

hammer t. Deformity of a toe marked by dorsiflexion of the proximal phalanx with plantar flexion of the second phalanx; the second toe is most often affected.

mallet t. Deformity of a toe marked by plantar flexion of the distal phalanx.

pigeon t. See intoe.

webbed t.'s Adjacent toes abnormally connected by a fold of tissue at their base; a form of syndactyly.

toenail (tō-nāl) A horny plate on the dorsal surface of the tip of each toe. See also nail.

ingrown t., ingrowing t. Condition in which an edge of the toenail is overgrown by the nail fold, producing a pyogenic granuloma; tight shoes, shrunken socks, and improper paring of the nail corners are common etiologic factors; trauma may also be a predisposing cause.

Togaviridae (to-gă-vir´ĭ-de) A large family of viruses (40 to 70 nm in diameter) that contain single-stranded RNA and replicate in cytoplasm; includes viruses causing yellow fever, encephalitis and German measles (rubella).

toilet (toi´let) Local care and cleansing (e.g., of a tracheostomy tube, of a wound and surrounding skin, of a patient after childbirth).

tolbutamide (tol-bu´tă-mīd) An oral hypoglycemic drug (sulfonamide derivative), used in the management of certain cases of diabetes; it stimulates the release of endogenous insulin; Orinase®.

tolerance, toleration (tol´er-ans, tol-er-a´shun) **1.** The capacity to assimilate a drug continuously or in large doses. **2.** Ability to withstand increased physiologic activities without experiencing unfavorable effects. **3.** Specific immunologic unresponsiveness.

acoustic t. The maximum sound pressure level (SPL) that can be endured without harmful effects.

cross t. Resistance to the effects of one drug resulting from an acquired tolerance to another, pharmaceutically related, drug.

drug t. Condition of decreased responsiveness to a drug acquired by repeated intake of the drug; characterized by the necessity to increase the size of successive doses in order to produce effects of equal magnitude or duration; it is the inability of the same dose to be as effective as the preceding one. See also drug dependence, under dependence.

g-t. Tolerance to certain forces resulting from either acceleration or deceleration.

glucose t. See glucose tolerance test, under test.

immunologic t. Unresponsiveness to stimulation of a specific antigen that under other conditions is capable of inducing an immune response; may occur in the primary lymphoid organs (bone marrow and thymus), or at any other location in the body.

impaired glucose t. Abnormal result of an oral glucose tolerance test although the abnormality is not sufficient to be diagnostic of diabetes mellitus. Also called latent diabetes mellitus; preclinical diabetes

T

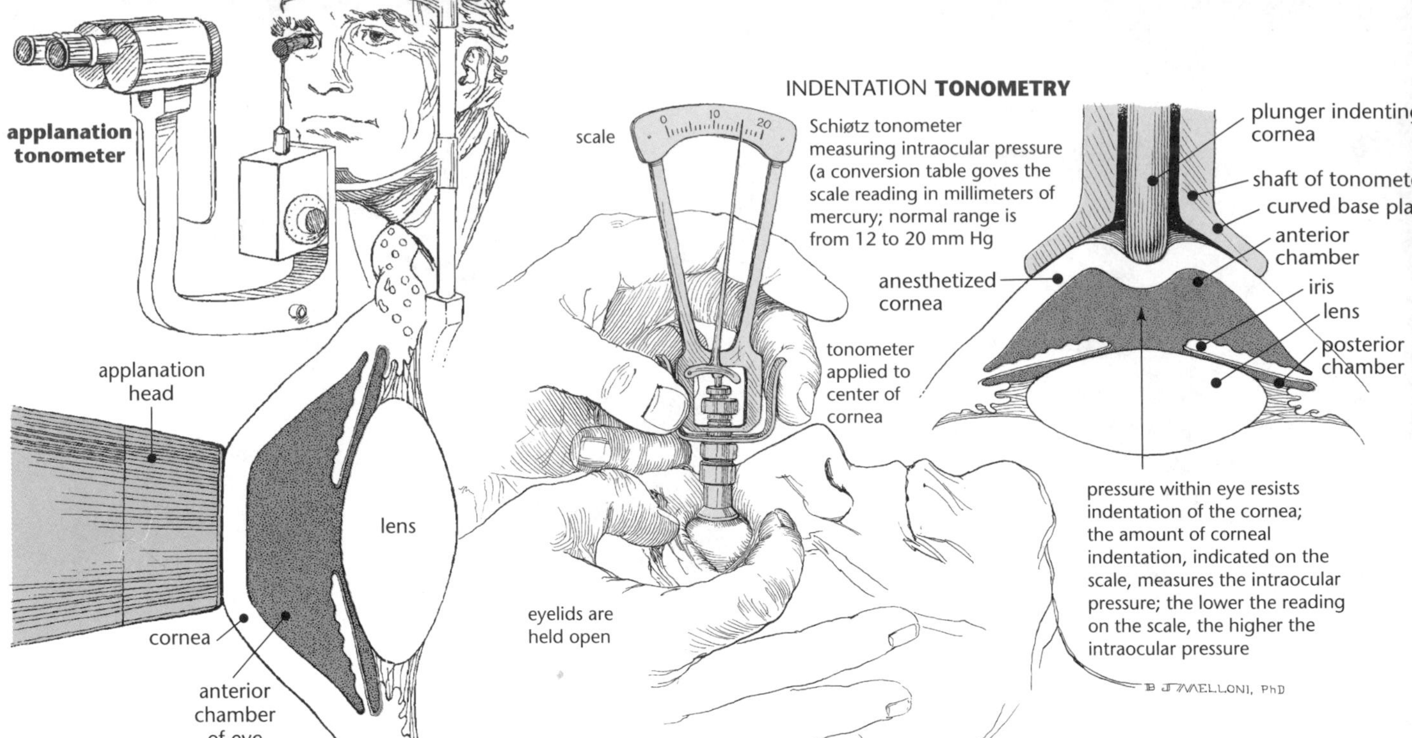

mellitus; subclinical diabetes mellitus.

natural t. See self tolerance.

pain t. The maximum degree of pain a person can endure.

self t. Lack of immune activity against the body's own antigens. Also called natural tolerance.

species t. Unresponsiveness to a drug existing as a characteristic of a particular species.

vibration t. The maximum vibratory movements that a person can endure without pain.

tolerogen (tol'er-o-jen) An antigen that causes the immune mechanisms of an organism to be unresponsive to itself, resulting in a state known as tolerance; the opposite of immunogen.

tolnaftate (tol-naf´tāt) A topical antifungal agent effective against those species of *Epidermophyton, Microsporum,* and *Trichophyton* that cause dermatophytic infections (ringworms) in man; Tinactin®.

toluene (tol´u-ēn) A colorless volatile liquid, $C_6H_5{\cdot}CH_3$, used in organic synthesis and the manufacture of explosives and dyes. Also called toluol; methylbenzene.

toluidine (tol-u´ĭ-din) A derivative of toluene.

toluidine blue (tol-u´ĭ-din bloo) Methylene blue.

toluol (tol´u-ol) See toluene.

tomogram (to´mo-gram) A roentgenogram made by tomography.

tomograph (to´mo-graf) An x-ray machine designed to take sectional roentgenograms (tomograms) of the body.

computed t. A tomograph that utilizes a computer to reconstruct a section of the patient's body from scanned x-ray profiles. Also called computerized axial tomograph.

tomography (to-mog´ră-fe) The radiographing of a selected level of the body while blurring structures in front of and behind this level; the x-ray tube and film move in opposite directions during exposure so that the roentgenographic shadow of a selected body plane remains stationary while the shadows of all other planes are in motion during exposure and therefore blurred. Also called body-section radiography; sectional radiography.

computed t. (CT) Tomography utilizing a computer-assisted tomograph. Also called computed axial tomography (CAT).

computed axial t. (CAT) See computed tomography.

helical computed t. See spiral computed tomography.

positron emission t. (PET) Direct visualization of physiologic and metabolic activities of living organs after administration of a biochemical substance (e.g., deoxyglucose) to which positron-emitting isotopes have been added; a computer interprets and produces data in the form of a color image; different shades of color indicate different concentrations of the substance.

single photon emission computed t. (SPECT) A method of computed tomography using radioactive substances that decay by emitting a single gamma ray (photon) of a given energy. The camera is rotated 180° or 360° around the patient to obtain images at multiple positions; the computer is then used to construct images (sagittal, coronal, and cross-sectional) from the three-dimensional distribution of the radioactive substance in the organ of concern. By using SPECT, it is possible to observe biochemical and physiologic processes and the size and volume of the organ. Also called SPECT imaging.

spiral computed t., spiral CT Computed tomography in which the x-ray tube rotates around the patient who, at the same time, is moved longitudinally. Also called helical tomography.

tomomania (to-mo-man´e-ă) **1.** The tendency of certain surgeons to perform operations for minor ailments. **2.** A morbid desire to be operated upon.

tone (tōn) **1.** The tension of a muscle or state of an organ. **2.** See pitch.

tongue (tung) The extremely mobile mass of striated muscle covered by mucous membrane that arises from the floor of the mouth; it serves as the principal organ of taste and aids in mastication, deglutition, and the articulation of sound.

bifid t. A tongue that is split in its anterior portion by a longitudinal fissure. Also called cleft tongue.

black t. Tongue with yellowish, brownish, or black furry patches on its dorsal aspect, made up of matted, overdeveloped papillae; the dark pigmentation is believed to be caused by microorganisms or by certain drugs. Also called furry tongue.

cleft t. See bifid tongue.

coated t. One having a whitish appearance due to deposits of food particles, inflammatory exudates, sloughed epithelial cells, or fungus growths; occurring when secretion of saliva is insufficient, or when special diets eliminate chewing or certain vitamins.

fissured t. See furrowed tongue.

furrowed t. A tongue with several longitudinal grooves. Also called fissured tongue.

furry t. See black tongue.

geographic t. Tongue with patches of papillary atrophy which fuse at their borders suggesting the appearance of a map.

hairy t. See black tongue.

magenta t. A tongue with a magenta coloration; occurring in riboflavin deficiency.

strawberry t. A tongue with a whitish coat and enlarged red papillae, occurring in scarlet fever.

tongue-tie (tung´ti) Condition in which tongue movements are restricted due to an abnormally short frenum. Also called ankyloglossia.

tonic (ton´ik) **1.** A state of sustained muscular contraction. **2.** A remedy that is supposed to restore vigor.

tonicity (to-nis´ĭ-te) **1.** The normal condition of tension, as the slight continuous contraction of skeletal muscles. Also called tonus. **2.** The effective osmotic pressure, usually compared to the osmotic pressure of plasma.

tonoclonic, tonicoclonic (ton-o-klon´ik, ton-ĭ-ko-klon´ik) Denoting muscular spasms that are both tonic and clonic.

tonofibril (ton´o-fi´bril) One of the fine fibrils found in the cytoplasm of epithelial cells which gives a supporting framework to the cell.

tonofilament (ton-o-fil´ă-ment) A structural cytoplasmic protein, bundles of which form a tonofibril.

tonography (to-nog´ră-fe) The continuous measuring and recording of changes in intraocular pressure with a tonometer.

tonometer (to-nom´ĕ-ter) An instrument for measuring tension or pressure.

applanation t. Tonometer consisting of a flat disk (applanation head) mounted on a light source that is equipped with a magnifier viewer (slit lamp biomicroscope). The disk is applied to the anesthetized cornea. The force needed to flatten a corneal surface of constant size, indicated on a calibrated knob on the tonometer, is a measure of the pressure within the eye.

Schiøtz t. Tonometer that measures the intraocular pressure by determining the indentability of the cornea by a weighted plunger.

tonometry (to-nom´ĕ-tre) The determination of tension of a part, as of pressure within the eyeball by means of an instrument (tonometer).

tonsil (ton´sil) **1.** A small mass of lymphoid tissue, especially the palatine tonsil. **2.** Any structure resembling a palatine tonsil.

cerebellar t. A lobule on the undersurface of each cerebellar hemisphere.

Gerlach's t. See tubal tonsil.

lingual t. An aggregation of lymphoid tissue on the posterior part of the tongue.

Luschka's t. See pharyngeal tonsil.

palatine t. One of two oval masses of lymphoid tissue, one on each side of the oral pharynx, between the pillars of the fauces.

pharyngeal t. A collection of lymphoid tissue on the posterior wall of the nasopharynx; when enlarged it is known as adenoids. Also called Luschka's tonsil.

tubal t. A collection of lymphoid tissue near the

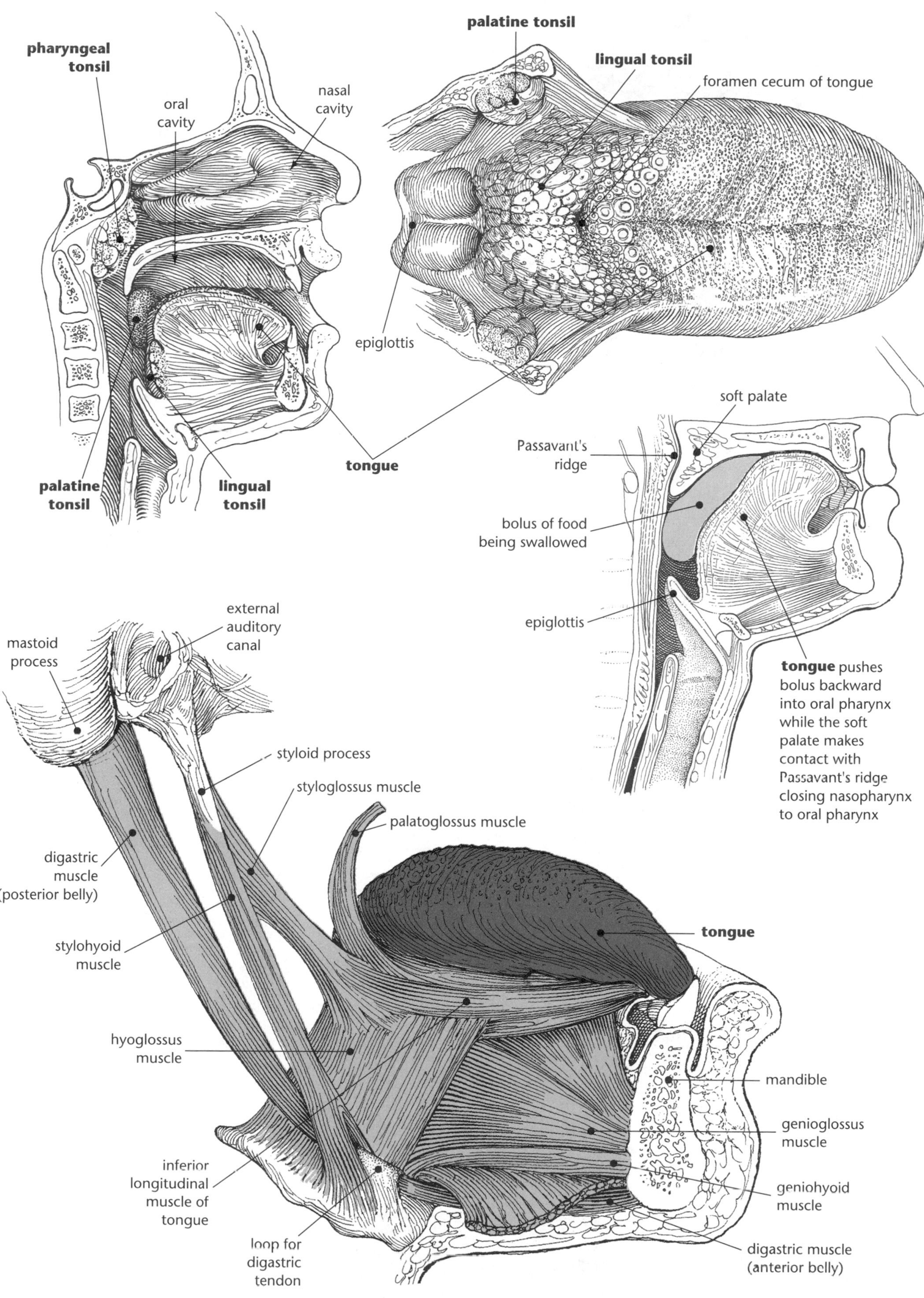
pharyngeal tonsil
oral cavity
nasal cavity
palatine tonsil
lingual tonsil
tongue
palatine tonsil
lingual tonsil
foramen cecum of tongue
epiglottis
soft palate
Passavant's ridge
bolus of food being swallowed
epiglottis
tongue pushes bolus backward into oral pharynx while the soft palate makes contact with Passavant's ridge closing nasopharynx to oral pharynx
external auditory canal
mastoid process
styloid process
styloglossus muscle
palatoglossus muscle
digastric muscle (posterior belly)
stylohyoid muscle
tongue
hyoglossus muscle
mandible
genioglossus muscle
inferior longitudinal muscle of tongue
geniohyoid muscle
loop for digastric tendon
digastric muscle (anterior belly)

T

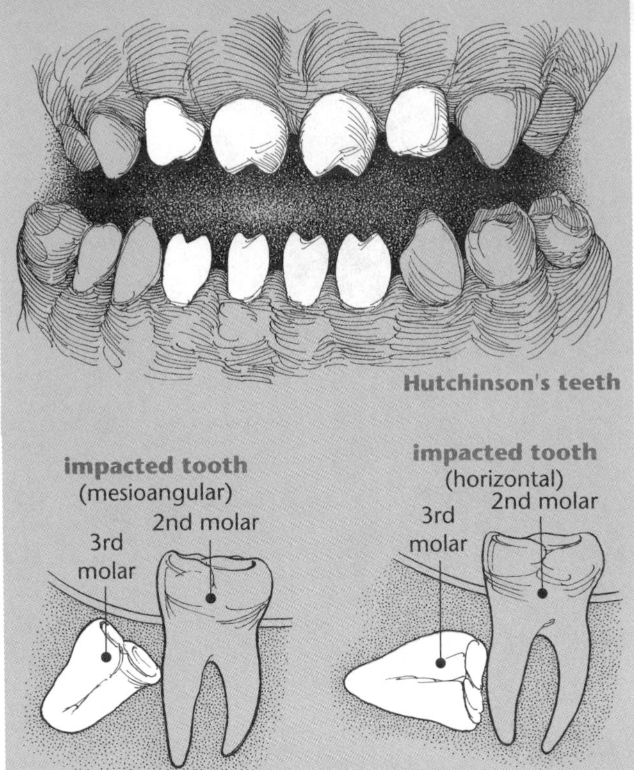

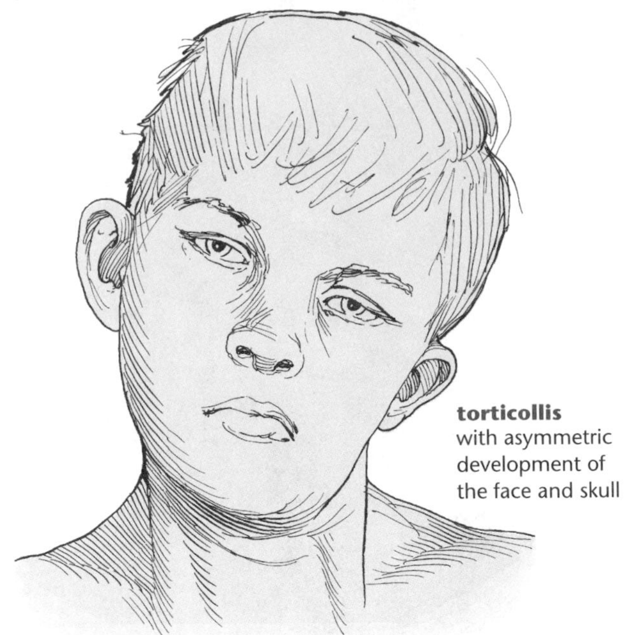

contracture of the left sternocleidomastoid muscle has caused tilting of the head to the left and turning of the chin to the right

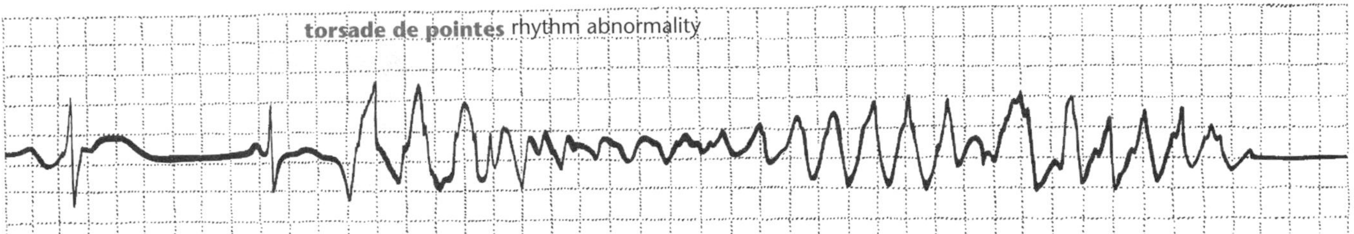

pharyngeal orifice of the auditory (eustachian) tube. Also called Gerlach's tonsil.

tonsillar (ton´sĭ-lar) Relating to a tonsil, especially the palatine tonsil.

tonsillectomy (ton-sĭ-lek´to-me) Surgical removal of the tonsils.

tonsillitis (ton-sĭ-li´tis) Inflammation of a tonsil or tonsils.

tonsilloadenoidectomy (ton-sil-o-ad-ĕ-noi-dek´to-me) (T&A) The surgical removal of both the palatine tonsils and the adenoids.

tonsillolith (ton-sil´o-lith) A concretion or calculus in a tonsil.

tonsillotome (ton-sil´o-tōm) An instrument, sometimes designed after a guillotine, for surgically removing a portion of a hypertrophied tonsil.

tonsillotomy (ton-sĭ-lot´o-me) The surgical removal of a portion of a hypertrophied tonsil.

tonus (to´nus) See tonicity (1).

T

tooth (to͞oth), *pl.* **teeth** One of the bonelike structures embedded in sockets in the jaws, used for chewing.

abutment t. See abutment.

buck teeth Prominent projecting maxillary anterior teeth; horizontal overlap in labioversion.

canine t. See cuspid.

dead t. Nonvital tooth.

deciduous teeth The 20 teeth that generally erupt between the 6th and 24th months of life, and are later replaced by the permanent teeth; they calcify partly before and partly after birth. Also called primary teeth; temporary teeth; milk teeth.

dog t. See cuspid.

eye t. See cuspid.

Hutchinson's teeth Permanent incisors in which the edge is notched and narrow; considered a sign of congenital syphilis. Also called notched teeth.

impacted t. A tooth that, due to its position in the jaw, is unable to erupt or to attain its normal position after it has erupted.

milk teeth See deciduous teeth.

natal t. Tooth that has erupted prior to birth.

nonvital t. A tooth from which the pulp has been removed or one in which the pulp has died.

notched teeth See Hutchinson's teeth.

permanent teeth The 32 teeth that generally erupt from the ages of 6 to 21 years, belonging to the second or permanent dentition; they include 4 incisors, 2 cuspids, 4 bicuspids, and 6 molars in each jaw. Sometimes called succedaneous teeth.

primary teeth See deciduous teeth.

snaggle t. A tooth out of proper line in relation to the others in the arch.

spaced teeth Teeth that have shifted and lost proximal contact with adjacent teeth.

succedaneous teeth See permanent teeth.

temporary teeth See deciduous teeth.

unerupted t. A tooth prior to eruption through the gingiva.

wisdom t. Third permanent molar; erupts between the ages of 17 and 21 years.

toothache (to͞oth´āk) An aching pain in or about a tooth, usually due to caries, infection, or trauma. Also called odontalgia.

toothpick (to͞oth´pik) A wood sliver used to remove food particles from between the teeth.

balsa wood t. A triangular wedge of balsa wood used to stimulate the interdental gingival tissues and to cleanse the interproximal surfaces of the teeth.

topagnosis (top-ag-no´sis) Inability to identify the exact place where the body is touched.

topalgia (to-pal´jă) Pain localized at one spot without any lesion or trauma to account for it; a symptom sometimes occurring in neuroses.

topesthesia (top-es-the´zhă) Ability to determine which part of the skin is touched.

tophaceous (to-fa´shus) **1.** Gritty. **2.** Having the features of a tophus.

tophus (to´fus), *pl.* **to´phi** An accumulation of urate crystals usually deposited in the articular and periarticular tissues in gout; it has a firm gritty consistency; the areas most vulnerable are those of the elbows, feet, hands, and the helix of the ear.

topical (top´ĭ-kal) Relating to a definite area.

topoanesthesia (top-o-an-es-the´zhă) Inability to determine the location of a cutaneous sensation.

topognosis (top-og-no´sis) The ability to recognize the location of a sensation.

topogometer (top-o-gom´ĕ-ter) A movable fixation target attached to the front of a keratometer for measuring the curvature of the cornea in its periphery.

topography (to-pog´ră-fe) In anatomy, description of a limited area of the surface of the body.

toponarcosis (top-o-nar-ko´sis) Loss of sensation on a localized area of the skin.

torpor (tor´por) Sluggishness and slow response to stimuli.

torque (tork) A rotary force capable of producing torsion and rotation about an axis, as one applied to a denture base; a twisting force.

torsades de pointes (tor-sahd dĕ pwant´) "Twisting of the points"; a form of ventricular tachycardia in which the QRS complexes of the electrocardiogram are of changing amplitude and appear to twist around an electrically neutral (isoelectric) point.

torsion (tor´shun) The act of turning or twisting, or the condition of being turned or twisted, as the twisting of the spermatic cord.

torso (tor´so) The trunk.

torticollis (tor-tĭ-kol´is) Spasmodic contraction of the muscles of one side of the neck, causing the head to be drawn and usually rotated to that side. Commonly called stiff neck; wryneck.

spasmodic t. See cervical dystonia, under dystonia.

torulopsosis (tor-u-lop´so-sis) Yeast infection caused by *Torulopsis glabrata*; usually seen as an opportunistic disease in severely debilitated or AIDS patients.

torulus (tor´u-lus) A small projection; a papilla.

torus (to´rus) **1.** A protuberance or projection. **2.** A benign, localized exostosis.

t. mandibularis A torus located on the lingual surface of the mandible in the cuspid-bicuspid region.

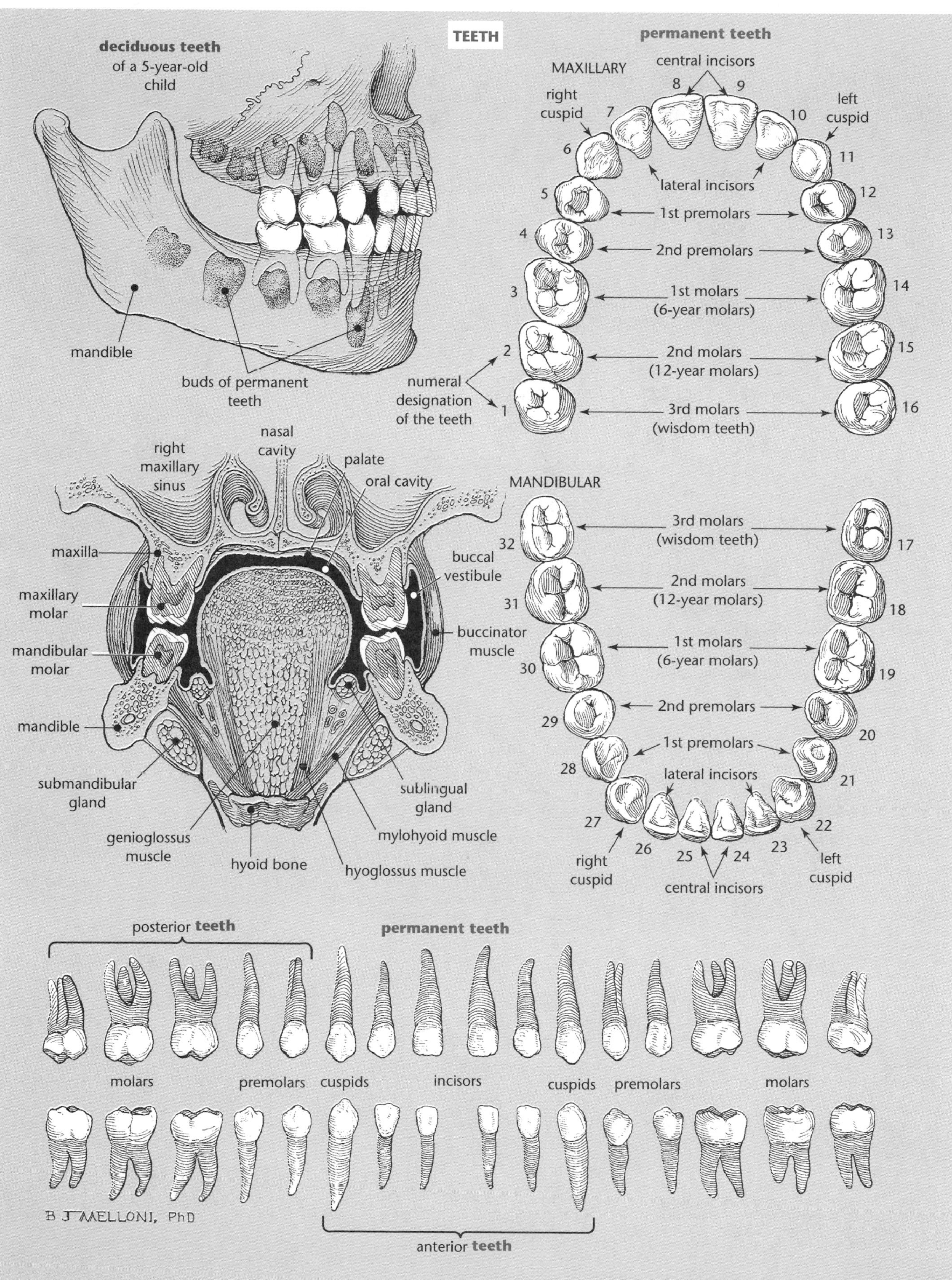
TEETH
deciduous teeth
of a 5-year-old
child
mandible
buds of permanent
teeth
permanent teeth
MAXILLARY
central incisors
8
9
right
cuspid
7
10
left
cuspid
6
11
lateral incisors
5
12
1st premolars
4
13
2nd premolars
3
14
1st molars
(6-year molars)
2
15
2nd molars
(12-year molars)
numeral
designation
of the teeth
1
16
3rd molars
(wisdom teeth)
nasal
cavity
right
maxillary
sinus
palate
oral cavity
maxilla
maxillary
molar
mandibular
molar
mandible
buccal
vestibule
buccinator
muscle
submandibular
gland
sublingual
gland
genioglossus
muscle
hyoid bone
mylohyoid muscle
hyoglossus muscle
MANDIBULAR
32
17
3rd molars
(wisdom teeth)
31
18
2nd molars
(12-year molars)
30
19
1st molars
(6-year molars)
29
20
2nd premolars
28
21
1st premolars
lateral incisors
27
22
26
23
25
24
right
cuspid
central incisors
left
cuspid
posterior teeth
permanent teeth
molars
premolars
cuspids
incisors
cuspids
premolars
molars
anterior teeth
B J MELLONI, PhD

T

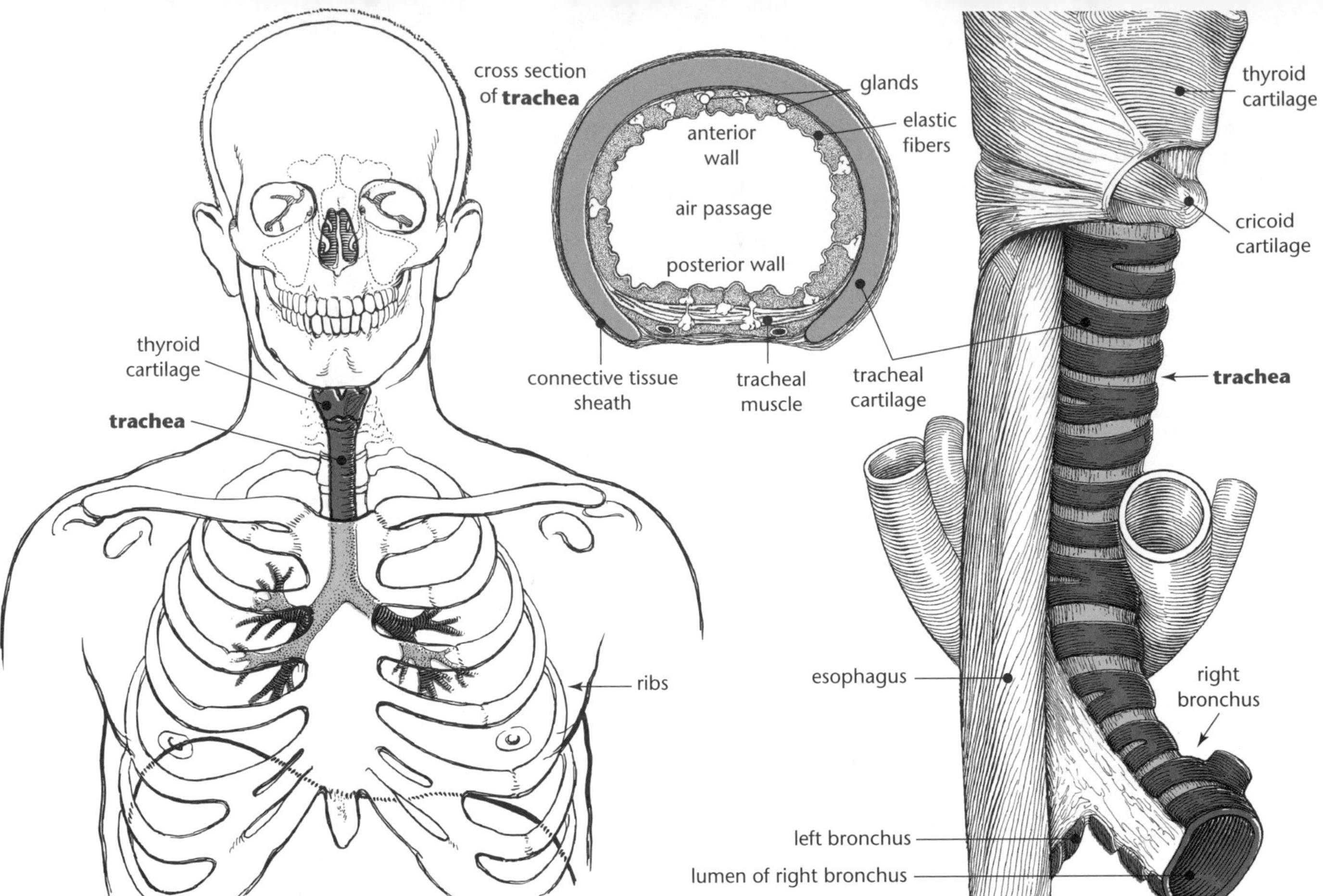

t. palatinus An overgrowth of bone usually located in the midline of the hard palate.

t. tubarius A ridge posterior to the pharyngeal opening of the auditory (eustachian) tube. Also called eustachian cushion.

totipotency (to-te-po´ten-se) The ability to regenerate a whole organism from a part, or the ability of a cell to differentiate into any type of cell.

touch (tuch) **1.** Special sense through which anything that comes in contact with the skin or mucous membrane is perceived. Also called the tactile sense. **2.** To palpate or feel with the hands.

Tourette's disease (too-retz dĭ-zēz´) See Gilles de la Tourette's syndrome.

Tourette's syndrome (too-retz sin´drōm) See Gilles de la Tourette's syndrome.

tourniquet (toor´nĭ-ket) Any device or constrictive wide band applied to an arm or leg for temporary compression of the blood vessels; used to stop arterial bleeding, prevent entry of a toxin into the body, or to distend the veins prior to venipuncture.

toxemia (tok-se´me-ă) The presence of bacterial poisons (toxins) in the blood.

t. of pregnancy See preeclampsia.

toxic (tok´sik) **1.** Poisonous; harmful. **2.** Pertaining to a toxin. **3.** Caused by a poison.

t. blood level See under level.

toxicant (toks´ĭ-kant) **1.** Poisonous. **2.** Any poisonous agent.

toxicity (tok-sis´ĭ-te) The quality of being poisonous.

acute t. Toxicity that occurs when exposure to a chemical or drug is sudden and severe and when absorption is rapid.

cumulative t. Toxicity caused by accumulation of a substance in the body as a result of repeated exposure to small amounts of the substance over a period of time.

subacute t. Toxicity resulting from frequent, repeated exposure over a period of several hours or days to a dose of drug that does not produce toxic effects when taken as a single dose.

Toxicodendron (tok-sĭ-ko-den´dron) *Rhus.*

toxicoderma (tok-sĭ-ko-der´mă) Any skin disease produced by a poison.

toxicodermatitis (tok-sĭ-ko-der-mă-ti´tis) Skin inflammation produced by a poison.

toxicogenic (tok-sĭ-ko-jen´ik) **1.** Producing a poison. **2.** Produced by a poison.

toxicoid (tok´sĭ-koid) Producing effects like those of a poison.

toxicologist (tok-sĭ-kol´o-jist) An expert on poisons and their antidotes.

toxicology (tok-sĭ-kol´ŏ-je) The study of the toxic or harmful effects of chemicals on the body; deals with the symptoms and treatment of poisoning as well as the identification of the poison.

forensic t. Diagnosis and treatment of intentional and accidental poisoning and the attendant legal implications.

toxicopathy (tok-sĭ-kop´ă-the) Any disease caused by a poison.

toxic shock syndrome (tok´sik shok sin´drōm) Sudden onset of fever, muscle ache, vomiting, and diarrhea, accompanied by a peeling rash (especially of the palms and soles) and followed by low body temperature and shock; multiple organ involvement is common and may include kidneys, liver, mucous membranes, and central nervous system; caused by staphylococcal endotoxin, especially from infection of the vagina associated with tampon use.

toxin (tok´sin) A poisonous substance produced by certain microorganisms.

extracellular t. See exotoxin.

intracellular t. See endotoxin.

toxipathy (tok-sip´ă-the) Any disease caused by a poison.

TOXLINE Toxicology information online; a computerized system of data that includes bibliographic references covering pharmacologic, biochemical, physiologic, environmental, and toxicologic effects of drugs and other chemicals. It is one of the databases of MEDLARS, based at the National Library of Medicine. See also MEDLARS.

Toxocara (tok-so-ka´ră) A genus of parasitic roundworms of the family Ascaridae.

toxocariasis (tok-so-kăr-i´ă-sis) Infection with larvae of dog and cat parasites of the genus *Toxocara*. Also called visceral larva migrans.

toxoid (tok´soid) A toxin that has been rendered nonpoisonous by chemicals or other agents but is still capable of producing immunity.

tetanus t. The toxin from the tetanus bacillus, rendered nontoxic and used for immunization against the toxin produced by tetanus infection.

toxophore (tok´so-fōr) The group of atoms in the toxin molecule that is responsible for its poisonous action.

Toxoplasma gondii (tok-so-plaz´mă gon´dĭ-i) Intracellular protozoan parasite of the genus *Toxoplasma* causing toxoplasmosis in humans.

toxoplasmosis (tok-so-plaz-mo´sis) Disease caused by infection with *Toxoplasma gondii*; it may resemble a mild cold or infectious mononucleosis in adults; a disseminated form may lead to hepatitis, pneumonitis, myocarditis, or meningoencephalitis; involvement of the eyes occurs in another form; an infected pregnant woman can spread the disease to her unborn child, causing eye or brain damage or even death; eating raw meat from infected animals is the most common way in which the disease is acquired.

trabecula (tră-bek´u-lar), *pl.* **trabec´ulae** A supporting, anchoring fiber of connective tissue; a dividing band.

septomarginal t. The moderator band that connects the septal band with the anterior papillary muscle and the parietal wall of the right ventricle of the heart.

trabeculae carneae cordis Thick muscular bands on the inner walls of the ventricles of the heart.

trabecular (tră-bek´u-lar) Relating to, or marked by, the presence of trabeculae.

trabeculation (tră-bek-u-la´shun) The formation or the presence of trabeculae in a part.

trabeculectomy (tră-bek-u-lek´tŏ-me) Microsurgery of the eye in which a small portion of the trabeculum and adjacent Schlemm's canal (scleral venous sinus) is removed to enhance drainage of aqueous humor, thus relieving intraocular pressure caused by open-angle glaucoma.

trabeculoplasty (tră-bek´u-lo-plas-te) Operation for the treatment of glaucoma in which small openings are made on the trabecular meshwork of the eye to improve aqueous humor flow and relieve intraocular pressure.

laser t. Trabeculoplasty using a laser beam.

tracer (trās´er) **1.** A substance that can be readily identified, such as a radioactive isotope, used to gain information. **2.** A device for recording the movements of the lower jaw.

trachea (tra´ke-ă) A cartilaginous and membranous

T

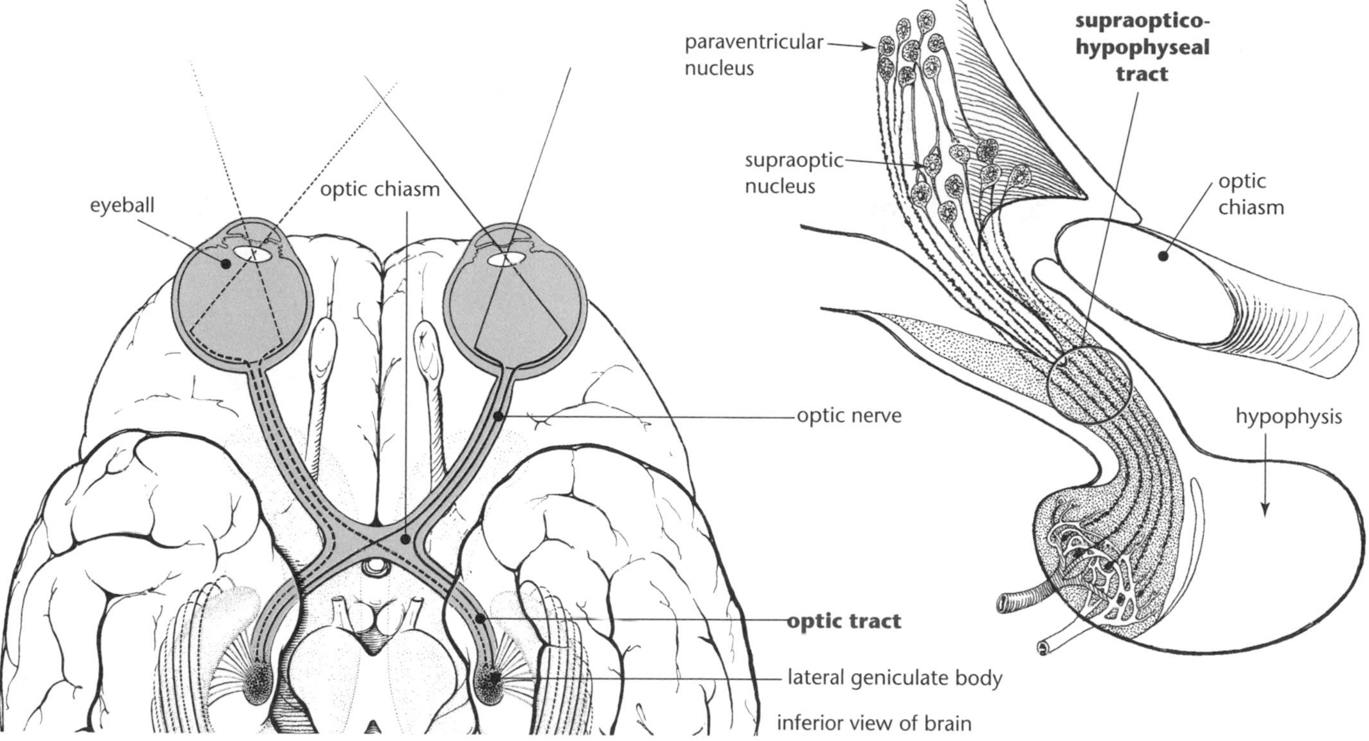

tube extending from, and continuous with, the lower part of the larynx to the bronchi. Commonly called windpipe.

tracheal (tra´ke-al) Relating to the trachea.

trachealgia (tra-ke-al´jă) Pain in the trachea.

tracheitis (tra-ke-i´tis) Inflammation of the trachea.

trachelectomy (tra-kĕ-lek´tŏ-me) See cervicectomy.

trachelism, trachelismus (tra´kĕ-liz-m, tra-kĕ-liz´mus) Spasmodic backward bending of the neck.

trachelorrhaphy (tra-ke-lor´ă-fe) Repair of the uterine cervix, as from lacerations.

tracheobronchial (tra-ke-o-brong´ke-al) Relating to the trachea and a bronchus or the bronchi.

tracheobronchitis (tra-ke-o brong-ki´tis) Inflammation of the mucous membrane of the trachea and bronchi.

tracheobronchoscopy (tra-ke-o-brong-kos´ko-pe) Visual inspection of the interior of the trachea and bronchi.

tracheocele (tra´ke-o-sēl) Hernial protrusion of the mucous membrane through a defect in the wall of the trachea.

tracheoesophageal (tra-ke-o-e-sof´ă-je-al) Relating to the trachea and the esophagus.

tracheolaryngeal (tra-ke-o-lă-rin´je-al) Relating to both the trachea and the larynx.

tracheomalacia (tra-ke-o-mă-la´shă) Softening and degeneration of the connective tissue of the trachea.

tracheopathy (tra-ke-op´ă-the) Any disease of the trachea.

tracheophony (tra-ke-of´o-ne) The hollow sound heard on auscultation over the trachea.

tracheoplasty (tra´ke-o-plas-te) Plastic surgery of the trachea.

tracheorrhagia (tra-ke-o-ra´jă) Bleeding from the trachea.

tracheoscopy (tra-ke-os´ko-pe) Visual examination of the interior of the trachea by means of a tracheoscope.

tracheostenosis (tra-ke-o-stĕ-no´sis) Constriction of the trachea.

tracheostoma (tra-ke-os´to-mă) An opening into the trachea through the neck.

tracheostomy (tra-ke-os´tŏ-me) **1.** A direct opening into the trachea through the neck to facilitate breathing or removal of secretions. **2.** The artificial opening or stoma so produced.

tracheotome (tra´ke-o-tōm) Tracheostomy knife.

tracheotomy (tra-ke-ot´ŏ-me) See tracheostomy.

trachoma (tră-ko´mă) Contagious infection of the conjunctiva and cornea caused by *Chlamydia trachomatis*; marked by inflammation and formation of numerous follicles in the conjunctiva of the upper eyelid; after about six weeks these turn to large, red, hard papillae that last from several months to one or more years, ending with scar tissue formation; the eyelid turns inward, causing the conjunctiva and cornea to become dry. The disease is one of the chief causes of blindness in some parts of the world, especially the Middle East.

tracing (trās´ing) A line or a pattern of lines made by a pointed instrument on thin paper or plate representing movement (e.g., cardiovascular activity, mandibular movements) or pertinent landmarks of a cephalometric x-ray picture.

tracks (traks) A slang expression for a series of tattoo-like needle scars from frequent narcotics injections.

tract (trakt) **1.** A system of structures, arranged in series, that perform one common function; e.g., the respiratory tract. **2.** A collection of nerve fibers possessing the same origin, termination, and function.

alimentary t. See digestive tract.

ascending t. Any band of nerve fibers conveying impulses toward the brain.

corticospinal t.'s Tracts composed of nerve fibers that originate from the cerebral cortex, pass through the medullary pyramid, and descend in the spinal cord. *Anterior corticospinal t.*, the portion of the corticospinal tracts that descends through the cervical segments adjacent to the anterior median fissure of the spinal cord (the fibers decussate at their level of innervation). Also called ventral corticospinal tract. *Lateral corticospinal t.*, the portion of the corticospinal tracts that upon decussation (at the junction of the medulla and spinal cord) descends the length of the lateral part of the spinal cord. Also called crossed pyramidal tract.

descending t. Any band of nerve fibers conveying impulses from the brain downward.

digestive t. The mucous membrane-lined passage from the mouth to the anus.

dorsolateral t. Poorly myelinated nerve fibers at the tip of the dorsal horn between the posteromarginal nucleus and the surface of the spinal cord, medial to the incoming dorsal roots; composed in part of primary pain and temperature fibers; they are a continuation of the dorsal fibers that ascend and descend over two segments before terminating in the substantia gelatinosa. Also called dorsolateral fasciculus; tract of Lissauer.

gastrointestinal t. The stomach and intestines.

geniculocalcarine t. Nerve fibers that pass through the posterior limb of the internal capsule and terminate on the visual cortex of the occipital lobe. Also called optic radiation.

genitourinary t. The urinary passageway from the pelvis of the kidney to the urinary orifice through the ureters, bladder, and urethra. Also called urogenital tract.

iliotibial t. A strong, wide, thickened portion of the fascia lata of the thigh extending from the tubercle of the iliac crest to the lateral condyle of the tibia; it receives the greater part of the insertion of the gluteus maximus muscle.

intestinal t. The part of the digestive tract between the pyloric end of the stomach and the anus.

t. of Lissauer See dorsolateral tract.

mamillotegmental t. Nerve fibers that arise from the mamillary nucleus and descend into the reticular formation of the brainstem, terminating in the dorsal and ventral tegmental nuclei.

mamillothalamic t. Nerve fibers in the brain connecting the mamillary body to the anterior thalamic nuclear complex.

olfactory t. A narrow band on the undersurface of the frontal lobe of the brain that connects the olfactory bulb to the cerebral hemisphere.

optic t. A band of nerve fibers that extends from the optic chiasm to the lateral geniculate body, with some reflex fibers going to the spinal cord.

pyramidal t. A term generally used to designate the corticospinal projections arising from the cerebral cortex and descending in the internal capsule, cerebral peduncle, and pens to the medulla oblongata; the term is restricted to mean nerve fibers that pass through the pyramid.

respiratory t. The conducting airway consisting of the nose, mouth, pharynx, larynx, trachea, bronchi, bronchioles, and alveoli.

rubrospinal t. A band of nerve fibers arising from the red nucleus (oval cell mass in the central part of the midbrain tegmentum); the fibers cross (decussate) and descend the length of the spinal cord.

solitary t. of medulla oblongata A tract that begins in the upper medulla and extends to the cervical junction; it terminates along the course of the solitary nucleus; formed primarily by visceral afferent and taste fibers from the vagus, glossopharyngeal, and facial (intermediate) nerves. Also called tractus solitarius.

spinal t. of trigeminal nerve Afferent trigeminal root fibers that extend from the middle of the pons to the uppermost cervical spinal segments, where they terminate in the adjacent spinal trigeminal nucleus which forms a long cell column medial to the tract.

T

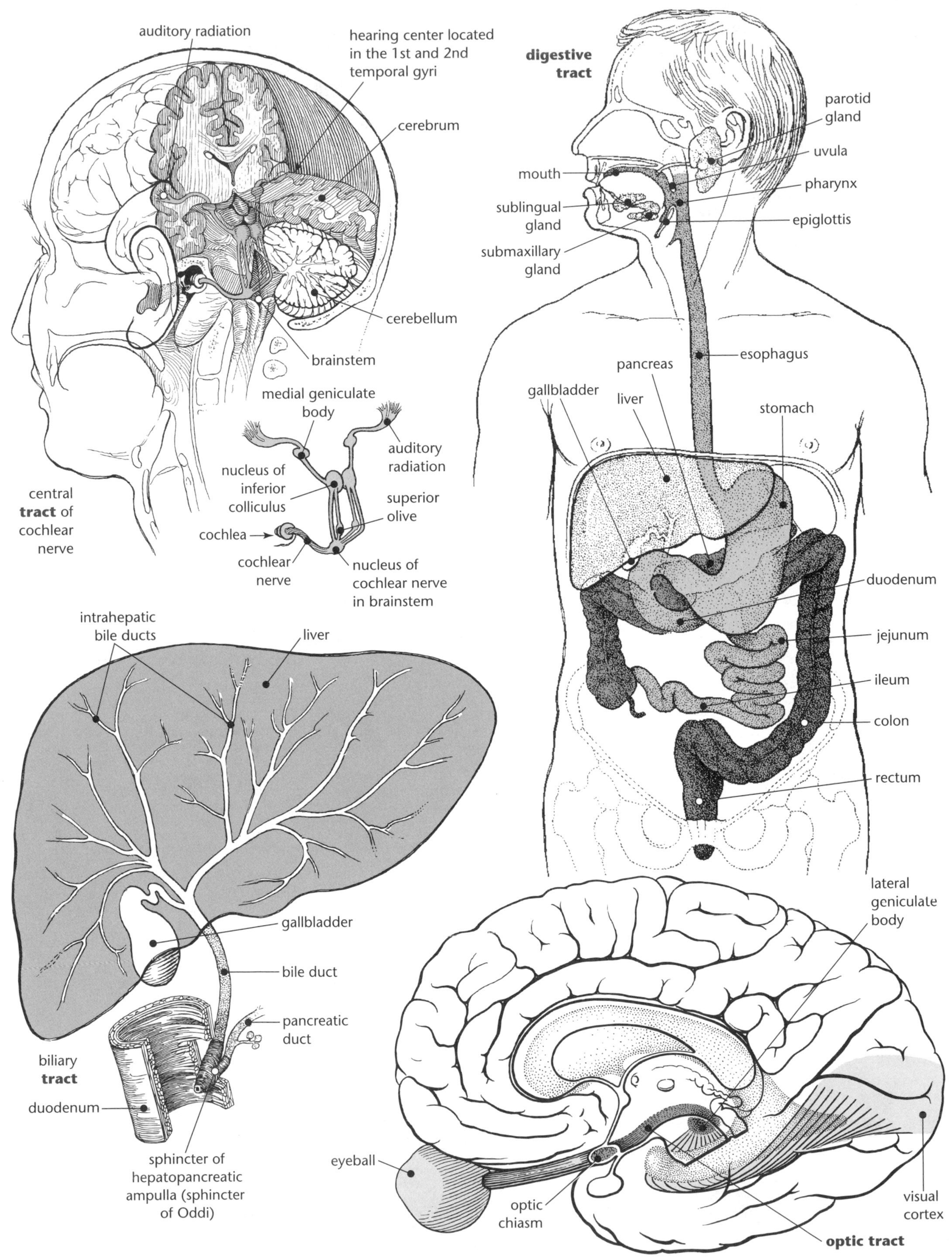

auditory radiation
hearing center located in the 1st and 2nd temporal gyri
cerebrum
cerebellum
brainstem
medial geniculate body
auditory radiation
nucleus of inferior colliculus
superior olive
cochlea
cochlear nerve
nucleus of cochlear nerve in brainstem
central **tract** of cochlear nerve
digestive tract
parotid gland
uvula
mouth
pharynx
sublingual gland
epiglottis
submaxillary gland
esophagus
pancreas
gallbladder
liver
stomach
duodenum
jejunum
ileum
colon
rectum
intrahepatic bile ducts
liver
gallbladder
bile duct
pancreatic duct
biliary **tract**
duodenum
sphincter of hepatopancreatic ampulla (sphincter of Oddi)
lateral geniculate body
eyeball
optic chiasm
visual cortex
optic tract

T

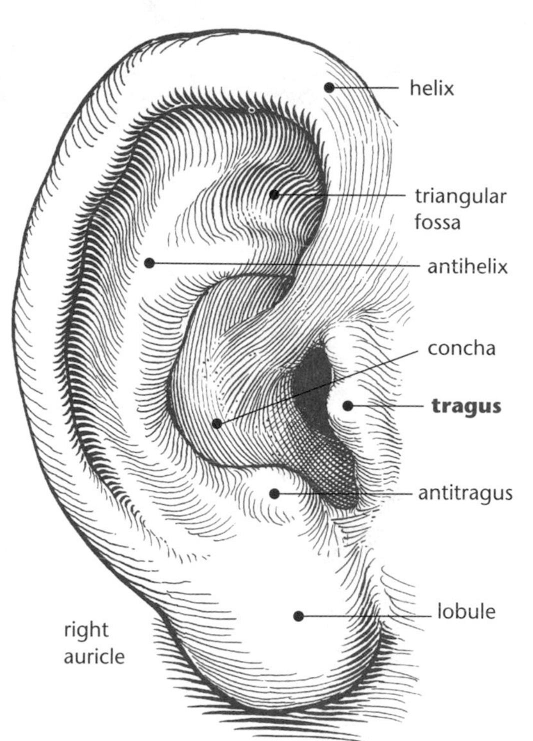

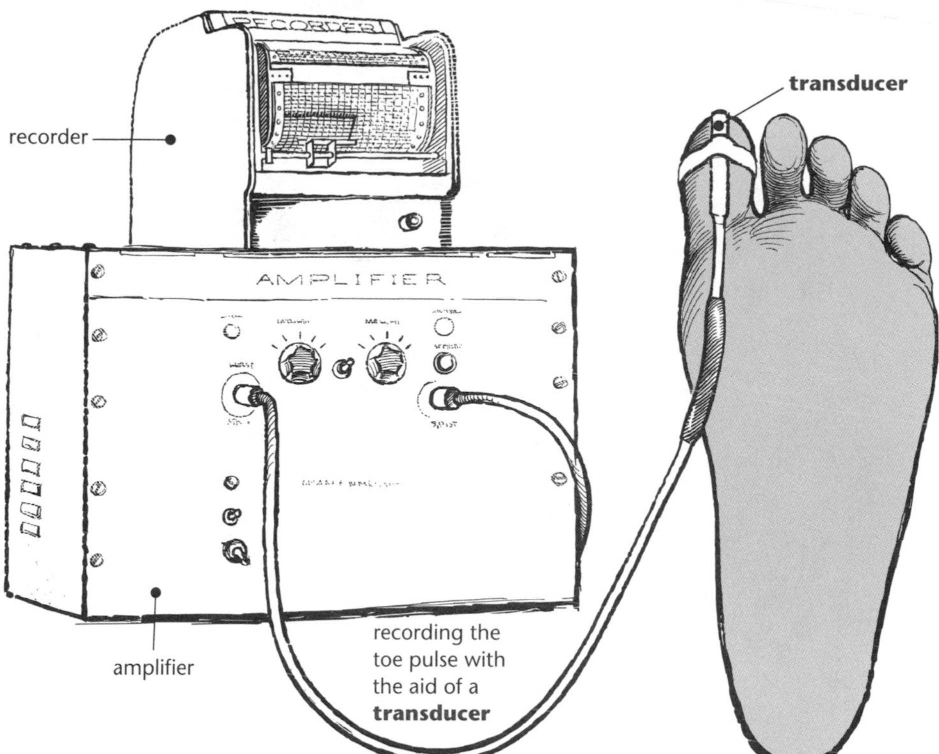

spinocerebellar t.'s *Anterior*, a band of nerve fibers that ascends along the lateral funiculus of the spinal cord to the cerebellum, via the superior cerebellar peduncle. Also called ventral spinocerebellar tract. *Posterior,* a tract that lies in the lateral funiculus of the spinal cord and conveys nerve fibers from the thoracic nucleus to the cerebellum, via the inferior cerebellar peduncle. Also called dorsal spinocerebellar tract.

spinothalamic t.'s *Anterior,* a band of nerve fibers in the anterolateral funiculus of the spinal cord that crosses over in the anterior white commissure before ascending to the ventral posterolateral (VPL) nucleus of the thalamus. Also called ventral spinothalamic tract. *Lateral,* a band of nerve fibers in the anterolateral funiculus of the spinal cord that ascends to the ventral posterolateral (VPL) nucleus of the thalamus, with some branches going to the reticular formation.

supraopticohypophysial t. A bundle of nerve fibers arising from the supraoptic and paraventricular nuclei of the hypothalamus and descending to the posterior lobe of the hypophysis (neurohypophysis), where these fibers branch profusely and form most of the bulk of the lobe.

tuberohypophysial t. A bundle of nerve fibers arising from small cells (arcuate nucleus) around the floor of the third ventricle and projecting to the infundibular stem of the hypophysis. Also called tuberoinfundibular tract.

tuberoinfundibular t. See tuberohypophysial tract.

urinary t. The urinary passageway from the pelvis of the kidney to the urinary orifice through the ureters, bladder, and urethra.

urogenital t. See genitourinary tract.

uveal t. See uvea.

traction (trak'shun) Application of tension to a body part to correct displacement, especially of bones.

skeletal t. Heavy traction delivered to a broken bone by pulling directly on a metal pin or wire inserted into or through a bone; capable of delivering a traction force of approximately 40 lb.

skin t. Light traction delivered to a bone by pulling on adhesive strips attached to the skin of an extremity; capable of delivering a traction force of approximately 10 lb; used frequently for the reduction of fractures in young children.

tractotomy (trak-tot'ŏ-me) Surgical severing of a nerve tract in the brainstem or spinal cord, usually performed to relieve pain.

spinothalamic t. Division of the spinothalamic tract to eradicate pain distal to the level of the division; may be performed in the spinal cord, medulla oblongata, or brainstem.

trigeminal t. Severing of the descending root of the trigeminal nerve.

tractus (trak'tus) Latin for tract.

tragacanth (trag'ă-kanth) The dried gummy exudation from the thorny shrubs of the genus *Astragalus*, especially *Astragalus gummifer*; used as an emulsifier in foods, cosmetics, and pharmaceuticals. Also called gum tragacanth.

tragal (tra'gal) Relating to the tragus.

tragus (tra'gus) The small projection of cartilage in front of the opening of the external ear.

trait (trāt) **1.** In genetics, any inherited gene-determined characteristic; applied to any normal variation or to a disease, whether occurring in a recessive or a dominant condition. **2.** A particular pattern of behavior.

autosomal t. Trait determined by a gene that is present on any chromosome other than a sex chromosome.

β-thalassemia t. See β thalassemia minor, under thalassemia.

dominant t. Trait occurring when the responsible gene is present in a heterozygous state or single dose (i.e., having dissimilar alleles in corresponding loci of a pair of chromosomes).

recessive t. Trait occurring when the responsible gene is present in a homozygous state or double dose (i.e., having identical alleles at corresponding loci of a pair of chromosomes).

sickle cell t. Term used in clinical medicine to denote a condition in which there is a tendency for the red blood cells to assume a sickle-like shape due to the presence of hemoglobin AS (the heterozygous state for hemoglobin S); individuals with the trait are usually asymptomatic but may manifest some of the complications of sickle cell disease.

trajector (tră-jek'tor) A device for following the path of a bullet in a wound.

trance (trans) A state of detachment from one's physical surroundings, characterized by diminished activity and consciousness, resembling sleep (e.g., the state seen in hypnosis).

tranquilizer (tran-kwī-līz'er) A drug that allays anxiety and calms the patient.

transacetylation (trans-as-ĕ-til-a'shun) Metabolic reaction involving the transfer of an acetyl group.

transaction (tran-sak'shun) The reciprocal interaction between two or more individuals involving simultaneous stimulation and response.

transaminase (trans-am'ĭ-nās) See aminotransferase.

transamination (trans-am-i-na'shun) The reversible process of amino group transfer, catalyzed by enzymes that have been called transaminases, aminopherases, and aminotransferases.

transcription (trans-krip'shun) **1.** The process of transcribing, as in the transfer of the genetic code information from DNA to messenger RNA. **2.** See signature.

reverse t. The synthesis of DNA on an RNA template.

transdiaphragmatic (trans-di-ă-frag-mat'ik) Across or through the diaphragm.

transducer (tran-doo'ser) A device that converts energy from one form to another.

Doppler ultrasonic t. A device that detects shift in sound (Doppler effect) from change in ultrasonic signal reflected from a bodily structure such as a blood vessel.

piezoelectric t. A transducer that transforms electric to mechanical energy; used in ultrasound procedures.

pressure t. A device that converts pressure differences into electric current, which can then be readily amplified and recorded.

transducin (trans-doo'sin) A G protein in the rod cells of the retina that interacts with activated rhodopsin (the photosensitive pigment in the rods) to initiate a cascade of reactions important in vision.

transduction (trans-duk'shun) **1.** The change in the genetic makeup of a cell by transfer of DNA from a virus to the cell. **2.** The conversion of energy from one form to another.

transection (tran-sek'shun) **1.** Cutting across. **2.** A cross section.

transfection (trans-fek'shun) Introduction of DNA into the genome of a cell.

stable t. Introduction of DNA into a recipient eukaryotic cell with incorporation into the chromosomal DNA (genome) of the recipient; it is then expressed in other generations.

transient t. Transfection in which the introduced DNA (transgene) is not incorporated into the genome.

transfer (trans'fer) A passage from one place to another.

embryo t. (ET) Procedure in which an embryo at the blastocyst stage (acquired through *in vitro* or *in vivo* fertilization) is transferred to the recipient's uterus through the vagina. The embryo may also be transferred to one of the recipient's fallopian (uterine) tubes via an abdominal incision.

gamete intrafallopian t. (GIFT) The placement of ova and spermatozoa together in the distal end of one or both fallopian (uterine) tubes. The placement is performed with a laparoscope through the abdominal wall.

***in vitro* fertilization and embryo t.** (IVF-ET) Fertilization by placing ova and spermatozoa together in a Petri dish and then placing the embryos within the recipient's uterus.

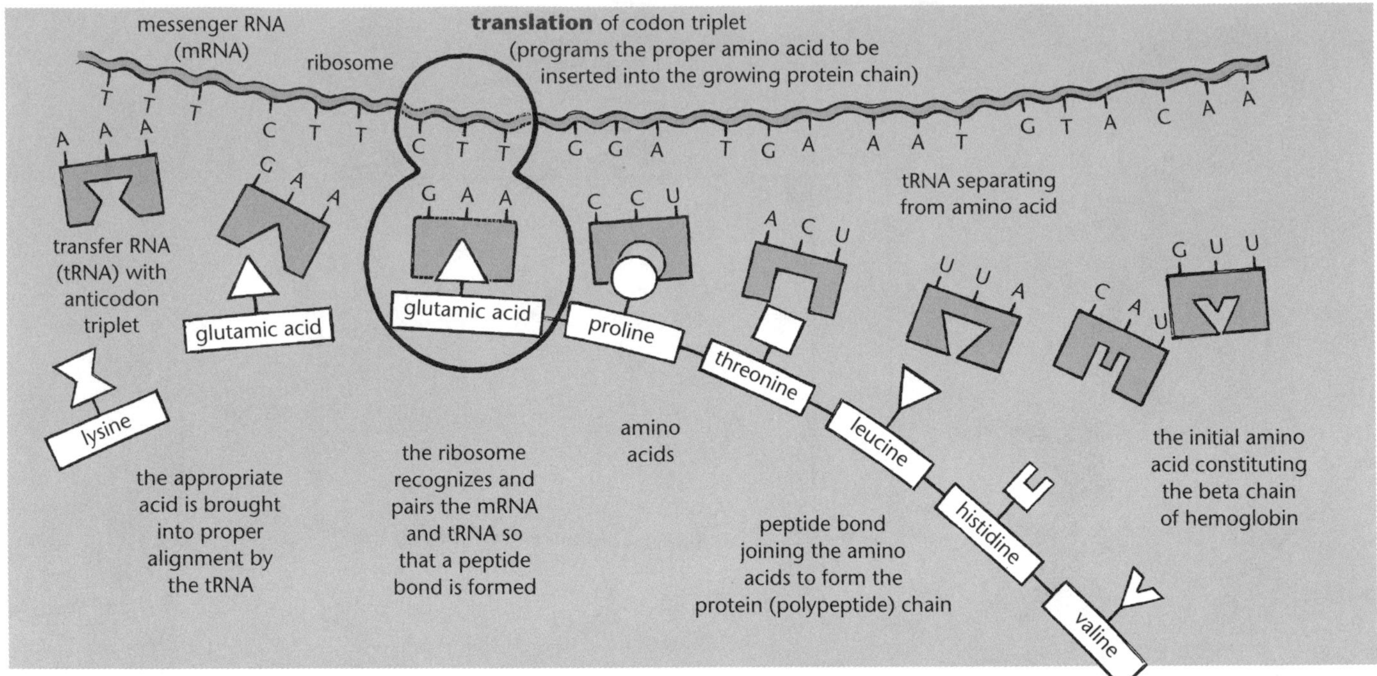
messenger RNA
(mRNA)
ribosome
translation of codon triplet
(programs the proper amino acid to be
inserted into the growing protein chain)
transfer RNA
(tRNA) with
anticodon
triplet
glutamic acid
glutamic acid
proline
threonine
leucine
histidine
valine
lysine
tRNA separating
from amino acid
amino
acids
the appropriate
acid is brought
into proper
alignment by
the tRNA
the ribosome
recognizes and
pairs the mRNA
and tRNA so
that a peptide
bond is formed
peptide bond
joining the amino
acids to form the
protein (polypeptide) chain
the initial amino
acid constituting
the beta chain
of hemoglobin

peritoneal oocyte and sperm t. (POST) Procedure in which oocytes and spermatozoa are transvaginally injected into the rectouterine pouch under ultrasound guidance.

tubal embryo t. (TET) The placement of 2- to 8-cell (cleaving) embryos in a fallopian (uterine) tube.

zygote intrafallopian t. (ZIFT) Procedure in which oocytes are fertilized *in vitro* and 24 hours later are transferred into the fallopian (uterine) tube.

transferase (trans´fer-ās) A class of enzymes that transfer a chemical group from one compound to another. Also called transferring enzyme.

transference (trans-fer´ens) **1.** The shifting of symptoms from one part of the body to another. **2.** In psychiatry, the unconscious shifting to others of feelings and attitudes that were originally experienced in significant early relationships.

transferrin (trans-fer´rin) Iron-binding beta globulin; it facilitates the transportation of iron to the bone marrow and tissue storage areas. Also called siderophilin.

transfer RNA (trans´fer ăr ĕn ā) A type of RNA (ribonucleic acid) that binds and transports amino acids to the ribosome; see under ribonucleic acid.

transfix (trans´fiks) **1.** To pierce through with a pointed instrument. **2.** To immobilize as with terror.

transformation (trans-for-ma´shun) **1.** In chemistry, a change of form or structural arrangement of atoms. **2.** In molecular biology, genetic changes incurred by a cell through incorporation of DNA from another species.

malignant t. The process by which a normal cell is converted into one that exhibits the four characteristics of cancer, i.e., a single cell that has undergone genetic changes and proliferates to form clones, unregulated growth, uncoordinated cell differentiation, and capacity for discontinuous growth and dissemination to other parts of the body.

transfusion (trans-fu´zhun) The introduction of a fluid, such as blood or plasma, into the bloodstream.

autologous blood t. (ABT) Transfusion of the patient's own blood, retrieved and antiseptically prepared, to maintain circulating blood volume subsequent to blood loss at surgery.

direct t. The transfer of blood directly from one person (donor) to another (recipient) without exposing it to air. Also called immediate transfusion.

exchange t. Removal of blood containing a toxic substance (e.g., removal of blood containing high levels of bilirubin from a newborn with erythroblastosis fetalis) coupled with blood replacement using donor blood. Also called substitution transfusion.

immediate t. See direct transfusion.

indirect t. Transfer of blood from a donor to a suitable container and thence to the recipient. Also called mediate transfusion.

intrauterine t. Exchange transfusion of the fetus within the uterus conducted by umbilical vein catheterization through the mother's abdominal wall under ultrasound guidance; performed to maintain an effective red blood cell mass within the fetal circulation and to maintain the pregnancy.

mediate t. See indirect transfusion.

reciprocal t. The transfer of blood from a person who has recovered from a contagious disease to a patient suffering with the same infection; an equal amount of blood is returned from the patient to the donor; used to confer passive immunity.

substitution t. See exchange transfusion.

transgene (trans´jēn) A gene introduced into a cell by transection.

transgenic (trans-jen´ik) In genetic engineering, containing genes that have been inserted from a set of chromosomes of another species.

transient (trans´shĕnt, trans´zē-ĕnt) Short-lived.

transiliac (trans-il´e-ak) Extending from one ilium to the other, as the transiliac diameter.

transillumination (trans-ĭ-lu-mĭ-na´shun) The examination of a body cavity by the passage of light through its walls; passage of light through a mass may indicate the presence of fluid, as in a cyst.

translation (trans-la´shun) Process by which the genetic data present in a messenger RNA (mRNA) molecule direct the order of the specific amino acids during protein synthesis.

translocation (trans-lo-ka´shun) The transfer (often reciprocal) of segments of one chromosome to another, nonhomologous, chromosome.

translucent (trans-lu´sent) Partially transparent; permitting light to pass through with sufficient diffusion to obliterate distinct images.

transluminal (trans-lu´mĭ-nal) Through a lumen (e.g., of a blood vessel).

transmethylase (trans-meth´ĭ-lās) See methyltransferase.

transmethylation (trans-meth-ĭ-la´shun) The process in which methyl groups are transferred to the precursors of methylated compounds (e.g., creatine, choline, and adrenaline).

transmigration (trans-mi-gra´shun) The normal passage of blood cells through the capillary walls.

transmissible (trans-mis´ĭ-bl) Capable of being passed from one person to another, as a disease.

transmission (trans-mish´un) **1.** Transfer (e.g., disease) from one person to another. **2.** Conveyance.

duplex t. Conveyance of impulses in both directions through one nerve trunk.

iatrogenic t. Transmission of infectious microorganisms through medical or dental interference (e.g., by contaminated instruments or equipment).

vertical t. Prenatal transmission from mother to child.

transmural (trans-mu´ral) Through or across a wall of a hollow organ or cyst.

transmutation (trans-mu-ta´shun) A change of a chemical element into another, resulting from radioactive decay or nuclear bombardment.

transpeptidase (trans-pep´tĭ-dās) Enzyme that promotes the transfer of an amino acid residue or a peptide residue from one amino compound to another.

transphenoidal (trans-fe-noi´dal) Through the sphenoid bone.

transphosphorylation (trans-fos-for-ĭ-la´shun) Chemical reaction in which a phosphate group is transferred from one organic phosphate to another.

transpiration (tran-spĭ-ra´shun) The passage of water or air through the skin or other tissue.

pulmonary t. The passage of water from the circulating blood into the airways within the lungs.

transpire (tran-spīr´) To give off moisture through the skin or mucous membrane.

transplacental (trans-plă-sen´tal) Denoting the movement of a substance through or across the placenta.

transplant (trans-plant´) **1.** To transfer from one part to another, as in grafting. **2.** The piece of tissue removed from the body for transplantation.

Gallie t. Narrow strip of fascia lata from the thigh, used as suture material.

transplantar (trans-plan´tar) Extending across the sole of the foot; denoting muscular or ligamentous structures.

transplantation (trans-plan-ta´shun) The transfer of tissue (graft) from one site to another.

bone marrow t. Infusion of bone marrow tissue, usually obtained from the donor's hipbone.

corneal t. See keratoplasty.

heart t. Replacement of a severely damaged heart with an entire organ from another person who has recently died.

heart-lung t. Transplantation of the heart and lungs as a unit.

heterotopic t. Transfer of tissue from one area of the body of the donor to another site in the recipient.

homotopic t. Orthotopic transplantation.

kidney t. The transplantation of a kidney from one individual to another; the kidney transplant is usually obtained from a living relative with the same blood type or from a cadaver. Also called renal transplantation.

liver t. Transplantation of a liver in cases of irreversible, progressive liver disease or to correct

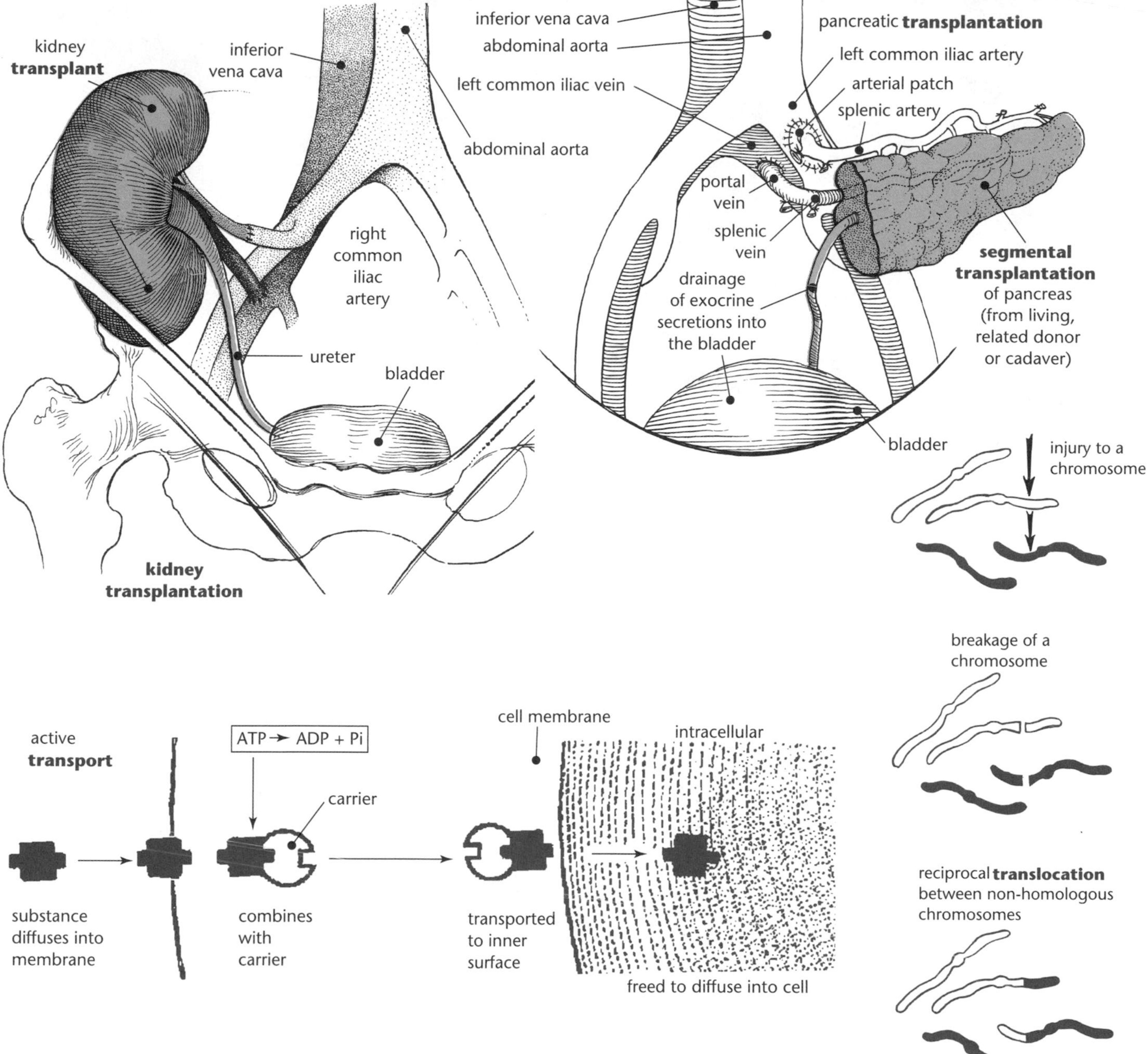

congenital enzyme deficiencies or inborn error of metabolism.

orthotopic t. Transfer of tissue from an area of the body of the donor to an identical recipient site.

renal t. See kidney transplantation.

segmental t. Transplantation of only a portion of an organ (e.g., of a pancreas or liver).

stem-cell t. Transplantation of stem cells, which may be autologous or allogeneic, for the treatment of certain disorders (e.g., sickle cell anemia, thalassemias, leukemias, and various immunodeficiencies).

syngeneic t. Transplantation of tissues between genetically identical or near-identical animals, such as identical twins or highly inbred animals.

syngenesioplastic t. The grafting of tissue to a recipient who is closely related to the donor, as from a mother to her child.

tendon t. The insertion of a slip from the tendon of a sound muscle into the tendon of a nonfunctioning (paralyzed) muscle.

tooth t. The insertion of a tooth or tooth germ into a dental alveolus.

xenogeneic t. Transplantation of tissue between two different species, such as the transplantation of a chimpanzee kidney into a human.

transport (trans´port) The conveyance of biochemical substances across cell membranes.

facilitated t. Movement of substances across cell membranes by a protein carrier without expending metabolic energy.

paracellular t. Movement of a substance in solution through the tight junctions between the cells of a layer of epithelium.

transcellular t. Movement of a substance in solution through the cells of a layer of epithelium.

transposition (trans-po-zish´un) **1.** The moving of tissues or structures from one place to another. **2.** The presence of an organ on the wrong side of the body.

transposon (tranz-po´zon) Any DNA sequence that may be transferred from one cell to another, resulting in rearrangement of the recipient cell's DNA.

transrectal (trans-rek´tal) Through the rectum (e.g., prostatic biopsy).

transseptal (trans-sep´tal) Across a septum, as the transseptal fibers of the periodontal membrane, which go from the cementum of one tooth across the bony septum to the cementum of the adjacent tooth.

transsexual (trans-seks´u-al) **1.** Relating to the surgical or hormonal intervention to alter an individual's external characteristics so that they resemble those of the opposite sex. **2.** Relating to transsexualism.

transsexualism (trans-seks´u-a-lizm) The overpowering desire to be of the opposite sex and desiring corrective surgery.

transsynaptic (trans-sĭ-nap´tik) Denoting the transmission of a nerve impulse across a synapse.

transthoracic (trans-tho-ras´ik) Across the chest or performed through the chest wall.

transtracheal (trans-tra´ke-al) Performed through the tracheal wall.

transudate (trans´u-dāt) A fluid that passes through a membrane, such as a capillary wall, as a result of differences in hydrostatic pressure.

transudation (trans-u-da´shun) The passage of a fluid through a membrane, as when parts of the plasma pass through the capillary walls into the tissue spaces; it differs from osmosis in that the fluid passes with most of the substances held in solution or suspension.

transurethral (trans-u-re´thral) Via or through the urethra.

transvaginal (trans-vaj´ĭ-nal) Through the vagina.

transverse (trans-vers´) Crosswise.

transversion (trans-ver´zhun) **1.** The eruption of a tooth in the wrong place or order. **2.** In genetics, mutation in which a purine is substituted for a pyrimidine, or vice versa.

transvestism (trans-ves´tiz-m) The persistent desire and practice of dressing in clothing of the opposite sex; especially by a male and usually for sexual gratification. Also called cross-dressing.

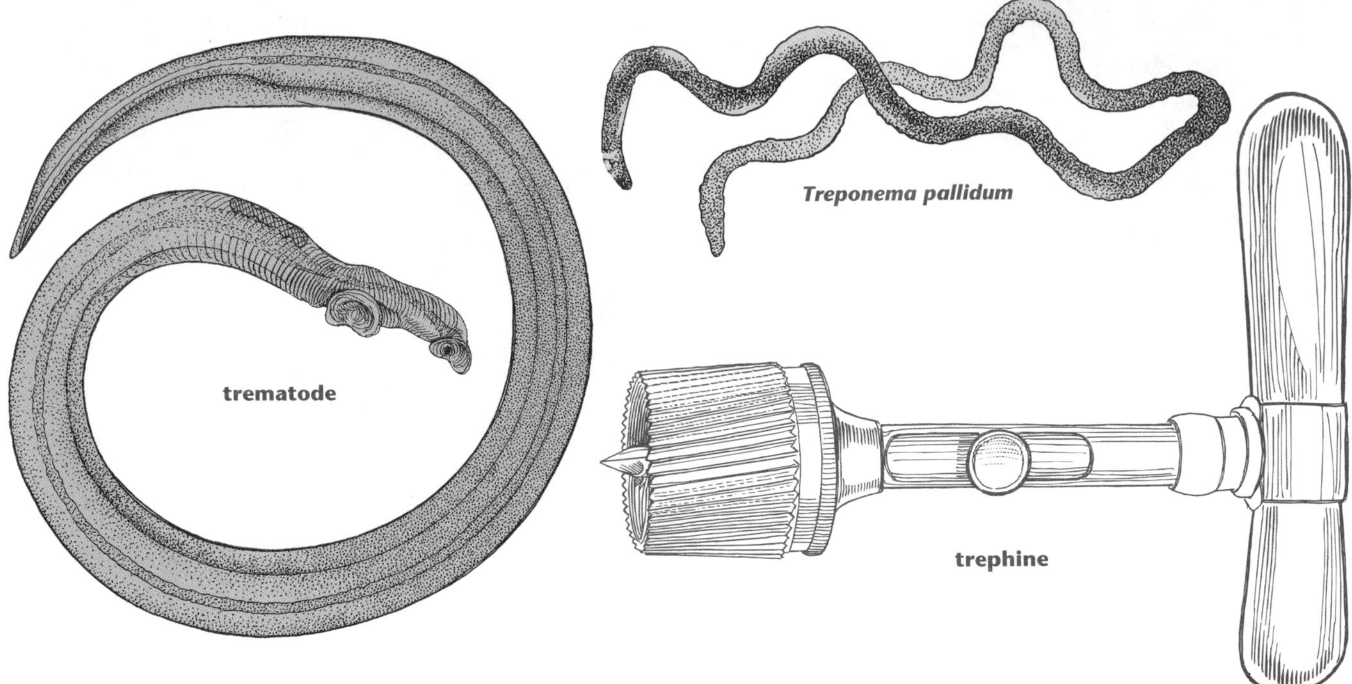

transvestite (trans-ves´tīt) An individual who practices transvestism.

trapezium (tră-pe´ze-um) Name given to certain anatomic structures generally having a four-sided shape with no parallel sides. See table of bones.

trauma (trou´mă, traw´mă) Injury or damage, physical or mental.

cumulative t. Damage to tissues by repetitive minor injuries, which would not otherwise cause significant damage. Also called cumulative injury.

occlusal t. Abnormal stresses and resulting pathologic changes on a tooth and surrounding tissues, caused by improper alignment of the teeth.

psychic t. A painful emotional experience.

t. X Colloquialism for the physical signs of child abuse.

traumatic (trou-mat´ik) Caused by, or related to, injury.

traumatize (trou´mă-tīz) To injure or wound either physically or psychologically.

traumatogenic (trou-mă-to-jen´ik) Capable of causing injury or a wound.

traumatologist (trou-mă-tol´ŏ-jist) A physician with special knowledge in traumatology.

traumatology (trou-mă-tol´ŏ-je) A surgical subspecialty concerned with the care and treatment of victims of violence or accidents.

tray (tra) A flat, shallow receptacle with raised edges used for carrying or holding various items.

acrylic resin t. In dentistry, a custom-made impression tray of autopolymerizing acrylic resin for the individual patient.

impression t. In dentistry, a metallic or acrylic receptacle consisting of a flanged body and a handle for use in carrying impression material to the mouth and holding it in position against the teeth or oral tissues while the material sets.

surgical t. A tray for holding instruments in the operating room during a surgical operation.

Treacher Collins' syndrome (tre´cher kol´inz sin´drōm) See mandibulofacial dysostosis, under dysostosis.

treadmill (tred´mil) A moving belt mechanism that permits individuals to walk or run in a stationary location under controlled conditions; used in studies of physiologic functions, particularly cardiac stress testing.

treat (trēt) To give medical aid to an individual by medicinal, surgical, dietary, or other measures.

treatment (trēt´ment) The course of action adopted to care for a patient or to prevent disease.

breast conservation t. See segmental mastectomy, under mastectomy.

conservative t. Treatment in which any radical therapeutic or surgical measures are avoided.

drug t. Treatment with medicines.

electroconvulsive t. (ECT) See electroconvulsive therapy, under therapy.

electroshock t. (EST) See electroconvulsive therapy, under therapy.

empirical t. Treatment based on experience rather than scientific data.

expectant t. Treatment aimed at the relief of symptoms until the nature of the illness is known. Also called symptomatic treatment.

futile t. Treatment that has no apparent therapeutic benefit.

heroic t. The use of aggressive measures to preserve the life of the patient.

maintenance t. Treatment aimed at stabilizing the patient's condition, especially when no cure is available.

medical t. **1.** Treatment that employs medicines rather than surgical procedures. **2.** Treatment rendered by medical personnel.

megavitamin t. The use of huge doses (megadoses) of vitamins in treating disorders, such as the use of vitamin B_3 (nicotinic acid) for the treatment of schizophrenia. Also called orthomolecular treatment.

orthomolecular t. See megavitamin treatment.

palliative t. Treatment aimed at mitigating symptoms rather than curing the disease.

preventive t., prophylactic t. Treatment instituted to prevent a person from acquiring a disease after exposure to the disease, or when expected to be exposed.

root canal t. Removal of the pulp of a tooth followed by obliteration of the root canal.

shock t. See electroconvulsive therapy, under therapy.

supportive t., supporting t. Treatment aimed at maintaining the patient's strength.

surgical t. Treatment by any cutting operation.

symptomatic t. See expectant treatment.

Trematoda (trem-ă-to´dă) A class of flatworms (including flukes) of the phylum Platyhelminthes; parasitic in humans and animals.

trematode, trematoid (trem´ă-tōd, trem´ă-toyd) **1.** A member of the class Trematoda; a fluke. **2.** Relating to a fluke.

tremens (tre´mens) See delirium tremens, under delirium.

tremor (trem´or, tre´mor) Rhythmic, involuntary, alternating contraction of opposing muscle groups; fairly uniform in frequency and amplitude.

coarse t. Tremor in which muscle contractions are slow (4 to 5 per second) and of large amplitude.

essential t. A fine tremor, especially of the extremities, occurring during voluntary movement or when limbs are outstretched; tremor disappears when limbs are relaxed; occurs in several members of the same family; inherited as an autosomal dominant inheritance. It is not associated with disease. Also called heredofamilial tremor.

fine t. Tremor characterized by rapid muscle vibrations (10 to 12 per second).

flapping t. See asterixis.

heredofamilial t. See essential tremor.

intention t. Tremor that is induced or intensified by a voluntary movement.

pill-rolling t. The rubbing of index finger and thumb together as if rolling a small object, as seen in parkinsonism. Also called coin-counting.

postural t. See static tremor.

resting t. Rhythmic movements, usually of the hands and forearms, occurring when the limbs are relaxed and disappearing with voluntary motion. Seen in Parkinson's disease.

static t. A coarse rhythmic tremor occurring when the person tries to hold a limb in a certain position. Also called postural tremor.

tremulous (trem´u-lus) Quivering, trembling.

Trendelenburg's sign (tren-del´en-bergz sīn) See Trendelenburg's test, under test.

trepanation (trep-ă-na´shun) See trephination.

trephination (tref-ĭ-na´shun) Removal of a circular piece of skull with a trephine. Also called trepanation.

trephine (trĕ-fīn´, trĕ-fēn´) A cylindrical saw for cutting a circular piece of bone or other tissue (e.g., the cornea).

trephining (trĕ-fīn-ing) The cutting of a circular portion of tissue with a trephine.

Treponema (trep-o-ne´mă) A genus (family Treponemataceae) of spiral bacteria; several species cause disease.

T. pallidum The cause of syphilis in man.

T. pertenue The cause of yaws.

treponeme (trep´o-nēm) An organism of the genus *Treponema*.

treponemiasis (trep-o-ne-mi´ă-sis) Infection with bacteria of the genus *Treponema*.

triad (tri´ad) A group of three closely related structures, signs, or symptoms.

adrenomedullary t. The symptoms produced by excessive activation of the adrenal medulla: tachycardia, vasoconstriction, and perspiration.

Charcot's t. (a) Fever, pain in the right upper area of the abdomen, and jaundice; usually seen in bile duct inflammation. (b) Nystagmus, tremor, and scanning speech, seen (rarely) in advanced stages of multiple sclerosis.

hepatic portal t. A triad at the angle of the liver lobule, consisting of a branch of the portal vein, a

T

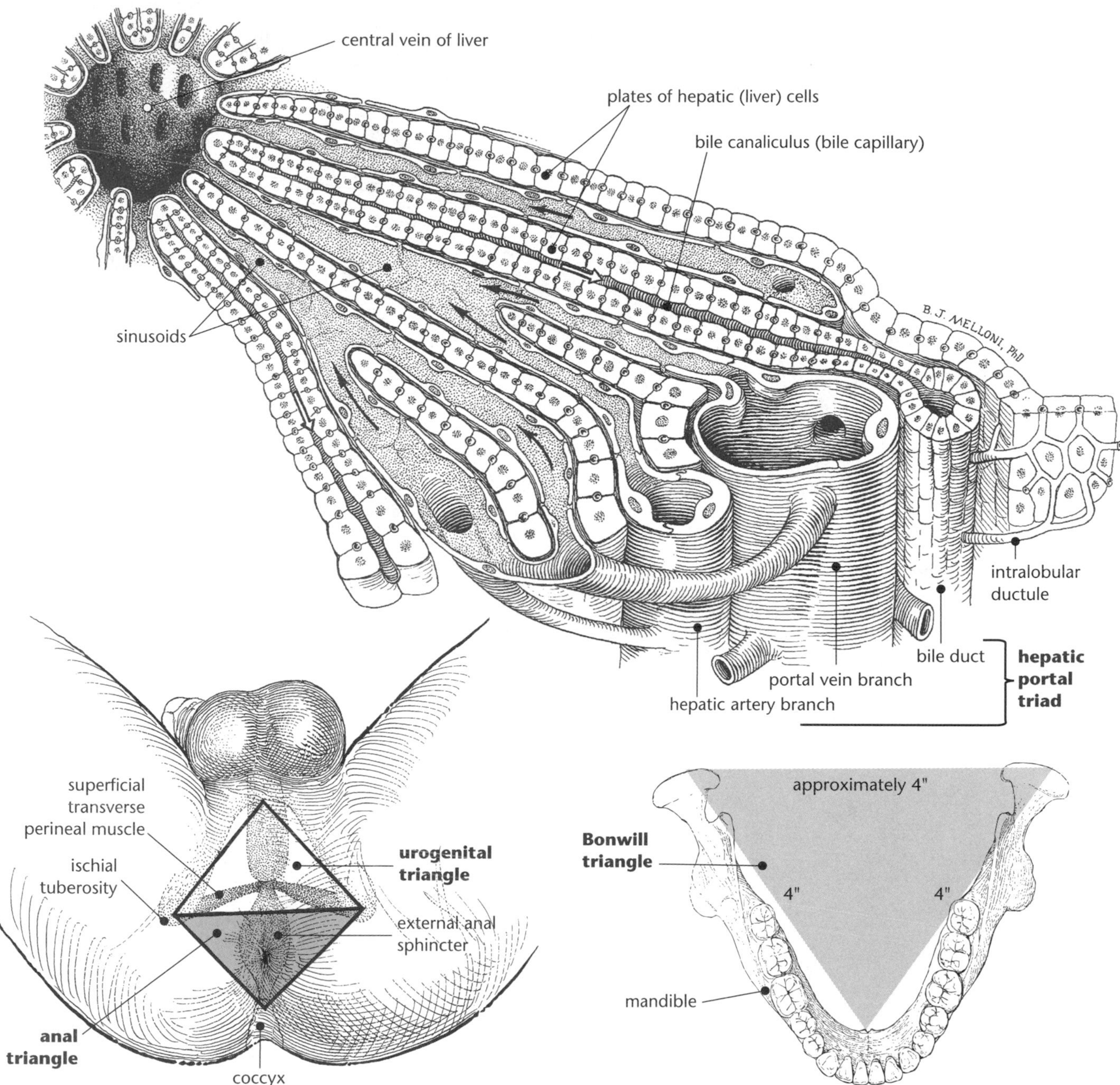

branch of the hepatic artery, and an interlobular bile ductule.

Hutchinson's t. Parenchymatous keratitis, labyrinthine disease, and Hutchinson's teeth, seen in congenital syphilis.

t. of Luciani Manifestations of cerebellar disease: weakness (astenia), lack of normal tone (atony), and inability to stand (astasia).

Saint's t. Hiatal hernia, diverticulosis, and gallstones.

triage (tre-ahzh´) The sorting of patients (as in a battlefield) to determine their priority for treatment.

trial (tri´ăl) An experiment or exploratory activity.

blind t. A trial in which either the experimenter or the subject does not know to which group the subject has been assigned (e.g., whether a patient is in the group receiving a medication or the one receiving a placebo). Also called blind experiment; blind study.

clinical t. Controlled study on human volunteers for the safety, efficacy, or optimal dosage (if appropriate) of a diagnostic, therapeutic, or prophylactic drug, device, or technique; the subjects are selected according to predetermined criteria and observed for predefined evidence of both favorable and unfavorable effects; in some trials one treatment modality may be compared with another for efficacy and side effects.

double-blind t. A trial in which both investigator and subject do not know which group of subjects is exposed to the variable (e.g., a drug) being tested. Also called double-blind experiment; double-blind study.

triamcinolone (tri-am-sin´o-lōn) A white crystalline powder, $C_{21}H_{27}FO_6$, used as an anti-inflammatory agent.

triamterene (tri-am´ter-ēn) A drug that acts directly on renal tubules, producing sodium loss with potassium retention; when used in combination with thiazides, it enhances their hypotensive and diuretic effects; used to reduce edema associated with congestive heart failure, hepatic cirrhosis, and the nephrotic syndrome; Dyrenium®.

triangle (tri´ang-gl) A figure or area formed by connecting three points with straight lines; a three-cornered area.

Alsberg's t. A triangular space formed by a line through the long axis of the femoral neck, a second through the center of the diaphysis, and a third transversely at the level of the base of the femoral head.

anal t. A triangular space with the angles placed at both ischial tuberosities and at the tip of the coccyx.

anterior cervical t. A triangular area in the neck, bounded by the mandible, the sternocleidomastoid muscle, and the midline of the neck.

t. of auscultation Space bounded by the lower border of the trapezius muscle, the latissimus dorsi muscle, and the vertebral border of the scapula.

axillary t. The triangular area formed by the inner aspects of the arm, the axilla, and the pectoral region.

Bonwill t. An equilateral triangle with the angles placed at the center of each mandibular condyle and at the mesial contact areas of the mandibular central incisors.

Bryant's t. A triangle whose base is from the anterior-superior iliac spine to the top of the greater trochanter; its sides are formed, respectively, by a horizontal line from the anterior-superior iliac spine and a vertical line from the top of the greater trochanter.

Calot's t. See cystohepatic triangle.

carotid t. The triangle of the neck, bounded above by the stylohyoid muscle and posterior belly of the digastric muscle, behind by the sternocleidomastoid muscle, and below by the omohyoid muscle.

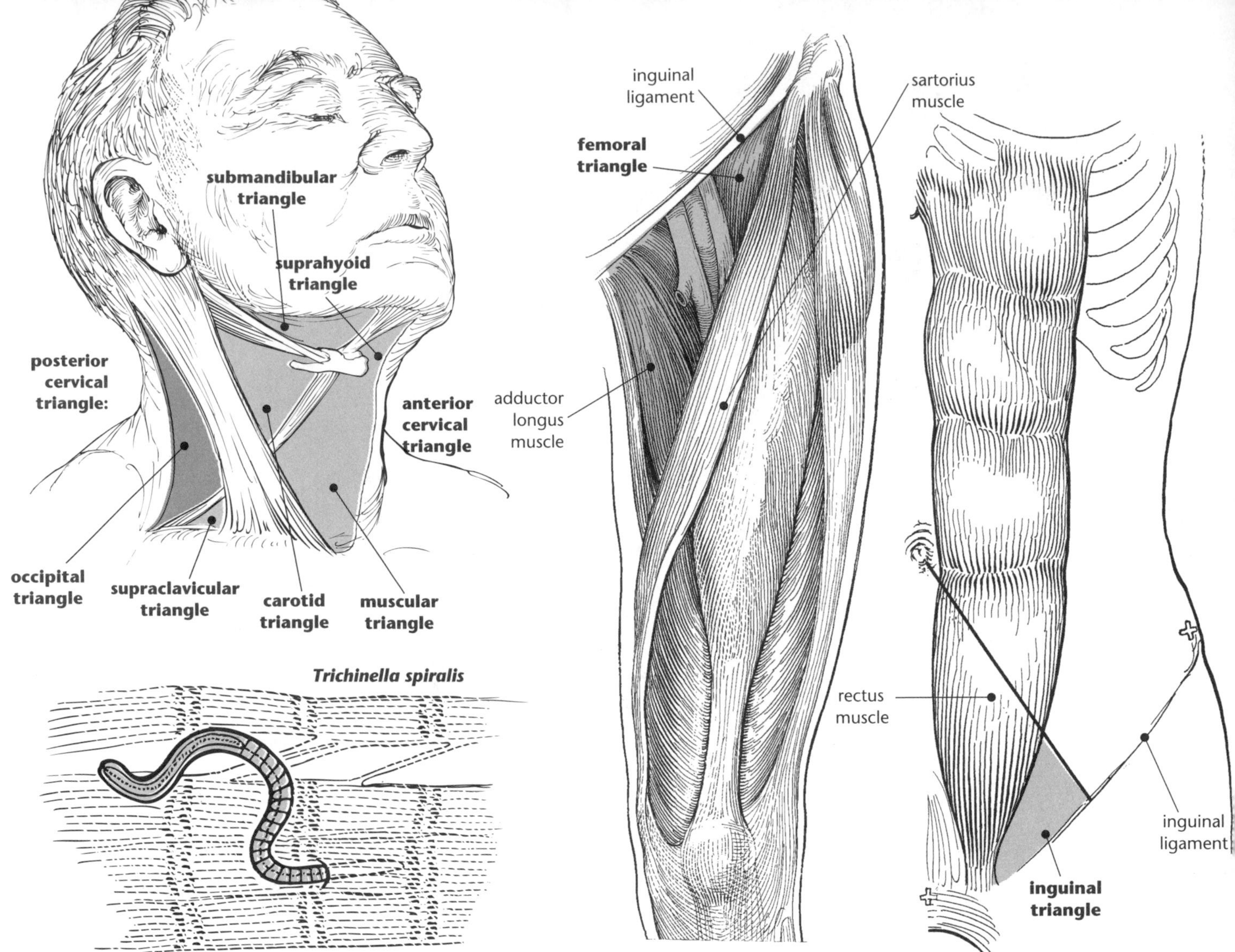

crural t. The triangular area formed by the inner aspect of the thigh and the lower abdominal, inguinal, and genital regions, with the base traversing the umbilicus.

cystohepatic t. The triangular area formed by the liver, the cystic duct, and the hepatic duct. Also called Calot's triangle.

Einthoven t. An imaginary equilateral triangle surrounding the heart, formed by lines representing the three standard limb leads of the electrocardiogram.

femoral t. A triangular space at the upper and inner part of the thigh, bounded by the sartorius and adductor longus muscles and the inguinal ligament; it is divided into two nearly equal parts by the femoral vessels. Also called Scarpa's triangle.

Hesselbach's t. See inguinal triangle.

inguinal t. A triangular area formed by the medial half of the inguinal ligament, the lateral edge of the abdominal rectus, and a line midway between the anterior-superior iliac spine and the pubic symphysis to the umbilicus; important area relating to inguinal hernia. Also called Hesselbach's triangle.

lumbar t. An area bounded by the edges of the latissimus dorsi and external oblique muscles and the crest of the ilium. Also called lumbar triangle of Petit.

lumbar t. of Petit See lumbar triangle.

muscular t. Triangle limited anteriorly by the median line of the neck from the hyoid bone to the sternum and posteriorly (above) by the superior belly of the omohyoid muscle and (below) by the anterior margin of the sternocleidomastoid muscle.

occipital t. The triangular area of the posterior neck formed by the sternocleidomastoid, trapezius, and omohyoid muscles; the larger division of the posterior triangle.

olfactory t. See olfactory trigone, under trigone.

omoclavicular t. See subclavian triangle.

posterior cervical t. A triangular area of the neck formed by the sternocleidomastoid muscle, the anterior margin of the trapezius muscle, and the middle third of the clavicle.

Scarpa's t. See femoral triangle.

subclavian t. The triangular area of the lower neck formed by the inferior belly of the omohyoid muscle, the clavicle, and the posterior border of the sternocleidomastoid muscle; the smaller division of the posterior triangle. Also called omoclavicular triangle.

submandibular t. The triangular area formed by the mandible, the stylohyoid muscle and posterior belly of the digastric muscle, and the anterior belly of the digastric muscle; it contains the submandibular gland.

submental t. See suprahyoid triangle.

suprahyoid t. Region bounded laterally by the anterior belly of the digastric muscle, medially by the middle of the neck from the hyoid bone to the mental symphysis, and inferiorly by the body of the hyoid bone. Also called submental triangle.

urogenital t. A triangular space with the angles placed at both ischial tuberosities and at the pubic symphysis.

vesical t. A triangular area in the bladder formed by the internal orifice of the urethra and the two orifices of the ureters. Also called trigonum vesicae.

triatomic (tri-ă-tom´ik) **1.** Denoting a molecule made up of three atoms. **2.** Possessing three replaceable atoms or radicals.

tribasic (tri-ba´sik) Denoting a molecule with three replaceable hydrogen atoms; denoting an acid with a basicity of three.

tribe (trīb) A taxonomic classification ranking just below the family, above the genus.

triceps (tri´seps) Having three sites of origin (e.g., the triceps muscle). See table of muscles.

trichatrophy, trichatrophia (tri-kă-tro´fe, tri-kă-tro´fī-ă) Atrophy of the hair bulbs, causing hair loss.

trichiasis (trĭ-ki´ă-sis) Inversion of hairs about an orifice (e.g., as eyelashes that turn in, causing irritation of the cornea).

trichina (trĭ-ki´nă) A larval worm of the genus *Trichinella*.

Trichinella (trik-ĭ-nel´ă) A genus of nematode parasites in the aphasmid group, i.e., those lacking postanal phasmids (chemoreceptors); the cause of trichinosis in humans.

T. spiralis An off-white, cylindroid worm about 1.5 mm in length; found coiled in a cyst in the striated muscle of various infected mammals, including humans. Also called trichina worm; pork worm.

trichiniasis, trichinelliasis (trik-ĭ-ni´ă-sis, trik-ĭ-nel-li´ă-sis) See trichinosis.

trichinosis (trik-ĭ-no´sis) A disease caused by the parasite *Trichinella spiralis*, usually ingested with raw meat, especially infested pork; the parasites become lodged in muscle, producing muscular stiffness and painful swelling, accompanied by nausea, diarrhea, fever, and sometimes prostration. Also called trichiniasis; trichinelliasis.

trichloroethylene (tri-klo-ro-eth´ĭ-lēn) A sweet-smelling, nonflammable, volatile liquid with potent analgesic properties; used primarily as an analgesic in minor diagnostic surgical procedures and in obstetrics and dentistry; Trilene®.

trichloromethane (tri-klo-ro-meth´ān) Chloroform.

trichobezoar (trik-o-be´zōr) A compact mass of hair in the intestinal tract, frequently occurring in cats.

trichoclasia, trichoclasis (trik-o-kla´zhă, trik-

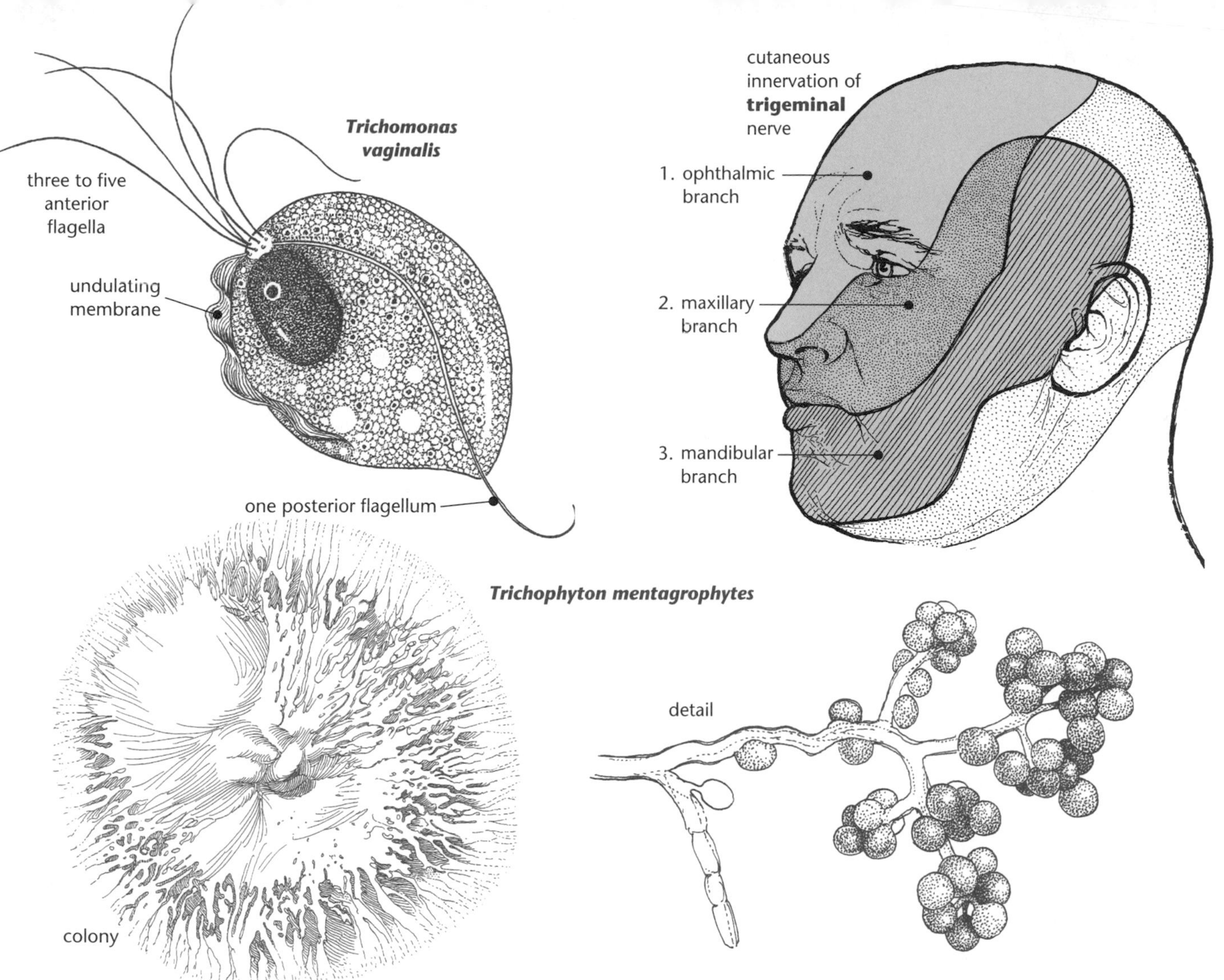

ok'lă-sis) Brittleness and eventual breakage of hair, as in monilethrix and trichorrhexis nodosa.

trichocryptosis (trik-o-krip-to´sis) **1.** Ingrown hairs. **2.** Any disease of the hair follicles.

trichocyst (trik'o-sist) One of the minute elongated cysts, arranged radially around the periphery of certain protozoans, capable of ejecting a bristle-like extension.

trichoepithelioma (trik-o-ep-ĭ-the-le-o´mă) A benign skin tumor originating in hair follicles; usually occurs on the face.

trichoesthesia (trik-o-es-the´zhă) The sensation felt when one of the hairs of the skin is touched.

trichogen (trik'o-jen) Anything that stimulates hair growth.

trichoglossia (trik-o-glos´e-ă) See black tongue, under tongue.

trichoid (trik'oid) Resembling hair.

trichologia (trik-o-lo´jă) Compulsive plucking of the hair.

trichology (tri-kol'ŏ-je) The scientific study of hair; its anatomy, growth, and diseases.

Trichomonas (trik-o-mo'nas) A genus of parasitic protozoan flagellates (class Mastigophora); some species have three to five anterior flagella, a posterior flagellum, and an undulating membrane.

T. vaginalis Species found in the vagina and in the male genital tract; the cause of trichomoniasis, a sexually transmitted disease (STD).

trichomoniasis (trik-o-mo-ni´ă-sis) Infection of the genital tract with *Trichomonas vaginalis* almost always acquired through sexual intercourse; in females, it usually causes varying degrees of vulvar and vaginal irritation and itching, profuse vaginal discharge, and inflammation of the vaginal epithelium. Infected males are usually asymptomatic; a few experience urethritis, prostate enlargement, and epididymitis; the organism can be detected following prostatic massage.

trichomycosis (trik-o-mi-ko'sis) Any infection of the hair with an organism that is an intermediate between a fungus and a bacterium.

t. axillaris Infection of the axillary (and occasionally pubic) hair with *Corynebacterium tenuis*; it affects the cortex of the hair, but not the roots or surrounding skin, and occurs in persons past puberty. Formerly thought to be a fungal infection.

trichonodosis (trik-o-no-do'sis) A hair condition characterized by knots or bulges; results from inability of new hairs to grow naturally from their follicles. Also called beaded hair.

trichopathy (trĭ-kop'ă-the) Any disease of hair.

trichophobia (trik-o-fo'be-ă) **1.** A morbid revulsion at the sight of loose hair on the clothing or elsewhere. **2.** An unwarranted fear of hair growth in excess of that considered normal for the area, or (especially) on the face of women.

trichophytobezoar (trik-o-fi-to-be´zōr) A hard ball composed of hair and vegetable fibers sometimes found in the stomach of humans and animals.

Trichophyton (tri-kof'ĭ-ton) A genus of pathogenic ringworm fungi (order Moniliales) possessing hyaline single-celled spores; parasitic in the skin, nails, and hair follicles of humans and some animals.

T. mentagrophytes A superficial dermatophyte that causes ectothrix infections of scalp and beard hair (hyphae grow within and on the surface of hair shafts), and also of skin and nails; microconidia are numerous and occur in clusters at the ends of hyphae or singly alongside hyphae.

T. rubrum A fungus with violet pigmentation of aerial mycelium; the cause of superficial infections in skin and nails.

T. schonleini A fungus that causes favus, a severe form of chronic ringworm of the scalp, with destruction of hair follicles and permanent loss of hair in the infected area; in culture, the hyphae resemble reindeer horns and are sometimes referred to as favic chandeliers.

T. tonsurans A yellowish fungus causing a seborrhea-like ringworm infection of hair; the hyphae grow only within the hair shaft, causing it to break at the scalp surface, leaving stubble that looks like black dots (black dot fungus).

trichophytosis (trik-o-fi-to'sis) A fungal infection caused by species of *Trichophyton*. See also tinea.

trichorrhea (trik-o-re'ă) Abnormal shedding of hair.

trichorrhexis (trik-o-rek´sis) Condition in which the hair breaks easily.

t. nodosa Nodular appearance of the hairs of the scalp, beard, and pubic area caused by transverse breakage of the shaft's cortex with subsequent longitudinal splitting into fine strands.

trichosis (tri-ko'sis) Any disease of the hair.

Trichosporon (tri-kos'po-ron) A genus of fungi that are the normal inhabitants of the skin and intestinal and respiratory tracts; some may cause disease in debilitated patients.

T. beigelii Pathogenic species causing white piedra or trichosporosis.

trichosporosis (trik-o-spo-ro´sis) Any mycotic infection of the hair caused by a pathogenic *Trichosporon*.

trichostasis spinulosa (trĭ-kos´tă-sis spin-u-lo'sa) A common condition in which the hair follicle opening contains a dark plug of from 10 to 50 short fine hairs in a horny mass; usually seen in persons with acne and seborrheic dermatitis.

Trichostrongylus (trik-o-stron'jĭ-lus) A genus of worms (class Nematoda) that are intestinal parasites of herbivorous animals; they infest man only rarely and accidentally.

trichotillomania (trik-o-til-o-ma'ne-ă) A compulsion to pull out or pluck one's own hair.

trichuriasis (trik-u-ri´ă-sis) Infestation of the intestine with the whipworm *Trichuris trichiura*.

Trichuris (trik-u'ris) A genus of worms of the class

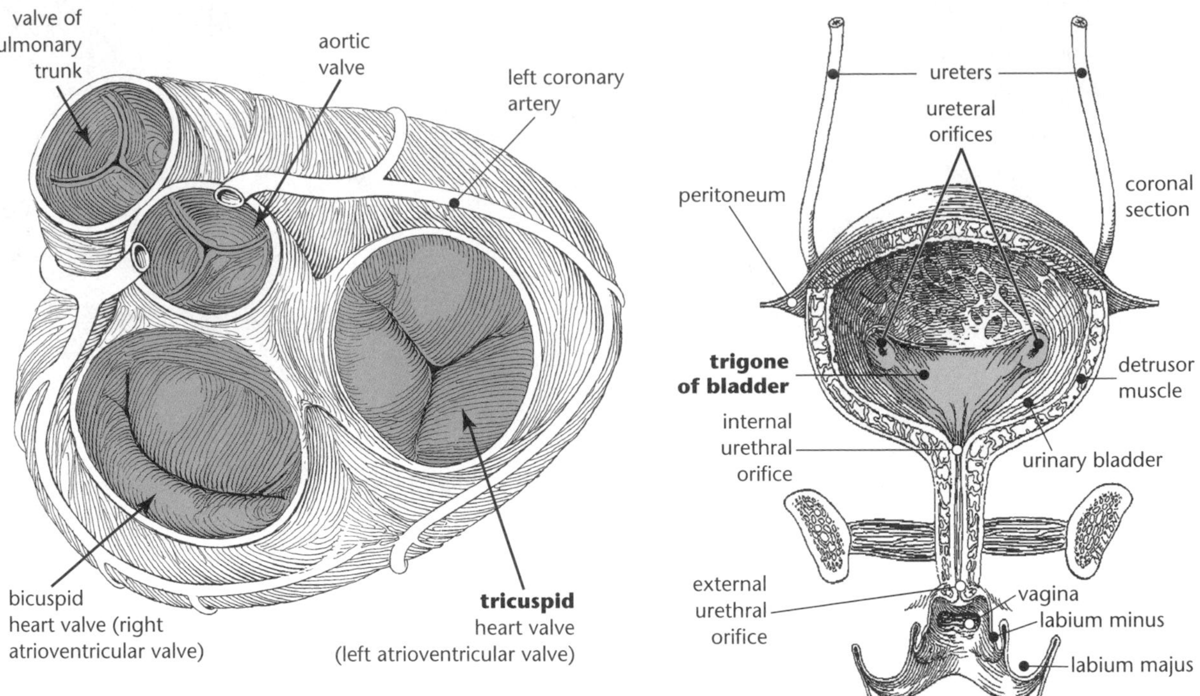

Nematoda.

T. trichiura An intestinal parasite of humans; the anterior three-fifths of the worm is whiplike, the posterior two-fifths is thicker; eggs are brownish and lemon-shaped with pluglike translucent polar prominences; infection is acquired by direct finger-to-mouth contact or by ingestion of food, water, or soil containing larvae. Also called whipworm.

tricuspid (tri-kus´pid) Having three cusps or points, applied to a valve in the heart or a tooth.

tricyclic (tri-si´klik) Possessing three rings in the molecular structure; refers to one or more of a class of antidepressant drugs, such as imipramine, amitriptyline, and doxepin hydrochloride.

triethylene glycol (tri-eth´ĭ-lēn gli´kol) A compound, $C_6H_{14}O_4$, used as an air disinfectant.

triethylenemelamine (tri-eth-ĭ-lēn-mel´ă-mēn) (TEM) A crystalline compound, $C_3N_3(NC_2H_4)_3$, used in the treatment of leukemia.

trifocal (tri-fo´kal) Having three focal lengths.

trifoliate (tri-fo´le-āt) Having three leaflike parts.

trifurcation (tri-fur-ka´shun) Division into three branches or portions, as seen in the area of maxillary molars where the roots divide into three distinct portions.

trigastric (tri-gas´trik) Denoting a muscle with three bellies.

trigeminal (tri-jem´ĭ-nal) **1.** Triple. **2.** Denoting the fifth cranial nerve.

trigeminy (tri-jem´ĭ-ne) A disturbance of the cardiac rhythm in which two premature beats follow each normal beat, or two normal beats are followed by a premature beat. Also called trigeminal rhythm.

T

triglyceride (tri-glis´er-īd) (TG) The most important of three groups of neutral fats; the basic unit consists of a molecule of glycerol in an ester bond with three molecules of fatty acid; it serves as the major storage form of fatty acids and is practically the exclusive constituent of adipose tissue.

trigonal (tri´go-nal) **1.** Relating to a trigone. **2.** Triangular.

trigone (tri´gōn) Triangle; a triangular space, eminence, or fossa.

t. of bladder A triangular, smooth area at the base of the bladder, whose apices are the openings of the ureters and the internal urethral orifice; in this area the mucosa is closely adherent to the muscular layer or the bladder wall. Also called vesical trigone.

collateral t. A somewhat triangular dilatation of the lateral ventricle of the brain between the posterior and descending horns.

fibrous t.'s The two somewhat triangular masses of fibrous tissue that lie between the aortic arterial ring and the right and left atrioventricular rings.

habenular t. A depressed triangular area of the brain between the habenula and the thalamus, rostral to the superior colliculus on each side.

interpeduncular t. The fossa at the base of the brain between the two cerebral peduncles.

olfactory t. The small grayish triangular eminence just above the optic nerve near the chiasm, forming the posterior extremity of the olfactory tract, where it diverges into three roots.

vesical t. See trigone of bladder.

trigonitis (trig-o-ni´tis) Inflammation of the urinary bladder, localized in the mucous membrane of the trigone; it usually follows an uncomplicated course and in most instances responds well to antibacterial agents.

trihydrate (tri-hi´drāt) Compound with three molecules of water.

trihydric (tri-hi´drik) Having three replaceable hydrogen atoms.

triiodothyronine (tri-i-o-do-thi´ro-nēn) (T_3) One of the two principal hormones secreted by the thyroid gland (the other being thyroxine); it aids in regulating the body's metabolism. Also called liothyronine.

reverse t. reverse T3 (rT_3) A product of the peripheral degradation of thyroxine; present in elevated levels in certain disease states; useful as an aid for diagnosis of fetal and infantile hypothyroidism.

trilaminar (tri-lam´ĭ-nar) Composed of three layers.

trill (tril) In speech, a sound produced by the vibration of a fluttering speech organ, most often the tongue; it causes a succession of closures and openings of the oral passage.

trilogy (tril´o-je) A group of three related symptoms.

t. of Fallot The combination of atrial septal defect, pulmonary stenosis, and ventricular hypertrophy.

trimer (tri´mer) A compound or complex made up of three units.

trimester (tri-mes´ter) A period of three months.

first t. The period of pregnancy from the first day of the last menstrual period before conception to the 98th day; the first 14 weeks of gestation.

second t. The term of pregnancy from the 15th through the 28th week of gestation.

third t. The term of pregnancy from the 29th through the 42nd week of gestation.

trimethoprim (tri-meth´o-prim) An antibacterial compound used, usually in conjunction with a sulfonamide, in the treatment of infections of the urinary tract, shigellosis, otitis media, and respiratory tract infections including those with *Pneumocystis carinii.*

trimethylene (tri-meth´ĭ-lēn) See cyclopropane.

trimorphous (tri-mor´fus) Occurring in three forms.

trinitroglycerin (tri-ni-tro-glis´er-in) See nitroglycerin.

trinitrophenol (tri-ni-tro-fe´nol) See picric acid.

trinitrotoluene (tri-ni-tro-tol´u-ēn) (TNT) Explosive obtained by nitrating toluene.

triolein (tri-o´le-in, tri-o´lēn) See olein.

triose (tri´ōs) A three-carbon sugar; a monosaccharide containing three carbon atoms in the molecule (e.g., glyceraldehyde, dihydroxyacetone); represents the smallest carbohydrate molecule.

trip (trip) Term used by drug abusers meaning (a) to take a narcotic or a hallucinogenic drug; (b) the effects produced by such drugs.

acid t. A hallucinatory experience following ingestion of LSD (acid).

ego t. Anything done to boost one's self-esteem.

tripe (trīp) The muscular wall of the stomach of cattle, used as food.

tripeptidase (tri-pep´tĭ-dās) Any of a class of enzymes of different specificities that promote the hydrolysis of tripeptides, producing a dipeptide and an amino acid.

tripeptide (tri-pep´tid) Compound composed of three amino acids linked by peptide bonds.

triphosphopyridine nucleotide (tri-fos-fo-pir´ĭ-dēn noo´kle-o-tid) (TPN) Old term for nicotinamide-adenine dinucleotide phosphate (NADP).

triplet (trip´let) **1.** One of three individuals born at one birth. **2.** Three lenses cemented or mounted together as a single lens system to correct aberration. **3.** Three consecutive premature contractions of the heart. **4.** In molecular biology, a unit of three successive bases in DNA or RNA coding for a specific amino acid.

triploblastic (trip-lo-blas´tik) Containing tissue derived from all three embryonic layers.

triploid (trip´loid) A cell having three haploid sets of chromosomes in its nucleus.

triplopia (trip-lo´pe-ă) Visual defect in which one object is perceived as three instead of one.

tripoli (trip´o-le) A mild abrasive derived from certain porous rocks, suspended in a greaselike medium; used in dentistry for finishing dental restorations.

triradius (tri-ra´de-us) In dermatoglyphics, a point from which the dermal ridges course in three directions.

trisaccharide (tri-sak´ă-rid) A carbohydrate with three monosaccharides in its molecule that upon hydrolysis yields three simple sugars (e.g., raffinose).

tris(hydroxymethyl)aminomethane (tris-hi-drok-se-meth-il-am-ĭ-no-meth´ān) (Tris) A buffer used in biologic preparations for *in vitro* studies, as with enzymes.

trismus (triz´mus) Difficulty in opening the mouth due to tonic spasm of the muscles of mastication;

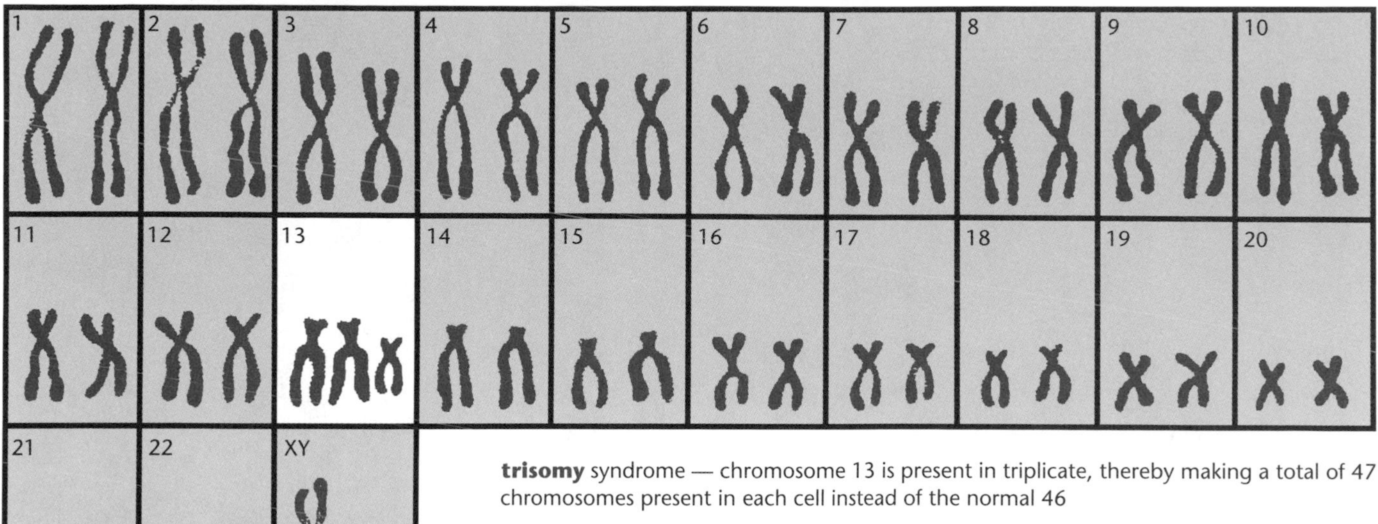

trisomy syndrome — chromosome 13 is present in triplicate, thereby making a total of 47 chromosomes present in each cell instead of the normal 46

karyotype of a male with **trisomy** syndrome

usually the first symptom of tetanus. Also called lockjaw.

trisomic (tri-so′mik) Denoting a cell or an individual having an extra chromosome.

trisomy (tri′so-me) Abnormality in which an additional chromosome is present in the cells (i.e., 47 instead of 46); the extra chromosome is a copy of one of an existing pair, so that one particular chromosome is present in triplicate. The consequences of trisomy can range from early fetal death and spontaneous abortion to numerous abnormalities in the live-born child.

trisomy 8 syndrome Mental retardation, short stature, congenital heart disease, and urinary tract anomalies.

trisomy 9 syndrome Mental retardation, congenital heart disease, and urinary tract anomalies.

trisomy 13 syndrome Cleft lip and palate, extra fingers or toes, abnormalities of the heart, abdominal organs, and genitalia and defects of the central nervous system associated with mental retardation; the extra chromosome (the 13th) is a member of the D group. Also called trisomy D; Patau syndrome.

trisomy 18 syndrome The presence of chromosome 18 (group E) in triplicate rather than duplicate; characterized by mental retardation, skull deformities, abnormally small chin, low set ears, webbed neck, deafness, heart defects, and Meckel's diverticulum. Also called trisomy 18; Edwards' syndrome.

trisomy 21 syndrome See Down syndrome.

trisomy 22 syndrome Mental and growth retardation; abnormally small head (microcephaly) and jaws (micrognathia), congenital heart disease, cleft palate, and deformed thumbs and lower extremities.

tritanopia (tri-tă-no′pe-ă) Inability to perceive the color blue and reduced ability to perceive its combined forms (bluegreens and greens), except the violets; congenital tritanopia is rare; it occurs usually as a result of disease or detachment of the retina. Also called blue blindness.

tritium (trit′e-um) See hydrogen-3.

triturable (trich′ūr-ă-bl) Having the capability of being triturated.

trituratio (trich-ūr-ra′she-o) (trit) Latin for triturate.

trituration (trich-ūr-a′shun) **1.** The process of reducing a solid to a fine powder by continuous rubbing, as in the reduction of a drug to a fine powder (usually mixed thoroughly with milk sugar). **2.** In dentistry, the mixing of amalgam alloy either by itself or with mercury.

triturium (trich-ūr-e′um) A device used to separate immiscible liquids by virtue of their different densities.

trivalent (tri-va′lent) Denoting an atom or radical with a valence of three.

trocar (tro′kar) A sharp-pointed metal rod, used in a metal tube (cannula) for piercing the wall of a body cavity, after which it is withdrawn, leaving the cannula in place to permit evacuation of the fluid from the cavity.

trochanter (tro-kan′ter) One of two prominences (major and minor) on the upper part of the femur.

troche (tro′kē) See lozenge.

trochlea (trok′le-ă) Any pulley-like structure, especially the fibrous loop in the orbital cavity through which passes the tendon of the superior oblique muscle of the eyeball.

trochlear (trok′le-ar) **1.** Relating to a trochlea or pulley. **2.** Denoting the trochlear (4th cranial) nerve. See table of nerves.

Trombicula (trom-bik′u-lă) A genus of mites (family Trombiculidae) whose larvae can infest humans.

T. akamushi The kedani mite, a parasite of rodents; vector of rickettsial diseases.

T. alfreddugesi A chigger; the larvae are human parasites, causing intensely irritating itching due to the injection of secretions into the skin.

trombiculiasis (trom-bik-u-li′ă-sis) Infestation with mites of the genus *Trombicula.* Also called trombiculosis.

Trombiculidae (trom-bik′u-li-de) A family of mites whose six-legged larvae (chiggers, red bugs, scrub mites, etc.) are parasitic on vertebrates, causing an irritating rash.

trophic (trof′ik) Relating to nutrition.

trophoblast (trof′o-blast) The outer layer of cells forming the wall of the blastocyst; it differentiates into two layers (cytotrophoblast and syncytiotrophoblast) at the time of attachment to the uterus and eventually enters into formation of the placenta, but not the embryo.

trophoblastoma (trof-o-blast-o′mă) See choriocarcinoma.

trophoneurosis (trof-o-nōō-ro′sis) Alteration of any tissue due to interruption of nerve supply to the part.

facial t. See facial hemiatrophy, under hemiatrophy.

trophopathy, trophopathia (tro-fop′ă-the, trof-o-path′e-ă) Any disorder of nutrition.

trophotropism (tro-fo-tro′piz-m) Movement of living cells toward or away from nutritive material.

trophozoite (trof-o-zo′īt) The young, ameboid, undivided stage of a sporozoan organism, such as the malarial parasite, after it has been transmitted to man; the younger forms are ring-shaped; they eventually mature to form schizonts (the adult forms).

tropia (tro′pe-ă) Deviation of the eyes from their normal position. See also strabismus.

tropine (tro′pin) A poisonous alkaloid, 3α-tropanol; the major constituent of atropine and scopolamine, from which it is derived on hydrolysis; it possesses a tobacco odor and has medicinal value.

tropism (tro′piz-m) Tendency for parts of a living organism (e.g., leaves) to turn toward or away from a stimulus.

tropocollagen (tro-po-kol′ă-jen) The fundamental unit of collagen fibrils consisting of symmetric molecules with three helically arranged polypeptide chains.

tropoelastin (tro-po-e-las′tin) A precursor to elastin.

tropometer (tro-pom′ĕ-ter) **1.** A device for measuring the degree of rotation of the eyeball. **2.** A device for measuring the torsion of the shaft of a long bone.

tropomyosin B (tro-po-mi′o-sin bē) A fibrous protein concentrated in the Z line of muscle that can be extracted from dry powdered muscle; it has a different molecular weight from myosin.

troponin (tro′po-nin) One of the protein components of muscle; it has an affinity for calcium and participates in regulation of muscle contraction. Elevated levels in the blood are found early after damage to cardiac muscle, as in a heart attack.

trough (trof) **1.** A narrow shallow depression. **2.** The minimum serum concentration of a drug (administered at regular intervals); used in monitoring of therapeutic drugs to ascertain that a minimum affective level of the drug is present at all times.

Trousseau's sign (troo-sōz′ sīn) Muscular spasm of the hand elicited by compression of the upper arm (as with a blood pressure cuff); a sign of latent tetany.

Trousseau's syndrome (troo-sōz′ sin′drōm) See migratory thrombophlebitis, under thrombophlebitis.

truncal (trun′kal) Relating to the trunk of the body or to any main branch.

truncate (trun′kāt) Cut at right angles to the main axis.

truncus (trun′kus) Latin for trunk or stem.

t. arteriosus The main arterial trunk of the embryonic heart that gives rise to the aortic and pulmonary arteries.

persistent t. arteriosus Congenital cardiovascular defect due to failure of the pulmonary trunk and aorta to separate during embryonic development; it results in a single blood vessel that takes origin astride a ventricular septal defect, receiving blood from both right and left ventricles.

trunk (trungk) **1.** The human body excluding the head and the extremities. Also called torso. **2.** The main part, usually short, of a nerve or vessel before its division. **3.** The main axis. **4.** A large collection

T

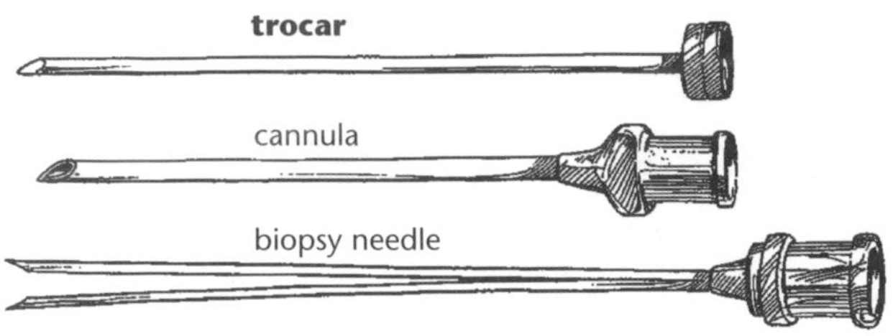

trocar
cannula
biopsy needle

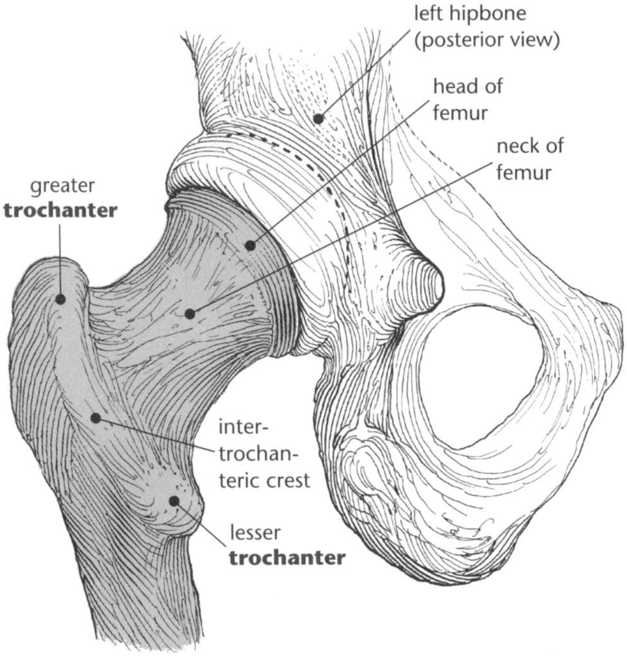

left hipbone (posterior view)
head of femur
neck of femur
greater **trochanter**
inter-trochan-teric crest
lesser **trochanter**

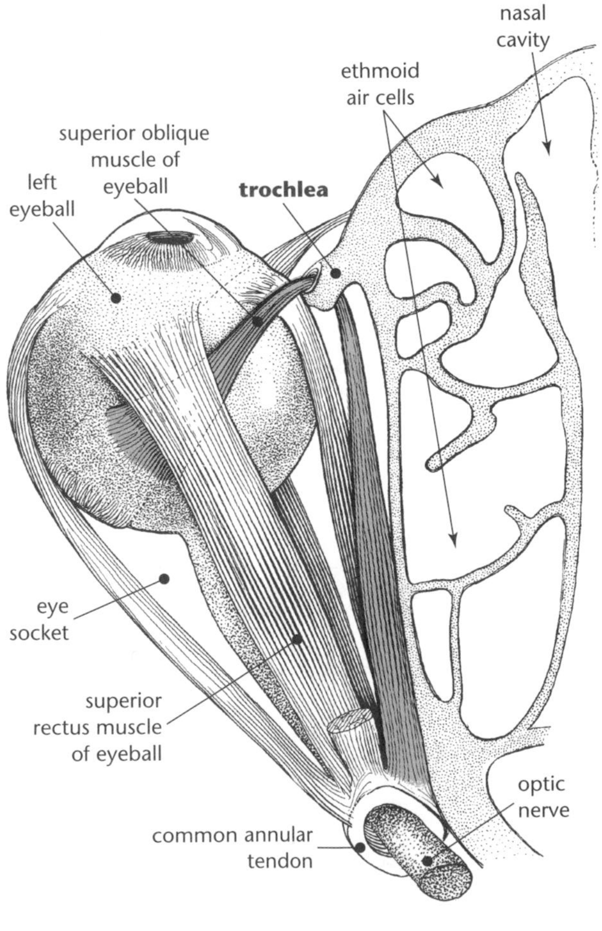

nasal cavity
ethmoid air cells
superior oblique muscle of eyeball
left eyeball
trochlea
eye socket
superior rectus muscle of eyeball
optic nerve
common annular tendon

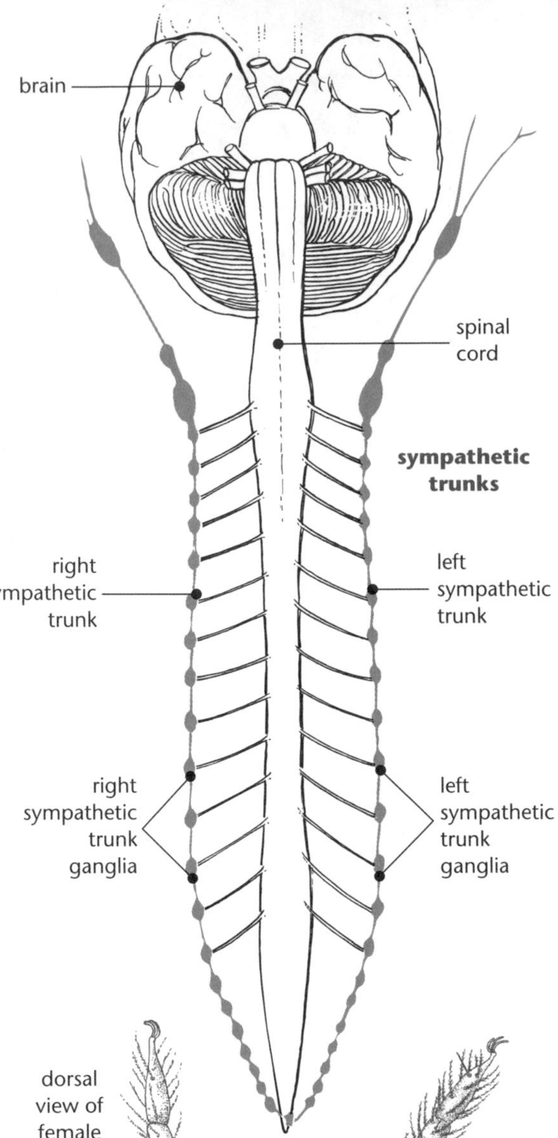

brain
spinal cord
sympathetic trunks
right sympathetic trunk
left sympathetic trunk
right sympathetic trunk ganglia
left sympathetic trunk ganglia

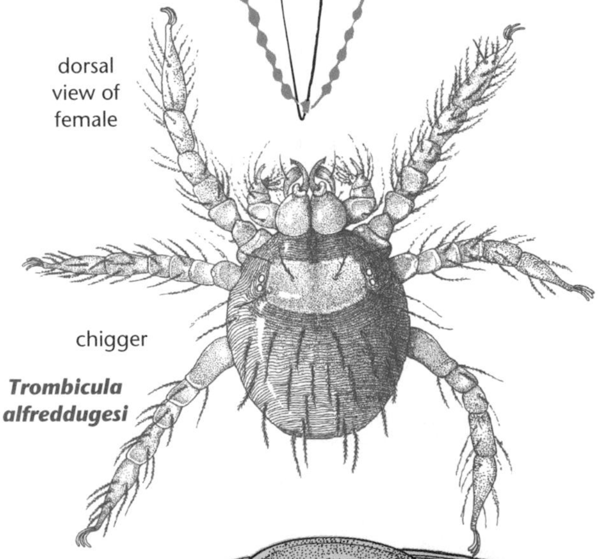

dorsal view of female
chigger
Trombicula alfreddugesi

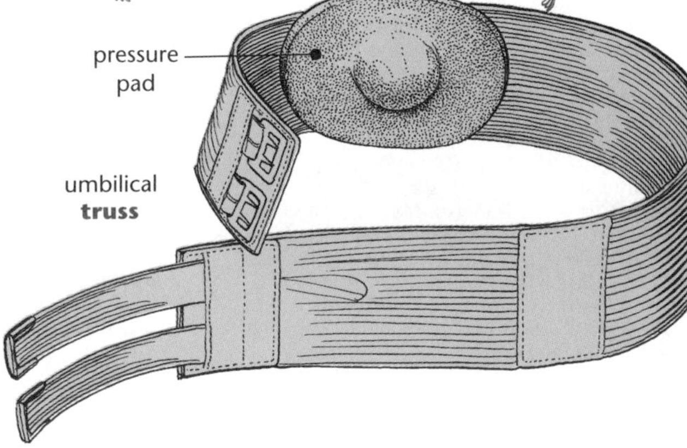

pressure pad
umbilical **truss**

T

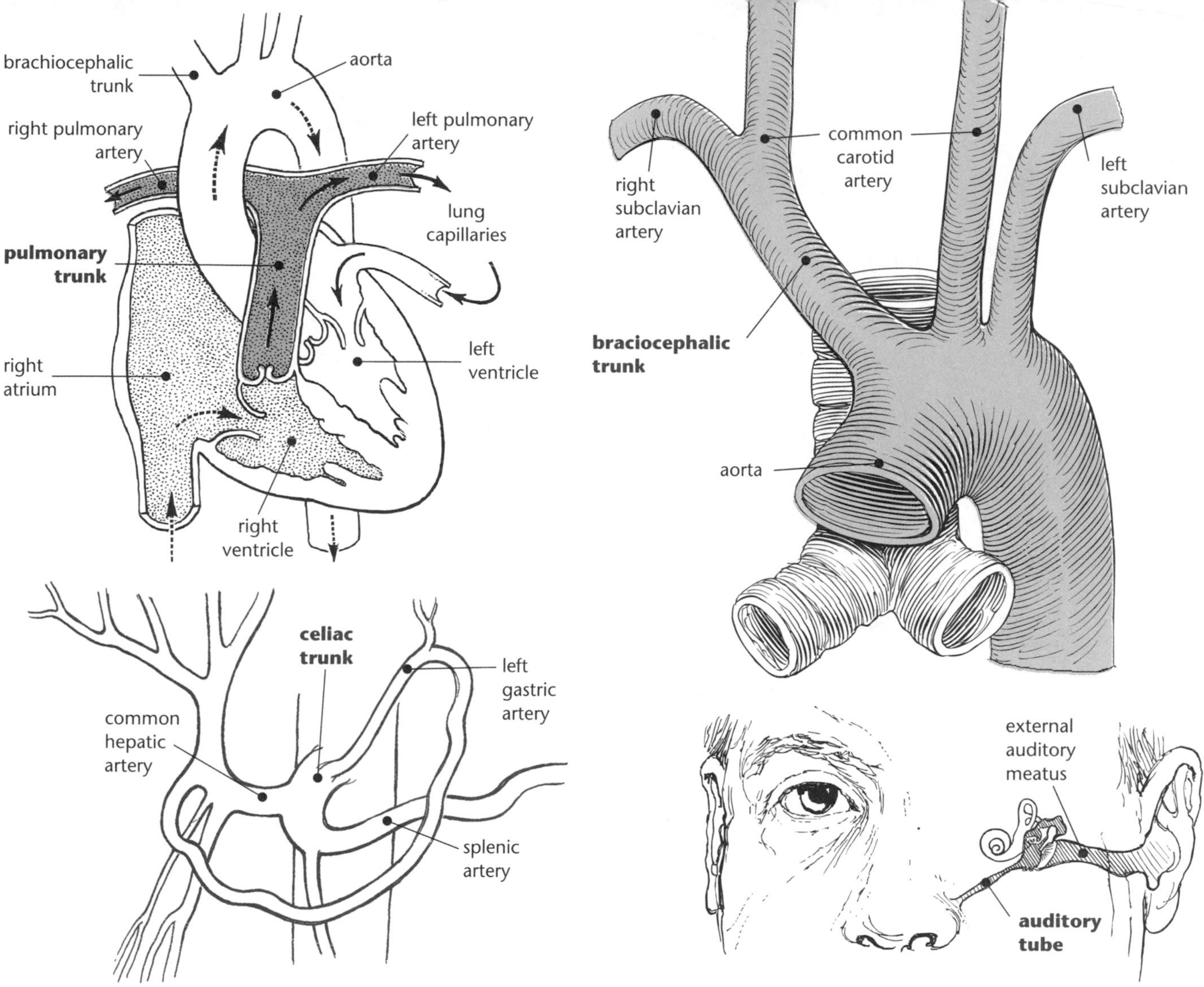

of lymphatic vessels.

brachial plexus t.'s The three trunks of the brachial plexus. See table of nerves.

brachiocephalic t. The large artery coming off the aortic arch that divides into the right subclavian and right common carotid arteries.

celiac t. The large artery arising from the abdominal aorta just below the diaphragm; it divides into the left gastric, common hepatic, and splenic arteries.

intestinal lymphatic t. A short lymphatic vessel that drains lymph from the gastrointestinal tract and empties into the cisterna chyli.

lumbar lymphatic t's Two large collecting lymphatic vessels, right and left, that drain lymph upward from the lumbar lymph nodes to the cisterna chyli.

lumbosacral t. A large nerve formed by the union of the smaller part of the fourth and the entire fifth lumbar nerves; it enters into the formation of the sacral plexus.

pulmonary t. A great vessel, about 5 cm in length and 3 cm in diameter, that arises from the base of the right ventricle of the heart and divides into right and left pulmonary arteries; it conveys unoxygenated blood from the heart to the lungs.

root t. The part of the multirooted posterior tooth situated between the cervical line and the points of bifurcation or trifurcation of the tooth.

sympathetic t.'s Two long chains of sympathetic ganglia on either side of the vertebral column extending from the base of the skull to the coccyx.

truss (trus) A device consisting of a belt and a pressure pad, used to retain a hernia in place after reduction or to prevent the increase in size of an irreducible hernia.

Trypanosoma (tri-pan-o-so´mă) A genus of parasitic protozoan flagellates (family Trypanosomidae), some of which are pathogenic.

T. brucei gambiense A subspecies causing Gambian or West African trypanosomiasis (African sleeping sickness), transmitted by tsetse flies, especially *Glossina palpalis*. Also called *Trypanosoma gambiense*.

T. brucei rhodesiense Subspecies causing Rhodesian trypanosomiasis, transmitted by tsetse flies, especially *Glossina morsitans*. Also called *Trypanosoma rhodesiense*.

T. cruzi The species that causes Chagas' disease; endemic in Central and South America, especially in Brazil, Chile, Argentina, and Venezuela; found also in vectors in California, Arizona, and Texas.

T. gambiense See *Trypanosoma brucei gambiense*.

T. rhodesiense See *Trypanosoma brucei rhodesiense*.

trypanosomiasis (tri-pan-o-so-mi´ă-sis) Any disease caused by infection with a protozoan parasite of the genus *Trypanosoma*; transmitted by the bite of the tsetse fly or by contamination of the bite wound of the kissing bug.

African t. Disease of the central nervous system occurring in two forms: Gambian, a chronic disease causing sleeping sickness and ending in death in approximately two years; and Rhodesian, an acute febrile form that is usually fatal within one year. Also called African sleeping sickness.

American t. See Chagas' disease.

trypsin (trip´sin) One of the protein-splitting (proteolytic) enzymes in the pancreatic juice derived from trypsinogen.

trypsinogen, trypsogen (trip-sin´o-jen, trip´so-jen) A substance secreted by the pancreas and converted, in the intestine, into trypsin by the enzyme enterokinase.

tryptic (trip´tik) Relating to the proteolytic enzyme trypsin.

tryptophan (trip´to-fān) (Trp) An essential amino acid present in varying quantities in common proteins; deficiency may result in the development of pellagra.

tsutsugamushi disease (soot-soo-gă-mu´shĭ dĭ-zēz´) Infectious disease occurring in Southeast Asia; caused by *Rickettsia tsutsugamushi* and transmitted by mites; characterized by painful swelling of the lymphatic glands, fever, headache, eruption of dark red papules with blackish scabs on the genitals. Also called mite-borne typhus; scrub typhus; tropical typhus; island fever; tsutsugamushi fever; Japanese river fever.

tubal (too´bal) Relating to a tube, especially a uterine tube.

tube (tōōb) **1.** A hollow cylinder. **2.** A channel or canal.

auditory t. A channel connecting the cavity of the middle ear with the upper part of the throat (nasopharynx); it equalizes the pressure in the middle ear chamber with the atmospheric pressure. Also called eustachian tube.

Cantor t. A 3.3 m rubber tube with a mercury-filled bag at the extreme end, used for intestinal intubation; it is usually introduced via the nose and directed into the stomach; with proper positioning of the patient, the weight of the mercury bag helps to lead the tube through the pyloric sphincter and into the small intestine beyond.

cathode ray t. (CRT) A vacuum tube containing a filament that, when a low-voltage electric current is passed through it, becomes incandescent and produces a beam of electrons.

Chaoul t. A low-voltage x-ray tube used for superficial x-ray therapy; designed so the anode can be placed close to the patient's body, thereby permitting intense but superficial tissue penetration of an x-ray beam.

Coolidge t. A hot-cathode x-ray tube that develops its electrons from a heated filament.

T

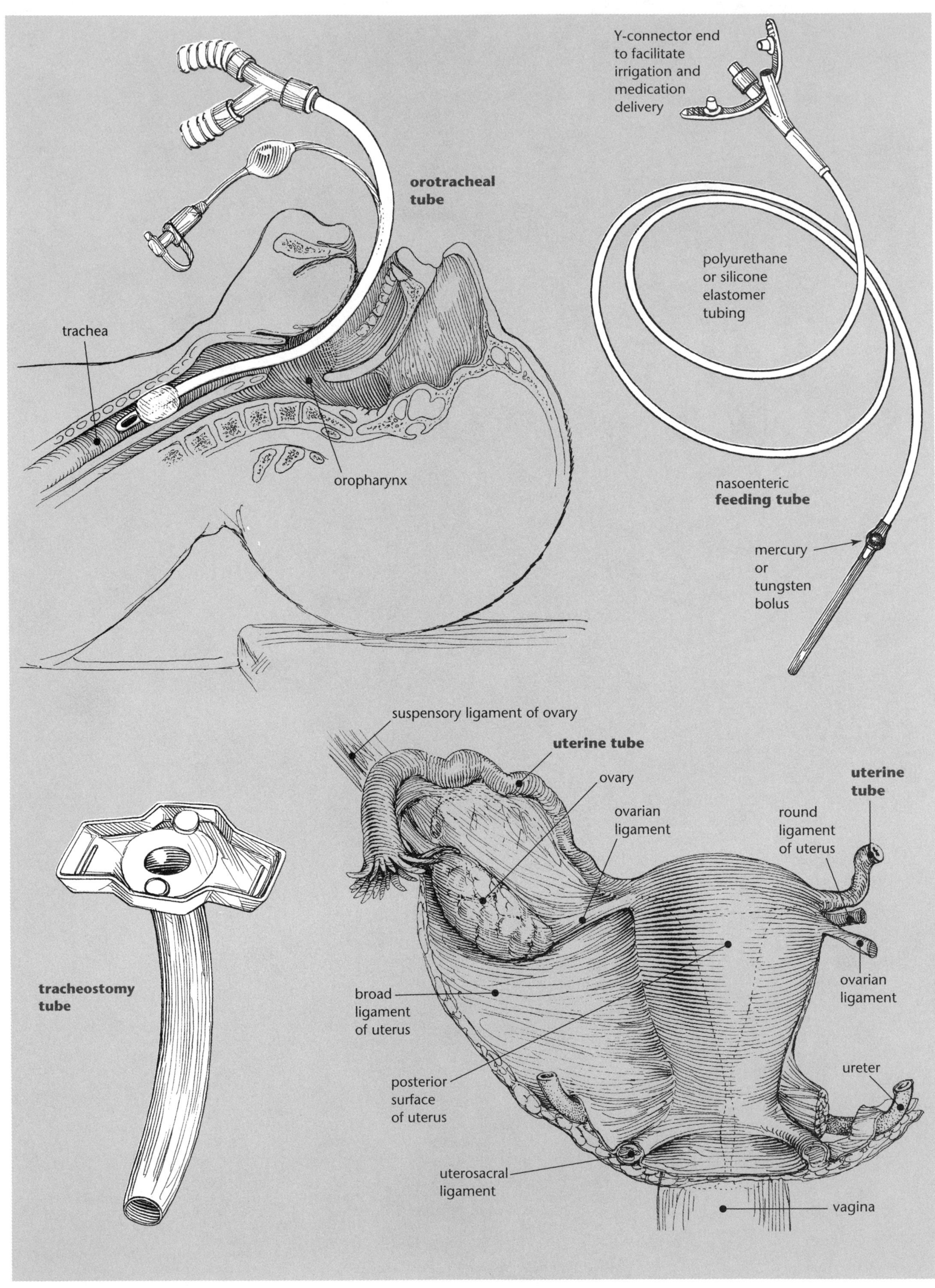
Y-connector end
to facilitate
irrigation and
medication
delivery
orotracheal
tube
polyurethane
or silicone
elastomer
tubing
trachea
oropharynx
nasoenteric
feeding tube
mercury
or
tungsten
bolus
suspensory ligament of ovary
uterine tube
ovary
ovarian
ligament
uterine
tube
round
ligament
of uterus
ovarian
ligament
tracheostomy
tube
broad
ligament
of uterus
posterior
surface
of uterus
ureter
uterosacral
ligament
vagina
T

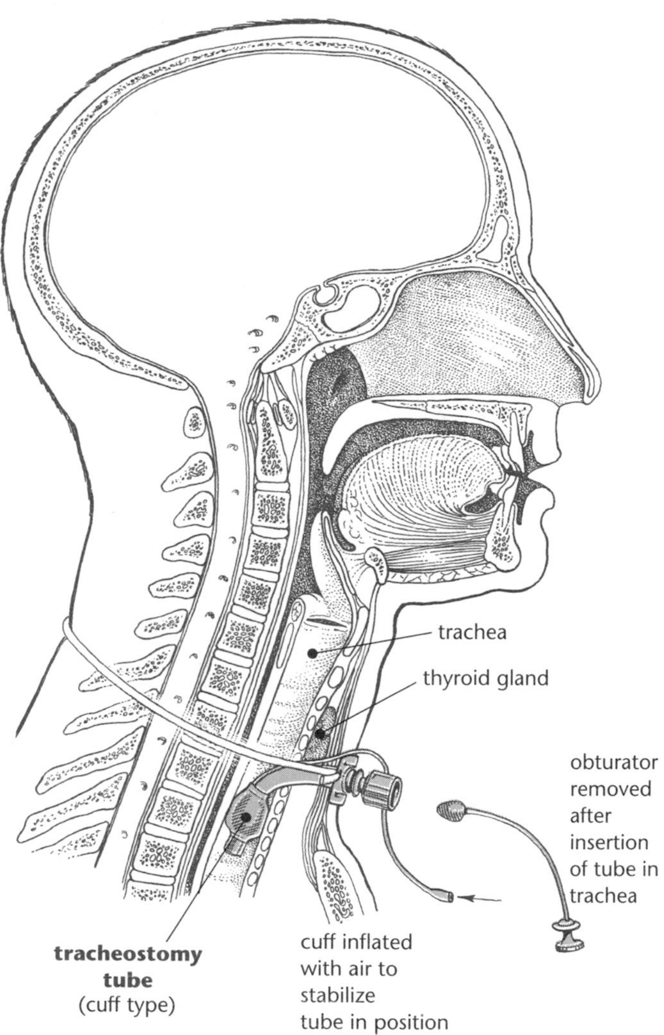

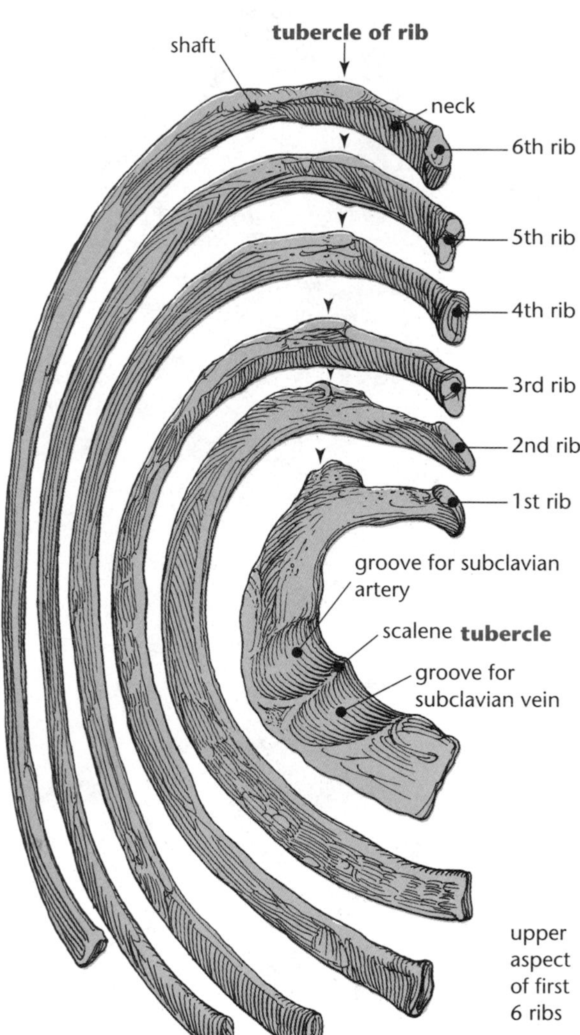

Dominici t. A tube that allows the passage of only beta and gamma rays; used for the therapeutic application of radium.

drainage t. Tube placed in a wound or cavity to allow the escape of fluids.

endotracheal t. A rubber tube inserted in the trachea as an airway in endotracheal intubation.

eustachian t. See auditory tube.

fallopian t. See uterine tube.

feeding t. A soft flexible tube for introducing high caloric liquids into the stomach.

Geiger t., Geiger-Müller t. (GM) A gas-filled tube containing a cylindrical cathode and axial wire electrode, used to detect radioactivity; radioactive particles penetrate the tube's shell and produce momentary current pulsations in the gas.

Levin t. A flexible tube introduced into the stomach or duodenum, usually through the nose, after an operation.

Miller-Abbott t. A double lumen 3.3 m intestinal tube, used for diagnosing and treating obstructions of the small intestine.

nasogastric t. (NG) A pliable plastic tube passed through the nose into the stomach for removal of stomach secretions or the introduction of solutions.

neural t. The epithelial tube of the early embryo formed by the closure of the neural groove; it develops into the brain and spinal cord.

orotracheal t. An endotracheal tube inserted through the mouth into the trachea.

photomultiplier t. Apparatus used to amplify images of low intensity.

pressure-equalizing t. See tympanostomy tube.

Sengstaken-Blakemore t. Device consisting of three tubes, two with an inflatable balloon and the third one attached to a suction apparatus; used to stop bleeding from the esophagus.

stomach t. A flexible 40 cm tube used for feeding or for washing out the stomach.

test t. Tube made of thin glass and closed at one end; used in a variety of laboratory procedures.

tracheostomy t. A metal or glass tube inserted into the trachea through a tracheotomy opening to facilitate breathing. Also called tracheotomy tube.

tracheotomy t. See tracheostomy tube.

tympanostomy t. A tiny tube inserted through an incision in the eardrum (tympanic membrane); the tube acts as an auxillary eustachian (auditory) tube for aerating the middle ear chamber; used in treating serous otitis media that is unresponsive to antibiotic and decongestant therapy. Also called pressure-equalizing tube.

uterine t. One of two slender tubes, about 10 cm long, on either side leading from the uterus to the area of the ovary; it conveys the ovum from the ovary to the uterus and is usually where conception occurs. Also called fallopian tube; oviduct.

vacuum t. Glass tube from which air has been almost completely removed.

x-ray t. A vacuum tube used for the production of x rays; the enclosed electrodes accelerate electrons and direct them to an anode, where their impacts produce high energy photons.

tubectomy (too-bek´to-me) See salpingectomy.

tube housing (to͞ob hou´zing) A lead-shielded container that provides radiation protection; it holds the x-ray tube, transformers, and insulating oils.

diagnostic protective t.h. One that reduces leakage radiation to 0.1 roentgens per hour at a distance of 1 m from the tube target when the tube is operating at its maximum rated voltage and current.

therapeutic protective t.h. One that reduces leakage radiation to 1 roentgen per hour at a distance of 1 m from the tube target when the tube is operating at its maximum rated voltage and current.

tuber (too´ber), *pl.* **tu´bera** A prominence.

t. cinereum The small portion of the hypothalamus that protrudes into the floor of the third ventricle of the brain.

tubercle (too´ber-kl) **1.** The specific lesion of tuberculosis. **2.** A rounded elevation on a bone. **3.** A nodule on the skin.

adductor t. of femur A small projection on the medial condyle of the lower end of the femur, near the knee joint; provides attachment to the tendon of the great adductor muscle.

anterior t. of calcaneus A small rounded tubercle on the bottom of the front part of the heel bone (calcaneus); marks the distal limit of the attachment of the long plantar ligament.

carotid t. The large anterior tubercle on either side of the sixth cervical vertebra; the common carotid artery lies anteriorly to it and can be compressed against it.

costal t. See tubercle of rib.

genial t.'s Small bony elevations on the lower part of the inner surface of the chin (mental protuberance); they provide attachment for the geniohyoid and genioglossus muscles. Also called mental spines.

Ghon's t. See Ghon's primary lesion, under lesion.

gracile t. One of two elevations on the dorsal surface of the medulla oblongata on either side of the posterior median sulcus (at the lower end of the fourth ventricle); it overlies the nucleus gracilis. Also called clava.

greater t. of humerus A large prominence on the lateral side of the upper end of the humerus; provides attachment for the supraspinatus, infraspinatus, and teres minor muscles; it is the most lateral bony prominence of the shoulder region and responsible for the rounded contour of the shoulder. Also called greater tuberosity of humerus.

t. of iliac crest A prominence on the outer lip of the iliac crest of the hipbone, approximately two inches above and behind the anterior superior iliac spine.

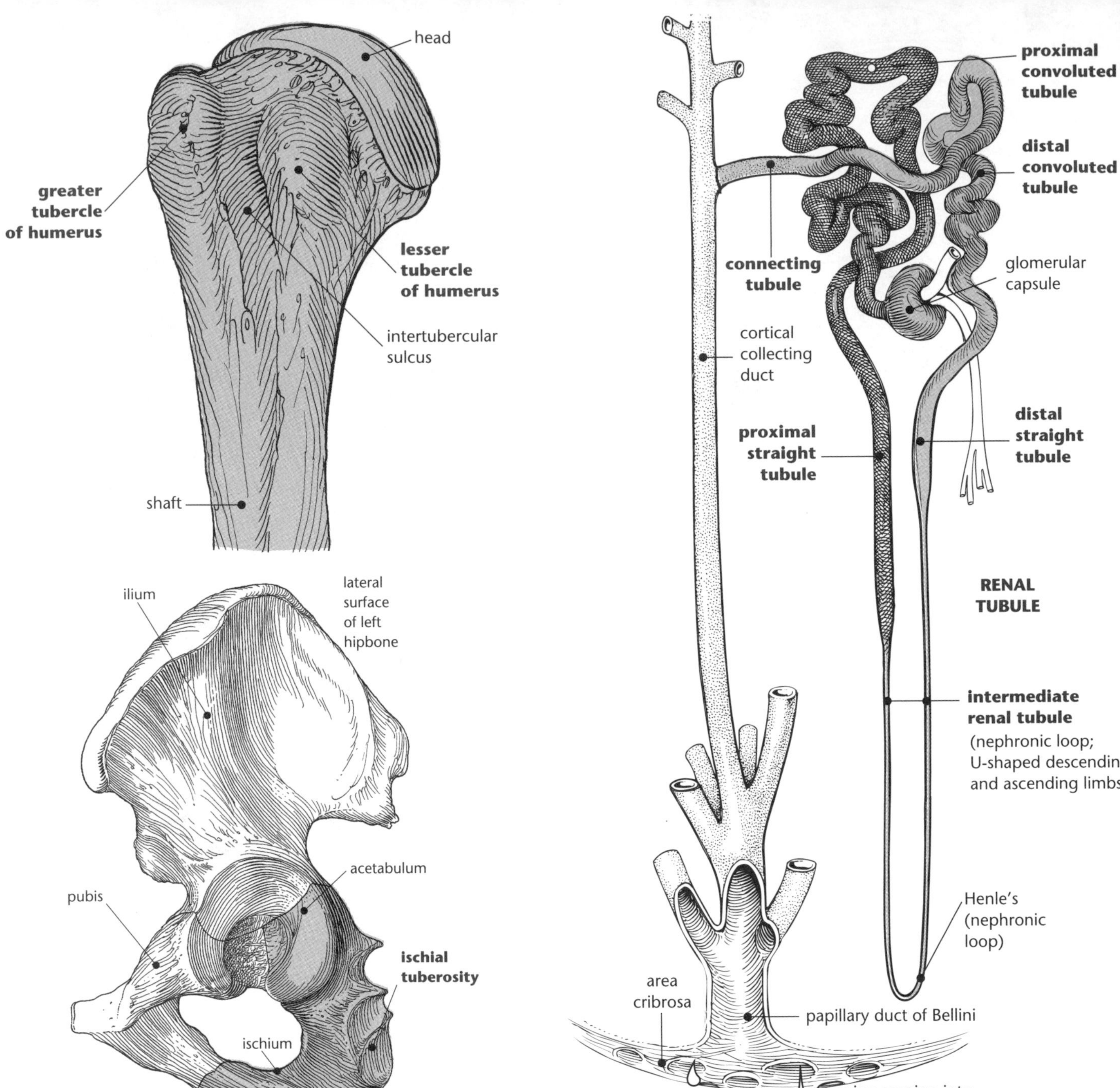

T

lesser t. of humerus A prominence on the anterior surface of the humerus just beyond its anatomical neck, near the shoulder joint; provides attachment for the subscapular muscle. Also called lesser tuberosity of humerus.

pubic t. A small tubercle at the lateral end of the pubic crest, on either side, about three-quarters of an inch from the pubic symphysis; provides attachment to the tendons of the straight muscle of abdomen (rectus abdominis muscle) and the pyramidal muscle. Also called pubic spine.

t. of radius See radial tuberosity, under tuberosity.

t. of rib A knoblike eminence on the posterior surface of a rib at the junction of its neck and shaft; articulates with the transverse process of the corresponding thoracic vertebra. Also called costal tubercle.

t. of tibia See tibial tuberosity, under tuberosity.

tubercular (too-ber´ku-lar) Relating to or having tubercles; erroneously used instead of tuberculous to describe a person afflicted with tuberculosis.

tuberculate, tuberculated (too-ber´ku-lāt, too-ber´ku-lāt-ed) Having nodules or tubercles.

tuberculation (too-ber-ku-la´shun) The formation or presence of nodules.

tuberculid (too-ber´ku-lid) A noninfectious skin lesion caused by hypersensitivity to tubercle bacilli; occurs in people previously exposed to the microorganisms.

tuberculin (too-ber´ku-lin) A substance made from the toxins of the tubercle bacillus, used in the diagnosis of tuberculosis; originally developed by Koch for the treatment of tuberculosis.

old t. (OT) A concentrated filtrate made from a six-week-old culture of tubercle bacilli in glycerol broth; it contains only the soluble substance produced by the bacilli during growth, not the microorganisms.

purified protein derivative of t. (PPD) An extract from tubercle bacilli prepared in the protein-free liquid medium.

tuberculoid (too-ber´ku-loid) **1.** Resembling tuberculosis. **2.** Resembling a tubercle.

tuberculoma (too-ber-ku-lo´mă) A tumor-like mass of tuberculous origin.

tuberculosis (too-ber-ku-lo´sis) (TB) A communicable disease caused by the bacterium *Mycobacterium tuberculosis*, which causes a distinctive ulcerating lesion in the affected tissues; human infections are most commonly caused by *Mycobacterium hominis* and *bovis*, acquired by inhaling airborne droplets of the coughing and sneezing from infected persons and, only rarely, by drinking infected milk; people most at risk are those with debilitating or immunosuppressive conditions, including malnutrition, alcoholism, diabetes, chronic lung disease, extensive corticosteroid use, and AIDS.

atypical t. A tuberculosis-like disease of the lungs caused by atypical organisms of the genus *Mycobacterium* (either *Mycobacterium avium-intracelluare* or *Mycobacterium kansasii*); occurs primarily in people with an underlying lung disease or as an opportunistic infection in immunodepressed patients.

cutaneous t. A rare group of skin diseases caused either by the presence of microorganisms in the subcutaneous tissues or by hypersensitivity reactions to a previous infection.

disseminated t. Acute miliary tuberculosis.

miliary t. A form of tuberculosis in which the tubercle bacilli are carried in the bloodstream throughout the body, thus affecting several organs simultaneously. Also called disseminated tuberculosis.

postprimary t. See secondary tuberculosis.

primary t. The usually asymptomatic phase of

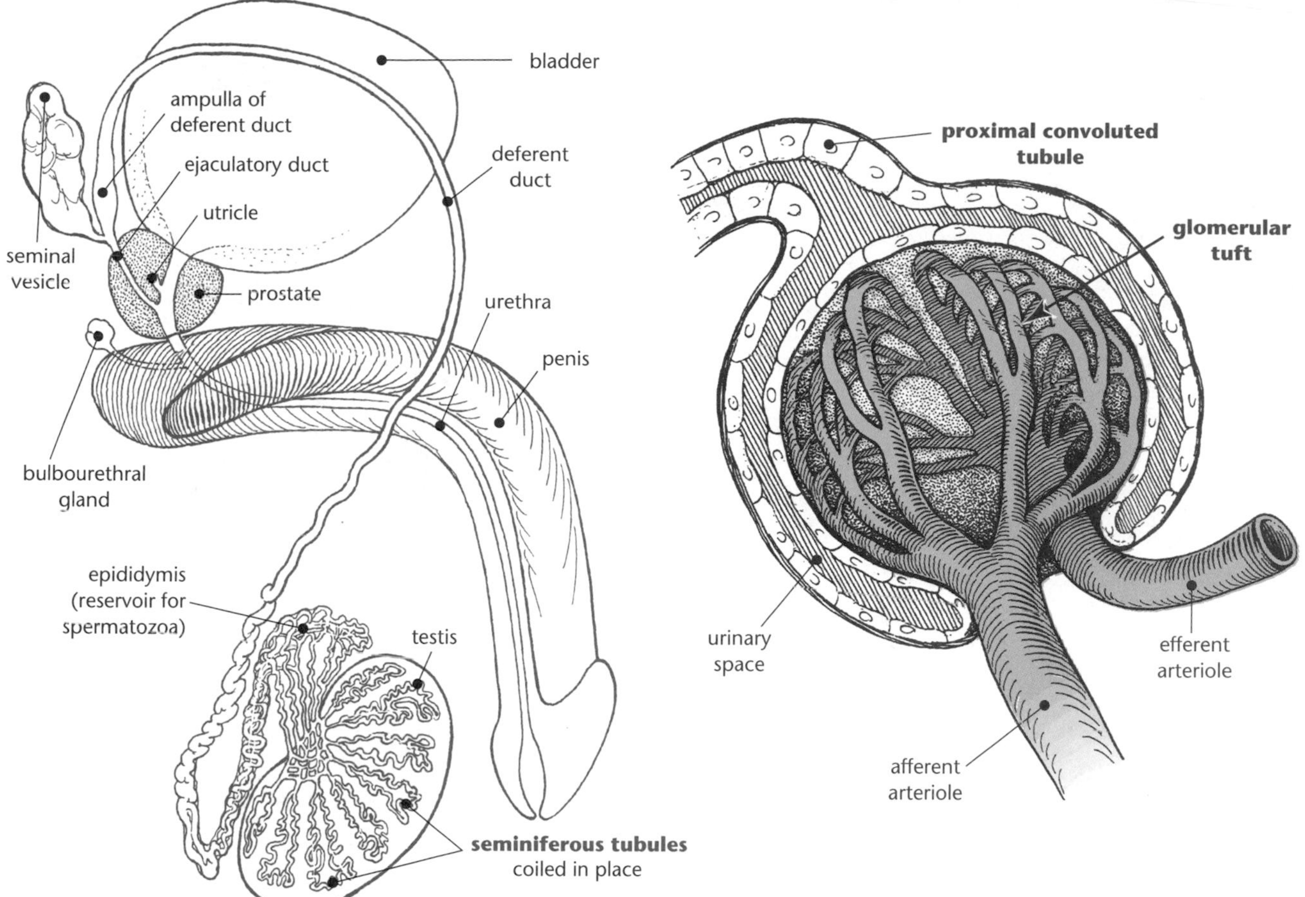

tuberculosis immediately following invasion of tissues by tubercle bacilli; occurs in people who did not have previous contact with the organism.

pulmonary t. Tuberculosis of the lungs, marked by ulceration and formation of cavities in the lungs, attended by fever and cough; infection may be arrested, leaving scars containing dormant bacilli, or may progress and spread to lymph nodes of the neck or throughout the body via the bloodstream.

reinfection t. See secondary tuberculosis.

secondary t. Active tuberculosis in a person who has been sensitized by previous contact with tubercle bacilli; mostly it is a reactivation of dormant organisms from a primary infection; occasionally it represents a new infection. Also called postprimary tuberculosis; reinfection tuberculosis.

tuberculostatic (too-ber-ku-lo-stat´ik) **1.** Denoting an agent that inhibits the growth of the tubercle bacillus. **2.** Arresting the growth of the tubercle bacillus.

tuberculous (too-ber´ku-lus) Afflicted with tuberculosis.

tuberculum (too-ber´ku-lum), *pl.* **tuber´cula** Latin for tubercle.

tuberosity (too-bĕ-ros´ĭ-te) A rounded protuberance from the surface of a bone or cartilage.

calcaneal t. The prominent posterior plantar extremity of the calcaneus that forms the projection of the heel; it bears lateral and medial processes.

deltoid t. A linear, raised area on the lateral surface of the middle part of the humerus; provides attachment for the deltoid muscle.

ischial t. The rough lower part of the ischium (of the hipbone); divided by a transverse ridge into an upper and lower area; the upper part provides attachment for the hamstring muscles and the inferior gemellus muscle; the lower part (on which the body rests in the sitting position) affords attachment to the great adductor muscle and the sacrotuberous ligament.

greater t. of humerus See greater tubercle of humerus, under tubercle.

lesser t. of humerus See lesser tubercle of humerus, under tubercle.

radial t. A broad bony prominence on the medial surface of the radius just below its neck, which affords attachment to the biceps muscle of arm (biceps brachii). Also called tubercle of radius.

tibial t. A broad triangular projection on the front of the upper end of the tibia; the upper portion of the tuberosity provides attachment for the ligament of the patella and the lower portion is associated with the infrapatellar bursa. Also called tubercle of tibia.

tuberous (too´ber-us) Having many small rounded projections; lumpy; nodular.

tubocurarine chloride (too-bo-ku-ră´rin klōr´īd) An active alkaloid derived from *Chondodendron tomentosum* that produces skeletal muscle paralysis by occupying the receptors at the neuromuscular junction, thereby blocking the action of the neurotransmitter acetylcholine; used to produce muscular relaxation during surgical operations and to reduce the severity of muscle spasms in severe tetanus.

tubocornual (too-bo-kor´nu-al) Relating to a fallopian (uterine) tube and one of the upper elongated portions (cornua) of the uterus.

tubo-ovarian (too´bo-o-va´re-an) Relating to a uterine (fallopian) tube and an ovary.

tubo-ovaritis (too´bo-o-vă-ri´tis) See salpingo-oophoritis.

tuboplasty (too´bo-plas-te)–See salpingoplasty.

tubular (too´bu-lar)–Relating to, shaped like, or consisting of a tube or tubes.

tubule (too´bul) A small tube or canal.

collecting t.'s See collecting ducts, under duct.

connecting t. (CNT) A nephron tubule connecting the distal convoluted tubule and the cortical collecting duct.

dental t.'s Minute tubes or canals in the dentin of the tooth containing the dentinal fibers and extending radially from the pulp to the dentoenamel junction.

distal convoluted t. (DCT) The tortuous segment of the renal tubule leading from the straight distal tubule to the connecting tubule.

distal straight t. (DST) The distal straight segment of the renal tubule connecting the thin ascending part of the intermediate tubule to the distal convoluted tubule. Also called thick-ascending limb.

intermediate renal t. (IRT) The thin tubule connecting the proximal straight tubule (PST) and the distal straight tubule (DST).

malpighian t.'s Slender tubular structures that emerge from the alimentary canal of some insects, usually between the midgut and hindgut.

mesonephric t.'s The tubules comprising the excretory organ (mesonephros) of the embryo; retained in the male beyond embryonic life as the epididymis and the deferent duct.

proximal convoluted t. (PCT) The tortuous segment of the renal tubule leading from the glomerular (Bowman's) capsule to the straight proximal tubule.

proximal straight t. (PST) The proximal straight segment of the renal tubule connecting the proximal convoluted tubule to the thin descending part of the intermediate tubule (loop of Henle). Also called thick descending limb.

renal t. The part of the nephron responsible for conveying the glomerular filtrate to the collecting duct and transforming the filtrate into urine; composed of the glomerular (Bowman's) capsule, proximal convoluted tubule, proximal straight tubule, intermediate renal tubule, nephronic or Henle's loop (between the ascending and descending limbs of the intermediate renal tubule), distal straight tubule, distal convoluted tubule, and connecting tubule.

seminiferous t.'s Long, threadlike, twisted tubules loosely packed in each lobule of the testis; the channels in which the spermatozoa develop and through which they are conveyed to the rete testis.

transverse t.'s Invaginations of the sarcolemma.

tubulin (too´bu-lin) A protein subunit of cytoplasmic microtubules, composed of two polypeptides.

tubulization (too-bu-li-za´shun) Protection of an injured or sutured nerve with an absorbable cylinder to promote healing.

tubulorrhexis (too-bu-lo-rek´sis) Localized disintegration of epithelium and basement membrane of renal tubules; a characteristic lesion of acute tubular necrosis.

tuft (tuft) A cluster.

glomerular t. The small cluster of capillaries projecting into the expanded end of the proximal convoluted tubule of the kidney, which encloses the tuft forming the Bowman's (glomerular) capsule. Formerly called malpighian tuft.

malpighian t. See glomerular tuft..

tularemia (too-lă-re´me-ă) Infectious disease caused by the bacterium *Francisella tularensis*, transmitted to humans from infected animals usually by the bite of insects; marked by a prolonged or recurrent fever and swelling of the lymph nodes. Also called rabbit fever; deer-fly fever.

T

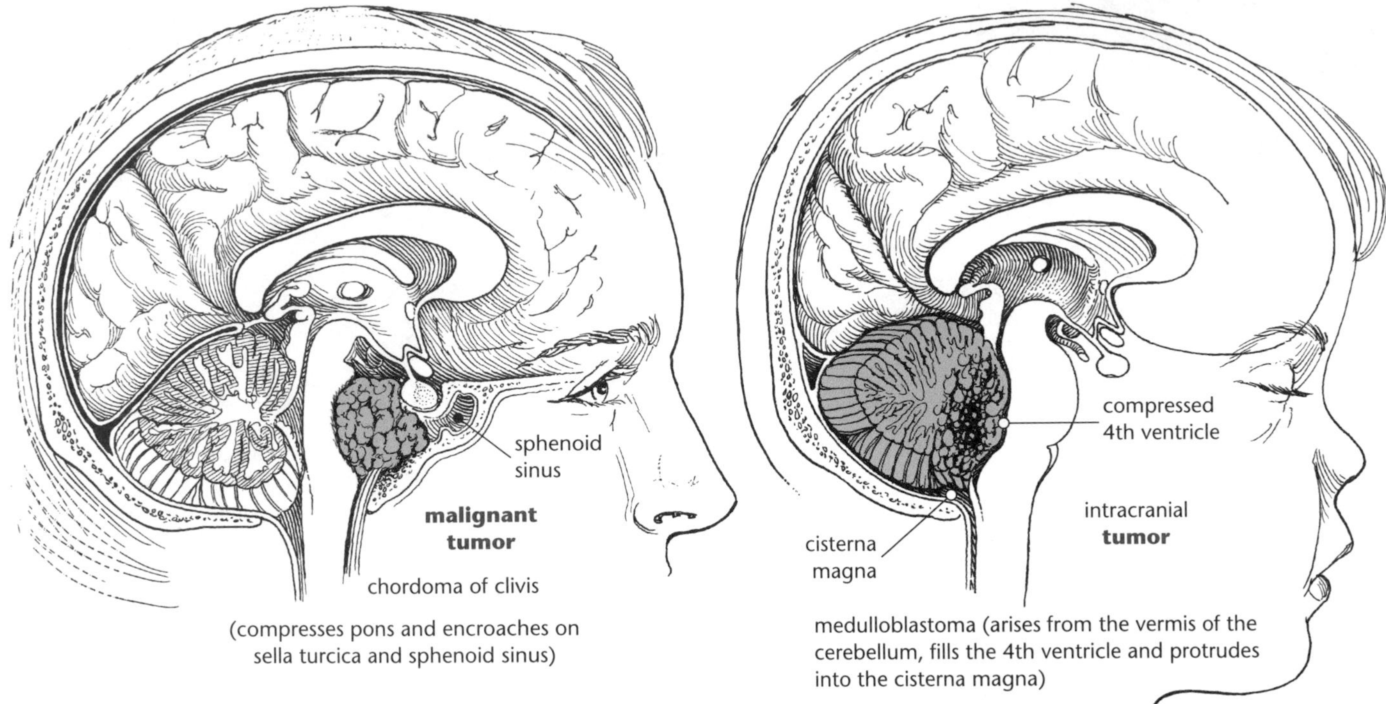

TULIP Acronym for transurethral ultrasound-guided laser induced prostatectomy.

tumefacient (too-me-fa′shent) Causing a swelling.

tumefaction, tumescence (too-me-fak′shun, too-mes′ens) **1.** A swollen condition. **2.** The process of swelling.

tumid (too′mid) Swollen; engorged.

tumor (too′mor) **1.** Any swelling. **2.** A neoplasm, an overgrowth of tissue.

adenomatoid t. Benign, slow growing, gray-white nodules of uncertain origin, occurring in both male and female genital tracts.

adipose t. See lipoma.

benign t. Tumor that does not metastasize or infiltrate and is unlikely to recur after its removal.

blood t. A swelling containing blood; term is sometimes used to denote an aneurysm, a hemangioma, or a hematoma.

Brenner's t. A yellow-brown solid tumor of the ovary that is typically benign but (rarely) may undergo malignant transformation; usually occurs unilaterally in postmenopausal women.

carcinoid t. A small, usually benign but potentially malignant growth in the lining of the intestinal tract, especially of the appendix; also found in the lung. Also called argentaffinoma; frequently call carcinoid.

carotid body t. See chemodectoma.

collision t. Synchronous squamous cell carcinomas and adenocarcinomas that infiltrate each other.

desmoid t. See desmoid.

embryonal t. General term for any tumor (usually malignant) believed to be derived from embryonic tissues. Also called embryoma.

endodermal sinus t. (EST) See yolk-sac tumor of ovary.

endometrioid t. of ovary Malignant tumor composed of a combination of solid and cystic masses, microscopically resembling endometrial adenocarcinoma; may occur bilaterally (40%) or unilaterally.

Ewing's t. See Ewing's sarcoma, under sarcoma.

fibroid t. See leiomyoma.

gas t. See pneumatocele (3).

germ-cell t. of ovary Any of a group of ovarian tumors derived from cell types of the endoderm, mesoderm, or ectoderm (i.e., the germ layers); they include dermoids, dysgerminomas, malignant teratomas, and yolk-sac tumors.

giant cell t. of bone A soft, reddish-brown, usually benign tumor of long bones, composed chiefly of multinucleated giant cells and ovoid or spindle-shaped cells. Also called giant cell myeloma; osteoclastoma.

giant cell t. of tendon sheath See nodular tenosynovitis, under tenosynovitis.

glomus t. An extremely painful, small, bluish-red benign tumor in the skin, arising from cells of a glomus body. Also called glomangioma.

granular cell t. A benign, usually small tumor of uncertain origin, often involving peripheral nerves in skin, mucosa, or connective tissue. Also called myoblastoma; granular cell myoblastoma.

granulosa cell t. An uncommon, benign (potentially malignant) tumor of the ovary that typically secretes large amounts of estrogen; may occur in any age group, usually confined to one ovary; causes vaginal bleeding in postmenopausal women; when occurring in young girls, it is commonly associated with pseudoprecocious puberty. Also called granulosa-theca cell tumor; folliculoma.

granulosa-theca cell t. See granulosa cell tumor.

Grawitz' t. See renal adenocarcinoma, under adenocarcinoma.

heterologous t. A tumor composed of tissue different from the one in which it grows.

homologous t. Tumor made up of the same kind of tissue as the one from which it grows.

Krukenberg t. A malignant, usually bilateral, tumor of the ovary, secondary to a mucous carcinoma of the stomach.

malignant t. Tumor that forms metastases, may recur after removal, and eventually causes death if not treated early and appropriately. Often called cancer.

melanotic neuroectodermal t. Benign tumor of the anterior portion of the upper jaw (maxilla) usually seen in infants younger than six months; causes displacement of tooth buds. Also called melanoameloblastoma.

mixed t. Tumor composed of more than one tissue or cell type.

mixed t. of salivary gland Tumor containing epithelial cells and cells of salivary glands, all arising from epithelial cells of salivary ducts; most frequently seen in the parotid gland. Also called pleomorphic adenoma.

papillary t. See papilloma.

phantom t. A circumscribed accumulation of fluid in the interlobar spaces of the lung and seen in chest x-ray pictures as opacities suggestive of a tumor; associated with congestive heart failure.

phyllodes t. A bulky, slow-growing, usually benign tumor of the breast most commonly seen in premenopausal women although it may occur at any age; it is composed chiefly of proliferative ducts and supportive tissues (stroma) of the breast; some have a malignant potential; those that become malignant metastasize to the lungs via the bloodstream. Formerly called cystosarcoma phyllodes.

Pincus t. See fibroepithelioma.

pontine angle t. Tumor located in the proximal portion of the acoustic nerve.

Pott's puffy t. A circumscribed swelling of the scalp resulting from osteitis of the skull or from an extradural abscess.

Sertoli-Leydig t. An uncommon benign tumor of the testis or the ovary, composed of Sertoli cells or a mixture of Leydig and Sertoli cells in varying proportions and degrees of differentiation; on rare occasions, it may turn malignant. Also called androblastoma.

sex cord-stromal t.'s A group of ovarian tumors derived either from the sex cords of the embryonic gonad or from the supporting tissues (stroma) of the ovary (e.g., fibromas, granulosa-theca cell tumors, Sertoli-Leydig cell tumors).

theca cell t. See thecoma.

theca lutein cell t. See thecoma.

Warthin's t. See adenolymphoma.

Wilm's t. A malignant tumor of the kidney, occurring mostly in young children; composed of embryonic elements. Also called embryoma of kidney; nephroblastoma.

yolk-sac t. of ovary A highly malignant tumor that grows rapidly and aggressively; it affects only one ovary and occurs mainly in young women (under 20 years of age) and children. Most secrete alpha-fetoprotein (AFP). Also called endodermal sinus tumor.

Zollinger-Ellison t. Tumor of the pancreas causing the Zollinger-Ellison syndrome.

tumor burden (too′mor burd′n) The total mass of tumor tissue in a patient with cancer.

tumorigenesis (too-mor-ĭ-jen′ĕ-sis) The formation of a new growth.

tumorigenic (too-mor-ĭ-jen′ik) Causing tumors.

tumorous (too′mor-us) Resembling a tumor.

tungsten (tung′sten) (W) A chemical element with a very high melting point used as the target material of an x-ray tube as well as in electric light filaments; symbol W, atomic number 74, atomic weight 183.85.

tunica (too′nĭ-kă) A coat or enveloping layer of tissue.

t. adventitia The fibrous outer layer of a blood vessel. Also called tunica externa; tunica fibrosa.

t. albuginea of ovary A delicate collagenous covering of the ovary between the outer germinal epithelium and the cortex; it increases in density with passing age.

t. albuginea of penis A fibrous envelope consisting of superficial and deep layers surrounding the corpora cavernosa and corpus spongiosum of the penis; the deep fibers envelope each corpus

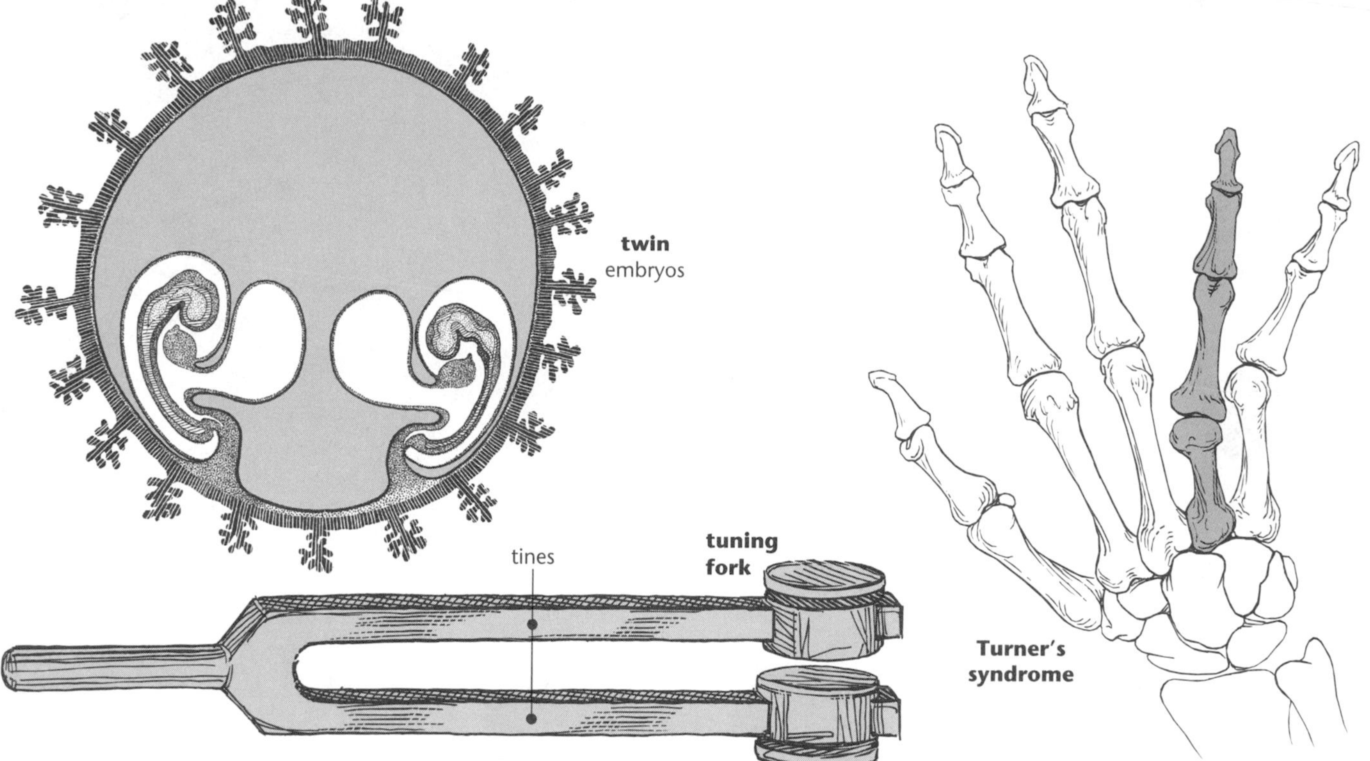

cavernosum separately and form by their junction the septum of the penis; the superficial fibers envelope both corpora cavernosa as a single tube; the corpus spongiosum is surrounded by a separate fibrous envelope.

t. albuginea of testis The thick, fibrous, bluish white membrane covering the testis.

t. dartos The highly vascular layer of smooth muscle in the scrotum; its deeper fibers form a septum which divides the scrotum into two halves.

t. externa See tunica adventitia.

t. interna See tunica intima.

t. fibrosa See tunica adventitia.

t. intima The inner, serous layer of a blood vessel. Also called tunica interna.

t. media The middle muscular layer of a blood vessel.

t. vaginalis of testis A closed serous pouch investing the testis; it consists of a parietal and a visceral layer.

tuning fork (toon′ing fork) A forklike metal instrument with two prongs that, when struck, produce a sound of fixed pitch; used for testing hearing and vibratory sensation.

turbidimetric (tur-bid-ĭ-met′rik) Relating to the measurement of turbidity.

turbidimetry (tur-bĭ-dim′ĕ-tre) Measurement of turbidity or cloudiness of a fluid.

turbidity (tur-bid′ĭ-te) Cloudiness caused by the stirring up of sediment or suspended foreign particles, resulting in a loss of transparency.

turbinate (tur′bĭ-nāt) **1.** Shaped like an inverted cone or a scroll. **2.** A turbinate bone. See table of bones.

turbine (tur′bīn, tur′bin) A rotary instrument activated by a stream of water.

turbinectomy (tur-bĭ-nek′to-me) Surgical removal of a turbinate bone.

Turcot syndrome (tur′kot sin′drom) The presence of polyps in the colon combined with brain tumors; transmitted as an autosomal recessive trait.

turgescence (tur-jes′ens) The process of swelling; the state of being swollen.

turgid (tur′jid) Congested; bloated.

turgor (tur′gor) Fullness.

turista (tu-rēs′tă) Colloquial term for traveler's diarrhea.

turn (turn) To move a fetus in the uterus from a malposition to one that will facilitate normal delivery.

Turner's sign Areas of discoloration about the navel and the loins occurring in acute hemorrhagic pancreatitis.

Turner's syndrome (tur′nerz sin′drōm) Condition due to a chromosomal anomaly (only one X chromosome); absence of ovaries or possession of only rudimentary structures, infantile female genitalia, short stature, and webbed neck are some of the symptoms.

TURP Acronym for transurethral resection of prostate.

tussis (tus′is) A cough.

tussive (tus′iv) Relating to or caused by a cough.

twin (twin) **1.** One of two children born at one birth. **2.** Double; growing in pairs.

conjoined t.'s Twins having varying degrees of connection or fusion with each other.

dizygotic t.'s See fraternal twins.

fraternal t.'s Twins developed from two separate ova fertilized at the same time; they may or may not be of the same sex. Also called dizygotic twins; heterozygous twins.

heterozygous t.'s See fraternal twins.

identical t.'s Twins resulting from a single fertilized egg that splits at an early stage of development; they are always of the same sex, have the same genetic constitution, and have pronounced resemblance to one another. Also called monozygotic twins; uniovular twins.

locked t.'s Twins whose heads become simultaneously impacted in the pelvis during delivery; while one twin descends through the birth canal in a breech presentation, the other follows in a vertex presentation, and the chin of the first locks in the neck and chin of the second.

monozygotic t.'s See identical twins.

uniovular t.'s See identical twins.

vanishing t. Colloquial term for the spontaneous release of amniotic fluid occurring in the first trimester of pregnancy, with the pregnancy usually continuing normally to term; cause is unknown; believed to be due to a twin pregnancy in which the second fetus and its amniotic sac are liquefied by enzymatic action (probably from the second fetus itself) early in the pregnancy, with consequent release of the amniotic fluid.

twinge (twinj) A sudden, short, sharp physical or mental pain.

twin-twin transfusion syndrome (twin-twin trans-fu′zhun sin′drōm) Syndrome diagnosed in identical (monozygotic) twins when there is a hemoglobin difference greater than 5g/dL between the twins; occurs when the fetuses share a single (monochorionic) placenta and there is a blood vessel communication between the two umbilical circulations, with a deep artery-to-vein flow from one twin to the other without a compensatory return flow. The donor twin tends to be pale, anemic, dehydrated, of low birth weight and decreased blood volume; it may die of heart failure. The recipient twin frequently has an abnormally large number of red blood cells, a high birth weight, increased organ mass, and an enlarged heart; although ruddy and apparently healthy, it may die of heart failure within 24 hours. Also called third circulation.

twitch (twich) **1.** A brief involuntary or spasmodic contraction of a muscle fiber; usually phasic. **2.** To move sharply and suddenly; to jerk.

two-carbon fragment (too′kar′bon frag′ment) The acetyl group CH_3CO–.

tyloma (ti-lo′mă) Heavy callus formation.

t. conjunctivae A localized cornification of the conjunctiva.

tylosis (ti-lo′sis) **1.** The formation of a callus. **2.** A callosity.

tympanectomy (tim-pă-nek′tŏ-me) Removal of the tympanic membrane (eardrum).

tympanic (tim-pan′ik) Relating to the chamber of the middle car.

tympanites (tim-pă-ni′tēz) Distention of the abdomen due to accumulation of gas in the intestines. Also called meteorism.

tympanitic (tim-pă-nit′ik) **1.** Relating to tympanites, as the sound produced by percussing over the distended abdomen. **2.** Tympanic or resonant.

tympanocentesis (tim-pă-no-sen-te′sis) Aspiration of fluid from the middle ear chamber with a needle inserted through the tympanic membrane; procedure used to identify organisms causing persistent middle ear infections.

tympanogram (tim-pan′o-gram) A graph made while testing the degree of conductive hearing impairment by means of impedance audiometry; the deflection pattern on the chart reveals the extent of elasticity of the eardrum and ear ossicles.

tympanomastoiditis (tim-pă-no-mas-toi-di′tis) Inflammation of the middle ear and the mastoid cells.

tympanometry (tim-pă-nom′ĕ-tre) The measurement of the flow of sound energy in the external auditory meatus; a means of detecting middle ear disease.

tympanoplasty (tim-pă-no-plas′te) A general term denoting any of several operative procedures designed to restore hearing in patients with middle ear or conductive hearing loss.

type I t. See myringoplasty.

tympanosclerosis (tim-pă-no-sklĕ-ro′sis) Scarring of the tympanic membrane (eardrum), causing hearing impairment.

tympanosquamosal (tim-pă-no-skwah-mo′sal) Pertaining to the tympanic and squamous portions of the temporal bone.

tympanotomy (tim-pă-not′o-me) See myringotomy.

tympanum (tim′pă-num) The chamber of the middle ear, a cavity in the temporal bone housing the chain of ossicles.

T

THE PROCESS OF PRODUCING **DNA TYPING**

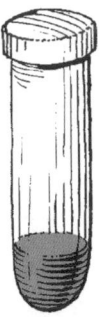

1 Sample of nucleated cells is collected, usually from blood, semen, or hair roots.

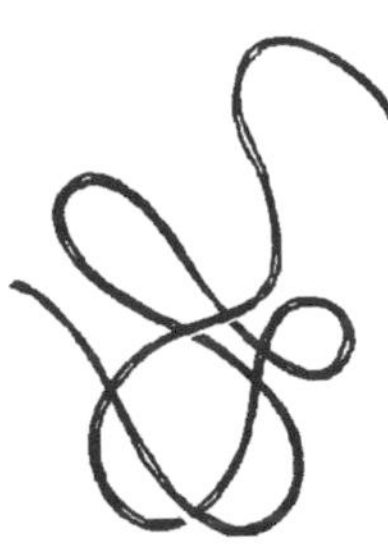

2 DNA is extracted from the nuclei of the cells.

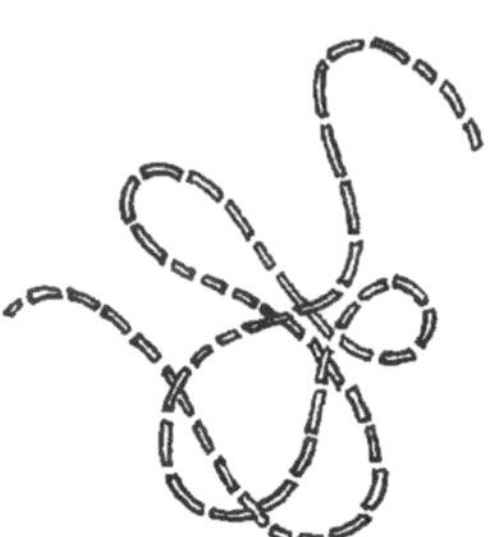

3 DNA is fragmented at specific sequences by a *restriction enzyme.*

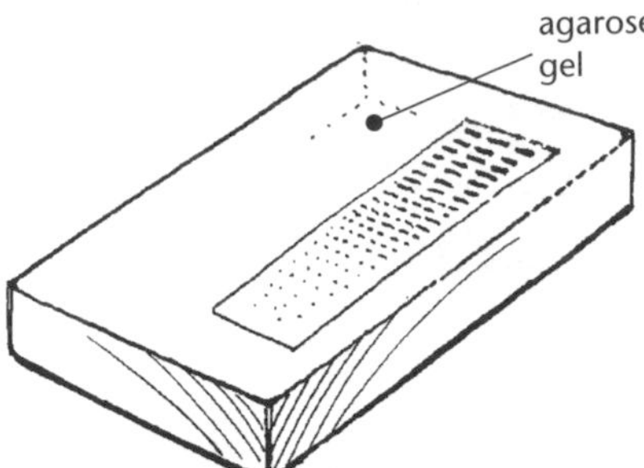

4 Using electrophoresis, the DNA fragments are separated. The fragments migrate by size into invisible bands. Then the double strands of DNA separate into single strands (denaturation).

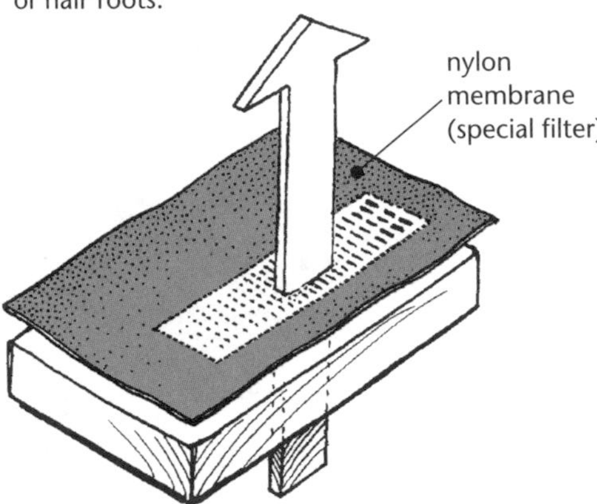

5 To preserve the band pattern, the DNA is transferred to a nylon membrane by a technique called *Southern blotting.*

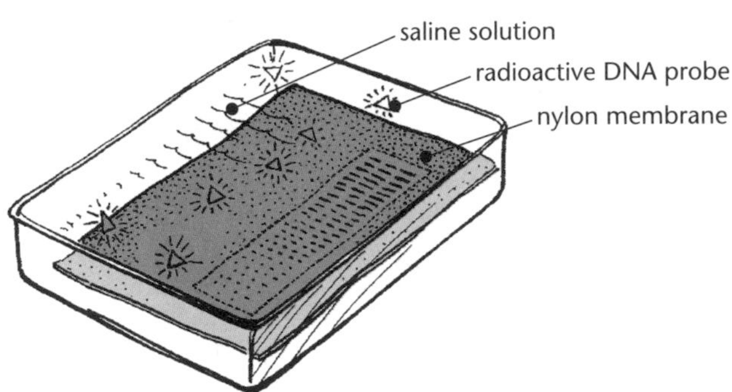

6 Radioactive DNA probe is added to a saline solution in which the nylon membrane is immersed. The probe binds to specific complementary bands of repetitive DNA sequences on the membrane.

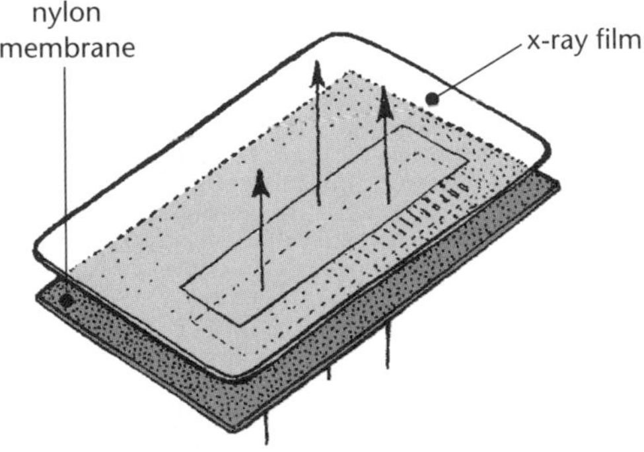

7 X-ray film is placed on the nylon membrane to detect where the radioactive DNA probe has bound.

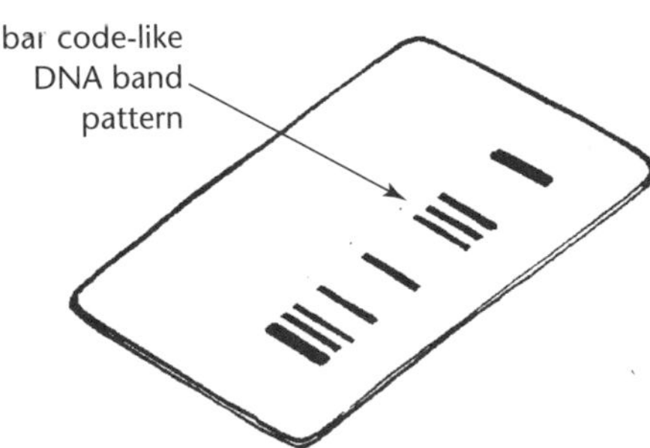

8 The pattern of DNA bands becomes visible when the x-ray film is developed. Each band occurs where the probe has unerringly located and zipped-up with its correct partner strand (repetitive sequence).

after CELLMARK DIAGNOSTICS

T

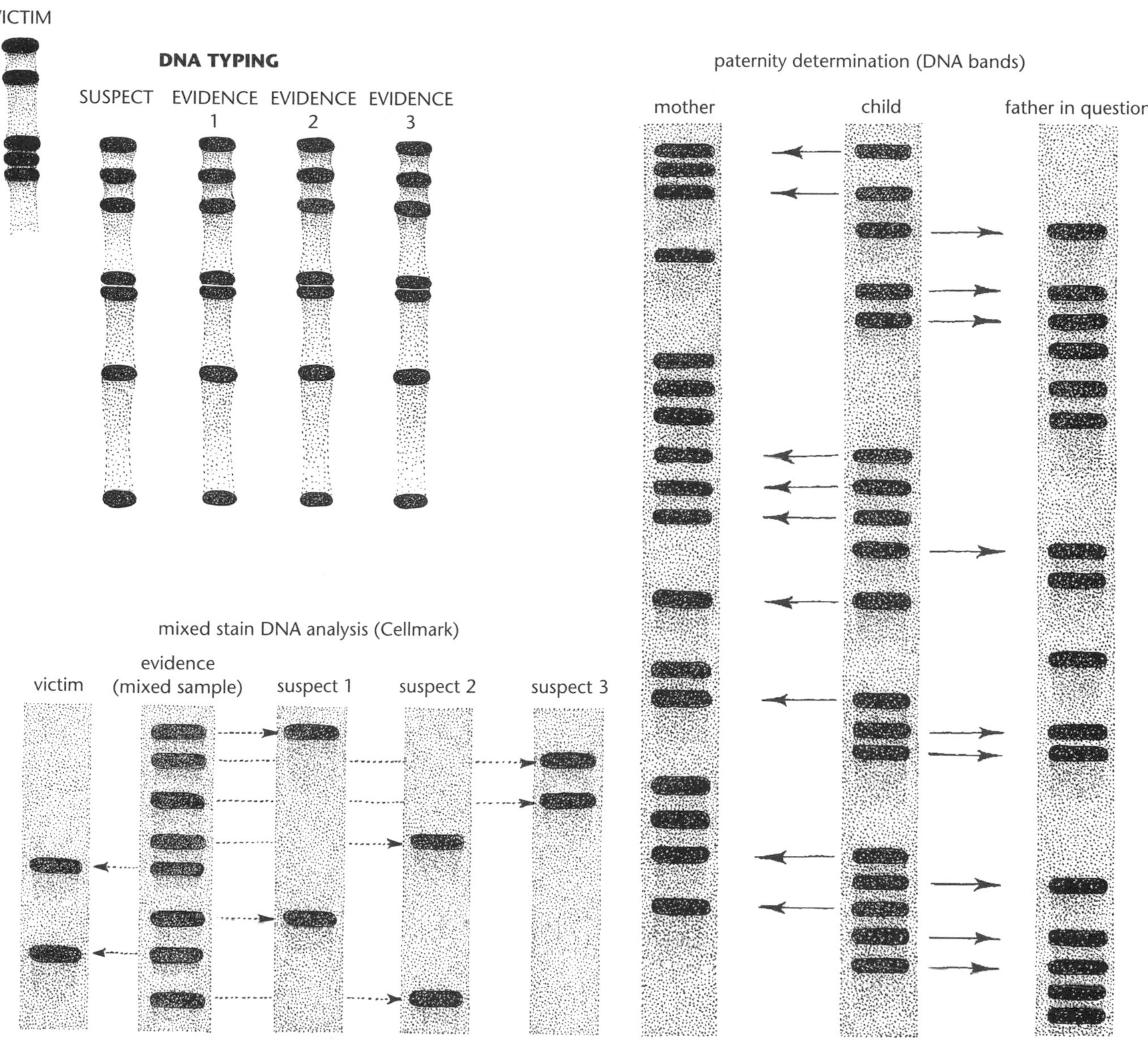

Each single locus probe produces a pattern of at most two bands per person. An eight band pattern indicates the sample was from at least four individuals. Matching of the suspects' band patterns with those of the evidence confirms their involvement.

The paternal DNA bands show a biologic relationship to the child.

tympany (tim′pă-ne) A drumlike percussion sound.

type (tīp) A pattern of characteristics common to a number of individuals, chemical substances, diseases, etc.

blood t. The specific reaction pattern of red blood cells of a person to the antisera of a blood group. See also blood group.

wild t. In genetics, the most frequently observed form of an organism, or the one arbitrarily designated as normal.

typhlitis (tif-li′tis) Inflammation of the cecum. Also called cecitis.

typhlo-, typhl- Prefixes denoting (a) the cecum; (b) blindness.

typhoid (ti′foid) Resembling typhus.

typhous (ti′fus) Relating to typhus.

typhus (ti′fus) An acute infectious and contagious disease caused by a rickettsia and marked by sustained high fever, severe headache, and a characteristic rash.

endemic t. See murine typhus.

epidemic t. Typhus caused by *Rickettsia prowazekii* and transmitted by body lice.

flea-borne t. See murine typhus.

mite-borne t. See tsutsugamushi disease.

murine t. Typhus caused by *Rickettsia mooseri* and transmitted by the rat flea. Also called endemic or flea-borne typhus.

recrudescent t. See Brill-Zinsser disease.

scrub t. See tsutsugamushi disease.

tropical t. See tsutsugamushi disease.

typing (tīp′ing) Determination of the type category to which any entity belongs.

blood t. See blood grouping.

DNA t. Test on a nucleated cell (e.g., of semen, blood, hair roots) to detect characteristics in genetic structure that are as unique to an individual as fingerprints. Also called DNA fingerprinting; DNA profiling.

HLA t. (human leukocyte antigen typing) Test to determine the HLA makeup of an individual; used to identify compatibility between transplant donors and recipients, to establish paternity, and in forensic investigations.

tyramine (ti′ră-mēn) An amine that produces effects similar to those of epinephrine; it is a product of the decarboxylation of the amino acid tyrosine and can have harmful effects on patients undergoing therapy with inhibitors of amine oxidase. It has been used as a provocative agent in the diagnosis of pheochromocytoma.

tyroid (ti′roid) Having the texture of cheese.

tyrosinase (ti-ro′sin-ās) See monophenol monooxygenase.

tyrosine (ti′ro-sēn) (Tyr) A crystallizable amino acid, $C_9H_{11}NO_3$, that is sparingly soluble in water; present in most proteins; an essential constituent of any diet; a precursor of melanin and thyroxin.

tyrosinemia (ti-ro-si-ne′me-ă) Disorder characterized by elevated blood concentration of tyrosine, increased urinary excretion of tyrosine and tyrosol compounds, enlargement of the liver and spleen, and defects of renal tubules.

hereditary t. A form occurring as an autosomal recessive inheritance.

t. of newborn A form occurring in newborn infants, especially premature; characterized by failure to thrive, diarrhea, and vomiting; the urine has a characteristic odor of decaying cabbage. The condition usually resolves spontaneously within three months and almost always without after effects.

tyrosinosis (ti-ro-sĭ-no′sis) An uncommon hereditary disorder of tyrosine metabolism, marked by excessive excretion of para-hydroxyphenylpyruvic acid.

T

U

ubiquinone (u-bik′wĭ-nōn) 2,3-Dimethoxybenzoquinone, a hydrophobic compound that plays a role in electron transport in tissues. Also called coenzyme Q (for quinone).

udder (ud′er) The baglike mammary gland of animals such as cows, sheep, and goats.

ulcer (ul′ser) A depressed lesion on the skin or mucous membrane.

aphthous u.'s Small whitish ulcers surrounded by a red border, occurring on the mucosa of the mouth in aphthous stomatitis.

Curling's u. Ulcer occurring in the duodenum as a result of severe burns or body injuries. Also called stress ulcer.

Cushing's u. One or multiple small ulcers occurring throughout the stomach and duodenum after severe head trauma.

decubitus u. Ulcer of the skin, and sometimes muscles, occurring in pressure areas of bedridden patients allowed to lie in the same position for long periods of time. Also called bedsore; pressure sore.

dendritic u., dendriform u. Superficial ulcer of the cornea that spreads in a branching pattern; caused by the herpes simplex virus.

dental u. Lesion on the oral mucosa resulting from biting or friction from a rough edge on a tooth.

diabetic u. Ulcer associated with diabetes, occurring most frequently in the lower extremities, especially the toes.

duodenal u. Ulceration of the mucous lining of the duodenum.

esophageal u. Ulcer generally located at the lower end of the esophagus, frequently due to chronic regurgitation of gastric juice.

gastric u. Ulcer of the stomach usually on or near the lesser curvature.

gummatous u. Ulcer appearing on the skin during the late stage of syphilis.

indolent u. Ulcer that does not respond to treatment.

penetrating u. Ulcer extending into the deep tissues of an organ.

peptic u. Gastrointestinal ulcer, especially of the stomach or duodenum, caused by the aggressive actions of acid-pepsin juices; it develops mainly from a *Helicobacter pylori* infection, also as a result of treatment with nonsteroidal anti-inflammatory drugs, or rarely from excessive acid secretion caused by a gastrinoma.

perforated u. Ulcer that has eroded through the wall of an organ (e.g., of the stomach).

rodent u. Basal cell carcinoma of the skin.

roentgen u. Ulcer caused by overexposure to x rays.

soft u. See chancroid.

stercoral u. Ulcer of the colon caused by impacted feces.

stomal u. Ulcer in jejunal mucosa following (and occurring near) the surgical union of the jejunum and stomach.

stress u. See Curling's ulcer.

transparent u. Ulcer occurring on the cornea and healing without opacity.

trophic u. Ulcer due to impaired circulation to the part.

tropical u. Sloughing ulcer occurring usually on the legs as a bacterial infection superimposed on a scratch or insect bite; seen in tropical climates.

varicose u. Ulcer due to and overlying a varicose vein.

venereal u. See chancroid.

ulcerate (ul′sĕ-rāt) To form an ulcer.

ulceration (ul-sĕ-ra′shun) **1.** The formation of an ulcer. **2.** An ulcer.

ulcerative (ul′ser-a-tiv) **1.** Causing the formation of ulcers. **2.** Marked by ulceration.

ulcerogenic (ul-ser-o-jen′ik) Causing the formation of ulcers.

ulcerous (ul′ser-us) Characterized by the presence of ulcers.

ulerythema (u-ler-ĭ-the′mă) An inflammatory process that ultimately results in atrophy or scarring.

u. ophryogenes Folliculitis of the eyebrows leaving scars after healing.

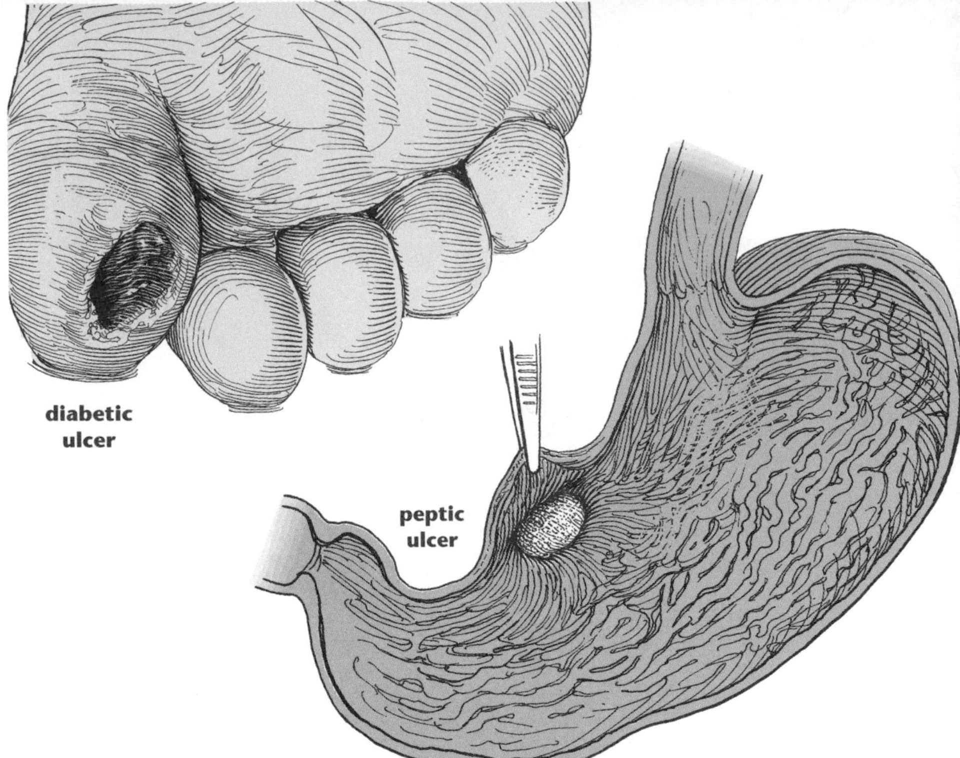

ulna (ul′nă) The larger of the two bones of the forearm, extending from the elbow to the wrist on the side opposite to the thumb. Popularly called elbow bone. See table of bones.

ulnar (ul′nar) Relating to the ulna.

ulnoradial (ul-no-ra′de-al) Relating to the ulna and radius (bones of the forearm).

ulotomy (u-lot′ŏ-me) The cutting or sectioning of contracting scar tissue to relieve tension or deformity.

ultracentrifuge (ul-tră-sen′trĭ-fūj) A convection-free high speed centrifuge (up to 100,000 rpm); used in the separation of large molecules and for determinations of molecular weight.

ultradian (ul-tra′de-an) Relating to biorhythms that occur in cycles more frequent than 24 hours. Also called ultradian rhythm.

ultrafilter (ul-tră-fil′ter) A semipermeable membrane (e.g., collodion, fish bladder, or filter paper impregnated with gels) capable of removing all but the smallest particles, such as viruses.

ultrafiltration (ul-tră-fil-tra′shun) **1.** Filtration using an ultrafilter. **2.** Filtration through a semipermeable membrane for the separation of colloids from their dispersion medium and dissolved crystalloids.

ultraligation (ul-tră-li-ga′shun) Ligation or tying of a blood vessel beyond the point where a branch is given off.

ultramicrometer (ul-tră-mi-krom′ĕ-ter) A micrometer with an extremely accurate gauge, capable of measuring to one millionth of a centimeter.

ultramicroscope (ul-tră-mi′kro-skōp) A darkfield microscope with high-intensity refracted illumination for viewing very minute objects or particles of colloidal size; the horizontal beam of light striking the particles is retracted and appears as bright spots against a black background.

ultramicroscopic (ul-tră-mi-kro-skop′ik) Too small to be visible under the ordinary microscope.

ultramicrotome (ul-tră-mi′kro-tōm) An instrument for cutting tissue into very thin sections (0.1 µm thick or less in thickness) for electron microscopy.

ultrasonic (ul-tră-son′ik) Relating to sound waves above 30,000 cycles per second, not perceptible to the human ear.

ultrasonogram (ul-tră-son′o-gram) A record made by ultrasonography. Also called sonogram; echograph.

ultrasonograph (ul-tră-son′o-graf) An apparatus that sends sound impulses (at frequencies above the range audible to the human ear) toward an organ, which in turn bounces back or echoes the sounds; the patterns produced are graphically displayed on a fluorescent screen for interpretation. Also called sonograph; echograph.

ultrasonography (ul-tră-son-og′ra-fe) The delineation of deep bodily structures by measuring the reflection of ultrasonic waves directed into the tissue. Also called sonography; echography.

Doppler u. Diagnostic technique to measure and visually record changes in the frequency of a continuous ultrasonic wave, indicative of the change in a moving target (e.g., velocity of the blood flow in underlying vessels).

endoscopic u. Ultrasonography performed via a small high-frequency transducer incorporated into the tip of a fiberoptic endoscope. Also called endosonography.

gray-scale u. Amplification and processing of echoes (by a television video-scan converter) into a visual image ranging from white to different shades of gray, white representing the strongest echoes.

ultrasonoscope (ul-tră-son′o-skōp) See ultrasonograph.

ultrasonosurgery (ul-tră-son-o-sur′jer-e) The use of ultrasound (high frequency sound waves) to disrupt tissues or tracts, especially in the central nervous system.

ultrasound (ul′tră-sound) Sound waves of frequency higher than the range audible to the human ear, especially in the 1- to 10-MHz range; the waves are propagated at a speed determined by the physical properties of the medium through which they travel.

ultrastructure (ul′tră-struk-chur) The ultimate structure or organization of protoplasm, as seen with the aid of the electron microscope. Also called fine structure; submicroscopic structure.

ultraviolet (ul-tră-vi′o-let) (UV) Denoting a range of invisible radiation extending from the visible violet portion of the spectrum out to the low-frequency x-ray region of the electromagnetic spectrum.

u. A (UVA) Ultraviolet radiation from 320 to 400 nm; a very weak producer of sunburn and cancer; causes tanning.

u. B (UVB) Ultraviolet radiation from 290 to 320 nm; causes tanning and sunburn; excessive exposure causes cancer of fair skin.

u. C (UVC) Ultraviolet radiation from 200 to 290 nm; does not reach surface of the earth; used as germicide and in mercury arc lamps; may cause sunburn and inflammation of the cornea.

ululation (ŭl-yu-lā′shun) **1.** The loud, inarticulate crying of emotionally disturbed persons, especially hysterical ones. **2.** Loud lamentation.

umbilical (um-bil′ĭ-kal) Relating to the navel. Also called omphalic.

umbilicated, umbilicate (um-bil′ĭ-kāt-ed, um-bil′ĭ-kāt) Dimpled; having a pit or depression that resembles the navel.

umbilication (um-bil-ĭ-ka′shun) A depression or pit resembling the navel.

U

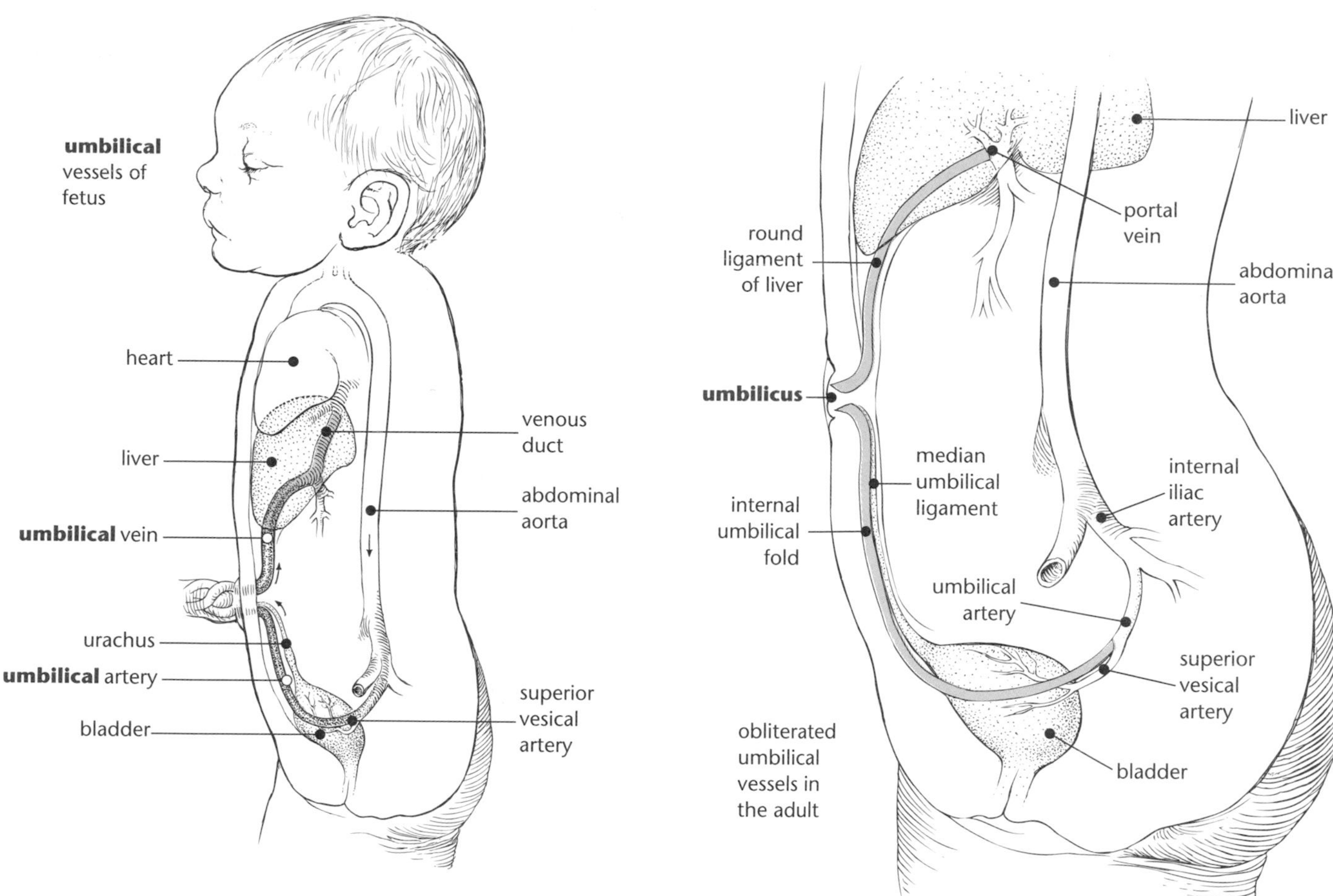

umbilicus (um-bil'ĭ-kus) The depressed area of the abdominal wall where the umbilical cord was attached to the fetus. Popularly called navel.

umbo (um´bo), *pl.* **umbo´nes** **1.** A projection at the center of a rounded surface. **2.** The most depressed point on the outer surface of the tympanic membrane, formed by traction of the malleus on the inner surface of the membrane to which it is attached.

uncal (ung'kal) Relating to the uncus (in the brain).

unciform (un´sĭ-form) See uncinate.

Uncinaria (un-sĭ-na´re-ă) A genus of hookworms (class Nematoda) that infect some mammals.

uncinariasis (un-sin-ă-ri´ă-sis) See ancylostomiasis.

uncinate (un´sĭ-nāt) **1.** Hooked or shaped like a hook. Also called unciform. **2.** Relating to an uncus.

unconscious (un-kon'shus) **1.** Inability to respond to sensory stimuli. **2.** In psychoanalytical theory, the part of the mind containing feelings, urges, and experiences of which the individual is only briefly or never aware.

uncoupler (un-kup´ler) Any substance (such as dinitrophenol) that uncouples the usual linkage between oxidation and phosphorylation.

uncus (ung'kus) The hooked anterior portion of the hippocampal gyrus.

undecylenic acid (un-de-sil-en'ik as'id) An antifungal proprietary agent, $CH_2CH(CH_2)_8COOH$, used in treating dermatophytic infections.

underachiever (un-der-ă-chēv´er) An individual, especially a student, who manifestly performs below his capacity as determined by tests of intelligence, aptitude, or ability.

undercut (un'der-kut) **1.** The portion of a prepared tooth cavity that mechanically locks the restorative filling, such as amalgam, into place. **2.** The portion of a tooth that lies between the gingiva and the crest of contour. **3.** The contour of a dental arch which prevents the proper insertion of a denture.

undernutrition (un-der-nu-trish'un) Any deviation below good nutrition; a condition resulting from a negative nutritive balance that occurs when metabolic utilization plus excretion of one or more essential nutrients exceeds the supply.

undescended (un-dĭ-sen'ded) Not descended to a normal position (e.g., a testis). See also cryptorchidism.

undifferentiated (un-dif-er-en-she-a´ted) Not differentiated, usually applied to cells.

undo (un´doo) Psychoanalytically, to act out in reverse an unacceptable prior action (a defense mechanism).

undulate (un´jŏŏ-lāt) **1.** To fluctuate in wavelike patterns (e.g., a fever). **2.** Having an irregular, wavy border or appearance (e.g., certain bacterial colonies).

unerupted (un-e-rup´ted) In dentistry, denoting a normal developing tooth or an impacted tooth that has not emerged or perforated the oral mucosa.

ungual (ung'gwal) Relating to the nails. Also called unguinal.

unguent (ung'gwent) Ointment.

unguentum (ung-gwen'tum) (ung., ungt.) Latin for ointment.

unguiculate (ung-gwik´u-lāt) Having nails or claws.

unguinal (ung´gwi-nal) See ungual.

unguis (ung´gwis), *pl.* **un´gues** Latin for nail (either a fingernail or a toenail).

uniaxial (u-ne-ak'se-al) **1.** Having but one axis (e.g., a hinge joint). **2.** Developing chiefly in only one direction.

unicameral (u-nĭ-kam'er-al) See monolocular.

unicellular (u-nĭ-sel´u-lar) Consisting of one cell (e.g., a protozoan).

unicuspid (u-nĭ-kus'pid) Denoting a tooth with one cusp.

uniform (u´nĭ-form) Consistent in appearance; without variation in form.

unigravida (u-nĭ-grav'ĭ-dă) See primigravida.

unilaminar (u-nĭ-lam'ĭ-nar) Having only one layer.

unilateral (u-nĭ-lat´er-al) Occurring only on one side.

unilocular (u-nĭ-lok´u-lar) Having only one compartment.

uninuclear, uninucleate (u-nĭ-nu'kle-ar, u-nĭ-nu´kle-āt) Having only one nucleus.

uniocular (u-nĭ-ok'u-lar) Relating to or having one eye.

union (yōōn´yun) The process of joining together of tissues. Also called healing.

delayed u. Healing of a fractured bone that appears to be unduly slow.

faulty u. Condition in which tissues have united but not in their proper positions.

fibrous u. Formation of a fibrous callus on a bone at the site of a fracture without development of bone tissue.

primary u. See healing by first intention, under healing.

secondary u. See healing by second intention, under healing.

syngamic nuclear u. The uniting of the nuclei of spermatozoon and ovum during fertilization.

vicious u. A faulty union that produces a deformity.

unipara (u-nip'ă-ră) See primipara.

uniparental (u-nĭ-pă-ren'tal) Relating to one parent only.

unipennate (u-nĭ-pen'āt) Resembling one half of a feather; said of certain muscles with a tendon on one side. Also called demipenniform.

unipolar (u-nĭ-po´lar) Having, produced by, or located at one pole.

uniport (u'nĭ-port) Transport of one substance across a cell membrane by a protein carrier.

unit (u'nit) (u) An entity regarded as an elementary constituent of a larger whole.

Angström u. (Å) See angstrom.

antigen u. The smallest amount of antigen that, in the presence of specific antiserum, will fix one unit of complement so as to prevent hemolysis.

antitoxin u. The unit for expressing the amount of antitoxin that will neutralize 100 minimal lethal doses of toxin.

base u. Any one of the fundamental units of a system of measurement, such as those of the International System of Units (SI); i.e., the meter (m), kilogram (kg), second (s), ampere (A), kelvin (K), mole (mol), and candela (cd).

British thermal u. (BTU) The amount of heat required to increase the temperature of 1 pound of water from 3.9°C to 4.4°C.

U

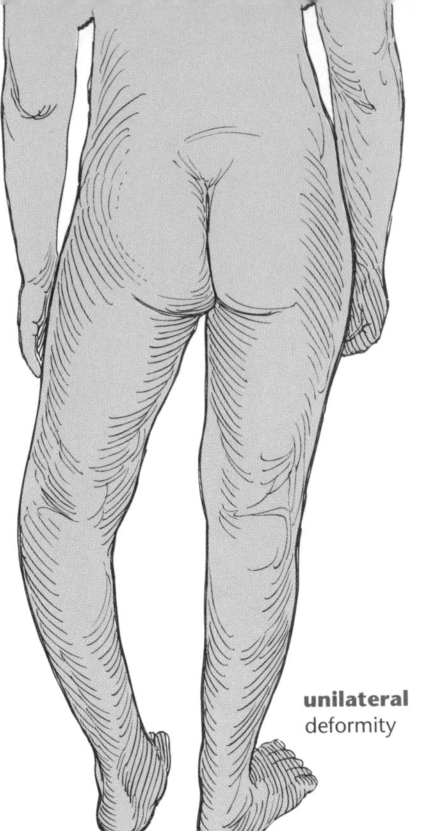

unilateral deformity

UNITS OF MEASUREMENT AND THEIR ABBREVIATIONS

Units of Concentration	
molar (mol/liter)	M
parts per million	ppm
Units of Length	
meter	m
micrometer	µm
Angstrom (0.1 nm)	Å
Units of Volume	
milliliter	ml
microliter	µl
Units of Mass	
gram	g
microgram	µg
Units of Time	
hour	hr
minute	min
second	s, sec
Units of Electricity	
ampere	amp
milliampere	mA
volt	V
ohm	
Units of Energy and Work	
joule	J
calorie	cal
Units of Temperature	
degree centigrade	°
thermodynamic temperature (Kelvin)	K
Units of Radioactivity	
counts per minute	cpm
curie(s)	Ci
Miscellaneous **Units**	
revolutions per minute	rpm
cycles per second (hertz)	Hz
pascal (newton/meter^2)	Pa
lux	lx
candela	cd
lumen	lm

Prefixes to Names of **Units**

Prefix	Factor	Symbol	Prefix	Factor	Symbol
exa	10^{18}	E	milli	10^{-3}	m
peta	10^{15}	P	micro	10^{-6}	µ
tera	10^{12}	T	nano	10^{-9}	n
giga	10^{9}	G	pico	10^{-12}	p
mega	10^{6}	M	femto	10^{-15}	f
kilo	10^{3}	k	atto	10^{-18}	a
centi	10^{-2}	c			

centimeter-gram-second u., CGS u. A metric unit denoting a rate of work.
coronary care u. (CCU) A facility designed to provide maximal surveillance and optimal therapy for patients suspected of having acute myocardial infarctions and other acute cardiac disorders requiring intensive and continuous monitoring.
critical care u. See intensive care unit (ICU).
dental u. An operative unit in which are assembled items used in dental procedures, such as saliva ejector, compressed air, dental engine, operative light, water supply, cuspidor, etc.
electromagnetic u. (emu) A unit in an absolute system of units that uses the magnetic effects of current (e.g., abampere).
electrostatic u. (esu) A unit in an absolute system of units that uses static electricity (e.g., statampere)
u. of force See dyne.
G u. A coupling protein in the plasma membrane, between the hormone receptor and adenyl cyclase, which facilitates transmission of a hormonal signal.
gravitational u. A unit equal to 1 pound of force divided by 1 pound of mass.
u. of heat In the centimeter-gram-second (CGS) system, the calorie; the amount of heat required to raise one milliliter of water from 14.5 to 15.5°C.
heparin u. The quantity of heparin required to keep 1 ml of cat's blood fluid for 24 hr at 0°C; equivalent to about 0.002 mg of pure heparin.
Hounsfield u. Unit of x-ray attenuation used for CT scans, based on a scale in which air is –1000, water is 0, and bone is +1000.
insulin u. See international insulin unit.
intensive care u. (ICU) A specially equipped facility in a hospital operated by trained personnel for the care of critically ill persons requiring immediate and continuous attention. Also called critical care unit.
international u. (IU) A unit of biologic substance (e.g., vitamins) established by the World Health Organization (WHO).
international insulin u. A unit of 0.045 milligram of pure international standard zinc-insulin crystals.
International System of U.'s See under system.
international u. of vitamin A The biologic activity of 0.3 micrograms of vitamin A (alcohol form).
international u. of vitamin D The antirachitic activity of 0.025 micrograms of a standard preparation of crystalline vitamin D.
map u. See centimorgan.
motor u. A motor nerve cell and the muscle fibers it innervates.
u. of oxytocin The oxytocic activity of 0.5 milligram of the USP Posterior-pituitary Reference Standard; 1 milligram of synthetic oxytocin corresponds to 500 international units of oxytocin activity.
u. of penicillin The penicillin activity of 0.6 microgram of penicillin G.
photofluorographic u. (PF unit) An apparatus consisting of an x-ray tube and a generator coupled to a photographic camera to record miniature radiographs.
rat u. (RU) The amount of a substance that under standardized conditions is just enough to produce a specified result in experimental rats.
SI u. Système International d'Unités; international system of units. See under system.
Svedberg u. (S) A unit of time and velocity measuring the sedimentation constant of a colloid solution, equal to 10^{-13} seconds.
USP u. A United States Pharmacopeia measure of the potency of any pharmacologic preparation.
u. of vasopressin The pressor activity of 0.5 milligram of the USP Posterior-pituitary Reference Standard.

United States Adopted Name Council (USAN) An enterprise that gives nonproprietary names to new drugs; it replaced the older AMAUSP Nomenclature Committee.

univalent (u-nĭ-va´lent) Having a valence of one; having the combining power of one hydrogen atom. Also called monovalent.

unmyelinated (un-mi´ĕ-lĭ-nāt-ed) Having no myelin sheath; a characteristic of some nerve fibers.

Unna's boot (oon´ăz bo͞ot) A flexible and porous occlusive dressing, similar to a plaster cast but consisting of gauze bandage impregnated with a gelatinous substance and a paste; applied primarily to the foot and leg, especially in treating dermatitides and ulcerated conditions.

unsaturated (un-sat´u-rāt-ed) **1.** Not saturated; denoting a solution capable of dissolving more solute at a given temperature. **2.** Denoting an organic compound possessing double or triple bonds, such as ethylene. **3.** Denoting a chemical compound in which all the affinities are not satisfied, thereby allowing other atoms or radicals to be added to it.

unsex (un-seks´) To deprive of gonads or sexual attributes; to castrate.

unstable (un-sta´bl) **1.** Readily changing in physical state. **2.** Tending to become spontaneously radioactive.

unstriated (un-stri´āt-ed) Lacking striations; denoting the structure of the smooth muscle.

untoward (un-tord´) Resistant to treatment.

upper (ŭp´er) Slang expression meaning an amphetamine pill or other substance which acts as a mood elevator.

up-regulation (up reg-u-la´shun) An increase in the number of active receptors on the cell surface in response to deficiency of a homologous hormone or neurotransmitter.

uptake (ŭp´tāk) The amount of a substance, especially a radionuclide, absorbed by any tissue; e.g., radioiodine (^{131}I) by the thyroid gland.

urachal (u´ră-kal) Relating to the urachus.

urachus (u´ră-kus) A canal present in the fetus between the umbilicus and the apex of the bladder; it obliterates early in intrauterine life, remaining thereafter as a fibrous cord (the median umbilical ligament).
patent u. A urachus which remains open after birth. Also called urachal fistula.

uracil (u´ră-sil) 2,4-Dioxypyrimidine, a prevalent pyrimidine (base) found in nucleic acid.

uranium (u-ra´ne-um) A heavy silvery-white, radioactive metallic element, occurring in several minerals, especially pitchblende; it has a half-life of 4.5×10^9 years; symbol U, atomic number 92, atomic weight 238.03.

uranium-235 (^{235}U) A uranium isotope with a half-life of 713 million years; the first substance shown capable of supporting a self-sustaining chain reaction.

uranium-238 (^{238}U) The most common uranium isotope, with a half-life of 4.51 billion years.

uranostaphyloplasty (u-ră-no-staf´ĭ-lo-plas-te) A surgical procedure for repairing a defect (usually a cleft) of both the soft and the hard palate. Also called uranostaphylorrhaphy.

uranostaphylorrhaphy (u-ră-no-staf´ĭ-lor-ă-fe) See uranostaphyloplasty.

uranostaphyloschisis (u-ră-no-staf-ĭ-los´kĭ-sis) Fissure or cleft of the soft and hard palates.

uranyl (u´ră-nil) The UO_2^{++} ion, as in such salts as uranyl nitrate, $UO_2(NO_3)_2$, and uranyl sulfate, UO_2SO_4.

urate (ūr´āt) A salt of uric acid; occurs commonly in urinary deposits and calculi.

urea (u-re´ă) **1.** $CO(NH_2)_2$; chief end product of mammalian protein metabolism, formed in the liver

U

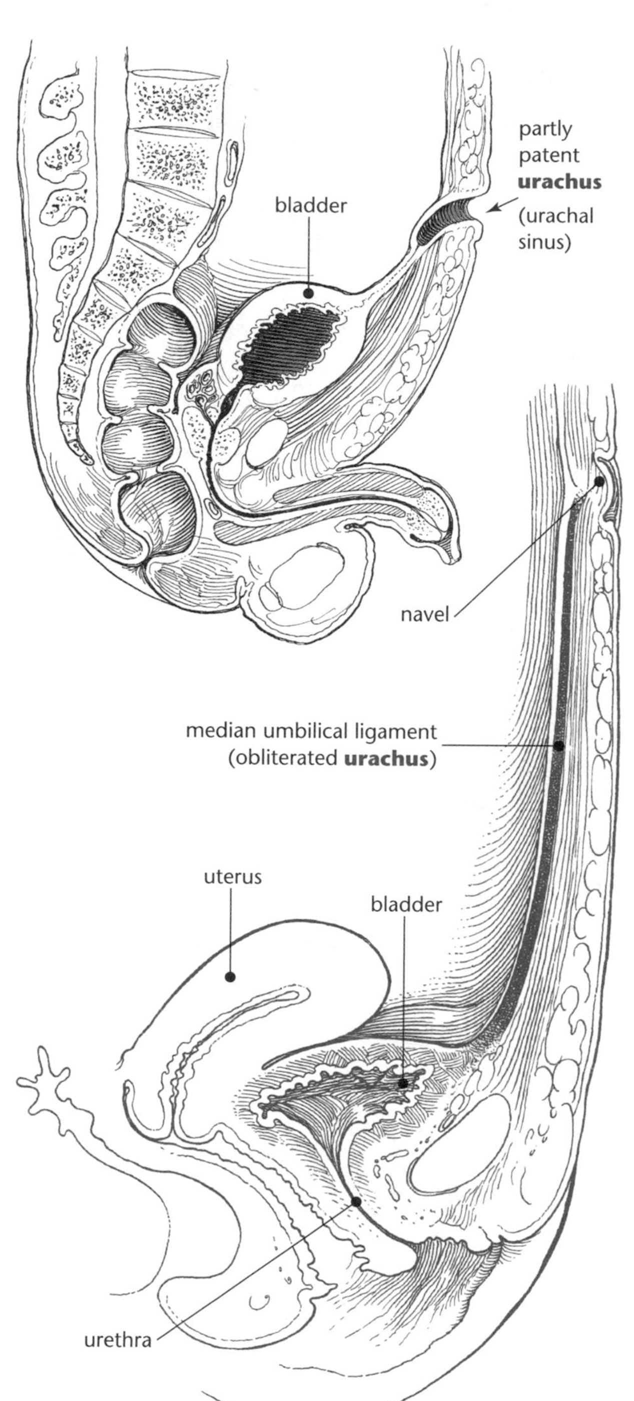

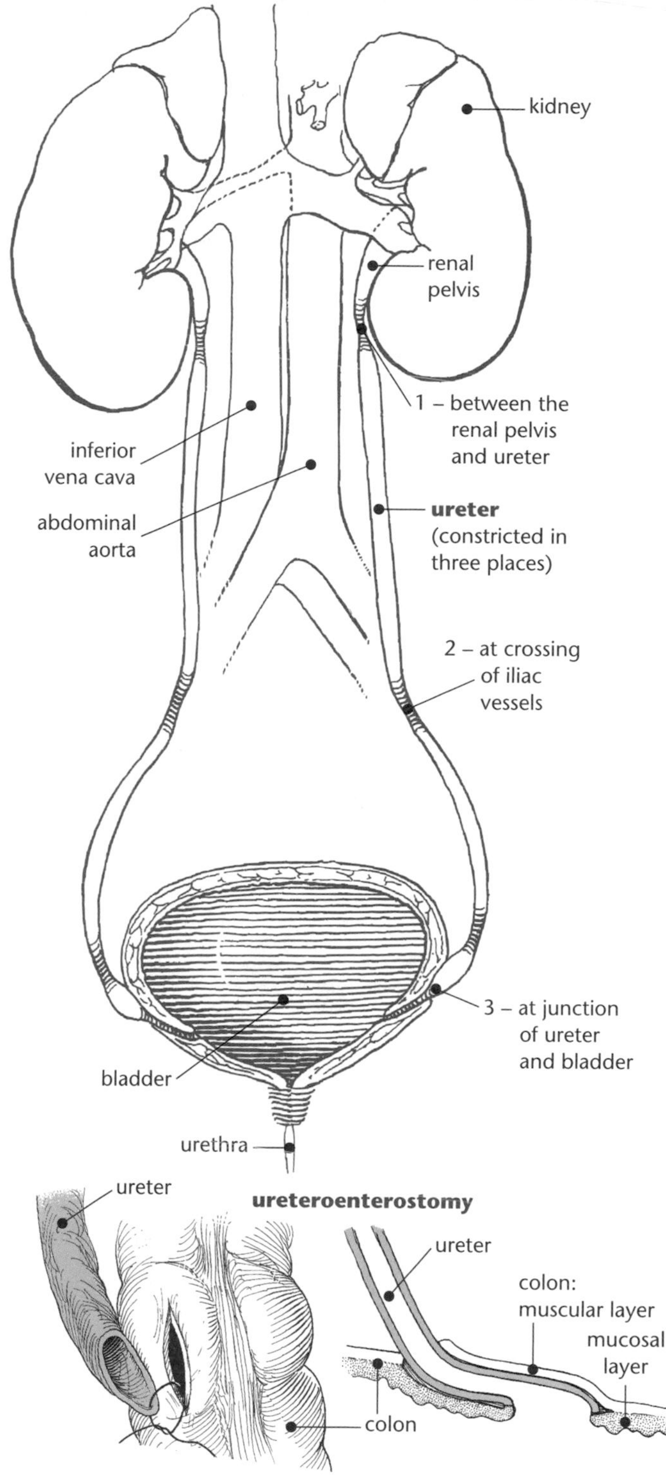

suturing ureteral transplant

from amino acids and compounds of ammonia; the chief nitrogenous component of urine; an average person, in steady state and consuming average amounts of dietary protein, excretes about 30 g of urea per day. **2.** A preparation of hypertonic urea (30%) used intravenously to temporarily reduce intracranial or cerebrospinal pressure in the control of cerebral edema; Ureaphil®.

ureal (u´re-al) Relating to urea.

Ureaplasma (u-re-ă-plaz´mă) A genus of gram-negative bacteria (family Mycoplasmataceae), which lack a cell wall and hydrolyze urea with production of ammonia.

U. urealyticum A sexually transmitted species causing disease of the genitourinary system; implicated in causing infertility in both males and females.

urease (u´re-ās) An enzyme that promotes the breakdown of urea into ammonia and carbon dioxide; present in certain seeds and produced by certain microorganisms, especially *Proteus* bacteria.

urecchysis (u-rek´ĭ-sis) Escape of urine into the tissues; e.g., in rupture of the bladder.

uredema (u-rĕ-de´mă) A swollen or edematous condition resulting from infiltration of extravasated urine into the tissues.

uredo (u-rē´do) **1.** See urticaria. **2.** A burning or itching sensation in the skin.

urelcosis (u-rel-ko´sis) Ulceration of any part of the urinary passage.

uremia (u-re´me-ă) A toxic condition caused by retention in the blood of waste substances normally excreted in the urine; the principal wastes that accumulate are products of protein metabolism; symptoms may include lethargy, loss of appetite, vomiting, anemia, blood clotting disorders, an abnormal mental state, pericarditis, and colitis.

uremic (u-re´mik) Relating to uremia.

ureolysis (u-re-ol´ĭ-is) The breaking down of urea into carbon dioxide and ammonia.

uresis (u-re´sis) Urination.

ureter (ūr´ĕter) The long, slender, muscular tube that conveys urine from the pelvis of the kidney to the base of the bladder.

ureteral (u-re´ter-al) Relating to a ureter or ureters. Also called ureteric.

ureterectasia (u-re-ter-ek-ta´zhă) Distention of a ureter.

ureterectomy (u-re-ter-ek´tŏ-me) Surgical removal of a ureter or a segment of it.

ureteric (u-rĕ-ter´ik) See ureteral.

ureterocele (u-re´ter-o-sēl) A cystlike dilatation at the lower end of a ureter, usually protruding into the bladder.

ureterocystostomy (u-re-ter-o-sis-tos´tŏ-me) See ureteroneocystostomy.

ureteroenterostomy (u-re-ter-o-en-ter-os´tŏ-me) The surgical procedure of forming an anastomosis between a ureter and the intestine.

ureterogram (u-re´ter-o-gram) A roentgenogram

U

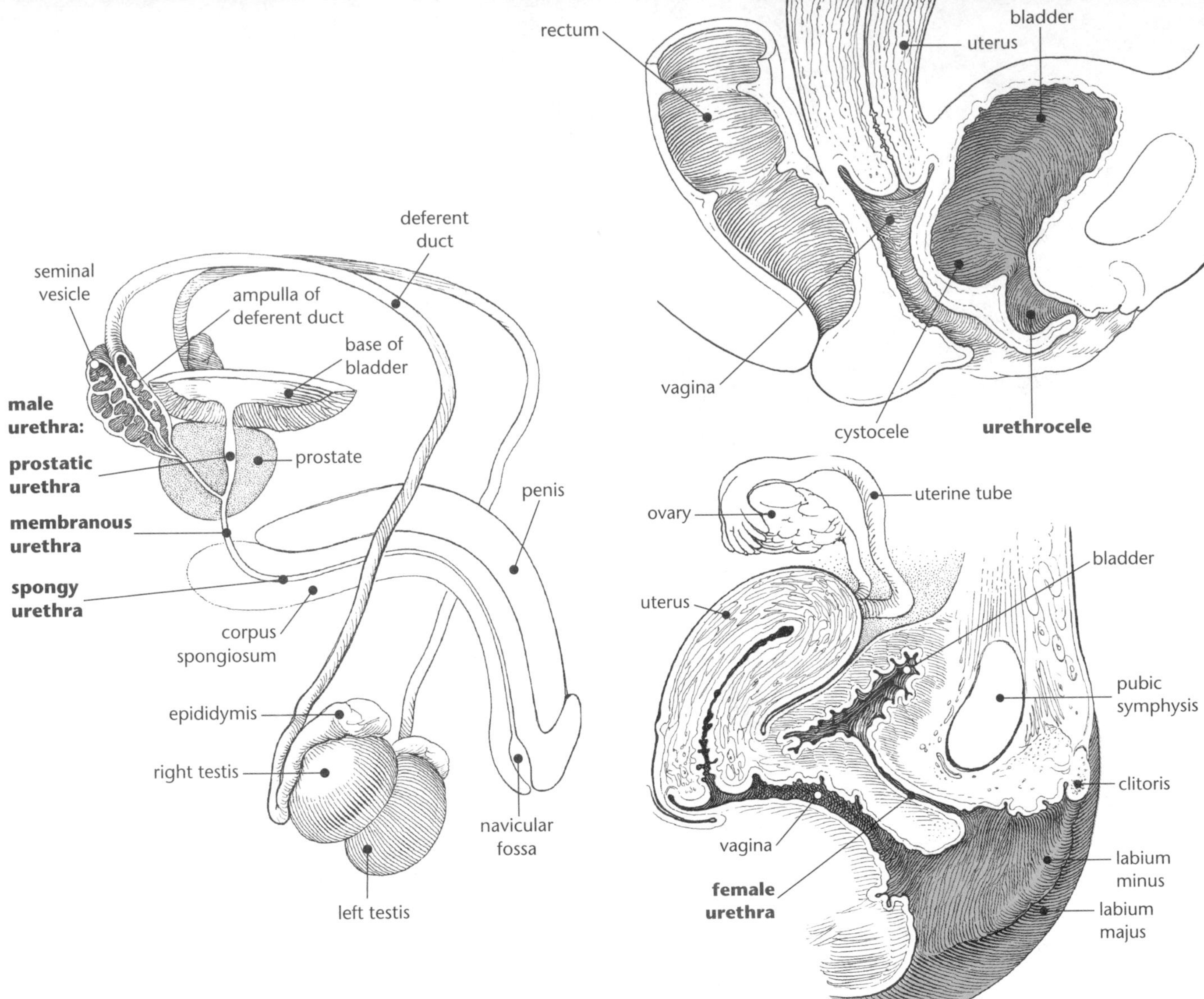

of a ureter after injection of a radiopaque substance.

ureterography (u-re-ter-og´ră-fe) The practice of x-raying the ureter after injection of a radiopaque substance.

ureterolith (u-re´ter-o-lith) A stone in the ureter.

ureterolithiasis (u-re-ter-o-lĭ-thi´ă-sis) The presence of a calculus in a ureter.

ureterolithotomy (u-re-ter-o-lĭ-thot´ŏ-me) Surgical removal of a stone from a ureter.

ureterolysis (u-re-ter-ol´ĭ-sis) Rupture of a ureter.

ureteroneocystostomy (u-re-ter-o-ne-o-sis-tos´tŏ-me) Transplantation of the distal part of the ureter to a site in the bladder other than the normal one. Also called ureterocystostomy.

ureteronephrectomy (u-re-ter-o-nĕ-frek´tŏ-me) Surgical removal of a kidney and its ureter.

ureteropelvic (u-re-ter-o-pel´vik) Pertaining to a ureter and the adjoining renal pelvis.

U

ureteropyelitis (u-re-ter-pi-ĕ-li´tis) Inflammation of a ureter extending up to and including the pelvis of the kidney.

ureteropyelogram (u-re-ter-o-pi´ĕ-lo-gram) See pyelogram.

ureteropyeloneostomy (u-re-ter-o-pi-ĕ-lo-ne-os´to-me) A surgical procedure for excising a portion of the ureter and inserting the remaining part through a new opening into the pelvis of the kidney.

ureteropyeloplasty (u-re-ter-o-pi´ĕ-lo-plas-te) Reparative surgery of the ureter and pelvis of the kidney.

ureteropyosis (u-re-ter-o-pi-o´sis) Accumulation of pus in a ureter.

ureteroscope (u-re´ter-o-skōp) Optical instrument introduced through the bladder for visual examination of the interior of a ureter.

ureterosigmoid (u-re-ter-o-sig´moid) Pertaining to the ureter and the sigmoid colon.

ureterosigmoidostomy (u-re-ter-o-sig-moi-dos´to-me) Surgical implantation of the ureters into the sigmoid colon.

ureterostenosis (u-re-ter-o- stĕ-no´sis) Abnormal stricture of a ureter.

ureterostomy, cutaneous (u-re-ter-os´tŏ-me, ku-ta´ne-us) Attachment of the divided distal end of a ureter to the skin of the lower abdomen to create an external opening through which urine may be discharged when the bladder has been removed.

ureterotomy (u-re-ter-ot´ŏ-me) Any surgical division of a ureter.

ureteroureterostomy (u-re-ter-o-u-re-ter-os´to-me) Surgical connection of the two ureters or of two sections of a ureter.

ureterovaginal (u-re-ter-o-vaj´ĭ-nal) Relating to or communicating with a ureter and the vagina.

ureterovesical (u-re-ter-o-ves´ĭ-kal) Relating to a ureter and the bladder, as the junction of the two structures.

ureterovesicostomy (u-re-ter-o-ves-ĭ-kos´to-me) Surgical division of a ureter and its implantation to another site in the bladder.

urethra (u-re´thră) The canal leading from the bladder and conveying urine to the exterior of the body.

female u. A channel extending from the neck of the bladder to the urinary opening, inferior and posterior to the clitoris.

male u. A channel extending from the neck of the bladder to the opening at the tip of the glans penis; divided into three parts as it passes through the prostate (prostatic part), urogenital diaphragm (membranous part), corpus spongiosum (spongy part); it conveys spermatic fluid as well as urine.

urethral (u-re´thral) Relating to the urethra.

urethralgia (u-rĕ-thral´je-ă) Pain in the urethra.

urethratresia (u-re-thră-tre´zhă) Congenital imperforation or occlusion of the urethra.

urethrectomy (u-rĕ-threk´tŏ-me) Surgical removal of the urethra, or a segment of it.

urethrism, urethrismus (u´re-thriz-m, u-re-thriz´mus) Irritability or chronic spasm of the urethra, usually associated with inflammation that may involve also the lower portion of the bladder. Also called urethrospasm.

urethritis (u-rĕ-thri´tis) Inflammation of the urethra.

chlamydial u. Sexually transmitted disease caused by the bacterium *Chlamydia trachomatis*. See also nongonococcal urethritis.

gonococcal u. Urethritis caused by gonococci; a form of gonorrhea; appears 2 to 7 days after sexual intercourse with an individual afflicted with gonorrhea.

nongonococcal u. (NGU) Asexually transmitted disease caused by various organisms, most commonly chlamydia; in males it usually produces a mild burning sensation on urination and a slight, grayish discharge, most commonly apparent before the first urination of the day; in females, it produces no symptoms although the organisms may be present in the cervix; a pregnant woman may transmit the infection to her newborn with serious complications. Also called nonspecific urethritis.

non-specific u. (NSU) See nongonococcal urethritis.

urethrocele (u-re´thro-sēl) Prolapse of the female urethra into the vagina, commonly associated with a cystocele; often associated with (not the cause of) urinary incontinence.

urethrocystitis (u-re-thro-sis-ti´tis) Inflammation of the urethra and bladder.

urethrocystopexy (u-re-thro-sis´to-pek-se) Any operation for the relief of stress urinary incontinence

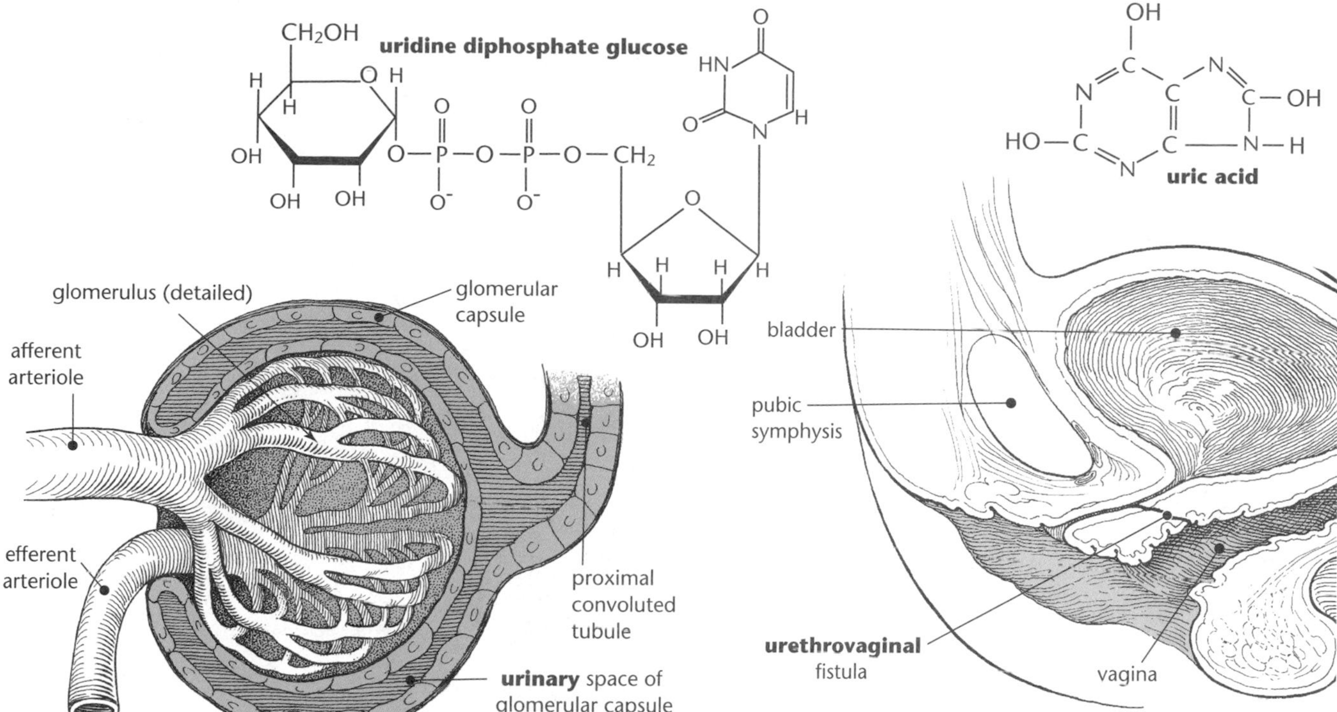

(SUI). Also called colpourethropexy; cystourethropexy.

Burch suprapubic u. Procedure in which the bladder neck is sewn to the Cooper's (pectineal) ligaments in the space of Retzius (retropubic space).

Marshall-Marchetti-Krantz u. Procedure in which the bladder neck is sewn to the periosteum of the symphysis pubis in the space of Retzius (retropubic space).

urethrography (u-rĕ-throg´ră-fe) X-ray examination of the urethra after introduction of a radiopaque substance.

urethrometer (u-rĕ-throm´ĕ-ter) An instrument for measuring the caliber of the urethra.

urethropenile (u-re-thro-pe´nīl) Relating to the urethra and the penis.

urethrophyma (u-re-thro-fi´mă) Any circumscribed swelling or tumor of the urethra.

urethroplasty (u-re´thro-plas-te) Surgical repair of a wound or a defect of the urethra.

urethroprostatic (u-re-thro-pros-tat´ik) Relating to the urethra and the prostate gland.

urethrorectal (u-re-thro-rek´tal) Relating to or communicating with the urethra and the rectum.

urethrorrhagia (u-re-thro-ra´je-ă) Bleeding from the urethra.

urethrorrhea (u-re-thro-re´a) Abnormal discharge from the urethra.

urethroscope (u-re´thro-skōp) An instrument for inspecting the interior of the urethra.

urethroscopy (u-rĕ-thros´ko-pe) Visual examination of the urethra with a urethroscope.

urethrospasm (u-re´thro-spazm) See urethrism.

urethrostenosis (u-re-thro-ste-no´sis) Abnormal narrowing or stricture of the urethra.

urethrostomy (u-re-thros´to-me) Surgical formation of an opening into the urethra for temporary or permanent diversion of urine.

urethrotome (u-re´thro-tōm) An instrument for dividing a urethral stricture.

urethrotomy (u-rĕ-throt´o-me) Incision into the urethra.

urethrovaginal (u-re-thro vaj´ĭ-nal) Relating to the urethra and vagina.

urethrovesical (u-re-thro-ves´ĭ-kal) Relating to the urethra and the bladder.

urgency (ur´jen-se) Colloquialism for a strong urge to urinate.

uric (u´rik) Relating to urine.

uric acid (u´rik as´id) A white crystalline compound, $C_5H_4O_3$; a normal constituent of urine. Also called lithic acid.

uricolysis (u-rĭ-kol´ĭ-sis) The splitting up of uric acid molecules.

uricosuria (u-rĭ-ko-su´re-ă) The passage of excessive amounts of uric acid in the urine.

uricosuric (u-rĭ-ko-su´rik) An agent that tends to increase the excretion of uric acid in the urine.

uridine (u´rĭ-dēn) (Urd) $C_9H_{12}N_2O_6$, a ribonucleoside containing uracil; important in carbohydrate metabolism; 1-β-D-ribofuranosyluracil.

u. diphosphate (UDP) A nucleotide important in glycogen and galactose metabolism and in nucleic acid synthesis.

u. diphosphate galactose (UDP-galactose) A nucleotide derivative of galactose, resulting from the reaction of uridine diphosphate glucose (UDP-glucose) and galactose-1-phosphate.

u. diphosphate glucose (UDP-glucose) A nucleotide derivative of glucose intermediary in glycogen synthesis; formed from the reaction of glucose-1-phosphate and uridine triphosphate (UTP). Also called uridine diphosphoglucose (UDPG).

u. triphosphate (UTP) A high-energy nucleotide that participates in glycogen metabolism.

uridrosis (u-rĭ-dro´sis) The presence of urea or uric acid in the perspiration, sometimes deposited on the skin as minute crystals. Also written urhidrosis.

uridyl transferase (u´rĭ-dil trans´fer-ās) See hexose-1-phosphate uridylyltransferase.

urinalysis (ur-ĭ-nal´ĭ-sis) Analysis of urine.

routine u., screening u. Testing of the urine to determine pH and the presence of blood, protein, or sugar.

microscopic u. Microscopic examination of the sediment from a centrifuged sample of urine; may reveal the presence of casts and crystals.

urinary (u´rĭ-năr-e) Relating to urine.

urinate (ur´ĭ-nāt) To pass urine, to micturate.

urination (u-rĭ-na´shun) The passing of urine. Also called micturition.

urine (u´rin) The fluid excreted by the kidneys, stored in the bladder, and discharged through the urethra; composed of approximately 96% water and 4% solid matter, chiefly urea and sodium chloride and including many metabolic wastes.

residual u. The urine left over in the bladder after urination.

uriniferous (u-rĭ-nif´er-us) Conveying urine, as the tubules in the kidney.

urinogenous (u-rĭ-noj´ĕ-nus) Producing urine.

urinometer (u-rĭ-nom´ĕ-ter) A device used for determining the specific gravity of urine. Also called urometer; urogravimeter.

urinous (u´rĭ-nus) Relating to, or of the nature of, urine.

uroacidimeter (u-ro-as-ĭ-dim´ĕ-ter) An apparatus for estimating the degree of acidity of a sample of urine.

urobilin (u-ro-bi´lin) A pigment normally found in small amounts in urine, formed by the oxidation of urobilinogen.

urobilinemia (u-ro-bil-ĭ-ne´me-ă) The presence of urobilin in the blood.

urobilinogen (u-ro-bi-lin´ŏ-jen) A colorless compound present in large amounts in feces and in small amounts in urine; formed in the intestines by the reduction of bilirubin; upon oxidation it forms urobilin.

urocele (u´ro-sēl) Distention of the scrotal sac with extravasated urine.

urochrome (u´ro-krōm) A yellow or brownish substance that imparts the characteristic color to urine.

urocystic (u-ro-sis´tik) Relating to the urinary bladder.

urodilatin (u-ro-di-la´tin) A 32-amino acid polypeptide found in urine, believed to facilitate sodium excretion.

urodynamics (u-ro-di-nam´ĭks) The study of the activities of the urinary bladder, urethral sphincter muscle, and pelvic musculature by means of various pressure devices.

urodynia (u-ro-din´e-ă) Urination accompanied by pain or discomfort.

uroerythrin (u-ro-er´ĭ-thrin) A pigment sometimes present in urine; believed to be derived from melanin metabolism.

uroflometer (u-ro-flo´me-ter) An instrument for measuring and graphically recording the rate of urine flow by weighing it during voiding; rate of urination indicator.

urogastrone (u-ro-gas´trōn) A polypeptide extractable from normal urine in man and dog which, when injected into the body, inhibits gastric secretions.

urogenital (u-ro-jen´ĭ-tal) See genitourinary.

urogram (u´ro-gram) An x-ray image of a part of the urinary tract.

urography (u-rog´ră-fe) The process of making x-ray images of any part of the urinary tract that has been rendered opaque by a radiopaque substance (contrast medium).

antegrade u. Urography in which the contrast medium is injected directly into the kidney pelvis through a percutaneus needle puncture. Also called antegrade pyelography.

intravenous u. (IVU) Urography of the kidneys, ureters, and bladder following injection of contrast medium into a peripheral vein. Formerly called intravenous pyelography (IVP).

retrograde u. Urography after injection of a contrast medium into the ureters through the bladder. Also called retrograde pyelography.

urogynecology (u-ro-gi-nĕ-kol´ŏ-je) The study,

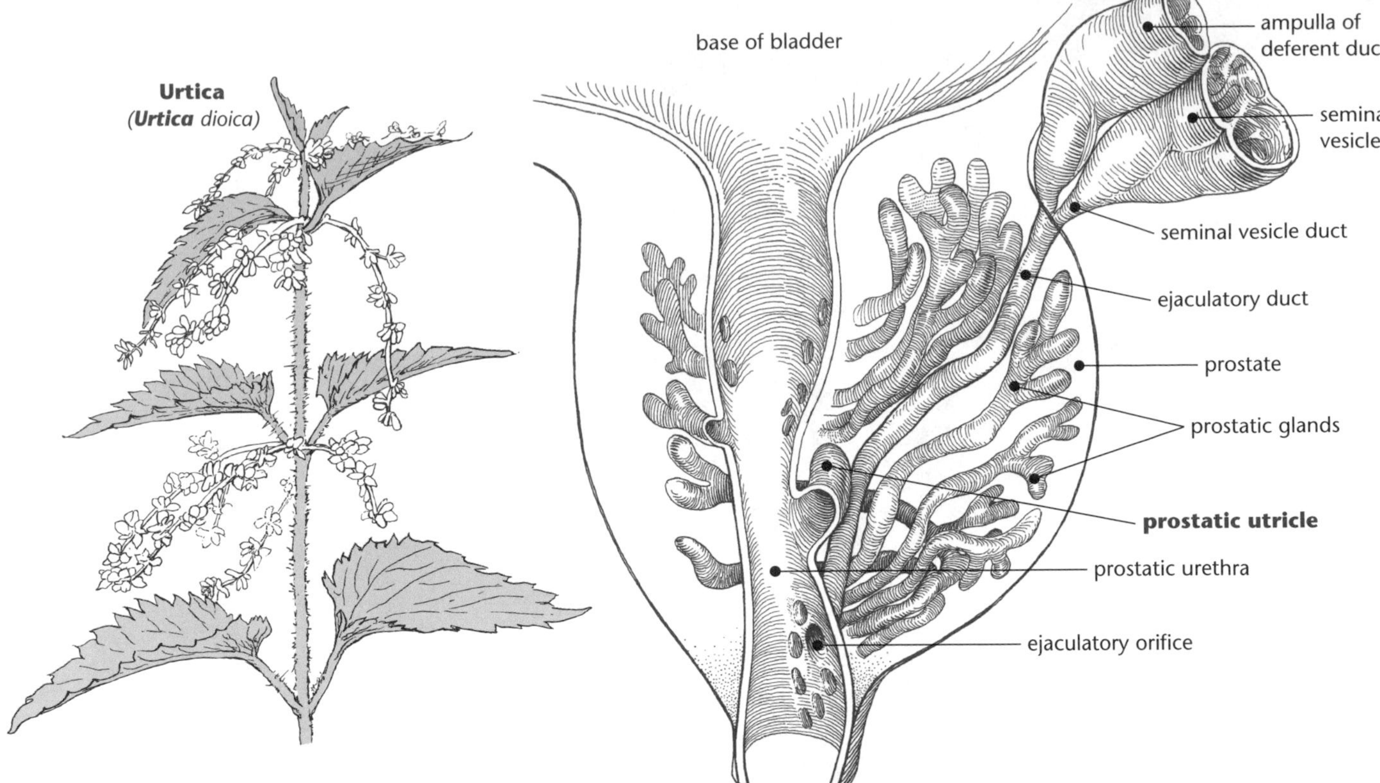

diagnosis, and treatment of diseases of the female urinary tract.

urokinase (u-ro-ki´nās) A proteolytic enzyme in blood and urine that activates the fibrinolytic system by converting plasminogen to plasmin; used to dissolve blood clots.

urolith (u´ro-lith) See urinary stone, under stone.

urolithiasis (u-ro-lĭ-thi´ă-sis) The formation of urinary stones and the resulting disease condition.

urologic (u-ro-loj´ik) Relating to urology.

urologist (u-rol´ŏ-jist) A specialist in urology.

urology (u-rol´ŏ-je) The branch of medicine concerned with the study, diagnosis, and treatment of diseases (especially by surgical techniques) of the urinary tract of both male and female, and of the genital organs of the male.

gynecologic u. Urology of the female reproductive system and lower urinary tract.

uropathy (u-rop´ă-the) Any disease of the urinary tract.

uroplania (u-ro-pla´ne-ă) The escaping or extravasation of urine into the tissues.

uropod (ur´o-pod) An enlarged cytoplasmic extension from the surface of a cell; it is usually capable of developing microspikes and pinocytotic vesicles.

uropoiesis (u-ro-poi-e´sis) The formation of urine.

uropontin (u-ro-pon´tin) A hormone-like protein that tends to inhibit crystallization of calcium oxalate (a kidney stone constituent). Also called urinary osteopontin.

uroporphyrin (u-ro-por´fĭ-rin) A porphyrin, usually found in small amounts in the urine; excretion of an excessive amount may be seen in heavy metal poisoning or in cutaneous porphyria or congenital erythropoietic porphyria.

uroschesis (u-ros´kĕ-sis) Urinary retention or suppression.

urosepsis (u-ro-sep´sis) Sepsis resulting from the absorption and decomposition of extravasated urine in the tissues.

urothelium (u-ro-the´le-um) Epithelium lining the interior of the urinary tract.

ursodeoxycholic acid (ur-so-de-ok-se-ko´lik as´id) Drug prepared from the bile acid chenodiol; used to destroy gallstones.

Urtica (ur-tĭ´kă) A genus of plants that have stinging hairs and secrete a poisonous fluid.

urticant (ur´tĭ-kant) **1.** Any agent that causes itching or stinging. **2.** Producing an itching or stinging sensation.

urticaria (ur-tĭ-kār´e-ă) Eruption of transitory itchy wheals, often due to hypersensitivity to foods or drugs or to emotional factors. Also called hives; uredo.

cholinergic u. Clusters of tiny itchy papules usually brought on by exercise or stress.

cold u. Wheal formed upon exposure to cold.

giant u. See angioneurotic edema, under edema.

u. medicamentosa Urticaria occurring as a reaction to a drug.

papular u. A common and troublesome skin disease of childhood, characterized by the appearance of a wheal followed by a papule; although food allergy is widely accepted as a cause of the eruption, recent evidence favors a parasitic origin, such as bites from cat fleas and bedbugs.

u. pigmentosa A form of mastocytosis characterized by mast cell infiltration of the skin, forming reddish brown pruritic macules or papules; may be accompanied by bone pain. Also called diffuse cutaneous mastocytosis.

Usher's syndrome (ush´ĕrz sin´drōm) Profound childhood hearing impairment with retinitis pigmentosa; inherited as an autosomal recessive trait.

ut dictum (ŭt dik´tum) Latin for as directed.

uterine (u´ter-in, u-tĕ-rīn´) Relating to the uterus.

uterocystostomy (u-ter-o-sis-tos´tŏ-me) Surgical establishment of a communication between the cervix of the uterus and the bladder.

uteroglobin (u-ter-o-glob´in) A protein present in epithelial cells of the inner lining of the uterus (endometrium).

utero-ovarian (u´ter-o o-va´re-an) Relating to the uterus and an ovary.

uteroplacental (u-ter-o-plă-sen´tal) Relating to the uterus and the placenta.

uteroplasty (u´ter-o-plas-te) Reparative surgery of the uterus.

uterosacral (u-ter-o-sa´kral) Relating to the uterus and the sacrum.

uterotomy (u-ter-ot´ŏ-me) See hysterotomy.

uterotonic (u-ter-o-ton´ik) **1.** Overcoming relaxation of the uterine muscle. **2.** An agent having such an effect.

uterotonin (u-ter-o-ton´in) General term for any substance that increases the tone, or induces contraction, of uterine smooth muscle (e.g., oxytocin, prostaglandins, endothelin 1).

uterotropic (u-ter-o-trop´ik) Denoting a substance that has an affinity for the uterus.

uterotropin (u-ter-o-tro´pin) Any substance that activates the functional elements of the uterus in preparation for labor (i.e., by facilitating contractile effectiveness of the myometrium and softening of the cervix).

uterotubal (u-ter-o-too´bal) Relating to the uterus and a fallopian (uterine) tube.

uterovaginal (u-ter-o-vaj´ĭ-nal) Relating to the uterus and the vagina.

uterovesical (u-ter-o-ves´ĭ-kal) Relating to the uterus and the bladder.

uterus (u´ter-us) A hollow, muscular organ of the female mammal situated in the pelvis between the bladder and rectum; its function is the nourishment of the developing young prior to birth; the mature human uterus is pear-shaped, thick-walled, and about 76 mm long, reaching adult size by the 15th year and diminishing after the menopause; the upper portion of the uterus opens on either side into the uterine tubes and the lower portion opens into the vagina. Also called womb.

anomalous u. A malformed uterus.

bicornuate u., u. bicornis A uterus that has a vascular fibromuscular partition indenting the fundus, forming two distinct uterine horns.

Couvelaire u. A purplish hard uterus that has lost a great deal of its contractile power; caused by blood infiltration of the uterine muscle (myometrium) from a partially detached placenta. Also called uteroplacental apoplexy.

u. didelphys A uterus separated throughout its length by a fibrous partition; each side having one separate uterine horn with a corresponding fallopian (uterine) tube. Also called double uterus.

double u. See uterus didelphys.

gravid u. A pregnant uterus.

inverted u. A uterus that is, in effect, turned inside out, with its fundus prolapsed toward or through the cervix into the vagina. See also inversion of the uterus, under inversion.

pubescent u. An underdeveloped adult uterus.

tipped u. Popular term for a retrodisplaced uterus (i.e., one that is tilted in a backward direction).

unicornuate u., u. unicornis A uterus with one normal horn on one side and a rudimentary horn on the opposite side; the lumen of the rudimentary horn may or may not be continuous with the uterine cavity.

utricle (u´trĭ-kl) **1.** A small sac. **2.** The larger of the two sacs of the membranous labyrinth in the vestibule of the inner ear.

prostatic u. A small pouch (about 6 mm long) in the prostate, with its opening on the crest of the seminal colliculus; it is the analog of the uterus and upper vagina, being the remains of the fused caudal ends of the paramesonephric ducts of the embryo.

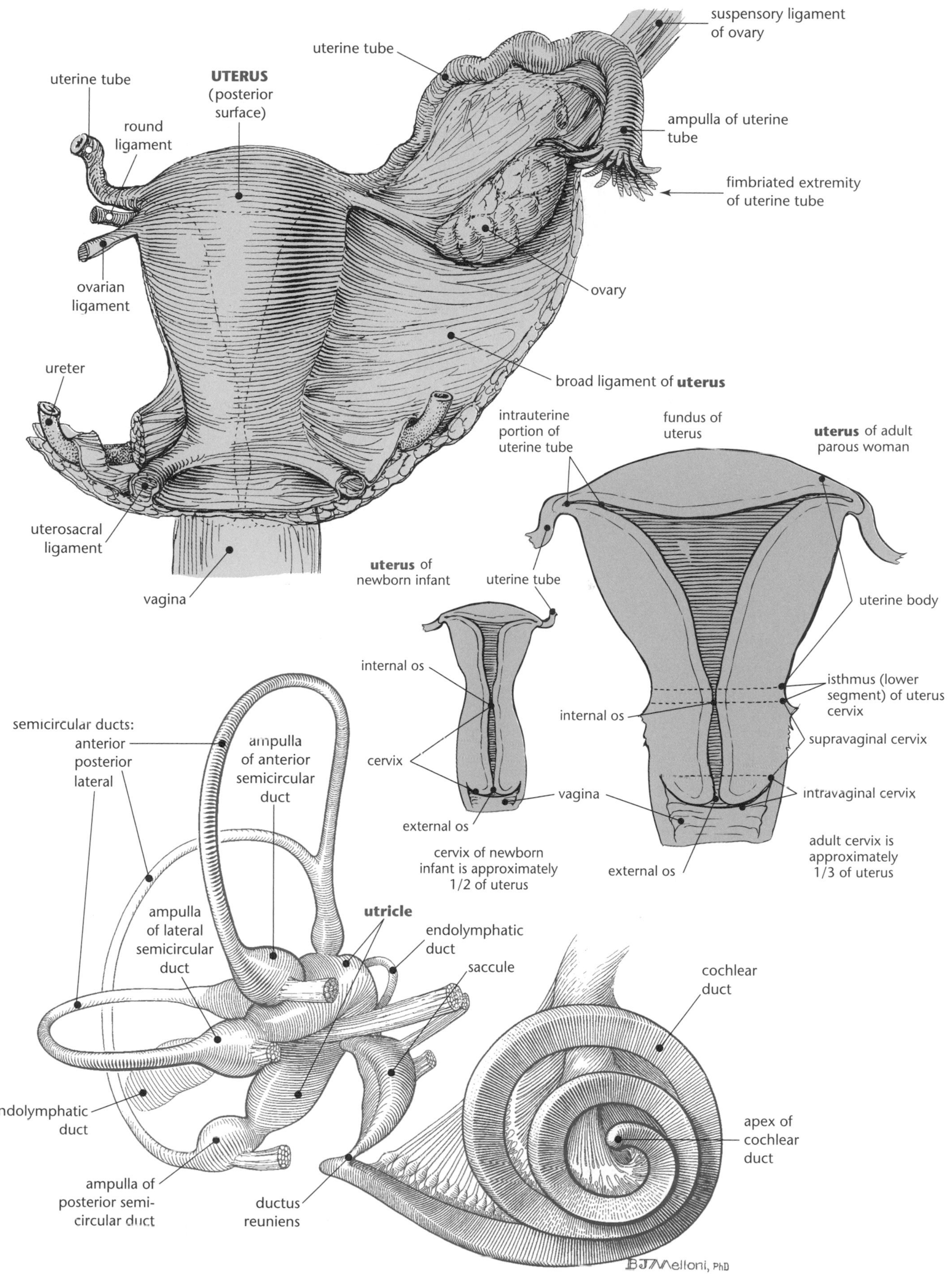
uterine tube
uterine tube
UTERUS
(posterior
surface)
round
ligament
suspensory ligament
of ovary
ampulla of uterine
tube
fimbriated extremity
of uterine tube
ovarian
ligament
ovary
ureter
broad ligament of uterus
uterosacral
ligament
vagina
intrauterine
portion of
uterine tube
fundus of
uterus
uterus of adult
parous woman
uterus of
newborn infant
uterine tube
uterine body
internal os
internal os
isthmus (lower
segment) of uterus
cervix
supravaginal cervix
cervix
vagina
intravaginal cervix
external os
cervix of newborn
infant is approximately
1/2 of uterus
external os
adult cervix is
approximately
1/3 of uterus
semicircular ducts:
anterior
posterior
lateral
ampulla
of anterior
semicircular
duct
ampulla
of lateral
semicircular
duct
utricle
endolymphatic
duct
saccule
cochlear
duct
endolymphatic
duct
apex of
cochlear
duct
ampulla of
posterior semi-
circular duct
ductus
reuniens
BJMelloni, PhD

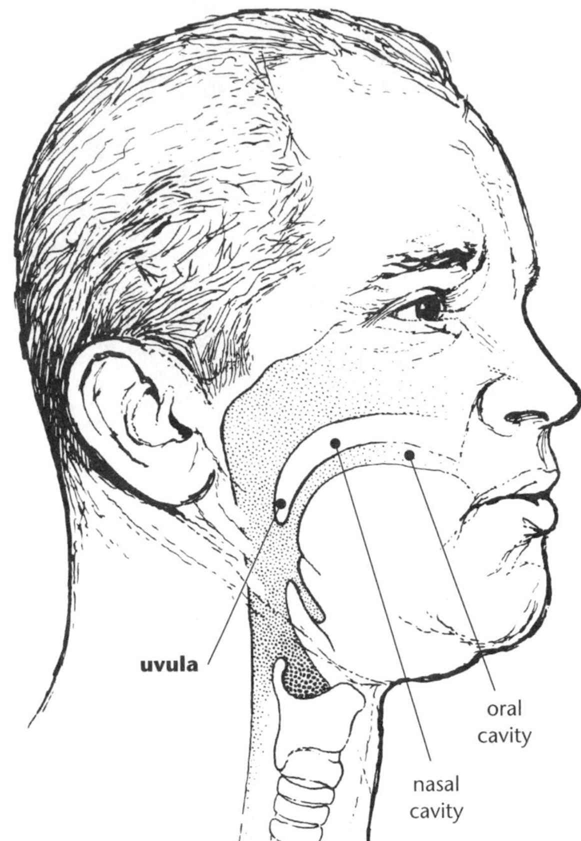

utricular (u-trik´u-lar) Relating to or resembling a utricle.

utriculosaccular (u-trik-u-lo-sak´u-lar) Relating to the utricle and the saccule of the inner ear.

uvea (u´ve-ă) The middle, pigmented, vascular layer of the eye consisting of the choroid, the ciliary body, and the iris. Also called uveal tract.

uveal (u´ve-ăl) Relating to the uvea.

uveitis (u-ve-i´tis) Inflammation of the uvea (choroid, ciliary body, and iris).

anterior u. See iridocyclitis.

sympathetic u. See sympathetic ophthalmia, under ophthalmia.

uveoparotitis (u-ve-o-par-o-ti´tis) Vascular inflammation of the uvea (middle coat of eye) and the parotid gland; a manifestation of sarcoidosis. Also called uveoparotid fever.

uviform (u´vĭ-form) Resembling grapes.

uvula (u´vu-lă) From Latin, a small grape; any anatomic structure resembling a small grape; when used alone, the term designates the palatine uvula.

palatine u. The conical, fleshy mass of tissue suspended from the free edge of the soft palate above the back of the tongue.

vesical u. A mucosal ridge of the bladder just behind the internal urethral orifice, formed by the underlying median lobe of the prostate gland in the male.

uvulectomy (u-vu-lek´to-me) Surgical removal of the uvula.

uvulitis (u-vu-li´tis) Inflammation of the uvula.

uvulopalatoplasty (u-vu-lo-pal´ă-to-plas-te) See palatopharyngoplasty.

uvulotomy (u-vu-lot´ŏ-me) Incision of the uvula or removal of a portion of it.

U

V v

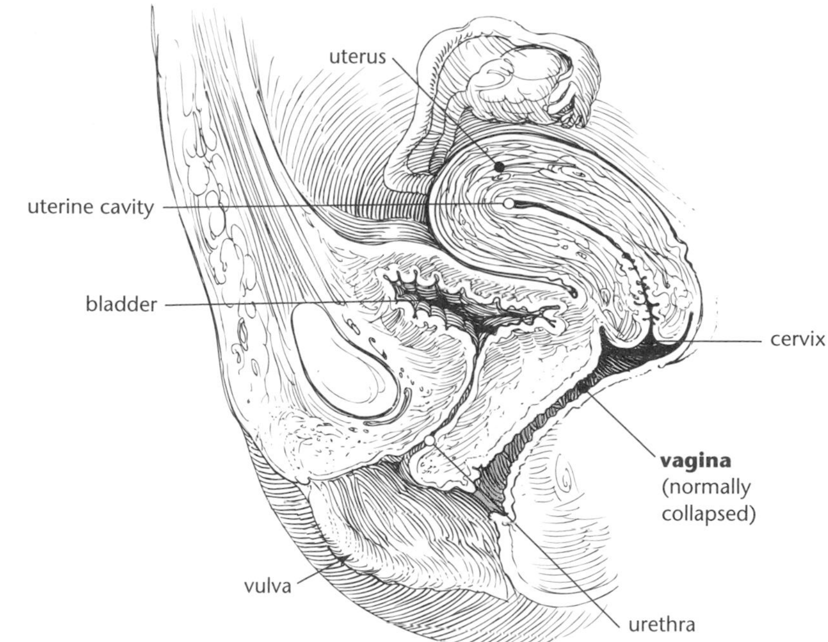

V1, V2, V3, V4, V5, V6 Precordial leads; see under lead.
vaccinate (vak´sĭ-nāt) To inoculate with a vaccine for the purpose of producing active immunity against a given infectious disease.
vaccination (vak-sĭ-na´shun) The act of vaccinating.
vaccinator (vak´sĭ-na-tor) **1.** One who vaccinates. **2.** Instrument used in vaccination.
vaccine (vak´sēn) A preparation of dead, or live attenuated viruses or bacteria for use in the prevention of infectious diseases by inducing active immunity.
attenuated v. See live vaccine.
autogenous v. Vaccine made from organisms obtained from the individual to be inoculated.
bacillus Calmette-Guérin v. See BCG vaccine.
BCG v. An attenuated viable strain of *Mycobacterium tuberculosis*, bovine type that provides immunity to tuberculosis. Also called bacillus Calmette-Guérin vaccine; Calmette-Guérin vaccine.
Calmette-Guérin v. BCG vaccine.
cholera v. A sterile suspension of killed *Vibrio cholerae* organisms containing 8 billion organisms per milliliter; given intramuscularly or subcutaneously in two doses one week to one month apart.
diphtheria and tetanus toxoids and pertussis v. (DTP) A triple vaccine against diphtheria, tetanus, and whooping cough for infants, usually administered in three intramuscular injections one to three months apart; diphtheria and tetanus toxoids, without pertussis, are used for a booster dose in adults.
hepatitis B v. Vaccine containing a formalin-inactivated hepatitis B surface antigen obtained from plasma of human carriers of the virus, or a genetically engineered (recombinant) subunit of the virus.
human diploid cell v. (HDCV) A vaccine against rabies prepared from rabies virus grown in human diploid cell culture and then inactivated with tri-*n*-butyl phosphate. Also called rabies vaccine.
inactivated v. Any vaccine in which the nucleic acid components in the core of the infectious microorganism have been destroyed by chemical or physical means (e.g., formaldehyde or gamma radiation) without affecting the immunogenicity of the outer coat proteins.
inactivated poliovirus v. (IPV) See poliovirus vaccine.
influenza virus v. A sterile, aqueous suspension of inactivated influenza virus grown in egg allantoic fluid and killed usually with formalin. The vaccine is reformulated annually, based on strains of the virus present in the previous years or anticipated for the upcoming season.
live v. Vaccine prepared from live organisms that have been made to undergo physical changes by submission to either radiation or unfavorable temperatures, or to serial passage in laboratory animals or infected tissue/cell cultures; the result is a living avirulent, mutant strain capable of inducing protective immunity against the original organisms. Live vaccines are contraindicated in febrile or immunosuppressed patients or in pregnant women. Also called attenuated vaccine.
measles v. Live, attenuated measles virus vaccine, given subcutaneously to children 1 year of age or older.
mixed v. Vaccine containing killed cultures of more than one species.
MMR v. A combination of live measles, mumps, and rubella vaccines.
MR v. A combination of live measles and rubella vaccines.
mumps v. A suspension of live attenuated mumps virus, given subcutaneously.
oral poliovirus v. See poliovirus vaccine.
poliovirus v., poliomyelitis v. Vaccine providing immunity against poliomyelitis; available in two forms: *Inactive poliovirus v.* (IPV), an aqueous suspension of formaldehyde-inactivated strains of poliomyelitis virus, administered subcutaneously. Also called Salk vaccine. *Oral poliovirus v.* (OPV), an aqueous suspension of live, attenuated strains of poliomyelitis virus, administered orally. Also called Sabin vaccine.
rabies v. See human diploid cell vaccine.
rubella v. A live attenuated vaccine containing either a strain of the virus alone, or combined with measles vaccine (MR) or with measles and mumps vaccines (MMR).
Sabin v. See poliovirus vaccine.
Salk v. See poliovirus vaccine.
typhoid v. (a) A suspension of chemically- or heat-killed *Salmonella typhi*, the organism causing typhoid fever, administered subcutaneously. (b) A live attenuated vaccine for oral administration.
typhus v. A suspension of formaldehyde-inactivated *Rickettsia prowazekii*, the organism causing typhus, administered subcutaneously.
smallpox v. A suspension of live attenuated vaccinia virus.
varicella virus v. A live attenuated vaccine containing the varicella virus, used to induce immunity to varicella (chickenpox). Pregnancy should be avoided for 3 months after vaccination.
yellow fever v. Vaccine containing live attenuated yellow fever virus, grown in chick embryos and then freeze-dried, administered subcutaneously as a reconstituted solution.
vaccinia (vak-sin´e-ă) **1.** The cutaneous lesion found at the site of vaccination with smallpox (vaccinia) virus. **2.** See cowpox.
v. gangrenosa See progressive vaccinia.
generalized v. Condition of secondary lesions of the skin following smallpox vaccination.
progressive v. Widespread vaccinal lesions following vaccination; a severe, often fatal condition occurring in individuals who fail to produce antibodies. Also called vaccinia gangrenosa.
vaccinial (vak-sin´e-al) Relating to vaccinia.
vaccinid (vak´sĭ-nid) Allergic reaction to vaccination marked by localized eruption of vesicles or papules.
vacciniform, vaccinoid (vak-sin´ĭ-form, vak´sĭ-noid) Resembling vaccinia.
vaccinogen (vak-sin´ō-jen) A source of vaccine.
VACTERL Acronym for vertebral, anal, cardiac, tracheal, esophageal, renal, and limb; a pattern of congenital anomalies.
vacuant (vak´u-ant) An agent that promotes emptying of the bowels.
vacuolate, vacuolated (vak´u-o-lāt, vak´u-o-lāt-ed) Containing vacuoles.
vacuolation (vak-u-o-la´shun) The formation of vacuoles.
vacuole (vak´u-ōl) **1.** A small space or cavity in the protoplasm of a cell. **2.** A small space in tissue.
vacuum (vak´u-um) A space devoid of gas or air; an empty space.
vagal (va´gal) Relating to the vagus (10th cranial) nerve.
vagectomy (va-jek´tŏ-me) Removal of a portion of the vagus (10th cranial) nerve.
vagina (vă-ji´nă) **1.** The musculomembranous tubular structure extending from the vulva to the uterine cervix. **2.** Any sheathlike structure.
vaginal (vaj´ĭ-nal) **1.** Relating to the vagina. **2.** Relating to any sheath.
vaginalitis (vaj-ĭ-nă-li´tis) Inflammation of the tunica vaginalis testis.
vaginate (vaj´ĭ-nāt) **1.** To form a sheath. **2.** Enclosed in a sheath.
vaginectomy (vaj-i-nek´tŏ-me) Partial or total removal of the vagina.
vaginismus (vaj-ĭ-niz´mus) Painful spasmodic contraction of the vaginal walls on slightest touch. Also called colpospasm.
vaginitis (vaj-ĭ-ni´tis) Inflammation of the vagina.
atrophic v. Thinning and dryness of the vaginal lining and loss of the vaginal folds (rugae) due to estrogen deficiency; commonly occurs during or after menopause. Also called senile vaginitis.
candidal v. Vaginitis caused by a candida species of the family Cryptococcaceae, most commonly *Candida albicans;* predisposing conditions include poorly controlled diabetes mellitus and systemic antibiotic treatment.
desquamative inflammatory v. Diffuse vaginitis, sometimes with superficial hemorrhagic spots in the upper vagina, occurring in the absence of estrogen deficiency.
emphysematous v. Vaginitis characterized by the presence of numerous small gas-filled cysts in the upper vagina and cervix; usually associated with *Gardnerella* and *Tricho-monas* infections.
***Gardnerella* v.** See bacterial vaginosis, under vaginosis.
nonspecific v. See bacterial vaginosis, under vaginosis.
senile v. See atrophic vaginitis.
trichomonas v. Vaginitis caused by the flagellated parasite *Trichomonas vaginalis,* a sexually transmitted organism; often coexists with bacterial vaginosis.
vaginodynia (vaj-ĭ-no-din´e-ă) Neuralgic vaginal pain. Also called colpodynia.
vaginofixation (vaj-ĭ-no-fik-sa´shun) See colpopexy.
vaginolabial (vaj-ĭ-no-la´be-al) Relating to the vagina and the labia.
vaginomycosis (vaj-ĭ-no-mi-ko´sis) Any fungal infection of the vagina.
vaginopathy (vaj-ĭ-nop´ă-the) Any vaginal disorder.

V

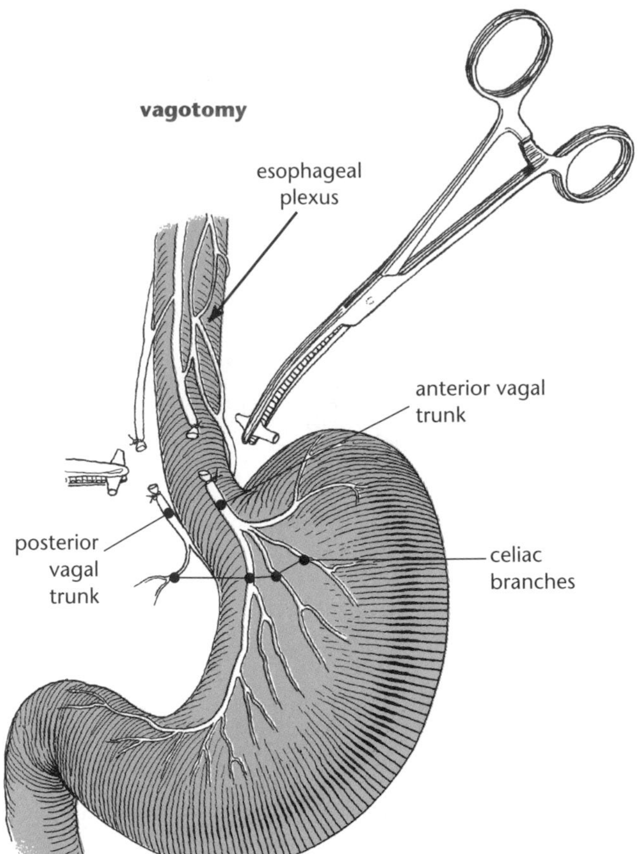

NORMAL **VALUES** OF BLOOD PLASMA

BASE	
sodium (Na^+)	142 mEq/l
potassium (K^+)	4 mEq/1
calcium (Ca^{++})	5 mEq/1
magnesium (Mg^{++})	2 mEq/1
ACID	
HCO_3-	27 mEq/1
Cl_	103 mEq/1
HPO_4	2 mEq/1
SO_4	1 mEq/1
organic acids	4 mEq/1
protein	16 mEq/1

THRESHOLD LIMIT VALUES OF SOME ENVIRONMENTAL CONTAMINANTS

SUBSTANCE	
ammonia	50 ppm
carbon monoxide	50 ppm
carbon dioxide	5000 ppm
hydrogen sulfide	10 ppm
ozone	0.1 ppm
mercury	0.1 mg/m^3
cement dust	30 mppcf

vaginoperineal (vaj-ĭ-no-per-ĭ-ne´al) Relating to the vagina and perineum.
vaginoperineorraphy (vaj-ĭ-no-per-ĭ-ne-or´a-fe) See colpoperineorraphy.
vaginopexy (vaj´ĭ-no-pek-se) See colpopexy.
vaginoplasty (vaj´ĭ-no-plas-te) Surgical repair of the vagina. Also called colpoplasty.
vaginoscope (vaj-ĭ-no-skōp) See colposcope.
vaginoscopy (vaj-ĭ-nos´kŏ-pe) See colposcopy.
vaginosis (vaj-ĭ-no´sis) Disease of the vagina.
bacterial v. (BV) Alteration of the normal vaginal flora, permitting overgrowth of multiple aerobic and anaerobic bacteria (e.g., *Gardnerella, Mycoplasma, Ureaplasma, Chlamydia);* may be asymptomatic or cause a gray-white discharge. BV is implicated as a risk factor for pelvic inflammatory disease (PID) and perinatal complications. Formerly called *Gardnerella* vaginitis; nonspecific vaginitis.
vaginotomy (vaj-ĭ-not´ŏ-me) See colpotomy.
vaginovesical (vaj-ĭ-no-ves´ĭ-kal) Relating to the vagina and the bladder.
vaginovulvar (vaj-ĭ-no-vul´var) See vulvovaginal.
vagitis (vă-ji´tus) Inflammation of the vagus (10th cranial) nerve.
vagitus uterinus (va-ji´tus u-ter-i´nus) Crying of a fetus while still in the uterus; a rare phenomenon thought to occur when the fetus inspires air entering the amniotic cavity after the membranes rupture.
vagolysis (va-gol´ĭ-sis) The surgical destruction of a portion of the vagus (10th cranial) nerve, usually the esophageal branch for the relief of cardiospasm.
vagolytic (va-go-lit´ik) **1.** Causing destruction of the vagus nerve. **2.** Any agent causing such an effect.
vagomimetic (va-go-mi-met´ik) Having an action similar to that of the vagus nerve.
vagotomy (va-got´ŏ-me) Interruption of the function of the vagus nerve.
medical v. Interruption of the activity of the vagus nerve by drugs.
surgical v. Surgical division of the vagus nerve.
vagotonia (va-go-to´ne-ă) Overaction or hyperexcitability of the vagus nerve.
vagus (va´gus) See table of nerves.
valence, valency (va´lens, va´len-se) The combining power of one atom or group of atoms, using the hydrogen atom as the unit of comparison.
valgus (val´gus) Bent outward, or away from, the midline.
valine (val´in) (Val) A naturally occurring amino acid, $C_5H_{11}NO_2$, constituent of many proteins; one of the amino acids essential for optimal growth.
vallate (val´āt) A depression bounded by a circular elevation; cupped.
vallecula (vă-lek´u-lă) In anatomy, a shallow groove, depression, or fossa.
v. cerebelli A deep hollow separating the inferior surface of the cerebellar hemispheres in which rests the medulla oblongata.
v. epiglottica The depression between the epiglottis and the root of the tongue, on either side of the median glossoepiglottic fold.
vallum (val´um) Any raised surface surrounding a circular depression.
valproic acid (val-pro´ik as´id) An anticonvulsant used in the treatment of seizure disorders.
value (val´u) A particular quantitative determination; a calculated numerical quantity; a number expressing a property.
caloric v. The measured heat evolved by a food when metabolized.
globular v. See color index, under index.
threshold limit v. (TLV) The amount of a potentially noxious material to which individuals may be exposed without adverse effects; some values have been determined for a variety of atmospheric contaminants.
valvate (val´vāt) Containing valves or valvelike parts.
valve (valv) A fold of the lining membrane of a tube or other hollow organ, so placed as to permit passage of fluid in one direction only.
anterior urethral v. A crescenteric valve in the male urethra, near the junction of the scrotum and penis.
aortic v. The valve between the left ventricle and the ascending aorta normally consisting of three semilunar cups.
Bianchi's v. The valve at the lower end of the nasolacrimal duct.
Bjork-Shiley v. Mechanical heart valve; consists of a cage containing a disk tilting at a 60° angle.
Carpentier-Edwards v. Heart valve made from preserved porcine valves mounted on a stent.
eustachian v. See valve of the inferior vena cava.
ileocecal v. The valve at the junction of the small and large intestines which regulates the flow of intestinal contents and prevents their backward flow. Also called ileocolic valve.
ileocolic v. See ileocecal valve.
v. of inferior vena cava The valve at the opening of the inferior vena cava in the right atrium of the heart. Also called eustachian valve.
v. of Kerckring See plica circularis.
left atrioventricular v. The bicuspid valve between the left atrium and the left ventricle of the heart. Also called mitral valve.
mitral v. See left atrioventricular valve.
posterior urethral v.'s Abnormal congenital folds of mucous membrane found in the distal prostatic urethra; they constitute the most common obstructive lesions in the urethra of male newborn and older infants.
prosthetic v. Any artificial valve designed to replace a diseased human heart valve.
v. of pulmonary trunk The valve located at the opening of the pulmonary trunk.
rectal v.'s See transverse folds of the rectum, under fold.
right atrioventricular v. The valve between the right atrium and the right ventricle of the heart. Also called tricuspid valve.
semilunar v. Valve composed of crescent-shaped segments or cusps (e.g., aortic valve and pulmonary valve).
Starr-Edwards v. Mechanical heart valve; consists of a ball contained within a cage.
tricuspid v. See right atrioventricular valve.
venous v. One of a number of small cup-shaped valves found in many of the veins preventing backward flow of blood.
valviform (val´vĭ-form) Shaped like a valve.
valvoplasty (val´vo-plas-te) Surgical reconstruction of a heart valve. Also called valvuloplasty.
valvotomy (val-vot´ŏ-me) Surgical incision of a valve, such as one of the heart. Also called valvulotomy.
valvula (val´vu-lă), *pl.* **val´vulae** A small valve.
valvular (val´vu-lar) Relating to valves.
valvular disease of heart (val´vu-lar dĭ-zēz´ ŭv hart) (VDH) Any disease caused by abnormalities of the heart valves.

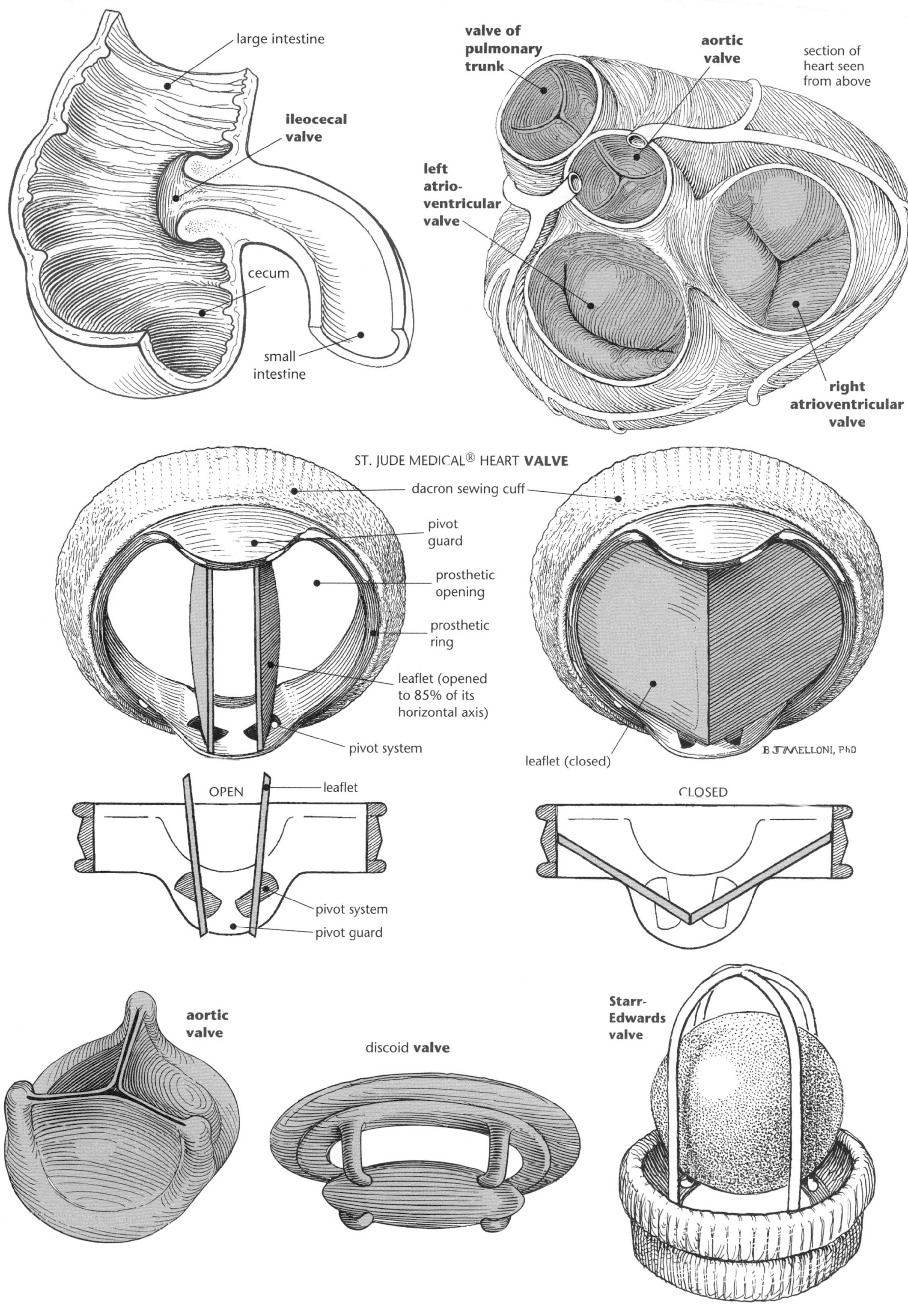
large intestine
ileocecal valve
cecum
small intestine
valve of pulmonary trunk
aortic valve
section of heart seen from above
left atrio-ventricular valve
right atrioventricular valve
ST. JUDE MEDICAL® HEART VALVE
dacron sewing cuff
pivot guard
prosthetic opening
prosthetic ring
leaflet (opened to 85% of its horizontal axis)
pivot system
leaflet (closed)
B J MELLONI, PhD
OPEN
leaflet
pivot system
pivot guard
CLOSED
aortic valve
discoid valve
Starr-Edwards valve

V

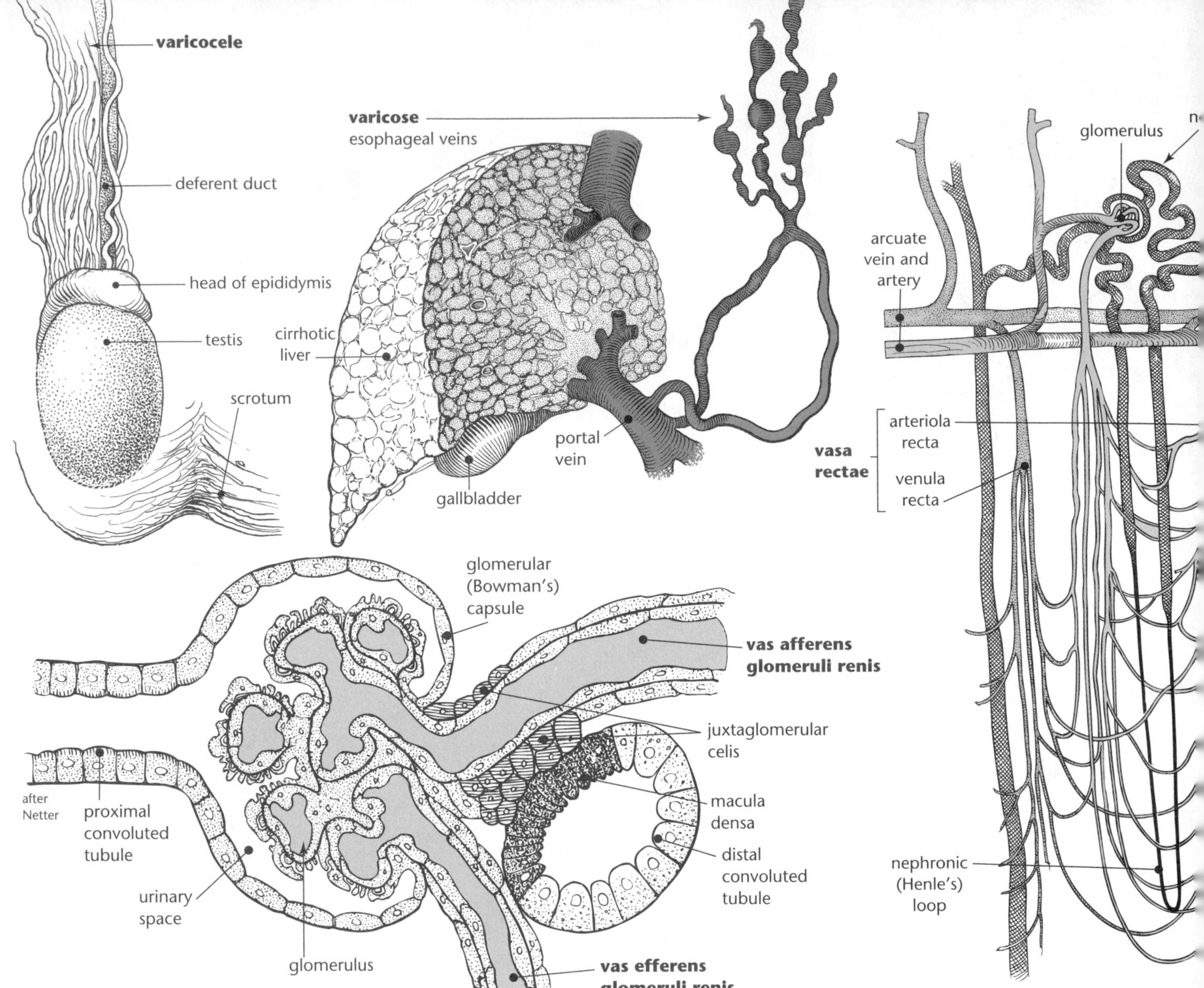

valvule (val′vyo͞ol) A small valve.
valvulitis (val-vu-li′tis) Inflammation of a valve, especially a valve of the heart.
valvuloplasty (val′vu-lo-plas-te) See valvoplasty.
valvulotome (val′vu-lo-tōm) Instrument for cutting a valve.
valvulotomy (val-vu-lot′ŏ-me) See valvotomy.
valyl (val′il, va′lil) The radical of valine.
vanadium (vă-na′de-um) Metallic element; symbol V, atomic number 23, atomic weight 50.95.
vanilla (vă-nil′ă) **1.** Any of several tropical orchids. **2.** The fruit of such plants, especially *Vanilla planifolia*, which yields the aromatic substance vanillin.
vanillin (vă-nil′in, van′ĭ-lin) Flavoring agent, $C_8H_8O_3$, derived from vanilla or prepared synthetically.

V

vanillylmandelic acid (vă-nil-il-man-del′ik as′id) (VMA) 3-Methoxy-4-hydroxymandelic acid, the major urinary metabolite of adrenal and sympathetic catecholamines; the normal range for excretion is 2 to 10 mg per day; elevated levels of excretion suggest a pheochromocytoma.
vapor (va′por) The gaseous state of any substance that is liquid or solid at ordinary temperatures.
vaporize (va′por-īz) To change into a vapor by heating.
vaporizer (va-por-ī′zer) An apparatus for reducing fluids to vapor for inhalation.
vapotherapy (va-po-ther′ă-pe) The treatment of any disorder with vapor, steam, or spray.
variance (văr′e-ans) **1.** A difference. **2.** The state of being different. **3.** In statistics, a measure of the variation evident in a set of observations.
ball v. The changes occurring in the ball of a ballvalve prosthesis.
variant (văr′e-ant) Tending to deviate from a standard.
L-phase v. A strain of bacteria with defective cell walls that has nutritive requirements similar to the strain from which it originated and is capable of reverting to its parental form. Also called L-form.
variceal (var-ĭ-se′al) Relating to a varix.
varicella (var-ĭ-sel′ă) See chickenpox.
varicelliform (var-ĭ-sel′ĭ-form) Resembling chickenpox.
varices (var′ĭ-sēz) Plural of varix.
varicocele (var′ĭ-ko-sēl) Dilatation of the veins of the spermatic cord in the scrotum.
varicocelectomy (var-ĭ-ko-sē-lek′tŏ-me) Operation for removal of dilated veins of the spermatic cord (varicocele).
varicography (var-ĭ-kog′ră-fe) Roentgenologic visualization of varicose veins achieved by introducing a radiopaque substance.
varicophlebitis (var-ĭ-ko-fle-bi′tis) Inflammation of varicose veins.
varicose (var′ĭ-kōs) Denoting abnormally dilated and tortuous vessels.
varicosity (var-ĭ-kos′ĭ-te) **1.** The state of being abnormally swollen. **2.** A varicose vein.
varicotomy (var-ĭ-kot′tŏ-me) An operation for the removal of a varicose vein.
varicula (vă-rik′u-lă) A varicose condition of small veins, especially of the conjunctiva.
varicule (var-ĭ-kyo͞ol) A small varicose vein.
variola (vă-ri′o-lă) See smallpox.
v. minor See alastrim.
variolar (vă-ri′o-lar) Relating to smallpox.
varioliform (va-re-o′lĭ-form) In the shape or form of smallpox.
varioloid (va′re-o-loid) A mild case of smallpox occurring in partially immune persons.
varix (var′iks), *pl.* **va′rices** A dilated and tortuous vessel, usually a vein.
aneurysmal v. Varix resulting from the direct communication between a vein and an adjacent artery.
esophageal varices Varicosities of the mucosal veins of the esophagus, usually the lower portion.
varnish (var′nish) A solution of a resin in a suitable solvent and an evaporating binder that, when applied in a thin layer, forms a hard, glossy, thin film.
dental v. A solution of natural resins and gums in an organic solvent; it is applied over the walls and floor of the prepared tooth cavity; when the solvent evaporates, a thin film is left that protects the underlying tooth structure against the constituents of the restorative material and thermal shock.
varus (va′rus) Bent inward or toward the midline.
vas (vas), *pl.* **va′sa** A duct or canal through which a liquid, such as blood, lymph, chyle, or semen, is conveyed; a vessel.
v. aberrans hepatis Any of the numerous, irregularly coursing, blind-ending bile ducts located in the coronary ligament, capsule, or fibrous appendix of the liver.
v. afferens glomeruli renis See afferent glomerular arteriole, under arteriole.
v. brevia Short gastric arteries. See table of arteries.
v. deferens See deferent duct, under duct.

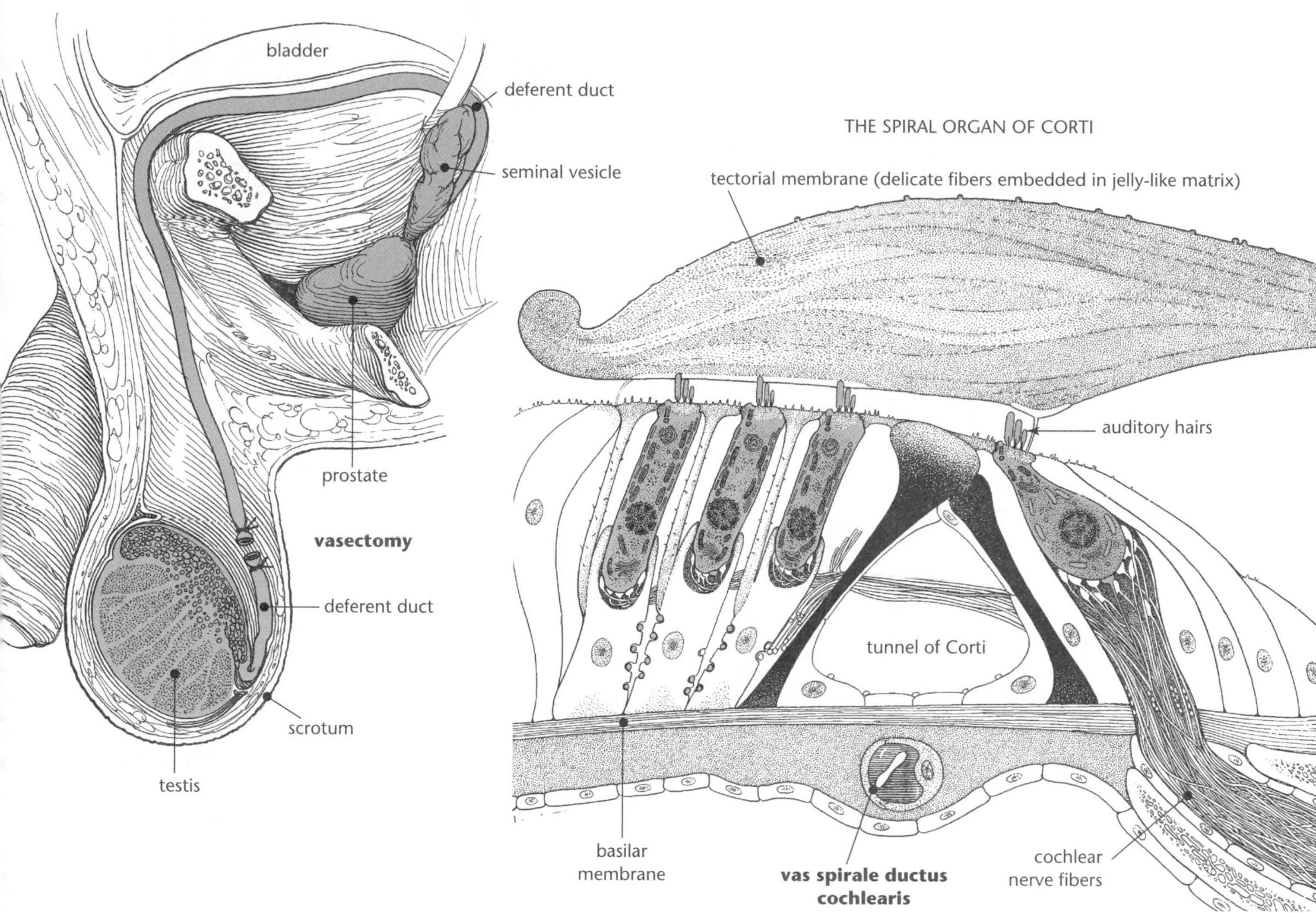

v. efferens glomeruli renis See efferent glomerular arteriole, under arteriole.

v. lymphaticum See lymph vessel, under vessel.

v. previa In obstetrics, a configuration of fetal blood vessels that traverse the lower uterine segment and appear across the internal cervical os ahead of the presenting part. It is associated with velamentous insertion of the umbilical cord and is clinically important because when membranes rupture, rupture of a fetal blood vessel may occur resulting in exsanguination of the fetus. See also velamentous cord insertion, under insertion.

vasa rectae The arterioles and venules that descend and ascend parallel to the nephronic (Henle's) loop in the pyramid of the kidney; the wider ascending limbs are often referred to as venulae rectae and the descending limbs are generally called arteriolae rectae.

v. spirale ductus cochlearis The largest blood vessel in the basilar membrane just beneath the tunnel of Corti in the inner ear.

v. vasorum One of many small blood vessels in the walls of larger arteries and their corresponding veins.

vascular (vas´ku-lar) Relating to vessels.

vascularity (vas-ku-lar´ĭ-te) The state of containing blood vessels.

vascularization (vas-ku-lar-ĭ-za´shun) The formation of blood vessels.

vasculature (vas´ku-lă-chur) The system of blood vessels of an organ.

vasculitis (vas-ku-li´tis) Inflammation of a blood vessel or vessels.

vasculogenesis (vas-ku-lo-jen´ĕ-sis) Formation of the system of blood vessels.

vasectomy (vă sek´tŏ-me) Removal of a segment of the deferent duct; a means of male sterilization. Also called deferentectomy; male sterilization.

vasiform (vas´ĭ-form) Tubular.

vasoactive (vas-o-ak´tiv) Having an effect on blood vessels.

vasocongestion (vas-o-kon-jes´chun) The state of being filled with blood.

vasoconstriction (vas-o-kon-strik´shun) Narrow-ing of the lumen of blood vessels, especially of arterioles.

vasoconstrictor (vas-o-kon-strik´tor) A drug or nerve that causes narrowing of the lumen of blood vessels.

vasodilatation (vas-o-dil-ă-ta´shun) Widening of the lumen of the blood vessels, especially of the lumen of arterioles, leading to increased blood flow to a part.

reflex v. Dilatation of a blood vessel due to a reflex response to a stimulus.

vasodilator (vas-o-di-lāt´or) A drug or nerve that causes widening of the lumen of blood vessels.

vasoganglion (vas-o-gang´gle-on) A glomus; a dense mass of blood vessels.

vasogenic (vas-o-gen´ik) **1.** Originating from blood vessels. **2.** Roentgenography of the deferent duct.

vasography (vă-sog´ră-fe) Roentgenography of blood vessels.

vasohypertonic (vas-o-hi-per-ton´ik) Causing increased tonicity in the smooth muscles of blood vessels; denoting increased arteriolar tension.

vasohypotonic (vas-o-hi-po-ton´ik) Causing reduced tonicity in the smooth muscles of blood vessels; denoting reduced arteriolar tension.

vasoinhibitor (vas-o-in-hib´ĭ-tor) A drug that depresses the action of vasomotor nerves.

vasoinhibitory (vas-o-in-hib´ĭ-tor-e) Reducing the action of the vasomotor nerves.

vasoligation (vas-o-li-ga´shun) Surgical ligation of the deferent duct (vas deferens).

vasomotion (vas-o-mo´shun) Dilatation and constriction of blood vessels. Also called angiokinesis.

vasomotor (vas-o-mo´tor) Causing constriction or dilatation of blood vessels; denoting the nerves that produce this action.

vasoneuropathy (vas-o-nōō-rop´ă-the) Any disease affecting the blood vessels and nerves.

vasoparalysis (vas-o-pă-ral´ĭ-sis) Hypotonia of blood vessels. Also called vasomotor paralysis.

vasopressin (vas-o-pres´in) (VP) A hormone produced by the posterior part of the pituitary (neurohypophysis) and also prepared synthetically; it has a constrictive action on blood circulation of the viscera, including the uterus. Also called antidiuretic hormone.

vasopressor (vas-o-pres´or) An agent that causes constriction of blood vessels and a rise in blood pressure.

vasorelaxant (vas-o-re-lak´sant) An agent that elicits a reduction of tension in blood vessel walls. Produced from a variety of tissues.

vasosensory (vas-o-sen´so-re) Denoting sensory nerves going to the blood vessels.

vasospasm (vas´o-spaz-m) Spastic contraction of the muscular coats of blood vessel walls. Also called angiospasm; angiohypertonia.

vasostimulant (vas-o-stim´u-lant) **1.** Exciting nerves that cause dilatation or constriction of blood vessels. **2.** Any agent having such property.

vasotomy (vă-sot´ŏ-me) Cutting into the deferent duct (vas deferens).

vasotonic (vas-o-ton´ik) Relating to the tone of a blood vessel; an agent that increases tension of blood vessels.

vasotrophic (vas-o-trof´ik) See angiotrophic.

vasotropic (vas-o-trop´ik) Tending to act on blood vessels.

V

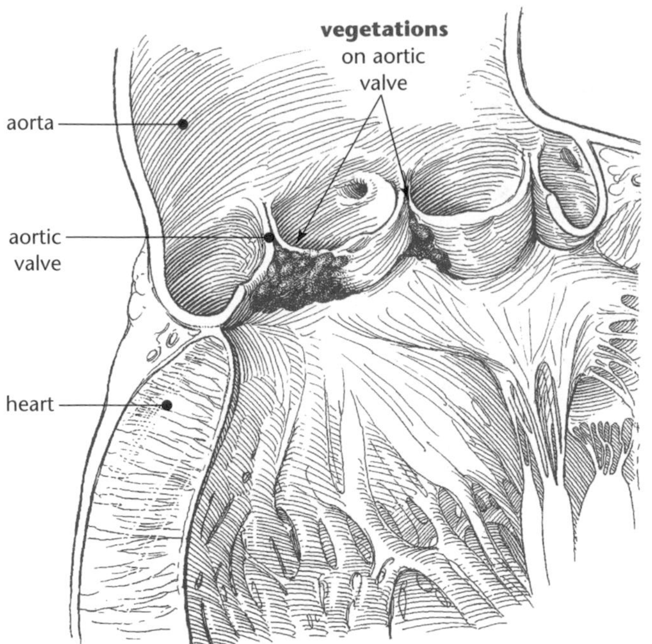

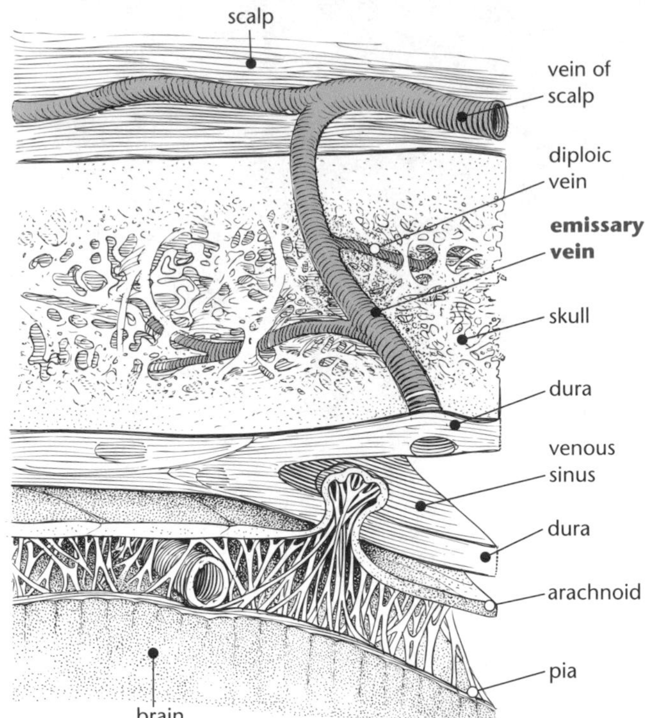

vasovagal (vas-o-va´gal) Relating to the action of the vagus nerve upon blood vessels. See also vasovagal attack, under attack.

vasovasostomy (vas-o-vă-sos´tŏ-me) Surgical union of the ends of a severed deferent duct.

vasovesiculectomy (vas-o-ve-sik-u-lek´tŏ-me) Surgical removal of a deferent duct and seminal vesicles.

VATER Acronym for vertebral, anal, tracheal, esophageal, and renal; a pattern of associated congenital anomalies.

vault (vawlt) Any arched anatomic structure resembling a dome.

vection (vek´shun) Transmission of causative agents of disease.

vector (vek´tor) **1.** An organism carrying pathologic microorganisms from one host to another. **2.** Anything (electromotive force, velocity, etc.) that has a magnitude and a direction. **3.** A plasmid or a bacteriophage used to carry a cloned segment of DNA.

biological v. Vector (such as the *Anopheles* mosquito) in whose body an infective organism must develop before becoming infective to its primary host.

cloning v. An autonomously replicating plasmid or bacteriophage into which DNA can be inserted and which then replicates as a normal component of the vector.

expression v. A vector used to experimentally introduce an exogenous DNA segment into a dividing host cell to replicate and amplify the added DNA as a recombinant molecule.

mechanical v. Vector (such as the housefly) that simply transports an infective organism on its feet or mouth parts from one host to another and is not essential to the life cycle of the parasite.

recombinant v. Vector into which an exogenous DNA segment has been inserted.

V

vectorcardiogram (vek-tor-kar´de-o-gram) (VCG) A graphic record of the magnitude and direction of the heart's action currents, displayed as a three-dimensional or spatial voltage loop.

vectorcardiography (vek-tor-kar-de-og´ră-fe) Determination of the direction and magnitude of the heart's electric forces at any time; represented by vector loops.

spatial v. Three-dimensional voltage loop produced by the heart's action current and projected on the frontal, horizontal, and sagittal reference planes.

vegan (vej´an, ve´gan) One who does not eat food derived from animals (meat, milk, eggs, etc.).

vegetarian (vej-e-tār´e-an) One whose diet excludes most animal products.

lacto-v. Vegetarian who eats dairy products but no eggs or animal flesh.

lacto-ovo-v. Vegetarian who eats dairy products and eggs but no animal flesh.

pesco-v. Vegetarian who eats dairy products, eggs, and fish but not other animal flesh.

vegetations (vej-e-ta´shuns) An abnormal plantlike outgrowth of tissue; specifically, growth composed of fibrin and fused blood platelets adherent to a diseased heart valve; circulating bacteria or fungi of blood-borne infections tend to plant at these sites.

vegetative (vej´e-ta-tiv) Having a role in the processes of growth and nutrition.

vehicle (ve´ĭ-kl) **1.** In pharmacology, an inactive substance in which an active drug is dissolved or suspended; an excipient. **2.** Any inanimate carrier of an infectious agent from one host to another.

veil (vāl) Colloquial term for caul.

Veillonella (va-yon-el´ă) A genus of anaerobic, gram-negative bacteria normally found in the mouth and intestinal, respiratory, and urogenital tracts of apparently healthy individuals.

vein (vān) (v) A vessel that carries blood toward the heart or one in the heart wall that returns blood to the right atrium. For specific veins, see table of veins.

aqueous v.'s Minute vessels that transport aqueous humor from the venous sinus of the sclera (canal of Schlemm) out of the eyeball to the episcleral, conjunctival, and subconjunctival veins.

cardinal v.'s The major embryonic vessels that drain the cephalic part (anterior cardinal vein) and caudal part (posterior cardinal vein) and empty into the heart (via the common cardinal vein).

emissary v.'s Veins that drain the intracranial venous sinuses and transport the blood to a vessel outside the skull; they serve as drainage channels in case of increased intracranial pressure.

large v. A vein, such as the inferior vena cava, characterized by having a tunica adventitia which is thicker than the tunica media and has many bundles of muscular fibers arranged longitudinally; the tunica media is thin or may be absent.

medium v. A vein that characteristically has a thick tunica media composed of connective tissue with elastic fibers intermingled with circularly arranged muscle fibers; the tunica adventitia contains longitudinal elastic fibers.

pulmonary v.'s The four veins that return oxygenated blood from the lungs to the left atrium of the heart. See table of veins.

small v. A vein whose walls are thin, with poorly defined tunica that contain a network of longitudinal elastic fibers; some contain a few fibers of smooth muscle arranged circularly.

systemic v.'s All the veins that return venous blood to the right atrium of the heart; may be categorized into three groups: (a) veins of the heart; (b) veins of the head, neck, thorax, and upper extremities, all of which carry blood to the superior vena cava; (c) veins of the abdomen, pelvis, and lower extremities, all of which carry blood to the inferior vena cava.

varicose v.'s Abnormally dilated, tortuous veins produced by prolonged, increased intraluminal pressure; most commonly seen in the superficial veins of the leg; varicose veins along with phlebothrombosis account for approximately 90 percent of clinical venous disease.

vitelline v.'s Veins that return blood from the yolk sac of an early embryo; they form an anastomotic network around the duodenum and in the liver and empty directly into the sinus venosus of the primitive heart.

vela (ve´lă) Plural of velum.

velamentous (vel-ă-men´tus) Resembling a curtain or veil; applied to certain body structures and membranes.

vellus (vel´us) Fine, soft, nonpigmented downy hair that replaces the lanugo hair (primary hair) of the neonate; it begins to appear in the early months of postnatal life. Also called vellus hair; secondary hair.

velocimetry (ve-lo-sim´ĕ-tre) Measurement of speed.

laser-Doppler v. Measurement of the flow of red blood cells in microcirculation by means of a laser beam directed to the area of interest and detected by a fiberoptic probe.

velopharyngeal (vel-o-fă-rin´je-al) Relating to the soft palate and the pharynx.

velum (vel´um), *pl.* **vel´a** Any structure resembling a curtain.

inferior medullary v., posterior medullary v. A thin sheet forming part of the roof of the cerebral fourth ventricle; composed of the cellular lining of the ventricle on the inside and pia mater on the outside.

superior medullary v., anterior medullary v. A thin layer of white matter between the cerebellar peduncles, forming the anterior portion of the roof of the cerebral fourth ventricle.

vena (ve´nă), *pl.* **ve´nae** Latin for vein.

v. cava See table of veins.

venae comitantes, *sing.* **v. comitans** Veins (usually two) accompanying the corresponding artery.

venation (ve-na´shun) The distribution of veins.

venectomy (ve-nek´tŏ-me) See phlebectomy.

veneer (vĕ-nēr´) In dentistry, a porcelain or resin facing applied to a gold crown or pontic for esthetic purposes.

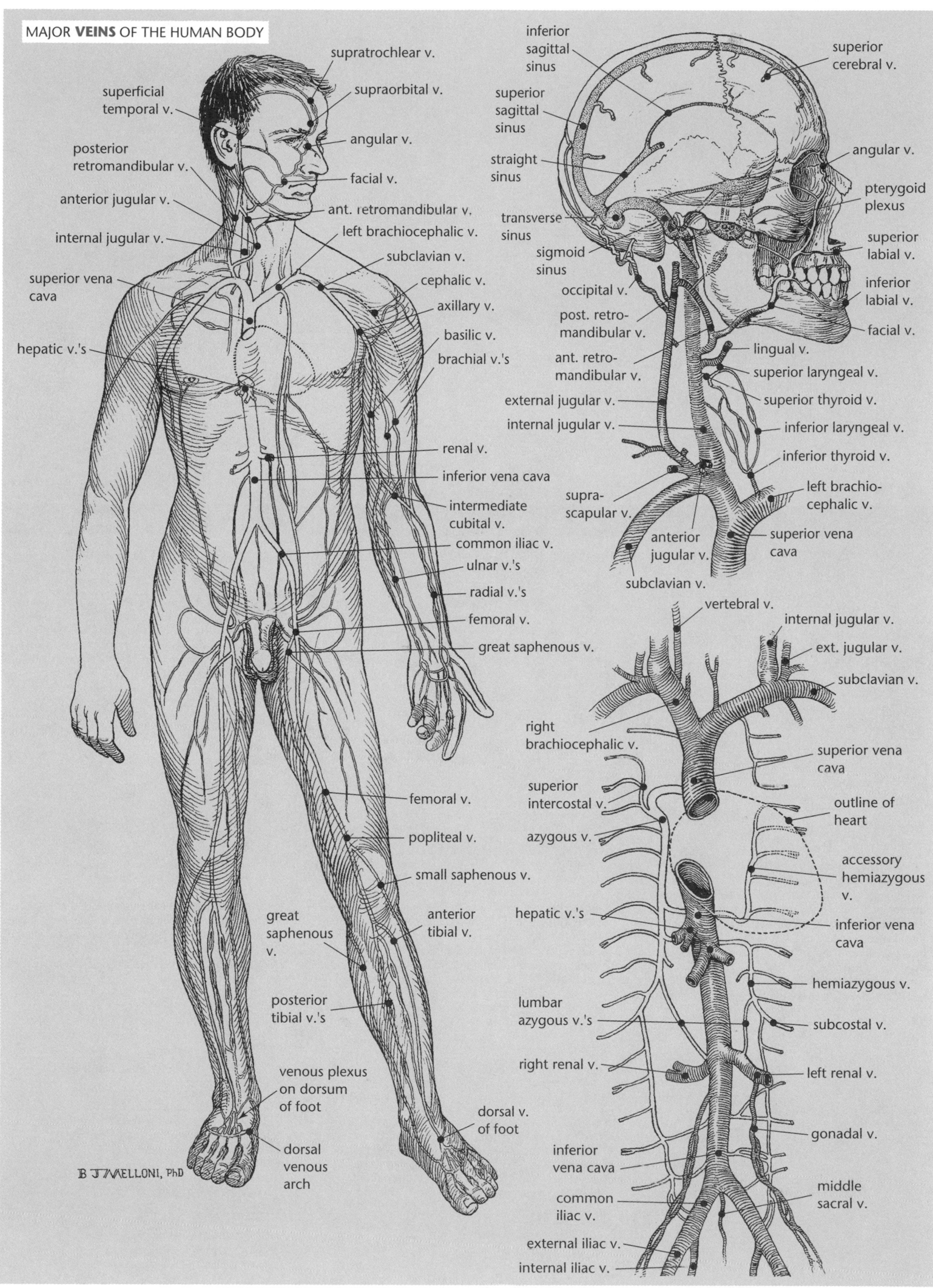
MAJOR VEINS OF THE HUMAN BODY
supratrochlear v.
superficial temporal v.
supraorbital v.
angular v.
posterior retromandibular v.
facial v.
anterior jugular v.
ant. retromandibular v.
left brachiocephalic v.
internal jugular v.
subclavian v.
superior vena cava
cephalic v.
axillary v.
basilic v.
hepatic v.'s
brachial v.'s
renal v.
inferior vena cava
intermediate cubital v.
common iliac v.
ulnar v.'s
radial v.'s
femoral v.
great saphenous v.
femoral v.
popliteal v.
small saphenous v.
great saphenous v.
anterior tibial v.
posterior tibial v.'s
venous plexus on dorsum of foot
dorsal v. of foot
dorsal venous arch
B J MELLONI, PhD
inferior sagittal sinus
superior cerebral v.
superior sagittal sinus
straight sinus
angular v.
pterygoid plexus
transverse sinus
sigmoid sinus
superior labial v.
occipital v.
inferior labial v.
post. retro-mandibular v.
facial v.
ant. retro-mandibular v.
lingual v.
superior laryngeal v.
external jugular v.
superior thyroid v.
internal jugular v.
inferior laryngeal v.
inferior thyroid v.
supra-scapular v.
left brachio-cephalic v.
anterior jugular v.
superior vena cava
subclavian v.
vertebral v.
internal jugular v.
ext. jugular v.
subclavian v.
right brachiocephalic v.
superior vena cava
superior intercostal v.
outline of heart
azygous v.
accessory hemiazygous v.
hepatic v.'s
inferior vena cava
hemiazygous v.
lumbar azygous v.'s
subcostal v.
right renal v.
left renal v.
gonadal v.
inferior vena cava
middle sacral v.
common iliac v.
external iliac v.
internal iliac v.

V

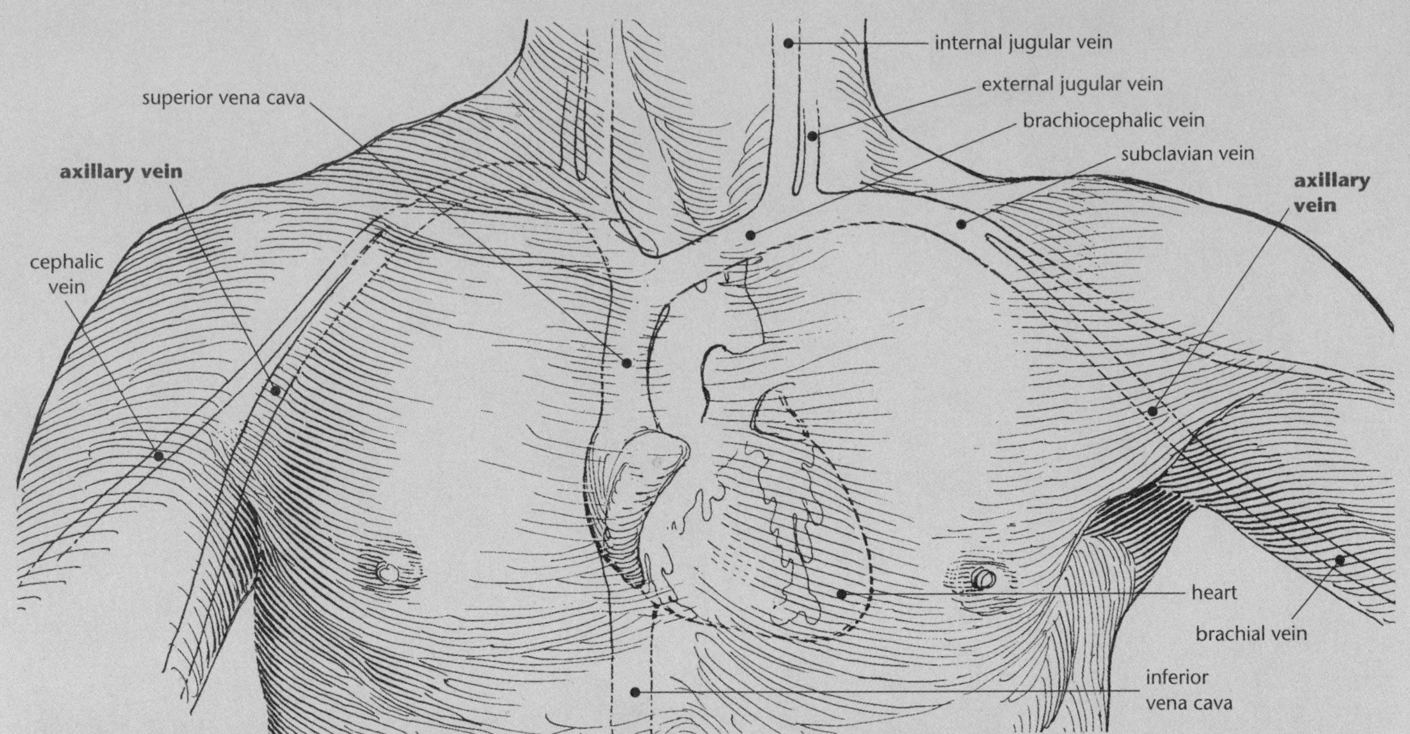

VEINS	LOCATION	DRAINS	EMPTIES INTO
alveolar v., inferior inferior dental v. *v. alveolaris*	from mandibular canal it passes up the ramus of lower jaw	teeth and body of lower jaw; lower lip	pterygoid plexus, facial v., retromandibular v.
anastomotic v., inferior v. of Labbé *v. anastomotica inferior*	courses over posterior part of temporal lobe of brain	superficial middle cerebral v., temporal lobe	transverse sinus
anastomotic v., superior v. of Trolard *v. anastomotica superior*	from lateral sulcus of brain across parietal lobe	superficial middle cerebral v., parietal lobe	superior sagittal sinus
angular v. *v. angularis*	anterior angle of orbit and root of nose	formed by union of frontal and supraorbital v.'s; receives infraorbital, superior and inferior palpebral and external nasal v.'s	facial v. (behind facial artery) at junction with superior labial v.'s
antebrachial v., median		see median v. of forearm	
appendicular v., *v. appendicularis*	along mesentery of vermiform appendix	appendix	ileocolic v.
v. of aqueduct of vestibule *v. aquaeductus vestibuli*	through aqueduct of vestibule (accompanied by endolymphatic duct)	semicircular ducts of inner ear, utricle, saccule	superior petrosal sinus or inferior petrosal sinus
arcuate v.'s of kidney *vv. arcuatae renis*	in corticomedullary zone of kidney	interlobular v.'s, venulae rectae	interlobar v.
auditory v.'s, internal		see labyrinthine v.'s	
auricular v.'s, anterior *vv. auriculares anteriores*	front part of ear	external ear	superficial temporal v.
auricular v., posterior *v. auricularis posterior*	side of head in back of ear	plexus on side of head, tributaries from back of ear, stylomastoid v.	external jugular v. in union with retromandibular v.
axillary v. *v. axillaris*	upper limb from lower border of teres major muscle to outer border of first rib	function of basilic and brachial v.'s; cephalic v., deep brachial comitans	subclavian v. (at outer border of first rib)
azygos v. *v. azygos*	from front of first lumbar vertebra it passes to right side of fourth thoracic vertebra where it arches over roots of right lung	ascending lumbar, right subcostal, intercostal, hemiazygos, esophageal, mediastinal, pericardial, and right bronchial v.'s	superior vena cava, near its entrance into pericardium
azygos v., left		see hemiazygos v.	
basal v. *v. basalis*	from anterior perforated substance it passes posteriorly around cerebral peduncle	anterior perforated substance; anterior cerebral v., deep middle cerebral v., inferior striate v.'s	internal cerebral v. in union with great cerebral v. (just under splenium of corpus callosum)

V

VEINS	LOCATION	DRAINS	EMPTIES INTO
basilic v. *v. basilica*	from ulnar part of hand it passes up forearm and continues along medial border of the biceps	dorsal venous network of hand; tributaries from ulnar side of forearm	joins brachial v. to form axillary v.
basivertebral v.'s *vv. basivertebrales*	tortuous channels in substance of vertebral bodies	vertebral bodies	anterior external, and internal vertebral venous plexuses
brachial v.'s *vv. brachiales*	from neck of radius, courses upward to lower border of teres major muscle	radial and ulnar v.'s, superior and inferior ulnar collateral v.'s, deep brachial v.	axillary v. in union with basilic v.
brachiocephalic v.'s *innominate v.'s* vv. brachiocephalicae	root of neck, medial end of clavicle	*right side:* internal jugular, subclavian, internal thoracic and inferior thyroid v.'s; *left side:* internal jugular, subclavian, and left highest intercostal v.'s	superior vena cava
bronchial v.'s *vv. bronchiales*	near bronchi	larger bronchi and roots of lungs	*right side:* azygos v.; *left side:* left highest intercostal or accessory hemiazygos v.'s
v. of bulb of penis *v. bulbi penis*	penis	expanded posterior part of the corpus spongiosum penis (bulb of penis)	internal pudendal v.
v. of bulb of vestibule *v. bulbi vestibuli*	vestibule	mass of erectile tissue on either side of vagina	internal pudendal v.
cardiac v.'s, anterior (three to four in number) *vv. cordis anteriores*	ventral side of heart	ventral side of right ventricle	right atrium
cardiac v., great left coronary v. *v. cordis magna*	from apex of heart it ascends to front of heart	tributaries from left atrium and both ventricles; left marginal v.	left extremity of coronary sinus
cardiac v., middle *v. cordis media*	ascends up back of heart from apex	tributaries from both ventricles	right extremity of coronary sinus
cardiac v., small right coronary v. *v. cordis parva*	ascends up heart from back of right atrium and ventricle	back of right atrium and ventricle; right marginal v.	right extremity of coronary sinus or right atrium
cardiac v.'s, smallest (many minute v.'s) v.'s of Thebesius *vv. cordis minimae*	in muscular wall of heart	muscular wall of heart	mostly in atria, some in ventricles
cavernous v.'s of penis *vv. cavernosae penis*	penis	cavernous venous spaces in the erectile tissue of the penis (corpora cavernosae)	deep dorsal v. of penis, prostatic plexus
central v.'s of liver *vv. centrales hepatis*	liver	sinusoids in liver substance	sublobular v.
central v. of retina *v. centralis retinae*	from eyeball it passes out in optic nerve	retinal v.'s	superior ophthalmic v., cavernous sinus
cephalic v. *v. cephalica*	from radial part of hand it passes up forearm to groove along lateral border of biceps muscle of arm and more proximally between deltoid and pectoralis major muscles	radial side of dorsal venous plexus of hand; palmar and dorsal tributaries in forearm; thoracoacromial v.	axillary v. just caudal to clavicle
cephalic v., accessory *v. cephalica accessoria*	radial side of forearm	dorsal venous network of hand	cephalic v. at elbow
cerebellar v.'s, inferior *vv. cerebelli inferiores*	bottom of cerebellum	inferior surface of cerebellum	inferior petrosal sinus, transverse and sigmoid sinuses, straight sinus
cerebellar v.'s, superior *vv. cerebelli superiores*	top of cerebellum (superior vermis)	upper surface of cerebellum	transverse sinus, superior petrosal sinus, great cerebral v. of straight sinus
cerebral v., anterior *v. cerebri anterior*	from upper surface of corpus callosum down through longitudinal fissure, above optic nerve to lateral cerebral sulcus	anterior perforated substance, lamina terminalis, rostrum of corpus callosum, septum pellucidum, striate v.	basal v. in union with deep middle cerebral v.
cerebral v., deep middle deep Sylvian v. *v. cerebri media profunda*	lower part of lateral cerebral sulcus	tributaries from insula, neighboring gyri	basal v. in union with anterior cerebral v.

V

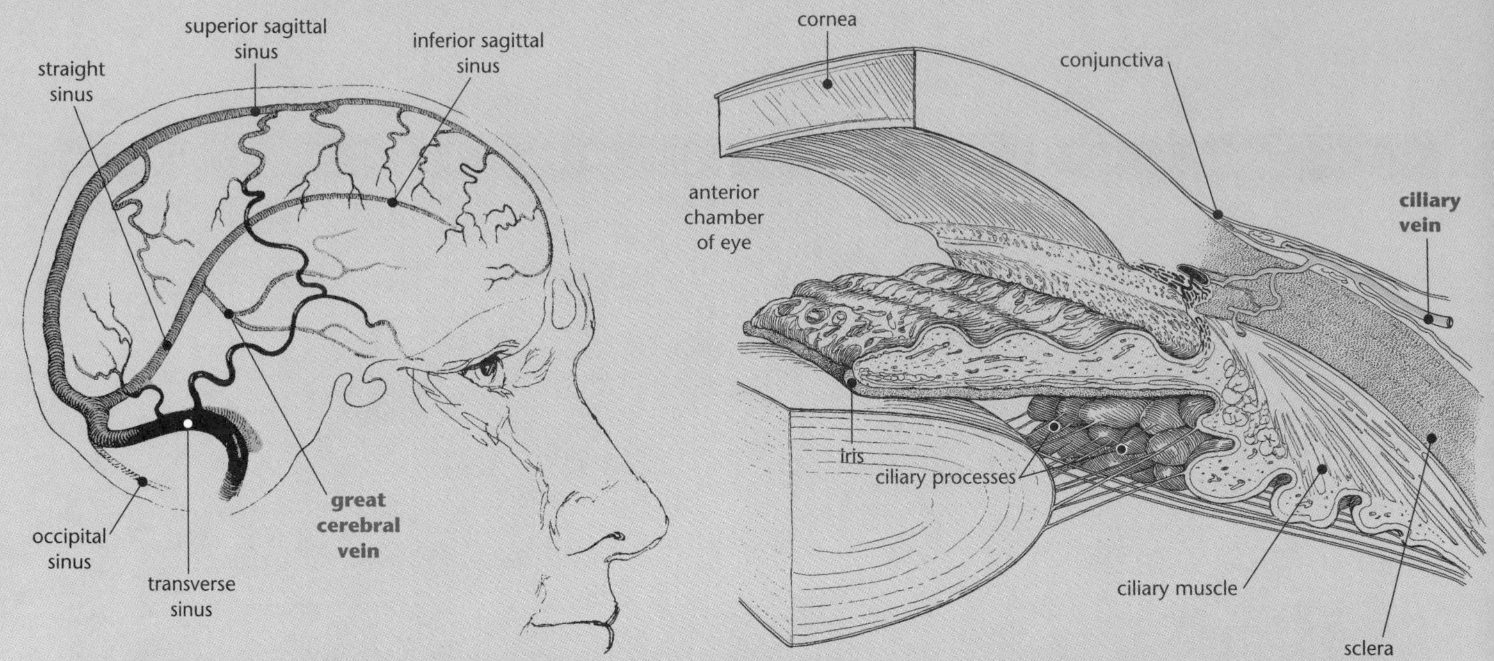

VEINS	LOCATION	DRAINS	EMPTIES INTO
cerebral v., great great v. of Galen *v. cerebri magna*	around back part of corpus callosum of brain	internal cerebral v.'s	anterior extremity of straight sinus, in union with inferior sagittal sinus
cerebral v.'s, inferior *vv. cerebri inferiores*	bottom of brain	inferior surface of cerebral hemispheres	*frontal lobe portion:* superior sagittal sinus; *temporal lobe portion:* cavernous, superior petrosal, and transverse sinuses: *occipital lobe portion:* straight sinus
cerebral v.'s, internal (two in number) v.'s of Galen deep cerebral v.'s *vv. cerebri internae*	from interventricular foramen they pass backward between the layers of the tela choroidea of the third ventricle	the deep parts of the cerebral hemispheres; thalamostriate, choroid, and basal v.'s	great cerebral v. in union with basal v.'s
cerebral v., superficial middle superficial Sylvian v. *v. cerebri media superficialis*	lateral surface of brain	lateral surface of cerebral hemispheres, corpus striatum, internal capsule	cavernous and sphenoparietal sinuses
cerebral v.'s, superior (8–12 in number) *vv. cerebri superiores*	sulci between gyri of brain	superior, lateral, and medial surfaces of cerebral hemispheres	superior sagittal sinus
cervical v., deep posterior deep cervical v. posterior vertebral v. *v. cervicalis profunda*	from suboccipital region it follows deep cervical artery down neck to level of first rib	plexus in suboccipital triangle, occipital v., deep muscles of back of neck, plexuses around spinal processes of cervical vertebrae	inferior part of vertebral v. or brachiocephalic v.
cervical v.'s, transverse *vv. transversae colli*	posterior triangle of neck	trapezius muscle and neighboring structures	subclavian v. or external jugular v.
choroid v. *v. choroidea*	lateral ventricle of brain	lateral ventricle, choroid plexus, corpus callosum	internal cerebral v.
ciliary v.'s (anterior and posterior) *vv. ciliares*	from outer surface of choroidal layer of eyeball they pass through sclera	ciliary body, scleral venous sinus, conjunctiva, iris, choroid	ophthalmic v.'s, superior and inferior
cochlear v.'s *v. cochleares*	from lamina spiralis and basilar membrane to base of modiolus	cochlea	labyrinthine v.
colic v., left *v. colica sinistra*	alongside descending colon	descending colon and left colic (splenic) flexure	inferior mesenteric v.
colic v., middle *v. colica media*	just behind transverse colon	transverse colon	superior mesenteric v.
colic v., right *v. colica dextra*	alongside ascending colon	ascending colon and right colic (hepatic) flexure	superior mesenteric v.
conjunctival v.'s *vv. conjunctivales*	eye	bulba conjunctiva	superior ophthalmic v.

VEINS	LOCATION	DRAINS	EMPTIES INTO
coronary v. gastric v. *v. gastrica dextra et sinistra*		see gastric v.	
coronary v., left		see cardiac v., great	
coronary v., right		see cardiac v., small	
coronary sinus (wide venous channel about 2.25 cm in length) *sinus coronarius*	posterior part of coronary sulcus (covered by muscular fibers from left atrium)	great, small, and middle cardiac v.'s, posterior v. of left ventricle, oblique v. of left atrium	right atrium between opening of inferior vena cava and atrioventricular aperture
cubital v., median *v. mediana cubiti*	passes obliquely across bend of elbow	cephalic v. below elbow	basilic v.
cystic v. *v. cystica*	in liver accompanying cystic duct	gallbladder	right branch of portal v.
digital v.'s, plantar *vv. digitales plantares*	plantar surface of toes	plexuses on the plantar surface of toes	unite to form four plantar metatarsal v.'s
diploic v., anterior temporal *v. diploica temporalis anterior*	middle layer (diploë) of frontal bone and parts of parietal bones of cranium	frontal bone and anterior part of parietal bones	sphenoparietal sinus and deep temporal v.
diploic v., frontal *v. diploica frontalis*	middle layer (diploë) of frontal bone of cranium	frontal bone	supraorbital v. and superior sagittal sinus
diploic v., occipital (largest of the four diploic v.'s) *v. diploica occipitalis*	middle layer (diploë) of occipital bone of cranium	parietal bone	occipital v. or transverse sinus
diploic v., posterior temporal *v. diploica temporalis posterior*	middle layer (diploë) of parietal bone of cranium	parietal bone	transverse sinus
dorsal v. of clitoris, deep (unpaired) dorsal v. of clitoris *v. dorsalis clitoridis profunda*	dorsal midline of clitoris; it passes under the public symphysis	body and glans of clitoris	primarily into the vesical venous plexus, internal pudendal v.
dorsal v.'s of clitoris, superficial *vv. dorsales clitoridis superficiales*	dorsal midline of clitoris	subcutaneous layers of clitoris, prepuce	external pudendal v.'s or femoral v.
dorsal v. of penis, deep (unpaired) dorsal v. of penis *v. dorsalis penis profunda*	dorsal midline of penis; it passes under the pubic symphysis	body and glans of penis	prostatic venous plexus, internal pudendal v.
dorsal v.'s of penis, superficial *vv. dorsales penis superficiales*	dorsal midline of penis	skin and subcutaneous layers of penis, prepuce	external pudendal v.'s or superficial epigastric v.
dorsal v.'s of tongue		see lingual v.'s, dorsal	
emissary v., condylar *v. emissaria condylaris*	through condylar canal of cranium	area of foramen magnum	deep v.'s of neck
emissary v.'s, foramen lacerum (two or three in number) *vv. emissariae foraminis lacerum*	through foramen lacerum of cranium	cavernous sinus	pterygoid plexus
emissary v., foramen of Vesalius *v. emissaria foraminis Vesalii*	through foramen of Vesalius (when present)	cavernous sinus	pterygoid plexus
emissary v., mastoid *v. emissaria mastoidea*	through mastoid foramen of cranium	transverse sinus	posterior auricular v. or occipital v.
emissary v., parietal *v. emissaria parietalis*	through parietal foramen of cranium	scalp	superior sagittal sinus
epigastric v., inferior deep epigastric v. *v. epigastrica inferior*	from area of umbilicus it descends to deep inguinal ring area	abdominal wall; *in male:* ductus deferens; *in female:* round ligament	external iliac v. about 1.25 cm proximal to inguinal ligament
epigastric v., superficial *v. epigastrica superficialis*	from umbilicus it runs downward and laterally toward inguinal ligament	cutaneous part of lower and medial part of abdominal wall	great saphenous v. or femoral v.
epigastric v.'s, superior *vv. epigastricae superiores*	from abdomen they ascend toward diaphragm	rectus muscle of abdomen; xiphoid process, diaphragm	internal thoracic v.'s
episcleral v.'s *vv. episclerales*	in sclera close to corneal margin	angle of eye, sclera, conjunctiva	anterior ciliary v.'s
esophageal v.'s (several in number) *vv. esophageae*	along the esophagus	esophagus	azygos, hemiazygos, left gastric, and left brachiocephalic v.'s

V

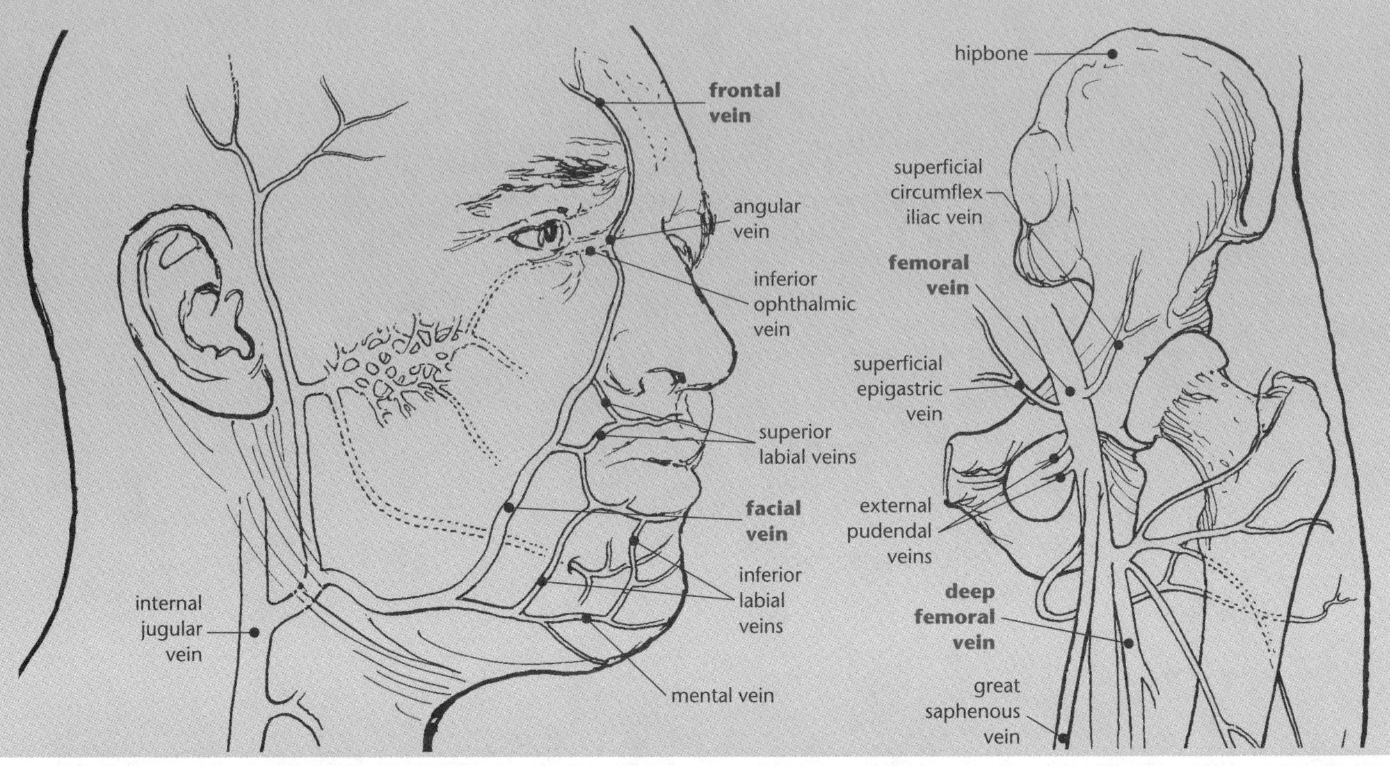

VEINS	LOCATION	DRAINS	EMPTIES INTO
ethmoidal v.'s *vv. ethmoidales*	ethmoidal sinuses	ethmoidal sinuses, frontal sinus, dura mater, walls and septum of nasal cavity	superior ophthalmic v.
facial v. anterior facial v. *v. facialis*	from medial angle of eye across face to neck, crossing lower margin of body of mandible	superficial structures of face; *tributaries include:* frontal, supraorbital, deep facial, superficial temporal, posterior auricular, occipital, and retromandibular v.'s	internal jugular v. or common facial v.
facial v., common	former term for the lower trunk of the facial v. (sometimes joined by retromandibular v.) which empties into the internal jugular v.		
facial v., deep *v. facialis profunda*	face, from infratemporal fossa, courses downward on maxilla just below zygomatic bone	pterygoid plexus; small tributaries from buccinator, zygomatic, and masseter muscles	facial v.
facial v., transverse *v. facialis transversa*	from cheek it passes backward (just below zygomatic arch) to front of ear	muscles and related structures near the zygoma	superficial temporal v.
femoral v. *v. femoralis*	proximal two-thirds of thigh up to inguinal ligament	popliteal v., great saphenous v., deep femoral v., muscular tributaries	external iliac v. at level of inguinal ligament
femoral v., deep profunda femoris v. *v. profunda femoris*	accompanies deep femoral artery	medial and lateral femoral circumflex v.'s; through muscular tributaries it anastomoses with popliteal v. distally and inferior gluteal v. proximally	femoral v.
femoral circumflex v.'s, lateral *vv. circumflexae femoris laterales*	winds around lateral side of upper femur	muscles of thigh, especially posterior muscles; lateral half of hip	femoral v. or deep femoral v.
femoral circumflex v.'s, medial *vv. circumflexae femoris mediales*	winds around medial side of upper femur	muscles of upper thigh, especially posterior muscles; hip joint	femoral v. or deep femoral v.
fibular v.'s		see peroneal v.'s	
frontal v. *v. frontalis*	from forehead to root of nose	plexus of forehead and scalp	facial v.
gastric v. coronary v. *v. gastrica*	from right to left along lesser curvature of stomach down peritoneum of lesser sac (omental bursa)	tributaries from both surfaces of stomach	portal v.
gastric v.'s, short (four or five in number) *vv. gastricae breves*	greater curvature of stomach, between fundus of stomach and spleen	fundus and left part of greater curvature of stomach	splenic v.

VEINS	LOCATION	DRAINS	EMPTIES INTO
gastroepiploic v., left *v. gastroepiploica sinistra*	from right to left along upper part of greater curvature of stomach	tributaries from ventral and dorsal surfaces of stomach and greater omentum	splenic v.
gastroepiploic v., right *v. gastroepiploica dextra*	from left to right along lower part of greater curvature of stomach	tributaries from greater omentum and parts of stomach	superior mesenteric v.
gluteal v.'s, inferior sciatic v.'s *vv. gluteae inferiores*	from the proximal part of posterior thigh they enter the pelvis through the greater sciatic foramen	skin and muscles of buttock and back of thigh; medial femoral circumflex and first perforating v.'s	internal iliac v.
gluteal v.'s, superior gluteal v.'s *vv. gluteae superiores*	from buttock through greater sciatic foramen to pelvis	tributaries from buttock, skin over sacrum	internal iliac v.
hemiazygos v. left azygos v. inferior minor azygos v. *v. hemiazygos*	in thorax, it ascends on left side of vertebral column to ninth thoracic vertebra before horizontally crossing over vertebral column to join the azygos v.	left ascending lumbar v.'s, caudal four or five intercostal v.'s, left subcostal v., esophageal and mediastinal v.'s	azygos v.
hemiazygos v., accessory superior minor azygos v. *v. hemiazygos accesoria*	descends on left side of vertebral column in thorax and usually crosses over vertebral column at eighth thoracic vertebra	fourth to seventh posterior intercostal v.'s, mediastinum, bronchus	azygos v. or hemiazygos v.
hemorrhoidal v.'s		see rectal v.'s	
hepatic v.'s *vv. hepaticae*	posterior surface of right, left, and caudate lobes of liver	substance of liver; central, intralobular, and sublobular v.'s	*upper group:* three large v.'s drain into the inferior vena cava below the diaphragm; *lower group:* several small v.'s drain into the inferior vena cava lower down
hypogastric v.		see iliac v., internal	
ileocolic v. *v. ileocolica*	right iliac fossa	terminal ileum, appendix, cecum, lower part of ascending colon	superior mesenteric v.
iliac v., common *v. iliaca communis*	from sacroiliac articulation, ascends to fifth lumbar vertebra	internal and external iliac v.'s; iliolumbar and lateral sacral v.'s (in addition, left common iliac v. receives middle sacral v.)	unites with its member of opposite side to form inferior vera cava at level of fifth lumbar vertebra
iliac v., external *v. iliaca externa*	from under inguinal ligament, along brim and lesser pelvis, to sacroiliac articulation	lower limb and lower abdominal wall; inferior epigastric, deep circumflex and pubic v.'s	common iliac v. in union with external iliac v.
iliac v., internal hypogastric v. *v. iliaca interna*	from greater sciatic foramen it passes upward to brim of pelvis	pelvic viscera, superior gluteal, inferior gluteal, internal pudendal, obturator, lateral sacral, middle sacral, dorsal v.'s of penis, vesical, uterine, vaginal	common iliac v. in union with external iliac v.
iliac circumflex v., deep *v. circumflexa ilium profunda*	inner aspect of ilium in lower abdomen	venae comitantes of deep iliac circumflex artery, internal oblique, transverse abdominal, iliac, psoas, and sartorius muscles	external iliac v. about 2 cm above inguinal ligament
innominate v.'s		see brachiocephalic v.'s	
intercostal v.'s, anterior (12 pairs) *vv. intercostales anteriores*	lower border of each rib	ribs, intercostal and pectoral muscles, breast, skin of chest	internal thoracic and musculophrenic v.'s
intercostal v., left highest left superior intercostal v. *v. intercostalis suprema sinistra*	first intercostal space	first left intercostal space	left brachiocephalic v. or vertebral v.
intercostal v., left superior *v. intercostalis superior sinistra*	from the upper left intercostal spaces, courses obliquely to area of left side of aortic arch	left second, third, and fourth intercostal v.'s	left brachiocephalic v. or accessory hemiazygos v.

V

interlobular vein of kidney
arcuate vein of kidney
nephron
interlobar vein of kidney
interlobar artery of kidney
collecting duct
loop of Henle

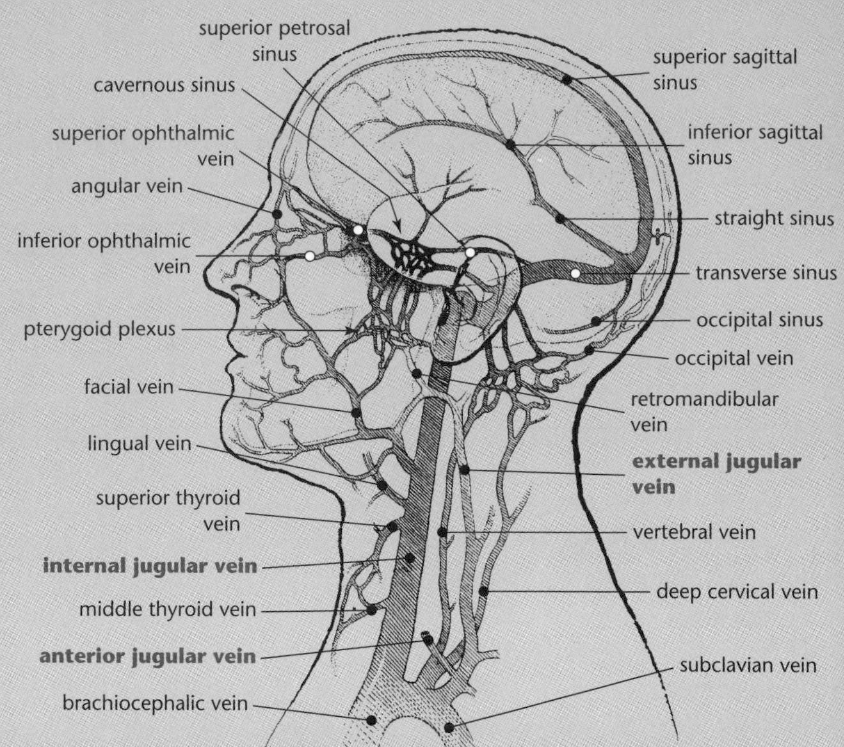

VEINS	LOCATION	DRAINS	EMPTIES INTO
intercostal v., right highest right superior intercostal v. *v. intercostalis suprema dextra*	posterior wall of upper thorax	first right intercostal space	azygos v.
intercostal v.'s, posterior *vv. intercostales posterior*	one in each intercostal space	skin and muscles of back and spinal tributary from vertebral plexuses	*right side:* azygos v., right highest intercostal v.; *left side:* left brachiocephalic v., hemiazygos v.
intercostal v., right superior *v. intercostalis superior dextra*	posterior mediastinum	right second, third, and fourth intercostal spaces	azygos v.
interlobar v.'s of kidney *vv. interlobares renis*	between pyramids of kidney	arcuate v.'s, venous arcades of kidney	renal v.
interlobular v.'s of kidney *vv. interlobulares renis*	cortex of kidney	cortex of kidney; stellate, capsular, and perforating v.'s	arcuate v.'s of kidney
interlobular v.'s of liver *vv. interlobulares hepatis*	in substance of liver between lobules	central or intralobular and sublobular v.'s	hepatic v.'s
intervertebral v.'s *vv. intervertebrales*	intervertebral foramen	internal and external vertebral plexuses; v.'s from spinal cord	vertebral, intercostal, lumbar, and lateral sacral v.'s
intestinal v.'s (usually 10–15 in number) jejunal and ileal v.'s *vv. intestinales*	run parallel with superior mesenteric artery between layers of mesentery	walls of jejunum and ileum	superior mesenteric v.
jejunal and ileal v.'s		see intestinal v.'s	
jugular v., anterior (usually two in number) *v. jugularis anterior*	from near hyoid bone it passes down anterior part of neck	laryngeal and thyroid v.'s, neck muscles	external jugular or subclavian v.
jugular v., external *v. jugularis externa*	from substance of parotid gland it runs perpendicularly down neck	deep parts of face, exterior of cranium, retromandibular and posterior auricular v.'s	subclavian v., internal jugular v., or brachiocephalic v.
jugular v., internal *v. jugularis interna*	from jugular fossa it descends side of neck lateral to internal carotid artery, and then lateral to common carotid artery	brain, face, and neck; transverse sinus, inferior petrosal sinus, facial, lingual, pharyngeal, superior and middle thyroid and at times the occipital v.'s	brachiocephalic v., after union with subclavian v.
jugular v., posterior external *v. jugularis externa posteriores*	from occipital region down to middle third of external jugular	skin and superficial muscles of back of head and neck	external jugular v.
labial v.'s, anterior *vv. labiales anteriores*	vulva	anterior portion of labia majora; mons pubis	external pudendal v.

VEINS	LOCATION	DRAINS	EMPTIES INTO
labial v.'s, inferior *vv. labiales inferiores*	edge of lower lip to angle of mouth	labial glands, mucous membrane and muscles of lower lip	facial v. or submental v.
labial v.'s, posterior *vv. labiales posteriores*	vulva	posterior portion of labia majora; vestibule, labia minora	internal pudendal v.
labial v.'s, superior *vv. labiales superiores*	edge of upper lip between mucous membrane and muscle	upper lip, tributaries from nose, nasal septum	facial v.
labyrinthine v.'s internal auditory v.'s *vv. labyrinthi*	from inner ear through internal acoustic meatus	inner ear (utricle, saccule, semicircular canals, lamina spiralis, basilar membrane)	inferior petrosal sinus or sigmoid sinus
lacrimal v. *v. lacrimalis*	orbit	lacrimal glands, eyelids, conjunctiva	superior ophthalmic v.
laryngeal v., inferior *v. laryngea inferior*	dorsal part of larynx	muscles and mucous membrane of larynx	inferior thyroid v.
laryngeal v., superior *v. laryngea superior*	larynx	glands, mucous membrane, and muscles of larynx	superior thyroid v.
lingual v. *v. lingualis*	tongue	tongue by way of two or three tributaries, sublingual gland, tonsil, gums, epiglottis	internal jugular or lower part of facial v.
deep lingual v. ranine v. *profunda v. linguae*	tongue	tip and deep part of tongue	vena comitans of deep lingual artery
lingual v.'s, dorsal dorsal v.'s tongue *vv. dorsales linguae*	tongue	posterior part of tongue	lingual v.
lumbar v.'s (usually four in number on each side) *vv. lumbales*	lumbar walls	dorsal tributaries from skin and muscles of loin and by abdominal tributaries from abdominal wall; vertebral plexus	first and second drain into ascending lumbar v.; third and fourth drain into inferior vena cava
lumbar v., ascending *v. lumbalis ascendens*	ventral to transverse process of lumbar vertebrae	sacral and lumbar v.'s	*right side:* azygos v. in union with subcostal v.; *left side: hemiazygos v. in union with subcostal v.*
maxillary v. *v. maxillaris*	short trunk between condyle of mandible and sphenomandibular ligament	pterygoid plexus, ear sinuses, auditory tube, pterygoid and temporal muscles, temporomandibular joint	retromandibular v. in union with superficial temporal v.
median v. of forearm median antebrachial v. *v. mediana antebrachii*	from base of thumb to middle of palmar forearm	venous plexus on palmar surface of hand	basilic v. and/or cephalic v., or median cubital v.
mediastinal v.'s anterior mediastinal v.'s *vv. mediastinales*	mediastinum	areolar tissue and lymph nodes of anterior mediastinum; pericardium	azygos v., brachiocephalic v., or superior vena cava
meningeal v.'s, anterior *vv. meningeae anteriores*	over small wing of sphenoid bone in endosteal layer of dura mater	dura mater of anterior cranal fossa; cranium	ethmoidal and diploic v.'s, venous sinuses
meningeal v.'s, middle *vv. meningeae mediae*	from endosteal layer of dura mater it leaves cranium via foramen spinosum of sphenoid bone	dura mater, internal surface of cranium, trigeminal ganglion, tensor tympani muscle	pterygoid venous plexus or parietosphenoidal sinus
mesenteric v., inferior *v. mesenterica inferior*	from rectum it ascends under cover of peritoneum to level of pancreas	upper rectum; sigmoid and descending parts of colon	splenic v. or junction of splenic v. and superior mesenteric v.
mesenteric v., superior *v. mesenterica superior*	from right iliac fossa it ascends between two layers of mesentery to the level of pancreas	small intestine, cecum, appendix, and ascending and transverse parts of colon	portal v. in union with splenic v.
metacarpal v.'s, dorsal *vv. metacarpeae dorsales*	on dorsum of hand over distal two-thirds of metacarpus	dorsal metacrapal region	dorsal venous rete of hand
metacarpal v.'s, palmar *vv. metacarpeae palmares*	palmar surface of hand	palmar metacarpal region	deep palmar venous arch
metatarsal v.'s, dorsal dorsal interosseous v.'s of foot *vv. metatarseae dorsales*	run proximally in metatarsal spaces of dorsal surface of foot	dorsal digital v.'s at clefts of toes; metatarsal bones and neighboring muscles	dorsal venous arch of foot
metatarsal v.'s, plantar *vv. metatarseae plantares*	between metatarsal bones of plantar surface of foot	plantar digital v.'s at clefts of toes; metatarsal bones and neighboring muscles	deep plantar venous arch of foot

V

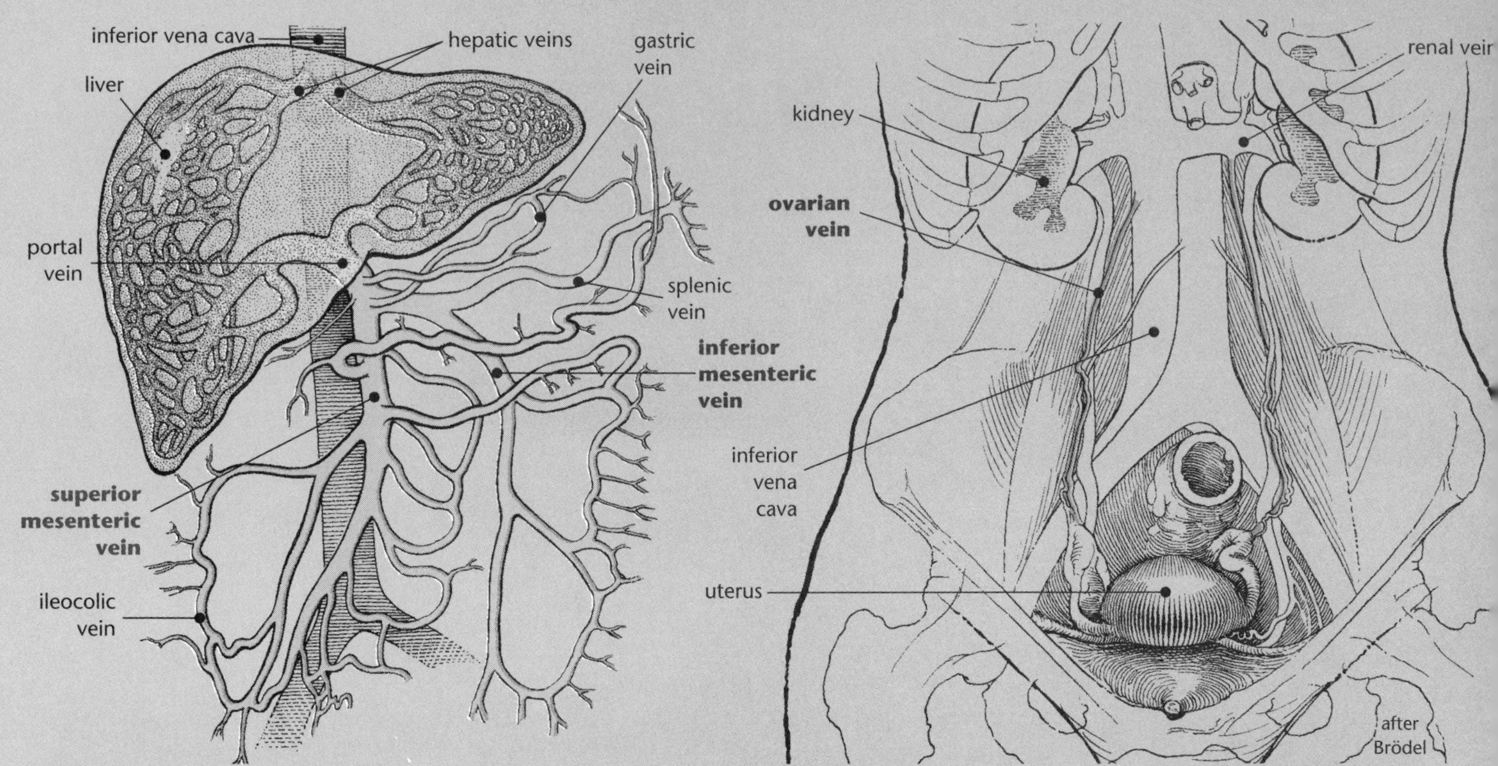

VEINS	LOCATION	DRAINS	EMPTIES INTO
musculophrenic v.'s *vv. musculophrenicae*	from diaphragm, along inner surface of costal cage at attachment of diaphragm, to sixth costal cartilage	diaphragm and lower intercostal spaces, abdominal wall	internal thoracic v.
nasal v.'s, external (several in number) *vv. nasales externae*	from nose extending upward	external aspect of nose	angular and facial v.'s
nasofrontal v. *v. nasofrontalis*	anterior medial part of orbit	supraorbital and angular v.'s	superior ophthalmic v.
oblique v. of left atrium *v. obliqua atrii sinistri*	posterior wall of left atrium of heart	heart wall	coronary sinus
obturator v. *v. obturatoria*	from proximal portion of adductor region of thigh to pelvis through obturator foramen	hip joint and regional muscles	internal iliac v., sometimes the inferior epigastric or common iliac v.
occipital v. *v. occipitalis*	from back part of scalp it passes to suboccipital triangle of neck	plexus on posterior part of head; tributaries from posterior auricular and superficial temporal v.'s; parietal emissary, mastoid emissary, and occipital diploic v.'s	deep cervical v. and vertebral v., occasionally the internal jugular v.
ophthalmic v., inferior *v. ophthalmica inferior*	from floor of orbit it passes posteriorly through superior orbital fissure	lower eyelid, lacrimal sac, muscle of eyeball	cavernous sinus or superior opthalmic v.
ophthalmic v., superior *v. ophthalmica superior*	from inner angle of orbit, through superior orbital fissure into cavernous sinus	eyeball, eye muscles, and eyelid	cavernous sinus
ovarian v.'s *vv. ovaricae*	in broad ligament near ovary and uterine tube	pampiniform plexus of broad ligament, ovary, uterus	*right side:* inferior vena cava; *left side:* left renal v.
palatine v., external *v. palatina externa*	palate region	tonsils and soft palate, pharyngeal wall	pterygoid and tonsillar plexuses; facial v.
palpebral v.'s, inferior *vv. palpebrales inferiores*	from lower eyelid, downward over cheek	lower eyelid, conjunctiva, nasolacrimal duct	facial v. or angular v.
palpebral v.'s, superior *vv. palpebrales superiores*	upper eyelid	upper eyelid, conjunctiva	angular v. and superior ophthalmic v.
pancreatic v.'s *vv. pancreaticae*	at pancreas	tributaries from body and tail of pancreas	splenic v.
pancreaticoduodenal v.'s *vv. pancreaticoduodenales*	head of pancreas and proximal part of duodenum	pancreas and duodenum	upper part of superior mesenteric v., portal v.

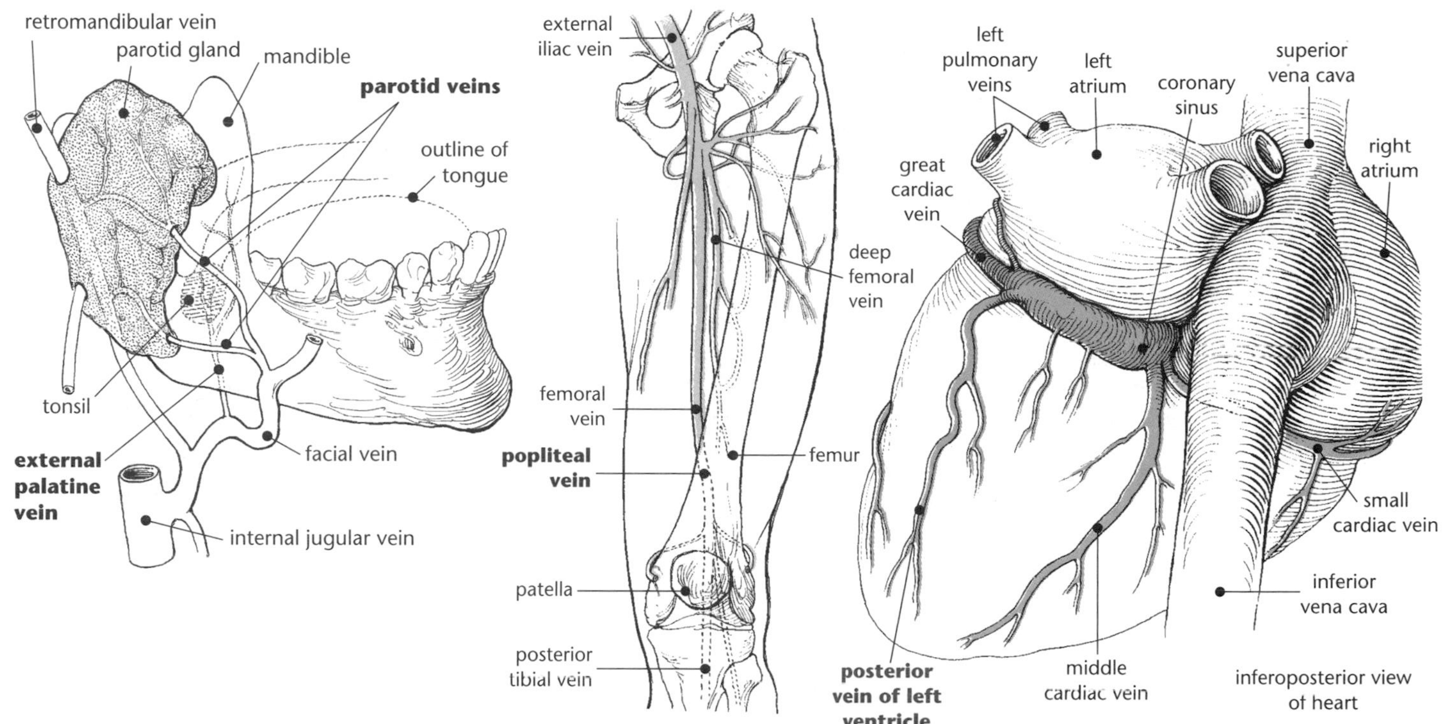

VEINS	LOCATION	DRAINS	EMPTIES INTO
paraumbilical v.'s parumbilical v.'s Sappey's v.'s *vv. paraumbilicales*	from umbilical area they pass along round ligament to liver and medial umbilical ligament to bladder	cutaneous v.'s about the umbilicus	accessory portal v.'s in liver
parotid v.'s *vv. parotideae*	parotid gland	part of parotid gland and overlying skin	facial v. or retromandibular v.
peforating v.'s *vv. perforantes*	perforate great adductor muscle to reach back of thigh	thigh muscles, especially hamstrings	deep femoral v.
pericardiac v.'s (several in number) *vv. pericardiaceae*	membranous capsule of heart (pericardium)	pericardium	brachiocephalic v., or superior vena cava, or internal thoracic v.
pericardiacophrenic v.'s superior phrenic v.'s *vv. pericardiocophrenicae*	parallel to phrenic nerve between pleura and pericardium	diaphragm; tributaries from pericardium; pleura	brachiocephalic v., superior vena cava, or azygos v.
peroneal v.'s fibular v.'s *vv. peroneae*	from lateral side of heel up back of leg just below knee	calcaneus, leg muscles, tibiotibular syndesmosis	posterior tibal v. after uniting with popliteal v.
petrosal sinus, inferior *sinus petrosus inferior*	inferior petrosal sulcus	cavernous sinus, internal auditory v.'s, v.'s from medulla oblongata, pons, and inferior surface of cerebellum	bulb of internal jugular v.
petrosal sinus, superior *sinus petrosus superior*	superior petrosal sulcus in head	cavernous sinus	transverse sinus or sigmoid sinus
pharyngeal v.'s (several in number) *vv. pharyngeae*	outer surface of pharynx	posterior meningeal v.'s and v. of the pterygoid canal; pharyngeal plexus	internal jugular v. occasionally the facial v.
phrenic v.'s, inferior *vv. phrenicae inferior*	undersurface of diaphragm	substance of diaphragm	*right side:* inferior vena cava; *left side:* left suprarenal v. (often a second v. on left side enters inferior vena cava)
popliteal v. *v. poplitea*	from lower border of popliteal muscle, through popliteal fossa to adductor hiatus	anterior and posterior tibial v.'s, skin and muscles of thigh and calf	femoral v. at adductor hiatus
portal v. (about 8 cm in length) *v. portae*	in abdomen behind neck of pancreas at level of second lumbar vertebra	superior mesenteric, splenic, gastric, pyloric, cystic, and paraumbilical v.'s	right and left terminal branches in liver
posterior v. of left ventricle *v. posterior ventriculi sinistri*	from apex of heart it travels parallel to posterior interventricular sulcus	diaphragmatic surface of left ventricle	coronary sinus of great cardiac v.
prepyloric v. v. of Mayo *v. prepylorica*	pyloric end of stomach	pylorus	right gastric v.

V

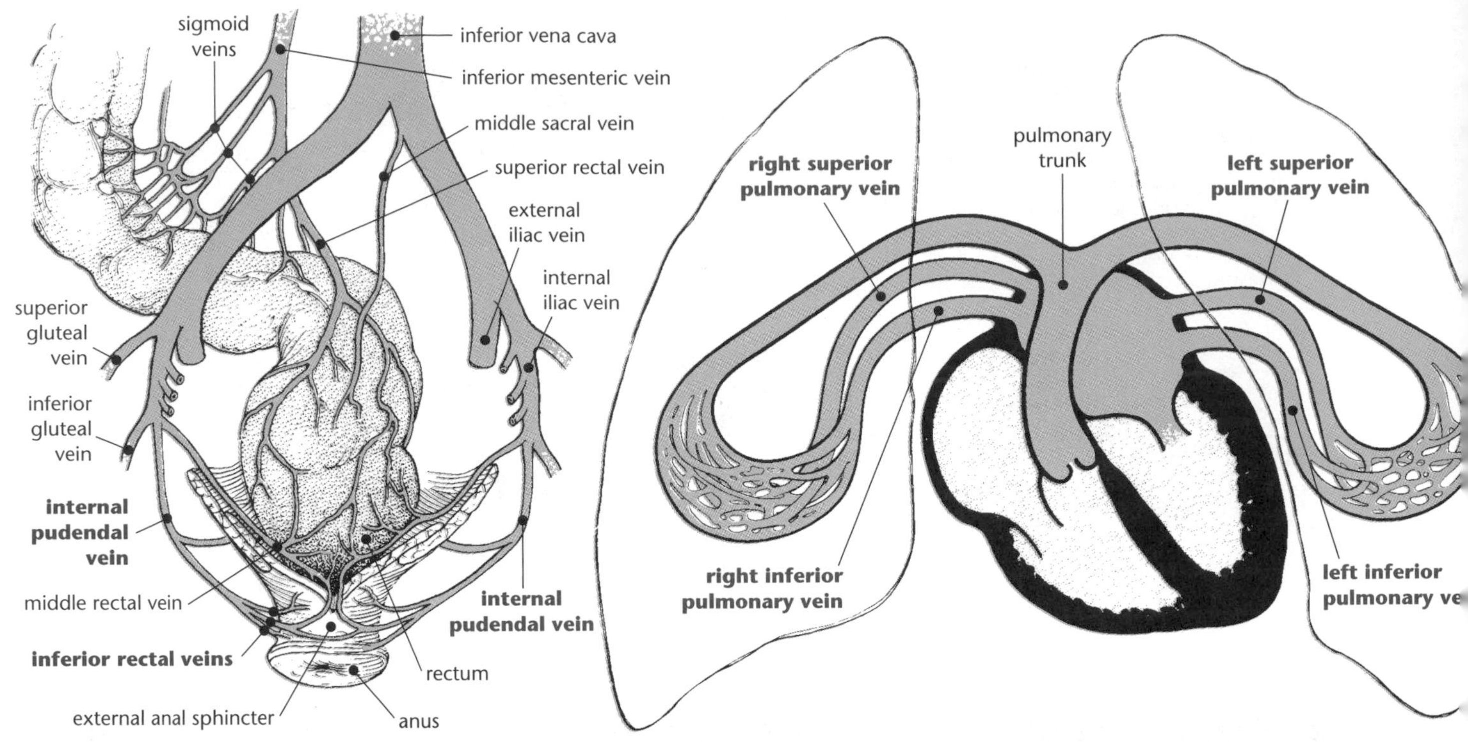

VEINS	LOCATION	DRAINS	EMPTIES INTO
profunda femoris v.		see femoral v., deep	
profunda linguae v.		see lingual v., deep	
v. of pterygoid canal vidian v. *v. canalis pterygoidel*	from ear and throat through pterygoid canal	sphenoid sinus	pterygoid plexus or cavernous sinus
pterygoid plexus *plexus pterygoideus*	infratemporal fossa	*tributaries from:* inferior alveolar, middle, meningeal, deep temporal, masseter, buccal, posterior superior alveolar, pharyngeal, descending palatine, infraorbital, pterygoid canal, and sphenopalatine v.'s	maxillary v.
pubic v. *v. pubis*	from dorsum of penis through obturator foramen to pelvis	pubic area	external iliac v.
pudendal v.'s, external external pudic v.'s *vv. pudendae externae*	from lower abdomen and genitalia to upper thigh	skin of lower part of abdomen; *in male:* anterior scrotal and superficial dorsal v.'s of penis; *in female:* anterior labial and superficial dorsal v. 's of clitoris	great saphenous v. or femoral v.
pudendal v.'s, internal internal pudic v.'s *vv. pudendae internae*	from perineum and genitalia to pelvis through greater sciatic foramen	perineum and genitalia	internal iliac v. (distal part)
pulmonary v., left inferior *v. pulmonalis inferior sinistra*	from left lung to heart	left lower lobe	left atrium of heart
pulmonary v., left superior *v. pulmonalis superior sinistra*	from left lung to heart	left upper lobe	left atrium of heart
pulmonary v., right inferior *v. pulmonalis inferior dextra*	from right lung to heart	right lower lobe	left atrium of heart
pulmonary v., right superior *v. pulmonis superior dextra*	from right lung to heart	right upper and middle lobe	left atrium of heart
pyloric v. *v. pylorus*	along pyloric portion of lesser curvature of stomach	pylorus and lesser omentum	portal v.
radial v.'s *vv. radiales*	from hand, winds around lateral side of carpus up forearm tofront of elbow	dorsal metacarpal v.'s, muscles of forearm, wrist, and hand; radius, ulna, elbow joint	brachial v.'s after uniting with ulnar v.'s
ranine v.		see lingual v., deep	
rectal v.'s inferior inferior hemorrhoidal v.'s *vv. rectales inferiores*	near anal canal and rectum	lower part of external rectal plexus and anal canal	internal pudendal v.

VEINS	LOCATION	DRAINS	EMPTIES INTO
rectal v., middle middle hemorrhoidal v. *v. rectalis media*	middle of rectum in lesser pelvis	rectal plexus; tributaries from bladder, prostate gland, and seminal vesicle	internal iliac v. or inferior gluteal v.
rectal v.'s, superior superior hemorrhoidal v.'s *vv. rectales superiores*	upper rectum to brim of pelvis	upper part of rectal plexus	inferior mesenteric v.
renal v.'s *vv. renales*	at right angle to hilum of kidneys	kidneys; testicular, inferior phrenic, and suprarenal v.'s	inferior vena cava (right renal v. opens into inferior vena cava at a slightly lower level than left)
retromandibular v. posterior facial v. *v. retromandibularis*	from substance of parotid gland it passes alongside ramus of lower jaw	superficial temporal, maxillary and tributaries from parotid gland and masseter muscle	external jugular v. in union with posterior auricular v; facial v.
sacral v.'s, lateral *vv. sacrales laterales*	anterior surface of sacrum	skin and muscles of dorsum of sacrum and coccyx	internal iliac v. or superior gluteal v.'s
sacral v., middle *v. sacralis media*	front of sacrum	region of posterior surface of rectum	left common iliac v.
saphenous v., accessory *v. saphena accessoria*	medial and posterior parts of thigh	inner and posterior parts of superficial thigh	great saphenous v.
saphenous v., great (longest vein in body) long saphenous v. *v. saphena magna*	from medial aspect of foot to 3 cm below inguinal ligament	tributaries from sole of foot; small saphenous v., anterior and posterior tibia v.'s, accessory saphenous v., superficial epigastric v., superficial iliac circumflex v., superficial external pudendal v.	femoral v.
saphenous v., small short saphenous v. *v. saphena parva*	from lateral ankle to middle of back of leg to 5 cm above knee joint	lateral marginal v., deep v.'s of dorsum of foot, large tributaries from back of leg	popliteal v. or great saphenous v.
scrotal v.'s, anterior *vv. scrotales anteriores*	scrotum	front part of scrotum	external pudendal v.
scrotal v.'s, posterior *vv. scrotales posteriores*	scrotum	back part of scrotum	vesical venous plexus or internal pudendal v.'s
sigmoid v.'s (several in number) *vv. sigmoideae*	lower left side of colon	sigmoid colon and descending colon	inferior mesenteric v.
spinal v.'s *vv. spinales*	in pia mater of spinal cord where it forms a tortuous venous plexus	spinal cord and pia matter	internal vertebral venous plexus
spiral v. of modiolus *v. spiralis modioli*	modiolus of cochlea	cochlea	labyrinthine v.'s
splenic v. lienal v. *v. lienalis*	from hilum of spleen to vicinity of neck of pancreas	short gastric, left gastroepiploic, pancreatic, and inferior mesenteric v.'s	portal v.
stellate v.'s of kidney *vv. stellatae renis*	cortex of kidney near capsule	superficial part of cortex of kidney	interlobular v.'s of kidney
sternocleidomastoid v. sternomastoid v. *v. sternocleidomastoidea*	neck	sternocleidomastoid, omohyoid, sternohyoid, sternothyroid, and platysma muscles, skin of neck	internal jugular v.
striate v.'s, inferior vv. thalamostriatae inferiores	corpus striatum	anterior perforated substance of cerebrum	basal v.
stylomastoid v. *v. stylomastoidea*	descends vertically from stylomastoid foramen	mastoid cells, middle ear chamber, semicircular canals	retromandibular v. or posterior auricular v.
subclavian v. *v. subclavia*	from outer border of first rib to sternal end of clavicle	continues from axillary v.; external jugular v., anterior jugular v. (occasionally)	joined by internal jugular to form brachiocephalic v.
subcostal v. *v. subcostalis*	in abdominal wall along caudal border of 12th rib	lower abdominal wall below 12th rib	*right side:* azygos v.; *left side:* hemiazygos v.
subcutaneous v.'s of abdomen *vv. subcutaneae obdominis*	abdominal wall	superficial layers of abdominal wall	thoracoepigastric, superficial epigastric, or deep v.'s of abdominal wall
sublingual v. *v. sublingualis*	below tongue	sublingual gland, mylohyoid and neighboring muscles, mucous membranes of mouth and gums, alveolar process of mandible	lingual v. or facial v.

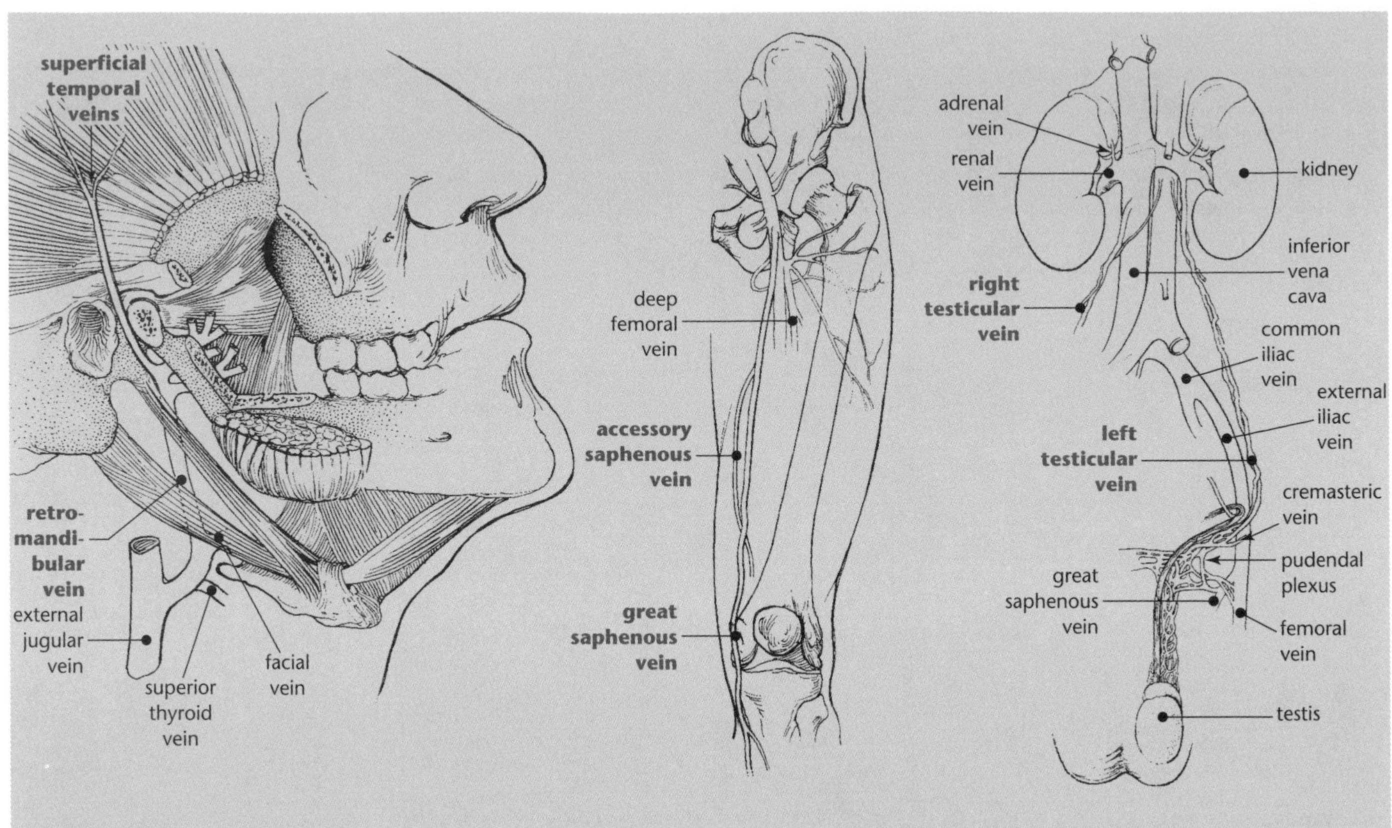

VEINS	LOCATION	DRAINS	EMPTIES INTO
submental v. *v. submentalis*	below margin of mandible	submandibular gland; mylohyoid, digastric, and platysma muscles	facial v.
supraorbital v. *v. supraorbitalis*	courses medially and downward to medial angle of eye	frontal muscle, frontal diploic v., superior rectus and levator palpebral muscles, frontal sinus	angular v. (beginning of facial v.), in union with supratrochlear v.
suprarenal v., left *v. suprarenalis sinistra*	hilium of left adrenal gland	left adrenal gland	left renal v. or left inferior phrenic v.
suprarenal v., right *v. suprarenalis dextra*	hilium of right adrenal gland	right adrenal gland	inferior vena cava
suprascapular v. transverse scapular v. *v. suprascapularis*	from posterior surface of scapula it passes through scapula notch, runs parallel with clavicle and then crosses over brachial plexus and subclavian artery	acromioclavicular and shoulder joints, scapula, clavicle, and neighboring muscles and skin	external jugular v. or subclavian v.
supratrochlear v.'s (usually two in number) *vv. supratrochleares*	front and top of head; course to medial angle of orbit	venous plexus of forehead, scalp of medial forehead, dorsum of nose	in union with angular v.
temporal v.'s, deep *vv. temporales profundae*	from side of head, course down behind zygomatic arch	deep areas of temporal muscle	pterygoid venous plexus
temporal v., middle *v. temporalis media*	from lateral angle of orbit, it passes to side of ear	temporal muscle; zygomaticoorbital v.	retromandibular v. or superficial and deep temporal v.'s
temporal v.'s, superficial *vv. temporales superficiales*	from scalp on side of head down to parotid gland front of ear	plexus on side of head; transverse facial, anterior auricular, and middle temporal v.'s	retromandibular v. in union with maxillary v.
temporomandibular v.'s *vv. temporomandibulares*	temporomandibular joint (TMJ)	area surrounding temporomandibular joint; tympanic v.'s	retromandibular v. or maxillary v.
testicular v., left left spermatic v. *v. testicularis sinistra*	from testis it ascends along spermatic cord through deep inguinal canal into abdomen	testis, epididymis, ureter, cremaster muscle	left renal v.
testicular v., right right spermatic v. *v. testicularis dextra*	from testis it ascends along spermatic cord through deep inguinal canal into abdomen	testis, epididymis, ureter, cremaster muscle	inferior vena cava
thalamostriate v. *v. thalamostriata superior*	deep part of brain	corpus striatum, thalamus, and corpus callosum	internal cerebral v.

VEINS	LOCATION	DRAINS	EMPTIES INTO
thoracic v., internal internal mammary v. *v. thoracica interna*	thorax	superior phrenic, superior epigastric, musculophrenic, perforating, anterior intercostal, sternal, thymic, mediastinal, and pericardiacophrenic v.'s	brachiocephalic v.
thoracic v., lateral long thoracic v. *v. thoracica lateralis*	lateral thoracic wall	lateral thoracic wall; mammary gland; axillary lymph nodes; costoaxillary v.'s	axillary v.
thoracoacromial v.'s acromiothoracic v.'s *vv. thoracoacromiales*	top of shoulder	acromion, coracoid process, sternoclavicular joint, tributaries from deltoid, subclavius, pectoralis major and minor muscles	subclavian v. or axillary v.
thoracoepigastric v. *v. thoracoepigastrica*	anterior and lateral aspect of trunk (in subcutaneous tissue)	skin and subcutaneous tissue of anterolateral aspect of trunk	*superiorly:* lateral thoracic v.; *inferiorly:* superficial epigastric v.
thymic v.'s *vv. thymicae*	thymus gland	substance of thymus gland	left brachiocephalic and thyroid v.'s
thyroid v.'s, inferior (two to four in number) *vv. thyroideae inferiores*	lower neck, anterior to fifth, sixth, and seventh tracheal rings	venous plexus of thyroid gland; esophageal, tracheal, and inferior laryngeal v.'s	brachiocephalic v.'s (occasionally just the left brachiocephalic v.)
thyroid v.'s, middle *vv. thyroidea mediae*	from thyroid gland they pass laterally over common carotid artery	lower part of thyroid gland; tributaries from trachea and larynx	lower part of internal jugular v. just below level of cricoid cartilage
thyroid v.'s, superior *v. thyroidea superiores*	from thyroid gland it passes up toward head	superior part of thyroid gland; superior laryngeal and cricothyroid v.'s	upper part of internal jugular v.
tibial v.'s, anterior *vv. tibiales anteriores*	from foot and ankle joint up front of leg between tibia and fibula about 5 cm below knee joint	venae comitantes of dorsal artery of foot; muscles and bones of anterior leg	popliteal v. in union with posterior tibial v.
tibial v.'s, posterior (usually two in number) *vv. tibiales posteriores*	from sole of foot to tibial side of leg where it ascends obliquely to back of leg just below bend of knee	muscles and bones of posterior leg	popliteal v. in union with anterior tibial v.
tracheal v.'s (several in number) *vv. tracheales*	trachea	substance of trachea	thyroid venous plexus, brachiocephalic v., or superior vena cava
v. of tympanic cavity *v. cavum tympani*	middle ear chamber	middle ear chamber (cavity), tympanic membrane, mastoid cells, auditory tube	pterygoid plexus and superior petrosal sinus
v.'s of tympanic membrane *vv. tympanicae membranae*	tympanic membrane (eardrum)	tympanic membrane	v.'s of middle ear chamber and external ear canal
ulnar v.'s *vv. ulnares*	from hand it runs along medial border of wrist, up forearm to bend of elbow	deep palmar venous arches; superficial v.'s at wrist; palmar and dorsal interosseous v.'s	brachial v.'s in union with radial v.'s
umbilical v. *v. umbilicalis*	accompanying umbilical cord	placenta	fetus
uterine v.'s *vv. uterinae*	sides and superior angles of uterus between two layers of broad ligament	uterine plexus	internal iliac v.
vaginal v.'s *vv. vaginales*	sides of vagina	vaginal plexus	internal iliac v. occasionally uterine v.
vena cava, inferior (largest v. in body) *vena cava inferior*	from level of fifth lumbar vertebra it ascends along vertebral column to right side of heart	both common iliac v. 's; lumbar, renal, testicular (male), ovarian (female), suprarenal, inferior phrenic, and hepatic v.'s	lower part of right atrium of heart
vena cava, superior (second largest v. in body) *vena cava superior*	from close behind sternum to upper portion of right side of heart	cranial half to body via brachiocephalic v.'s	upper part of right atrium
vertebral v. *v. vertebralis*	from suboccipital triangle through transverse foramina of first six cervical vertebrae	suboccipital venous plexus, occipital v., internal and external vertebral venous plexuses, anterior cerebral v., deep cervical v.'s, first intercostal v. (occasionally)	brachiocephalic v.

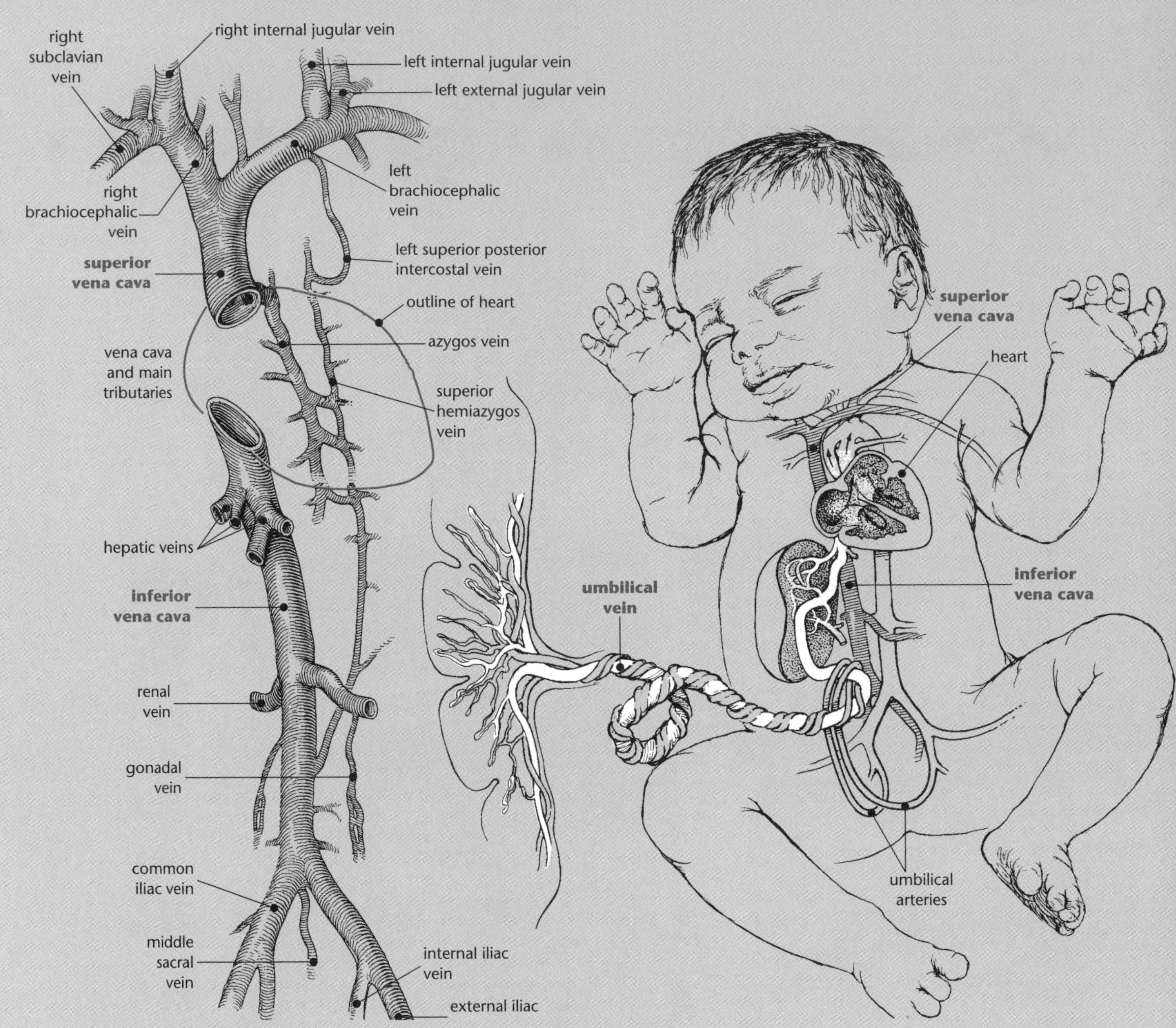

VEINS	LOCATION	DRAINS	EMPTIES INTO
vertebral v., accessory *v. vertebralis accessoria*	when present it accompanies vertebral v. and emerges through transverse foramen of seventh cervical vertebra	venous plexus of vertebral artery, suboccipital venous plexus	brachiocephalic v.
vertebral v., anterior ascending cervical v. *v. vertebralis anterior*	from transverse processes of cervical vertebrae it descends between anterior scalene and longus capitis muscles (it accompanies ascending cervical artery)	plexus around transverse processes of cervical vertebrae; muscles of neck	terminal part of vertebral v.
vesical v.'s *vv. vesicales*	back part of bladder	vesical venous plexus	internal iliac v.
vestibular v.'s *vv. vestibulares*	vestibule of inner ear	utricle, saccule, semicircular ducts	labyrinthine v.'s and v.'s of vestibular aqueduct
vorticose v.'s (usually four or five in number) vortex v.'s *vv. vorticosae*	eyeball, midway between cribosa and sclerocorneal junction	choroid layer of eyeball	superior or inferior ophthalmic v.'s

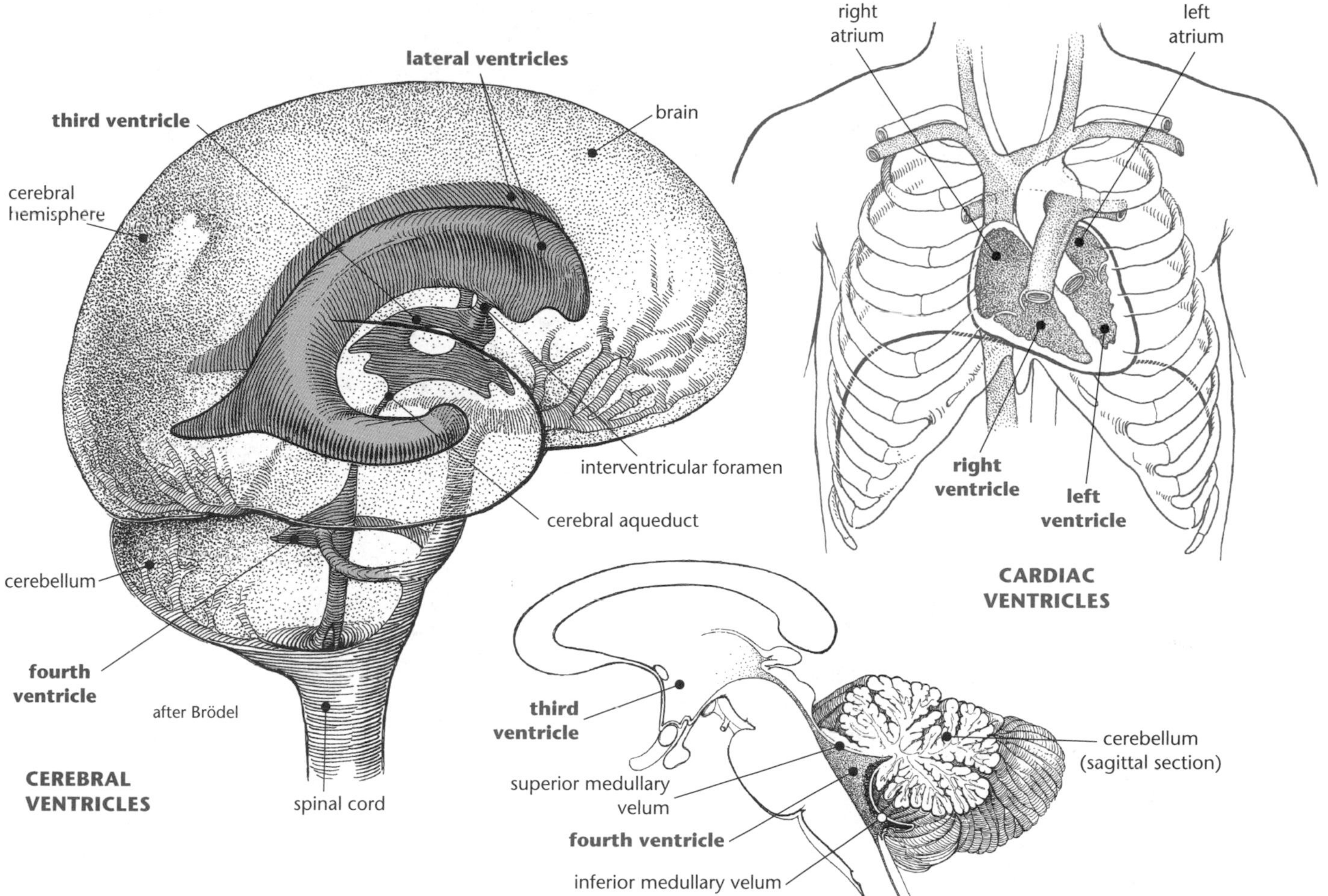

venenation (ven-ĕ-na´shun) Poisoning.
veneniferous (ven-ĕ-nif´er-us) Bearing poison.
venereal (vĕ-ne´re-al) Relating to, or resulting from, sexual intercourse; the term is derived from the Latin *venereus*, love.
venereology (vĕ-nēr-e-ol´ŏ-je) The study of venereal disease.
venesection (ven-ĕ-sek´shun) Withdrawing of blood through an incision of a vein. Also called phlebotomy.
venipuncture (ven´ĭ-punk-chur) The insertion of a needle into a vein.
venisuture (ven-ĭ-soo´chur) See phleborrhaphy.
venoclysis (ve-nok´lĭ-sis) The continuous injection into a vein of a medicinal or nutritive fluid; intravenous infusion of fluids by slow gravity flow or intravenous drip.
venogram (ve´no-gram) A roentgenogram of a vein or veins made after intravenous injection of a radiopaque substance.
venography (ve-nog´ră-fe) The making of a venogram.
venom (ven´um) A poisonous substance secreted by snakes or other animals.
venomotor (ve-no-mo´tor) Causing changes in the internal diameter of veins.
venomous (ven´ĕ-mus) Poisonous; toxic.
venopressor (ve-no-pres´or) An agent that increases venous blood pressure by stimulating constriction of veins (venoconstriction).
venostasis (ven-o-sta´sis) See phlebostasis.
venotomy (ve-not´ŏ-me) See phlebotomy.
venous (ve´nus) Relating to a vein.
venovenostomy (ve-no-ve-nos´tŏ-me) Surgical connection of two veins.
ventilation (ven-tĭ-la´shun) Physiologic process in which air in the lungs is exchanged with atmospheric air; a cyclic process of inspiration and expiration in which alternately fresh air enters the respiratory tract and an equal amount of pulmonary gas is exhaled.
alveolar v. The amount of inspired gas which enters the alveoli each minute.
artificial v. The maintenance of respiratory movements by manual or mechanical means. Also called artificial respiration.
assisted v. Respiration in which the patient's own breathing effort initiates the cycle but the volume of air entering the lungs is increased by mechanical means. Also called assisted respiration.
continuous positive pressure v. (CPPV) Administration of air or mixture of gases to the lungs under continuously positive pressure applied by a life-supporting machine (ventilator) The pressure in the airways fluctuates to allow air or gases to flow in and out of the lungs. Also called continuous positive pressure breathing; positive pressure respiration.
controlled v. In anesthesiology, artificial respiration requiring no effort by the patient; each inspiration is initiated by a timing mechanism of the respirator. Also called controlled respiration.
controlled mechanical v. (CMV) (a) See continuous positive pressure ventilation. (b) See intermittent positive pressure ventilation.
intermittent positive pressure v. (IPPV) Administration of air or a mixture of gases to the lungs under intermittent positive pressure applied by a life-supporting machine (ventilator) during each inspiration. Also called intermittent positive pressure breathing; positive pressure respiration.
maximum voluntary v. (MVV) The maximum volume of air that a person can voluntarily breathe as deeply and as quickly as possible in a given period of time (e.g., 12 seconds). Also called maximum breathing capacity (MBC).
ventilation/perfusion mismatch (ven-tĭ-la´shun / per-fu´zhun mis-măch´) Imbalance between alveolar ventilation and blood flowing through capillaries in the lungs.
ventrad (ven´trad) Toward the ventral side.
ventral (ven´tral) **1.** Relating to the belly. **2.** Denoting the anterior part of a structure.
ventricle (ven´trĭ-kl) A cavity, especially in the heart or the brain.
cardiac v. One of the two lower and larger chambers of the heart.
cerebral v.'s The cavities within the brain (two lateral, the third, and the fourth ventricles).
left v. (LV) The left lower chamber of the heart.
right v. (RV) The right lower chamber of the heart.
ventricular (ven-trik´u-lar) Relating to any ventricle.
ventriculitis (ven-trik-u-li´tis) Inflammation of the lining of the ventricles of the brain.
ventriculocisternostomy (ven-trik-u-lo-sis-ter-nos´to-me) Surgical creation of an opening between the ventricles of the brain and the cisterna magna.
ventriculocordotomy (ven-trik-u-lo-kor-dot´ŏ-me) Removal of a portion of each vocal cord of a dog to reduce the sound of its bark.
ventriculogram (ven-trik´u-lŏ-gram) A roentgenogram of the brain following the direct introduction of air or an opaque medium into the cerebral ventricles.
ventriculography (ven-trik-u-log´ră-fe) X-ray visualization of the cerebral ventricles following injection of a gas or radiopaque substance.
ven triculomegaly (ven-trĭ-ku-lo-meg´ă-le) An abnormally expanded state of a ventricle, especially a cerebral ventricle as seen in hydrocephalus.
ventriculoplasty (ven-trik´u-lo-plas-te) Surgical repair of a defect in a ventricle of the heart.
ventriculostomy (ven-trik-u-los´to-me) Surgical creation of an opening into a ventricle of the brain (e.g., in the treatment of hydrocephalus).
ventriculopuncture (ven-trik´u-lo-punk-chur) Introduction of a needle into a ventricle.
ventriculotomy (ven-trik-u-lot´ŏ-me) Incision into a ventricle.
ventroscopy (ven-tros´ko-pe) Laparoscopy.
ventrotomy (ven-trot´ŏ-me) Laparotomy.
venula (ven´u-lă), *pl.* **ven´ulae** Venule.
venulae rectae The numerous ascending venules that drain the medullary pyramids of the kidney and empty into arcuate veins.
venulae stellatae The stellate venules in the renal cortex near the capsule.
venule (ven´yōōl) A minute vein; usually one less than 100 µm in diameter.
high endothelial v.'s See postcapillary venules.
postcapillary v.'s Unique venules situated in the lymph node cortex and gut-associated lymphoid tissue, composed of elongated endothelial cells that allow lymphocytes to pass from the blood to the lymph. Also called high endothelial venules.

V

The head is turned in the direction of the occiput and the breech is turned in the direction of the feet (backward somersault).
EXTERNAL VERSION (technique for changing a breech to cephalic presentation).
The head is moved downward in the direction of the occiput and the breech is moved upward.
It is held in a transverse position to rest before continuing the procedure.
After completion of the version, the head is directed into the pelvis.
operator
patient
baby
vermis cerebelli
anterior lobe
fissura prima
superior aspect of cerebellum
postiunate fissure
middle lobe
axillary vein

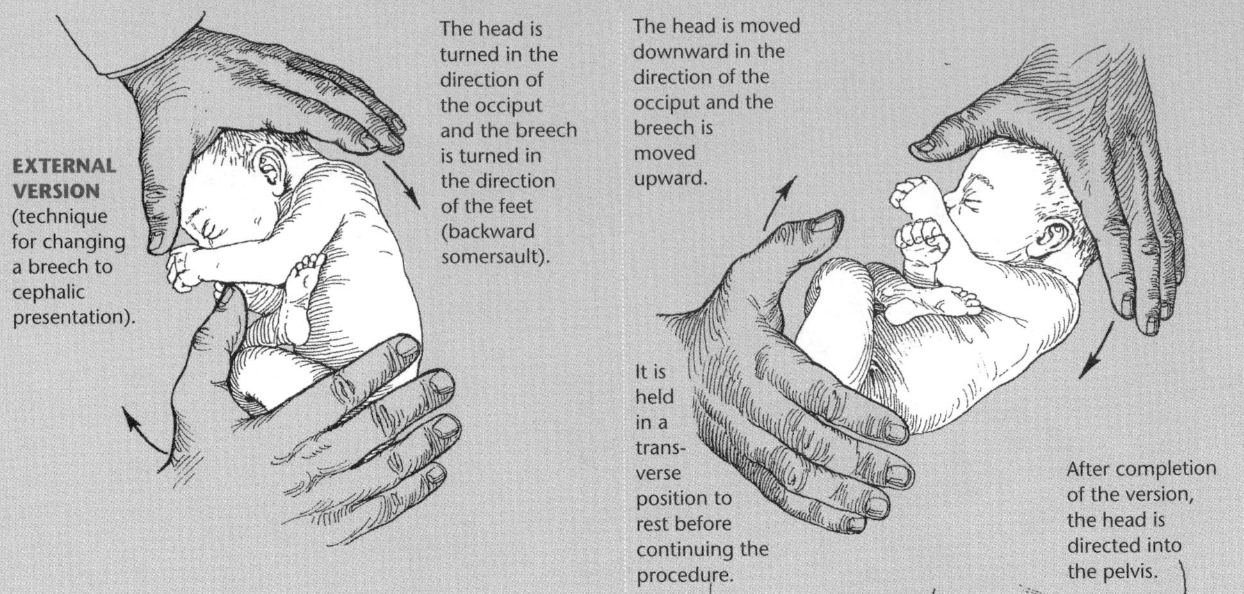

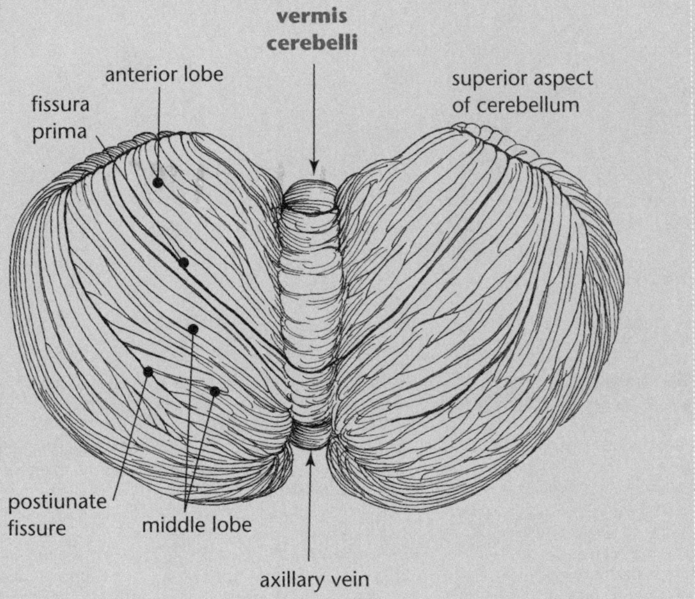

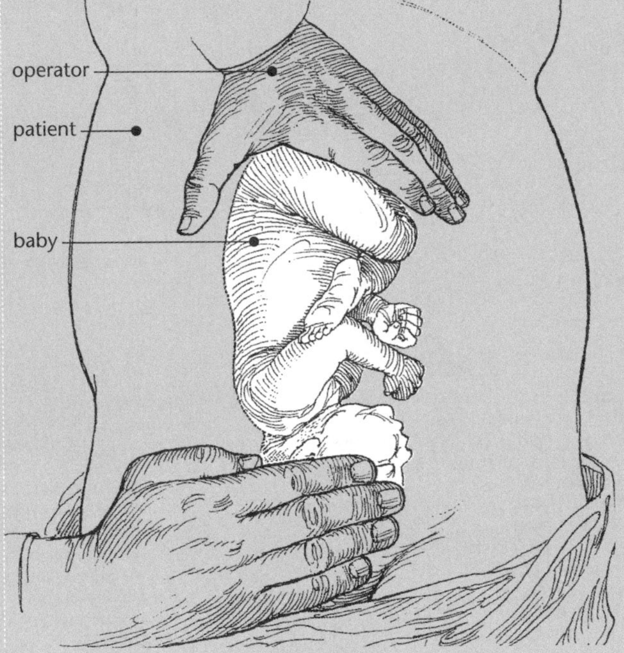

V

verapamil (ver-ap´ă-mil) A calcium channel blocking agent used in the treatment of angina pectoris, especially variant angina and hypertension.
verbigeration (ver-bij-er-a´shun) Repetition of meaningless words or phrases. Also called oral stereotypy.
verge (verj) Margin.
anal v. Area between the perianal skin and the anal canal.
vergence (ver´jens) Movement of the eyes in opposite directions.
vermicide (ver´mĭ-sīd) An agent that kills intestinal worms.
vermicular (ver-mik´u-lar) Wormlike.
vermiculation (ver-mik-u-la´shun) A wormlike motion.
vermicule (ver´mĭ-kūl) A small wormlike body structure.
vermiculous, vermiculose (ver-mik´u-lus, ver-mik´u-lōs) **1.** Infected with worms. **2.** Wormlike.
vermiform (ver´mĭ-form) Having the shape of a worm.
vermifuge (ver´mĭ-fūj) An agent that expels intestinal worms.
vermilionectomy (ver-mil-yon-ek´tŏ-me) Excision of the vermilion border of the lip; the exposed area is generally resurfaced by advancing the undermined labial mucosa.
vermin (ver´min) Parasitic insects.
verminous (ver´mĭ-nus) Infested with or caused by worms or any parasite.
vermis (ver´mis) Latin for worm.
v. cerebelli The narrow median part of the cerebellum that connects the two cerebellar hemispheres.
vermix (ver´miks) The vermiform appendix.
vernix Latin for varnish.
v. caseosa A fatty or cheesy substance on the skin of a newborn, consisting of stratum corneum, sebaceous secretions, and remnants of epithelium.
verruca (vĕ-roo´kă) Wart.
v. acuminata Obsolete term. See condyloma acuminatum, under condyloma.
verruciform (vĕ-roo´sĭ-form) In the shape of warts; wartlike projections.
verrucosis (ver-oo-ko´sis) A condition characterized by the presence of multiple warts or wartlike elevations.
verrucous, verrucose (ver´oo-kus, ver´oo-kōs) Resembling or covered with warts or wartlike roughness; denoting wartlike projections or elevations.
verruga (vĕ-roo´gă) Verruca.
verruga peruana (vĕ-roo´gă pĕ-roo-a´nă) The chronic form of bartonellosis; it usually, but not always, follows the anemic stage (Oroya fever); marked by a profuse skin eruption, chiefly on the face and limbs, which may persist from one month to two years. See also bartonellosis.
versicolor (ver-sĭ-kol´or) Marked by a variety of color; denoting turning or changing color.
version (ver´zhun) **1.** The manual turning of a fetus in the uterus to alter its position to one more favorable for delivery. **2.** The state of an organ of being turned from its normal position. **3.** In ophthalmology, similar movement of the two eyes in the same direction.
bimanual v; bipolar v. Turning of the fetus with two hands; may be external or combined.
Braxton Hicks v. Seldom used procedure in which the forefinger and/or middle finger are introduced into the uterus to displace the presenting part of the fetus (often the shoulder) while the head is guided toward the birth canal by the operator's external hand placed on the maternal abdomen.
cephalic v. Version used to turn the fetal presenting part from breech to cephalic presentation; performed in modern obstetrics only by external manipulations and before 38 weeks of gestation, usually with the aid of ultrasonographic scanning. With hands on the patient's abdomen, the operator locates each pole of the fetus and gently but firmly displaces the breech upward and lateralward while moving the fetal head downward toward the birth canal (like a forward somersault).
combined v. Version in which one hand is introduced into the uterus and the other is placed on the abdominal wall.
external v. Version conducted entirely by placing the hands on the patient's abdomen and applying force gently and intermittently.
external cephalic v. See cephalic version.
Hicks v. Braxton Hicks version.
internal v. Direct turning of the fetus by

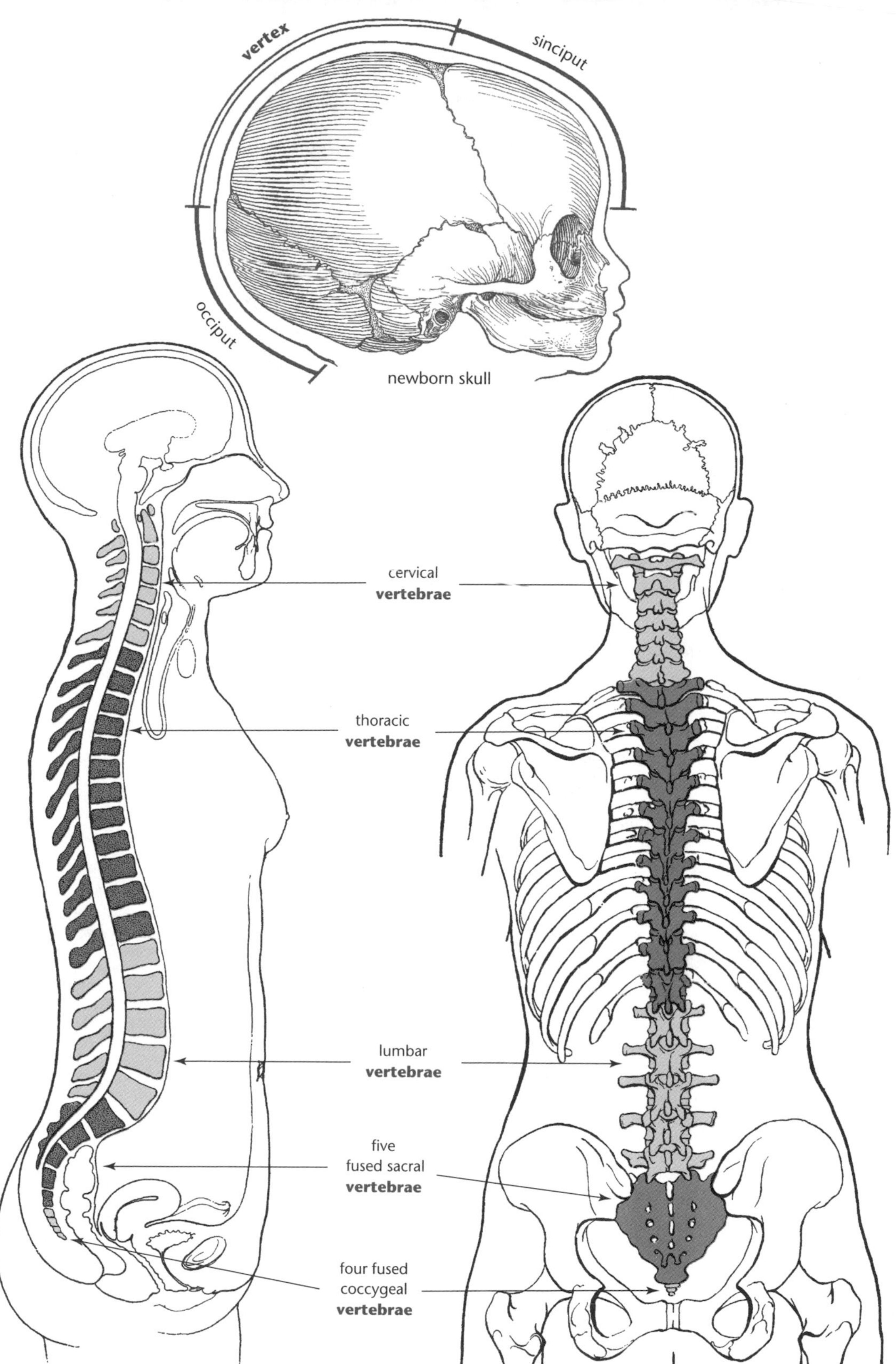

introducing a hand into the uterus.
internal podalic v. See podalic version.
podalic v. Internal version performed only rarely (e.g., for a second twin with fetal distress or for a small dead fetus in a transverse lie); a hand is introduced into the uterus through the fully dilated cervix; the fetus is turned by seizing both feet and drawing them through the cervix; a total breech extraction is then performed.
spontaneous v. Version effected by contraction of the uterus alone.

vertebra (ver´tĕ-bră), *pl.* **ver´tebrae** One of the 33 bones that form the spinal column; they are divided into 7 cervical, 12 thoracic, 5 lumbar, 5 sacral, and 4 coccygeal vertebrae.

vertebral (ver´te-bral) Relating to a vertebra.

vertebrate (ver´tĕ-brāt) **1.** Having a backbone (vertebral column). **2.** Any member of the subphylum Vertebrata, characterized by having a segmented vertebral column.

vertebrectomy (ver-tĕ-brek´tŏ-me) Surgical removal of a portion of a vertebra.

vertebroplasty (ver-te´bro-plas-te) Operative repair of a vertebra.
percutaneous v. A minimally invasive procedure used to treat vertebral compression fractures (e.g., those caused by osteoporosis).

vertex (ver´teks) **1.** The uppermost point of the skull. **2.** In obstetrics, the crown of the fetal head.

vertical (ver´tĭ-kal) Straight up and down; perpendicular, or at right angles, to the horizon.

verticil (ver´tĭ-sil) A whorl or circular arrangement; a collection of similar parts radiating about a point on an axis.

verticillate (ver-tis´ĭ-lāt) Forming a whorl or whorls; circularly arranged.

vertigo (ver´tĭ-go) Illusion of revolving motion, either of oneself or of one's surroundings.
auditory v. See Ménière's disease.
aural v. Vertigo caused by disease of the inner ear.
benign positional v. Brief attacks of vertigo accompanied by nystagmus; precipitated by certain

V

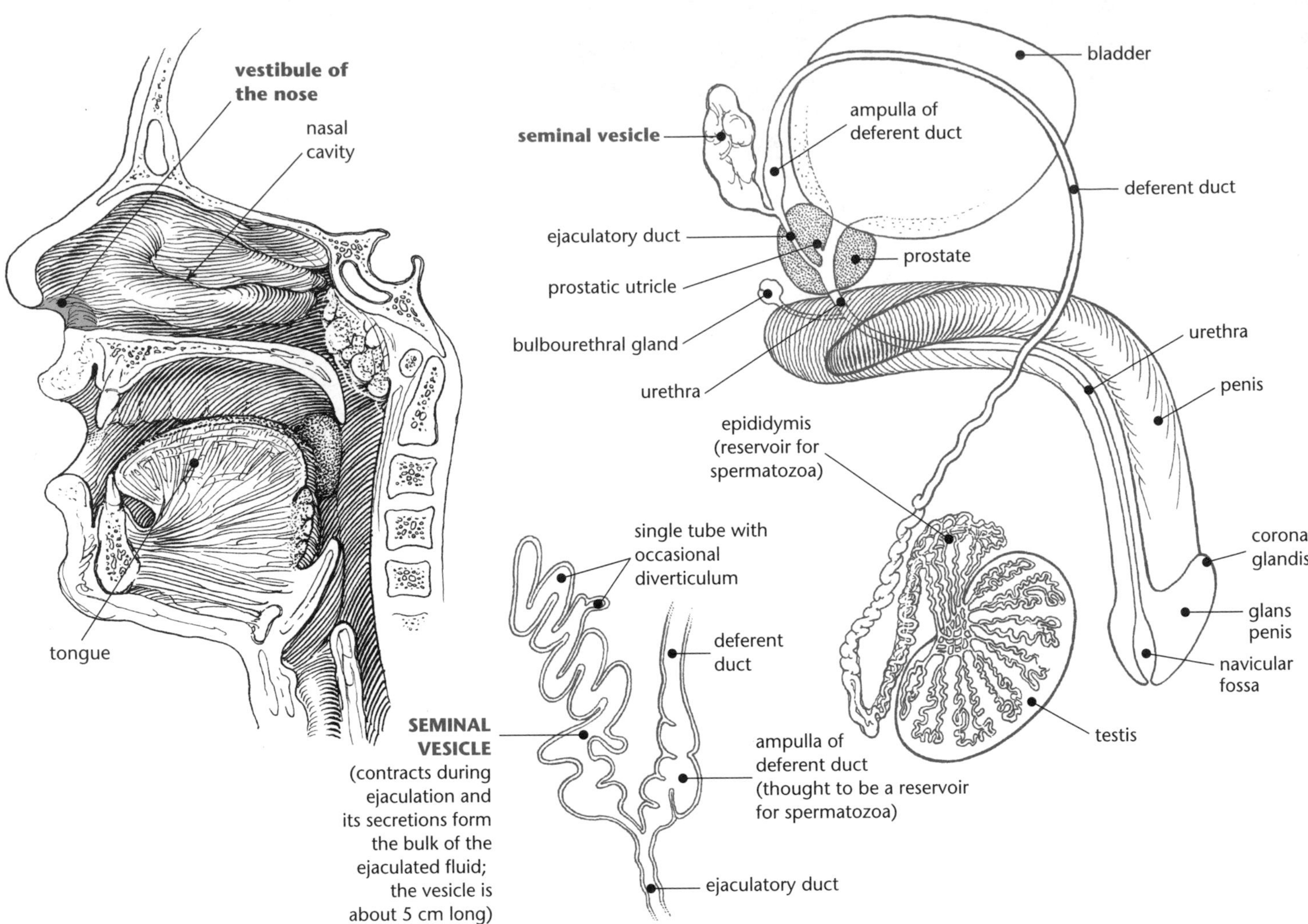

critical positions of the head (e.g., leaning backward, or turning over while lying down).

ocular v. Vertigo caused by errors in the refractive system of the eye or imbalance in the eye muscles.

organic v. Vertigo caused by brain damage.

verumontanitis (ve-ru-mon-tă-ni´tis) Inflammation of the verumontanum (seminal colliculus). Also called colliculitis.

verumontanum (ve-ru-mon-ta´num) An elevation in the prostatic portion of the urethra, on either side of which open the prostatic and ejaculatory ducts. Also called seminal colliculus.

vesica (vĕ-sĭ´kă) Latin for bladder and blister.

vesical (ves´ĭ-kal) Relating to the urinary bladder.

vesicant (ves´ĭ-kant) Any agent that produces blisters.

vesicate (ves´ĭ-kāt) To blister.

vesication (ves-ĭ-ka´shun) **1.** The formation of a blister. **2.** A blister or blistered surface.

vesicle (ves´ĭ-kl) **1.** A sac or hollow structure containing fluid or gas. **2.** A blister or circumscribed elevation on the skin containing serous fluid and ranging in size up to one centimeter (e.g., as in early chickenpox). COMPARE: bulla.

blastodermic v. See blastocyst.

seminal v. One of the two saclike glandular structures situated behind the bladder; its secretion is one of the components of semen.

synaptic v.'s A profusion of small spherical membrane-bound organelles in presynaptic nerve terminals that contain packages of protein-bound humoral transmitter substance; when released through the presynaptic membrane into the intercellular space, they cause changes in permeability and electric potential.

vesicobullous (ves-ĭ-ko-bul´us) Describing blisterlike lesions containing serum.

vesicocele (ves´ĭ-ko-sēl) See cystocele.

vesicocervical (ves-ĭ-ko-ser´vĭ-kal) Relating to the bladder and uterine cervix.

vesicoclysis (ves-ĭ-kok´lĭ-sis) Washing out of the bladder.

vesicolithiasis (ves-ĭ-ko-lĭ-thi´ă-sis) See cystolithiasis.

vesicolithotomy (ves-ĭ-ko-lĭ-thot´ŏ-me) See cystolithotomy.

vesicoprostatic (ves-ĭ-ko-pros-tat´ik) Relating to the bladder and prostate gland.

vesicopubic (ves-ĭ-ko-pu´bic) Relating to the bladder and pubic bone.

vesicorectal (ves-ĭ-ko-rek´tal) Relating to the urinary bladder and the rectum.

vesicostomy (ves-ĭ-kos´tŏ-me) See cystostomy.

vesicotomy (ves-ĭ-kot´ŏ-me) See cystotomy.

vesicoureteral (ves-ĭ-ko-u-re´ter-al) Relating to the bladder and the ureters.

vesicourethral (ves-ĭ-ko-u-re´thral) Relating to the bladder and the urethra.

vesicouterine (ves-ĭ-ko-u´ter-in) Relating to the bladder and the uterus.

vesicouterovaginal (ves-ĭ-ko-u-ter-o-vaj´ĭ-nal) Relating to the bladder, uterus, and vagina.

vesicovaginal (ves-ĭ-ko-vaj´ĭ-nal) Relating to the bladder and vagina.

vesicovaginorectal (ves-ĭ-ko-văj-ĭ-no-rek´tal) Relating to the bladder, vagina, and rectum.

vesicula (vĕ-sik´u-lă), *pl.* **vesic´ulae** A small bladderlike structure.

vesicular (vĕ-sik´u-lar) **1.** Relating to vesicles. **2.** Containing vesicles.

vesiculation (vĕ-sik-u-la´shun) The formation of vesicles or the condition of having numerous vesicles.

vesiculectomy (vĕ-sik-u-lek´tŏ-me) Removal of a seminal vesicle.

vesiculiform (vĕ-sik´u-lĭ-form) Having the shape of a vesicle.

vesiculitis (vĕ-sik-u-li´tis) Inflammation of a seminal vesicle.

vesiculopapular (vĕ-sik-u-lo-pap´u-lar) Relating to superficial blisters (vesicles) and small, solid elevations (papules).

vesiculoprostatitis (vĕ-sik-u-lo-pros-tă-ti´tis) Inflammation of the urinary bladder and the prostate.

vesiculopustular (vĕ-sik-u-lo-pus´tu-lar) Relating to superficial blisters (vesicles) and small accumulations of pus (pustules).

vesiculotomy (vĕ-sik-u-lot´ŏ-me) Incision into a seminal vesicle.

vessel (ves´el) Tubular structure that conveys fluids.

blood v. An artery, arteriole, capillary, venule, or vein.

chorionic v.'s Branches of the umbilical blood vessels that fan out throughout the connective tissue layer of the chorionic plate (placental tissues on the fetal side). Also called placental surface vessels.

great v.'s The aorta and venae cavae.

lymph v. A vessel conveying lymph.

placental surface v.'s See chorionic vessels.

vestibular (ves´tib´u-lar) Relating to a vestibule.

vestibule (ves´tĭ-būl) A small chamber or space at the entrance to a canal.

buccal v. The space between the teeth and gums and the cheek.

labial v. The space between the teeth and gums and the lips.

v. of aorta A small space within the left ventricle just below the aortic opening. Also called Sibson's aortic vestibule.

v. of ear The oval cavity in the middle of the bony labyrinth of the inner ear.

v. of mouth The space in the oral cavity between the cheeks and lips and the gums and teeth.

v. of nose The area just inside the nares.

Sibson's aortic v. See vestibule of aorta.

v. of vagina The space between the labia minora into which open the vagina, urethra, and the ducts of the greater and lesser vestibular glands. Also called vestibule of vulva.

v. of vulva See vestibule of vagina.

vestibulitis (ves-tĭ-bu-li´tis) Inflammation of a vestibule.

vulvar v. Condition marked by redness and [illegible] in the vestibule of the vagina, with small

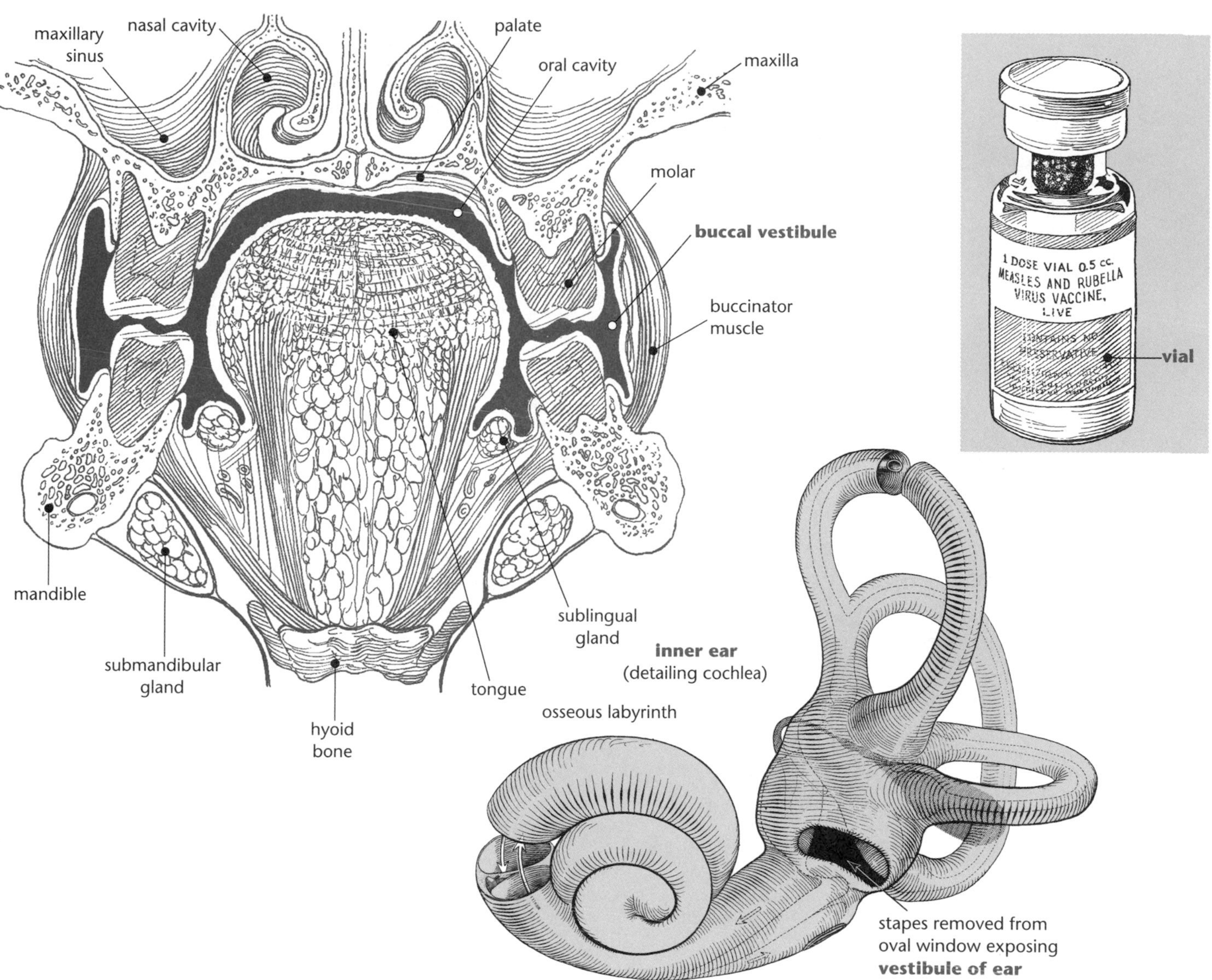

red patches on the vulvar region; causes are varied, ranging from abrasions (e.g., from sexual intercourse, use of tampons, bike riding, wearing tight-fitting pants), to recurrent yeast infection and trauma (e.g., from caustic chemicals or laser surgery used to treat genital warts); often the cause is unknown.

vestibulopathy (ves-tib´u-lo-pa-the) Any abnormal condition of the vestibular apparatus of the inner ear.

vestibuloplasty (ves-tib´u-lo-plas-te) Operative procedure to deepen the labial sulcus (especially of the maxilla) and increase ridge height.

vestibulotomy (ves-tib-u-lot´ŏ-me) Surgical opening into the vestibule of the ear (labyrinth).

vestibulourethral (ves-tib-u-lo-u-re´thral) Relating to the vestibule of the vagina and the urethra.

vestibulum (ves-tib´u-lum), *pl.* **vestib´ula** A vestibule.

vestige (ves´tij) **1.** A rudimentary anatomic structure, usually the remnant of a structure that was functional in, and normally part of, the embryo. **2.** An imperfectly developed organ that has ceased to function.

vestigial (vĕ-stij´e-al) Pertaining to a vestige.

vestigium (vĕ-stij´e-um), *pl.* **vestig´ia** Latin for vestige.

veterinarian (vet-er-ĭ-năr´e-an) A person trained and licensed to diagnose and treat the diseases of animals, both domestic and wild.

veterinary (vet´er-ĭ-ner-e) Relating to the diagnosis and treatment of diseases of animals.

via (vi´ă), *pl.* **vi´ae** Passage.

viability (vi-ă-bil´ĭ-te) The condition of being viable.

viable (vi´ă-bl) Capable of living (e.g., a fetus that has developed enough to be able to live outside of the uterus).

vial (vi´al) A small glass container for holding liquid medicines.

vibration (vi-bra´shun) A rapid back-and-forth movement; the rapid movement in alternately opposite directions of an elastic solid or a particle about an equilibrium position.

sonic v. Sound waves of ultrasonic frequencies used for disrupting cell structures in an aqueous medium.

vibrator (vi´bra-tor) A device that vibrates or causes vibrations.

Vibrio (vib´re-o) A genus of motile, gram-negative bacteria, occurring in salt and fresh water and in soil.

V. cholerae A comma-shaped rod causing Asiatic cholera in man. Also called *Vibrio comma*; (formerly) Koch's bacillus.

V. comma See *Vibrio cholerae*.

vibrio (vib´re-o) Any bacterium of the genus *Vibrio*.

El Tor v. A strain of cholera bacteria isolated from six pilgrims who died of dysentery and gangrene of the colon at the El Tor Quarantine Station on the Sinai peninsula.

vibrissa (vi-bris´ă), *pl.* **vibris´sae** One of the hairs within the nostrils.

vibrotherapeutics (vi-bro-ther-ă-pu´tiks) Therapeutic use of vibrating devices.

vicarious (vi-kar´e-us) Acting as a substitute; occurring in a part of the body not normally associated with that specific function.

vicinal (vi´sin-al) (v) Relating to the adjoining or neighboring position of radicals in an organic compound (e.g., 1, 2, 3 positions in the benzene ring).

Victoria green (vik-tōr´ē-ă grēn) See malachite green.

view (vyo͞o) See projection (4).

vigilambulism (vij´il-am´bu-liz-m) Condition, resembling sleepwalking but occurring in the wakeful state, in which the individual is unaware of his surroundings.

vigilance (vij´ĭ-lans) A state of watchfulness; marked alertness.

villi (vil´i) Plural of villus.

villikinin (vil-ĭ-ki´nin) One of a group of gastrointestinal hormones believed to be responsible for the contraction of villi during digestion.

villoma (vi-lo´mă) See papilloma.

villositis (vil-o-si´tis) Inflammation of the villous aspect of the placenta.

villosity (vi-los´ĭ-te) An aggregation of villi.

villous (vil´us) Covered with minute hairlike projections (villi).

villus (vil´us), *pl.* **vil´li** A minute, vascular, hairlike projection from the surface of a membrane, such as the mucous membrane of the intestines.

arachnoid villi See arachnoid granulations, under granulation.

chorionic villi Slender vascular projections of the chorion forming part of the placenta and through which all substances are exchanged between maternal and fetal circulations.

intestinal villi Small projections on the surface of the mucosa of the small intestine; they are leaf-shaped in the duodenum and become finger-shaped, shorter, and sparser in the ileum; the sites of absorption of fluids and nutrients.

vinblastine sulfate (vin-blas´tēn sul´fāt) A salt of an antineoplastic alkaloid extracted from the periwinkle plant, *Vinca rosea*; Velban®.

Vinca rosea (vin´kă ro´ze-ă) See periwinkle.

V

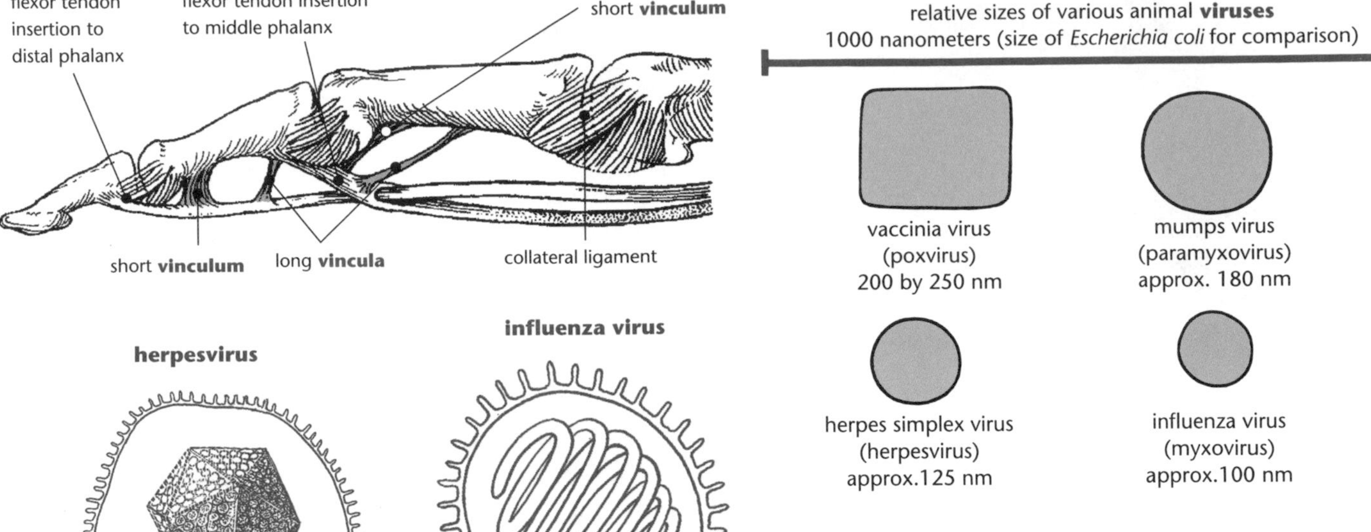

vincristine sulfate (vin-kris´tēn sul´fāt) A salt of an antineoplastic alkaloid extracted from the periwinkle plant, *Vinca rosea*; used primarily in the treatment of acute leukemias, lymphomas, and solid tumors in children; Oncovin®.

vinculum (ving´ku-lum), *pl.* **vincula** A frenum or restricting bandlike structure.

vinegar (vin´e-gar) An impure, dilute (approximately six percent) solution of acetic acid formed by the fermentation of alcoholic liquids (wine, cider, malt, etc.), or by the distillation of wood.

vinegaroon (vin-e-gă-ro͞on´) The nonvenomous whip-scorpion, *Mastigoproctus giganteus*, of southern United States and Mexico that emits a vinegary odor when disturbed.

vinic (vi´nik) Relating to wine.

violaceous (vi-o-lā´shus) Denoting a violet or purple discoloration, usually of the skin.

viper (vi´per) A venomous snake of the family Viperidae and sometimes of the closely related Crotalidae.

European v. A common European viperine snake (*Vipera berus*), about 61 cm long with black markings patterned over a brownish-red to gray body. Also called adder.

pit v. Any of various venomous snakes of the family Crotalidae, characterized by a hollow, heat-sensitive pit between the eye and nostril; includes rattlesnakes, copperheads, and water moccasins.

Viperidae (vi-per´ĭ-de) A family of snakes that includes many venomous species, characterized by movable, hollow, front fangs; included are the vipers and adders.

viral (vi´ral) Relating to a virus.

viremia (vi-re´me-ă) The presence of viable virus in the blood.

virgin (vir´jin) **1.** A person who has never had sexual intercourse. **2.** Term used in reference to a part of the body or a pathologic condition that has not been previously treated by a surgical procedure (e.g., virgin lumbar anatomy, virgin disk herniation).

virginity (vir-jin´ĭ-te) The state of not having experienced sexual intercourse.

virile (vir´il) **1.** Relating to male sexual functions. **2.** Having male characteristics.

virilism (vir´ĭ-liz-m) The presence of male secondary sex characteristics in the female, caused usually by excessive amounts of androgenic hormones.

virility (vĭ-ril´ĭ-te) Masculine potency; manhood.

virilization (vir-ĭ-lĭ-za´shun) The abnormal appearance of secondary male characteristics, especially in the female. Also called masculinization.

virion (vi´re-on) A structurally complete virus.

viroid (vi´roid) Any of a group of microorganisms comprising the smallest known agents to cause disease in higher plants; they are unencapsulated and composed of single-stranded RNA.

virologist (vi-rol´o-jist) A specialist in virology.

virology (vi-rol´ŏ-je) The study of viruses and diseases caused by them.

viromicrosome (vi-ro-mi´kro-sōm) An incompletely formed virus released during the premature disruption of the host cell.

viropexis (vi-ro-pek´sis) A process of phagocytosis in which cells engulf virus particles.

virucide (vi´ru-sīd) Any agent destructive to viruses.

virulence (vir´u-lens) The degree of disease-producing capability of a microorganism once it infects the host; the state of being poisonous.

viruliferous (vir-u-lif´er-us) Conveying viruses.

viruria (vīr-u´re-ă) The presence of viruses in the urine.

virus (vi´rus) An intracellular, infectious parasite, capable of living and reproducing only in living cells; virus particles usually range in size from 10 to 300 nm, are visible under the electron microscope, and are spherical, polyhedral, or rod-shaped in form; each particle is composed of a protein shell which usually encloses a single nucleic acid, either ribonucleic acid (RNA) or deoxyribonucleic acid (DNA).

adeno-associated v. (AAV) See *Dependovirus.*

adeno-pharyngeal-conjunctival v., A-P-C v. See *Dependovirus.*

adenosatellite v. See *Dependovirus.*

attenuated v. A virus so modified as to be incapable of producing a disease.

common cold v. Any virus, especially of the genus *Rhinovirus*, associated with the common cold.

coxsackie v. See coxsackievirus.

dengue v. The causative agent of dengue, belonging to a group B arbovirus.

DNA v.'s A class of viruses having an inner core of DNA and multiplying chiefly in the nuclei of cells; included are those causing herpes simplex, herpes zoster, chickenpox, smallpox, warts, and certain malignant tumors.

Ebola v. A virus of the genus *Filovirus* (family Filoviridae); the cause of Ebola virus disease, a hemorrhagic fever for which there is no known cure; transmitted by contact with infected blood and other body secretions.

ECHO v. See echovirus.

enteric v. See *Enterovirus.*

epidemic gastroenteritis v. The causative agent of epidemics of nonbacterial diarrhea.

epidemic keratoconjunctivitis v. A type 8 adenovirus causing epidemic inflammation of the conjunctiva at the border of the cornea (shipyard eye); also associated with swimming pool conjunctivitis.

Epstein-Barr v., EB v. (EBV) See human herpesvirus 4, under herpesvirus.

equine encephalomyelitis v. A virus (genus *Alphavirus*, family Togaviridae) causing encephalomyelitis in horses and humans; named by the region where it occurs, as eastern (EEE) virus, Venezuelan (VEE) virus, and western (WEE) virus.

filtrable v. One small enough to pass through a porcelain filter or a filter of diatomaceous earths.

hepatitis A v. (HAV) A 27-nm RNA virus (genus *Enterovirus,* family Picornaviridae) causing hepatitis A, often as self-limited outbreaks in day-care centers and residential institutions; spread by contaminated food and water. Also called infectious hepatitis virus.

hepatitis B v. (HBV) A 42-nm DNA virus (family Hepadnoviridae) causing hepatitis B; found in body fluids, including saliva; spreads via transfusion, needle-stick accidents, shared needles, sexual route, or in childbirth. Also called serum hepatitis virus.

hepatitis C v. (HCV) A 50-nm RNA virus (family Flaviviridae), the cause of hepatitis C; spreads chiefly through transfusion and shared needles.

hepatitis D v. (HDV) A 37-nm RNA virus that requires the presence of the HBV to survive; spreads by infected blood or sexual contact. Also called delta agent.

hepatitis E. v. (HEV) A 30-nm RNA virus (family Caliciviridae); causes hepatitis E, mainly by contaminated water, via the gastrointestinal tract.

herpes v. See herpesvirus.

human immunodeficiency v. (HIV) A virus (subfamily Lentivirinae, family Retroviridae) causing acquired immune deficiency syndrome (AIDS); two types are known (HIV-1, HIV-2). Also called human T-cell lymphoma/leukemia virus type III; human T-cell lymphotropic virus type III.

human papilloma v. (HPV) See human papillomavirus, under papillomavirus.

human T-cell lymphotropic v. (HTLV) A virus (subfamily Oncovirinae, family Retroviridae) causing T-cell leukemia or lymphoma; two types are known (HTLV-I, HTLV-II). Also called human T-cell lymphoma/leukemia virus.

infectious hepatitis v. See hepatitis A virus.

influenza v. A virus (genus *Influenzavirus*, family Orthomyxoviridae) causing influenza (flu).

JC v. A virus of the genus *Polyomavirus* (family Papovaviridae) causing progressive multifocal leukoencephalopathy; named after the patient identified by the initials JC in whom it was discovered.

lymphocytic choriomeningitis v., LCM v. A virus (genus *Arenavirus*, family Arenaviridae) causing congenital lymphocytic choriomeningitis in mice; believed to be associated with other inapparent and influenza-like infections.

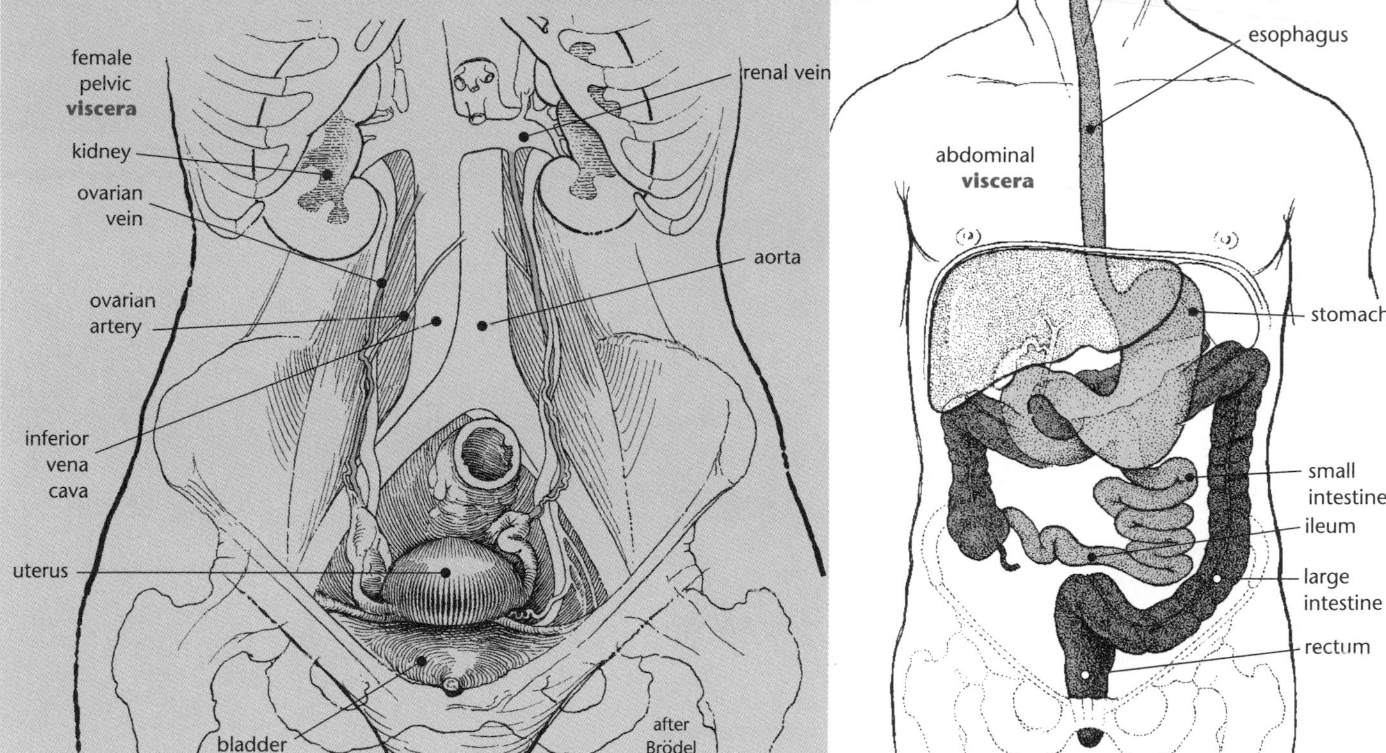

measles v. A virus (genus *Morbillivirus*, family Paramyxoviridae) that causes measles. Also called rubeola virus.

neurotropic v. One that thrives in nervous tissue.

Newcastle disease v. Virus of the genus *Paramyxovirus* causing Newcastle disease in poultry and other birds; human infection is mild, restricted to the eyes (conjunctivitis) and lymph nodes (lymphadenitis).

Norwalk v. A 27 to 32 nm round particle, the cause of epidemic gastroenteritis; transmitted via the oral-fecal route with an incubation period of 18 to 72 hours; symptoms include abrupt nausea, abdominal cramps, vomiting, and sometimes diarrhea; the illness lasts 24 to 48 hours.

oncogenic v. Any of a variety of DNA and RNA viruses that are known to cause cancer, including the human papillomavirus (HPV), human herpesvirus 4, hepatitis B virus (HBV), and human T-cell leukemia virus (HTLV). Also called tumor virus.

orphan v. A virus that has been isolated but not yet identified with any disease.

poliomyelitis v. See poliovirus.

rabies v. A virus (genus *Lyssavirus*, family Rhabdoviridae) that causes rabies.

REO v. See respiratory enteric orphan virus.

respiratory enteric orphan v. Virus of the family Reoviridae frequently found in the respiratory tract and intestines; has not been associated with disease, hence the name "orphan." Also called REO virus.

respiratory syncytial v., RS v. (RSV) A virus (genus *Pneumovirus*, family Paramyxoviridae) that causes pneumonia and bronchiolitis in infants; derives its name from its capacity to fuse cells into a multinucleated mass (syncytium).

Rift Valley fever v. Virus of the genus *Phlebovirus* causing severe disease in cattle, sheep, and goats in southern and central Africa, and a dengue-like infection in humans; transmitted by mosquitoes and contact with tissues and secretions of infected animals.

RNA v.'s A large class of viruses having an inner core of RNA and multiplying chiefly in the cytoplasm of cells; included are those causing poliomyelitis, meningitis, yellow fever, encephalitis, mumps, measles, rabies, German measles, and the common cold. Also called riboviruses.

rubella v. A virus (genus *Rubivirus*, family Togaviridae) causing German measles (rubella).

rubeola v. See measles virus.

serum hepatitis v. See hepatitis B virus.

simian v.'s Viruses isolated from monkeys.

slow v. Any virus causing a disease (such as subacute inclusion-body encephalitis) that is characterized by a long unremitting course and, once symptoms appear, a gradual progression.

smallpox v. See variola virus.

small round-structured v. (SRSV) Virus of the family Caliciviridae causing viral gastroenteritis, transmitted through contaminated food and water.

St. Louis encephalitis v. Virus of the family Flaviridae causing encephalitis; transmitted by *Culex* mosquitoes; seen in the eastern and midwestern regions of the USA, usually in the late summer months.

tumor v. See oncogenic virus.

vaccinia v. The poxvirus used for vaccination against smallpox.

varicella-zoster v. See human herpesvirus 3, under herpesvirus.

variola v. Poxvirus of the genus *Orthopoxvirus*, the cause of smallpox in humans.

West Nile v. Virus of the genus *Flavivirus* causing West Nile encephalitis; transmitted by *Culex* mosquitoes; wild birds such as crows serve as reservoir.

viscance (vis´kans) A measure of the dissipation of energy in the flow of bodily fluids within cells and tissues or in tubes.

viscera (vis´er-ă), *sing.* **vis´cus** The large organs in the thoracic, abdominal and pelvic cavities.

visceral (vis´er-al) Pertaining to the internal organs.

visceral larva migrans (vis´er-al lar´vă mi´granz) See toxocariasis.

visceroinhibitory (vis-er-o-in-hib´ĭ-tor-e) Restricting the function of the viscera.

visceromegaly (vis-er-o-meg´ă-le) Abnormal enlargement of the viscera.

visceromotor (vis-er-o-mo´tor) Causing functional activity of the viscera.

visceroparietal (vis-er-o-pă-ri´ĕ-tal) Relating to the abdominal organs and the abdominal wall.

visceroptosia, visceroptosis (vis-er-op-to´se-ă, vis-er-op-to´sis) Downward displacement of the abdominal organs.

viscerosensory (vis-er-o-sen´so-re) Relating to sensations in the viscera.

viscerotropic (vis-er-o-trop´ik) Affecting the organs.

viscid (vis´id) Sticky and thick.

viscidity (vĭ-sid´ĭ-te) Stickiness.

viscoelastic (vis-ko-ĕ-las´-tik) Both viscous and elastic.

viscosimeter (vis-ko-sim´ĕ-ter) Apparatus for measuring the viscosity of a fluid.

viscosity (vis-kos´ĭ-te) The resistance to flow by a substance caused by molecular cohesion.

viscosurgery (vis-ko-sur´jer-e) Surgery of structures in front of the anterior chamber of the eye, performed after injecting a viscous fluid into the chamber; the fluid facilitates the operation by maintaining the shape of the chamber.

viscous (vis´kus) Having a relatively high resistance to flow. Also called sticky; glutinous.

viscus (vis´kus), *pl.* **vis´cera** See viscera.

visile (viz´il) Relating to vision; applied to the ability to comprehend or remember most easily what has been seen, as opposed to what has been heard. COMPARE: audile.

vision (vizh´un) (V) Sight.

binocular v. Vision in which both eyes contribute to the formation of one fused image.

central v. Vision elicited when the area of greatest visual acuity on the retina (fovea centralis) is stimulated. Also called direct vision.

direct v. See central vision.

double v. See diplopia.

indirect v. See peripheral vision.

multiple v. See polyopia.

night v. See scotopic vision.

peripheral v. Ability to see objects outside of the direct line of vision. Also called indirect vision.

red v. See erythropsia.

scotopic v. Inability to distinguish colors and small details, without diminution of the ability to detect motion and low luminous intensities (i.e., vision that is adapted to low levels of illumination). Also called scotopia; twilight vision.

stereoscopic v. See stereopsis.

tritanopic v. See tritanopia.

tubular v. See tunnel vision.

tunnel v. Vision in which the visual field is severely contracted. Also called tubular vision.

twilight v. See scotopic vision.

yellow v. See xanthopsia.

visna (vis´nă) Disease affecting the central nervous system of sheep; caused by a retrovirus (subfamily Lentivirinae) similar to HIV, the virus causing acquired immune deficiency syndrome (AIDS) in humans.

visual (vizh´u-al) Relating to vision.

visualize (vizh´u-al-īz) **1.** To make a mental image. **2.** To view.

visual purple (vizh´u-al pur´pl) See rhodopsin.

visual violet (vizh´u-al vi´ŏ-lit) See iodopsin.

visual yellow (vizh´u-al yel´ō) All-*trans*-retinal; see retinaldehyde.

visuoauditory (vizh-u-o-aw´dĭ-tor-e) Relating to both vision and hearing.

visuopsychic (vizh-u-o-si´kik) Relating to the visual association areas of the occipital cortex of the brain, concerned with the interpretation or judgment of visual impressions.

visuosensory (vizh-u-o-sen´sor-e) Relating to

V

VITAMIN	SOURCES	FUNCTIONS	DEFICIENCY
A	green and yellow vegetables, liver, eggs, dairy products	helps maintain normal body growth and health of specialized tissues especially retina	nightblindness, skin lesions, xerophthalmia (keratinization and dryness of tissues of the eye)
B_1 (thiamine)	yeast, meat, bran coat of cereals	involved in carbohydrate metabolism	beriberi
B_2 (riboflavin)	milk, egg yolk, fresh meat	hydrogen transfer from metabolites to blood stream	proliferation of blood vessels around cornea, abnormal reddening of lips, ulceration of corners of mouth, inflammation of tongue
B_6 (pyridoxine)	meat, vegetables	involved in protein metabolism	convulsions, muscular weakness, dermatitis of face
B_{12}	foods of animal source	involved in nucleic acid metabolism	pernicious anemia
C (ascorbic acid)	citrus fruits, green leafy vegetables, new potatoes	development of normal bones, cartilage and collagen	scurvy
D	fish liver oil	essential in formation of bone	rickets in children, osteomalacia in adults
E	green leafy vegetables, wheat germ, rice	antioxidant	impairment of fat absorption
K	fish, cereal	involved in clotting of blood	tendency to hemorrhage

perception of visual impressions.

visuscope (vizh´u-skōp) Instrument designed to identify the fixation characteristics of a partially blind (amblyopic) eye.

vita (vi´tă) Latin for life.

vital (vi´tal) Relating to life.

vitality (vi-tal´ĭ-te) **1.** Vigor; energy. **2.** The capacity to live, grow, or develop.

Vitallium (vi-tal´e-um) Trademark for a platinum-white, extremely hard cobalt-chromium alloy; used in orthopedic appliances, instruments, and dentures.

vitalometer (vi-tă-lom´ĕ-ter) An electrical device for determining the vital condition of a dental pulp, it could be of either high or low frequency. Also called pulp tester.

vitals (vi´tals) See viscera.

vital signs (vi´tal sīns) (VS) Breathing, heartbeat, and blood pressure; the signs of life.

vitamer (vi´tă-mer) Substance performing a vitamin function.

vitamin (vi´tă-min) (V) General term for any of several organic substances essential for normal metabolic processes and which, when absent in the diet, produce deficiency states.

v. A A fat-soluble vitamin necessary for normal bone development and the health of certain specialized epithelial tissues, especially the retina for production of visual purple; present in green and yellow vegetables as a provitamin or precursor, which the body transforms into its active form; occurs in its preformed state in animal products (liver, eggs, and dairy products).

v. A_1 See retinol.

v. B A member of the vitamin B complex.

v. B_1 See thiamine.

v. B_2 See riboflavin.

v. B_6 See pyridoxine.

v. B_{12} A protein complex occurring in foods of animal source; lack of vitamin B_{12} causes pernicious anemia. Also called cobalamin.

v. B complex A group of water-soluble compounds found together in foodstuffs; some are believed to be chiefly concerned with release of energy from food (e.g., nicotinamide, riboflavin, thiamine, and biotin), others with the formation of red blood cells (e.g., vitamin B_{12}).

v. C See ascorbic acid.

v. D A group of fat-soluble sterols that promote retention of calcium and phosphorus, thus aiding in bone formation; lack of vitamin D causes rickets in children and osteomalacia in adults; present primarily in fish liver oils; can be formed in the body upon exposure of the skin to sunlight.

v. D_2 An irradiation product of ergosterol used as an antirachitic vitamin. Also called ergocalciferol; calciferol.

v. D_3 A sterol of the vitamin D group formed in the skin by ultraviolet irradiation of the provitamin 7-dehydrocholesterol. The liver adds a hydroxyl group to form 25-hydroxyvitamin D_3 and the kidney adds another hydroxyl group to form 1,25-dihydroxyvitamin D_3, which is the most potent of the vitamin D forms. Also called cholecalciferol.

v. E A group of naturally occurring fat-soluble substances that have antioxidant properties; in experimental animals, a lack of vitamin E may lead to sterility and muscular degeneration. Also called alpha-tocopherol.

v. K A group of fat-soluble compounds essential for clotting of blood; produced in the body by normal intestinal bacteria.

vitaminic (vi-tă-min´ik) Relating to vitamins.

vitellin (vi-tel´in) The main protein present in the yolk of eggs.

vitelline (vi-tel´in) Relating to, or resembling, the yolk of an egg.

vitellogenesis (vi-tel-o-jen´ĕ-sis) Formation of yolk.

vitellus (vi-tel´us) The yolk of an egg.

vitiliginous (vit-ĭ-lij´ĭ-nus) Characterized by vitiligo.

vitiligo (vit-ĭ-lī´go) Sharply demarcated, milky white patches on the skin, usually on the face, neck, hands, lower abdomen, and thighs, caused by absence of melanin. Also called acquired leukoderma.

vitrectomy (vĭ-trek´tŏ-me) The surgical removal of the formed vitreous body from the eye.

closed v. Vitrectomy performed via minute incisions; a miniaturized surgical instrument is introduced to gain access to the diseased vitreous body. Also called pars plana vitrectomy.

radical anterior v. The surgical removal of the vitreous body within the eye's anterior half, usually performed during a full-thickness corneal graft procedure.

vitreoretinopathy (vit-re-o-ret´ĭ-nop´ă-the) Disease of the eye involving the vitreous body and the retina.

vitreous (vit´re-us) **1.** Glassy. **2.** See vitreous body, under body.

vitrification (vĭ-trĭ-fi-ka´shun) Conversion of dental porcelain into a glassy substance.

vitriol (vit´re-ol) **1.** Any of various sulfates of heavy metals. **2.** Sulfuric acid.

blue v. Cupric sulfate.

green v. Ferrous sulfate.

oil of v. Sulfuric acid.

salt of v. Zinc sulfate.

white v. Zinc sulfate.

vivarium (vī-var´ē-um) Quarters in which animals are kept for observation or medical research. Popularly called animal house.

vividialysis (viv-ĭ-di-al´ĭ-sis) Dialysis through a living membrane, as in lavage of the peritoneal cavity.

vividiffusion (viv-ĭ-dĭ-fu´zhun) The passage of blood through a membrane and its return to the living body without exposure to air; the principle used in the artificial kidney.

vivification (viv-ĭ-fi-ka´shun) See revivification.

viviparous (vi-vip´ă-rus) Giving birth to living young developed within the maternal body.

viviperception (viv-ĭ-per-sep´shun) Study of vital processes in a living organism.

vivisection (viv-ĭ-sek´shun) The performance of surgery on living animals for the purpose of experimentation.

vocal (vo´kal) Relating to the voice.

voice (vois) The sound produced by air passing through the larynx, upper respiratory tract, and oral structures of vertebrates, especially humans.

v. box See larynx.

void (void) **1.** The act of voiding. **2.** Empty. **3.** Having no legal or binding effect or force; null.

voiding (void´ing) Discharging a body waste, especially urine.

double v. Popular term for the act of urinating a second time several minutes after the first; a method of fully emptying the bladder by individuals with a large cystocele.

vola (vo´lă) Latin for the palm of the hand or the sole of the foot.

volar (vo´lar) Denoting the palmar surface of the hand or the plantar surface of the foot.

volatile (vol´ă-til) Having a tendency to evaporate rapidly at normal temperatures and pressures.

volatilization (vol-ă-til-i-za´shun) Evaporation.

volatilize (vol-ă-til-īz) To cause evaporation or to pass off in vapor.

volley (vol´e) A group of synchronous impulses.

volt (vōlt) (v) A unit of measure of electricity; a unit of electric potential necessary to cause one ampere of current to flow against one ohm of resistance on a conducting wire; named after the Italian physicist Alessandro Volta.

voltage (vōl´tij) Electromotive force expressed in volts.

voltameter (vōl-tam´ĕ-ter) Apparatus for measuring the strength and quantity of a current.

voltampere (vōlt-am´pēr) A unit of electric power, equal to 1 volt times 1 ampere; one watt.

voltmeter (vōlt´mē-ter) An electronic apparatus for measuring the potential differences in volts between two points.

volume (vol´ūm) (v, V) The space occupied by matter in any state or form.

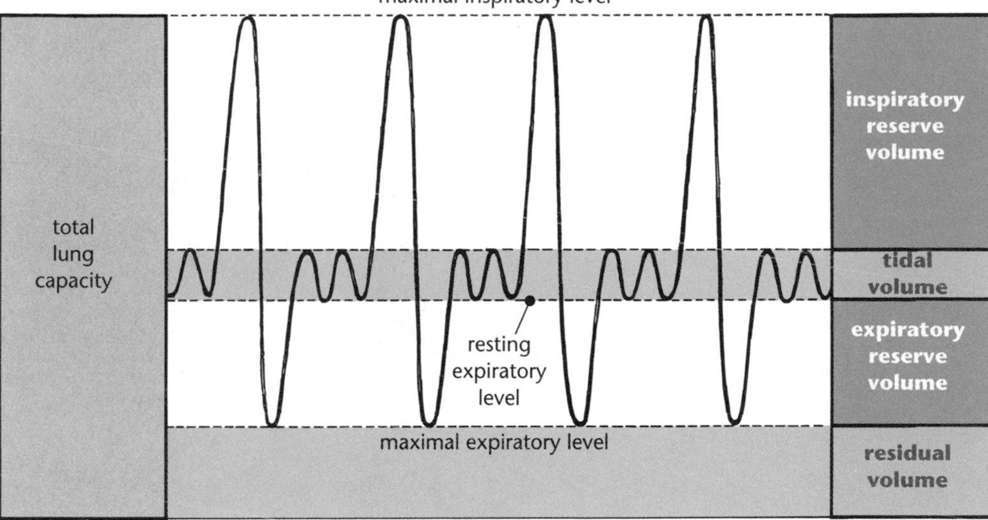

blood v. The quantity of blood present in the vascular compartment of the body.

closing v. (CV) Lung volume at which airways at the bases of the lungs begin to close during expiration and airflow from the lungs is mainly from the upper portions (apices).

v. of distribution (Vd) The volume of fluid in which a test substance is evenly distributed. By measuring the concentration of the test substance after equilibrium, an estimate can be made of the volume of a fluid compartment (e.g., extracellular fluid).

expiratory reserve v. (ERV) The quantity of air that can be expelled from the lungs after a normal expiration. Formerly called supplemental air; reserve air.

extracellular fluid v. (ECFV) The portion of total body water outside of cells. Approximately 20% of body weight.

forced expiratory v. (FEV) Maximal volume of air exhaled from the lungs during a particular time interval, starting from maximal inspiration.

inspiratory reserve v. (IRV) The quantity of air that can be inspired after a normal inspiration. Formerly called complemental air.

intracellular fluid v. (ICFV) The portion of total body water contained within cells. Approximately 40% of body weight.

minute v. (a) The volume of air expelled from the lungs per minute. (b) The volume of blood pumped by the left ventricle in one minute, normally 4 to5 liters at rest.

packed cell v. (PCV) See hematocrit (l).

plasma v. The total volume of blood plasma.

residual v. (RV) The quantity of air remaining in the lungs after a maximal expiration. Also called residual air; residual capacity.

standard v. The volume of a perfect gas at standard temperature and pressure, measured at 22.414 liters.

stroke v. The quantity of blood expelled from each cardiac ventricle with each heartbeat.

tidal v. (V_T) The volume of air inspired and expired in a normal breath. Also called tidal air.

volumenometer (vol-ūm-nom´ĕ-ter) Instrument for measuring the volume of a body.

volumetric (vol-u-met´rik) Relating to measurement of, or by, volume.

voluntary (vol´un-tăr-e) Initiated by one's own free will.

volute (vo-lūt´) Rolled up.

volvulosis (vol-vu-lo´sis) See onchocerciasis.

volvulus (vol´vu-lus) Twisting of a segment of intestine, causing obstruction.

vomer (vo´mer) See table of bones.

vomica (vom´ĭ-kă) A pus-containing cavity, as in the lung.

vomit (vom´it) **1.** To expel the contents of the stomach forcibly through the mouth. **2.** The matter expelled from the stomach. Also called vomitus.

vomiting (vom´it-ing) The forceful expulsion of the stomach contents through the mouth. Also called emesis.

cyclic v. Periodic or recurrent vomiting.

pernicious v. Persistent, uncontrollable vomiting.

projectile v. Expulsion of the stomach contents with great force, often not preceded by nausea.

v. of pregnancy Vomiting occurring during pregnancy usually at 2 to 12 weeks of gestation; occurs at any time, especially in the early morning.

vomitus (vom´ĭ-tus) Vomited material.

von Gierke's disease (von-gĕr´kez dĭ-zēz´) See type I glycogenosis, under glycogenosis.

von Graefe's sign (von-gĕr´kez sīn) See Graefe's sign.

von Hippel-Lindau disease (von hip´el-lin´dow dĭ-zēz´) An autosomal dominant disorder marked by angiomas of the retina and hemangioblastomas of the cerebellum, medulla oblongata, and spinal cord; sometimes associated with hemangiomas and cysts of several organs, especially the kidneys and pancreas and with renal cell carcinoma and pheochromocytoma. Also called von Hippel-Lindau syndrome; Lindau's disease; cerebelloretinal angiomatosis.

von Recklinghausen's disease (von-rek´ling-how-zenz dĭ-zēz´) See neurofibromatosis.

von Willebrand's disease (von-vil´ĕ-brahntz dĭ-zēz) (vWD) Hemorrhagic disease transmitted as an autosomal inheritance; marked by spontaneous bleeding from mucous membranes, excessive bleeding from wounds, and profuse or prolonged menstrual flow; platelet count and clot retraction are normal; caused by partial and variable deficiency of factor VIII, a blood clotting factor.

vortex (vor´teks), *pl.* **vor´tices** Latin for whirlpool; a general anatomic term designating a pattern involving rotation about an axis; a whorled design.

v. coccygeus The whorl of hairs sometimes present in the coccygeal region.

v. cordis The whorl of muscular fiber bundles at the apex of the heart.

v. lentis The whorl or star-shaped pattern of light lines visible on the surface of the lens of the eye.

vortices pilorum Hair growth arranged about an axis (e.g., at the crown of the head).

vorticose (vor´tĭ-kōs) Having a whorled appearance, as the vorticose veins of the choroid layer of the eye.

vox (voks) Latin for voice.

voyeur (voi-yer´) One who practices voyeurism; French for one who sees.

voyeurism (voi´yer-iz-m) The practice of deriving sexual gratification from watching people who are nude, undressing, or engaged in sexual acts.

vulcanize (vul´kă-nīz) To combine rubber with sulfur or other additives under high temperature and pressure in order to improve its strength and resiliency.

vulgaris (vul-ga´ris) Of the usual type; belonging to the multitude. Also called ordinary; common.

vulva (vul´vă) The external female genitalia; consists of the prominence over the pubic bone (mons pubis), the labia majora and minora, clitoris, vestibule of the vagina, bulb of the vestibule, greater and lesser vestibular glands, and the vaginal orifice. Also called pudendum.

vulvar, vulval (vul´var, vul´val) Relating to the vulva.

vulvectomy (vul-vek´tŏ-me) Partial or complete removal of the vulva.

vulvitis (vul-vi´tis) Inflammation of the vulva.

atrophic v. See lichen sclerosis, under lichen.

diabetic v. Vulvitis associated with diabetes mellitus; caused by a chronic vulvovaginal infection by the yeastlike fungus *Candida albicans*.

gonorrheal v. Vulvitis caused by infection of the glandular structures of the vulva by *Neisseria gonorrhoeae*.

leukoplakic v. See lichen sclerosus, under lichen.

vulvocrural (vul-vo-kroo´ral) Relating to the vulva and the crura of the clitoris.

vulvodynia (vul-vo-din´e-ă) Chronic pain or burning sensations of the vulva without evidence of disease or abnormalities, usually causing sexual dysfunction; thought to be a form of peripheral neuralgia.

vulvouterine (vul-vo-u´ter-in) Relating to the vulva and the uterus.

vulvovaginal (vul-vo-vaj´ĭ-nal) Relating to the vulva and the vagina. Also called vaginovulvar.

vulvovaginitis (vul-vo-vaj-ĭ-ni´tis) Inflammation of the vulva and vagina.

vulvovaginoplasty (vul-vo-vaj-ĭ-no-plas´ty) Reparative or reconstructive surgery of the vulva and vagina.

Williams' v. Surgical construction of an artificial vagina using the labia majora to form the vaginal pouch.

V

W

Waardenburg's syndrome (var´den-bergz sin´drōm) A genetic defect characterized by anomalies of certain facioskeletal structures, congenital deafness, and pigmentary disorders. Several clinical types are known.

wadding (wŏd´ing) A soft layer of fibrous cotton or wool, used for surgical dressings.

waddle (wŏd´l) To walk with short steps that cause the body to sway from side to side, as a duck; occurring in pseudohypertrophic muscular dystrophy and certain other nervous conditions.

waist (wāst) The part of the trunk between the bottom of the rib cage and the hips.

w. of the heart The middle part of the heart as seen in an x-ray picture; it contains the pulmonary salient.

waisting (wāst´ing) Shape of a bone in which the middle is narrower than the ends in transverse diameter.

Waldenström's syndrome (vahl´den-strermz sin´drōm) See Waldenström's macroglobulinemia, under macroglobulinemia.

walk (wok) **1.** To move on foot. **2.** The manner in which one moves when going on foot. See also gait.

wall (wawl) A structure that serves to enclose, divide, or protect an anatomic part; a part enclosing a cavity or space.

cavity w. One of the enclosing surfaces bounding a prepared cavity in a tooth.

enamel w. The part of the wall of a prepared cavity consisting of enamel.

walleye (wawl´ī) **1.** A dense, whitish opacity (leukoma) of the cornea. **2.** See exotropia.

walleyed (wawl´īd) Having exotropia.

ward (wawrd) **1.** A large room in a hospital usually with several beds for patients. **2.** A section of the hospital for special care and treatment of a particular group of patients.

isolation w. A ward in a hospital or institution where persons having or suspected of having a contagious disease are placed in quarantine.

locked w. A ward in which mental patients are confined by locked doors.

open w. A ward which is not locked.

psychopathic w. A ward in a general hospital for the reception and treatment of mental patients.

warfarin (war´fă-rin) A colorless crystalline compound, 3-(α-acetonylbenzyl)-4-hydroxycoumarin, widely used as an anticlotting drug and rat poison; an acronym for Wisconsin Alumni Research Foundation + (Coum)arin.

warm-blooded (wŏrm´blud´īd) Having a relatively high and constant body temperature independent of surrounding temperature. Also called homothermal.

warp (worp) To distort out of shape.

wart (wort) A small horny outgrowth on the skin, usually of viral origin. Also called verruca.

anorectal w. See condyloma acuminatum.

common w. A rough horny lesion varying in size from 1 mm to 2 cm in diameter; usually occurring on the hands. Also called verruca vulgaris.

digitate w. A wart resembling a skin tag, seen most commonly on the neck.

fig w. See condyloma acuminatum.

filiform w. A long, horny, fingerlike projection, usually occurring in multiples; seen most commonly in adult males, in the bearded area of the face; also occurring on the eyelids and the neck.

flat w. A small, smooth, skin-colored wart occurring in clusters; commonly seen on the face, neck, and dorsum of the hands.

genital w. See condyloma acuminatum.

moist w. See condyloma acuminatum.

pointed w. See condyloma acuminatum.

plantar w. A wart occurring on the sole of the foot. Also called verruca plantaris.

telangiectatic w. See angiokeratoma.

venereal w. See condyloma acuminatum.

wash (wŏsh) **1.** In chemistry, to remove particulate matter in a liquid suspension. **2.** A lotion, often containing solid matter in suspension.

eye w. See eyewash.

mouth w. See mouthwash.

red w. A lotion of zinc sulfate in compound tincture of lavender.

yellow w. A suspension of mercuric oxide derived by precipitating a solution of mercuric chloride with calcium hydroxide.

washing (wosh´ing) The act of removing particulate matter in a liquid suspension.

cell w. Instillation of a solution into a body cavity or tube (e.g., uterine cavity, stomach, bronchi) to loosen exfoliated cells from crevices, followed by aspiration of the solution for study and diagnosis.

sperm w. An adjunct to intrauterine insemination in which the semen sample is diluted and centrifuged prior to introduction into the uterus.

wasp (wosp) An insect of the superfamilies Vespoidea and Sphecoidea, having a slender spindle-shaped body with elongated waist; it is second only to the bumblebee in frequency of reported fatalities from its sting.

waste (wāst) **1.** To emaciate; to grow thin. **2.** The undigested residue of food voided from the bowels. Also called feces.

wasting (wāst´ing) Emaciation.

watchful waiting (wach´ful wāt´ing) An option that involves not intervening in a disease process (or changing treatment) but closely monitoring its progress.

water (wŏ´ter, waw´ter) A clear, colorless liquid, H_2O, present in all organic tissues and essential for life.

alkaline w. Water that contains appreciable amounts of the bicarbonates of calcium, lithium, potassium, or sodium.

bound w. Water in bodily tissues tenaciously held to colloids.

w. of combustion See water of metabolism.

w. of crystallization Water in chemical combination with a crystal, necessary for the maintenance of crystalline properties but capable of being separated by adequate heat.

distilled w. Water purified by the heat-dependent process of distillation.

free w. (a) Water in the body that is not attached to colloids; it can be removed by ultrafiltration. (b) The amount of dilute urine formed per minute that can be considered free of dissolved substances (solute), assuming that the remainder of the urine is isotonic; CH_2O (free water clearance) = V (urine flow in ml/min – C_{osm} (osmolar clearance).

hard w. Water containing ions, such as Mg^{++} and Ca^{++}, that form insoluble salts with fatty acids, especially water containing more than 90 parts per million of calcium carbonate; it generally resists the action of soap to form a lather.

heavy w. A compound analogous to water in which most of the hydrogen atoms are deuterium (heavy hydrogen); it differs from ordinary water in having higher boiling and freezing points. Also called deuterium oxide (D_2O).

w. of hydration Water chemically united with a substance to form a hydrate, which can be removed (e.g., by heating) without substantially changing the chemical composition of the substance.

w. of injection Water purified by distillation for parenteral use.

lime w. A solution of calcium hydroxide.

metabolic w. See water of metabolism.

w. of metabolism The water in the body derived from the oxidation of the hydrogen of a food element such as starch, glucose, or fat; the largest amount is produced in the metabolism of fat, approximately 117 g per 100 g of fat. Also called metabolic water; water of combustion.

mineral w. Water that has appreciable amounts of mineral salts in solution.

potable w. Drinkable water free from contamination.

saline w. Water that contains neutral salts (chlorides, bromides, iodides, sulfates) in appreciable amounts.

soft w. Water that contains few or no ions that form insoluble salts with fatty acids, especially water with less than 80 parts per million of calcium carbonate; ordinary soap can lather in it easily.

total body w. (TBW) The total water content of the adult human body; equal to 50% to 70% of the body weight.

water-borne (wŏ´ter-born) Conveyed by drinking water; describing certain diseases transmitted by contaminated water, such as cholera and typhoid fever.

water brash (wŏ´ter brash) The filling of the mouth with refluxed fluid from the esophagus, usually associated with heartburn.

Waterhouse-Friderichsen syndrome (wŏ´ter-hous-frid-er-ik´sen sin´drōm) A disorder of rapid onset marked by an extensive purpuric rash, bilateral adrenal hemorrhage, shock, and circulatory collapse. Also called acute fulminating meningococcemia.

water-on-the-brain (wo´ter ŏn thĕ-brān) Colloquialism for hydrocephalus.

water-on-the-knee Colloquialism for accumulation of fluid within or around the knee joint, usually caused by bursitis.

waters, water (wŏ´ters, wŏter) Colloquial terms for amniotic fluid, the fluid that surrounds the fetus.

watershed (wŏ´ter-shed) The region of diminished blood circulation around a vascular bed.

watt (wot) (W) The amount of electrical power produced by 1 volt with 1 ampere of current.

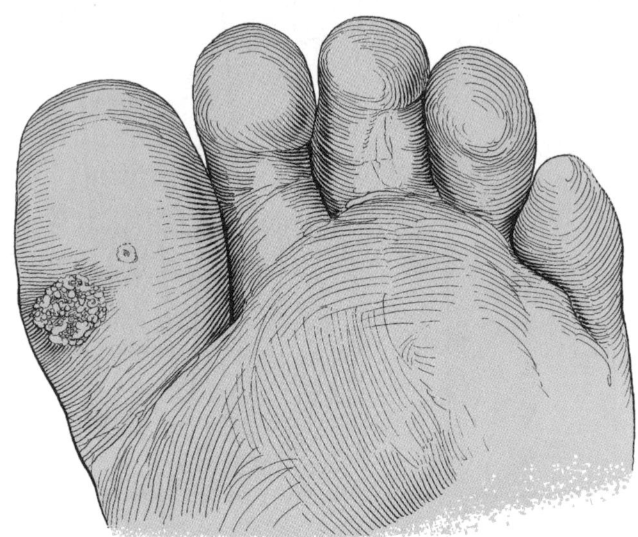

plantar wart
(mosaic type)

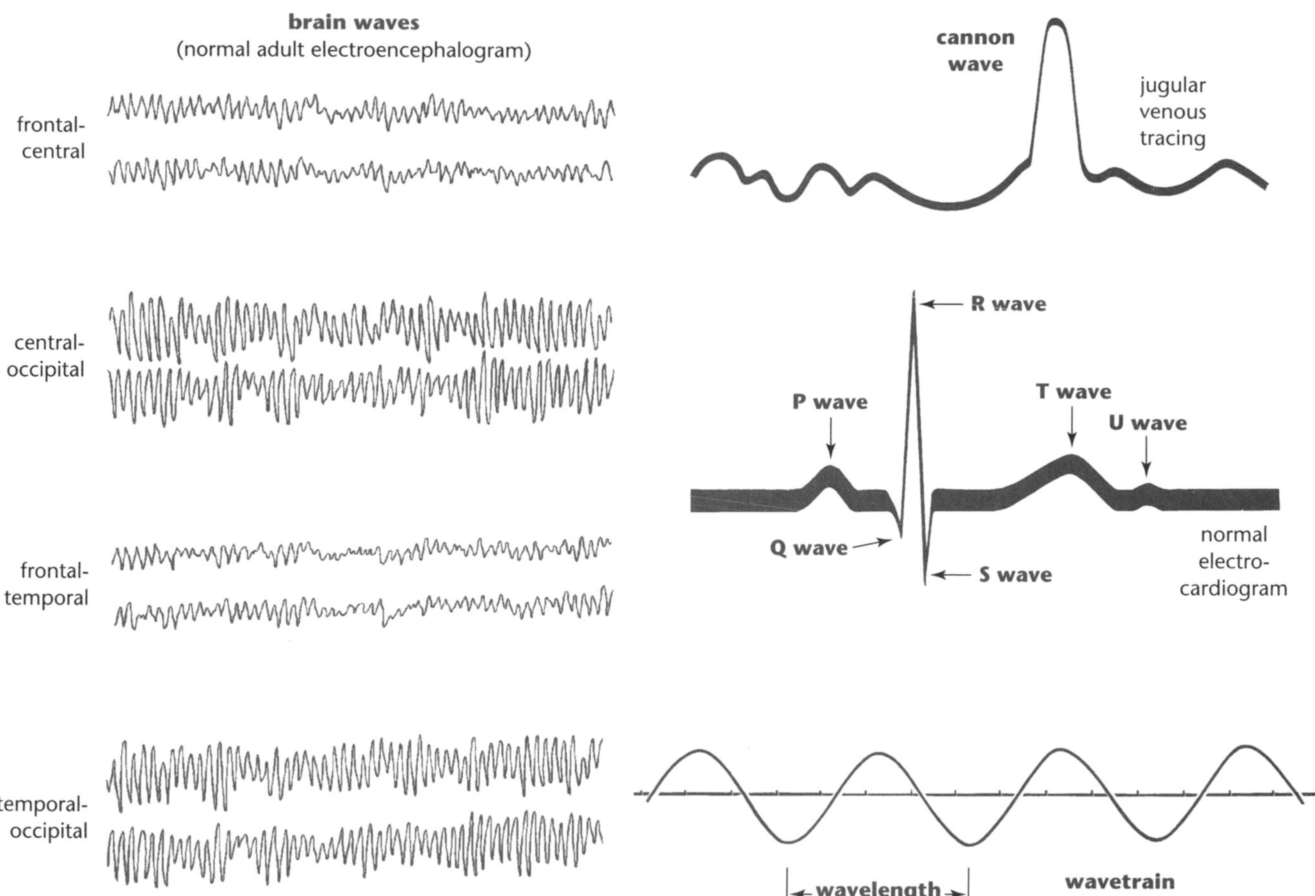

wattage (wot´ij) Amperage multiplied by voltage.
wave (wāv) A periodic increase and subsidence; as an oscillation propagated from point to point in a medium, characterized by alternate elevations and depressions.
alkaline w. See alkaline tide, under tide.
alpha (α) **w.'s** Waves in the electroencephalogram (EEG) with a frequency band from 8 to 13 Hz. Also called alpha rhythm.
arterial w. A wave in the jugular phlebogram due to the vibration produced by the carotid pulse.
beta (β) **w.'s** Waves in the electroencephalogram (EEG) that have a frequency band from 18 to 30 Hz. Also called beta rhythm.
brain w.'s Electrical potential waves of the brain.
cannon w. A large positive venous pulse wave produced by atrial contraction; it occurs when the right atrium contracts at the same time the tricuspid valve is closed by right ventricular systole, as in complete heart block and ventricular premature beats.
delta (δ) **w.'s** (a) Waves in the electroencephalogram (EEG) that have a frequency band from 1/2 to 3 cycles per second. Also called delta rhythm. (b) The slow-rising, slurred, initial portion of the upstroke of the electrocardiographic R wave seen in the Wolff-Parkinson-White (W-P-W) syndrome, caused by preexcitation of a part of the ventricular myocardium.
dicrotic w. The second notch in the tracing of the normal arterial pulse.
excitation w. An electrical wave propagated along a muscle just prior to its contraction.
f w.'s Small irregular waves or oscillations of the atria, characteristically seen in atrial fibrillation.
F w.'s Regular rapid undulating atrial waves seen in atrial flutter, thought to represent the manifestation of atrial depolarization and repolarization occurring in rapid succession from an ectopic focus.
fluid w. A sign of free fluid in the abdominal cavity; percussion on one side of the abdomen transmits a wave that is felt on the opposite side.
microelectric w. See microwave.
P w. The initial deflection of the electrocardiogram, representing depolarization of the atria; if retrograde or ectopic, it is labeled P´.
pulse w. A wave originated by the impact of ejection of blood from the left ventricle into the full aorta and propagated to the periphery through the column of blood and the arterial walls.
Q w. The initial deflection of the QRS complex when such deflection is downward (negative).
R w. The first upward deflection of the QRS complex in the electrocardiogram (ECG).
radio w.'s Electromagnetic waves with wavelengths between 1 mm and 30 km. Also called hertzian rays.
random w.'s Brain waves in the encephalogram produced by irregular changes of electric potential.
retrograde w. A distorted P wave pattern in the electrocardiogram (ECG), inverted in several leads where it should be upright; caused by an ectopic impulse from the ventricle spreading backward into the atria.
S w. A downward (negative) deflection of the QRS complex following an R wave.
sine w. A wave characterized by a rise from zero to maximum positive potential, then descending back to zero and to maximum negative potential.
sound w. System of longitudinal pressure waves passing through any medium; may or may not be audible.
T w. The deflection of the normal electro-cardiogram which follows the QRS complex; it represents ventricular repolarization.
theta (θ) **w.** Brain wave in the encephalogram having a frequency between 4 and 7 cycles per second. Also called theta rhythm.
tidal w. The second and lesser of the two waves forming the main systolic arterial pulse wave.
U w. A minor deflection of the normal electro-cardiogram which occasionally occurs in early ventricular diastole following the T wave; especially prominent in persons with electrolyte imbalance.
ultrasonic w. A high frequency sound wave, greater than 20,000 Hz; it cannot be heard by humans; used therapeutically and in diagnostic imaging.
x w. Downward deflection of the graphic curve of the venous pulse, denoting relaxation of the cardiac atria.
y w. Downward deflection of the graphic curve of the venous pulse, produced by rapid filling of the ventricles just after the atrioventricular valves open.
waveform (wāv-form) The mathematical graphic representation of a wave.
wavelength (wāv´length) (λ) One of three measurements of the vibration of a sound wave (others are amplitude and frequency); the longitudinal distance between the crests of two successive sound waves.
wavetrain (wāv´trān) A series of waves sent along the same axis by a vibrating body.
wax (waks) A plastic, heat-sensitive substance secreted by insects, or obtained from plants or petroleum; consists essentially of high molecular weight hydrocarbons or esters of fatty acids; characteristically insoluble in water but soluble in most organic solvents.
baseplate w. A hard wax used in dentistry for making baseplates and occlusion rims.
bone w. Wax used for filling sterile bone cavities.
boxing w. A soft wax for boxing impressions for dental prostheses.
carnauba w. A hard wax with a high melting point used for the control of the melting range of various waxes; it is derived from the fine powder on the leaves of certain tropical palms.
casting w. A compound of various waxes with controlled properties of thermal expansion and contraction, used in making patterns which represent the exact reproduction of the missing tooth structure; it allows a mold to be made, into which the alloy is cast.
ear w. See cerumen.
grave w. See adipocere.
inlay w. Wax used in making patterns for dental restoration from which an inlay is cast.
paraffin w. A white or colorless wax derived from the high-boiling fractions of petroleum; composed chiefly of a complex mixture of hydrocarbons of the methane series. Also called paraffin.
sticky w. An adhesive wax used in dentistry for attaching a sprue pin to a wax restoration pattern.

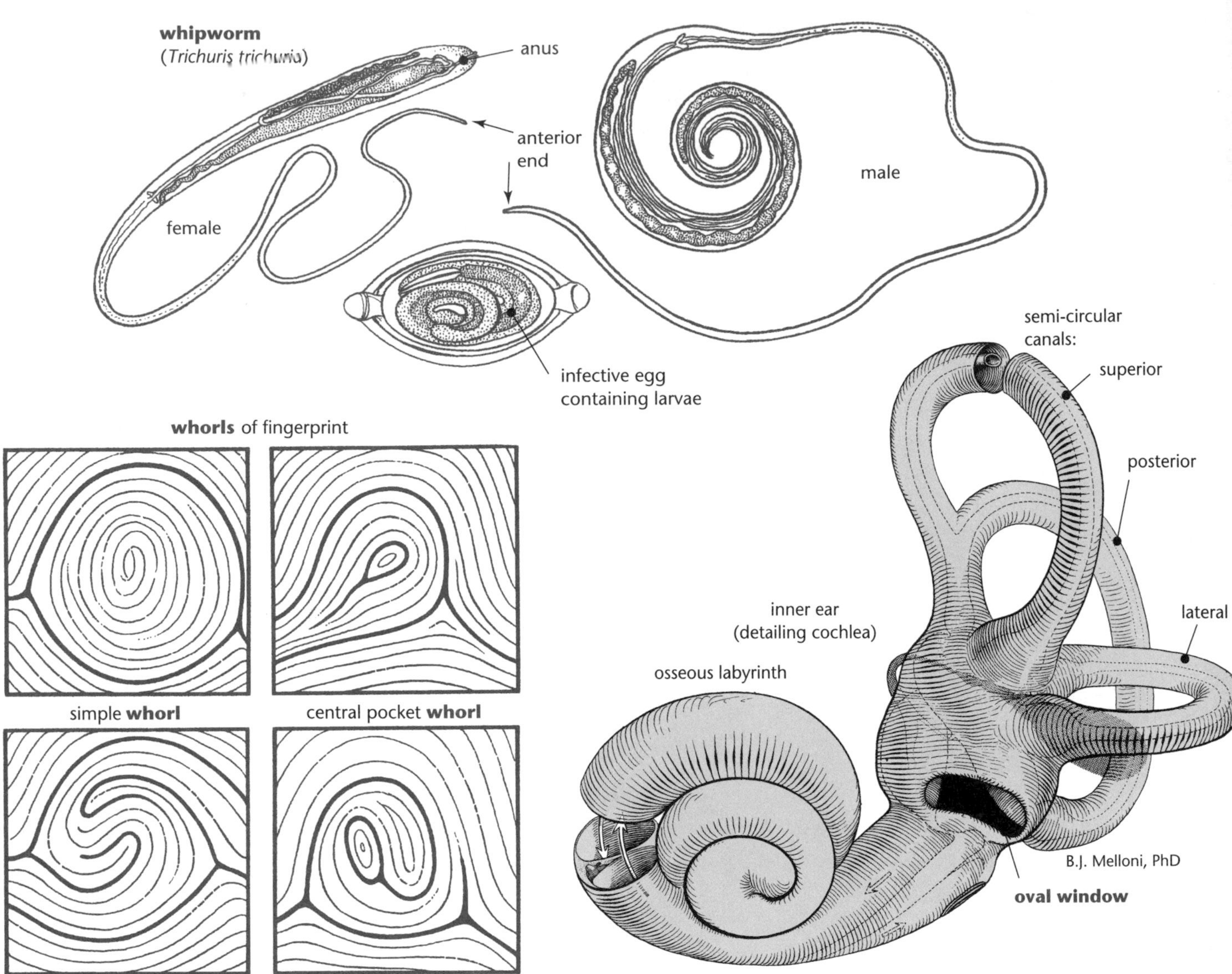

wean (wēn) **1.** A gradual substitution (e.g., of formula for breast feeding, or of solid food for formula in an infant's diet). **2.** Withdrawal (e.g., of a medication or a life support system).

web (web) A membrane or membranous fold.

esophageal w. A condition marked by the presence of one or more membranous wedge-like folds within the esophagus. Also called upper esophageal rings.

Weber-Christian disease (web′ber-kris′chan dĭ-zēz′) See relapsing febrile nodular nonsuppurative panniculitis, under panniculitis.

weight (wāt) (wt.) The measured heaviness of a specific object; the force with which a body is pulled toward the earth by gravity.

atomic w. (at wt) The weight of an atom of any element compared with the weight of an atom of carbon-12 (^{12}C), which is taken as 12.00000; tables of atomic weights list a value of the element's isotopic weights.

avoirdupois w. A system of weights and measures in which 1 pound equals 16 ounces, 7000 grains, or 453.59 grams.

dry w. The weight of a material after removal of all water content.

combining w. See gram equivalent, under equivalent.

equivalent w. See gram equivalent, under equivalent.

gram-molecular w. The numerical molecular weight of a substance expressed in grams; an amount of substance containing a weight in grams numerically equal to its molecular weight.

molecular w. (mol wt, MW) The sum of the atomic weights of all the atoms that make up a molecule.

weightlessness (wāt′lis-nis) The state of experiencing no gravitational pull.

Weil's disease (vīlz dĭ-zēz′) Severe leptospirosis caused by the bacterium *Leptospira icterohemorrhagiae,* transmitted to humans by rats; characterized primarily by continued fever and liver disturbances associated with jaundice, renal manifestations, and congestion of the conjunctiva. Also called infectious spirochetal jaundice; icterohemorrhagic fever; leptospirosis icterohemorrhagia.

welt (welt) See wheal.

wen (wen) Sebaceous cyst, especially of the scalp.

Werdnig-Hoffmann disease (verd′nig-hof′mahn dĭ-zēz′) See infantile spinal muscular atrophy (ISMA), under atrophy.

Wernicke-Korsakoff syndrome (ver′nĭ-kĕ-kor′să-kof sin′drōm) Disorder of the central nervous system caused by abusive intake of alcohol and nutritional depletion, especially of thiamine; characterized primarily by sudden weakness and paralysis of eye muscles, double vision, and inability to stand or walk unaided; followed by derangement of mental functions (e.g., confusion, apathy, loss of retentive memory, and confabulation); it may terminate in death.

Western blot (west′ern blot) See Western blot analysis, under analysis.

wet nurse (wet′nurs) A woman who breast-feeds another woman's child.

wheal (hwēl) A round or ridgelike transitory swelling on the skin.

wheeze (hwēz) **1.** To breathe with difficulty, producing a whistling sound, usually due to bronchiolar constriction as in asthma. **2.** The sound thus produced.

whey (hwā) The watery part of milk that separates from the casein or coagulated part. Also called serum lactis.

whiplash (hwip′lash) See whiplash injury, under injury.

Whipple's disease (hwip′elz dĭ-zēz′) A rare systemic disorder characterized by anemia, increased skin pigmentation, arthritis, steatorrhea, and other signs of malabsorption; the intestinal wall and lymphatics are infiltrated by macrophages filled with glycoproteins; occurs predominantly among middle-aged men. Also called lipophagic intestinal granulomatosis; intestinal lipodystrophy.

whipworm (hwip′werm) See *Trichuris trichiura,* under *Trichuris.*

whitehead (hwīt′hed) Popular term for milium.

whites (hwīts) See leukorrhea.

whiting (hwīt′ing) A pure grade of chalk, $CaCO_3$; used in polishing metal and plastic structures, especially dental prosthetics.

whitlow (hwit′lo) Painful, suppurative inflammation of a finger tip, especially under or around the nail.

herpetic w. A recurrent cluster of blisters caused by a herpesvirus transmitted through abrasions on the finger.

melanotic w. See acral lentiginous melanoma,

W

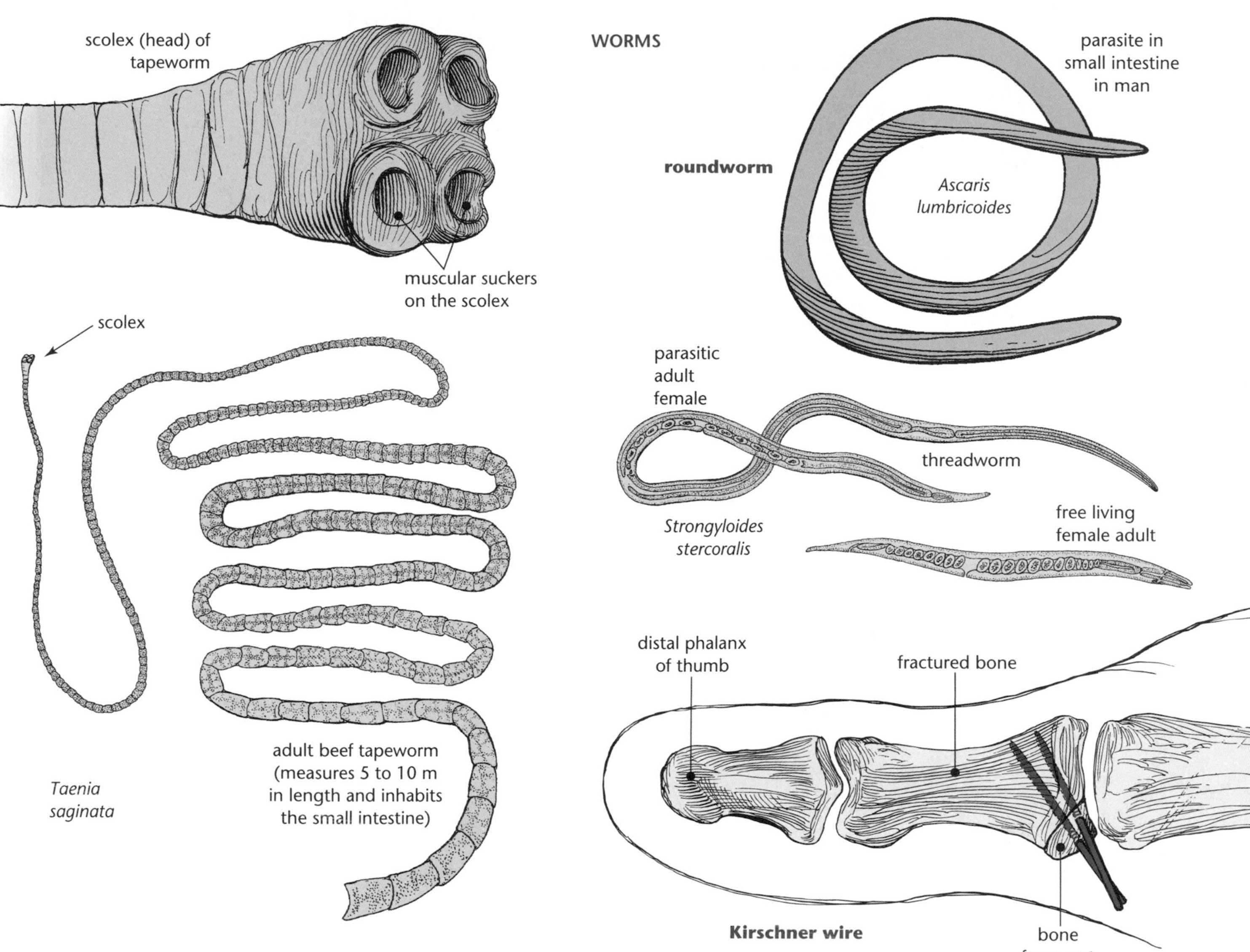

under melanoma.

thecal w. Infection of the distal phalanx of a finger, involving the synovial sheath of the flexor tendon.

whoop (hōōp) The shrill, noisy, paroxysmal gasp characteristic of whooping cough.

systolic w. See systolic honk, under honk.

whooping cough (hōōp′ing kawf) See pertussis.

whorl (hwerl) A spiral twist, such as any of the circular ridges of a fingerprint, the arrangement of muscular fibers at the apex of the heart, or the hairs growing in a radial manner.

Wilson's disease (wil′sunz dĭ-zēz′) An autosomal recessive disease marked by a defect in copper metabolism, resulting in toxic accumulation of copper deposits primarily in the liver, lenticular nucleus of the brain, and around the cornea, which acquires a green-brown discoloration (Kayser-Fletcher ring); eventually may cause cirrhosis of the liver and degenerative changes in the brain. Also called hepatolenticular degeneration.

windage (win′dij) Injury to internal organs caused by a sudden impact of the pressure of compressed air. Also called wind contusion.

windburn (wind′burn) Skin irritation due to excessive exposure to wind.

window (win′do) **1.** In anatomy, an opening in any partition-like structure or membrane. **2.** In radiology, a clear (radiolucent) area in an x-ray picture. **3.** In pharmacology, a range of drug concentration in the blood. **4.** A time interval (e.g., between ingestion of a poison and the production of irreversible organ damage).

aortic w. A radiolucent area below the aortic arch formed by the bifurcation of the trachea and traversed by the left pulmonary artery, visible in the left anterior oblique roentgenogram.

cochlear w. See round window.

implantation w. The time period during which the uterine wall will allow implantation of the fertilized ovum; its length in humans has been estimated to be between one and four days.

oval w. An oval opening in the medial wall of the middle ear chamber, which leads into the vestibule of the inner ear; it houses the baseplate of the stapes. Also called fenestra vestibuli; vestibular window.

round w. A round opening in the lateral wall of the inner ear, which leads from the scala tympani of the cochlea to the middle ear chamber; it is closed by the secondary tympanic membrane. Also called cochlear window; fenestra cochleae.

therapeutic w. The range of a drug's concentration within which a desired effect is most probable to occur; it may vary among individual patients.

vestibular w. See oval window.

windpipe (wind′pīp) Common term for trachea.

wing (wing) Any anatomic structure resembling the wing of a bird.

winking (wingk′ing) The rapid closing and opening of the eyelids.

Winterbottom's sign (win′ter-bot-umz sīn) Swelling of the posterior cervical lymph nodes; indicative of early stages of African sleeping sickness.

wintergreen (win′ter-grēn) A low-growing evergreen plant of eastern North America, *Gaultheria procumbens*.

oil of w. See under oil.

wire (wīr) **1.** A slender, pliable, metallic strand, used in surgery and dentistry. **2.** To bind structures with a wire or wires.

arch w. An orthodontic wire attached to molar bands positioned around the dental arch; used to provide tooth stabilization and/or maintain controlled pressure for tooth movement.

guide w. A fine flexible wire used to introduce and position a catheter within a blood vessel (e.g., in angiographic procedures).

Kirschner w. A heavy-gauge steel wire used for applying traction and fixation of a fractured bone.

ligature w. A soft slender wire used to tie an arch wire to the band attachment around a tooth.

wiring (wīr′ing) Fixation of the ends of broken bones by means of wire.

Wiskott-Aldrich syndrome (vis′kot-awl′drik sin′drōm) (WAS) Eczema, low platelet count, bloody diarrhea, and increased susceptibility to infections due to a defect in cellular immunity; a recessive inheritance affecting males (primarily infants and young children); Also called Aldrich syndrome.

witch hazel (wich hā′zel) A liquid extract obtained from the dried bark and leaves of the plant *Hamamelis virginiana*; used as an astringent.

withdrawal (with-draw′ăl) **1.** The act of removing, relinquishing, or discontinuing. **2.** A pathologic detachment or retreat from emotional involvement with people or the environment; seen in its extreme in schizophrenics. **3.** See withdrawal symptoms, under symptom.

withdrawal syndrome (with-draw′ăl sin′drōm) See withdrawal symptoms, under symptoms.

Wolff-Parkinson-White (WPW) **syndrome** (woolf-pahr′kin-son-hwīt sin′drōm) Congenital

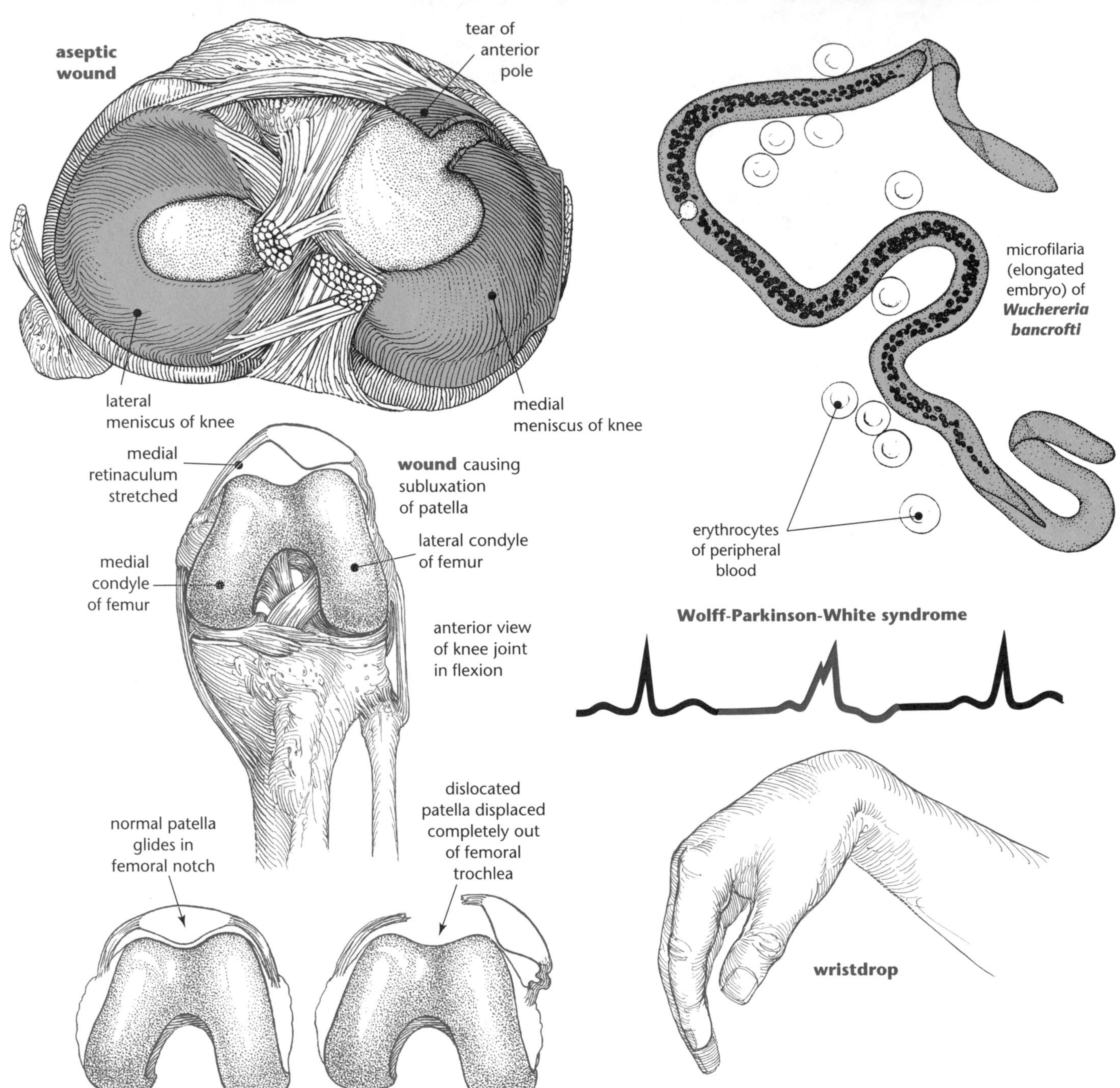

heart condition that has as its main feature an anomalous atrioventricular excitation; marked by irregular heartbeat and distorted patterns of the electrocardiogram (shortened P-R interval and prolonged QRS complex). Also called preexcitation syndrome.

womb (woom) See uterus.

falling of w. See prolapse of uterus, under prolapse.

neck of w. See uterine cervix, under cervix.

wool fat (wo͝ol fat) The fatlike substance obtained from sheep's wool, used in the preparation of ointments. Also called anhydrous lanolin.

wool-sorters' disease See pulmonary anthrax, under anthrax.

W

working through (wer´king thro͞o) In psychoanalysis, the process through which a problem is actively explored by patient and therapist until a satisfactory solution has been found or until a symptom has been traced to its unconscious sources; it generally involves the recapture of infantile, repressed, unconscious material and its conversion into conscious thoughts and strivings.

World Health Organization (wurld helth or-gă-ni-za´shun) (WHO) An agency of the United Nations concerned with health on an international level.

worm (werm) Common name for any of various elongated invertebrates of the phyla Annelida (segmented worms), Nematoda (roundworms), or Platyhelminthes (flatworms).

eye w. See *Loa loa*.

flat w. See flatworm.

guinea w. See *Dracunculus medinensis*, under *Dracunculus*.

heart w. See *Dirofilaria immitis*, under *Dirofilaria*.

lung w. See lungworm.

Medina w. See *Dracunculus medinensis*, under *Dracunculus*.

pin w. See pinworm.

pork w. See *Trichinella spiralis*, under *Trichinella*.

seat w. See pinworm.

serpent w. See *Dracunculus medinensis*, under *Dracunculus*.

trichina w. See *Trichinella spiralis*, under *Trichinella*.

wound (wo͞ond) Injury or trauma in any tissue.

aseptic w. (a) A wound made under sterile conditions (e.g., a surgical incision). (b) A wound that is free of infective microorganisms.

incised w. A cut made with a knife or any sharp instrument.

lacerated w. A wound with jagged edges caused by a tearing.

open w. One with an exposed opening.

penetrating w. One that enters a body cavity.

puncture w. A narrow wound made by a spiked instrument or weapon.

septic w. An infected wound.

wrinkle (ring´kl) **1.** A crease in the skin, such as one caused by habitual frowning or by atrophy of the corium, as in old age. **2.** A furrow or crevice on a normally smooth surface.

wrist (rist) The carpal bones and adjoining structures between the hand and the forearm.

wristdrop (rist´drop) Paralysis of the extensor muscles of the hand and digits.

wrist sign (rist sīn) The distal phalanges of the first and fifth fingers of one hand overlap when wrapped around the opposite wrist, as seen in individuals with the Marfan syndrome.

wryneck (ri´nek) See torticollis.

Wuchereria (voo-ker-e´re-ă) A genus of parasitic nematode roundworms (family Onchocercidae).

W. bancrofti Parasite of the lymph vessels and the cause of elephantiasis; transmitted by mosquitoes.

wuchereriasis (voo-ker-e-ri´ă-sis) Infection with worms of the genus *Wuchereria*.

X

xanthelasma (zan-thel-az ´mă) A form of xanthoma; yellow, wrinkled, slightly raised patches on the skin, occurring on the eyelid, usually bilaterally near the inner angle of the eye. Also called xanthelasma palpebrarum.
xanthemia (zan-the´me-ă) See carotenemia.
xanthene (zan´then) A crystalline compound that is the basic structure of many dyestuffs.
xanthic (zan´thik) **1.** Yellow. **2.** Relating to xanthine.
xanthine (zan´thēn) A white purine base present in most of the body tissues; sometimes found in urinary stones; converted to uric acid by xanthine oxidase.
xanthinuria (zan-thin-u´re-ă) Passage of excessive amounts of xanthine in the urine.
xanthochromia (zan-tho-kro´me-ă) A yellow discoloration of spinal fluid, usually an indication of a previous bleeding episode within the central nervous system.
xanthochromic, xanthochromatic (zan-tho-kro´mik, zan-tho-kro-mat´ik) Yellow colored.
xanthocyanopsia (zan-tho-si-ă-nop´se-ă) Abnormal color vision marked by inability to perceive red and green hues; vision is limited to yellow and blue.
xanthodont (zan´thō-dont) A person who has yellowish teeth.
xanthogranuloma (zan-tho-gran-u-lo´mă) Infiltration of tissue by lipid-laden macrophages.
juvenile x. Benign condition of infants and children, most commonly seen in infants during the first months of life; marked by the presence of yellowish nodules on the skin (which regress spontaneously), with an occasional ocular involvement. Also called nevoxanthoendothelioma.
xanthoma (zan-tho´mă) Slightly raised, yellow skin plaque, due to a disorder of fat metabolism.
eruptive x. Clusters of small xanthomas that appear suddenly on the elbows, knees, back, and buttocks, associated with high serum lipid levels and, occasionally, with severe diabetes.
x. multiplex See xanthomatosis.
plane x. Yellow bands occurring in skin folds or creases, especially on the palms; occasionally associated with primary cirrhosis of the liver.
tendinous x. Yellowish nodules occurring over the Achilles tendon (tendo calcaneus) and extensor tendons of the fingers.
tuberous x. Eruption of yellow nodules of varying size chiefly on the knees, elbows, palms, and soles.
xanthomatosis (zan-tho-mă-to´sis) The presence of multiple xanthomas. Also called lipid granulomatosis; lipoid granulomatosis; xanthoma multiplex.
cerebrotendinous x. Genetic disorder transmitted as an autosomal recessive inheritance; characterized by the formation of cholesterol deposits in tendons, lungs and the brain, causing pulmonary insufficiency and neurologic dysfunction; it usually develops after puberty.

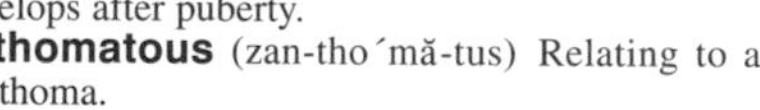

xanthomatous (zan-tho´mă-tus) Relating to a xanthoma.
Xanthomonas (zan-tho-mo´nas) Genus of gram-negative, aerobic bacteria, family Pseudomonadaceae.
X. maltophilia A species causing infections in hospitalized and immunocompromised patients.
xanthophyll (zan´tho-fil) A yellow carotenoid pigment in plants and egg yolk; also seen in human plasma as a result of ingesting food containing the pigment.
xanthopsia (zan-thop´se-ă) Condition in which everything appears yellow. Also called yellow vision.
xanthopterin (zan-thop´ter-in) A yellow pigment present in many sources including butterfly wings and the integument of wasps and hornets; an inhibitor of xanthine oxidase.
xanthosine (zan´tho-sēn) A nucleoside, xanthine-9-ribofuranoside, $C_{10}H_{12}O_6N_4$; formed by the deamination of guanosine.
xanthosis (zan-tho´sis) A yellow discoloration of the skin, sometimes seen in cancer patients.
xanthous (zan´thus) Yellowish.
xanthurenic acid (zanth-u-ren´ik as´id) 4,8-Dihydroquinaldic acid, large amounts of which are excreted during pregnancy and by pyridoxine-

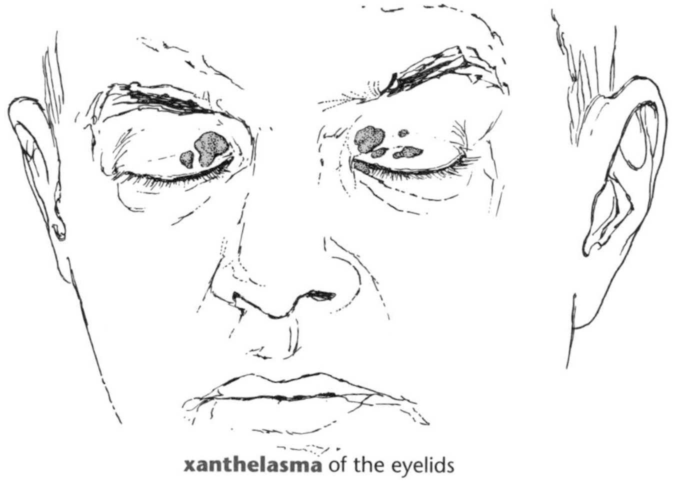

xanthelasma of the eyelids

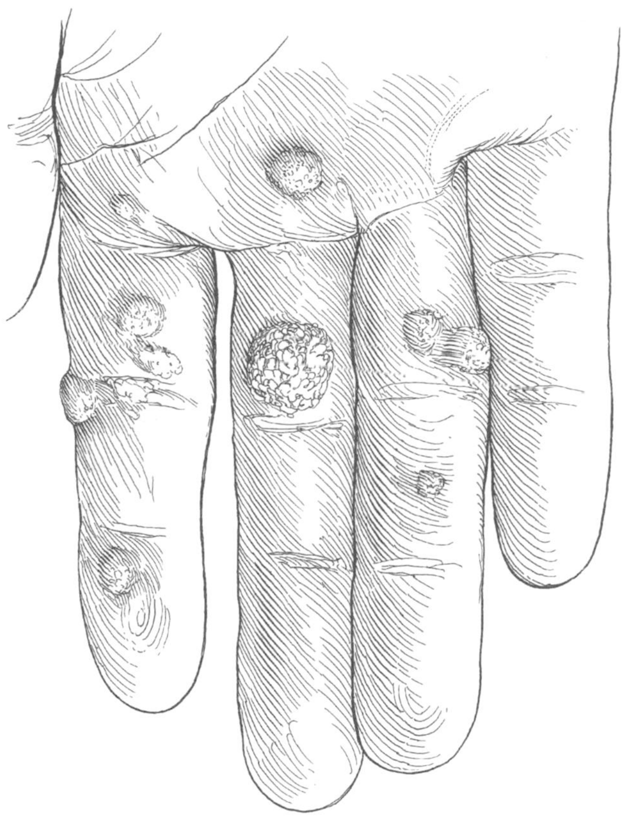

tuberous xanthoma of the foot

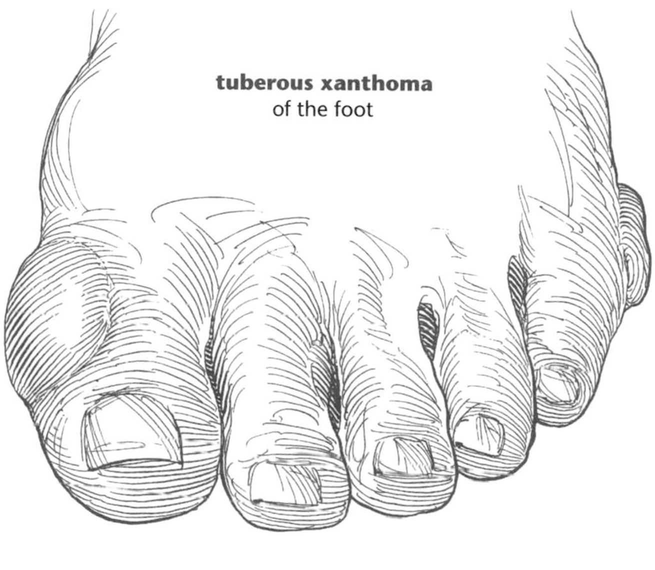

tuberous xanthoma of the hand

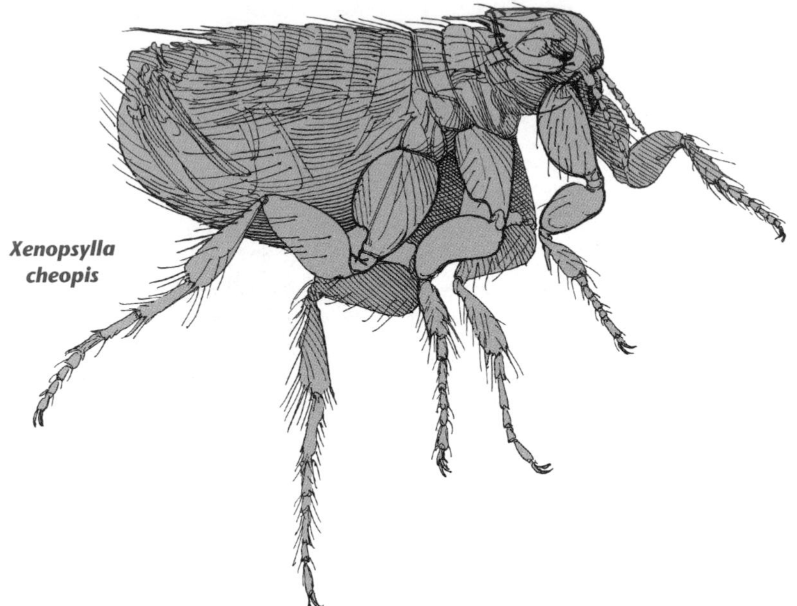

deficient individuals.

xanthyl (zan´thil) The monovalent radical $C_{13}H_9O$ which occurs in xanthene.

xenobiotic (zen-o-bi-ot´ik) Any chemical substance not produced by, therefore foreign to, living organisms (e.g., carcinogens, drugs, insecticides).

xenogeneic (zen-o-jen-a´ik) Relating to individuals of different species; applied to tissue grafting. Also called heterologous.

xenogenic (zen-o-jen´ik) Originating outside the body or in a foreign substance within the body.

xenograft (zen´o-graft) A graft derived from a species different from that receiving it. Also called xenogeneic graft; heterotransplant.

xenology (ze-nol´ŏ-je) The study of the relationship between a parasite and its host.

xenon (ze´non) An odorless inert gaseous element present in minute proportions in the atmosphere; symbol Xe, atomic number 54, atomic weight 131.3.

xenon-133 (^{113}Xe) A gamma-emitting radioactive inert gas with a physical half-life of 5.27 days; used to measure blood flow and regional pulmonary ventilation.

xenophobia (zen-o-fo´be-ă) Irrational fear of strangers or foreigners.

xenophthalmia (zen-of-thal´me-ă) Inflammation of the transparent covering of the eye (conjunctiva) due to injury or to the presence of a foreign body.

Xenopsylla (zen-op-sil´ă) A genus of fleas.

X. cheopis The rat flea; vector of *Pasteurella pestis*, the causative bacillus of plague.

xeransis (zē-ran´sis) Loss of moisture in the tissues.

xerantic (zē-ran´tik) Causing dryness.

xerocheilia (zēr-o-kī´le-ă) Dryness of the lips.

xeroderma (zēr-o-der´mă) A skin disease marked by roughness, dryness, and discoloration of the skin.

x. pigmentosum (XP) A congenital condition of the skin marked by extreme sensitivity to light, which causes skin inflammation, freckles, superficial ulcerations, glossy white spots due to thinning of the skin, and keratoses that become malignant. Also called atrophoderma pigmentosum.

xerography (zēr-og´ră-fe) See xeroradiography.

xeromammography (zēr-o-mam-og´ră-fe) A dry, totally photoelectric process of producing x-ray images of the female breast.

xeromenia (zēr-o-me´ne-ă) Occurrence of the usual general symptoms of menstruation but without a blood flow.

xerophthalmia (zēr-of-thal´me-ă) Degenerative condition marked by extreme dryness and thickness of the transparent covering of the eye (conjunctiva) with diminished secretion of tears. Also called ophthalmoxerosis.

xeroradiography (zēr-o-ra-de-og´ră-fe) The making of nontransparent black and white prints of densities produced by x rays on a specially coated plate.

xerosis (zēr-o´sis) Abnormal dryness of the skin, conjunctiva, or mucous membranes.

xerostomia (zēr-o-sto´me-ă) Abnormal dryness of the mouth, caused by diminished or arrested secretion of saliva. Popularly called dry mouth.

xerotic (zēr-ot´ik) Affected with abnormal dryness of the skin, conjunctiva, or mucous membranes.

xerotocia (zēr-o-to´se-ă) See dry labor, under labor.

Xg blood group Erythrocyte antigen controlled by a gene located on the X chromosome.

xiphisternum (zif-ĭ-ster´num) The xiphoid process or cartilage.

xiphocostal (zif-o-kos´tal) Relating to the xiphoid cartilage and the ribs.

xiphodynia (zif-o-din´e-ă) Pain in the area of the xyphoid cartilage.

xiphoid (zif´oid) Sword-shaped. See table of bones.

X linkage (eks-lingk´ij) See under linkage.

X-linked (ĕks´linkt) Determined by a gene located on the X chromosome.

x ray (ĕks rā) See under ray.

XXY syndrome (ĕks-ĕks-wī sin´drōm) See Klinefelter's syndrome.

xylene (zi´lēn) A flammable hydrocarbon obtained from wood and coal tar, used as a solvent. Also called xylol.

xylitol (zi´lĭ-tol) A five-carbon sugar alcohol used as a sugar substitute in diabetic diets.

xylometazoline (zi-lo-met-ă-zo´lēn) Compound used to reduce congestion of the nasal mucosa.

xylose (zi´lōs) A pentose sugar (its molecule has five carbon atoms, $C_5H_{10}O_5$), found in beechwood, straw, and vegetable gums; intestinal xylose absorption is used as a test in suspected cases of malabsorption.

xylulose (zi´lu-lōs) A pentose sugar found in two forms: *D-xylulose,* an intermediate in pentose metabolism; and *L-xylulose,* an abnormal constituent of urine seen in essential pentosuria.

xylyl (zi´lil) The hydrocarbon radical, $C_6H_4(CH_3)CH_2$, consisting of xylene minus a hydrocarbon atom.

X

Y

yabapox (yab´ă-poks) Smallpox of nonhuman primates. Also called tanapox; monkeypox.
yaw (yaw) One of the lesions of the eruption of yaws.
yawn (yawn) A deep inspiration, usually involuntary, through the open mouth.
yaws (yawz) An infectious skin disease of tropical regions, marked by papular eruptions on the face, hands, and feet, and around the external genitals; caused by a spirochete, *Treponema pertenue*. Also called frambesia; pian.
yeast (yēst) **1.** Any of several fungi of the genus *Saccharomyces* capable of fermenting carbohydrates. **2.** A commercial preparation, in either dry or moist form, used as a leavening agent or as a dietary supplement.
brewer's y. A by-product of the brewing of beer; used as a source of protein and vitamin B complex.
yellow fever (yel´o fe´ver) See under fever.
yellow jacket (yel´o jak´et) Any of various small wasps of the family Vespidae, having yellow and black markings and usually constructing round, paper-like nests in the ground under logs or rocks; their stings can cause severe and lethal allergic reactions in hypersensitive people.
Yersinia (yer-sin´e-ă) Genus of coccoid, oval, or rod-shaped, gram-negative bacteria (family Enterobacteriaceae).
Y. enterocolitica Species found in wild and domestic animals; causes yersiniosis in humans.
Y. pestis Causative organism of plague in humans and rodents; transmitted by fleas from infected animals (e.g., rats, squirrels, prairie dogs). Formerly called *Pasteurella pestis*.
Y. pseudotuberculosis A gram-negative, aerobic, non-spore-forming bacillus that is coccobacillary when virulent and bacillary when avirulent; a ubiquitous animal pathogen, now recognized as causing mesenteric lymphadenitis in humans.
yersiniosis (yer-sin-ē-o´sis) Infection with *Yersinia enterocolitica*, characterized by diarrhea, inflammation of lymph nodes, especially in the abdomen, and arthritis of several joints.
yield (yēld) **1.** The amount produced. **2.** The number of individuals having a disease identified by a screening test.
Y linkage (wī lingk´ij) See under linkage.
Y-linked (wī-linkt) Determined by a gene located on the Y chromosome.
yoga (yō´gă) A system of exercises aimed at promoting the control of the body and mind.
yogurt (yō´go͝ort) Curdled milk produced by the combined action of *Lactobacillus acidophilus* and *Streptococcus thermophilus*.
yohimbine (yo-him´bēn) An alkaloid, the active principle of the bark of the African tree *Corynanthe yohimbi*, similar in structure to reserpine; a relatively selective inhibitor of alpha$_2$-adrenergic receptors.
yolk (yōk) **1.** The nutrient portion of an ovum, especially conspicuous as the yellow mass of the egg of a bird or a reptile. Also called vitellus. **2.** The fatty substance present in the unprocessed wool of sheep which, when purified, becomes lanolin.
yolk sac (yōk sak) The highly vascular umbilical vesicle enveloping the nutritive yolk of an embryo. Also called vitelline sac.
yolk stalk (yōk stawk) The narrowed passage between the midgut of the embryo and the yolk sac.
ytterbium (ĭ-ter´be-um) A bright silvery rare-earth element that has the ability to vary its valence in different environments; symbol Yb, atomic number 70, atomic weight 173.04.
yttrium (ĭ´tre-um) A silvery metallic element; symbol Y, atomic number 39, atomic weight 88.90; always occurs with the rare earth minerals.
yttrium-90 (^{90}Y) An artificial radioactive isotope of yttrium (radioyttrium); has been used in the treatment of breast and prostatic cancer.

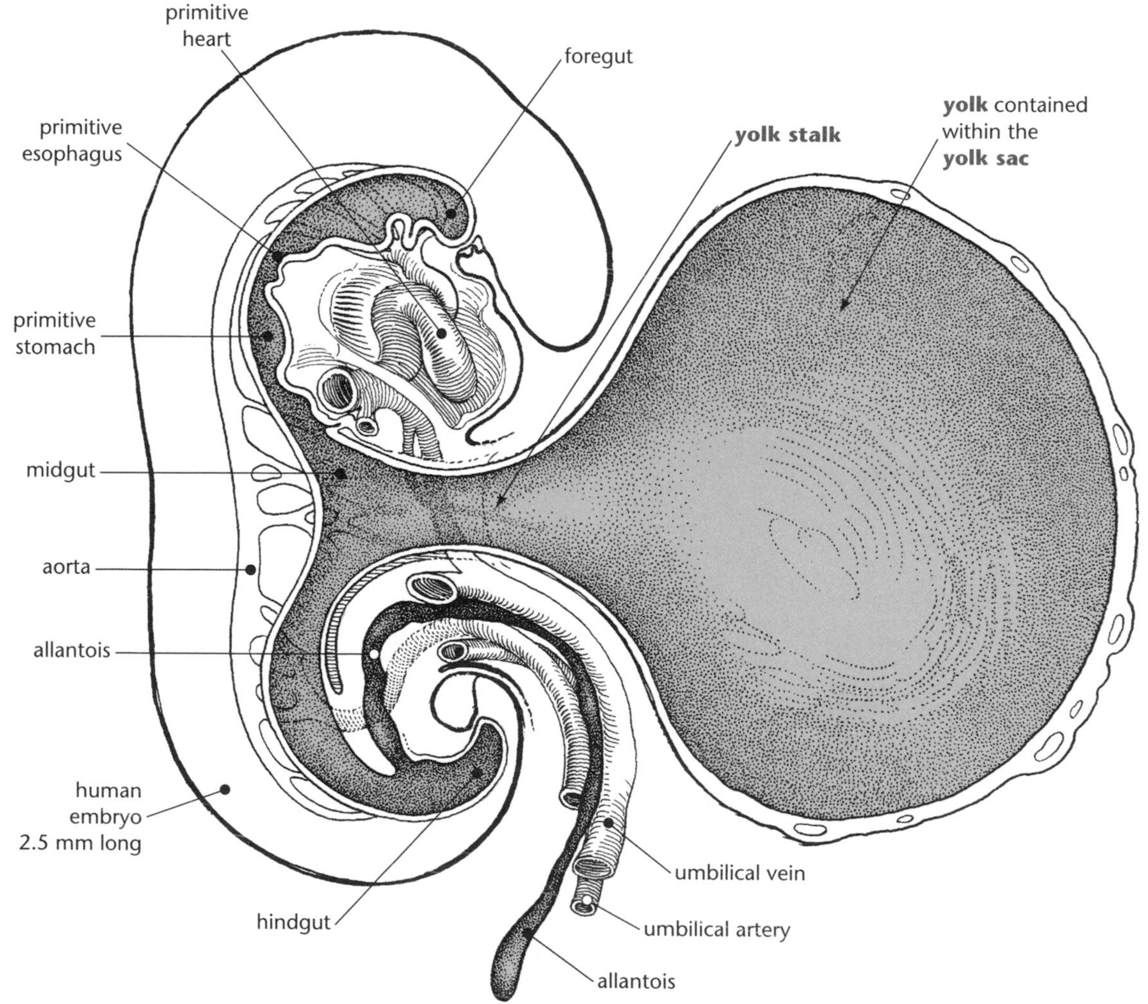

Y

Z z

zeaxanthin (ze-ă-zan´thin) A carotinoid found in yellow corn, egg yolk, and certain seaweed (*Fucus vesiculosus*) of the North Atlantic Ocean; used as a coloring agent.

zeolite (ze´o-lit) A hydrated sodium aluminum silicate occurring naturally; an ion exchanger used for softening of hard water by exchanging its Na^+ for the Ca^{++} of the water. Zeolites have no chemical relationship with synthetic ion exchangers.

zero (ze´ro) (z) The point on a thermometer scale from which the graduations are numbered in either direction; in the centrigrade scale, the freezing point for distilled water.

absolute z. The hypothetical point in a temperature scale in which there is complete absence of heat; in kinetic theory, absence of relative linear molecular motion, postulated as –273.2°C.

zeta (zā´tă, zē´tă) The sixth letter of the Greek alphabet, ζ; used to denote the sixth in a series.

zidovudine (zi-do´vu-dēn) A drug used in the management of acquired immune deficiency syndrome (AIDS); adverse effects include anemia and gastrointestinal intolerance. Formerly called azidothymidine (AZT).

ZIFT Acronym for zygote intrafallopian transfer. See under transfer.

zinc (zingk) A malleable and ductile metallic element; symbol Zn, atomic number 30, atomic weight 65.38.

z. carbonate A white amorphous powder with mild astringent properties; chief constituent of calamine lotion.

z. chloride A water-soluble caustic powder, $ZnCl_2$; used locally to destroy tissues.

z. gelatin See under gelatin.

z. ointment A compound made of 20% zinc oxide with beeswax and petrolatum; used as a salve.

z. oxide A white powder, ZnO, insoluble in water; a mild astringent and antiseptic incorporated in ointments, lotions, and dusting powders; used to prevent sunburn and to treat skin disorders (eczema, ringworm, psoriasis, varicose ulcers, and ivy poisoning); the main ingredient of calamine lotion.

z. oxide and augenol (ZOE) Compound used widely as a base material beneath tooth restorations, a temporary filling, an impression paste, and root canal filling; also used as a hardening agent for demineralized dentin.

z. permanganate Dark brown, water-soluble crystals, used in solution as a germicide.

z. peroxide (ZPO) A yellowish powder, ZnO_2, insoluble in water; used as a wash for oral infections (suspended in four parts of water) and to disinfect, deodorize, and promote healing of wound infections.

z. peroxide, medicinal A mixture of zinc peroxide, zinc carbonate, and zinc hydroxide; used as a local disinfectant, astringent, and deodorant.

z. stearate White greasy granules, insoluble in water; an antiseptic in dusting powder form, used to protect epithelial surfaces and wounds.

z. sulfate White water-soluble powder, used in solution as an eyewash to treat mild eye irritations and as a lotion (white lotion) to treat skin diseases and infections (acne, impetigo, and ivy poisoning). Also called salt of vitriol, white vitriol.

z. white See zinc oxide.

zinciferous (zing´kif´er-us) Containing zinc.

zirconium (zir-ko´ne-um) A metallic element, symbol Zr, atomic number 40, atomic weight 91.22.

zoacanthosis (zo-ak-an-tho´sis) Any dermatitis following skin implantation of foreign materials such as animal bristles, hairs, and stingers.

zoanthropic (zo-an-throp´ik) Relating to zoanthropy.

zoanthropy (zo-an´thro-pe) The delusion of being an animal.

zoetic (zo-et´ik) Relating to life.

zoic (zo´ik) Relating to animal life.

Zollinger-Ellison syndrome, Z-E syndrome (zol´in-jer-el´ĭ-son sin´drōm) Syndrome caused by a gastrin-secreting tumor of the pancreas, producing a high concentration of hydrochloric acid in the stomach; ulcers are formed in the esophagus and upper intestinal tract; symptoms include malabsorption, diarrhea, pain, and nausea; often associated with other endocrine abnormalities, especially hyperparathyroidism.

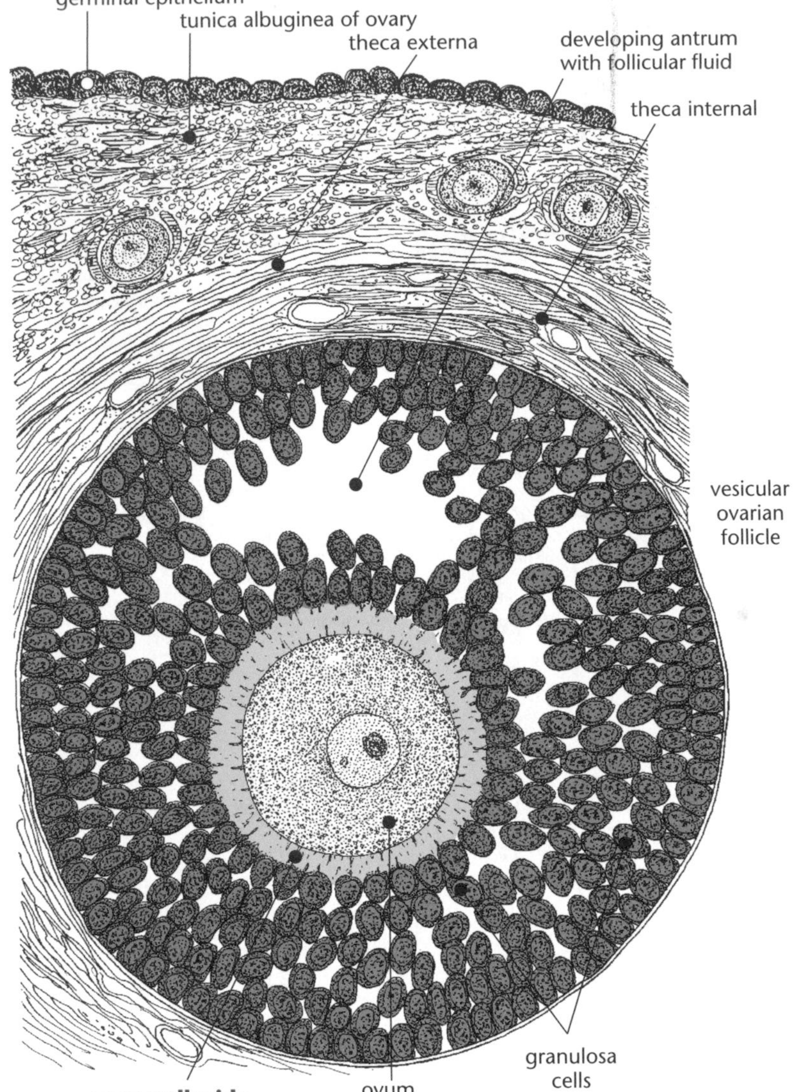

zona (zo´nă) A zone, especially an encircling region distinguished from adjacent parts by some distinctive feature.

z. adherens See zonula adherens.

z. dermatica An area of thick, elevated skin surrounding the protrusion of a meningocele.

z. fasciculata The intermediate layer of radially arranged cell cords in the cortex of the adrenal gland, between the zona glomerulosa and zona reticularis; together with the zona reticularis, it is the site of formation of adrenal steroids other than aldosterone.

z. glomerulosa The thin outermost layer of the cortex of the adrenal gland just below the capsule; the site of aldosterone production.

z. granulosa A mass of stratified cuboidal epithelium surrounding the ovum within a vesicular ovarian (graafian) follicle.

z. hemorrhoidalis The part of the anal canal that contains the rectal (hemorrhoidal) venous plexus.

z. incerta The narrow zone of gray matter between the lateral nucleus of the thalamus and the subthalamic nucleus.

z. occludens See tight junction, under junction.

z. orbicularis of the hip joint The deeper, circularly arranged fibers of the articular capsule of the hip joint which encircle the neck of the femur.

z. pellucida A refractile, gel-like neutral glycoprotein formed around the developing ovum; it is about 4 μm thick and formed by the mutual interaction of the ovum and follicular granulosa cells; it degenerates and disappears just prior to im-plantation to the endometrium.

z. reticularis The inner layer of the cortex of the adrenal gland where the cell cords form an irregular network; together with the zona fasciculata, the site of production of adrenal steroids other than aldosterone.

z. vasculosa of Waldeyer The highly vascular stroma in the center of the ovary. Also called medullary substance.

zone (zōn) (Z) Any area or space with specific characteristics.

ciliary z. The peripheral region of the anterior surface of the iris. COMPARE: pupillary zone.

comfort z. A range of environmental temperature in which the body heat is maintained in equilibrium, without sweating or shivering; 28° to 30°C (82° to 86°F) for the naked body and 13° to 21°C (55° to 70°F) for the clothed body.

erogenous z., erotogenic z. An area of the body which on appropriate stimulation produces sexual sensations.

extravisual z. The anterior portion of the retina outside the visual zone; it is too far forward for images to fall upon it.

functional z. See functional layer of endometrium, under layer.

Golgi z. The portion of the cytoplasm, near the cell nucleus, that contains the Golgi apparatus; in a secretory cell it is the area between the nucleus and the luminal side of the cell through which expulsion of the secretion takes place.

visual z. The area of the retina that receives light rays passing through the center of the pupil without any significant spherical aberration.

optical z. of cornea The central third of the cornea of the eye.

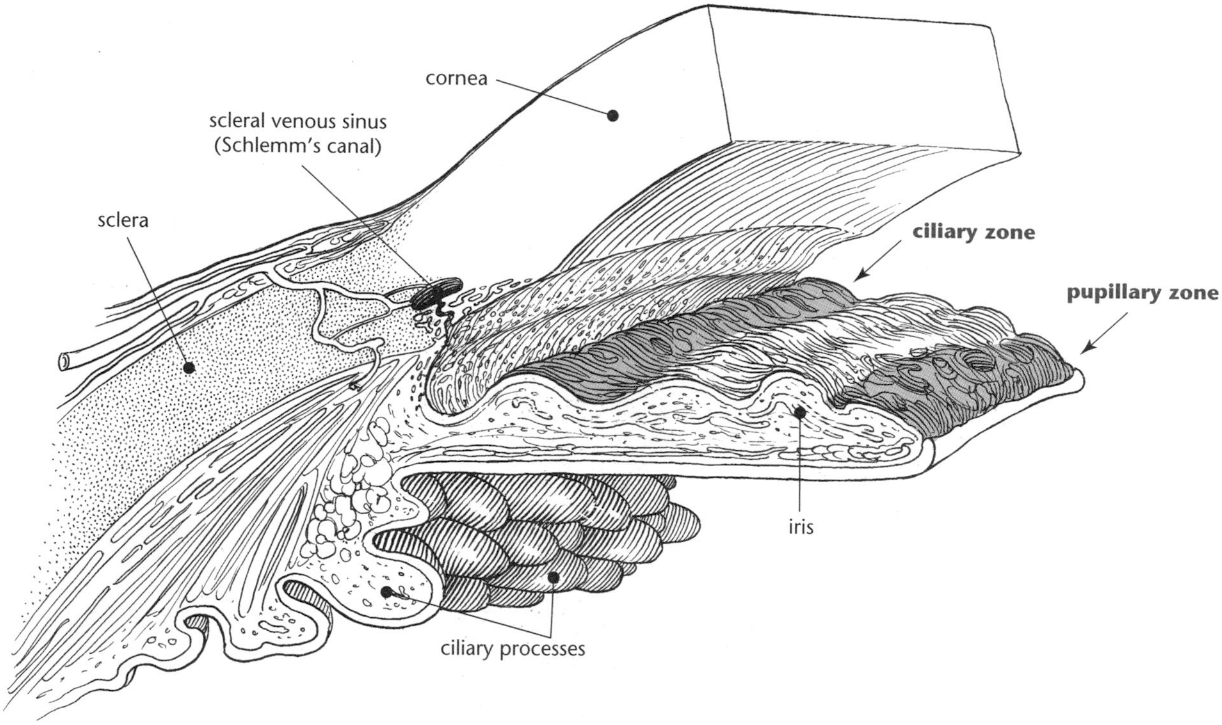

cornea
scleral venous sinus
(Schlemm's canal)
sclera
ciliary zone
pupillary zone
iris
ciliary processes

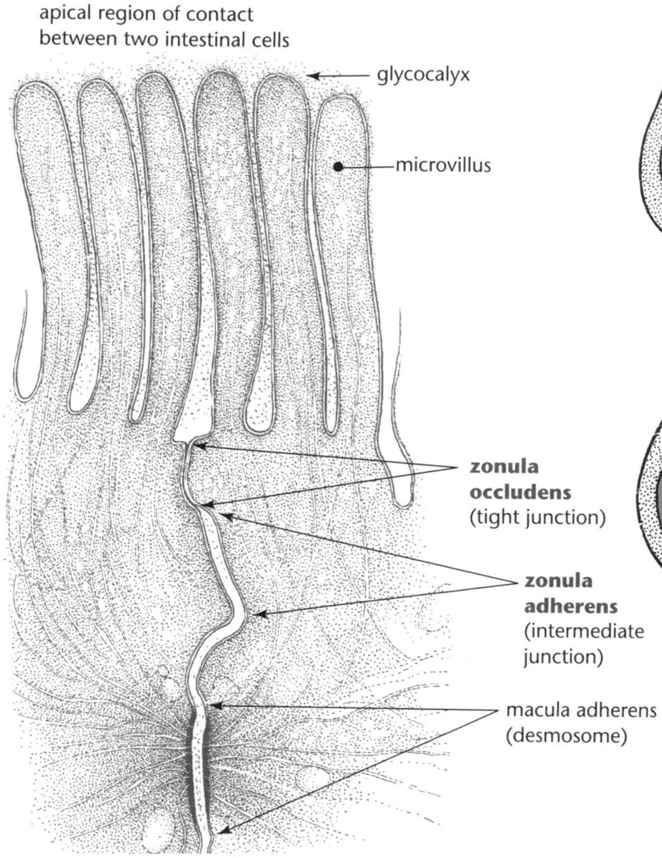

apical region of contact
between two intestinal cells
glycocalyx
microvillus
zonula occludens
(tight junction)
zonula adherens
(intermediate junction)
macula adherens
(desmosome)

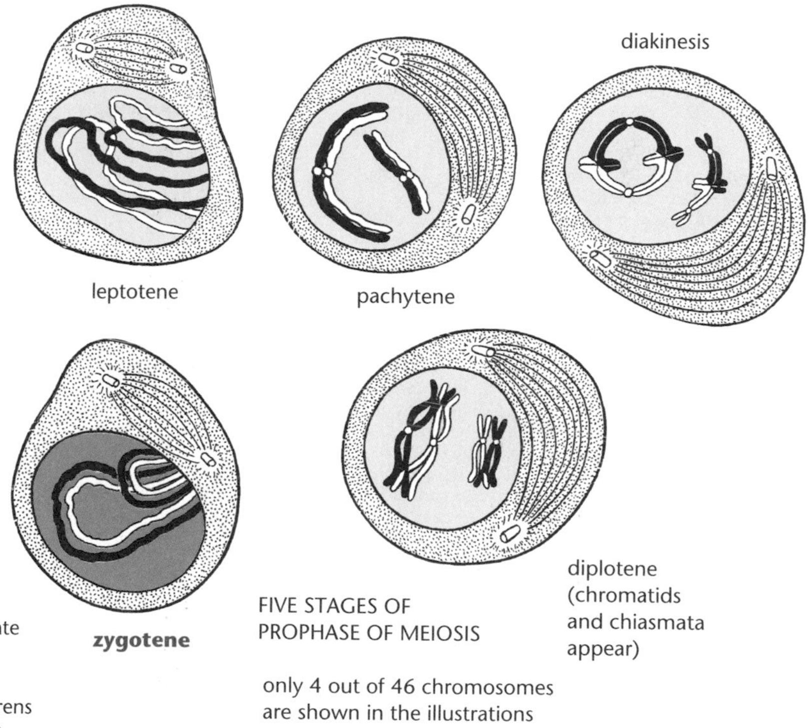

leptotene
pachytene
diakinesis
zygotene
diplotene
(chromatids
and chiasmata
appear)

FIVE STAGES OF
PROPHASE OF MEIOSIS

only 4 out of 46 chromosomes
are shown in the illustrations

pupillary z. The central region of the anterior surface of the iris, around the pupil. COMPARE: ciliary zone.

transformation z. (TZ) Area surrounding the external opening (external os) of the uterine cervix, between the columnar epithelium of the cervical canal and the squamous epithelium of the vaginal portion of the cervix; it changes in response to hormonal action and is the area in which cervical intraepithelial neoplasia (CIN) usually develops.

transitional z. **1.** The region of the lens of the eye where the anterior epithelial capsule cells develop into the fibers that constitute the lens substance. **2.** The border of a scleral contact lens that joins the scleral and corneal sections.

z.'s of discontinuity Concentric zones of varying optical density seen in the lens of the eye with the aid of the slit lamp.

zonesthesia (zo-nes-the´zhă) A constricting sensation, as by a girdle.

zonography (zo-nog´ră-fe) A type of tomography in which the plane of focus is relatively thick.

zonula (zōn´u-lă) A small zone or zonule.

z. adherens The part of the junctional complex of epithelial cells where the adjacent cells have a narrow (~200 Å) space between apposing membranes. Also called zona adherens.

ciliary z. The suspensory apparatus of the lens of the eye, consisting of numerous delicate fibers that originate in the ciliary body and attach to the anterior and posterior surface of the capsule of the lens; as the ciliary muscle contracts, the tension of the fibers accomodates, thus determining the degree of convexity of the lens. Also called suspensory ligament of lens; zonula of Zinn.

z. occludens See tight junction, under junction.

z. of Zinn See ciliary zonula.

zonular (zon´u-lă) Relating to a zonula.

zonule (zo´nūl) A small zone.

zonulolysis (zon-u-lol´ĭ-sis) Dissolving of the ciliary zonule by an enzyme, such as chymotrypsin, to facilitate removal of the lens in some cases of cataract extraction.

zooanthroponosis (zo-o-an-thro-po-no´sis) A disease usually occurring in humans that is trans-

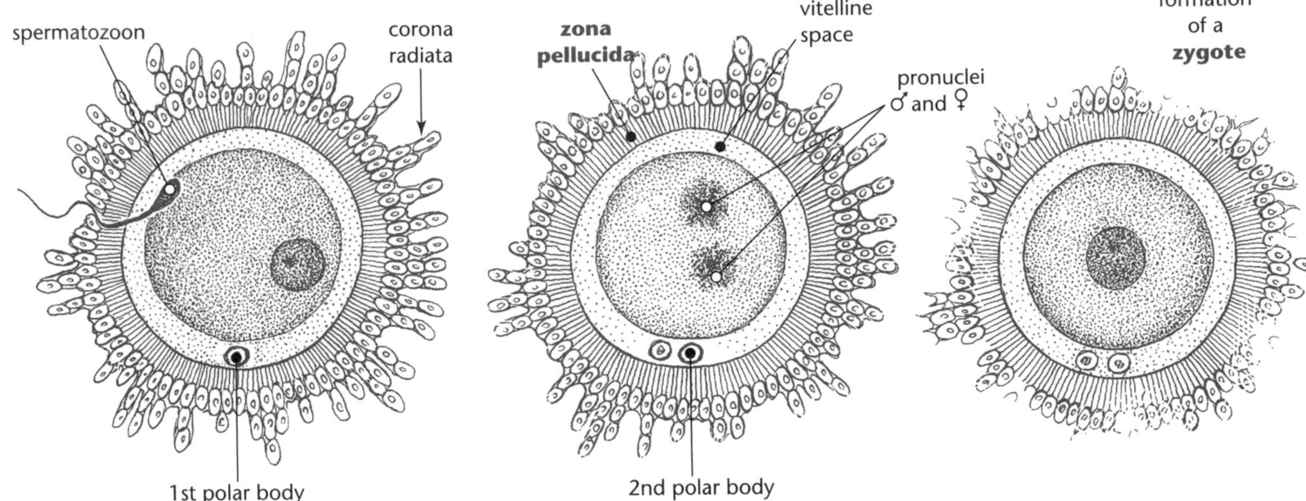

missible to animals. COMPARE: anthropozoonosis; amphixenosis.

zoochemistry (zo-o-kem´is-tre) The chemistry of animal tissues.

zoogenic, zoogenetic (zo-o-jen´ik, zo-o-jĕ-net´ik) Caused by animals.

zoogonous (zo-og´o-nus) See viviparous.

zooid (zo´oid) **1.** An animal cell capable of independent movement within a living organism (e.g., spermatozoon and ovum). **2.** Resembling an animal.

zoological (zo-o-loj´ĭ-kal) **1.** Relating to animals. **2.** Relating to the science of zoology.

zoologist (zo-ol´ŏ-jist) One who specializes in zoology.

zoology (zo-ol´ŏ-je) The branch of biology concerned with the study of animals.

comparative z. The comparative study of the structure and function of different animals.

zoonosis (zo-o-no´sis) Any disease acquired from animals, or shared by humans and other vertebrates.

zoonotic (zo-o-not´ik) **1.** Pertaining to zoonosis. **2.** Describing a disease transmitted to humans from an animal.

zooparasite (zo-o-par´ă-sīt) An animal parasite.

zoopathology (zo-o-pă-thol´ŏ-je) Veterinary pathology; the study of diseases that affect animals.

zoophilic (zo-o-fil´ik) Denoting a preference for animals; applied to parasites.

zoophobia (zo-o-fo´be-ă) Abnormal fear of animals.

zoophyte (zo´o-fīt) An invertebrate animal that superficially resembles a plant (e.g., a sponge).

zoospermia (zo-o-sper´me-ă) The presence of live spermatozoa in ejaculated sperm.

zoospore (zo´o-spōr) A motile, flagellated, asexual spore, as of certain fungi. Also called swarm spore.

zootoxin (zo-o-tok´sin) A substance elaborated by certain animals that has poisonous or antigenic properties (e.g., snake venom; secretions of certain insects).

zoster (zos´ter) An encircling belt or pattern; a girdle.

herpes z. See under herpes.

zosteroid (zos´ter-oid) Resembling herpes zoster.

Z-plasty (ze-plas´te) A technique for repairing contracted scar tissue.

zwitterion (tsvit´er-i-on) See dipolar ion, under ion.

zygal (zi´gal) Shaped like a yoke.

zygodactyly (zi-go-dak´tĭ-le) Fusion of the skin and connective tissue between fingers or toes without fusion of bones.

zygoma (zi-go´mă) **1.** The zygomatic process of the temporal bone. **2.** See zygomatic arch, under arch. **3.** Term sometimes applied to the zygomatic bone (cheekbone).

zygomatic (zi-go-mat´ik) Relating to the zygoma.

zygomycetes (zi-go-mi-se´tēz) A class of fungi that reproduce by the union of gametes of equal size.

zygomycosis (zi-go-mi-ko´sis) See phycomycosis.

zygosis (zi-go´sis) Fusion of two unicellular organisms, including exchange of nuclear material.

zygosity (zi-gos´ĭ-te) A state relating to the fertilized egg (zygote). Often used as a word termination, e.g., *monozygosity* (development of twins from one zygote) or *dizygosity* (from two zygotes) and *homozygosity* (identical genetic characteristics) or *heterozygosity* (different genetic characteristics).

zygote (zi´gōt) The single fertilized cell formed by the union of two gametes.

zygotene (zi´go-tēn) In meiosis, the second stage of prophase in which the homologous chromosomes approach each other and begin to pair.

zymogen (zi´mo-jen) See proenzyme.

zymogenesis (zi-mō-jen´ĕ-sis) The formation of an active enzyme from a proenzyme (inactive precursor).

zymogenic, zymogenous (zi-mo-jen´ik, zi-moj´ĕ-nus) **1.** Pertaining to a proenzyme or to zymogenesis. **2.** Producing a fermentation.

zymogram (zi´mo-gram) A graphic representation of electrophoretically separated enzymes.

zymoid (zi´moid) Resembling an enzyme.

zymology (zi-mol´ŏ-je) See enzymology.

zymolysis (zi-mol´ĭ-sis) Chemical process or fermentation brought about by means of an enzyme.

zymolytic (zi-mo-lit´ik) Fermentative.

zymophore (zi´mo-fōr) The active portion of an enzyme molecule.

zymoplastic (zi-mo-plas´tik) Participating in the formation of enzymes.

zymosan (zi´mo-san) An insoluble anticomplementary factor derived from the walls of yeast cells and used in the assay of the protein properdin; composed of lipids, polysaccharides, proteins, and ash of variable concentrations.

zymose (zi´mos) Invertase.

zymosis (zi-mo´sis) **1.** Fermentation. **2.** The development of infectious diseases.

zymotic (zi-mot´ik) **1.** Relating to fermentation. **2.** Denoting any infectious disease.

zyxin (ziks´in) A cytoplasmic protein that may participate in the organization of cell membrane-cytoskeletal attachments.

Abbreviations

A

A alveolar gas (as a subscript); mass number
a accommodation; recessive allele
a. *ante* [Latin] before
AAA acute anxiety attack; abdominal aortic aneurysm
AAS aortic arch syndrome
AAV adeno-associated virus
A/B acid/base (ratio)
Ab abortion; antibody
abbr abbreviated
ABC antigen binding capacity
ABE acute bacterial endocarditis
ABG arterial blood gas
ABMT autologous bone marrow transplant
ABO blood groups A, B, AB, and O
ABP arterial blood pressure
ABR auditory brainstem response; absolute bed rest
abs. absent
abs. feb. *absente febre* [Latin] while fever is absent
abstr abstract
ABT autologous blood transfusion
ABX antibiotics
Ac actinium
a.c. *ante cibum* [Latin] before meals
ACC ambulatory care center
ACE angiotensin converting enzyme
ace acetone
ACEI angiotensin converting enzyme inhibitor
ACh acetylcholine
AChE acetylcholinesterase
AChR acetylcholine receptor
ACJ acromioclavicular joint
ACL anterior cruciate ligament
ACLS advanced cardiac life support
ACP aspirin-caffeine-phenacetin
ACT activated clotting time
ACTH adrenocorticotropic hormone
ACV acyclovir
AD addict; Alzheimer's disease; analgesic dose; autosomal dominant
a.d. *alternis diebus* [Latin] every other day; *auris dextra* [Latin] right ear
ADA adenosine deaminase
ADC AIDS dementia complex
AdC adrenal cortex
ADD attention deficit disorder
ADEM acute disseminating encephalomyelitis
ADH antidiuretic hormone; alcohol dehydrogenase
ADHD attention deficit hyperactivity disorder
ADI acceptable daily intake
ad. lib. *ad libitum* [Latin] as desired
adm admission
Ado adenosine
ADP adenosine diphosphate
ADPase adenosine diphosphatase
ADR adverse drug reaction
adr adrenalin
ADS anonymous donor's sperm
adst. feb. *adstante febre* [Latin] when fever is present
ad us. ext. *ad usum externum* [Latin] for external use
ADV adenovirus
AF atrial fibrillation
AFAFP amniotic fluid alpha-fetoprotein
AFB acid-fast bacteria; acid-fast bacillus
AFC antibody-forming cells
AFE amniotic fluid embolism
aff afferent
AFL atrial flutter
AFP alpha-fetoprotein
AFX atypical fibroxanthoma
AG atrial gallop
A/G albumin/globulin ratio
Ag antigen; silver
AGA appropriate for gestational age
AGE angle of greatest extension
AGF angle of greatest flexion
AGG agamma-globulinemia
agit. ante sum. *agita ante sumendum* [Latin] shake before taking
AGL acute granulocytic leukemia
AGN acute glomerulonephritis
A/G r albumin/globulin ratio
agt agent
AH abdominal hysterectomy
AHA American Heart Association; autoimmune hemolytic anemia
AHC acute hemorrhagic conjunctivitis
AHD arteriosclerotic heart disease
AHF antihemophilic factor; acute heart failure
AHG antihemophilic globulin
AI aortic insufficiency; artificial insemination; artificial intelligence
AID acute infectious disease; artificial insemination by donor
AIDS acquired immune deficiency syndrome
AIH artificial insemination-husband (homologous insemination)
AIHA autoimmune hemolytic anemia
AL acute leukemia
Al aluminum
Ala alanine
alb albumin
ALD alcoholic liver disease
ALG antilymphocyte globulin
alk alkaline
ALL acute lymphoblastic leukemia
ALM acral lentiginous melanoma
ALP alkaline phosphatase
ALS advanced life support; amyotrophic lateral sclerosis
ALT alanine transaminase; argon laser trabeculoplasty
alt. dieb. *alternis diebus* [Latin] every other day
alt. hor. *alternis horis* [Latin] every other hour
AMA against medical advice
amb ambulatory
AMI acute myocardial infarction
AML acute myeloblastic leukemia; anterior mitral leaflet
AMP adenosine monophosphate
amp ampule; amputation
AN anesthesia; aneurysm; anorexia nervosa
ANA antinuclear antibody
AND anterior nasal discharge
anes. anesthesia
ANF antinuclear factor
ANG angiogram
ANLL acute nonlymphoblastic leukemia
ANOVA analysis of variance
ANP atrial natriuretic peptide
ANS anterior nasal spine; autonomic nervous system
ANSI American National Standards Institute
ant. anterior
ANUG acute necrotizing ulcerative gingivitis
AOAP as often as possible
AOB alcohol on breath
AOD arterial occlusive disease
AOHS angio-osteohypertrophy syndrome
AOM acute otitis media
AON acute optic neuritis
AP acid phosphatase; alkaline phosphatase; angina pectoris; antepartum; appendix;

anteroposterior (view)

A&P auscultation and palpation; auscultation and percussion

a.p. *ante prandium* [Latin] before dinner

APACHE acute physiology and chronic health evaluation system

APB atrial premature beat

APC acetylsalicylic acid, phenacetin, and caffeine; atrial premature contraction

APE acute psychotic episode;

APH antepartum hemorrhage; anterior pituitary hormone

APKD adult polycystic kidney disease

APL acute promyelocytic leukemia

APM aspartame

APN acute pyelonephritis

APO apoenzyme; apolipoprotein

appx appendix

6-APS 6-aminopenicillanic acid

APSGN acute poststreptococcal glomerulonephritis

aPTT activated partial thromboplastin time

APUD amine precursor uptake and decarboxylation

aq aqueous

AQP aquaporin

AQP1 aquaporin1

AR aortic regurgitation; artificial respiration

Ar argon

A&R advised and released

Ara arabinose

ARBD alcohol-related birth defects

ARC AIDS-related complex

ARD acute respiratory disease

ARDS acute respiratory distress syndrome

ARF acute renal failure; acute respiratory failure; acute rheumatic fever

Arg arginine

ARLD alcohol-related liver disease

ARM artificial rupture of membranes

AROM active range of motion

Arry arrhythmia

ART acid reflux test; acoustic reflex test

art. artery

AS aortic stenosis; arteriosclerosis; atherosclerosis

As arsenic; astigmatism

a.s. *auris sinistra* [Latin] left ear

ASA acetylsalicylic acid (aspirin); antisperm antibody

ASAP as soon as possible

ASB anesthesia standby

ASCUS atypical squamous cells of undetermined significance

ASCVD arteriosclerotic cardiovascular disease

ASD atrial septal defect

ASDH acute subdural hematoma

ASH asymmetrical septal hypertrophy

ASHD arteriosclerotic heart disease

ASIS anterosuperior iliac spine

Asn asparagine

ASO antistreptolysin O; arteriosclerosis obliterans

Asp aspartic acid

AST antibiotic sensitivity test; aspartate transaminase

Ast astigmatism

as tol. as tolerated

ASU acute stroke unit

ASV antisnake venom

ASX asymptomatic

AT Achilles tendon; atrial tachycardia

AT 10 dihydrotachysterol

ATC anterior tibial compartment (syndrome)

ATFL anterior talofibular ligament

ATG antithymocyte globulin

ATL adult T cell leukemia

ATN acute tubular necrosis

at no atomic number

ATP adenosine triphosphate

ATPase adenosine triphosphatase

ATS antitetanus serum; anxiety tension state

at wt atomic weight

a.u. *auris uterque* [Latin] each ear

Au gold

AUDIT alcohol use disorders identification test

AV aortic valve

A-V arteriovenous; atrioventricular

AVD aortic valve disease

AVF arteriovenous fistula

Avg average

AVH acute viral hepatitis

AVM arteriovenous malformation

AVN atrioventricular node; avascular necrosis

AVP arginine vasopressin (human antidiuretic hormone)

AVRT atrioventricular reciprocating tachycardia

AWS alcohol withdrawal syndrome

Ax. axis

AZT azidothymidine

B

B bacillus; blood type B+, B-; bel; boron

b blood (as a subscript); born

b. *bis* [Latin] twice

BA backache; blood alcohol; bone age; boric acid; bronchial asthma

BAC blood alcohol concentration

Ba barium

BaEn barium enema

BAER brainstem auditory evoked response

BAL blood alcohol level; British antilewisite (dimercaprol); bronchoalveolar lavage

BALT bronchus-associated lymphoid tissue

BAT blunt abdominal trauma

BAVP balloon aortic valvuloplasty

BB belly button; blood bank; breast biopsy

BBA born before arrival (of physician or midwife)

BBB blood-brain barrier; bundle-branch block

BBBB bilateral bundle branch block

BBD brittle bone disease

BBT basal body temperature

BC birth control; blood culture

Be beryllium

BCA balloon catheter angioplasty

BCC basal call carcinoma

BCD basal cell dysplasia

BCG bacillus Calmette-Guérin (vaccine)

BCP birth control pill

BCS battered child syndrome

BD behavioral disorder; belladonna; below diaphragm; birth defect; brain dead

b.d. *bis die* [Latin] twice a day

BDT bronchodilator therapy

BE barium enema; breast examination

b.e. bacterial endocarditis; barium enema

Be beryllium

BEAM brain electrical activity mapping

BFPR biologic false-positive reaction

BG blood glucose; bone graft

bGH bovine growth hormone

BHN Brinell harness number

Bi bismuth

BID brought in dead

b.i.d. *bis in die* [Latin] twice a day

BIH benign intracranial hypertension

bil bilirubin

b.i.n. *bis in nocte* [Latin] twice a night

BJ Bence Jones (protein); biceps jerk

Bk berkelium

blad bladder

BLD black lung disease

Bld blood

Bld Bk blood bank

BLS basic life support; blind loop syndrome

BM basal metabolism; basement membrane; bone marrow; bowel movement

BMD bone mineral density

BMG benign monoclonal gammopathy

BMI body mass index

bmk birthmark

BMR basal metabolic rate

BMT bone marrow transplant

BNA Basle Nomina Anatomica

BNS benign nephrosclerosis

BO bowel obstruction

BOA born on arrival

BOOP bronchiolitis obliterans with organizing pneumonia
BOW bag of water (s)
BP bathroom privileges; blood pressure; bypass
BPD bronchopulmonary dysplasia
BPH benign prostatic hyperplasia;
BPM beats per minute; breaths per minute
BPP biophysical profile
BPS binge-and-purge syndrome
Bq becquerel
BR bed rest
Br bromine
BRBPR bright red blood per rectum
BS blood sugar; breath sounds; bowel sounds
BSA body surface area; bovine serum albumin
BSE breast self examination
BSER brainstem evoked response
BSL blood sugar level
BSP Bromsulphalein,
BSPT Bromsulphalein test,
BT bedtime; biuret test; blind test; blood transfusion; body temperature
BTL bilateral tubal ligation
BUN bleeding of unknown origin; blood, urea, nitrogen;bruising of unknown origin
BV blood vessel; blood volume
BVAD biventricular assist device
BW birth weight; body weight
BWS battered woman syndrome
Bx biopsy

C

C calculus; carbohydrate; carbon; cathode; Celsius; centigrade; cervical (vertebrae); cesarean; complement; concentration;
contraction; coulomb; large calorie
c curie; cycle; cylinder; small calorie
c. *cum* [Latin] with
C1 first cervical spinal nerve;
first cervical vertebra
C2 second cervical spinal nerve;
second cervical vertebra
C3 third cervical spinal nerve;
third cervical vertebra
C4 fourth cervical spinal nerve;
fourth cervical vertebra
C5 fifth cervical spinal nerve;
fifth cervical vertebra
C6 sixth cervical spinal nerve;
sixth cervical vertebra
C7 seventh cervical spinal nerve;
seventh cervical vertebra
CA cancer; cardiac arrest; chronologic age
CA-125 cancer antigen 125(test)
Ca calcium; cancer; carotid artery; cathode; cerebral aqueduct; chronological age
ca cancer
ca. *circa* [Latin] about
CABG coronary artery bypass graft
CABS coronary artery bypass surgery
CAD computer-assisted diagnosis; coronary artery disease
CAH chronic active hepatitis;
congenital adrenal hyperplasia
CAHD coronary artery heart disease
Cal large calorie
cal small calorie
calef. *calefac* [Latin] make warm
CALLA common acute lymphoblastic
leukemia antigen
CAM cell adhesion molecule
cAMP cyclic adenosine monophosphate
CAN cord (umbilical) around neck
CAO chronic airflow obstruction
cap. *capiat* [Latin] let him (the patient) take
CAPD chronic ambulatory peritoneal dialysis
CAS carotid artery stenosis; cerebral arteriosclerosis
CASA computer-assisted semen analysis
CAT cataract; computerized axial tomography
cath. catheter; catheterize
cath'd catheterized
CATSCAN computer-assisted tomography scanner
CAVB complete atrioventricular block
CAVS calcified aortic valve stenosis
CB catheterized bladder; cesarean birth; chronic bronchitis; code blue
C&B crown and bridge
Cb columbium
CBC complete blood count
CBD closed bladder drainage
CBE clinical breast examination
CBF cerebral blood flow
CBG capillary blood gases;
corticosteroid-binding globulin
CBH cutaneous basophil hypersensitivity
CBR complete bed rest
CBS closed building syndrome
CBT cognitive-behavioral therapy
CC cardiac catheterization; cardiac cycle; cerebral concussion; chief complaint; chronic complainer; creatinine clearance; critical care
cc cubic centimeter
CCA common carotid artery
CCB calcium channel blocker
CCCR closed-chest cardiac resuscitation
CCF congestive cardiac failure
CCG cholecystogram
CCI chronic coronary insufficiency
CCJ costochondral junction
CCK cholecystokinin
CCMS clean-catch midstream (urine specimen)
CCPD chronic cyclic peritoneal dialysis
Ccr creatinine clearance
CCRU critical care recovery unit
CCS costoclavicular syndrome
CCU cardiac care unit; coronary care unit; critical care unit
CD cadaver donor; cardiac disease; cesarean delivery; cluster designation; cluster determinant; cluster of differentiation (system); communicable disease; consanguineous donor; contact dermatitis; contagious disease; curative dose
c.d. *conjugata diagonalis* [Latin] diagonal conjugate
CD3 antigenic marker on T cell associated with T cell receptor
CD4 antigenic marker of helper/inducer T cells
CD8 antigenic marker of suppressor/cytotoxic T cells
Cd cadmium
cd candela
CDC Centers for Disease Control (and Prevention)
CDH congenital diaphragmatic hernia;
congenital dislocation of the hip;
cDNA complementary deoxyribonucleic acid
CDP cytidine diphosphate
CDR continuing disability review
CDS cervical disk syndrome
CDT carbon dioxide therapy
CE continuing education; cardiac emergency
Ce cerium
CEA carcinoembryonic antigen
CEP congenital erythropoietic porphyria
CER conditioned emotional response
CE & R central episiotomy and repair
cerv cervical; cervix
CES cauda equina syndrome
CF cancer-free; cystic fibrosis; cardiac failure; citrovorum factor; complement fixation; complement-fixing (antibody); counting fingers (used in ophthalmology)
Cf californium; *confer* [Latin] compare
CFA colonization factor antigens
CFL calcaneofibular ligament (of the ankle joint)
CFT capillary fragility test
CFU colony-forming unit
CG cholecystogram; chorionic gonadotropin; chronic glomerulonephritis
cg centigram
CGB chronic gastrointestinal bleeding
CGD chronic granulomatous disease
CGL chronic granulocytic leukemia
cGMP cyclic guanosine monophosphate
CGN chronic glomerulonephritis
CGRP calcitonin gene related peptide

CGS centimeter-gram-second (system of units)
CH child; cholesterol; cluster headache
C-H crown-heel (applied to the length of a fetus)
CHA chronic hemolytic anemia
CHD congenital heart disease; congenital hip dislocation; coronary heart disease
ChE cholinesterase
CHF congestive heart failure
CHIP channel-forming integral protein
CHN congenital hairy nevus
CHO carbohydrate
chol. cholesterol
chpx chickenpox
chr chronic
CHS Chediak-Higashi syndrome
Ci curie
cib. *cibus* [Latin] food
CIBD chronic inflammatory bowel disease
CIC clean intermittent catheterization
CID cytomegalovirus inclusion disease
CIDS continuous insulin delivery system
CIg cytoplasmic immunoglobulin
Cin insulin clearance
CIN cervical intraepithelial neoplasia
CIN I cervical intraepithelial neoplasia (with mild dysplasia)
CIN II cervical intraepithelial neoplasia (with moderate dysplasia)
CIN III cervical intraepithelial neoplasia (with severe dysplasia)
CIPD chronic intermittent peritoneal dialysis
CIS carcinoma *in situ*
CIT Casoni intradermal test
CJD Creutzfeldt-Jakob disease
CK creatine kinase; cytokinin
CL corpus luteum; critical list
Cl chlorine
cl centiliter
clav clavicle
CLL chronic lymphocytic leukemia
CLP cleft lip and palate
CM cardiac monitor; cardiomyopathy; common migraine; continuous murmur
Cm curium
cM centimorgan
cm centimeter
C-max maximum concentration
CMC carpometacarpal; chronic mucocutaneous candidiasis
CMCC chronic mucocutaneous candidiasis
CME continuing medical education; cystic macular edema
CMI cell-mediated immunity
chronically mentally ill
CMID cytomegalic inclusion disease
c/min cycles per minute
CML cell-mediated lympholysis;
chronic myeloid leukemia
cmm cubic millimeter
CMN cystic medial necrosis
CMP cardiomyopathy; cytidine monophosphate
CMPGN chronic membrano-proliferative
omerulonephritis
CMR cerebral metabolic rate
CMV controlled mechanical ventilation; cytomegalovirus
CN Charge Nurse; cranial nerve
CNM Certified Nurse-Midwife
CNP continuous negative pressure
CNS central nervous system
CO carbon monoxide; cardiac output; cervical orthosis
Co cobalt; coenzyme
Co I coenzyme I (now called NAD)
Co II coenzyme II (now called NADP)
Co III coenzyme III
c/o complains of
CoA coarctation of the aorta; coenzyme A
COAD chronic obstructive airway disease; chronic obstructive arterial disease
coc coccygeal
coch. mag. *chochleare magnum* [Latin] tablespoon
COD cause of death
COLD chronic obstructive lung disease
collat collateral
comp complication; compound; compress
C-ONC cellular oncogene
consult consultant; consultation
cont containing; content; continue
contin. *continuetur* [Latin] let it be continued
COPD chronic obstructive pulmonary disease
cor coronary
CORD chronic obstructive respiratory disease
COX cyclooxygenase
CP cerebral palsy; chemically pure; chest pain; chronic pain; cleft palate; cor pulmonale; creatine phosphate
CPAP continuous positive air pressure; continuous positive airway pressure
CPC clinicopathological conference
CPDD calcium pyrophosphate disposition disease (pseudogout)
CPE cardiogenic pulmonary edema; chronic pulmonary emphysema
CPGN chronic proliferative glomerulonephritis
CPH chronic persistent hepatitis
CPID chronic pelvic inflammatory disease
CPK creatine phosphokinase
CPKD childhood polycystic kidney disease
cpl complete
CPM cardiac pacemaker; central pontine myelinolysis; continue present management; continuous passive motion; counts per minute; cycles per minute
cpm counts per minute; cycles per minute
CPN chronic pyelonephritis
CPP cerebral perfusion pressure
CPPB continuous positive pressure breathing
CPPD calcium pyrophosphate dihydrate
CPPV continuous positive pressure ventilation
CPR cardiopulmonary resuscitation
cps counts per second; cycles per second
CPTH chronic post traumatic headache
CPUE chest pain of undetermined etiology
CPX complete physical examination
CR cardiorespiratory; chest radiograph; closed reduction (of a fracture); code red; colon resection; complete remission; conditioned reflex; creatinine
C-R crown-rump (applied to length of fetus)
Cr chromium; creatinine
CRC colorectal cancer
CRD chronic renal disease;
chronic respiratory disease
CRE cumulative radiation effect
creat creatine
CREST calcinosis, Raynaud's phenomenon, esophageal motility disorders, sclerodactyly, telangiectasia
CRF chronic renal failure
CRH corticotropin-releasing hormone
CRL crown-rump length (of fetus)
CRO cathode ray oscilloscope
CRP C-reactive protein; cAMP receptor protein
CRS Chinese restaurant syndrome
CRT cardiac resuscitation team; cathode ray tube
CS carotid sinus; cesarean section; cigarette smoker; congenital syphilis
Cs cesium
CSA colony-stimulating activity
CSAP Center for Substance Abuse Prevention
CSD cat-scratch disease
C section cesarean section
CSF cerebrospinal fluid; colony-stimulating factor
CSII continuous subcutaneous insulin infusion
CSM cerebrospinal meningitis
CSOM chronic serous otitis media
CSP criminal sexual psychopath
C-spine cervical spine
CSR corrected sedimentation rate
CST contraction stress test
CT calcitonin; carpal tunnel; cerebral thrombosis; clotting time; coagulation time; computed tomography; connective tissue; corneal transplant
ct count

CTD connective tissue disease
CTL cytotoxic T lymphocyte; cytotoxic lymphocyte
CTR carpal tunnel release
CTS carpal tunnel syndrome
CTT cytotoxicity test
CTZ chemoreceptor trigger zone
CU cause unknown; convalescent unit
Cu copper
cu cubic
CUC chronic ulcerative colitis
CUT carbohydrate utilization test
CV cardiovascular; closing volume (of lung); coefficient of variation
CVA cardiovascular accident; cerebrovascular accident;
CVC central venous catheter
CVD cardiovascular disease
CVID common variable immunodeficiency
CVM cardiovascular monitor
CVP central venous pressure
CVS chorionic villus sampling
CUSA cavitron ultrasonic surgical aspirator
CWP childbirth without pain
Cx cervix; convex
CXR chest x-ray
cyc cycle
cyclic AMP cyclic adenosine monophosphate
cyclic GMP cyclic guanosine monophosphate
Cyd cytidine
cyl cylinder
CYS cystoscopy
Cys cysteine
Cyt cytosine

D

D day; deceased; deciduous (teeth); deuterium; diagnosis; diopter; donor; dorsal; dose; drug
d day; deceased; density
D/3 distal third
DA delayed action; developmental age; disability assistance; drug addict; ductus arteriosus
DAD dispense as directed
DAF delayed auditory feedback.
DAG diacylglycerol
dag decagram
DAI diffuse axonal injury
DAT delayed action tablet
DAW disperse as written
DB date of birth; disability
Db diabetic
dB decibel
dbl double
DBT double-blind test
DBW desirable body weight
DC dendritic cells; diagonal conjugate; diagnostic center; direct current; discharge; discontinue
DCA deoxycorticosterone acetate
D&C dilatation and curettage
DC&B dilatation, curettage, and biopsy
DCB dichlorobenzedine
DCIS ductal carcinoma *in situ*
DCT direct Coombs' test; distal convoluted tubule
DD dangerous drug; differential diagnosis
d.d. *detur ad* [Latin] let it be given to
D&D diarrhea and dehydration
DDAVP deamino D-arginine vasopressin (desmopressin acetate)
DDI dideoxyinosine
DDS dialysis disequilibrium syndrome
DDT dichlorodiphenyl-trichloroethane
DDx differential diagnosis
DE dermoepidermal
D&E dilatation and evacuation
def defecation
dehyd dehydration
DEN dienestrol
depr depressed
DES diethylstilbestrol
DESI direct egg sperm injection
DET diethyltryptamine
detox detoxify
d. et s. *detur et signetur* [Latin] let it be given and labeled
DFP diisopropyl fluorophosphate
DFS dead fetus syndrome
DFU dead fetus *in utero*
DGI disseminated gonococcal infection
DH delayed hypersensitivity; dermatitis herpetiformis; diaphragmatic hernia
DHEA dihydroepiandrosterone
DHEAS dihydroepiandrosterone sulfate
DHT dihydrotestosterone
DI diabetes insipidus
dias. diastolic
DIB disability insurance benefits
DIC disseminated intravascular coagulation
DIE died in emergency room
dieb. alt. *diebus alternis* [Latin] every other day
digit I big toe; first digit; thumb
digit II index finger; second digit; second toe
digit III middle finger; third digit; third toe
digit IV fourth digit; fourth toe; ring finger
digit V fifth digit; little finger; little toe
dil. dilute
dilat dilatation; dilated
dim. *dimidus* [Latin] one-half
DIP desquamative interstitial pneumonia; distal interphalangeal (joint)
diph diphtheria
DIPJ distal interphalangeal joint
dis disability; disease; dislocation
disc discontinue
disch discharge
DISH diffuse idiopathic skeletal hyperostosis
DISI dorsiflexed intercalated segment instability
disl dislocation
distal/3 distal third
DIT diiodotyrosine
DJD degenerative joint disease
DKA diabetic ketoacidosis
DL danger list; diffuse lymphoma; disabled list
dl deciliter
DLE dialyzable leukocyte extract; discoid lupus erythematosus; disseminated lupus erythematosus
DLMP date of last menstrual period
DM diabetes mellitus; diastolic murmur
dM decimorgan
dm decimeter
DMD Duchenne's muscular dystrophy
DMOOC diabetes mellitus out of control
DMSA dimercaptosuccinic acid
DMSO dimethyl sulfoxide
DMT dimethyltryptamine
DNA deoxyribonucleic acid; does not apply
DNase deoxyribonuclease
DNC did not come
DND died a natural death
DNI do not intubate
DNP dinitrophenol
DNR do not resuscitate (order); do not report
DNS deviated nasal septum
DOA date of admission; dead on arrival
DOB date of birth
DOC deoxycholate; deoxycorticosterone
DOCA deoxycorticosterone acetate
DOE dyspnea on exertion
DOI date of injury
DOM dominance
DOOR deafness, onycho-osteodystrophy, (mental) retardation
DOPA dopamine
DOS date of surgery
DOT died on (operating room) table
DP diastolic pressure; displaced person; distal phalanx; donor's plasma
DPA dual-photon absorptiometry
DPG diphosphoglycerate
DPM discontinue previous medication
DPN diphosphopyridine nucleotide
DPT diphtheria-pertussis-tetanus (vaccine)
DR delivery room; diabetic retinopathy
dr dram
DRE digital rectal examination
DRG diagnosis-related group
DS decompression sickness; discharge summary; donor's serum; dry socket; Down syndrome
DSA digital subtraction angiography

DSBL disabled

DSD dry sterile dressing

DSM *Diagnostic and Statistical Manual (of Mental Disorders)*

DSMO dimethyl sulfoxide

DST distal straight tubule; donor-specific (blood) tranfusion

DT delirium tremens; diphtheria and tetanus (vaccine); duration of tetany

DTH delayed-type hypersensitivity

DTP diphtheria (toxoid), tetanus (toxoid), pertussis (vaccine)

DTR deep tendon reflex

DU decubitus ulcer; diagnosis undetermined; duodenal ulcer

DUB dysfunctional uterine bleeding

DUCT differential ureteral catherization test

DUI driving under the influence

dur. dolor. *durante dolor* [Latin] while the pain lasts

D&V diarrhea and vomiting

DVT deep vein thrombosis

DW distilled water

D/W dextrose in water

Dx diagnosis

Dy dysprosium

DZ disease; dizygotic (twins); dizziness

E

E edema; electrode potential; enema; enzyme; epinephrine; erythrocyte; esophagus; eye

e electron

EA early antigens; erythrocyte amboceptor

ea each

EAA essential amino acid

EAC erythrocyte amboceptor complement; external auditory canal

ead. *eadem* [Latin] the same

EAHF eczema-asthma-hay fever

EB elementary body

EBF erythroblastosis fetalis

EBL estimated blood loss

EBM expressed breast milk

EBV Epstein-Barr virus

EC entering complaint

ECC emergency cardiac care

ECCE extracapsular cataract extraction

ECF eosinophil chemotactic factor; extended care facility; extracellular fluid

ECFV extracellular fluid volume

ECG echocardiogram; electrocardiogram;

ECH extended care hospital

ECHO echocardiogram; echoencephalogram; enteric cytopathogenic human orphan (virus)

ECM extracellular matrix

ECMO extracorporeal membrane oxygenation

E. coli *Escherichia coli*

ECS electrocerebral silence; electroconvulsive shock

ECT electroconvulsive therapy; electroconvulsive treatment; enteric-coated tablet

ECW extracellular water

ED effective dose; electrodialysis; epidural; evidence of disease

ED50 dose producing desired effect in 50% of subjects tested

EDB ethylene dibromide

EDC estimated date of confinement

EDD effective drug duration; expected date of delivery

EDR effective direct radiation

EDRF endothelium-derived relaxing factor

EDS Ehlers-Danlos syndrome

EDTA ethylenediaminetetra-acetic acid

EDU eating disorder unit

EEE eastern equine encephalitis; eastern equine encephalomyelitis

EEG electroencephalogram; electroencephalograph

EENT eye, ear, nose, and throat

EFA essential fatty acid

EFE endocardial fibroelastosis

EFM electronic fetal monitoring

EGD esophago-gastroduodenoscopy

EGF epidermal growth factor

EGOT erythrocyte glutamic oxaloacetic transaminase

EGF epidermal growth factor

EH enlarged heart; essential hypertension

EHBF estimated hepatic blood flow

EHBP essential high blood pressure

EHEC enterohemorrhagic *Escherichia coli*

EHO extrahepatic obstruction

EI enzyme inhibitor

EIA enzyme immunoassay; exercise-induced asthma

EIB exercise-induced bronchospasm

EIEC enteroinvasive *Escherichia coli*

EKG electrocardiogram; electrocardiograph

EKY electrokymogram

EL exercise limit

E-LAM endothelial leukocyte adhesion molecule

elev elevated

ELISA enzyme-linked immunosorbent assay

elix elixir

ELND elective lymph node dissection

ELOS estimated length of stay

ELP electrophoresis

ELSS Emergency Life Support System

EM electron micrograph; electron microscope; emergency medicine; external monitor

EMB endometrial biopsy

EMC endometrial curettage

EMF electromotive force

EMG electromyogram

EMIT enzyme-multiplied immunoassay technique

e.m.p. *ex modo prescripto* [Latin] in the manner prescribed

EMS early morning specimen; emergency medical service

emu electromagnetic unit

En enema

ENA extractable nuclear antigen

ENBS early neurobehavioral score

ENDO endoscopy

ENG electronystagmogram

ENT ear, nose, and throat

enz enzyme

EOG electro-oculogram; electro-olfactogram

EOM extraocular movement; extraocular muscle

EP ectopic pregnancy; electrophoresis; emergency procedure; erythropoietin

EPEC enteropathogenic *Escherichia coli*

EPI epinephrine; evoked potential index

epis episiotomy

epith epithelium

EPM electronic pacemaker

EPO eosinophil peroxidase

EPS exophthalmos-producing substance

EPSP excitatory postsynaptic potential

Eq equivalent

ER emergency room; endoplasmic reticulum; estrogen receptor; evoked response

Er erbium

ERA evoked response audiometry

ERBF effective renal blood flow

ERCP endoscopic retrograde cholangiopancreatography

ERE external rotation in extension

ERF external rotation in flexion

ERG electroretinogram

ERPF effective renal plasma flow

ERT estrogen replacement therapy

ERV expiratory reserve volume

ES extrasystole

Es einsteinium

ESEP extreme somatosensory evoked potential

ESF erythropoiesis-stimulating factor (erythropoietin)

ESKD end-stage kidney disease

ESP eosinophil stimulator promoter; extrasensory perception

ESR electron spin resonance; erythrocyte sedimentation rate

ESRD end stage renal disease

ESRD-DM end stage renal disease-diabetes mellitus

ESRF end stage renal failure

ESRT erythrocyte sedimentation rate test

EST electroshock therapy

Est estrogen
esu electrostatic unit
ESV end-systolic volume
ESWL extracorporeal shock wave lithotripsy
ET embryo transfer; endotracheal tube; etiology; eustachian tube
ETC estimated time of conception
ETEC enterotoxigenic *Escherichia coli*
E tO ethylene oxide
ETS environmental tobacco smoke
ETT endotracheal tube; exercise tolerance test
EU excretory urography
Eu europium
EUS external urethral sphincter
eV electron-volt
exog exogenous
EXP exploration
exp experiment; expired
expir expiration; expiratory
ext external; extraction
extens extension; extensor
extr extremity
Ez eczema

F

F factor; Fahrenheit; family; farad; fat; feces; female; fertility;flow; fluorine; formula; fracture; visual field
F1 first filial generation
F2 second filial generation
F3 third filial generation
F4 fourth filial generation
f fluid; focal length; frequency
FA false aneurysm; far advanced; fatty acid; fetal age; first aid; folic acid
FAAT fluorescent antinuclear antibody test
Fab antigen-binding fragment
FACS fluorescence-activated cell sorter
FAD familial Alzheimer's disease; flavin adenine dinucleotide
FAE fetal alcohol effects
FAM-M familial atypical mole and melanoma (syndrome)
FANA fluorescent antinuclear antibody
FAS fetal alcohol syndrome
FB feedback; foreign body
FBP femoral blood pressure
FBS fasting blood sugar; fetal blood sample
Fc crystallizable fragment (of immunoglobulin); footcandle
Fcath Foley catheter
FCC familial colorectal cancer
FCD fibrocystic disease
FCI flow cytometric immunophenotyping
FCIS Flint Colon Injury Scale
FCM flow cytometry
FCR fractional catabolic rate
FCS fetal cocaine syndrome
FD fatal dose; forceps delivery
FDIU fetal death *in utero*
FDLMP first day of last menstrual period
FDP fibrin degradation product; fibrinogen degradation product
FDS for duration of stay
Fe iron
feb. dur. *febre durante* [Latin] while the fever lasts
FECG fetal electrocardiogram
FEF forced expiratory flow
FES functional electrical stimulation
FET forced expiratory time
FEV forced expiratory volume
FEV1 forced expiratory volume in one second
FF fat free; flat feet; force fluids
FFA free fatty acids
FFC fixed flexion contracture
FFI free from infection
FFP fresh frozen plasma
FG fibrinogen
FGF fibroblast growth factor
FGT female genital tract
FH family history
FHCM familial hypertrophic cardiomyopathy
FHH fetal heart heard
FHNH fetal heart not heard
FHR fetal heart rate
FHT fetal heart tone
FHx family history
FICU fetal intensive care unit
FIGLU formiminoglutamic acid
fist fistula
FIUO for internal use only
fl fluid
fld field; fluid
fld rest fluid restriction
flex flexion
flex sig flexible sigmoidoscopy
flu influenza
fluoro fluoroscopy
FM face mask; fetal monitor; fetal movements; forensic medicine
Fm fermium
FMC fetal movement count
FMD foot-and-mouth disease
FMF familial Mediterranean fever; fetal movement felt
FMG foreign medical graduate
FMN flavin mononucleotide
FMP first menstrual period
FMX full mouth x-ray
FN false-negative
FNA fine needle aspiration
FNAB fine-needle aspiration biopsy
FOB fecal occult blood; fiberoptic bronchoscopy
FOD free of disease
FP false-positive; family physician; family planning; food poisoning; frozen plasma
fp freezing point
FPC familial polyposis coli
fps foot-pound-second (system of units)
fPt fasting patient
F&R force and rhythm (of pulse)
FR flocculation reaction
Fr francium
fract fracture
fract. dos. *fracta dosi* [Latin] in divided doses
FRC functional residual capacity
FRJM full range of joint movement
Fru fructose
FSGN focal sclerosing glomerulonephritis; focal segmental glomerulosclerosis
FSH follicle-stimulating hormone
FSH-LH follicle-stimulating hormone-luteinizing hormone
FSH-RF follicle-stimulating hormone-releasing factor
FSH-RH follicle stimulating hormone-releasing hormone
FSP fibrin split product
FST foam stability test
FT family therapy; full term
FTA fluorescent titer antibody
FTG full thickness graft
FTND full term normal delivery
FTR for the record
FTA-ABS fluorescent treponema antibody-absorption (test)
FTT failure to thrive
FTTS failure to thrive syndrome
FU follow up
FUDR floxuridine; fluorodeoxyuridine
FUE fever of undetermined etiology
FUO fever of undetermined origin; fever of unknown origin
FVC forced vital capacity
FWB full weight-bearing
Fx fracture
Fx-dis fracture-dislocation
FXS fragile X syndrome

G

G gas; gauge; gauss; gingiva; glucose; glycine; glycogen; gram; guanosine
g gender; gram; gravitational constant; gravity; group
GA gastric analysis; general anesthesia; gestational age
Ga gallium
GABA gamma-aminobutyric acid
GALT gut-associated lymphoid tissue
gang ganglion
gast fl gastric fluid
GB gallbladder
GBM glomerular basement membrane
GBG glycine-rich beta-glycoprotein
GC gas chromatography; geriatric

care; gonococcus; gonorrheal cervicitis

GCS Glasgow Coma Scale

G-CSF granulocyte colony-stimulating factor

GCT giant cell tumor

G & D growth and development

Gd gadolinium

GDM gestational diabetes mellitus

GDS gradual dosage schedule

GE gastroenterology; gel electrophoresis

Ge germanium

GEJ gastroesophageal junction

GEN gender; generic; genetics; genital

gen'l general

GEPH gestational edema with proteinuria and hypertension

GER gastroesophageal reflux; geriatrics

GERD gastroesophageal reflux disease

GF gastric fluid; germ-free; growth factor

GFR glomerular filtration rate

GGG glycine-rich gammaglycoprotein

GH growth hormone; general hospital

GHD growth hormone deficiency

GH-RH growth hormone-releasing hormone

GHT glycosylated hemoglobin test

GI gastrointestinal; gingival index

GIF glycosylation inhibition factor

GIFT gamete intrafallopian transfer

GIP gastric inhibitory polypeptide

GIS gas in stomach; gastrointestinal series

GIT gastrointestinal tract

GJ gap junction; gastrojejunostomy

GL gastric lavage

gl. gland

g / l grams per liter

GLC gas-liquid chromatography

glc glaucoma

Gln glutamine

Glu glucose; glutamic acid

Gly glycine

gm gram

GM-CSF granulocyte-macrophage colony-stimulating factor

GMP guanosine monophosphate (guanylic acid)

GN glomerulonephritis; gram-negative

Gn gonadotropin

GN-RH gonadotropin-releasing hormone

GOT glutamic-oxaloacetic transaminase

GP general paresis; gram-positive

gp glycoprotein

G6PD glucose-6-phosphate dehydrogenase

GPI gingival-periodontal index

GPT glutamic pyruvic transaminase

gr grain

GRAS generally regarded as safe

grav gravid

GS general surgery; glomerular sclerosis

GSC gas-solid chromatography

GSD-1 glycogen storage disease, type 1

GSE grip strong and equal

GSH growth-stimulating hormone

GST genetic screening test

GSW gunshot wound

GT glucose tolerance; guaiac test

gt. *gutta* [Latin] a drop

GTD gestational trophoblastic disease

GTP guanosine triphosphate

GTT glucose tolerance test

gtt. *guttae* [Latin] drops

GU gastric ulcer; genitourinary

GUS genitourinary system

GV gingivectomy

GVH graft-versus-host (disease or reaction)

GVHD graft-versus-host disease

GVHR graft-versus-host reaction

GXT graded exercise test

GYN gynecology

H

H heart; hemisphere; henry; hernia; heroin; hot; hydrogen; hyperopia

H+ hydrogen ion

1H hydrogen-1

2H hydrogen-2

3H hydrogen-3

h height; horizontal; hour; hundred

h Planck's constant

HA headache; hearing aid; hemolytic anemia; hepatitis A; high anxiety; hospital admission

H/A headache

HAA hepatitis-associated antigen

HAAg hepatitis A antigen

HAC hyperactive child

HAE hereditary angioneurotic edema

HAI hospital-acquired infection

HAL hyperalimentation

HANE hereditary angioneurotic edema

HAP hospital-acquired pneumonia

HAPE high altitude pulmonary edema

HAPS hepatic arterial perfusion scintigraphy

HAQ Headache Assessment Questionnaire; Health Assessment Questionnaire

HARM hypertension, anemia, renal, malabsorption

HAS hypertensive arteriosclerosis

HASHD hypertensive arteriosclerotic heart disease

HAV hepatitis A virus

HB bundle of His; heart block; hepatitis B;

Hb hemoglobin

HbA adult hemoglobin; hemoglobin A

HBAb hepatitis B antibody

HBAg hepatitis B antigen

HbAS heterozygosity for hemoglobin A and hemoglobin S

HBB hospital blood bank

HBc hepatitis B core

HBcAb antibody to hepatitis B core antigen

HBcAg hepatitis B core antigen

HbCO carboxyhemoglobin

HBe hepatitis B e

HbE hemoglobin E

HBeAb antibody to hepatitis B e antigen

HBeAg hepatitis B e antigen

HbF fetal hemoglobin; hemoglobin F

HBGM home blood glucose monitoring

HbH hemoglobin H

HBIG hepatitis B immune globulin

HbO_2 oxyhemoglobin

HBOT hyperbaric oxygen therapy

HBP high blood pressure

HbS hemoglobin S

HBs hepatitis B surface

HBsAb antibody to the hepatitis B surface antigen

HBsAg hepatitis B surface antigen

HBV hepatitis B virus

HBW high birth weight

HC head circumference; hydrocortisone

HCC hepatocellular carcinoma

HCD heavy chain disease

hCG human chorionic gonadotropin

HCL hairy-cell leukemia; hard contact lens

HCM hypertrophic cardiomyopathy

HCO_3 bicarbonate

HCP health care provider

hCS human chorionic somatomammotropin

Hct hematocrit

HCV hepatitis C virus

HCVD hypertensive cardiovascular disease

HD herniated disk; high dose; Hodgkin's disease; hospital day; Huntington's disease

h.d. *heloma durum* [Latin] hard corn; *hora decubitus* [Latin] at bedtime

HDCV human diploid-cell vaccine

HDL high-density lipoprotein

HDL-C high-density lipoprotein cholesterol

HDN high-density nebulizer

HDRV human diploid cell rabies vaccine

HDU hemodialysis unit

HDV hepatitis D (Delta) virus

H&E hematoxylin and eosin (stain); heredity and environment

He helium

HEENT head, ears, eyes, nose, and throat

HELLP hemolysis, elevated liver function, low platelets

hem hemorrhage; hemorrhoid

hep heparin; hepatitis

HEV hepatitis E virus; high endothelial venules

HF hay fever; heart failure

Hf hafnium

HFD	high forceps delivery
HFHL	high-frequency hearing loss
HFMD	hand-foot-and-mouth disease
HFPPV	high-frequency positive pressure ventilation
Hfr	high frequency
HG	herpes genitalis
Hg	hemoglobin; mercury
Hgb	hemoglobin
hG	human gonadotropin
hGH	human growth hormone
hgt	height
HH	hard of hearing; hiatal hernia
HHN	hand-held nebulizer
HHV	human herpesvirus
HI	head injury; health insurance
HIDA	dimethyl iminodiacetic acid
His	histidine
HIV	human immunodeficiency virus
HIV-1	human immunodeficiency virus type 1
HIV-2	human immunodeficiency virus type 2
HIVD	herniated intervertebral disk
HL	hearing level; hearing loss
HLA	human leukocyte antigen
HLD	herniated lumbar disk
hLH	human luteinizing hormone
HM	heart murmur; human milk
Hm	manifest hyperopia
HMD	hyaline membrane disease
hMG	human menopausal gonadotropin
HMG-CoA	b-hydroxy-b-methylglutaryl-CoA
HMO	health maintenance organization
HNP	herniated nucleus pulposus
HNV	has not voided
Ho	holmium
HOCM	hypertrophic obstructive cardiomyopathy
HOH	hard of hearing
HOPA	hospital-based organ procurement agency
hor. decub.	*hora decubitus* [Latin] at bedtime
hor. som.	*hora somni* [Latin] at bedtime
HP	handicapped person; hot pack; house physician
Hp	*Helicobacter pylori*
H&P	history and physical (examination)
HPA	hypothalamic-pituitary-adrenal
HPD	high protein diet; home peritoneal dialysis
hPL	human placental lactogen
HPLC	high-pressure liquid chromatography; high performance liquid chromatography
HPV	human papillomavirus
HPVD	hypertensive pulmonary vascular disease
HR	heart rate; hospital record
H&R	hysterectomy and radiation
HRCT	high-resolution computed tomography
HRF	homologous restriction factor
HRIG	human rabies immune globulin (vaccine)
HRP	horseradish peroxidase
HRT	hormone replacement therapy
HRV	human rotavirus
HS	half-strength; hazardous substance; heart sounds; herpes simplex
h.s.	*hora somni* [Latin] at bedtime
HSA	human serum albumin
HSAS	hypertrophic subaortic stenosis
HSE	herpes simplex encephalitis
HSV	herpes simplex virus
HT	hammertoe; Hashimoto's thyroiditis; height; high temperature; hypertension; hypertropia
Ht	heart; height; total hyperopia
HTL	hearing threshold level
HTLV-I	human T-cell leukemia virus-type I
HTLV-II	human T-cell leukemia virus-type II
HTLV-III	human T-cell leukemia virus-type III
HTN	hypertension
hTSS	human toxic shock syndrome
HUGO	Human Genome Organization
HUS	hemolytic-uremic syndrome
HV	has voided; herpes virus; hyperventilation
HVA	hemovanillic acid
HVD	hypertensive vascular disease
HVGR	host-versus-graft reaction
Hx	history; hospitalization
Hy	hyperopia
Hyg	hygiene
hypno	hypnosis
hypo	hypodermic syringe
hyst	hysterectomy
HZ	herpes zoster
Hz	hertz

I

I	intensity of electric current; intensity of magnetism; iodine
^{125}I	radioactive isotope of iodine, with a half-life of 57.4 days
^{131}I	radioactive isotope of iodine, with a half-life of 8.05 days
IA	image amplification; incurred accidently; infected area
I& A	irrigation and aspiration
IABC	intra-aortic balloon catheter
IABP	intra-aortic balloon pump
IAO	immediately after onset
IAP	intermittent acute porphyria
IASD	interatrial septal defect
IAT	impedance audiometry test; intraoperative autologous transfusion
IB	inclusion body; infectious bronchitis
IBC	iron-binding capacity
IBD	inflammatory bowel disease
IBI	intermittent bladder irrigation
IBS	irritable bowel syndrome
IC	indwelling catheter; inspiratory capacity; intensive care; intermittent catheterization; intracranial; irritable colon
i.c.	*inter cibos* [Latin] between meals
ICA	internal carotid artery; intracranial aneurysm
ICAO	internal carotid artery occlusion
ICC	intensive coronary care
ICCE	intracapsular cataract extraction
ICCU	intensive coronary care unit
ICD	immune complex disease; *International Classification of Diseases of the World Health Organization;* intrauterine contraceptive device
ICD 9 CM	*International Classification of Diseases, Ninth Revision, Clinical Modification*
ICF	intermediate care facility; intracellular fluid
ICH	intracranial hemorrhage
ICIDH	International Classification of Impairments, Disabilities, and Handicaps
ICN	intensive care nursery
ICP	intracranial pressure
ICPP	intubated continuous positive pressure
ICS	intercostal space
ICSH	interstitial cell-stimulating hormone
ICT	indirect Coombs' test; insulin coma therapy
ICU	intensive care unit
ICW	intracellular water
ID	idiotype; immunodeficiency; infectious disease; infective dose; initial dose
id.	*idem* [Latin] the same
I&D	incision and drainage; irrigation and drainage
IDA	iron deficiency anemia; iminodiacetic acid
IDAM	infant of drug-abusing mother
IDDM	insulin-dependent diabetes mellitus
IDIPF	idiopathic diffuse interstitial pulmonary fibrosis
IDK	internal derangement of the knee
IDM	infant of diabetic mother
IDP	intraductal papilloma
IDU	idoxuridine; injecting-drug user
IE	infective endocarditis
IEL	intraepithelial lymphocyte
IEM	inborn error of metabolism
IF	interferon; interstitial fluid; intrinsic factor
IFA	indirect fluorescent antibody (test)
IFE	immunofixation electrophoresis
IFN	interferon
IFN-a	interferon alpha

IFN-b interferon beta
Ig immunoglobulin
IgA immunoglobulin A (gamma A globulin)
IgD immunoglobulin D (gamma D globulin)
IGDM infant of gestational diabetic mother
IgE immunoglobulin E (gamma E globulin)
IGF insulin-like growth factor
IgG immunoglobulin G (gamma G globulin)
IgM immunoglobulin M (gamma M globulin)
IGT impaired glucose tolerance
IGTT intravenous glucose tolerance test
IH immediate hypersensitivity; inguinal hernia
IHB incomplete heart block
IHD ischemic heart disease
IHSS idiopathic hypertrophic subaortic stenosis
IICU infant intensive care unit
IL interleukin
IL 1 interleukin 1
IL 2 interleukin 2
IL 3 interleukin 3
IL 4 interleukin 4
IL 5 interleukin 5
IL 6 interleukin 6
IL 7 interleukin 7
IL 8 interleukin 8
IL 9 interleukin 9
IL 10 interleukin 10
IL 11 interleukin 11
IL 12 interleukin 12
IL 13 interleukin 13
IL 14 interleukin 14
IL 15 interleukin 15
ILD inflammatory lung disease; interstitial lung disease
Ile isoleucine
IM infectious mononucleosis; intramuscular
im intramuscular
IMB intermenstrual bleeding
ImD50 median immunizing dose
IMR individual medical record; infant mortality rate
IMV intermittent mandatory ventilation
IN internist; interstitial nephritis
In indium
INC incontinence
in d. *in dies* [Latin] daily
IndMed *Index Medicus*
INF interferon; intravenous nutritional feeding
inf infection; inferior
INFH ischemic necrosis of femoral head
inj injection
Ino inosine
inop inoperable
IN-PT inpatient
INR international normalized ratio
Ins insulin; insurance
INT intermittent; internal; internist
int. cib. *inter cibos* [Latin] between meals
int. noct. *inter noctem* [Latin] during the night
int obst intestinal obstruction
I&O intake and output
IODAM infant of drug-addicted mother
IODM infant of diabetic mother
IOF intraocular fluid
IOP intraocular pressure
IOV initial office visit
IP incubation period; inpatient; interphalangeal (joint); intraperitoneal
IPA invasive pulmonary aspergillosis
IPCD infantile polycystic disease
IPD inflammatory pelvic disease; intermittent peritoneal dialysis
IPJ interphalangeal joint
IPP inflatable penile prosthesis; intermittent positive pressure
IPPA inspection, palpation, percussion, and auscultation
IPPB intermittent positive pressure breathing
IPPV intermittent positive pressure ventilation
IPSID immunoproliferative small intestinal disease
IPSP inhibitory postsynaptic potential
IPT immunologic pregnancy test
IPV inactivated poliovirus vaccine
IQ intelligence quotient
i.q. *idem quod* [Latin] the same as
IR immune response; infrared; insulin reaction; insulin resistance; insulin resistant
Ir iridium
IRC inspiratory reserve capacity
IRDS infant respiratory distress syndrome
IRMA immunoradiometric assay
IRV inspiratory reserve volume
IS immunosuppressive; inguinal syndrome; intercostal space
ISA intrinsic sympathomimetic activity
ISD iron-storage disease
ISF interstitial fluid
ISG immune serum globulin
i.s.q. *in status quo* [Latin] unchanged
IT immunity test; inhalation therapy
ITP idiopathic thrombocytopenic purpura
IU immunizing unit; International Units; intrauterine
IUD intrauterine (contraceptive) device
IUI intrauterine insemination
IV interventricular; intravenous
i.v. *in vitro* [Latin] within glass; *in vivo* [Latin] within a living body
IVC inferior vena cava; inspiratory vital capacity
IVD intervertebral disk
IVDA intravenous drug abuse; intravenous drug abuser
IVF *in vitro* fertilization
IVF-ET *in vitro* fertilization and embryo transfer
IVH intraventricular hemorrhage
IVIg intravenous immunoglobulin
IVP intravenous pyelogram
IVT intravenous transfusion
IVU intravenous urogram

J

J joint; joule; journal; juvenile
JA juvenile atrophy
JAMA *Journal of the American Medical Association*
JAMG juvenile autoimmune myasthenia gravis
jc juice
JCA juvenile chronic arthritis
JCML juvenile chronic myelocytic leukemia
jct junction
JCV JC virus
JD juvenile diabetes
JDC Joslin Diabetes Center
JDM juvenile-onset diabetes mellitus
jej jejunum
JG juxtaglomerular
JGA juxtaglomerular apparatus
JGC juxtaglomerular complex
j-g complex juxtaglomerular complex
JLP juvenile laryngeal papilloma
jnt joint
JOD juvenile-onset diabetes
JODM juvenile-onset diabetes mellitus
Jour journal
JPB junctional premature beat
JPS juvenile polyposis syndrome
JRA juvenile rheumatoid arthritis
J seg joining segment (of DNA encoding immunoglobulins)
junct junction
JV jugular vein
JVD jugular venous distention
JVP jugular venous pressure; jugular venous pulse
JXG juvenile xanthogranuloma

K

K constant; kidney; kilogram; potassium; lysine; coefficient of sclera rigidity
k constant; Kelvin; reaction rate
KA ketoacidosis
ka cathode
KB ketone bodies
kb kilobase
KC keratoconus; Kupffer cells
kc kilocycle

kcal large calorie
K cell killer cell
KCS keratoconjunctivitis sicca
KD knee disarticulation; kilodalton
KDA known drug allergies
keV kiloelectron-volt
Kg kilogauss; kilogram
KJ knee jerk
kl kiloliter
km kilometer
Kn knee
KNO keep needle open
KO keep open; knee orthosis
KOH potassium hydroxide
Kr krypton
KS Kaposi's sarcoma; ketosteroid
17-KS 17-ketosteroids
KS/OI Kaposi's sarcoma and opportunistic infections
KT kidney transplant
KTU kidney transplant unit
KUB kidney, ureter, and bladder
KUF kidney ultrafiltration rate
kv kilovolt
KVO keep vein open
kw kilowatt

L

L inductance; *Lactobacillus*; lambert; lethal; lidocaine; light; liter; lumbar vertebra; lumen; lung; lymphocyte; lysosome
l left; length; lethal; ligament; long
L1 first lumbar spinal nerve; first lumbar vertebra
L2 second lumbar spinal nerve; second lumbar vertebra
L3 third lumbar spinal nerve; third lumbar vertebra
L4 fourth lumbar spinal nerve; fourth lumbar vertebra
L5 fifth lumbar spinal nerve; fifth lumbar vertebra
LA left arm; left atrium; left auricle; local anesthesia; long acting; low anxiety
L&A light and accommodation (reaction of the pupil); living and active
La labial; lanthanum
lab laboratory
LAC laceration; long-arm cast
LADCA left anterior descending coronary artery
LAE left atrial enlargement
LAF leukocyte-activating factor
LAG lymphangiogram
LAH left atrial hypertrophy
LAK lymphokine-activated killer (cells)
LAL left axillary line
LAM late ambulatory monitoring; left atrial myxoma
lam laminectomy; laminogram
LAMB lentigines, atrial myxoma, mucocutaneous myxomas, and blue nevi
lami laminotomy
LAO left anterior oblique (view)
LAP laparotomy; left arterial pressure; leukocyte alkaline phosphatase
laryn. laryngitis
LAS laxative abuse syndrome; long-arm splint; lower abdominal surgery
LASER light amplification by stimulated emission of radiation
LASH left anterosuperior hemiblock
LASIK laser-assisted *in situ* keratomileusis
L-ASP L-asparaginase
lat latent; lateral; latex
lat men lateral meniscectomy
LATS long-acting thyroid stimulator
LAV lymphadenopathy-associated virus
lax. laxative
LB large bowel; left breast; left buttock; live birth
LBAT leukocyte bactericidal assay test
LBB left breast biopsy
LBBB left bundle branch block
LBH length, breadth, and height
LBM lean body mass
LBO large bowel obstruction
LBP low back pain; low blood pressure
LBW low birth weight
LC lethal concentration; low calorie
LCA left coronary artery; left carotid artery
LCCA left circumflex coronary artery; left common carotid artery
LCCS low cervical cesarean section
LCD liquid crystal display
LCIS lobular carcinoma *in situ*
LCL lateral capsular ligament; lymphocytic leukemia
LCLC large cell lung carcinoma
LCM lymphocytic choriomeningitis
LCMV lymphocytic choriomeningitis virus
LCR laser correlational spectroscopy; late cutaneous reaction
LCS low continuous suction
LD learning disability; lethal dose; levodopa; living donor; low dosage; Lyme disease
LD_{50} median dose that will kill within a stated time 50% of the animals inoculated
L&D labor and delivery
LDH lactate dehydrogenase
LDL low-density lipoprotein; loudness discomfort level
LDL-C low-density lipoprotein cholesterol
L-dopa levodopa
LDR labor, delivery, and recovery (room)
LE left eye; lower extremity; lupus erythematosus
LE cell lupus erythematosus cell
LEEP loop electrosurgical excision procedure
leio. leiomyoma
LEL lowest effect level
LE prep lupus erythematosus preparation
LES Lambert-Eaton syndrome; local excitatory state; lower esophageal sphincter
Leu leucine
leuk. leukemia
LF low forceps; low frequency
LFA left femoral artery; left frontoanterior (fetal position); low friction arthroplasty; lymphocyte functional antigen
LFD lactose-free diet; low fat diet
LFH left femoral hernia
LFP left frontoposterior (fetal position)
LFT left frontotransverse (fetal position)
LG laryngectomy
lg large
LGA large for gestational age
LGL large granular lymphocyte
lgth length
LGV lymphogranuloma venereum
LH left hand; luteinizing hormone
LHC left hypochondrium
LHF left heart failure
LH-RH luteinizing hormone-releasing hormone
Li lithium
LIC left iliac crest
LICA left internal carotid artery
LICM left intercostal margin
LICS left intercostal space
LIF left iliac fossa; leukocyte inhibiting factor
lig. *ligamentum* [Latin] ligament
ligg ligature
LIH left inguinal hernia
LIP lymphocytic interstitial pneumonia
liq liquid
LIS locked-in syndrome
litho lithotripsy
LK left kidney
LL large lymphocyte; lymphoblastic lymphoma
LLC long-leg cast
LLD leg length discrepancy
LLE left lower extremity
LLL left long leg (brace); left lower limb; left lower lobe (of lung)
LLQ left lower quadrant (of abdomen)
LLS long-leg splint
LLWC long-leg walking cast
LM light microscopy
lm lumen
LMA left mentoanterior (fetal position)
LMCA left main coronary artery
LME left mediolateral episiotomy
LMI leukocyte migration inhibition
L/min liters per minute

LMM lentigo maligna melanoma
LMN lower motor neuron
LMP last menstrual period; left mentoposterior
(fetal position); lumbar puncture
LMT left mentotransverse (fetal position)
LN lymph node
LNB lymph node biopsy
LNMP last normal menstrual period
LOA left occipito-anterior (fetal position)
LOC laxative of choice; level of care; level of consciousness; loss of consciousness
loc. dol. *loco dolenti* [Latin] to the painful spot
LOI level of injury
LOM left otitis media; limitation of movement
LoNa low sodium
LOP left occipitoposterior (fetal position)
LOS length of stay
LOT left occipitotransverse (fetal position)
lot. *lotio* [Latin] lotion
LP light perception; lipoprotein; lumbar puncture
Lp(a) lipoprotein (a)
LPA lysophosphatidic acid
L proj. light projection
LPS last Papanicolaou smear; lipopolysaccharide
LPV left pulmonary vein; lymphotropic papovavirus
lq liquid
LR labor room; light reaction
Lr lawrencium
LRA left renal artery
LRD living related donor; living renal donor
LRH luteinizing hormone-releasing hormone
LRI lower respiratory infection
LRR labor room
LRV left renal vein
LS lichen sclerosis; lumbosacral
L/S lecithin/sphingomyelin (ratio)
LSA left sacroanterior (fetal position)
LSCS lower segment cesarean section
LSCV left subclavian vein
LSD life-sustaining device; lysergic acid
diethylamide
LSH lutein-stimulating hormone
LSK liver, spleen, and kidneys
LSO lumbosacral orthosis
LSV left subclavian vein
LT left; leukotriene; long term; low temperature
lt left
LTC long-term care
LTCS low transverse cesarean section
LTG long-term goal
LTM long-term memory
Lu lutetium
LUE left upper extremity
LUL left upper limb; left upper lobe (of lung)
lum lumbar
LUQ left upper quadrant (of abdomen)
LV left ventricle; leukemia virus; live vaccine; lung volume
Lv leave
LVA left ventricular aneurysm
LVAD left ventricular assist device
LVD left ventricular dysfunction
LVE left ventricular enlargement
LVET left ventricular ejection time
LVF left ventricular failure
LVH left ventricular hypertrophy
LVI left ventricular insufficiency
LVM left ventricular mass
LVSP left ventricular systolic pressure
LW lacerating wound
LX local irradiation
lym lymphocyte
Lys lysine

M

μ micron
M echomotion; male; malignant; married; mass; massage; maximum; median; memory; meter; minimum; mol; molar; murmur; muscle; myopia
m meter; molar; motile; murmur; muscle
m. *misce* [Latin] mix; *musculus* [Latin] muscle
mm millimicron
M/3 middle third
MA menstrual age; mental age; milliampere
mA milliampere
ma milliampere
MAA macroaggregated albumin
Mab monoclonal antibody
MABP mean arterial blood pressure
MAC maximum allowable concentration (of hazardous substance); membrane-attack complex; *Mycobacterium avium* complex; macrophage-activating factor
Mac-1 macrophage-1 glycoprotein
MAD mind-altering drug
MAIDS murine acquired immune deficiency syndrome
MAL midaxillary line
malig malignant
MALT mucosa-associated lymphoid tissue
mammo mammogram
mand mandible
man. pr. *mane primo* [Latin] early in the morning
MAO monoamine oxidase; maximal acid output
MAOI monoamine oxidase inhibitor
MAP mean airway pressure; mean arterial pressure; muscle action potential
MAS meconium aspiration syndrome
mas masculine
MASER microwave amplification by stimulated emission of radiation
MASH mobile army surgical hospital
MAST medical antishock trousers
mast mastoid
MAT multifocal atrial tachycardia
max maxillary; maximum
m.b. *misce bene* [Latin] mix well
Mb myoglobin
MBC maximum breathing capacity
MBD minimal brain damage; minimal brain dysfunction
MBL menstrual blood loss
MBM mother's breast milk
MBP myelin basic protein; mean blood pressure
MBPS Munchausen-by-proxy syndrome
MC mast cell; maximum concentration; metacarpal; miscarriage
M&C morphine and cocaine
mCi millicurie
MCA middle carotid artery; middle cerebral artery; multiple congenital abnormalities
McB pt McBurney's point
MCC midstream clean-catch (urine sample)
MCD minimal change disease
mcg microgram
MCH mean corpuscular hemoglobin
MCHC mean corpuscular hemoglobin concentration
MCL maximum contamination level; midclavicular line
MCP membrane cofactor protein;
metacarpophalangeal (joint)
M-CSF macrophage colony- stimulating factor
MCT mean circulating time; medium-chain triglycerides; mucin clot test
MCTD mixed connective tissue disease
MCU maximum care unit
MCV mean corpuscular volume
MD manic-depressive; mean deviation; mental deficiency; muscular dystrophy
Md mendelevium
MDD male development disorder; major depressive disorder; mean daily dose
MDF myocardial depressant factor
MDI manic depressive illness
MDMA 3,4-methylene dioxymeth-amphetamine
mdn median
MDR multidrug resistance
MDRI multidrug-resistant infection
MDY month, date, and year
ME macular edema; medial episiotomy; ediastinalemphysema; middle ear
Me methyl

mec	meconium
MED	medicine; medium; minimal effective dose
med	medial; medicine
MEDLARS	MEDical Literature Analysis and Retrieval System
MEDLINE	MEDlars on-LINE
med men	medial meniscectomy
MEE	middle ear effusion
MEFR	maximal expiratory flow rate
MEN	multiple endocrine neoplasia
mEq	milliequivalent
MESA	microsurgical epididymal sperm aspiration
MET	metastasis
Met	methionine
MetHb	methemoglobin
m. et n.	*mane et nocte* [Latin] morning and night
m. et sig.	*misce et signa* [Latin] mix and label
MeV	megavolt; million electron volts
MF	mitogenic factor; mycosis fungoides
M&F	male and female; mother and father
MFD	mid-forceps delivery; minimum fatal dose
MFW	multiple fragment wounds
MG	mammary gland; myasthenia gravis
Mg	magnesium
mg	milligram
MH	medical history; menstrual history
MHA	major histocompatibility antigen
MHC	major histocompatibility complex
MHD	minimum hemolytic dilution; minimum hemolytic dose
NHL	non-Hodgkin's lymphoma
M Hx	medical history
MHz	megahertz
MI	mitral insufficiency; myocardial infarction
MIC	minimal inhibitory concentration
MICU	medical intensive care unit
MID	minimal infecting dose; minimal inhibiting dose; multi-infarct dementia
mid/3	middle third
min	minimal; minor; minute
MIO	minimal identifiable odor
MIP	minimal invasive procedure
misc	miscarriage; miscellaneous
MIT	monoiodotyrosine
mIU	milli-International Unit
mks	meter-kilogram-second (system)
ML	malignant lymphoma
ml	milliliter
MLC	mixed leukocyte culture
MLD	minimal lethal dose
MLE	midline episiotomy
MLNS	mucocutaneous lymph node syndrome
MLR	mixed leukocyte reaction
MLS	mean life span; middle lobe syndrome
MM	medial malleolus; mucous membrane
mM	millimole; millimolar
mm	millimeter; mucous membrane
mm.	*musculi* [Latin] muscles
MMEF	maximal midexpiratory flow
MMFR	maximal midexpiratory flow rate
mmHg	millimeters of mercury
MMI	macrophage migration inhibition
mmol	millimole
MMPI	matrix metalloprotease inhibitor
mmpp	millimeters partial pressure
MMR	measles, mumps, rubella (vaccine)
MMT	manual muscle testing
MMWR	*Morbidity and Mortality Weekly Report*
MN	mononuclear
MND	motor neuron disease
Mn	manganese
MNJ	myoneural junction
MNM	motile (sperm) with normal morphology
MO	medulla oblongata; mineral oil
Mo	molybdenum
MOAb	monoclonal antibody
mod	moderate
MODS	multiple organ dysfunction syndrome
MODY	maturity-onset diabetes of youth
MOF	multiple organ failure
mol	mole; molecule
mol wt	molecular weight
MOM	milk of magnesia
MONAb	monoclonal antibody
monos	monocytes
MOPD	multiple oocytes per disk
MOR	morphine; morphology
mor. dict.	*moro dicto* [Latin] as directed
mOsm	milliosmole
MOTT	mycobacterium other than tubercle bacilli
MP	mean pressure; menstrual period; metacarpophalangeal (joint); middle phalanx; multiparous
mp	melting point
MPB	male pattern baldness
MPC	maximum permissible concentration
MPD	maximal permissible dose; multiple personality disorder
MPE	malignant pericardial effusion
MPS	meconium plug syndrome; mononuclear phagocyte system; mucopolysaccharidosis
MPV	mean platelet volume
MR	may repeat; medical record; Moro's reflex; mental retardation; mitral regurgitation
mR	milliroentgen
mrad	millirad
MRD	minimal reactive dose
mrem	millirem
MRI	magnetic resonance imaging
MPJ	metaphalangeal joint
mRNA	messenger ribonucleic acid
MRSA	methicillin-resistant *Staphylococcus aureus*
MRSE	methicillin-resistant *Staphylococcus epidermidis*
MS	mitral stenosis; morphine sulfate; multiple sclerosis; musculoskeletal
Ms	murmurs
ms	millisecond
MSAFP	maternal serum alfa-fetoprotein
msec	millisecond
MSG	monosodium glutamate
MSH	melanocyte-stimulating hormone
MSL	midsternal line
MSN	mildly subnormal
MST	mean survival time
MSUD	maple syrup urine disease
MT	major tranquilizer; mammary tumor
MT bar	metatarsal bar
MTD	maximal tolerated dose
MTDDA	Minnesota Test for Differential Diagnosis of Aphasia
mtDNA	mitochondrial deoxyribonucleic acid
MTF	modulation transfer function
MTJ	midtarsal joint
MTP	metatarsophalangeal (joint)
MTV	metatarsus varus
mu	million units; mouse unit
MUC	maximum urinary concentration
MUDDLES	miosis, urination, diarrhea, defecation, lacrimation, excitation, and salivation
multi-CSF	multi-colony-stimulating factor
multip	multiparous
MV	megavolt; mitral valve
mV	millivolt
MVC	maximum vital capacity
MVI	multiple vitamin infusion
MVP	mitral valve prolapse
MVS	mitral valve stenosis
MVV	maximal voluntary ventilation
MW	molecular weight
MWD	microwave diathermy
My	myopia
MZ	monozygotic (twins)

N

N	nasal; negative; nerve; nitrogen; normal
	(solution); normal concentration; number
n	nasal; neutron; refractive index
n.	*nervus* [Latin] nerve
Na	sodium
NAA	no apparent abnormalities
NABS	normoactive bowel sounds
NAD	nicotinamide adenine dinucleotide; no apparent distress; nothing abnormal detected
NADP	nicotinamide adenine dinucleotide phosphate

NAME nevi, atrial myxoma, myxoid neurofibroma, and ephilides
NANA N-acetylneuraminic acid
NANB non-A, non-B (hepatitis)
Narc narcotic
Narco narcolepsy
NAS no added salt
NB needle biopsy; newborn
Nb niobium
NBM no bowel movement; nothing by mouth
NBT nitroblue tetrazolium
NBTE nonbacterial thrombotic endocarditis
NBW normal birth weight
NC no change; no charge; no complaints; noncompliance; not completed
nCi nanocurie
NCT nerve conduction time
NCV nerve conduction velocity
ND natural death; neonatal death; new drug; no disease; normal delivery; notifiable disease
Nd neodymium
NE nerve ending; norepinephrine
Ne neon
NEC necrotizing enterocolitis
NED no evidence of disease; no expiration date
neg negative
NEFA nonesterified fatty acids
NEJM *New England Journal of Medicine*
NEO neonatology
NER no evidence of recurrence
NF *National Formulary;* neurofibromatosis
NFAR no further action required
NF-ET *in vitro* fertilization and embryo transfer
NFTD normal full-term delivery
NG nitroglycerin
ng nanogram; nasogastric
NGU nongonococcal urethritis
NHGRI National Human Genome Research Institute
NHL non-Hodgkin's lymphoma
NI neonatal isoerythrolysis; no improvement
Ni nickel
NICC neonatal intensive care center
NICU neonatal intensive care unit
NIDDM non-insulin dependent diabetes mellitus
NIH National Institutes of Health
NIHL noise-induced hearing loss
NIL nothing in light microscopy (disease)
NK natural killer (cells); no ketones
NKA no known allergies
NKDA no known drug allergies
NL normal limits
NLMC nocturnal leg muscle cramp
NM neuromuscular; nodular melanoma
nm nanometer
NMJ neuromuscular junction
NMP normal menstrual period
NMR nuclear magnetic resonance
NMS neuroleptic malignant syndrome
NMSC nonmelanoma skin cancer
nn. nerves
NNACS neonatal neurologic and adaptive capacity score
NND *New and Nonofficial Drugs*
NO nitric oxide
No nobelium; number
noct. maneq. *nocte maneque* [Latin] at night and in the morning
non rep. *non repetatur* [Latin] no refill
NOR noradrenaline
NO syntase nitric oxide syntase
NP nasopharynx; no pain; not pregnant
Np neptunium
NPC nasal point of conversion; no previous complaint
NPCC National Poison Control Center
NPH neutral protamine Hagedorn (insulin); no previous history; normal-pressure hydrocephalus
NPhx nasopharynx
NPN nonprotein nitrogen
n.p.o. *nulla per os* [Latin] nothing by mouth
NPT nocturnal penile tumescent
NR normal range; not recorded
NREM non-rapid eye movement (sleep)
nRNA nuclear ribonucleic acid
NRT nicotine replacement therapy
NS nephrosclerosis; nephrotic syndrome; nonsymptomatic; normal saline
NSA no significant abnormality
nsa no salt added
NSAIA nonsteroidal anti-inflammatory analgesic
NSAID nonsteroidal anti-inflammatory drug
NSC no significant change
NSD no significant defect
NSR normal sinus rhythm
NST nonstress test
NSU nonspecific urethritis
NT nasotracheal; nephrostomy tube; not tested
NTG nitroglycerin
NTMI nontransmural myocardial infarction
NTP normal temperature and pressure
NTS nucleus tractus solitarii
NTT nasotracheal tube
Nuc nucleoside
NUG necrotizing ulcerative gingivitis
NV neurovascular; next visit; nonvenereal
N&V nausea and vomiting
NVD nausea, vomiting, and diarrhea
nWA normal when awake
NWB non-weight-bearing
NYD not yet diagnosed

O

O opium; oxygen
o oral
o. *oculus* [Latin] eye
O^3 ozone
OA ocular albinism; old age; osteoarthritis
OAA oxaloacetic acid
OAD obstructive airway disease
OAS opiate abstinence syndrome
OB obstetrics; occult bleeding
OBD organic brain disease
OB/GYN obstetrics and gynecology
obl oblique
OBN occult blood negative
OBP occult blood positive
OBS organic brain syndrome
obs observation
OC on call; only child; oral contraceptive
OCA oculocutaneous albinism
OCCC oocyte-cumulus-corona complex
OCCM open chest cardiac massage
OCD obsessive-compulsive disorder; osteochondritis dissecans
OCT oxytocin challenge test
OD overdose
o.d. *omni die* [Latin] every day; *oculus dexter* [Latin] right eye
ODA right occipito-anterior (fetal position)
ODP right occipitoposterior (fetal position)
ODT right occipitotransverse (fetal position)
OGTT oral glucose tolerance test
OFA oncofetal antigen
OFC occipital frontal circumference
o.h. *omni hora* [Latin] every hour
OHA oral hyperglycemia agent
17-OHCS 17-hydroxycorticosteroid
OHS open heart surgery
OI opportunistic infection; osteogenesis imperfecta
OLD occupational lung disease
olf olfactory
OLP left occipitoposterior (fetal position)
OLT left occipitotransverse (fetal position)
OM osteomalacia; osteomyelitis; otitis media
omn. bih. *omni bihors* [Latin] every two hours
omn. hor. *omni hora* [Latin] every hour
omn. man. *omni mane* [Latin] every morning

omn. quar. hor. *omni quadrante hora* [Latin] every quarter of an hour
OMPA octamethyl pyrophosphoramide
OMS osteomalacia senile
ON overnight
ONCO oncology
ONTR order not to resuscitate
OOC out of control
OPD outpatient department
OPO organ procurement organization
OP operative procedure; osteoporosis
OPD outpatient department
OPt outpatient
OPTN Organ Procurement and Transportation Network
OPV oral poliovirus vaccine
OR open reduction (of a fracture); operating room
ORIF open reduction/internal fixation
Orn ornithine
ORT oral rehydration therapy
Ortho orthopedics
OS osteogenic sarcoma; osteosclerosis
Os osmium
o.s. *oculus siniste* [Latin] left eye
Osm osmole
OT occupational therapy; oral temperature; oxytocin
OTC over the counter (drugs)
o.u. *oculus uterque* [Latin] each eye
Ov ovary; ovum
OW open wedge
OXT oxytocin
oz ounce

P

P pain; passive; peripheral; phosphate; pint; placebo; plasma; positive; progesterone; pulse; pupil; short arm of chromosome
Palv alveolar pressure
Pao pressure at airway opening
Ppl pleural pressure
^{32}P phosphorus-32
p page; papilla; pint; pulse; pupil; short arm of chromosome
P1 first parental generation; first pulmonic heart sound
P2 second pulmonic heart sound
P/3 proximal third
PA paralysis agitans; pernicious anemia; posteroanterior; prior to admission; pulmonary artery
P-A posteroanterior
P&A percussion and auscultation
pA picoampere
PABA para-aminobenzoic acid
PAC premature atrial contraction
PAD peripheral arterial disease
p. ae. *partes aequale* [Latin] in equal parts
PAF platelet-activating factor; platelet-aggregating factor
PAH para-aminohippuric (acid); pulmonary artery hypertension; pulmonary artery hypotension
PAI-1 plasminogen activator inhibitor 1
PAL posterior axillary line
PALS periarteriolar lymphatic sheath
PAMP pulmonary arterial mean pressure
PAN polyarteritis nodosa
PAOD peripheral arterial occlusive disease
PAP Papanicolaou (test); peroxidase antiperoxidase (complex); prostatic acid phosphatase
Pap smear Papanicolaou smear
Pap test Papanicolaou test
P&PD percussion and postural drainage
PAR population attributable risk; postanesthesia room; pulmonary arteriolar resistance
paracent. paracentesis
part. aeq. *partes aequales* [Latin] in equal parts
PARR postanesthetic recovery room
PAS para-aminosalicylic (acid); periodic acid-Schiff (stain); pulmonary artery stenosis
PASA para-aminosalicylic acid
PAT paroxysmal atrial tachycardia; platelet aggregation test;preadmission testing
Path pathogenic; pathologic
PATI penetrating abdominal trauma index
PB paraffin bath; phenobarbital; premature birth
Pb lead
PBC primary biliary cirrhosis
PBD proliferative breast disease
PBG porphobilinogen
PBI protein-bound iodine
PBLC premature-birth living child
PBV percutaneous balloon valvuloplasty
PBZ pyribenzamine
PC platelet count; postcoital; premature contraction
p.c. *post cibum* [Latin] after a meal
PCA passive cutaneous anaphylaxis; patient-controlled anesthesia; posterior cerebral artery
PCAN potential child abuse and neglect
PCB polychlorinated biphenyl; postcoital bleeding
PCC Poison Control Center
PCCU postcoronary care unit
PCE physical capacities evaluation
PCG phonocardiogram
pCi picocurie
PCKD polycystic kidney disease
PCL persistent corpus luteum; posterior cruciate ligament
PCLD polycystic liver disease
PCM protein-calorie malnutrition
pCO_2 partial pressure of carbon dioxide
PCOS polycystic ovary syndrome
PCP phencyclidine pill (phencyclidine hydrochloride); *Pneumocystis carinii* pneumonia; primary care physician; principal care provider
PCR polymerase chain reaction; protein catabolic rate
PCT porphyria cutanea tarda; proximal convoluted tubule
pct percent
PCU pain control unit
PCV packed cell volume
PD patent ductus; periodontal disease; peritoneal dialysis; postnasal drainage; postnasal drip
PDA patent ductus arteriosus
PDGF platelet-derived growth factor
PDI periodontal disease index
PDLL poorly differentiated lymphocytic lymphoma
PDM periodontal membrane
PDR *Physicians' Desk Reference;* proliferative diabetic retinopathy
pdr powder
PDS peritoneal dialysis system
PE physical examination; pleural effusion; probable error; pulmonary edema; pulmonary embolism
PED pre-existing disease
PEEP positive end-expiratory pressure
PEFR peak expiratory flow rate
PEL permissible exposure limit
PEMF pulsating electromagnetic fields
Per permission
PERRLA pupils equal, round, and react(ive) to light and accommodation
PET positron emission tomography; pre-eclamptic toxemia
PETT positron emission transaxial tomography
PF peak factor; posterior fontanelle; pulmonary fibrosis; push fluids
Pf platelet factor
PFC pelvic flexion contracture; persistent fetal circulation; plaque-forming cell
PFFD proximal femoral focal deficiency
PFO patent foramen ovale
PFT pulmonary function test
PFU plaque-forming unit
PG postgraduate; pregnant; prostaglandin
pg page; picogram
PGA prostaglandin A
PGB prostaglandin B
PGH pituitary growth hormone
PGM phosphoglucomutase
PGU postgonococcal urethritis
PGY-1 first year postgraduate training
PGY-2 second year postgraduate training
PGY-3 third year postgraduate training
PGY-4 fourth year postgraduate training
PH past history; personal history; poor health
pH hydrogen-ion concentration
Ph 1 Philadelphia chromosome

PHA phytohemagglutinin
phal phalanges; phalanx
PHC posthospital care
PhD Doctor of Philosophy
Phe phenylalanine
phono phonocardiogram
PHP pseudo-hypoparathyroidism
PHT pulmonary hypertension
PhysTh physical therapy
PI periodontal index; physician intervention; pulmonary infarction; pulmonary insufficiency
PICU pediatric intensive care unit
PID pelvic inflammatory disease; prolapsed intervertebral disk
PIE pulmonary interstitial emphysema
PIF prolactin-inhibiting factor
PIH pregnancy-induced hypertension
PIP peak inspiratory pressure; proximal interphalangeal (joint); phosphatidylinositol 4-phosphate
PIP2 phosphatidylinositol 4,5-biphosphate
PIPJ proximal interphalangeal joint
PIVD protruded intervertebral disk
PJ Peutz-Jeghers (syndrome)
PK pyruvate kinase
PKD polycystic kidney disease
PKU phenylketonuria
PL placebo
Plfl pleural fluid
PLN pelvic lymph node
Plt platelet
plx plexus
PM pacemaker; petit mal; pneumomediastinum; presystolic murmur; prostatic massage
pM picomolar
PMB postmenopausal bleeding
PMBV percutaneous mitral balloon valvotomy
PMD progressive muscular dystrophy
PMF progressive massive fibrosis
PMHx past medical history
PMI past medical illness; point of maximum impulse
PML progressive multifocal leukoencephalopathy
PMN polymorphonuclear neutrophil
PMO postmenopausal osteoporosis
pmol picomole
PMP plasma membrane protein
PMR polymyalgia rheumatica
PM&R physical medicine and rehabilitation
PMS passive maternal smoking; premenstrual syndrome
PMT premenstrual tension
PN peripheral neuropathy; pyelonephritis
Pn pneumonia
PNB prostatic needle biopsy
PNC prenatal care
PND paroxysmal nocturnal dyspnea; postnasal drainage; postnasal drip
PNF proprioceptive neuromuscular facilitation
PNH paroxysmal nocturnal hemoglobinuria
PNI peripheral nerve injury
PNP peripheral neuropathy
PNPB positive-negative pressure breathing
PNS peripheral nervous system
Pnx pneumothorax
PO postoperative
Po polonium
p.o. *per os* [Latin] by mouth; postoperative
POA pancreatic oncofetal antigen
POC point of care; postoperative care
POD podiatry; postoperative day
POEMS polyneuropathy, organomegaly, endocrinopathy, monoclonal gammopathy, and skin changes (syndrome)
POL premature onset of labor
polio poliomyelitis
polys polymorphonuclear neutrophils
POMC pro-opiomelanocortin
POMR problem-oriented medical record
POP plaster of Paris
POR problem-oriented record
POS polycystic ovary syndrome; point of service
pos positive
POST peritoneal oocyte and sperm transfer
post posterior
post op postoperative
post-stim post-stimulation
pot. AGT potential abnormality of glucose tolerance
PP pink puffer; pin prick; postprandial; proximal phalanx; pyrophosphate
PPA phenylpropanolamine
PPBS postprandial blood sugar
PPCA proserum prothrombin conversion accelerator
PPD purified protein derivative (TB skin test); postpartum day
PPH primary pulmonary hypertension
PPHP pseudo-pseudohypoparathyroidism
PPLO pleuropneumonia-like organisms
ppm parts per million
PPMS postpoliomyelitis syndrome
PPO preferred-provider organization
PPPPPP pain, pallor, paresthesia, pulselessness,paralysis, prostration (mnemonic of 6 symptoms of acute arterial occlusion)
ppt precipitate
PR partial remission; peer review
Pr presbyopia
p.r. *per rectum* [Latin] through the rectum
PRA plasma renin activity
PRBC packed red blood cells
PRCA pure red cell aplasia
PRE progressive resistive exercise
pre-op preoperative
prep preparation (for surgery); prepare for
prev AGT previous abnormality of glucose tolerance
PRF prolactin-releasing factor
primip. primiparous
PRK photorefractive keratectomy
PRL prolactin
p.r.n. *pro re nata* [Latin] as needed
Pro proline
PROG progesterone
prog prognosis
PROM premature rupture of membranes
pron pronator; pronation
prot protein
pro time prothrombin time
prox proximal
prox/3 proximal third
PRP platelet-rich plasma
PRRE pupils round, regular, and equal
PS paradoxical sleep; pulmonary stenosis
P&S pain and suffering
PSA prostate-specific antigen
PSAT prostate-specific antigen test
PSC primary sclerosing cholangitis
PSGN poststreptococcal glomerulonephritis
psi pounds per square inch
PSIS posterosuperior iliac spine
PSO provider-sponsor organization
PSP phenolsulfonphthalein
PSRO Professional Standard Review Organization
PSS progressive systemic sclerosis
PT parathyroid; paroxysmal tachycardia; physical therapy; prothrombin time
Pt platinum
pt patient; pint
PTA plasma thromboplastin antecedent; phosphotungstic acid; percutaneous transluminal angioplasty; pretreatment anxiety; prior to admission
PTB patellar-tendon-bearing (base or prosthesis); prior to birth
PTC plasma thromboplastin component
PTCA percutaneous transluminal coronary angioplasty
PTD permanent and total disability; prior to discharge
PTH parathyroid hormone; posttransfusion hepatitis
PTP posterior tibial pulse
PTSD posttraumatic stress disorder
PTT partial thromboplastin time; patellar tendon transfer
PTU propylthiouracil
PTX pneumothorax; parathyroidectomy
PU peptic ulcer; pressure ulcer
Pu plutonium
PUBS percutaneous umbilical blood sampling
PUD peptic ulcer disease

PUE pyrexia of unknown etiology
PUL percutaneous ultrasonic lithotripsy
PUO pyrexia of unknown origin
PUPPP pruritic urticarial papules and plaques of pregnancy
PUVA psoralen (plus) ultraviolet A
PV polycythemia vera; portal vein
p.v. *per vaginam* [Latin] through the vagina
PVC polyvinyl chloride; premature ventricular contraction
PVD peripheral vascular disease
PVE prosthetic valvular endocarditis
PVL periventricular leukomalacia
PVP polyvinylpyrrolidone
PVS persistent vegetative state
pvt private
PW plantar wart
PWA person with AIDS
PWB partial weight-bearing
PWM pokeweed mitogen
Px physical examination; pneumothorax; prognosis
PXE pseudoxanthoma elasticum
PYLL potential years of life lost
PZI protamine zinc insulin

Q

Q coulomb; electric quantity; quadrant; quantity; question; quotient; volume of blood
q long arm of chromosome
q. *quaque* [Latin] every
QA quality assurance
q.a.m. *quaque ante meridiem* [Latin] every morning
QC quality control
QCT quantitative computed tomography
q.d. *quaque die* [Latin] every day
q.d.s. *quater die sumendum* [Latin] to be taken four times daily
QF quick freeze
q.h. *quaque hora* [Latin] every hour
q.2h. *quaque secunda hora* [Latin] every 2 hours
q.3h. *quaque tertia hora* [Latin] every 3 hours
q.h.s. *quaque hora somni* [Latin] at bedtime
q.i.d. *quater in die* [Latin] four times a day
q.l. *quantum libet* [Latin] as much as desired
q.m. *quaque mane* [Latin] every morning
q.n. *quaque nocte* [Latin] every night
q.p. *quantum placeat* [Latin] as much as desired
QPC quality of patient care
q.q.h. *quaque quarta hora* [Latin] every four hours
QR quick recovery
QS quiet sleep
q.s. *quantum sufficit* [Latin] sufficient amount
q. suff. *quantum sufficit* [Latin] sufficient amount
QT quiet
quad quadriceps; quadriplegic
quant quantity
quotid. *quotidie* [Latin] daily
q.v. *quo vide* [Latin] which see

R

R arginine; gas constant; organic radical; race; rate; reaction; rectum; regular; resident; resistance; respiratory rate/min; review; right (eye); roentgen; rough; rub
Raw airway resistance (resistance of tracheo-bronchial tree to flow of air into lungs
r oxidation-reduction potential; roentgen
RA radioactive; radium; ragweed antigen; residual air; rheumatoid arthritis; right atrium
Ra radium
RAD right axis deviation
rad radiation absorbed dose
RAE right atrium enlargement
RAI radioactive iodine
RAIU radioactive iodine uptake (test)
RAM random access memory
RANA rheumatoid agglutinin nuclear antigen
RAO right anterior-oblique (view)
RAS reticular activating system; rheumatoid arthritis serum
RA slide rheumatoid arthritis slide (test)
RAST radioallergosorbent test
RAU recurrent aphthous ulceration
RAV Rous-associated virus
RB right bronchus; right buttock
Rb rubidium
RBA rescue breathing apparatus
RBB right breast biopsy
RBBB right bundle branch block
RBC red blood cell; red blood count
rbc red blood cell
RBE relative biological effectiveness
RBF renal blood flow
RBN retrobulbar neuritis
RBOW ruptured bag of waters
RBP resting blood pressure
RBS random blood sugar
rBST recombinant bovine somatotropin
RC radial-carpal; red cell; Red Cross; retention catheter; root canal; rotator cuff
RCA right coronary artery
RCC rape crisis center; red cell count; renal cell carcinoma
RCG radiocardiography
R/CS repeat cesarean section
RCT root canal therapy
RCV red cell volume
RD reaction of degeneration; renal dialysis; retinal detachment; ruptured disk
RDA recommended dietary allowance
rDNA recombinant deoxyribonucleic acid
RDS respiratory distress syndrome
RDT regular dialysis treatment
RDVT recurrent deep vein thrombosis
RE rectal examination; regional enteritis; reticuloendothelial; retinol equivalent; retrograde ejaculation; right eye
Re rhenium
REC radioelectrocardiogram
Rec recommendation
rec'd received
redox reduction oxidation
REG radioencephalogram
REL recommended exposure limit
REM rapid eye movement
rem roentgen-equivalent-man
REM sleep rapid eye movement sleep
ren. sem. *renovetum semel* [Latin] renewable only once
REO respiratory enteric orphan (virus)
rep. *repetatur* [Latin] let it be renewed; report
RER rough endoplasmic reticulum
RES research; reticuloendothelial system
REVL reviewed by laboratory (pathologist)
RF renal failure; respiratory failure; rheumatic fever; riboflavin; risk factor
Rf rutherfordium
RFA right frontoanterior (fetal position)
RFB retained foreign body (in surgery)
RFLP restriction fragment length polymorphism
RFP right frontoposterior (fetal position)
RFT right frontotransverse (fetal position)
RH relative humidity; releasing hormone;
Rh Rhesus factor; rhodium
RHC respiration has ceased
RHD rheumatic heart disease
RHF right heart failure
RhIg Rh immunoglobulin
RI radiation intensity; radioisotope; regional ileitis; regular insulin
RIA radioimmunoassay
Rib ribose
RICS right intercostal space
RID radial immunodiffusion
RIH right inguinal hernia
RIND reversible ischemic neurologic deficit
RISA radioiodinated serum albumin
RIST radioimmunosorbent test
RIU radioactive iodine uptake
RK radial keratoplasty
RLE right lower extremity

RLF retrolental fibroplasia
RLL right lower limb; right lower lobe (of lung)
RLN recurrent laryngeal nerve; regional lymph nodes
RLQ right lower quadrant (of abdomen)
RLS restless legs syndrome
RLX relaxin
RM radical mastectomy
Rm remission
RMI repetitive motion injury
RML right middle lobe (of lung)
RMP right mentoposterior (fetal position)
RMSF Rocky Mountain spotted fever
RMT right mentotransverse (fetal position)
Rn radon
RNA ribonucleic acid
RNase ribonuclease
PNL percutaneous nephrolithotomy
RNP ribonucleoprotein
RO reality orientation
R/O rule out
ROM range of motion (of a joint); read only memory; rupture of membranes
ROMI rule out myocardial infarction
ROP retinopathy of prematurity
ROS review of (organ) systems
ROT right occipitotransverse (fetal position)
RP radial pulse; Raynaud's phenomenon;
relapse prevention; retinitis pigmentosa
RPF relaxed pelvic floor; renal plasma flow (rate)
RPLND retroperitoneal lymph node dissection
rpm revolutions per minute
RPR rapid plasma reagin
RPRTs rapid plasma reagin tests
rps revolutions per second
RQ respiratory quotient
RR recovery room; relative risk; respiratory rate
RR-1 first recovery room
RR-2 second recovery room
RRE round, regular, and equal
rRNA ribosomal ribonucleic acid
RRR relative risk reduction
RS rectal sinus; rheumatoid spondylitis;
RSD reflex sympathetic dystrophy (syndrome); relative standard deviation
RSDS reflex sympathetic dystrophy syndrome
RSR regular sinus rhythm
RSV respiratory syncytial virus; Rous sarcoma virus
RT radiation therapy; rectal temperature; renal transplant; rubella titer
RTA renal tubular acidosis
RTx radiation therapy
RU radial-ulnar; residual urine; roentgen unit
Ru ruthenium
RUE right upper extremity
RUL right upper limb; right upper lobe (of lung)
RUQ right upper quadrant (of abdomen)
RV residual volume; right ventricle; rubella vaccine; rubella virus
RVF recto-vaginal fistula
RVH right ventricular hypertrophy
RVT renal vein thrombosis
RVU retroversion of uterus
Rx drug; medication; prescription

S

S heart sound; sacral vertebrae (S1 through S5); saline; saturated; section; sedimentation coefficient; selection coefficient; septum; serum; solid; soluble; spherical (lens); spleen; sulfur; Svedberg unit; systolic
s. *semis* [Latin] half; *sinister* [Latin] left; *sine* [Latin] without
S1 first sacral spinal nerve; first sacral vertebra
S2 second sacral spinal nerve; second sacral vertebra
S3 third sacral spinal nerve; third sacral vertebra
S4 fourth sacral spinal nerve; fourth sacral vertebra
S5 fifth sacral spinal nerve; fifth sacral vertebra
SI first heart sound
S2 second heart sound
S3 third heart sound
S4 fourth heart sound
SA salicylic acid; salt added; sarcoma; semen analysis; serum albumin; sinoatrial; sinus arrhythmia; surface antigen
S-A sinoatrial
SAA severe aplastic anemia
SAB spontaneous abortion
SAC short-arm cast
SACT sinoatrial conduction time
SAD seasonal affective disorder
SADS sudden arrhythmia death syndrome
SAH subarachnoid hemorrhage
sal saliva; salt
SAN sinoatrial node
S-A node sinoatrial node
SAP systemic arterial pressure
SART sinoatrial recovery time
SAS scalenus anterior syndrome; short-arm splint; supravalvular aortic stenosis
SAT streptococcal antibody test
sat saturated
SB shortness of breath; spina bifida; stillborn
Sb antimony; strabismus
SBE subacute bacterial endocarditis
SBP subacute bacterial peritonitis
SBR strict bed rest
SBS shaken baby syndrome
SC sclerocorneal; secretory component; self-care; sternoclavicular (joint); subclavian; subcutaneous; sugar coated
Sc scandium
sc subcutaneous
SCA sickle-cell anemia; sudden cardiac arrest
SCAN scintiscan; suspected child abuse or neglect
SCB strictly confined to bed
SCC squamous cell carcinoma; squamous skin
cancer
SCD sudden cardiac death
SCFE slipped capital femoral epiphysis
SCI spinal cord injury
SCID severe combined immunodeficiency
SCJ sclerocorneal junction
SCOP scopolamine
SCT sickle-cell trait; sugar-coated tablet
SD senile dementia; septal defect; standard deviation; sterile dressing; sudden death
SDA specific dynamic action
SDAT senile dementia, Alzheimer type
SDD sterile dry dressing
SDH subdural hematoma
SDR surgical dressing room
SDS same-day surgery
SE side effect; standard error
Se selenium
sec second
SEH subependymal hemorrhage
SEM scanning electron microscopy; standard error of the mean; systolic ejection murmur
sem semen
SER somatosensory evoked response; smooth endoplasmic reticulum
Ser serine
SF seminal fluid; spinal fusion; symptom-free; synovial fluid
SG skin graft
SGA small for gestational age (infant)
SGOT serum glutamic oxaloacetic transaminase
SGPT serum glutamic pyruvic transaminase
SH short; shoulder; shower
SHCS second hand cigarette smoke
SHM self-help method
SHTS second hand tobacco smoke
SI International System of Units; sacroiliac (joint); stress incontinence
Si silicon
SIA stress-induced anesthesia; sulfite-induced asthma

SIADH syndrome of inappropriate secretion of antidiuretic hormone
sib sibling
SICU surgical intensive care unit
SIDS sudden infant death syndrome
SIF somatotropin release-inhibiting factor
SIG sigmoidoscopy
SIg surface immunoglobulin
sig. *signa* [Latin] let it be labeled (directions)
sigmo sigmoidoscopy
SIH somatotropin release-inhibiting hormone
SIJ sacroiliac joint
SIMV spontaneous intermittent mandatory ventilation; synchronized intermittent mandatory ventilation
SIO sacroiliac orthosis
si op. sit *si opus sit* [Latin] if needed
SIRS soluble immune response suppressor; systemic inflammatory response syndrome
SIW self-inflicted wound
SK seborrheic keratosis; streptokinase
SKSD streptokinase-streptodornase
s.l. *secundum legem* [Latin] according to the law
SLC short-leg cast
SLE systemic lupus erythematosus
SLL small lymphocytic lymphoma
SLN sentinel lymph node (biopsy); superior laryngeal nerve
SLS short-leg splint
SM simple mastectomy; small; smoker; smooth muscle; systolic murmur
Sm samarium
SMA sequential multichannel autoanalyzer; smooth-muscle antibody
SMD senile macular degeneration
SMP sympathetically maintained pain
SMR standardized mortality ratio; submucous resection
SMS sperm motility study
Sn tin
SNagg serum normal agglutinator
SNHL sensorineural hearing loss
SO second opinion; sex offender; standing order
SOAP subjective, objective, assessment, plan
SOB shortness of breath
SOD superoxide dismutase
Sod sodomy
soln solution
solv. *solve* [Latin] dissolve
SOM serous otitis media
sono sonogram
SOP standard operating procedure
S.O.S. *si opus sit* [Latin] if needed
SP sodium pentothal; speech pathology
sp species; specific
SpA staphylococcal protein A
SPA single-photon absorptiometry; spermatozoa penetration assay; suprapubic aspiration
SPBT suprapubic bladder tap
SPC salicyamide, phenacetin, and caffeine; standard platelet count
SPCA serum prothrombin conversion accelerator
sp cd spinal cord
SPE serum protein electrophoresis
SPECT single photon emission computerized tomography
SPF specific-pathogen free; sun-protection factor
sp fl spinal fluid
spg sponge
sp gr specific gravity
SPH severely and profoundly handicapped
Sph spherical (lens)
SPL sound pressure level
SPM synchronous pacemaker
SPROM spontaneous premature rupture of membranes
sp tap spinal tap
sput sputum
SQ subcutaneous
SR sarcoplasmic reticulum; sedimentation rate; sinus rhythm; stomach rumble
Sr strontium
s-r stimulus-response (psychology)
SRH somatotropin-releasing hormone
sRNA soluble ribonucleic acid (RNA)
SRS slow-reacting substance
SRS-A slow-reacting substance of anaphylaxis
SRSV small round-structured virus
SRT sedimentation rate test
SRU side rails up
SS saline solution; saliva sample; salt substitute; Sezary syndrome; short stay; somatostatin; standard score; sterile solution
S&S signs and symptoms
ss. *semis* [Latin] one-half
SSc systemic sclerosis
SSE soap suds enema
SSKI saturated solution of potassium iodide
SSM superficial spreading melanoma
SSPE subacute sclerosing panencephalitis
SSRO sagittal split ramus osteotomy
SSS soluble specific substance; subclavian steal syndrome
SSSS staphylococcal scalded skin syndrome
s.s.v. *sub signo veneni* [Latin] under a poison label
ST scar tissue; sinus tachycardia; smokeless tobacco; stable toxin; survival time
STAG split thickness autogenous graft
staph. *Staphylococcus* (usually implies *Staphylococcus aureus)*
stat. *statim* [Latin] at once; immediately
stats statistics
STB stillborn
ST BY stand by
STD sexually transmitted disease; standard test dose
std standard
STEL short-term exposure limit
STH somatotrophic hormone
STI soft tissue injury
STJ subtalar joint
STM short-term memory
STP supracondylar tibial prosthesis
strep. streptococcal; *Streptococcus*
STS serologic test for syphilis
STSG split-thickness skin graft
STU shock trauma unit
STUMP smooth-muscle tumor of undetermined malignant potential
subcu subcutaneous (injection)
SUD sudden unexpected death; sudden unexplained death
SUID sudden unexpected infant death; sudden unexplained infant death
sum. *sumantur* [Latin] take
sup superior
surg surgery
SV severe; simian virus; snake venom
SVBPG saphenous vein bypass graft
SVC superior vena cava
SVD sudden vaginal delivery
SVG saphenous vein graft
SVT supraventricular tachycardia
SW stab wound
SWD shortwave diathermy
SWS slow wave sleep (non-rapid eye movement sleep); Sturge-Weber syndrome
sympt symptom
synd syndrome
syn. fl. synovial fluid
sx surgery

T

T tablespoon; temperature; tension; term; tesla thorax; thyroid; time; tissue; tocopherol; total; toxicity; trace; tritium; type
T absolute temperature
t teaspoon; temperature; tertiary; tocopherol;translocation
T1/2 biologic half-life
T1 first thoracic spinal nerve; first thoracic vertebra
T2 second thoracic spinal nerve; second thoracic vertebra
T2 diiodotyrosine
T3 third thoracic spinal nerve; third thoracic vertebra
T3 triiodothyronine
T4 fourth thoracic spinal nerve; fourth thoracic vertebra
T4 thyroxine
T5 fifth thoracic spinal nerve; fifth thoracic vertebra

T6	sixth thoracic spinal nerve; sixth thoracic vertebra
T7	seventh thoracic spinal nerve; seventh thoracic vertebra
T8	eighth thoracic spinal nerve; eighth thoracic vertebra
T9	ninth thoracic spinal nerve; ninth thoracic vertebra
T10	tenth thoracic spinal nerve; tenth thoracic vertebra
T11	eleventh thoracic spinal nerve; eleventh thoracic vertebra
T12	twelfth thoracic spinal nerve; twelfth thoracic vertebra
TA	toothache; toxin-antitoxin; truncus arteriosus; transplantation antigen; tricuspid atresia
Ta	tantalum
T&A	tonsillectomy and adenoidectomy
TAA	thoracic aortic aneurysm; tumor-associated antigen
tab.	tablet
Tac	T cell activation receptor
tachy	tachycardia
TAE	total abdominal eventration
TAF	tumor-angiogenesis factor
TAH	total abdominal hysterectomy
TAO	thromboangiitis obliterans
TAP	titanium acetabular prosthesis
TAR	thrombocytopenia and absent radius (syndrome)
TAT	tetanus antitoxin; thematic appreciation test
TATA	tumor-associated transplantation antigen
TB	tracheobronchitis; tuberculin; tuberculosis
Tb	terbium
TBG	thyroid-binding globulin; thyroxine-binding globulin
TBI	traumatic brain injury
TBII	thyroid-binding inhibitory immunoglobulin
TBLC	term birth, living child
TBM	tubular basement membrane
TBP	thyroxine-binding protein
TBR	total bed rest
TBSA	total burn surface area
tbsp	tablespoon
TBV	total blood volume
TBW	total body water
TC	thoracic cage; throat culture; tissue culture; total cholesterol
Tc	technetium
^{99}Tc	technetium-99
TCA	terminal cancer; transluminal coronary angioplasty; trichloroacetic acid
TCAB	triple coronary artery bypass
TCDD	tetrachlorodibenzo-p-dioxin
TCGF	T cell growth factor
TCI	transient cerebral ischemia
TCMI	T cell-mediated immunity
TCR	T cell receptor
TCT	thrombin-clotting time; total cholesterol test
TD	tardive dyskinesia; temporary disability; tetanus and diphtheria; thymus-dependent; total disability; traveler's diarrhea
Td	tetanus and diphtheria toxoids, adult type
TDD	telecommunication device for the deaf
TDI	toluene diisocyanate; therapeutic donor insemination
TDM	therapeutic drug management
tDNA	transfer deoxyribonucleic acid (DNA)
t.d.s.	*ter die sumendum* [Latin] to be taken three times a day
TdT	terminal deoxynucleotidyl transferase
TE	tennis elbow; thromboembolism; tooth extracted; total ejaculate (number of sperm); treadmill exercise
Te	tellurium; tetanus
TEBG	testosterone-estradiol-binding globulin
TEC	total eosinophil count
TED	threshold erythema dose
TEE	transesophageal echocardiography
TEF	tracheoesophageal fistula
TEM	transmission electron microscope; triethylenemelanine
TEN	toxic epidermal necrolysis
TENS	transcutaneous electrical nerve stimulation
TEPA	triethylene-phosphoramide
TEPP	tetraethyl pyrophosphate
TESD	total end-systolic diameter
TEST	tubal embryo stage transfer
TET	tubal embryo transfer; treadmill exercise test
TEV	talipes equinovarus
TF	tetralogy of Fallot; tracheal fistula; transfer factor; tube feeding; tuning fork
TG	tendon graft; thyroglobulin; triglyceride
TGC	time-varied gain control
TGE	transmissible gastroenteritis
TGF	transforming growth factor
TGFα	transforming growth factor alpha
TGFA	triglyceride fatty acid
TGFβ	transforming growth factor beta
TGSI	thyroid growth-stimulating immunoglobulin
TGV	thoracic gas volume
TH	thyroid hormone; total hysterectomy
Th	thorium
THA	total hip arthroplasty
THAM	trishydroxy-methylaminomethane
THAN	transient hyperammonemia of newborn
THC	tetrahydrocannabinol; transhepatic cholangiography
THIO	thiopental sodium
thor	thoracic; thorax
THR	total hip replacement
Thr	threonine
thromb	thrombosis
Thy	thymine
TI	tricuspid insufficiency
Ti	titanium
TIA	transient ischemic attack
TIBC	total iron-binding capacity
TID	therapeutic insemination, donor
t.i.d.	*ter in die* [Latin] three times a day
TIG	tetanus immune globulin
TIH	therapeutic insemination, husband
TIL	tumor-infiltrating lymphocyte
t.i.n.	*ter in nocte* [Latin] three times nightly
tinc	tincture
TIPS	transjugular intrahepatic portosystemic shunts
TIS	tumor *in situ*
TITh	triiodothyronine
TJR	total joint replacement
TKA	total knee arthroplasty
TKD	tokodynamometer
TKG	tokodynagraph
TKR	total knee replacement
TL	temporal lobe; thymic lymphocyte; time lapse; total lipids; tubal ligation
Tl	thallium
TLC	thin-layer chromatography; total lung capacity; total lymphocyte count
TLE	thin-layer electrophoresis
TLI	total lymphoid irradiation
TLSO	thoracolumbosacral orthosis
TLV	threshold limit value
TM	transmetatarsal (amputation); tropical medicine; tympanic membrane
Tm	thulium; transport maximum
TMI	transmandibular implant
TMJ	temporomandibular joint
TMJS	temporomandibular joint syndrome
TMST	treadmill stress test
TMT	tarsometatarsal (joint)
TN	trigeminal neuralgia
T&N	tar and nicotine
Tn	normal intraocular tension
TNDS	transdermal nicotine delivery system
TNF	tumor necrosis factor
TNI	total nodal irradiation
TNM	tumor-node-metastasis (staging)
TNS	transcutaneous nerve stimulation
TNT	trinitrotoluene
TO	target organ
TOA	time of arrival; tubo-ovarian abscess
TOD	target organ disease
TOF	tetralogy of Fallot
tomo	tomogram
TOP	termination of pregnancy
TORCH	toxoplasmosis, other infections, rubella, cytomegalovirus infection, and herpes (simplex)
TORCHS	toxoplasmosis, other infections, rubella, cytomegalovirus infection, herpes (simplex), and syphilis

TOS thoracic outlet syndrome
TOT total operating time
tox toxic
TP terminal phalanx; trigger point; tubal pregnancy
Tp precursor T cells
T&P temperature and pressure
tPA tissue plasminogen activator
TPC thromboplastic plasma component; total patient care
TPE therapeutic plasma exchange
TPH transplacental (fetal) hemorrhage
TPHA *Treponema pallidum* hemagglutination assay
TPI *Treponema pallidum* immobilization (test)
TPM temporary pacemaker
TPN total parenteral nutrition
TPP thiamine pyrophosphate
TPR temperature, pulse, and respiration; testosterone production rate; total peripheral resistance
TQ tourniquet
TR tricuspid regurgitation; tubular reabsorption
tr tincture
TRA thyrotropin receptor antibody
Trach trachea
TRAP tartrate-resistant acid phosphatase
TRBF total renal blood flow
TRF thyrotropin-releasing factor
trf transfer
TRH thyrotropin-releasing hormone
TRHST thyrotropin-releasing hormone stimulation test
TRIC trachoma inclusion cojunctivitis
TRIS tris(hydroxymethyl)-aminomethane
tRNA transfer ribonucleic acid
Trp tryptophan
trt treatment
TRUS transrectal ultrasonography
TS test solution; toxic substance; transsexual; tricuspid stenosis
Ts suppressor T cells
TSA total shoulder arthroplasty; tumor-specific antigen
TSAS total severity assessment score
TSE testicular self-examination; total skin examination
TSF triceps skinfold
TSH thyroid-stimulating hormone
TSH-RH thyroid-stimulating hormone-releasing hormone
TSI thyroid-stimulating immunoglobulin
tsp teaspoon
T-spine thoracic spine
TSS toxic shock syndrome
TST treadmill stress test
TSTA tumor-specific transplantation antigen
TT tendon transfer; thrombin time
TTD tissue tolerance dose
TTN transient tachypnea of the newborn
TTP thrombotic thrombocytopenic purpura
TTS temporary threshold shift; through the skin; transdermal therapeutic system
TTTS twin-twin transfusion syndrome
TU toxic unit; tuberculin unit
TUBD transurethral balloon dilatation
tub lig tubal ligation
TUIP transurethral incision of prostate
TULIP transurethral ultrasound-guided laser-induced prostatectomy
TUR transurethral resection
TURP transurethral resection of prostate
TV total volume; tricuspid valve
TVC total vital capacity
TVH total vaginal hysterectomy
TW tapwater
TWZ triangular working zone
Tx thromboxane; traction; transplant; treatment
typ typical
Tyr tyrosine

U

U unit; upper; uracil; uranium; uridine; urine
u unit
UA unstable angina; uric acid; urinalysis
U/A urinalysis
UAC umbilical artery catheterization
UAO upper airway obstruction
UC ulcerative colitis; urea clearance; urine culture; uterine contraction
UCO urinary catheter out
ucs unconscious
u.d. *ud dictum* [Latin] as directed
UDCA ursodeoxycholic acid
UDE undetermined etiology
UDO undetermined origin
UDP uridine diphosphate
UDPG uridine diphosphate glucose
UF unknown factor
UG urogenital
UGA under general anesthesia
UGI upper gastrointestinal
UI unidentified; urinary incontinence
u.i.d. *uno in die* [Latin] once every day
umb umbilicus
UMCD uremic medullary cystic disease
UMI unstable myocardial ischemia
UN ulnar nerve; urea nitrogen
ung. *unguentum* [Latin] ointment
unk unknown
uns unsatisfactory
UO under observation; urinary output
UP upright position
UPJ ureteropelvic junction
UQ upper quadrant
URD upper respiratory disease
Urd uridine
urg urgent
URI upper respiratory (tract) infection
url unrelated
URR urea reduction ratio
US ultrasonography; ultrasound
USI urinary stress incontinence
USP *The United States Pharmacopeia*
USPHS United States Public Health Service
UT urinary tract; uterus
ut dict. *ut dictum* [Latin] as directed
UTI urinary tract infection
UTV unable to void
UV ultraviolet
UVA ultraviolet A
UVB ultraviolet B
UVC ultraviolet C; umbilical vein catherization
UVL ultraviolet light
UVR ultraviolet radiation

V

V vanadium; virus; volt
v valve; ventilation; ventral; vision; vitamin; voice; volt; volume; vomiting
v. *vena* [Latin] vein
V1,V2 vasopressin receptors
V max maximum velocity (in an enzymatic reaction)
vacc vaccination
VACTERL vertebral, anal, cardiac, tracheal, esophageal, renal, limb (a pattern of associatedcongenital anomalies)
VAD ventricular assist device
Vag vagina
Val valine
vas vas deferens
vasc vascular
VATER vertebral defects, anal atresia, tracheoesophageal fistula, esophageal atresia, renal anomalies (a pattern of associated congenital anomalies)
VATS video-assisted thoracic surgery
VB vertebral body; viable birth
VBAC vaginal birth after (previous) cesarean section
VBG venous blood gas
VC vasoconstriction; vena cava; visual cortex; vital capacity
VCG vectocardiogram
VCT venous clotting time

VD	vasodilator; venereal disease; viral diarrhea; voided
Vd	volume of distribution
VDDR	vitamin D-dependent rickets
VDG	venereal disease - gonorrhea
VDRR	vitamin D-resistant rickets
VDS	venereal disease - syphilis
VE	vaginal examination; visual efficiency
VEE	Venezuelan equine encephalomyelitis
vel	velocity
vent	ventricular
vent fib	ventricular fibrillation
VEP	visually evoked potential
VER	visually evoked response
VF	ventricular fibrillation; visual field
VFl	ventricular flutter
VG	vein graft
VH	vaginal hysterectomy; ventricular hypertrophy; viral hepatitis; visually handicapped
VHD	valvular heart disease
VHDL	very high density lipoprotein
VI	vaginal irritation
VIN	vulvar intraepithelial neoplasia
VIN I	vulvar intraepithelial neoplasia, mild (with mild dysplasia)
VIN II	vulvar intraepithelial neoplasia, moderate (with moderate dysplasia)
VIN III	vulvar intraepithelial neoplasia, severe (with severe dysplasia)
VIP	vasoactive intestinal polypeptide
VIS	vaginal irrigation smear
VISI	volar-flexed intercalated segment instability
VLA	very late activation (antigen)
VLBW	very low birth weight
VLDL	very low-density lipoprotein
VLP	virus-like particle
VMA	vanillylmandelic acid
VMAT	vanillylmandelic acid test
VO	verbal order
VOD	venous occlusive disease
V-ONC	viral oncogene
VP	variegate porphyria; vasopressin; venipuncture; venous pressure
VPB	ventricular premature beat
VPC	ventricular premature contraction
VR	valve replacement; vascular resistance; vocal resonance
VRE	vancomycin resistant enterococci
VRI	viral respiratory infection
VS	vital sign; volumetric solution; voluntary sterilization
VSD	ventricular septal defect; virtual safe dose
VSS	vital signs stable
VT	venous thrombosis; ventricular tachycardia; vitality test
V tach.	ventricular tachycardia
VV	varicose veins; vesicovaginal
vv	veins
v/v	volume (of solute) per volume (of solvent)
VVF	vesicovaginal fistula
VW	vessel wall
VZ	varicella zoster
VZIG	varicella-zoster immune globulin
VZV	varicella zoster virus

W

W	tungsten; watt; week; weight; white; width
w	week; white; with
WA	when awake; while awake
WAS	Wiskott-Aldrich syndrome
WB	water bottle; whole blood
WBC	white blood cell; white blood count
wbc	white blood cell
WBCT	whole blood clotting time
WBS	whole body shower
WC	white (blood) cell; whooping cough
WCC	white (blood) cell count
WD	wallerian degeneration; warm and dry; watery diarrhea; well developed; wet dressing; wrist dislocation
WDHA	watery diarrhea, hypokalemia, achlorhydria (syndrome)
WDLL	well differentiated lymphocytic lymphoma
WDWN	well developed, well nourished
W/E	wound of entry (of a bullet)
WEE	western equine encephalomyelitis
WEST	work evaluation systems technology
WFE	Williams flexion exercise
wgt	weight
WH	walking heel (cast)
whp	whirlpool
wk	week
WL	waiting list; wavelength
WLI	whiplash injury
WMX	whirlpool, massage, and exercise
WN	well nourished
WNL	within normal limits
WO	wrist orthosis; written order
WOP	without pain
WPB	whirlpool bath
WPW	Wolff-Parkinson-White (syndrome)
WR	Wassermann reaction; water retention
WRE	whole ragweed extract
WS	withdrawal syndrome
WT	Wada test
wt	weight
WtB	weight bearing
W/U	work up
w/v	weight (of solute) per volume (of solvent)
W/X	wound of exit (of a bullet)

X

X	crossed with; except; extra; removal; times
x	axis (of cylindric lens); except; mean value
Xaa	unknown amino acid
X&D	examination and diagnosis
XCCE	extracapsular cataract extraction
Xe	xenon
^{133}Xe	xenon-133
XL	extra large; X-linked
XLR	X-linked recessive
X match	cross match
XMP	xanthosine monophosphate
XO	extraction of
XP	xeroderma pigmentosum
XR	roentgen ray; xray
XRT	x-ray therapy
XS	cross section
xs	excess
XT	exotropia
XU	excretory urogram
46XX	normal number of female chromosomes
46XY	normal number of male chromosomes
Xylo	xylocaine

Y

Y	yellow; yttrium
y	year
Yb	ytterbium
YF	yellow fever
YJV	yellow jacket venom
YOB	year of birth
YPLL	years of potential life lost
YS	yolk sac
YST	yeast

Z

Z	standard score; zero; zone
z	atomic number; standardized device; zone
ZD	zero defects
ZDV	zidovudine
ZIFT	zygote intrafallopian (tube) transfer
ZIG	zoster immune globulin
Zn	zinc
ZOE	zinc oxide and eugenol
ZPO	zinc peroxide
ZPG	zero population growth
Zr	zirconium
ZSR	zeta sedimentation ratio

Illustration credits

The authors acknowledge the following publications as sources from which the listed original illustrations for this dictionary were derived by permission.

American Family Physician, American Academy of Family Physicians, Kansas City, MO.

Adrenal glands, ampulla, anesthsia, antibody, bone cement, tables of bones (lunate), constrictor muscles of pharynx, descensus testes, dialysis, diverticulum, dog tick, ductus arteriosus, fetal membrane, flexion, glaucoma, hookworm, hymenopterans, Jackson-Pratt® drain, omphalomesenteric cyst, ovary, pancreas, pleura, proglottid, prostatic message, Pyemotes ventricosus, rheumatoid arthritis, spur, strain, tooth designation.

Bellanti JA. *Immunology* (II), 2nd edn. Philadelphia: WB Saunders Co, 1978.

Afferent, hilum, lumph node.

Dorland's Illustrated Medical Dictionary, 25th edn. Philadelphia: WB Saunders Co. 1974.

Auricle.

Dox IG, *et al. Melloni's Illustrated Dictionary of Obstetrics and Gynecology*. London: Parthenon Publishing, 2000.

Abruptio placentae, cervical caps, chorionic villus sampling, diameters of pelvis, external version, inferior hypogastric plexus, limb buds, nuchal arm, punch forceps, tubal sterilization, types of pessaries, urinary bladder.

Dox IG, *et al. Attorney's Illustrated Medical Dictionary*, West Publishing Group, 1997.

Balloon catheterization, breast implant, carpal tunnel syndrome, closed urinary drainage system, complement-fixing antibody, coronary arteriography, DNA analysis, DNA typing, embolism, endometriosis, *in vitro* fertilization, major veins of the human body, penile prosthesis, percutaneous transluminal angioplasty, replantation of severed finger, rotator cuff.

Grollman S. *The Human Body: Its Structure and the Physiology,* 3rd edn. New York: McMillan Publishing Co. Inc, 1974.

Nerve (vestibular and cochlear), osseous labyrinth, pathway, retina.

Kruger GO. *Textbook of Oral Surgery*. 4th edn. St. Louis: The CV Mosby Co, 1974.

Alveolectomy, impaction.

Langley L, Telford I, Christian J. *Dynamic Anatomy and Physiology*, 4th edn. New York: McGraw-Hill Book Co, 1974.

Acromion, aperture of sinus (sphenoid and maxillary), table of bones (femur and sphenoid), calvaria, chamber, ciliary body, ethmoidal infundibulum, navicular bone, optic axis, sacrum, vertebral arch, vertebral body.

Melloni BJ, *et al. Anatomy and Physiology* (I and III). New York: McGraw-Hill Books Co, 1971.

Air cells, basion, table of bones (ethmoid), canaliculus, cephalic index, cochlear duct, concha, conjunctiva, crista ampullaris, lacrimal gland, lacrimal sac, mastoid, nasal septum, opisthion, orbit, ossicles, scala, spinal ganglia of cochlea, visual pathways.

Melloni BJ. The internal ear. *What's New* 1957;199:14-19.

Ear, semicircular canals.

Melloni BJ. Anatomy of hearing. *What's New* 1960;219:26.

Cochlear duct.

Melloni BJ. Anatomy of sight. *What's New* 1961;222: 25-28.

Retina, optic chiasm.

Melloni BJ. How the aqueous humor circulates. *Am Fam Phys* 1972;5:2.

Chambers of the eye (anterior and posterior).

Melloni BJ. Plants of medical importance. *Am Fam Phys* 1973;8:6.

Hemlock; jimsonweed; poison ivy, oak, and sumac; marijuana; ragweed.

Melloni BJ. Focus on cells: osteocytes. *Am Fam Phys* 1974;10:3.

Osteocyte.

Melloni BJ. *Melloni's Illustrated Dictionary of the Musculoskeletal System*. London: Parthenon Publishing, 1998.

Bursae, external sphincter muscles of anus, ligaments, musculoskeletal system, osteoporosis, sinuses, skeleton, tendons and ligaments of hand and wrist.

Melloni JL, *et al. Melloni's Student Atlas of Human Anatomy*, London: Parthenon Publishing, 1997.

Cervical and brachial plexuses, parotid veins, pharyngeal aponeurosis, quadriceps, trigeminal ganglion.

Smith DR. *General Urology*, 10th edn. Los Altos: Lange Medical Publishers, 1981.

Benign.

Vidic B, Melloni BJ. Applied anatomy of the oral cavity and related structures. In Kornblut AD, deFries HO, eds. *The Otolaryngological Clinics of North America* 12:1, Philadelphia: WB Saunders Co, 1979.

Buccal vestibule, facial vein, retromandibular vein.

The authors

Ida Dox, PhD, listed in Marquis *Who's Who in America* and *Who's Who in the World*, is the senior author of several reference books in the medical sciences, including *Melloni's Illustrated Dictionary of Obstetrics and Gynecology* (Parthenon Publishing) and *Attorney's Illustrated Medical Dictionary* (West Group), and is a co-author of the award-winning book *Illustrated Review of Human Anatomy* (J.B. Lippincott) and *Melloni's Illustrated Student Atlas of Human Anatomy* (Parthenon Publishing). Her many consulting services in medical communication and human anatomy have included working for the U.S. House of Representatives on the medical panel of the Select Committee on Assassinations, investigating the assassinations of President John F. Kennedy and Dr Martin Luther King, Jr. She testified with the medical panel before the congressional hearing about her involvement in the investigation. Her detailed study of the anatomical evidence and resulting illustrations are housed in the National Archives. Dr Dox was employed at Georgetown University School of Medicine and her scientific articles appear in professional journals. She resides near the National Institutes of Health and the National Library of Medicine in Bethesda, Maryland, where she consults their voluminous medical literature and resources.

B. John Melloni, PhD, is the author and co-author of several books, including *Anatomy and Physiology* (four volumes, McGraw-Hill); *Databases: A Primer for Retrieving Information by Computer* (Prentice-Hall); *Melloni's Illustrated Review of Human Anatomy* (J.B. Lippincott) recipient of the Award of Excellence from the AMI; *Melloni's Illustrated Student Atlas of Human Anatomy* (Parthenon Publishing); *Melloni's Illustrated Dictionary of Medical Abbreviations* (Parthenon Publishing); *Attorney's Illustrated Medical Dictionary* (West Group), and *Melloni's Illustrated Dictionary of the Musculoskeletal System* (Parthenon Publishing), selected by Doody's Rating Service as one of the 250 Best Health Sciences Books of 1999.
Over the years, Dr Melloni has served as a professorial lecturer in human anatomy at Georgetown University School of Medicine and was founder and chairman of the School's Department of Medical-Dental Communication. He was director of medical visual information for the American Family Physician (AFP), published by the American Academy of Family Physicians and was Editor-in-Chief of *Visual Medicine*, Journal of Visual Communication in the Medical and Dental Sciences. In private consulting, he was initial reviewer of grant proposals for the U.S. Department of Public Health and has served the AMA, VA, Human Research Resources Organization (HUMRRO), pharmaceutical companies (Abbott Laboratories, Chas. Pfizer, and Glaxo SmithKline), and publishers (W.B. Saunders Company, Williams & Wilkins, and HarperCollins). He has held offices in national professional organizations and received a number of awards for his contribution to illustrated books in medicine. Now retired from the National Institutes of Health, where he served as Special Expert in Biomedical Communication, he continues in his post as co-director of the Archives of Medical Visual Resources of the Francis A. Countway Library of Medicine at Harvard Medical School.

Gilbert M. Eisner, MD, is a graduate of Harvard College, cum laude, and Yale Medical School. He served as an intern at the Grace New Haven Hospital in New Haven Connecticut, spent 2 years in the U.S. Army as a Captain in the Medical Corps, then was a resident and a fellow in renal disease at Mt. Sinai Hospital in New York City. Dr Eisner completed his medical residency at Georgetown University Hospital in Washington, DC. Since 1962, he has been on the part-time faculty of Georgetown University Medical Center and in the private practice of internal medicine and nephrology. He served for 25 years as Assistant Editor of *American Family Physicians* and his bibliography includes 60 scientific papers. He has held offices in numerous local and national professional organizations.

June L. Melloni, PhD, is senior author of the award-winning book *Melloni's Illustrated Review of Human Anatomy* (J.B. Lippincott) and of *Melloni's Illustrated Student Atlas of Human Anatomy* (Parthenon Publishing). She is co-author of *Attorney's Illustrated Medical Dictionary* (West Group); *Melloni's Illustrated Dictionary of Obstetrics and Gynecology* (Parthenon Publishing); and *Melloni's Illustrated Dictionary of Medical Abbreviations* (Parthenon Publishing). Dr Melloni specializes in qualitative evaluation and instructional design targeted towards disciplines in the medical and allied health fields and has conducted multiple studies, using qualitative research techniques, for organizations in both the public and private sectors. Her research has included analyses of interactive videodiscs in medical education and a nationwide study on visual-based instruction in medicine. She designed and implemented computer-based educational programs in collaboration with medical scientists and educators at Human Research Resources Organization (HUMRRO). She maintains an active consulting service for a clientele that includes fortune 500 companies and medical schools. Dr Melloni resides in Potomac Falls near the 'Silicon Valley' of Northern Virginia.